MW01505012

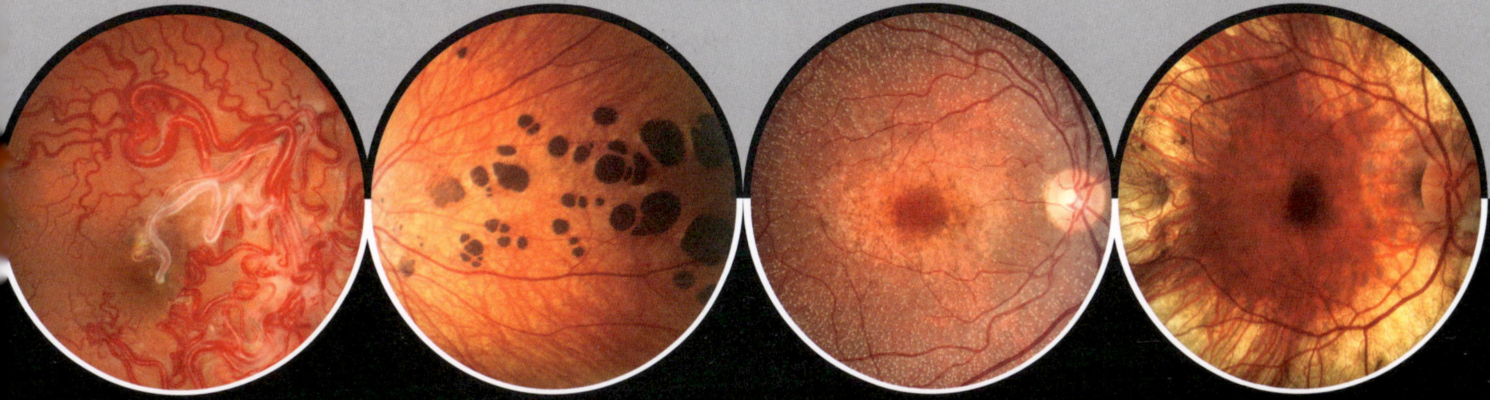

Gass' Atlas of MACULAR DISEASES

Dedication

To my parents, grandmother and siblings

Vimala Chandraiah
Daksha Chandraiah
M.C. Chandraiah
B. S. Puttamma
Dinesh, Suchita, Vinuta and Mamata
for their unending love and faith in me

To my teachers

J. Donald M. Gass
Amod Gupta
for their inspiration and teaching

and to their spouses and children
Margy Ann Gass and Gunita Gill Gupta
John, Carlton, Media, Dean and Sumedha
for supporting their careers and allowing me to borrow their time

To my colleagues and friends
for selflessly sharing their cases and knowledge

To our patients
for giving us the privilege of learning through them

Commissioning Editor: Russell Gabbedy
Development Editor: Sharon Nash
Editorial Assistant: Kirsten Lowson
Project Manager(s): Jess Thompson/Andrew Riley
Design: Stewart Larking
Illustration Manager: Gillian Richards
Illustrator: Martin Woodward
Multimedia Producer: Nathan Wiles
Marketing Manager(s) (UK/USA): Gaynor Jones/Helena Mutak

VOLUME ONE

FIFTH EDITION

Gass' Atlas of MACULAR DISEASES

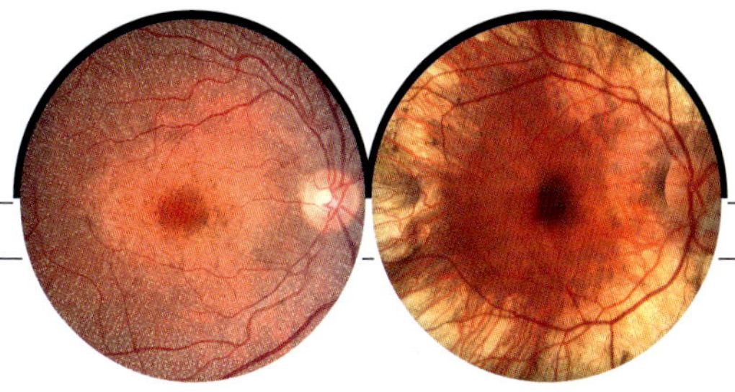

ANITA AGARWAL, MD

Associate Professor of Ophthalmology

Vanderbilt Eye Institute

Vanderbilt University School of Medicine

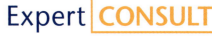

Nashville, TN

USA

ELSEVIER
SAUNDERS

ELSEVIER
SAUNDERS

SAUNDERS is an imprint of Elsevier Inc.

First edition 1970
Second edition 1977
Third edition 1987
Fourth edition 1997
Fifth edition 2012

Notices
Knowledge and best practice in this field are constantly changing. As new research and experience broaden our understanding, changes in research methods, professional practices, or medical treatment may become necessary. Practitioners and researchers must always rely on their own experience and knowledge in evaluating and using any information, methods, compounds, or experiments described herein. In using such information or methods they should be mindful of their own safety and the safety of others, including parties for whom they have a professional responsibility.

With respect to any drug or pharmaceutical products identified, readers are advised to check the most current information provided (i) on procedures featured or (ii) by the manufacturer of each product to be administered, to verify the recommended dose or formula, the method and duration of administration, and contraindications. It is the responsibility of practitioners, relying on their own experience and knowledge of their patients, to make diagnoses, to determine dosages and the best treatment for each individual patient, and to take all appropriate safety precautions.

To the fullest extent of the law, neither the Publisher nor the authors, contributors, or editors, assume any liability for any injury and/or damage to persons or property as a matter of products liability, negligence or otherwise, or from any use or operation of any methods, products, instructions, or ideas contained in the material herein.

Saunders

British Library Cataloguing in Publication Data
Agarwal, Anita.
Gass' atlas of macular diseases. – 5th ed.
1. Macula lutea Diseases Atlases.
I. Title II. Gass, J. Donald M. (John Donald M.), 1928-2005
Stereoscopic atlas of macular diseases.
617.7'3-dc22

Library of Congress Cataloging in Publication Data
A catalog record for this book is available from the Library of Congress

ISBN: 978-1-4377-1580-4

Printed in China
Last digit is the print number: 9 8 7 6 5 4 3 2 1

CONTENTS

VOLUME ONE

Figures with 3D indicate bonus stereoscopic images available online at www.expertconsult.com

Figures with 3D indicate bonus stereoscopic images available online at www.expertconsult.com

6 Macular Dysfunction Caused by Retinal Vascular Diseases 437

Anita Agarwal

Figures with 3D indicate bonus stereoscopic images available online at www.expertconsult.com

CONTENTS

VOLUME TWO

Acknowledgements

First, I want to express my thanks to my chairman, Dr. Paul Sternberg, for his confidence in allowing me to work on the 5th edition of the Gass Atlas. His counsel, support, and periodic overseeing helped keep the project in line and on to conclusion. The strength of any work is its contents. Towards this end, I am indebted to Dr. Arun D. Singh for his talent and time in updating the tumor section of the book. I am also deeply grateful to all my colleagues and friends, who have unhesitatingly shared their patients' case histories and images. Their generous contributions have enhanced immeasurably the content and quality of the Atlas. The Atlas helped me make several new friends around the world; to my immense surprise and pleasure, not one retinal specialist declined to contribute cases when I approached them, often as a complete stranger. I am particularly grateful to Dr. Amod Gupta, Chairman of Ophthalmology at my *alma mater*, PGI, Chandigarh and Dr. Vishali Gupta for the images and cases they contributed, and the knowledge they shared that made the Atlas truly international. My colleagues at Vanderbilt gave me a free hand to select any of their cases; I sincerely respect their confidence. I also wish to thank my vitreoretinal colleagues for taking on some additional clinical responsibilities while I devoted time to this project. I feel fortunate to have developed a close friendship with several leading retinal specialists who have welcomed me into their community, thus enhancing and enriching my knowledge. Dr. Lee Jampol's review of some of the chapters was timely and encouraging. Overall, the information in this book originates not only from my clinical experience and publications of experts, but also knowledge gained through my long association with faculty, fellows and residents at Vanderbilt and other institutions.

I am deeply indebted to the always-positive Russell Gabbedy, commissioning editor for Elsevier, and the prompt and ever available Sharon Nash, development editor. They both were the backbones of the production of the Atlas. I acknowledge Gillian Richards, the illustration manager, and Martin Woodward, the talented illustrator who has skillfully converted all of Don Gass' hand drawn cartoons into illustrations. Stewart Larking designed the elegant cover and pages and Kristen Lowson was the editorial assistant. Nathan Wiles was the multimedia producer. I thank Jess Thompson and Andrew Riley, the project managers who coordinated the various arms of production, even across continents and smoothed and polished the final product. I thank students Jose Garcia, Paige Munn and Patrick Donahue for their help in downloading loads of articles and PDFs and painstakingly extracting images from presentations and labeling them. I acknowledge the talented photographers at Vanderbilt for their abilities and their help in enhancing the quality of images. In addition, this Atlas would not be in its present form without the ever-dependable Lynne Siesser, my administrative assistant who can find a solution to almost any problem.

Finally, I want to again thank the inspiration for this project, Dr. J. Donald M. Gass. It has been a privilege and honor to continue the work of my mentor, colleague, and friend.

Anita Agarwal

Contributors

Arun D Singh MD

Professor of Ophthalmology
Director, Department of Ophthalmic Oncology
Cole Eye Institute
Cleveland Clinic
Cleveland, OH, USA

Forewords

This fifth edition of the Gass Atlas of Macular Diseases by Dr. Anita Agarwal brilliantly combines the best of the previous editions with new technical advances, new entities and international perspective. The Atlas is a guide to help the clinician to arrive at a diagnosis of both common and uncommon diseases and to understand the pathogenesis. The online version continues the tradition for viewing stereo photographs. A hallmark of Dr. Gass' teaching style is a simple yet detailed description of clinical observations. This technique is preserved in the current edition and enhanced through electronic illustrations and Optical Coherence Tomography (OCT) which frequently depicts precisely what Dr. Gass envisaged.

The table of contents is reorganized to reflect the explosion of information, particularly in areas such as inflammatory and infectious diseases and tumors addressed in separate chapters. Updates on manifestations of tuberculosis and syphilis are included along with new viral diseases such as Epstein–Barr and West Nile virus. Chapter 11 contains a description of some new diagnostic entities including acute idiopathic maculopathy and persistent and relentless placoid pigment epitheliopathy. Tumors are presented in three chapters – Retinal Pigment Epithelium (12), Retina (13) and Choroid (14).

Dr. Agarwal and her co-author, Dr. Arun D Singh, have updated and extended the extraordinary work of Dr. J. Donald M. Gass, an individual recognized as one of the outstanding ophthalmologists of the 20th century, and helped to catapult his work into the future. In a time of increasing paperless communication this wonderful text will serve all physicians interested in macular disease as a continuing reference to improve their diagnostic acumen and provide better care for their patients.

John G. Clarkson, MD
Professor, Chair and Dean Emeritus
Bascom Palmer Eye Institute, Miami, FL

What a task it would be to rewrite the Bible! What about the Bible of retinal disease – Donald Gass' stereoscopic atlas? For the last three decades this book has informed us, helped us in the diagnosis and treatment of difficult cases, and served as the foundation for the evolution of the entire field of medical retina. The brilliant pattern recognition, memory, and synthesizing skills of Donald Gass allowed him to document an unimaginable amount of important information in his book. He described for the first time scores of new diseases and physical findings. His photographic collection – built over years of seeing patients, providing mail consultations, and attending innumerable meetings, is unparalleled. His knowledge of ocular pathology added to the value of these archives. Even today, time and time again, when we suspect we have a new observation, perusal of the atlas shows us to be way behind Don.

As expected, the Atlas aged and illness prevented Don from completing a new edition. In most circumstances an editor or many editors, (but not a single author) would try to live up to the original and usually not succeed. Fortunately one of Don's most talented disciples has stepped into the breach.

Anita Agarwal was a fellow with Don and worked side by side with him at Vanderbilt University. Since his death, at conferences and in her publications, she has shown immense grasp of Don's knowledge base and has taken his place in educating us about the diseases that Don had mastered. She has an excellent knowledge of systemic diseases, genetics and many aspects of internal medicine very rare in ophthalmology. Now we are grateful that she has devoted years of her life to updating this precious text. Using Don's original files and her encyclopedic knowledge of the retina, a new version of the Bible appears. (Dr. Arun D. Singh has assisted her on the chapters on tumors.) The figures, including colour photographs, OCTs, angiographies, X-rays, and histopathologic specimens are still unparalleled; multiple images are often available of the same entity, demonstrating the variability of these diseases. Anita has also added an international flavour to the book with discussions of diseases rarely or not seen in the USA. The book covers common diseases (e.g. age-related macular degeneration) in detail, but also discusses very rare entities (e.g. diffuse unilateral subacute neuroretinitis).

There are other great books and atlases of medical retina but this book remains the Bible. Thank you Anita

Lee M. Jampol, MD
Louis Feinberg Professor and Chair Emeritus
Northwestern University, Chicago, IL

Of all my ophthalmology books, the Gass Atlas of Macular Diseases has been the most treasured, and most dog-eared, possession. Since I first acquired my copy of the second edition as a resident, I avidly awaited the publication of the more recent version, then immediately purchased it to replace my worn copy of the previous edition. When Dr. Gass became too ill to write a fifth edition, I made a personal commitment to ensure that the legacy of this impactful book would not pass away as well. Thus, it is with great pride that I write this foreword, celebrating the continuance of the Gass Atlas, acknowledging the importance of careful clinical examination in the diagnosis of retinal disease, and recognizing the "passing of the baton" to the next generation.

Most of the ophthalmic community links J. Donald M. Gass to the Bascom Palmer Eye Institute. Dr. Gass was one of the founding physicians there, and forever changed our understanding of the macula. He opened our eyes to the complexity of macular diseases, by creating logical, well-defined classifications, based on carefully made clinical observations and a remarkable recollection of patients with similar histories and examinations. He passed on this knowledge to a world of residents, fellows, and colleagues across the globe. In fact, virtually every retina specialist considers himself or herself to be a student of Dr. Gass, even if they never had the opportunity to meet him. Fortunate were those who trained at BPEI and had the privilege of seeing patients with him and attending the weekly fluorescein conferences. It is no coincidence that Bascom Palmer became the breeding ground for many of the future leaders of the retina community.

However, the rest of us still learned from him. For some, it was attending lectures at conferences like the Annual Meeting of the American Academy of Ophthalmology. For others, they had the good fortune to work beside him as part of multicenter collaborative trials. I vividly remember my first meeting as an investigator in the Macular Photocoagulation Study in the 1980s. As the day concluded, they held a session where the Reading Center shared cases that were more difficult or confusing. The various experts would put forward their thoughts; however, the case was not settled until Dr. Gass weighed in. Even in a room filled with the "giants" in our field, Dr. Gass had the final word.

Here at Vanderbilt, we feel privileged to share some of the credit for the legacy of Dr. Gass' impact on ophthalmology. While J. Donald M. Gass was born in Canada, he was raised in Nashville, Tennessee when his father accepted a job in the state department of public health. He attended Vanderbilt as an undergraduate and as a medical student, winning the Founder's Medal as the top student in his graduating class. He married his high school sweetheart, Margy Ann, and it was anticipated that they would return to Nashville when he completed his training.

However, his return to Nashville was delayed for over 30 years until 1995 when he retired from his long-time faculty position as Professor of Ophthalmology at the University of Miami. Fortunately, his retirement was short-lived. Dr. Denis O'Day, the chair at Vanderbilt at that time, was able to convince Dr. Gass to join the faculty here. He returned to clinical practice, writing, and teaching. Dr. O'Day writes, "The image that will forever endure for me is the one I saw every week. It is of a man sitting, surrounded by colleagues, residents, students, and fellows. All are peering at photographs of the retina and the conversation is animated: all are engaged. As I walk by, I recognize our singular good fortune in having such a true academician in our midst."

One of those individuals surrounding Dr. Gass is Dr. Anita Agarwal. Drawn to Vanderbilt for a medical retina fellowship to learn under Dr. Gass, Anita developed an almost photographic memory of the Gass Atlas, and an encyclopedic knowledge of the retina literature. She came to evaluate a case in a brilliant Gass-like manner. Over time, her interest in the diversity of retinal diseases and her ability to make challenging diagnoses led her to earn a position of respect among the small community of similar experts.

It is highly appropriate that Dr. Anita Agarwal should be authoring this fifth edition. As well as any retina specialist in the world, she knows the previous editions from cover to cover. She has had the good fortune to have daily access to the Gass Archives: Dr. Gass' slides, patient charts, and personal notes that were bequested to the Vanderbilt Eye Institute upon his death. In fact, much of her writing has been conducted in a faculty office devoted to the Gass material: a room in which Dr. Gass' white coat hangs on the door and where the space is dominated by the large wooden cabinet with sliding trays that Dr. Gass would use to prepare his lectures and his manuscripts.

Dr. Agarwal has spent the better part of two years preparing this magnificent fifth edition. While she has restructured the chapters, updated the material to include newer conditions and new testing modalities like OCT, and engaged her talented friend and colleague, Dr. Arun D. Singh to write the chapters on intraocular tumors, this new edition retains the format of the previous editions. Most importantly, she has retained "the voice" of Dr. Gass. The words may be new or the condition may have been described subsequent to Dr. Gass's death, but Dr. Gass still speaks to us in this new edition.

I am hopeful that the Gass Atlas will live on through many future generations. The editors and publishers at Elsevier have done the ophthalmic community a wonderful service by investing in the creation of this fifth edition. I am grateful for their confidence in Dr. Agarwal, and certain that the readers will agree that this is a worthy successor to the previous editions.

Paul Sternberg, Jr., M.D.
G. W. Hale Professor and Chair,
Vanderbilt Eye Institute, Nashville, TN

World Map

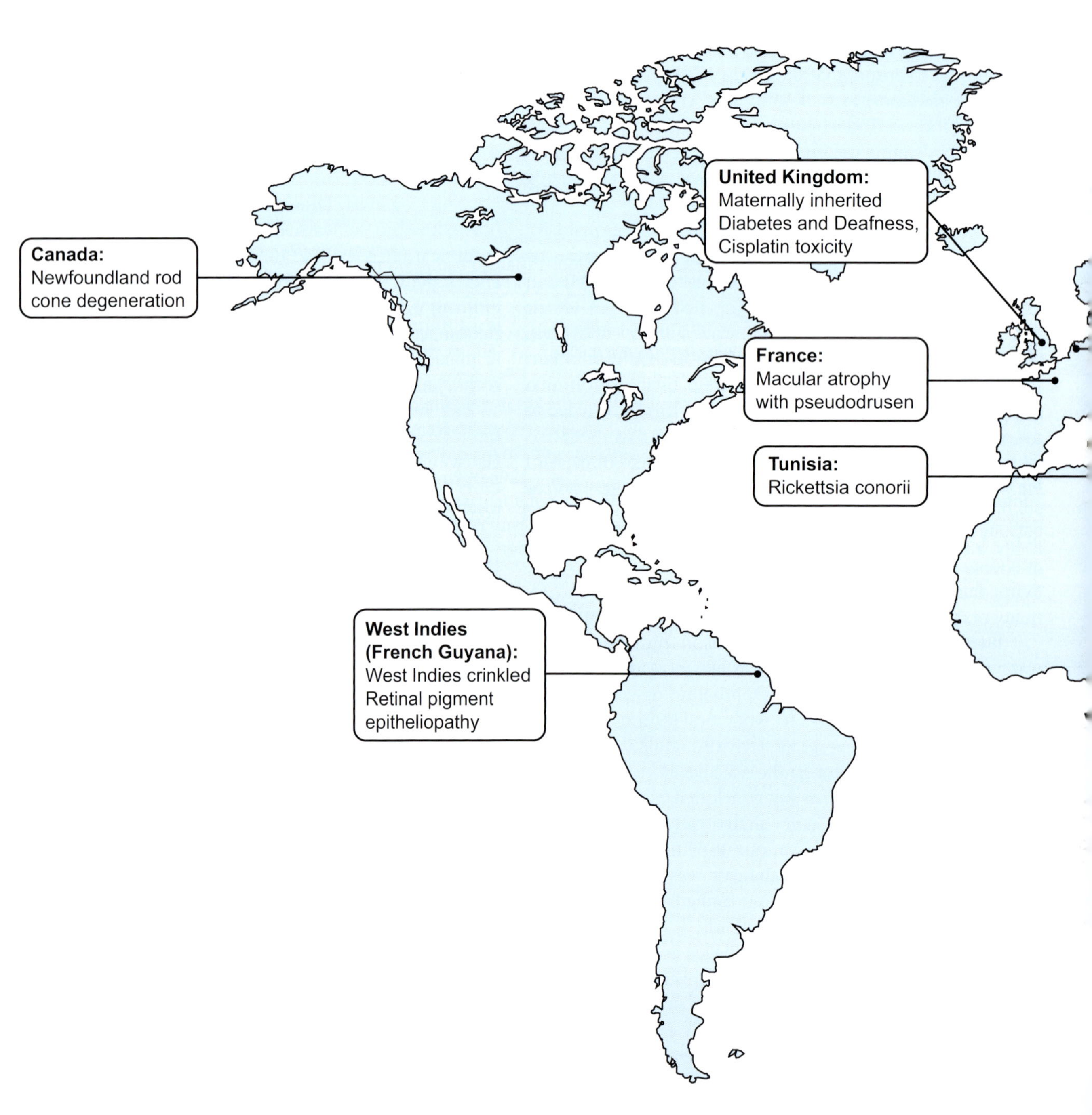
International Cases Presented in the Fifth Edition
Canada:
Newfoundland rod cone degeneration
United Kingdom:
Maternally inherited Diabetes and Deafness, Cisplatin toxicity
France:
Macular atrophy with pseudodrusen
Tunisia:
Rickettsia conorii
West Indies (French Guyana):
West Indies crinkled Retinal pigment epitheliopathy

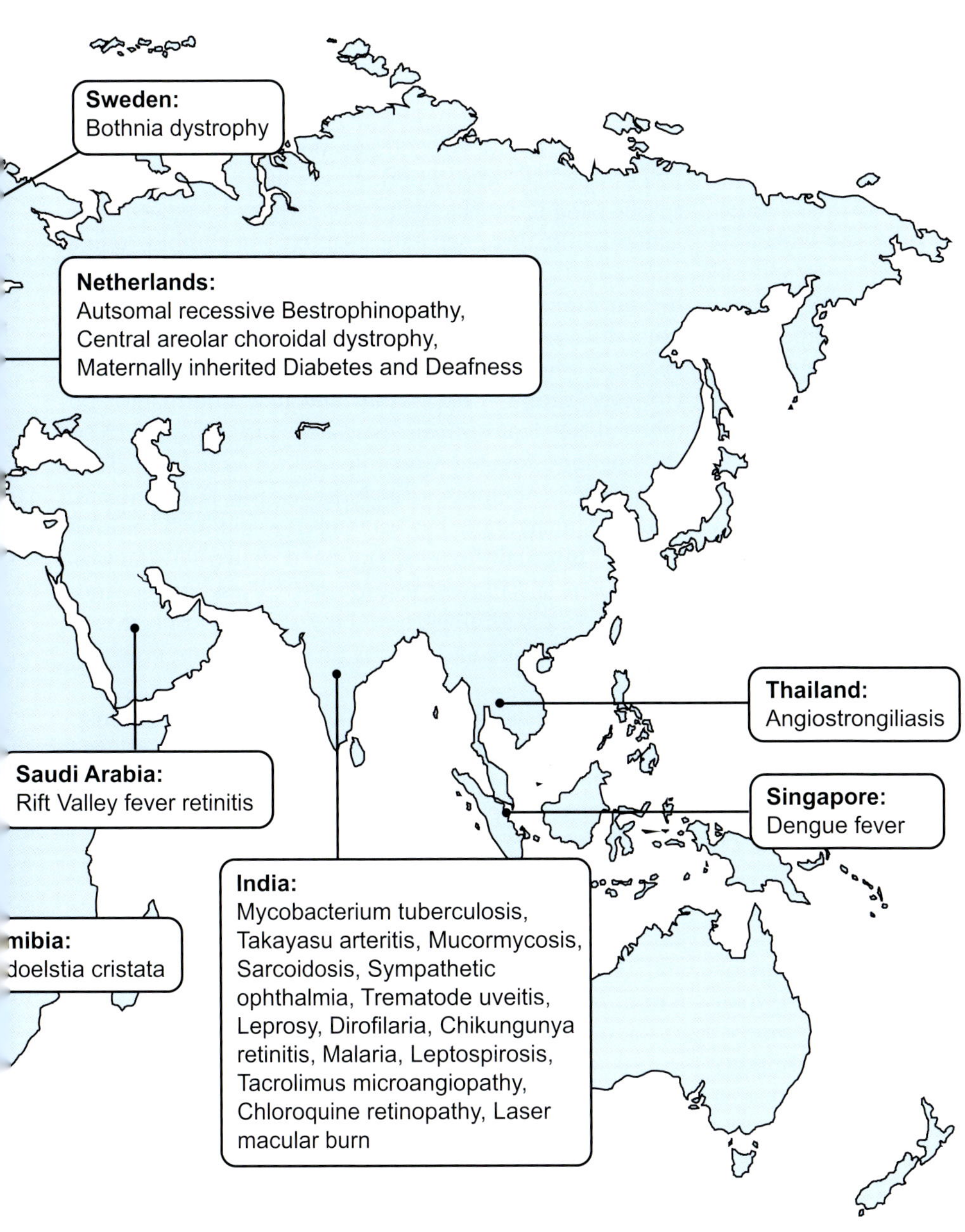

Sweden:
Bothnia dystrophy
Netherlands:
Autsomal recessive Bestrophinopathy,
Central areolar choroidal dystrophy,
Maternally inherited Diabetes and Deafness
Thailand:
Angiostrongiliasis
Singapore:
Dengue fever
Saudi Arabia:
Rift Valley fever retinitis
India:
Mycobacterium tuberculosis,
Takayasu arteritis, Mucormycosis,
Sarcoidosis, Sympathetic
ophthalmia, Trematode uveitis,
Leprosy, Dirofilaria, Chikungunya
retinitis, Malaria, Leptospirosis,
Tacrolimus microangiopathy,
Chloroquine retinopathy, Laser
macular burn
mibia:
doelstia cristata

Preface to the Fifth Edition

One of the most fortunate turns in life landed me square in front of J. Donald M. Gass, my idol from a distance, whose work I had read, studied and admired since the beginning of my ophthalmology training in India. In 1997, I entered my medical retina fellowship, initiating an unending, rewarding lesson from this giant. As known to the entire world of retinal physicians, Don Gass has had a truly profound impact on our understanding of retinal and macular diseases. His keen observation skills, photographic memory of ocular features, and ability to integrate clinical findings with pathological changes led him to describe several diseases for the first time and help us understand the pathogenic mechanisms of many other previously described conditions. Two of his singularly important qualities – meticulous attention to clinical details and analysis of stereoscopic images of the retina – became the hallmark of his defining publication, his 'Stereoscopic Atlas of Macular Diseases'. The evolution of the Atlas over its multiple editions has captured and illustrated the tremendous growth our field has experienced over the decades between the first and fourth version.

It is the greatest privilege of my professional life to be selected to edit this new 5th edition of Gass' Atlas of Macular Diseases . In this publication, I have tried to retain the "voice" of Dr. Gass, and continue his work, presenting new disease entities, consolidating known diseases, and discussing new concepts in the pathogenesis of existing conditions.

This edition incorporates a number of structural modifications.

First, each chapter includes an expanded table of contents to facilitate locating the individual conditions. The contents of the Atlas in Chapters 3, 5, 7, 10 and 11 of the 4th edition have been reorganized. Previously, Chapter 3 was quite exhaustive and lengthy, containing all disorders that caused a serous or hemorrhagic retinal detachment, be it inflammatory (such as VKH and sympathetic ophthalmia), infectious (such as Toxocara or certain fungal diseases), neoplastic (such as choroidal tumors), degenerative (such as age-related macular degeneration) or inherited (such as Malattia levantinese and Sorsby's dystrophy). The various infectious, inflammatory, neoplastic and inherited disorders have been moved to individual chapters, with the current Chapter 3 discussing only idiopathic, degenerative and miscellaneous causes of serous and hemorrhagic retinal detachment. The contents of Chapter 7, that included both infectious and inflammatory retinal diseases, have been split into two separate chapters, one on infectious diseases (Chapter 10) and a second on inflammatory diseases (Chapter 11). Chapter 5 addresses heredo-dystrophic conditions of the retina, choroid and pigment epithelium; it includes several new disorders including Bothnia dystrophy, Newfoundland rod cone degeneration, and pattern dystrophy associated with newly identified systemic diseases such as maternally inherited mitochondrial diseases and hereditary spastic paraplegia. The neoplastic diseases have been reorganized into three separate chapters for choroid, retina and retinal pigment epithelium and include the various benign tumors and hamartomas. The chapter on infectious diseases (Chapter 10) includes previously discussed bacterial followed by fungal, parasitic and viral diseases. However, various new entities and new information on tuberculosis, leptospirosis, parasites, and viruses such as chikungunya, dengue, west nile and rift valley fever have been added. Attempts to include diseases prevalent outside the United States has been made to aid in diagnosing rare and unusual diseases. The hand drawn illustrations, which were a hallmark feature of Dr. Gass' understanding of disease pathology, have been skillfully converted to electronic artwork, and fundus photographs are now presented in color.

The Atlas has maintained the case descriptive format of Gass' teaching method, encompassing history, clinical exam and follow up when available. The online version features stereoscopic images that are notated by a 3D sign. A stereo viewer accompanies the book.

Overall, the Atlas emphasizes clinical features, pathogenesis, information about genetics and its role in disease pathogenesis where known, differential diagnosis, and limited information on treatment. Extensive elaboration on results of clinical trials, controversies on medical management and surgery are not discussed; the Atlas is designed to be an exhaustive guide in arriving at the proper diagnosis of common and uncommon diseases and understanding their pathogenesis.

Anita Agarwal

Preface to the First Edition

The accessibility of the tissues of the inner eye to close scrutiny by the physician is unequaled by any other organ of the body. Having acquired a knowledge of ocular pathology and the skills of ophthalmoscopy and biomicroscopy, the physician is able to record his in vivo observations of the ocular fundus in gross pathologic terms with reasonable accuracy. This becomes of particular importance in evaluating the patient with loss of central vision resulting from alterations in the structure of the macula. The physician should attempt to determine as far as possible the anatomic changes present, such as choroidal atrophy, choroidal thickening, choroidal wrinkling, change in color of the pigment epithelium, serous detachment of the pigment epithelium, serous detachment of the retina, hemorrhagic detachment of the pigment epithelium and retina, cystoid retinal edema, intraretinal hemorrhage, loss of retinal transparency, retinal wrinkling, and preretinal membrane. He should also attempt to determine the locus of the primary disease process–choroid, retinal pigment epithelium, retinal, or vitreous. Only after making these determinations can the physician evaluate the significance of the patient's ocular, medical, and family history in arriving at a diagnosis, prognosis, and course of therapy.

A variety of ancillary studies may be helpful in certain instances. The use of intravenous fluorescein is of particular value in detecting and defining certain physiologic as well as anatomic changes in the ocular fundus.

The purpose of this atlas is to utilize black and white fundus photographs, stereo color fundus photographs, fluorescein angiographs, and photomicrographs to illustrate some of the anatomic and physiologic alterations produced by a variety of intraocular disease processes affecting the macular region.

After a discussion of the normal macular region (Chapter 1), the diseases affecting this region will be considered in the following order according to the primary tissue involved: diseases of the choroid (Chapters 2 to 4), pigment epithelium (Chapter 5), retina (Chapters 6 to 10), vitreous (Chapter 11), and congenital pit of the optic nerve head (Chapter 12). This subdivision is somewhat arbitrary in that it is not possible in some instances to know which of the ocular tissues is primarily involved by a particular disease process. Stereophotographs of some of the fundus photographs are included in fifteen reels, each containing seven views, attached to the back cover of the book. The appropriate reel number (Roman numeral) and view number (Arabic numeral) are indicated in the lower right-hand corner of the black and white photographs.

All fundus photographs were made with the Zeiss fundus camera. Fluorescein angiography was done utilizing modifications[1,2] of the technique described by Novotny and Alvis.[3] Kodak Kodachrome II and Kodak Tri-X film was used.

With a single exception, the fundus photographs used in this atlas were obtained from the photographic files of the Bascom Palmer Eye Institute of the University of Miami. Most of the patients were examined by me.

I wish to thank Dr. Edward W.D. Norton, Chairman of the Department of Ophthalmology, the members of the full-time and resident staff, and the many other physicians whose patients are illustrated in this book. I am particularly indebted to Mr. Johnny Justice, Jr. and his assistants, Mr. Kenneth Peterson, Mrs. Dixie Sparks Gilbert, and Mr. Earl Choromokos for their skill in fundus photography, and to Mr. Joseph Goren and Miss Barbara French for preparation of the illustrations. Finally, I wish to thank Mrs. Margaret Bertolami, Dr. Alexander R. Irvine, Mrs. Reva Hurtes, and Miss Beth Railinshafer for their help in preparing and editing the manuscript.

J. Donald M. Gass

In Remembrance of Dr Gass

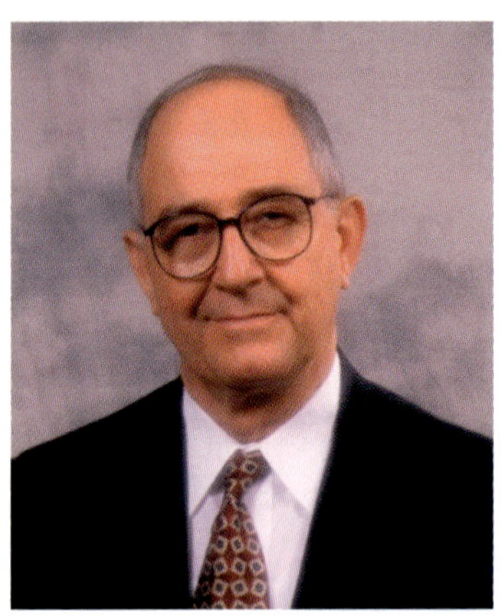

As a teenager growing up on Key Biscayne, I would awake on school days and leave the house in time to catch a 6:15 a.m. school bus into town. On the way out, I would find my father, up since before dawn, hard at work in the downstairs den of our home. The images of him pecking away on his electric typewriter with his four finger technique, peering up at slides, rummaging through piles of index cards, and painstakingly drawing illustrations of the macula remain imprinted in my memory. This scene repeated itself for many years beginning in the late sixties. "The book", as we called it around the house (we didn't know it as the "Atlas" back then), was taking shape. In those days, we were always aware of the presence of the book in the background of daily life around the Gass household. My father was usually careful not to let it intrude on other family priorities, but from time to time an increased sense of urgency to meet some deadline would become evident. My mother would often wonder out loud, sometimes with a tinge of irritation, if the book would ever be finished. As it turned out, the answer was not for at least forty years and I am now honored to contribute this foreword for the fifth edition of **Gass' Atlas of Macular Diseases** by Anita Agarwal MD.

I'm not sure when I became fully aware of the profound impact on the world of ophthalmology that my father's work at Bascom Palmer was having. The family received hints of this from time to time, hearing stories about my father from his colleagues and friends who would appear at our house. A modest and unassuming person, we would never hear a thing about any of this directly from him. Not being a doctor myself, it took me some years to piece together the full picture, but over time I became cognizant of the fact that the man I called "Dad" had become a giant in his field.

My job has taken me all over the world and I have lived on five continents. Over the years and until now, I have been amazed by the number of encounters I have had around the world with former colleagues, residents, fellows, students or patients who knew my father personally or were somehow influenced by his work, in many cases via the Gass Atlas. There are always the comments about the impact of his research, his skill as a teacher, or the brilliance of his scientific insights. But I also find, without exception, that the comments from those who knew him personally are accompanied by a story about some kindness my father had shown them or an anecdote about how he had somehow touched their lives. They always want to tell me something that I already know... that in addition to being a renowned physician, Don Gass was a very special human being.

Indeed, my father was an extraordinary person apart from all of his contributions to ophthalmology. He was first and foremost a loving husband, father, and grandfather who cherished his family. To my brothers and sister and me, he was "Dad". To everyone else in the family, including his five grandchildren, he was "Don". Growing up, there was nothing I wanted more than to be doing something with him. I can remember him teaching me how to fly a kite, ride a bike, throw a spiral, shoot a free throw underhanded, and how to fish. He took me to baseball games, taught me how to read a box score, and turned me into a lifelong Orioles fan. More importantly, I learned from him what it means to live one's life well, by observing over the years the most powerful example of this I have ever seen. Whether one knew my father as a physician, colleague, mentor, friend, neighbor or family, he was respected and loved for his kindness, his gentleness, his patience, his sense of humor, his integrity, his steadfast faith in the Lord, and a genuine humility rarely seen in others.

When I was younger, I often thought about what motivated my father to get up every day before dawn to write a book. I knew it was not a desire for fame or recognition or money. I could always see the constancy of purpose and his passion for what he was doing that remained unabated until the day he died. I could also sense the personal responsibility he felt for the continued stewardship of his work, including the Gass Atlas, because he understood it was important. But as I observed my father over the years, I came to understand there was also something else that made him tick. It was the simple yet deep satisfaction and joy that he got from creating something, solving a problem, and completing a task well. In his later years, I watched him become an accomplished wood craftsman by applying the same creativity, curiosity, dexterity, attention to detail, and patience that made him a great doctor. He spent much of his spare time in his wood shop crafting toys for the grandchildren, furniture for the house, or incredibly detailed model sailing ships. Some of these projects took hours; others took several years to complete. I loved seeing the smile on his face and the twinkle in his eyes which gave away the pure joy and sense of accomplishment he felt after completing even the simplest of these projects. I am certain that is the same feeling he had in completing each successive edition of the Gass Atlas.

I am delighted and grateful that Dr. Anita Agarwal who worked with my father in his final years at

Vanderbilt agreed to take on the challenge of authoring the fifth edition of the Gass Atlas more than four decades after the first edition was published. I know that my father would be very proud of her. The Gass Atlas represents a significant piece of my father's life's work and an important part of his legacy. However, the most enduring legacy of Dr. J. Donald M. Gass is the one that lives on in the lives, the careers, and the memories of the people touched by this remarkable man over the course of a lifetime.

John D. Gass on behalf of my mother Margy Ann, my brothers Carlton and Dean, and my sister Media

J. Donald M. Gass

Gentleman, Scholar and Genius

John Donald McIntyre Gass was born on Prince Edward Island, Canada on August 2nd 1928. At 2 weeks of age, he rode on a train with his mother from Canada to Nashville to join his father, a chest physician who had been named to direct the tuberculosis hospitals in Tennessee. He attended the two-room Grassland primary school, which housed 3 grades in each room. Being exposed to the same lessons for 3 years, Don Gass mastered 3rd grade while still in first grade, leaving himself plenty of time to learn more. He always fondly recalled his 1st grade teacher, who loaded her station wagon every month with books from the library for her students to read. Thus, was born his interest in reading. Several years later, he met his first and only love, Margy Ann Loser, on their high school bus; they were married in 1950. He attended Vanderbilt University for his undergraduate education and was deployed to Korea soon after being married. On his return, he began medical school at Vanderbilt, graduating with the highest honor: the Founder's medal.

Much to his father's puzzlement, Don Gass chose ophthalmology, a field then in its infancy. He spent his internship at the University of Iowa, and went on to be a resident at the Wilmer Eye Institute at the Johns Hopkins Hospital. There, he idolized Dr. Frank Walsh; whom he recognized the instant Dr. Walsh walked in for morning rounds on day one. While a resident, he wrote several papers on topics ranging from the optic chiasm to corneal iron lines. Between his senior residency and year as Chief Resident, he completed a fellowship in ophthalmic pathology at the Armed Forces institute of Pathology. This experience gave him an insight into disease pathology that he used skillfully through his entire career. He became quite facile in describing and postulating the pathogenesis of many diseases, most often accurately. Many of these insights were confirmed subsequently, using sophisticated tests such as OCT and autofluorescence imaging.

His numerous clinical contributions resulted from a unique combination of keen observation skills including the evaluation of stereoscopic images, attention to details, ability to comprehend and explain symptoms, and an uncanny memory for clinical findings among patients that he may have seen decades apart. He could not rest until he figured out all aspects of a new disease. Dr. Gary Abrams once told me that when Don Gass came upon a new disease, he talked about it incessantly till he figured it out completely in his mind. His excitement on seeing a new or rare disease was palpable and spread to his trainees. I recall the twinkle in his eyes and the excitement in his voice when he found the 250 micron DUSN worm coiled up in the midst of several retinal scars. His approach to understanding findings was simple and straightforward, and he used common objects to describe the analogy: a bagel for ring shaped sub RPE neovascularization and the petalloid appearance of fluorescein staining in cystoid macular edema. Fluorescein angiography was just introduced as Don Gass began his career in Miami, his study and interpretation of this investigative modality in retinal and choroidal diseases has helped us understand a majority of them. To this end, the talented photographer Johnny Justice at Bascom Palmer Eye Institute aided him.

Don Gass had a *simple but diligent* method to make notes about the various patients' findings. He carried 4×6″ note cards in his pocket and wrote down salient information about a hitherto undescribed condition that he saw. He cataloged them alphabetically. When he saw a few more patients with similar findings, he gathered all his cards and began deciphering the findings. In this manner, he described more than 30 original diseases and new features of several others. The descriptive names he gave to these diseases such as acute posterior multifocal placoid pigment epitheliopathy, acute exudative polymorphous vitelliform maculopathy, and acute zonal occult outer retinopathy would provide the clinician insight towards their pathogenesis or pattern of involvement. His understanding of disease pathology was cemented by his drawings. Many of his drawings are exact replica of what we now see on OCT imaging; a feat that Don Gass achieved several decades before the availability of OCT imaging. Renderings of the pathogenesis of a macular hole, vitreofoveal traction, type 1 and type 2 choroidal neovascularization, and the appearance of RPE detachments are just a few examples.

This giant in our field was kind, humble and generous. The transcriptionist at Vanderbilt told me of the largest fruit basket that she had ever seen in her life arrive at her doorstep when she was ill, sent by Dr. Gass. He enjoyed simple pleasures, such as fishing and woodworking. His knowledge and interest in sports was evident during animated discussions on Monday at lunch about the weekend's various sporting events and results. Most of all, he was a healer and teacher, who made each one of us a better doctor, a better teacher and a better human being. We were so privileged to have known him.

Written on behalf of all his students, past, present and future.

Anita Agarwal

CHAPTER 1

Normal Macula

ANATOMIC SUBDIVISIONS

The retina is a delicate transparent tissue of maximal thickness (approximately 0.55 mm) at the foveal margin and minimal thickness (0.13 mm) at the umbo. Anatomically the macula (macula lutea or central retina) is defined as that portion of the posterior retina that contains xanthophyll and two or more layers of ganglion cells. It measures approximately 5.5 mm in diameter and is centered approximately 4 mm temporal to and 0.8 mm inferior to the center of the optic disc (Figure 1.01).[1] On the basis of microscopic anatomy, the macular area can be further subdivided into several zones. The fovea (fovea centralis) is a depression in the inner retinal surface in the center of the macula. It measures approximately 1.5 mm (1500 μm) or one disc diameter in size. The central floor of the fovea is called the foveola. It measures approximately 0.35 mm in diameter. It lies within the capillary-free zone or foveal avascular zone, which measures approximately 0.5 mm (500 μm) in diameter in most patients. A small depression in the center of the foveola is called the umbo. A 0.5-mm-wide ring zone where the ganglion cell, inner nuclear layer, and outer plexiform layer of Henle are the thickest is called the parafoveal area. This zone is in turn surrounded by a 1.5-mm zone referred to as the perifoveal area.

1.01 Normal macula.

A–C: Topographic anatomy and histopathology of the macula. A, Fovea containing the foveola (a), capillary-free zone (cfz), and umbo (u). B, Parafovea. C, Perifovea.
D: Optical coherence tomography image of the normal macula corresponding to the histology seen in C.

1.02 Variations in appearance of normal macula.

A: Brunette fundus showing moderate to heavy concentration of pigment in the retinal pigment epithelium that obscures most of the choroidal vessels. Note the greater density of pigment in the macular area, the cilioretinal artery (black arrow), a first-order arteriole (upper black and white arrow), and a second-order arteriole (lower black and white arrow).
B: Blond fundus. Choroidal vessels are visible everywhere except in the macular area. The oval light reflex in the macula of this young child is located at the margin of the fovea.
C: Tesselated fundus in older patient. Large choroidal vessels are visible in the macular area because of relative hypopigmentation of retinal pigment epithelium.
D: Heterochromia of the fundus.

(A, from Gass.[42],)

CLINICAL APPEARANCE

Ophthalmoscopically, the anatomic subdivisions of the macula are ill defined (Figure 1.02). The center of the macula appears as a poorly defined, one-fourth to one disc diameter size zone of greater pigmentation that is maximum in the foveolar area. The foveal reflex, which is present in most normal eyes, appears to lie just in front of the center of the foveola and therefore overlies the anatomic umbo. There are no consistent ophthalmoscopic landmarks to indicate the margins of either the 0.35-mm diameter foveola or the 1.5-mm diameter fovea. The margins of the capillary-free zone of the retina that in most patients measures approximately 500 μm in diameter angiographically can only be estimated biomicroscopically because the perifoveolar capillary network is not visible. In younger patients an oval or round halo light reflex at the inner retinal surface may correspond with the foveal margin (Figure 1.02B). The foveal depression can be visualized with the narrow slit-lamp beam.

BLOOD SUPPLY

Retina

The blood supply to the inner half of the retina is by way of the central retinal artery, which usually divides into a superior and inferior trunk within the optic nerve head. These trunks divide into two branches, one supplying the nasal and the other the temporal quadrant of the retina. The corresponding retinal venous branches have much the same distribution as the arteries. These major blood vessels lie in the nerve fiber layer close to the internal limiting membrane of the retina. They give off arteriolar and venular branches that posteriorly occur primarily at right angles to the parent vessel. The branching is predominantly dichotomous as they course peripherally. The right-angle branches are referred to as first-order arterioles and venules (Figure 1.02A). In approximately 20% of patients Justice and Lehmann[2] found that a variable portion of the papillomacular area was supplied by one or more cilioretinal arteries derived from the ciliary circulation (Figure 1.02A). Occasionally a large cilioretinal artery may supply virtually the entire macula. The retinal arterial circulation is ordinarily an end-artery system that does not communicate with the blood vessels of the choroid or ciliary body. The retinal arteries and veins are interconnected via an extensive capillary network that extends outward to the external border of the inner nuclear layer. The blood vessel walls are normally transparent.[3] The postcapillary venules join to become retinal veins that accompany the retinal arteries and exit through the lamina cribrosa and drain into the superior ophthalmic vein. The retinal pigment epithelium (RPE) and the photoreceptors are nourished by diffusion from the choriocapillaris.

Choroid

The ophthalmic artery, the first branch of the internal carotid artery, divides into medial and lateral posterior ciliary arteries. Before entering the sclera each of these divides into one long posterior ciliary (LPCA) and 5–10 short posterior ciliary arteries (SPCA). A total of two LPCA and 15–20 SPCAs are thus formed. The LPCAs pierce the sclera 3–4 mm from the optic nerve and course between

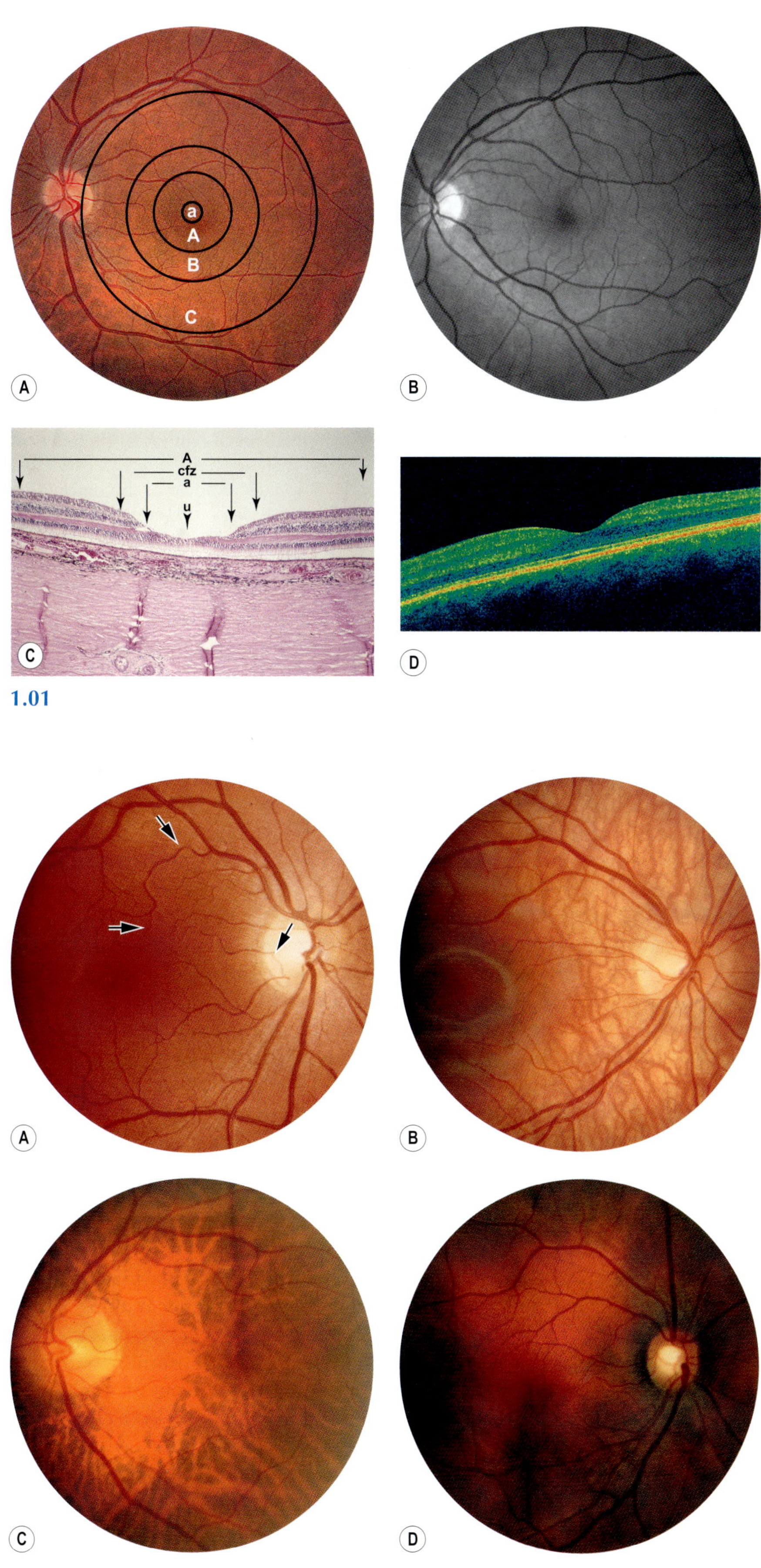

1.01

A
B
C
D

1.02

the choroid and the sclera along the 3 and 9 o'clock meridians till they branch at the ora serrata. Three to five branches bend posteriorly and supply the choroid till the equator. The SPCA enter the sclera around the optic nerve and course for a short distance in the suprachoroidal space, then enter the peripapillary choroid and branch anteriorly and posteriorly to supply the choroid up to the equator. There are seven anterior ciliary arteries (ACA) that accompany the four rectus muscles, about 8–12 recurrent branches of the ACA supply the anterior choriocapillaris, and the rest of the ACA form the major circle of the iris.

The venous drainage of the choroid is mostly through the vortex veins and a small anterior portion occurs through the anterior ciliary veins. Postchoriocapillaris venules form afferent veins that converge into the ampulla of the vortex veins (2 mm wide and 5 mm long) in each quadrant. Each quadrant has one vortex vein; occasionally more than one is present. They are situated 3–3.5 mm behind the equator (Figure 1.06D) and drain into the superior and inferior ophthalmic veins. The superior ophthalmic vein drains a major part of the globe and enters the cavernous sinus after passing through the superior orbital fissure while the inferior ophthalmic vein enters the pterygoid plexus via the inferior orbital fissure.[4]

Choriocapillaris

The choriocapillaris have unique features compared to capillaries elsewhere in the human body. They are 40–60 μm in diameter, as opposed to other capillaries that are 5–10 μm in size, and have thin walls with fenestrations measuring 600–800 Å. The fenestrations have a thin covering diaphragm and are more numerous on the internal side than the external side, which has the endothelial cell nuclei. Three to four red blood cells can pass through the choriocapillaris at a time. Pericytes are seen occasionally and gap junctions are present. Connective tissue, fibroblasts, and nerve fibers are present between the capillaries and provide support. There is a rapid transition from the arterioles to the capillaries, hence the large blood flow in the choroid. There is a central precapillary arteriole that breaks up into a lobule of choriocapillaris and empties into a peripheral postcapillary venule. There is regional variation in the choriocapillaris architecture. The lobular pattern of the choriocapillaris is seen in the posterior pole, whereas near the equator the precapillary arteriole and postcapillary venule have a more direct connection through the capillaries, and anteriorly the choriocapillaris connects the arterioles and venules at right angles, creating a ladder-like pattern.

The RPE is more highly pigmented in the central macular area than elsewhere. Whereas the amount of melanin in the RPE is similar in all races, the number of melanocytes and the amount of melanin in the choroid are greater in more highly pigmented races.[5] In caucasians the combination of the pigment in the RPE and the choroid imparts an orange or orange-red color to the fundus. In most pigmented individuals the RPE and choroidal pigment impart a brown color that obscures most or all

1.03 Gross dissection of a fresh human eye.

A: Fundus of the eye after removal of the anterior segment showing partial loss of the normal retinal transparency. The dark foveolar spot (arrow) is caused by the densely concentrated xanthophyll and the retinal pigment epithelium (RPE), which is visible through the thin portion of the foveolar retina. A halo of yellowish color (xanthophyll) in the retina surrounds the dark spot.
B: Slightly magnified view of the same eye. Following removal of the semiopaque retina, the orange color of the RPE, which is denser in the foveal area (arrow), is visible.
C: Same eye following incomplete removal of the RPE. Compare greater density of RPE remnant in the macular area (arrow) with that surrounding the optic disc and elsewhere. Note that in this particular eye the darkness of the macular area is primarily caused by the difference in the density of the RPE and not by the difference in concentration of the uveal melanocytes.
D: Eye after removal of the choroid. Approximately 12 short ciliary arteries (arrowheads) perforate the sclera in the mid peripheral macular area. Two branching short ciliary arteries are evident nasal to the optic nerve head. Note the long ciliary artery and nerve (arrow) temporal to the macula.

1.04 Retinal xanthophyll.

Location and relative concentration of xanthophyll pigment (dots) in the retina in the macula area. RPE, retinal pigment epithelium.

of the choroidal vascular details throughout the posterior fundus. Even in very blond individuals, in whom much of the choroidal vasculature is visible, the choroidal blood vessels in the macular region usually are obscured by the greater density of the RPE centrally (Figure 1.02B). RPE becomes less pigmented with age, and in brunette patients the greater contrast between the larger choroidal vessels and the surrounding melanocytes gives a tesselated appearance to the fundus (Figure 1.02C). Often there is less pigmentation of the choroid and RPE in a segmental area of the fundus inferior to the disc in the area of closure of the fetal fissure. Uneven distribution of melanocytes in the uvea may occasionally give a distinct heterochromic appearance to the fundus (Figure 1.02D).

GROSS ANATOMY

Examination of the macular area with a dissecting microscope is possible after making a coronal section through the pars plana of a fresh eye (Figure 1.03). The retina begins to lose its normal transparency within hours of death. Yellow pigment is apparent in the center of the macula. It is highly concentrated in the foveolar area (Figure 1.03A). If the central macular area of a fresh human retina is viewed in cross-section, the concentration of the xanthophyll appears to be maximal in the outer nuclear and outer plexiform layers. Xanthophyll is also present, however, within the inner plexiform layer inside the foveal area (Figure 1.04). In monkeys the yellow

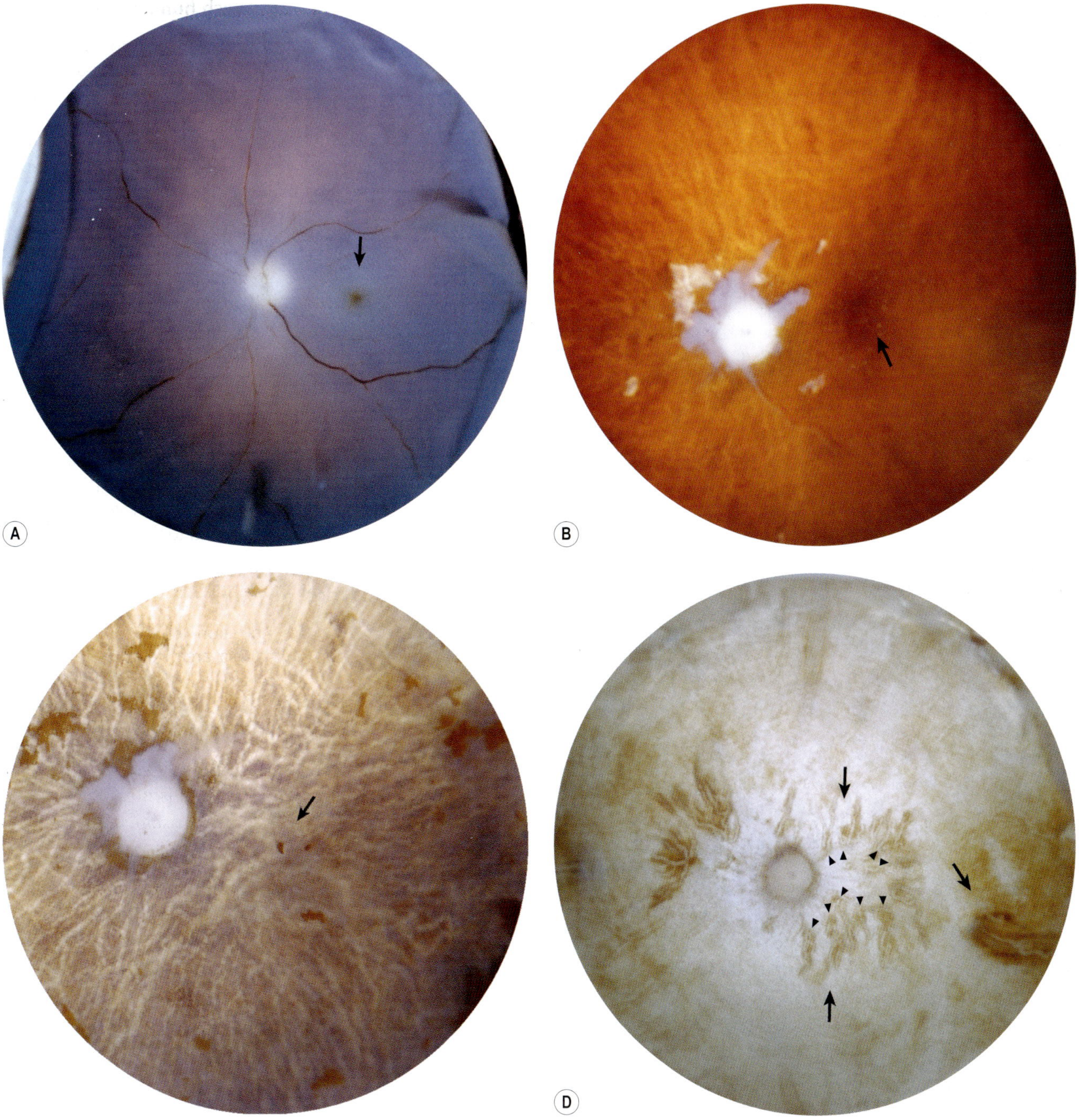

1.03

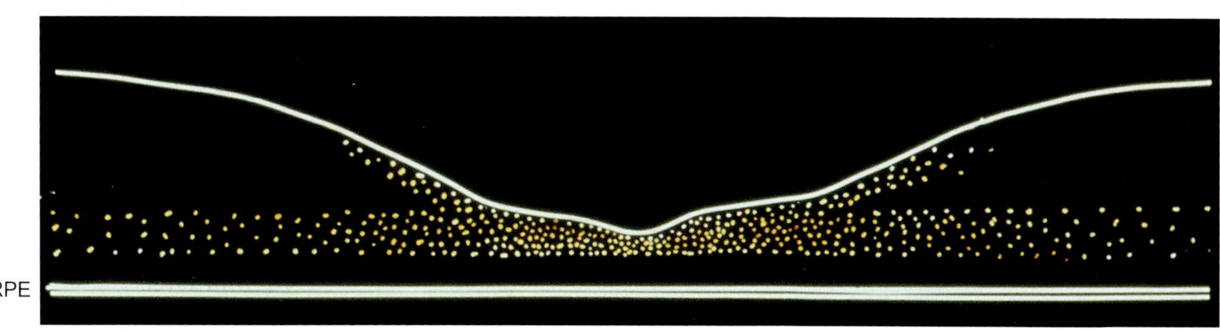

1.04

pigment has been localized by spectrophotometric analysis to all layers from the outer nuclear layer inward but with the greatest concentration in the outer and inner plexiform layer centrally.[6–10] Microdensitometry of retinal sections of primate retinas suggests that the greatest concentration is in the cones axons centrally.[9] Stereochemical analysis has demonstrated evidence that xanthophyll comprises two carotenoids with properties identical to those of zeaxanthin and lutein.[10,11] After removal of the semitransparent retina, the normal orange-red appearance of the fundus is restored (Figure 1.03B). This color results primarily from the melanin within the RPE cells and not, as often implied, from the blood within the choroidal vessels. The relatively dark area in the foveal region is probably caused primarily by the increased pigment content of the RPE cells. The relative darkness of this area, along with the normal orange-red color of the surrounding fundus, largely disappears after the RPE is removed with a cotton applicator (Figure 1.03C). Some of the relative darkness of the central macular area remains, however, because of the greater concentration of choroidal melanocytes in this area. The large choroidal vessels in older patients appear as yellowish white cords coursing through the macular area. This loss of choroidal vessel wall transparency in older patients, although often referred to as "choroidal sclerosis," probably represents a normal aging change in the choroidal vessel wall and is not associated with significant narrowing of its lumen.

After removal of the choroid, the entrance sites of the short and long posterior ciliary arteries are visualized (Figure 1.03D). The short posterior ciliary arteries are concentrated in the macular area, particularly along the temporal margin of the fovea and the peripapillary area. In the choroid they branch frequently and course outward toward the periphery. Several short posterior ciliary arteries enter nasal to the optic disc. The temporal long posterior ciliary artery and ciliary nerve enter about 1½ disc diameters temporal to the center of the fovea. Melanocytes are concentrated along either side of both of these structures.

HISTOLOGY

The specialized structure in the macular region accounts for the predilection of certain disease processes to involve this area and for the variety of ophthalmoscopic changes peculiar to this area. In the macula we find the thickest portion of the retina (Figure 1.01B) surrounding the thinnest portion, the foveolar area. The normal retina is composed of a mass of interwoven neural cells with little extracellular space. The relative lack of extracellular space is apparent only with electron microscopy, which demonstrates cell membranes not visible with ordinary histologic techniques. In the inner half of the retina there is extensive intertwining of horizontally and vertically coursing neural cell processes and blood vessels, all of which are enveloped by lateral extensions of the Müller cell processes. In the outer plexiform layer of Henle, however, the long Müller and receptor cell processes radiate in an almost horizontal and then oblique direction away from the central foveal area and are not interconnected by intertwining neural processes and blood vessels. The Müller cells are modified glial cells that provide the structural framework supporting the neural elements of the retina. Their nuclei lie in the inner nuclear layer. Anteriorly their basal cell processes constitute the inner retinal surface, which is lined anteriorly by the so-called internal limiting membrane, basement membrane, or basal lamina of the Müller cells (Figure 1.05). This membrane is relatively thick in the macular region except in the area of the foveola, where it is visible only by electron microscopy. The internal limiting membrane serves as an anchoring structure for the collagen framework of the vitreous. The apical or outer cell processes of the Müller cells extend external to the outer nuclear layer, where they are connected to the visual cells by a system of terminal bars that constitute the external limiting membrane (Figure 1.05B).[12] This row of tight junctions probably provides at least a partial barrier to the passage of large molecules in either direction. It probably functions on the one hand to protect the retinal extracellular compartment from encroachment by subretinal exudate and on the other hand to prevent intraretinal exudate from spreading into the subretinal space.

An overlooked part of the fovea is the inverted cone-shaped zone of specialized Müller cells composing the floor of the fovea – Müller cell cone, first reported by Yamada in 1969.[13,14] This cone of Müller cells is likely a reservoir for concentrated xanthophyll and the primary structural support for the foveola (Figure 1.05C). The apex of the cone was close to the outer limiting membrane and the base formed the floor of the fovea centralis and extended into the area of the clivus in the perifoveal region. The cytoplasm towards the apex of the Müller cells appeared scant and optically empty. It was denser towards the base of the Müller cells; this is in contrast to the greater density of cytoplasm of the Müller cells elsewhere in the retina. The internal limiting membrane lining the inner surface of the Müller cell cone was thin (10–20 nm) compared with that in the peripheral foveal area (1.5 μm).[14]

1.05 Histology of macular and paramacular retina.

Peripheral macula, **A**: and paramacular retina, **B**: showing internal limiting membrane (i), ganglion cell layer (g), inner plexiform layer (ip), inner nuclear layer (in), outer plexiform layer of Henle (n), outer nuclear layer (o), external limiting membrane (ELM), and receptor elements (r).
C: Schematic depiction of the Müller cell cone (Mcc). g, ganglion cell layer; H, Henle nerve fiber layer.

(C, adapted from Gass.[13],)

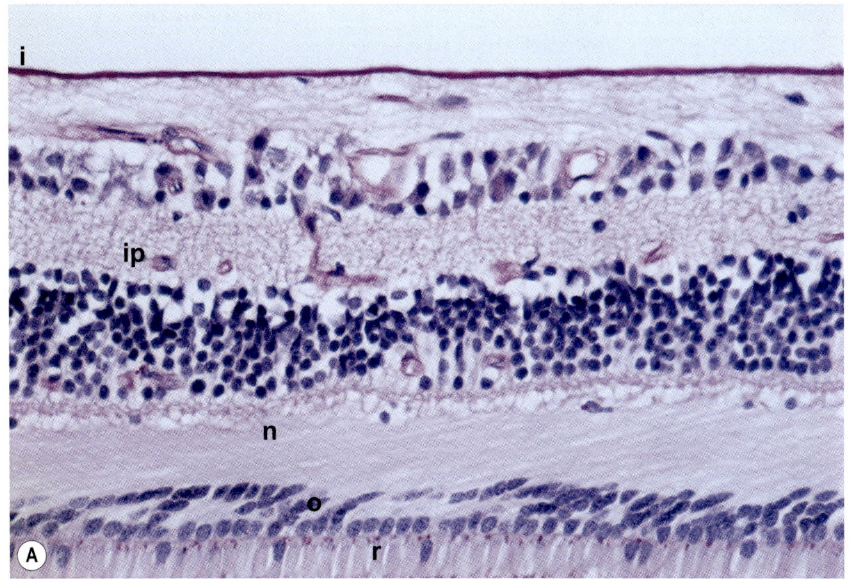
i
ip
n
o
r
A

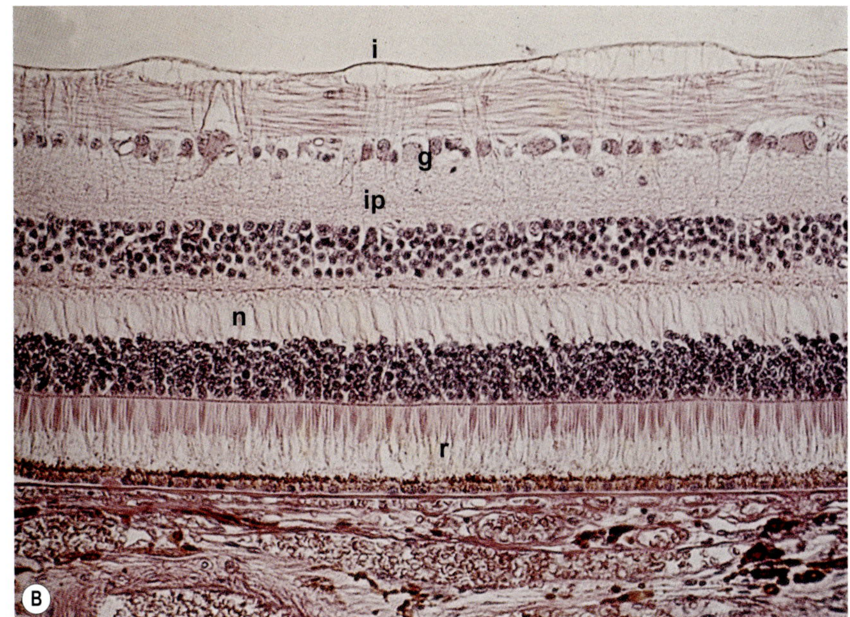
i
g
ip
n
r
B

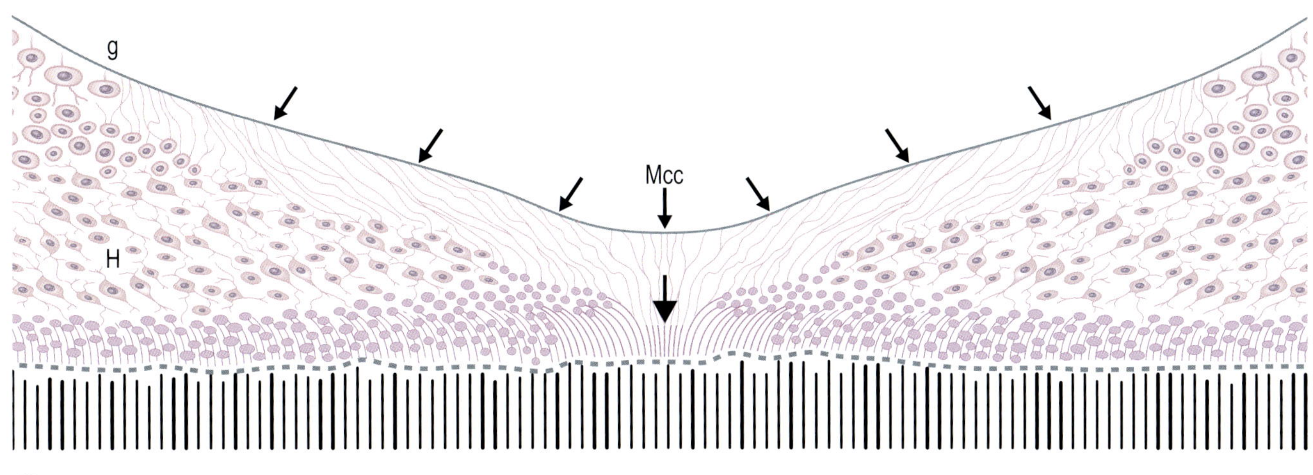
g
Mcc
H
C

The retinal blood vessels are confined to the inner half of the retina. Electron microscopy has revealed that all of the major branches of the retinal arterial system have the structure of small arteries that persists even beyond the equator.[4] Retinal arteries differ in their structure from muscular arteries of the same size in other organs in their lack of an internal elastic lamina and their well-developed muscularis. Posteriorly the arterial wall consists of five to seven layers of smooth-muscle cells; peripherally this is reduced to one or two layers. The retinal veins near the optic disc have three to four layers of smooth-muscle cells. The muscularis disappears, however, a short distance from the optic disc and is replaced by fibroblasts. There is controversy concerning the pattern of distribution of the capillary network in the retina. Retinal trypsin digest studies suggest a diffuse arrangement[1,15,16] whereas injected whole mounts suggest a two- or three-tier arrangement.[17] The superficial network is predominantly postarteriolar and the deep network prevenular. There is a distinct radial peripapillary capillary network that arises at the optic disc and extends along an arcuate course within the nerve fiber layer. This network richly interconnects with the inner retinal capillary layer.[17] In the perifoveolar area, the capillary network is reduced to a single layer of capillaries that surround a capillary-free zone, which varies in size but which usually measures 0.4–0.5 mm in diameter (see Figure 1.09F, below). The capillary-free zone is an important fluorescein angiographic landmark in evaluating patients with macular disease. There is experimental evidence to suggest that the capillary-free zone is normally vascularized during the prenatal development of the retina. Just before or shortly after birth the capillary-free zone develops as a result of spontaneous capillary obliteration.[18] In a few patients with normal visual function, all or part of this prenatal capillary network may persist into adulthood. The retinal blood vessels, as well as all of those within the central nervous system, are lined by an endothelium with tight cellular junctions demonstrable in electron micrographs. This peculiar endothelial structure constitutes the inner part of the blood–retinal and blood–brain barrier system that is responsible for maintaining the extracellular spaces of the retina and brain relatively free of extracellular fluid.

The RPE is a monolayer of hexagonal cells densely adherent to one another by a system of tight cellular junctions or terminal bars that comprise the outer blood–retinal barrier, which maintains the subretinal space in a state of deturgescence. The intercellular cohesiveness of the RPE is not easily disrupted. Interdigitation of the apical processes of the RPE cells with the rod and cone outer segments of the retina provides only a tenuous adhesion of the RPE to the sensory retina. The RPE cells are taller and contain a greater concentration of melanin pigment in the macular region than elsewhere.[5,19] There is an inverse relationship between melanin and lipofuscin pigment concentration in the pigment epithelium. Lipofuscin concentration increases initially during the first two decades of life and then again in the sixth decade of life. The concentration of lipofuscin in the pigment epithelium is significantly greater in white than in black persons, whereas the concentration of melanin in the pigment epithelium is similar in black and white persons. The melanin content of the pigment epithelium and choroidal melanocytes declines with age. In young and middle-aged individuals the RPE is tightly adherent to the underlying Bruch's membrane by means of its own basement membrane. This adherence decreases with advancing age. In this book the term "Bruch's membrane" is used only to refer to the sheet-like condensation of the innermost portion of the choroidal stroma that consists of two layers of collagen, one on either side of a layer of elastic tissue (Figure 1.06). Its inner surface is smooth, whereas its outer surface is composed of a series of waffle-like collagenous protrusions that extend externally to form the pillars separating and supporting the choriocapillaris. The inclusion of the submicroscopic basement membrane layers of the RPE and the choriocapillaris endothelium as part of Bruch's membrane by some authors is unfortunate for several reasons. First, Bruch could not have seen these latter two structures with light microscopy, and second, and more important from the pathophysiologic point of view, it is logical to consider Bruch's membrane as being part of the choroidal stroma. The condensation of mesodermal connective tissue that composes Bruch's membrane is similar in its relationship to the stroma of the choroid, as Bowman's membrane is in its relationship to the stroma of the cornea. As an integral part of the stroma surrounding the endothelial walls of the choriocapillaris, Bruch's membrane does not represent a distinct tissue layer capable of being separated physically from the choriocapillary bed. Because of its porous structure it probably plays a minimal role in regulating movement of substances across it.

1.06 Normal choroid.

A: Histologic sagittal section. Retinal pigment epithelium (left arrow), Bruch's membrane (right arrow), choriocapillaris (cc), choroidal melanocyte (m), precapillary arteriole (p), and choroidal artery (ca).

B: Three-dimensional schematic representation. Note the lobular patterns of the choriocapillaris with each lobule supplied by an arteriole. ca, choroidal artery; cv, choroidal vein.

C, D: Vortex vein ampulla seen under the macula in this high myope, normally seen 14–15 mm from the limbus (D)

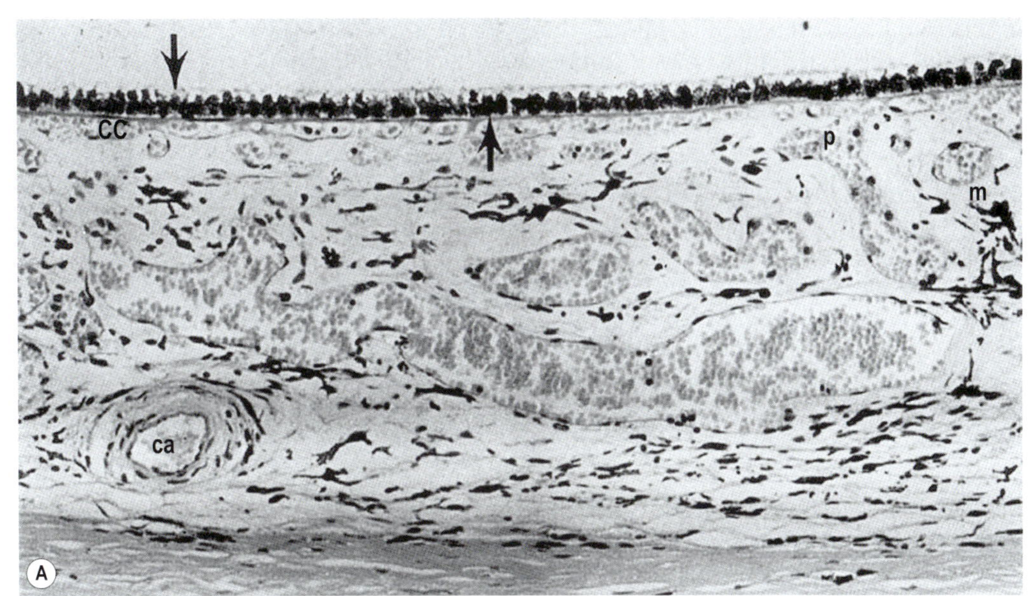

1.06

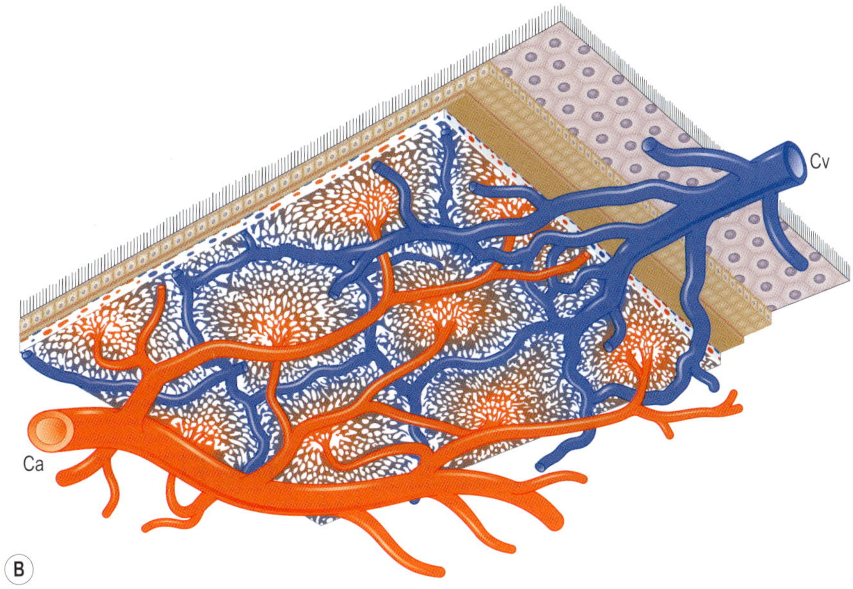

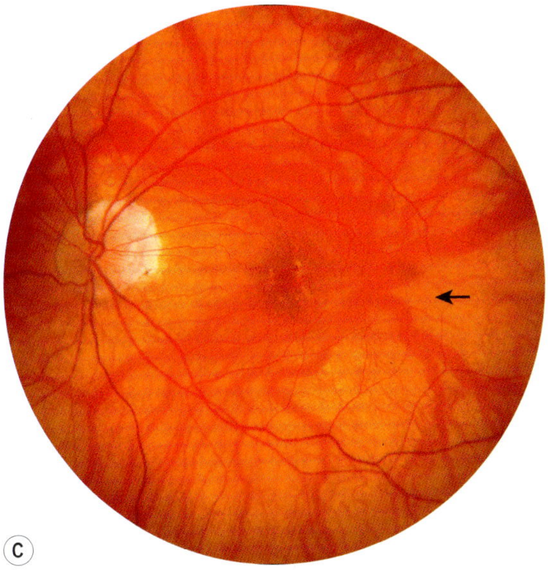

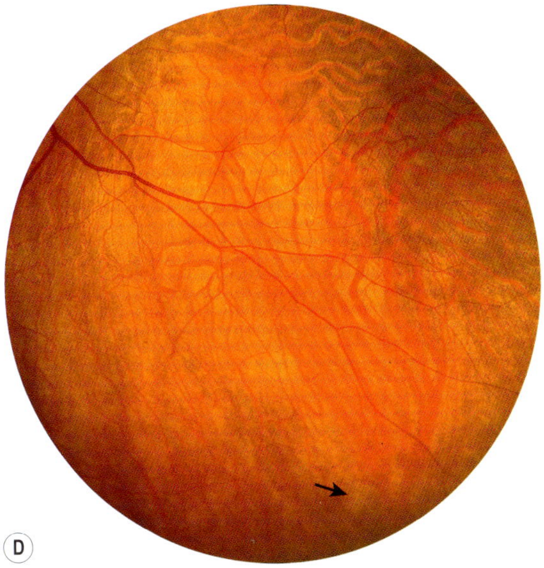

B
Cv
Ca

C

D

The choroid is supplied by the short ciliary or choroidal arteries that are concentrated in the macula and peripapillary region. Posteriorly, these arteries form a rich anastomotic network that quickly empties large quantities of blood into the sinusoidal network, referred to as the choriocapillaris, that is encased within the outer part of Bruch's membrane.[17,20–24] These wide interconnecting capillary spaces are lined by a fenestrated endothelium that is attached by its basement membrane to the outer collagenous zone of Bruch's membrane. The choriocapillaris is arranged in a segmental pattern that varies with its location.[21,25–28] In the macula there is a lobular pattern of highly concentrated interconnecting capillaries supplied by a central arteriole and drained by circumferential venules (Figure 1.06B).[26,29–32]

The peripapillary branches of the short posterior ciliary arteries supply the majority of the capillaries in the prelaminar part of the optic nerve.[23] Although occasional arterial branches from the choroid supply the optic disc, the choriocapillaris does not communicate directly with the optic disc capillaries. The prelaminar capillaries freely anastomose at the disc margin with those of the retina. Both capillary systems drain into the venules leading to the central retinal vein.[23,26,32,33]

The nutrition of the inner half of the retina is supplied by the retinal blood vessels. The tight cellular junctions of the retinal capillary endothelium (blood–inner retinal barrier) and the RPE (blood–outer retinal barrier), although permitting free exchange of water, nutrients, and waste products between the blood and the retina, form a barrier that prevents passage of large molecules, including proteins and lipids, into the extracellular space of the retina and into the subretinal space. The oncotic pressure, exerted primarily by the high concentration of intravascular proteins, together with intracellular physiologic pumping mechanisms within the RPE and retinal capillary endothelium, are important in maintaining the retinal extracellular space and subretinal space relatively free of water. The RPE is involved also in the photochemistry of vision, the phagocytosis of degenerated outer segments of the retinal elements, and the transport of metabolic wastes from the retina into the choriocapillaris.

The peculiar structure of the choroidal vascular tree in the macula provides this area with the highest rate of blood flow of any tissue in the body. This is greatly in excess of that needed to meet the nutritional demands of the retina[34] and probably functions to stabilize the temperature environment of the retina, particularly in the macular area.[35] The choriocapillaris is the major source of nutrition for the RPE and outer retinal layers. Although rapid-sequence angiography has demonstrated some degree of segmentation of the blood supply to the choroid in both normal humans and experimental animals, the availability of many pathways of collateral blood flow in the choroid is responsible for the infrequent demonstration of loss of visual function caused by obstruction

1.07 Schematic diagram showing relationship of choroidal circulation, retinal pigment epithelium (RPE), and retina.

Fluorescein enters by way of the ophthalmic artery (OA) and the short ciliary arteries (CA) into the blood vessels of the choroid and small capillaries supplying the optic nerve head. The dye passes in a more circuitous route by way of the central retinal artery (CRA) into the retinal circulation. In the macula the more densely pigmented pigment epithelium and the retinal xanthophyll act as filters to obscure the underlying choroidal vessels from view.

(From Hayreh.[21],)

1.08 Technique of fluorescein angiography.

Patient (left), photographer, and physician.

of large choroidal arteries, particularly in the posterior fundus. The choriocapillaris, like the rest of the capillary system outside the central nervous system, has an endothelium with a pore size sufficient to allow some larger molecules, including proteins, to escape into the extravascular space. Outside the eye, extracellular protein returns to the intravascular system via the lymphatic system. In the eye there are no lymphatic channels, and the perivascular and perineural spaces in the sclera probably function as lymphatic channels to provide a pathway for extracellular protein to exit the eye and to gain entrance into the lymphatic system. Thus the choriocapillaris endothelium is of primary importance in controlling the amount of extracellular fluid normally present in the choroid.

NORMAL FLUORESCEIN ANGIOGRAPHIC FINDINGS

Sodium fluorescein in solution when excited by a blue light (465–490 nm) will fluoresce and emit a yellow-green light (peak wave length of 520–530 nm). Its molecular weight of 376 is such that it diffuses freely out of all the body capillaries except those in the central nervous system, including the retina. It diffuses throughout the extracellular compartment, and it stains collagen, but it does not enter the intracellular compartment in concentrations sufficient to be visualized. Approximately 80% of the dye is bound to plasma proteins, mostly albumin. It is predominantly the unbound fluorescein in the plasma layer lying between the retinal blood vessel wall and the column of flowing erythrocytes that is detected angiographically.

In the eye the retinal circulation and the choroidal circulation are separated by a filter of irregular and variable density, the RPE (Figure 1.07). Fluorescein injected rapidly into the antecubital vein of the normal patient (Figure 1.08) enters the choroidal circulation by way of the short ciliary arteries about 10–15 seconds after injection

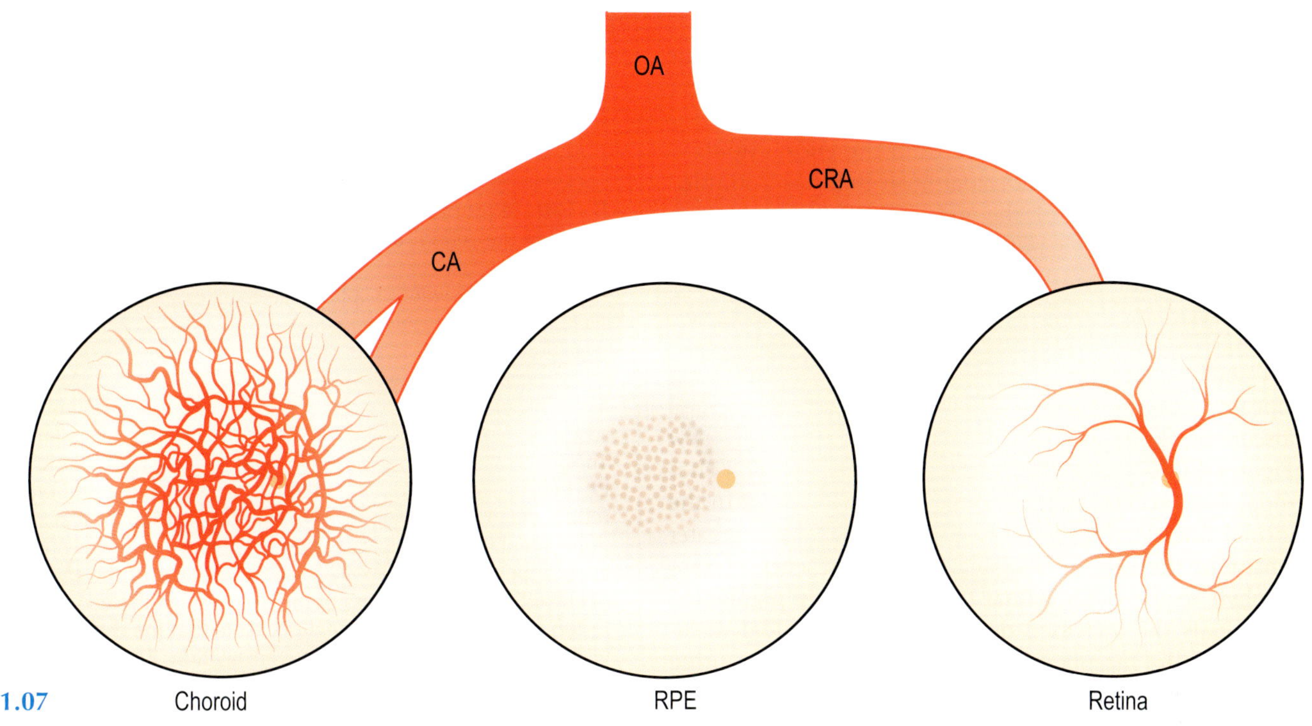

1.07

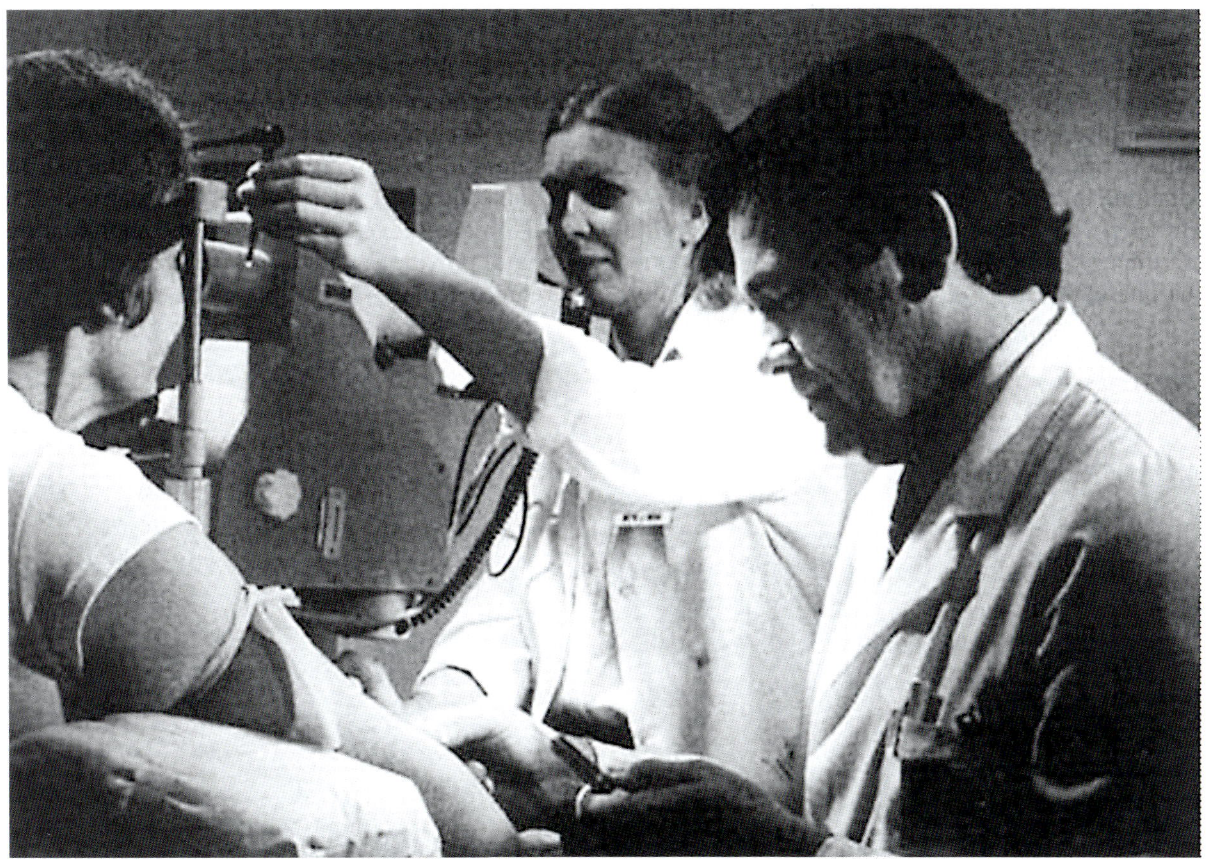

1.08

In many patients, particularly in those with a brunette fundus, the fine retinal capillary network, including that surrounding the central avascular zone, can be visualized angiographically using the ordinary techniques of intravenous injection into the antecubital vein (Figure 1.09F). The diameter of the capillary-free zone is variable and is usually 400–500 μm (one-third disc diameter). Serial photography permits detection of major flow alterations, whether caused by arterial, capillary, or venous obstruction. The detection of minor flow alterations is difficult without the use of cinematographic techniques. The blood vessels of the central nervous system, including those of the retina, appear impermeable to the fluorescein molecule. This is not true of blood vessels outside the central nervous system, including those of the choroid. The dye leaks out of the choriocapillaris, stains Bruch's membrane, diffuses into the extravascular spaces of the choroid, and eventually stains the sclera (Figure 1.10). Just as the retinal vascular endothelium is a barrier to the diffusion of dye into the retina, so the RPE is a barrier to the diffusion of dye from the choroid into the retina. As the dye diffuses into the body tissues and is rapidly excreted in the kidneys and liver, the intravascular concentration of fluorescein decreases and dye begins to diffuse back into the choroidal vessels. The large choroidal vessels lying in the pool of extravascular dye appear relatively hypofluorescent during the later stages of angiography (Figure 1.09D). This is partly because of a delay in the return of extravascular dye into the choriocapillaris, but more importantly, it is a result of the greater amount of dye in the extravascular spaces compared with the thin layer of intravascular fluorescein surrounding the central column of erythrocytes.

In evaluating diseases of the macula, fluorescein angiography can be of value in detecting: (1) alterations in blood flow; (2) alterations in permeability of the retinal blood vessels; (3) alterations in the retinal vascular pattern; (4) alterations in the density of the pigment epithelium; and (5) other changes affecting the normal angiographic pattern in this area.

In 1969 indocyanine green (ICG) was introduced as a supplement to fluorescein as another dye for angiographic study of the ocular fundus.[36–38] The weak fluorescent efficiency of ICG limited its usefulness, however, until the recent development of digital video imaging systems.[39,40] ICG is a water-soluble tricarbocyanine dye containing 5% or less of sodium iodide. It has a molecular weight of 775. When injected intravenously it is tightly bound to plasma globulins and is excreted solely by the liver. It has been widely used medically since 1956 with minimal adverse reactions.[37,41] It should not be used in patients with a history of allergy to iodine. The principal advantages of ICG over fluorescein are its spectral absorption and fluorescent characteristics in the near-infrared wavelengths. ICG in blood absorbs and emits light in the near-infrared range (805 and 835 nm, respectively). Thus ICG angiography allows greater visualization through exudate, lipid, melanin, and hemoglobin and provides a greater view of the choroidal circulation than is possible with fluorescein angiography. Being more highly protein-bound than fluorescein, it escapes more slowly from the choriocapillaris and new vessels into serous tissue spaces and, therefore, in some circumstances is better able to detect and localize areas of neovascularization lying beneath serous detachment of the pigment epithelium and retina.[40] In spite of the increased use of ICG angiography over the past two decades, there still exist some gaps in our knowledge concerning the interpretation of ICG angiograms.

1.10 Fluorescein angiographic study of normal fundus. Perfusion of normal choroid during angiography. Compare angiogram (left) with schematic diagram (right). Black dots indicate fluorescein molecules.

A1 and **A2**: early perfusion of short ciliary arteries (sca) and choriocapillaris (cc) produces early background choroidal fluorescence and fills capillaries of the optic disc. RPE, retinal pigment epithelium; bm, basement membrane; BM, Bruch's membrane.

B1 and **B2**: Arteriovenous phase showing increase in background choroidal fluorescence caused by dye molecules escaping from the choriocapillaris to stain Bruch's membrane and the extravascular tissues of the choroid. The dye does not penetrate the cell membrane of the retinal pigment epithelium, which is adherent to Bruch's membrane by means of the basement membrane.

C1 and **C2**: Later stages of angiography. Note the large choroidal vessels are relatively hypofluorescent (arrow). The dye is diffusing back into the choriocapillaris as the intravascular dye concentration decreases. The large amount of dye in the extravascular spaces and sclera in comparison to that intravascularly causes the larger vessels to appear hypofluorescent.

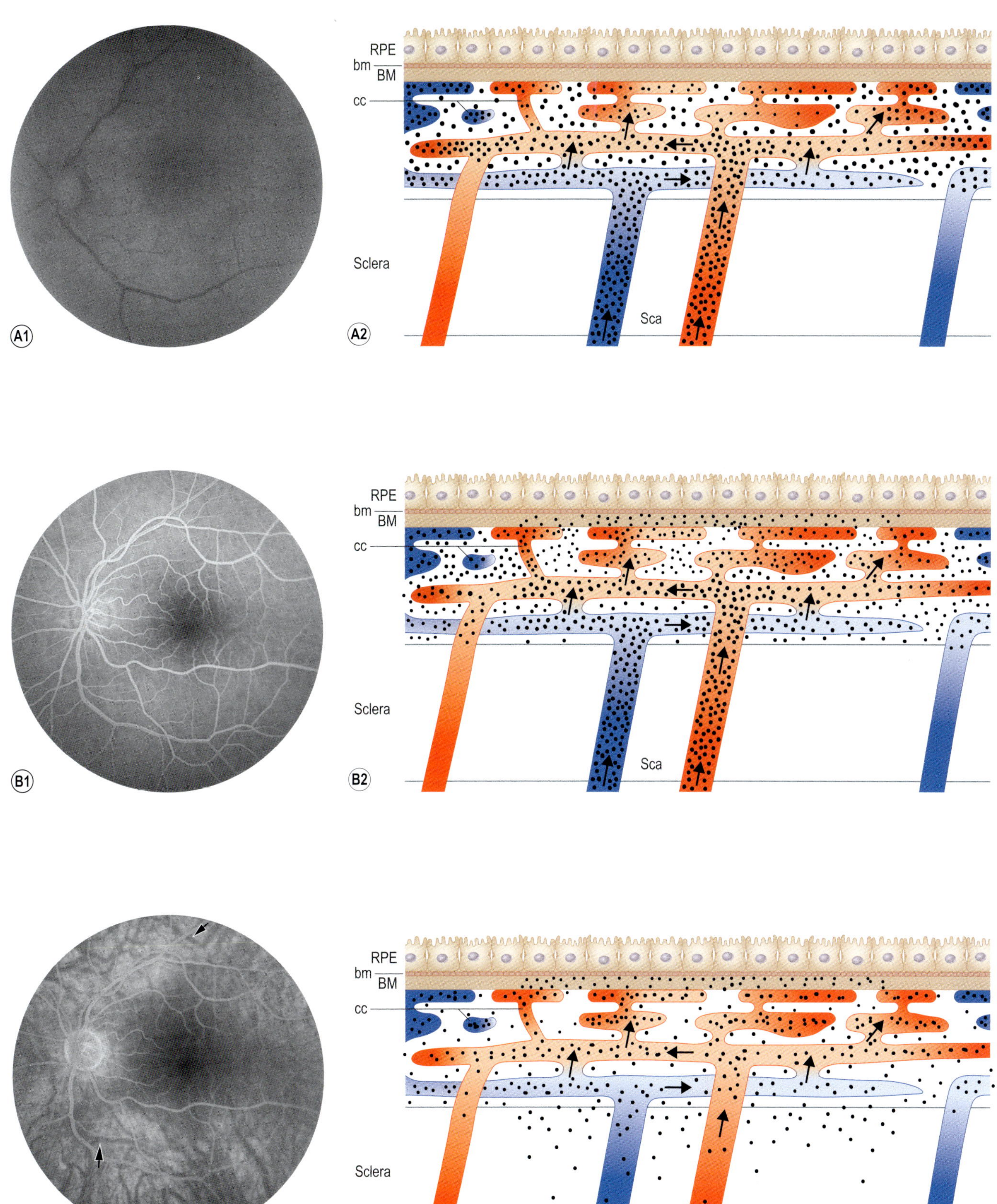
RPE
bm
BM
cc
Sclera
Sca
A1
A2
B1
B2
C1
C2

References

1. Hogan MJ, Alvarado JA, Weddell JE. Histology of the human eye: an atlas and textbook. Philadelphia: WB Saunders; 1971. p. 508–19.
2. Justice Jr J, Lehmann RP. Cilioretinal arteries: a study based on review of stereo fundus photographs and fluorescein angiographic findings. Arch Ophthalmol 1976;94:1355–8.
3. Michaelson IC, editor. Retinal circulation in man and animals. Springfield, IL: Charles C Thomas; 1954.
4. Hogan MJ, Alvarado JA, Weddell JE. Histology of the human eye: an atlas and textbook. Philadelphia: WB Saunders; 1971.
5. Weiter JJ, Delori FC, Wing GL, et al. Retinal pigment epithelial lipofuscin and melanin and choroidal melanin in human eyes. Ophthalmol Vis Sci 1986;27:145–52.
6. Auran J. Localization and optical density determination of the macular pigment within the layers of monkey retinas. Harvard, MA: Harvard College; 1979.
7. Nussbaum JJ, Pruett RC, Delori FC. Historic perspectives: macular yellow pigment; the first 200 years. Retina 1981;1:296–310.
8. Snodderly DM, Auran J, Delori FC. Localization of the macular pigment. ARVO Abstracts. Invest Ophthalmol Vis Sci 1979;18(Suppl.):80.
9. Snodderly DM, Auran JD, Delori FC. The macular pigment. II. Spatial distribution in primate retinas. Invest Ophthalmol Vis Sci 1984;25:674–85.
10. Wald G. Human vision and the spectrum. Science 1945;101:653–8.
11. Bone RA, Landrum JT, Hine GW, et al. Stereochemistry of the human macular carotenoids. Invest Ophthalmol Vis Sci 1993;34:2033–40.
12. Fine BS. Limiting membranes of the sensory retina and pigment epithelium: an electron microscopic study. Arch Ophthalmol 1961;66:847–60.
13. Gass JD. Muller cell cone, an overlooked part of the anatomy of the fovea centralis: hypotheses concerning its role in the pathogenesis of macular hole and foveomacualr retinoschisis. Arch Ophthalmol 1999;117:821–3.
14. Yamada E. Some structural features of the fovea centralis in the human retina. Arch Ophthalmol 1969;82:151–9.
15. Marquardt R. Ein Beitrag zur Topographie und Anatomie der Netzhautgefässe des menschlichen Auges. Klin Monatsbl Augenheilkd 1966;148:50–64.
16. Toussaint D, Kuwabara T, Cogan DG. Retinal vascular patterns. Part II. Human retinal vessels studied in three dimensions. Arch Ophthalmol 1961;65:575–81.
17. Shimizu K, Ujiie K. Structure of ocular vessels. Toyko: Igaku Shoin; 1978.
18. Henkind P, Bellhorn RW, Murphy ME, et al. Development of macular vessels in monkey and cat. Br J Ophthalmol 1975;59:703–9.
19. Tso MOM, Friedman E. The retinal pigment epithelium. I. Comparative histology. Arch Ophthalmol 1967;78:641–9.
20. Araki M. Observations on the corrosion casts of the choriocapillaris. Acta Soc Ophthalmol Jpn 1976;80:315–26.
21. Hayreh SS. Submacular choroidal vasculature pattern: experimental fluorescein fundus angiographic studies. Albrecht von Graefes Arch Klin Exp Ophthalmol 1974;192:181–96.
22. Itotagawa S, Fukumi K, Doi H. Observations on the plastic cast of the choroidal vasculature. Part 1. Vascular characteristics in the submacular area. Acta Soc Ophthalmol Jpn 1977;81:678–87.
23. Risco JM, Grimson BS, Johnson PT. Angioarchitecture of the ciliary artery circulation of the posterior pole. Arch Ophthalmol 1981;99:864–8.
24. Torczynski E, Tso MOM. The architecture of the choriocapillaris at the posterior pole. Am J Ophthalmol 1976;81:428–40.
25. Amalric PM. Choroidal vessel occlusive syndromes – clinical aspects. Trans Am Acad Ophthalmol Otolaryngol 1983;77:OP291–OP299.
26. Hayreh SS. The choriocapillaris. Albrecht von Graefes Arch Klin Exp Ophthalmol 1974;192:165–79.
27. Hayreh SS. Segmental nature of the choroidal vasculature. Br J Ophthalmol 1975;59:631–48.
28. Krey HF. Segmental vascular patterns of the choriocapillaris. Am J Ophthalmol 1975;80: 198–206.
29. Dollery CT, Henkind P, Kohner EM, et al. Effect of raised intraocular pressure on the retinal and choroidal circulation. Invest Ophthalmol 1968;7:191–8.
30. Hayreh SS. Recent advances in fluorescein fundus angiography. Br J Ophthalmol 1974;58: 391–412.
31. Perry HD, Hatfield RV, Tso MOM. Fluorescein pattern of the choriocapillaris in the neonatal rhesus monkey. Am J Ophthalmol 1977;84:197–204.
32. Weiter JJ, Ernest JT. Anatomy of the choroidal vasculature. Am J Ophthalmol 1974;78:583–90.
33. Ernest JT, Stern WH, Archer DB. Submacular choroidal circulation. Am J Ophthalmol 1976;81:574–82.
34. Alm A, Bill A. Ocular and optic nerve blood flow at normal and increased intraocular pressures in monkeys (*Macaca irus*): a study with radioactively labelled microspheres including flow determinations in brain and some other tissues. Exp Eye Res 1973;15:15–29.
35. Parver LM, Auker CR, Carpenter DO. The stabilizing effect of the choroidal circulation on the temperature environment of the macula. Retina 1982;2:117–20.
36. Flower RW, Hochheimer BF. Indocyanine green dye fluorescence and infrared absorption choroidal angiography performed simultaneously with fluorescein angiography. Johns Hopkins Med J 1976;138:33–42.
37. Fox IJ, Wood EH. Indocyanine green: physical and physiologic properties. Proc Staff Mtgs Mayo Clin 1960;35:732–44.
38. Kogure K, David NJ, Yamanouchi U, et al. Infrared absorption angiography of the fundus circulation. Arch Ophthalmol 1970;83:209–14.
39. Guyer DR, Puliafito CA, Monés JM, et al. Digital indocyanine-green angiography in chorioretinal disorders. Ophthalmology 1992;99:287–91.
40. Yannuzzi LA, Slakter JS, Sorenson JA, et al. Digital indocyanine green videoangiography and choroidal neovascularization. Retina 1992;12:191–223.
41. Hope-Ross M, Yannuzzi LA, Gragoudas ES, et al. Adverse reactions due to indocyanine green. Ophthalmology 1994;101:529–33.
42. Gass JDM. A. fluorescein angiographic study of macular dysfunction secondary to retinal vascular disease. I. Embolic retinal artery obstruction. Arch Ophthalmol 1968;80:535–49.

CHAPTER 2

Imaging and Electrophysiological Studies

PATHOPHYSIOLOGIC AND HISTOPATHOLOGIC BASES FOR INTERPRETATION OF FLUORESCEIN ANGIOGRAPHY

The anatomy and physiology of the choroid and retina and their relationship to the normal fluorescein angiographic findings were presented in Chapter 1 and are fundamental to understanding the principles of interpretation of fluorescein angiography in patients with ocular fundus abnormalities. In this regard the following facts are most important:

1. The choroidal vasculature and its extracellular compartment are similar to that of the body outside the central nervous system in that ultrastructurally the capillary endothelial cells have a pore size that permits escape of relatively large molecules, including sodium fluorescein and some smaller proteins, into the choroidal extracellular compartment, which is normally partly expanded by extracellular fluid.
2. The retinal vasculature and its greatly contracted extracellular compartment are similar to that of the brain in that the capillary endothelial cells are separated by tight junctions (blood–inner retinal barrier) that do not permit escape of large molecules, including sodium fluorescein and protein, into the retinal extracellular compartment, which is normally maintained in a state of relative deturgescence.
3. The choroidal circulation and its expanded extracellular compartment, which are normally stained with fluorescein, are separated from the subretinal space and retinal extracellular compartment, which are not stained with fluorescein, by the retinal pigment epithelium (RPE; blood–outer retinal barrier). The RPE is a monocellular layer of cells connected by tight junctions that prevent escape of large molecules, including fluorescein and protein, from the choriocapillaris into the subretinal space, which is maintained in a state of relative deturgescence. To assist in the regulation of the extracellular environment, the choroidal and retinal vascular endothelia, as well as the RPE, probably have intracellular physiologic mechanisms that permit movement of molecules and water against an osmotic gradient. In addition to these functions, the RPE acts as an optical filter of irregular density to obscure the choroid partly from view.

This chapter briefly describes some of the basic pathophysiologic and histopathologic changes occurring in the posterior ocular fundus and illustrates how fluorescein angiography can assist in the detection and definition of these changes. Additional details concerning specific diseases are given in subsequent chapters.

In general, fluorescein angiography is useful in detecting (1) abnormalities of blood flow to or within the choroid, optic nerve head, and retina and (2) lesions that alter the normal pattern of fundus fluorescence.

2.01 Angiographic demonstration of blood flow abnormalities in the eye.

A: Delayed appearance of fluorescein (20.2 seconds) in retinal and choroidal circulation in patient with obstruction of the right carotid artery.
B: Branch retinal artery obstruction (arrow).
C: Branch retinal vein obstruction (arrow).
D: Perifoveolar retinal capillary occlusion.
E: Delayed perfusion of the choroid (dark area) caused by ciliary arterial occlusion following krypton red photocoagulation in papillomacular bundle area. Collateral circulation to the choriocapillaris was adequate to prevent loss of visual acuity.
F: Contrast E with normal patchy areas (arrows) of delayed choroidal perfusion by the short ciliary arteries during early phases of angiography.

(E, from Cohen et al.[1])

ABNORMALITIES OF BLOOD FLOW

With severe obstruction of either the carotid or the ophthalmic artery, there is usually evidence of delay in appearance of fluorescein in both the choroidal and the retinal circulation (Figure 2.01A). Because of the end-artery arrangement of the retinal circulation and its high visibility angiographically, severe obstruction of its circulation at any level from the central retinal artery to the central retinal vein is readily detected angiographically (Figure 2.01B–D).

Because of multiple posterior short ciliary arteries supplying the choroidal circulation and the rich arterial anastomosis within the choroid, angiographic demonstration of obstruction of one or more of the major choroidal arteries is infrequently demonstrated. Even when obstruction occurs, collateral circulation is usually sufficient to prevent infarction of the overlying retina, as illustrated in Figure 2.01E in a patient with ciliary artery obstruction caused by krypton red laser.[1] Rapid-sequence angiography used in normal eyes often shows patchy areas of delayed choroidal perfusion in the posterior pole caused by minor variations in the length and diameter of the short ciliary arteries (Figure 2.01F). It may be difficult to differentiate these changes from those caused by pathologic obstruction of the posterior ciliary arteries. Peripherally, fewer pathways for anastomosis are available and occlusion of a major choroidal artery may cause a wedge-shaped area of ischemic infarction of the RPE and outer retina (Amalric's triangle). After the disappearance of the white ischemic retina, angiography usually demonstrates evidence of arterial obstruction as the cause of the wedge-shaped area of RPE atrophy (see Figures 3.56K and L, and 9.15E and F). Acute obstruction of the precapillary arterioles and choriocapillaris is usually accompanied by ischemic whitening of the RPE and outer retina and a corresponding area of patchy loss of choroidal fluorescence (Figure 9.15C–F). It is difficult to differentiate these lesions biomicroscopically and angiographically from similar changes that are unrelated to choroidal vascular obstruction (such as blocked fluorescence due to opacification of the RPE (see discussion of acute posterior multifocal placoid pigment epitheliopathy, chapter 11).

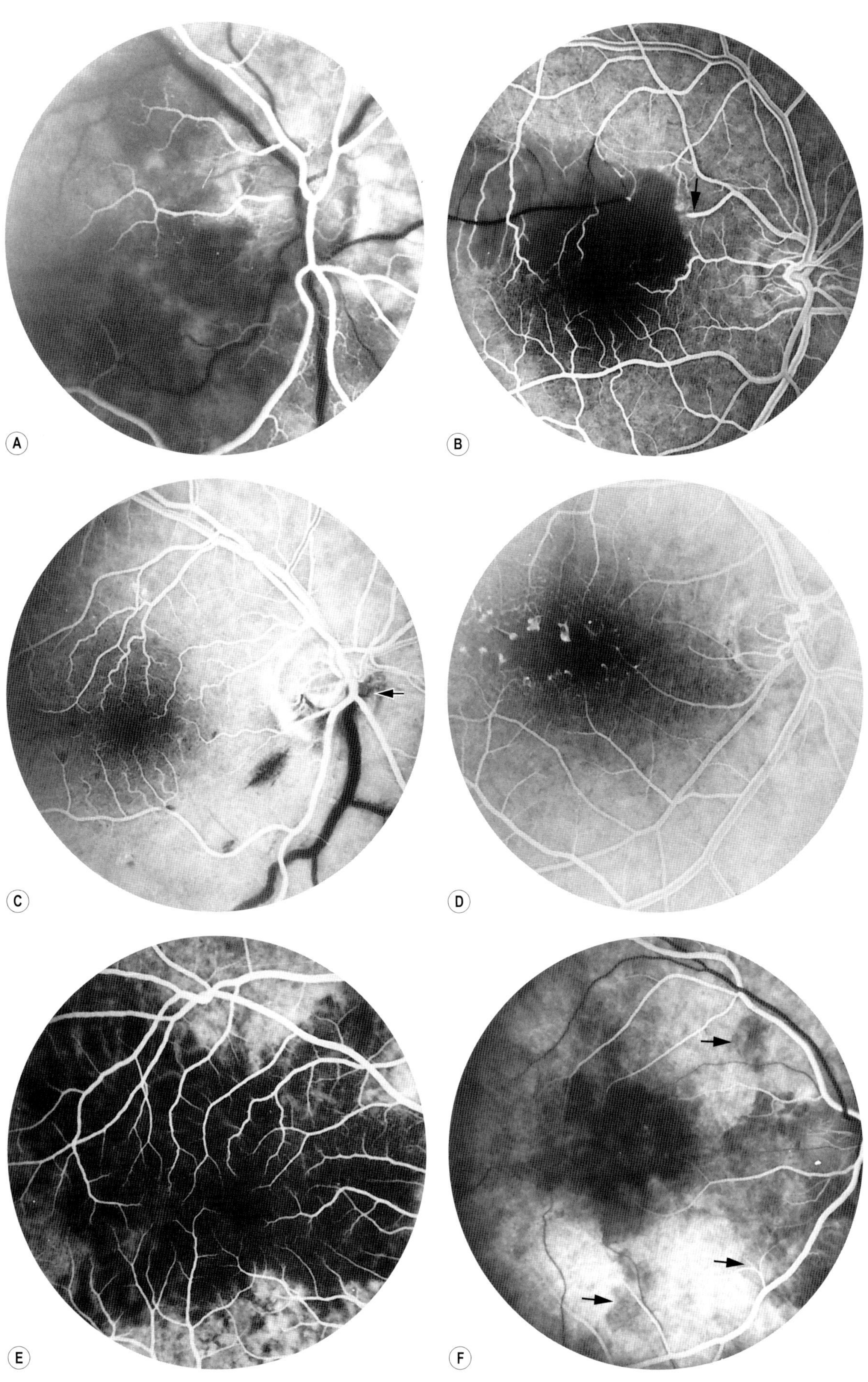
A
B
C
D
E
F

Angiography is helpful in detecting a focal area of chronic obstruction of the choriocapillaris that is accompanied by atrophy of the overlying RPE and retina. Fluorescein leakage in the normal choroid occurs primarily from the choriocapillaris. If the choriocapillaris is obstructed, angiography may demonstrate perfusion of the large choroidal vessels but will show a delay in choriocapillaris perfusion and late choroidal and scleral staining within the area of overlying RPE atrophy (Figure 2.02E–H). Early staining along the periphery of such lesions occurs from leakage of fluorescein from the intact surrounding choriocapillaris. Angiography is helpful in differentiating these focal areas of RPE, retinal, and choriocapillaris atrophy from focal or geographic areas of depigmentation of the RPE that biomicroscopically may appear similar (Figure 2.02A–D). In these latter instances angiography may show that the choriocapillaris is relatively intact (see discussion of chloroquine maculopathy, chapter 9).

2.02 Hyperfluorescence caused by "window" defect in the retinal pigment epithelium (RPE).

A–C: Fifty-one-year-old woman with lupus erythematosus and bull's-eye pattern of depigmentation of the RPE caused by chloroquine. Note evidence of early perfusion of the relatively intact choriocapillaris (cc) in B.
D: Diagram of vertical histopathologic section through the macula of A showing focal depigmentation of RPE (arrows) surrounding the central area of normally pigmented RPE, and intact underlying choriocapillaris.
E–G: Forty-six-year-old patient with severe atrophy and loss of the RPE caused by Sorsby's central areolar choroidal dystrophy. Note delayed choroidal perfusion in F indicative of atrophy of the choriocapillaris, and late fluorescein staining of choroid and sclera in area of RPE atrophy in G.
H: Histopathologic changes, including atrophy of RPE and choriocapillaris.

"WINDOW" DEFECTS (TRANSMISSION HYPERFLUORESCENCE) IN THE RETINAL PIGMENT EPITHELIUM CAUSING FOCAL HYPERFLUORESCENCE

Focal areas of hypopigmentation, or thinning of the RPE, when associated with minimal or no alterations in the underlying choriocapillaris, will appear hyperfluorescent during the early phases of angiography because of the greater amount of inciting blue light reaching the choroid and the greater visibility of the choroidal fluorescence (Figure 2.02A–D). Stereoscopically, the area of the hyperfluorescence appears flat or depressed and remains relatively constant in size throughout the study. The changes in intensity of the fluorescence parallel that of the normal choroidal fluorescence (Figure 2.02A–D). Areas of focal atrophy or loss of the RPE and choriocapillaris will cause a delay in the early development of hyperfluorescence (Figure 2.02E–H).

EXUDATION AND FLUORESCEIN STAINING

Water and electrolytes are free to move back and forth across the capillary endothelium. Large molecules, particularly protein and lipids, are not, however, because of the small capillary pore size. The amount of water that is present in the extracellular space is determined osmotically primarily by the pore size of the capillary endothelium and the amount of protein within the extracellular space. The amount of protein normally present there represents a balance between that escaping from the vascular compartment and that returning to the circulation by way of the lymphatic system. When either elevation of the intracapillary pressure or pathologic alteration in the capillary endothelium occurs, protein and in some cases larger lipoproteins and lipids escape into the extracellular space and bring water with them (exudation).

Intrachoroidal Exudation

Since fluorescein escapes normally from the choriocapillaris, angiography is of little value in detecting changes in capillary permeability in the choroid unless these changes are associated with either loss of adherence of the RPE to Bruch's membrane or damage to the RPE blood–outer retinal barrier.

Choroidal Exudation Causing Localized (Disciform) Retinal Detachment

Localized detachment of the retina, often referred to as disciform detachment, that is caused by exudate derived from the choroidal circulation occurs primarily by three mechanisms: (1) detachment of the RPE; (2) choroidal neovascularization; and (3) devitalization of the RPE.

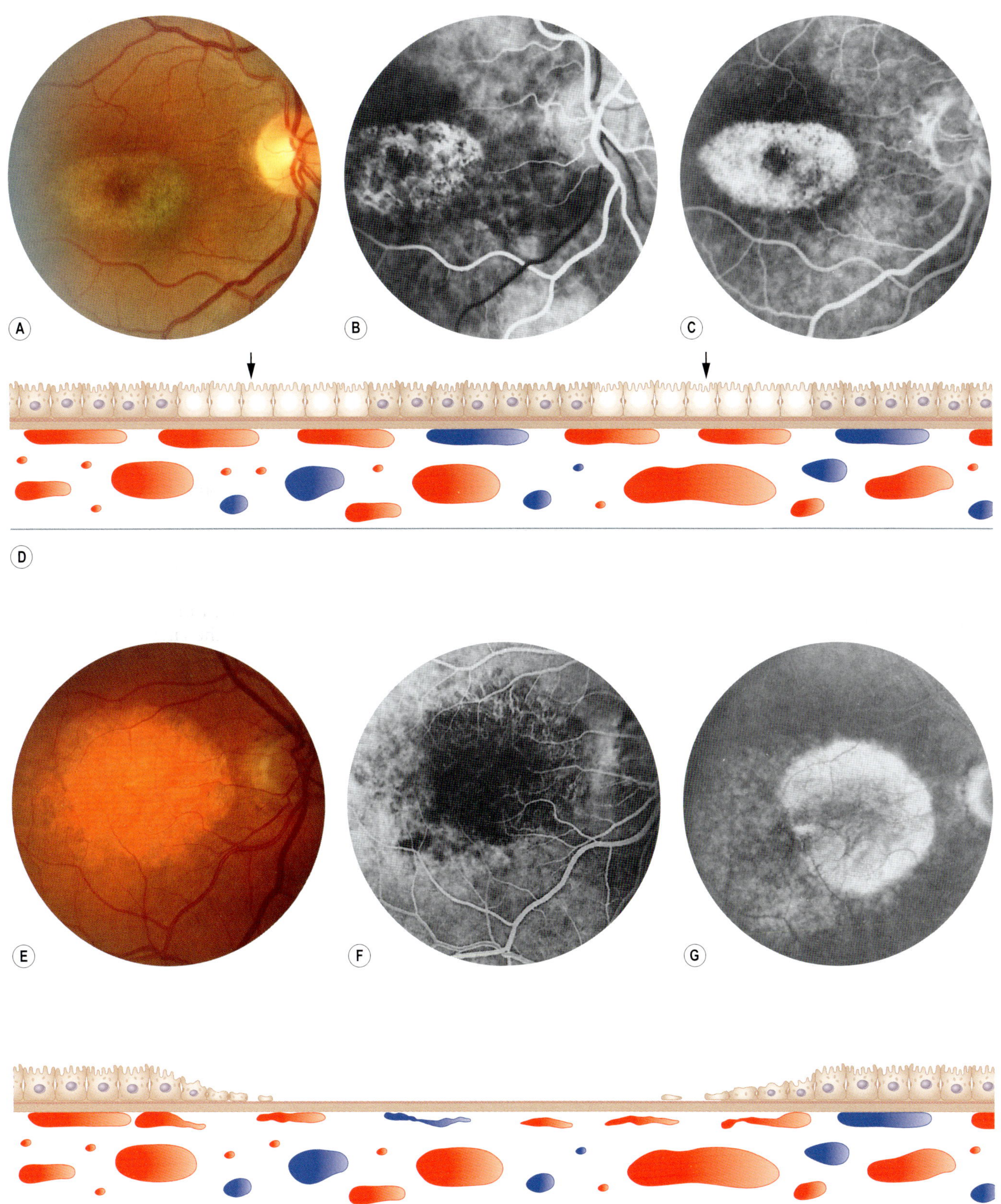
A
B
C
D
E
F
G
H

Detachment of the RPE

The normal adherence of the RPE basement membrane to the inner collagenous zone of Bruch's membrane may be disrupted by a variety of causes, including increased permeability of the choriocapillaris, degeneration of Bruch's membrane, degeneration of the RPE and its basement membrane, and exudation from sub-RPE choroidal neovascularization. Whatever the cause, serous exudation from the choriocapillaris or from sub-RPE new vessels may produce a sharply defined, often blister-like, detachment of the RPE (Figure 2.03).[2] Its size varies from subbiomicroscopic to several disc diameters or larger. When the RPE detachment is not caused by choroidal neovascularization, it is usually round or oval in shape and less than one disc diameter in size. It appears solid, and its color varies from that of the normal orange-brown RPE to yellow-gray. There may be a pinkish rim of subretinal fluid around the edge of the RPE detachment (Figure 2.03). When small, an RPE detachment may be seen best in side illumination with the slit lamp. When caused by choroidal neovascularization the serous RPE detachment often has a kidney or notched configuration and biomicroscopically and angiographically demonstrates features suggesting the presence of choroidal neovascularization (see discussion in the next section). In nonvascularized serous RPE detachments fluorescein molecules rapidly diffuse from the choriocapillaris across the full extent of the normally permeable Bruch's membrane into the sub-RPE exudate to produce the pathognomonic stereo angiographic picture of a sharply localized area of fluorescein staining (Figure 2.03). The fluorescence typically appears slightly later than the background choroidal fluorescence and becomes maximally intense later and persists longer than the surrounding choroidal fluorescence. Even when the RPE is detached, its blood–outer retinal barrier may remain intact and prevent exudation into the subsensory retinal space (Figure 2.04).

2.03 Angiography showing sequence of events in a 37-year-old man with a large serous detachment of retinal pigment epithelium (RPE) surrounded by a marginal serous detachment of the retina.

A1: Note light-colored, oval, serous detachment of the RPE surrounded by the darker halo of serous retinal detachment that extends inferiorly to the inferotemporal artery. Arrow indicates several small paramacular serous detachments of the RPE.
A2: Schematic diagram depicting serous detachment of the RPE and retina (R). Soon after injection of fluorescein, dye molecules (black dots) enter the choroidal circulation and begin to diffuse out of the choriocapillaris (cc) into the extravascular spaces of the choroid and across Bruch's membrane (BM) into the sub-RPE space (sRs).
B1 and **B2**: The dye pools in the sub-RPE space but does not enter the subretinal space (sRs).
C1 and **C2**: Later the dye outlines the area of detachment of the RPE. Although the fluorescence of the sub-RPE exudate begins to fade as the dye diffuses back into the choriocapillaris, it is still easily visible 1 hour after dye injection.

(A1, B1, and C1 from Gass et al.[2])

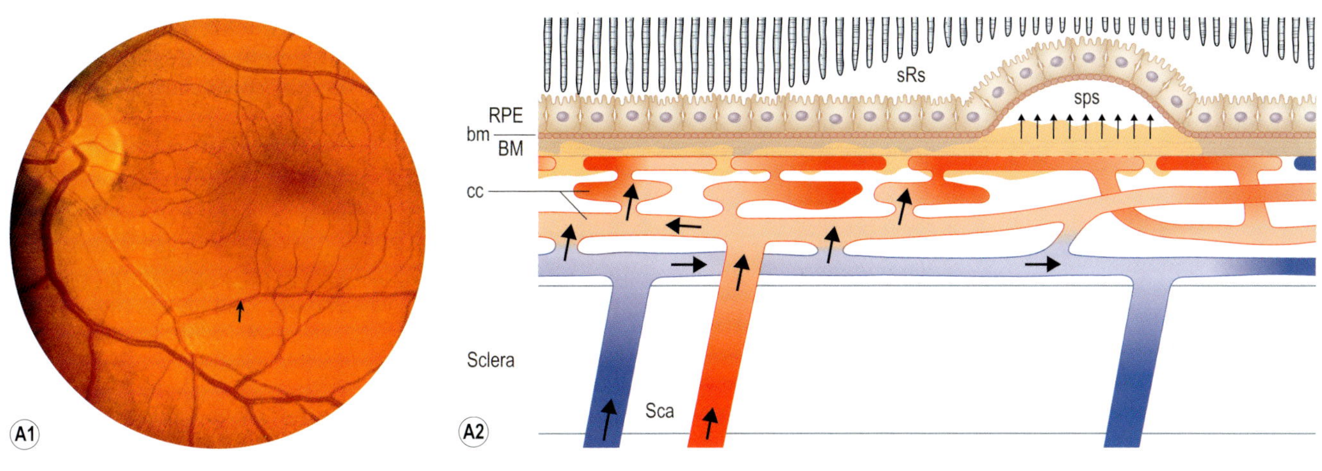
sRs
sps
RPE
bm
BM
cc
Sclera
Sca
A1
A2

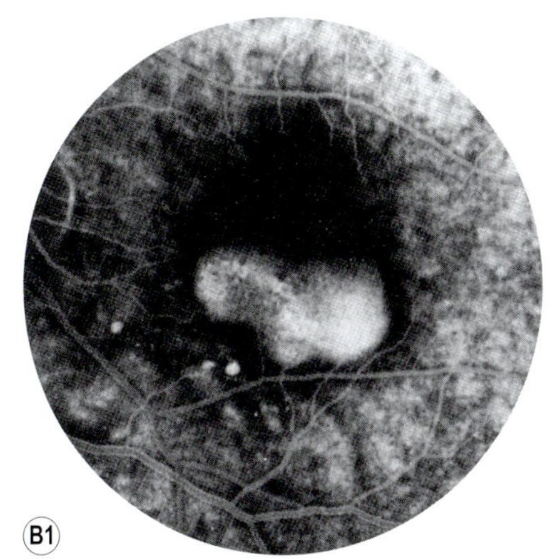
B1

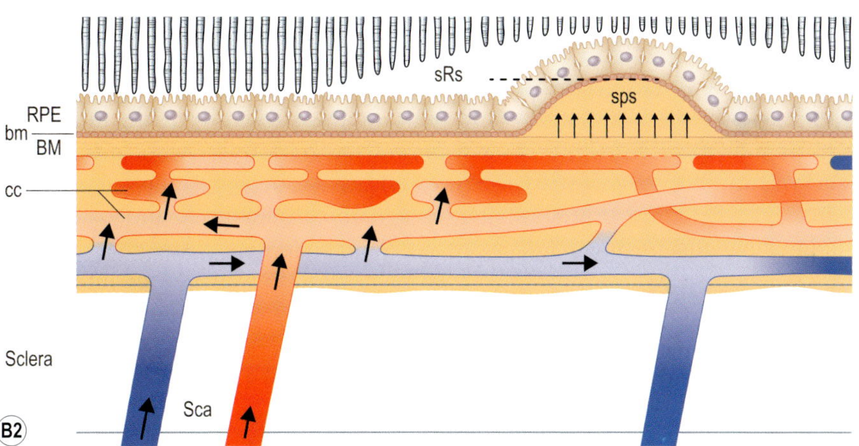
sRs
sps
RPE
bm
BM
cc
Sclera
Sca
B2

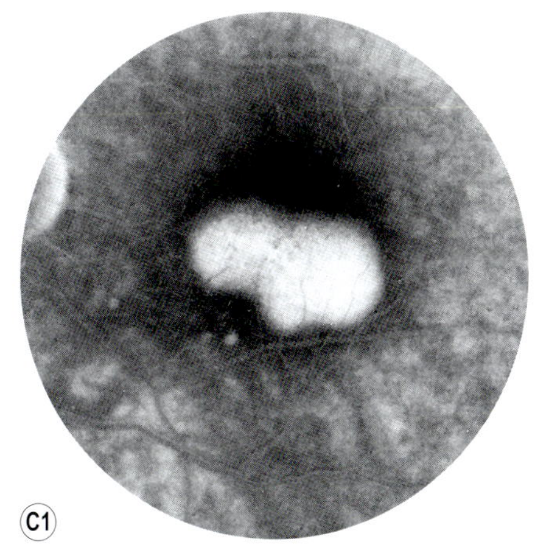
C1

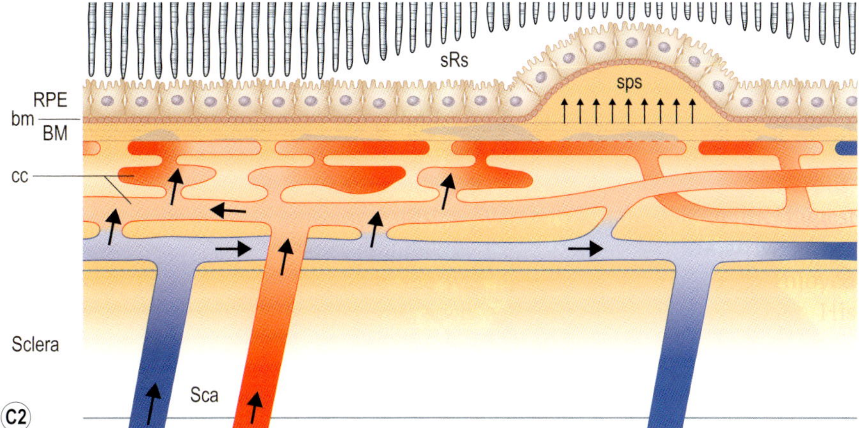
sRs
sps
RPE
bm
BM
cc
Sclera
Sca
C2

A serous RPE detachment may cause loss of central vision in two ways. It may enlarge concentrically until it extends beneath the center of the macula (Figures 2.03 and 2.04), or the detached RPE may decompensate and permit large molecules and water to enter the subretinal space and detach the retina (Figure 2.04). If the breakdown in the RPE barrier is low-grade and not associated with a physical break in the continuity in the RPE, fluorescein molecules may not be able to diffuse across the detached RPE into the subretinal exudate in concentrations sufficient to be visible angiographically (see Figures 2.03 and 3.03A–C). In the presence of a break, however, fluorescein streams into the subretinal exudate (see Figure 3.03 D–I).

2.04 Disciform macular detachment. Exudative detachment of the retinal pigment epithelium (RPE) and retina without choroidal neovascularization.

2.05 Developmental stages of occult type I sub-retinal pigment epithelium (RPE) choroidal neovascularization before retinal detachment.

A: Choriocapillary (cc) invasion of Bruch's membrane (BM). B: Perforation of Bruch's membrane and growth beneath the retinal pigment epithelium.

Choroidal Neovascularization

Under a great variety of circumstances, neovascular tufts arising from the choroid may either invade and perforate Bruch's membrane or grow through defects in Bruch's membrane and proliferate in either the sub-RPE space (type I choroidal neovascularization) or in the subsensory retinal space (type II choroidal neovascularization).[3] The location and growth pattern of the neovascular proliferation are determined primarily by the age of the patient and the pre-existing disease.

Type I Sub-RPE Neovascularization

As part of the normal aging process as well as in certain degenerative and dystrophic disorders (e.g., age-related macular degeneration and pseudoxanthoma elasticum), the firm attachment of the RPE and its basement membrane to the inner collagenous zone of Bruch's membrane becomes loosened. In these patients new vessels extending from the choroid through Bruch's membrane find little resistance to their lateral growth into the sub-RPE space (Figures 2.05 and 2.06).[3] Their pattern of growth often simulates that of a sea fan or cartwheel with radial arterioles and venules supplying and draining a circumferential dilated capillary sinus (Figure 2.07). As neovascularization of the sub-RPE space occurs, the new vessels establish a relatively firm adhesion to the overlying RPE. Initially, the blood flow through the neovascular network is sluggish and there is little or no exudation (Figure 2.06). During this period of occult neovascularization, the overlying retina and RPE may be minimally affected, and the network may not be detectable biomicroscopically or angiographically (Figure 2.06A and B). These occult neovascular complexes may be one disc diameter or larger and may be irregularly or focally elevated into a mound by virtue of proliferation of accompanying fibroblastic cells and new vessels before development of evidence of the escape of exudate from the blood vessels (Figure 2.06C). With an increase in blood flow through the network, the endothelium decompensates, particularly at the outer margin of the network, and exudation extends into the subpigment epithelial space around the network. In such cases when the overlying RPE is thinned and only slightly detached by serous fluid, details of the neovascular network may be easily detected angiographically, even though biomicroscopically the network may be hidden from view by cloudiness of the exudate (Figure 2.08). The exudation may extend through the RPE and detach the overlying retina (Figure 2.09A and B).

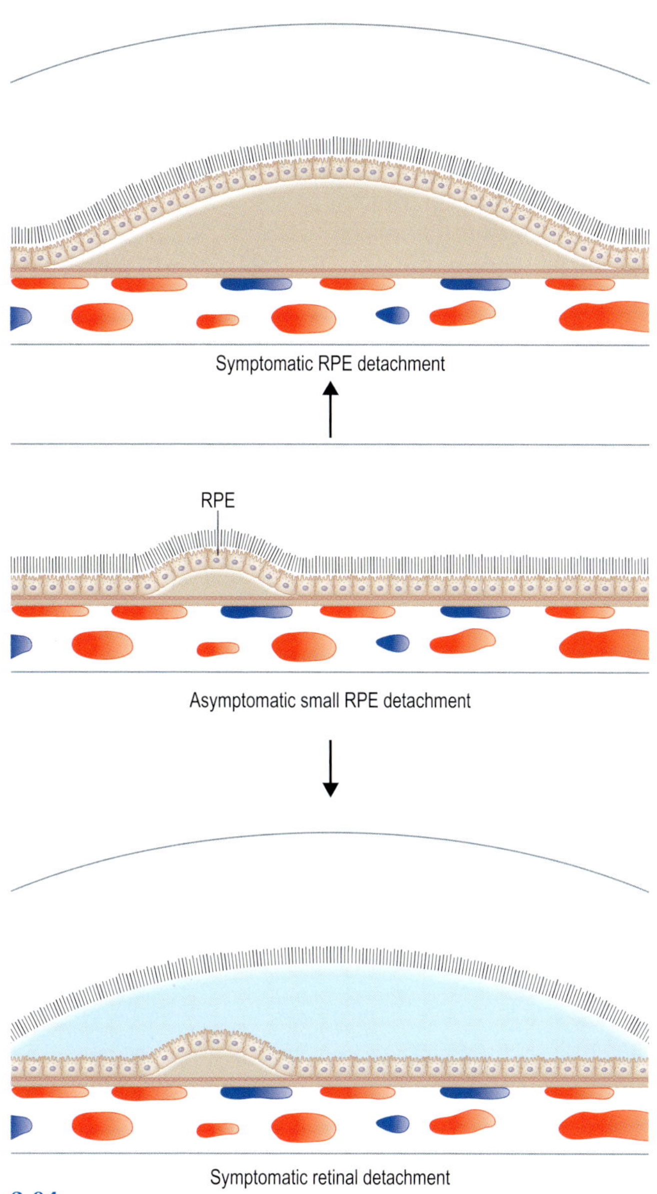
Symptomatic RPE detachment
RPE
Asymptomatic small RPE detachment
Symptomatic retinal detachment

2.04

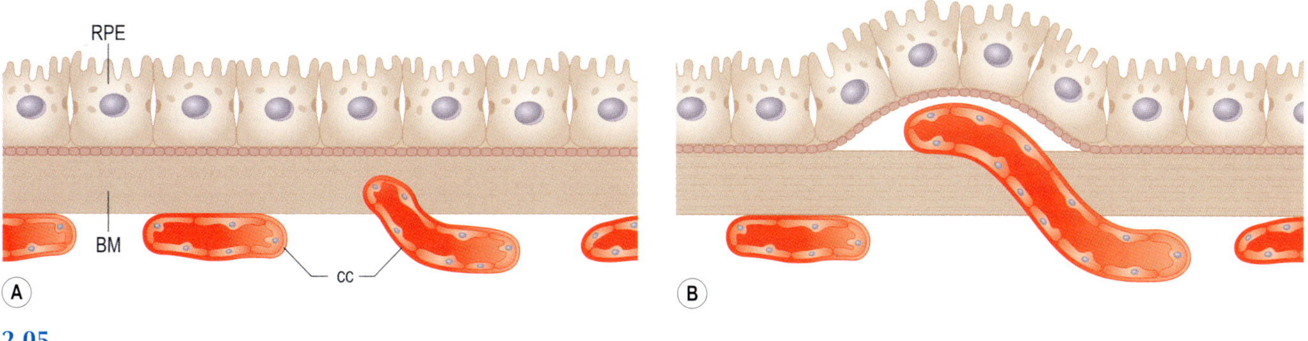
RPE
BM
cc
A
B

2.05

In other patients, exudation may begin at one margin of the neovascular network and cause serous detachment of a large adjacent area of RPE. Because of the relatively firm attachment of the RPE to the neovascular membrane, these serous detachments of the RPE typically have a reniform or notched shape as a result of their development around the margin of the network, most of which lies outside the area of RPE detachment within the notch (Figures 2.09C–E and 2.10A–C). The presence of the new vessel membrane within the notch may or may not be evident angiographically as a mottled area of early hyperfluorescence with or without some evidence of ill-defined late staining. If the detachment extends away from the entire border of the membrane, it may assume a doughnut configuration (Figures 2.09E and 2.10II). If a highly elevated serous detachment of the overlying as well as surrounding RPE occurs, the choroidal neovascular network will be completely obscured biomicroscopically and angiographically by the RPE detachment, which usually has an oval or round configuration (Figure 2.09F).

2.06 Pre-exudative stages of development of occult type I sub-retinal pigment epithelium (RPE) choroidal neovascularization.

A: Early stage. BM, Bruch's membrane.
B: Flat neovascular membrane.
C: Elevated fibrovascular complex.

2.07 Growth pattern of choroidal neovascular membrane, frontal view.

Growth begins with small capillary loop (1) extending beneath either the retinal pigment epithelium (type I) or sensory retina (type II) and expands into a large sea fan-shaped complex (4) with well-differentiated radial retinal arteries and veins and a dilated circumferential capillary network.

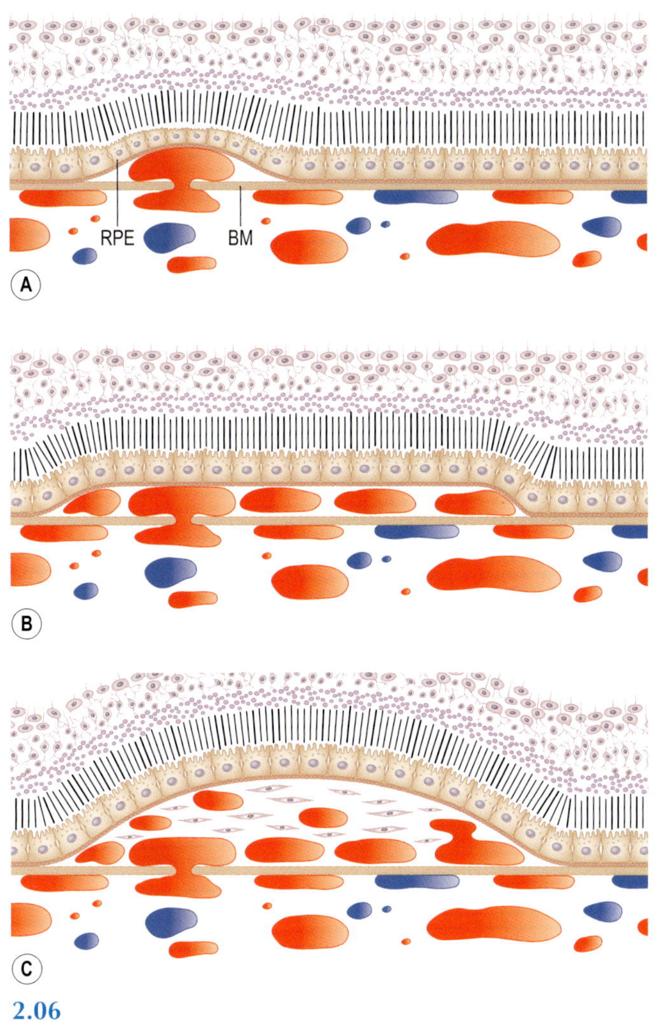

2.06

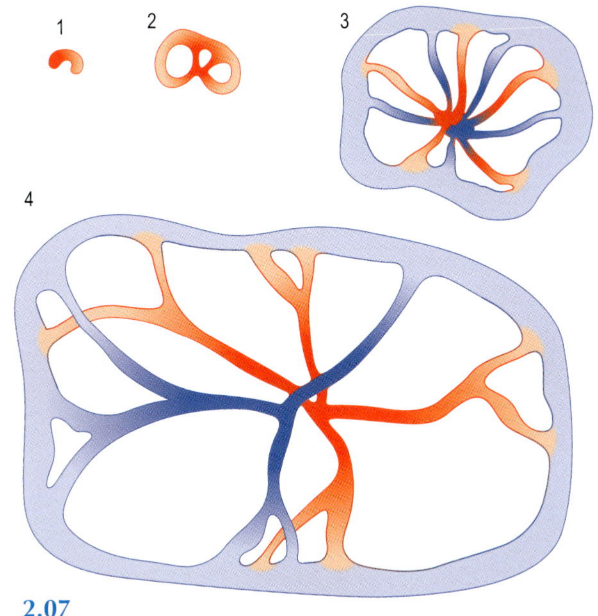

2.07

Leakage of large proteins and extravasation of erythrocytes from the neovascular complex, causing large serous RPE detachments, often produce other biomicroscopic and angiographic clues to the presence of neovascularization. Biomicroscopic clues include yellow subretinal and intraretinal exudate or blood near the margin of the detachment (see Figure 3.02D), dark sub-RPE "fluid level" at the inferior edge of the detachment (see Figure 3.19G), and uneven elevation of the detached RPE not explained by gravity. Angiographic clues to the presence of occult neovascularization include delayed and incomplete staining of the sub-RPE exudate (see Figure 3.21). The neovascular membrane is most likely to be located in the less fluorescent zone of greatest opacification of the sub-RPE exudate. Accurate localization of new vessel membranes lying beneath large serous RPE detachments, however, is not possible with fluorescein angiography because of rapid movement of the dye through Bruch's membrane throughout the extent of the detached RPE. In these types of RPE detachments computer-enhanced indocyanine green (ICG) angiography appears to provide a more accurate means of localizing the sub-RPE new vessel membranes.[4] ICG dye is tightly bound to the serum proteins and gradually stains the choroidal neovascular membranes (CNVMs) but does not, as occurs with fluorescein, diffuse rapidly into the sub-RPE exudate.

2.08 Sequence of events during angiography in a 70-year-old man with loss of central vision caused by a type I sub-retinal pigment epithelium (RPE) choroidal neovascular membrane (CNVM).

A1: The arrows indicate the location of the faintly gray CNVM. There is a small amount of blood beneath the RPE at the margin of the CNVM.
A2: Schematic diagram depicting serous detachment of the retina overlying a CNVM lying in the sub-RPE space. Soon after injection of fluorescein, dye molecules (black dots) enter the choroidal circulation and begin to perfuse the CNVM lying in the sub-RPE space.
B1 and **B2**: Details of the CNVM are outlined by fluorescein.
C1 and **C2**: Dye leaks from the CNVM and stains the exudate but not the blood (nonfluorescent areas) in the sub-RPE space.

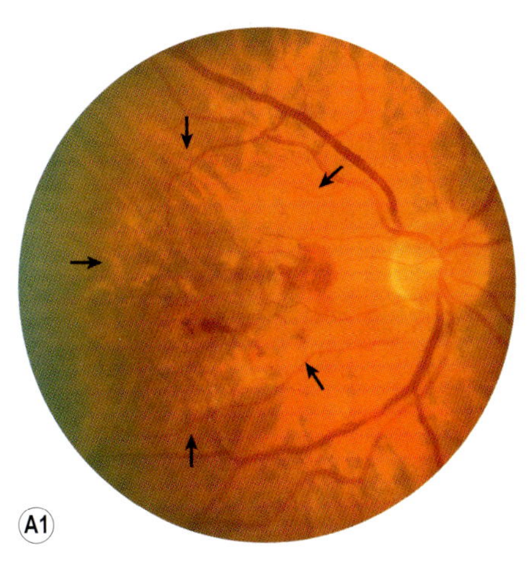

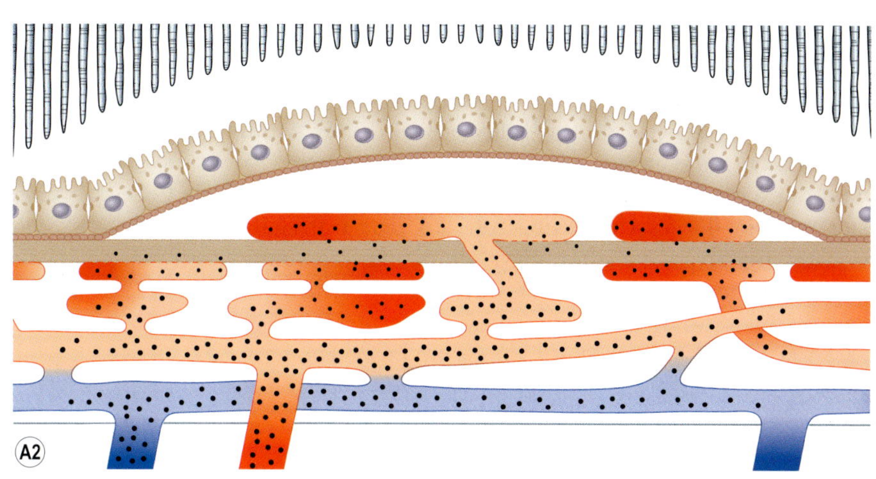

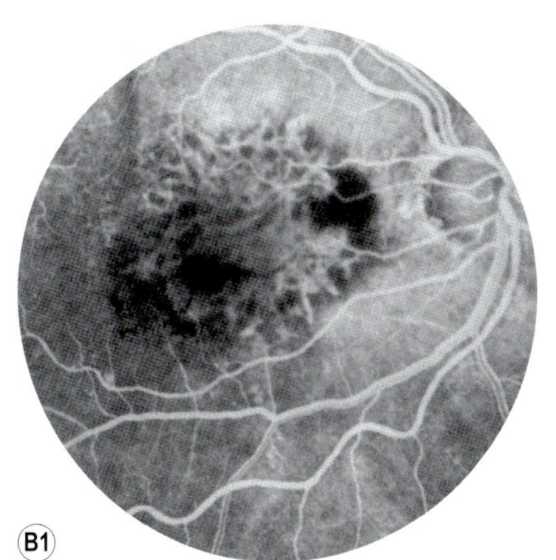

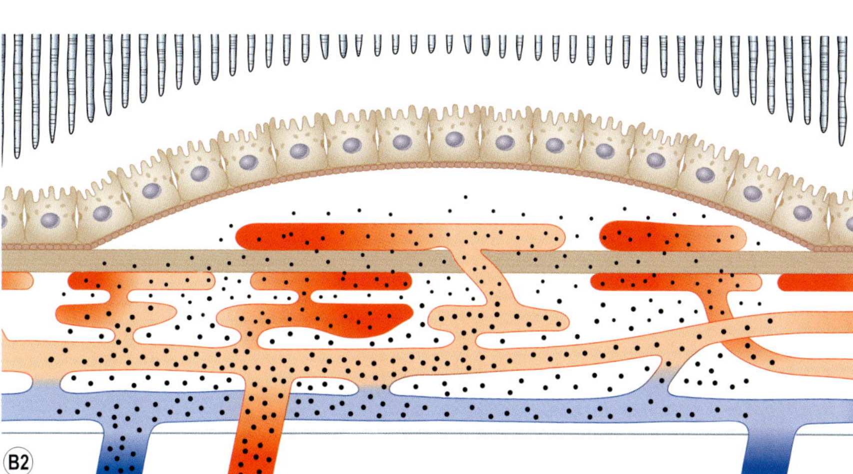

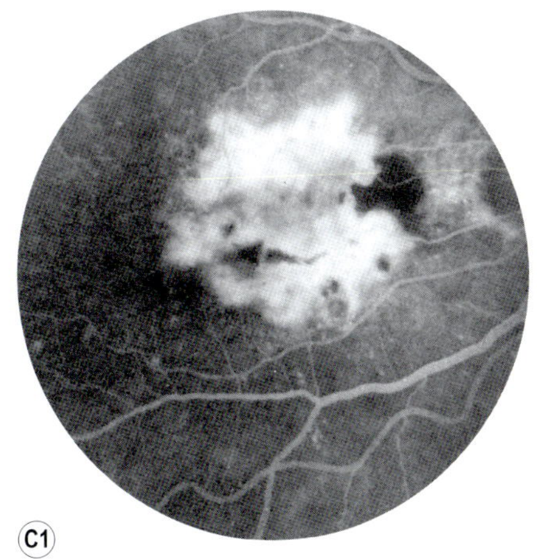

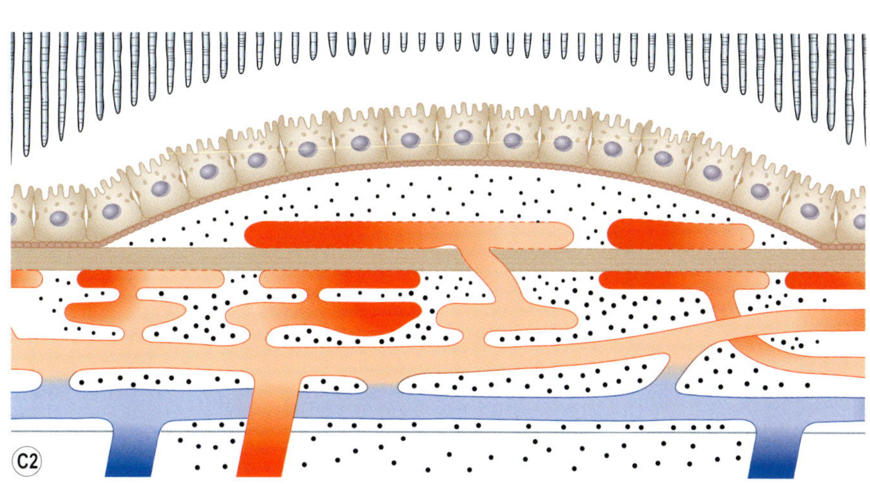

2.08

Detection and accurate localization of choroidal neovascular networks may be difficult because of rapid diffusion of fluorescein into the exudate overlying and surrounding the network, variability of blood flow within the network, and partial obscuration of the network by cloudy exudate, blood, or melanin pigment. The use of stereoscopic fluorescein angiography to detect irregular nonstaining areas of shallow elevation of the RPE caused by occult neovascularization, and detection of other biomicroscopic and angiographic clues to the presence and location of CNVMs are important to the proper management of the patient.

2.09 Disciform exudative macular detachment caused by type I sub-retinal pigment epithelium (RPE) choroidal neovascularization.

A: Early serous retinal detachment.
B: Serous retinal detachment.
C: Serous detachment of the adjacent RPE.
D: Fibrovascular detachment of RPE and exudative detachment of adjacent RPE.
E: Multilobed or ring serous RPE detachment.
F: Serous detachment of the overlying RPE.

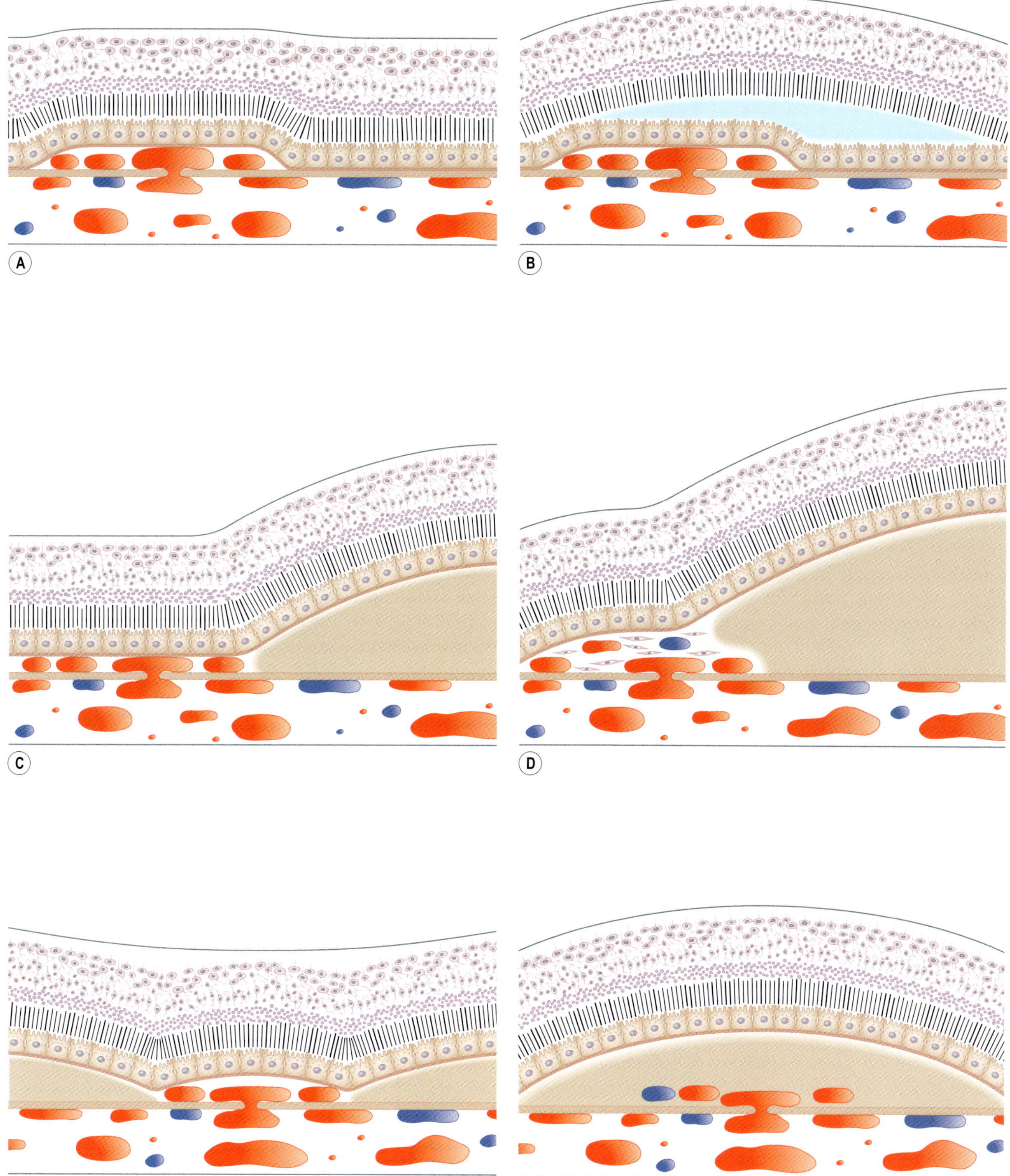
A
B
C
D
E
F

Type II Subretinal Choroidal Neovascularization

Type II subretinal choroidal neovascularization occurs primarily in younger and middle-aged patients with acquired damage to the choriocapillaris–Bruch's membrane–RPE complex caused by focal choroiditis (presumed ocular histoplasmosis syndrome, punctate inner choroiditis, serpiginous choroiditis, toxocariasis), retinochoroiditis (toxoplasmosis), trauma (choroidal rupture), choroidal hamartomas (osteomas), optic disc anomalies (optic disc drusen, optic disc pits, and colobomas), and retinal dystrophies (Best's disease).[3] In these patients, new blood vessels extending from the choroid through the acquired defects in Bruch's membrane as they grow laterally in the subretinal space encounter the firm adherence of the surrounding RPE to the underlying Bruch's membrane. The path of the advancing neovascular complex is therefore directed anteriorly beneath the sensory retina rather than beneath the RPE (Figures 2.11 and 2.12). As the capillary network enters the space between the retinal receptor cells and the apical processes of the RPE, it stimulates the RPE cells to proliferate and to attach themselves by their cell bases to the advancing sheet of new vessels in an effort to envelop them. This reactive RPE proliferation initially results in a zone of hyperplasia of the RPE at the advancing border of the membrane, often producing a hyperpigmented ring ophthalmoscopically. As the fibrovascular membrane continues to expand laterally into the subretinal space, a monolayer of inverted, variably pigmented RPE cells with their base directed toward the new vessels grows along the posterior surface of the membrane. This inverted layer of RPE cells is firmly attached by the base of the RPE cells to the posterior surface of the membrane, and is loosely attached by the apical processes of the RPE to the apical processes of the native RPE. Anteriorly the proliferating layer of RPE cells has more difficulty keeping pace with the advancing neovascular membrane that is usually separated from the overlying retinal receptor cells by a layer of subretinal exudate (see chapter 3 for clinicopathologic correlations of type II membranes). Biomicroscopically this expanding fibrovascular membrane typically produces a gray or partly pigmented subretinal sheet or mound of tissue extending away from the edge of the pigment ring. This is usually accompanied by varying amounts of subretinal exudate and/or blood. Except for the tendency for the new vessels to grow in a sea fan configuration in both type I and type II neovascularization, their pattern of growth otherwise is distinctly different histopathologically. In spite of these histopathologic differences, however, biomicroscopically and angiographically the two types of neovascularization are not always easy to differentiate from each other. The presence of a black or slate-colored subretinal halo or mound at the site of origin of the new vessel and the absence of evidence of either solid or serous RPE detachment suggest type II neovascularization. With further fibrovascular proliferation, exudation, and hemorrhage the pigment halo or mound may be obscured and there may be no biomicroscopic clues to differentiate type I from type II neovascularization. In such cases the age of the patient and the nature of the underlying eye disease are most important in determining which type of neovascularization is present. Patients under 50 years of age without evidence of retinal dystrophies affecting the RPE–Bruch's membrane complex, e.g., pseudoxanthoma elasticum and pattern dystrophy, are most likely to have type II neovascularization. Determination of the type is of relatively little importance in regard to indications and techniques used for laser photocoagulation treatment of the membranes. Differentiating the two types, however, is important if surgical excision of the new vessel membrane is contemplated (Figures 2.11, 2.12, and 3.52).[3] Excision of type II membranes allows the sensory retina to reattach to the underlying native RPE, and in some cases there may be excellent recovery of visual acuity (Figures 2.12 and 3.52).[3] Excision of type I membranes, on the other hand, results in loss of the native RPE and an absolute scotoma corresponding to the site of the membrane (Figure 2.13). Thus surgical removal of type I subfoveal membranes appears to offer no advantages over laser photocoagulation in regard to visual rehabilitation or preservation and has the disadvantage of risks associated with one, and in most cases two, intraocular operative procedures.

2.10 Patterns of serous detachments of the retinal pigment epithelium (RPE) caused by type I sub-RPE choroidal neovascular membrane (CNVM: stippled area).

I: RPE detachments occurring at the margin of the CNVM. (Compare A, B, and C with Figure 2.09C, and D, and D with Figure 2.09E.)
II: RPE detachment overlying the CNVM (compare with Figure 2.09F).

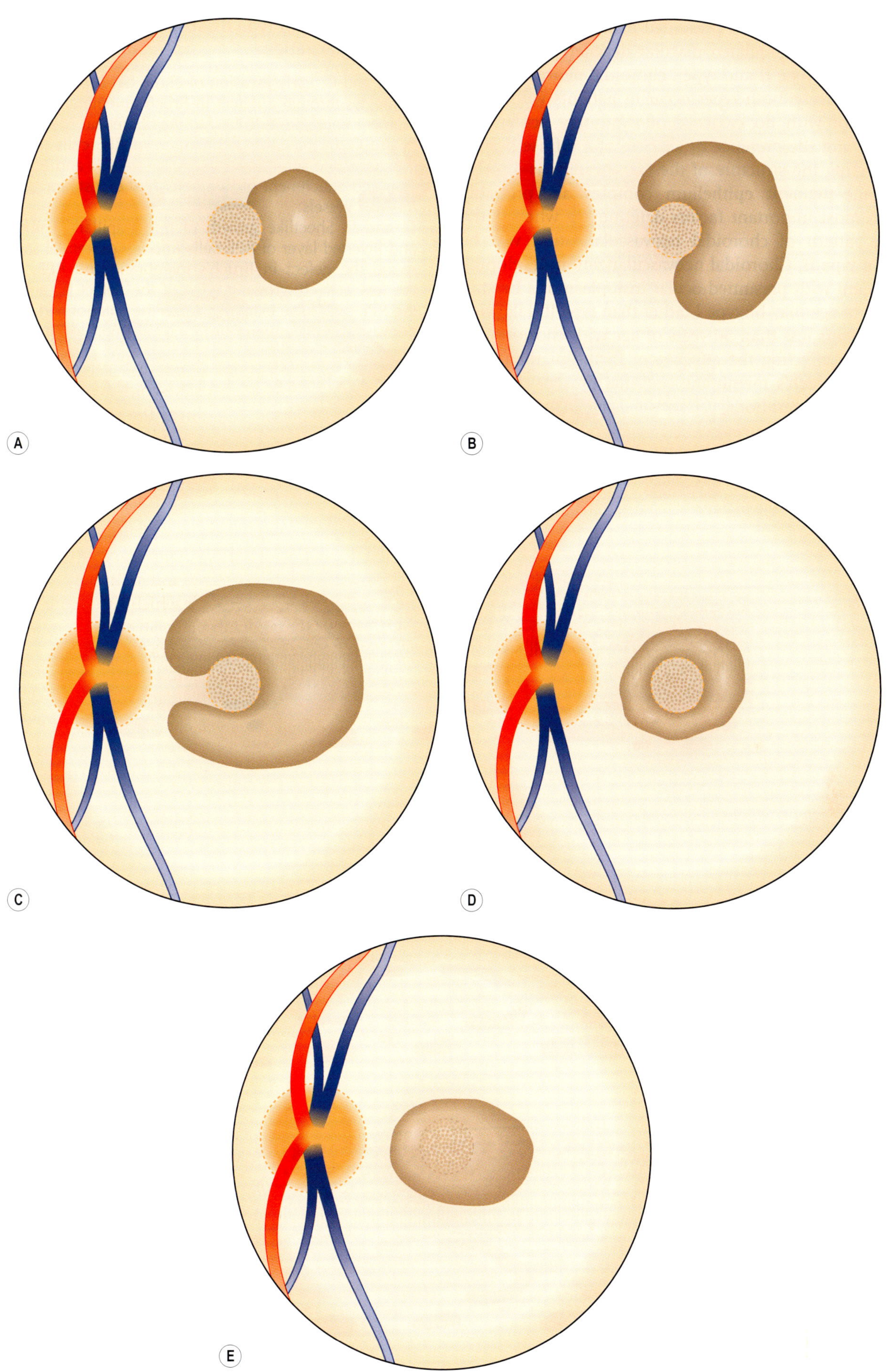
A
B
C
D
E

Chronic choroidal congestion associated with increased extravascular protein and water (ciliochoroidal edema and detachment) may overwhelm the ability of the RPE to prevent passage of protein and water into the subretinal space. Initially, this may occur in the absence of any biomicroscopic or angiographic evidence of RPE damage. The transport of protein across the RPE is apparently so slow and widespread that angiographic evidence of leakage of fluorescein dye across the RPE cannot be demonstrated in most patients with combined ciliochoroidal retinal detachments, at least during the early phases of the detachment. Later, hyperfluorescence caused by RPE atrophy and by irregular areas of fluorescein staining at the level of the RPE may occur in patients with long-standing detachment (see discussion of idiopathic uveal effusion, see Chapter 3).

2.12 Surgical excision of type II subretinal neovascular membrane.

A: Type II neovascular membrane has extended through a defect in Bruch's membrane (Bm: arrows), is covered on its posterior surface by an adherent inverted layer of retinal pigment epithelium (RPE) cells, and is loosely adherent to the underlying native RPE cells and the overlying sensory retina except at the site of Bruch's membrane defect. cc, choroidal capillaries.
B and **C**: The surgeon has grasped with forceps (open arrow) the neovascular membrane that includes the inverted RPE attached to its outer surface with forceps (open arrow), has detached it from its site of origin, and is sliding it through a retinotomy.
D: This allows the retinal receptors to be re-approximated to the native RPE cells postoperatively. See Figure 3.52 for fundus photographs and photomicrographs of type II membranes and their surgical excision. Compare this figure with diagrams of surgical excision of type I membranes in Figure 2.13.

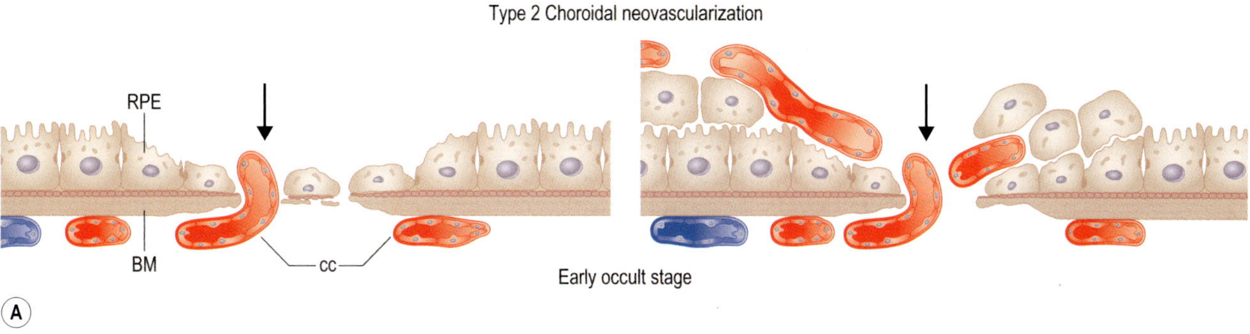
Type 2 Choroidal neovascularization
RPE
BM
CC
Early occult stage
A

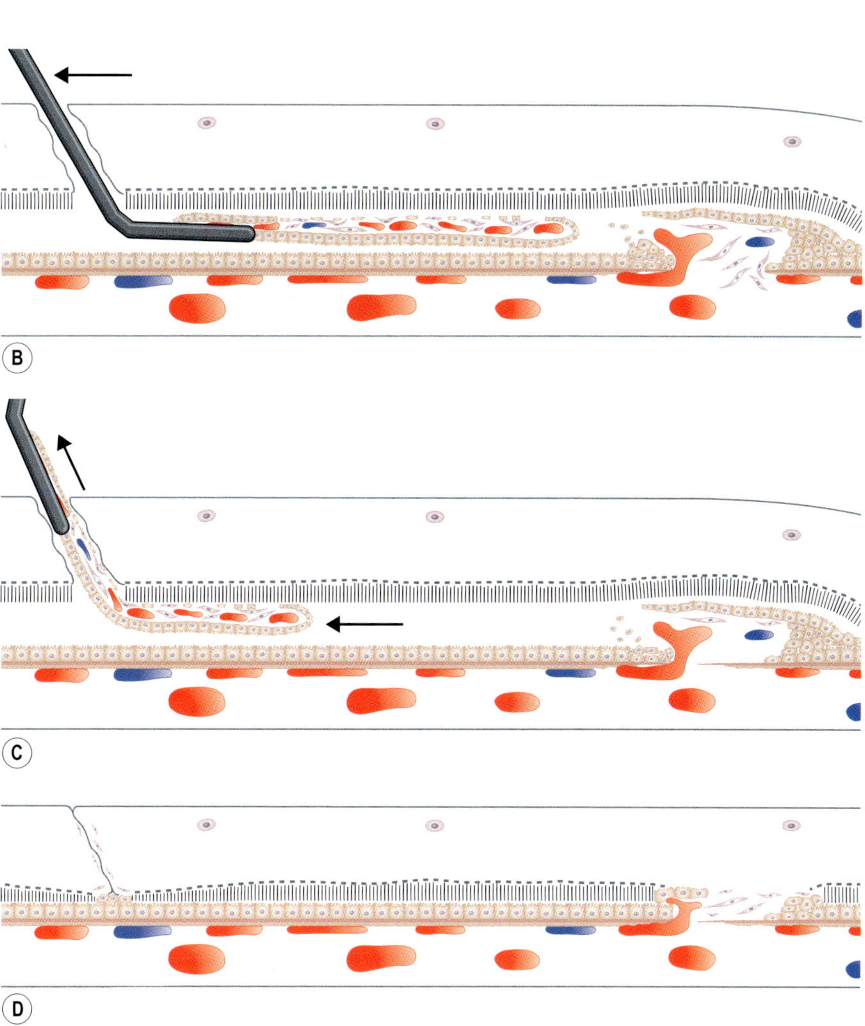
B
C
D

2.13 Surgical excision of type I sub-retinal pigment epithelium (RPE) neovascular membrane.

A and **B**: Type I neovascular membrane has invaded and extended through Bruch's membrane (arrows) and beneath the RPE. The membrane is loosely adherent to the inner surface of Bruch's membrane but is firmly attached on its anterior surface to the native RPE, which in turn is loosely adherent to the overlying sensory retina.
C: The surgeon's forceps (open arrow) extends through a retinotomy and has grasped the neovascular membrane that lies beneath and is firmly attached to the native RPE.
D: Following removal of the membrane, which includes the native RPE through the retinotomy, the surviving retinal receptors will lie against the inner surface of Bruch's membrane and visual function in this area will be lost.

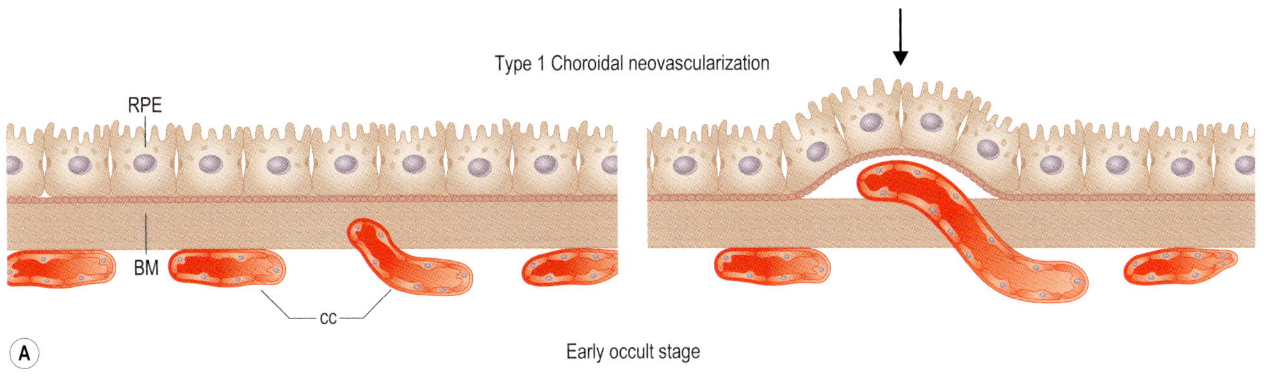
Type 1 Choroidal neovascularization
RPE
BM
CC
A
Early occult stage

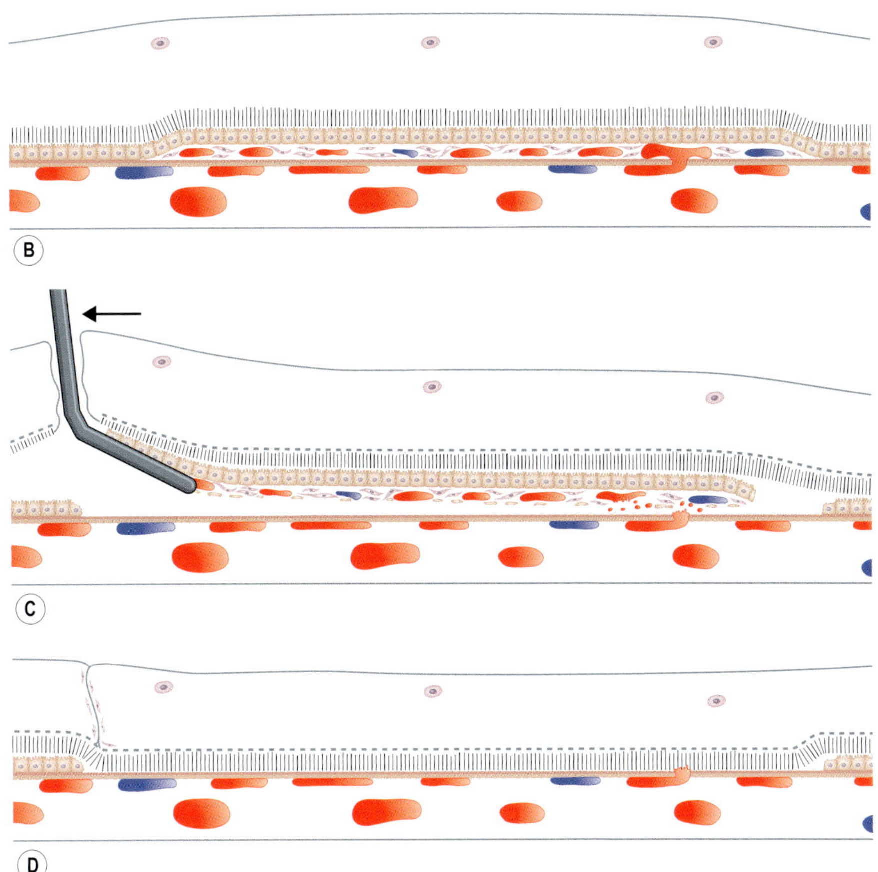
B
C
D

Devitalization of the RPE

Breakdown of the RPE blood–outer retinal barrier and exudative retinal detachment may be caused by either acute or chronic devitalization of the RPE. A variety of acute, inflammatory, ischemic, toxic, or traumatic insults to the RPE may cause exudative detachment of the retina (Figure 2.14). These include inflammatory cell infiltration of the choroid (e.g., Harada's disease, sympathetic uveitis and posterior scleritis; see Figures 11.27 and 11.28), neoplastic infiltration of the choroid (e.g., melanoma (see Figure 14.12), metastatic carcinoma (see Figure 14.30), and leukemia (see Figure 14.34)), acute occlusion of the choriocapillaris (e.g., disseminated intravascular coagulopathy, accelerated hypertension), toxemia of pregnancy (see Figure 3.59), collagen vascular diseases (Figure 2.14), and contusion necrosis of the pigment epithelium (see Figure 8.03). Fluorescein angiography typically reveals multiple progressively enlarging pinpoint areas of fluorescein leakage at the level of the pigment epithelium and late staining of the subretinal exudate.

There is some experimental as well as clinical evidence to suggest that alteration of the RPE metabolism may be associated with changes in the structure and permeability of the retinal capillaries.[5–7] Photoirradiation of the RPE with minimal doses of long-wavelength laser may produce endothelial proliferative changes in the overlying retinal capillary bed.[6] Some authors believe that some of the diffuse retinal edema and staining of the outer retina with fluorescein in patients with bilateral juxtafoveolar telangiectasis, diabetic retinopathy, and tapetoretinal dystrophies may be caused by alteration of the blood–outer retinal barrier.[8]

2.14 Serous retinal detachment caused by devitalization of the retinal pigment epithelium (RPE).

A–C: Serous detachment of the macula in a 14-year-old girl with acute disseminated lupus erythematosus. Note multifocal areas of leakage of fluorescein through infarcted RPE into the subretinal exudate.
D: Focal infarction of the RPE (arrows) caused by focal occlusion of choriocapillaris. Fine black dots indicate fluorescein molecules. Bm, Bruch's membrane; cc, choroidal capillaries.
E, F, and G: Serous retinal detachment caused by diffuse granulomatous infiltration of the choroid in a woman with Harada's disease. Note multiple pinpoint foci of leakage of fluorescein dye through damaged RPE.
H: Multifocal damage to the RPE (arrows) by choroidal inflammatory cells (coarse black dots).

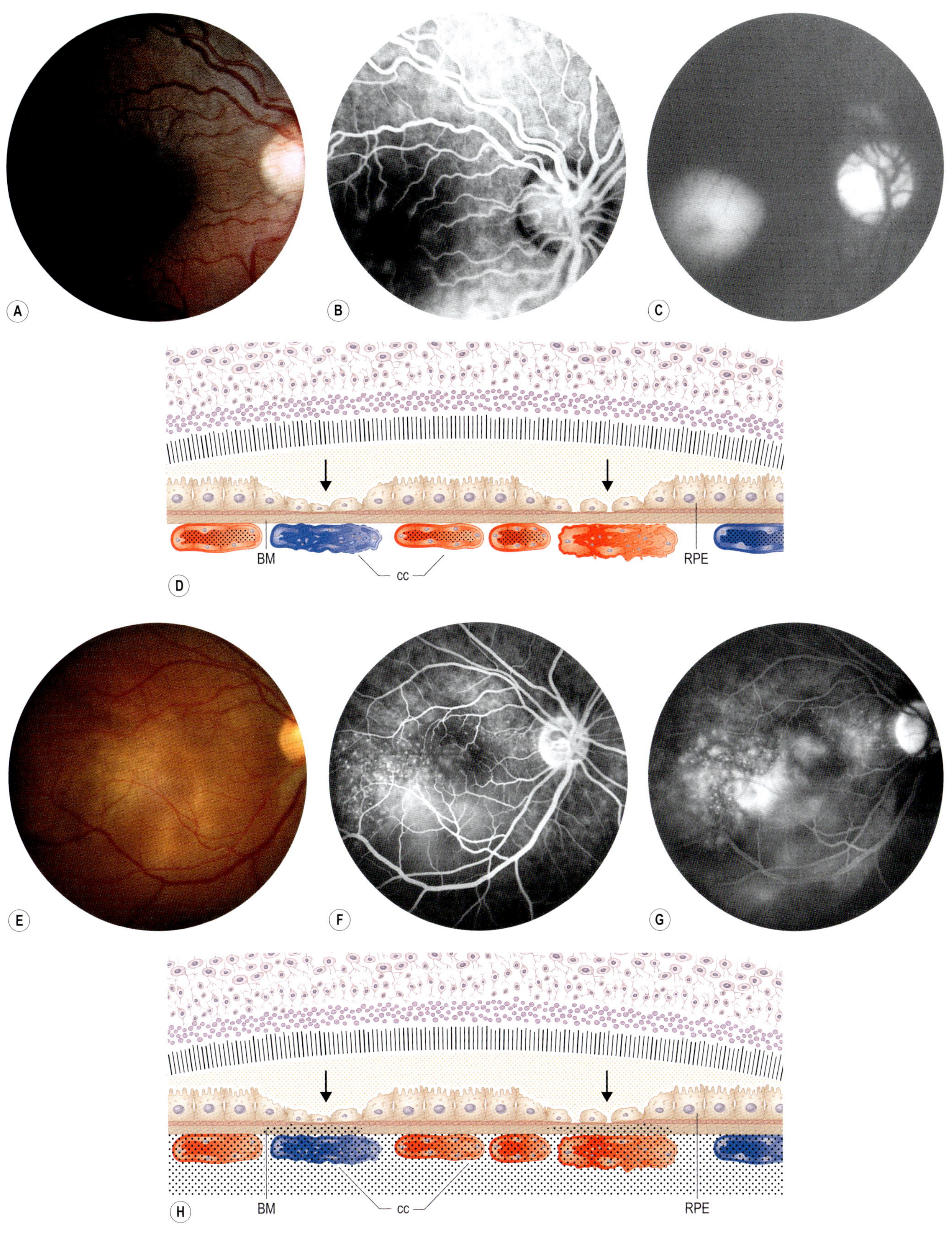
A
B
C
BM
cc
RPE
D
E
F
G
BM
cc
RPE
H

Intraretinal Exudation Caused by Damage to the Blood–Inner Retinal Barrier

Damage to the retinal vascular endothelium may involve primarily arteries, veins, or capillaries or any combination of the three. When it is confined to the arteries or veins, the exudation is largely restricted to the extracellular space surrounding these large vessels (e.g., arteritis or phlebitis).

In many diseases the endothelial damage is largely confined to the capillary bed. The endothelial decompensation may be focal or widespread. The severity of capillary endothelial damage determines the composition and the location of the extracellular fluid. If the decompensation is mild, only relatively small molecules, including small proteins, escape into the extracellular space, and clear serous exudate may be confined to the inner retinal layers, where it is not visible biomicroscopically and is detected angiographically as diffuse mild staining of the inner retina. If the capillary damage is moderate, and particularly if the deeper plexus of capillaries is affected, the serous fluid spreads posteriorly and laterally where it accumulates within the inner nuclear and outer plexiform layers. There the paucity of horizontally coursing interconnecting cell processes permits large polycystic expansion of the extracellular space. The polycystic pattern of exudation may spread laterally away from the site of the endothelial decompensation. When the capillaries near the center of the macula are involved, expansion of the large extracellular space available in the outer plexiform layer of Henle causes the typical biomicroscopic picture of cystoid macular edema. There is swelling of the retina and loss of the foveal depression caused by development of three or four large central cysts that are surrounded by a series of progressively smaller cysts (Figure 2.16). Angiographically, fluorescein molecules diffuse out of the damaged capillaries, stain the extracellular serous exudate, and produce a stellate pattern of fluorescein staining (Figure 2.16). Compression of Henle's layer that contains a high concentration of xanthophyll pigment by the large cystic areas of serous exudation is probably the cause of the central yellow spot seen biomicroscopically in the outer retina as well as the prominent nonfluorescent central star figure seen angiographically (Figure 2.16C1).

2.16 Aphakic cystoid macular edema.

A1 and A2: There is thickening of the central macula associated with multiple cystoid spaces filled with serous exudate.
B1, and B2: Early leakage of fluorescein (dots) out of perifoveolar retinal capillaries into serous exudate.
C1 and C2: Complete staining of intraretinal exudate 1 hour after fluorescein injection.

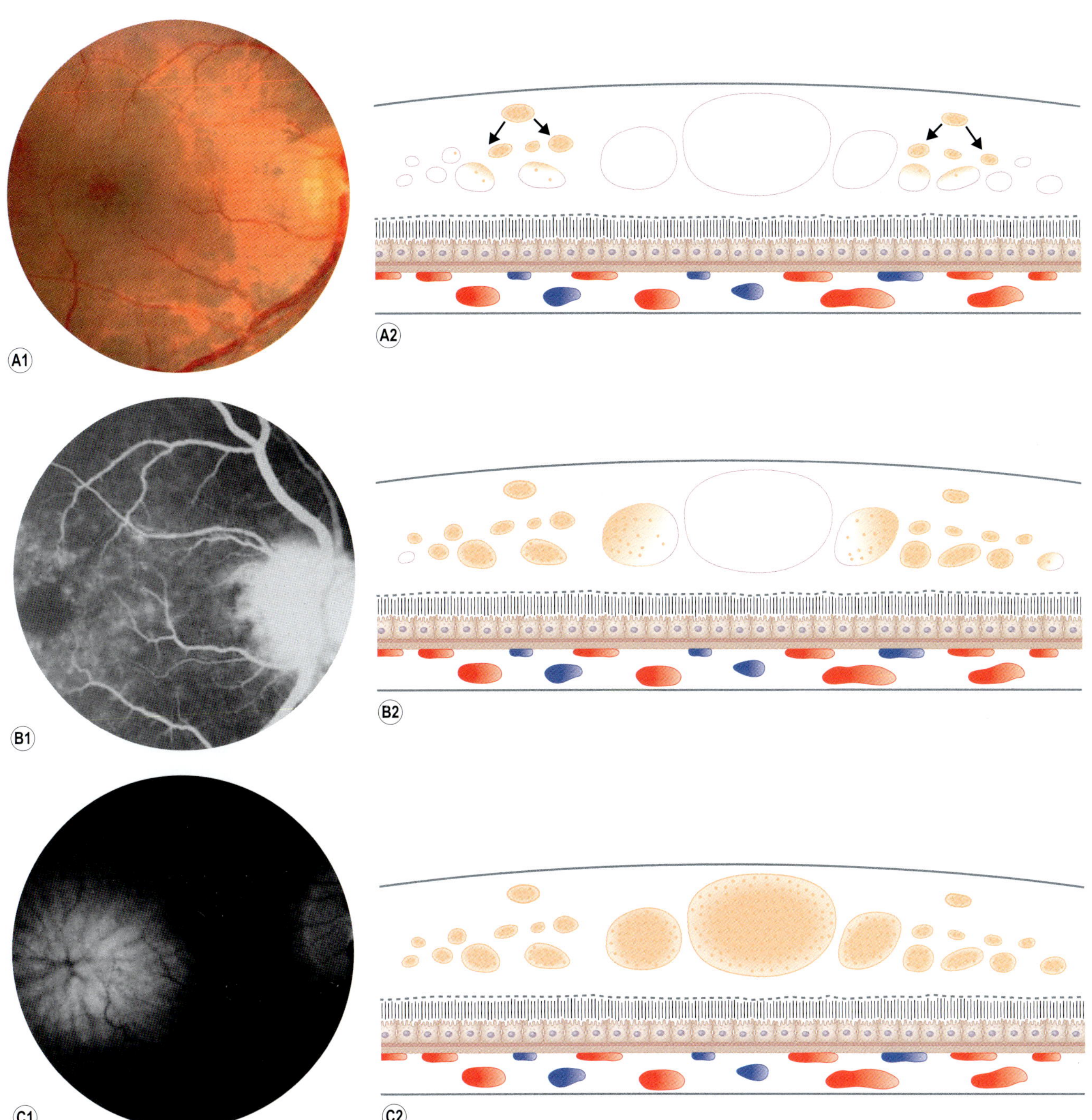
A1
A2
B1
B2
C1
C2

LESIONS THAT OBSCURE THE NORMAL RETINAL AND CHOROIDAL FLUORESCENCE

Any lesion that interferes with transmission of either the exciting blue light or the emitted yellow-green light will appear either hypofluorescent or nonfluorescent angiographically. If it is located anterior to the level of the retinal vessels, it will obscure both the retinal and the background choroidal fluorescence (Figure 2.18).

FLUORESCENCE OF LESIONS UNRELATED TO CHANGES IN VASCULAR PERMEABILITY

"Pseudofluorescent" Lesions

When angiography is done with poorly matched exciting and barrier filters, the blue light reflected from the surface of any white or light-colored nonfluorescent lesion in the fundus may bypass the barrier filter and angiographically appear to be fluorescent.

Reflected Fluorescence

Even when the exciting and barrier filters are carefully matched, light-colored, nonfluorescent lesions may exhibit fluorescence during the late stages of angiography because of reflection from their surface of the yellow-green light generated by the dye that normally escapes into the ocular media.

Autofluorescent Lesions

Some fundus lesions before the administration of fluorescein are capable of emitting yellow-green light when irradiated with blue light. Examples of this "autofluorescence" are calcified drusen of the optic nerve head and large deposits of lipofuscin.

2.17 Circinate maculopathy caused by congenital retinal telangiectasis in a 48-year-old man with cystoid macular edema.

A–C: Note angiographic evidence of dilated capillaries and late polycystic pattern of staining centrally, and absence of staining in the areas of lipid exudate outside the area of telangiectasis.
D: Escape of protein (P) and lipid-rich exudate (L) out of damaged retinal vessel into the extracellular compartment of the retina and into the subretinal space. The protein molecules are transported across the choroid and sclera into the extrascleral space. The water component of the exudate is drained into the choriocapillaris and surrounding normal retinal vessels. The lipid molecules precipitate to form yellow exudate (coarse stippling) within and beneath the retina in the peripheral area, where maximum dehydration of the exudate occurs.

2.18 Obstruction of normal choroidal and retinal fluorescence.

A: Obstruction of choroidal fluorescence by subretinal blood.
B: Obstruction of choroidal and retinal fluorescence by blood lying between the internal limiting membrane of the retina and the nerve fiber layer of the retina.

Conclusion

Although for purposes of analysis and instruction the various components of the pathologic fluorescein angiogram have been divided, the reader should recognize that multiple components often occur together and that at times it may be difficult to determine which component is dominant. Further, we still have much to learn about the pathophysiology of chorioretinal diseases and some of the concepts used in angiographic interpretations at this time may prove to be wrong. Nevertheless, these guidelines should assist readers as they explore other sections in this book and as they begin to interpret angiograms of their patients.

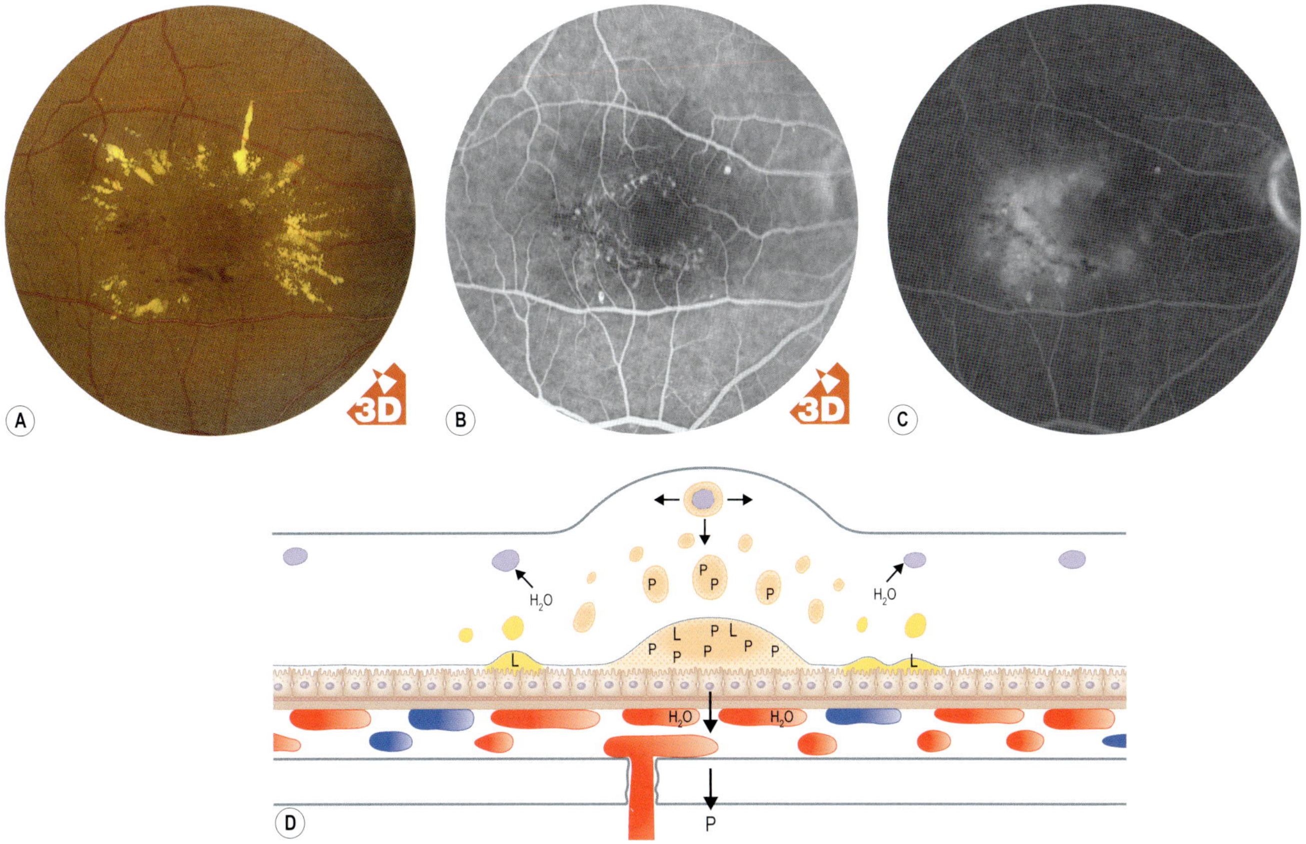

2.17

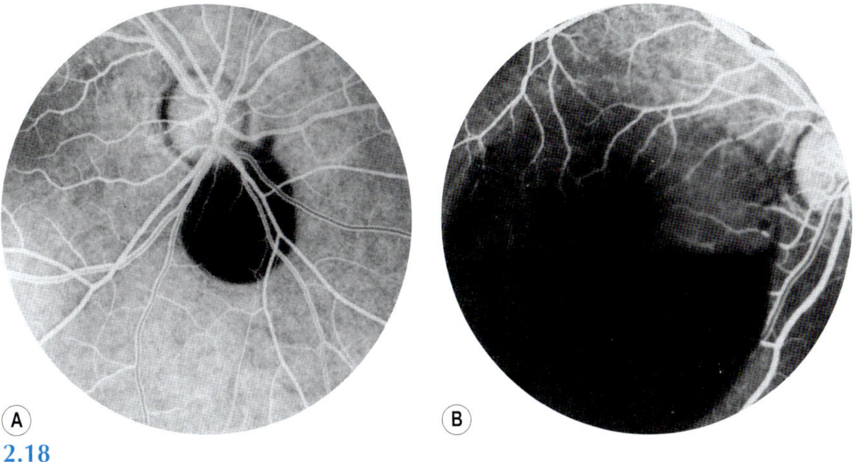

2.18

INDOCYANINE GREEN ANGIOGRAPHY

ICG is a water-soluble tricarbocyanine dye with both hydrophilic and lipophilic characteristics. It absorbs light in the near-infrared range of 790–805 nm. It emits light in the 770–880-nm range with peak emission at 835 nm. The RPE and choroid absorb 60–75% of the blue green light used in fluorescein angiography (500 nm), and only 20–38% of the near infrared light (800 nm) used in ICG angiography; hence ICG can be used to visualize structures under the RPE.[9]

ICG is 98% protein-bound, mostly to globulins such as alpha-lipoproteins, hence less of the dye escapes through the fenestrations of the choriocapillaris, thus allowing for imaging the choroidal vessels, unlike fluorescein that rapidly escapes into the extravascular space, preventing delineation of the choroidal anatomy.[10–14] However, some amount of ICG slowly diffuses through the choroidal vessels, staining the choroidal stroma in about 12 minutes. Images should be captured up to 30 minutes during the study.[15] The digital imaging system has an excitation filter that allows passage of only near-infrared light which excites the ICG molecule and the emitted light is captured via a barrier filter that blocks wavelength below 825 nm, thus capturing only light emitted from the excited ICG dye. Real-time, wide-angle, digital subtraction, and high-speed angiography using scanning laser ophthalmoscope are all possible.

ICG contains a small amount of iodine and has to be used with caution in patients with iodine allergy. Nausea, vomiting, and urticaria are less common than with fluorescein. ICG comes packaged as a 25-mg dry powder and is reconstituted with 5 ml sterile water.

Principles of Interpretation of ICG Angiography

Fluorescein angiography is still the mainstay in the evaluation of most retinal and chorioretinal disorders. ICG angiography has a role in certain conditions. With presently available technology and knowledge, ICG angiography can be specific for: (1) identification of polypoidal choroidal vasculopathy; (2) occult choroidal neovascularization; (3) neovascularization associated with pigment epithelial detachments; and (4) recurrent CNVMs. ICG angiography has a clear edge over fluorescein in delineating these lesions. ICG has some role as a guide in diagnosis or treatment – in identifying feeder vessels in age-related macular degeneration, CNVMs, chronic central serous retinopathy, multiple evanescent white-dot syndrome, acute multifocal placoid pigment epitheliopathy, Vogt–Koyanagi–Harada syndrome, macular lesions associated with angioid streaks, and birdshot chorioretinopathy. Fluorescein angiography is sufficient in most of these conditions to make the diagnosis; ICG helps to corroborate some additional evidence.[16]

Schematic interpretations are similar to fluorescein angiography with hyperfluorescence and hypofluorescence relative to the surrounding area of presumed normal fluorescence (Figure 2.19). Hypofluorescence can be from blocked fluorescence by thick blood or melanin pigment, or due to vascular filling defect. Similar to fluorescein angiography, the study has to be interpreted by reviewing images at various time points, since some areas that are initially hypofluorescent may turn hyperfluorescent late, such as plaque staining in occult CNVM (Figure 2.19G–I), and chronic central serous chorioretinopathy. In others, hyperfluorescence seen in the early frames may turn iso- or hypofluorescent late in the study, as in "washout" phenomenon of choroidal hemangioma. Pooling of ICG dye can be seen in the late frames of serous RPE detachments. In addition certain anatomic changes in the choroidal vessels can be seen such as polypoidal vessels (Figure 2.19C and D) and feeder vessel(s) of a CNVM on high-speed angiography. Areas of occluded or missing choroidal vessels can be seen in arteritic ischemic optic neuropathy. Individual examples are described as and when they appear in various chapters in the text.

2.19 Indocyanine green (ICG) angiography.

A–E: Left fundus of a 32-year-old African American woman with bilateral polypoidal choroidal vasculopathy (A). Note the orange nodules in the juxtapapillary retina and temporal fovea (arrows). A small juxtafoveal disciform is seen. Midframes of the fluorescein angiogram and ICG delineate the polyps (B–D). Autofluorescence imaging (E) shows decreased autofluorescence and the fluorescein angiogram shows a transmission defect corresponding to the foveal scar. The outlines of the polyps are visible on autofluorescence imaging.

F–L: A 55-year-old woman with serous detachment of the macula (F). Early ICG shows the individual choroidal vessels and the late frames a hot spot or staining at the nasal edge (G–I). The fluorescein angiogram also shows staining of the same region though the staining pattern in the two differ (J and K). The lesion seen on the fluorescein angiogram and ICG shows decreased autofluorescence; however the proteinaceous SRF in the macula shows hyper autofluorescence (L).

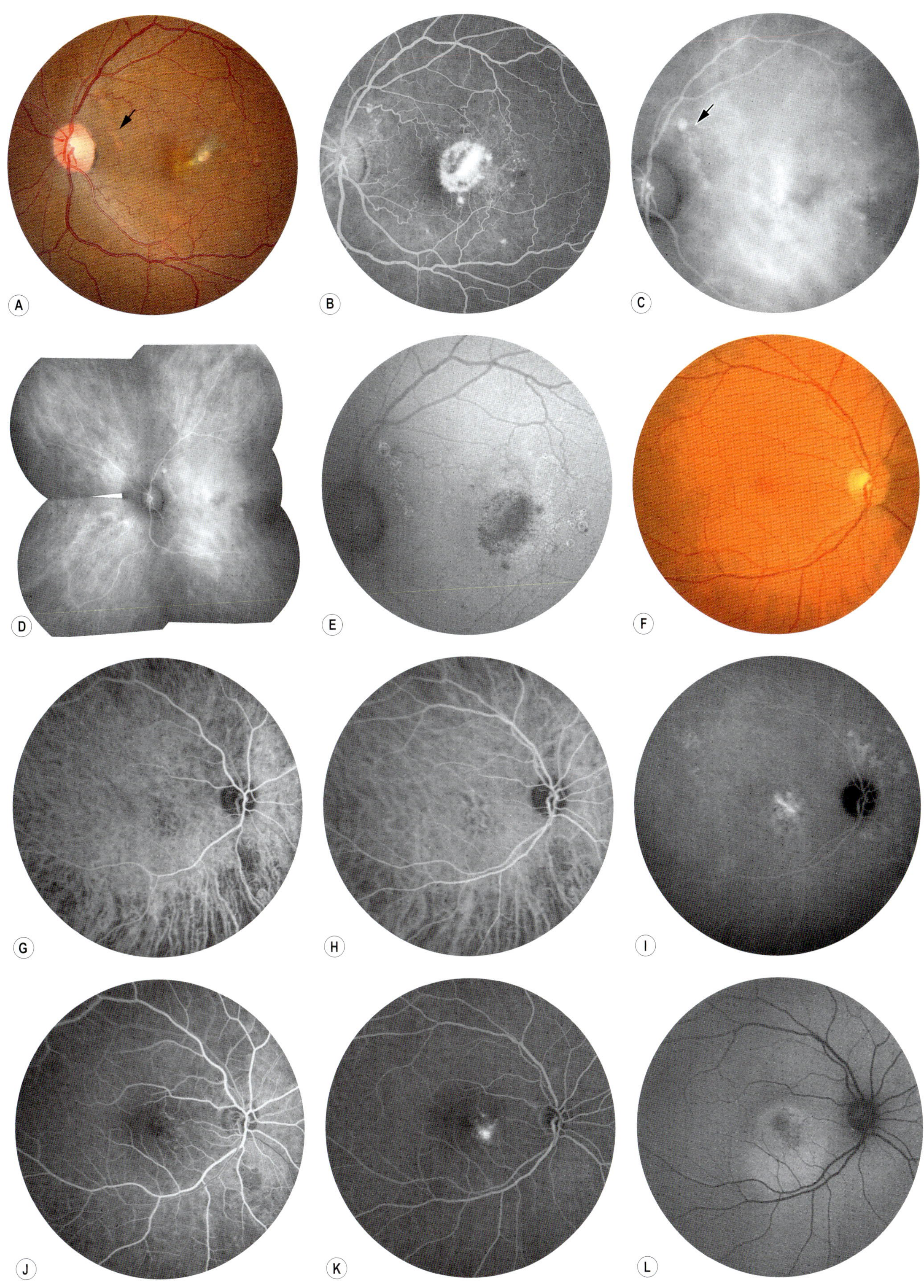
A
B
C
D
E
F
G
H
I
J
K
L

AUTOFLUORESCENCE

Lipofuscin is a pigment that autofluoresces when excited by blue light or an ultraviolet light. The RPE accumulates lipofuscin and melanolipofuscin over time and this gives a background autofluorescence to the retina.[17–20] In certain disease states the autofluorescence increases or decreases, and this can be imaged by autofluorescence imaging.

The Heidelberg machine uses a 488-nm exciting and barrier filter for capturing autofluorescence. However, the Topcon uses 512 nm for exciting and 488 nm for capturing the autofluorescence. In addition to the lipofuscin, A2E and other products can also exhibit autofluorescence.[21–23] One has to remember that autofluorescence is masked by increasing nuclear sclerosis of the lens. The lens absorbs some of the blue-wavelength light, which decreases both the excitation of the autofluorescing material at the pigment epithelial level and capture of the return autofluorescence.

Both the scanning laser ophthalmoscope and a video fundus camera can be used for capturing autofluorescence images. The fluorophores other than lipofuscin and A2E are iso-A2E, A2-PE-H2, A2PE, and A2-rhodopsin, all of which are precursors of A2E, and which are formed in the outer segments prior to phagocytosis by the RPE.[22,24–26] Lipofuscin fluorescence has a broader emission band ranging from 400 to 750 nm, hence the video fundus camera, which has excitation filter at 550 nm, picks up more autofluorescence than the Heidelberg scanning laser ophthalmoscope, which uses a 488-nm excitation filter.

Common conditions that show increased autofluorescence are flecks of Stargardt's disease/fundus flavimaculatus where the RPE cells are not atrophic (Figure 2.20I and J), RPE surrounding areas of atrophy (Figure 2.20), RPE surrounding the areas of photoreceptor disruption such as in cone dystrophy, adjacent to areas of atrophy in maculopathy associated with mitochondrial mutations and the vitelliform material in pattern dystrophy (Figure 2.20C and D) and Best disease (Figure 2.20E and F). Other examples of increased autofluorescence are patients who have had resolution of uveal effusion where the highly proteinaceous material is being reabsorbed by the RPE and is loaded with this fluorophore (Figure 2.20A and B) (see Chapter 3).

Autofluorescence imaging is especially useful when there is decreased autofluorescence in areas of RPE loss. This is of benefit in patients with geographic atrophy (Figure 2.20J and L) where the contrast on autofluorescence imaging is more distinct compared to color fundus photographs and helps in accurately monitoring for progression, especially in age-related macular degeneration and Stargardt's disease. Another good example is in patients with chronic central serous chorioretinopathy and MEWDS where the subtle RPE alteration may not be easily visible on a fundus photograph (Figures 3.06, 3.07 and 11.15, 11.16). Several examples are described in the various chapters.

2.20 Autofluorescence.

A and B: Post scleral windows in a patient with idiopathic uveal effusion shows resolution of the SRF with plump retinal pigment epithelium (RPE) cells filled with absorbed protein and reorganization of lipofuscin and intracellular pigment shows increased autofluorescence.
C and D: Focal increased autofluorescence corresponding to the vitelliform change in this patient with solitary vitelliform pattern dystrophy or adult-onset foveomacular dystrophy.
E and F: A 6-year-old girl with Best disease shows intense hyperautofluorescence of the vitelliform detachment.
G and H: Oval bull's-eye change in the macula in this 52-year-old woman with chloroquine toxicity shows decreased autofluorescence due to disruption of RPE cells.
I and J: This 40-year-old man with Stargardt's disease and fundus flavimaculatus shows increased autofluorescence corresponding to the yellow flecks and decreased autofluorescence corresponding to the areas of RPE atrophy and loss.
K and L: Autofluorescence imaging clearly shows the distinct margins of chorioretinal atrophic patches that are not as discernible on the color photograph in this 58-year-old woman with probable non-X-linked choroideremia. Note the flecks of increased autofluorescence in the intervening zones suggesting uptake of excess lipofuscin by the surviving RPE cells.

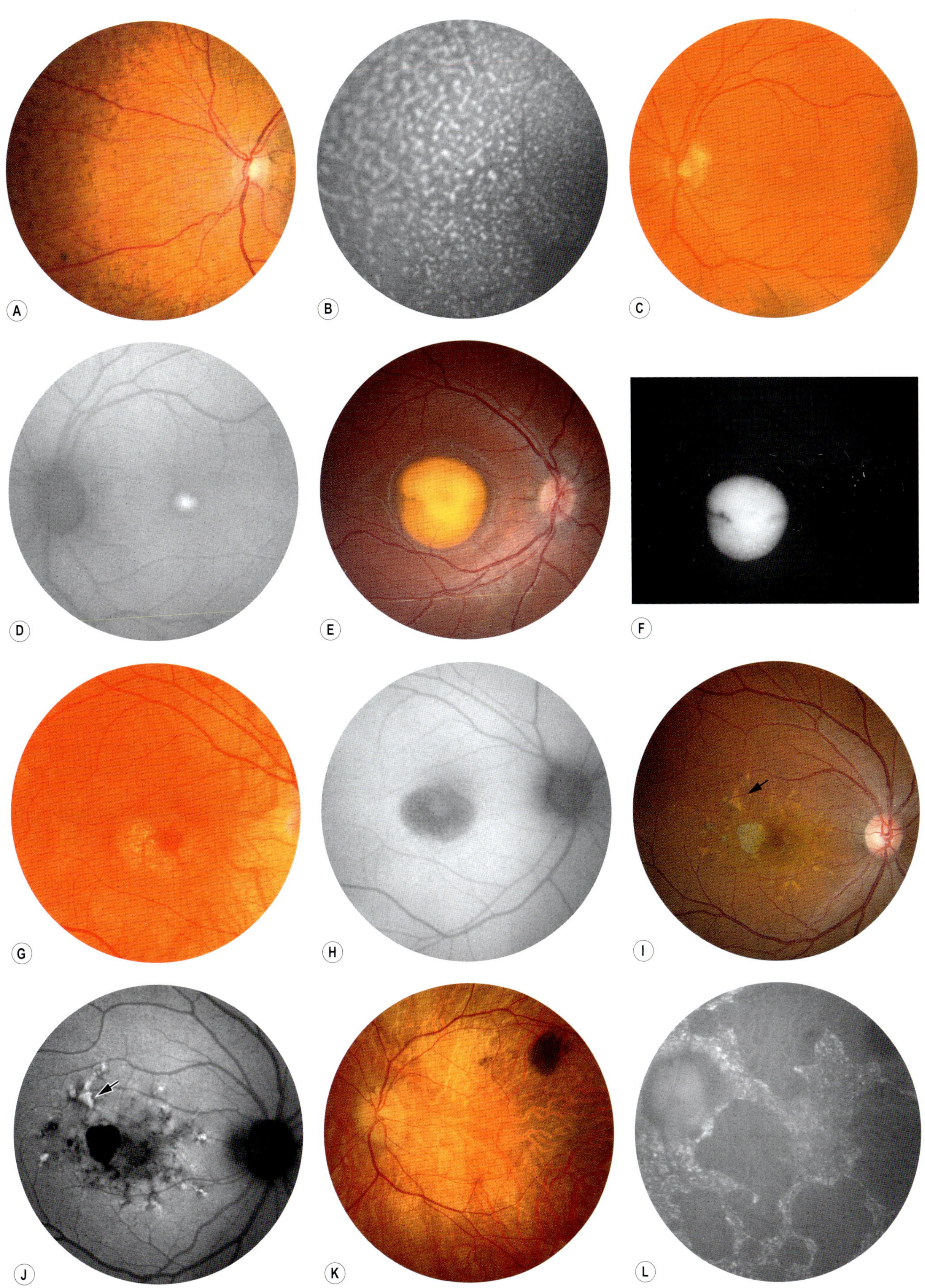
A
B
C
D
E
F
G
H
I
J
K
L

OPTICAL COHERENCE TOMOGRAPHY

Ocular coherence tomography (OCT) measures the echo time delay and intensity of back-reflected or back-scattered light. It provides real-time high-resolution cross-sectional images of the eye, and this enables identification of morphological alterations, and provides contour information and thickness measurements. Its principle is similar to ultrasound, except that it uses light instead of sound. Low-coherence interferometry is the principle on which OCT measurements are based.[27–29]

The interferometer has an 800-nm laser light source, which is projected on to a beam splitter (partially reflecting mirror) that splits the light into two paths, one that is transmitted into the eye and the other that is reflected. The light that is transmitted into the eye is reflected back to the beam splitter from various intraocular structures as multiple echoes based on their distance and thickness. The second beam is reflected from a reference mirror placed at a known spatial position back to the beam splitter where it combines with the beam reflected from the intraocular structures. The interferometer can precisely interpret the echo structure of the reflected light to make high-resolution measurements of distance and thickness of the various structures. The OCT allows:

1. imaging of retinal and choroidal layers (Figure 2.21A–F)
2. retinal thickness measurements
3. retinal topography mapping and analysis
4. retinal nerve fiber layer thickness measurements
5. retinal nerve fiber layer analysis
6. optic nerve head imaging and analysis
7. enhanced depth imaging of the choroid (Heidelburg Spectralis OCT).

Two principles of OCT imaging are currently used – time domain and spectral domain. Spectral domain (SD-SLO/OCT) uses a 840-nm diode light source and performs a sweep of 256 serial parallel OCT B-scans with an axial resolution of 5 μm, covering a 9 × 9-mm area in the transverse plane through the macula. Time domain stratus OCT (Stratus OCT, version 4.0.1, Carl Zeiss Meditec, Dublin, CA, USA) uses an 810-nm wavelength diode source and scans six consecutive radial B scans with a resolution of 10 μm. Spectral domain has several advantages over time domain imaging in that it has a faster acquisition speed (50 times faster, thereby decreasing motion artifacts from eye movements), scans a larger area, has higher resolution, and can reproduce the same point of reference each time.

2.21 Optical coherence tomography (OCT).

A and **B**: Swollen disc with dilated vessels on its surface with macular star in a patient with cat-scratch disease. OCT shows turbid subretinal fluid and intraretinal lipid in the outer plexiform layer (arrows).
C and **D**: Bull's-eye maculopathy in a patient with chloroquine toxicity. Corresponding OCT shows disruption of photoreceptors and loss of inner segment/outer segment (IS/OS) junction in the fovea.
E and **F**: Patient with vascularized retinal pigment epithelium (RPE) detachment secondary to occult choroidal neovascularization in the right eye. Stratus (time domain) OCT shows the elevated RPE and adjacent subretinal fluid (SRF) (arrow).

ULTRASONOGRAPHY

Ultrasound uses acoustic waves that are created from oscillation of particles within a medium. Ultrasound waves have a frequency greater than 20 000 oscillations per second or 20 kHz, rendering them inaudible to humans. The frequencies used in ophthalmic ultrasound range from 8 to 10 MHz for conventional A and B scan. The higher the frequency, the shorter the depth of penetration. An ultrasound biomicroscope uses a 50-MHz probe; hence the depth of penetration is low and limited to the anterior segment. The velocity of the wave is dependent on the medium through which it passes; hence the wave passing through water, vitreous, silicone oil, or a solid mass has different speeds. The more compressible the medium the slower the propagation, thus the sound waves move faster in a solid tumor than the liquid vitreous. Acoustic interfaces created at the junction of two media have different acoustic impedance. The angle of incidence of the sound beating against an interface is important in determining the strength of the returning echo. In addition, the size, shape, and smoothness of the interface play a role in the character of the returning echo. Some of the ultrasound is absorbed and converted to heat as it passes through a medium; however, this is extremely low and has no harmful effects on tissue.

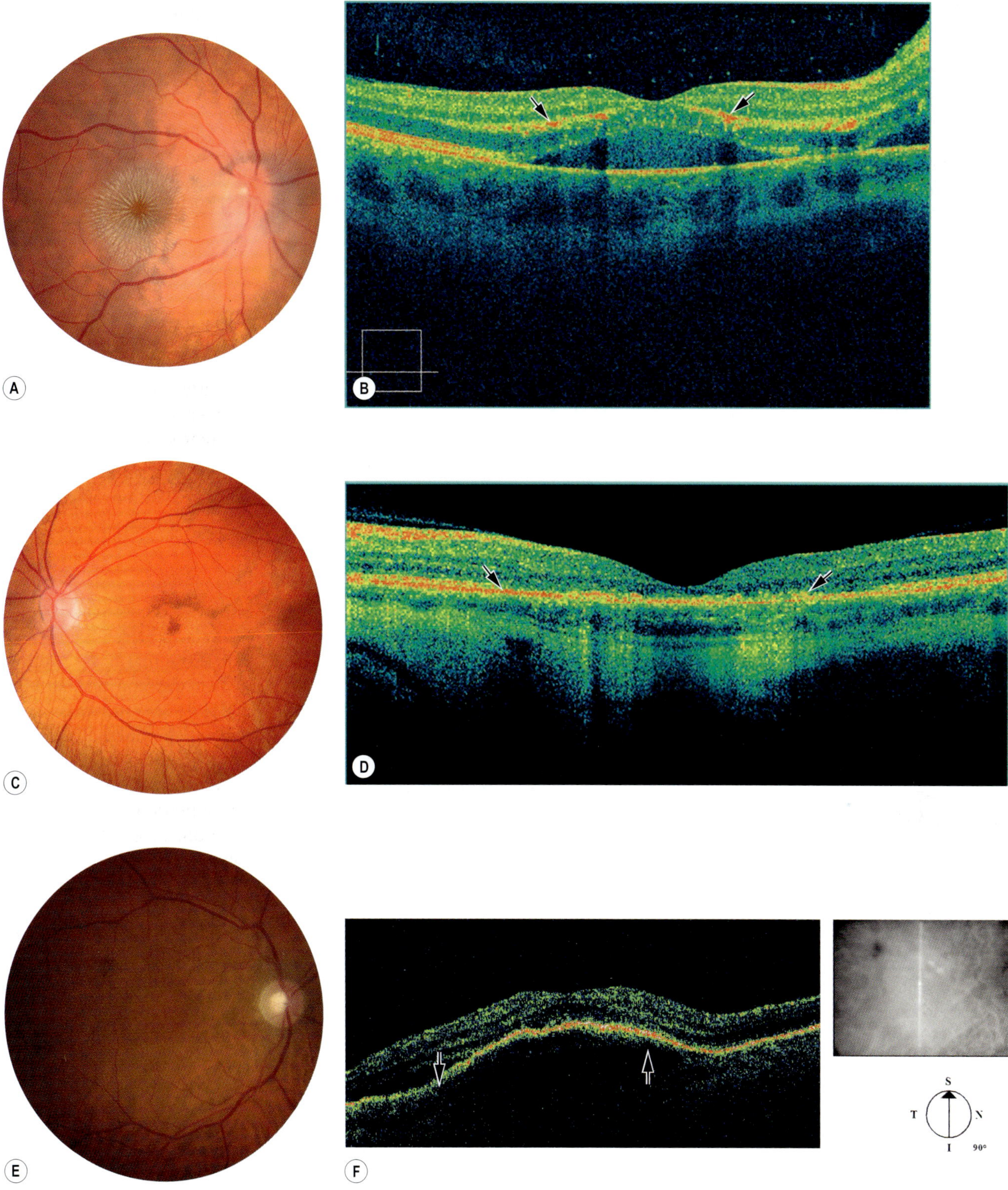
A
B
C
D
E
F
S
T
N
I
90°

Two American ophthalmologists, Drs. Mundt and Hughes, evaluated an intraocular tumor by using an amplitude mode (A-scan) ultrasound for the first time in ophthalmology in 1956.[30] In 1958 Baum and Greenwood developed the first two-dimensional immersion brightness mode (B-scan) ultrasonogram for ophthalmology.[31,32] Coleman and Weininger, in the late 1960s, developed the first commercial immersion B-scan ophthalmic instrument.[33] A contact B-scan machine was introduced by Bronson.[34,35]

Instrument and Technique

The transducer probe is the structure that produces the echo. A piece of the electro crystal is placed near the face of the probe and undergoes mechanical vibration when stimulated by electrical energy. This vibration causes a longitudinal ultrasound wave that is propagated through any medium. Certain terms need to be defined and understood in order to perform and interpret ocular ultrasonography.

Gain

All ultrasound instruments are created to adjust the amplification of the echo signals. Gain is measured in decibels and represents the relative units of ultrasound intensity. Adjusting the gain does not change the amount of energy emitted from the transducer; however, it changes the intensity of the returning echo that is displayed on the screen. The higher the gain, the greater the ability of the instrument to display weaker echoes, e.g., vitreous opacities. Conversely, if the gain is lowered only strong echoes of the retina are displayed, and thus eliminating low-intensity echoes from vitreous hemorrhage and other opacities, if present.

Shadowing

When the sound beam interfaces with solid tissue a significant portion of the echo of the beam is reflected back and only a small amount is transmitted. This creates a shadow behind the solid interface. Shadowing is prominent when sound waves interface with high-density substances such as calcium or bone.

Dampening

When the sound waves interface with a solid mass, some of the echoes are dampened, and this is especially seen in choroidal melanoma, where the reflected echoes drop in intensity as the wave passes through the tumor.

Important steps in performing a good ultrasound B-scan are based on the following.

The B-Scan Probe Orientation

The basic orientations are axial, longitudinal, and transverse. The ultrasound probe has a mark at the 12 o'clock hour, which signifies the superior pole of the displayed image. Turning this line to a specific clock hour allows images to be seen in an axial orientation in that clock hour. When evaluating an intraocular lesion, the following components are evaluated: the location, extent, shape, reflectivity, internal structure and attenuation, after movement, vascularity and convection movement.

2.21 Continued

Ultrasonography (USG).

G: Normal ultrasound B scan of the posterior segment. The optic nerve is normally echo-lucent.

H–J: A patient with choroidal hemangioma showing an orange elevation. The B scan shows a solid mass with smooth contour. A scan through the mass shows high internal reflectivity.

K and L: A patient with a retinal detachment on B scan (K) and a single spike on an A scan that denotes the detached retina (L).

Reflectivity

Reflectivity measures the reflectivity of all detected lesions. Depending on the number of interfaces present within the lesion, the reflectivity is altered. Those that have multiple interfaces such as a choroidal hemangioma display high internal reflectivity (Figure 2.21H–J). A solid mass such as a choroidal melanoma decreases the internal reflectivity as the sound waves pass through the compact lesion. Much more solid structures such as choroidal osteoma or a metallic foreign body will cause shadowing by preventing transmission of most of the sound waves through the solid structure.

An ultrasound B-scan is invaluable in evaluating features of choroidal tumors, choroidal osteoma, or a retinal detachment (Figure 2.21K and L) when associated with media opacities such as cataract or a vitreous hemorrhage. It is also invaluable in determining the presence of, or locating, a retinal tear in patients presenting with a dense vitreous hemorrhage. It is useful in locating an intraocular foreign body if associated with a vitreous hemorrhage that obscures fundus details. The start of, or presence of, a posterior vitreous separation can be seen in patients with traumatic vitreous hemorrhage to help time surgical intervention. Presence of a dislocated intraocular lens can be confirmed in eyes with trauma. A choroidal effusion in a postoperative glaucoma eye can be evaluated and monitored. Liquefaction of blood in suprachoroidal hemorrhage a few days after the event is useful in timing the draining of the suprachoroidal blood. Choroidal thickening can be evaluated in patients with uveal effusion and choroidal inflammation such as Vogt–Koyanagi–Harada syndrome and sympathetic ophthalmia. The presence of any mass in and around the ciliary body can be evaluated.

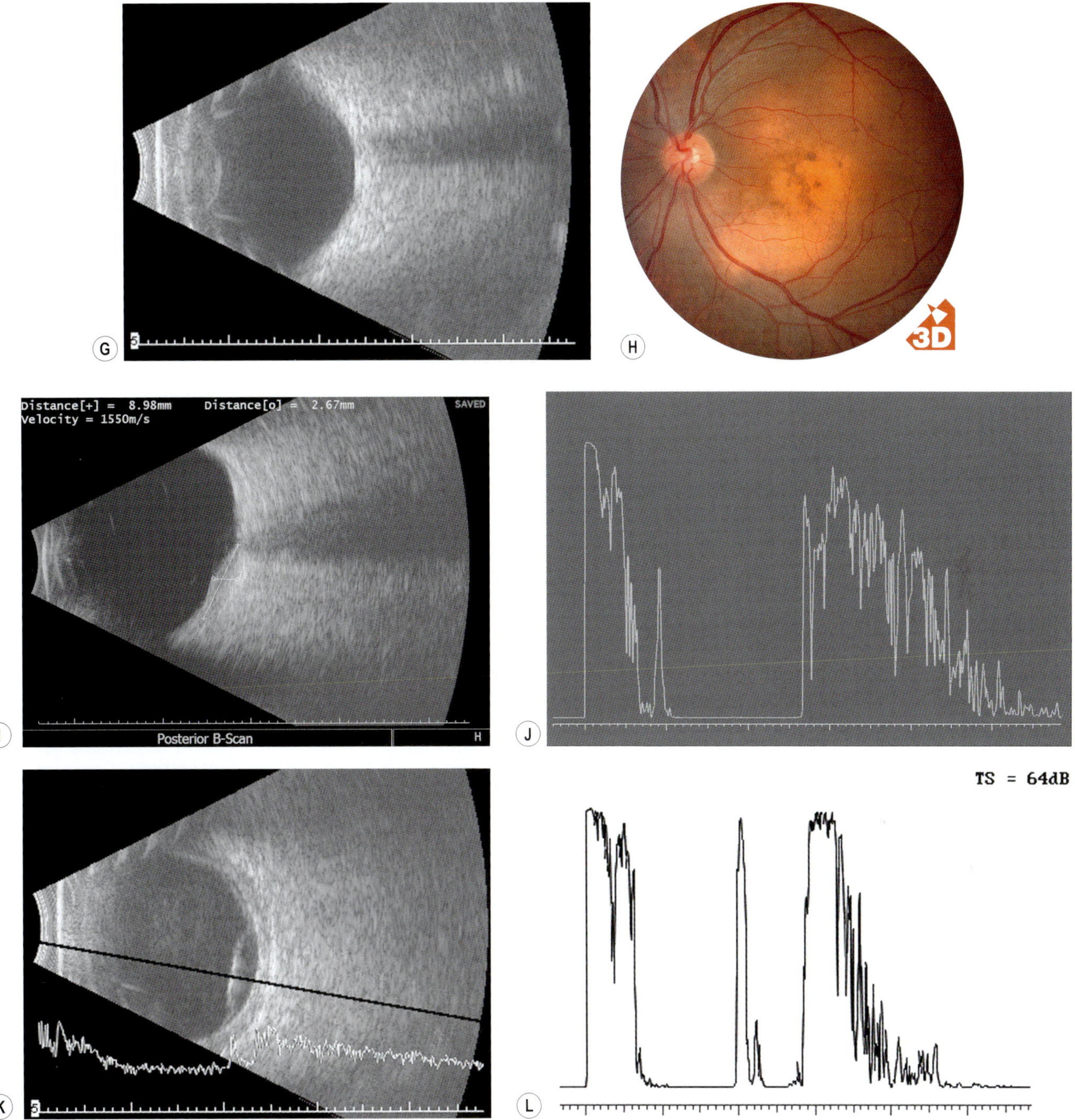
G
H
3D
Distance[+] = 8.98mm
Distance[o] = 2.67mm
SAVED
Velocity = 1550m/s
Posterior B-Scan
I
J
K
TS = 64dB
L

ADAPTIVE OPTICS

Scanning laser ophthalmoscope allows microscopic viewing of living tissue. The system has to overcome several aberrations beginning from the tear film, cornea, refractive indices of the lens and other structures and various accommodative status of the eye to be able to obtain a clear image of the retinal structures. Babcock,[36] Hubin and Noethe,[37] and Liang et al.[38] used adaptive optics to compensate for the monochromatic aberrations of the eye. AOSLO is a scanning laser ophthalmoscope that uses adaptive optics to measure and correct the high-order aberrations of the human eye. Adaptive optics increases both lateral and axial resolution, permitting axial sectioning of retinal tissue in vivo. The instrument is used to visualize photoreceptors, nerve fibers, and movement of cells through retinal capillaries.[39] The central 10–12° of cone mosaic can be imaged in the fovea,[40] and combining it with images obtained using high-resolution spectral domain OCT may be helpful in detecting photoreceptor changes, and their loss over time in understanding progressive macular dystrophies.[41,42]

2.22 Electroretinogram (ERG).

A–E: Normal ERG recordings in a 65-year-old woman. In the dark-adapted state a dim flash (24 db) stimulates the rods and is measured as a b wave (A). A stronger flash (0 db) in the dark-adapted state stimulates both the rods and cones generating larger a (first negative) and b (first positive) waves (B). The oscillatory potentials (OPs) are recorded next (C). In a light-adapted state a strong flash (0 db) stimulates only the cones generating both a and b waves (D). Continuous stimulation of the cones by a 30-Hz flicker light results in several negative and positive waves; only the b wave amplitude is measured and interpreted (E).
F–K: A 34-year-old woman with rapidly enlarging temporal field defect associated with photopsias in her left eye was diagnosed with acute zonal occult outer retinopathy (AZOOR). An ERG shows asymmetry between the two eyes both in rod and cone function (F–I). The right fundus is normal (J), the left shows peripapillary retinal pigment epithelium atrophy corresponding to the extent of the enlarged blind spot (K). The left eye's ERG amplitudes are lower than the right due to loss or dysfunction of the peripapillary photoreceptors.

ELECTRORETINOGRAM (ERG)

The ERG is an electrical potential generated by the retina in response to a flash of light. A standard ERG testing done in the clinic measures: (1) the ERG to weak flash or 24-dB flash, performed in scotopic or dark-adapted conditions that measure the rod photoreceptor potential; (2) followed by a very strong flash, 0 dB in the dark-adapted state, which measures combined rod and cone function; (3) the oscillatory potentials are next recorded; (4) the patient is light-adapted for approximately 10 minutes followed by ERG with a strong flash 0 dB to measure the potential arising from the cones; and (5) repeated stimulus – 30 Hz flicker is used to stimulate repeatedly the cones to pick up photopic responses to superstimulation. Specialized types of ERG include: multifocal ERG (mfERG), focal ERG, and pattern ERG.

Technique

The patient is asked to sit in front of a Ganzfeld bowl. Contact lenses are placed over both corneas and a ground electrode is placed over the ears. The patient is dark-adapted for 20–30 minutes prior to testing in usual cases. Longer dark adaptation is used in certain situations such as in stationary night blindness. In the dark-adapted state, a 24-dB photopic flash or a blue light is used; this is a weak flash that stimulates the rods (Figure 2.22A and F).

The origin of the a-wave is mainly associated with photoreceptors but also has a postreceptor contribution primarily from the retinal off pathway. The dark-adapted a-wave is the initial negative wave that occurs in response to the strong stimulus. This is only seen when both rod and cone functions are tested (Figure 2.22B and G). The a-wave from cones alone occurs in the light-adapted state using a strong stimulus. The b-wave is generated when the conduction of the receptor potential occurs from the photoreceptor onwards through the inner retina. The b-wave is contributed by the depolarizing activity of the bipolar cells (Figure 2.22B and G). Patients who have some amount of cone dysfunction may show adequate amplitude on the single flash photopic recording (Figure 2.22D and H). However, on repeated stimulation (Figure 2.22E and I), the amplitudes may fall off. The b-wave is a positive deflection at light offset that is characteristic of photopic ERG. Special cases of electronegative b-wave in patients with congenital stationary night blindness are due to the poor onward conduction of the receptor potential generated at the photoreceptors.

The oscillatory potentials are a series of high-frequency, low-amplitude wavelength superimposed on the b-wave that occur in response to strong stimulus. These are present in the light- and dark-adapted conditions with contribution from both rod (Figure 2.22C) and cone signals. The number of oscillatory potentials induced by one flash of light ranges between four and 10.

The oscillatory potentials are generated due to neuronal interactions and feedback circles and to intrinsic membrane properties of amacrine cells.

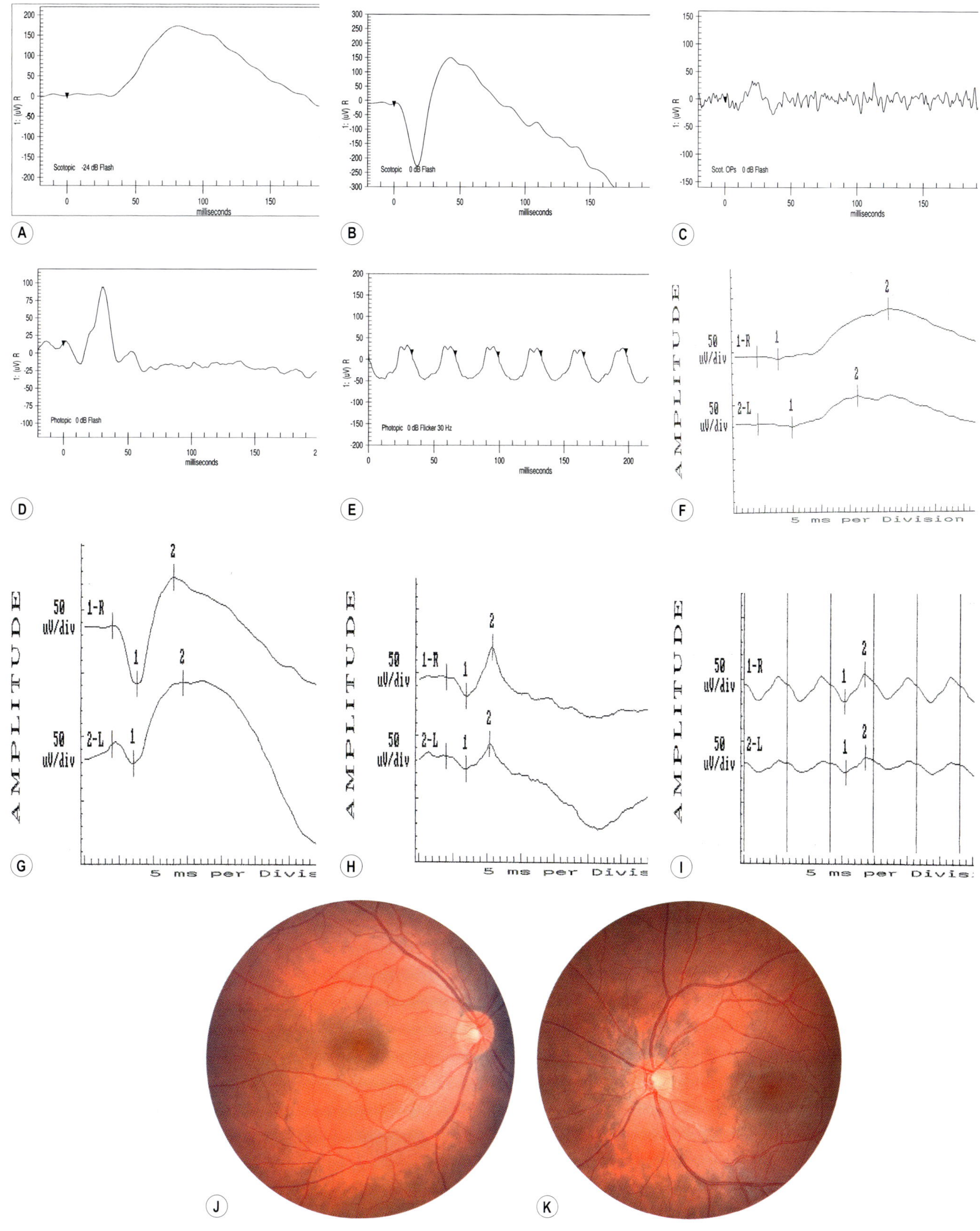

A
B
C
D
E
F
G
H
I
J
K
Scotopic -24 dB Flash
Scotopic 0 dB Flash
Scot. OPs 0 dB Flash
Photopic 0 dB Flash
Photopic 0 dB Flicker 30 Hz
milliseconds
1: (uV) R
AMPLITUDE
50 uV/div
1-R
2-L
5 ms per Division

not technically "little ERG responses." Therefore, the designations "a-wave" and "b-wave," used for the full-field ERG, are not appropriate to describe features of the mfERG waveform.[46]

Technique

The pupils should be dilated and pupil size noted. Fixation stability is important and can affect the quality of recordings and can be monitored. Refractive errors may alter the area of the retina stimulated due to diffraction of the light stimuli; hence refractive errors should be corrected. Preadaptation involves exposing the subject to ordinary room light for at least 15 minutes prior to testing. Moderate room lighting close to the illumination on the stimulus screen should be used. A total recording time of 4 minutes for the 61 stimuli and 8 minutes for the 103 stimuli is required.

The responses are displayed as trace arrays (wave forms) (Figure 2.23B and D) and three-dimensional response density plots (Figure 2.23C and E). Trace arrays are useful in comparing an area of low amplitude to another area in the same eye or a corresponding area in the fellow eye.[47] It can be compared against similar quadrants on a visual field.[48] The three-dimensional plot shows the overall signal strength per unit area of the retina. This should be interpreted in conjunction with the trace arrays and not by itself.

ELECTRO-OCULOGRAM (EOG)

When an electrode is placed on the cornea and another near the posterior pole of the eye (or elsewhere in the body), a positive resting potential is found.[49,50] The EOG displays this corneofundal potential, which renders the cornea 0.006–0.010 V positive compared to the posterior wall structures (retinal receptors and RPE) of the eye. The corneofundal potential is the result of metabolic activity of the epithelium of the cornea, lens, and retina. The potential from the RPE is photosensitive while that from the cornea and lens epithelium is not. The RPE loses the potential in the dark and recharges during light adaptation. This difference in the potential between dark and light, called the "light peak," is termed Arden ratio (Figure 2.23H).

The measurement is based on the eye movement-dependent voltage generated and recorded between electrodes placed at the inner and outer canthi of the eye. The patient is seated in front of the Ganzfield bowl and asked to look back and forth between two fixation lights placed 30° from each other. When the eye moves to the right the positive cornea becomes closer to one of the electrodes, thus rendering this electrode more positive than the other, and the opposite occurs when the eye moves to the left. The patient is preadapted in room light for 15 minutes. Fifteen minutes of the recording occurs in the dark, followed by 20-minute recording under standard light adaptation using the Ganzfield bowl. The test can be performed with the patient dilated or not. If the patient is dilated the intensity of the Ganzfield background light should be lower than if not dilated. The dark-adapted EOG reaches a minimum and then fluctuates. The light-adapted EOG gradually increases and reaches a maximum and then drops gradually. The Arden ratio is the difference in the amplitude between the "light peak" and the "dark trough" and the normal is at least 1.8, often around 2.5 (Figure 2.23H). The right and left eyes are recorded simultaneously.

The EOG is a function of the entire RPE–photoreceptor complex and not just the macular RPE and photoreceptors. Rod and cone mechanisms contribute to the generation of the potential.[51] EOG is abnormal whenever the ERG is abnormal but the reverse is not true, as in Best disease and chloroquine toxicity.[52]

In conclusion, a given patient should receive the necessary and appropriate studies for diagnosis and re-evaluation of treatment response. The principles and interpretation of fluorescein angiography have received the most attention in this chapter. Understanding fluorescein angiography should help the reader interpret other studies such as ICG angiography, autofluorescence, and OCT. Only the basic principles of the remaining studies have been touched upon, to assist the reader in quickly interpreting their results. For a more succinct understanding of the individual studies, the reader is directed to more elaborate sources.

References

1. Cohen SMZ, Fine SL, Murphy RP, et al. Transient delay in choroidal filling after krypton red laser photocoagulation for choroidal neovascular membranes. Retina 1983;3:284–90.
2. Gass JDM, Norton EWD, Justice Jr J. Serous detachment of the retinal pigment epithelium. Trans Am Acad Ophthalmol Otolaryngol 1966;70:990–1015.
3. Gass JDM. Biomicroscopic and histopathologic considerations regarding the feasibility of surgical excision of subfoveal neovascular membranes. Am J Ophthalmol 1994;118:285–98.
4. Guyer DR, Puliafito CA, Monés JM, et al. Digital indocyanine green angiography in chorioretinal disorders. Ophthalmology 1992;99:287–91.
5. Kirber WM, Nichols CW, Grimes PA, et al. A permeability defect of the retinal pigment epithelium; occurrence in early streptozocin diabetes. Arch Ophthalmol 1980;98:725–8.
6. Marshall J, Glover G, Rothery S. Some new findings on retinal irradiation by krypton and argon lasers. Doc Ophthalmol Proc Ser 1984;36:21–37.
7. Tso MOM, Cunha-Vaz JGF, Shih C-Y, et al. A clinicopathologic study of blood–retinal barrier in experimental diabetes. ARVO Abstracts. Invest Ophthalmol Vis Sci 1979;18:169.
8. Casswell AG, Chaine G, Rush P, et al. Paramacular telangiectasis. Trans Ophthalmol Soc UK 1986;105:683–92.
9. Flower RW, Hochheimer BF. Indocyanine green dye fluorescence and infrared absorption choroidal angiography performed simultaneously with fluorescein angiography. Johns Hopkins Med J 1976;138:33–42.
10. Chang AA, Morse LS, Handa JT, et al. Histologic localization of indocyanine green dye in aging primate and human ocular tissues with clinical angiographic correlation. Ophthalmology 1998;105:1060–8.
11. Orth DH, Patz A, Flower RW. Potential clinical applications of indocyanine green choroidal angiography – preliminary report. Eye Ear Nose Throat Mon 1976;55:15–28. [58.]
12. Flower RW, Hochheimer BF. A clinical technique and apparatus for simultaneous angiography of the separate retinal and choroidal circulations. Invest Ophthalmol 1973;12:248–61.
13. Geeraets WJ, Berry ER. Ocular spectral characteristics as related to hazards from lasers and other light sources. Am J Ophthalmol 1968;66:15–20.
14. Baker KJ. Binding of sulfobromophthalein (BSP) sodium and indocyanine green (ICG) by plasma alpha-1 lipoproteins. Proc Soc Exp Biol Med 1966;122:957–63.
15. Ho AC, Yannuzzi LA, Guyer DR, et al. Intraretinal leakage of indocyanine green dye. Ophthalmology 1994;101:534–41.
16. Stanga PE, Lim JI, Hamilton P. Indocyanine green angiography in chorioretinal diseases: indications and interpretation: an evidence-based update. Ophthalmology 2003;110:15–21. [quiz 2–3.]

17. Delori FC, Goger DG, Dorey CK. Age-related accumulation and spatial distribution of lipofuscin in RPE of normal subjects. Invest Ophthalmol Vis Sci 2001;42:1855–66.
18. Delori FC, Fleckner MR, Goger DG, et al. Autofluorescence distribution associated with drusen in age-related macular degeneration. Invest Ophthalmol Vis Sci 2000;41:496–504.
19. Yin D. Biochemical basis of lipofuscin, ceroid, and age pigment-like fluorophores. Free Radic Biol Med 1996;21:871–88.
20. Senba M. Autofluorescence of lipofuscin granules? Am J Clin Pathol 1985;83:134.
21. Kim DY, Hwang JC, Moore AT, et al. Fundus autofluorescence and optical coherence tomography of congenital grouped albinotic spots. Retina 2010;30:1217–22.
22. Sparrow JR, Kim SR, Cuervo AM, et al. A2E, a pigment of RPE lipofuscin, is generated from the precursor, A2PE by a lysosomal enzyme activity. Adv Exp Med Biol 2008;613:393–8.
23. Sparrow JR, Cai B, Jang YP, et al. A2E, a fluorophore of RPE lipofuscin, can destabilize membrane. Adv Exp Med Biol 2006;572:63–8.
24. Bakall B, Radu RA, Stanton JB, et al. Enhanced accumulation of A2E in individuals homozygous or heterozygous for mutations in BEST1 (VMD2). Exp Eye Res 2007;85:34–43.
25. Delori FC. Autofluorescence method to measure macular pigment optical densities fluorometry and autofluorescence imaging. Arch Biochem Biophys 2004;430:156–62.
26. Parish CA, Hashimoto M, Nakanishi K, et al. Isolation and one-step preparation of A2E and iso-A2E, fluorophores from human retinal pigment epithelium. Proc Natl Acad Sci USA 1998;95:14609–14613.
27. Huang D, Swanson EA, Lin CP, et al. Optical coherence tomography. Science 1991;254:1178–81.
28. Swanson EA, Izatt JA, Hee MR, et al. In vivo retinal imaging by optical coherence tomography. Opt Lett 1993;18:1864–6.
29. Fujimoto JG, Brezinski ME, Tearney GJ, et al. Optical biopsy and imaging using optical coherence tomography. Nat Med 1995;1:970–2.
30. Mundt Jr GH, Hughes Jr WF. Ultrasonics in ocular diagnosis. Am J Ophthalmol 1956;41:488–98.
31. Baum G, Greenwood I. The application of ultrasonic locating techniques to ophthalmology. II. Ultrasonic slit lamp in the ultrasonic visualization of soft tissues. AMA Arch Ophthalmol 1958;60:263–79.
32. Baum G. An evaluation of techniques used in the radiation of the eye with ultrasonic energy. Am J Phys Med 1957;36:212–20.
33. Coleman DJ, Weininger R. Ultrasonic M-mode technique in ophthalmology. Arch Ophthalmol 1969;82:475–9.
34. Bronson II NR. Intraocular foreign bodies. Ultrasonic localization. Int Ophthalmol Clin 1968;8:199–203.
35. Bronson NR. Techniques of ultrasonic localization and extraction. Am J Ophthalmol 1965;60:596–603.
36. Babcock HW. Adaptive optics revisited. Science 1990;249:253–7.
37. Hubin N, Noethe L. Active optics, adaptive optics, and laser guide stars. Science 1993;262:1390–4.
38. Liang J, Williams DR, Miller DT. Supernormal vision and high-resolution retinal imaging through adaptive optics. J Opt Soc Am A Opt Image Sci Vis 1997;14:2884–92.
39. Roorda A, Romero-Borja F, Donnelly Iii W, et al. Adaptive optics scanning laser ophthalmoscopy. Opt Express 2002;10:405–12.
40. Chui TY, Song H, Burns SA. Adaptive-optics imaging of human cone photoreceptor distribution. J Opt Soc Am A Opt Image Sci Vis 2008;25:3021–9.
41. Godara P, Rha J, Tait DM, et al. Unusual adaptive optics findings in a patient with bilateral maculopathy. Arch Ophthalmol 2010;128:253–4.
42. Yoon MK, Roorda A, Zhang Y, et al. Adaptive optics scanning laser ophthalmoscopy images in a family with the mitochondrial DNA T8993C mutation. Invest Ophthalmol Vis Sci 2009;50:1838–47.
43. Kretschmann U, Gendo K, Seeliger M, et al. Multifocal ERG recording by the VERIS technique and its clinical applications. Dev Ophthalmol 1997;29:8–14.
44. Chappelow AV, Marmor MF. Effects of pre-adaptation conditions and ambient room lighting on the multifocal ERG. Doc Ophthalmol 2002;105:23–31.
45. Hood DC. Assessing retinal function with the multifocal technique. Prog Retin Eye Res 2000;19:607–46.
46. Hood DC, Odel JG, Chen CS, et al. The multifocal electroretinogram. J Neuroophthalmol 2003;23:225–35.
47. Hood DC, Bach M, Brigell M, et al. ISCEV guidelines for clinical multifocal electroretinography (2007 edition). Doc Ophthalmol 2008;116:1–11.
48. Hood DC, Zhang X. Multifocal ERG and VEP responses and visual fields: comparing disease-related changes. Doc Ophthalmol 2000;100:115–37.
49. Francois J, Verriest G, De Rouck A. Modification of the amplitude of the human electro-oculogram by light and dark adaptation. Br J Ophthalmol 1955;39:398–408.
50. Monnier M, Hufschmid HJ. [Electro-oculogram (EOG) and electro-nystagmogram (ENG) in man.] Helv Physiol Pharmacol Acta 1951;9:348–66.
51. Elenius V, Aantaa E. Light-induced increase in amplitude of electro-oculogram. Evoked with blue and red lights in totally color-blind and normal humans. Arch Ophthalmol 1973;90:60–3.
52. Kolb H. Electro-oculogram findings in patients treated with antimalarial drugs. Br J Ophthalmol 1965;49:573–90.

CHAPTER 3

Diseases Causing Exudative and Hemorrhagic Detachment of the Choroid, Retina and Retinal Pigment Epithelium

SPECIFIC DISEASES CAUSING DISCIFORM MACULAR DETACHMENT

Idiopathic Central Serous Chorioretinopathy

Clinical Features

Idiopathic central serous chorioretinopathy (ICSC), previously referred to as central serous retinopathy, idiopathic flat detachment of the macula, and central angiospastic retinopathy, is a specific disease that typically affects young and middle-aged males with type A personalities between 20 and 45 years of age.[8–20] Unusual emotional stress frequently accompanies the onset of visual symptoms. There may be a history of headaches, which occasionally are of the migraine type. Males are affected more commonly than females by approximately 10 to 1. Before the onset of symptoms, most patients develop one or more small areas of serous detachment of the RPE in the macula or paramacular area (Figure 3.02A–C).[12,13,21] This may be followed by serous detachment of the overlying and surrounding retina (Figure 3.02D–F). If the detachment does not extend into the central macular area, the patient is usually asymptomatic (Figure 3.02A–C). The retinal detachment may resolve spontaneously (Figure 3.02G). When the detachment spreads into the central macular area, the patient typically develops metamorphopsia, a positive scotoma, and micropsia (Figures 3.02D, 3.03, and 3.04). An occasional patient will describe macropsia with the affected eye. Macropsia is the result of crowding of the photoreceptors in a unit area and micropsia is due to decrease in their number in a unit area. A relatively positive central scotoma and metamorphopsia can usually be demonstrated on Amsler grid testing. The micropsia may be unappreciated by the patient until demonstrated by confrontational comparison of image size of the examiner's head. Some describe the micropsia as "objects being farther away with the affected eye as compared with the normal eye." The visual acuity is often only moderately decreased and may be improved to near normal with the addition of a small hyperopic correction. There is a delay in retinal recovery time after exposure to bright light, loss of color saturation, and loss of contrast sensitivity. The patient's past medical history, family history, and general physical findings are usually unremarkable. The author has seen two instances of ICSC occurring in siblings.

3.02 Idiopathic central serous chorioretinopathy.

A–C: Localized serous detachment of the retinal pigment epithelium (RPE: arrows, A) with a small halo of surrounding retinal detachment in a 34-year-old man with a serous detachment of the macula in the right eye. He was asymptomatic in the left eye. Note that the detachment does not extend into the fovea. His visual acuity was 20/15. Angiography outlines the area of RPE detachment (B). Six months later spontaneous reattachment of the RPE occurred (C).

D–I: A 37-year-old woman with blurred vision secondary to serous detachment of the retina. Note slight cloudiness of the subretinal exudate and the moderately large underlying RPE detachment (arrows, D). The RPE is mottled where it is detached. There is a small RPE detachment outside the area of macular detachment superiorly. Stereoscopic angiograms (E and F) showed dye pooled in the region of the RPE detachment beneath the retinal detachment as well as beneath the smaller RPE detachment superiorly (arrow, F). Two months later there was spontaneous resolution of the retinal detachment and slight enlargement of the RPE detachment (G). In the right eye she had developed three paracentral RPE detachments (H and I). She was asymptomatic in both eyes.

J–L: This 40-year-old man had serous retinal detachment, multiple small subretinal precipitates, and a small serous detachment of the RPE (arrows, J and K). Angiography demonstrated the site of a serous detachment of the RPE (arrow, K). L is a diagram of J. The black dots represent fluorescein that stains the exudate beneath the detached RPE but does not enter the subretinal space. SRP, subretinal precipitates.

Ophthalmoscopically and biomicroscopically, a well-defined round or oval area of shallow elevation of the retina in the macular region is the typical finding (Figures 3.02–3.04). This area usually presents a slightly darker color than the surrounding normal retina. The foveal reflex is attenuated or absent. The detachment may be relatively inconspicuous ophthalmoscopically but is usually readily apparent on slit-lamp examination of the macula with a fundus lens. The stereopsis obtained by using a wide light beam directed from a few degrees off the visual axis is generally adequate to appreciate separation of the retina from the underlying RPE. Observation of the increased distance separating a retinal vessel from its shadow cast on the underlying RPE is another helpful clue to the presence of serous detachment of the retina. Separation of the narrow light-beam reflex traversing the retina from that striking the RPE, when demonstrable, is further evidence of a serous detachment. In some instances, particularly in the presence of a shallow detachment, this separation may be impossible to demonstrate.

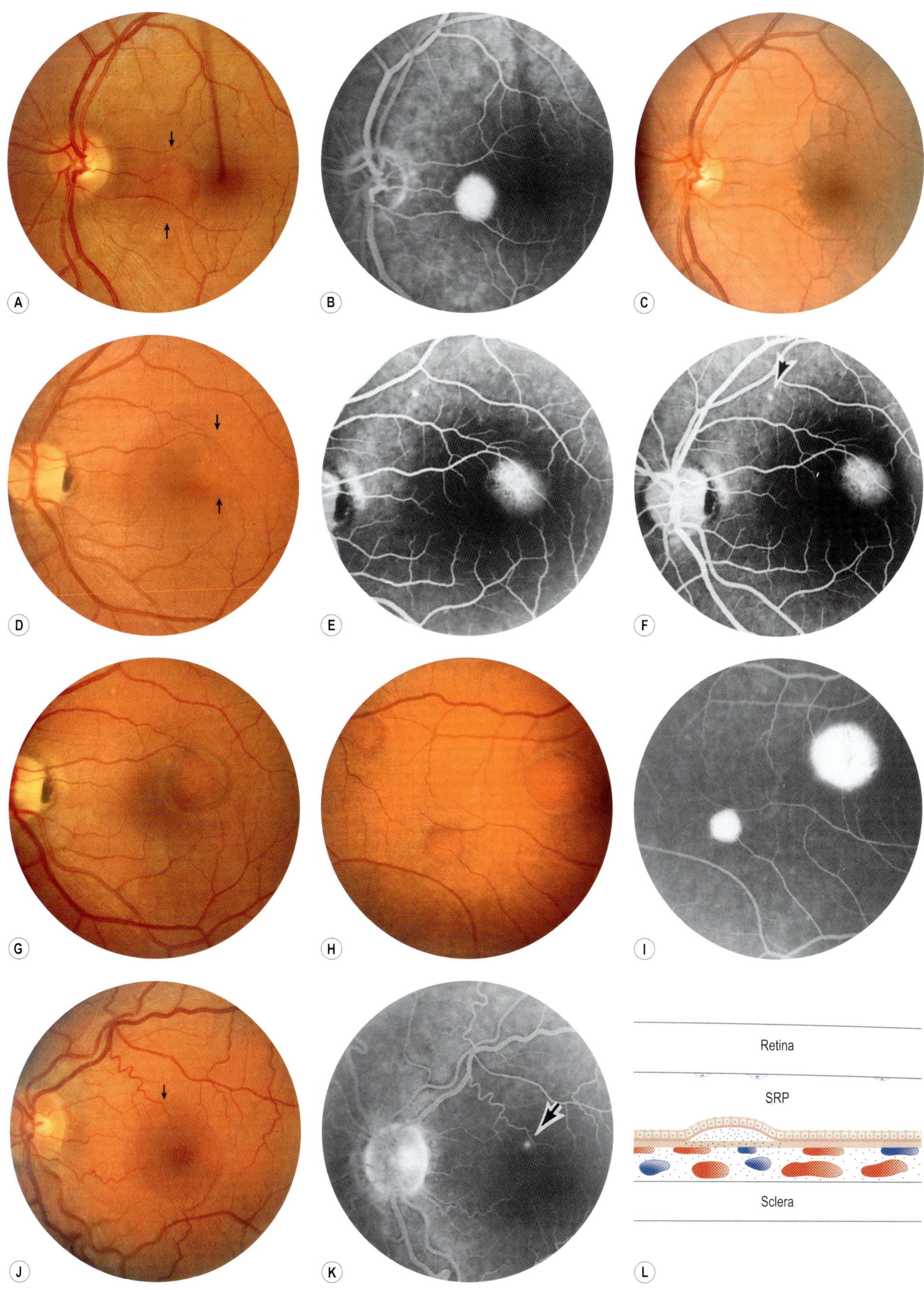
A
B
C
D
E
F
G
H
I
J
K
L
Retina
SRP
Sclera

The detached retina is usually transparent and of normal thickness. The subretinal serous fluid is usually clear. There may be a small round yellow spot, probably caused by increased visibility of the retinal xanthophyll, in the center of the fovea. This may be mistaken for a small RPE detachment. In some cases the posterior surface of the retina may be partly covered with multiple yellowish dot-like precipitates (Figure 3.02J). In approximately 10% of eyes the subretinal space may be partly filled with a gray-white serofibrinous exudate that may be misinterpreted as a focal area of acute retinitis, an ischemic infarction of the retina, or a subretinal neovascular membrane (Figure 3.03J).[22] Serofibrinous exudate is often associated with a larger area of retinal detachment as well as more prominent fluorescein leakage into the subretinal fluid (Figure 3.03A and L). The serous detachment of the RPE underlying the retinal detachment is variable in size and in some patients is often impossible to detect without the aid of fluorescein angiography (Figure 3.03A). Typically, it appears as a round or oval, yellowish or yellowish-gray lesion that is less than one-fourth disc diameter in size (Figure 3.02J). The surface of the RPE detachment may be finely mottled (Figure 3.02A, D, G, and H).

A small RPE detachment is easiest to detect in retroillumination adjacent to the slit beam of light focused on the RPE. It is usually located beneath the superior half of the area of retinal detachment. It occurs infrequently in the center of the fovea. In some cases the RPE detachment may appear to lie beyond the superior margin of the retinal detachment. Because of gravity the subretinal fluid tends to pool inferior to the area of serous detachment of the RPE. Positioning the patient may be required to demonstrate continuity of the areas of retinal and RPE detachment. Focal detachments of the RPE are difficult to visualize biomicroscopically when they are small in size, shallow in depth, or obscured by turbid subretinal exudate. Fluorescein angiography may be necessary to detect the site of RPE detachment.

Multiple RPE detachments may occur (Figures 3.02D and H, and 3.05). Occasionally one or several detachments of the RPE may lie outside the primary area of retinal detachment (Figure 3.02D). In lieu of a discrete RPE detachment there may be an irregular, round, or flask-shaped area of mottled depigmentation of the RPE beneath the retinal detachment (Figure 3.05H–J, 3.06, and 3.07). This occurs often in patients subject to recurrent serous elevation of the RPE and surrounding retina in the paracentral area before they become symptomatic from spread of retinal detachment into the central macular area.

Although RPE detachments are typically small in patients with ICSC, in some patients they may encompass a disc diameter or larger. When larger, the blisterlike RPE detachment may be surrounded by a reddish or salmon-pink halo caused by a marginal serous separation of the retina (Figures 3.02A, G, and H, and 3.04A).[12,13,23,24] Large RPE detachments are typically circumscribed, oval or round, dome-shaped, and orange or yellow-gray; they present a solid rather than a translucent appearance. It is these features that occasionally cause a misdiagnosis of a choroidal hemangioma, hypopigmented melanoma, or metastatic carcinoma of the choroid (Figure 3.04A).

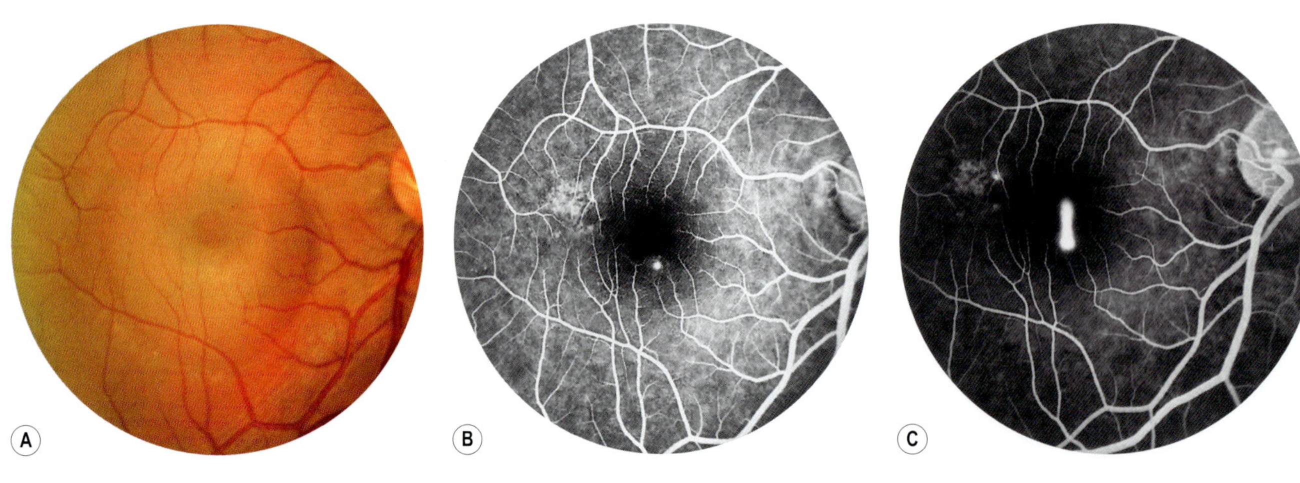

3.03 Idiopathic central serous chorioretinopathy.

A–F: Young woman with serous retinal detachment. Note small retinal pigment epithelium (RPE) leak inferonasally and window defect temporally in B. Angiograms B–D, including stereoangiograms D, show dye streaming superiorly into the subretinal space. Note evidence of small focal leak (arrow, D) in the area of the window defect temporally. E is a diagram illustrating diffusion of the dye (stippling) from the choroid into the sub-RPE space and then into the subretinal space through a break (arrow) in the RPE. F is a representative optical coherence tomography showing a small RPE detachment within the area of serous retinal detachment.

G–I: Serous retinal detachment overlying moderately large RPE detachment with fluorescein streaming through small defect (arrows, H and I) in dome of RPE detachment into subretinal space.

J–L: Serous detachment of retina with whitish subretinal fibrin surrounding small RPE detachment in a 40-year-old man. Note heavy fluorescein staining in area of fibrinous exudate as well as the serous exudate elsewhere in the subretinal space.

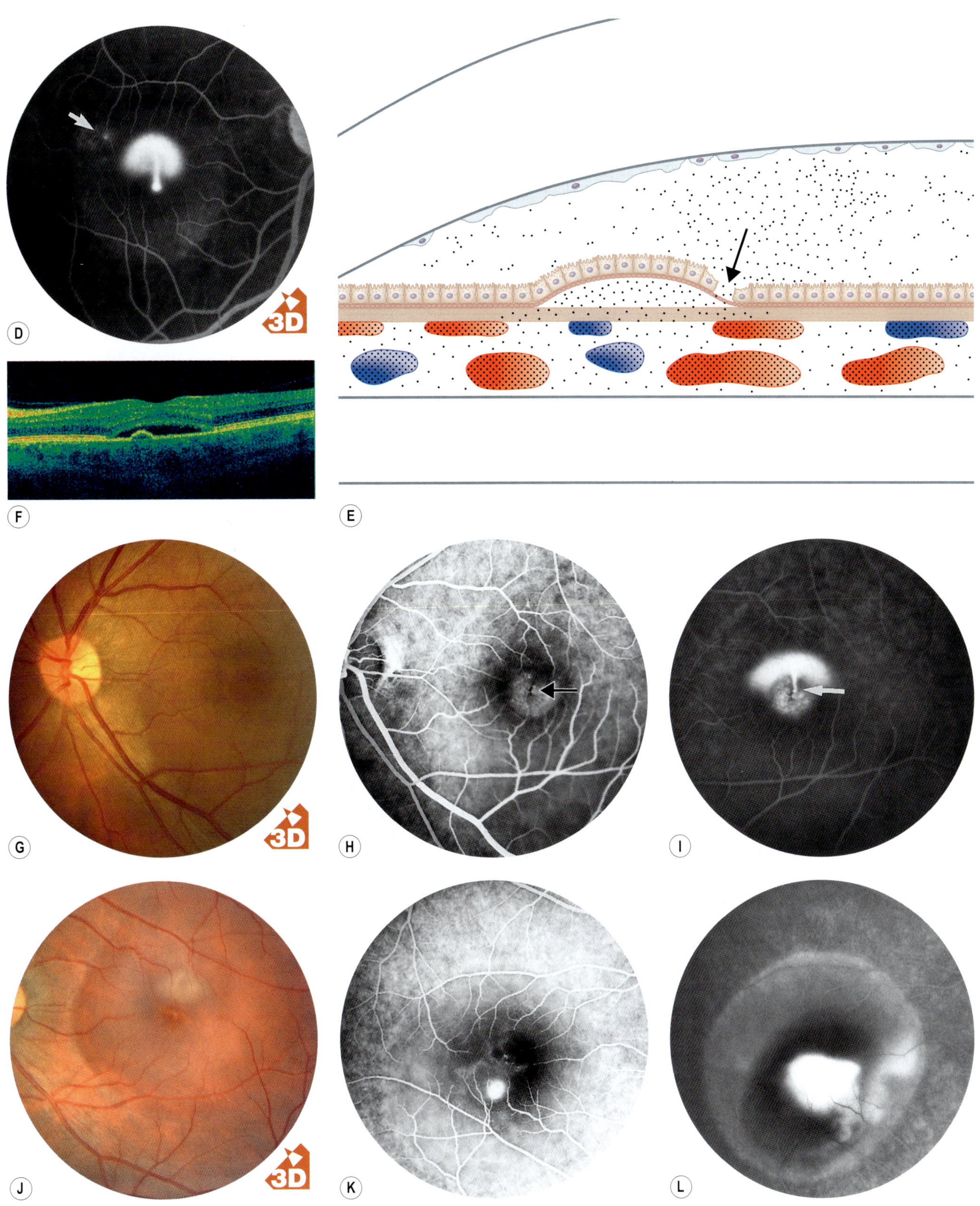
D
3D
F
E
G
3D
H
I
J
3D
K
L

The junction of the detached and attached RPE typically produces a discrete and circumscribed halo surrounding the base of the lesion, in contrast to the less discrete light reflex halo surrounding an area of serous detachment of the retina. The choroidal pattern that is often visible posterior to the serous detachment of the retina is usually not visible behind the serous detachment of the RPE, except in the rare case in which there is extensive thinning and depigmentation of the detached RPE. Fine mottling of the pigment and clumping of pigment on the surface of the detached RPE are common (Figures 3.02 and 3.04). This pigment clumping may produce a cruciate (hot cross bun) or triradiate pigment figure (Figure 3.04A and B). The vitreous in patients with ICSC contains no inflammatory cells.

Fluorescein Angiography

Angiography in patients with ICSC shows a variety of patterns. In the presence of serous detachment of the retina, fluorescein angiography identifies the area where the RPE is detached and where serous exudate derived from the choriocapillaris is gaining entrance into the subretinal space (see Chapter 2).[12,25–32] In those cases with a discrete blisterlike detachment of the RPE, fluorescein rapidly diffuses out of the choriocapillaris across Bruch's membrane and stains the exudate beneath the RPE, creating a discrete, often round spot of hyperfluorescence, corresponding to the size of the RPE detachment (Figures 3.02–3.04). In cases of a shallow detachment of the RPE, the spot of hyperfluorescence enlarges concentrically during the course of angiography. In some patients the dye is confined to the sub-RPE space (Figure 3.02B, E, F, I, and J). In others the dye may diffuse slowly through the detached RPE to produce a faint fluorescent haze in the subretinal exudate surrounding the RPE detachment. In less than 10% of cases the dye passes through a small hole in the RPE, often at the margin of, and occasionally within, the dome of the detached RPE, and streams upward in a smokestack configuration into the subretinal exudate to form an umbrella pattern of fluorescein staining (Figure 3.03A–I). This upward movement of the dye is probably caused both by convection currents and by the relatively higher specific gravity of the dependent subretinal exudate.[33] Eventually the entire subretinal exudate may stain and appear hyperfluorescent, except in the foveal area, where the luteal retinal pigment obstructs the pathway of the exciting blue as well as the emitted fluorescent light. Retinal detachments associated with "smokestack" leaks are generally larger in area than those with focal leaks.[25]

3.04 Idiopathic central serous chorioretinopathy.

A–C: This 48-year-old man had a large serous detachment of the retinal pigment epithelium (RPE). Seven years previously he had serous macular detachment in his left eye that resolved spontaneously within 2 months. Visual acuity in the right eye was 20/50. Note the sharp margin of the serous detachment of the RPE (A). There was no serous detachment of the surrounding retina. Note also the pigment figure on the surface of the detached RPE. Angiography showed diffuse leakage of dye across Bruch's membrane into the sub-RPE space (B). Note the pigment figure outlined on the background of fluorescein. The patient was observed at yearly intervals without change in his visual acuity or the appearance of the fundus. When he returned 9 years after the photograph in A, the serous detachment of the RPE had almost disappeared (C) and his visual acuity was 20/50.

D–I: Idiopathic central serous chorioretinopathy in a 34-year-old man with a persistent serous detachment of the macula for longer than 4 months (D). Arteriovenous phase revealed presence of either an RPE detachment or defect in the RPE, which is extremely minute (arrow, E). The dye leaked into the subretinal space and was carried superiorly (F). The dye pooled superiorly in the subretinal fluid in the dome of the detachment (G). One day after treatment the single application of low-intensity xenon photocoagulation was visible (lower arrow, H). The two small round spots are light reflex artifacts. Upper arrow indicates test spot. The retina was flat 3½ weeks after photocoagulation (I). Visual acuity was 20/15. The test spot was no longer visible.

J–L: Subretinal fibrin surrounding RPE detachment (arrows, J–L) in two pregnant women who developed idiopathic central serous chorioretinopathy during the seventh month of pregnancy. The detachment disappeared early postpartum in both patients.

(A–C from Gass et al.[13]; J and K from Gass.[22],)

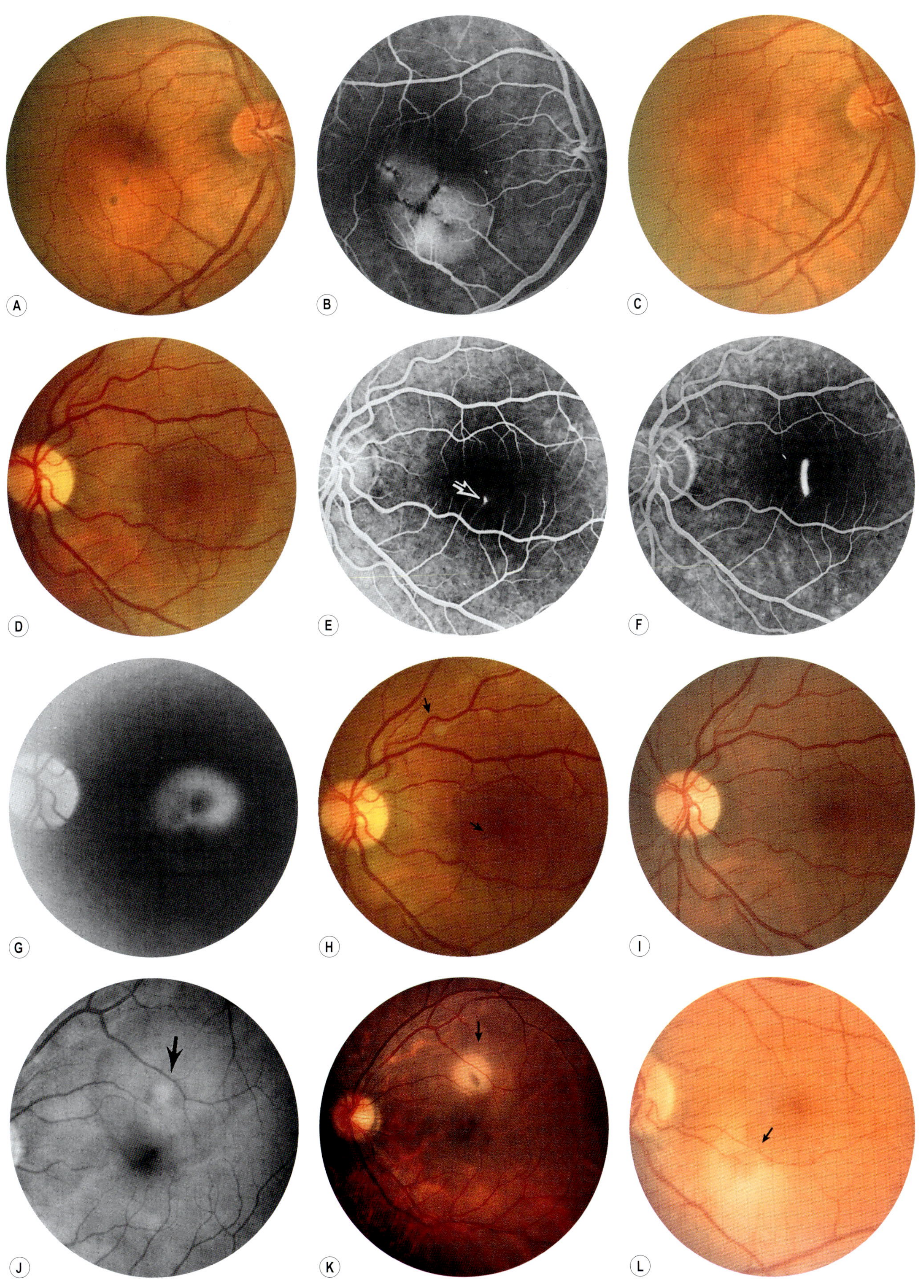
A
B
C
D
E
F
G
H
I
J
K
L

In patients with irregular RPE detachments and atrophy, the pattern of hyperfluorescence is correspondingly irregular, particularly during the early phases of angiography (Figure 3.05B and C). Patients with gray-white subretinal serofibrinous exudate usually show streaming of dye into the subretinal space near the exudate (Figures 3.03J–L, 3.06A–C, and 3.08A–D).[22,34,35] After resolution of the macular detachment, the angiographic findings may return to normal. However, angiographic evidence of the small RPE detachment may persist in some patients. Irregular loss of pigment from the RPE after prolonged retinal detachment will be evident angiographically as mottled areas of hyperfluorescence that tend to fade during the course of angiography. Angiography is helpful in detecting the large zones of extramacular depigmentation of the RPE caused by chronic retinal detachment in patients with a more severe chronic form of this disease (Figures 3.05 and 3.06).[34,36] In the majority of cases the leaking site is found within one disc diameter of the center of the fovea.[25] The foveolar area, however, is infrequently affected.[31]

Approximately 30% occur in the superior nasal quadrant and 25% in the papillomacular bundle area.[25] Angiography, however, should always include photographs of the paramacular areas as well as the macular regions of both eyes. It is particularly important to photograph those areas superior to the macula and optic disc on the side of the macular detachment to detect eccentric areas of leakage, which, because of gravity, may lie superior to the area of detachment. Scanning the fundus during the later phases of angiography may be necessary to detect extramacular areas of fluorescein leakage. Failure to find evidence of a leak angiographically in a patient with a serous detachment of the macula should suggest the following possibilities: (1) a leak has occurred outside the macular area, usually superiorly; (2) the leaking area has healed and the detachment will disappear within the next few days or weeks; (3) presence of a peripheral retinal hole or choroidal tumor (usually superiorly located); (4) a congenital pit of the optic nerve head is present; and (5) idiopathic uveal effusion syndrome (IUES) is present.

Studies of patients with ICSC with indocyanine green have shown congested and dilated choroidal vein and capillaries, choroidal staining, and leakage into the extracellular space that appears as areas of hyperfluorescence in the middle and late phases. This renders evidence of a broader area of choroidal involvement than that demonstrated by fluorescein angiography, hence the better name, ICSC.[37–40]

3.05 Multifocal and recurrent idiopathic central serous chorioretinopathy.

A–N: This 42-year-old woman with lupus nephropathy who had undergone a renal transplant 7 years previously noted a change in vision in her left eye in 2005. The right eye was uninvolved and saw 20/20 while vision in the left eye had dropped to 20/30. A single pocket of subretinal fibrosis (SRF) associated with orange flecks was seen extending temporally from the disc (A). An angiogram revealed leopard-spot change with transmission hyperfluorescence of the area not blocked by the orange pigment that remained dark. There were four hot spots of hyperfluorescence. She was observed and the serous detachment resolved spontaneously in 2 months. She returned 3½ years later with symptoms in her right eye from a pocket of SRF temporal to the fovea. An angiogram revealed patchy leopard-spot change in both eyes, five hot spots on the right, and a single one on the left. She underwent focal laser to the hot spots in the right eye with resolution of fluid in 2 months (K–N). Autofluorescence images show increased autofluorescence corresponding to the orange pigment and decreased autofluorescence corresponding to the retinal pigment epithelium loss (I and J).

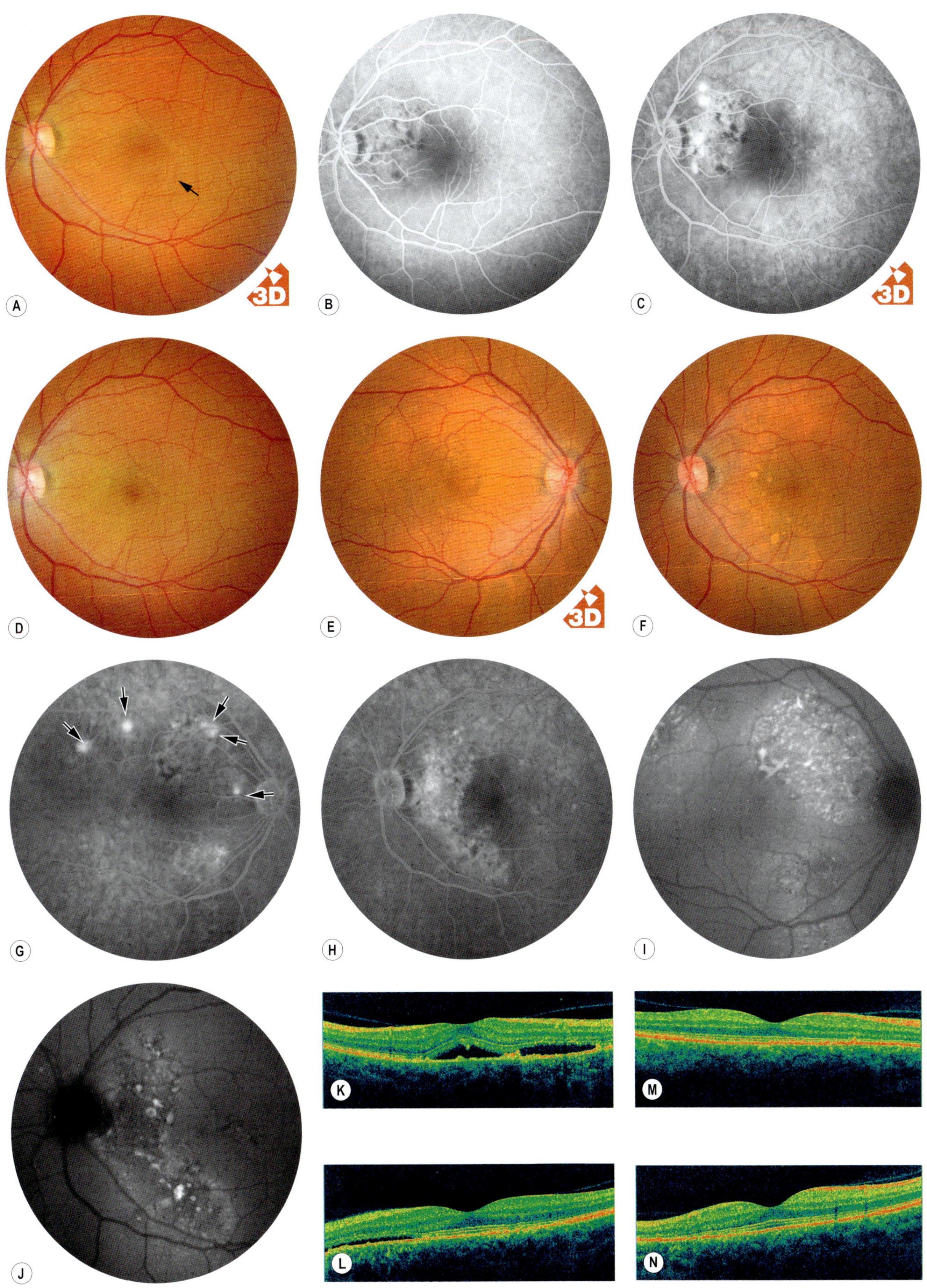
A
3D
B
C
3D
D
E
3D
F
G
H
I
J
K
M
L
N

Autofluorescence imaging depicts a variety of findings in ICSC. The orange spots seen in acute ICSC that may be sites of fibrin; the subretinal orange deposits within an area of serous detachment which could be fibrin alone or mixed with photoreceptor elements; and serofibrinous plaques that resemble retinitis all show increased autofluorescence (Figure 3.09D (arrow) and I).[41–43] In eyes with chronic and recurrent ICSC/steroid-related/organ transplant retinopathy, areas of RPE atrophy are seen as wide gutters of hypoautofluorescence, the edges of which show increased autofluorescence (Figures 3.06E and H, and 3.07C and D). Autofluorescence imaging with its mixed areas of increased and decreased autofluorescence is extremely typical and is a useful noninvasive technique in eyes suspected of chronic recurrent ICSC.

Choroidal congestion and thickening can be confirmed by ultrasound B scan, and more recently with enhanced depth imaging on optical coherence tomography (OCT) using Spectralis.[44] The patient's eye is brought closer to the OCT machine than during conventional retinal scanning, and this enables the choroid to be visualized. Eyes with ICSC have been found to have a thicker choroid as compared to normal eyes. High-resolution imaging of the cones in the posterior pole with adaptive optics scanning laser ophthalmoscope may prove to be useful in monitoring progression in eyes with chronic/steroid-associated ICSC.[45] The technology is still evolving and the instrument cost precludes its use routinely.

3.06 Chronic recurrent idiopathic central serous chorioretinopathy associated with large dependent zones of depigmentation of the retinal pigment epithelium (RPE) and migration of pigment into the overlying retina.

A–C: A 47-year-old man complained of bilateral loss of paracentral and superior fields of vision and difficulty driving at night of 4 years' duration. Note zones of atrophy of RPE (arrows, A and B). Angiography showed multiple zones of RPE atrophy and multiple leakage sites (arrows, C). Electroretinography was within normal limits.

D–I: Composite of fundi of a 64-year-old man with a long history of bilateral recurrent episodes of loss of vision caused by serous detachment of the retina. His vision could be corrected to 20/25– on the right and 20/50 on the left. Note prominent zones of RPE changes extending to the ora serrata inferiorly. The areas of RPE loss appear hypoautofluorescent (E and H). Increased autofluorescence is seen surrounding these areas, suggesting the neighboring RPE cells are ingesting broken down photoreceptor and other cellular material. The right eye was dry (F); the left showed shallow subretinal fluid (I), for which he received low-fluence photodynamic therapy. He did not recall steroid intake but may have received injections to his wrist joint.

(A–C from Gass.[34])

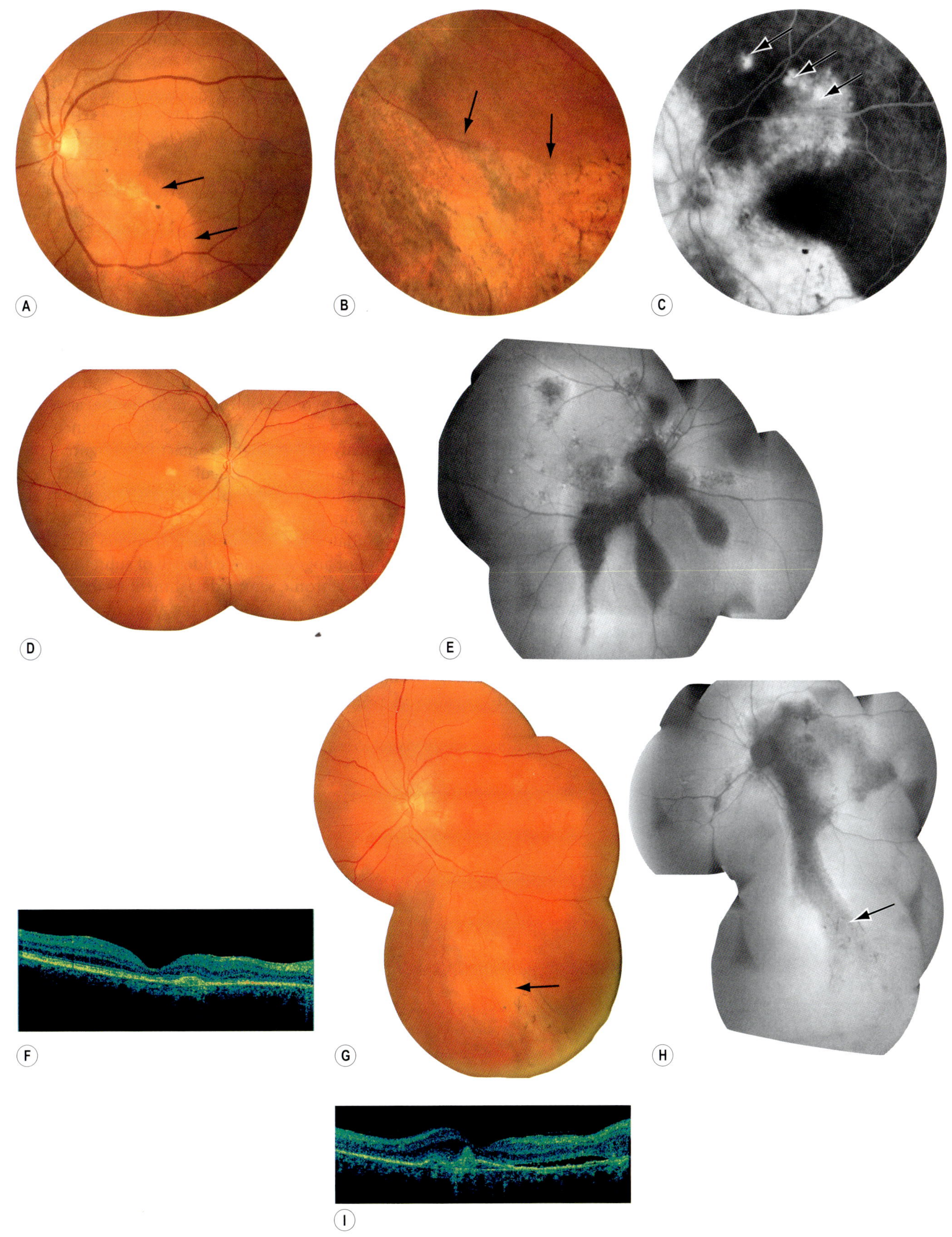
A
B
C
D
E
F
G
H
I

Acute Bullous Retinal Detachment

Multiple areas of serous detachment of the retina may occasionally develop rapidly in the same or both eyes of patients with ICSC.[11,52] These may occur in the midperiphery of the fundus as well as in the posterior pole. In a few patients these detachments may become confluent and result in a large bullous retinal detachment involving the lower half or more of the fundus (Figures 3.08A–C, and 3.10).[11,34,53–55] This acute severe form of ICSC is particularly likely to occur in otherwise healthy patients who, as the result of a misdiagnosis, receive systemic corticosteroids.[48] Multiple serous detachments of the RPE, often ½–1 disc diameter or larger in size, are typically present. They are frequently partly obscured by cloudy and at times gray-white fibrinous subretinal exudate. A similar picture often develops in the second eye within several days or weeks. These patients may be misdiagnosed as having a rhegmatogenous detachment, multifocal chorioretinitis, metastatic carcinoma, Harada's disease, or uveal effusion. The angiographic demonstration of multiple serous detachments of the RPE (Figures 3.08B and C) underlying shifting subretinal fluid permits an accurate diagnosis. Fluorescein characteristically streams through a hole in the pigment epithelium at the edge of the large RPE detachments into the subretinal exudate (Figures 3.08B and C, and 3.10C and D).[25,35,56] Occasionally, large RPE rips may occur at the edge of large RPE detachments (Figure 3.10H, J, and K).[48,57]

3.08 Severe idiopathic central serous chorioretinopathy (ICSC) with bullous retinal detachment in otherwise healthy patients receiving systemic corticosteroid therapy.

A–C: This 45-year-old man initially presented with a serous detachment of the macula in the right eye. It was attributed to choroiditis and the patient received oral prednisone. This was followed by bilateral bullous retinal detachment associated with multiple large serous retinal pigment epithelium (RPE) detachments, some of which were surrounded by a cloud of white fibrinous subretinal exudation (arrows, A). Fluorescein dye streamed through small breaks (arrows, B) in the dome of the RPE detachments into the subretinal space. Resolution of the subretinal exudate occurred after photocoagulation of RPE detachments and stopping the corticosteroids. The patient had no further episodes of macular detachment until 69 years of age, when he developed subretinal neovascularization at the site of treated RPE detachment superior to the right fovea.

D–L: This 27-year-old man developed bilateral serous detachment of the macula (D) in 1982. In 1990, in addition to a chronic complaint of subnormal vision, he developed floaters. Bilateral peripheral bullous retinal elevation inferiorly and several tufts of retinal neovascularization were noted (arrow, E). These changes were attributed to X-linked juvenile retinoschisis. In 1991, in spite of fluorescein angiographic findings that suggested chronic recurrent ICSC (F and G), the diagnosis was retinal vasculitis and treatment with systemic corticosteroids resulted in severe bilateral bullous retinal detachment, incorrectly attributed to uveal effusion syndrome. In 1993, bilateral scleral windows, vortex vein decompression, and larger doses of corticosteroids resulted in massive subretinal serofibrinous exudation (H and I). Arrows indicate foci of retinal neovascularization. Fluorescein angiography revealed multifocal areas of RPE elevation and decompensation posteriorly, leakage from several foci of retinal neovascularization (arrows, J), and a broad zone of retinal capillary nonperfusion inferiorly in both eyes (K). After discontinuance of the corticosteroids the retinal detachment resolved promptly, leaving subretinal fibrous bands in the macular region of both eyes.

(D–L from Gass and Little.[48])

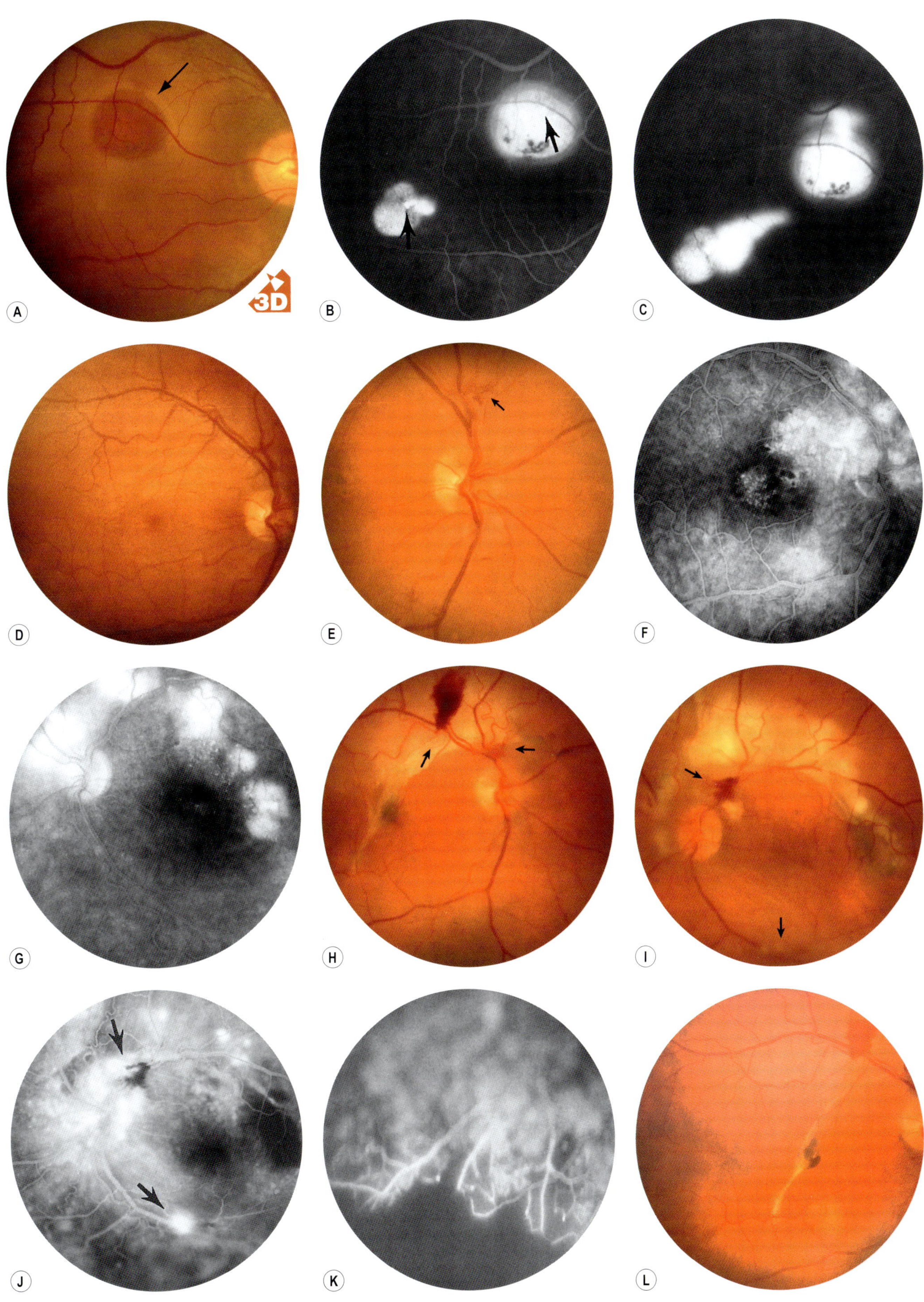
3D
A
B
C
D
E
F
G
H
I
J
K
L

All of the otherwise healthy patients with bullous retinal detachment complicating ICSC seen by Gass have been middle-aged men. By the time he examined them many of them had diagnoses other than ICSC and were receiving oral corticosteroids.[11,48] This same clinical and angiographic picture may, however, occur occasionally in women, particularly those receiving corticosteroids for systemic disease, e.g., disseminated lupus erythematosus,[58–63] Crohn's disease,[64] rheumatoid arthritis,[65] hemodialysis,[66] and renal transplantation (Figures 3.11 and 3.12).[67] In addition to these disorders Gass has seen this severe form of ICSC in women with hemolytic anemia, cryoglobulinemia, eosinophilic fasciitis, severe allergic bronchitis after commencement of systemic corticosteroid therapy, and in one woman with multiple peculiar cutaneous and mucous membrane vascular malformations infiltrated with mast cells (Figure 3.11A–F).

At the 1982 Eastern Ophthalmic Pathology Society meeting Dr. Gilbert de Venecia reported the histopathologic findings in one eye of a 40-year-old Native American man who soon presented after a kidney transplant with bilateral bullous retinal detachment and multiple serous RPE detachments surrounded by white subretinal exudate (Figure 3.12E and F).[22,68,69] He found histopathologic evidence that the whitish exudate beneath and surrounding the RPE detachment was fibrinous in type (Figure 3.12G and H).

ICSC Associated with Chorioretinal Folds

ICSC may occasionally occur in eyes with chorioretinal folds in the macular area secondary to choroidal congestion (Figure 3.09L and M).

ICSC in Women

ICSC in otherwise normal women is similar to that in males except that onset tends to be at an older age in women.[70] ICSC in women receiving exogenous corticosteroids is more likely to be associated with bilateral involvement and subretinal fibrin.

3.09 Central serous chorioretinopathy in the elderly.

Acute idiopathic central serous chorioretinopathy (ICSC) with sildanefil use.

A–F: This 84-year-old man presented with a drop in vision in his right eye to 20/30. There was a smooth serous retinal detachment without any drusen extending from the disc edge to the fovea (A). Angiogram showed a mild late hyperfluorescent spot temporal to the disc edge that was hyperautofluorescent (B–D). The serous detachment was smooth on optical coherence tomography (OCT) without evidence of drusen or other RPE abnormalities (E). Light laser to this spot caused resolution of most of the subretinal fluid (F) within 4 weeks and return of vision to 20/20.

New-onset steroid-induced ICSC with leopard-spot change in the elderly.

G–M: This 72-year-old male with no previous ocular history experienced fluctuating vision more in his left eye than right. His glasses prescription had to be corrected twice and he underwent cataract surgery in the left eye. Four weeks following cataract surgery he was noted to have cystoid macular edema on the left eye and received a sub-Tenon injection of triamcinalone. His vision dropped further. When examined a month later, his vision was correctable to 20/30 on the right and 20/50 on the left. In addition to the flask-shaped serous detachment in the left eye there were chorioretinal folds (G and H). No peripheral choroidal detachments were seen. Inner retinal fluid was present in both eyes and subretinal fluid in the left eye on OCT (J and K). Fluorescein showed only a leopard-spot change corresponding to the subretinal fluid without significant breakdown of the RPE (L and M). There was mild hyperfluorescence at the disc edge that was attributed to peripapillary atrophy. He denied steroid intake at any time, he was a well-controlled diabetic and hypertensive with a blood pressure of 130/78 mmHg in the office, and was in good health. His serum light chains were slightly elevated but M-protein spike was absent. On further questioning and speaking to his primary physician, he was found to have received three intramuscular injections of steroids over the previous 18 months for nasal congestion and used penile injections of papaverine, prostaglandin, and phentolamine for impotence for the previous 2 years.

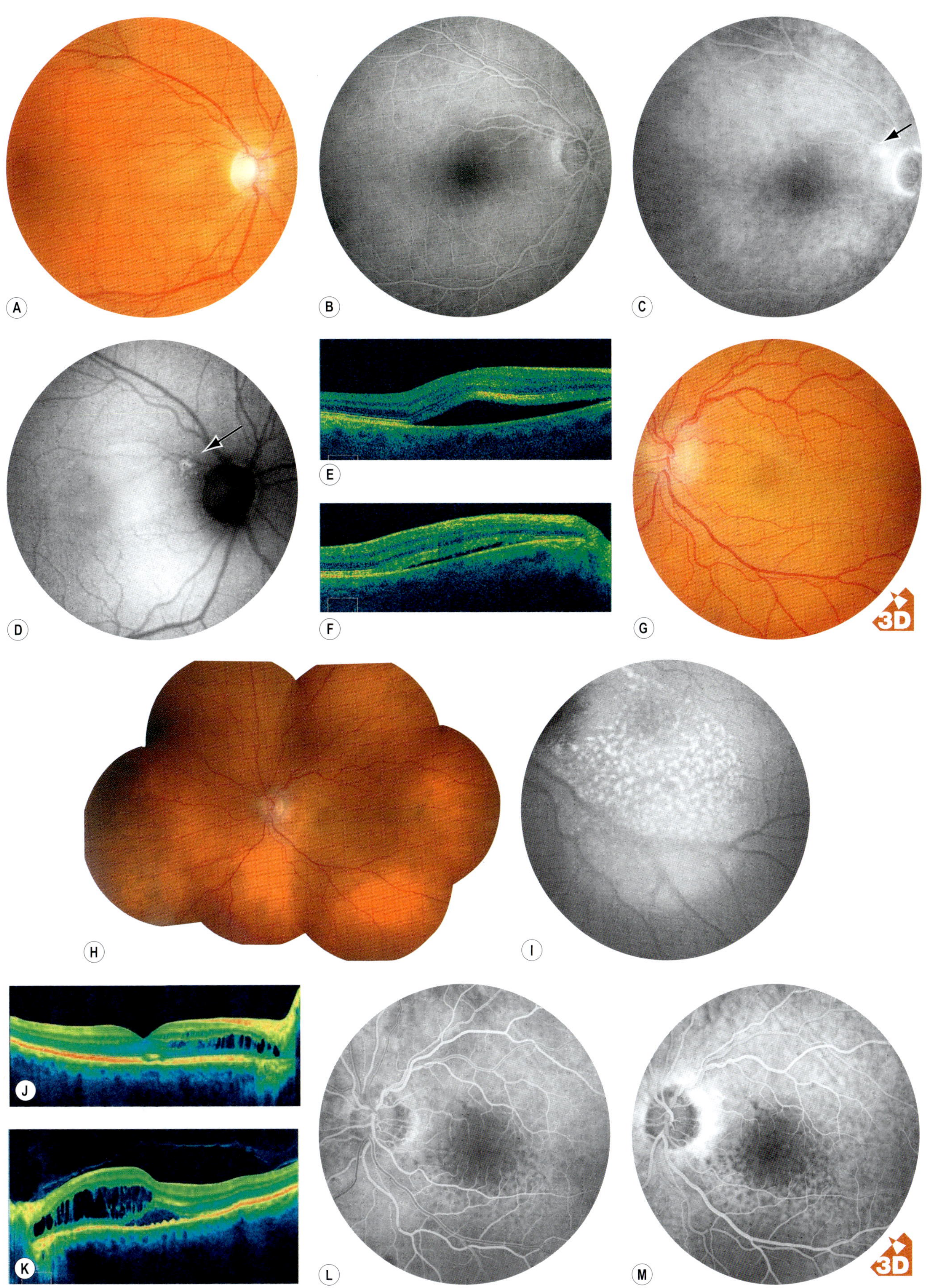
A
B
C
D
E
F
G
3D
H
I
J
K
L
M
3D

ICSC may occur in healthy women during the latter half of otherwise uncomplicated pregnancy.[22,71–76] For unknown reasons it is associated with white subretinal exudation surrounding the RPE detachment in over 90% of affected pregnant women.[22] It is important not to mistake this serofibrinous exudation for evidence of subretinal neovascularization, focal retinitis, or focal retinal infarction, all of which may suggest investigations including fluorescein angiography, which are usually unnecessary in the differential diagnosis. The detachment resolves spontaneously soon after delivery and the visual prognosis is excellent. ICSC may or may not recur during subsequent pregnancies.

ICSC in the Elderly

Although most patients with ICSC are young and middle-aged males, some first develop symptoms in the later decades of life (Figure 3.11C–H).[77,78] The clinical picture may be identical to that occurring in younger patients, although a larger percentage of the older patients will manifest fundoscopic evidence of previous episodes of subclinical eccentric retinal detachment, as described previously. In older patients there is more concern that the focal leak demonstrated angiographically may represent a focus of occult choroidal neovascularization. Although an occasional patient with ICSC will eventually develop evidence of AMD, there is no evidence that the two diseases are more than casually related.

ICSC associated with sildenafil

More older males are presenting with ICSC associated with use of agents for erectile dysfunction such as sildenafil (Figure 3.09A–F).[79–81] Unlike older patients with drusen and age-related macular degeneration (AMD), the smooth elevation of the photoreceptors and no areas of RPE bumps caused by drusen (Figure 3.09E) on OCT should prompt the diagnosis of ICSC. Cessation of sildenafil use caused resolution in most patients and some showed recurrence on resuming the medication.

3.10 Severe idiopathic central serous chorioretinopathy (ICSC) with bullous retinal detachment in otherwise healthy patients receiving systemic corticosteroid therapy.

A–F: This 31-year-old man developed detachment of the left macula associated with a focus of subretinal fibrin that was misinterpreted as acute retinitis. Treatment for toxoplasmosis, including prednisone, was given. One week later the patient had bullous serofibrinous retinal detachment in the right eye and juxtapapillary and macular retinal detachment in the left eye (A and B). Large serous detachments of the RPE surrounded by subretinal fibrin were present bilaterally. The detachment resolved completely within 2 weeks after all medications were stopped. He remained asymptomatic and at last examination, 11 years later, had 20/20 bilaterally.
G–K: This 54-year-old man maintained near normal visual acuity in spite of a 31-year history of recurrent episodes of ICSC, until he developed an epiretinal membrane in the right eye. One day before scheduled vitrectomy he developed ICSC in the fellow eye. He was started on a course of prednisone 100 mg/day preoperatively. Within several days of surgery he developed bilateral bullous retinal detachment. Postoperatively the oral prednisone was supplemented by retrobulbar injection of corticosteroids. Six weeks postoperatively his visual acuity was 20/400, right eye, and counting fingers at 2 feet (60 cm), left eye. There was total bullous retinal detachment associated with multiple large retinal pigment epithelium (RPE) detachments bilaterally associated with fibrinous exudation and subretinal fibrous band formation (G and H). In the left eye there was a 300° tear (arrows) along the edge of a large RPE detachment involving the superior macular region (H). Angiography confirmed the presence of multiple RPE detachments in the right eye (I) and the RPE tear in the left eye (J). Note the irregular retracted edge (arrow) of the torn RPE and the fluorescein staining within the area of missing RPE. Eighteen months later, after corticosteroids were stopped, and after multiple operative procedures, a tractional retinal detachment was still present in the right eye, but the retina in the left eye was reattached (K) and the visual acuity had returned to 20/30.

(G–K from Gass and Little.[48])

ICSC with leopard-spot retinopathy in elderly patients on systemic steroids

This fundus appearance of yellow deposits in a "reticulated leopard-spot fashion" was brought to attention by Iida et al.[82] in 2002 as a newly recognized finding in 5 older men between 68 and 81 years of age receiving systemic corticosteroids. However this same pattern was previously described by Gass et al. in 1992 in patients following renal, heart, and heart–lung transplant who were receiving systemic steroids (see Figure 3.60A–L). Corticosteroids seem to be the common factor linking these two groups of patients (Figure 3.09L and M).

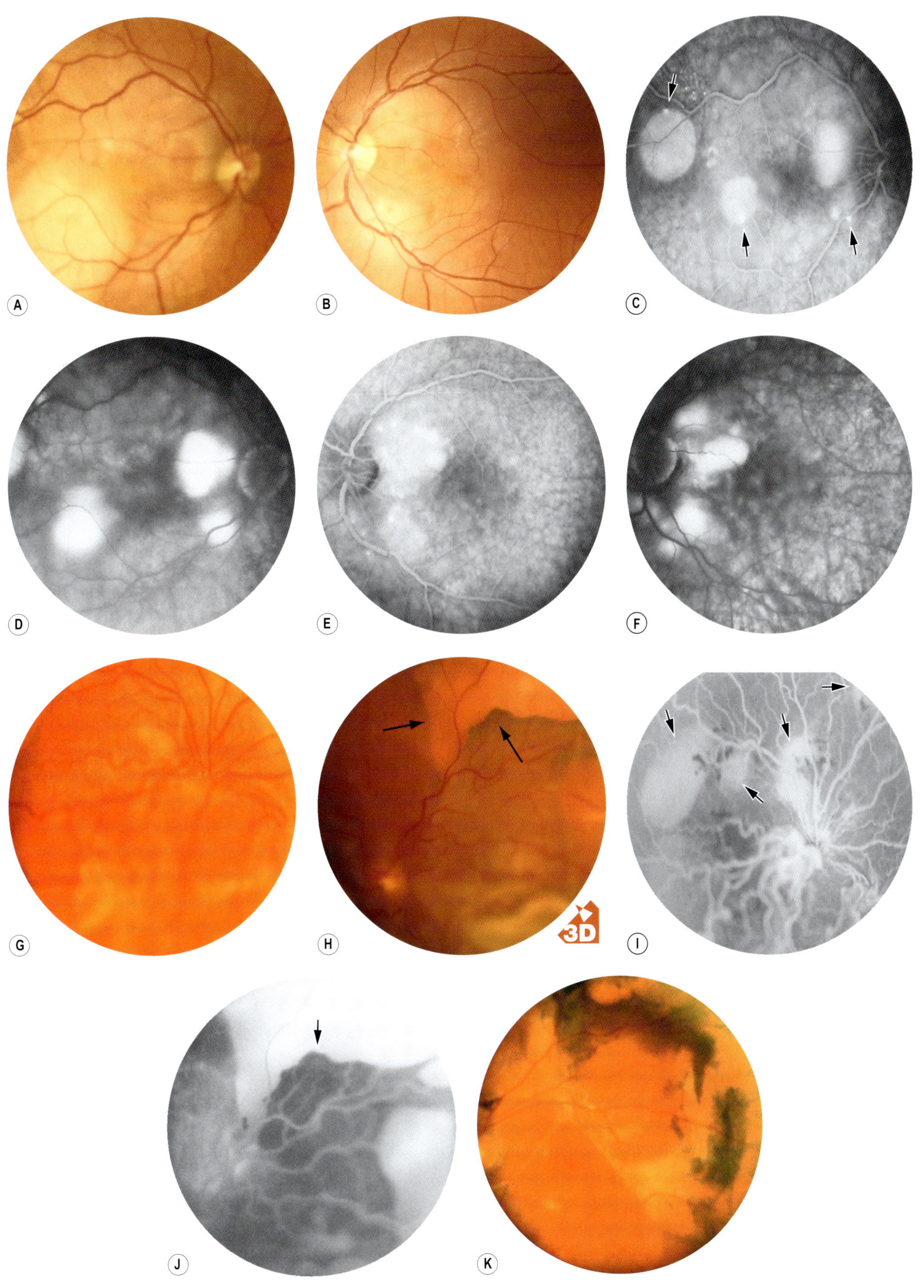
A
B
C
D
E
F
G
H
3D
I
J
K

ICSC Simulating Pattern Dystrophy

Patients presenting with the typical findings of ICSC may over a period of years develop multiple focal yellow lesions with pigmented centers in one or both eyes, simulating that seen in patients with pattern dystrophy. These lesions may also simulate Elschnig spots caused by fibrinoid necrosis associated with severe hypertension, collagen vascular disease, and disseminated intravascular coagulopathy (DIC).

Other Associations with ICSC

The author has seen ICSC occurring in 2 women in association with retinitis pigmentosa (see Figure 5.41A–C)[61,83] and with episcleritis.[69,84]

Prognosis

The prognosis for the majority of patients with ICSC for spontaneous resolution of macular detachment and return of visual acuity is excellent.[29,50,77,78,85–90] Improvement can continue for up to 6 months after reattachment of the retina. However, when tested carefully, many patients recovering 20/20 acuity will still have a mild permanent defect, such as a decrease in color sensitivity, loss of contrast sensitivity, relative scotoma, micropsia, metamorphopsia, or nyctalopia.[86,90–100] Approximately 5% will fail to recover 20/30 or better acuity. With prolonged and recurrent episodes of detachment the patient may develop permanent visual loss to levels of 20/200 or less. This is more likely to occur in patients with the multicentric chronic form of the disease.

The prognosis for reattachment of large serous detachments of the RPE is not as good as that for small detachments. Patients with large serous detachments of the RPE, however, usually maintain relatively good vision for months or years (Figure 3.04A–C).[21,23,24] There is great variability in the biomicroscopic appearance of the macula after resolution of retinal detachment. In some patients the fundus may regain a normal appearance. Most, however, will demonstrate some evidence of irregular depigmentation of the RPE, usually most noticeable in the area of the RPE detachment. Those with recurrent detachment may show extensive atrophy of the RPE throughout the central macular area.

The long-term visual prognosis for most patients with ICSC is good. Approximately 20–30% of patients will have one or more recurrences.[23,46,50,51,85,88,101] Although approximately one-third of patients will have biomicroscopic and angiographic evidence of one or more focal changes in the RPE in the opposite eye; fewer than 20% are destined to develop serous detachment of the macula in the opposite eye. Evidence to date suggests that only a small percentage, probably less than 5%, of these patients will ever develop choroidal neovascularization or chronic detachment with cystoid macular edema.[102]

3.11 Serofibrinous retinal pigment epithelium (RPE) and retinal detachment occurring in patients receiving corticosteroid treatment for systemic disease.

A–C: Bilateral multifocal RPE detachments surrounded by fibrinous subretinal exudate in a woman receiving systemic corticosteroids for treatment of lupus erythematosus.

D–F: Bilateral multifocal RPE detachments surrounded by fibrinous subretinal exudate in a patient receiving systemic corticosteroid treatment for lupus erythematosus.

G–I: Bilateral multifocal RPE detachments and subretinal fibrin in a woman receiving systemic corticosteroid treatment for nodular fasciitis.

J–L: This woman with a 6-year history of continuous prednisone therapy for lupus erythematosus and Sjögren's syndrome developed exudative detachment of the right macula associated with multiple serous RPE detachments (arrows), subretinal serofibrinous retinal detachment, and a pigment epitheliopathy resembling fundus flavimaculatus in her right eye. Her left eye had been enucleated following *Pseudomonas* endophthalmitis. Two years previously she had multiple amputations of the fingers and both legs (J). Laser photocoagulation of the RPE detachments failed to produce resolution of the macular detachment. There was progression of the pigment epitheliopathy to involve most of the fundus (J). Angiography revealed a leopard-spot pattern of nonfluorescence and multiple focal sites of leakage throughout the posterior fundus (L). Note persistent areas of RPE detachment (arrows).

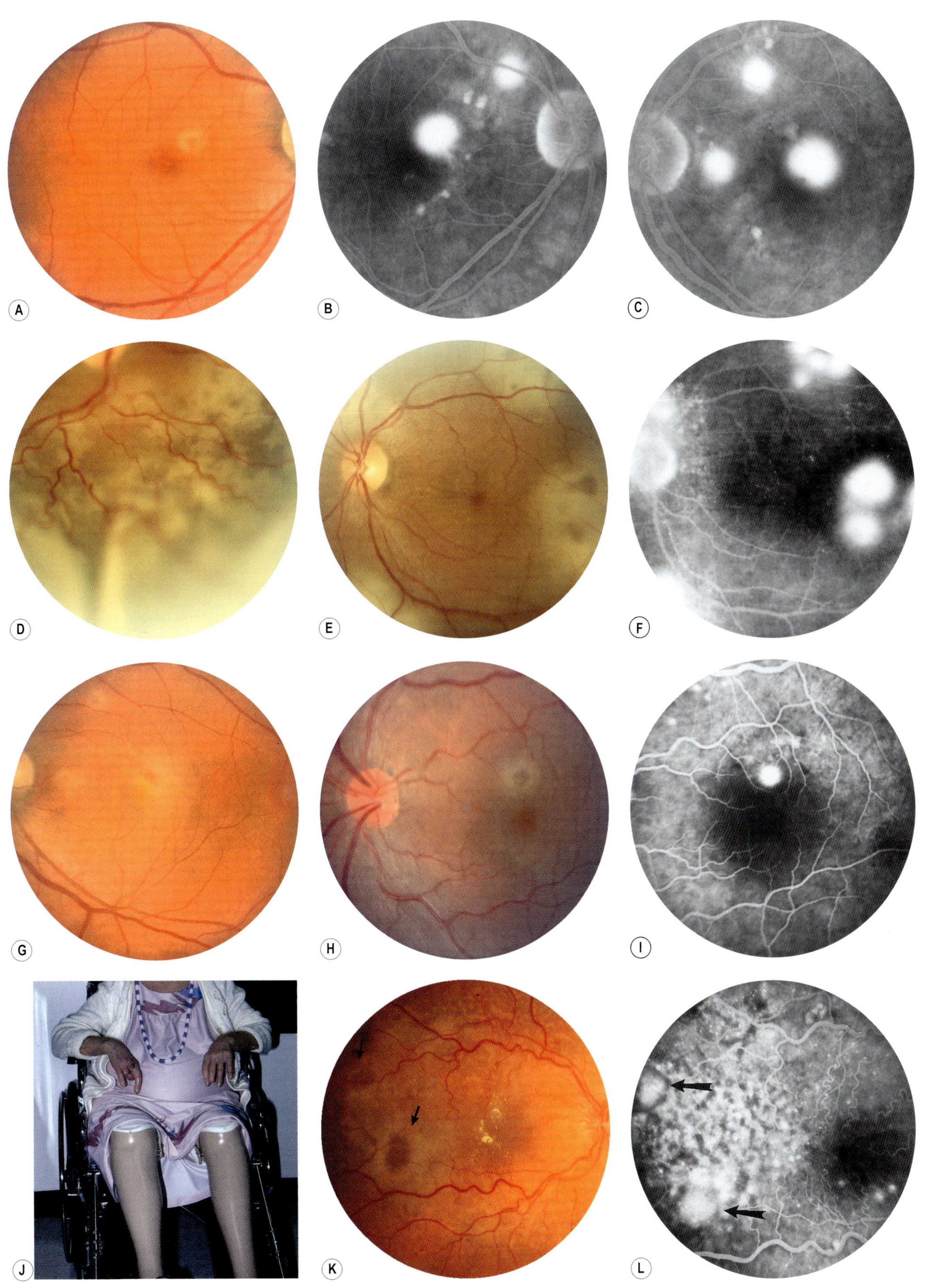
A
B
C
D
E
F
G
H
I
J
K
L

Pathology and Pathogenesis

There is limited information concerning the pathology of ICSC (Figures 3.12 and 3.13). Histopathologic examination of one eye obtained from a patient who died of a myocardial infarction showed no abnormality in the choriocapillaris underlying the RPE detachment (Figure 3.13).[103] Dr. de Venecia found no definite abnormality in the choriocapillaris in the case occurring in the patient with chronic renal failure previously cited (Figure 3.12).[68] His finding, however, that the gray-white exudate noted clinically contained fibrin provides evidence that a marked alteration occurring in the permeability of the choriocapillaris had permitted escape of serum proteins as large as fibrinogen. This white serofibrinous subretinal exudation occurs in the area of RPE detachment in 10–15% of all patients with ICSC.[22] This observation, together with other features of ICSC, including the frequent blister-like detachment of the RPE underlying the serous retinal detachment and the frequent presence of large amounts of subretinal fluid, is further evidence that increase in the permeability of the choriocapillaris is the primary cause of damage to the overlying RPE, focal loss of the RPE attachment to Bruch's membrane, and movement of plasma proteins and water into the subretinal space in patients with ICSC.[12,22,69] Indocyanine green videoangiography has provided additional evidence of abnormal choriocapillary permeability that may be more extensive than that indicated by fluorescein angiography.[104,105] Spitznas has suggested that a reversal of direction of ion secretion by the focally damaged RPE allows water to move toward the retina rather than the choroid.[106] Marmor postulates that patients with ICSC must have a more diffuse area of metabolic impairment of the RPE to explain the detachment that may persist for weeks or months.[107] There is experimental evidence that a focal injury to the choriocapillary wall as well as the RPE may be important in the pathogenesis of ICSC.[108] The pathogenesis of ICSC and the mechanisms explaining how photocoagulation accelerates resolution of retinal detachment are unclear.[12,13,28,107,109–111]

3.12 Bilateral serofibrinous retinal pigment epithelium (RPE) and bullous retinal detachment occurring in patients receiving renal dialysis and after renal transplantation.

A–D: A 37-year-old Native American woman receiving renal dialysis developed bilateral serofibrinous retinal detachment. She had well-controlled hypertension. Note the fibrin enveloping the RPE detachments (arrows, A and B). Angiograms (C and D) show multiple RPE detachments in right eye.
E–H: Inferior bilateral bullous detachment in a 40-year-old Native American man 1 month after receiving a renal transplant. He was receiving systemic corticosteroids and antimetabolites. He had well-controlled hypertension. Note white fibrinous exudation surrounding RPE detachments (arrows, E and F). Angiography revealed "smokestack" leaks from the areas of RPE detachment. Nine days later he developed rapid loss of vision in the left eye. Within 4 weeks visual loss progressed to no light perception. Computed tomography revealed evidence of thickening of the left optic nerve and orbital tissue. The left eye was enucleated. Histopathologic examination revealed fibrinous exudate in the sub-RPE space (arrows) and subretinal space (G and H). No definite pathologic changes in the choriocapillaris were identified. Separate tissue removed from the orbital apex revealed aspergillosis of the optic nerve and orbit.

(From de Venecia.[68])

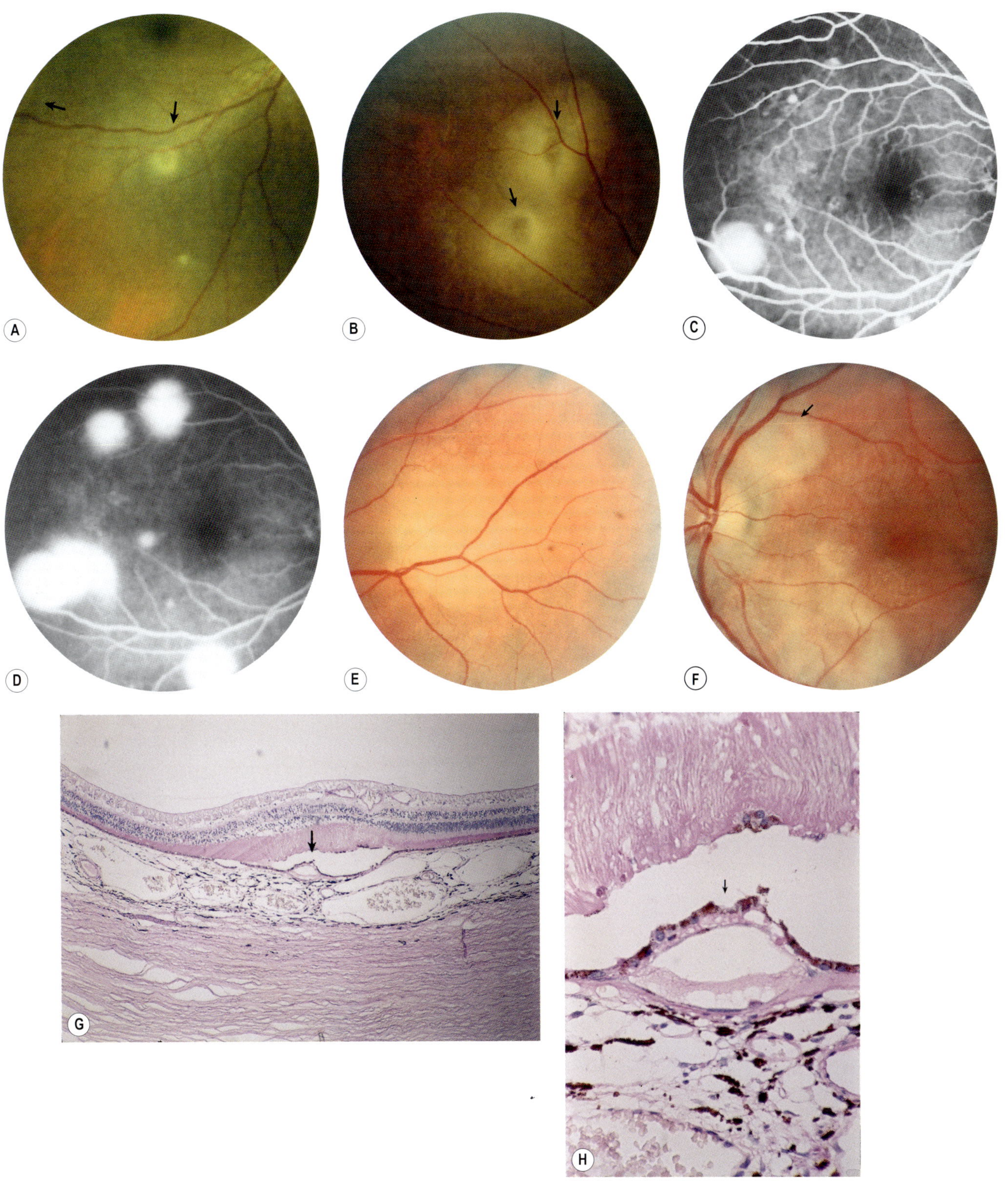
A
B
C
D
E
F
G
H

Although patients with ICSC typically have no systemic disease, they often are highly competitive and compulsive workaholics who relate the onset of their symptoms to unusual stress, such as a change in job, demanding deadlines, marital problems, family death or sickness, or accidental injury.[14,112–115] Yannuzzi has demonstrated a high association of type A behavior pattern in patients with ICSC compared to control groups of patients.[115] There is no convincing evidence that ICSC is either infectious or inflammatory in nature[116] or that it represents a diffuse RPE dystrophy.[28]

A picture similar to ICSC has been produced experimentally by intrascleral injection of indomethacin in rabbits, and by repeated intravenous administration of epinephrine in monkeys and rabbits.[117–119] This work lends credence to the theory that stress may play an important role in causing focal permeability changes in the choriocapillaris and loss of adherence of the RPE to Bruch's membrane in patients who are predisposed to macular detachment. The observations that: (1) systemic corticosteroid administration may precipitate and aggravate ICSC; (2) patients with Cushing's disease may develop ICSC; and (3) pregnant women show a predilection for developing ICSC suggest that elevated serum cortisol levels may be of importance in the pathogenesis of ICSC.[48,58,61,65,103,120–122]

There is some evidence to suggest that the prevalence and severity of ICSC are related to race. ICSC, along with most other disorders associated with exudative detachment of the macula, occurs infrequently in black persons. ICSC occurs commonly in Latins, Orientals, Asian Indians and Caucasians. The severe recurrent form of the disease may be more common in the Latin population, Asian Indians, and in Orientals.

3.13 Histopathology of idiopathic central serous chorioretinopathy.

A: Histopathology of serous detachment of the retinal pigment epithelium (RPE) and retina in a 52-year-old man who died because of acute coronary thrombosis. The patient apparently had no visual complaints. The detachment was found on routine examination of the eye at autopsy. Note exudative detachment of the macula. The choroid and pigment epithelium were normal.

B: Serial sections through the macula revealed a small area of serous detachment of the RPE beneath the peripheral part of the detachment (arrow). The underlying choriocapillaris was normal.

C–H: Probable idiopathic central serous chorioretinopathy occurring in a 69-year-old man who developed a large area of serous retinal detachment of the left macula (small arrows, C). Superiorly there was subretinal whitish-gray exudate (large arrow, C) that blocked fluorescence early and stained late angiographically (arrow, D). There were scattered drusen in the peripheral fundus but only a few in the macular areas. The retinal detachment resolved spontaneously within several months. Four years later his visual acuity was 20/20, right eye, and 20/25, left eye, just before his death as a result of complications of laryngeal surgery. Histopathological examination revealed a small focus of type I sub-RPE neovascularization beneath one drusen in the right macula (see Figure 3.18) and in the juxtapapillary region of the left optic disc (H). In the area of fluorescein leakage in the left eye there was a focal loss of the retinal receptors and RPE (E). The thinned RPE was irregularly elevated by a deposit of eosinophilic (E), periodic acid–Schiff-positive (F), phosphotungstic acid-positive (G) material with a fine brushlike pattern, suggesting that the sub-RPE material included fibrin. In this area there was some migration of RPE cells into the subretinal space (arrows, E and F).

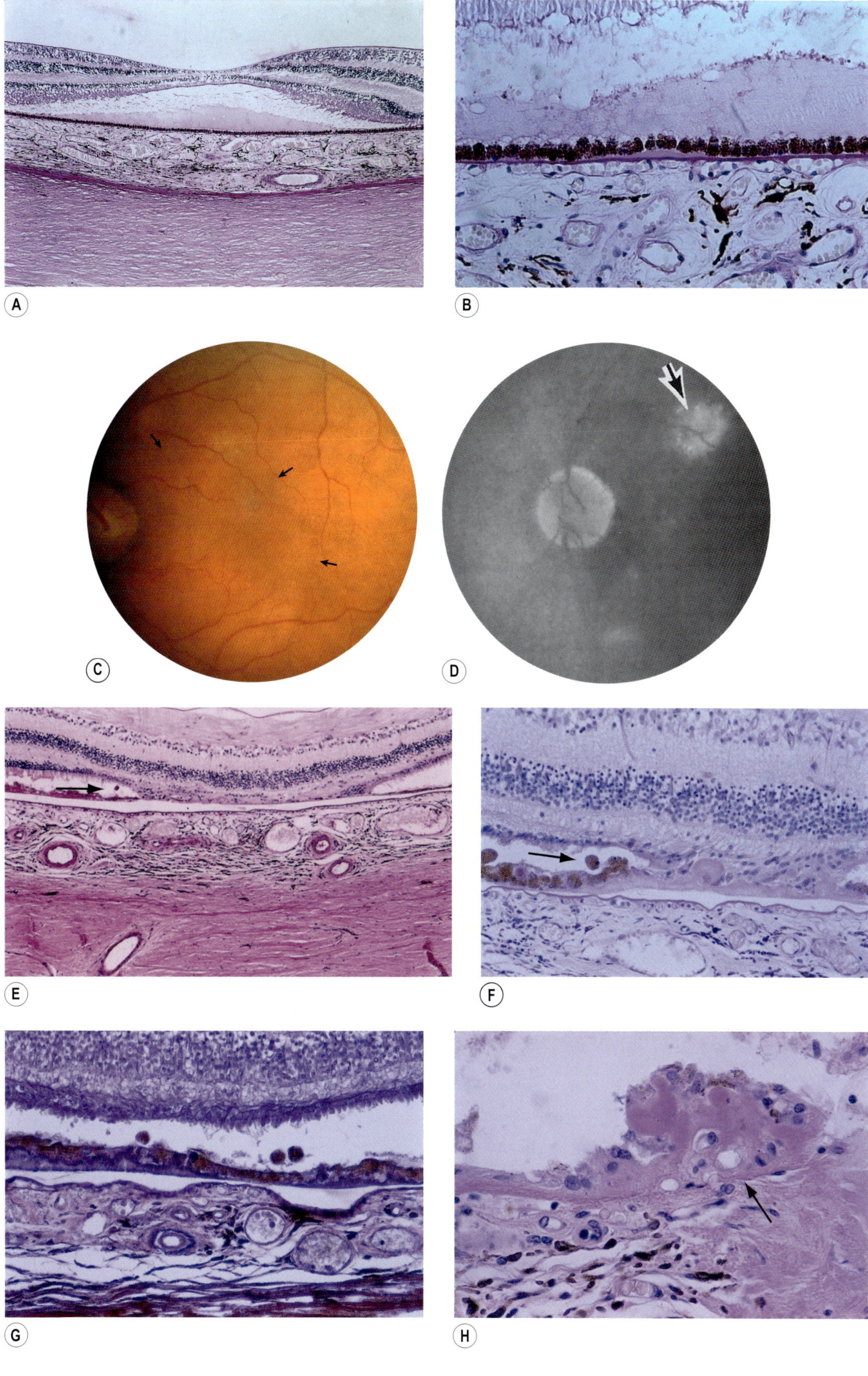
A
B
C
D
E
F
G
H

Differential Diagnosis

Other diseases that may cause localized serous detachment of the macula include: (1) congenital pit of the optic nerve; (2) choroidal tumors, located in either the macula or peripheral areas, particularly superiorly, for example, hemangiomas, metastatic carcinoma, leukemia, melanoma, and osteoma; (3) retinal hole in either the macula or paramacular area of patients with high myopia with posterior staphylomata or in the peripheral fundus superiorly; (4) malignant hypertension, toxemia of pregnancy, collagen vascular diseases, or other diseases associated with DIC; (5) choroidal inflammatory diseases, either focal, for example, presumed ocular histoplasmosis or sarcoidosis, or diffuse, for example, Harada's disease, sympathetic ophthalmia, benign reactive lymphoid hyperplasia of the uveal tract, and posterior scleritis; (6) idiopathic uveal effusion; (7) ocular contusion; (8) traction maculopathy caused by incomplete posterior vitreous separation; and (9) senile macular degeneration and idiopathic polypoidal choroidal vasculopathy (IPCV). Long-standing inferior peripheral exudative retinal detachment in patients with chronic ICSC may be mistaken for retinoschisis, uveal effusion, rhegmatogenous detachment, or Eales' disease if the patients develop retinitis proliferans and retinal capillary closure in the area of chronic retinal detachment.[48,49] (See discussion of atypical presentations of ICSC.) In patients older than 50 years of age and with a few small drusen in the macula, or in patients with one or two small chorioretinal scars, it may be impossible to exclude senile macular degeneration in the former and the presumed ocular histoplasmosis syndrome (POHS) in the latter as the cause of the serous macular detachment. In such cases there is a greater risk that the focal leak may represent a small neovascular complex rather than a serous detachment of the RPE. In some cases the association of a systemic disease with serous macular detachment may be coincidental.[123]

Patients following scleral buckling procedures in the early postoperative course may have one or more round or oval areas of exudative retinal detachment that simulate serous detachments of the RPE in the macula (see Figure 7.29G–I).

Treatment

There is no evidence that medical treatment, abstinence from smoking, or the administration of beta-blockers has proved useful in the treatment of ICSC.[124] There is good evidence that photocoagulation of the site of RPE detachment or the RPE leak produces resolution of the retinal detachment usually within 3–4 weeks in most of these patients (Figure 3.04D–I).[11,34,47,49,50,84,87,90,96,98,125–149] There is no evidence, however, that prompt photocoagulation reduces the chances of permanent loss of visual function.[27,34,85,86,90,132,143] There is no value of placement of photocoagulation into areas other than those showing evidence of leakage angiographically.[101,138,139,145]

Although the complications of photocoagulation, such as accidental coagulation of the foveola, retinal distortion, and choroidal neovascularization,[34,150,151] are few, it is probably not advisable to recommend immediate photocoagulation treatment in all of these patients. The following criteria for photocoagulation are utilized by Gass:

- Allow 4 months for spontaneous resolution if the patient has had no previous history or ophthalmoscopic evidence of previous detachment.
- Wait 6 months or longer before photocoagulation if the RPE leak is less than one-fourth disc diameter from the fovea.
- Allow 1 month for spontaneous resolution in patients with a history of several episodes of detachment in the same eye, if after each episode the patient has regained normal macular function.
- When the leak is at least one-fourth disc diameter from the center of the fovea, prompt photocoagulation is justified: (1) if detachment has been present for 4 months or longer; (2) if the patient has evidence of permanent loss of acuity or paracentral visual field in either eye secondary to previous episodes of detachment; or (3) if for occupational reasons the patient cannot work because of the visual dysfunction caused by the detachment.

Light- to moderate-intensity applications of all modalities of photocoagulation including argon, krypton, and dye laser photocoagulation to the area of RPE detachment or RPE leakage are effective in treating ICSC.[47,101,134,141]

Laser debridement of the RPE in the area of the leakage, permitting ingrowth of surrounding RPE, is probably all that is required to cause resolution of the detachment (Figures 3.05 and 3.09A–F).[119,152] It is important to look for any of the biomicroscopic or angiographic signs of choroidal neovascularization when evaluating the leaking area in these patients. Minimal-intensity photocoagulation applications of a size tailored to the area of RPE detachment should be used. If there is any evidence to suggest the leak may be caused by choroidal neovascularization, then more intense treatment is indicated. Even in cases where no evidence of neovascularization is evident, probably 2–5% of these patients will develop evidence of choroidal neovascularization within several weeks or months of treatment.[34,102,150,151] This is one of the most important complications occurring after photocoagulation in these patients. In some, it is probably caused by the treatment, and in others, it may exist before treatment. Careful monitoring of the size of the treatment scotoma on the Amsler grid by the patient after treatment is important in the early detection and treatment of this complication.

Chronic and Recurrent ICSC

Lowering or discontinuing systemic steroids in those receiving steroids should be tried as the first step. Failure of resolution of fluid should prompt light focal laser to the leaks (Figure 3.05) if demonstrated on an angiogram. In those eyes with widespread chorioretinal involvement as seen on fluorescein or indocyanine green angiography, photodynamic therapy is beneficial in most cases.[153–158] Both full- and reduced-fluence treatments and full- and half-dose have been used; more recently reduced fluence has been advocated to reduce toxic effects of the therapy. The spot size is determined by the area of staining on the angiograms. An extra 500-μm zone is not necessary, as in treating choroidal neovascularization. Care must be taken to avoid including the foveal center if no significant subfoveal fluid is present.

Jampol et al.[159] have shown resolution of subretinal fluid by the use of mifepristone, an antiglucocorticoid and antiprogesterone medication used as an abortifacient. A daily dose of 200 mg caused dramatic resolution of subretinal fluid, but it recurred once the drug was discontinued. The drug works by blocking the glucocorticoid receptors via negative-feedback control of adrenocorticotropic hormone and cortisol, causing an increase of both in the serum.

AGE-RELATED MACULAR DEGENERATION†

AMD is a chronic degenerative or dystrophic disease affecting primarily the choriocapillaris, Bruch's membrane, and the RPE.[160–175] It is the commonest cause of legal blindness in the USA and UK. The large number of names used in the old literature to describe the various stages of the disorder have served to obscure the fact that it is probably a single disease that in many cases is familial and inherited as an autosomal-dominant trait.[176–183] The presently most widely accepted name, age-related macular degeneration, is unfortunate in some respects because it suggests that all affected patients are elderly and that its root cause is aging. Although the average age of patients when they lose central vision in the first eye is 65 years of age, some patients develop evidence of the disease in the fourth and fifth decades of life. As of 2004, it was estimated that about 8 million individuals are affected by AMD in the USA and 1.75 million of them have advanced disease.[184] It mostly affects white blue-eyed individuals and is rarely responsible for visual loss in black persons.[185] AMD should be distinguished from the following diseases: (1) dominantly inherited progressive juvenile foveal dystrophy associated with drusenlike changes and macular staphyloma, a disease that is endemic in western North Carolina (see p. 296); (2) basal laminar drusen and macular degeneration (see p. 132); and (3) pattern dystrophy (see Chapter 5).

†Also known as senile macular degeneration, senile macular choroidal degeneration, senile disciform macular degeneration, Kuhnt-Junius disciform detachment, familial drusen, dominantly inherited drusen, Hutchinson-Tays central guttate choroiditis, Doyne's honeycombed choroiditis, and Holthouse-Batten superficial choroiditis.

3.14 Typical or exudative drusen.

A–C: Macular, peripapillary, and peripheral drusen in a 24-year-old man with 20/20 visual acuity in both eyes (A). Angiograms showed hyperfluorescent spots corresponding with drusen (B and C).

D–F: Multiple variably sized drusen in a 42-year-old man with 20/20 visual acuity.

G–I: Confluence of multiple large drusen in a 68-year-old man. Note the irregular pattern of staining of the larger drusen centrally. Visual acuity was 20/80.

J: Schematic diagram showing variations in the fluorescent pattern of exudative drusen in which the retinal pigment epithelium (RPE) basement membrane (bm, arrow) is of normal or near normal thickness. Black dots represent fluorescein molecules. A hyalinized drusen (1) may transmit the intrachoroidal fluorescence because of thinning of the overlying RPE but may be sufficiently dense that diffusion of dye across Bruch's membrane (BM) into the sub-RPE material does not occur. In the case of drusen with less dense material beneath the RPE (2, 3), the dye may diffuse into the sub-RPE material and cause intensification of fluorescence of the drusen during the later stages of angiography.

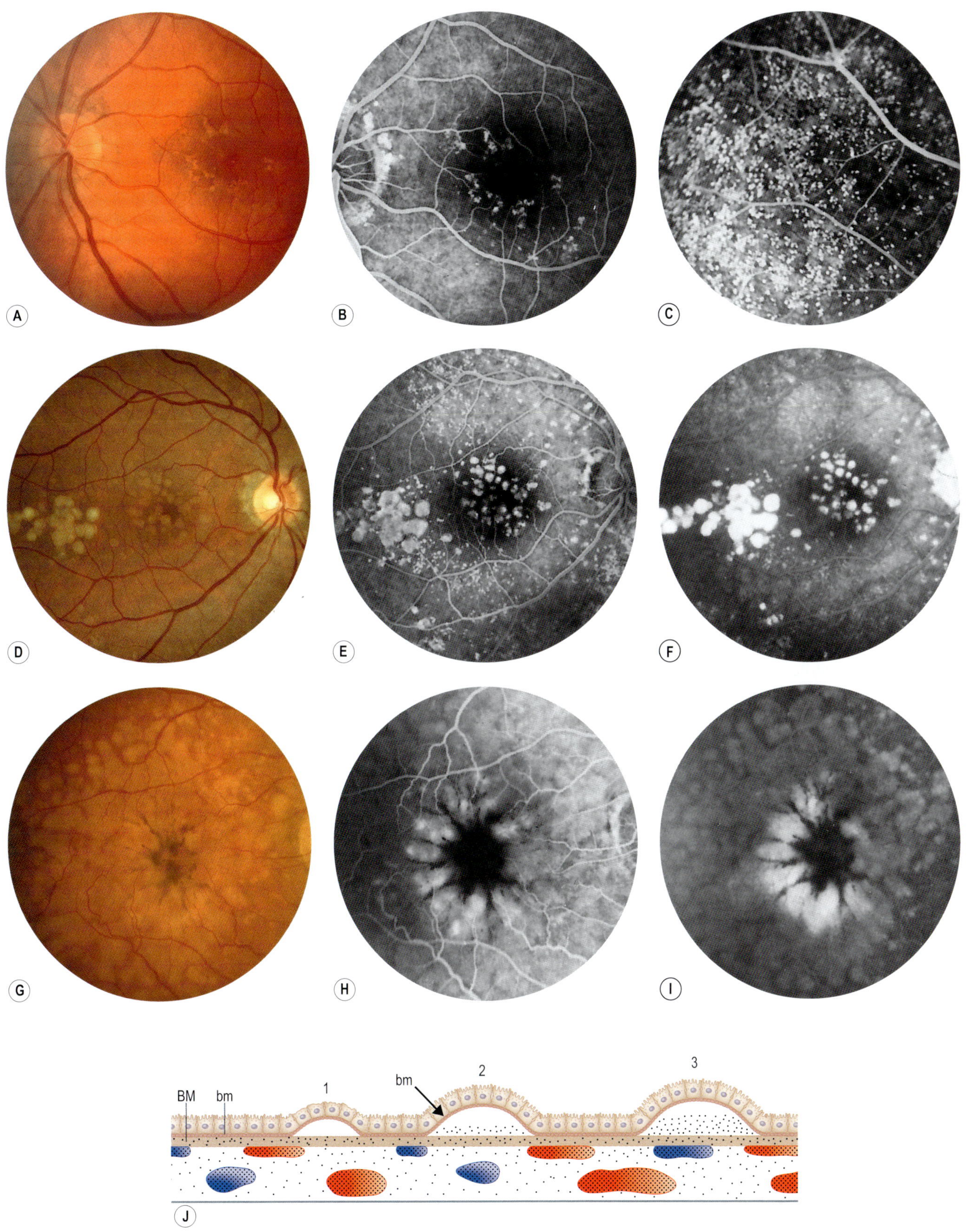
A
B
C
D
E
F
G
H
I
BM
bm
1
bm
2
3
J

Predisciform Stage

Typical or Exudative Drusen

The earliest sign of AMD is the development of multiple, usually discrete, round, slightly elevated, variably sized, sub-RPE deposits in the macula and elsewhere in the fundus of both eyes (Figures 3.14–3.16).[186–198] These deposits are called drusen. The German word "druse" (plural "drusen") means nodule, referring in particular to areas of clear crystallization within stones. The term "typical" or "exudative" drusen is used here to differentiate these variably sized deposits of extracellular material lying between the basement membrane of the RPE and the inner collagenous zone of Bruch's membrane from uniformly small, round, nodular thickenings of the RPE basement membrane (basal laminar drusen, cuticular drusen) that probably have a different pathogenesis (see p. 132). Typical or exudative drusen may develop in early adulthood but infrequently are visible biomicroscopically until middle life or later. Early in their development drusen may be inapparent ophthalmoscopically because of their small size and relatively normal overlying RPE. Usually, however, they can be detected in retroillumination with the slit lamp as semitranslucent bodies.

As the deposit enlarges and the overlying RPE thins, drusen assume a yellow or gray color and are more easily detected. They vary widely in size from yellow punctate nodules ("hard" drusen; Figure 3.14A) to large, pale yellow or gray-white, placoid or dome-shaped structures indistinguishable from localized serous detachments of the RPE ("soft" drusen; Figures 3.14D and G and 3.15A). Drusen are often clustered in the macular or paramacular area. Whether centrally or eccentrically located, their distribution is usually symmetric in both eyes.[199] Drusen change in size, shape, distribution, color, and consistency with the passing years (Figure 3.15).[200] Although they tend to increase in number and size (Figure 3.15C and D), drusen may also fade from view and decrease in number (Figure 3.15A and B). In some cases, areas of geographic atrophy of the pigment epithelium may remain following disappearance of drusen (Figure 3.15E and F). Drusen may become calcified and crystalline in appearance (Figure 3.15A, and see Figure 3.29). This change suggests dehydration of the drusen and often precedes the development of geographic atrophy of the RPE. Occasionally drusen develop a polychromatic or golden sparkling appearance indicative of cholesterol deposits. Some drusen may become ossified and assume a white appearance. A few may appear pink secondary to choroidal neovascular tufts growing through Bruch's membrane into the drusen. In some patients the sub-RPE deposits are distributed diffusely rather than focally and are evident ophthalmoscopically only as an ill-defined area of slightly mottled yellow color of the RPE in the macula.

3.15 Natural course of typical (exudative) drusen.

A and **B**: Multiple large drusen, some of which are confluent, in a 65-year-old woman with a visual acuity of 20/40. Several drusen are partly calcified (arrows, A). Same patient 4 years later (B) showing fading and disappearance of drusen. Visual acuity was still 20/40.

C and **D**: Note the change in distribution, shape, and size of the drusen in this 73-year-old patient over a period of 3 years. Visual acuity in C was 20/25 and in D was 20/30.

E and **F**: This 73-year-old patient developed multiple focal areas of geographic atrophy of the retinal pigment epithelium (RPE) over a period of 2 years. Her initial visual acuity was 20/30. Her visual acuity when last seen (F) was 20/40.

G–L: Progression of large drusen to "drusenoid" RPE detachments of the RPE (arrows, I and L) in a 67-year-old woman. Left eye, July 1986 (G), April 1991 (H), February 1993 (I and J). Right eye, July 1986 (K), and February 1993 (L).

Most patients with the predisciform stage of the disease have excellent visual acuity and are asymptomatic. Some with many drusen centrally complain of decreased ability to read, particularly in dimmed illumination, and mild metamorphopsia. Loss of contrast sensitivity is common and may be out of proportion to loss of Snellen acuity.[201–206] This loss may involve the entire macula and is not confined to the areas with drusen.[207] Early loss of sensitivity may be a predictor of severe visual loss.[208] Patients frequently experience difficulty with driving an automobile at night. Electrophysiologic tests in most patients are normal.[209–211] Some may have mild to moderate reduction in electro-oculographic responses.

Drusen are not always confined to the macular area. In some patients they may be present nasal to the optic disc. In others they may be largely confined to the peripheral macular area, particularly in the areas of the major vascular arcades. Drusen in this latter distribution may have a somewhat granular, less discrete appearance and may be seen in black patients, who infrequently develop drusen in the macular area.[212] Many widely scattered drusen are usually visible with a three-mirror gonioprism in the peripheral fundus. In contrast to drusen in the posterior pole, these drusen often have a halo of pigment at their base. In some patients these drusen are arranged in a confluent, linear, and triradiate pattern to produce a prominent pigmented network visible ophthalmoscopically in the midperiphery of the fundus (Figure 3.17). This is usually most evident nasally and is referred to as senile reticular pigmentary degeneration.[191,213–218] A narrow, indistinct, yellow or gray zone caused by the deposition of sub-RPE drusen material often surrounds the temporal half or more of the optic disc.

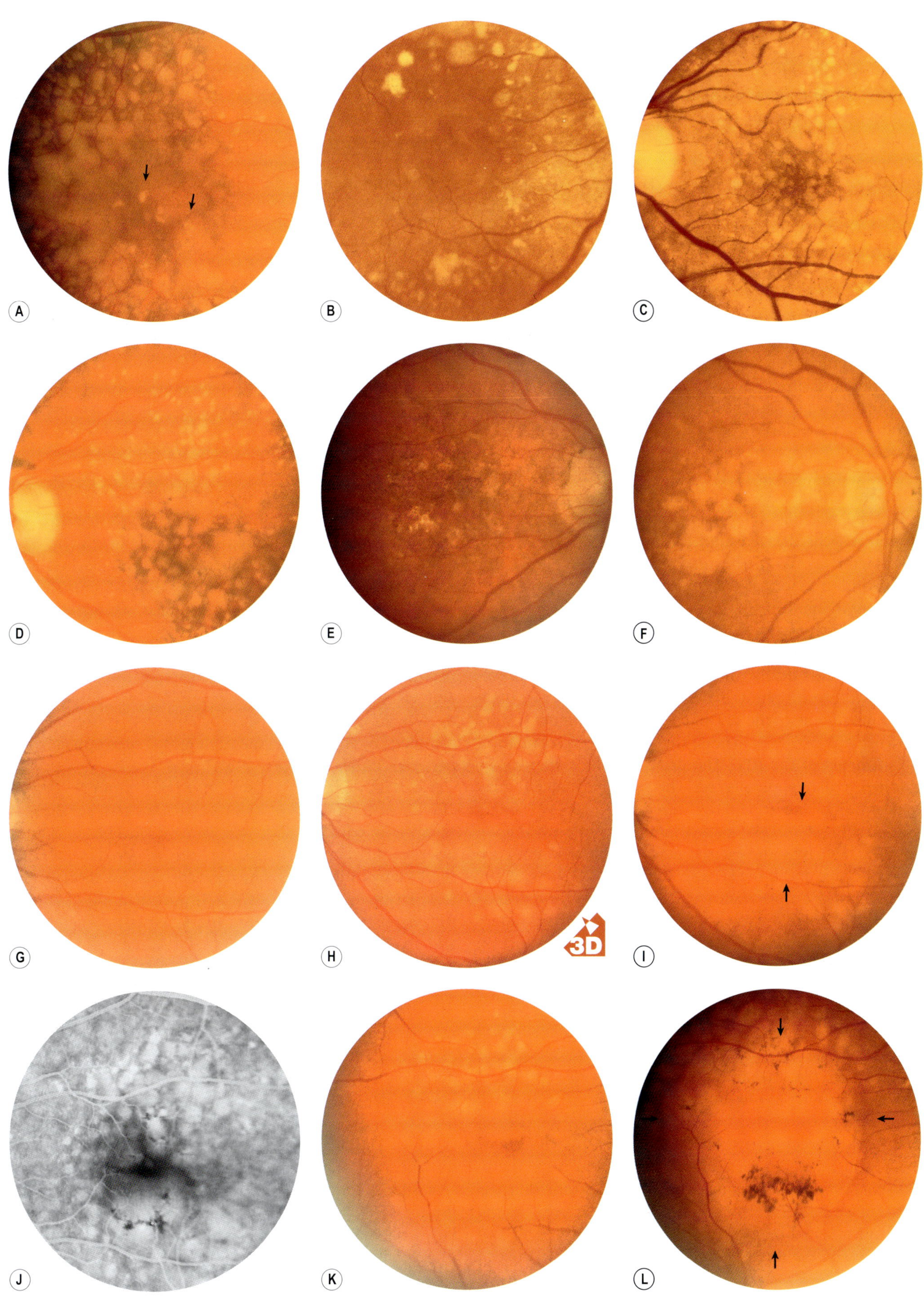
A
B
C
D
E
F
G
H
3D
I
J
K
L

Patients with multiple large drusen and with focal areas of hyperpigmentation in the macular area are at greater risk of developing subretinal neovascularization.[202,219,220] Fluorescein angiographic findings in drusen are variable and depend upon their size, height, degree of pigmentation of the RPE on their surface, and the contents and consistency of the material lying between the RPE and Bruch's membrane. Most drusen cause focal well-defined hyperfluorescence. The time of appearance of their early fluorescence depends upon the rate of staining of Bruch's membrane and the sub-RPE material, and their translucency. The intensity of their later staining with fluorescein depends primarily on their consistency (Figure 3.14). Although a delay in the appearance of the background choroidal fluorescence occurs in some patients with drusen, it is probable that this is caused by a delay in staining of Bruch's membrane and the sub-RPE material, both of which in some patients may have a higher lipid content, rather than a delay in perfusion of the choroidal blood vessels.[221–225] Smaller nodular ("hard") drusen typically show a peak fluorescence within several minutes of injection, and fading paralleling that of the background choroidal fluorescence. Fluorescence of medium and large drusen may be delayed until the later stages of angiography (Figure 3.14G–J). This may be caused by the thickness of the drusen as well as the lipid content of the drusen and the underlying Bruch's membrane (Figure 3.14G–J).[226] Angiography may reveal the presence of more drusen than are apparent ophthalmoscopically.

Histopathologically, most drusen consist of focal collections of eosinophilic material lying between the basement membrane of the RPE and Bruch's membrane (Figure 3.16).[189,197,200,227–233] They therefore represent focal detachments of the RPE. The detached RPE cells may be thinned and hypopigmented. The sub-RPE material may appear homogeneous and hyalinized (Figure 3.16A), finely granular (Figure 3.16B), or a combination of both (Figure 3.16C).[197,200] In some cases it may contain calcium, cholesterol clefts, and bone (Figure 3.16D).[197,200] The variable histopathologic appearance and composition of drusen suggest that their consistency probably varies from watery or mushy in the case of the large placoid drusen (Figure 3.16B), to firm in the case of the nodular hyalinized periodic acid–Schiff (PAS)-positive drusen (Figure 3.16A), to hard in the case of calcified or ossified white drusen (Figure 3.16D).[197,200] It is these histopathologic variations that have given rise to physicians' use of the terms "hard" and "soft" to describe the clinical appearance of small, discrete and larger, often placoid drusen, respectively.

As might be expected from the variability of the clinical and histopathologic appearance of drusen, there is heterogeneity in regard to their ultrastructural and histochemical makeup. There is evidence in monkeys and humans that the earliest development of some drusen involves the outward evagination of portions of the basal cell wall and cytoplasm of the RPE cell into the sub-RPE space between the inner collagenous portion of Bruch's membrane and the RPE cell.[227,234–236] These vesicles of cytoplasm become pinched off, degenerate, and form a nidus for the accumulation of an admixture of metabolic products and substances derived from the surrounding RPE, retina, and choriocapillaris. Histochemical and electron microscopic studies of typical or exudative drusen reveal a variety of substances and materials accumulating between the relatively normal basement membrane of the detached RPE and the inner collagenous zone of Bruch's membrane. These include sulfated and nonsulfated glycoconjugates; lipid material; plasma membranelike material; vesicles; amorphous material; types I, III, IV, and V collagen; fibronectin; immunoglobulins; degenerated RPE organelles; and viable cell processes.[190,197,231,232,235–239] Some investigators have attributed these viable cell processes surrounded by basement membrane to macrophages, or pericytes, rather than RPE cells.[240]

Histopathologically there may be minimal degeneration of the retinal receptor elements overlying drusen. Many eyes with focal drusen show, in addition, a thin layer of fine granular eosinophilic material separating the RPE from Bruch's membrane throughout most of the macular region (Figure 3.16E). Ultrastructurally this sub-RPE deposit may lie between the RPE plasma membrane and its basement membrane (basal laminar deposit) or between the inner collagenous zone of Bruch's membrane and the basement membrane of the RPE (basal linear dep osit).[197,231,233,241–243] The basal laminar deposit is composed primarily of wide-spaced collagen; the basal linear deposit is composed of vesicular and granular electron-dense, lipid-rich material. Some authors believe that basal laminar deposit, which is primarily type IV collagen, is a unique feature found in eyes predisposed to the development of AMD,[197,233,244] whereas others have presented evidence that it, along with the thickening of Bruch's membrane and drusen, is an aging change and is not unique for AMD.[243,245] Both types of deposit are particularly noticeable in eyes with multiple large so-called "soft" drusen and disciform detachments.[242]

3.16 Morphologic variations of typical or exudative drusen.

A: Multiple hyalinized "firm" nodular drusen.
B: Granular "soft" drusen.
C: Combined granular and hyalinized drusen (arrow).
D: Calcified "crystalline" drusen. Note new vessel (arrow) beneath the retinal pigment epithelium.
E: Diffuse deposition of granular drusen material (probably both basal laminar and basal linear deposits) in macular area. Note focal calcification (arrows) of Bruch's membrane, widening of the intercapillary pillars of the choriocapillaris, and partial obstruction of the choriocapillaris.
F: Extramacular area of same eye. Note relatively normal Bruch's membrane and choriocapillaris.

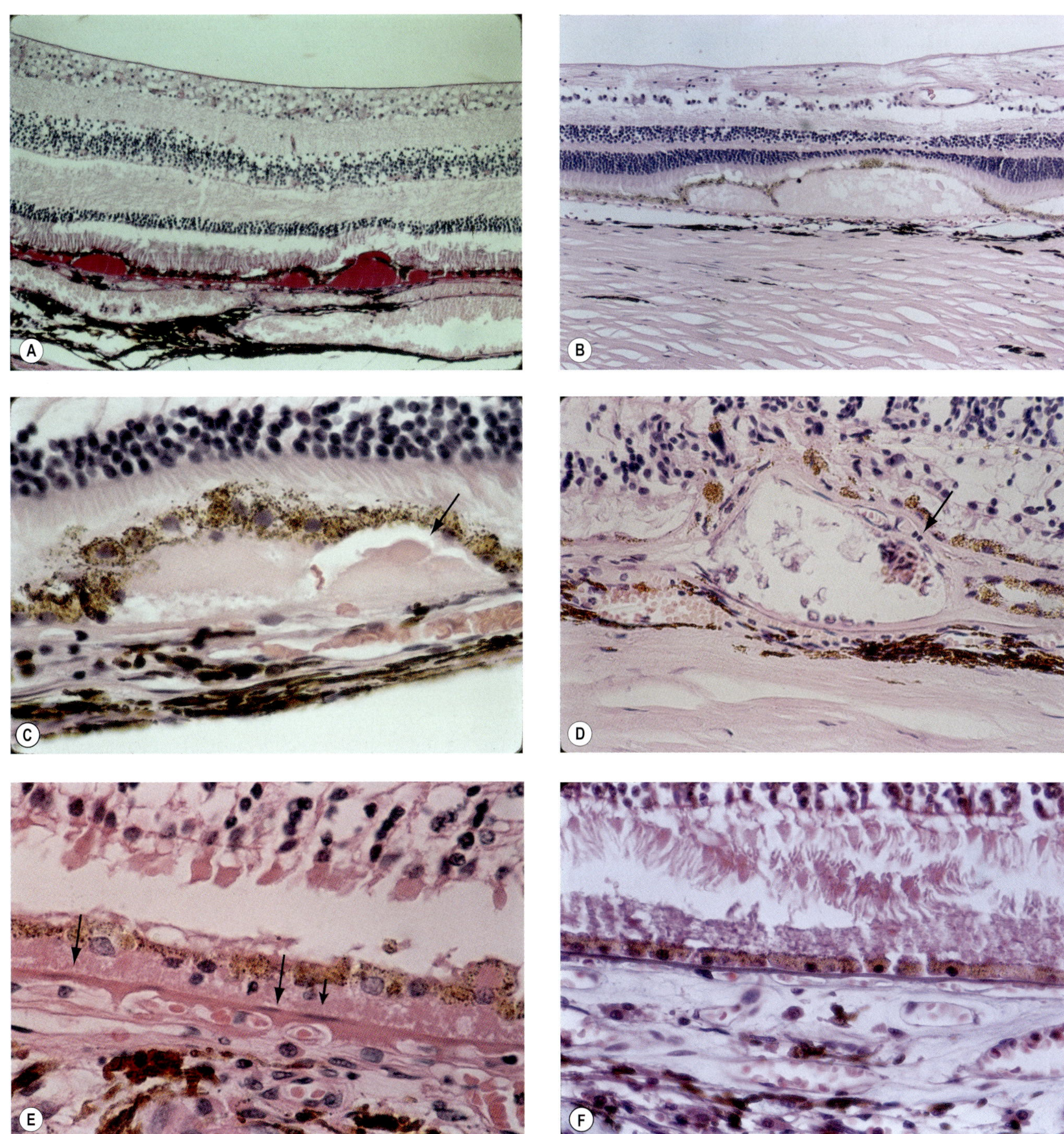
A
B
C
D
E
F

Other important histopathologic changes in the macula accompany drusen.[197,200,231–233,246–253] There is irregular thickening and thinning of Bruch's membrane associated with calcific degeneration of the elastic and collagen tissue comprising this structure.[200,231,237,246,247,254] In the underlying choriocapillaris there is thickening and hyalinization of the intercapillary stromal pillars secondary to the deposition of a PAS-positive material that effectively reduces the surface area of the capillary bed (Figure 3.16E).[200,231,255] The large choroidal vessels are unaffected. There is no indocyanine green angiographic or rheologic evidence of impaired choroidal perfusion in patients with drusen.[224,256] The changes in Bruch's membrane and the choriocapillaris that accompany macular drusen have been referred to previously as senile macular choroidal degeneration.[200] It is uncertain, however, whether these changes are manifestations of a dominantly inherited dystrophy or are merely degenerative changes secondary to aging.

Histopathologically, a few scattered drusen are found frequently in the peripheral fundus, particularly in the aging eye of white patients.[257] When numerous they are arranged in a reticular pattern and are associated with hyperplasia of the RPE between drusen that produces a reticular pattern of pigmentation ophthalmoscopically that may be mistaken clinically for that in retinitis pigmentosa (Figure 3.17).[210,213,218,257] In all, 80–90% of patients with many peripheral drusen show evidence of age-related macular changes.[218,257]

The pathogenesis of typical or exudative drusen is unknown. Although most recent authors have favored the view that aging or dystrophic changes in the RPE are primarily responsible for the accumulation of abnormal material beneath its basement membrane, it is uncertain whether the primary locus of the disease resides in one or a combination of the retina and RPE, Bruch's membrane, or choriocapillaris.[191,197,200,227,232,235,236,255,258–264] The demonstration of viable cell processes within drusen in their early development[227,236,265] and the later finding of incompletely digested RPE and retinal cell organelles within the sub-RPE material suggest that the posterior evagination of buds of RPE cell basal cytoplasm and basement membrane is an important stage in the development of drusen.[190,227,229,234,236,266] Accumulation of lipids in Bruch's membrane is part of the aging process of Bruch's membrane and makes it to some degree a hydrophobic barrier to the movement of water and ions toward the choroid.[267,268] This may be an important factor in fostering enlargement of drusen (conversion from hard to soft drusen), and confluence of drusen to form serous detachments of the pigment epithelium.[219,266,269–271] Although there is much evidence to suggest that typical or exudative drusen may be inherited as an autosomal-dominant characteristic, the role of heredity in the causation of drusen in most patients is uncertain.[177,188,210,272] Drusen have been produced experimentally in animals with intravitreal injection of aminoglycosides.[273]

Other retinal flecks that may clinically simulate drusen include those occurring in patients with cuticular or basal laminar drusen (see p. 132), Stargardt's disease (see p. 278), North Carolina fundus dystrophy (see p. 296), fundus albi punctate dystrophy (see p. 326), Alport's disease (see p. 316), and ring-17 chromosome retinopathy (see p. 320). In monkeys and humans focal lipidization of RPE cells may cause fundus lesions that resemble small drusen.[274–276] These punctate, yellow lesions usually are not evident angiographically. A few of them are often found in the central macular area of otherwise normal fundi in adults of all ages. Their pathogenesis and their relationship to drusen formation are unknown.

The primary cause of significant loss of central vision in patients with AMD is serous and hemorrhagic detachment of the RPE and retina caused by choroidal neovascularization.

3.17 Peripheral senile reticular pigmentary degeneration.

A–F: Macular drusen, choroidal neovascularization, and peripheral reticular pigmentary degeneration (A–C). Angiography revealed a triradiate pattern of peripheral drusen at the equator peripherally (D–F).

G–I: Note the peripheral drusen and pigment changes in this 75-year-old man whose eye was enucleated because of a small malignant melanoma of the choroid. Angiography showed evidence of multiple drusen and irregular loss of pigment from the retinal pigment epithelium (RPE) (H). Note the reticular pattern of nonfluorescent pigment. Histopathologic section of G showed multiple drusen, irregular thinning of the RPE, and clumps of large pigment-laden cells (arrow, I). The retina (not shown) showed mild loss of the receptor elements.

J and **K**: Peripheral cross-hatch-like pigment changes of senile reticular pigment degeneration show up as triradiate hyperautofluorescent changes.

(G–I from Gass.[216])

Occult Choroidal Neovascularization

The ingrowth of new vessels extending from the choroid into the sub-RPE space in one or more areas occurs frequently and is the most important histopathologic change that predisposes patients with drusen to macular detachment and loss of central vision (see discussion of type I choroidal neovascularization in Chapter 2).[21,192,200,210,216,231,249,251,263,277–294] Neovascular buds invade and penetrate the degenerated Bruch's membrane and proliferate beneath the RPE (Figures 2.05–2.07 and 3.18).[282,295,296] In addition, capillaries may invade the sub-RPE drusenlike deposits adjacent to the optic disc by extension through or around the edge of Bruch's membrane (Figure 3.18D).[200,297] It is not known whether the granulomatous inflammatory response to degenerated Bruch's membrane found in some cases is an important factor in the process of subretinal neovascularization.[249,254,298] The accumulation of phospholipid-containing membranes in the outer collagenous zone of Bruch's membrane and of lipid within drusen may be responsible for attracting these macrophages.[254]

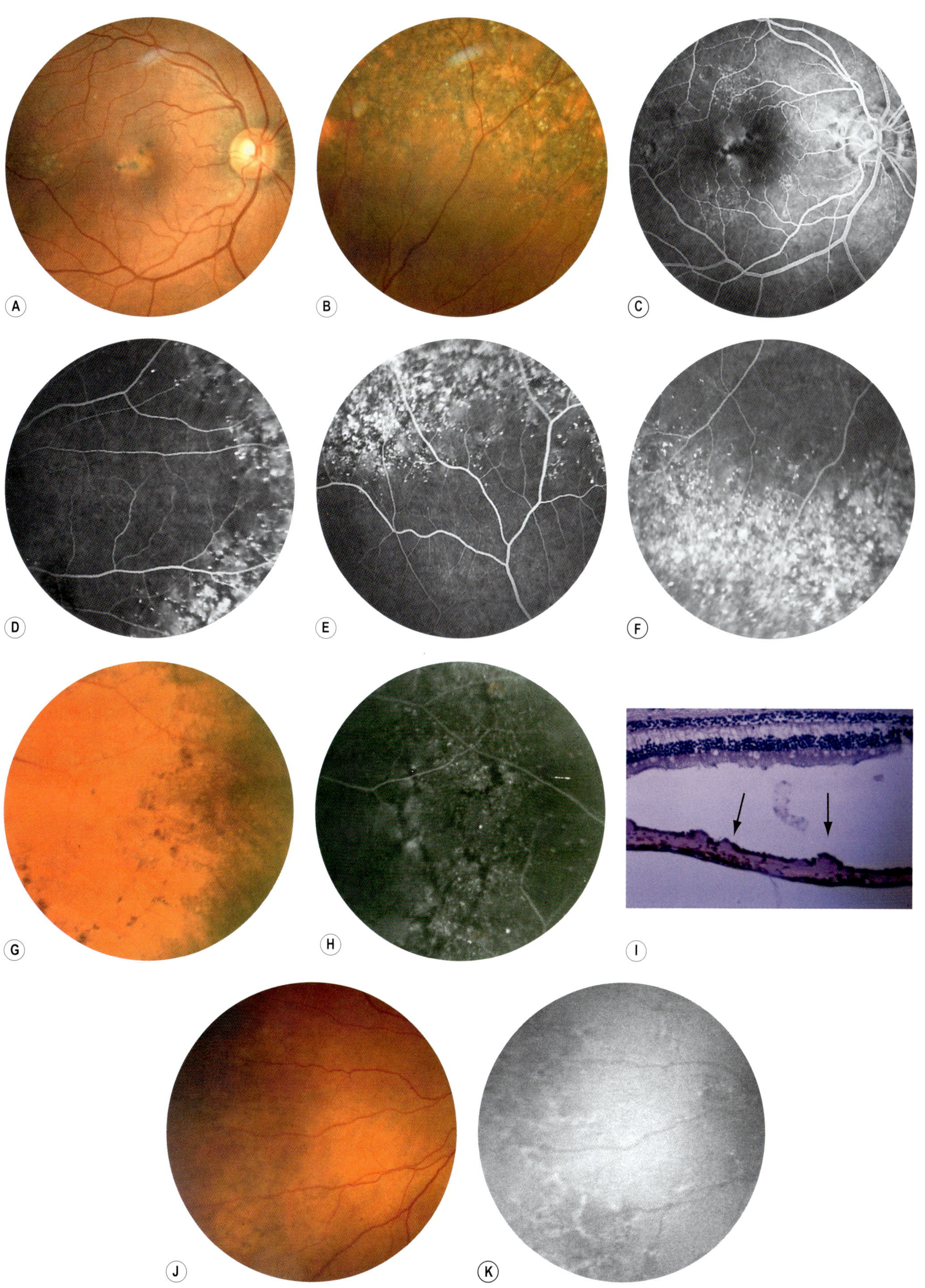
A
B
C
D
E
F
G
H
I
J
K

The new capillaries that penetrate Bruch's membrane grow in a flat cartwheel or seafan configuration away from their site of entry into the sub-RPE space (see Figure 2.07). The retinal blood flow in these vessels initially is slow, and the integrity of the capillary endothelium is adequate to prevent exudation (Figure 3.18E). In some cases the slow proliferation of new vessels and fibroblastic proliferation may produce a solid elevation of the RPE (see Figure 2.06). These organized RPE detachments or mounds may vary in size and shape and are often irregular in elevation (see Figure 3.22A and D). Because the fine biomicroscopic details of the elevated RPE and drusen look much the same as the surrounding RPE, and because of the minimal angiographic changes in the area of these organized RPE mounds, they may be easily overlooked without careful contact lens examination and good-quality stereoscopic fluorescein angiograms. Occasionally these organized RPE detachments may assume tumorlike proportions and simulate choroidal hemangiomas clinically (see Figure 3.28E). Failure to recognize areas of organized RPE detachment adjacent to areas of high-flow choroidal neovascular membranes (CNVMs) or adjacent to large serous detachments of the RPE is responsible for many of the poor results of photocoagulation.[285,299,300] The structure and function of the RPE and retina overlying these occult CNVMs or mounds may be minimally affected (Figure 3.18). During this occult stage of choroidal neovascularization the patient is usually asymptomatic and the new vessels may not be apparent either ophthalmoscopically or angiographically.[295] The stimulus causing neovascular invasion of the sub-RPE space and the explanation for its more frequent occurrence near the center of the macula and the peripapillary region is unknown. The histopathologic observation of choriocapillary atrophy in the vicinity of neovascular ingrowth suggests that ischemia may be an important factor. Experimentally, type II subretinal choroidal neovascularization can be produced by photocoagulation damage to the choriocapillaris–Bruch's membrane–RPE complex.[5–7,301–305] There is no experimental model for type I sub-RPE choroidal neovascularization that occurs in AMD.

3.18 Occult choroidal neovascularization in patients with drusen.

A–D: This 69-year-old man with a few drusen (arrows, A) in the macula of the right eye presented with a large serous detachment of the retina in the macula of the left eye (see Figure 3.10). He died of complications of laryngeal surgery and serial sections of the right macula at the site of one drusen (temporalmost arrow in A) revealed six round breaks in Bruch's membrane. Through each of these breaks passed a small capillary tuft from the choriocapillaris into the subretinal pigment epithelium (RPE) space (arrows, B and C). Similar sub-RPE capillary tufts were found beneath the temporal margin of the right optic disc (arrow, D).

E: Large sub-RPE occult choroidal neovascular membrane (CNVM; arrows). Note relatively normal RPE and retina as well as absence of exudation.

(E from Green and Key.[231])

Disciform Detachment Stages

Although most patients with AMD are in their seventh decade at the time of onset of symptoms, loss of acuity in some patients may occur in the fifth decade or earlier. Significant loss of central vision in these patients occurs primarily by three mechanisms: (1) confluence of drusen to form multilobulated exudative RPE detachments (5% or fewer of cases); (2) geographic atrophy of the RPE and retina (5–10%); and (3) subretinal neovascularization with serous and hemorrhagic detachment of the RPE and retina (80–90%).[192,210,269,294,297,306–318]

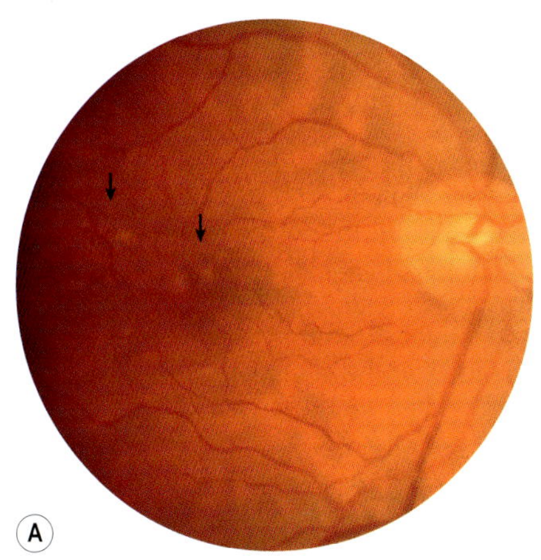

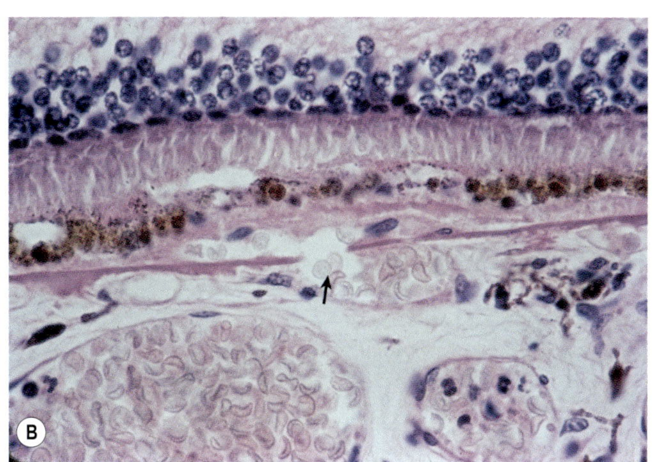

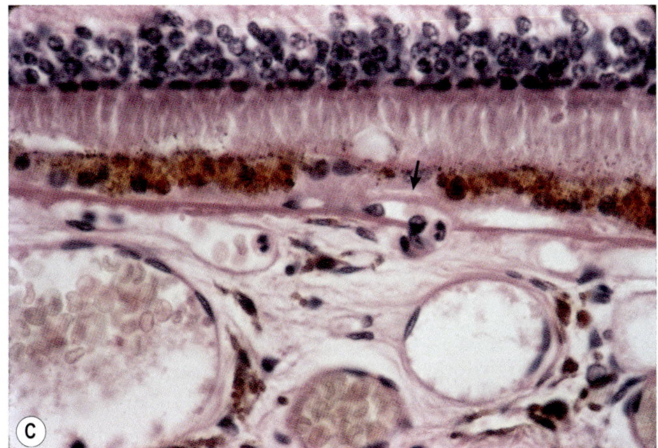

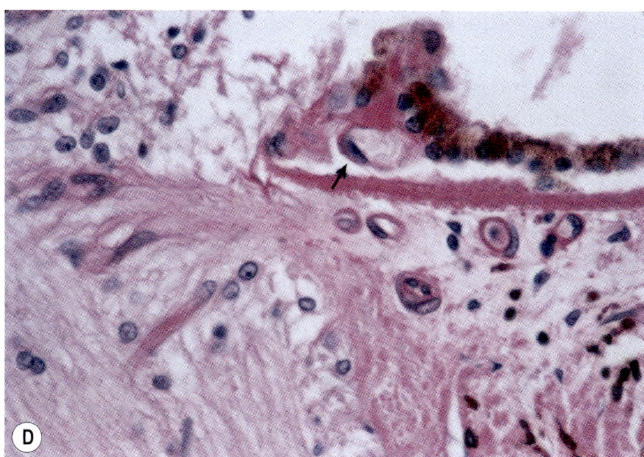

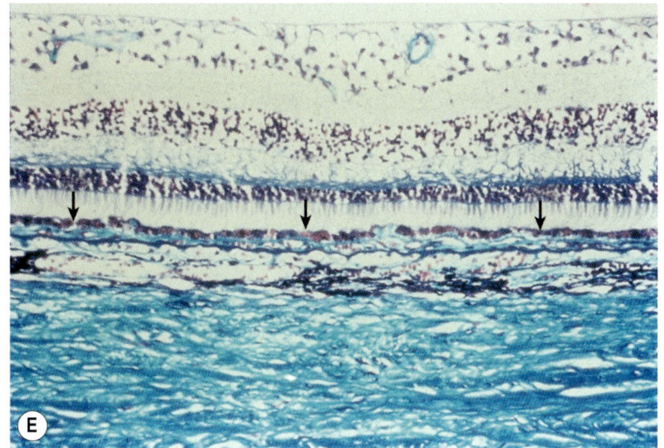

Exudative Detachment of the Retinal Pigment Epithelium Unassociated with Choroidal Neovascularization (Avascular Serous RPE Detachment)

Unlike patients with ICSC, patients with drusen infrequently develop large areas of serous retinal detachment overlying small serous RPE detachments, but they frequently present with large serous RPE detachments and minimal serous retinal detachment (Figures 2.04, 2.09, and 3.19). The normal aging changes in the inner zones of Bruch's membrane as well as those that may be peculiar to AMD cause loosening of the adherence of the RPE basement membrane to Bruch's membrane. Increased lipidization of Bruch's membrane renders it hydrophobic and a barrier to normal movement of fluid by the RPE into the choroid.[221,271] This predisposes patients with AMD to the formation of soft drusen and to progressive enlargement and confluence of drusen to form a focal area of RPE detachment, often with scalloped borders, a slightly irregular surface, and a triradiate pattern of orange or gray pigmentation on its surface. These avascular RPE detachments, referred to by some as drusenoid RPE detachments, typically develop slowly and initially may cause minimal complaints of blurring and metamorphopsia (Figures 3.14G–I and 3.15G–L). Angiography in these slowly developing avascular serous RPE detachments shows a gradual staining of the sub-RPE exudate and outlines the nonfluorescent pigment figure on its surface (Figures 3.14H and I and 3.15J). There may be some irregularity of the late staining pattern caused by irregular density of the sub-RPE material. A few patients may experience abrupt visual loss and distortion caused by a more rapidly developing, round or oval, smooth-surfaced, dome-shaped area of serous detachment of the RPE in the absence of any evidence of occult neovascularization (Figure 3.19A–D). These rapidly developing avascular RPE detachments show a pattern of rapid even fluorescein staining (Figure 3.19B) that is unlike that seen with most serous RPE detachments caused by choroidal neovascularization (see discussion of vascularized RPE detachments, p. 106) as well as those lesions that may simulate serous RPE detachment, such as metastatic carcinoma, amelanotic melanomas, or other solid tumors.

Because of prognostic and therapeutic implications, it is important to look for signs of choroidal neovascularization, which usually is the cause of these rapidly developing detachments of the RPE.[295] The vision of patients with subfoveal serous RPE detachments can usually be corrected to 20/25–20/40 with the addition of plus lenses. When there is no choroidal neovascularization there may be only minimal progression of visual loss over many months or years. The detachment may enlarge slowly and occasionally may spontaneously flatten. The value of photocoagulation (Figure 3.19) is uncertain.[210,216,319–324]

3.19 Serous detachment of the retinal pigment epithelium (RPE) in patients with age-related macular degeneration.

A–D: This 64-year-old man experienced the onset of metamorphopsia in the right eye. Visual acuity was 20/30. A serous detachment of the RPE was present (A). Drusen were present in the left macula. Angiography revealed rapid, even staining of the sub-RPE exudate (B). The dark zone centrally is caused by the retinal xanthophyll. Argon laser applications were placed straddling the margin of the RPE detachment (C). Nine months later the detachment had resolved (D). Visual acuity was 20/30.

E and **F**: A 60-year-old woman with serous detachment of the RPE (arrows, E). One month after ruby laser treatment to the margins of the RPE detachment, it had resolved (F). Visual acuity was 20/40.

G: Histopathology of serous detachment of the RPE in a 68-year-old woman with macular drusen. This lesion was misdiagnosed as a malignant melanoma. Arrow indicates small drusen that are detached along with the RPE. Sub-RPE exudate extends through a small microrip in the RPE into the subretinal space near the left end of the photomicrograph.

(G from Zscheile.[264],)

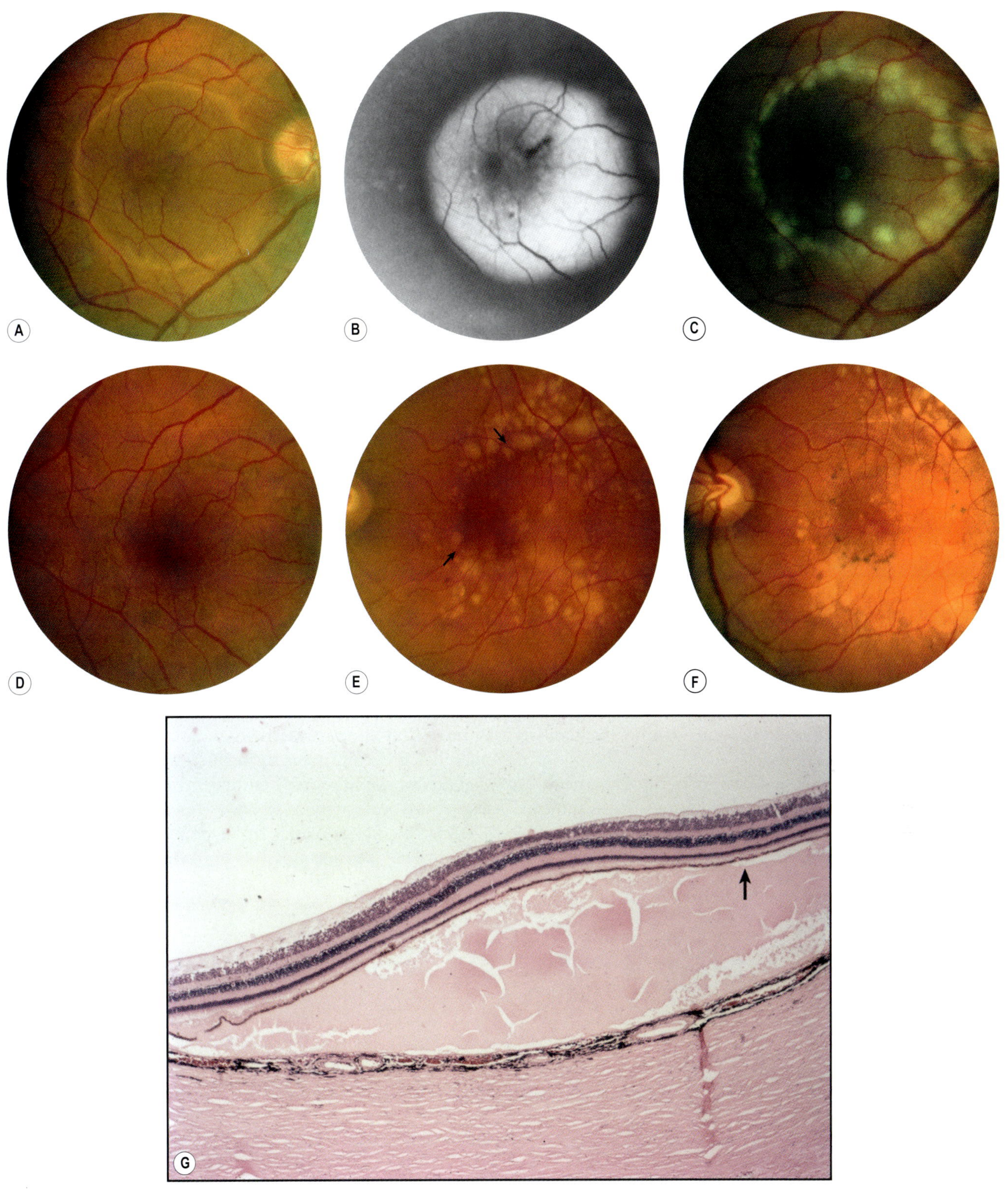
A
B
C
D
E
F
G

Serous and Hemorrhagic Detachment of the Retina Caused by Choroidal Neovascularization

At any stage in the development of an occult CNVM beneath the RPE, blood flow may become sufficient to cause leakage of serous exudate and diapedesis of red cells into the subpigment space around the CNVM. This may progress to produce a variety of ophthalmoscopic pictures of exudative and hemorrhagic detachment of the macula. The most frequent sequence of events giving rise to symptoms is the decompensation of the RPE overlying the CNVM and serous detachment of the overlying and surrounding retina (Figure 3.20). A light-grayish discoloration usually occurs in the area of the CNVM. The blood vessels comprising the CNVM may or may not be visible biomicroscopically (Figure 3.20). Small foci of subretinal blood or yellow, lipid-rich exudate may occur near the margins of the CNVM. In cases where the neovascular membrane extends beneath the retinal capillary-free zone, cystoid macular edema may occur. The reasons for the accumulation of intraretinal exudate in this instance are uncertain, but it may be caused in part by disruption of the retinal outer limiting membrane–receptor cell barrier to the intraretinal migration of subretinal exudate and the paucity of the retinal capillaries in this area to remove it (see Figure 2.15 and discussion in Chapter 2). The ability of stereoscopic fluorescein angiography to localize a CNVM accurately depends primarily on the rate of blood flow through the membrane and the presence or absence of material anterior to the membrane that may obstruct the view of the fluorescence within the capillary network.[210,295,299,325]

The typical cartwheel or seafan pattern of the new vessels is visible in high-flow membranes with minimal extravasated blood, cloudy exudate, or fibrous tissue anterior to it (Figure 3.20). In some membranes with only a moderate blood flow rate, an ill-defined ooze of fluorescein appears late in the area of the membrane (Figure 3.21).[326] When the serous retinal detachment is caused by leakage of exudate from the surface of an occult sub-RPE neovascular complex, angiography may show only a multifocal pinpoint or irregular pattern of staining at the surface of the organized RPE detachment (Figure 3.22B and C).[281,295,326,327] The accurate localization of choroidal neovascularization in such cases is difficult. It is also difficult or impossible if part of the CNVM is obscured by blood located beneath either the RPE or the retina. Stereoscopic angiograms are essential to the detection and localization of most CNVMs, particularly that part of the CNVM complex that is occult. Areas of irregular elevation of the RPE that do not stain probably harbor occult new vessels. Once exudation begins, most CNVMs progressively enlarge to 1–2 disc diameters in size or larger and cause progressive loss of visual function.

3.20 Sub-retinal pigment epithelium (RPE) neovascularization in patients with drusen.

A–C: This elderly woman complained of mild blurring of vision. The new-vessel membrane was largely obscured by the grayish-yellow exudate (arrows) in the sub-RPE space (A). A few red capillaries were visible near the upper margin of the membrane. Note dye perfusing the sub-RPE vessels that were arranged in a seafan pattern (B and C). The dye leaked from these vessels and stained the surrounding exudate in the sub-RPE space.

D and **E**: Another patient with choroidal neovascularization (D). Angiogram showed seafan configuration of new vessels (E).

F: Large choroidal neovascular membrane (arrows) that extended through break in Bruch's membrane (left arrow).

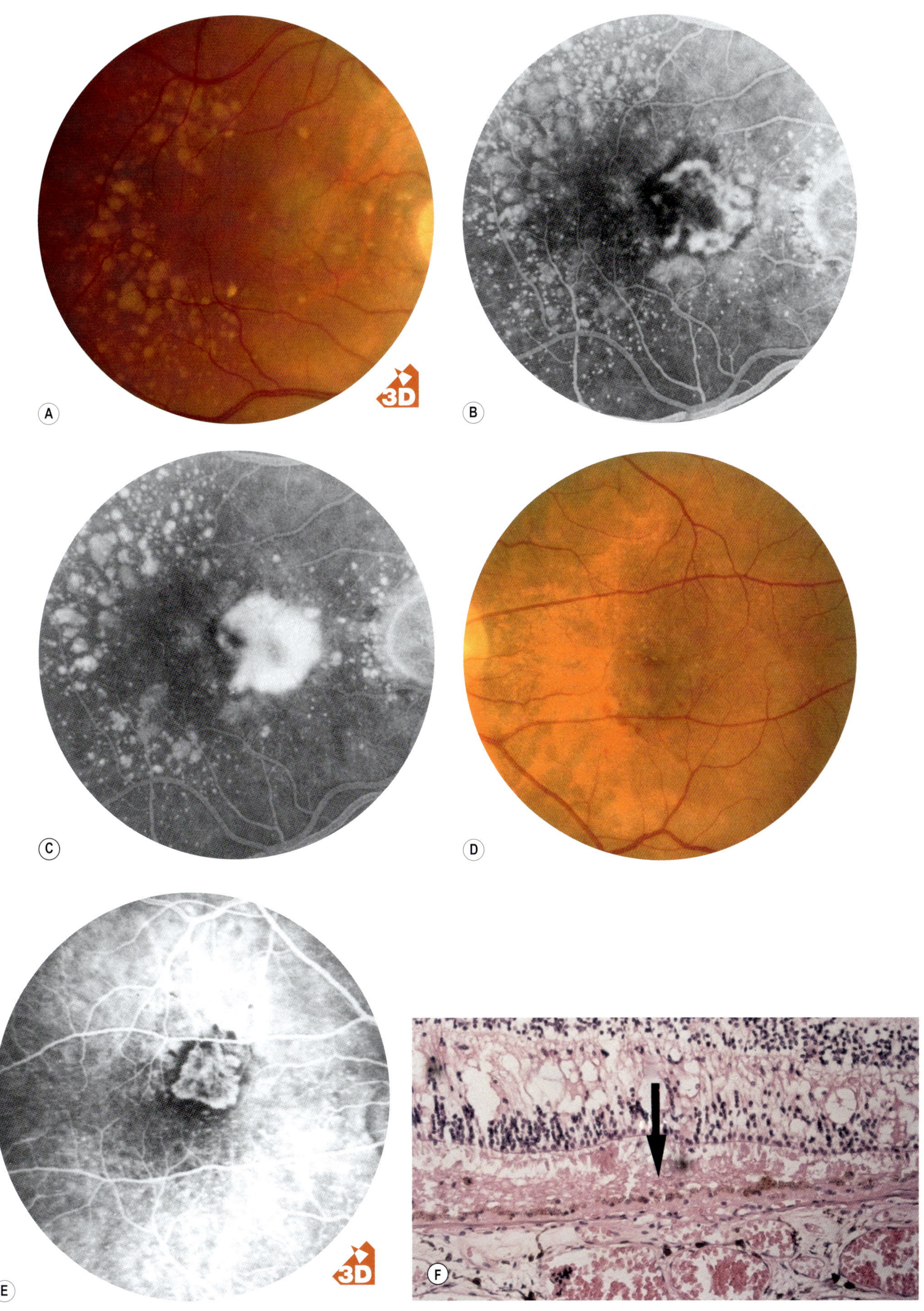
A
3D
B
C
D
E
3D
F

Serous Detachment of the Retinal Pigment Epithelium Caused by Choroidal Neovascularization (Vascularized RPE Detachment)

In patients with AMD, acute visual loss is caused by a large, sharply circumscribed, smooth-surfaced, serous detachment of the RPE in approximately 10% of cases.[216] In the majority of cases, this detachment is caused by choroidal neovascularization.[13,200,295,328–330] Because of the cartwheel or seafan pattern of sub-RPE CNVM and because of the relatively firm connection established between the new capillaries and the base of the overlying RPE, there is a predilection for serous exudation and/or hemorrhage to occur near the margin of the CNVM. This results in detachment of the adjacent RPE around the margin of the CNVM, and production of a variety of shapes of large RPE detachments (see Figures 2.09, 2.10, 3.21, and 3.22).[295] If the detachment occurs at one segment of the edge of the CNVM, a flat-sided, reniform, or notched RPE detachment is the result (Figures 3.21 and 3.22).[295] If the detachment extends away from the entire margin of the CNVM, a doughnut-shaped RPE detachment may occur. Any of these irregularly shaped RPE detachments should suggest the probable presence of a CNVM that for the most part lies outside the area of RPE detachment, within either the notch or the central depressed area of the RPE detachment (Figures 3.21 and 3.22). Biomicroscopically there may or may not be any other evidence of the presence of the CNVM in these areas. If serous detachment of the RPE overlying the CNVM occurs, a round or oval, dome-shaped detachment identical to an avascular RPE detachment may result. If serous detachment of the RPE develops adjacent to an organized sub-RPE detachment, an irregularly elevated, oval or dumbbell-shaped RPE detachment develops (Figures 3.22A–C and 3.23A). The details of the RPE and drusen are better preserved in the less-elevated, organized part of the detachment (Figure 3.22D). The presence of a dark meniscus (blood or blood pigment) at the dependent part of the serous RPE detachment (Figure 3.21G) or of subretinal blood or yellow exudate near its margin is evidence of the presence of a CNVM located either just outside of the edge of, or beneath, the RPE detachment.

3.21 Notched serous detachments of the retinal pigment epithelium (RPE) caused by choroidal neovascularization.

A–F: A 74-year-old woman with an RPE detachment caused by two occult choroidal neovascular membranes (CNVMs: arrows, C) within notched zones (A). Stereoscopic view of the late angiogram (B and C) and early angiogram (D). Argon laser treatment was applied to the two neovascular membranes, and two focal laser burns were placed at the 4:30 margin of the RPE detachment (E). Twelve days later the retina and RPE were reattached (F). Subretinal blood was present at the sites of photocoagulation of the CNVMs.

G–L: A 56-year-old man with a large RPE detachment, dark fluid level (small arrow, G), and notch (large arrow, G). Six months later the RPE detachment was larger (H). Note slow staining of sub-RPE fluid, nonfluorescent fluid level, and late fluorescein staining in the area of the notch (J, arrows). Argon laser treatment was placed along the margin of the detachment and at the site of occult neovascularization (arrow, K). Note dark blood that appeared just above new-vessel membrane (arrow) during treatment. Four weeks later the retinal and RPE detachments had resolved (L). Visual acuity was 20/40.

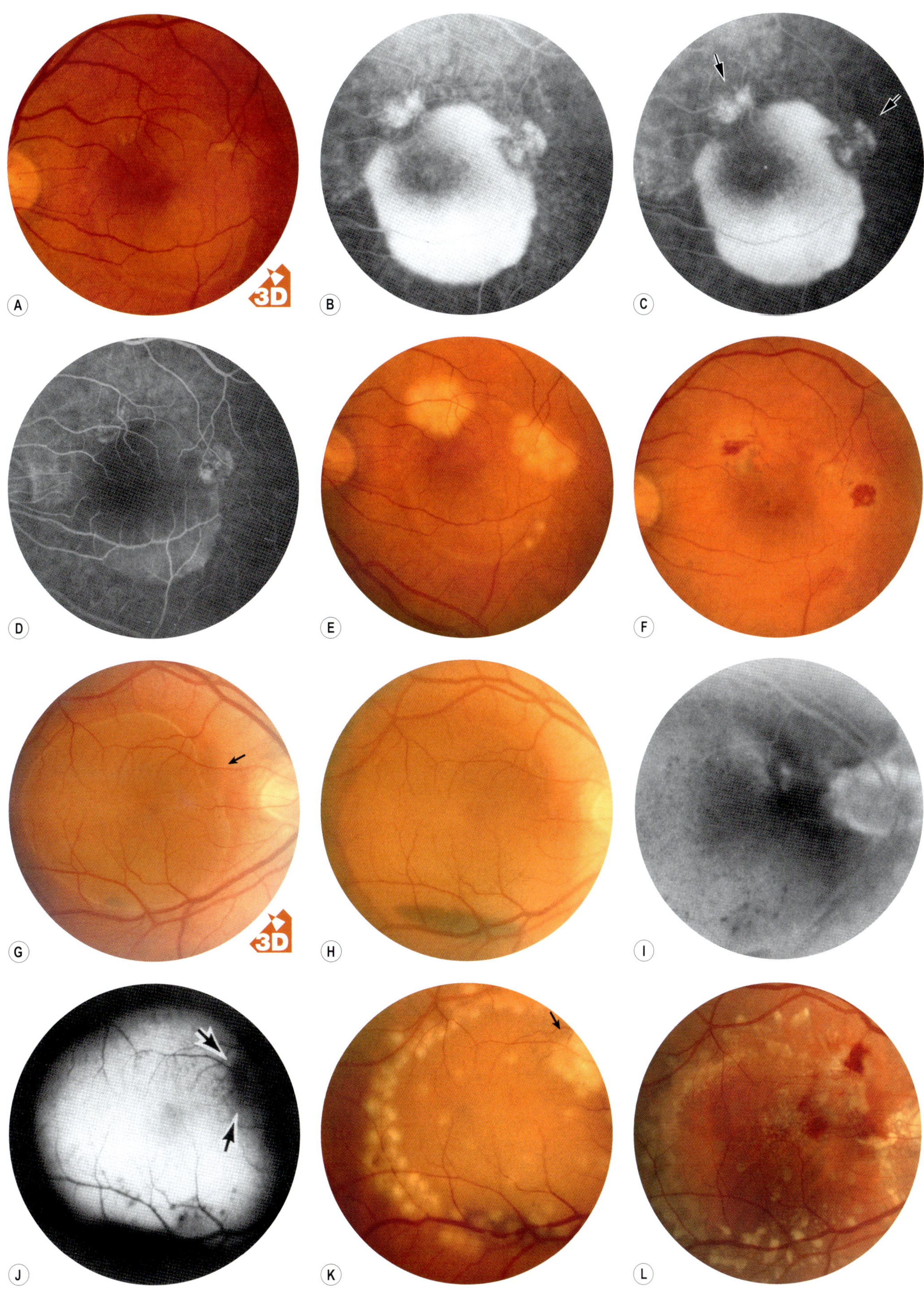
A
3D
B
C
D
E
F
G
3D
H
I
J
K
L

The fluorescein angiographic findings are important in differentiating vascularized from nonvascularized serous RPE detachments.[295,299] In vascularized serous RPE detachments, the sub-RPE exudate usually stains more slowly, presumably because of the presence of a large amount of protein and blood pigment within the exudate, and incompletely because of an uneven distribution of blood or a mound of fibrovascular tissue present beneath the RPE detachment (Figures 3.21 and 3.22). When a serous RPE detachment arises at one edge of either a flat or elevated organized CNVM, angiography often shows early fluorescein staining of the sub-RPE serous exudate in the area of serous detachment but delayed and uneven or, occasionally, no staining in the area of the CNVM. In some cases, however, there may be an intensification of the staining of the sub-RPE exudate adjacent to the CNVM (Figure 3.21I). When exudate from the CNVM detaches the overlying as well as adjacent RPE to produce a round or oval detachment, slow or uneven staining of the sub-RPE exudate in the area of the neovascular complex may be the only clue to the presence of the underlying CNVM.

Serous RPE detachments caused by choroidal neovascularization are likely to be large, to develop evidence of hemorrhage and organization (sub-RPE fibrovascular proliferation), and to cause significant loss of central vision soon after onset of symptoms. Because portions of the CNVM are nearly always hidden from view beneath the RPE detachment, treatment with photocoagulation is difficult and of uncertain value.[192,216,320,322–324,331,332]

3.22 Partly organized retinal pigment epithelium (RPE) detachments.

A–B: Two notched serous RPE detachments surrounding an elevated organized RPE detachment. The latter stained irregularly with fluorescein (B, stereo; arrows).

C–H: RPE tear occurring in partly organized serous RPE detachment in an 85-year-old man. Note drusen and pigment epithelial markings evident overlying nasal organized half of RPE detachment (arrows, C). Note uneven and incomplete staining of nasal part of RPE detachment (D and E). Several weeks later a tear has occurred along the temporal margin of the detachment (F). The edge of the tear has curled under and retracted nasally against the organized part of the detachment (arrow). Angiography showed minimal staining within the pigmented mound, indicating presence of choroidal new vessels (G). Several weeks later there was subretinal bleeding from the choroidal new vessels within the pigmented mound (arrows, H).

RPE tear posttreatment with ranibizumab.

I–L: This 65-year-old woman with a strong family history of age-related macular degeneration developed a fibrovascular pigment epithelial detachment that was asymptomatic (I) and found during follow-up of cataract surgery. She received intravitreal ranibizumab and noted distortion of vision after the second injection. A tear in the RPE was found and her vision had dropped to 20/40, quickly worsening to 20/400 in 3 weeks due to further retraction of the pigment epithelium (K). Four years later a large disciform scar with chronic subretinal fluid and blood in the eye could be seen.

Retinal Pigment Epithelial Tear

Patients who develop a serous RPE detachment extending away from one part of an organized RPE detachment are at some risk of developing an RPE tear spontaneously, during or following photocoagulation, and even following anti-VEGF therapy (Figures 3.19G, 3.22, and 3.23).[270,271,300,333–348] Typical pretear findings are: (1) a large, round, oval, or slightly dumbbell-shaped elevation of the RPE with one area less elevated than the other; (2) preservation of the RPE details, including drusen in the smaller, less elevated, organized portion of the RPE elevation; and (3) irregular and incomplete fluorescein staining in the area of less elevation, and delayed but even more intense staining of the sub-RPE exudate in the more elevated serous portion of the RPE detachment (Figures 3.22 and 3.23).[336,338] There may be no other biomicroscopic signs of underlying choroidal neovascularization. Either spontaneously or following treatment, an acute RPE tear may occur at or along the border of the serous RPE detachment on the side opposite the location of the new vessels. These patients usually notice an abrupt increase in visual loss caused by the passage of serous exudation from beneath the RPE into the subretinal space. Occasionally, however, patients may retain excellent visual acuity in spite of extension of the rip beneath the foveal center (Figure 3.23A–F, I, and J).[333,344] Only if seen within 24 hours after the tear will the free edge of the RPE be seen before it rolls under and retracts toward the area of subretinal neovascular tissue.

By the time most patients present there is a crescent-shaped geographic zone of absent RPE adjacent to an elevated hyperpigmented mound composed of the retracted and rolled-under RPE collapsed against the surface of the fibrovascular tissue (Figures 3.22G and K). The retinal detachment resolves soon after development of the tear, presumably because of regrowth of hypopigmented RPE cells across the defect and perhaps also because of partial closure of the choriocapillaris (Figures 3.22 and 3.23).[344] In some patients this new growth of RPE is visible biomicroscopically as a blunting of the edges of the tear by ingrowth of a faintly opaque layer of tissue into the area of the tear. In some cases a prominent layer of fibrous metaplastic RPE grows into and obliterates evidence of the tear. Subretinal blood and lipid exudate frequently appear soon after development of the tear. Angiography done after the tear usually shows evidence of early nonfluorescence and mottled late staining in the area of the retracted and organized RPE mound, as well as marked diffuse early and late hyperfluorescence in the area of absent or hypopigmented RPE and staining of any subretinal fluid that is present (Figure 3.22).

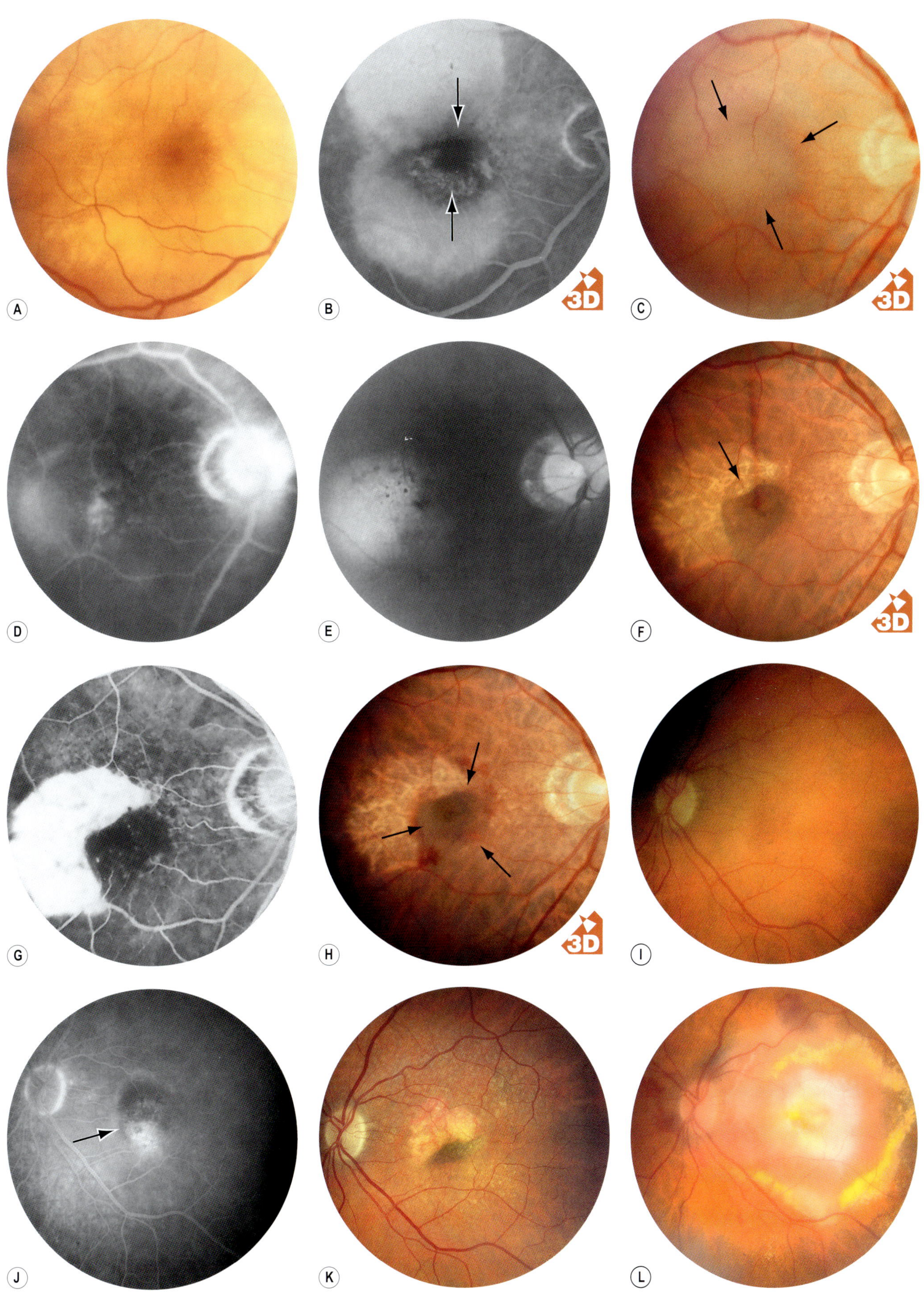
3D
3D
3D
3D
A
B
C
D
E
F
G
H
I
J
K
L

Hoskin and associates[341] suggested that the pretear picture was best explained by separation of the RPE from its basement membrane in the area of maximum elevation, predisposing it to tear. This explanation, however, is unlikely because of the tight adhesion of the RPE to its basement membrane in normal as well as pathologic conditions,[349] and because it does not explain the clinical and angiographic findings that suggest that underlying choroidal neovascularization is the primary cause of both the pretear and posttear appearance.[338] Chuang and Bird[270] and Bird and Marshall[271] have stressed the importance of the hydrophobic nature of the lipidized Bruch's membrane acting as a barrier to passage to fluid into the choroid in the pathogenesis of RPE tears in patients with AMD. The biomicroscopic and angiographic findings, however, strongly suggest that hydrostatic pressure generated by leakage of exudate from the margin of occult sub-RPE new vessels is the primary precipitating cause of most of the large, smooth-surfaced, blisterlike serous RPE detachments as well as the acute RPE tears that occur in patients with AMD (Figure 3.20G).[338,350] Occasionally, however, rents developing in the thinned RPE at the edge of long-standing avascular serous RPE detachments are responsible for their spontaneous collapse. Patients with large RPE tears associated with AMD are at high risk of developing RPE tears in the fellow eye.[335]

3.23 Retinal pigment epithelium (RPE) tears in patients with age-related macular degeneration.

A–F: This 59-year-old woman developed metamorphopsia in the left eye. Arrowheads indicate angiographic evidence of partly organized portion of a bilobate RPE detachment (A and B) in April 1984. Note delay in complete staining of the inferonasal part of the RPE detachment (stereoscopic views B and C). In May 1984 she developed a rip in the RPE that extended beneath the center of the fovea (D and stereoscopic views E and F). Two months later, in spite of the subfoveal rip and serous detachment of the retina, her visual acuity corrected to 20/20. Ten months later the acuity was reduced to 20/200.

G: Diagram showing pathogenesis of RPE tear. Stage 1, Organized RPE detachment (arrow). Stage 2, Serous detachment of the adjacent RPE. Stage 3, Tear in the RPE and serous detachment of the retina. Stage 4, Free edge of torn RPE has rolled toward fibrovascular tissue and nonpigmented RPE has grown across the defect, causing resolution of the serous retinal detachment that occurred following the tear. Rr, retinal receptors; RPE, retinal pigment epithelium; cc, choriocapillaris.

H–K: This 88-year-old male developed an RPE detachment with subretinal and intraretinal fluid in his left eye (H). A rip occurred after his second intravitreal ranibizumab injection but the vision remained at 20/40 (I). A vertical section on optical coherence tomography reveals the discontinuity of the pigment epithelium (J) and the dark zone bereft of RPE on autofluorescence imaging (K).

(A–F case presented at Fluorescein Club Meeting November 11, 1984; G from Gass.[338])

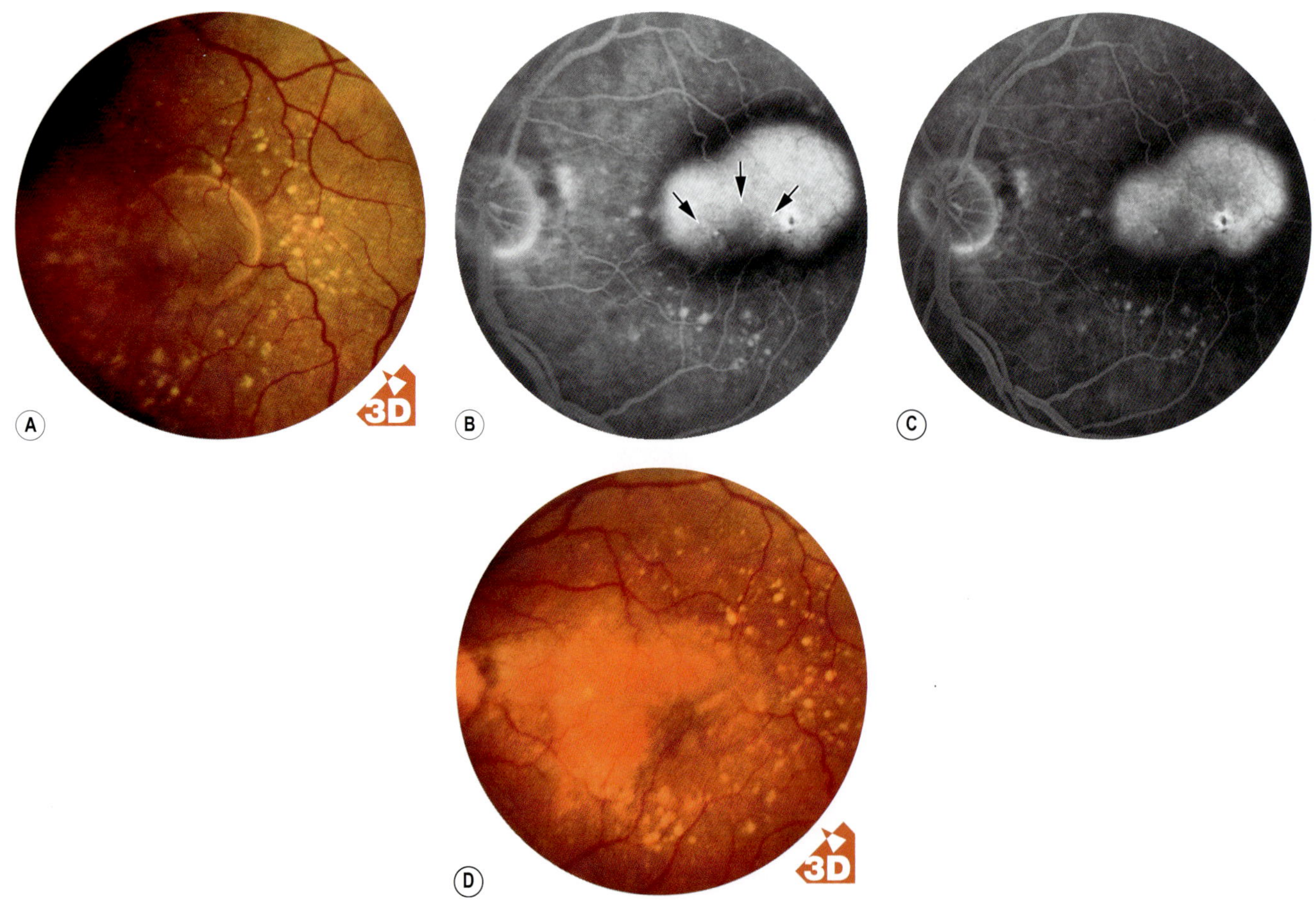

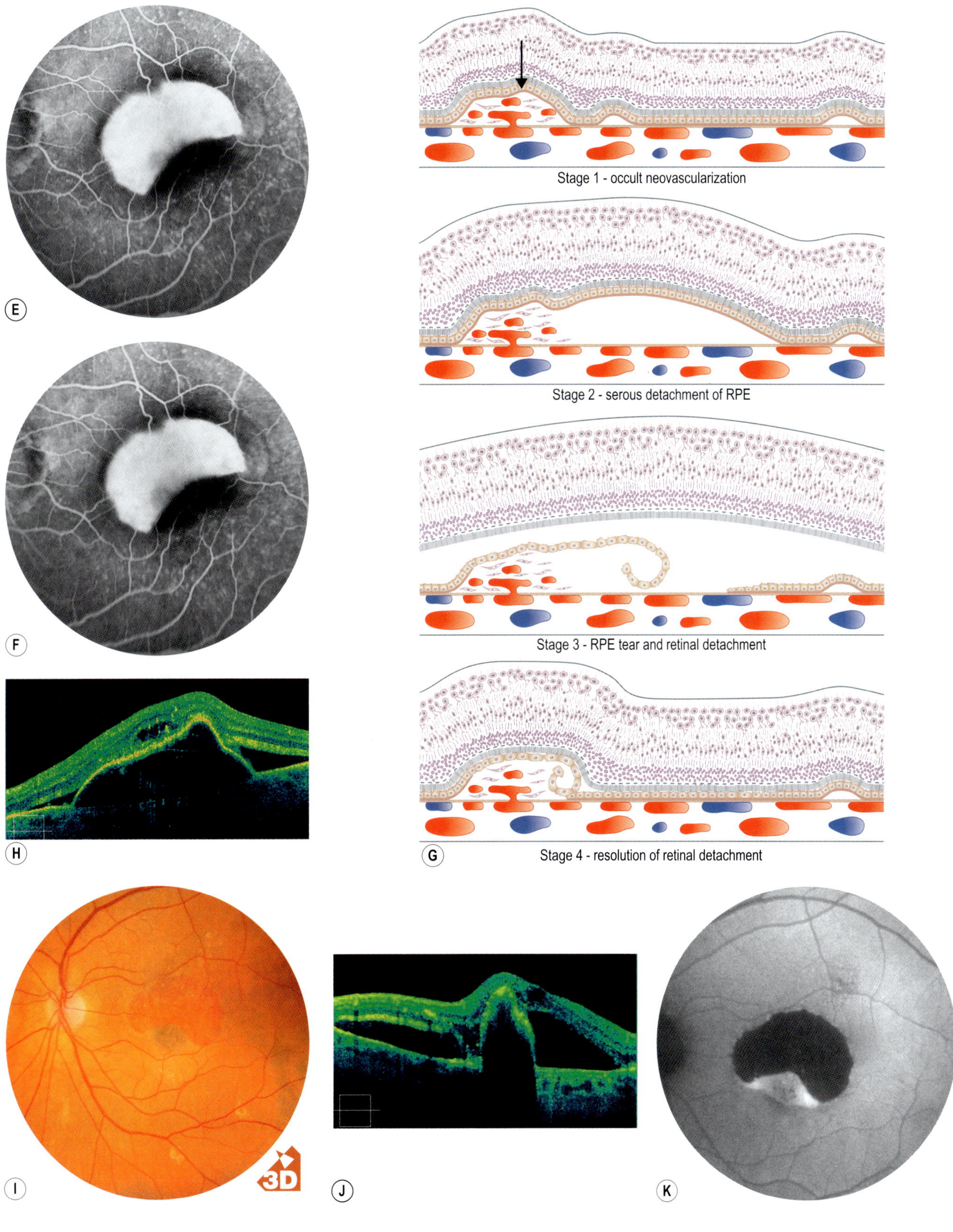
E
F
H
Stage 1 - occult neovascularization
Stage 2 - serous detachment of RPE
Stage 3 - RPE tear and retinal detachment
Stage 4 - resolution of retinal detachment
G
I
3D
J
K

Angiographic evidence of microrips at the edge of smaller RPE detachments, with streaming of fluorescein dye into the subretinal space similar to that seen in patients with ICSC, occasionally occurs in patients with AMD.[300,342] Likewise, large RPE tears similar to those associated with AMD occasionally occur in otherwise healthy patients with ICSC with large, often multifocal serofibrinous RPE detachments, and in patients with systemic lupus erythematosus and the same findings (Figure 3.10). The RPE tears in these patients are presumably caused by hydrostatic pressure generated by severe focal damage to the permeability of the choriocapillaris (see discussion in earlier section on ICSC).

Tears in the RPE may occur along the juncture of fibrovascular elevation of the RPE and serous RPE detachment during applications of photocoagulation to the neovascularization.[300,343] These tears occur most frequently during treatment of hypopigmented, thick subretinal neovascular membranes with krypton red laser and are caused by contraction of the fibrovascular tissue comprising the membrane.

3.24 Hemorrhagic disciform detachment stages occurring in patients with drusen.

A and B: Hemorrhagic detachment in a 68-year-old man with drusen. Most of the blood is in the subretinal space and was derived from a choroidal neovascular membrane in the papillomacular bundle region (arrows, A). Visual acuity in this eye was 20/50. There was spontaneous resolution of subretinal blood and return of visual acuity to 20/25. B was taken 3 years after A.

C and D: Spontaneous resolution of large black hemorrhagic detachment of retinal pigment epithelium (RPE) and retina (C). The disciform scar (D) extended to the inferior edge of the foveal center.

E and F: This patient was referred for treatment of a choroidal melanoma. The irregular brown color change in the sub-RPE and subretinal blood was responsible for the misdiagnosis. Angiography showed no evidence of fluorescence within the lesion (F).

G: Large hemorrhagic detachment of the RPE in a patient with macular drusen. Bleeding occurred from new vessels lying beneath the RPE (arrow).

(From Gass.[200])

Radiating Chorioretinal Folds Surrounding Partly Organized RPE Detachments

Spontaneous contraction of the fibrovascular tissue often hidden beneath serous RPE detachments may pucker Bruch's membrane and cause a series of radiating chorioretinal folds around the base of the RPE detachment (see Figure 4.04).[351] The radial pattern of yellow rays seen ophthalmoscopically and the hyperfluorescent rays seen angiographically are produced by the linear ridges of infolding of the RPE and choroid. This pattern of folds may be the only ophthalmoscopic sign of occult choroidal neovascularization detectable in some patients with large serous detachments of the RPE. It is curious that this radiating pattern of folds does not occur more often in response to photocoagulation of CNVM. The forces producing this radiating pattern of chorioretinal folds are similar to those responsible for a finer pattern of superficial inner retinal folds radiating outward from a contracted epiretinal fibrocellular membrane.

Linear Chorioretinal Folds Associated with Organized RPE Detachments

A series of slightly irregular chorioretinal folds may develop on the surface of organized RPE detachments if the superficial portion of the sub-RPE fibrovascular tissue undergoes shrinkage.[352]

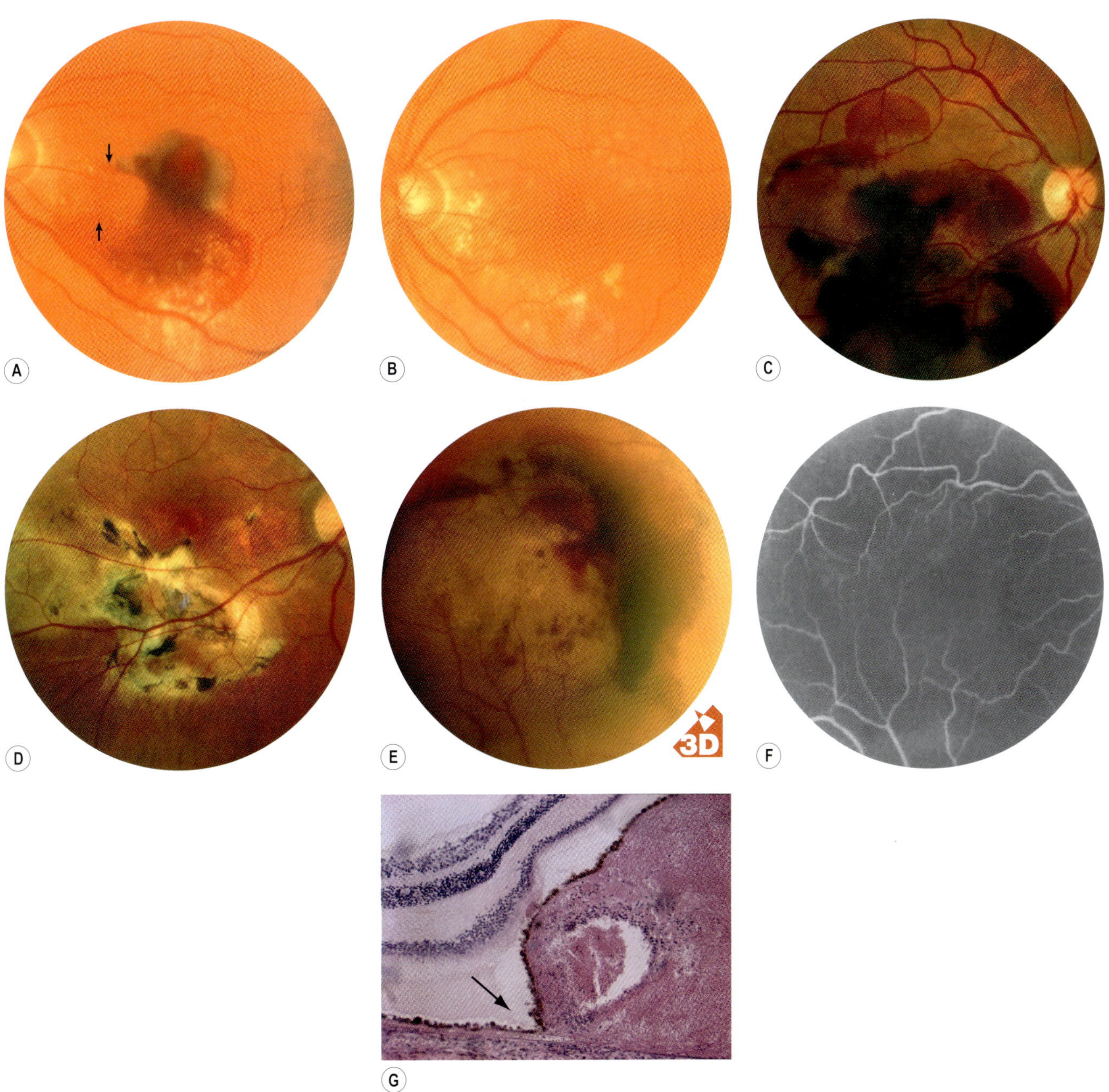
A
B
C
D
E
3D
F
G

Hemorrhagic Detachment of the RPE and Retina

Bleeding from the margin of a CNVM may be mild and cause only mild blurring of vision. Spontaneous rupture of a blood vessel usually near one margin of a CNVM, however, may cause sudden loss of central vision secondary to a large hemorrhagic detachment of the RPE and retina (Figures 3.24 and 3.25).[200] Initially the blood may be confined to the sub-RPE space and ophthalmoscopically may cause a dark, almost black, discretely elevated mound beneath the retina. Drusen are often evident on the surface of this mound. At the time of the hemorrhage or within a few days or weeks the blood dissects through the edge of the RPE detachment and spreads in a shallow layer into the subretinal space, where it often appears as a reddish halo at the margin of the RPE detachment (Figure 3.24). The dark appearance of blood beneath the RPE is caused by the moundlike collection of blood and not by its mere presence beneath the RPE. The reddish appearance of the surrounding subretinal blood is caused by the absence of the filtering effect of the RPE but also by the thinness of the layer of blood. Large mounds of blood, whether beneath the RPE or the retina or within the vitreous cavity, often have a black appearance. In a few patients during the early weeks after the bleeding episode there may be remarkable retention of visual function in spite of a large subfoveal hematoma.

3.25 Severe intraocular hemorrhage caused by age-related macular degeneration (AMD).

A–E: Three months after a large hemorrhagic detachment of the retina and retinal pigment epithelium (RPE) (A) in the left eye, this elderly man returned with blood staining of the vitreous (B) and iris (arrow, C). Over a 6-month period the vitreous cleared and the iris returned to its normal blue color (D). A large disciform scar was present in the macula (E).

F: Secondary subretinal hemorrhage occurring at the temporal edge of a disciform scar. Compare with J.

G and H: Extensive subretinal, suprachoroidal, and intravitreal bleeding occurring spontaneously in the left eye of an elderly patient with AMD and a disciform lesion in the right eye.

I: Massive subretinal and intravitreal hemorrhage caused by bleeding from a focal area of sub-RPE neovascularization in the macular area (arrow). This occurred in a 66-year-old man with essential hypertension, chronic lymphatic leukemia, and drusen in the macula of the opposite eye.

J: Secondary sub-RPE hemorrhage occurring at the temporal margin of an old disciform scar (arrow) in the macula of an elderly patient whose eye was misdiagnosed as having a malignant melanoma of the choroid.

(I and J from Gass.[200])

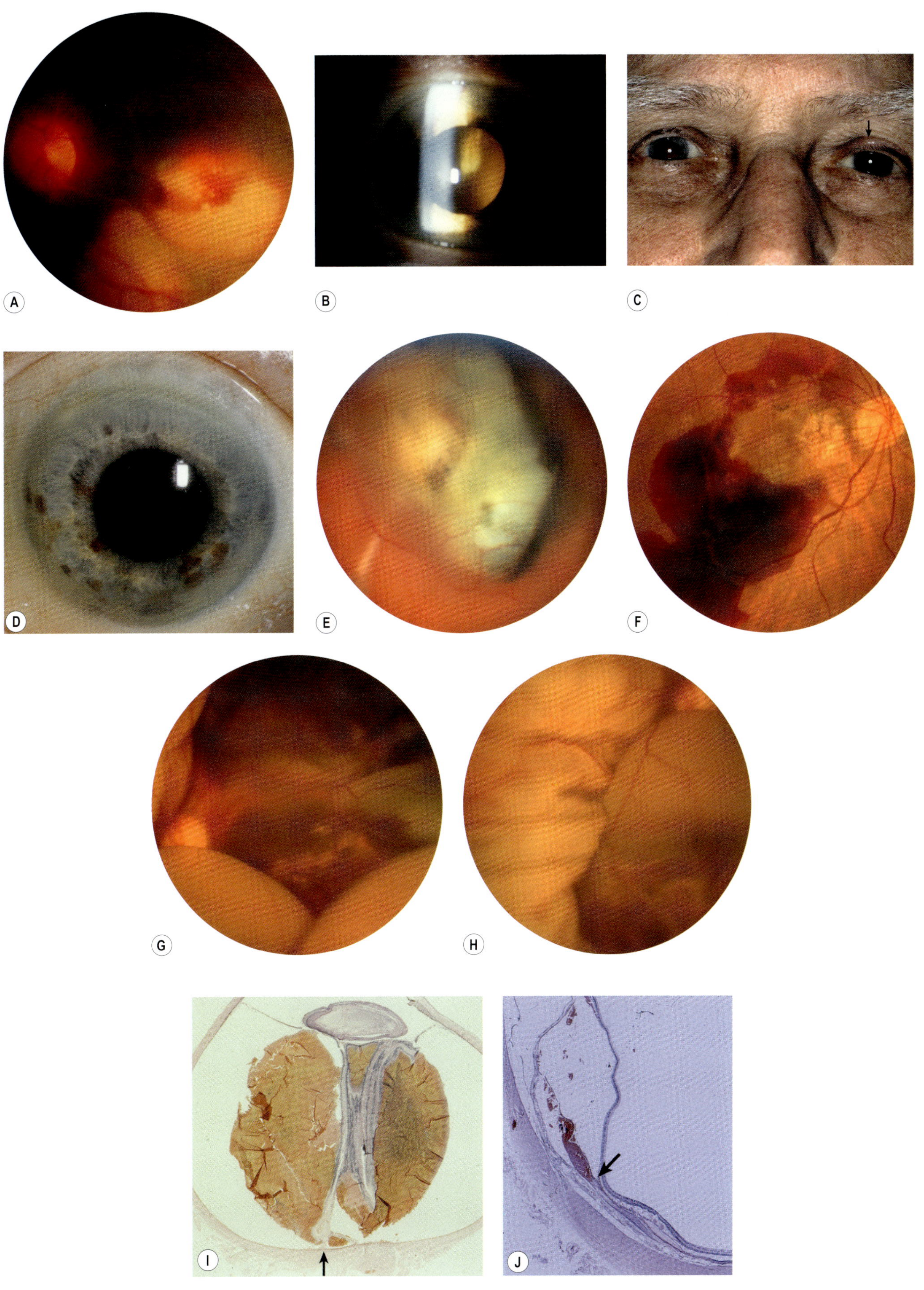
A
B
C
D
E
F
G
H
I
J

Blood in the subretinal and sub-RPE space typically obscures completely the underlying choroidal fluorescence and most or all of the fluorescein leaking from the neovascular complex (Figure 3.24). The absence of subretinal fluorescence serves to differentiate a dark mound of blood from a choroidal melanoma, which always shows evidence of late staining because of blood vessels near its surface (Figure 3.24E and F). Once bleeding occurs in the sub-RPE space, varying degrees of organization of the blood occur and there is usually extensive degeneration of both the overlying pigment epithelium and retina. Conversely, blood present in the subretinal space may reabsorb completely with variable and often minimal permanent damage to the structure and function of the overlying retina (Figure 3.24A and B).[353,354]

Many patients who develop large hemorrhagic macular detachments will experience transient loss of peripheral vision that in most cases is caused by diffusion of hemoglobin, rather than whole blood, into the vitreous several weeks or months after the hemorrhagic detachment occurs.[200] The fundus may be completely obscured from view for many months (Figure 3.26A–E). This process of anterior diffusion of hemoglobin across the relatively intact retina after damage to the outer barrier structures of the retina by the subretinal blood is similar to that which occurs in some patients after a massive hyphema with hemoglobin diffusing across damaged corneal endothelium and Descemet's membrane to cause blood staining of the cornea. The breakdown products of blood may stain not only the vitreous but also the iris stroma. This causes a yellow-brown discoloration of the vitreous and a noticeable heterochromia in lightly pigmented individuals (Figure 3.26B and C). Usually after 3–6 months or longer, as the blood pigment is phagocytosed, the iris regains its normal color, the vitreous clears, and the peripheral vision returns. Poor central vision and a large disciform scar are usually the end result (Figure 3.26E). In elderly patients presenting with intravitreal blood, AMD should always be considered as a possible cause.[200,355,356] Evidence of AMD in the opposite eye is an important clue to the correct diagnosis. Ultrasonographic demonstration of a mass of variable reflectivity in the macular area of these patients is helpful in excluding some of the other causes of vitreous hemorrhage.

3.26 Massive exudative and hemorrhagic detachment of the retinal pigment epithelium (RPE) and retina caused by pre-equatorial type I sub-RPE neovascularization.

A–C: This 83-year-old woman with macular drusen developed loss of central vision bilaterally because of posterior extension of subretinal lipid exudation arising in a large peripheral exudative and hemorrhagic subretinal neovascular complex (A and B). Laser photocoagulation and transscleral cryopexy were successful in destroying the new vessels and causing resolution of the submacular exudation (C).

D–F: Multiple areas of peripheral hemorrhagic detachment of the RPE and retina in an 87-year-old man with minimal evidence of macular degeneration.

G–J: Histopathologic findings in an elderly woman who initially had the same ophthalmoscopic findings seen in D–F. She developed massive sub-RPE, subretinal, and vitreous hemorrhage just before death while in the hospital. Arrow (G) indicates site of sub-RPE neovascular network and hemorrhage. Bleeding from a neovascular network lying along the inner side of Bruch's membrane (white arrows, H) near the equator was responsible for the hemorrhagic detachment of the RPE (black and white arrows). Note rupture of blood vessels in sub-RPE neovascular network (black arrows, I) internal to Bruch's membrane (white arrows). J shows sub-RPE neovascular network (black arrows) on the inner surface of the Bruch's membrane (white arrows) in another area of the same eye.

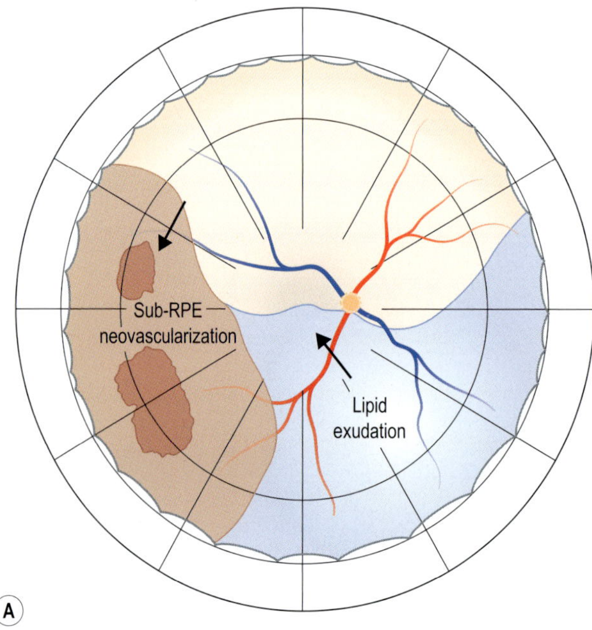

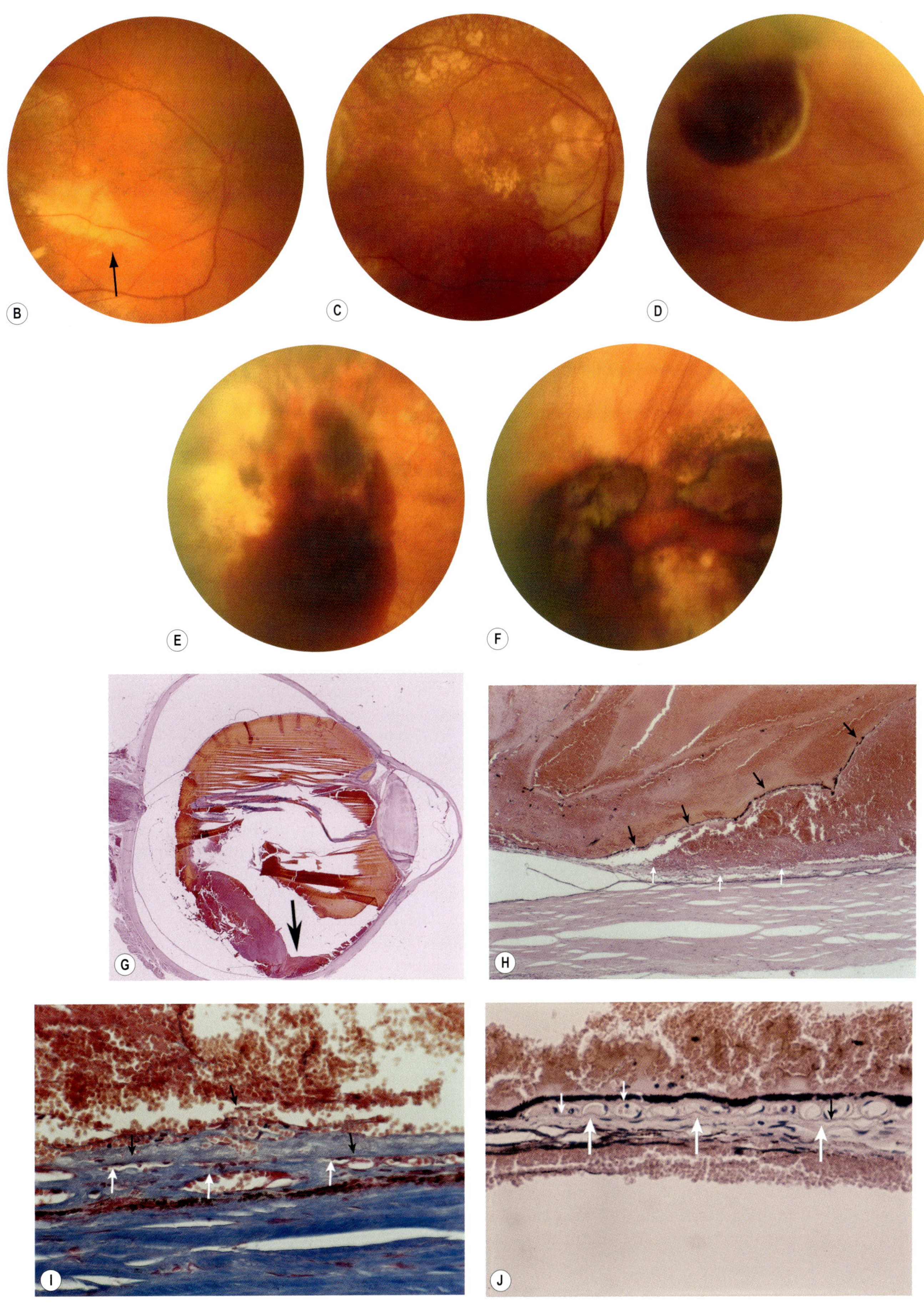
B
C
D
E
F
G
H
I
J

In patients with moderate to large areas of hemorrhagic detachment of the RPE and retina, photocoagulation is often not effective because the blood obscures at least part of the CNVM from view. In cases where the bleeding appears to have occurred from one edge of the CNVM and where the configuration of the CNVM suggests that it does not extend far beneath the blood, photocoagulation of the CNVM with a long-wavelength laser may be of some value.

Chronic Exudative and Hemorrhagic Stages

Once the process of exudation and hemorrhage begins, the CNVM usually continues to enlarge, often in a concentric manner. Oozing of blood cells from the outer dilated margin of the CNVM occurs frequently and is responsible for the flecks of subretinal blood that may intermittently appear at its margins (Figure 3.27A). The dark irregular areas often seen angiographically at the edge of these sub-RPE membranes, even in the absence of biomicroscopic evidence of blood, are probably caused by breakdown products of blood accumulating there. The yellow exudate that occurs in the outer retinal layers and subretinal space peripheral to the area of choroidal neovascularization is caused by precipitation of the lipid component of the exudate as water is drawn into the normal blood vessels of the retina and choroid (see pp. 46–47). The expanding neovascular complex causes nutritional damage to the outer layers of the overlying retina, and once the membrane has grown beneath the center of the fovea, loss of useful central vision is usual, but not always a certainty. Involution of this neovascular process may occur at any stage of its development and typically occurs within several years. Approximately 70% of eyes that develop detachment caused by a CNVM extending into the capillary-free zone of the retina will have a visual acuity of 20/200 or less within 1 year.[308]

Cicatricial Stage

Involution of the neovascular complex eventually occurs and is associated with varying degrees of subretinal scar tissue, depending primarily on the duration and extent of hemorrhage and exudation (Figure 3.27). In some cases, neovascularization extending throughout the macula may be associated with minimal reactive hyperplasia and fibrous metaplasia of the RPE, and the large neovascular membrane after involution may be difficult or impossible to demonstrate biomicroscopically or angiographically. In some cases the larger radial vascular trunks of the involuted membranes may be visible as red vessels superimposed over the usually partly yellow-colored larger choroidal vessels (Figure 3.27D–F). The slow rate of blood flow in these involuted neovascular membranes may prevent their demonstration angiographically. Angiography may demonstrate nothing more than a circular area of mottled or early hyperfluorescence and minimal or no staining. In some cases, cystoid macular edema and degeneration may be present overlying flat, difficult-to-detect, involuted neovascular membranes that extend into the center of the fovea (see pp. 42–43).

Following development of a large hemorrhagic detachment of the RPE and retina, degradation of the blood beneath the RPE usually causes a brown or yellowish sub-RPE mass to form (Figure 3.24E). The blood in the subretinal space surrounding the RPE detachment often requires a longer period of time before a color change is noted and before the blood is degraded (Figure 3.27A). There is a gradual organization of the sub-RPE blood and exudate by further ingrowth of new vessels and fibroblasts from the choroid (Figure 3.27G). Eventually the exudative mass may be replaced by fibrous tissue containing varying degrees of hyperplastic RPE (Figure 3.27B, C, and H). The cicatricial lesions vary in color from white to brown or even to black and may be mistaken for choroidal melanomas (Figure 3.27B). Often anastomosis between the retinal circulation and underlying choroidal circulation develops within these old disciform scars (Figure 3.27C).[200,357,358] There is a general tendency for the development of a similar pattern and size of disciform detachment in the fellow eye.[359] Fluorescein angiography in the cicatricial stages of disciform detachment demonstrates a wide variety of pictures, some of which may be similar to that produced by choroidal neoplasms.

3.27 Reparative and cicatricial stages of disciform macular detachment in patients with drusen.

A: Partial resolution of hemorrhagic detachment of the retinal pigment epithelium (RPE) and retina. Note evidence of degradation of the blood lying beneath the RPE (arrows). There has been little change in the subretinal blood that surrounds the RPE detachment (see G).

B: Partly organized, pigmented subretinal disciform mass (arrows) stimulating a melanoma.

C: Large, white fibrovascular disciform scar with retinochoroidal anastomosis (arrow).

D–F: Bilateral patchy fibrous proliferation and diffuse atrophy of the retinal pigment epithelium with extracellular pigment clumps (D and E). The autofluorescence image reveals the diffuse loss of RPE resulting partly from atrophy and partly from retraction by the fibrovascular tissue (F).

G: Photomicrograph of hemorrhagic detachment of the RPE and retina in a patient similar to A. Blood in the sub-RPE space has undergone greater degradation than that in the subretinal space.

H: Photomicrograph of a pigmented vascularized subretinal scar following hemorrhagic detachment of the RPE and retina. Note degeneration of the outer retinal layers and degeneration and proliferation of the RPE overlying fibrovascular scar. Arrows indicate Bruch's membrane.

(C from Gass[283]; G and H from Gass.[200])

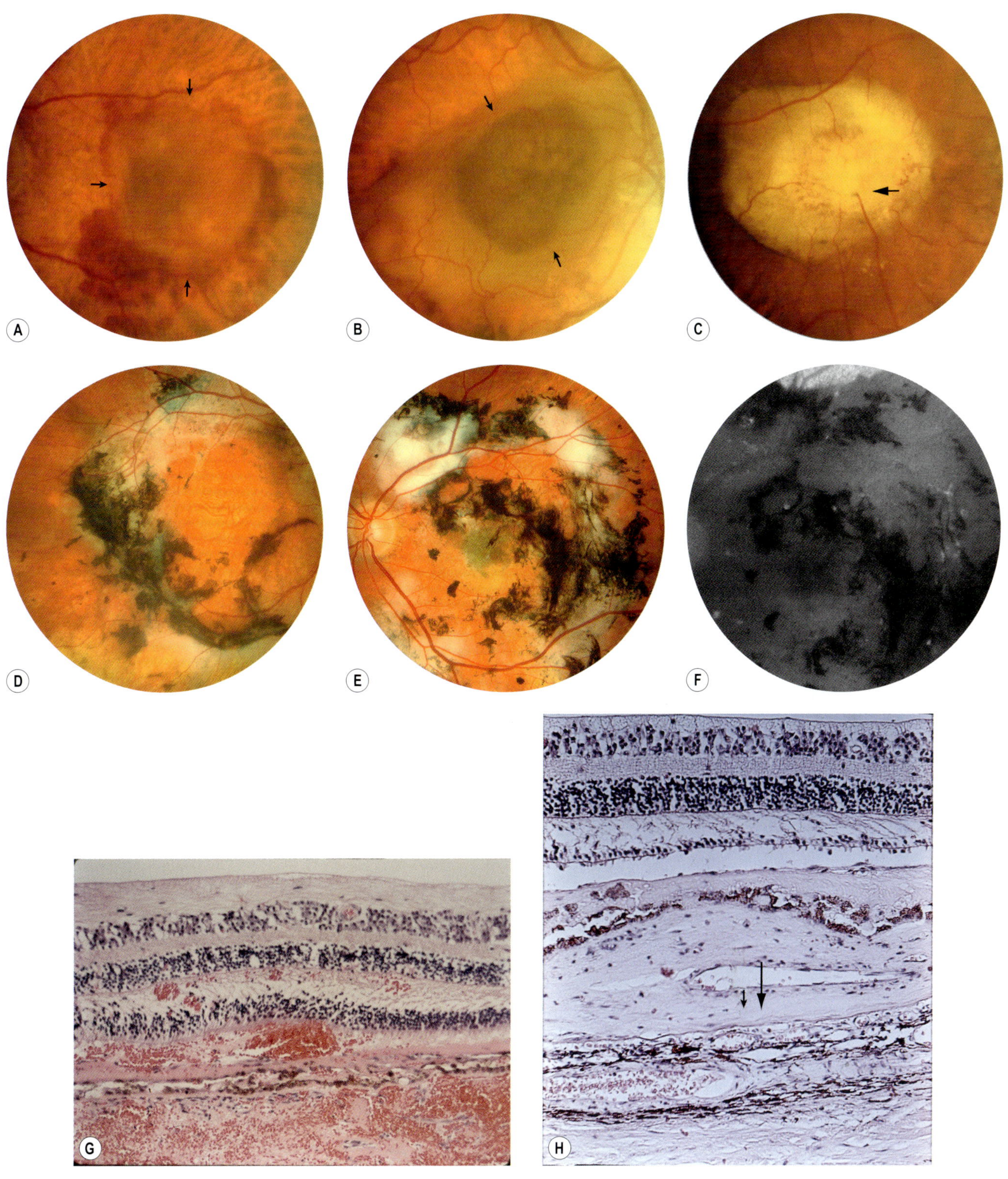
A
B
C
D
E
F
G
H

Massive Exudative Detachment of the Retina (Senile Coats' Syndrome)

In most patients with drusen, the area of disciform detachment is confined to the macular area and peripheral vision is maintained. A few patients, however, show progressive exudative detachment of the retina that spreads far beyond the macular region and may cause severe loss of peripheral as well as central vision (Figure 3.28D–J).[200,360,361] Multifocal areas of eccentric choroidal neovascularization and serous detachment of the RPE and retina may occur.[200,362] Extensive deposition of yellowish exudate occurs in the subretinal space and in the outer layers of the retina. It typically spreads initially in an inferior direction. The fundus may resemble that usually seen in younger patients with massive yellowish exudative detachment of the retina secondary to congenital telangiectasis of the retinal vessels (the most common cause of Coats' syndrome in young patients). The cause of this unusual degree of exudation from the choroid in these elderly patients is unknown. The exudate may eventually resolve spontaneously, but it leaves in its wake marked widespread degenerative changes in the RPE and retina. Retinal neovascularization and vitreous hemorrhage may arise as complications of the chronic exudative detachment.

Bullous Serous Retinal Detachment

Rarely these patients will develop massive bullous serous detachment of the retina caused by chronic leakage of serous exudate from large, highly vascularized RPE detachments or disciform mounds that are usually located in or near the macular area (Figure 3.28D–J). Long-duration, moderately intense, large-size applications of laser photocoagulation to these fibrovascular RPE detachments, occasionally photodynamic therapy and anti-VEGF therapy may cause reattachment of the retina and return of ambulatory vision (Figure 3.28).

Secondary Hemorrhage from a Disciform Scar

A secondary exudative or hemorrhagic detachment of the RPE can develop around the edge of an old disciform scar and produce a lesion adjacent to the scar that on occasion may cause the physician to remove the eye because of a suspected melanoma (Figure 3.25F and J).[200]

Other Complications of Choroidal Neovascularization

Vitreous Hemorrhage

The initial hemorrhage from CNVMs may dissect its way into the retina where it is visible biomicroscopically as a focal intraretinal hemorrhage. The bleeding may be sufficiently intense that blood may break through the retina into the vitreous and cause a massive vitreous hemorrhage (Figure 3.01).[200,355,356] This process of dissection of blood through a defect in the retina is different from that of blood staining of the vitreous, which occurs more frequently in these patients as a delayed phenomenon following large hemorrhagic detachments of the RPE and retina (see previous discussion).

3.28 Massive exudative retinal detachment (Coats' syndrome) caused by age-related macular degeneration.

A and **B**: Right eye of patient with large disciform detachment and subretinal and intraretinal lipid exudation that extended to the ora serrata inferiorly.

C: Histopathology of massive lipoproteinaceous subretinal exudation overlying a large macular and juxtapapillary choroidal neovascular complex in an elderly patient with age-related macular degeneration.

D–J: Massive exudative bullous retinal detachment caused by a large, orange, organized extramacular retinal pigment epithelium (RPE) detachment (arrows, D–H) in the right eye of a 74-year-old man whose left eye was blind from rubeotic glaucoma caused by a similar massive exudative retinal detachment complicating age-related macular degeneration. Note that the organized RPE detachment located temporal to a white disciform scar showed minimal evidence of fluorescein staining (arrows, E–G). Argon photocoagulation was placed on the surface of the organized RPE detachment (arrows, I) and was successful in causing resolution of the bullous retinal detachment and restoration of ambulatory vision 4 months after treatment (J).

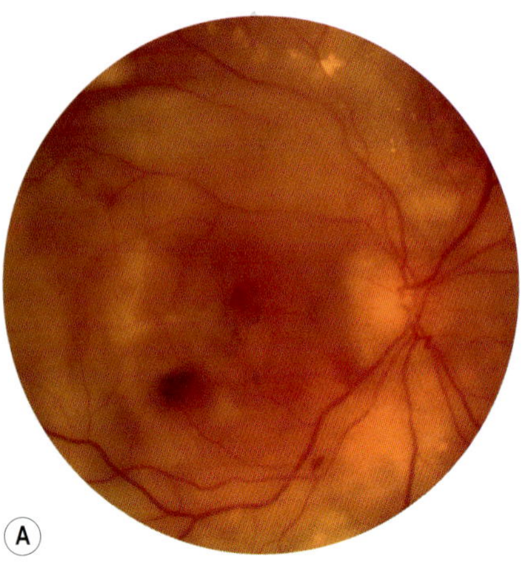

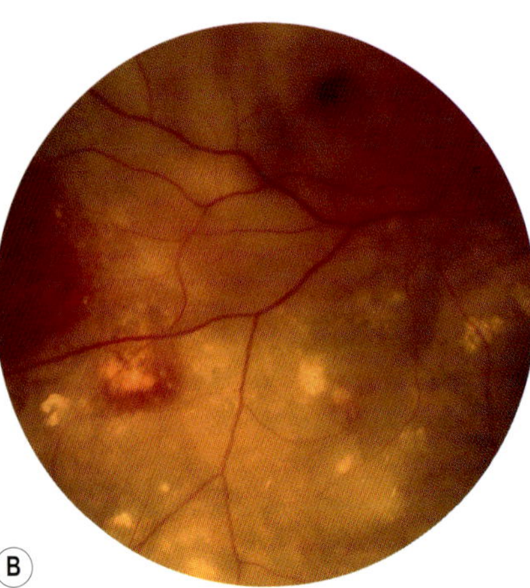

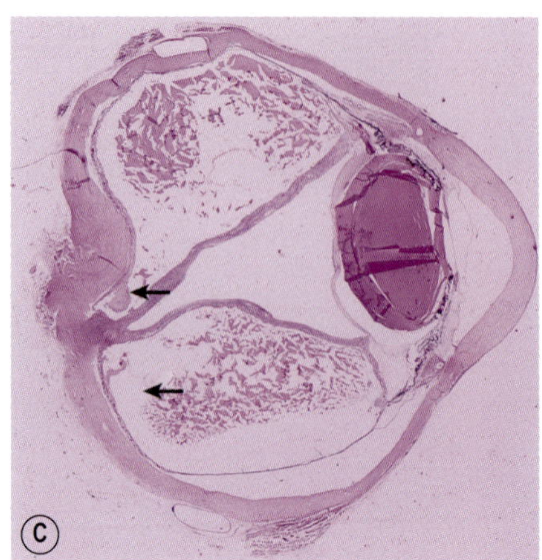

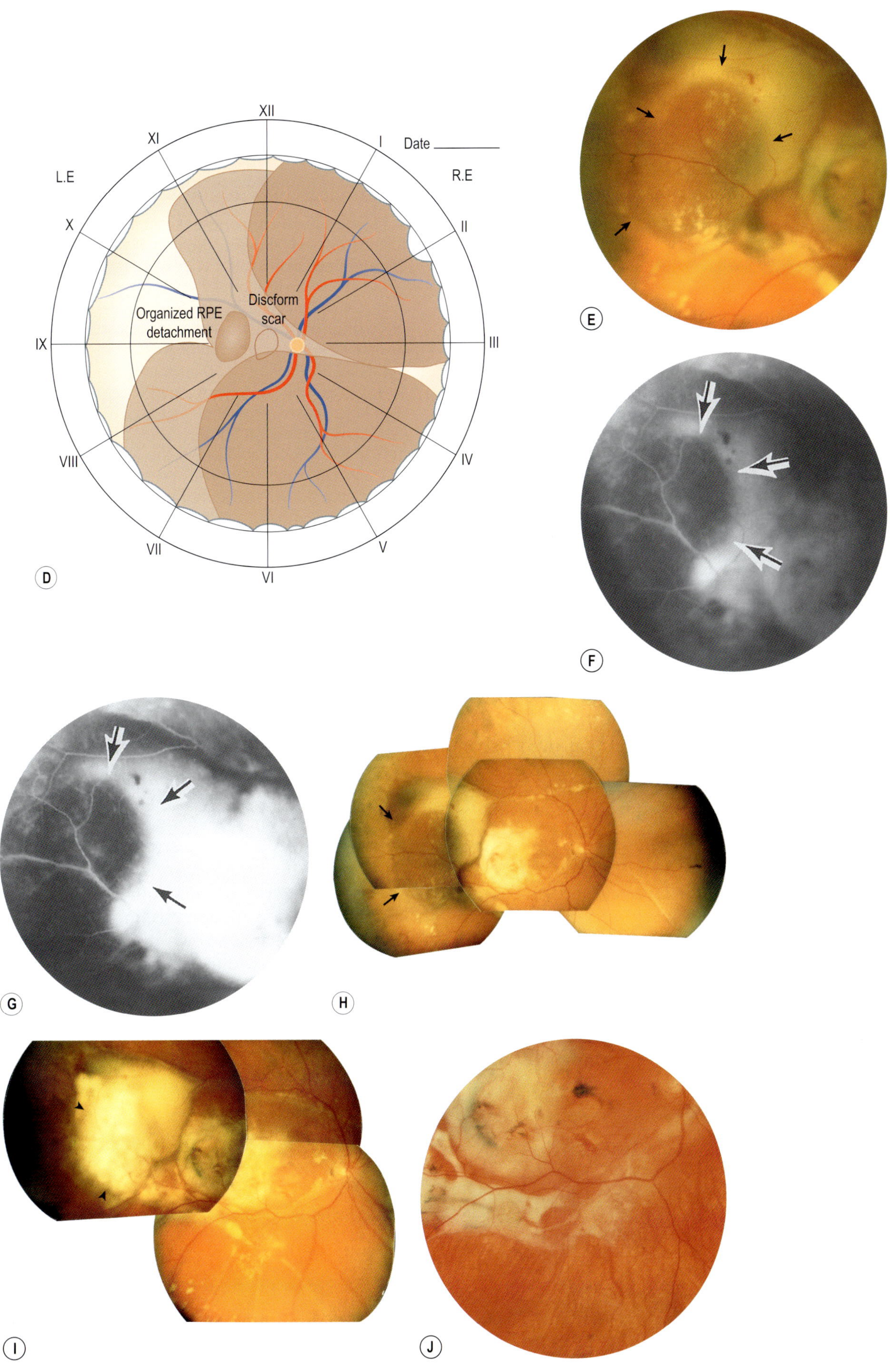
XII
I
Date
XI
L.E
R.E
X
II
Organized RPE
detachment
Discform
scar
IX
III
VIII
IV
VII
V
VI
D
E
F
G
H
I
J

Massive Hemorrhagic Detachment of the RPE and Retina

Rarely hemorrhage from a CNVM in the macular region may produce a massive detachment of the RPE, retina, and choroid, as well as vitreous hemorrhage, closed-angle glaucoma, and loss of the eye.[363] This is more likely to occur in patients receiving anticoagulant therapy or with a systemic disease affecting the clotting mechanism (Figure 3.25G–I).[200]

Peripheral Exudative and Hemorrhagic Disciform Detachment

Elderly patients with macular drusen or without evidence of AMD may develop serous and hemorrhagic detachment of the retina secondary to one or more sites of sub-RPE neovascularization in the equatorial or pre-equatorial area, usually in the temporal half of the eye (Figure 3.26). Large areas of serous or dark-colored hemorrhagic detachment of the RPE in the periphery may be mistaken for a choroidal melanoma because of the detachment's unusual peripheral location.[200,362,364] Many of these patients will show some evidence of peripheral sub-RPE neovascularization in the temporal portion of the opposite eye. These detachments will usually resolve spontaneously without treatment. In those cases complicated either by bullous exudative retinal detachment or by extension of yellowish exudate derived from the neovascular network into the macula, photocoagulation or cryotherapy may be beneficial (Figure 3.26A–C). Peripheral sub-RPE neovascularization frequently develops as part of the normal aging process in the peripheral fundus and is derived primarily from the ciliary body rather than the choroid (Figure 3.26).[251,255,365] (See discussion of peripheral idiopathic choroidal neovascularization, p. 140.)

Geographic or Central Areolar RPE Atrophy

Although most patients with drusen lose useful central vision because of complications of choroidal neovascularization, approximately 5–10% lose central vision as a result of the development of one or occasionally more sharply circumscribed geographic areas of atrophy of the RPE and retina in the posterior pole (Figure 3.29).[200,250,252,307,317,320,366,367] Dehydration and calcific crystallization of drusen are often the forerunners of geographic atrophy that may begin either centrally or paracentrally. Loss of central vision occurs slowly and progressively as the area of atrophy concentrically enlarges. A similar pattern of atrophy is often seen in the second eye. Approximately 20% of these patients, however, who develop geographic atrophy in one eye will develop choroidal neovascularization and its complications in the second eye.[200] Fluorescein angiography shows varying degrees of loss of the choriocapillaris within the area of geographic atrophy (Figure 3.29G and H). Histologically the area of geographic atrophy is associated with focal loss of the retinal receptor cells and RPE and varying degrees of atrophy of the choriocapillaris (Figure 3.29K and L).

3.29 Geographic atrophy in patients with macular drusen.

A–C: Gradual enlargement of area of geographic atrophy occurred in a 63-year-old man over a 6-year period. Visual acuity in A was 20/60 and in C was 20/200. Note changing pattern of drusen, some of which are calcified (arrows).
D–F: In 1970 this 61-year-old woman presented with bilateral large drusen and a serous detachment of the retinal pigment epithelium (RPE) (arrows, D) in both eyes. Note the scalloped border of the RPE detachment resulting from confluence of large drusen. Visual acuity was 20/30 bilaterally. The right eye was treated with laser applications to the margin of the RPE detachment. The RPE detachment in the left eye spontaneously collapsed and was replaced by a pattern of geographic atrophy that changed very little between 1974 (E) and 1985 (F), at which time both fundi looked similar and the visual acuity was 20/50 bilaterally.
G–J: Geographic atrophy of the RPE in a 71-year-old woman with large drusen. Similar changes were present in the fellow eye. Early angiogram showed evidence of partial preservation of the choriocapillaris in the area of geographic atrophy (H). Late angiogram showed staining of the choroid (I). Several years later many of the drusen have faded and the area of geographic atrophy has enlarged. Note calcification of some of the drusen (arrows).
K and L: Geographic atrophy in a 65-year-old man with drusen. His visual acuity was 3/200 in the right eye and 20/80 in the left eye 4 months before he died. Histopathologic examination revealed a sharp margin between the relatively normal retina and choroid and a zone of absence of the outer retinal layers and RPE (L). There was partial closure of the choriocapillaris in the region of the geographic atrophy.

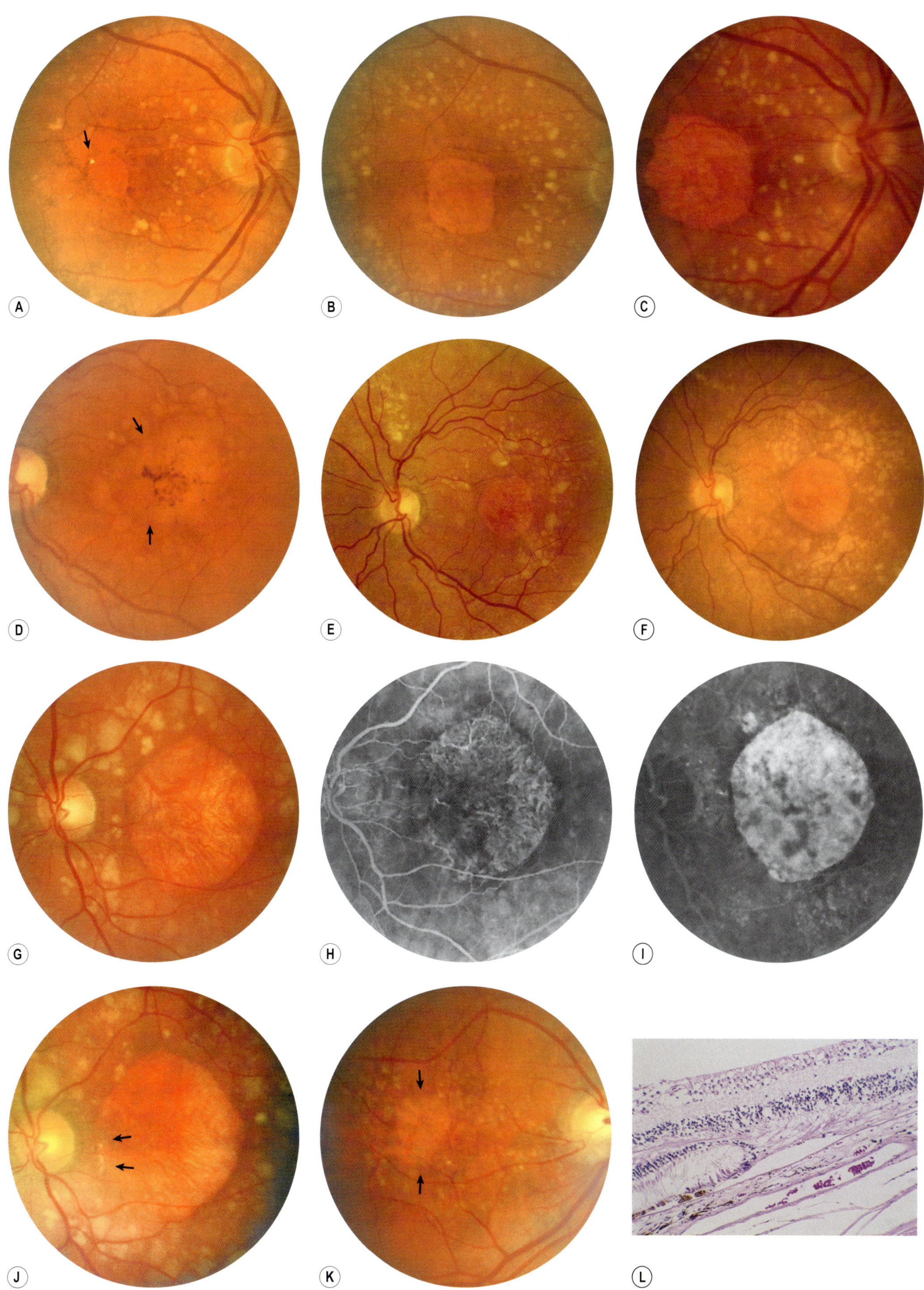
A
B
C
D
E
F
G
H
I
J
K
L

The pathogenesis of these sharply circumscribed areas of atrophy is not understood. It is not known whether the partial obstruction and atrophy of the choriocapillaris are the primary cause of, or the result of, the overlying RPE and retinal atrophy. Geographic atrophy of the RPE, retina, and choriocapillaris is an ophthalmoscopic finding that occurs in association with many other diseases, including Sorsby's central areolar choroidal sclerosis, basal laminar drusen, Stargardt's disease, Best's vitelliform macular dystrophy, cone dystrophies, rod–cone dystrophies, chloroquine retinopathy, ICSC, and traumatic maculopathy. In patients with AMD, geographic atrophy may develop in at least the following three ways: (1) with no precursor lesion other than macular drusen; (2) following an acute tear in the RPE (see pp. 108–111); and (3) following collapse of a long-standing serous RPE detachment.

Prognosis

Most patients with macular drusen never experience significant loss of central vision. The average age when they develop loss of central vision in the first eye is approximately 65 years.[210,259,318,368] These patients will lose central vision in the second eye at a rate of approximately 5–10% each year thereafter. Thus many patients who have visual loss in one eye will never experience visual loss in the second eye. Nevertheless, AMD is the leading cause of legal blindness not amenable to surgery in the USA and the UK.

Etiology and Pathogenesis

Our lack of knowledge concerning the cause of AMD and macular degeneration parallels our inability to alter its natural course. The only established factors of importance regarding causation of this disease relate to age, race, and heredity.[185,212,369] The breakthrough in relating genetics to AMD occurred in 2005 with the discovery of complement factor H (*CFH*) variant in 43–50% of patients with AMD by three groups.[370–372] Since then, other genetic risk factors, including ARMS 2 (*HTRA1*), complement factor B (C2), and C3 have been found to be variously associated with the risk of AMD.[373–379] *Fibulin 5* and *ABCA4* render a risk in less than 5% of AMD patients.[380–386] The *CFH* variant has been studied extensively in various population groups and seems to be most commonly associated with AMD. However, preliminary data suggest that *ARMS2* may be more specific in rendering severity to the condition. Complement activation occurs as a result of inflammation and healing, which may be the underlying mechanism contributing to the constituents of drusen.[387,388]

3.30 Treatment of exudative age-related macular degeneration.

A–G: This 67-year-old man presented with a serous pigment epithelial detachment and a notch with a visual decline to 20/50 that could be corrected to 20/25 with a hyperopic shift. Angiogram confirmed the serous detachment with a hot spot at its superior edge (B and C). Optical coherence tomography revealed subretinal fibrosis (SRF) adjacent to the retinal pigment epithelium detachment (D). He subsequently underwent 26 Lucentis injections in this eye over 3 years. After injection 15 he developed *Staphylococcus epidermidis* endophthalmitis and received intravitreal antibiotics and dexamethasone. Persisting inflammation led to a pars plana vitrectomy and lensectomy 3 days later. Intravitreal Lucentis was continued for further 11 injections and a total of 26 for mild persistent SRF (E). Two and three years later his vision is still 20/25– with a persisting PED and no SRF (F and G). Note the good retinal thickness, which accounts for the 20/25 vision. In the meanwhile the left eye also developed a combined serous/fibrovascular pigment epithelial detachment and received 11 Lucentis injections. Vision remains at 20/20 in the left with a hyperopic shift in spite of an extrafoveal retinal pigment epithelium rip.

H–L: One week post pars plana vitrectomy and gas displacement of subretinal blood in this 82-year-old woman reveals an occult membrane with late punctate staining (I and J). Note the clearing of blood in the center (H). She was continued on anti-vascular endothelial growth factor injections, and developed a new larger subretinal hematoma after two further injections (K). A repeat vitrectomy with tissue plasminogen activator (tpa) injection displaced the blood temporally and inferiorly (L). She maintained moderate vision for a few months but eventually developed a disciform scar in spite of continued treatment.

Other environmental and health factors and biochemical alterations of possible importance as either causative or aggravating factors include: exposure to sunlight,[389–396] cigarette smoking,[397–399] female hormone replacement therapy,[400] systemic hypertension,[401] anticoagulation,[402,403] dermal elastosis of exposed skin surfaces,[404] low levels of serum carotenoids,[397,398] elevated serum cholesterol[397,398] and serum zinc and copper,[405] low levels of serum selenium[406] and serum ceruloplasm,[345,407] high hematocrit,[408] high white cell blood count,[408] hyperopia,[409] increased scleral rigidity,[410] autoantibodies to retina and retinal astrocytes,[411,412] decreased levels of catalase activity in the RPE,[244] decreased levels of hyaluronic acid in the chorioretinal complex,[413] and use of anticoagulants.[403] Much is being discovered and a lot remains to be understood regarding the pathogenesis of AMD in relation to genetic and environment risk factors, and is outside the scope of this clinical text.

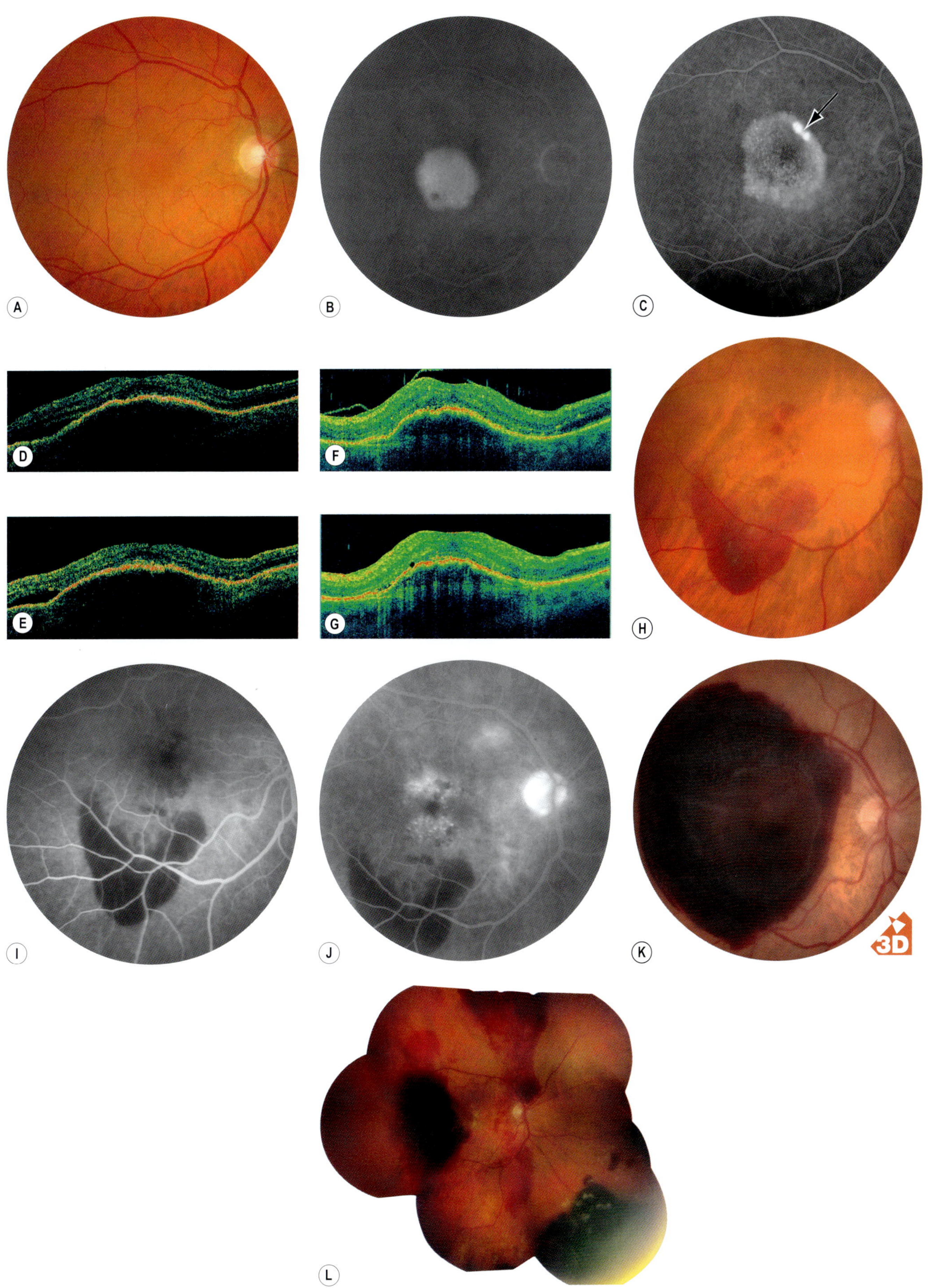
A
B
C
D
F
H
E
G
I
J
K
3D
L

Reticular Pseudodrusen

Reticular pseudodrusen (RPD) (Figure 3.31) is a yellowish interlacing pattern seen best in red-free or blue light, most often seen straddling the superotemporal arcades, but can be present through out the macula, across the infero-temporal arcade and nasal to the optic disc.[292,412a,412b,412c,412d] Early on, it is made up of several punctate yellow dots, that evolve into an interlacing pattern. It is not usually visible on fluorescein angiography, and correlation with autofluorescence and spectral domain OCT shows the deposits to lie between the retinal pigment epithelium and the photoreceptors (Figure 3.31L).[412e,412f,412g,412h] Even though pseudodrusen is seen most often in patients with ARMD, it can sometimes be seen in eyes with no other abnormality. Though several papers describe it to be a feature of advanced AMD, mostly neovascular, this author has seen pseudodrusen to be distributed over all grades of ARMD (Figure 3.31H to K), and even in eyes without ARMD. The incidence of RPD is underestimated as it can often be overlooked especially in eyes with some degree of cataract or subretinal fluid, and also early in its evolution before it has developed the interlacing pattern. At the present time, the complete significance of RPD in relation to severity of, and association with genetic markers of ARMD is not fully understood.

Figure 3.31 Reticular pseudodrusen.

Unilateral pseudodrusen.

A and B: 82-year-old male with mostly intermediate drusen in the fovea (grade 2 age-related macular degeneration (AMD)) and pseudodrusen in the superior half of the macula (A). The left eye had occult choroidal neovascular membrane (CNVM) (grade 5) with no pseudodrusen (B).

Bilateral symmetric pseudodrusen with advanced AMD.

C–E: This 77-year-old woman had a vision of 20/70 in the right and 20/50 in the left eye. Extensive pseudodrusen were seen symmetrically distributed in the two eyes (C and D). The right eye had a disciform scar and the left an occult CNVM. The red-free image of the left eye demonstrates the pseudodrusen well (E).

F and G: This 90-year-old woman has bilateral active choroidal neovascularization, the left eye demonstrating occult chorioretinal anastomosis (intraretinal hemorrhage, G). The pseudodrusen is distributed in the superior macula straddling the superotemporal arcade and extends nasal to the disc in both eyes (arrows).

H and I: Bilateral pseudodrusen with mild AMD (grade 1a). Both eyes show pseudodrusen that is symmetrically distributed superior to the disc with very few small punctate drusen in each eye.

J and K: Pseudodrusen visible on color photos and red-free images, with intermediate drusen visible only on the color photos.

L: Pseudodrusen localize to the photoreceptor layer on optical coherence tomography seen just anterior to the retinal pigment epithelium (arrows).

(A and B courtesy of Dr. Franco Recchia; C–E courtesy of Dr. Paul Sternberg.)

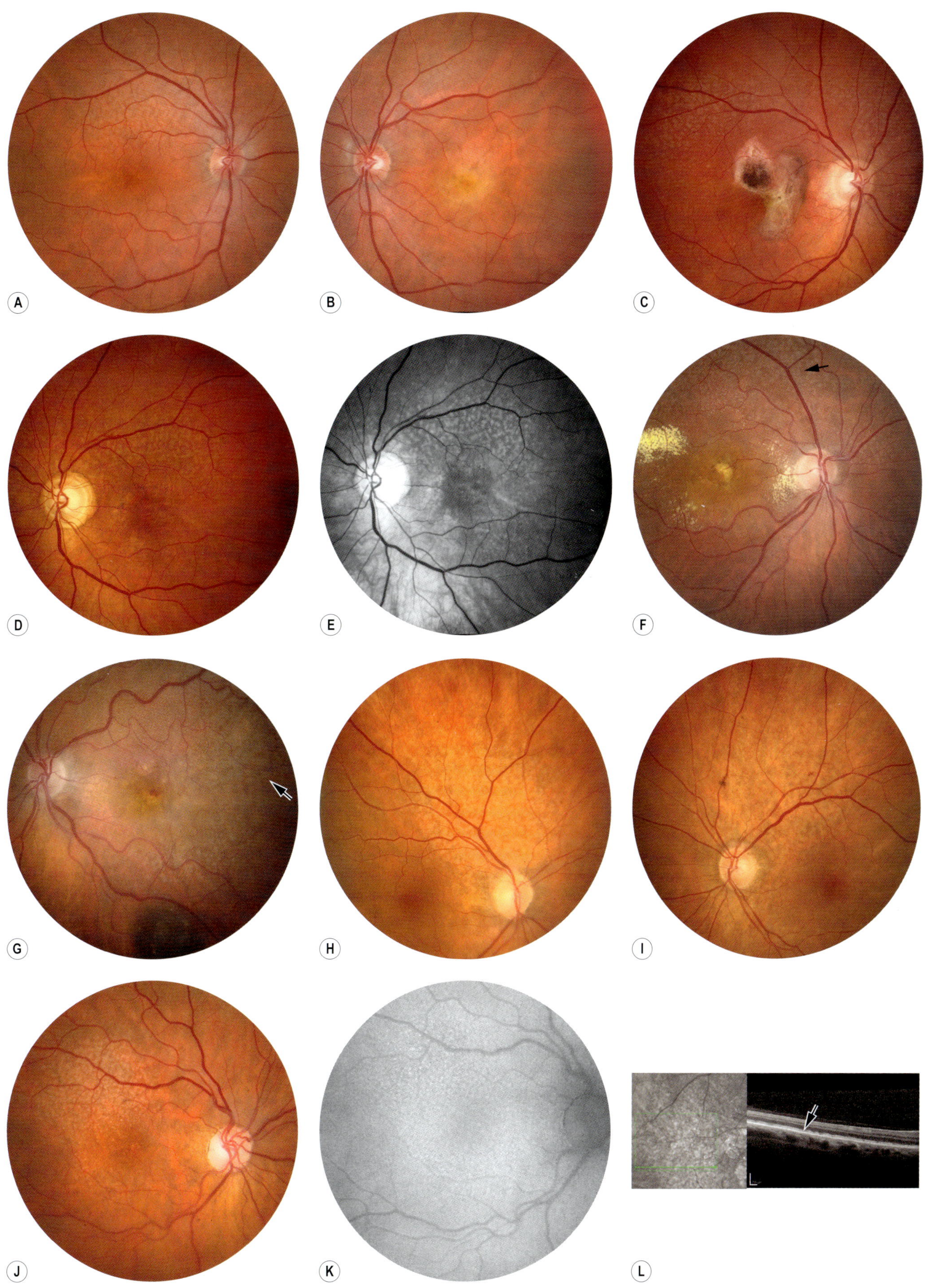
A
B
C
D
E
F
G
H
I
J
K
L

Occult Chorioretinal Anastamosis

The presence of small intraretinal hemorrhages in eyes with drusen and other features of agerelated macular degeneration as a sign of occult chorioretinal anastamosis was brought to attention by work of Soubrane and Coscas.[292] Debate has ensued about the site of origin and evolution of the chorioretinal anastamosis since Yannuzzi coined the term retinal angiomatous proliferation (RAP).[412i] He describes the vascular malformation to arise in the inner retina and grow vertically downwards towards the RPE and eventually reach the space between the RPE and Bruch's membrane where it spreads horizontally. At this stage, pigment epithelial detachment may be seen. Others believe that a loss in the photoreceptors from AMD brings the inner retinal vessels in closer proximity to diseased RPE/choriocapillaris complex that induces growth of bridging vessels to communicate with occult choroidal neovascular vessels possibly already present in that location.[412j] At our present understanding, it is likely both mechanisms play a role in different eyes, suffice to say that management of these eyes is difficult; laser photocoagulation, PDT and anti VEGF agents have all been used. It is likely that the best results are obtained if we recognize its presence early in the course and use anti VEGF agents (see case illustrated in Figure 3.32).[412k,412l,412m] Often the occult anastamosis is bilateral and looking for the small focal retinal hemorrhages in the fellow eye is vital.[412j]

3.32 Occult chorioretinal anastomosis (OCRA).

A–I: This 80-year-old woman was evaluated for metamorphopsia and decrease in her right eye vision to 20/200. She was found to have exudative age-related macular degeneration with an occult choroidal neovascular membrane in her right eye. The vision in the left eye was 20/20 and careful examination revealed two (one smaller than the other) intraretinal dot hemorrhages temporal to the foveal center that are also seen on the red-free image (A and B, arrows). Optical coherence tomography (OCT) through the red hemorrhage revealed an intraretinal channel extending towards the retinal pigment epithelium (C). Due to shadowing the remaining course of the channel is not visible. She was advised intravitreal bevacizumab, but did not receive it by the referring retina specialist. Three months later the hemorrhage appears more prominent and her vision is still stable at 20/20 (D, arrow). OCT reveals the communicating vessel. She was started on monthly injections of bevacizumab, and the red lesion became very small; the second one disappeared 4 months later (F). Six (G) and 18 months later (H) only the superficial intraretinal component remains on OCT. Two further years later she is still stable with vision of 20/25– from a cataract (I). A month after this picture was taken she developed active leakage and received intravitreal bevacizumab, the membrane and vision stabilized after six injections and her vision remains at 20/30–.

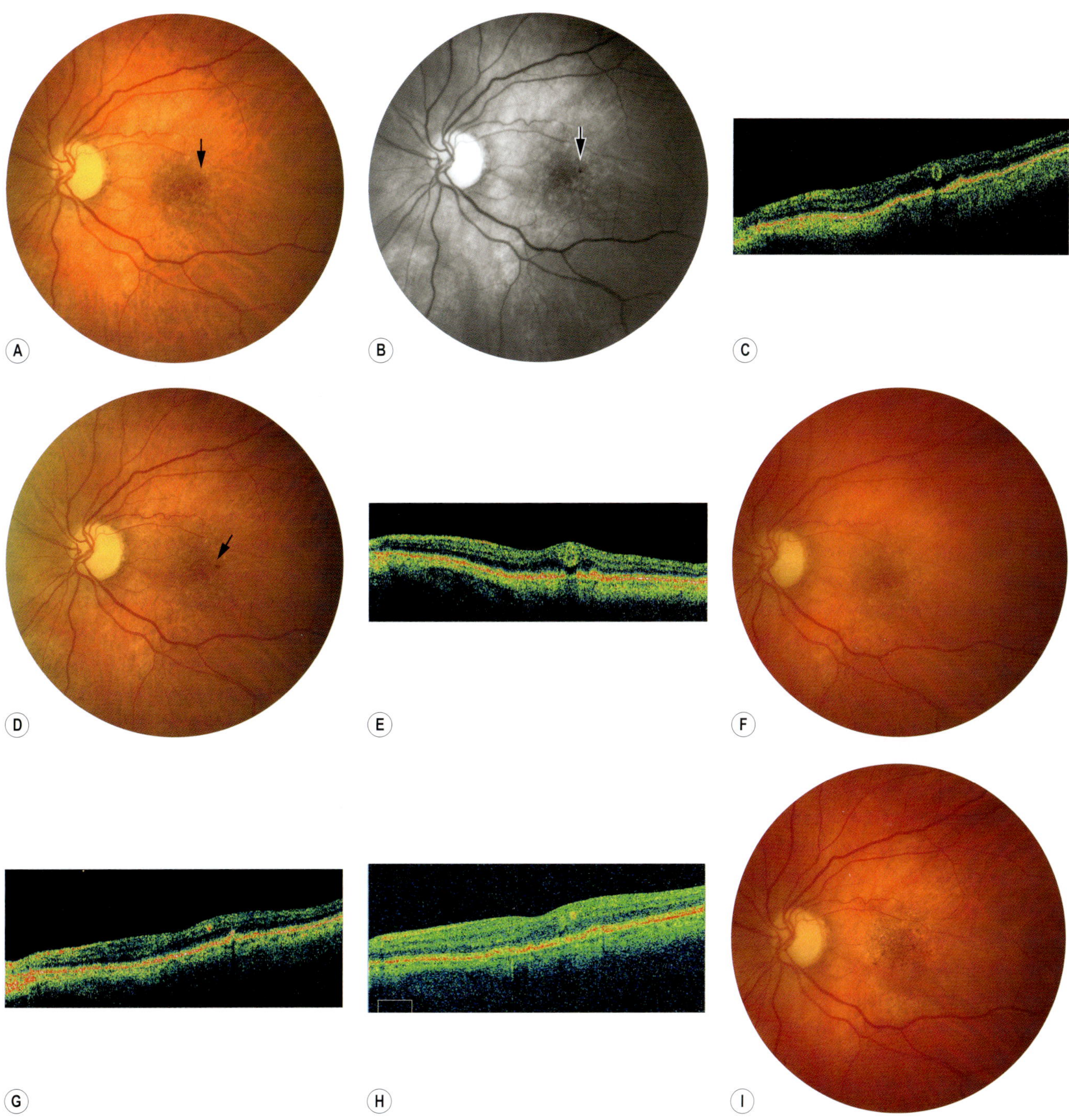
A
B
C
D
E
F
G
H
I

Treatment

Many authors have reported the possible benefit of photocoagulation in treating the neovascular complications of AMD.[127,128,133,175,210,246,284,319,324,331,358,365,414–439] Randomized controlled clinical trials have convincingly demonstrated that argon blue-green laser and krypton red laser treatment is of value in the treatment of well-defined CNVMs in the parafoveal (outside the capillary-free zone), juxtafoveal (inside but not beneath the center of the capillary-free zone), and subfoveal membranes in patients with AMD.[205,206,332,434,440–449] These studies have also demonstrated the value of laser photocoagulation in the treatment of persistent and recurrent CNVM.[422,450,451] Unfortunately the great majority of patients with AMD present because of loss of vision caused by ill-defined or extensive subretinal neovascular lesions where there are no guidelines for treatment.[278,452] In 2000, photodynamic therapy was introduced to treat classic subfoveal CNVM. Approximately 54% showed stabilization and less than 15 letters of visual loss (severe visual loss); however this treatment did not restore or improve vision in more than 7–9% of patients.

Since the introduction of intravitreal ranibizumab, a Fc component of anti-VEGF antibody, visual recovery and stabilization have been seen in up to 38% of patients with neovascular AMD at the end of 2 years. MARINA and ANCHOR trials established the success of this treatment in both classic and occult CNVM.[453–458] Since then bevacizumab, which is the complete antibody to VEGF, has shown equal success in improving and maintaining vision in neovascular AMD patients.[459–463] Use of ranbizumab and bevacizumab has become the standard of care for neovascular AMD at the present time. Some people use a combination of anti-VEGF injections with photodynamic therapy to reduce the frequency of intravitreal injections. The injections are being done at various intervals based on experience and results of several studies. Generally at least four monthly injections are given initially, and further injection intervals are based on individual physician preferences.

There is little evidence to support laser treatment to reduce or eradicate drusen, and there are no clinical trials regarding the effectiveness of such treatment.

Surgical Treatment for Complications of AMD

Pars plana vitrectomy has proved useful in removal of vitreous blood that fails to reabsorb spontaneously (Figure 3.30H–L).[464] It also appears to have some usefulness in the evacuation of large subretinal hematomas in the macular area, particularly when used in association with tissue plasminogen activator.[464–468] Surgical excision of CNVMs, which lie in the sub-RPE space in patients with AMD, appears to offer no advantages over laser photocoagulation in regard to restoration or preservation of visual function.[280,282,469–476] Both result in permanent loss of retinal function in the area of the neovascular membrane. (See discussion of surgical excision of types I and II choroidal neovascularization in Chapter 2.) There is hope that transplantation of RPE after surgical excision of subfoveal membranes, or other modifications of the surgical technique, will improve the visual results.[282,472,477] Surgical relocation of the macular retina has been suggested as another possible method of restoring central vision in patients with AMD.[478]

The high susceptibility of the retina to oxidative stress because of the close proximity of high concentrations of polyunsaturated fatty acids in the photoreceptor outer-segment membrane, where exposure to short-wavelength light may generate free radicals, has suggested the possible value of antioxidants in retarding the development of AMD.[479,480] There is evidence that increased serum levels of alpha-tocopherol, and an antioxidant index, including ascorbic acid, alpha-tocopherol, and beta-carotene, are protective for AMD. There is, however, no evidence to show that daily supplementation of vitamins or minerals is of any value in preventing or ameliorating AMD.[237,480–484] The Age-Related Eye Disease Study found retardation of progression of nonexudative AMD in approximately 29% of patients treated with antioxidant viatamins, zinc, and copper. Several pilot studies have suggested that low-dose external-beam irradiation treatment may be of value in the treatment of subfoveal neovascularization.[485,486] Recognition of the earliest symptoms of macular detachment by the patient and prompt examination (within several days after onset) by the ophthalmologist are the best means of preventing loss of vision in this disease. Patients should be instructed in regard to the use of the Amsler grid and near-vision chart and the importance of prompt examination.[487,488] The role of trauma, intraocular surgery, and anticoagulants in precipitating exudation and hemorrhage in these patients is uncertain.[489,490]

Most patients who have lost central vision in both eyes will benefit from the use of any one or several of the wide variety of low visual aids available.[473,491,492]

3.33 Basal laminar drusen.

A and **B**: A 28-year-old woman with 20/20 visual acuity. Early arteriovenous phase angiogram (B) reveals multiple punctate drusen not evident in A.
C–I: A 70-year-old woman seen because of metamorphopsia in both eyes. Visual acuity in the right eye was 20/40 and in the left eye was 20/40. Arrows indicate localized retinal detachment and yellow subretinal exudate (C). Similar findings were present in the left eye. Angiography showed prompt hyperfluorescence of innumerable uniformly small basal laminar drusen and late staining of larger variably sized typical drusen as well as the subretinal exudate in the right eye (D–F). Angiograms of left eye showed early focal staining (arrows, G) and late staining of subretinal exudate (G and H). Thirty-six months later, spontaneous resolution of the subretinal fluid in the right eye had occurred (I). Visual acuity was 20/30.
J–L: A 58-year-old woman with a 1-year history of decreased vision caused by similar vitelliform retinal detachment in both eyes (J). Note fluid level of yellowish subretinal exudate. Visual acuity was 20/200. Electro-oculography was normal. Angiography showed basal laminar drusen and staining of the subretinal exudate (K and L).

(From Gass et al.[494]; Published with permission from The American Journal of Ophthalmology; copyright by The Ophthalmic Publishing Co.)

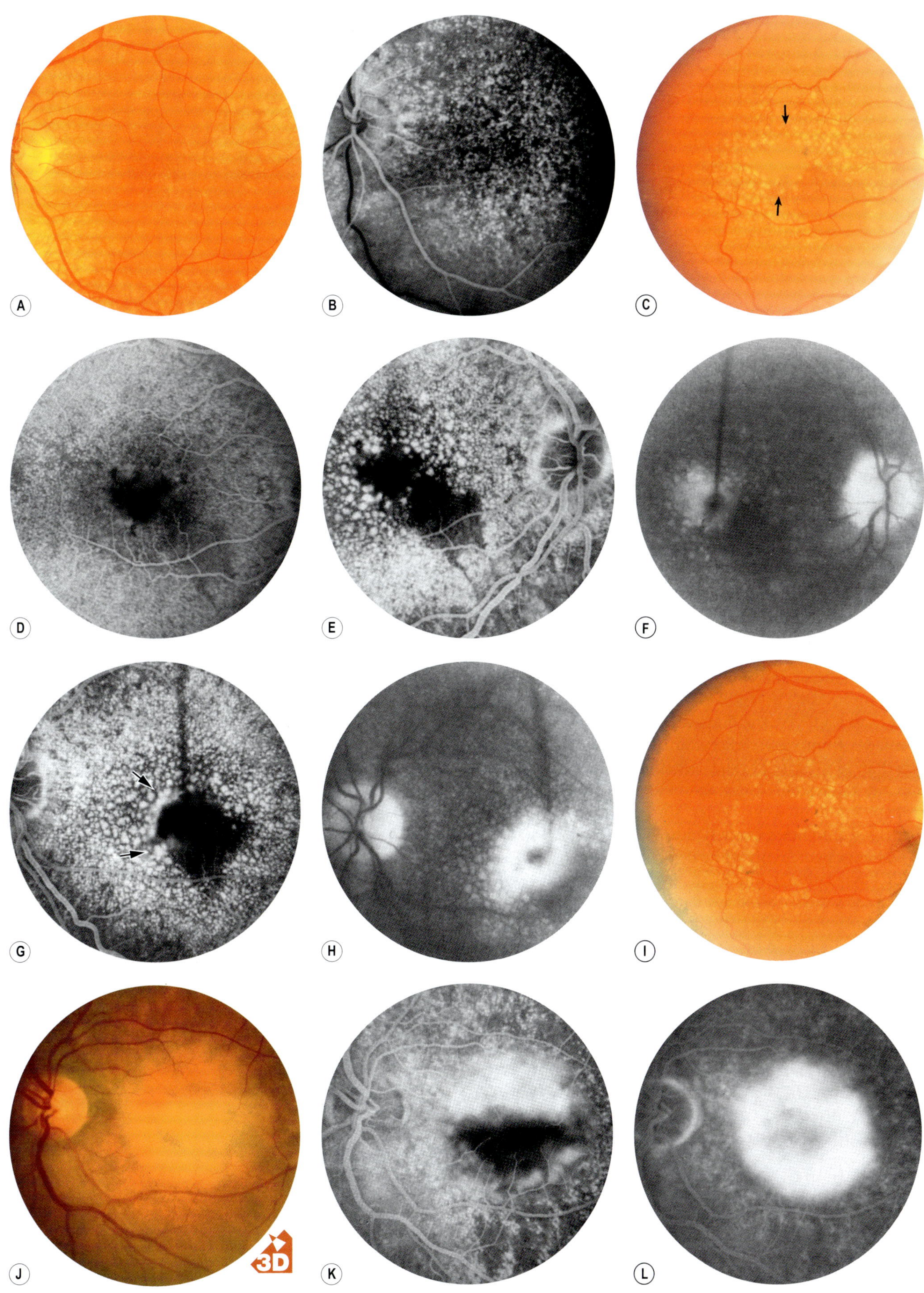
A
B
C
D
E
F
G
H
I
J
3D
K
L

BASAL LAMINAR DRUSEN AND MACULAR DEGENERATION

There is accumulating evidence to support the concept of nodular thickening of the basement membrane of the RPE as the cause for a distinctly different pattern of uniformly small round drusen that may appear in early adulthood and that occur with equal frequency in blacks, Latins, and whites (Figures 3.33, 3.34A–E, and 3.35A–J).[493–497] These peculiar basal laminar or cuticular drusen predispose patients, particularly white persons, to the development in the sixth decade and beyond of typical or exudative, larger, and variably sized drusen and occasional loss of central vision that is often caused by an unusual vitelliform exudative macular detachment (Figures 3.33, 3.34A, and 3.35F).[494] Basal laminar drusen are usually 25–75 μm in size and are discretely round, slightly raised, yellow, subretinal nodules that initially may be randomly scattered in the macular area of young adults, but later often become more numerous and in some patients are grouped in clusters of 15–20 drusen. These clusters, in turn, may be closely arranged in a tightly knit pattern giving the entire macular and paramacular area an orange-peel appearance biomicroscopically. This pattern is coarser and is composed of more discrete flecks than that seen in pseudoxanthoma elasticum (PXE). Basal laminar drusen are more easily seen in young patients with brunette fundi. They are more easily visualized angiographically than biomicroscopically. They fluoresce discretely during the early arteriovenous phase and in many patients give the fundus a "stars-in-the-sky" or "milky-way" picture (Figure 3.33B, D, E, and G).[493,494] The fluorescence in basal laminar drusen fades from view earlier and shows less intense staining than in the case of exudative drusen (Figure 3.33D–F). On autofluorescence imaging, these punctate drusen show a hypoautofluorescent center surrounded by a ring of increased autofluorescence (Figure 3.35A–J).

Patients, particularly white persons beyond age 50 years, with basal laminar drusen may begin to develop superimposed, variably sized exudative drusen usually in the central macular region. They may experience visual loss usually caused by yellow serous exudative detachment of the retina in one or both eyes (Figures 3.33C and J, 3.34A, and 3.35F). When discretely outlined and densely yellow, these detachments may simulate the lesions seen in Best's vitelliform dystrophy and some patients with adult vitelliform foveomacular or pattern dystrophy (Figures 3.33J and 3.34A). They may be mistaken for serous detachments of the RPE. In the early phases of angiography this

3.34 Basal laminar drusen.

A–C: Vitelliform macular detachment in this 54-year-old woman with a 2-year history of difficulty with adaption to changing lighting conditions. Her visual acuity was 20/30 bilaterally. Both eyes had similar vitelliform macular lesions and angiographic evidence of basal laminar drusen.

D: Diagram showing structure of: 1, typical or exudative drusen with detachment of the retinal pigment epithelium (RPE) and normal-thickness basement membrane (bm) from inner collagenous part of Bruch's membrane (BM) by extracellular material; 2, basal laminar drusen composed of nodular thickening of the basement membrane of the RPE; 3, combined basal laminar and typical or exudative drusen. cc, Choriocapillaris.

E: Electron micrograph of combined basal laminar and exudative drusen. The two adjacent areas of nodular thickening of the RPE basement membrane (bm, small arrows) and its normal-thickness basement membrane (large arrows) are detached from the collagenous and elastic part of Bruch's membrane by amorphous material (am).

Cuticular and calcified drusen in patients with type II membranoproliferative glomerulonephritis (MPG).

F–I: A 50-year-old man, who had a history of renal transplant at ages 36 and 39 years because of type II MPG, complained of blurred vision of 2 months' duration. Visual acuity in right eye was 20/200, left eye 20/20. Note variability of the size of the drusen, some of which appear calcified. Angiography revealed cuticular drusen (H and I).

J and K: A 19-year-old man with childhood-onset diabetes and nephrotic syndrome associated with type II MPG. Visual acuity in the right eye was 20/20 and of the left eye was 20/25. Note clusters of tiny basal laminar drusen (arrows) and mild background diabetic retinopathy.

L: Histology of an eye with basal laminar deposits shows the location at the base of the RPE (arrow).

(D and E from Gass et al.[494]; Published with permission from The American Journal of Ophthalmology; copyright by The Ophthalmic Publishing Co.; L courtesy of Ralph Eagle.)

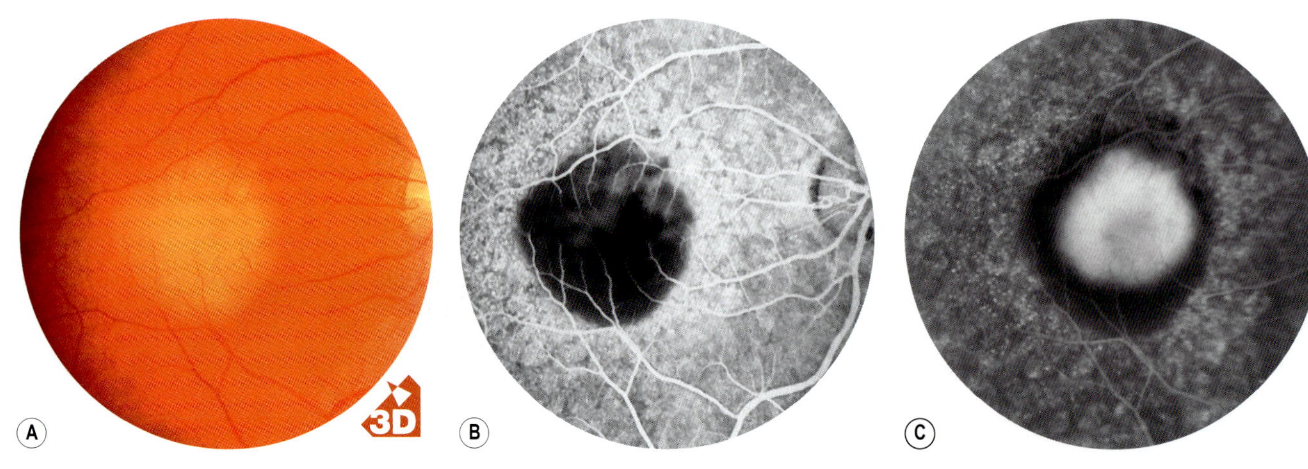

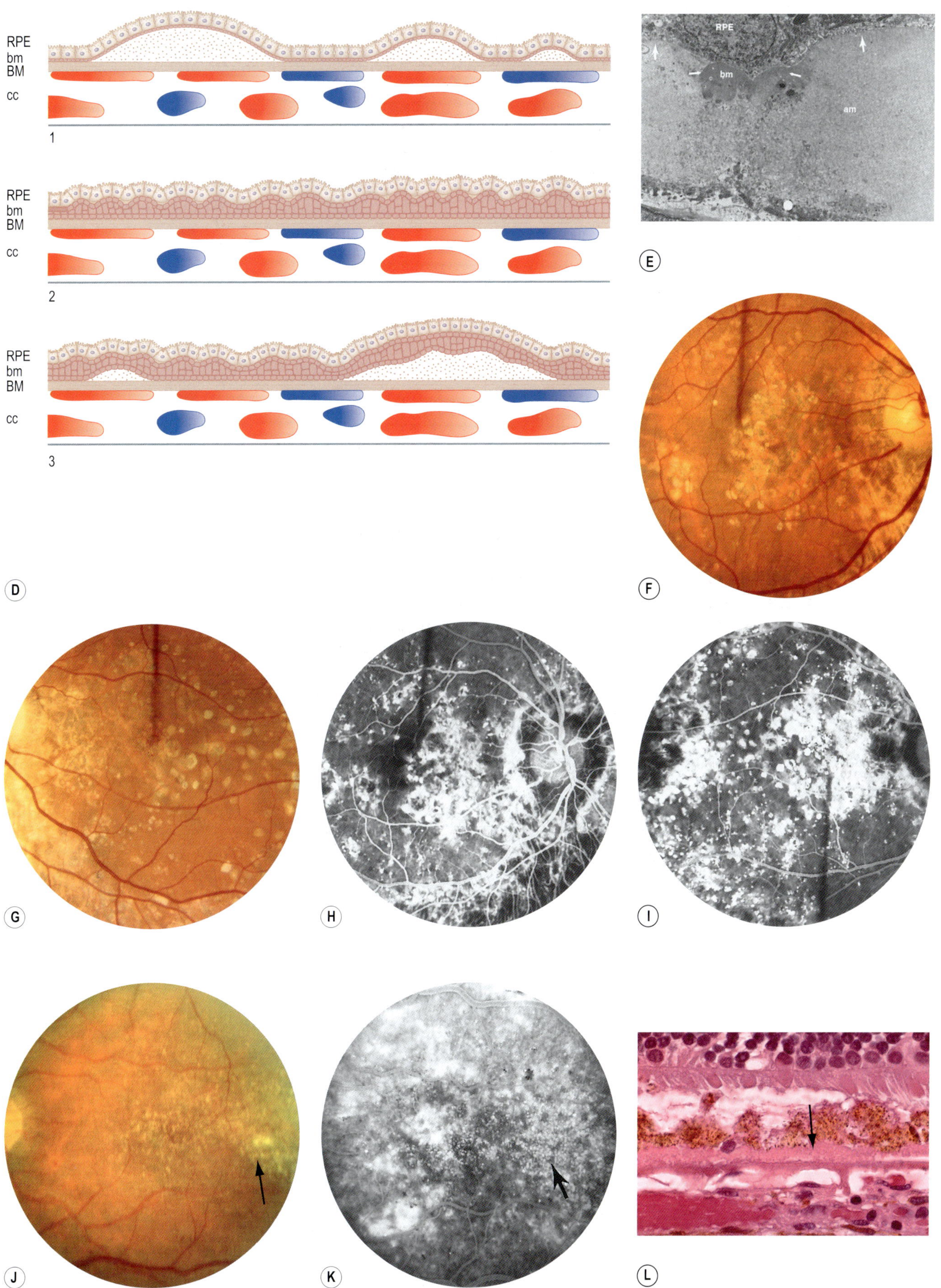
RPE
bm
BM
cc
1
RPE
bm
BM
cc
2
RPE
bm
BM
cc
3
D
RPE
bm
am
E
F
G
H
I
J
K
L

yellowish subretinal fluid obstructs the background choroidal fluorescence. Later, multiple progressively enlarging sites of movement of dye through the RPE into the subretinal fluid occur (Figures 3.33E–H, and 3.34B and C). This pattern may be mistakenly interpreted as choroidal neovascularization.

The older patients who develop yellowish detachment of the macula often maintain acuity of 20/30–20/50 for many months with no change in the appearance of the subretinal fluid. In some patients, the subretinal fluid disappears spontaneously and good acuity is restored (Figure 3.33I). The drusen in the area of the detachment often disappear or become less prominent after reattachment of the retina. In a significant number of patients geographic atrophy of the RPE and poor visual acuity develop after resolution of the detachment (Figure 3.35F–H). Choroidal neovascularization and serous and hemorrhagic disciform detachment may develop in some patients. This latter complication may occasionally occur in middle-aged patients who have not developed superimposed exudative drusen. The electro-oculogram and electroretinogram are normal. Most of the patients' siblings and offspring examined to date have shown no signs of the disease. It has, however, occurred in other family members in a few cases.[496] It probably will prove to be an inherited dystrophy, primarily causing progressive thickening and nodularity of the RPE basement membrane similar to changes occurring in the corneal endothelial basement membrane in Fuchs' dystrophy (Figure 3.34D). These nodules probably begin to develop early in life.

In addition to the frequency of development of yellowish subretinal exudate, other differences between these patients with basal laminar drusen and those with AMD include the following: (1) visual symptoms occur less frequently and they are detected on average 5–10 years earlier; (2) the rate of visual loss after onset of symptoms is slower; (3) spontaneous improvement in acuity is more likely to occur; (4) the incidence of development of geographic atrophy is higher; (5) the incidence of choroidal neovascularization and large exudative detachments of the RPE probably is lower; and (6) the prognosis for retention of useful central vision is better.

Clinicopathologic study of basal laminar drusen by light and electron microscopy has revealed that basal laminar drusen are caused by nodularity of a diffusely thickened RPE basement membrane (Figure 3.34E).[494,495] Though this is distinctly different in appearance on light microscopy from typical or exudative drusen that are focal detachments of the RPE and its relatively normal thickness basement membrane by amorphous and granular material, cytoplasmic processes, and bent fibers,[190,227,231] immunohistochemistry by Russell and coworkers has shown that the constituents of cuticular drusen resemble those of exudative drusen.[239] It is of historical interest that as early as 1856 Müller[497] and later Coats[498] and other light microscopists recognized that Bruch's membrane was composed of an inner cuticular zone and an outer elastic zone. They proposed that all drusen represented focal thickening of the cuticular or inner part of Bruch's membrane secreted by the RPE rather than the outer elastic zone. It was not until the advent of electron microscopy that it was realized that typical or exudative drusen were deposits of extracellular material lying between the relatively normal basement membrane (basal lamina) of the RPE and the inner collagenous part of Bruch's membrane.[190,227,232,499,500] It is likely that some of the uniformly small punctate yellow nodules that are seen in small numbers in the macular area of many patients of all ages are basal laminar drusen and that some of these patients go on to develop exudative drusen and visual loss later in life (Figure 3.35K and L). It is not possible biomicroscopically to differentiate one or several basal lamina drusen from small typical hard drusen or from focal lipidization of RPE cells.

Recent genetic studies in patients with basal laminar drusen have found heterozygous Tyr402His AMD risk variant of *CFH* gene in five families of 30 probands.[501] The association of the same variant in membranoproliferative glomerulonephritis type 2, which also has drusen as a feature (Figure 3.34 F to K), suggests that the *CFH* variant may confer a common risk for drusen formation, and that other genetic or environmental risk factors determine the occurrence of exudative drusen, versus drusen of membranoproliferative glomerulonephritis type 2 or cuticular drusen.[502]

Dominantly inherited disorders associated with cuticular drusen North Carolina Macular dystrophy and Malattia levantinese and Sorsby's fundus dystrophy are discussed in chapter 5.

3.35 Cuticular drusen and autofluorescence.

A–E: Well-demarcated edges of the cuticular drusen seen in the fovea and nasal to the disc in this 48-year-old woman with a vision of 20/20 in each eye. The compact drusen appear as rings with a dark center and a hyperautofluorescent outer ring in both eyes (B and C). High-power view shows the rings more vividly (D and E).

F–J: This 45-year-old man had extensive cuticular drusen in both eyes and a vitelliform detachment in the fovea. He had been treated with photodynamic therapy in this eye for a diagnosis of choroidal neovascularization. He was placed under observation and the vision dropped to 20/400 from the initial 20/100 over 4 years; meanwhile the yellow material was reabsorbed leaving a central geographic atrophy (G) Autofluorescence imaging shows innumerable hypoautofluorescent dots surrounded by hyperautofluorescent rings, except in the region of the geographic atrophy (H). Vision in the left eye decreased to 20/100 with patchy loss of retinal pigment epithelium in the fovea and a similar appearance of the drusen on the color photos and autofluorescent images.

K and **L**: This 84-year-old woman has exudative drusen some of which are very large (K). The autofluorescence images appear similar to the cuticular drusen, suggesting the "ring appearance" is likely related to the compactness of the drusen and its distinct edge rather than being typical of cuticular drusen alone (L). Note that the large drusen also have the ring appearance (arrow).

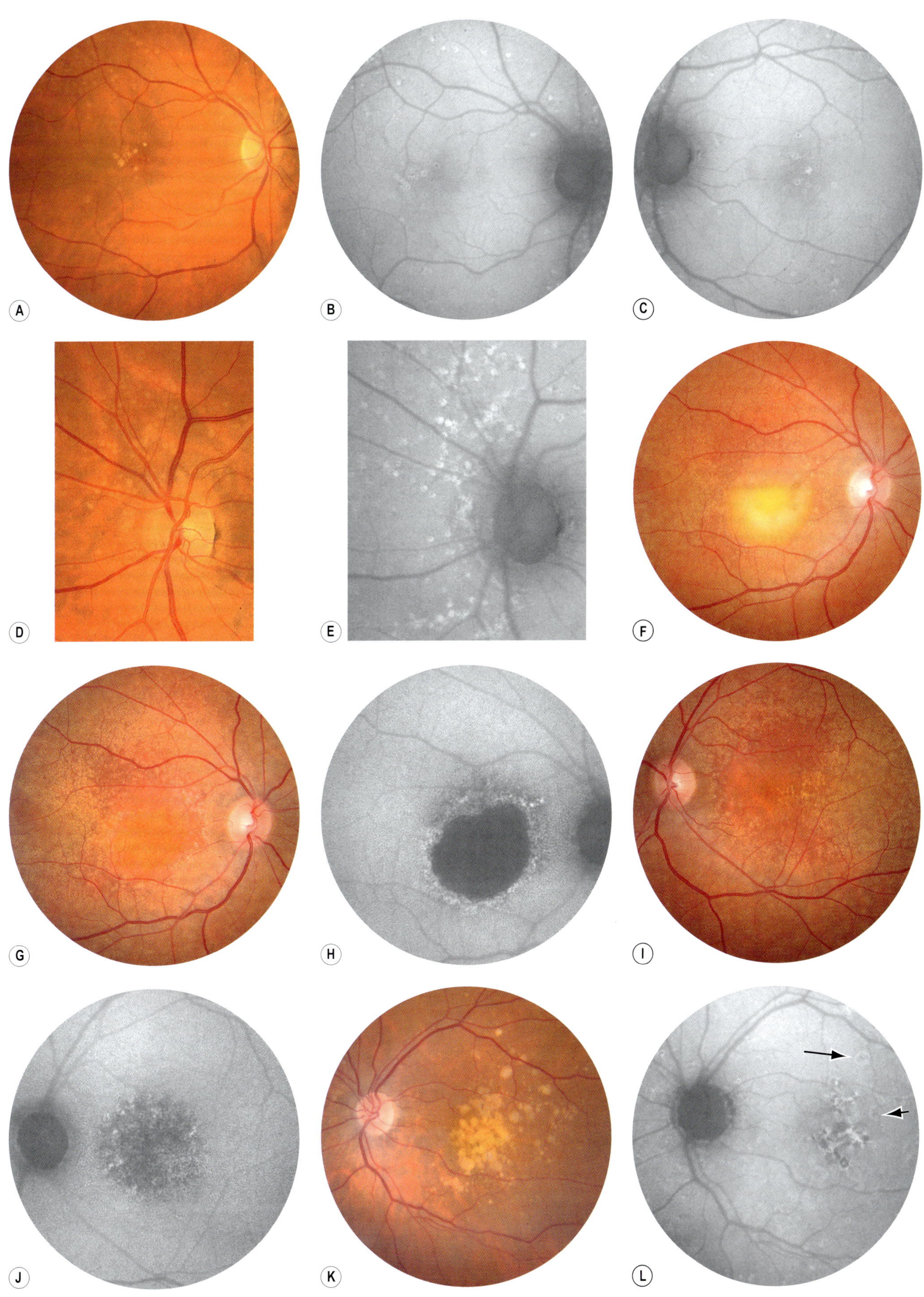
A
B
C
D
E
F
G
H
I
J
K
L

IDIOPATHIC CHOROIDAL NEOVASCULARIZATION

Patients may develop loss of central vision secondary to serous and hemorrhagic detachment of the macula caused by choroidal neovascularization arising in the macula (Figure 3.36A–C), at the margins of the optic disc (Figures 3.36D–F, 3.37, and 3.38), and less frequently in the paramacular (Figure 3.36G–K) or peripheral fundus (Figures 3.37 and 3.38) without any other evidence of intraocular disease.[503–512]

Macular Type

When the choroidal neovascularization develops in the macular region of a child or a young or middle-aged adult, it often occurs in association with a pigment ring or gray mound similar to that described in POHS (type II subretinal neovascularization) (Figure 3.36A–C). Gass noted no sex predilection for idiopathic membranes in the macular region. Although the cause of these neovascular membranes is unknown, it is probable that many of those located in the macula in younger individuals seen in the eastern half of the USA represent a forme fruste of POHS, whereas those occurring in patients 50 years of age or older are more likely to represent a forme fruste of senile macular degeneration.[513]

Ultrastructural features of three excised submacular idiopathic neovascular membranes were similar to that in patients with POHS.[511] Spitznas and Böker studied 151 eyes with idiopathic choroidal neovascularization, excluding all eyes with greater than 6 D of myopia. They found that the probability of developing neovascularization was proportional to the degree of myopia.[509]

3.36 Idiopathic subretinal neovascularization.

A–C: This healthy 45-year-old woman developed blurred vision in her right eye caused by a type II subretinal choroidal neovascular membrane of unknown cause (A). There were no peripheral scars and the left eye was normal. Angiography revealed a 1.5-disc diameter membrane (arrows, A and B) that probably extended into the center of the fovea. The patient was scheduled for surgical excision of the membrane but decided to postpone the operation. When she returned 6 months later, the vision had returned to 20/30, the subretinal blood and exudate had disappeared, and neovascular membrane had contracted to a small area outside the capillary-free zone (arrows, C).

D–F: Bilateral idiopathic juxtapapillary subretinal neovascularization (arrows) in a 66-year-old white woman. In her left eye there was evidence of a small juxtapapillary neovascular membrane and minimal evidence of macular degeneration. The exudative detachment resolved spontaneously. Seven years later she had developed a few drusen in the macula bilaterally, and visual acuity was 20/30 (E). Twelve years after her initial examination she developed a large recurrent new-vessel membrane (arrows, F).

G–K: A large elevated subretinal pigment epithelium–neovascular complex (arrows, G and H) of unknown cause centered in the extramacular area temporally was associated with exudative retinal detachment and loss of central vision in this 76-year-old woman. A large scar had been seen in that area 8 years previously. Her left eye was normal. Angiography showed evidence of widespread ill-defined subretinal neovascularization (I). After intense photocoagulation treatment (J) the exudative detachment resolved and 4 years later her visual acuity was 20/40 (K).

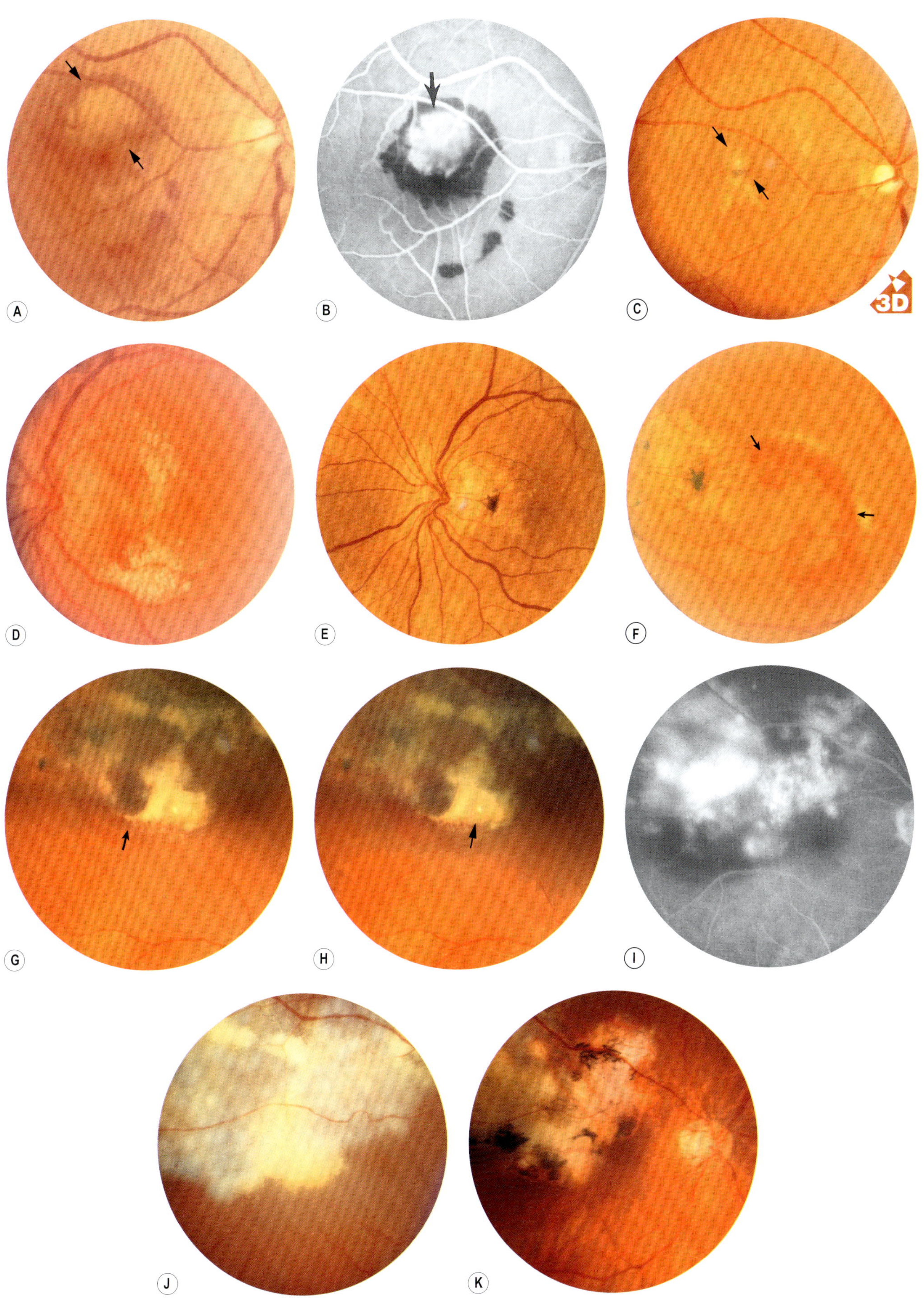
A
B
C
3D
D
E
F
G
H
I
J
K

Juxtapapillary Type

Although idiopathic juxtapapillary choroidal neovascularization may occur at all ages, it is seen most frequently in women in the sixth and seventh decades of life (Figure 3.36D–F).[192,507] In Caucasians it usually occurs as a single partly organized juxtapapillary neovascular network extending outward from the optic disc toward the macular area. It is often surrounded on its temporal aspect by serous or yellowish subretinal exudate with or without subretinal blood. In the opposite eye there is frequently biomicroscopic as well as angiographic evidence of small choroidal neovascular tufts at the margin of the optic disc. The visual prognosis for these latter patients is relatively good, since the process often spontaneously subsides. Nevertheless, they should be watched carefully and if they show progression of the neovascular membrane beyond the halfway point to the center of the fovea, they should be considered for laser therapy. Sub-RPE neovascularization in the absence of hemorrhage or exudation is found frequently in the pathology laboratory as an incidental finding in the juxtapapillary and peripheral areas temporarily in the eyes of elderly patients (Figures 3.18D and 3.26).[251,365] The new vessels, which might be considered as part of the normal aging process, are probably the source of many symptomatic juxtapapillary and peripheral idiopathic neovascular membranes.

The general guidelines for laser photocoagulation of extrafoveal and juxtafoveal choroidal neovascularization associated with AMD and POHS are used in patients with idiopathic choroidal neovascularization. More recently anti VEGF antibodies are being increasingly used to treat all types of choroidal neovascularization.[513]

3.36 Continued

L–Q: Large notched serous detachment of the retinal pigment epithelium (RPE) caused by an occult juxtapapillary sub-RPE new-vessel membrane (arrows, L) in a 50-year-old woman with skin changes compatible with pseudoxanthoma elasticum. She had angioid streaks in the right eye. Visual acuity was 20/30. Note finely mottled appearance of the elevated RPE and the sharp outline of the margin of the detachment of the RPE (L). There is minimal serous elevation of the retina surrounding the base of the RPE detachment. No definite angioid streak is visible. Several minutes following fluorescein injection there was faint staining of the sub-RPE exudate. One-hour angiogram showed diffuse staining of the sub-RPE exudate (N). This slow development of staining indicated the probable presence of high protein concentration and blood pigment in the sub-RPE space. Note absence of staining in the area of the notch (arrow, N). Six weeks later the patient developed circinate deposits along the margins of the RPE detachment (O). This was defi nite evidence of the presence of choroidal neovascularization somewhere beneath the RPE detachment. Eight days following the photograph in D the patient developed evidence of bleeding into the area of RPE detachment (P. Note the fl uid level of blood (arrows). Many months later there were prominent neovascular trunks (arrow, Q) and the RPE detachment had collapsed.

Eccentric Type

Solitary subretinal hematomas and disciform masses may develop anywhere in the extramacular region in one eye of patients whose eyes are otherwise normal (Figure 3.36G–K).[514,515] Many of these probably arise in old postinflammatory or traumatic scars that are hidden by the disciform detachment.

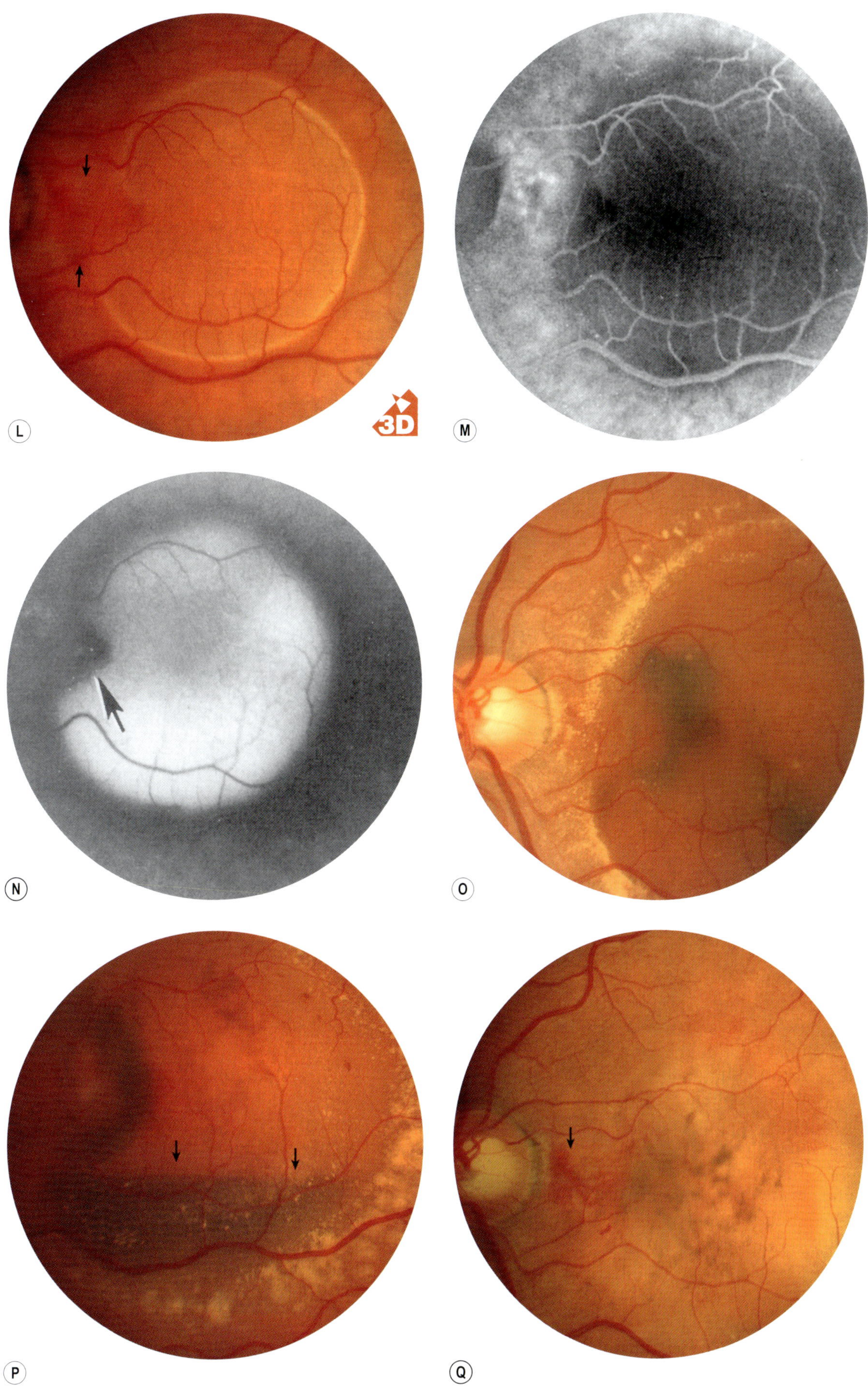
L
3D
M
N
O
P
Q

PERIPHERAL IDIOPATHIC SUB-RPE NEOVASCULARIZATION

Multifocal areas of bleeding beneath the pigment epithelium and retina may occur anterior to the equator, usually in the temporal half of the fundus in elderly patients.[355,362,504,505,514–518] These patients may or may not have evidence of AMD (Figures 3.28 and 3.37). These hemorrhages probably occur secondary to bleeding from neovascularization, which has been demonstrated in the sub-RPE region in the area of the inner collagenous portion of Bruch's membrane in approximately 43% of eyes at autopsy near the ora serrata, particularly in the temporal sectors.[251,365] These vessels emanate from the adjacent pars plana region.[365] Subretinal scarring caused by these peripheral hemorrhages is often discovered on routine eye examination. Large sub-RPE hematomas or fibrovascular masses may be mistaken for melanomas (Figures 3.26 and 3.37). Extension of the subretinal blood into the vitreous may cause the patient to seek an eye examination. Occasionally loss of central vision occurs because of gradual migration of subretinal exudation posteriorly into the macular region. Abrupt loss of vision may result from large serosanguineous RPE detachments extending from the posterior edge of the peripheral neovascular complex into the macular area where a rip in the RPE may occur (Figure 3.37).[338,339,504,505] Asymptomatic patients with no visual impairment can be followed with the expectation that most will eventually show resolution of the bleeding spontaneously. Transscleral cryopexy, laser photocoagulation, and anti-VEGF therapy are effective in controlling the hemorrhage and exudation if the condition progresses (Figure 3.37K and L).

3.37 Idiopathic peripheral choroidal neovascularization causing large tears in the retinal pigment epithelium and loss of central vision.

A–D: Large serous retinal pigment epithelium (RPE) detachment and RPE tear in the temporal macular area of the left eye of a 67-year-old woman with subretinal and sub-RPE hemorrhages in the temporal periphery of both eyes. Note equatorial hemorrhages in A that extended posteriorly to the temporal edge of the macula of the right eye. In the left eye along the temporal edge of the macula there was a serpentine RPE tear (arrows, B) at the posterior edge of a large peripheral serosanguineous RPE detachment. Angiography revealed striking hyperfluorescence in the area of the tear (C and D). Four years previously she had a renal transplant because of renal failure related to light-chain disease.

E–J: A 79-year-old man developed sudden loss of vision in the left eye. It was caused by rapid decompression of a large peripherally located serosanguineous detachment of the RPE through a large RPE rip in the nasal edge of the RPE detachment into the subretinal space in the macula (E and F). His visual acuity was 20/300. Note the early hyperfluorescence in the area of the large RPE tear (arrow, F) and the movement of dye through the hole (arrow, G) into the subretinal fluid in the macula. The subretinal fluid in the macula had resolved 2½ weeks later (H and I) but the large peripheral serosanguineous detachment of the RPE remained (arrows, J). Note absence of evidence of macular degeneration and rolled peripheral edge of RPE tear (I). The source of the bleeding and the serous exudation was probably a choroidal neovascular membrane in the vicinity of the equator temporally.

K and **L**: Idiopathic peripheral choroidal neovascularization associated with exudative retinal detachment extending into the macula (K) was successfully treated with photocoagulation (L).

(A–D courtesy of Dr. Nancy Kirk; E–J from Green and Yarian.[339])

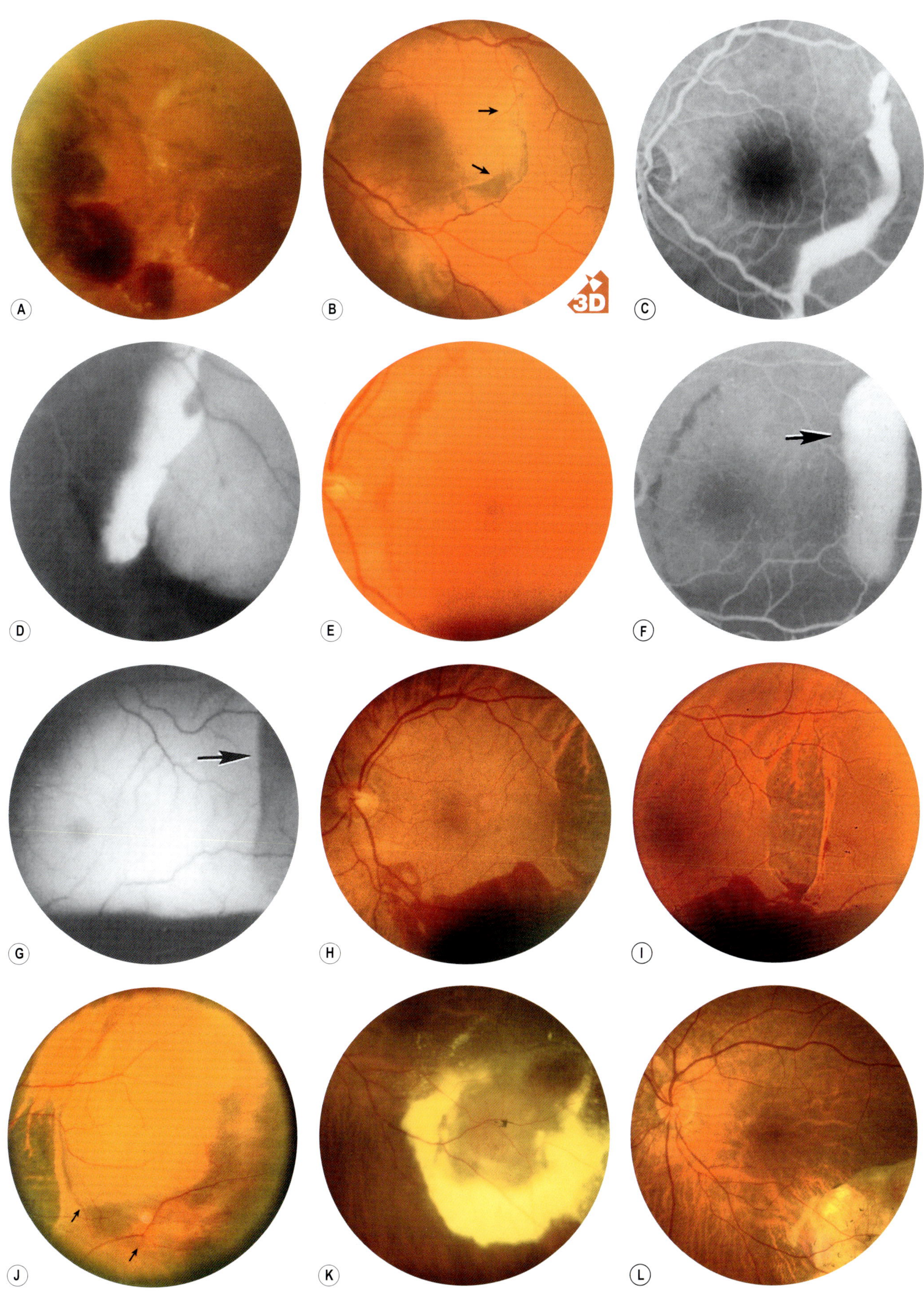
A
B
3D
C
D
E
F
G
H
I
J
K
L

ANGIOID STREAKS AND ASSOCIATED DISEASES

Angioid streaks are irregular, radiating, jagged, tapering lines that extend from the peripapillary area into the peripheral fundus.[519–524] The term "angioid" was chosen because of the ophthalmoscopic similarity of these streaks to blood vessels. They are caused by linear cracklike dehiscences in the collagenous and elastic portion of Bruch's membrane (Figures 3.38–3.43).[525,526] Near the optic disc, they are often interconnected by circumferential breaks in Bruch's membrane. Early in the disease the streaks are sharply outlined in color, varying from reddish orange to dark red or brown, depending on the pigmentary characteristics of the underlying choroid that becomes visible through the thinned RPE overlying the linear defects in Bruch's membrane. Fibrovascular proliferation from the choroid may grow through the breaks in Bruch's membrane and elevate the surrounding RPE (Figure 3.40G–I). This causes blurring and in some cases totally obscures the streak margins. The proliferative changes are often prominent along streaks extending into the macular region, and they may be associated with slowly progressive macular changes and loss of central vision. Abrupt loss of vision, however, is more frequently caused by serous and hemorrhagic detachment surrounding areas of choroidal neovascularization that have grown through the angioid streaks into the sub-RPE or subretinal space in or near the papillomacular bundle region (Figures 3.39A and G and 3.41A–C). Occasionally patients will develop large areas of serous detachment of the RPE adjacent to these neovascular membranes (Figure 3.42A).[527] Because of the brittleness of Bruch's membrane in patients with angioid streaks, they may develop loss of central vision secondary to choroidal rupture and submacular hemorrhage following insignificant trauma (Figure 3.39E and F).[521]

3.38 Angioid streaks and pseudoxanthoma elasticum.

A–C: This 25-year-old man's visual acuity was normal. Note the clump of pigment and multiple white subretinal crystalline bodies inferior to the optic disc (A and B, arrows). Angiography showed irregular hyperfluorescence along the course of the angioid streaks (C).

D and E: Large pigmented angioid streaks. Note peau d'orange temporal to the left macula (E).

F: Angioid streaks (top arrow), multiple calcified drusenlike structures (bottom arrow), and peau d'orange change.

G and H: Reticular macular dystrophy, angioid streaks, and crystalline bodies (arrow).

I: Angioid streaks and drusen of optic disc.

J and K: Pseudoxanthoma elasticum in antecubital fossa and neck.

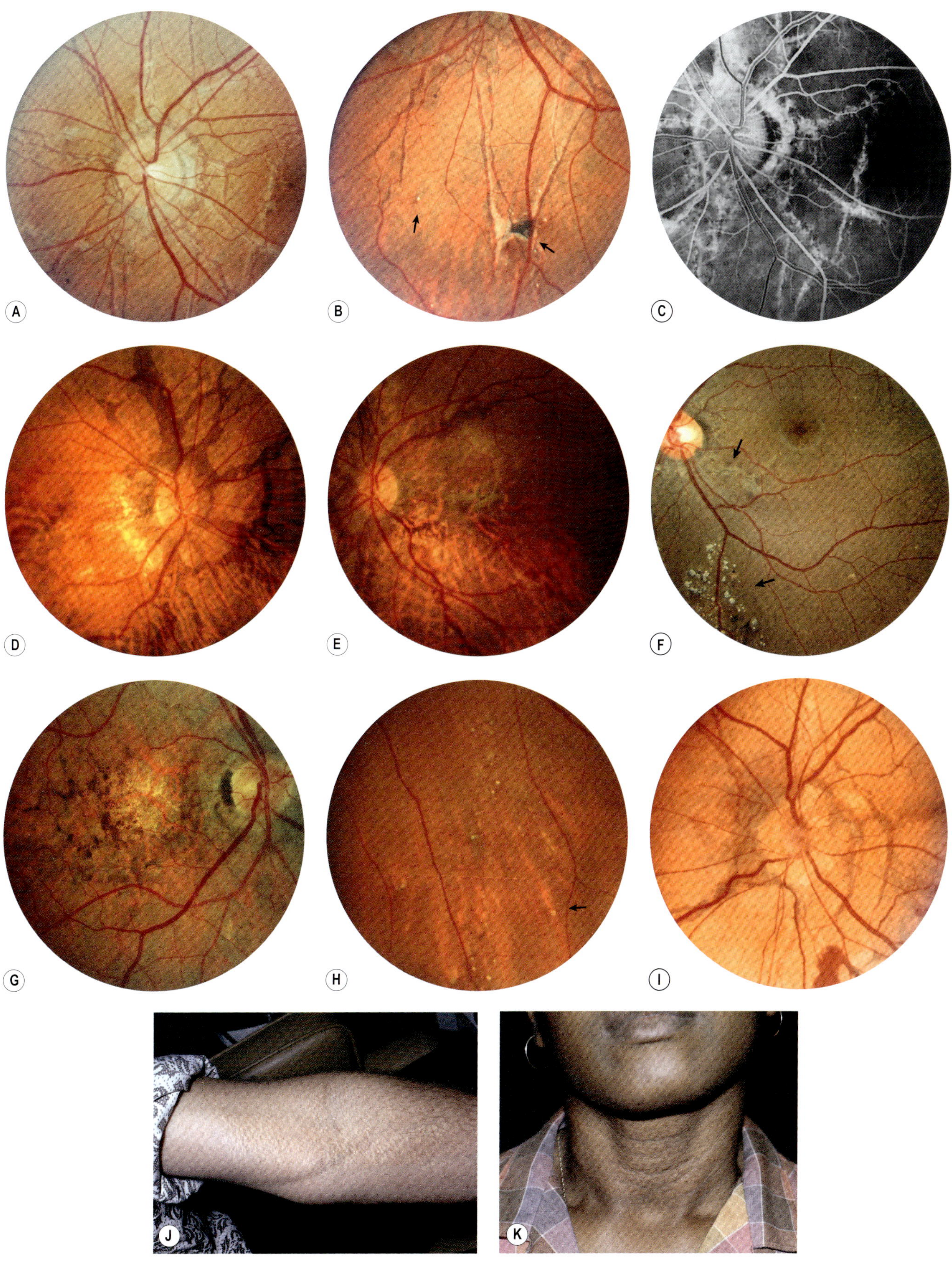
A
B
C
D
E
F
G
H
I
J
K

Angioid streaks may show irregular hyperfluorescence during the early phases of angiography and varying degrees of staining during the later phases (Figures 3.38C, 3.39F, 3.42H, and 3.43D).[524,528,529] In some patients with heavily pigmented choroids, however, well-defined angioid streaks may be barely visible angiographically (Figure 3.39D). In other patients, angiography may be helpful in detecting RPE alterations along small angioid streaks before they are visible ophthalmoscopically. Angiography is also of value in detecting choroidal neovascularization (Figures 3.39B, D, and I, and 3.41). In some cases of occult choroidal neovascularization, however, angiography may fail to show evidence of new vessels (Figure 3.42A–F).

Histopathologically, angioid streaks are discrete linear breaks in Bruch's membrane, which often shows extensive calcific degeneration (Figure 3.43G).[522,525,526,528] This may be associated with changes in the choriocapillaris similar to those seen in patients with macular drusen. Fibrous tissue alone, capillary proliferation, or both may grow from the choroid around the edge of the dehiscence in Bruch's membrane into the sub-RPE space. It is these capillaries that are the source of serous and hemorrhagic detachment in these patients.

Clarkson and Altman,[519] in a diagnostic workup of 50 patients with angioid streaks, were able to establish a related systemic diagnosis in 25 patients (50%). In 17 of these patients the diagnosis was PXE, 5 had Paget's disease, and 3 had sickle-cell hemoglobinopathy. There is evidence that angioid streaks may be pathogenetically related to Ehlers–Danlos syndrome.[530] The evidence is less convincing for many other diseases that have occasionally occurred in patients with angioid streaks.[531]

3.39 Angioid streaks and pseudoxanthoma elasticum.

A and B: Choroidal neovascularization (arrow, A) extending from the edge of angioid streak and causing submacular hemorrhage in a patient with pseudoxanthoma elasticum. Angiogram showed new-vessel network (arrows, B).

C and D: Prominent angioid streaks in a 35-year-old man with pseudoxanthoma elasticum and loss of central vision secondary to serous detachment of the macula (arrows, C). Angiogram showed evidence of a choroidal neovascular membrane (arrows, D) originating at the site of an angioid streak. Note in this patient that the angiogram showed minimal alterations of the angiographic pattern along the course of the streaks.

E and F: Subretinal hemorrhage after a minor blow to the left eye of a 28-year-old woman with multiple angioid streaks and pseudoxanthoma elasticum. Note vertical choroidal rupture on the nasal edge of the fovea and partly reabsorbed subretinal blood (E). Fluorescein angiography showed irregular fluorescence along the course of the angioid streaks and prominent fluorescence in the region of the choroidal rupture (F). The brittleness of Bruch's membrane caused by pseudoxanthoma elasticum was probably responsible for the development of a choroidal rupture following relatively minor trauma. This patient subsequently recovered normal visual acuity.

G–L: Subretinal neovascularization (arrows, G and I) in the right eye of this middle-aged woman with pseudoxanthoma elasticum, angioid streaks, and pattern dystrophy (G and H). Laser photocoagulation treatment (K) was successful in eradicating the neovascularization (L).

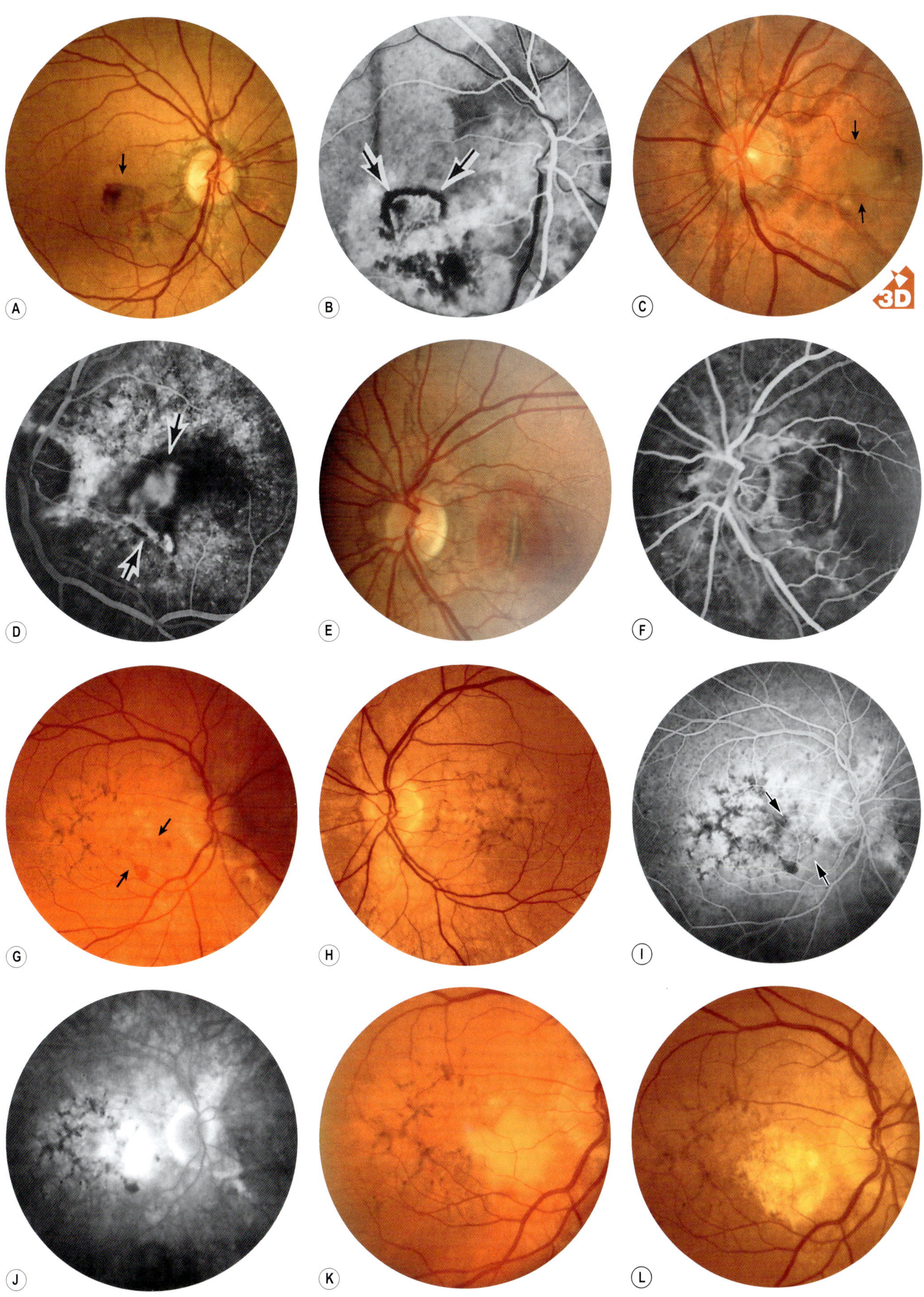
A
B
C
3D
D
E
F
G
H
I
J
K
L

PSEUDOXANTHOMA ELASTICUM (GRONBLAD–STRANDBERG)

PXE is a systemic disease named for its cutaneous counterpart, which is characterized by the development of confluent, yellowish papules that give the skin a "plucked chicken" appearance on the flexural surfaces in the neck, antecubital fossa, and periumbilical area.[519,532–536] Histologically, these changes are caused by degeneration and calcification of the elastic tissue of the dermis. These changes may be associated with premature calcification of the large arteries of the extremities and with gastrointestinal bleeding. PXE is a hereditary disease whose causal gene is the adenosine triphosphate-binding cassette, subfamily C (CFTR/MRP), member 6 (*ABCC6*) gene, which encodes multidrug resistance-associated protein-6 (MRP6).[537] In addition to streaks, other associated fundoscopic findings in these patients include the following:

- Peau d'orange pigmentary change. Widespread areas of mottling of the fundus caused by multiple, indistinct, confluent, yellowish lesions at the level of the RPE that have been likened to that of an orange skin (peau d'orange).[538–540] These may become prominent in the fundi in childhood before the development of angioid streaks (Figure 3.38E and F).[538,540] They are usually most apparent in the mid peripheral fundus, particularly on the temporal side in older patients with PXE. They are seen less often in patients with angioid streaks associated with Paget's disease and sickle-cell disease.[519]

3.40 Pseudoxanthoma elasticum and pattern dystrophy.

A and **B**: Appearance of punctate brown pigment spots of fundus pulverulentus type of pattern dystrophy in the macula of this male with angioid streaks and pseudoxanthoma elasticum (B).
C: Patient with pseudoxanthoma elasticum and angioid streaks shows butterfly type in the macula and fundus flavimaculatus type of pattern dystrophy near the arcades (arrows).

Transition from one type of pattern dystrophy to another.

D and **E**: Initial fundus pulverulentus type of pattern dystrophy with granular brown dots (D) progressed to develop yellow vitelliform type of dystrophy 5 years later (E).
F and **G**: Extensive distribution of the pattern dystrophy even outside the macula.
H–L: This 48-year-old male had optic nerve drusen, angioid streaks, butterfly pattern dystrophy and progressive spontaneous retinal pigment epithelium atrophy in both eyes. The flecks of pattern dystrophy show brilliant autofluorescence (I and K).

The histopathologic changes responsible for the peau d'orange appearance are unknown. These lesions cause minimal alterations on fluorescein angiography but may be associated with a diffuse speckled pattern of indocyanine green hyperfluorescence, a finding that suggests that the orange peel appearance may be caused by an alteration at the level of Bruch's membrane.[541]

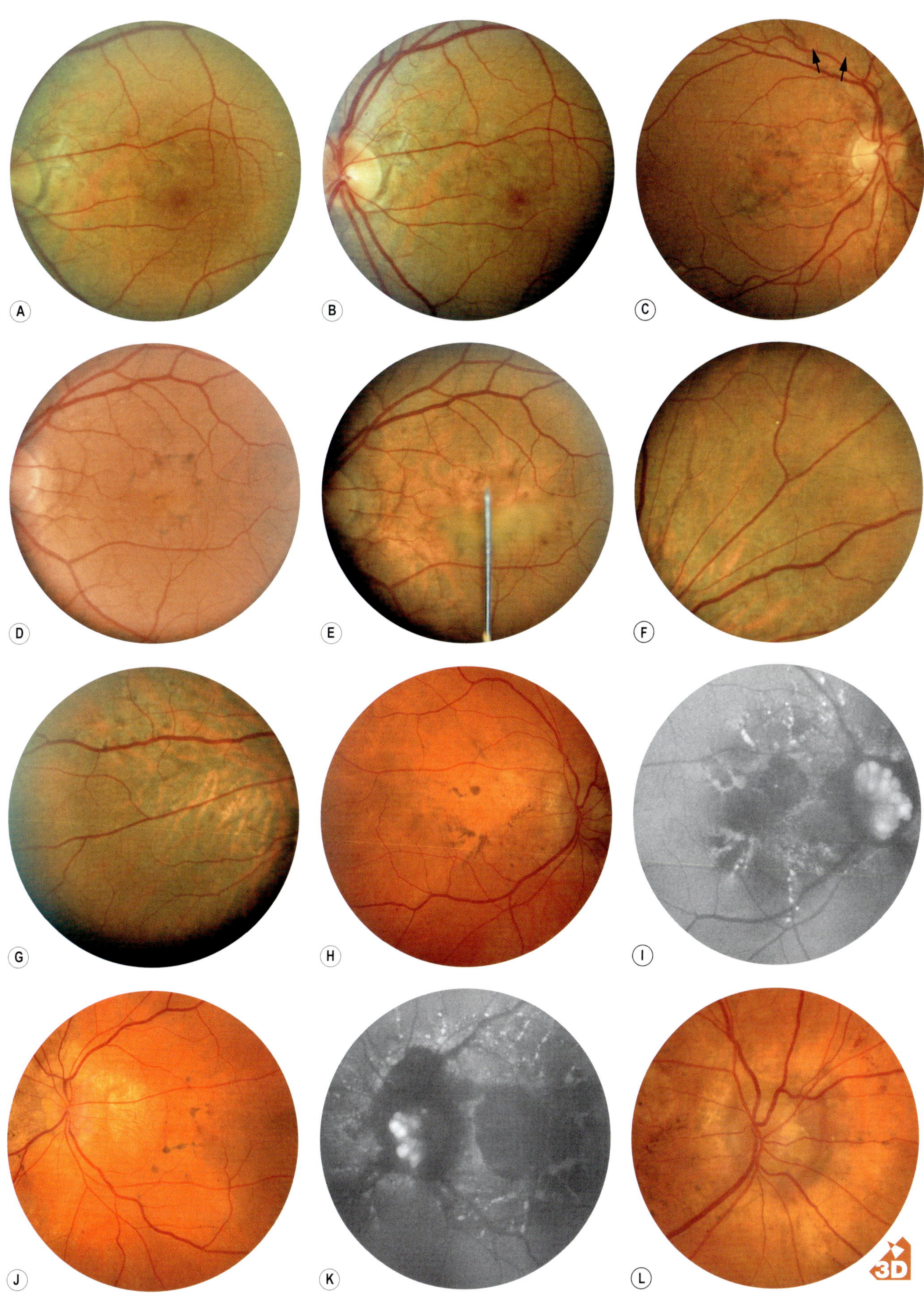
A
B
C
D
E
F
G
H
I
J
K
L
3D

- Pattern dystrophy of the macula. Approximately 65% of patients with PXE may develop a pattern dystrophy of macula bilaterally.[542] It is most frequently manifest as a reticular network or a combination of reticular network and multiple punctate pigment spots (fundus pulverulentus) (Figures 3.38G, 3.39G and H, and 3.40A–D).[543–545] (See pattern dystrophies, Chapter 5.) Other types of pattern dystrophy have also been noted, including vitelliform (Figure 3.40E), butterfly (Figure 3.40H–K), and fundus flavimaculatus type (Figure 3.40C, arrows), though less frequently.[542] Pattern dystrophy may appear during follow-up (Figure 3.40A and B) or progress from one type to another over time (Figure 3.40D and E). The pigmentary disturbance is often more apparent angiographically than ophthalmoscopically.
- Focal atrophic pigment epithelial lesions. Multiple small, round, yellow or slightly pink, RPE atrophic lesions as well as discretely punched-out white scars with varying amounts of pigment similar to those seen in POHS occur commonly in the peripheral fundus of these patients. These have occasionally been referred to as "salmon spots."[523]

3.41 Pseudoxanthoma elasticum: progression and choroidal neovascularization.

A–G: This 48-year-old male with pseudoxanthoma elasticum had previously undergone laser photocoagulation to two extrafoveal sites of choroidal neovascularization along the angioid streaks (arrowheads). He developed recurrence of the membrane (A–C) that required three sessions of photodynamic therapy. In the meantime spontaneous thinning and atrophy of the retinal pigment epithelium (RPE) were noted (arrows) away from the site of the neovascular membranes, that gradually increased in size (A–C, E and G). Autofluorescence imaging clearly delineates the area of RPE atrophy in G.

- Crystalline bodies. Multiple round, small, subretinal, crystalline bodies typically occur in the mid peripheral fundus or juxtapapillary area, particularly inferiorly, in as many as 75% of patients (Figure 3.38B, F, and H).[521,546] These are always associated with some atrophic changes of the RPE. In some cases a "tail" of RPE thinning lying posteriorly to a crystalline body gives it the appearance of a "comet" (Figure 3.38B and H).

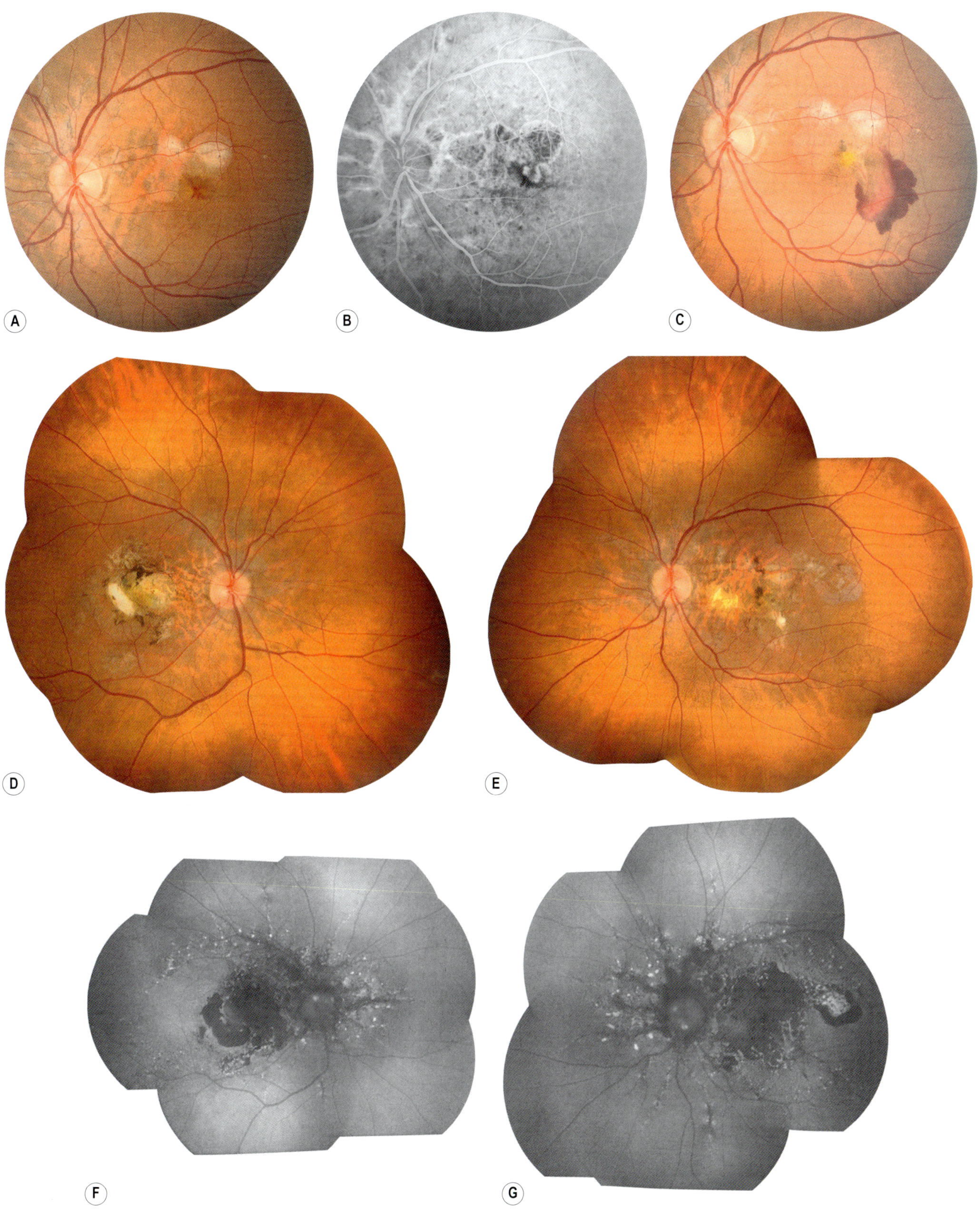
A
B
C
D
E
F
G

- Hyaline bodies of the optic disc. Hyaline bodies (drusen) of the optic discs occur in approximately 5% of patients with angioid streaks and PXE[543,546–548] (Figures 3.38I and 3.40H, J, and L). It is not as common as believed. Acute visual loss caused by an optic neuropathy may occur in these patients with hyaline bodies.[543]
- Progressive atrophy of the RPE. Spontaneous atrophy of the pigment epithelium occurs in the vicinity of the angioid streaks without evidence of, or contraction of, choroidal neovascularization (Figure 3.40A–C, E and F, arrows).

A PXE patient with congenital communication between a cilioretinal artery and retinal artery has been described.[549] The inheritance pattern of PXE may be either autosomal-dominant or recessive. Gass has seen one patient whose mother and two maternal uncles had Paget's disease of the bone.[550]

3.42 Angioid streaks.

A–C: This 42-year-old male complained of progressive visual loss in both eyes for 5 years. He had atypical streaks running in the middle of his macula (arrows A and B), fundus pulverulentus-type pattern dystrophy in both eyes and several areas of spontaneous subretinal fibrous proliferation without evidence of choroidal neovascularization (arrowheads B and C). The fluorescein angiogram helped in finding the angioid streaks and the pattern dystrophy (not shown). The skin on his neck showed the typical changes of pseudoxanthoma elasticum.

Angioid streaks in sickle cell disease

D and **E**: Angioid streaks in a black patient with sickle-cell C disease. Note tortuosity of veins.

F: Angioid streaks in a 41-year-old black woman with sickle-cell C disease.

Sickle-Cell Disease and Other Hemoglobinopathies

It has been estimated that 1–2% of patients with the sickle-cell hemoglobinopathies will develop angioid streaks (Figures 3.40J–L and 6.59E and F).[519,564–574] Streaks in these patients have rarely occurred under the age of 25 years. Serous and hemorrhagic detachment of the macula occurs infrequently in sickle-cell patients with streaks and in black patients in general (see Figure 3.55). Streaks have been reported in homozygous sickle-cell disease, sickle-cell hemoglobin C disease, sickle-cell thalassemia,[572,575,576] sickle-cell trait,[569,577] hemoglobin H disease,[578] homozygous beta-thalassemia major,[579,580] beta-thalassemia intermedia, beta-thalassemia minor,[581–583] congenital dyserythropoietic anemia type 1,[584] and hereditary spherocytosis.[531] Some patients with sickle thalassemia may have PXE as well as angioid streaks.[575]

Deposition of iron–calcium complexes in Bruch's membrane caused by excessive blood breakdown was suggested as a possible cause for the brittleness of the membrane and angioid streaks in sickle-cell disease.[523,573] However, this could not be confirmed histopathologically in the eyes of a 63-year-old man with homozygous sickle-cell disease and angioid streaks.[571] There was extensive calcification of Bruch's membrane but no iron deposition.

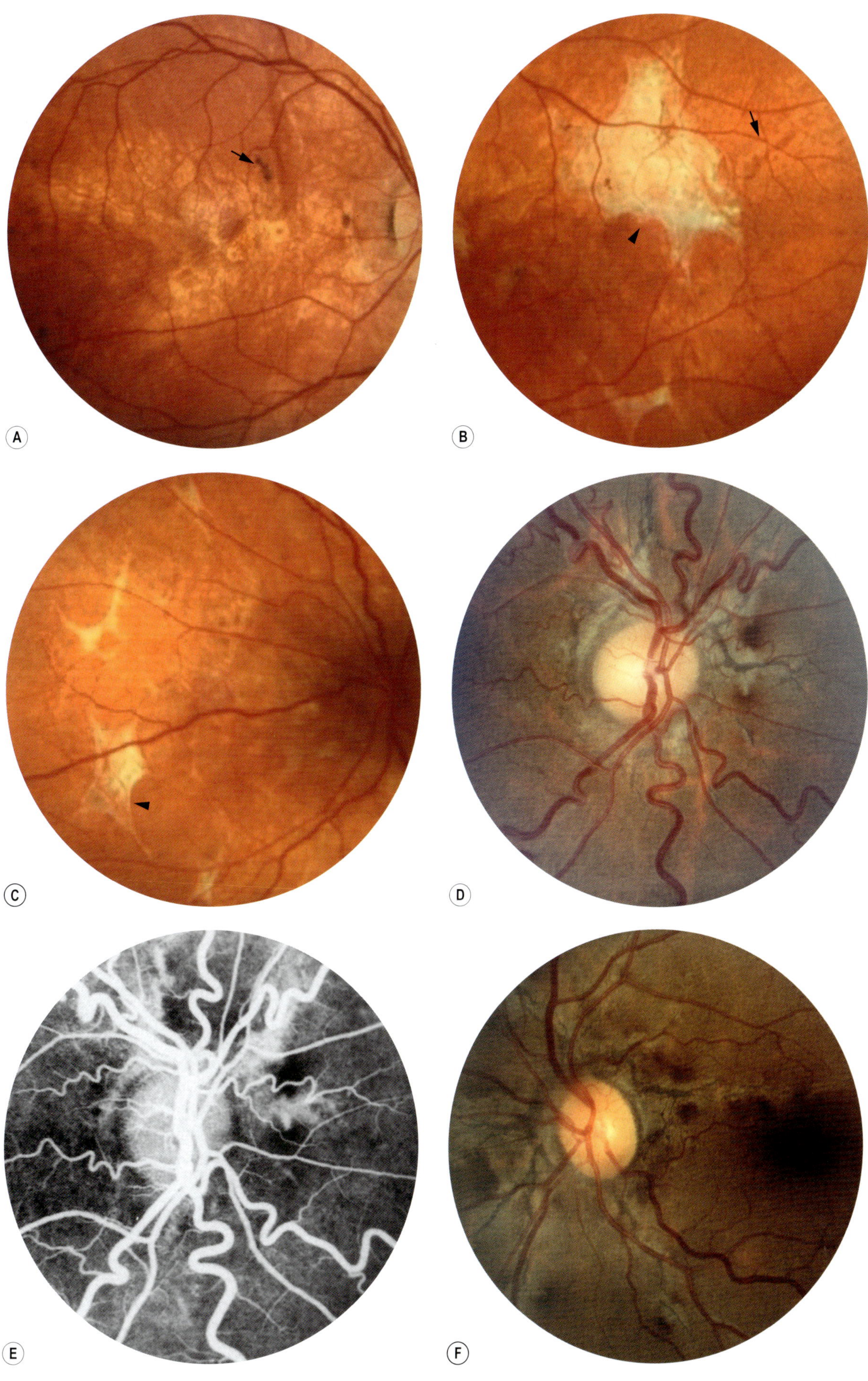
A
B
C
D
E
F

PAGET'S DISEASE

Paget's disease is a chronic, progressive, and in some cases hereditary disease characterized by thickening, rarefaction, and deformity of the bones. The disease may be confined to a few bones or may be generalized. In the latter case, usually after the age of 40 years, the patient develops enlargement of the skull, deformity of the long bones, kyphoscoliosis, and hearing loss (Figure 3.43). The axial skeleton is most affected. The condition is often asymptomatic but can be associated with bone pain, osteoarthritis, pathological fractures, and nerve compression syndromes. Exophthalmos and normal-pressure hydrocephalus are rare complications secondary to involvement of the skull.[551–554] These patients, particularly those with skull involvement, may develop extensive calcification of Bruch's membrane, an irregular pattern of angioid streaks, and severe choroidal neovascularization and disciform scarring (Figure 3.43).[519,525,555–559] Approximately 10% or less of patients with Paget's disease develop angioid streaks.[519,555,556,558] Those with the earliest onset of disease and severe bone involvement are most likely to develop angioid streaks and choroidal neovascularization. Some of these patients show mottling of the RPE in the midperiphery (peau d'orange) similar to that seen in PXE. Visual loss is caused most frequently by choroidal neovascularization but can also be caused by optic atrophy that cannot be explained solely on the basis of bony compression.[560] The choroidal neovascularization is type 2 that grows in the subretinal space, similar to that seen in PXE, POHS, and other chorioretinal scars, and unlike the neovascularization of AMD which grows under the RPE.

Paget's disease is more common in Caucasians, particularly in the UK and amongst British migrants to Australia, New Zealand, and South Africa, and in western and southern Europe. Though reported, the disease is rare in Scandinavia, India, China, Japan, and South-east Asia. Mutations have been identified in four genes: the most important is Sequestome 1 (*SQSTM1*), which is a scaffold protein in the nuclear factor-κB signaling pathway.[561] There is some evidence that a slow virus infection related to either measles (paramyxoma virus) or respiratory syncytial virus may act as a trigger for Paget's disease.[557] Other potential triggers include dietary deficiency of calcium and repetitive mechanical loading of the skeleton. Bisphosphonates decrease bone turnover and are helpful in alleviating bone pain.

An orbital osteoclastoma which was extraskeletal in origin was removed from the orbit of a 51-year-old with Paget's disease. Sarcomatous transformation of the orbital bone has also been reported.[562,563]

Rare Associations

Angioid streaks may occur in patients with abetalipoproteinemia.[585–587] Isolated case reports of angioid streaks associated with pituitary tumor, familial polyposis of the colon, congenital hypertrophy of the RPE, and Sturge–Weber syndrome with facial angiomatosis have been reported.[588–591]

Treatment

Patients with angioid streaks should be warned of the potential risk of choroidal rupture from relatively mild contusion to the eye. As patients with streaks reach the fifth decade, they are at risk of spontaneously developing serous and hemorrhagic detachment of the retina secondary to choroidal neovascularization. Laser treatment may be successful in obliterating the neovascularization if it has not extended inside the capillary-free zone (Figure 3.39G–L).[567,574,592–598] Because of the multiple breaks in Bruch's membrane, other neovascular membranes are likely to occur. More recently, anti-VEGF treatment with intravitreal bevacizumab and ranibizumab has been successful and may be safer by preventing further breaks in the Bruch's membrane from laser.[599–602]

3.43 Angioid streaks and Paget's disease: clinicopathologic correlation.

A–H: This 61-year-old man with Paget's disease was seen because of recent loss of central vision in his left eye. He had previously lost the central vision in his right eye following a macular hemorrhage. Note the enlarged cranium, dilated tortuous temporal artery, and hearing aid on the right side (A). There was a serous detachment of the macula secondary to choroidal neovascularization in the area of an angioid streak (B and C). Note the prominent streak in B (arrow). The histopathology of this streak at the site indicated by the arrow is illustrated in G. Angiography showed hyperfluorescence along the streaks and a large choroidal neovascular membrane (CNVM) in the papillomacular bundle region (arrows, D). Xenon photocoagulation was placed in the area of the CNVM (E). The subretinal fluid resolved. Fifteen weeks later (E), however, he developed further evidence of choroidal neovascularization (arrows, F). The patient subsequently died, and his eyes were obtained at autopsy. Histopathology of the angioid streak depicted in B showed a break in Bruch's membrane (arrow), thinning of the retinal pigment epithelium (RPE), sub-RPE deposition of fibrillar eosinophilic material, and herniation of the choroidal blood vessels into the area of the break (G). There was some atrophy of the choriocapillaris surrounding the break. Von Kossa's stain for calcium revealed extensive calcification of Bruch's membrane and collagen tissue surrounding the choriocapillaris (H). Note the atrophic retina and flat vascularized subretinal scar.

I and J: Pigmented angioid streaks and submacular choroidal neovascularization in 55-year-old physician with Paget's disease.

(A–H from Gass and Clarkson.[525])

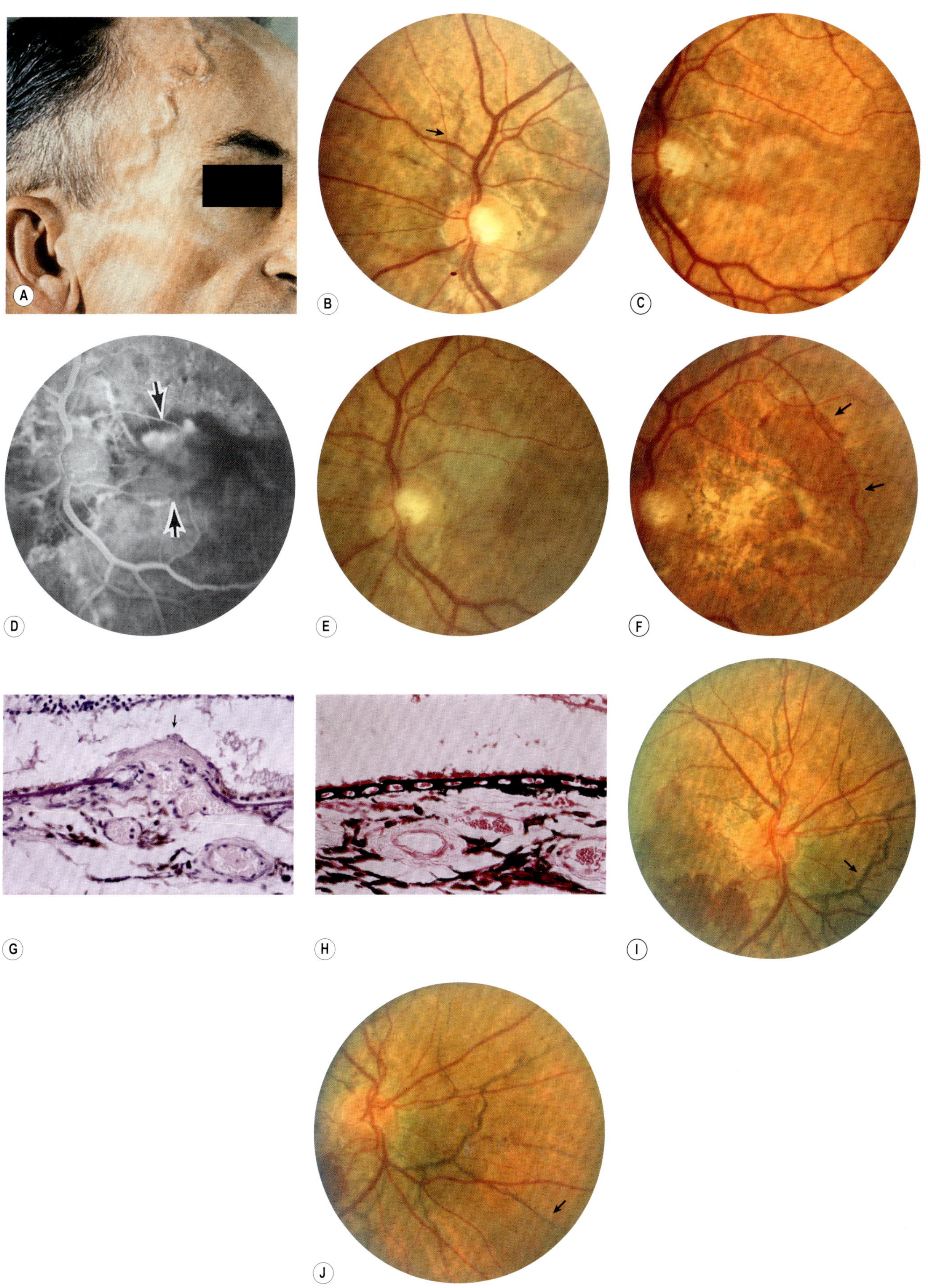
A
B
C
D
E
F
G
H
I
J

MYOPIC CHOROIDAL DEGENERATION

Patients with progressive elongation of the eye (pathologic myopia) develop thinning of the choroid and RPE in the macular area. This may be associated with the development of tilting of the optic disc, peripapillary chorioretinal atrophy, posterior staphylomata, gyrate areas of atrophy of the pigment epithelium and choroid, and lacquer cracks (Figures 3.44 and 3.45).[528,603–607] Lacquer cracks are caused by spontaneous focal linear breaks in Bruch's membrane. This rupture may be accompanied by a small subretinal hemorrhage unassociated with evidence of choroidal neovascularization (Figure 3.44D).[608–610] These subretinal hemorrhages are usually noted during routine examination of young patients either at the site of or immediately preceding the development of a lacquer crack. Lacquer cracks often radiate outward in a reticular pattern from one or several areas of choroidal pigment epithelial atrophy (Figure 3.44A and B).[611] Visual acuity may be excellent in spite of extensive atrophic changes in the RPE and choroid.

Most patients are in their fifth decade or beyond when they begin to experience slowly progressive loss of central acuity associated with myopic degenerative changes. Rapid loss of central vision is usually caused by exudative and hemorrhagic macular detachment overlying small areas of choroidal neovascularization (Figures 3.44C, E, and F, and 3.45A). This may occur adjacent to a lacquer crack, in an area of geographic atrophy of the RPE, or often in an area of generalized attenuation of the RPE and choroid. The new-vessel membrane and the area of detachment are usually small and located close to the central macular area. The new-vessel membrane characteristically appears biomicroscopically as a faintly gray semitranslucent plaque with a hyperpigmented border (Figures 3.44C and E, and 3.45A). If associated with subretinal bleeding, a small, relatively round mound of RPE proliferation may develop as the blood clears (Figure 3.44G and H). This pigmented mound may obscure the CNVM from view.[528]

The relatively small size of choroidal neovascular complexes in myopia is probably a function of the attenuated blood supply to the thin choroid. Because of the smallness of the disciform lesions, the chances for retaining 20/200 or better acuity is higher in these patients following choroidal neovascularization than in patients with emmetropia and senile macular degeneration.[608] Förster[612] and later Fuchs[604] described a raised, circular, pigmented lesion that frequently develops in the macula of middle-aged persons with myopia (Förster–Fuchs spot). Clinically and histopathologically, this lesion, which typically is approximately ½ disc diameter in size, consists of a localized ingrowth of fibrovascular tissue from the choroid and proliferation of the RPE (Figures 3.44G and 3.45D).[528] There is limited histopathologic information concerning choroidal neovascularization in myopic degeneration.[528,613,614]

3.44 Fundus changes in high myopia.

A: Lacquer cracks (arrow).
B and C: Small lacquer crack (arrow, B) 5 months prior to developing small type II subretinal neovascular membrane surrounded by a pigmented halo.
D: Small subretinal hemorrhage (arrow) that subsequently cleared without showing evidence of subretinal neovascularization.
E and F: Subretinal neovascularization (arrows).
G: Pigmented disciform scar (arrow) at edge of geographic atrophy of RPE and choroid.
H and I: Natural history of progression of juxtapapillary geographic atrophy of the retina and choroid over a 13-year period. Note disappearance of small pigmented disciform scar (white arrow) and the development of a focal staphyloma simulating an optic disc (black arrow).
J: Idiopathic retinal detachment with concave configuration within a macular staphyloma (arrows) in a patient who recently developed blurred vision in the right eye. Biomicroscopy and fluorescein angiography revealed no cause for the detachment, which may be related to vitreoretinal traction.
K: Rhegmatogenous macular detachment in the right eye caused by a macular hole (arrow) in a patient with bilateral juxtapapillary and macular staphylomata.
L: Rhegmatogenous detachment of the retina in the macula and paramacular area caused by a small round juxtapapillary retinal hole (arrow).

The infrequency of development of serous RPE detachments in these patients and the frequency of occurrence of choroidal neovascularization in middle-aged rather than older patients suggest that the new vessels from the choroid in most patients would be more likely to grow into the subretinal space (type II neovascularization) rather than into the sub-RPE space (type I) (Figure 3.45D). Fluorescein angiography may demonstrate abnormally slow choroidal and retinal blood flow in these patients. Angiography is helpful in identifying and locating the site of choroidal neovascularization in patients who develop serous and hemorrhagic macular detachment (Figures 3.44F, and 3.45B and C).

Exudative detachment of the macula must be clearly differentiated from a localized detachment caused by a macular hole or a minute, usually round, retinal hole that may be in the paramacular area in myopic persons with posterior staphylomata (Figure 3.44K and L). Biomicroscopy is usually required to find these holes. Fluorescein angiography is helpful in distinguishing this rhegmatogenous detachment from an exudative detachment. In the former case, no evidence of fluorescein leakage from the choroid is present. These detachments are relatively stable and in some cases may spontaneously resolve.[615] A chronic shallow serous detachment of the macula may also occur in some myopic patients with juxtapapillary and macular staphylomas in the absence of subretinal neovascularization, retinal hole, optic disc pit, or angiographic evidence of a leak at the level of the RPE (Figure 3.44J). The cause

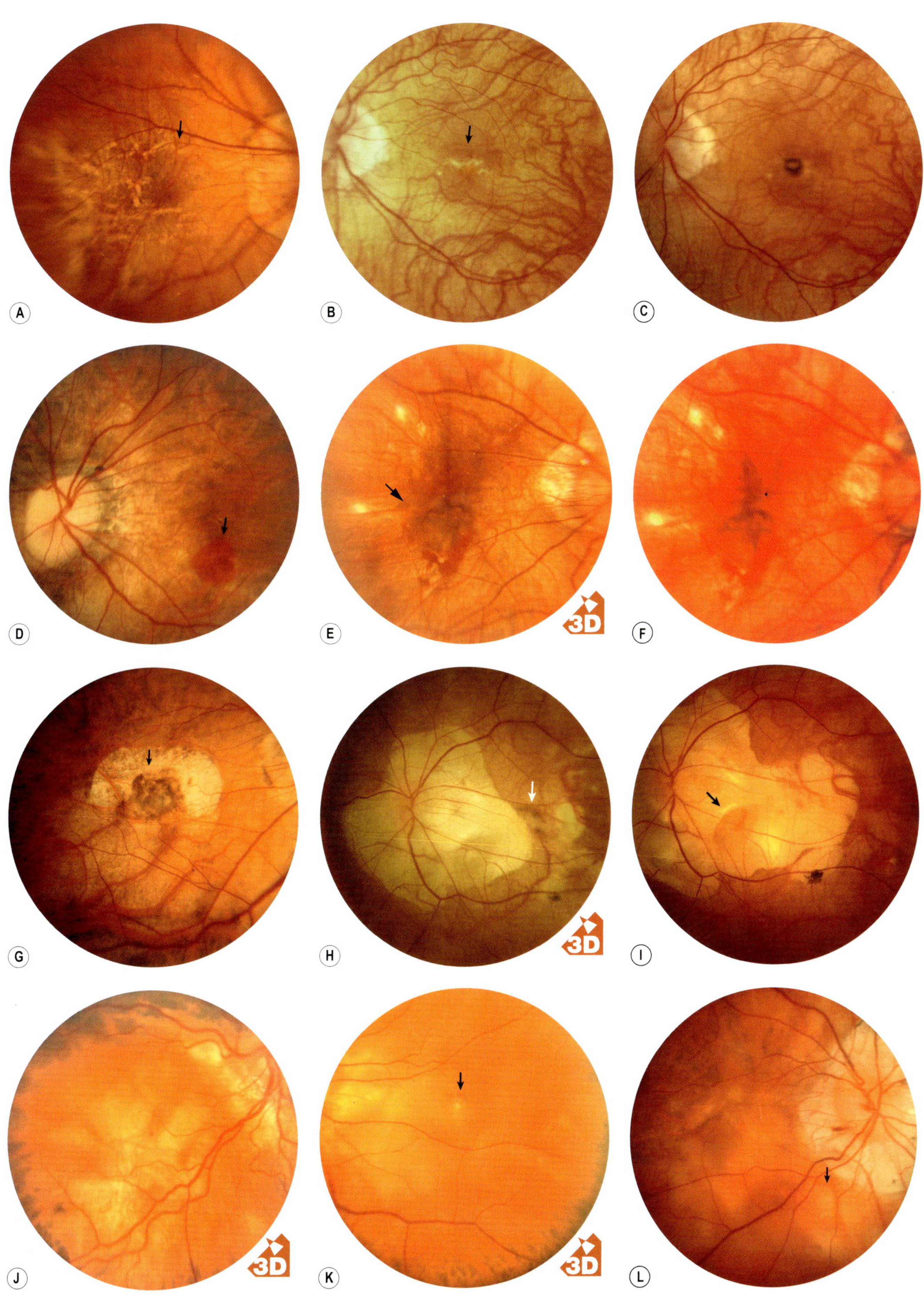
A
B
C
D
E
3D
F
G
H
3D
I
J
3D
K
3D
L

of this shallow, smooth-surfaced, and in some cases concave retinal detachment is uncertain, but it may be caused by occult vitreous traction in the presence of the staphyloma. That some of these may be a macular schisis rather than a retinal detachment or a combination of both has been identified with the use of high-resolution OCT (Figure 3.45H and I). Most recently, a localized choroidal excavation termed unilateral myopic choroidal excavation or ectasia has been noted in myopes who complained of metamorphopsias (Figure 3.45J–L). Spectral domain OCT demonstrates one of two appearances: the choroidal excavation involves the outer retinal layers up to the external limiting membrane (Figure 3.45K and L), or it involves only the RPE accompanied by an optically empty zone between the photoreceptors and the RPE.[616,617] The exact cause of these excavations is hitherto unknown; it is usually located in the vicinity of the fovea, not always under the foveal center.

The chorioretinal changes in high myopia may not be confined to the posterior pole. Cobblestone degeneration and lattice retinal degeneration may be present in approximately 15–30% of eyes.[614,618] Lattice degeneration is more common in eyes with mild than severe degrees of high myopia.[618]

It is still unclear whether the chorioretinal degenerative changes in progressive myopia are merely secondary biomechanical changes caused by progressive expansion of the scleral coats of the eye in response to normal intraocular pressure or whether they are an integral part of the genetically determined abiotrophy.[619] Myopic degenerative changes affecting the posterior pole may occur in some patients with only modest degrees of myopia and enlargement of the eye. Contrariwise, other patients with high degrees of ocular enlargement may show minimal degenerative changes. Although choroidal neovascularization is more likely to occur in eyes with some degree of myopic degenerative changes in the fundi, it is not solely related to the axial length of the eye or the presence of degenerative changes.[620] I have seen it occur in patients with only moderate myopia and minimal evidence of attenuation of the RPE or evidence of a posterior staphyloma. Spitznas and Böker have demonstrated that the predilection for developing idiopathic posterior subretinal neovascularization is directly proportional to the degree of myopia in patients with myopia of 6 D or less.[509] When focal atrophic lesions of the RPE in the macula accompany the neovascularization in the absence of other myopic degenerative changes in patients with high myopia, it may be impossible to determine whether the atrophic lesions and the new vessels are a product of focal myopic chorioretinal degenerative changes or a prior episode of asymptomatic multifocal choroiditis.

Funata and Tokoro induced axial myopia associated with scleral thinning experimentally in monkeys by occluding the ipsilateral eye.[621] They concluded that alteration of fibrillogenesis in the sclera is the key feature of scleral thinning in lid suture myopia, and that axial elongation of the eyeball probably results from a combination of altered fibrillogenesis and mechanical expansion.

The guidelines for laser photocoagulation treatment for subretinal neovascularization caused by other diseases are not necessarily applicable to treatment of this complication in patients with myopic degeneration. The extreme thinness of the choroid and Bruch's membrane in eyes with myopic degeneration (Figure 3.45H) makes them particularly vulnerable to mechanical effects, including those induced by photocoagulation. Attenuation of the choroid is probably also responsible for the tendency for subretinal neovascular membranes to remain relatively small. This, together with the predilection in these patients for photocoagulation scars to enlarge, suggests that photocoagulation treatment of subretinal neovascularization in these patients is of limited value.[622] Anti-VEGF agents work very well and cause prompt regression of myopic choroidal neovascularization and are the treatment of choice presently. Photodynamic therapy is also successful in most cases.

3.45 Choroidal neovascularization in high myopia.

A–C: Serous detachment of the macula caused by choroidal neovascularization at the margins of an area of chorioretinal atrophy in a 30-year-old man with high myopia. Note the pigment ring (arrow, A) at the superior margin of the atrophic choroidal lesion. Angiograms showed evidence of a small choroidal neovascular membrane (CNVM: arrow) on the temporal edge of the capillary-free zone of the foveal region (B). The CNVM and its feeding vessels were treated with argon laser photocoagulation (C). Two years after photocoagulation treatment the patient's visual acuity was 20/20.
D: Histopathology of subretinal type II fibrovascular membrane (Förster–Fuchs spot) in the macula of a highly myopic eye. Note that the fibrovascular plaque (arrow) is lined posteriorly by an inverted layer of retinal pigment epithelium (RPE) separating the membrane from the native RPE (type II).
E: Macular region and posterior staphyloma in a highly myopic eye. Note the extreme thinness of the choroid and relatively normal overlying sensory retina.

Myopic macular schisis.

F–I: Posterior staphyloma, lacquer cracks, and myopic crescent in a 48-year-old woman with 20/30 vision in the right eye and 20/50 + in the left eye (F–H). The left macula had myopic schisis with significant stretching of the outer plexiform region and ganglion cell layer (I). The posterior hyaloid was still attached without exerting significant traction. Optical coherence tomography findings and the visual acuity were unchanged a year later.

Choroidal excavation in myopia.

J–L: This 47-year-old, 6-D myopic Asian woman had a vision of 20/25. Several areas of choroidal excavation (ectasia) were seen (K and L). Some of these sites have been known to develop choroidal neovascularization that responds to anti-vascular endothelial growth factor treatment.

(J–L courtesy of Dr. K. Bailey Freund.)

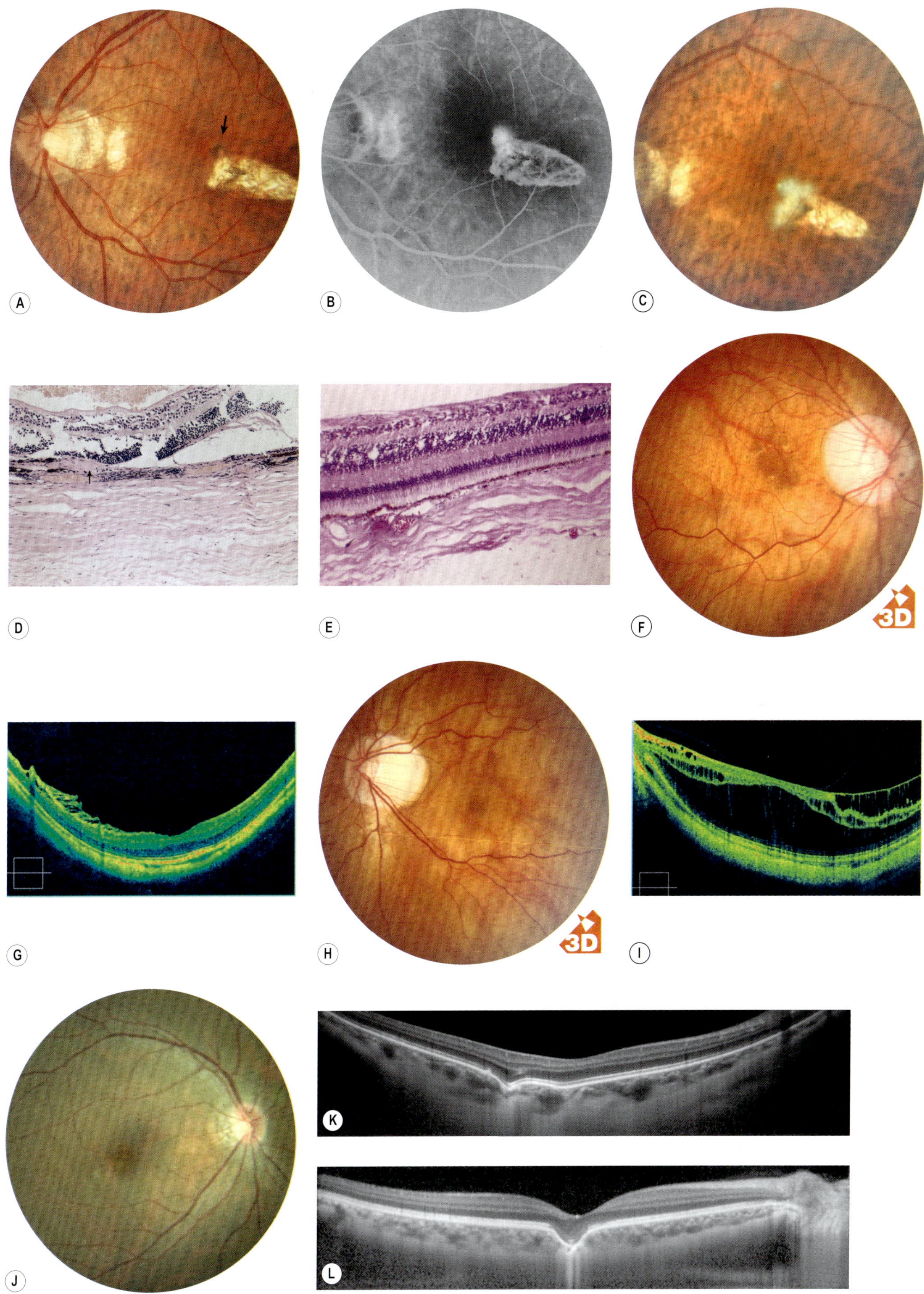
A
B
C
D
E
F
3D
G
H
3D
I
J
K
L

Successful repair of a macular detachment caused by a small posterior hole can be accomplished using a variety of special scleral buckling techniques, vitrectomy, and intravitreal injection of air or gas (Figure 3.44J–L).[623] There is little evidence that scleral reinforcement procedures prevent or lessen the effect of choroidal degeneration and neovascularization.[624]

PRESUMED OCULAR HISTOPLASMOSIS SYNDROME

Woods and Wahlen[625] described a clinical syndrome of serous and hemorrhagic detachment of the macula associated with multiple peripheral atrophic chorioretinal scars and peripapillary chorioretinal scarring that occurs usually in healthy patients between 20 and 50 years of age in the eastern half of the USA (Figures 3.46–3.53).[626] There is considerable evidence that the multiple chorioretinal scars are probably caused by a mild or subclinical systemic infection with *Histoplasma capsulatum* many years before the onset of macular detachment and visual symptoms. The loss of central vision is caused years later by choroidal neovascularization occurring at the site of one of these scars.[625,627–637] The average age of patients seen at the Bascom Palmer Eye Institute with symptoms in the first eye was 40 years and in the second eye approximately 44 years.[633,638] This syndrome occurs infrequently in black persons.[636,639]

The patient's general physical findings are typically normal. Approximately 90% of patients show a positive skin reaction to intracutaneous injection of 1:1000 histoplasmin. Most patients show a 3+−4+ reaction. Complement-fixing antibodies are demonstrable in only 16–68% of cases.[640] Check and associates[641] demonstrated that lymphocyte stimulation by the yeast phase of *Histoplasma* antigens was more sensitive than either the skin test or serum antibody test in these patients. Ganley and associates[642] have demonstrated evidence of a hyperactive cellular immune response to histoplasmin antigens by the lymphocyte transformation technique in patients who develop disciform complications. There is a higher frequency of the HLA-B7 and HLA-DRw2 antigens in these patients with disciform lesions compared to healthy persons. Patients with only peripheral atrophic scars also have a high occurrence of HLA-DRw2, but not HLA-B7.[643–647] This relationship of patients with POHS to HLA-DR2 is not found in patients with multifocal choroiditis and panuveitis (pseudo-POHS).[647] Chest roentgenogram evidence of healed histoplasmosis is a frequent finding. Focal calcification in the liver and spleen may occasionally be demonstrable. Rarely is there evidence of active pulmonary histoplasmosis.

Sudden blurring of vision, metamorphopsia, micropsia, and a positive scotoma in one eye are the initial symptoms in most patients. As many as 25% of patients note the onset of symptoms at times of unusual emotional stress.[630] The anterior segment and vitreous are free of evidence of inflammation. A localized serous or hemorrhagic detachment of the retina involving the macula is the most frequent finding (Figures 3.46B and C, 3.47A and G, 3.48F, I, and L, and 3.49C and G). Usually in the parafoveolar region there is a poorly defined, round or oval, slightly elevated, light gray, subretinal lesion that varies in appearance. Frequently a darker gray, round or oval ring of pigment is present within this light-gray area (Figures 3.47A and G). The hyperpigmentation that accompanies the choroidal neovascularization in patients with POHS is indicative of growth of the new vessels within the subretinal rather than the sub-RPE space. (See discussion of type I and II choroidal neovascularization in Chapter 2 and Figures 3.46 and 3.52.)

3.46 Pathogenesis of a disciform detachment caused by focal choroiditis.

Focal choroiditis, A, damages the choriocapillaris, retinal pigment epithelium (RPE), and Bruch's membrane and produces an exudative detachment of the retina, B, or type II subretinal neovascularization and hemorrhage into the subretinal space, C. Any of these three stages may resolve, leaving either a focal area of atrophy of the RPE, Bruch's membrane, and choroid (D) or, in the case of subretinal hemorrhage, a disciform scar, G. Either in the absence of further inflammation or under the influence of recurrent episodes of inflammation, the choroidal blood vessels surrounding an atrophic choroidal scar (D) may decompensate and cause serous exudation, choroidal neovascularization, and transient serous detachment of the retina (E). This in turn may result in hemorrhagic detachment of the retina (F) and a disciform scar (G).

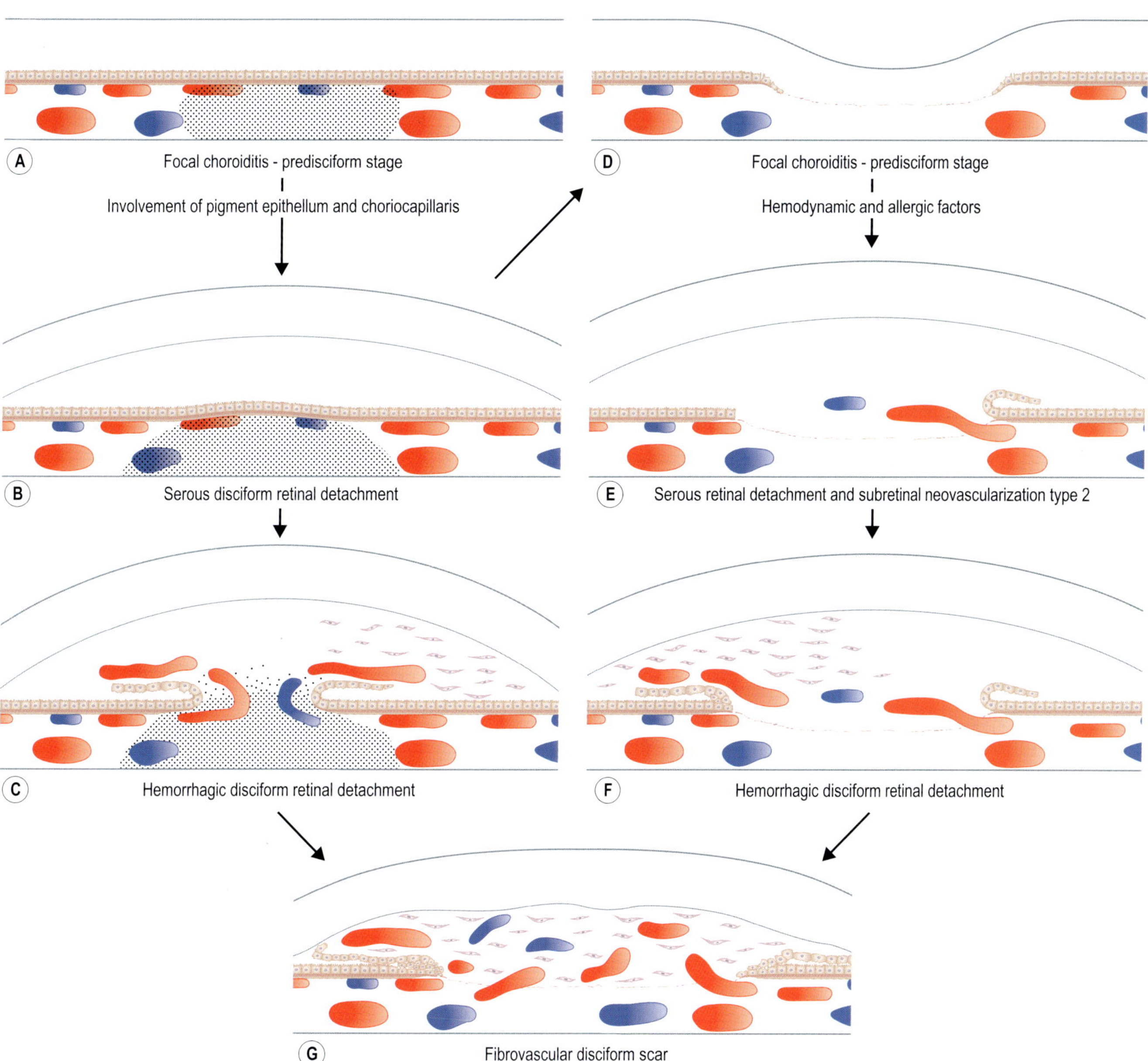
A
Focal choroiditis - predisciform stage
Involvement of pigment epithelium and choriocapillaris
D
Focal choroiditis - predisciform stage
Hemodynamic and allergic factors
B
Serous disciform retinal detachment
E
Serous retinal detachment and subretinal neovascularization type 2
C
Hemorrhagic disciform retinal detachment
F
Hemorrhagic disciform retinal detachment
G
Fibrovascular disciform scar

Varying amounts of subretinal blood may be present surrounding the margins of this dark halo. This pigment halo indicates the probable presence of a CNVM, the details of which are often obscured from biomicroscopic view by the presence of cloudy subretinal exudate. The chorioretinal scar from which the neovascularization arises is occasionally visible either beneath or at one margin of the lesion (Figures 3.47A and F, 3.48F, and 3.52A). In some cases a larger oval, round, or tongue-shaped diffusely greenish-gray membrane or mound is present in lieu of the pigment ring (Figure 3.47F). The pigment ring or mound is caused by reactive proliferation of the RPE as it attempts to surround and envelop the sheet of choroidal new vessels entering the subretinal space at the edge of a focal scar (see discussion of pathology in a later subsection). Exudative and hemorrhagic detachment of the RPE occurs infrequently in these patients. When it occurs, it is usually in patients 50 years of age or older. In POHS the exudation and bleeding occur primarily beneath the retina and not beneath the RPE. The CNVM may be confined to the area of the pigment ring, or it may extend outward from it into the surrounding subretinal space. This further extension of the neovascular membrane is usually evident as a gray-white semitranslucent or slightly pigmented membrane biomicroscopically surrounding the pigment halo. In a few patients the area of the choroidal scar and neovascularization may be so small that it cannot be visualized biomicroscopically beneath the serous retinal detachment. The angiographic findings may simulate that seen in patients with ICSC. In some cases the retinal detachment overlies an atrophic choroidal scar in the absence of a demonstrable new-vessel membrane (Figure 3.47D and E).[629,648] A tongue-shaped neovascular membrane arising at the site of peripapillary scarring (Figure 3.40L) may be the cause of macular detachment. Peripapillary retinal detachment and optic disc edema without evidence of subretinal neovascularization may occur occasionally.[649,650] Multiple sites of retinal detachment overlying CNVMs may be present in the same eye. Occasionally, serous and hemorrhagic retinal detachment develops at the edge of a peripherally located chorioretinal scar. Figure 3.50 (A and B) illustrates one such patient who was misdiagnosed as having a melanoma. The disciform macular scars that develop after the resolution of the subretinal blood and exudate vary in size, shape, and color. In general they are smaller in diameter than those occurring in older patients with drusen. Occasionally, however, they may exceed 2 disc diameters in size.

3.47 Serous and hemorrhagic detachment of the macula in the presumed ocular histoplasmosis syndrome.

A–C: Serosanguineous retinal detachment in left macula. Note faint pigment halo and blood around gray scar (A), subretinal neovascular membrane (arrow, B), and linear, confluent, equatorial distribution of peripheral chorioretinal scars (C).
D and E: Recurrent serous detachment of the retina (arrowheads, E) without other evidence of subretinal neovascularization surrounding a focal atrophic chorioretinal scar.
F: Serous retinal detachment caused by a large subfoveal hyperpigmented type II subretinal neovascular membrane (small arrows) arising from an extrafoveal chorioretinal scar (large arrow). This patient would be a good candidate for surgical excision of the membrane. (See Figure 3.52A–F.)
G–I: Spontaneous resolution of hemorrhagic detachment of the macula secondary to a choroidal neovascular membrane (CNVM) in the center of the macula in a 28-year-old woman (G and H). Visual acuity was 20/200. Twelve years later (I) the visual acuity was 20/30 in spite of the subfoveolar scar. (See Figure 3.53.)
J–L: Spontaneous resolution of serous and hemorrhagic detachment of the macula associated with a large extrafoveal CNVM (arrows, K) in a 45-year-old woman. The patient's visual acuity initially was 20/200. Eighteen months after resolution of the blood and exudate the visual acuity was 20/40 (L).

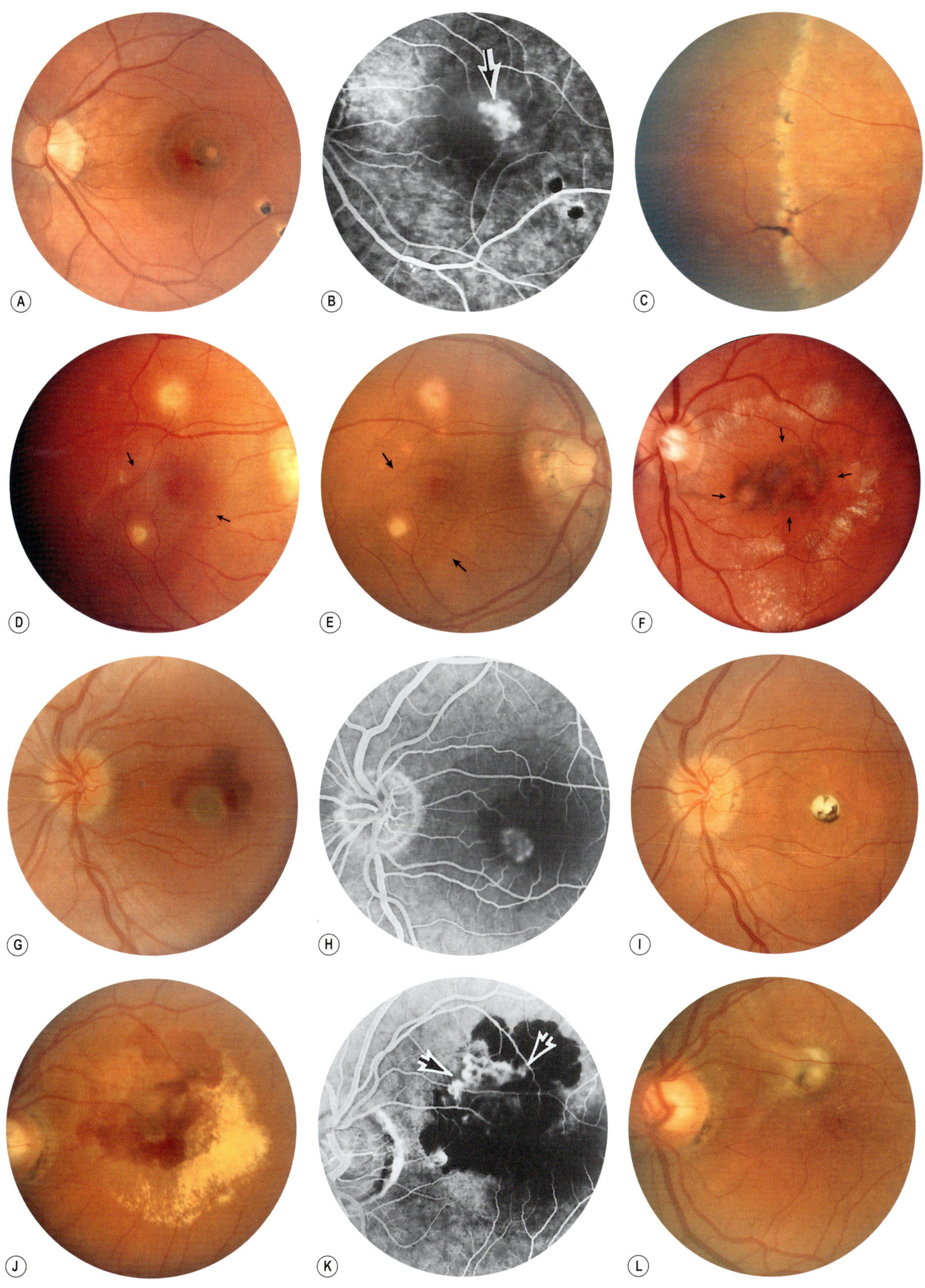
A
B
C
D
E
F
G
H
I
J
K
L

Other important features of POHS include peripapillary chorioretinal scarring and the presence of multiple, often sharply circumscribed, round or oval, focal, white, atrophic scars scattered throughout the fundi (Figures 3.47A and C, 3.48A and C, and 3.51F and G). The focal scars vary in size and degree of hyperpigmentation. Most are ¼–1 disc diameter in size or smaller. Some involve the full thickness of the choroid and RPE and present the biomicroscopic appearance of white, punched-out, atrophic lesions (Figure 3.48A and C). A large choroidal vessel may course through some of these lesions. Other lesions are more deeply located in the choroid and involve the RPE to a lesser degree. They have a more yellow or orange appearance and may be mistaken for focal nodules of choroidal infiltration. Some lesions show a combination of these two changes, that is, a focal atrophic lesion surrounded by an orange halo. Although RPE proliferation is often conspicuously absent in these lesions, black pigment may occur within or at the margins of the lesions (Figures 3.47A, 3.48C, and 3.51F). The lesions may be located anywhere in the fundus. Occasionally, they are arranged in a curvilinear row near the equator (Figure 3.47C).[627,651] In some patients a continuous band of depigmentation may extend around the equator in one or all quadrants. This equatorial distribution of lesions may occur in as many as 5% of patients with POHS. Similar streaks have been noted in patients with multifocal choroidal scars, vitritis, and no evidence of histoplasmosis (see discussion of pseudo-POHS, pp. 988–992).[652–655] Acute visual symptoms in a few patients with POHS may be associated with swelling of the optic disc and enlargement of the blind spot in the absence of any evidence of subretinal neovascularization.[649,650] The symptoms and disc edema usually resolve spontaneously and leave evidence of juxtapapillary scarring. (See discussion of reactive lesions simulating papilledema in a subsequent section.)

Fluorescein Angiography

Angiography typically reveals evidence of a cartwheel- or seafan-shaped CNVM in the area of the subretinal gray or pigment ring lesion (Figure 3.47B, H, and K). The neovascular membrane may be confined to the area of the pigment ring, or it may extend well beyond its border. Good-quality, early stereoangiograms are essential to determine accurately the location, size, and proximity of the CNVM to the center of the fovea. In some instances blood or cloudy exudate overlying the neovascular membrane prevents visualization of its capillary structure (Figure 3.47K) and its proximity to the fovea. The subretinal exudate that surrounds the neovascular membrane stains intensely with fluorescein. The various hemorrhagic and cicatricial disciform stages of macular detachment show fluorescein angiographic features similar to that described in patients with AMD. Angiographic evidence of serous detachment of the RPE occurs very infrequently in patients with POHS unless they are 60 years of age or older. Fluorescein diffuses from the choriocapillaris as well as from the retrobulbar vessels to stain the sclera and subretinal tissue within the focal and peripapillary atrophic chorioretinal scars (Figure 3.48D and E).[630,633,638]

3.48 Natural course of focal scars in the presumed ocular histoplasmosis syndrome.

A–C: Acquisition of a new focal chorioretinal scar. Note two peripheral atrophic choroidal scars in a patient with active pulmonary disease and hemorrhagic detachment of the macula (A). Angiography showed no evidence of other focal choroidal scars (B). Compare with photograph (C) taken 7 years later. Note increase in the pigmentation of old scars and presence of an additional scar (arrow, C) in 1971.

Choroidal neovascularization and hemorrhagic detachment of the macula occurring at the sites of previously observed chorioretinal scars in the presumed ocular histoplasmosis syndrome.

D–F: A perifoveal scar was present in 1965 when the visual acuity was 20/15 (D and E). Three years later the patient developed serous and hemorrhagic detachment of the macula (F).

G–I: A small perifoveal scar (arrow, G) was barely visible biomicroscopically in this patient when he was examined in January 1969. Visual acuity was 20/20. Angiography showed faint spotty hyperfluorescence (arrow, H). In July 1971 he developed serous and hemorrhagic disciform detachment (I); his visual acuity was 20/60.

J–L: A 27-year-old woman with visual acuity of 20/20 had mild chorioretinal changes between 4 and 6 o'clock at the edge of the optic disc in August 1968 (J). Angiography showed evidence of juxtapapillary scarring but no chorioretinal scarring in the macula (K). In September 1969 she developed serous and hemorrhagic detachment of the macula secondary to a choroidal neovascular membrane arising at the edge of the optic disc (L).

(A–L from Gass and Wilkinson.[630])

Natural Course and Prognosis

Over a period of 17 years the fundoscopic changes in a series of patients with POHS were studied and documented by means of fundus photographic maps and fluorescein angiography at the Bascom Palmer Eye Institute to determine the natural course of the macular lesions as well as the widely scattered atrophic chorioretinal scars.[630,633,638]

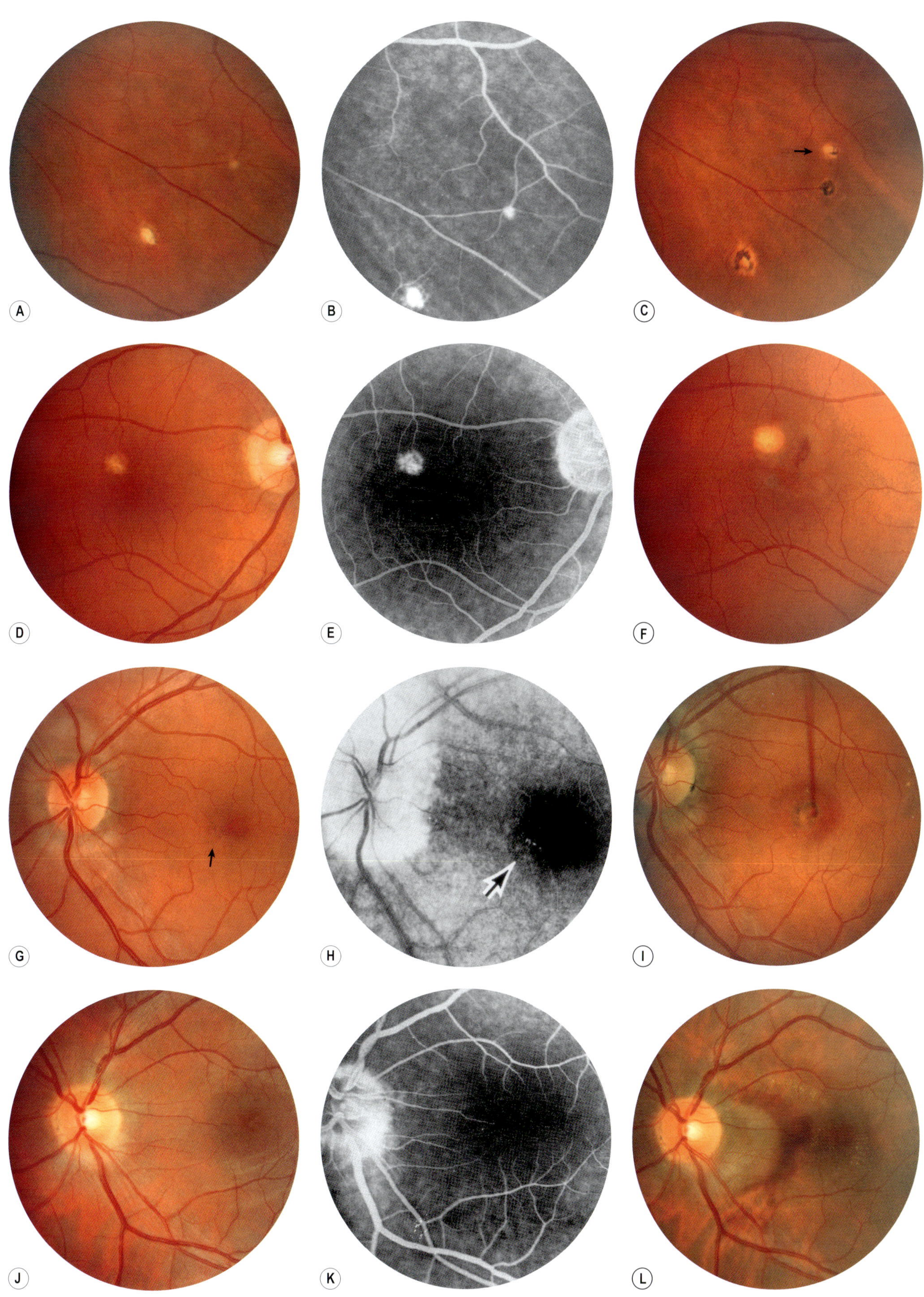
A
B
C
D
E
F
G
H
I
J
K
L

Once macular detachment has occurred, the visual prognosis depends on several factors. The proximity of the CNVM to the center of the fovea is the single most important factor. Following retinal detachment the CNVM may not grow or it may expand in a circular pattern or, less often, in a tonguelike projection from the defect in Bruch's membrane. Usually the membrane does not extend further than 1 disc diameter from the Bruch's membrane defect. As long as the subretinal CNVM does not grow beneath the fovea, the patient with either a serous or hemorrhagic macular detachment may regain good central vision following retinal reattachment, whether it occurs spontaneously (Figures 3.47G–I, 3.49K and L, and 3.53) or following photocoagulation treatment (Figure 3.49C–F and G–I). In general, patients whose CNVM arises from a point beyond 1 disc diameter from the center of the fovea have a relatively good short- and long-term prognosis. This includes those patients who develop macular detachment secondary to a sheet of subretinal new vessels growing temporally from the optic disc margins (Figure 3.48L).[656] Because recurrent detachment may occur and because it may be associated with further growth of the neovascular membrane, those patients with the origin of the new-vessel membrane within 1 disc diameter of the fovea have a more guarded prognosis even if they recover successfully from one episode of detachment. Some patients, however, may recover and retain excellent acuity for many years, even in the presence of a CNVM extending beneath the center of the fovea (Figures 3.47F and 3.53).[657,658] In some cases this recovery occurs over a period of many months.

The frequency of recurrent detachment and duration of detachment are also important factors in visual prognosis. The fundoscopic and fluorescein angiographic finding of a discrete zone of hyperfluorescence secondary to pigment epithelial atrophy that extends from the site of the CNVM into the central foveal area usually indicates permanent damage to the overlying retina caused by a previously prolonged serous or hemorrhagic macular detachment.

Prior to anti-VEGF therapy, multiple studies concerning the natural course have found that patients with serous detachment and with choroidal neovascularization that lies outside the capillary-free zone have a 60–70% chance of retaining 20/40 or better vision in the affected eye.[630,659–662] If the neovascular membrane extends inside the capillary-free zone, 15% or fewer retained 20/40 or better vision.

Follow-up studies have revealed that some of these patients continue to develop new scars as well as changes in the appearance and size of old scars (Figures 3.48A and C, and 3.49A and C).[627,630,633,636,638,660,663–669] In a few cases, small lesions may disappear. In the follow-up study in Miami approximately 20% of patients showed an increase in the size of one or more scars in the macular region, and over an average 8.4-year follow-up, 9% of patients with normal maculas by both biomicroscopy and angiography developed new atrophic scars in the macular region.[633,638]

3.49 Photocoagulation treatment in the presumed ocular histoplasmosis syndrome.

A–F: This 39-year-old patient was asymptomatic when seen initially. There was one inactive scar in the macula (arrow, A). He returned 5 years later with blurred vision caused by a de novo choroidal neovascular membrane (arrows, C and D). He responded to argon laser treatment (E and F). Visual acuity at the time of F was 20/20. Note the changes that occurred in the juxtapapillary scars during the course of observation.

G–I: This 26-year-old man with a perifoveal neovascular membrane (arrows, G) and an adjacent scar in the right eye had argon laser treatment (H). Thirty-eight months after treatment, his visual acuity was 20/15 (I). His visual acuity in the left eye improved spontaneously from 20/200 (K) to 20/50 (L) during the period of observation in the right eye.

J–M: This 48-year-old woman had received one session of photodynamic therapy to this subfoveal neovascular membrane 3 months before being seen. A pigmented ring of choroidal neovascularization located subfoveally with flecks of blood was noted. Peripapillary atrophy typical of presumed ocular histoplasmosis syndrome was also present and her vision was 20/80 (J). A classic pattern of lacy fluorescence was seen on angiography (K). The membrane regressed and remained inactive after three monthly injections of bevacizumab (L and M).

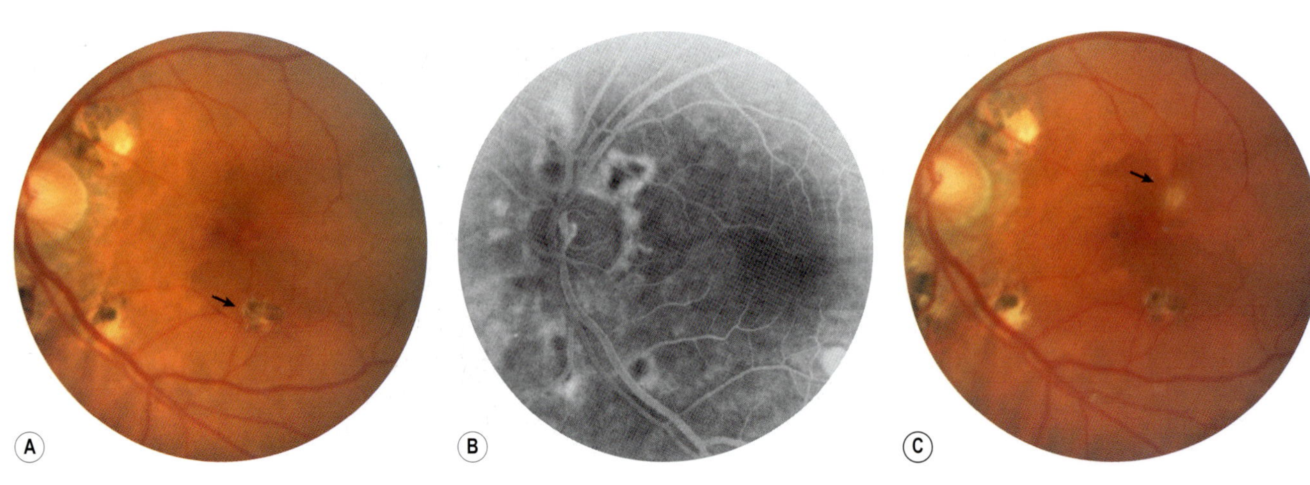

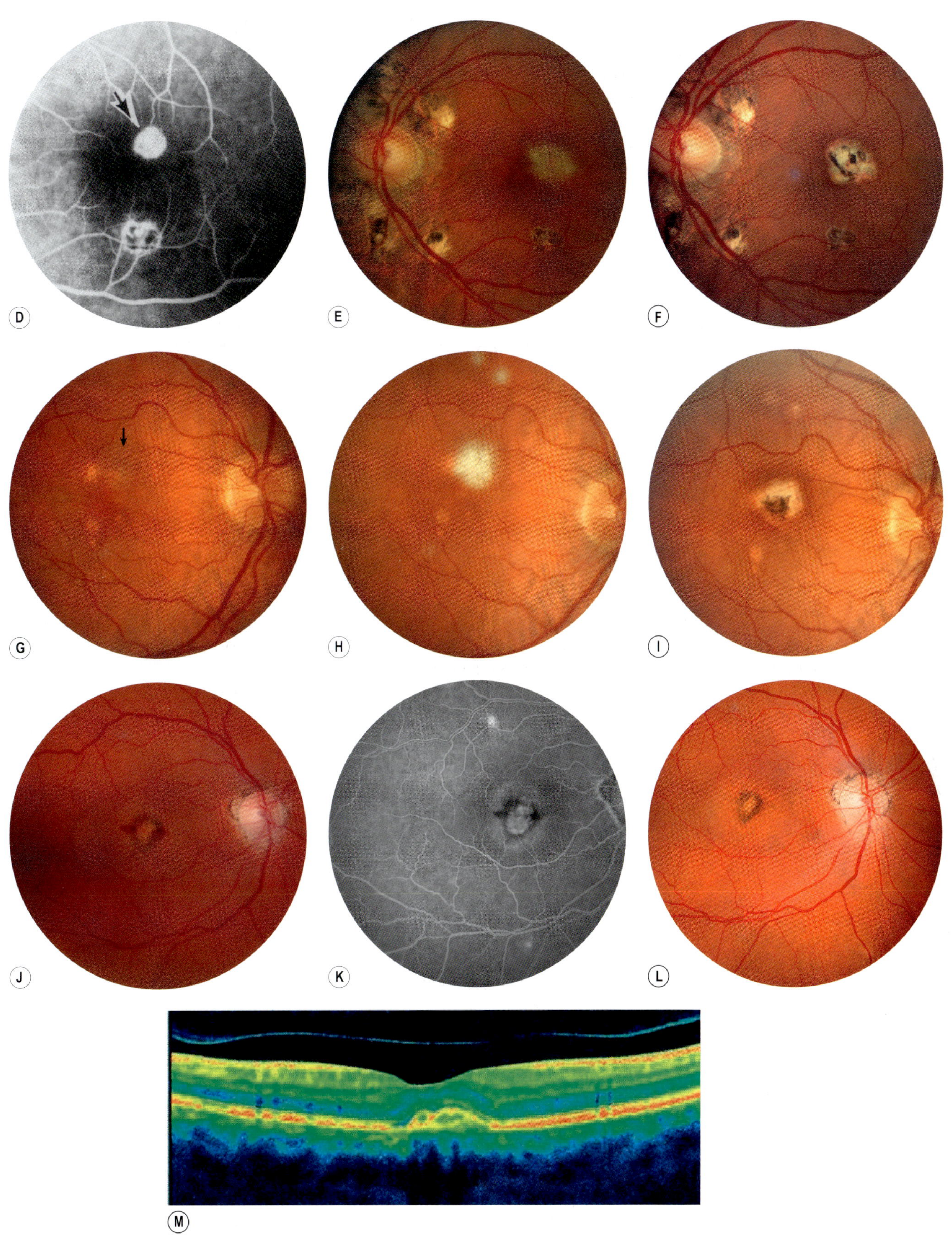
D
E
F
G
H
I
J
K
L
M

Life-table analyses of the patients observed in Miami revealed that 12% will develop symptoms in the second eye within 5 years and 22% will develop symptoms in the second eye within 10 years.[633] The relative risk of developing symptoms in the second eye caused by choroidal neovascularization developing in the juxtapapillary area or macula is twice as great in patients with macular scars compared to those with none. The risk of developing symptoms from a neovascular membrane arising in the macula (excluding the juxtapapillary origin) is 3.5 times as great. Patients with symptoms in their first eye should have several early angiographic views made of the opposite eye to exclude the presence of macular scars that may not be visible biomicroscopically. Of 42 patients without biomicroscopic or angiographic evidence of a scar at the time of initial presentation, only two have developed macular detachment from a de novo macular scar.

3.50 Pseudotumors caused by presumed ocular histoplasmosis syndrome.

A and **B**: Large black peripheral subretinal hemorrhage (A) that was initially misdiagnosed as a choroidal melanoma. It was caused by peripheral choroidal neovascular membrane (arrows, B) that became apparent several months after partial resolution of the blood.

C–F: This patient was being observed for a disciform scar (C) in the right eye when he returned because of further decrease in vision. The disciform lesion had enlarged and was associated with subretinal exudation. It continued to expand over a 6-month period of observation, and there was concern that a melanoma had arisen in the scar (D and E). Three months later the lesion began to shrink spontaneously (F).

G–J: Reactivation of an eccentric hypertrophic scar (G) discovered on a routine eye examination in March 1986 in a 23-year-old woman from Tennessee with multifocal chorioretinal scars in both eyes. The multiple white spots in G are artifacts. She was asymptomatic until March 1992 when she developed loss of central vision in the right eye. Her visual acuity was 20/400. Note the macular star and multilobular elevated chorioretinal lesion (large arrows, H and I) and multifocal chorioretinal scars (arrowheads) superonasal to the slightly swollen optic disc. The tissue comprising the upper right lobe (right large arrow, I) appears to be posterior to the retinal pigment epithelium. Following treatment with corticosteroids the macular star and retinal detachment surrounding the elevated lesion resolved. When last seen in September 1994 there was a multilobulated elevated white scar superonasally (J). The macula appeared normal but her visual acuity was 20/200.

K and **L**: Pseudo-capillary angioma optic disc in a patient with presumed ocular histoplasmosis syndrome.

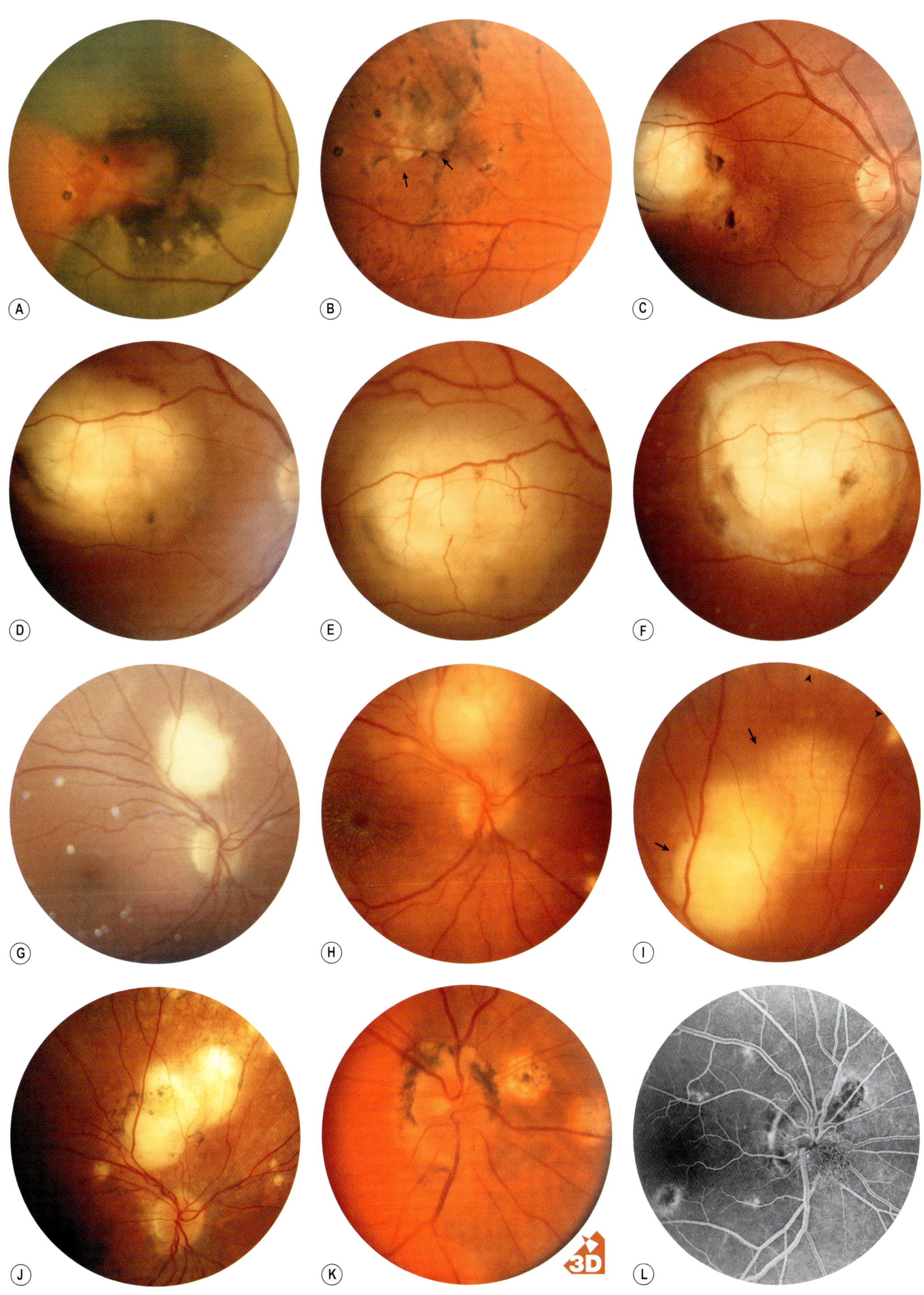
A
B
C
D
E
F
G
H
I
J
K
L
3D

Histopathology

Histoplasma capsulatum has been convincingly demonstrated histopathologically in the human eye of patients with systemic histoplasmosis on several occasions but in no patient who at the time of enucleation was known to have the typical clinical picture of POHS.[629,631,670–679] The organisms have been described in three eyes of patients with POHS, but there is some doubt that the structures found were *H. capsulatum*.[680–683] There is one report of exogenous histoplasmosis endophthalmitis developing in a patient with the vitreous wick syndrome after cataract extraction.[675] In some of the cases of histoplasmosis endophthalmitis the organisms have been found in the retina, the vitreous, and the ciliary body, but not the choroid.[671,672,675] In a patient with acquired immunodeficiency syndrome (AIDS) who presented with multifocal white retinal and subretinal lesions, the organisms were found in the retina and optic nerve as well as the uveal tract.[679] Figure 3.51 (A–C) depicts the clinical and histopathologic findings of multiple choroidal granulomas in a 14-year-old boy who died of widely disseminated histoplasmosis.[631] This represents the early granulomatous stage, which is rarely seen clinically. Figure 3.51D depicts a disciform macular detachment secondary to a large solitary *Histoplasma* choroidal granuloma in a healthy 18-year-old man whose eye was enucleated with the mistaken diagnosis of an intraocular neoplasm.[627,676] *H. capsulatum* organisms were found within the granuloma.[627,634,676] Examination of the opposite eye some years later revealed multiple atrophic chorioretinal scars typical of POHS.[676] One can only speculate as to whether or not the patient had active granulomas in both eyes at the time of enucleation. This patient probably was detected during the infectious stage of the disease only by virtue of the unusual size of the macular granuloma.

3.51 Histopathologic findings in disseminated systemic histoplasmosis and in the presumed ocular histoplasmosis syndrome.

A–C: Fundus painting of a 14-year-old boy with disseminated systemic histoplasmosis and two focal choroidal infiltrates (A). Histopathologic examination of the eye of the patient illustrated in A revealed a focal choroidal *Histoplasma* granuloma (B). Note destruction of the overlying retinal pigment epithelium and minimal evidence of inflammatory signs in the surrounding choroid and retina. Special stains showed *Histoplasma capsulatum* (arrows, C).

D: Large focal choroidal granuloma secondary to histoplasmosis in an 18-year-old boy whose eye was removed with the mistaken diagnosis of an intraocular tumor. Note that the granuloma had eroded through Bruch's membrane and pigment epithelium into the subretinal space. A rim of pigment-laden macrophages surrounds the subretinal portion of the granuloma (arrows). *Histoplasma capsulatum* organisms were identified within this lesion. Scars typical of the presumed ocular histoplasmosis syndrome were subsequently noted in the opposite eye.

E: Serous and hemorrhagic detachment of the retina arising from an area of focal nongranulomatous choroiditis (arrow) in a 32-year-old man. The eye was removed because of a suspected intraocular tumor. Ophthalmoscopic examination of the opposite eye revealed the presence of scattered lesions compatible with the presumed ocular histoplasmosis syndrome. No organisms were identified in this lesion.

F and G: Clinicopathologic correlation of focal atrophic chorioretinal scar in a 59-year-old man with typical findings in both eyes of the presumed ocular histoplasmosis syndrome. Note the lymphocytic infiltration surrounding the area of downgrowth of retinal cells, presumably astrocytes, into the underlying choroid (G).

(A–C from Klintworth et al.[631], D from Gass[627] and Maumenee and Ryan[705]; E from Gass.[628])

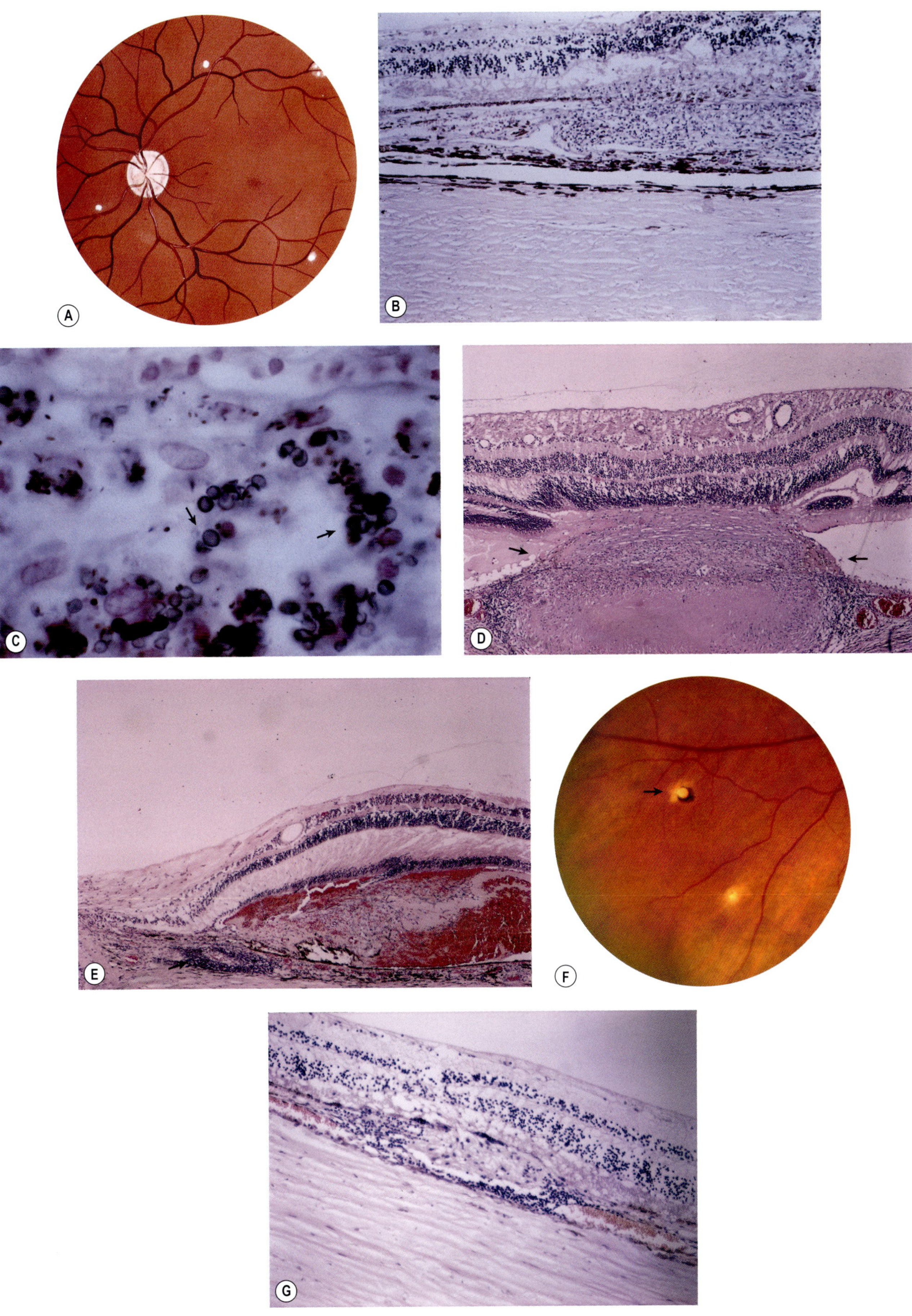
A
B
C
D
E
F
G

Figure 3.51 (F and G) depicts the clinical and histopathologic findings of an atrophic chorioretinal scar in an eye obtained at autopsy from a patient who had been treated with photocoagulation unsuccessfully several years previously for the typical fundus picture of POHS.[628] Histopathologic examination of several of the atrophic peripheral scars revealed focal lymphocytic infiltration surrounding a nodule of retinal tissue (presumably astrocytic proliferation) that had filled in a focal defect in the underlying choroid and RPE. There was only minimal inflammatory reaction in the area of the large disciform macular scars in both eyes (Figure 3.52G and H). Other authors have also demonstrated similar choroidal lymphocytic infiltrates around juxtapapillary and peripheral atrophic scars in these patients.[682,684–686]

Histopathologic examination of eyes of patients with POHS and actively growing CNVMs demonstrates type II subsensory retinal choroidal neovascularization. (See discussion of types of choroidal neovascularization in Chapter 2.) New capillaries and fibrocytes, originating within the choroid at the site of a chorioretinal scar and lymphocytic infiltration, grow through a defect in Bruch's membrane, choriocapillaris, and RPE into the subretinal space (Figures 2.11, 2.12, 3.46C, E, and F, and 3.52A–C). Because most of these patients are young or middle-aged adults with the RPE firmly adherent to Bruch's membrane, the fibrovascular membrane overrides the RPE and grows in a sheetlike fashion in the subretinal space. The new vessels induce reactive hyperplasia of the RPE at the site of the membrane's entry into the subretinal space and in front of its advancing border during the symptomatic stage of POHS. The RPE cells align themselves in a monolayer with their base attached to the outer surface of the expanding membrane. These active new vessels are associated with serous exudation or bleeding into the subretinal space. If the proliferating RPE cells succeed in covering the anterior surface of the membrane, exudation may cease and the membrane may undergo involution (Figure 3.53). Figure 3.51E depicts a large subretinal hematoma derived from choroidal neovascularization occurring within an area of Bruch's membrane and RPE destruction overlying a focal nodule of lymphocytes and plasma cells in the choroid. The nodule contained no organisms. Pigment-laden macrophages and proliferation of the RPE surrounded the defect in Bruch's membrane and an inverted layer of proliferating RPE cells extended along the outer surface of the neovascular complex. Several focal areas of lymphocytic choroiditis and overlying retinal atrophic scars were present in the peripheral fundus. This eye was enucleated because of the incorrect diagnosis of choroidal melanoma. Ophthalmoscopic examination of the opposite eye at a later date revealed the presence of scattered focal atrophic chorioretinal scars compatible with POHS.[676]

Choroidal lesions similar to those occurring in humans have been produced experimentally in animals infected with *H. capsulatum*.[687–692] Exacerbation of lymphocyte infiltration occurring in the vicinity of macular or juxtapapillary scars occasionally may cause reactive vascular and RPE hyperplasia and tumefaction simulating a choroidal melanoma (Figures 12.14H–L, 3.50C–J, and 3.52A–C) or benign hamartomas (Figures 3.50K and L, and 12.14F and G).

3.52 Clinicopathologic correlations in the presumed ocular histoplasmosis syndrome.

A–C: Hyperpigmented type II subretinal neovascular membrane mistaken for choroidal melanoma. Arrow (A and color plate V-1) indicates origin of new-vessel membrane at site of old scar surrounded by a pigmented halo. Histopathologic examination of horizontal section at the level of focal scar (arrow, A) shows ingrowth of new vessels from the choroid (curved arrow, B) into the subretinal space. Note hyperplastic retinal pigment epithelium (RPE) (straight arrows) at edge of fibrovascular membrane, which is covered on its anterior surface by thinned RPE (open arrow) and on its posterior surface by an inverted layer of RPE. Horizontal section at the level of the optic disc shows large subretinal fibrovascular membrane (arrows, C) lined on its posterior surface by a layer of inverted RPE. Note partial preservation of retinal receptors and tenuous adherence of the fibrovascular membrane to the overlying retina and underlying native RPE.
D–F: Surgical excision of a type II subfoveal neovascular membrane in this 30-year-old woman who noted loss of central vision caused by ingrowth of choroidal new vessels at the site of a focal chorioretinal scar (D). The visual acuity was 20/80. The neovascular membrane was grasped with forceps and dragged through a retinotomy site temporal to the macula (E). Note normal RPE (arrow) in the center of the macula. Several weeks later the visual acuity has returned to 20/20. Note old chorioretinal scar (arrow) and sclerotomy scar temporally.
G and **H**: Clinicopathologic correlation of pigmented disciform scar in patient with presumed ocular histoplasmosis syndrome (same patient illustrated in Figure 3.43F and G). Histopathologic examination revealed a subretinal fibrovascular scar separated from Bruch's membrane and remnants of the native RPE (lower arrows) by an inverted layer of RPE (upper arrows), evidence suggesting type II choroidal neovascularization.

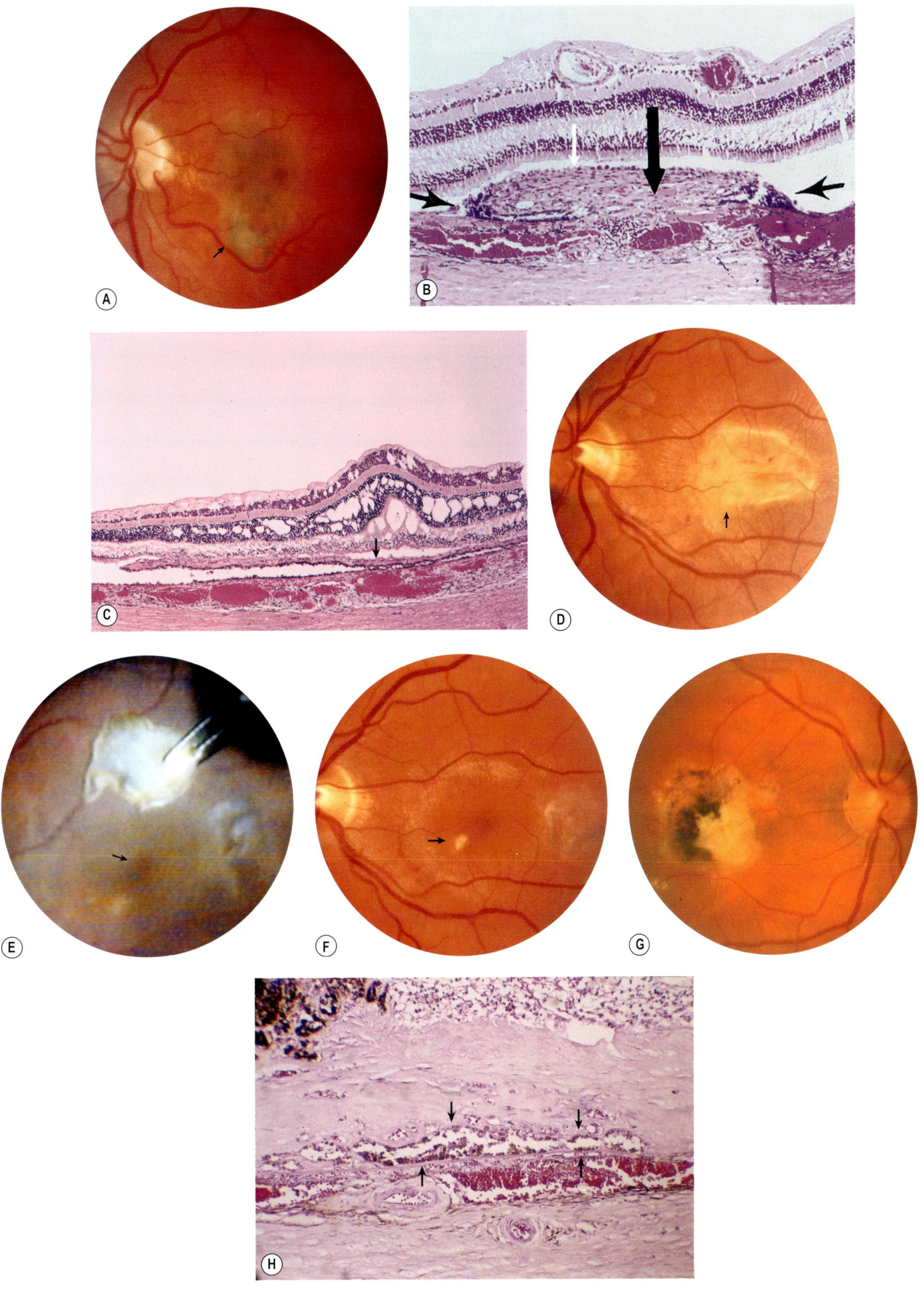
A
B
C
D
E
F
G
H

Pathogenesis

Evidence supporting the concept that *H. capsulatum* is a cause of this clinical syndrome in the USA includes: (1) 90–95% associated incidence with a positive histoplasmin skin test; (2) the high incidence of demonstrable lymphocyte stimulation and transformation to histoplasmin antigens in these patients; (3) good correlation between the prevalence of the disease in areas where histoplasmosis is endemic and where it is not; (4) frequency of radiographic findings of multiple pulmonary scars typical of histoplasmosis; (5) the Walkersville epidemiologic study[693]; (6) the identification of *Histoplasma* organisms in the eye of at least one patient who was subsequently observed to develop the typical POHS picture in the opposite eye (Figure 3.51D); (7) the finding of multifocal scars typical of POHS in six of eight patients who had systemic histoplasmosis some years previously[694]; and (8) the experimental production of POHS, including development of subretinal neovascularization, in subhuman primates following intracarotid injection of *H. capsulatum*.[627,628,630,642,673,694–698]

Although the pathogenesis of this disease is uncertain, the following is postulated: during an acute primary pulmonary infection with *H. capsulatum*, these patients develop dissemination of the organisms in the blood stream and multiple small granulomas throughout the body, including the choroid. Except for mild respiratory symptoms, the patient is asymptomatic during this phase of the disease. The primary choroidal lesions are sufficiently small that even when they occur near the central foveal area, they rarely produce visual symptoms. Because the human being is very resistant to this organism, it is rapidly destroyed, leaving minute atrophic scars surrounded by hyperimmune tissue. It is probable that most of these focal scars are subclinical initially. Over a period of years recurrent lymphocytic infiltration around these foci produces a gradual enlargement of these scars so that they become ophthalmoscopically visible. When they occur in the macular region and adjacent to the optic disc these scars represent a locus minoris resistentiae, where the choroidal circulation is exposed to the subretinal space. By virtue of the hemodynamic stress associated with the peculiar blood supply in the macula, these patients are predisposed to the development of serous exudation, choroidal neovascularization, and serous hemorrhagic disciform detachment. An exacerbation of the lymphocytic infiltration around these scars may be important in precipitating these complications.

The finding of focal lymphocytic choroiditis in the vicinity of apparently inactive focal chorioretinal scars (Figure 3.51F and G), as well as in scars associated with an actively growing subretinal neovascular membrane (Figures 3.51E and 3.52A–C), supports the theory that allergic phenomena may play an important role not only in gradual changes observed in the atrophic scars but also in stimulating choroidal neovascularization and macular detachment. The failure of most patients with early macular detachment to show an apparent response to intensive corticosteroid therapy is disconcerting if indeed allergic phenomena are important in the pathogenesis. By the time therapy is instituted, however, the proliferative vascular changes may be sufficiently advanced that suppression of the allergic reaction is insufficient to stop or slow the exudative and hemorrhagic complications.

Evidence supporting the concept that the macular lesions are caused by vascular decompensation and/or an allergic reaction at the site of a previous choroidal scar, rather than the direct result of an infectious granuloma, includes: (1) failure to find evidence of active histoplasmosis elsewhere in these patients; (2) failure to find ophthalmoscopic evidence of active choroidal infiltrates elsewhere in the eye; (3) failure of the lesions to respond to antifungal therapy[699]; (4) failure of the disease to worsen when treated with corticosteroids; and (5) occurrence of serous and hemorrhagic disciform detachment in the second eye at the site of a choroidal scar that was usually present at the time of detachment in the first eye. The development of macular detachment in some patients with POHS during pregnancy, usually during the last trimester, is further evidence in support of vascular decompensation.

3.53 Clinicopathologic correlation of spontaneous resolution of subfoveal type II neovascularization associated with good visual acuity in a young woman with presumed ocular histoplasmosis syndrome.

A–E: A 27-year-old woman noted loss of central vision caused by a juxtafoveal subretinal neovascular membrane (arrow, A). The subretinal blood and exudate resolved spontaneously. Eight years later she had a recurrent serous and hemorrhagic detachment of the left macula, and angiography showed evidence of subfoveal extension of the membrane (B and C). Her visual acuity was 20/70. The detachment cleared spontaneously and she recovered visual acuity of 20/25, which she maintained for 9 years when she died because of metastatic carcinoma. Histopathologic examination revealed a thin atrophic subfoveal fibrovascular membrane (arrows, D). The separation of the retina from the membrane is an artifact. Higher-power view of the membrane (E) shows encirclement of the membrane by an atrophic layer of retinal pigment epithelium (RPE) (arrowheads) except where it communicated with the choroid. Small arrows indicate native RPE separated from overlying inverted RPE cells attached to the membrane. Large arrow indicates sclerotic and occluded blood vessel in the membrane. There was some thinning of the receptor cell layer.

F: The diagram summarizes the sequence of events in this patient.

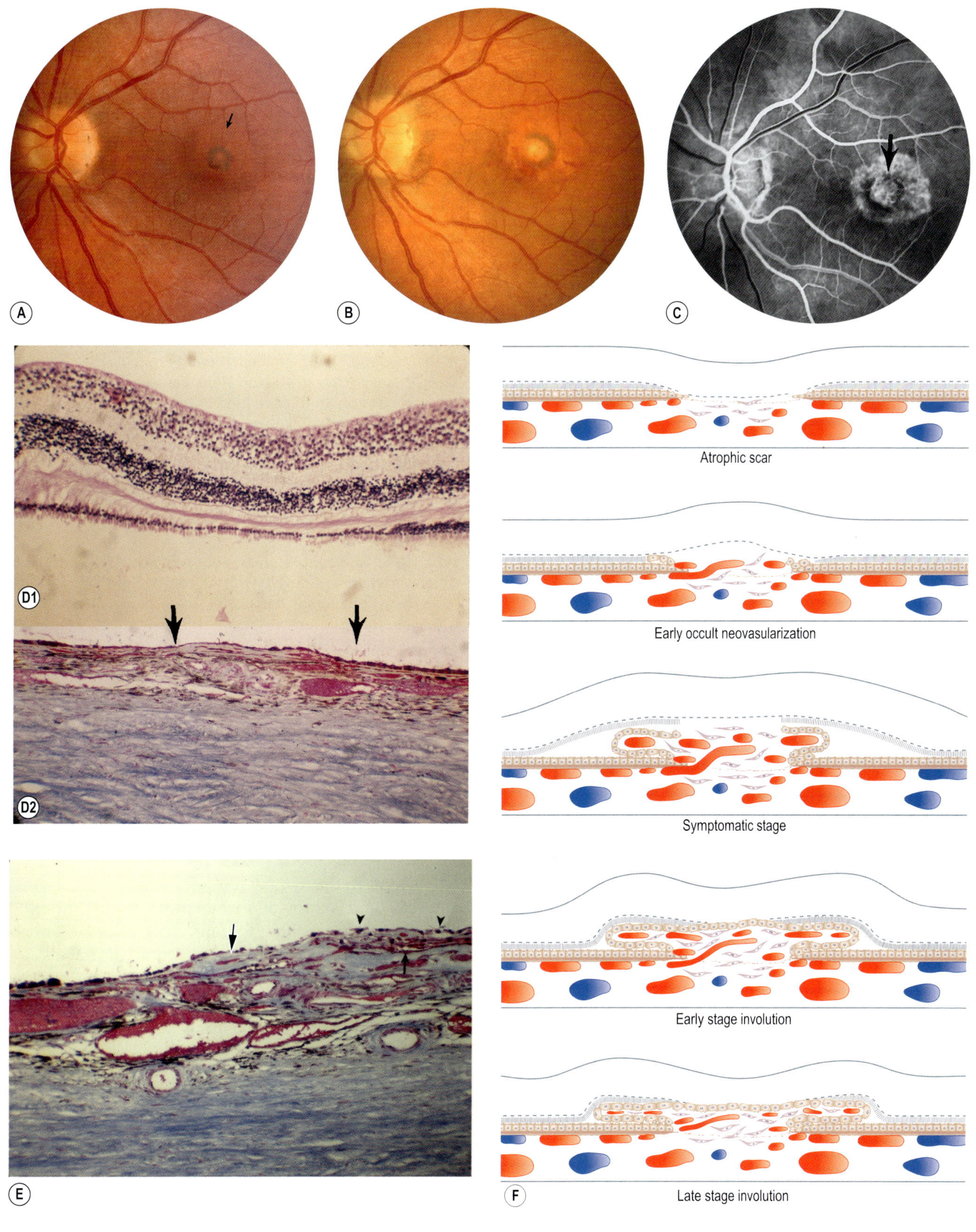
A
B
C
D1
D2
E
F
Atrophic scar
Early occult neovasularization
Symptomatic stage
Early stage involution
Late stage involution

Differential Diagnosis

The typical picture of POHS has been reported in patients from nonendemic areas of histoplasmosis and undoubtedly can be caused by other organisms, such as *Coccidioides* (Figures 10.17A–F and 10.18A–C).[700] The clinician must rely heavily on the extramacular findings to differentiate POHS from other diseases, such as panuveitis and multifocal choroiditis[654] (see discussion of pseudo-POHS, p. 988), diffuse unilateral subacute neuroretinitis (see p. 864), vitiliginous chorioretinitis (see p. 1038), and multiple scars caused by toxoplasmosis (see p. 848).

Diagnosis

The diagnosis of POHS is based on the clinical features. Cutaneous reaction to *Histoplasma* antigen and serologic tests, including complement fixation, immunodiffusion, and mycelial antigen identification, are limited to confirming the diagnosis in patients with unusual clinical presentations.

Treatment

The medical treatment of POHS is unsatisfactory. Although it is of some theoretical value, there is little evidence to date to support the practical value of oral and sub-Tenon's injections of corticosteroids. Their use should be limited to those patients with a relatively recent history of loss of central acuity whose lesion does not reveal the typical features of a CNVM. In such cases the author uses 40–100 mg prednisone per day for several weeks, and then on an alternate-day basis for several weeks. If no response is apparent, the dose should be rapidly tapered and discontinued. If apparently favorable responses occur, then a longer schedule of progressively decreasing dose may be used.

Photocoagulation has been advocated for the treatment of the neovascular component of POHS (Figure 3.49C–F, G–J).[127,444,635,701–712] The Macula Photocoagulation Study (MPS) has demonstrated the effectiveness of intense laser photocoagulation of CNVMs in preventing severe visual loss of six or more lines of visual acuity in the following groups of patients with POHS: (1) intense argon laser photocoagulation used to cover the entire area of CNVMs that lie outside the capillary-free zone; (2) krypton laser of juxtafoveal CNVMs that do not extend into the center of the macula; and (3) krypton laser of persistent or recurrent neovascularization following photocoagulation (Figure 3.49).[444,663,701,703,713,714] The long-term results of photocoagulation of juxtafoveal and extrafoveal neovascularization in patients with POHS are good.[444,703] The rate of persistence and recurrence of CNVMs after photocoagulation in the MPS study was 23% and 8%, respectively.[702] Both were associated with an increased incidence of severe visual loss.

Surgical excision of type II subretinal neovascular membranes that have extended beneath the fovea has restored excellent visual acuity in some patients with POHS (Figures 2.11, 2.12, 3.52A–F).[282,469,476,715–720] The best candidates for surgical excision are patients with recent subfoveal extension of the membrane that has arisen from an identifiable scar outside the capillary-free zone. Photodynamic therapy has also been successful in treating subfoveal membranes secondary to POHS.[721,722] However, a safer and more effective therapy has been the introduction of anti-VEGF therapy, in the treatment of most cases of extrafoveal, juxtafoveal, and subfoveal membranes.[723,724] A monthly treatment regimen of about four injections of bevacizumab or ranibizumab is first performed. Repeat treatments are necessary only in some cases and can be performed as needed. Surgical excision of a juxtapapillary membrane may still be considered in an occasional patient.[725]

Patients with retention of useful central vision in one or both eyes should be instructed in the frequent use of the Amsler grid and near-vision card and the importance of prompt examination if changes are detected.

Reactive Lesions Simulating Melanomas, Hamartomas, and Papilledema

As mentioned previously, large subretinal hematomas arising from subretinal neovascularization occurring within peripheral as well as centrally located chorioretinal scars may simulate a choroidal melanoma. Additionally, reactive

3.54 Idiopathic polypoidal choroidal vasculopathy – recurrent large subretinal hemorrhages.

A–F: This 50-year-old African American woman was seen for sudden loss of vision in her right eye to count fingers. A large macular subretinal hemorrhage was noted and an angiogram showed mostly blocked fluorescence, except for a small area of perfusion. She returned 6 months later with a vision of 20/400 in this eye and 20/200 in the fellow eye. The subretinal blood was mostly gone, but a fibrotic partly contracted polyp was seen in the superior macula. Subretinal lipid and chorioretinal starfold was also noted (C). She was poorly compliant with her follow-up and returned 2 years later with an improvement in the left eye vision to 20/40. Two years later she developed several polyps and subretinal blood in the inferior macula (D and E). Two more years later the blood and the polyps had disappeared and the vision was 20/150 in this eye and 20/40– in the left eye (F).

G–I: This 65-year-old African American woman with hypertension was known to have bled in the left eye 15 years previously and lost vision. Her vision was 20/20– on the right and 20/400 on the left. There were small orangish nodules temporal to the disc and several drusen superotemporally (G). Indocyanine green angiography confirmed the polyps (H); the left macula had a disciform scar (I).

Laser treatment of polyps.

J–L: This 58-year-old man of African American and Caucasian heritage developed progressive lipid and shallow subretinal fluid while the polyps were being observed (J). Moderate-intensity argon green laser (long-duration, low to intermediate power) was applied to the extrafoveal polyps. Three months later the fluid has resolved and the lipid exudates have decreased (L).

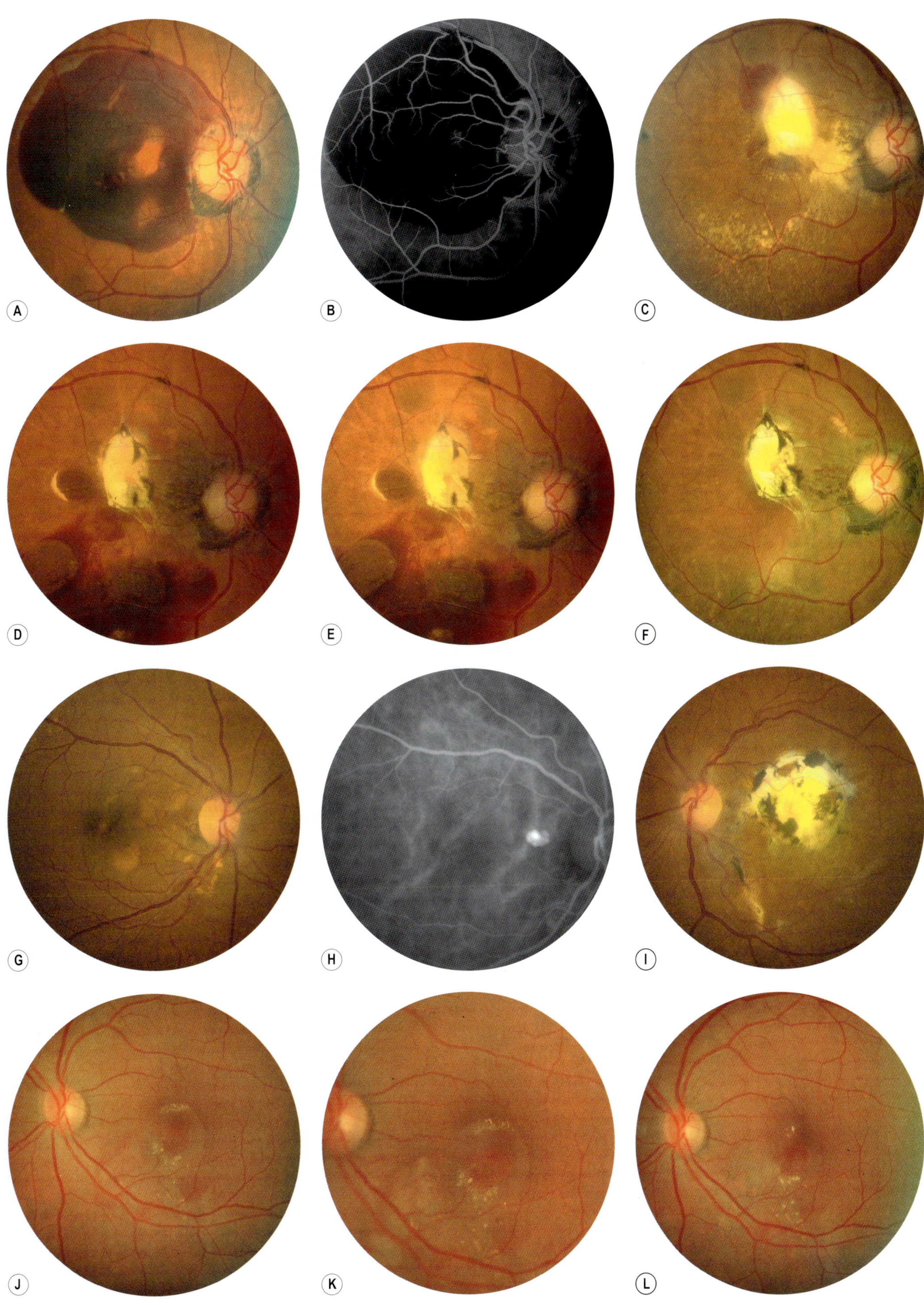
A
B
C
D
E
F
G
H
I
J
K
L

proliferation of subretinal fibrovascular, retinal glial vascular tissue, and retinal pigment epithelial cells may simulate choroidal melanomas (Figures 3.50A–J, and 12.14H–L); choroidal hamartomas, e.g., cavernous hemangiomas and osteomas (Figure 3.50G–J); and retinal hamartomas, e.g., capillary angiomas (Figure 3.50K), astrocytoma, and combined retinal and pigment epithelial hamartoma (see Figures 3.50K and L and 12.14F and G).[726–729] The stimulus for this exuberant reactive proliferation is presumed to be the same recurrent lymphocytic response that causes enlargement of the focal chorioretinal scars in POHS. Rarely, the mass lesion may be caused by proliferation of *H. capsulatum* within the mass.[726] As might be expected from the frequency of juxtapapillary scars in POHS, there is some predilection for these reactive tumors to develop in that region. In addition to the more slowly developing juxtapapillary pseudotumors, patients with POHS may present with acute visual symptoms, usually a temporal scotoma and optic disc swelling simulating papillitis, papilledema, or neoplastic infiltration of the optic nerve head.[649,650] These latter patients must be differentiated from patients with acute blind-spot enlargement associated with multifocal choroiditis and panuveitis that may simulate POHS. (See discussion of pseudo-POHS and acute zonal occult outer retinopathy in Chapter 11, pp. 988 and 980.)

HISTOPLASMOSIS RETINITIS AND CHOROIDITIS IN IMMUNE-INCOMPETENT PATIENTS

Multifocal active white retinal, subretinal, and choroidal lesions may occur in one or both eyes of patients with AIDS or other immune-incompetent states (see Chapter 10).

IDIOPATHIC POLYPOIDAL CHOROIDAL VASCULOPATHY (MULTIFOCAL IDIOPATHIC SUB-RPE NEOVASCULARIZATION OCCURRING IN DARKLY PIGMENTED INDIVIDUALS, POSTERIOR UVEAL BLEEDING SYNDROME)

Although neovascularization occurs much less commonly in black persons, Orientals, and darkly pigmented individuals, these patients, most of whom are black middle-aged women, may develop multiple and recurrent serosanguineous detachment of the pigment epithelium and retina associated with multifocal, often orange, nodular or plaquelike areas of sub-RPE neovascularization, that early in the course of the disorder are often most prominent in the juxtapapillary region (Figure 3.55).[505,506,510,512,730–732] Many of these sub-RPE angiomatous lesions show minimal evidence of perfusion and late-staining fluorescein angiographically (Figure 3.55).[510,732] In those who are subject to recurrent episodes of symptomatic bleeding, there is a predilection for development of vitreous hemorrhage. This disorder should be considered in the middle-aged or older black woman presenting with a dense vitreous hemorrhage. Since its original description in pigmented individuals, the disorder has been seen in all ethnic races, including Caucasians (Figure 3.54). It is more common among Japanese and Orientals and makes up a significant proprtion of their AMD patients.[733–737] The polyps can be few and confined to the posterior pole, or they are peripheral or extensive (Figure 3.55).

They are visualized well on indocyanine green angiography and can be located within the choriocapillaris or deeper in the choroid (Figures 3.54 and 3.55H). When in the deeper choroid or if the blood flow is slow within the aneurysmal dilatation, they are not easily visualized on the fluorescein angiogram. Other than the orange nodules, the presence of several pigment epithelial detachments, especially if associated with small or large subretinal hemorrhages, should prompt the diagnosis of IPCV (Figure 3.54). They can sometimes mimic central serous chorioretinopathy and should be suspected in persistent or recurrent ICSC.[733,738,739] Recently, high-resolution OCT has been able to isolate the polyp if in the choriocapillaris.[740,741] In eyes that present with vitreous hemorrhage, ultrasound may be helpful in detecting the extensive irregularly elevated sub-RPE fibrovascular plaques that may be present in the macular and extramacular areas of these patients.[732] Perkovich et al. found a high association of systemic hypertension in this group of patients.[732] One patient with biopsy-proven sarcoidosis became legally blind because of progressive subretinal fibrosis in both eyes.

3.55 Extensive idiopathic polypoidal choroidal vasculopathy.

A–H: A 70-year-old Caucasian woman was referred for worsening blurred vision in both eyes for 5 months. Her vision was 20/50 on the right and count fingers on the left. Both eyes had several pockets of retinal pigment epithelium (RPE) detachments, and areas of subretinal blood (A, C, D, G and H, arrows). There were areas of chorioretinal scars and subretinal fibrosis (SRF) more in the right than left eye (G and H). The left macula had subretinal fluid. Angiogram showed rapid filling of the RPE detachments in both eyes (B and F) and indocyanine green demonstrated polyps (E). Focal laser was done to the RPE detachment temporal to the fovea; 3 weeks later her vision had improved to 20/50 with resolution of SRF. Another month later she had new subretinal blood around this RPE detachment. Intravitreal bevacizumab was tried with no significant reduction in SRF. She was subsequently managed locally and no further information was available.

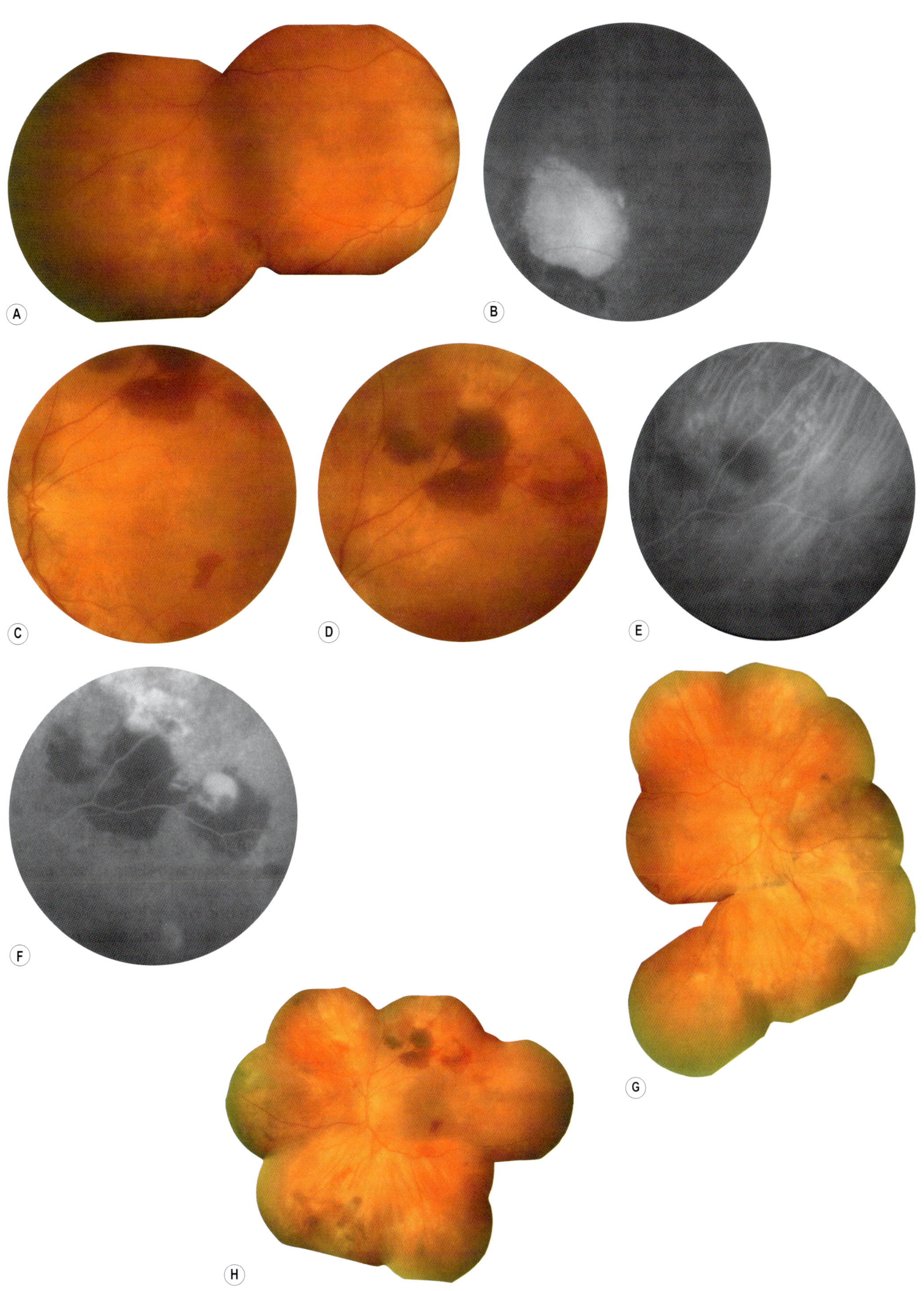
A
B
C
D
E
F
G
H

Treatment includes direct laser photocoagulation of the extrafoveal and extramacular polyps (Figure 3.55J–L). Care should be taken to use low-power and long-duration green laser to coagulate the polyp slowly and avoid bleeding. Photodynamic therapy has been more successful than anti-VEGF medications in shrinking the polyps located close to the foveal center. Large subretinal bleeds can be watched, as most resolve with no sequelae (Figure 3.55D–F).

Histopathologic examination of one eye of a white, 58-year-old man followed for 6 years because of multiple sites of idiopathic subretinal neovascularization, hemorrhagic pigment epithelial and retinal detachments revealed extensive subretinal fibrovascular proliferation and lymphocytic and plasma cell infiltration of the choroid.[731] A nonsynonymous variant I62V has recently been suggested as a possible candidate for causal polymorphism leading to IPCV in Japanese patients.[742]

UNUSUAL CAUSES OF CHOROIDAL NEOVASCULARIZATION

It is probable that any disease that damages the RPE is capable of causing choroidal neovascularization as a secondary response to the injury. Some unusual causes of choroidal neovascularization that are discussed elsewhere in this book are acute multifocal posterior placoid pigment epitheliopathy (see p. 956), rubella retinopathy (see p. 918), Best's disease (see p. 240), uveitis, demarcation lines caused by rhegmatogenous retinal detachment (see p. 686), chorioretinal folds (see p. 220), photocoagulation, optic disc colobomas and pits (see pp. 1260–1262), chronic papilledema (see pp. 1294–1296, fig. 15.17D–H), and hyaline bodies of the optic nerve head (see p. 1268).

ACUTE OCCLUSION OF THE SHORT CILIARY AND CHOROIDAL ARTERIES

We seldom have the opportunity to see patients with either functional or structural changes in the eye caused by localized occlusion of the short ciliary or major choroidal arteries because of the availability of many collateral pathways of blood flow. Occasionally, however, patients present with visual loss caused by ciliary arterial obstruction resulting from prolonged elevation of the intraorbital pressure (Figure 3.56A–F and J–L); systemic vascular disease, for example, giant cell arteritis (Figure 3.57),[743–748] periarteritis nodosa,[749] malignant hypertension (Figure 3.56G–I), or sickle-cell disease[750]; thrombotic infectious arteritis such as that caused by phycomycosis (mucormycosis)[751] and herpes zoster (see acute retinal necrosis, and Figures 10.43 and 10.46)[752–754]; embolization[755,756]; and hyperthermia.[757] Occlusion of the posterior ciliary arteries may occur as a complication of surgery involving the posterior sclera such as the Vasco–Posada sectioning of the scleral ring to alleviate central retinal vein obstruction.[758] Although the posterior ciliary artery blood supply generally has a temporal–nasal distribution on either side of the optic disc, in some cases the territorial division of the ciliary circulation may be horizontally based.[759] Because of the rich anastomosis of the choroidal vasculature, the area of delayed choroidal perfusion demonstrated by fluorescein angiography during the acute phase of the obstruction is much larger than the area of white outer retinal ischemia seen ophthalmoscopically (Figure 3.56G–L),[760,761] and in some cases this choroidal hypoperfusion may be associated with no visible changes in the fundus. The rich anastomotic network in the choroid explains why multifocal gray-white ischemic lesions affecting the pigment epithelium and outer retina caused by ciliary artery obstruction rarely occur clinically.[749]

3.56 Outer retinal ischemic whitening and infarction caused by transient occlusion of the choroidal circulation.

A–F: One day after phacoemulsification of a cataract this 37-year-old man noted a large central scotoma in the operated eye. Note the central cherry-red spot (B) and polygonal islands of outer retinal whitening (A and C) at the junction of the diffusely ischemic and nonischemic retina. A 30-second angiogram showed polygonal zones of staining of the retinal pigment epithelium (RPE) and outer retina (D). Fourteen months later visual acuity was 20/25. There was a dense paracentral scotoma to finger counting that corresponded with the areas of RPE derangement (E and F).

Inner and outer retinal infarction caused by transient occlusion of the choroidal and retinal circulation by an intraorbital hemorrhage.

G–J: Ischemic optic neuropathy (H), patchy areas of inner retinal ischemic whitening in the macula, and wedge-shaped areas of ischemic whitening of the outer retina (arrowheads, G and H) caused by ophthalmic artery obstruction in a woman with severe hypertension and atherosclerotic cardiovascular disease. Note delay in choroidal and retinal arterial perfusion at 48 seconds (I) and late staining of outer retinal ischemic areas (J).

K and **L**: After general anesthesia for a rhinoplasty, this 19-year-old healthy woman awoke with pain, severe lid swelling, and blindness in the right eye caused by obstruction of the choroidal and retinal circulation. At the time of these photographs 5 weeks later her visual acuity in the right eye was no light perception. Note optic atrophy, narrowing of retinal blood vessels and segmental wedge-shaped zones of severe mottling and atrophy of the RPE in the peripheral fundus. Angiography demonstrated an increased retinal circulation time and diffuse RPE changes.

(A–D from Rosenblum et al.[778]; E and F from Gass and Parrish.[776])

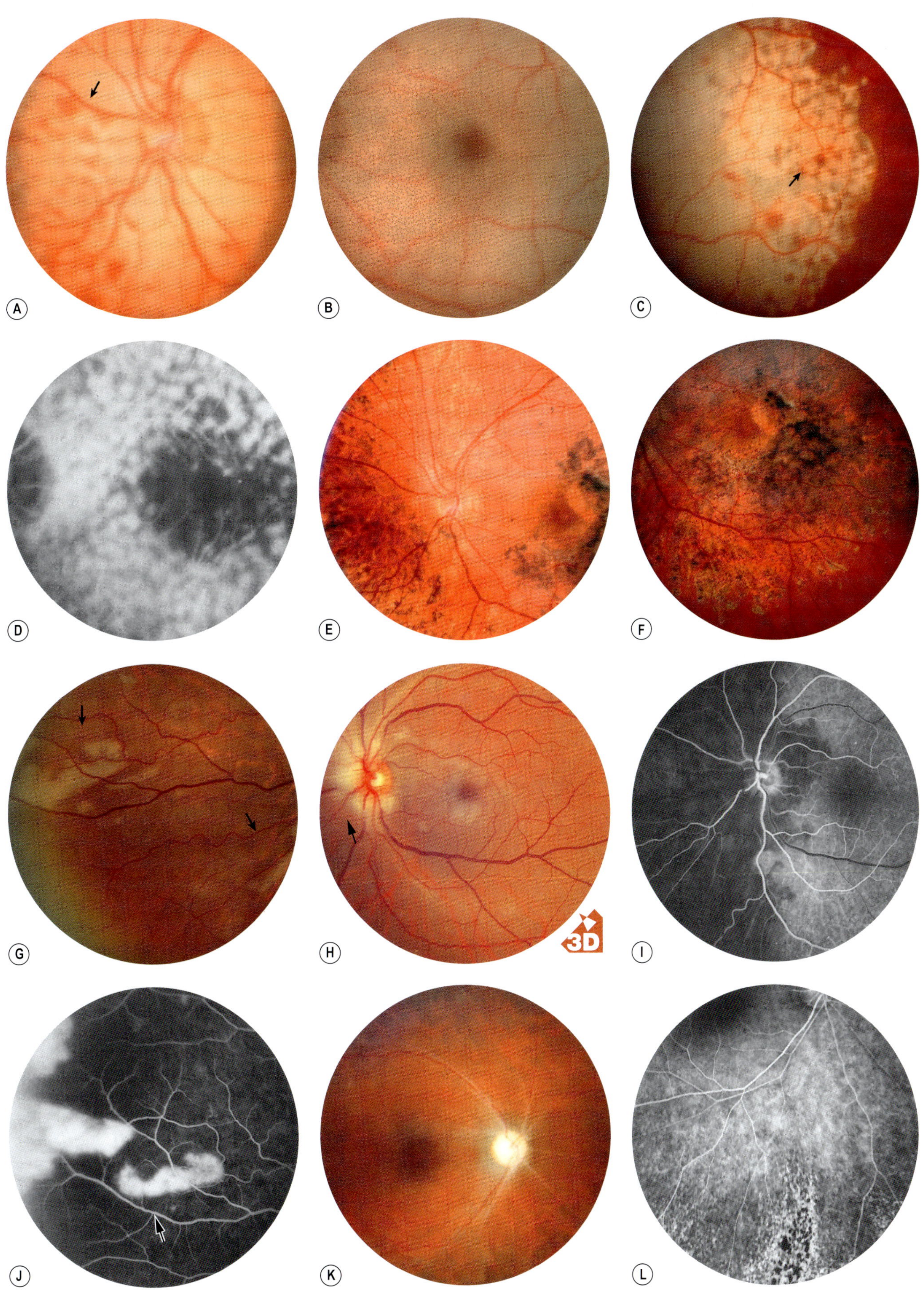
A
B
C
D
E
F
G
H
3D
I
J
K
L

A large zone of delayed choroidal perfusion may be seen adjacent to an area of krypton laser closure of one or more large choroidal arteries in the absence of any evidence of ischemic whitening of the outer retina or permanent damage to the retinal function in that area.[762–764] A triangular zone of solitary or multiple patches of outer retinal ischemic whitening followed by chorioretinal atrophy is more likely to occur after occlusion of a large choroidal artery in the midperiphery of the fundus, where there are fewer arterial anastomoses (Figure 3.56G–L) (see Chapter 6, and Figure 9.15A–F).[765–774]

A peculiar picture of acute outer retinal ischemic infarction of the posterior retina may occur in patients complaining of acute visual loss usually on the first postoperative day following phakoemulsification for cataract removal, vitrectomy procedures, or neurosurgery procedures in which prolonged pressure has been inadvertently placed on the eye (Figure 3.56A–C).[746,772,775–779] Fundoscopic examination reveals a picture that may be mistakenly diagnosed as a central retinal artery occlusion. The outer rather than the inner retinal layers are whitened. The whitening extends beyond the macula but does not reach the equator (Figure 3.56A–C). Multiple discrete patches of whitening separate the diffuse areas of whitening posteriorly from the relatively normal-appearing anterior half of the retina. A cherry-red spot is present. Fluorescein angiography may show no abnormalities of the retinal or choroidal circulation times, or it may show a late hexagonal or pentagonal pattern of fluorescein staining in the area of retinal whitening (Figure 3.56D). Mottled salt-and-pepper changes in the RPE become apparent as the retinal whitening clears (Figure 3.56E and F). The RPE in the foveola may remain normal. The patients may regain a small central island of vision and excellent visual acuity in addition to retaining a broad zone of their peripheral visual field. Although the pathogenesis of these changes is not certain, it has been hypothesized that they result from an extended period of elevation of the intraocular pressure just before or during the course of surgery. The duration of the pressure elevation and closure of the choroidal and retinal circulation is sufficient to cause ischemic infarction of the outer retina but not the inner retina. The outer retina, particularly in the posterior pole where it is thickest, is more sensitive to oxygen deprivation than is the inner retina and is more predisposed to infarction during an extended period of closure of both the choroidal and retinal circulation. The retina in the foveolar area, by virtue of its thinness, is less susceptible to transient oxygen deprivation. This hypothesis has been tested and verified experimentally in owl monkeys.[746] If the retinal and choroidal circulation are obstructed long enough, total irreversible blindness of the eye and a biomicroscopic picture of widespread profound ischemic whitening of both the inner and outer retinal layers and ischemic swelling of the optic disc occur. This picture of combined cilioretinal arterial occlusion is followed by optic atrophy and severe atrophic changes in the retina and RPE (Figures 3.56G–L).

3.57 Chorioretinal and optic nerve ischemia caused by giant cell arteritis occluding the major branches of the ophthalmic artery.

A–D: Ischemic optic neuropathy, cotton-wool patches in the distribution of cilioretinal arteries, and ischemic choroidopathy in a 73-year-old woman with acute loss of vision in both eyes (A). Angiography reveals delay in perfusion of the choroid (B and C) and late staining in the inner retina and at the level of the retinal pigment epithelium in the papillomacular bundle and macular areas (D). A temporal artery biopsy was positive for temporal arteritis.

E and **F**: Bilateral ischemic optic neuropathy, choroidopathy, and retinopathy in a 78-year-old man with malaise, weight loss, jaw claudication, and total loss of vision in both eyes. Two weeks prior to the fundus photographs (E and F), he developed sudden total loss of vision in the right eye and the following day became blind in the left eye. Note the severe optic disc ischemia and sludging of blood in the retinal vessels of the right eye (E) and the persistent cherry-red spot in the left eye (F).

Disseminated intravascular coagulopathy causing submacular choroidal hemorrhage.

G–J: This 27-year-old woman with anorexia, abdominal pain, arthralgia, fever, diarrhea, and bizarre neurologic symptoms noted visual loss associated with yellowish gray plaques and hemorrhage in the posterior choroid of both eyes (arrows, G). She developed progressive thrombocytopenia, hypofibrinogenemia, and accelerated fibrinolysis and died. Histopathologic examination of the eyes revealed choroidal thickening (arrows, H) caused by intrachoroidal hemorrhage involving the temporal half of the macula. There was extensive thrombotic occlusion of the choriocapillaris and larger choroidal arteries (arrows, I and J).

(G–J from Samples and Buettner.[810])

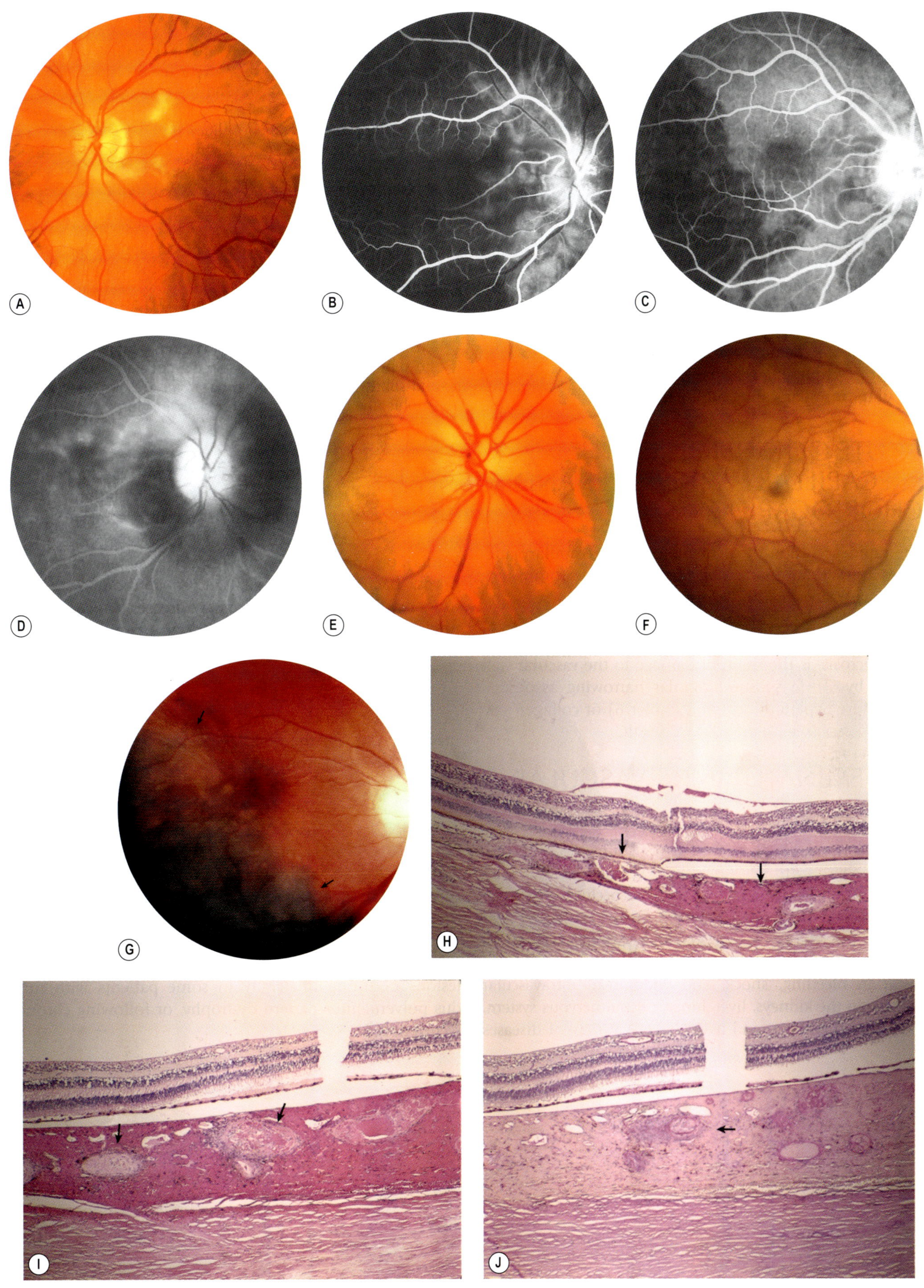
A
B
C
D
E
F
G
H
I
J

Malignant Hypertension

Patients with malignant hypertension may develop secondary detachment of the retina caused by acute multifocal areas of fibrin platelet occlusion and necrosis of choroidal arteries and choriocapillaris, and necrosis of the overlying RPE (Figures 3.58 and 6.26 to 6.28).[784,785,816] Elschnig spots, irregular areas of pigment epithelial atrophy, and angiographic evidence of choroidal vascular obstruction often remain after resolution of the detachment (Figures 3.58C, D, and H, and 6.28).[784,785,817]

3.59 Fundus changes caused by toxemia of pregnancy.

A: Massive preretinal hemorrhage and retinal detachment in a young woman who died several days later of complications of eclampsia.

B and C: This 42-year-old Haitian woman was hospitalized because of hypertension and generalized seizures during the 35th week of gestation. Three days after delivery by cesarean section she developed loss of vision caused by bilateral bullous retinal detachment. Note the patchy white areas of ischemic infarction of the retinal pigment epithelium (RPE) (arrows) beneath the retinal detachment (B). Angiograms showed multiple areas of leakage at the level of the RPE (C).

D and E: Acute bilateral loss of vision occurred in a 29-year-old mother soon after delivery of her baby. She had severe toxemia of pregnancy. Three days after delivery there were multiple white lesions at the level of the pigment epithelium and only minimal evidence of retinal detachment (D). Early angiograms showed a reticular pattern of nonfluorescence (E). Multifocal areas of staining (arrow) were evident later.

F and G: This asymptomatic 63-year-old woman was referred because of suspected heredomacular dystrophy. Visual acuity was 20/20. The multiple Elschnig spots (arrows) and branched pattern of yellow changes in both eyes were caused many years previously by severe toxemia that caused transient bilateral loss of vision just before birth of her second child.

H and I: Asymptomatic 50-year-old woman with RPE changes that were misinterpreted as heredomacular dystrophy. She had experienced bilateral visual loss associated with toxemia of pregnancy just before delivery of each of her last two children.

J–L: At age 18 years this 38-year-old woman had eclampsia and was blind in both eyes after delivery. She regained 20/400 visual acuity in both eyes. Note Elschnig spots (arrows, J and L), reticular network of pigment epithelial atrophy, narrowing of the retinal arteries, and peripheral intraretinal migration of pigment simulating a severe tapetoretinal dystrophy.

(A–L from Gass and Pautler.[819])

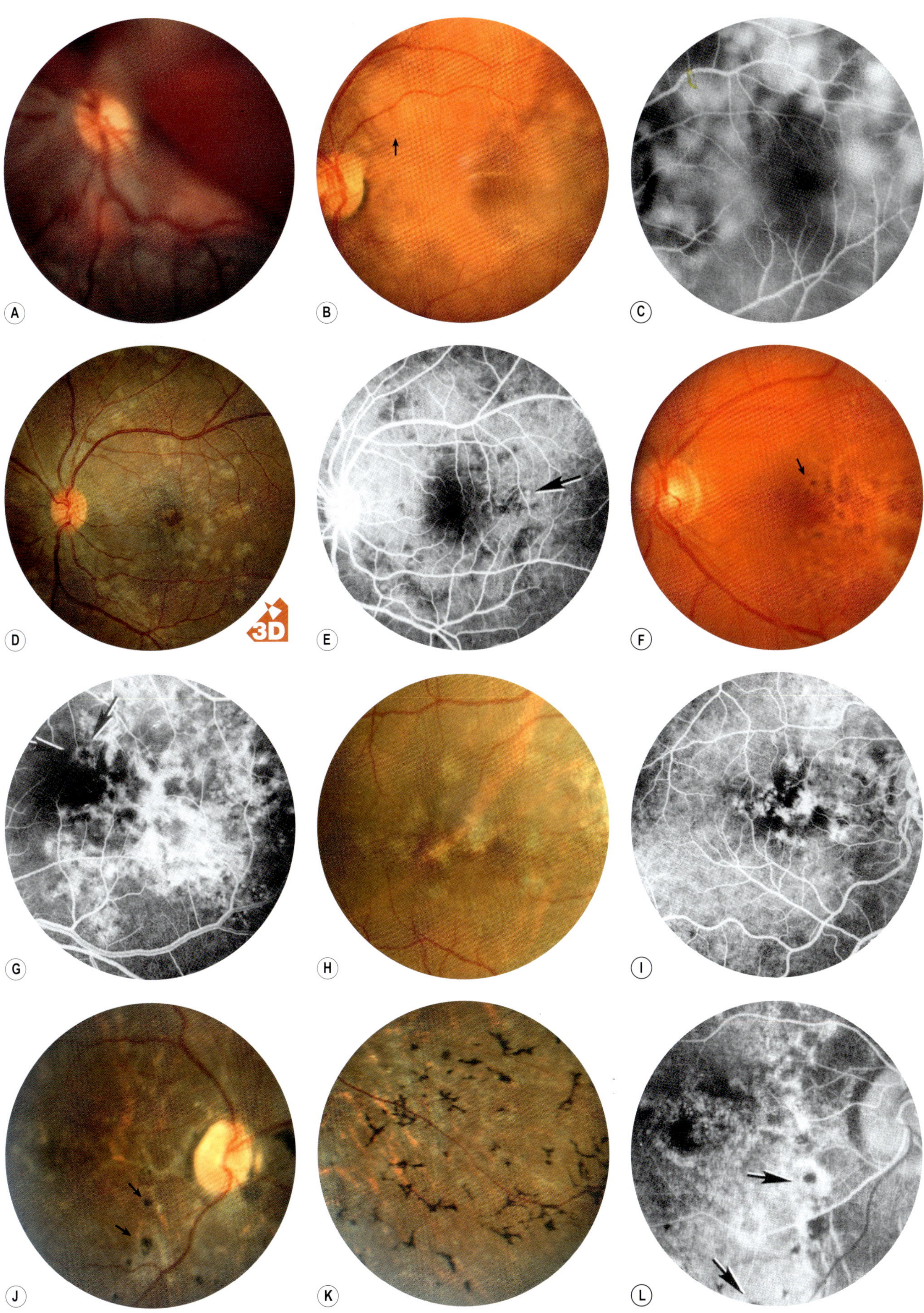
A
B
C
D
3D
E
F
G
H
I
J
K
L

TOXEMIA OF PREGNANCY

Approximately 1–2% of patients who develop severe hypertension, proteinuria, and edema during the third trimester of pregnancy develop loss of vision caused by serous retinal detachment (Figure 3.59A and B).[789,790,792–795,818–823] This usually occurs just before or immediately following delivery. A branching pattern of yellow-white patches caused by focal necrosis of the RPE and outer retina may or may not be evident (Figure 3.59B and D). The detachment may be confined to the macula or, particularly in patients with seizures (eclampsia), may involve the entire fundus and may rarely be associated with bleeding into the choroid, subretinal space, and vitreous (Figure 3.59A). These patients may or may not show evidence of cotton-wool patches and hemorrhages in the retina. Angiography may demonstrate evidence of delayed perfusion of segments of the choroid as well as multiple pinpoint areas of leakage of dye through the RPE in the region of the subretinal yellow-white patches (Figure 3.59C and E). After delivery and treatment of the hypertension, the detachment rapidly resolves and recovery of visual function is relatively complete in most patients. An irregular branching pattern of hyperpigmented dots (Elschnig spots), yellowish patches, and interconnecting lines of depigmentation of the RPE often remains in the juxtapapillary and macular area (Figure 3.59F, H, and J). These changes, caused by infarction of the RPE, are frequently symmetric in both eyes and, if initially detected on a routine eye examination years later, may be incorrectly interpreted as signs of a macular dystrophy.[818,819] They are often more evident angiographically than ophthalmoscopically (Figure 3.59E, G, I, and L). Patients with severe toxemia may develop profound visual loss and blindness secondary to total serous and hemorrhagic retinal detachment and be left following recovery with extensive degenerative changes in the RPE and retina that may simulate a diffuse tapetoretinal dystrophy (Figure 3.59J–L).[819] Correct diagnosis is important since the changes caused by toxemia are nonprogressive.

The cause of toxemia of pregnancy is unknown. Some patients presenting with bilateral retinal detachment may manifest other evidence of DIC, for example, hemolysis, elevated liver enzymes, low platelets, and upper abdominal pain (HELLP syndrome). Some of these patients may have normal or near-normal blood pressure.[824] HELLP syndrome has been associated with central retinal vein occlusion, serous and serosanguineous retinal detachment (Figure 3.60), vitreous hemorrhage, Purtscher-like retinopathy and occipital infarcts.[825–834] Increased VEGF levels have been noted in the serum of these women.[835]

3.60 HELLP syndrome (hemolysis, elevated liver enzymes, low platelets, and upper abdominal pain).

A–E: This 28-year-old Caucasian woman was diagnosed with HELLP (elevated liver enzymes and low platelets) syndrome at 37 weeks' gestation and underwent emergency cesarean section. She required temporary hemodialysis for renal failure that recovered. On the first day postpartum she noted blurred vision in her right eye. Ophthalmology consultation was not obtained. When examined 2 months later her vision had improved considerably to 20/25 in each eye. The retina was attached with interlacing subretinal fibrin plaques that had scalloped margins (A and B). Optical coherence tomography shows the material to be in the subretinal space. We presume she had extensive exudative retinal detachment when symptomatic, that since resolved leaving the proteinaceous material subretinally. Three weeks (D) and 3 months (E) later the subretinal fibrin has decreased and resolved almost completely.

(Courtesy of Dr. David Weinberg.)

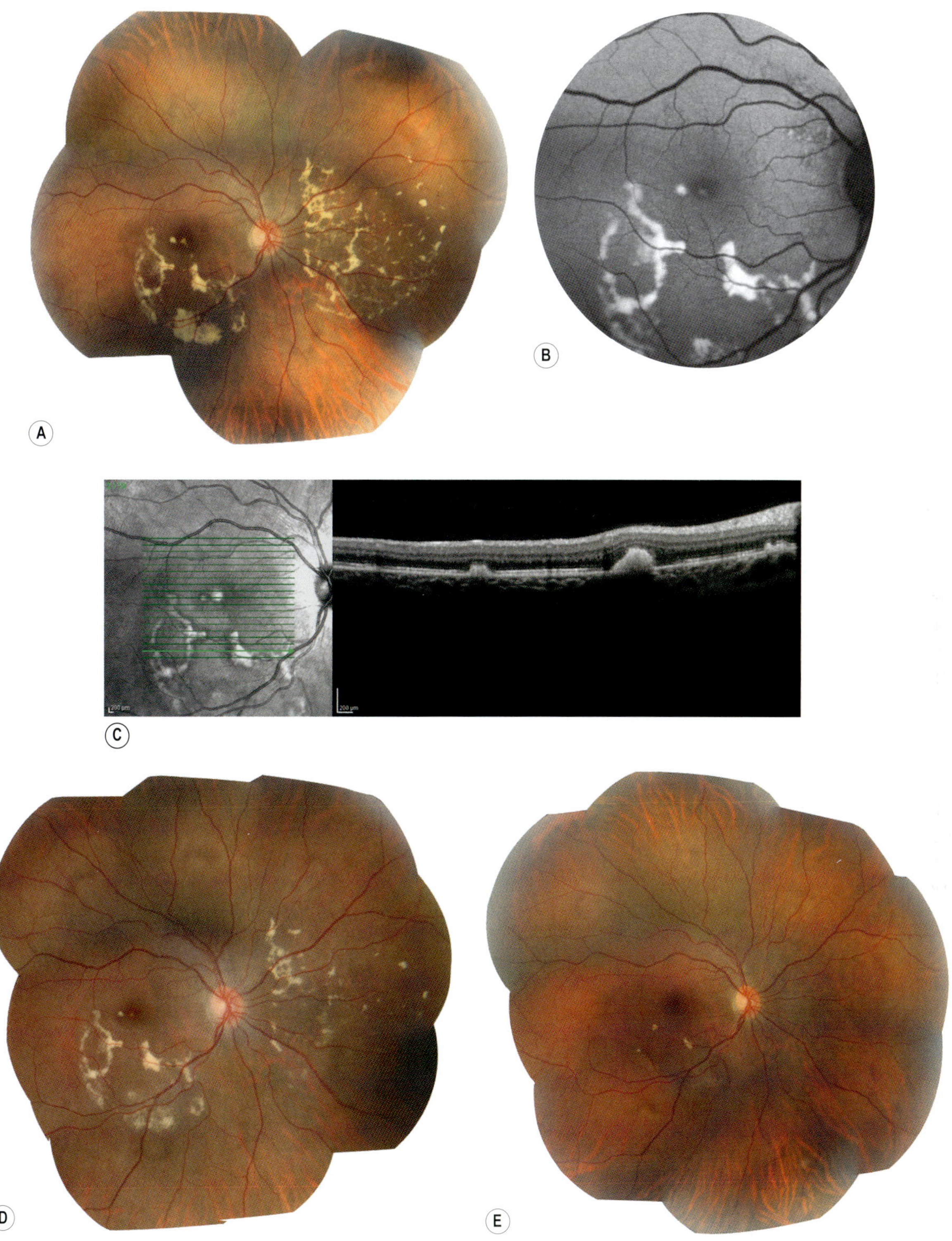

Collagen Vascular Disease

Patients with disseminated lupus erythematosus,[799,800] polyarteritis nodosa,[801,811] disseminated scleroderma, dermatomyositis, and relapsing polychondritis may develop serous detachment of the macula caused by fibrinoid necrosis of the choroidal vessels (see Figure 2.14). They may or may not show ophthalmoscopic evidence of retinal vascular involvement. They may or may not have systemic hypertension.

Goodpasture's Syndrome

Goodpasture's syndrome is characterized by the onset of signs and symptoms of hemorrhagic pulmonary disease (hemoptysis) and rapidly progressive glomerulonephritis (hematuria) leading to progressive pulmonary and renal failure. Deposition of immunoglobulin G occurs in a linear pattern in the basement membranes of the glomeruli, the lungs, and the choroidal blood vessels.[804] Circulating basement membrane antibodies are frequently demonstrated. The autoantibodies are directed against the Goodpasture antigen, which is part of the noncollagenous domain of the alpha 3(IV) collagen chain. Approximately 75% of patients die within the first year. Scattered retinal hemorrhages and exudates occur in approximately 10% of the patients; bilateral juxtapapillary subretinal neovascularization and peripheral retinoschisis have been seen in one patient.[836] Bullous retinal detachment secondary to fibrinoid necrosis of the choriocapillaris and overlying RPE may occur.[837,838]

Systemic Necrotizing Vasculitis (Wegener's Granulomatosis and Lymphoid Granulomatosis)

Visual loss associated with multiple outer white lesions at the level of the RPE similar to that occurring in acute posterior multifocal placoid pigment epitheliopathy in patients with Wegener's granulomatosis[839] and lymphoid granulomatosis[803] is seen occasionally. Retinal and choroidal artery occlusions, serous retinal detachments, branch and central retinal vein occlusions, severe retinitis and uveitis, scleritis, and sclerochoroidal granuloma mimicking a choroidal tumor are other posterior-segment manifestations in these patients.[839–848]

3.61 Organ-transplant chorioretinopathy and exudative retinal detachment.

A–C: Five months after a renal transplant, this 51-year-old man noted bilateral paracentral scotomas and blurred vision. After cataract extraction his visual acuity returned to 20/20 bilaterally, but his paracentral scotomas persisted. There were zones of yellowish flecks and retinal pigment epithelium (RPE) disruption paracentrally in both eyes (A). Angiography revealed within these zones a leopard-spot pattern of nonfluorescent flecks on a background of hyperfluorescence (C and D).

D–F: Two years after a heart transplant this 68-year-old man developed blurred vision and distortion of vision in the right eye associated with serous retinal detachment and progressively enlarging zones of RPE damage in a pattern similar to the patient in A–C. At the time of the photographs in D–F, his visual acuity had improved spontaneously from 20/60 to 20/30 and most of the subretinal fluid had resolved. The late-phase angiograms showed pinpoint leakage of fluorescein (arrow, F). The left eye was unaffected.

G–L: Two years after a heart–lung transplant, this 47-year-old man noted mild visual disturbance. Examination at that time revealed zones of paracentral disruption and clumping of the RPE associated with localized serous retinal detachment in the macula of both eyes (G and H). Angiography showed a leopard-spot pattern of fluorescence and pinpoint areas of focal staining in both eyes. Fourteen months later there was evidence of progression of the pigment epitheliopathy and inferior bullous retinal detachment that extended into the macular areas. There was a widespread pattern of yellow flecks resembling fundus flavimaculatus throughout the posterior fundi (J–L).

(A, C, and G–L from Gass et al.[797],)

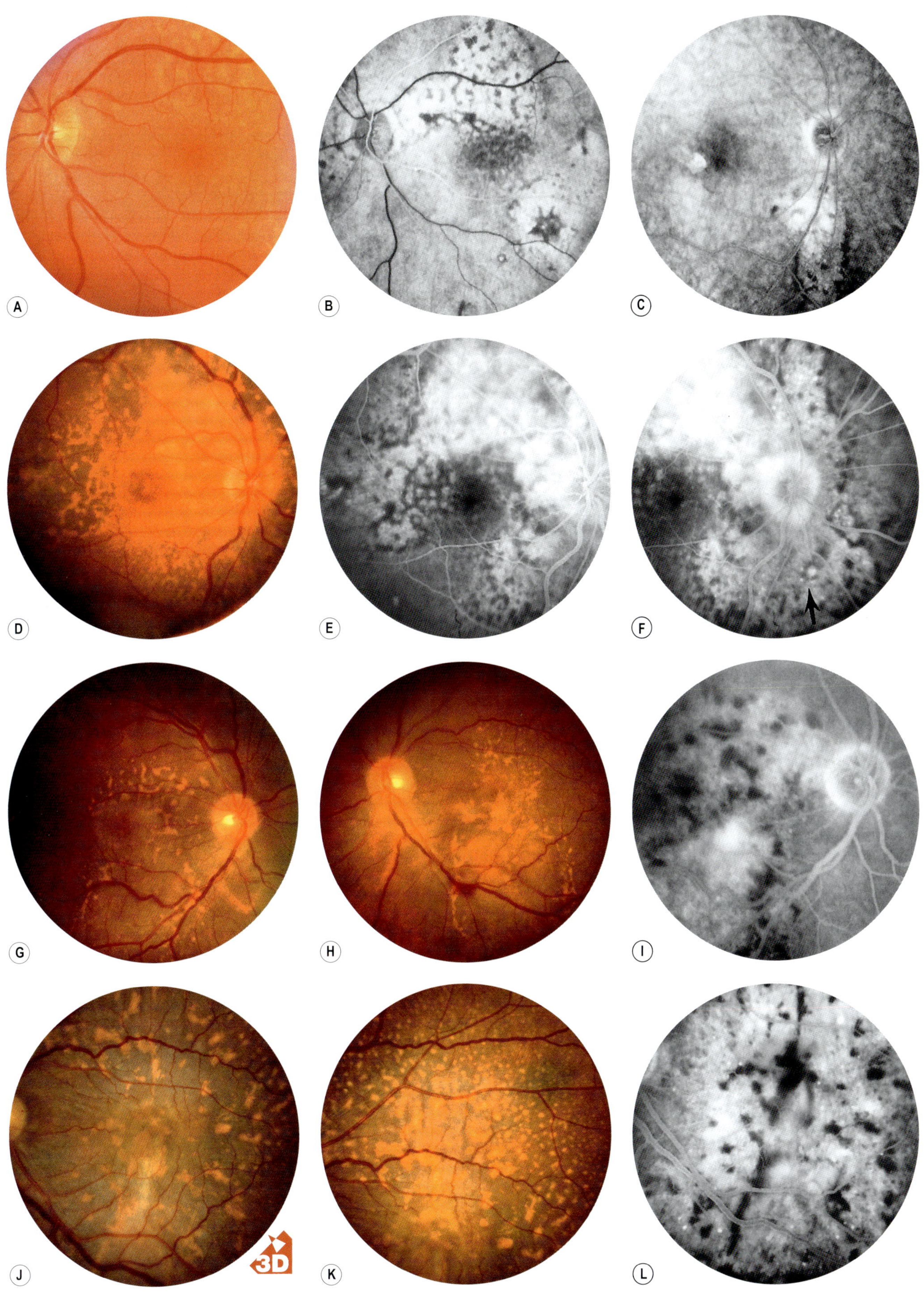
A
B
C
D
E
F
G
H
I
J
3D
K
L

ORGAN TRANSPLANTATION AND HEMODIALYSIS

Patients following renal, heart, and heart–lung transplantation may develop loss of vision caused by serous retinal detachment associated with geographic zones of leopard-spot pattern of clumping of orange RPE and RPE depigmentation in the posterior fundi of both eyes (Figure 3.61).[797] Fluorescein angiography accentuates these RPE changes and during the exudative phases of the disease demonstrates multiple pinpoint areas of fluorescein leakage within the zones of pigment epithelial damage (Figure 3.61B, C, E, F, I, and L). The subretinal fluid usually resolves spontaneously within several weeks or months. Recurrences are common. The episodes of exudative detachment do not coincide necessarily with clinical evidence of graft rejection. All of the patients were receiving a combination of oral corticosteroids, cyclosporine, and azathioprine. Any one or a combination of these drugs, particularly the corticosteroids, may be of pathogenetic importance.[48] The pattern of pigment epithelial changes suggests that acute damage to the RPE, perhaps by localized intravascular coagulopathy affecting the choriocapillaris, may be responsible.

Multifocal serofibrinous retinal pigment epithelial detachments and retinal detachment identical to that seen in patients with severe ICSC may occur, usually bilaterally in patients receiving hemodialysis because of renal failure,[66] and occasionally after renal transplantation.[48,67,68,798,818] (See previous discussion, ICSC, pp. 84–86.) When occurring after renal transplantation, the ocular symptoms have developed soon after the transplant in patients who presumably were receiving hemodialysis preoperatively. All but one of these patients who developed ocular symptoms while receiving hemodialysis and all of those who became symptomatic after renal transplantation were receiving systemic corticosteroids, which may either aggravate or cause ICSC.[48,66] Reduction of the dosage of corticosteroids and laser treatment of extrafoveal RPE detachments may be beneficial in causing resolution of retinal detachment.[66] Low-fluence photodynamic therapy is useful in eyes with widespread leakage.

EXTRINSIC AND INTRINSIC EMBOLIC OBSTRUCTION OF THE CHORIOCAPILLARIS

Because of the availability of multiple pathways of collateral blood flow, embolic obstruction of the choriocapillaris, whether caused by a shower of exogenous embolic material, such as corticosteroid preparations after periorbital injections, or fibrin platelet or cholesterol emboli from the carotid artery, rarely causes symptomatic damage to the retina.[756] Experimentally, it is difficult to produce retinal damage and retinal detachment by embolization of the choroidal vasculature alone. Injection of emboli retrograde via the vortex veins to obtain an element of venous obstruction, and photocoagulation to damage the RPE physically as well as occlude the choroidal blood vessels are techniques used to produce exudative retinal detachment experimentally.[849]

Serous macular detachment may be produced experimentally in cats by photodynamic injury produced by laser activation of intravascular rose Bengal.[850] Histopathologically the detachment is associated with occlusion of the choriocapillaris and retinal vessels.

3.62 Dysproteinemia and serous macular detachment.

A–D: A 63-year-old man with Waldenström's macroglobulinemia developed loss of central vision bilaterally associated with localized serous retinal detachment (arrows, B) in the macula of both eyes. There were scattered retinal hemorrhages in the periphery (A) but minimal evidence of retinal venous dilation. The visual acuity was 7/200 bilaterally. Angiography revealed some scattered foci of mild retinal microvascular changes, but no evidence of staining either in the retina or at the level of the retinal pigment epithelium (C and D). One week later, following plasmapheresis, the serous macular detachments had resolved and the visual acuity had improved to 20/200.

E–I: This woman with diabetes mellitus and multiple myeloma developed loss of central vision caused by serous retinal detachment in the macula (arrows, E) of both eyes. She had minimal background diabetic retinopathy. The detachment persisted and was associated with an increase in the diabetic retinopathy (F and G). Angiography revealed evidence of background retinopathy and intense staining of the subretinal fluid.

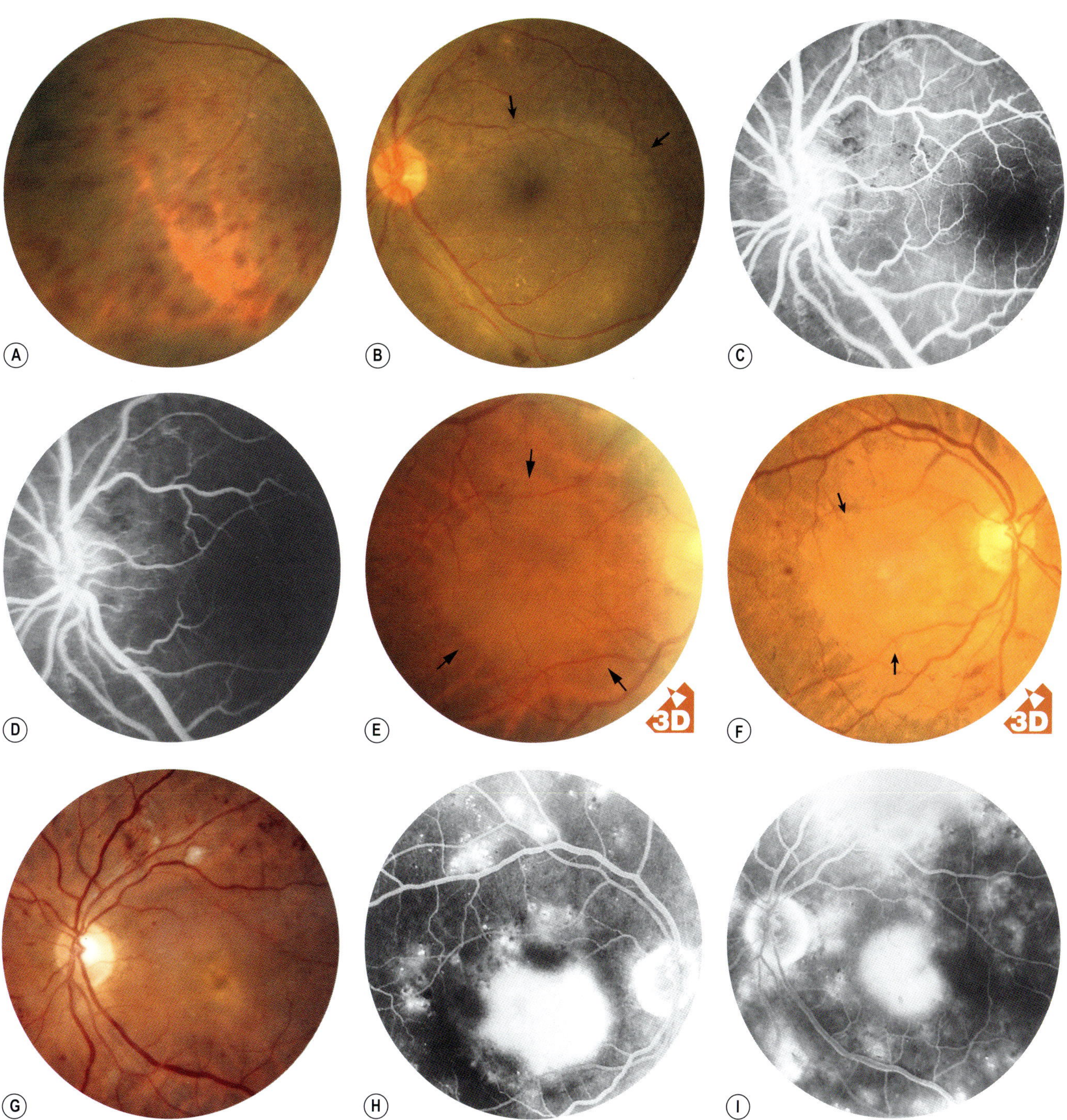
A
B
C
D
E
3D
F
3D
G
H
I

DYSPROTEINEMIA CAUSING SEROUS MACULAR DETACHMENT AND RETINOPATHY

A patient with Waldenström's macroglobulinemia developed bilateral loss of central vision caused by serous detachment of the retina in the macular area, unassociated with any fluorescein angiographic evidence of permeability alteration of either the inner or outer blood–retinal barrier (Figure 3.62A–D). One week after plasmapheresis the retina reattached bilaterally. Presumably the high levels of abnormal serum proteins in these patients may gain entrance into the subretinal space and cause the accumulation of water by osmosis. As demonstrated in the first case, this may occur in the absence of a demonstrable alteration of either the RPE or retinal vascular endothelium to fluorescein (Figure 3.62A–D). Similar serous retinal detachments that do not exhibit fluorescein leakage have also been seen in patients with multiple myeloma, POEMS syndrome (see below), and benign monoclonal gammopathy.[851–858] Many of these patients also have diabetic retinopathy and this additional mechanism for the serous detachment may be overlooked for diabetic vascular leakage. Other manifestations of hyperviscosity and secondary anemia in these patients include retinal hemorrhages, microaneurysms, venous dilation and tortuosity, and small-vessel occlusions (Figure 3.63A–E).[853,859,860]

3.63 Serous macular detachment and Waldenström's macroglobulinemia.

A–K: This diabetic male with moderate nonproliferative diabetic retinopathy was noted to have bilateral macular detachments (A and B). An angiogram showed microaneurysms but no reason for the subretinal fluid, which could be confirmed on optical coherence tomography (F and G). Observation was recommended, and a few months later, the macular fluid had increased in both eyes (H and I). Further increase in the exudative detachment 6 months later (J and K) prompted an evaluation for dysproteinemias. He was found to have Waldenström's macroglobulinemia and was started on chemotherapy and plasmapheresis.

(Courtesy of Dr. Karen Gehrs.)

Waldenström's macroglobulinemia is a B-cell lymphoproliferative disorder with lymphoplasmacytic infiltration of the bone marrow and lymphatic tissue, and secretion of a monoclonal immunoglobulin protein IgM into the serum. Clinical manifestations are secondary to infiltration of the bone marrow and extramedullary sites and elevated IgM levels. Pancytopenia, organomegaly, neuropathy, and effects of hyperviscosity characterize the clinical picture. Treatment strategies are complex and involve chemotherapeutic drugs such as cyclophosphamide, rituximab, dexamethasone, and eventually autologous stem cell transplant and supportive therapy for anemia, and plasmapheresis for hyperviscosity.

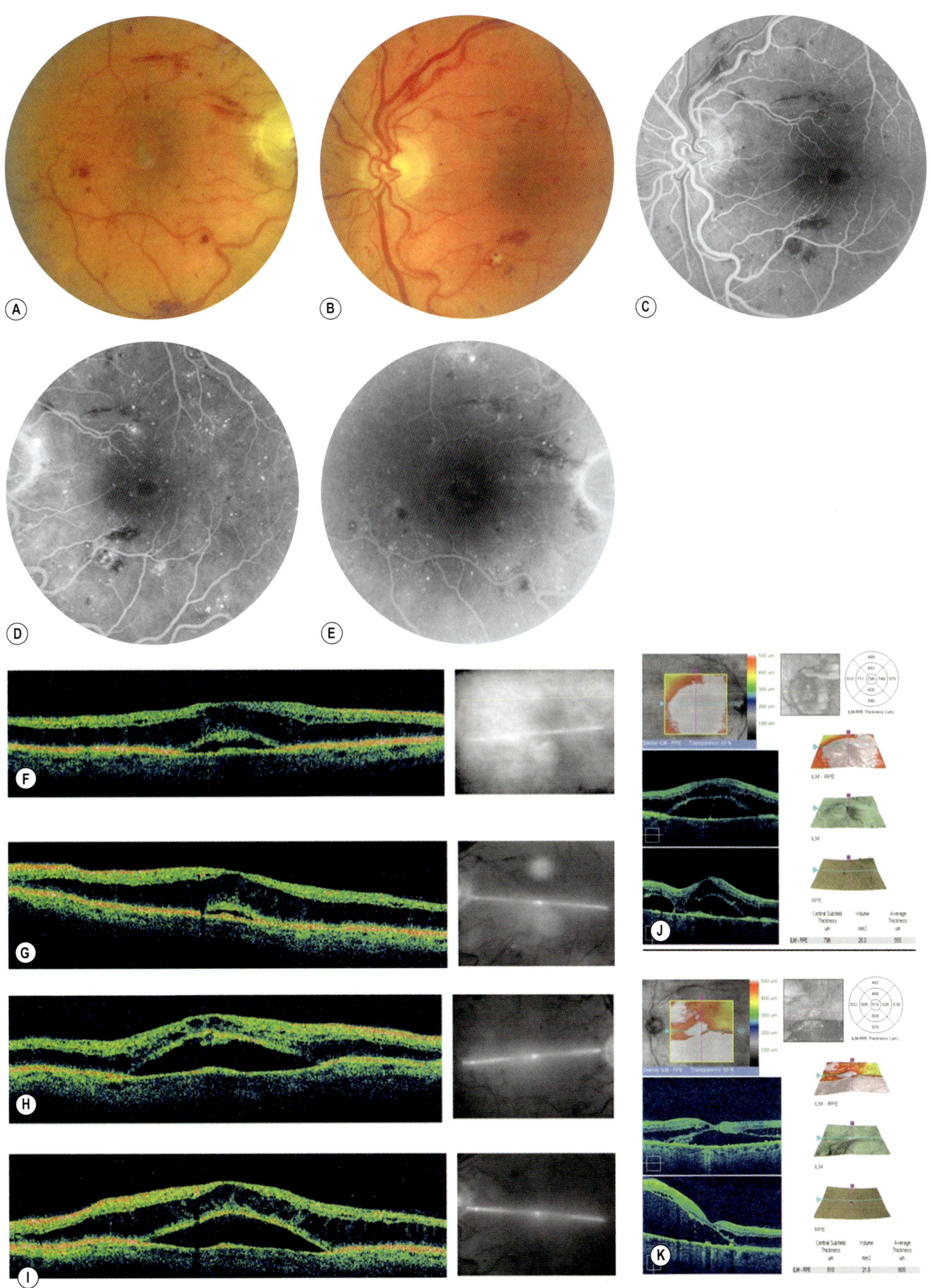
A
B
C
D
E
F
G
H
I
J
K

Multiple myeloma is a B-cell malignancy with a monoclonal expansion of abnormal plasma cells in the bone marrow that produce excess immunoglobulin. Clinical manifestations occur either secondary to the excess M protein, resulting in renal failure, systemic amyloidosis, or recurrent bacterial infection due to decrease in polyclonal immunoglobulins; or due to excess plasma cell proliferation resulting in lytic bone lesions, osteoporosis, bone fractures, anemia, and extramedullary plasmacytomas. Treatment includes high-dose chemotherapy and stem cell transplantation, and supportive therapy for anemia, and plasmapheresis for hyperviscosity.

POEMS is an acronym for a rare multisystem disorder of plasma cell dyscrasia featuring polyneuropathy, organomegaly (spleen, liver, lymph node), endocrinopathy (adrenal, thyroid, pituitary, parathyroid, gonadal, pancreatic), M protein and skin changes (hyperpigmentation, hypertrichosis, and hemangiomata). Secondary sclerotic bone lesions can occur. They have anasarca and bilateral optic disc edema and are known to have high systemic levels of VEGF. Bilateral retinal hemorrhages, serous retinal detachment, cystoid macular edema, and optic disc edema are ocular features.[854,861–864] Treatment by autologous peripheral blood stem cell transplantation reduces the VEGF level and the systemic manifestations. Perhaps, temporary stabilization may be expected after systemic or intraocular injection of anti-VEGF antibodies.[862]

Courtesy of Dr. Leonard Joffe, Gass reviewed the photographs of another patient with multiple myeloma and diabetes mellitus who developed chronic serous detachment of the retina in the macular region (Figure 3.61E–I). Unlike the former case, angiography revealed evidence of background diabetic retinopathy and intense staining of the subretinal fluid. It was not possible to determine the source of the fluorescein in the subretinal fluid.

3.64 Uveal effusion syndrome.

A–F: Dilated conjunctival vessels (A) and bullous retinal detachment (B) in a healthy 13-year-old girl who had peripheral ciliochoroidal detachment and leopard-spot mottling of the pigment epithelium (C). There were similar findings in the opposite eye (D). Visual acuity was counting fingers. Ultrasonography showed diffuse thickening of the posterior choroid (arrows, E and F).

G–L: This 42-year-old Hispanic man experienced recurrent episodes of serous detachment of the macula (G). Angiograms showed diffuse areas of hyperfluorescence and some staining (arrow, H). He was incorrectly diagnosed as having idiopathic central serous chorioretinopathy. Two years later note leopard-spot changes that were evident angiographically (I and J). There were now cells in the vitreous and peripheral ciliochoroidal detachments. Six months later he was legally blind because of bilateral bullous retinal and ciliochoroidal detachment (K). Ten weeks after lamellar sclerectomies and sclerostomies without drainage of subretinal fluid the detachments had resolved (L). Ten years later there had been no evidence of recurrence of detachment.

(A–G and J from Gass and Jallow[869]; I from Gass.[890])

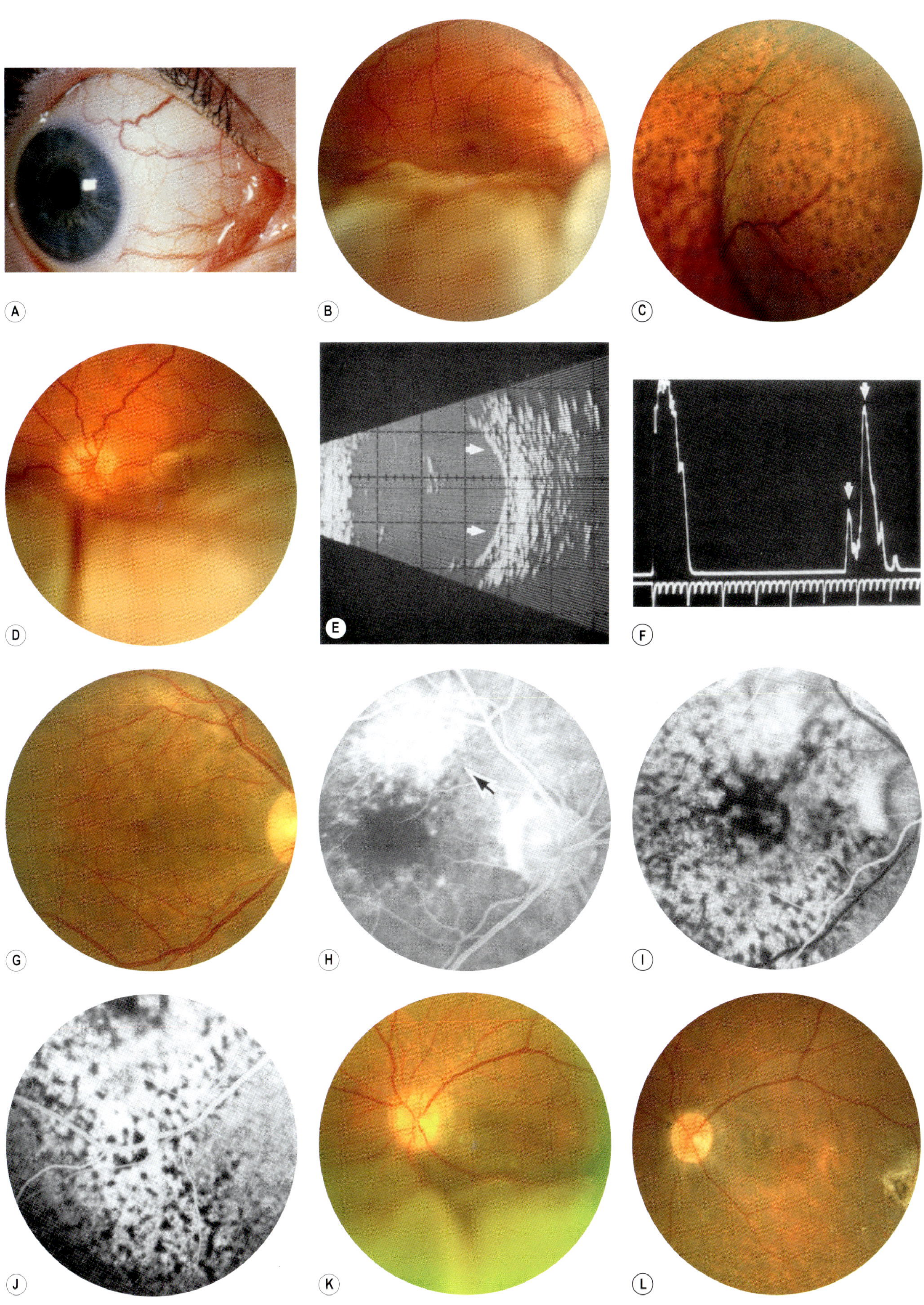
A
B
C
D
E
F
G
H
I
J
K
L

IDIOPATHIC UVEAL EFFUSION SYNDROME

Patients with IUES, most often healthy middle-aged men with normal-size eyes, develop loss of vision in one or both eyes, caused by serous detachment first of the choroid and ciliary body and then of the retina (Figures 3.64–3.67).[865–876] Patients may present either because of loss of their superior visual field secondary to an inferior retinal detachment or because of metamorphopsia and a positive scotoma secondary to a serous detachment of the macula. Dilation of the large conjunctival veins is often present (Figure 3.64A). The anterior segment otherwise is usually free of inflammatory signs. There may be blood in Schlemm's canal. Intraocular pressure is normal. There are usually some cells in the vitreous. Initially, the serous retinal detachment may be confined to the macular area and the choroidal and ciliary body detachment may be overlooked unless ultrasonography is done (Figures 3.64E and F, 3.65J and 3.66A and C). Other patients present with bullous detachment of the retina as well as serous elevation of the peripheral choroid and ciliary body (Figures 3.64B–D and K, 3.65 and 3.66). Typically there is marked shifting of the subretinal fluid that is caused by its very high protein content, which is 2.5–3 times that in the normal plasma.[876–879] Fluorescein angiography may show some evidence of mild changes in the RPE early but often does not show a discrete leak beneath the serous detachment of the retina. The disease may affect initially only one eye. Often a similar detachment occurs in the second eye weeks, months, or years later. These patients do not respond to systemic corticosteroid treatment or antimetabolite therapy. Scleral buckling and drainage of subretinal fluid often fail and may be complicated by hemorrhage. Decompression of the vortex veins in nanophthalmic eyes has proved to be successful.[880,881] Patients often have a prolonged course that is subject to remissions and exacerbations. They eventually develop a leopard-spot pattern of irregular clumping and thinning of the RPE that may be most easily detected angiographically (Figures 3.64B, C, H, I, and J, 3.65L and 3.66E, F, and H). The yellow-brown pigment clumping is brilliantly autofluorescent, suggesting the material is likely lipofuscin and other lipoprotein fluorophores (Figures 3.65 and 3.66). These are visible in pretreated eyes and become more prominent once surgical intervention has resulted in resolution of the choroidal and retinal detachments (Figures 3.65 and 3.66). In a few patients flecks of yellow subretinal and outer retinal lipid exudation may develop in the macular area. Severe chorioretinal degeneration and loss of visual field may develop in some patients. Most of these patients are hyperopic and if carefully reviewed will show gradual increase in their hyperopia over the preceding years.

3.65 Uveal effusion syndrome.

A–F: This +5 hyperopic 69-year-old male with history of exudative age-related macular degeneration in both eyes, treated previously with intravitreal bevacizumab, developed progressive exudative retinal detachment and the vision dropped to hand motions over 2 months. Peripheral choroidal detachments were seen all around in addition (A, C, and D). Autofluorescence imaging shows mottled increased and decreased autofluorescence in the attached retina and no fluorescence of the detached retina (B). Following three scleral windows the choroidal and retinal detachments resolved with increase in the hyperautofluorescent specks (E). They were present anterior to the retinal pigment epithelium as clumps of yellow brown pigmented material (F).

G–H: Montage color and autofluorescence images shows a reattached retina with yellow brown pigment clumps (G and H).

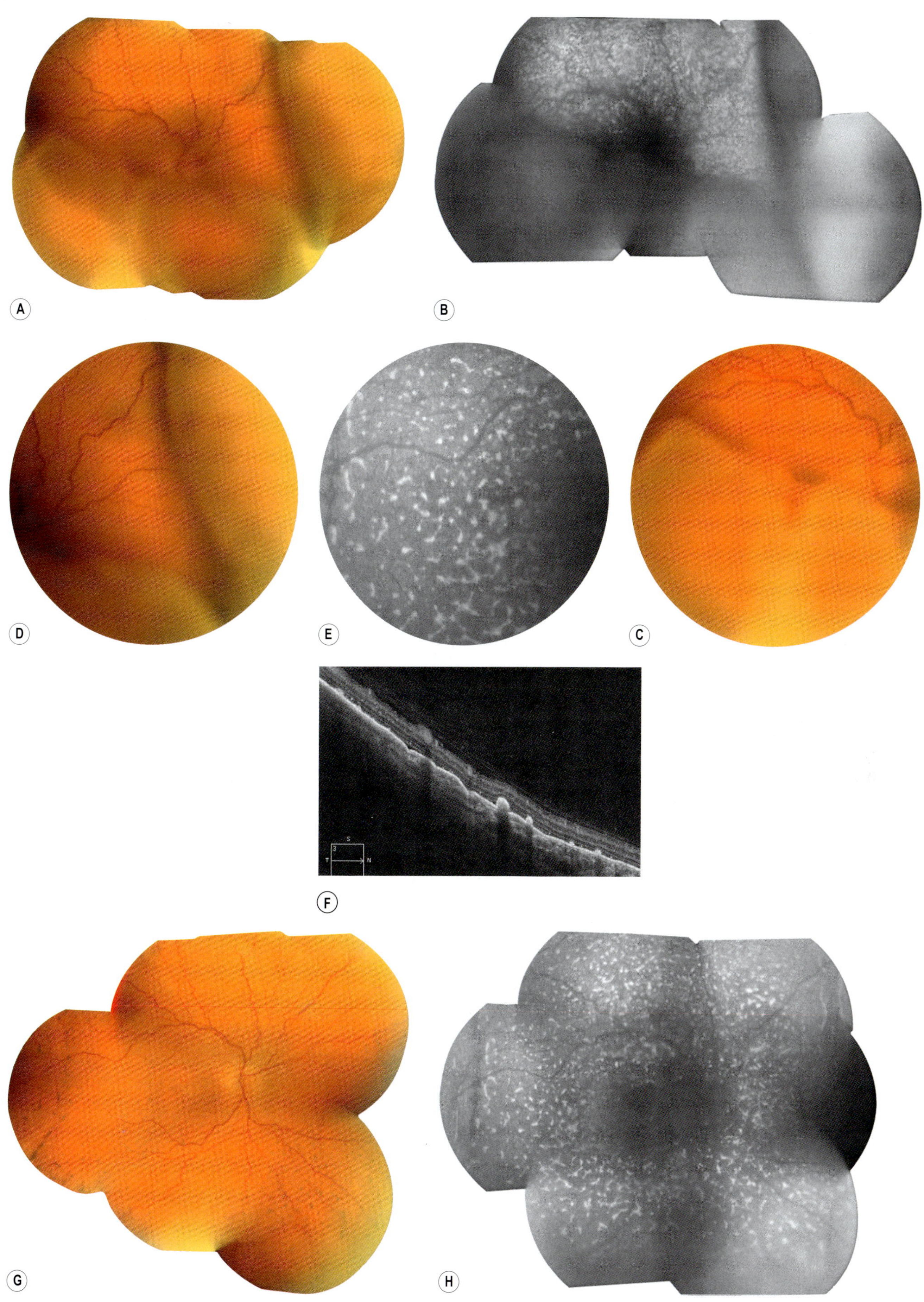
A
B
D
E
C
S
T
N
F
G
H

Histopathologically, the eyes show accumulation of protein-rich extracellular exudate within the choroid and ciliary body; serous detachment of the choroid, ciliary body, and retina; engorgement of the choroidal blood vessels; minimal evidence of inflammation; and expansion of the subarachnoid space around the optic nerve (Figure 3.67A–C).[869,874,882] Abnormal accumulation of glycoaminoglycans occurs between the scleral fibers.[882–884] Histochemically, in one case, this accumulation consisted primarily of proteodermatan sulfate and small amounts of proteochondroitin sulfate.[882] Scleral cell tissue culture has demonstrated intracellular glycogen-like deposits.[884] Abnormalities in scleral proteoglycans, increased scleral fibronectin, and twisting and fraying of scleral fibers have been described in nanophthalmic sclera.[883,885–889]

The cause of IUES is unknown. It is probably caused by a congenital abnormality of the scleral structure with intrascleral accumulation of abnormal amounts of extracellular glycosaminoglycans over years, and hypoplasia of the vortex veins.[867,869,890] Forrester et al. have suggested that IUES may be a form of ocular mucopolysaccharidosis with a primary defect in proteodermatan synthesis and/or degradation by scleral fibroblasts.[882] The observation of uveal effusion in a patient with Hunter's syndrome and Maroteaux–Lamy syndrome (MPS type VI) is further evidence to suggest that abnormalities in scleral mucopolysaccharides may be important in the causation of ciliochoroidal effusion in patients with IUES and nanophthalmos.[891] Thickened sclera and vortex vein obstruction in nanophthalmic eyes have been incriminated in the pathogenesis of uveal effusion.[877,880,881,892–896]

The following hypothesis has been suggested to explain the serous detachment of the uveal tract in idiopathic uveal effusion: as aging changes take place in the thickened, abnormal sclera, particularly in the male patient, the eye loses its ability to cope with protein that normally escapes in small quantities from the choroidal blood vessels into the extracellular space.[890] One of the primary functions of the lymphatic system is to provide a means of returning protein in the extravascular compartment to the vascular system.[897] In the eye the scleral emissary channels probably function as lymphatic channels for extravascular protein in the choroid and ciliary body to escape into the periocular tissue.[898] Encroachment on these channels by aging changes in the thick mucopolysaccharide-infiltrated sclera, as well as a hypoplastic vortex vein system, predisposes the eyes to vortex vein obstruction and excessive accumulation of extravascular protein and water in the uveal tract (Figure 3.67D3). When the extravascular protein concentration in the choroid and ciliary body approaches that in the vascular system, protein begins to move across the RPE into the subretinal space and bullous retinal detachment develops. The protein in the subretinal fluid becomes superconcentrated to levels 2–2½ times that in the vascular system. This is probably the cause of: (1) the marked shifting of the subretinal fluid; (2) the leopard-spot appearance of the RPE; (3) the occasional precipitation of yellow subretinal and intraretinal lipoproteins; and (4) elevation of the protein levels of the perioptic cerebrospinal fluid that causes secondary expansion of the perioptic subarachnoid space. Diffusion of the protein from this area posteriorly probably explains why lumbar puncture in these patients reveals elevation of the cerebrospinal fluid protein levels in approximately 50% of patients in the absence of pleocytosis. Dilation of the episcleral veins and blood in Schlemm's canal are anterior-segment manifestations of the chronic vortex vein obstruction that is usually present. The intraocular pressure in most diseases causing ciliochoroidal edema or detachment is lower than normal because of the lowered resistance to the uveoscleral outflow of aqueous humor.[893,899,900] The typically normal intraocular pressure in patients with idiopathic uveal effusion is probably caused by the greater than normal resistance to uveoscleral outflow.

3.66 Uveal effusion syndrome: pathology and treatment.

A and B: Histopathologic findings in a patient with the uveal effusion syndrome. Note serous detachment of the engorged peripheral choroid (A), absence of evidence of inflammation, serous retinal detachment, choroidal engorgement, and dilated subarachnoid space (arrow, B).

C: Histopathologic findings in another patient with uveal effusion. There are thickening of the sclera, thickening of the choroid by periodic acid–Schiff-positive proteinaceous exudate (arrows), and the folding of the inner choroid and retinal pigment epithelium beneath the proteinaceous subretinal exudate.

D: Diagrams of pathways (arrows) of transscleral movement of extravascular protein (stippling). 1, Focal vascular leak in an otherwise normal eye. 2, Aphakic eye with transient postoperative ciliochoroidal detachment that may require several days or weeks for resolution. 3, Idiopathic uveal effusion syndrome with increased resistance to protein outflow and uveal venous outflow caused by abnormal sclera.

E: Diagram of surgical technique for the treatment of chronic uveal effusion. Note the lamellar sclerectomies and sclerostomies (arrows) done without drainage of subretinal fluid in each quadrant, avoiding the meridian of the vortex veins.

(A and B from Verhoeff and Waite[874]; D and E from Gass.[890])

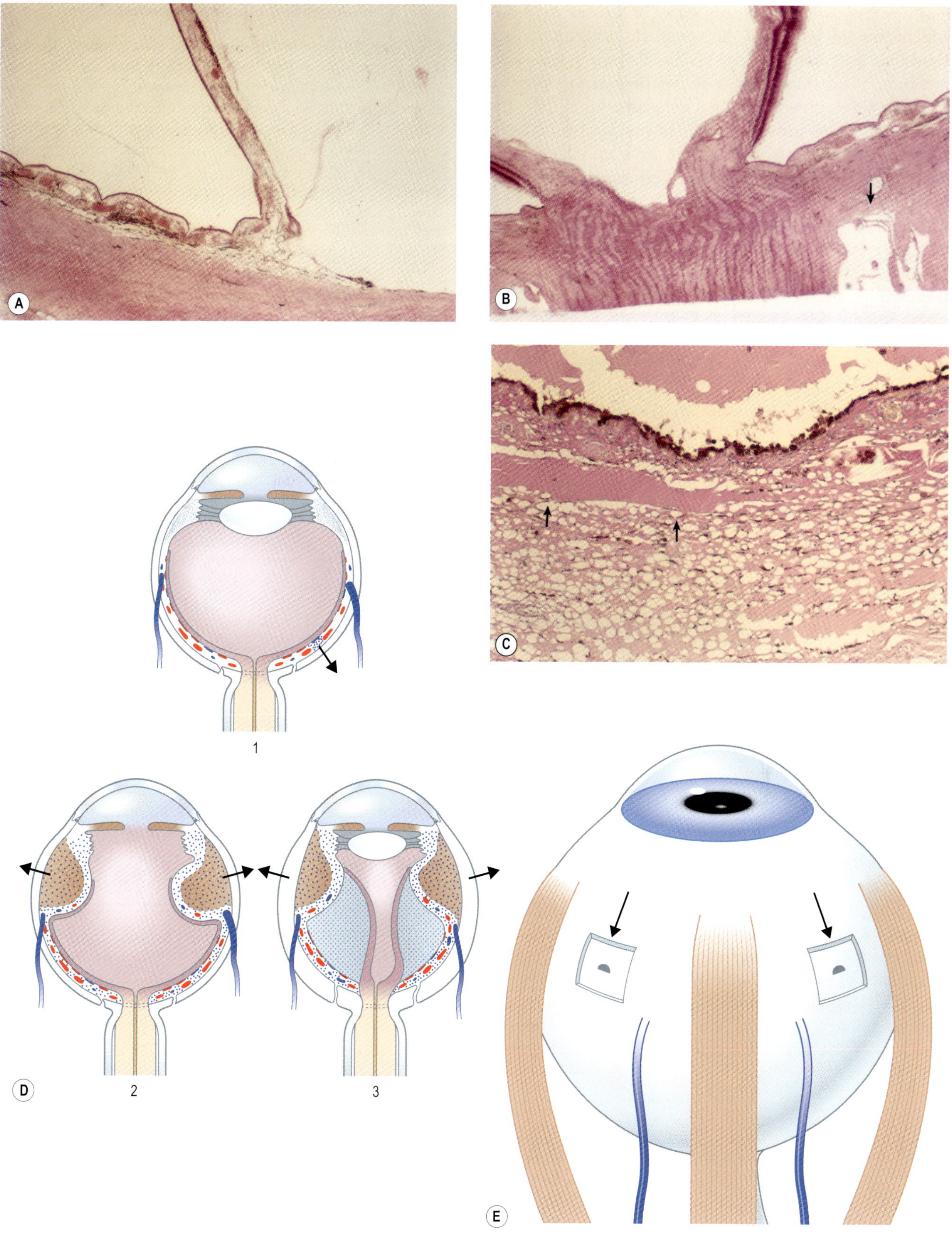
A
B
C
1
D
2
3
E

Ultrasonography in the early stages of the disease shows evidence of thickening of the sclera, choroid, and ciliary body that may antedate any visible changes in the ocular fundus. This thickening is always present just prior to and after development of retinal detachment.[890,901,902] The demonstration of ultrasonographic evidence of increased thickening of the posterior choroid by extracellar fluid is essential before a diagnosis of uveal effusion can be made and scleral windows can be done. Ultrasonography may also demonstrate evidence of expansion of the optic nerve sheaths (positive 30° test) (Figure 3.67B). The uveal thickening may also be detected in some cases by computed tomography, and more recently by enhanced depth imaging of the choroid on Spectralis OCT.[903]

Segmental, partial-thickness sclerectomies at or slightly anterior to the equator, avoiding the meridians of any existing vortex veins, followed by full-thickness sclerostomies without perforation of the underlying choroid within the sclerectomy sites, have been successful in the treatment of IUES and nanophthalmos (Figure 3.67E).[890,891,904–907] Use of episcleral instillation of corticosteroids in the area of the sclerectomies before closure of the conjunctiva probably reduces the chance of regrowth of tissue across the sclerectomies and recurrence of ciliochoroidal detachment.

Decompression of the vortex veins and scleral resection have proved successful in the treatment of uveal effusion in nanophthalmic eyes.[880,881,908] The author believes that the scleral resection alone is responsible for the beneficial effects of the operation, and that decompression of the vortex veins is unnecessary and adds to the morbidity of the procedure. This view is supported by the recent findings of Jin and Anderson.[906]

Secondary causes for uveal effusion include nanophthalmos,[880,881,892,893,896,901] dural arteriovenous fistulas,[909,910] scleritis,[911] Harada's disease, benign reactive lymphoid hyperplasia of the uveal tract, luetic chorioretinitis,[911] carotid artery obstruction (Figure 6.13D–I), orbital cellulitis, diffuse neoplasms of the uveal tract,[912] oxygen inhalation therapy,[913] wound leaks following surgical or other traumatic wounds of the eye,[870,878,906,914–916] serous choroidal detachment occurring during intraocular surgery,[916–918] and after photocoagulation.[919] Angle closure glaucoma may occur after ciliochoroidal detachment of any cause.[893] Uveal effusion may occur in family members with nanophthalmos and a tapetoretinal degeneration.[920] The author has seen two siblings with nanophthalmos, retinitis pigmentosa, and bilateral uveal effusion, and another patient with nanophthalmos and retinitis pigmentosa who was referred for consideration of sclerectomies because of suspected chronic uveal effusion. The patient had no clinical or ultrasonic evidence of uveal effusion. The patient's electroretinogram was virtually extinguished.

Long-term follow-up of some patients after scleral windows has revealed that some show evidence of progressive chorioretinal degenerative changes in the absence of evidence of recurrence of uveal effusion. It is not known whether this may be caused by mild chronic recurrent effusion or perhaps is caused by the same anomaly of mucopolysaccharide metabolism affecting the sclera in these patients.

3.67 Idiopathic uveal effusion syndrome

A–L: This 80-year-old Caucasian woman noted gradual decline in vision in both eyes, left more than the right over 3 months. She was started on oral prednisone 60 mg for a diagnosis of choroidal detachment in her left eye. She had a history of breast cancer that was treated with a mastectomy 5 years previously. Her visual acuity was 20/30 in the right eye and 20/100 in the left eye. The right eye had a few yellow orange punctate dots in the posterior pole and peripheral choroidal effusions (A). The left eye had several small punctate yellow dots throughout the fundus, 360° peripheral choroidal effusions and inferior exudative retinal detachment extending up to the inferior arcade (B, C, and J). Fluorescein angiogram showed diffuse leopard-spot change in the left eye and hypofluorescent lines corresponding to choroidal folds at the equator from the choroidal detachments (D and E, arrows) The yellow dots were brilliantly hyperautofluorescent and the choroidal and retinal detachments were hypoautofluorescent. An ultrasound confirmed the serous choroidal (G) and retinal detachments (F). Optical coherence tomography of the left macula showed intraretinal and subretinal fluid in the macula, and intraretinal fluid in the right macula. She underwent scleral windows in three quadrants in the left eye, the choroidals resolved overnight, but the serous retinal detachment resolved over 8 weeks. The fundus of the left eye 3 months post scleral windows shows no subretinal fibrosis, increased visibility of the orange brown pigment epithelial clumps (K), which are vividly hyperautofluorescent (L).

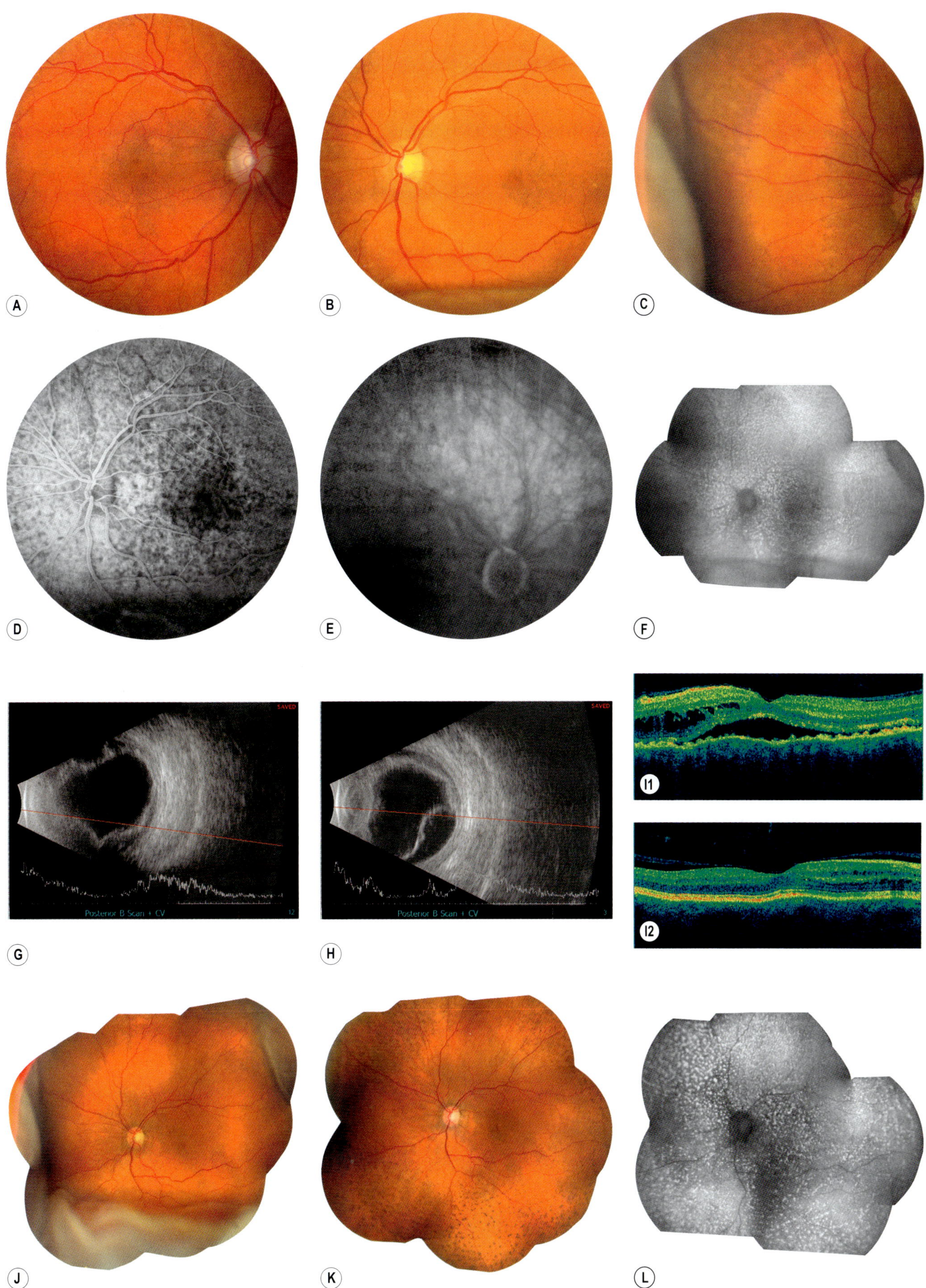
A
B
C
D
E
F
SAVED
Posterior B Scan + CV
G
SAVED
Posterior B Scan + CV
H
I1
I2
J
K
L

The differential diagnosis of IUES includes rhegmatogenous retinal detachment with associated cilioretinal detachment, inflammatory pseudotumor of the uveal tract, diffuse amelanotic melanoma or metastatic carcinoma, bilateral diffuse uveal melanocytic proliferation (see p. 1202), Harada's disease (see pp. 998–1002), ICSC, particularly if complicated by steroid therapy resulting in large exudative retinal detachment (see p. 78),[866] sympathetic uveitis (see p. 1004), and posterior scleritis (see p. 1016). Ultrasonography is particularly valuable in making the correct diagnosis. The leopard-spot pigmentation that frequently develops in patients with uveal effusion syndrome is similar in appearance to that occurring in some patients with systemic large cell lymphoma (see p. 1160, Fig. 13.34D–J), leukemia (see p. 1244), or bilateral diffuse uveal melanocytic proliferation (see pp. 1202–1204), and in patients with organ transplant chorioretinopathy (see p. 188).

Primary Pulmonary Hypertension

Primary pulmonary hypertension is a rare fatal disorder of idiopathic obliteration of the pulmonary capillaries that results in right heart failure. Ocular findings are not very common, but when present manifest as dilated conjunctival and episcleral vessels, exudative choroidal and retinal detachment (Figure 3.68), or venous stasis retinopathy progressing to central retinal vein occlusion at times.[921-925] One case of acute angle closure glaucoma has been reported.[926] The resistance in the typically low-resistance pulmonary vascular bed increases, resulting in right heart failure. This in turn translates higher venous pressure to the head and neck veins, liver vasculature, and peripheral veins. Stagnation of flow in the retinal and choroidal veins results in venous stasis retinopathy and choroidal effusions and prominent episcleral vessels.

Primary pulmonary hypertension is familial in 10% (familial pulmonary arterial hypertension); the rest are sporadic (idiopathic pulmonary arterial hypertension). A female preponderance is known and the average age at presentation is 36 years. Germline bone morphogenetic protein receptor type II gene mutations has been found in some of the familial and sporadic cases.[927] The lumen of the precapillary arterioles and small pulmonary arteries is obliterated by cellular and myofibroblast proliferation and in situ thrombosis, causing vascular remodeling that raises the pulmonary arterial pressure.[928] The secondary causes of pulmonary hypertension are more common and include connective tissue diseases such as scleroderma, lupus, rheumatoid arthritis, mixed connective tissue diseases, human immunodeficiency virus (HIV) infection, cirrhosis, portal hypertension, and the use of appetite suppressants.[929] Since the condition is common in women, a history of use of appetite suppressants should be sought. Death occurred within 2–3 years of diagnosis when treated medically alone, previously. Newer medical and support therapy has prolonged survival.[930,931] Recent success of lung transplants has improved morbidity and life expectancy.[932,933]

3.68 Primary pulmonary hypertension.

A–J: This 25-year-old white male with end-stage primary pulmonary hypertension presented 1 week before lung transplant with mild distortion in the left eye which was diagnosed as central serous chorioretinopathy. Two weeks post lung transplant, his vision decreased further to 20/400. The right eye remained at 20/20. The left fundus showed serous retinal detachment (A, B). A fluorescein and indocyanine green angiogram revealed mild window defect corresponding to the center of the fovea (C, D). Optical coherence tomography confirmed intraretinal and subretinal fluid (E). A diagnosis of possible central serous chorioretinopathy versus graft-versus-host disease was made. Steroids were decreased. His symptoms worsened to involve the right eye to 20/60 and further decreased to 20/200 in both eyes. The patient developed a skin rash and looked very ill. At this time, his oral steroid was increased. The vision improved to 20/50 and 20/70 in 2 weeks, and further to 20/20 in both eyes in about 6 weeks. The retinal and choroidal fluid resolved (F–I). A diagnosis of serous retinal and choroidal effusion secondary to primary pulmonary hypertension was made, since his symptoms began before the lung transplant and responded to corticosteroids.

(Courtesy of Dr. Colin McCannel. Also, Yannuzzi Lawrence J., The Retinal Atlas, Saunders 2010, 978-0-7020-3320-9, p.756.)

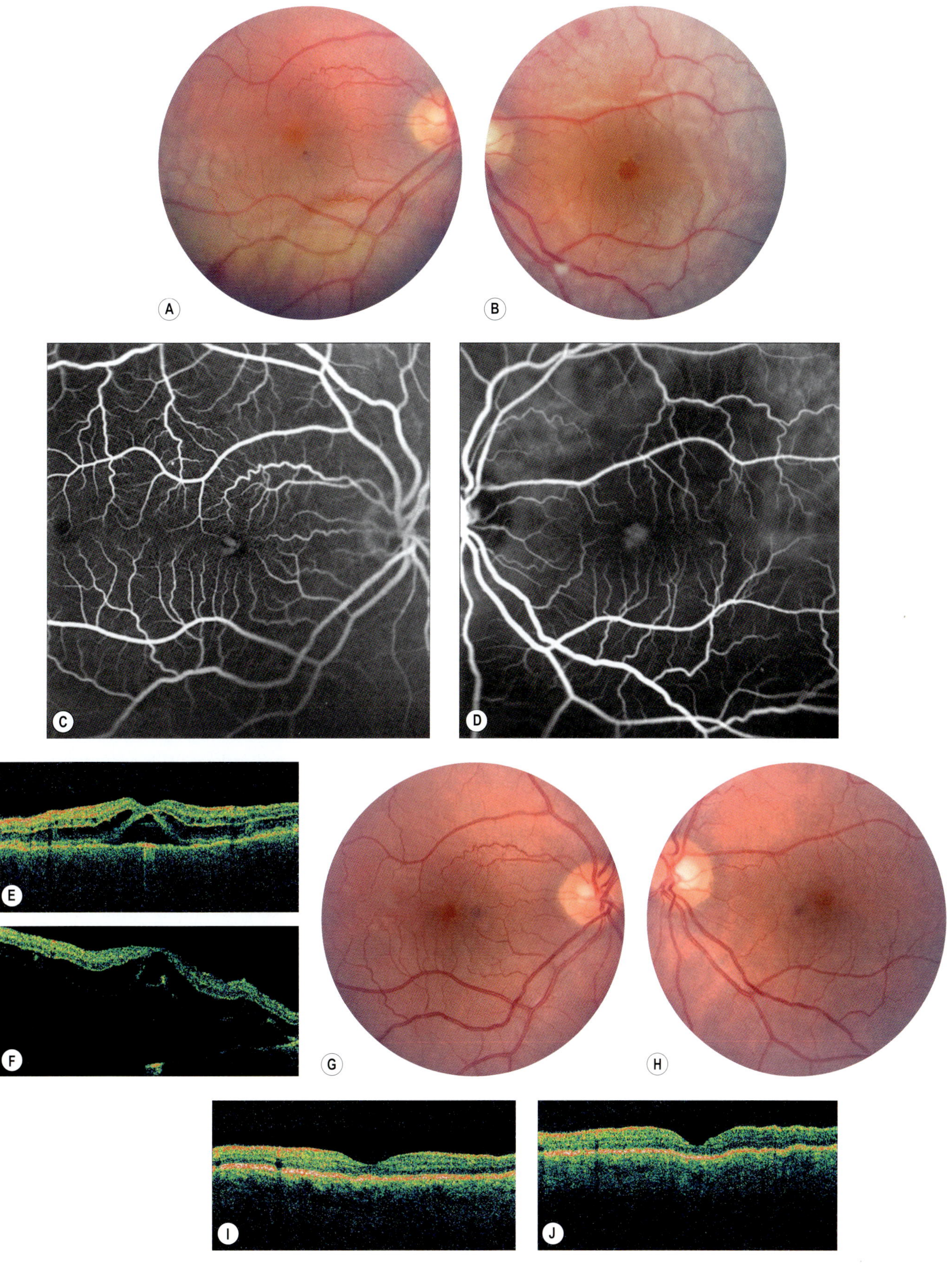
A
B
C
D
E
F
G
H
I
J

SUPRACHOROIDAL HEMORRHAGE

Spontaneous bleeding of a choroidal blood vessel may produce a variety of clinical pictures. When it occurs during the course of intraocular surgery, bleeding may be massive and produce an expulsive hemorrhage. Risk factors for the development of spontaneous intraoperative suprachoroidal hemorrhage are: history of glaucoma, increased intraocular pressure preoperatively, increased axial length of the eye, older age, aphakia, posterior-capsule rupture, generalized atherosclerosis, cardiovascular disease, diabetes mellitus, and elevated intraoperative pulse.[934] Clinical signs of suprachoroidal hemorrhage include pain, increased intraocular pressure, loss of red reflex, progressive shallowing of the anterior chamber and smooth bullous, dark elevated mass(es) in the fundus. If bleeding occurs postoperatively, often during a period of hypotony, the bleeding may produce a ciliochoroidal detachment of similar configuration to, but usually of darker color than, that of uveal effusion (Figure 3.69A–C).[935] Transillumination clearly differentiates serous from hemorrhagic detachment of the choroid and ciliary body. In some cases, particularly following cataract extraction, the suprachoroidal hemorrhage may remain localized and mimic a choroidal melanoma, a large choroidal nevus, or a subretinal pigment epithelial hematoma.[936–939] Fluorescein angiography shows no obstruction of background choroidal fluorescence over the center of the lesion, some relative nonfluorescence around its border, and usually some evidence of chorioretinal folds overlying the suprachoroidal hematoma. Ultrasonography shows acoustic hollowness of the lesion without choroidal excavation (Figure 3.69D, F–H).

The etiology and pathogenesis of suprachoroidal hemorrhage appear to be dependent upon the change in intraocular pressure. The primary event for initiation of the hemorrhage is thought to be hypotony resulting in effusion of serous fluid into the suprachoroidal space, which stretches and tears the long or short posterior ciliary arteries, resulting in hemorrhage. Subsequent stretching of the ciliary nerves due to rapid accumulation of blood is responsible for the patient's sensation of pain. It has been postulated that necrosis secondary to associated systemic vascular disease may result in weakening of the integrity of blood vessel walls and contribute to extravasation of blood as well.[935,940–942]

3.69 Suprachoroidal hemorrhage.

A–C: This 74-year-old woman bumped her eye one day after she underwent an intraocular lens exchange. While repositioning the displaced intraocular lens a change in the red reflex was noted. She had developed an intraoperative choroidal hemorrhage that was photographed the next day when her vision was hand motions (A–C). The hemorrhage resolved over time with conservative management and vision returned to 20/20 eventually.

D and **E**: A semilunar-shaped brown reflex was noted while this 79-year-old patient was undergoing cataract surgery. His posterior capsule had ruptured during the procedure and anterior-chamber lens was placed and wound closed quickly. When examined the next day he had a large temporal suprachoroidal hemorrhage that obscured his macula and could be confirmed on an ultrasound B scan (D). Ten days later the hemorrhage was drained, following which fundus photographs could be done. Autofluorescence image shows alternating dark and light lines corresponding to the chorioretinal folds at the posterior edge of the choroidal hemorrhage (E).

F and **G**: Postglaucoma surgery suprachoroidal hemorrhage (F) in this 80-year-old woman 4 days apart showing reduction in size by almost 50% (G).

H: Extensive choroidal hemorrhage in this 79-year-old male who underwent a vitrectomy and scleral buckle placement for a post traumatic cataract removal retinal detachment. His sclera was very thin in the superior half and the buckle sutures had to be placed carefully. The retina was flat at the end of the surgery and 20% SF_6 gas was placed. On post-op day 1, he complained of no overnight pain; the gas had completely disappeared and the globe was filled with choroidal blood (H). The eye did poorly with development of a new giant retinal tear superiorly.

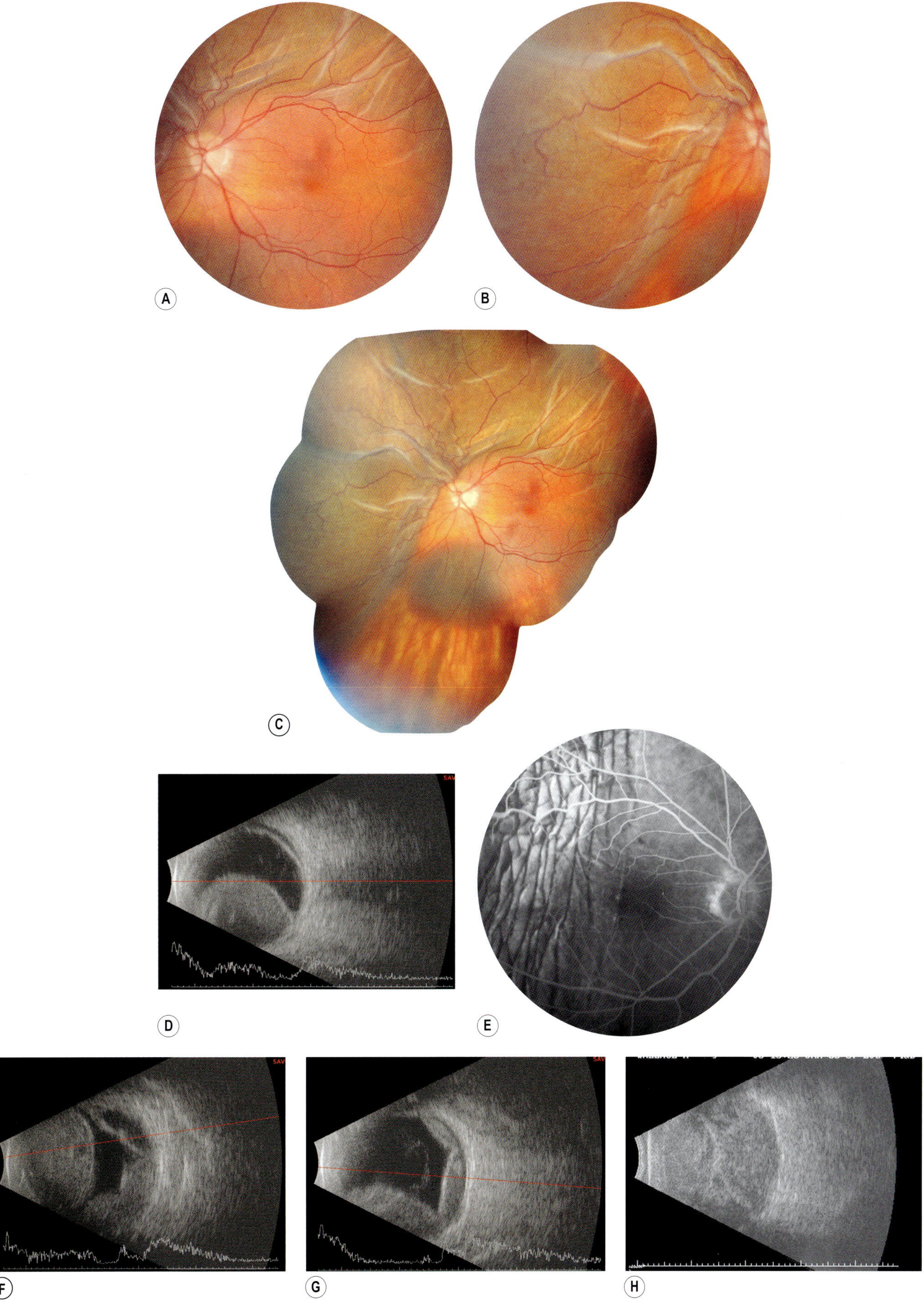
A
B
C
D
E
F
G
H

References

1. Archer DB. Neovascularization of the retina. Trans Ophthalmol Soc UK 1976;96:471–93.
2. Archer DB, Gardiner TA. Electron microscopic features of experimental choroidal neovascularization. Am J Ophthalmol 1981;91:433–57.
3. Archer DB, Gardiner TA. Morphologic, fluorescein angiographic, and light microscopic features of experimental choroidal neovascularization. Am J Ophthalmol 1981;91:297–311.
4. Miller M, Miller B, Ryan SJ. The role of retinal pigment epithelium in the involution of subretinal neovascularization. Invest Ophthalmol Vis Sci 1986;27:1644–52.
5. Ohkuma H, Ryan SJ. Experimental subretinal neovascularization in the monkey; permeability of new vessels. Arch Ophthalmol 1983;101:1102–10.
6. Ryan SJ. The development of an experimental model of subretinal neovascularization in disciform macular degeneration. Trans Am Ophthalmol Soc 1979;77:707–45.
7. Ryan SJ. Subretinal neovascularization after argon laser photocoagulation. Albrecht von Graefes Arch Klin Exp Ophthalmol 1980;215:29–42.
8. Bennett G. Central serous retinopathy. Br J Ophthalmol. 1955;39:605–18.
9. Burton TC. Central serous retinopathy. In: Blodi FC, editor. Current concepts in ophthalmology. St. Louis: CV Mosby; 1972. p. 1–28.
10. Edwards TS, Priestley BS. Central angiospastic retinopathy. Am J Ophthalmol 1964;57:988–96.
11. Gass JDM. Bullous retinal detachment: an unusual manifestation of idiopathic central serous choroidopathy. Am J Ophthalmol 1973;75:810–21.
12. Gass JDM. Pathogenesis of disciform detachment of the neuroepithelium. II. Idiopathic central serous choroidopathy. Am J Ophthalmol 1967;63:587–615.
13. Gass JD, Norton EWD, Justice Jr J. Serous detachment of the retinal pigment epithelium. Trans Am Acad Ophthalmol Otolaryngol 1966;70:990–1015.
14. Gelber GS, Schatz H. Loss of vision due to central serous chorioretinopathy following psychological stress. Am J Psychiatry 1987;144:46–50.
15. Gifford SR, Marquardt G. Central angiospastic retinopathy. Arch Ophthalmol 1939;21:211–28.
16. Klein BA. Symposium: macular diseases. Clinical manifestations. I. Central serous retinopathy and chorioretinopathy. Trans Am Acad Ophthalmol Otolaryngol 1965;69:614–22.
17. Mitsui Y, Sakanashi R. Central angiospastic retinopathy. Am J Ophthalmol 1956;41:105–14.
18. Straatsma BR, Allen RA, Pettit TH. Central serous retinopathy. Trans Pacif Cst Oto-Ophthalmol Soc 1966;47:107–27.
19. von Graefe A. Ueber centrale recidivirende Retinitis. Albrecht von Graefes Arch Ophthalmol 1866;12:211–5.
20. Walsh FB, Sloan LL. Idiopathic flat detachment of the macula. Am J Ophthalmol 1936;19: 195–208.
21. Gass JDM. Pathogenesis of disciform detachment of the neuroepithelium. I. General concepts and classification. Am J Ophthalmol 1967;63:573–85.
22. Gass JDM. Central serous chorioretinopathy and white subretinal exudation during pregnancy. Arch Ophthalmol 1991;109:677–81.
23. Laatikainen L, Hoffren M. Long-term follow-up study of nonsenile detachment of the retinal pigment epithelium. Eur J Ophthalmol 1991;1:79–84.
24. Lewis ML. Idiopathic serous detachment of the retinal pigment epithelium. Arch Ophthalmol 1978;96:620–4.
25. Friberg TR, Campagna J. Central chorioretinopathy: an analysis of the clinical morphology using image-processing techniques. Graefes Arch Clin Exp Ophthalmol 1989;227:201–5.
26. Fujisawa Y. Clinical studies on central serous chorioretinitis by fluorescein fundus photography. Jpn J Ophthalmol 1966;10:19–26.
27. Lyons DE. Conservative management of central serous retinopathy. Trans Ophthalmol Soc UK 1977;97:214–6.
28. Nadel AJ, Turan MI, Coles RS. Central serous retinopathy; a generalized disease of the pigment epithelium. Mod Probl Ophthalmol 1979;20:76–88.
29. Nørholm I. Central serous retinitis; a follow-up study. Acta Ophthalmol. 1969;47:890–9.
30. Norton EWD, Gass JD, Smith JL, et al. Symposium: macular diseases. Diagnosis; fluorescein in the study of macular disease. Trans Am Acad Ophthalmol Otolaryngol 1965;69:631–42.
31. Spitznas M, Huke J. Number, shape, and topography of leakage points in acute type I central serous retinopathy. Graefes Arch Clin Exp Ophthalmol 1987;225:437–40.
32. Yamada K, Hayasaka S, Setogawa T. Fluorescein-angiographic patterns in patients with central serous chorioretinopathy at the initial visit. Ophthalmologica 1992;205:69–76.
33. Shimizu K, Tobari I. Central serous retinopathy dynamics of subretinal fluid. Mod Probl Ophthalmol 1971;9:152–7.
34. Gass JDM. Photocoagulation treatment of idiopathic central serous choroidopathy. Trans Am Acad Ophthalmol Otolaryngol 1977;83:OP456–OP463.
35. Goldstein BG, Pavan PR. "Blow-outs" in the retinal pigment epithelium. Br J Ophthalmol 1987;71:676–81.
36. Yannuzzi LA, Shakin JL, Fisher YL, et al. Peripheral retinal detachments and retinal pigment epithelial atrophic tracts secondary to central serous pigment epitheliopathy. Ophthalmology 1984;91:1554–72.
37. Hayashi K, Hasegawa Y, Tokoro T. Indocyanine green angiography of central serous chorioretinopathy. Int Ophthalmol 1986;9:37–41.
38. Scheider A, Nasemann JE, Lund O-E. Fluorescein and indocyanine green angiographies of central serous choroidopathy by scanning laser ophthalmoscopy. Am J Ophthalmol 1993;115:50–6.
39. Guyer DR, Yannuzzi LA, Slakter JS, et al. Digital indocyanine green videoangiography of central serous chorioretinopathy. Arch Ophthalmol 1994;112:1057–62.
40. Spaide RF, Campeas L, Haas A, et al. Central serous chorioretinopathy in younger and older adults. Ophthalmology 1996;103:2070–9. [discussion 2079–2080]
41. Maruko I, Iida T, Ojima A, et al. Subretinal dot-like precipitates and yellow material in central serous chorioretinopathy. Retina 2010 Nov 3 [in press]
42. Imamura Y, Fujiwara T, Spaide RF. Fundus autofluorescence and visual acuity in central serous chorioretinopathy. Ophthalmology 2010 Nov 3 [in press]
43. Spaide RF, Klancnik Jr JM. Fundus autofluorescence and central serous chorioretinopathy. Ophthalmology 2005;112:825–33.
44. Imamura Y, Fujiwara T, Margolis R, et al. Enhanced depth imaging optical coherence tomography of the choroid in central serous chorioretinopathy. Retina 2009;29:1469–73.
45. Ooto S, Tsujikawa A, Mori S, et al. Thickness of photoreceptor layers in polypoidal choroidal vasculopathy and central serous chorioretinopathy. Graefes Arch Clin Exp Ophthalmol 2010;248:1077–86.
46. Castro-Correia J, Coutinho MF, Rosas V, et al. Long-term follow-up of central serous retinopathy in 150 patients. Doc Ophthalmol 1992;81:379–86.
47. Yannuzzi LA, Slakter JS, Kaufman SR, et al. Laser treatment of diffuse retinal pigment epitheliopathy. Eur J Ophthalmol 1992;2:103–14.
48. Gass JDM, Little HL. Bilateral bullous exudative retinal detachment complicating idiopathic central serous chorioretinopathy during systemic corticosteroid therapy. Ophthalmology 1995;102:737–47.
49. Akiyama K, Kawamura M, Ogata T, et al. Retinal vascular loss in idiopathic central serous chorioretinopathy with bullous retinal detachment. Ophthalmology 1987;94:1605–9.
50. Brancato R, Scialdone A, Pece A, et al. Eight-year follow-up of central serous chorioretinopathy with and without laser treatment. Graefes Arch Clin Exp Ophthalmol 1987;225:166–8.
51. Dickhoff KV, Hoffren M, Laatikainen L. Les modifications de l'épithélium pigmentaire rétinien en rapport avec la rétinopathie séreuse centrale. J Fr Ophtalmol 1989;12:877–81.
52. O'Connor PR. Multifocal serous choroidopathy. Ann Ophthalmol 1975;7:237–45.
53. Benson WE, Shields JA, Annesley Jr WH, et al. Idiopathic central serous chorioretinopathy with bullous retinal detachment. Ann Ophthalmol 1980;12:920–4.
54. Kayazawa F. Central serous choroidopathy with exudative retinal detachment. Ann Ophthalmol 1982;14:1035–42.
55. Tsukahara I, Uyama M. Central serous choroidopathy with bullous retinal detachment. Albrecht von Graefes Arch Klin Exp Ophthalmol 1978;206:169–78.
56. Weiler W, Foerster MH, Exsudative Netzhautablösung Wessing A. Pigmentepithelriss und subretinales Exsudat bei einem Fall von Retinopathia centralis serosa. Klin Monatstbl Augenheilkd 1991;199:450–3.
57. Menerath JM, Bacin F, Al-Odeh A, et al. Déchirure géante et périphérique de l'épithélium pigmentaire rétinien. J Fr Ophtalmol 1992;15:282–7.
58. Carpenter MT, O'Boyle JE, Enzenauer RW, et al. Choroiditis in systemic lupus erythematosus. Am J Ophthalmol 1994;117:535–6.
59. Diddie K, Aronson AJ, Ernest JT. Chorioretinopathy in a case of systemic lupus erythematosus. Trans Am Ophthalmol Soc 1977;75:122–31.
60. Eckstein MB, Spalton DJ, Holder G. Visual loss from central serous retinopathy in systemic lupus erythematosus. Br J Ophthalmol 1993;77:607–9.
61. Gass JDM. Stereoscopic atlas of macular diseases; diagnosis and treatment, 3rd ed. St. Louis: CV Mosby; 1987. p. 276–277.
62. Jabs DA, Hanneken AM, Schachat AP, et al. Choroidopathy in systemic lupus erythematosus. Arch Ophthalmol 1988;106:230–4.
63. Matsuo T, Nakayama T, Koyama T, et al. Multifocal pigment epithelial damages with serous retinal detachment in systemic lupus erythematosus. Ophthalmologica 1987;195:97–102.
64. Schreiber JB, Lakhanpal V, Nasrallah SM. Crohn's disease complicated by idiopathic central serous chorioretinopathy with bullous retinal detachment. Dig Dis Sci 1989;34:118–22.
65. Williamson J, Nuki G. Macular lesions during systemic therapy with depot tetracosactrin. Br J Ophthalmol 1970;54:405–9.
66. Gass JDM. Bullous retinal detachment and multiple retinal pigment epithelial detachments in patients receiving hemodialysis. Graefes Arch Clin Exp Ophthalmol 1992;230:454–8.
67. Friberg TR, Eller AW. Serous retinal detachment resembling central serous chorioretinopathy following organ transplantation. Graefes Arch Clin Exp Ophthalmol 1990;228:305–9.
68. de Venecia G, editor. Fluorescein angiographic smoke stack. Case presentation at Verhoeff Society Meeting, April 24–25,1982, Washington, DC.
69. Gass JDM. Stereoscopic atlas of macular diseases; diagnosis and treatment, 3rd ed. St. Louis: CV Mosby; 1987. p. 46–59.
70. Quillen DA, Gass JDM, Brod RD, et al. Central serous chorioretinopathy in women. Ophthalmology 1996;103:72–9.
71. Bedrossian RH. Central serous retinopathy and pregnancy. Am J Ophthalmol 1974;78:152–4.
72. Chumbley LC, Frank RN. Central serous retinopathy and pregnancy. Am J Ophthalmol 1974;77:158–60.
73. Cruysberg JRM, Deutman AF. Visual disturbances during pregnancy caused by central serous choroidopathy. Br J Ophthalmol 1982;66:240–1.
74. Fastenberg DM, Ober RR. Central serous choroidopathy in pregnancy. Arch Ophthalmol. 1983;101:1055–8.
75. Sunness JS. The pregnant woman's eye. Surv Ophthalmol 1988;32:219–38.
76. Sunness JS, Haller JA, Fine SL. Central serous chorioretinopathy and pregnancy. Arch Ophthalmol 1993;111:360–4.
77. Berger AR, Olk RJ, Burgess D. Central serous choroidopathy in patients over 50 years of age. Ophthalmic Surg 1991;22:583–90.
78. Schatz H, Madeira D, Johnson RN, et al. Central serous chorioretinopathy occurring in patients 60 years of age and older. Ophthalmology 1992;99:63–7.
79. Fraunfelder FW, Fraunfelder FT. Central serous chorioretinopathy associated with sildenafil. Retina 2008;28:606–9.
80. Quiram P, Dumars S, Parwar B, et al. Viagra-associated serous macular detachment. Graefes Arch Clin Exp Ophthalmol 2005;243:339–44.
81. Allibhai ZA, Gale JS, Sheidow TS. Central serous chorioretinopathy in a patient taking sildenafil citrate. Ophthalmic Surg Lasers Imaging 2004;35:165–7.
82. Iida T, Spaide RF, Haas A, et al. Leopard-spot pattern of yellowish subretinal deposits in central serous chorioretinopathy. Arch Ophthalmol 2002;120:37–42.
83. Lewis ML. Coexisting central serous choroidopathy and retinitis pigmentosa. South Med J 1980;73:77–80.

84. Fine SL, Owens SL. Central serous retinopathy in a 7-year-old girl. Am J Ophthalmol 1980;90:871–3.
85. Ficker L, Vafidis G, While A, et al. Long-term follow-up of a prospective trial of argon laser photocoagulation in the treatment of central serous retinopathy. Br J Ophthalmol 1988;72:829–34.
86. Klein ML, Van Buskirk EM, Friedman E, et al. Experience with nontreatment of central serous choroidopathy. Arch Ophthalmol 1974;91:247–50.
87. Leaver PK, Williams CM. Effects of central serous retinopathy on visual function. Trans Ophthalmol Soc UK 1977;97:655
88. Levine R, Brucker AJ, Robinson F. Long-term follow-up of idiopathic central serous chorioretinopathy by fluorescein angiography. Ophthalmology 1989;96:854–9.
89. Nanjiani M. Long-term follow-up of central serous retinopathy. Trans Ophthalmol Soc UK 1977;97:656–61.
90. Watzke RC, Burton TC, Leaverton PE. Ruby laser photocoagulation therapy of central serous retinopathy. I. A controlled clinical study. II. Factors affecting prognosis. Trans Am Acad Ophthalmol Otolaryngol 1974;78:OP205–OP211.
91. Chuang EL, Sharp DM, Fitzke FW, et al. Retinal dysfunction in central serous retinopathy. Eye 1987;1:120–5.
92. Folk JC, Thompson HS, Hand DP, et al. Visual function abnormalities in central serous retinopathy. Arch Ophthalmol 1984;102:1299–302.
93. Forsius H, Krause U, Eriksson A. Dazzling test in central serous retinopathy. Acta Ophthalmol 1964;41:25–32.
94. Koskela P, Laatikainen L, von Dickhoff K. Contrast sensitivity after resolution of central serous retinopathy. Graefes Arch Clin Exp Ophthalmol 1994;232:473–6.
95. Kovács B. Visual phenomena following light coagulation in central serous retinopathy (CSR). Doc Ophthalmol 1977;44:445–53.
96. Leaver P, Williams C. Argon laser photocoagulation in the treatment of central serous retinopathy. Br J Ophthalmol 1979;63:674–7.
97. Tsuneoka H, Kabayama T, Fukuda J, et al. Night visual acuity in patients with idiopathic central serous choroidopathy. Jpn J Ophthalmol 1980;24:178–87.
98. Uyama M, Uchida S. Central serous retinopathy and allied conditions: treatment with photocoagulation. In: Shimizu K, editor. Fluorescein angiography; proceedings of the international symposium on fluorescein angiography (ISFA), Tokyo, 1972. Tokyo: Igaku Shoin; 1974. p. 405–9.
99. Van Meel GJ, Smith VC, Pokorny J, et al. Foveal densitometry in central serous choroidopathy. Am J Ophthalmol 1984;98:359–68.
100. Kanis MJ, van Norren D. Delayed recovery of the optical Stiles-Crawford effect in a case of central serous chorioretinopathy. Br J Ophthalmol 2008;92:292–4.
101. Robertson DM. Argon laser photocoagulation treatment in central serous chorioretinopathy. Ophthalmology 1986;93:972–4.
102. Gomolin JES. Choroidal neovascularization and central serous chorioretinopathy. Can J Ophthalmol 1989;24:20–3.
103. Gass JDM. Stereoscopic atlas of macular diseases; diagnosis and treatment, 2nd ed. St. Louis: CV Mosby; 1977. p. 40.
104. Guyer DR, Yannuzzi LA, Slakter JS, et al. Digital indocyanine green videoangiography of central serous chorioretinopathy. Arch Ophthalmol 1994;112:1057–62.
105. Piccolino FC, Borgia L. Central serous chorioretinopathy and indocyanine green angiography. Retina 1994;14:231–42.
106. Spitznas M. Pathogenesis of central serous retinopathy: a new working hypothesis. Graefes Arch Clin Exp Ophthalmol 1986;224:321–4.
107. Marmor MF. New hypothesis on the pathogenesis and treatment of serous retinal detachment. Graefes Arch Clin Exp Ophthalmol 1988;226:548–52.
108. Yao X-Y, Marmor MF. Induction of serous retinal detachment in rabbit eyes by pigment epithelial and choriocapillary injury. Arch Ophthalmol 1992;110:541–6.
109. Behrendt T. Central serous retinopathy (CSR). In: Brockhurst RJ, Boruchoff SA, Hutchinson BT, editors. Controversy in ophthalmology. Philadelphia: WB Saunders; 1977. p. 698–705.
110. Negi A, Marmor MF. Experimental serous retinal detachment and focal pigment epithelial damage. Arch Ophthalmol 1984;102:445–9.
111. Piccolino FC. Central serous chorioretinopathy: some considerations on the pathogenesis. Ophthalmologica 1981;182:204–10.
112. Gross M, Froom P, Tendler Y, et al. Central serous retinopathy (choroidopathy) in pilots. Aviat Space Environ Med 1986;57:457–8.
113. Lipowski ZJ, Kiriakos RZ. Psychosomatic aspects of central serous retinopathy; a review and case report. Psychosomatics 1971;12:398–401.
114. Werry H, Arends C. Untersuchung zur Ohjektivierung von Persönlichkeitsmerkmalen bei Patienten mit Retinopathia centralis serosa. Klin Monatsbl Augenheilkd 1978;172:363–70.
115. Yannuzzi LA. Type-A behavior and central serous chorioretinopathy. Retina 1987;7:111–30.
116. Sie-Boen-Lian The etiological agent of serous central chorioretinitis. Ophthalmologica 1964;148:263–70.
117. Watanabe S, Ohtsuki K. Experimental serous choroidopathy. Acta Soc Ophthalmol Jpn 1979;83:808–17.
118. Yoshioka H. The etiology of central serous chorioretinopathy. Acta Soc Ophthalmol Jpn 1991;95:1181–95.
119. Yoshioka H, Katsume Y, Akune H. Experimental central serous chorioretinopathy in monkey eyes: fluorescein angiographic findings. Ophthalmologica 1982;185:168–78.
120. Bouzas EA, Scott MH, Mastorakos S, et al. Central serous chorioretinopathy in endogenous hypercortisolism. Arch Ophthalmol 1993;111:1229–33.
121. Wakakura M, Ishikawa S. An evaluation of corticosteroid treatment for central serous chorioretinopathy. Jpn J Clin Ophthalmol 1980;34:123–9.
122. Wakakura M, Ishikawa S. Central serous chorioretinopathy complicating systemic corticosteroid therapy. Br J Ophthalmol 1984;68:329–31.
123. Blair NP, Brockhurst RJ, Lee W. Central serous choroidopathy in the Hallermann–Streiff syndrome. Ann Ophthalmol 1981;13:987–90.
124. Browning DJ. Nadolol in the treatment of central serous retinopathy. Am J Ophthalmol 1993;116:770–1.
125. Annesley Jr WH, Tasman WS, Le Win DP, et al. Retrospective evaluation of photocoagulation for idiopathic central serous chorioretinopathy. Mod Probl Ophthalmol 1974;12:234–8.
126. Gass JDM. Options in the treatment of macular diseases. Trans Ophthalmol Soc UK 1972;92:449–68.
127. Gass JDM. Photocoagulation of macular lesions. Trans Am Acad Ophthalmol Otolaryngol 1971;75:580–608.
128. Gass JDM. Ruby laser and xenon photocoagulation of macular lesions. Concilium Ophthalmologicum XXI, Mexico, 1970. Acta Ophthalmol 1971;1:485–506.
129. Gass JDM, editor. Fluorescein angiography; proceedings of the international symposium on fluorescein angiography (ISFA), Tokyo, 1972. Tokyo: Igaku Shoin; 1974.
130. Heydenreich A, Lemke L, Jütte A. Lichtkoagulation bei Chorioretinitis centralis serosa. Klin Monatsbl Augenheilkd 1974;165:578–84.
131. Hirose I. Therapy of central serous retinopathy. Folia Ophthalmol Jpn 1969;20: 1003–34.
132. Landers III MB, Shaw Jr HE, Anderson Jr WB, et al. Argon laser treatment of central serous chorioretinopathy. Ann Ophthalmol 1977;9:1567–72.
133. L'Esperance Jr FA. Argon and ruby laser photocoagulation of disciform macular disease. Trans Am Acad Ophthalmol Otolaryngol 1971;75:609–25.
134. Makabe R. Krypton- und Argonlaserkoagulation bei Chorioretinitis centralis serosa. Klin Monatsbl Augenheilkd 1987;190:489–90.
135. Maumenee AE. Symposium: macular diseases. Pathogenesis. Trans Am Acad Ophthalmol Otolaryngol 1965;69:691–9.
136. Novak MA, Singerman LJ, Rice TA. Krypton and argon laser photocoagulation for central serous chorioretinopathy. Retina 1987;7:162–9.
137. Peabody RR, Zweng HC, Little HL. Treatment of persistent central serous retinopathy. Arch Ophthalmol 1968;79:166–9.
138. Piccolino FC. Laser treatment of eccentric leaks in central serous chorioretinopathy resulting in disappearance of untreated juxtafoveal leaks. Retina 1992;12:96–102.
139. Robertson DM, Ilstrup D. Direct, indirect, and sham laser photocoagulation in the management of central serous chorioretinopathy. Am J Ophthalmol 1983;95:457–66.
140. Shimizu K, Tobari I. Fluorography and photocoagulation of central serous retinopathy. Jpn J Clin Ophthalmol 1969;23:438–50.
141. Slusher MM. Krypton red laser photocoagulation in selected cases of central serous chorioretinopathy. Retina 1986;6:81–4.
142. Spalter HF. Photocoagulation of central serous retinopathy; a preliminary report. Arch Ophthalmol 1968;79:247–53.
143. Theodossiadis G, Tongos D. Treatment of central serous retinopathy; a comparative study with and without light coagulation. Ophthalmologica 1974;169:416–31.
144. Watzke RC, Burton TC, Leaverton P. Ruby laser photocoagulation therapy of central serous retinopathy; a preliminary report. Mod Probl Ophthalmol 1974;12:242–6.
145. Watzke RC, Burton TC, Woolson RF. Direct and indirect laser photocoagulation of central serous choroidopathy. Am J Ophthalmol 1979;88:914–8.
146. Wessing A. Zur Pathogenese und Therapie der sogenannten Retinitis centralis serosa. Ophthalmologica 1967;153:259–76.
147. Wessing A. Central serous retinopathy and related lesions. Mod Probl Ophthalmol 1971;9: 148–51.
148. Wessing A. Changing concept of central serous retinopathy and its treatment. Trans Am Acad Ophthalmol Otolaryngol 1973;77:OP275–OP280.
149. Zweng HC, Little HL, Peabody RR. Laser photocoagulation and retinal angiography: with current concepts in retinal and choroidal diseases. St. Louis: CV Mosby; 1969. p. 79.
150. Schatz H, Yannuzzi LA, Gitter KA. Subretinal neovascularization following argon laser photocoagulation treatment for central serous chorioretinopathy: complication or misdiagnosis? Trans Am Acad Ophthalmol Otolaryngol 1977;83:OP893–OP906.
151. François J, De Laey JJ, Cambie E, et al. Neovascularization after argon laser photocoagulation of macular lesions. Am J Ophthalmol 1975;79:206–10.
152. Gass JDM, editor. Fluorescein angiography; proceedings of the international symposium on fluorescein angiography (ISFA); 1972. Tokyo: Igaku Shoin; 1974.
153. Reibaldi M, Cardascia N, Longo A, et al. Standard-fluence versus low-fluence photodynamic therapy in chronic central serous chorioretinopathy: a nonrandomized clinical trial. Am J Ophthalmol 2010;149(307–315):e2.
154. Inoue R, Sawa M, Tsujikawa M, et al. Association between the efficacy of photodynamic therapy and indocyanine green angiography findings for central serous chorioretinopathy. Am J Ophthalmol 2010;149(441–446):e1–e2.
155. Chan WM, Lai TY, Lai RY, et al. Safety enhanced photodynamic therapy for chronic central serous chorioretinopathy: one-year results of a prospective study. Retina 2008;28:85–93.
156. Ober MD, Yannuzzi LA, Do DV, et al. Photodynamic therapy for focal retinal pigment epithelial leaks secondary to central serous chorioretinopathy. Ophthalmology 2005;112:2088–94.
157. Yannuzzi LA, Slakter JS, Gross NE, et al. Indocyanine green angiography-guided photodynamic therapy for treatment of chronic central serous chorioretinopathy: a pilot study. Retina 2003;23:288–98.
158. Tarantola RM, Law JC, Recchia FM, et al. Photodynamic therapy as treatment of chronic idiopathic central serous chorioretinopathy. Lasers Surg Med 2008;40:671–5.
159. Nielsen JS, Weinreb RN, Yannuzzi L, et al. Mifepristone treatment of chronic central serous chorioretinopathy. Retina 2007;27:119–22.
160. Bressler NM, Bressler SB, Gragoudas ES. Clinical characteristics of choroidal neovascular membranes. Arch Ophthalmol 1987;105:209–13.
161. Ferris III FL. Senile macular degeneration: Review of epidemiologic features. Am J Epidemiol 1983;118:132–51.
162. Ferris III FL, Fine SL, Hyman L. Age-related macular degeneration and blindness due to neovascular maculopathy. Arch Ophthalmol 1984;102:1640–2.

163. Ganley JP, Roberts J. Eye conditions and related need for medical care among persons 1–74 years of age United States, 1971–72. Washington, DC: U.S. Government Printing Office; 1983. Vital and Health Statistics, series 11 no 228, DHHS publication no (PHS) 83–1678
164. Hyman LG. Senile macular degeneration: an epidemiologic case control study (thesis). Baltimore: Johns Hopkins University; 1981.
165. Kahn HA, Leibowitz HM, Ganley JP, et al. The Framingham Eye Study. I. Outline and major prevalence findings. Am J Epidemiol 1977;106:17–32.
166. Kahn HA, Leibowitz HM, Ganley JP, et al. The Framingham Eye Study. II. Association of ophthalmic pathology with single variables previously measured in the Framingham Heart Study. Am J Epidemiol 1977;106:33–41.
167. Kahn HA, Moorehead HB. Statistics on blindness in the model reporting area, 1969–1970. Washington, DC: National Institutes of Health; 1973. DHEW publication (NIH) 73–427
168. Kini MM, Leibowitz HM, Colton T, et al. Prevalence of senile cataract, diabetic retinopathy, senile macular degeneration, and open-angle glaucoma in the Framingham Eye Study. Am J Ophthalmol 1978;85:28–34.
169. Klein BE, Klein R. Cataracts and macular degeneration in older Americans. Arch Ophthalmol 1982;100:571–3. [correction p. 1333]
170. Leibowitz HM, Krueger DE, Maunder LR, et al. The Framingham Eye Study monograph: an ophthalmological and epidemiological study of cataract, glaucoma, diabetic retinopathy, macular degeneration, and visual acuity in a general population of 2631 adults, 1973–1975. Surv Ophthalmol 1980;24:335–610.
171. MacDonald AE. Causes of blindness in Canada: an analysis of 24 605 cases registered with the Canadian National Institute for the Blind. Can Med Assoc J 1965;92:264–79.
172. Martinez GS, Campbell AJ, Reinken J, et al. Prevalence of ocular disease in a population study of subjects 65 years old and older. Am J Ophthalmol 1982;94:181–9.
173. McGuinness R. The Framingham Eye Study. Am J Ophthalmol 1978;86:852–3.
174. Sorsby A. The incidence and causes of blindness in England and Wales 1948–1962. London: Her Majesty's Stationery Office; 1966. Reports in public health and medical subjects, no.114
175. Wessing A. Photocoagulation in the treatment of macular lesions. Concilium Ophthalmologicum XXI, 1970, Mexico. Acta 1971;1:507–12.
176. Donders FC. Beiträge zur pathologischen Anatomie des Auges. Albrecht von Graefes Arch Ophthalmol 1855;1:106–18.
177. Doyne RW. Peculiar condition of choroiditis occurring in several members of the same family. Trans Ophthalmol Soc UK 1899;19:71
178. Forni S, Babel J. Etude clinique et histologique de la malattia leventinese; affection appartenant au groupe des dégénérescences hyalines du pôle postérieur. Ophthalmologica 1962;143: 313–22.
179. Holthouse EH, Batten RD. A case of superficial choroidoretinitis of peculiar form and doubtful causation. Trans Ophthalmol Soc UK 1897;17:62–3.
180. Hutchinson J. Symmetrical central choroido-retinal disease occurring in senile persons. R Lond Ophthalmic Hosp Rep 1876;8:231–44.
181. Junius P, Kuhnt H. Die scheibenformige Entartung der Netzhautmitte (Degeneratio maculae luteae disciformis). Berlin: Karger; 1926.
182. Oeller JN. In: Bergmann J, editor. Atlas seltener ophthalmoskopischer Befunde Zugleich Ergänzungstafeln zu dem Atlas der Ophthalmoskopie, Section C, Tab XII. Wiesbaden 1900–1924.
183. Ormond AW. Four cases of disc-like degeneration of the macula lutea. Guys Hosp Rep 1927;77:16–21.
184. Seddon JM, Chen CA. The epidemiology of age-related macular degeneration. Int Ophthalmol Clin 2004;44:17–39.
185. Gregor Z, Joffe L. Senile macular changes in the black African. Br J Ophthalmol 1978;62: 547–50.
186. Bonnet M. Beitrag zur Klinik der Maculadrusen. Klin Monatsbl Augenheilkd 1973;162: 326–31.
187. Deutman AF. Rümke AML. Reticular dystrophy of the retinal pigment epithelium; dystrophia reticularis laminae pigmentosa retinae of H. Sjögren. Arch Ophthalmol 1969;82:4–9.
188. Farkas TG. Drusen of the retinal pigment epithelium. Surv Ophthalmol 1971;16:75–87.
189. Farkas TG, Krill AE, Sylvester VM, et al. Familial and secondary drusen: Histologic and functional correlations. Trans Am Acad Ophthalmol Otolaryngol 1971;75:333–43.
190. Farkas TG, Sylvester V, Archer D. The ultrastructure of drusen. Am J Ophthalmol. 1971;71: 1196–205.
191. Friedman E, Smith TR. Senile changes of the choriocapillaris of the posterior pole. Trans Am Acad Ophthalmol Otolaryngol 1965;69:652–61.
192. Gass JDM. Choroidal neovascular membranes–their visualization and treatment. Trans Am Acad Ophthalmol Otolaryngol 1973;77:OP310–OP320.
193. Gold D, Friedman A, Wise GN. Predisciform senile macular degeneration. Am J Ophthalmol 1973;76:763–8.
194. Klein R, Klein BEK, Linton KLP. Prevalence of age-related maculopathy. The Beaver Dam Eye Study. Ophthalmology 1992;99:933–43.
195. Pauleikhoff D, Barondes MJ, Minassian D, et al. Drusen as risk factors in age-related macular disease. Am J Ophthalmol 1990;109:38–43.
196. Pearce WG. Doyne's honeycomb retinal degeneration; clinical and genetic features. Br J Ophthalmol 1968;52:73–8.
197. Sarks SH. Drusen and their relationship to senile macular degeneration. Aust J Ophthalmol 1980;8:117–30.
198. Tanenbaum HL, Eshagian M. Senile disciform degeneration of the macula: The other eye–a fluorescein angiographic study. Can J Ophthalmol 1972;7:280–4.
199. Barondes M, Pauleikhoff D, Chisholm IC, et al. Bilaterality of drusen. Br J Ophthalmol 1990;74:180–2.
200. Gass JDM. Pathogenesis of disciform detachment of the neuroepithelium. III. Senile disciform macular degeneration. Am J Ophthalmol 1967;63:617–44.
201. Alexander MF, Maguire MG, Lietman TM, et al. Assessment of visual function in patients with age-related macular degeneration and low visual acuity. Arch Ophthalmol 1988;106:1543–7.
202. Eisner A, Stoumbos VD, Klein ML, et al. Relations between fundus appearance and function; eyes whose fellow eye has exudative age-related macular degeneration. Invest Ophthalmol Vis Sci 1991;32:8–20.
203. Kleiner RC, Enger C, Alexander MF, et al. Contrast sensitivity in age-related macular degeneration. Arch Ophthalmol 1988;106:55–7.
204. Lennerstrand G, Ahlström CO. Contrast sensitivity in macular degeneration and the relation to subjective visual impairment. Acta Ophthalmol 1989;67:225–33.
205. Macular Photocoagulation Study Group. Laser photocoagulation of subfoveal neovascular lesions in age-related macular degeneration; results of a randomized clinical trial. Arch Ophthalmol 1991;109:1220–31.
206. Macular Photocoagulation Study Group. Subfoveal neovascular lesions in age-related macular degeneration; guidelines for evaluation and treatment in the Macular Photocoagulation Study. Arch Ophthalmol 1991;109:1242–57.
207. Sunness JS, Johnson MA, Massof RW, et al. Retinal sensitivity over drusen and nondrusen areas; a study using fundus perimetry. Arch Ophthalmol 1988;106:1081–4.
208. Sunness JS, Massof RW, Johnson MA, et al. Diminished foveal sensitivity may predict the development of advanced age-related macular degeneration. Ophthalmology 1989;96:375–81.
209. Fishman GA, Carrasco C, Fishman M. The electro-oculogram in diffuse (familial) drusen. Arch Ophthalmol 1976;94:231–3.
210. Gass JDM. Drusen and disciform macular detachment and degeneration. Arch Ophthalmol 1973;90:206–17.
211. Marcus M, Merin S, Wolf M, et al. Electrophysiologic tests in assessment of senile macular degeneration. Ann Ophthalmol 1983;15:235–8.
212. Jampol LM, Tielsch J. Race, macular degeneration, and the macular photocoagulation study. Arch Ophthalmol 1992;110:1699–700.
213. Bastek JV, Siegel EB, Straatsma BR, et al. Chorioretinal juncture; pigmentary patterns of the peripheral fundus. Ophthalmology 1982;89:1455–63.
214. Daiker B. Lineare Degenerationen des peripheren retinalen Pigmentepithels; Eine pathologisch-anatomische Studie. Albrecht von Graefes Arch Klin Exp Ophthalmol 1973;186:1–12.
215. Deutman AF, Jansen LMAA. Dominantly inherited drusen of Bruch's membrane. Br J Ophthalmol 1970;54:373–82.
216. Gass JDM. Drusen and disciform macular detachment and degeneration. Trans Am Ophthalmol Soc 1972;70:409–36.
217. Humphrey WT, Carlson RE, Valone Jr JA. Senile reticular pigmentary degeneration. Am J Ophthalmol 1984;98:717–22.
218. Lewis H, Straatsma BR, Foos RY, et al. Reticular degeneration of the pigment epithelium. Ophthalmology 1985;92:1485–95.
219. Bressler NM, Bressler SB, Seddon JM, et al. Drusen characteristics in patients with exudative versus nonexudative age-related macular degeneration. Retina 1988;8:109–14.
220. Bressler SB, Maguire MG, Bressler NM, et al. Relationship of drusen and abnormalities of the retinal pigment epithelium to the prognosis of neovascular macular degeneration. Arch Ophthalmol 1990;108:1442–7.
221. Bird AC. Bruch's membrane change with age. Br J Ophthalmol 1992;76:166–8.
222. Pauleikhoff D, Chen JC, Chisholm IH, et al. Choroidal perfusion abnormality with age-related Bruch's membrane change. Am J Ophthalmol 1990;109:211–7.
223. Piguet B, Palmvang IB, Chisholm IH, et al. Evolution of age-related macular degeneration with choroidal perfusion abnormality. Am J Ophthalmol 1992;113:657–63.
224. Scheider A, Neuhauser L. Fluorescence characteristics of drusen during indocyanine-green angiography and their possible correlation with choroidal perfusion. Ger J Ophthalmol 1992;1:328–34.
225. Sheraidah G, Steinmetz R, Maguire J, et al. Correlation between lipids extracted from Bruch's membrane and age. Ophthalmology 1993;100:47–51.
226. Pauleikhoff D, Harper CA, Marshall J, et al. Aging changes in Bruch's membrane; a histochemical and morphologic study. Ophthalmology 1990;97:171–8.
227. Burns RP, Feeney-Burns L. Clinico-morphologic correlations of drusen of Bruch's membrane. Trans Am Ophthalmol Soc 1980;78:206–25.
228. Coffey AJH, Brownstein S. The prevalence of macular drusen in postmortem eyes. Am J Ophthalmol 1986;102:164–71.
229. Fenney-Burns L, Burns RP, Gao CL. Age-related macular changes in humans over 90 years old. Am J Ophthalmol 1990;109:265–78.
230. Frank RN, Green WR, Pollack IP. Senile macular degeneration; clinicopathologic correlations of a case in the predisciform stage. Am J Ophthalmol 1973;75:587–94.
231. Green WR, Key III SN. Senile macular degeneration: histopathologic study. Trans Am Ophthalmol Soc 1977;75:180–254.
232. Hogan MJ. Bruch's membrane and disease of the macula; role of elastic tissue and collagen. Trans Ophthalmol Soc UK 1967;87:113–61.
233. Sarks SH. Ageing and degeneration in the macular region: a clinico-pathological study. Br J Ophthalmol 1976;60:324–41.
234. Fenney-Burns L, Gao CL, Tidwell M. Lysosomal enzyme cytochemistry of human RPE, Bruch's membrane and drusen. Invest Ophthalmol Vis Sci 1987;28:1138–47.
235. Ishibashi T, Patterson R, Ohnishi Y, et al. Formation of drusen in the human eye. Am J Ophthalmol 1986;101:342–53.
236. Ishibashi T, Sorgente N, Patterson R, et al. Pathogenesis of drusen in the primate. Invest Ophthalmol Vis Sci 1986;27:184–93.
237. Newsome DA, Hewitt AT, Huh W, et al. Detection of specific extracellular matrix molecules in drusen, Bruch's membrane, and ciliary body. Am J Ophthalmol 1987;104:373–81.
238. Hageman GS, Luthert PJ, Victor Chong NH, et al. An integrated hypothesis that considers drusen as biomarkers of immune-mediated processes at the RPE–Bruch's membrane interface in aging and age-related macular degeneration. Prog Retin Eye Res 2001;20:705–32.
239. Russell SR, Mullins RF, Schneider BL, et al. Location, substructure, and composition of basal laminar drusen compared with drusen associated with aging and age-related macular degeneration. Am J Ophthalmol 2000;129:205–14.

240. Duvall J, Tso MOM. Cellular mechanisms of resolution of drusen after laser coagulation; an experimental study. Arch Ophthalmol 1985;103:694–703.
241. Bressler NM, Silva JC, Bressler SB, et al. Clinicopathologic correlation of drusen and retinal pigment epithelial abnormalities in age-related macular degeneration. Retina 1994;14:130–42.
242. Green WR, Enger C. Age-related macular degeneration histopathologic studies. Ophthalmology 1993;100:1519–35.
243. van der Schaft TL, Mooy CM, de Bruijn WC, et al. Immunohistochemical light and electron microscopy of basal laminar deposit. Graefes Arch Clin Exp Ophthalmol 1994;232:40–6.
244. Loeffler KU, Lee WR. Is basal laminar deposit unique for age-related macular degeneration? Arch Ophthalmol 1992;110:15–16.
245. van der Schaft TL, de Bruijn WC, Mooy CM, et al. Is basal laminar deposit unique for age-related macular degeneration? Arch Ophthalmol 1991;109:420–5.
246. Hogan MJ. Electron microscopy of Bruch's membrane. Trans Am Acad Ophthalmol Otolaryngol 1965;69:683–90.
247. Hoshino M, Mizuno K, Ichikawa H. Aging alterations of retina and choroid of Japanese: Light microscopic study of macular region of 176 eyes. Jpn J Ophthalmol 1984;28:89–102.
248. Kornzweig AL. Changes in the choriocapillaris associated with senile macular degeneration. Ann Ophthalmol 1977;9:753–64.
249. Penfold P, Killingsworth M, Sarks S. An ultrastructural study of the role of leucocytes and fibroblasts in the breakdown of Bruch's membrane. Aust J Ophthalmol 1984;12:23–31.
250. Sarks SH. Senile choroidal sclerosis. Br J Ophthalmol. 1973;57:98–109.
251. Sarks SH. New vessel formation beneath the retinal pigment epithelium in senile eyes. Br J Ophthalmol 1973;57:951–65.
252. Sarks SH. Drusen patterns predisposing to geographic atrophy of the retinal pigment epithelium. Aust J Ophthalmol 1982;10:91–7.
253. Small ML, Green WR, Alpar JJ, et al. Senile macular degeneration; a clinicopathologic correlation of two cases with neovascularization beneath the retinal pigment epithelium. Arch Ophthalmol 1976;94:601–7.
254. Killingsworth MC, Sarks JP, Sarks SH. Macrophages related to Bruch's membrane in age-related macular degeneration. Eye 1990;4:613–21.
255. Friedman E, Smith TR, Kuwabara T. Senile choroidal vascular patterns and drusen. Arch Ophthalmol 1963;69:220–30.
256. Inhoffen W, Nüssgens Z. Rheological studies on patients with posterior subretinal neovascularization and exudative age-related macular degeneration. Graefes Arch Clin Exp Ophthalmol 1990;228:316–20.
257. Lewis H, Straatsma BR, Foos RY. Chorioretinal juncture; multiple extramacular drusen. Ophthalmology 1986;93:1098–112.
258. Fenney L. Lipofuscin and melanin of human retinal pigment epithelium; fluorescence, enzyme cytochemical, and ultrastructural studies. Invest Ophthalmol Vis Sci 1978;17:583–600.
259. Friedman E, Van Buskirk EM, Fineberg E, et al. Pathogenesis of senile disciform degeneration of the macula. Concilium Ophthalmologicum XXI, Mexico, 1970. Acta 1971;1:454–8.
260. Gragoudas ES, Chandra SR, Friedman E, et al. Disciform degeneration of the macula. II. Pathogenesis. Arch Ophthalmol. 1976;94:755–7.
261. Potts AM. An hypothesis on macular disease. Trans Am Acad Ophthalmol Otolaryngol 1966;70:1058–62.
262. van der Schaft TL, Mooy CM, de Bruijn WC, et al. Histologic features of the early stages of age-related macular degeneration. Ophthalmology 1992;99:278–86.
263. Verhoeff FH, Grossman HP. Pathogenesis of disciform degeneration of the macula. Arch Ophthalmol 1937;18:561–85.
264. Zscheile FP. Disciform lesion of the macula simulating a melanoma. Arch Ophthalmol 1964;71:505–7.
265. Ishibashi Y, Watanabe R, Hommura S, et al. Endogenous Nocardia asteroides endophthalmitis in a patient with systemic lupus erythematosus. Br J Ophthalmol 1990;74:433–6.
266. Holz FG, Sheraidah G, Pauleikhoff D, et al. Analysis of lipid deposits extracted from human macular and peripheral Bruch's membrane. Arch Ophthalmol 1994;112:402–6.
267. Anderson DH, Talaga KC, Rivest AJ, et al. Characterization of beta amyloid assemblies in drusen: the deposits associated with aging and age-related macular degeneration. Exp Eye Res 2004;78:243–56.
268. Mullins RF, Russell SR, Anderson DH, et al. Drusen associated with aging and age-related macular degeneration contain proteins common to extracellular deposits associated with atherosclerosis, elastosis, amyloidosis, and dense deposit disease. FASEB J 2000;14:835–46.
269. Hartnett ME, Weiter JJ, Garsd A, et al. Classification of retinal pigment epithelial detachments associated with drusen. Graefes Arch Clin Exp Ophthalmol 1992;230:11–19.
270. Chuang EL, Bird AC. The pathogenesis of tears of the retinal pigment epithelium. Am J Ophthalmol 1988;105:285–90.
271. Bird AC, Marshall J. Retinal pigment epithelial detachments in the elderly. Trans Ophthalmol Soc UK 1986;105:674–82.
272. Meyers SM, Zachary AA. Monozygotic twins with age-related macular degeneration. Arch Ophthalmol 1988;106:651–3.
273. Tabatabay CA, D'Amico DJ, Hanninen LA, et al. Experimental drusen formation induced by intravitreal aminoglycoside injection. Arch Ophthalmol 1987;105:826–30.
274. El Baba F, Green WR, Fleischmann J, et al. Clinicopathologic correlation of lipidization and detachment of the retinal pigment epithelium. Am J Ophthalmol 1986;101:576–83.
275. Fenney-Burns L, Malinow MR, Klein ML, et al. Maculopathy in cynomolgus monkeys; a correlated fluorescein angiographic and ultrastructural study. Arch Ophthalmol 1981;99:664–72.
276. Fine BS. Lipoidal degeneration of the retinal pigment epithelium. Am J Ophthalmol 1981;91:469–73.
277. Baudouin C, Peyman GA, Fredj-Reygrobellet D, et al. Immunohistological study of subretinal membranes in age-related macular degeneration. Jpn J Ophthalmol 1992;36:443–51.
278. Bressler NM, Frost LA, Bressler SB, et al. Natural course of poorly defined choroidal neovascularization associated with macular degeneration. Arch Ophthalmol 1988;106: 1537–42.
279. Bressler SB, Silva JC, Bressler NM, et al. Clinicopathologic correlation of occult choroidal neovascularization in age-related macular degeneration. Arch Ophthalmol 1992;110:827–32.
280. Das A, Puklin JE, Frank RN, et al. Ultrastructural immunocytochemistry of subretinal neovascular membranes in age-related macular degeneration. Ophthalmology 1992;99:1368–76.
281. Frederick Jr AR, Morley MG, Topping TM, et al. The appearance of stippled retinal pigment epithelial detachments; a sign of occult neovascularization in age-related macular degeneration. Retina 1993;13:3–7.
282. Gass JDM. Biomicroscopic and histopathologic considerations regarding the feasibility of surgical excision of subfoveal neovascular membranes. Am J Ophthalmol 1994;118:285–98.
283. Gass JDM. Pathogenesis of disciform detachment of the neuroepithelium. IV. Fluorescein angiographic study of senile disciform macular degeneration. Am J Ophthalmol 1967;63: 645–59.
284. Gass JDM. Present indications and future promise of the krypton laser. In: March WF, editor. Ophthalmic lasers: current clinical uses. Thorofare, NJ: Charles B. Slack; 1984. p. 133.
285. Gass JDM. Stereoscopic atlas of macular dis eases; diagnosis and treatment, 3rd ed. St. Louis: CV Mosby; 1987. p. 19–35, 789.
286. Gehrs KM, Heriot WJ, de Juan Jr E. Transmission electron microscopic study of a subretinal choroidal neovascular membrane due to age-related macular degeneration. Arch Ophthalmol 1992;110:833–7.
287. Green WR. Clinicopathologic studies of treated choroidal neovascular membranes; a review and report of two cases. Retina 1991;11:328–56.
288. Green WR, McDonnell PJ, Yeo JH. Pathologic features of senile macular degeneration. Ophthalmology 1985;92:615–27.
289. Grossniklaus HE, Martinez JA, Brown VB, et al. Immunohistochemical and histochemical properties of surgically excised subretinal neovascular membranes in age-related macular degeneration. Am J Ophthalmol 1992;114:464–72.
290. Lopez PF, Grossniklaus HE, Lambert HM, et al. Pathologic features of surgically excised subretinal neovascular membranes in age-related macular degeneration. Am J Ophthalmol 1991;112:647–56.
291. Maumenee AE. Serous and hemorrhagic disciform detachment of the macula. Trans Pacif Cst Oto-Ophthalmol Soc 1959;40:139–60.
292 Soubrane G, Coscas G, et al. Occult subretinal new vessels in age-related macular degeneration. Natural History and early laser treatment. Ophthalmology 1990;97(5):649–57.
293. Teeters VW, Bird AC. A clinical study of the vascularity of senile disciform macular degeneration. Am J Ophthalmol 1973;75:53–65.
294. Teeters VW, Bird AC. The development of neovascularization of senile disciform macular degeneration. Am J Ophthalmol 1973;76:1–18.
295. Gass JDM. Serous retinal pigment epithelial detachment with a notch; a sign of occult choroidal neovascularization. Retina 1984;4:205–20.
296. Patel BCK, Barondes M, Hamilton AMP. Acute tear of the retinal pigment epithelium. Int Ophthalmol 1992;16:7–13.
297. Kies JC, Bird AC. Juxtapapillary choroidal neovascularization in older patients. Am J Ophthalmol 1988;105:11–19.
298. Dastgheib K, Green WR. Granulomatous reaction to Bruch's membrane in age-related macular degeneration. Arch Ophthalmol 1994;112:813–8.
299. Gass JDM. Pathogenesis of macular detachment and degeneration. Ophthalmic Forum 1984;2:8–17.
300. Gass JDM. Retinal pigment epithelial rip during krypton red laser photocoagulation. Am J Ophthalmol 1984;98:700–6.
301. Dobi ET, Puliafito CA, Destro M. A new model of experimental choroidal neovascularization in the rat. Arch Ophthalmol 1989;107:264–9.
302. El Dirini AA, Ogden TE, Ryan SJ. Subretinal endophotocoagulation; a new model of subretinal neovascularization in the rabbit. Retina 1991;11:244–9.
303. Uyama M. Choroidal neovascularization, experimental and clinical study. Acta Soc Ophthalmol Jpn 1991;95:1145–80.
304. Zhu Z-R, Goodnight R, Sorgente N, et al. Experimental subretinal neovascularization in the rabbit. Graefes Arch Clin Exp Ophthalmol 1989;227:257–62.
305. Zhu Z-R, Goodnight R, Sorgente N, et al. Morphologic observations of retinal pigment epithelial proliferation and neovascularization in the rabbit. Retina 1989;9:319–27.
306. Berkow JW. Subretinal neovascularization in senile macular degeneration. Am J Ophthalmol 1984;97:143–7.
307. Blair CJ. Geographic atrophy of the retinal pigment epithelium; a manifestation of senile macular degeneration. Arch Ophthalmol 1975;93:19–25.
308. Bressler SB, Bressler NM, Fine SL, et al. Natural course of choroidal neovascular membranes within the foveal avascular zone in senile macular degeneration. Am J Ophthalmol 1982;93:157–63.
309. Bressler SB, Bressler NM, Fine SL, et al. Subfoveal neovascular membranes in senile macular degeneration; relationship between membrane size and visual prognosis. Retina 1983;3:7–11.
310. Chandra SR, Gragoudas ES, Friedman E, et al. Natural history of disciform degeneration of the macula. Am J Ophthalmol 1974;78:579–82.
311. Gregor Z, Bird AC, Chisholm IH. Senile disciform macular degeneration in the second eye. Br J Ophthalmol 1977;61:141–7.
312. Hyman LG, Lilienfeld AM, Ferris III FL, et al. Senile macular degeneration: a case-control study. Am J Epidemiol 1983;118:213–27.
313. Klein ML, Jorizzo PA, Watzke RC. Growth features of choroidal neovascular membranes in age-related macular degeneration. Ophthalmology 1989;96:1416–21.
314. Smiddy WE, Fine SL. Prognosis of patients with bilateral macular drusen. Ophthalmology 1984;91:271–7.
315. Strahlman ER, Fine SL, Hillis A. The second eye of patients with senile macular degeneration. Arch Ophthalmol 1983;101:1191–3.
316. Vander JF, Morgan CM, Schatz H. Growth rate of subretinal neovascularization in age-related macular degeneration. Ophthalmology 1989;96:1422–9.

317. Willerson Jr D, Aabert TM. Senile macular degeneration and geographic atrophy of the retinal pigment epithelium. Br J Ophthalmol 1978;62:551–3.
318. Wiznia RA. Natural history of senile disciform macular dystrophy. Ophthalmology 1979;86: 1620–8.
319. Bird AC. Treatment of pigment epithelial detachments in the elderly. Trans Ophthalmol Soc NZ 1983;35:73–5.
320. Braunstein RA, Gass JDM. Serous detachments of the retinal pigment epithelium in patients with senile macular disease. Am J Ophthalmol 1979;88:652–60.
321. Ho PC, Namperumalsamy P, Pruett RC. Photocoagulation of serous detachments of the retinal pigment epithelium in patients with senile macular disease. Ann Ophthalmol 1984;16:213–8.
322. The Moorfields Macular Study Group. Retinal pigment epithelial detachments in the elderly: a controlled trial of argon laser photocoagulation. Br J Ophthalmol 1982;66:1–16.
323. Tornambe PE. Treatment of retinal pigment epithelial detachments. Ann Ophthalmol 1984;16:884–8.
324. Versteeg-Tijmes NT, de Jong PTVM, Bos PJM, et al. Argon laser treatment of pigment epithelial detachments and of subretinal neovascular membranes in Junius-Kuhnt's senile disciform macular degeneration; a prospective, randomized study. Graefes Arch Klin Exp Ophthalmol 1982;218:271–4.
325. Chamberlin JA, Bressler NM, Bressler SB, et al. The use of fundus photographs and fluorescein angiograms in the identification and treatment of choroidal neovascularization in the Macular Photocoagulation Study. Ophthalmology 1989;96:1526–34.
326. Boldt HC, Folk JC. Slow leakage from the retinal pigment epithelium (ooze) in age-related macular degeneration. Retina 1990;10:244–50.
327. Bressler NM, Bressler SB, Alexander J, et al. Loculated fluid; a previously undescribed fluorescein angiographic finding in choroidal neovascularization associated with macular degeneration. Arch Ophthalmol 1991;109:211–5.
328. Meredith TA, Braley RE, Aaberg TM. Natural history of serous detachments of the retinal pigment epithelium. Am J Ophthalmol 1979;88:643–51.
329. Poliner LS, Olk RJ, Burgess D, et al. Natural history of retinal pigment epithelial detachments in age-related macular degeneration. Ophthalmology 1986;93:543–51.
330. Singerman LJ, Stockfish JH. Natural history of subfoveal pigment epithelial detachments associated with subfoveal or unidentifiable choroidal neovascularization complicating age-related macular degeneration. Graefes Arch Clin Exp Ophthalmol 1989;227:501–7.
331. Bird AC, Grey RHB. Photocoagulation of disciform macular lesions with krypton laser. Br J Ophthalmol 1979;63:669–73.
332. Macular Photocoagulation Study Group. Visual outcome after laser photocoagulation for subfoveal neovascularization secondary to age-related macular degeneration. The influence of initial lesion size and initial visual acuity. Arch Ophthalmol 1994;112:480–8.
333. Bressler NM, Finklestein D, Sunness JS, et al. Retinal pigment epithelial tears through the fovea with preservation of good visual acuity. Arch Ophthalmol 1990;108:1694–7.
334. Cantrill HL, Ramsay RC, Knobloch WH. Rips in the pigment epithelium. Arch Ophthalmol 1983;101:1074–9.
335. Chuang EL, Bird AC. The bilaterality of tears of the retinal pigment epithelium. Br J Ophthalmol 1988;72:918–20.
336. Coscas G, Koenig F, Soubrane G. The pretear characteristics of pigment epithelial detachments; a study of 40 eyes. Arch Ophthalmol 1990;108:1687–93.
337. Decker WL, Sanborn GE, Ridley M, et al. Retinal pigment epithelial tears. Ophthalmology 1983;90:507–12.
338. Gass JDM. Pathogenesis of tears of the retinal pigment epithelium. Br J Ophthalmol 1984;68:513–9.
339. Green SN, Yarian D. Acute tear of the retinal pigment epithelium. Retina 1983;3:16–20.
340. Heriot WJ, Machemer R. Pigment epithelial repair. Graefes Arch Clin Exp Ophthalmol 1992;230:91–100.
341. Hoskin A, Bird AC, Sehmi K. Tears of detached retinal pigment epithelium. Br J Ophthalmol 1981;65:417–22.
342. Ie D, Yannuzzi LA, Spaide RF, et al. Microrips of the retinal pigment epithelium. Arch Ophthalmol 1992;110:1443–9.
343. Koenig F, Soubrane G, Coscas G. Déchirures de l'épithélium pigmentaire après photocoagulation au cours de la dégénérescence maculaire liée à l'age. J Fr Ophtalmol 1989;12:775–80.
344. Machemer R, Heriot W. Retinal pigment epithelial tears through the fovea with preservation of good visual acuity. Arch Ophthalmol 1991;109:1492–3.
345. Newsome DA, Huh W, Green WR. Bruch's membrane age-related changes vary by region. Curr Eye Res 1987;6:1211–21.
346. Schoeppner G, Chuang EL, Bird AC. The risk of fellow eye visual loss with unilateral retinal pigment epithelial tears. Am J Ophthalmol 1989;108:683–5.
347. Swanson DE, Kalina RE, Guzak SV. Tears of the retinal pigment epithelium; occurrence in retinal detachments and a chorioretinal scar. Retina 1984;4:115–8.
348. Hannan SR, Madhusudhana KC, Lotery AJ, et al. Retinal pigment epithelial tear following intravitreal bevacizumab for choroidal neovascular membrane due to age-related macular degeneration. Br J Ophthalmol 2007;91:977–8.
349. Goldbaum MH, Madden K. A new perspective on Bruch's membrane and the retinal pigment epithelium. Br J Ophthalmol 1982;66:17–25.
350. Yeo JH, Marcus S, Murphy RP. Retinal pigment epithelial tears; patterns and prognosis. Ophthalmology 1988;95:8–13.
351. Gass JDM. Radial chorioretinal folds; a sign of choroidal neovascularization. Arch Ophthalmol 1981;99:1016–8.
352. Schatz H, McDonald HR, Johnson RN. Retinal pigment epithelial folds associated with retinal pigment epithelial detachment in macular degeneration. Ophthalmology 1990;97:658–65.
353. Bennett SR, Folk JC, Blodi CF, et al. Factors prognostic of visual outcome in patients with subretinal hemorrhage. Am J Ophthalmol 1990;109:33–7.
354. Nasrallah F, Jalkh AE, Trempe CL, et al. Subretinal hemorrhage in atrophic age-related macular degeneration. Am J Ophthalmol 1989;107:38–41.
355. Bloome MA, Ruiz RS. Massive spontaneous subretinal hemorrhage. Am J Ophthalmol 1978;86:630–7.
356. Tani PM, Buettner H, Robertson DM. Massive vitreous hemorrhage and senile macular choroidal degeneration. Am J Ophthalmol 1980;90:525–33.
357. Green WR, Gass JDM. Senile disciform degeneration of the macula; retinal arterialization of the fibrous plaque demonstrated clinically and histopathologically. Arch Ophthalmol 1971;86: 487–94.
358. Jalkh AE, Avila MP, Trempe CL, et al. Choroidal neovascularization in fellow eyes of patients with advanced senile macular degeneration; role of laser photocoagulation. Arch Ophthalmol 1983;101:1194–7.
359. Lavin MJ, Eldem B, Gregor ZJ. Symmetry of disciform scars in bilateral age-related macular degeneration. Br J Ophthalmol 1991;75:133–6.
360. Blair CJ, Aaberg TM. Massive subretinal exudation associated with senile macular degeneration. Am J Ophthalmol 1971;71:639–48.
361. Woods AC, Duke JR. Coats's disease. I. Review of the literature, diagnostic criteria, clinical findings, and plasma lipid studies. Br J Ophthalmol 1963;47:385–412.
362. Silva VB, Brockhurst RJ. Hemorrhagic detachment of the peripheral retinal pigment epithelium. Arch Ophthalmol 1976;94:1295–300.
363. Pesin SR, Katz LJ, Augsburger JJ, et al. Acute angle-closure glaucoma from spontaneous massive hemorrhagic retinal or choroidal detachment; an updated diagnostic and therapeutic approach. Ophthalmology 1990;97:76–84.
364. Gass JDM. Stereoscopic atlas of macular diseases; diagnosis and treatment, 2nd ed. St. Louis: CV Mosby; 1977. p. 66.
365. Foos RY, Trese MT. Chorioretinal juncture; vascularization of Bruch's membrane in peripheral fundus. Arch Ophthalmol 1982;100:1492–503.
366. Maguire P, Vine AK. Geographic atrophy of the retinal pigment epithelium. Am J Ophthalmol 1986;102:621–5.
367. Schatz H, McDonald HR. Atrophic macular degeneration; rate of spread of geographic atrophy and visual loss. Ophthalmology 1989;96:1541–51.
368. Holz FG, Wolfensberger TJ, Piguet B, et al. Bilateral macular drusen in age-related macular degeneration; prognosis and risk factors. Ophthalmology 1994;101:1522–8.
369. Klein ML, Mauldin WM, Stoumbos VD. Heredity and age-related macular degeneration; observations in monozygotic twins. Arch Ophthalmol 1994;112:932–7.
370. Klein RJ, Zeiss C, Chew EY, et al. Complement factor H polymorphism in age-related macular degeneration. Science 2005;308:385–9.
371. Haines JL, Hauser MA, Schmidt S, et al. Complement factor H variant increases the risk of age-related macular degeneration. Science 2005;308:419–21.
372. Edwards AO, Ritter III R, Abel KJ, et al. Complement factor H polymorphism and age-related macular degeneration. Science 2005;308:421–4.
373. Tong Y, Liao J, Zhang Y, et al. LOC387715/HTRA1 gene polymorphisms and susceptibility to age-related macular degeneration: A HuGE review and meta-analysis. Mol Vis 2010;16:1958–81.
374. Marioli DI, Pharmakakis N, Deli A, et al. Complement factor H and LOC387715 gene polymorphisms in a Greek population with age-related macular degeneration. Graefes Arch Clin Exp Ophthalmol 2009;247:1547–53.
375. Deangelis MM, Ji F, Adams S, et al. Alleles in the HtrA serine peptidase 1 gene alter the risk of neovascular age-related macular degeneration. Ophthalmology 2008;115(1209–1215):e7.
376. Leveziel N, Souied EH, Richard F, et al. PLEKHA1-LOC387715-HTRA1 polymorphisms and exudative age-related macular degeneration in the French population. Mol Vis 2007;13:2153–9.
377. Kondo N, Honda S, Ishibashi K, et al. LOC387715/HTRA1 variants in polypoidal choroidal vasculopathy and age-related macular degeneration in a Japanese population. Am J Ophthalmol 2007;144:608–12.
378. DeWan A, Bracken MB, Hoh J. Two genetic pathways for age-related macular degeneration. Curr Opin Genet Dev 2007;17:228–33.
379. Spencer KL, Olson LM, Anderson BM, et al. C3 R102G polymorphism increases risk of age-related macular degeneration. Hum Mol Genet 2008;17:1821–4.
380. Mullins RF, Olvera MA, Clark AF, et al. Fibulin-5 distribution in human eyes: relevance to age-related macular degeneration. Exp Eye Res 2007;84:378–80.
381. Stone EM, Braun TA, Russell SR, et al. Missense variations in the fibulin 5 gene and age-related macular degeneration. N Engl J Med 2004;351:346–53.
382. Shastry BS. Evaluation of the ABCR and glutathione peroxidase-3 genes in familial and sporadic cases of exudative age-related macular degeneration. Int J Mol Med 2004;14:753–7.
383. Allikmets R. Further evidence for an association of ABCR alleles with age-related macular degeneration. The International ABCR Screening Consortium. Am J Hum Genet 2000;67: 487–91.
384. De La Paz MA, Guy VK, Abou-Donia S, et al. Analysis of the Stargardt disease gene (ABCR) in age-related macular degeneration. Ophthalmology 1999;106:1531–6.
385. Stone EM, Webster AR, Vandenburgh K, et al. Allelic variation in ABCR associated with Stargardt disease but not age-related macular degeneration. Nat Genet 1998;20:328–9.
386. Allikmets R, Shroyer NF, Singh N, et al. Mutation of the Stargardt disease gene (ABCR) in age-related macular degeneration. Science 1997;277:1805–7.
387. Hageman GS, Hancox LS, Taiber AJ, et al. Extended haplotypes in the complement factor H (CFH) and CFH-related (CFHR) family of genes protect against age-related macular degeneration: characterization, ethnic distribution and evolutionary implications. Ann Med 2006;38:592–604.
388. Hageman GS, Anderson DH, Johnson LV, et al. A common haplotype in the complement regulatory gene factor H (HF1/CFH) predisposes individuals to age-related macular degeneration. Proc Natl Acad Sci U S A 2005;102:7227–32.
389. Cruickshanks KJ, Klein R. Klein BEK. Sunlight and age-related macular degeneration; the Beaver Dam eye study. Arch Ophthalmol 1993;111:514–8.
390. Taylor HR, Muñoz B, West S, et al. Visible light and risk of age-related macular degeneration. Trans Am Ophthalmol Soc 1990;88:163–78.
391. Taylor HR, West S, Muñoz B, et al. The long-term effects of visible light on the eye. Arch Ophthalmol 1992;110:99–104.

392. Tso MOM. Pathogenetic factors of aging macular degeneration. Ophthalmology 1985;92:628–35.
393. van Norren D, Vos H. Sunlight and age-related macular degeneration. Arch Ophthalmol 1990;108:1670–1.
394. West SK, Rosenthal FS, Bressler NM, et al. Exposure to sunlight and other risk factors for age-related macular degeneration. Arch Ophthalmol 1989;107:875–9.
395. Young RW. Pathophysiology of age-related macular degeneration. Surv Ophthalmol 1987;31:291–306.
396. Young RW. Solar radiation and age-related macular degeneration. Surv Ophthalmol 1988;32:252–69.
397. The Eye Disease Case-Control Study Group Antioxidant status and neovascular age-related macular degeneration. Arch Ophthalmol 1993;111:104–9.
398. The Eye Disease Case-Control Study Group Risk factors for neovascular age-related macular degeneration. Arch Ophthalmol 1992;110:1701–8.
399. Klein R, Klein BEK, Linton KLP, et al. The Beaver Dam Eye Study: the relation of age-related maculopathy to smoking. Am J Epidemiol 1993;137:190–200.
400. Edwards DR, Gallins P, Polk M, et al. Inverse association of female hormone replacement therapy with age-related macular degeneration and interactions with ARMS2 polymorphisms. Invest Ophthalmol Vis Sci 2010;51:1873–9.
401. Jampol LM. Hypertension and visual outcome in the macular photocoagulation study. Arch Ophthalmol 1991;109:789–90.
402. Kingham JD, Chen MC, Levy MH. Macular hemorrhage in the aging eye: the effects of anticoagulants. N Engl J Med 1988;318:1126–7.
403. Lewis H, Sloan SH, Foos RY. Massive intraocular hemorrhage associated with anticoagulation and age-related macular degeneration. Graefes Arch Clin Exp Ophthalmol 1988;226:59–64.
404. Blumenkranz MS, Russell SR, Robey MG, et al. Risk factors in age-related maculopathy complicated by choroidal neovascularization. Ophthalmology 1986;96:552–8.
405. Silverstone BZ, Landau L, Berson D, et al. Zinc and copper metabolism in patients with senile macular degeneration. Ann Ophthalmol 1985;17:419–22.
406. Tsang NCK, Penfold PL, Snitch PJ, et al. Serum levels of antioxidants and age-related macular degeneration. Doc Ophthalmol 1992;81:387–400.
407. Newsome DA, Swartz M, Leone NC, et al. Macular degeneration and elevated serum ceruloplasmin. Invest Ophthalmol Vis Sci 1986;27:1675–80.
408. Klein R, Klein BEK, Franke T. The relationship of cardiovascular disease and its risk factors to age-related maculopathy. The beaver dam eye study. Ophthalmology 1993;100:406–14.
409. Sandberg MA, Tolentino MJ, Miller S, et al. Hyperopia and neovascularization in age-related macular degeneration. Ophthalmology 1993;100:1009–13.
410. Friedman E, Ivry M, Ebert E, et al. Increased scleral rigidity and age-related macular degeneration. Ophthalmology 1989;96:104–8.
411. Gurne DH, Tso MOM, Edward DP, et al. Antiretinal antibodies in serum of patients with age-related macular degeneration. Ophthalmology 1991;98:602–7.
412. Penfold PL, Provis JM, Furby JH, et al. Autoantibodies to retinal astrocytes associated with age-related macular degeneration. Graefes Arch Clin Exp Ophthalmol 1990;228:270–4.
412a Mimoun G, Soubrane G, et al. Significance of the digital image in the diagnosis and classification of macular drusen. Ophtalmologie 1990:48–50.
412b Arnold JJ, Sarks SH, et al. Reticular pseudodrusen. A risk factor in age-related maculopathy. Retina 1995:183–91.
412c Maguire MG, Fine SL. Reticular pseudodrusen. Retina 1996:167–8.
412d Smith RT, Chan JK, et al. Autofluorescence characteristics of early, atrophic, and high-risk fellow eyes in age-related macular degeneration. Invest Ophthalmol Vis Sci 2006:5495–504.
412e Spaide RF, Curcio CA. Drusen characterization with multimodal imaging. Retina 2010;30(9):1441–54.
412f Zweifel SA, Imamura Y, et al. Prevalence and significance of subretinal drusenoid deposits (reticular pseudodrusen) in age-related macular degeneration. Ophthalmology 2010;117(9):1775–81.
412g Switzer DW, Engelbert M, et al. Spectral domain optical coherence tomography macular cube scans and retinal pigment epithelium/drusen maps may fail to display subretinal drusenoid deposits (reticular pseudodrusen) in eyes with non-neovascular age-related macular degeneration. Eye (Lond) 2011 [Epub ahead of print]
412h Zweifel SA, Imamura Y, et al. Multimodal fundus imaging of pseudoxanthoma elasticum. Retina 2011;31(3):482–91.
412i Yannuzzi LA, Negrao S, et al. Retinal angiomatous proliferation in age-related macular degeneration. Retina 2001;21(5):416–34.
412j Gass JD, Agarwal A, et al. Focal inner retinal hemorrhages in patients with drusen: an early sign of occult choroidal neovascularization and chorioretinal anastomosis. Retina 2003:741–51.
412k Mahmood S, Kumar N, et al. Early response of retinal angiomatous proliferation treated with intravitreal pegaptanib: a retrospective review. Eye (Lond) 2009:530–5.
412l Atmani K, Voigt M, et al. Ranibizumab for retinal angiomatous proliferation in age-related macular degeneration. Eye (Lond) 2010:1193–8.
412m Scott AW, Bressler SB. Retinal angiomatous proliferation or retinal anastomosis to the lesion. Eye 2010:491–6.
413. Tate Jr DJ, Oliver PD, Miceli MV, et al. Age-dependent change in the hyaluronic acid content of the human chorioretinal complex. Arch Ophthalmol 1993;111:963–7.
414. Bird AC. Recent advances in the treatment of senile disciform macular degeneration by photocoagulation. Br J Ophthalmol 1974;58:367–76.
415. Bird AC. Macular disciform response and laser treatment. Trans Ophthalmol Soc UK 1977;97:490–3.
416. Cleasby GW, Fung WE, Fiore Jr JV. Photocoagulation of exudative senile maculopathy. Arch Ophthalmol 1971;85:18–26.
417. Cleasby GW, Nakanishi AS, Norris JL. Prophylactic photocoagulation of the fellow eye in exudative senile maculopathy; a preliminary report. Mod Probl Ophthalmol 1979;20:141–7.
418. Coscas G. Le laser à krypton en ophtalmologie; premiers essais expérimentaux et cliniques. Bull Mem Soc Fr Ophtalmol 1981;93:100–6.
419. Coscas G, Soubrane G. Photocoagulation des néovaisseaux sous-rétiniens dans la dégénérescence maculaire sénile par laser à argon; résultats de l'étude randomisée de 60 cas. Bull Mem Soc Fr Ophtalmol 1982;84:149–54.
420. Coscas G, Soubrane G. The effects of red krypton and green argon laser on the foveal region; a clinical and experimental study. Ophthalmology 1983;90:1013–22.
421. Folk JC. Aging macular degeneration; clinical features of treatable disease. Ophthalmology 1985;92:594–602.
422. Folk JC, Blackhurst DW, Alexander J, Macular Photocoagulation Study Group. Pretreatment fundus characteristics as predictors of recurrent choroidal neovascularization. Arch Ophthalmol 1991;109:1193–4.
423. Grey RHB, Bird AC, Chisholm IH. Senile disciform macular degeneration: features indicating suitability for photocoagulation. Br J Ophthalmol 1979;63:85–9.
424. Harris GS. Photocoagulation of macular lesions following fluorescein angiography. Can J Ophthalmol 1969;4:16–19.
425. Jepson CN, Wetzig PC. Photocoagulation in disciform macular degeneration. Am J Ophthalmol 1969;67:920–30.
426. L'Esperance Jr FA. Clinical photocoagulation with the krypton laser. Arch Ophthalmol 1972;87:693–700.
427. Marshall J, Bird AC. A comparative histopathological study of argon and krypton laser irradiations of the human retina. Br J Ophthalmol 1979;63:657–68.
428. Marshall J, Hamilton AM, Bird AC. Intra-retinal absorption of argon laser irradiation in human and monkey retinae. Experientia 1974;30:1335–7.
429. McPherson A, Sabates F, Trempe CL. Macular disease experience sharing project. (American Academy of Ophthalmology exhibit 17 abstract). Ophthalmology 1982;89:173.
430. Patz A, Maumenee AE, Ryan SJ. Argon laser photocoagulation in macular diseases. Trans Am Ophthalmol Soc 1971;69:71–83.
431. Peyman GA, Li M, Yoneya MF, et al. Fundus photocoagulation with the argon and krypton lasers: a comparative study. Ophthalmic Surg 1981;12:481–90.
432. Schatz H. The senile maculopathies and the retinal pigment epithelium. Int Ophthalmol Clin 1975;15:169–80.
433. Schatz H, Patz A. Exudative senile maculopathy. I. Results of argon laser treatment. Arch Ophthalmol 1973;90:183–96.
434. Soubrane G, Coscas G, Baudouin C, et al. Long-term follow-up of the randomized argon blue/green trial in senile macular degeneration. Int Ophthalmol 1985;8:83.
435. Watzke RC, Snyder WB. Light coagulation for hemorrhagic disciform degeneration of the macula. Trans Am Acad Ophthalmol Otolaryngol 1968;72:389–95.
436. Yannuzzi LA. Krypton red laser photocoagulation for subretinal neovascularization. Retina 1982;2:29–46.
437. Yannuzzi LA, Shakin JL. Krypton red laser photocoagulation of the ocular fundus. Retina 1982;2:1–14.
438. Yassur Y, Axer-Siegel R, Cohen S, et al. Treatment of neovascular senile maculopathy at the foveal capillary free zone with red krypton laser. Retina 1982;2:127–33.
439. Zweng HC, Little HL, Peabody RR. Laser photocoagulation of macular lesions. Trans Am Acad Ophthalmol Otolaryngol 1968;72:377–88.
440. Fine SL. Macular photocoagulation study. Arch Ophthalmol 1980;98:832.
441. Fine SL, Murphy RP, Macula Photocoagulation Study Group. Photocoagulation for choroidal neovascularization. Ophthalmology 1983;90:531–3.
442. Macular Photocoagulation Study Group. Age-related macular degeneration. Am J Ophthalmol 1984;98:376–7.
443. Macular Photocoagulation Study Group. Argon laser photocoagulation for senile macular degeneration; results of a randomized clinical trial. Arch Ophthalmol 1982;100:912–8.
444. Macular Photocoagulation Study Group. Argon laser photocoagulation for neovascular maculopathy; three-year results from randomized clinical trials. Arch Ophthalmol 1986;104:694–701.
445. Macular Photocoagulation Study Group. Krypton laser photocoagulation for neovascular lesions of age-related macular degeneration; results of a randomized clinical trial. Arch Ophthalmol 1990;108:816–24.
446. Macular Photocoagulation Study Group. Argon laser photocoagulation for neovascular maculopathy; five-year results from randomized clinical trials. Arch Ophthalmol 1991;109: 1109–14.
447. Macular Photocoagulation Study Group. Five-year follow-up of fellow eyes of patients with age-related macular degeneration and unilateral extrafoveal choroidal neovascularization. Arch Ophthalmol 1993;111:1189–99.
448. Macular Photocoagulation Study Group. Laser photocoagulation of subfoveal neovascular lesions of age-related macular degeneration; updated findings from two clinical trials. Arch Ophthalmol 1993;111:1200–9.
449. The Moorfields Macular Study Group. Treatment of senile disciform degeneration: a single-blind randomised trial by argon laser photocoagulation. Br J Ophthalmol 1982;66:745–53.
450. Macular Photocoagulation Study Group. Laser photocoagulation of subfoveal recurrent neovascular lesions in age-related macular degeneration; results of a randomized clinical trial. Arch Ophthalmol 1991;109:1232–41.
451. Macular Photocoagulation Study Group. Persistent and recurrent neovascularization after laser photocoagulation for subfoveal choroidal neovascularization of age-related macular degeneration. Arch Ophthalmol 1994;112:489–99.
452. Freund KB, Yannuzzi LA, Sorenson JA. Age-related macular degeneration and choroidal neovascularization. Am J Ophthalmol 1993;115:786–7891.
453. Boyer DS, Heier JS, Brown DM, et al. A phase IIIb study to evaluate the safety of ranibizumab in subjects with neovascular age-related macular degeneration. Ophthalmology 2009;116:1731–9.
454. Boyer DS, Antoszyk AN, Awh CC, et al. Subgroup analysis of the MARINA study of ranibizumab in neovascular age-related macular degeneration. Ophthalmology 2007;114:246–52.
455. Sorensen TL, Kemp H. Ranibizumab treatment in patients with neovascular age-related macular degeneration and very low vision. Acta Ophthalmol 2011;89:e97.

456. Mones J. A review of ranibizumab clinical trial data in exudative age-related macular degeneration and how to translate it into daily practice. Ophthalmologica 2011;225:112–9.
457. Raja MS, Saldana M, Goldsmith C, et al. Ranibizumab treatment for neovascular age-related macular degeneration in patients with good baseline visual acuity (better than 6/12): 12-month outcomes. Br J Ophthalmol 2010;94:1543–5.
458. Querques G, Azrya S, Martinelli D, et al. Ranibizumab for exudative age-related macular degeneration: 24-month outcomes from a single-centre institutional setting. Br J Ophthalmol 2010;94:292–6.
459. Suzuki M, Gomi F, Sawa M, et al. Bevacizumab treatment for choroidal neovascularization due to age-related macular degeneration in Japanese patients. Jpn J Ophthalmol 2010;54:124–8.
460. Subramanian ML, Abedi G, Ness S, et al. Bevacizumab vs ranibizumab for age-related macular degeneration: 1-year outcomes of a prospective, double-masked randomised clinical trial. Eye (Lond) 2010;24:1708–15.
461. Spaide RF, Laud K, Fine HF, et al. Intravitreal bevacizumab treatment of choroidal neovascularization secondary to age-related macular degeneration. Retina 2006;26:383–90.
462. Avery RL, Pieramici DJ, Rabena MD, et al. Intravitreal bevacizumab (Avastin) for neovascular age-related macular degeneration. Ophthalmology 2006;113(363–372):e5.
463. Rosenfeld PJ, Schwartz SD, Blumenkranz MS, et al. Maximum tolerated dose of a humanized anti-vascular endothelial growth factor antibody fragment for treating neovascular age-related macular degeneration. Ophthalmology 2005;112:1048–53.
464. de Juan Jr E, Machemer R. Vitreous surgery for hemorrhagic and fibrous complications of age-related macular degeneration. Am J Ophthalmol 1988;105:25–9.
465. Kimura AE, Reddy CV, Folk JC, et al. Removal of subretinal hemorrhage facilitated by preoperative intravitreal tissue plasminogen activator. Retina 1994;14:83–4.
466. Toth CA, Morse LS, Hjelmeland LM, et al. Fibrin directs early retinal damage after experimental subretinal hemorrhage. Arch Ophthalmol 1991;109:723–9.
467. Vander JF, Federman JL, Greven C, et al. Surgical removal of massive subretinal hemorrhage associated with age-related macular degeneration. Ophthalmology 1991;98:23–7.
468. Wade EC, Flynn Jr HW, Olsen KR, et al. Subretinal hemorrhage management by pars plana vitrectomy and internal drainage. Arch Ophthalmol 1990;108:973–8.
469. Berger AS, Kaplan HJ. Clinical experience with the surgical removal of subfoveal neovascular membranes. Short-term postoperative results. Ophthalmology 1992;99:969–76.
470. Lambert HM, Capone Jr A, Aaberg TM, et al. Surgical excision of subfoveal neovascular membranes in age-related macular degeneration. Am J Ophthalmol 1992;113:257–62.
471. Lopez PF, Lambert HM, Grossniklaus HE, et al. Well-defined subfoveal choroidal neovascular membranes in age-related macular degeneration. Ophthalmology 1993;100:415–22.
472. Peyman GA, Blinder KJ, Paris CL, et al. A technique for retinal pigment epithelium transplantation for age-related macular degeneration secondary to extensive subfoveal scarring. Ophthalmic Surg 1991;22:102–8.
473. Peyman GA, Koziol J. Age-related macular degeneration and its management. J Cataract Refract Surg 1988;14:421–30.
474. Russell SR, Crapotta JA, Zerbolio Jr DJ. Surgical removal of subfoveal neovascularization. Ophthalmology 1993;100:795–6.
475. Thomas MA, Dickinson JD, Melberg NS, et al. Visual results after surgical removal of subfoveal choroidal neovascular membranes. Ophthalmology 1994;101:1384–96.
476. Thomas MA, Grand MG, Williams DF, et al. Surgical management of subfoveal choroidal neovascularization. Ophthalmology 1992;99:952–68.
477. Bhatt NS, Newsome DA, Fenech T, et al. Experimental transplantation of human retinal pigment epithelial cells on collagen substrates. Am J Ophthalmol 1994;117:214–21.
478. Machemer R, Steinhorst UH. Retinal separation, retinotomy, and macular relocation. II. A surgical approach for age-related macular degeneration?. Graefes Arch Clin Exp Ophthalmol 1993;231:635–41.
479. De La Paz M, Anderson RE. Region and age-dependent variation in susceptibility of the human retina to lipid peroxidation. Invest Ophthalmol Vis Sci 1992;33:3497–9.
480. West S, Vitale S, Hallfrisch J, et al. Are antioxidants or supplements protective for age-related macular degeneration?. Arch Ophthalmol 1994;112:222–7.
481. Liles MR, Newsome DA, Oliver PD. Antioxidant enzymes in the aging human retinal pigment epithelium. Arch Ophthalmol 1991;109:1285–8.
482. Newsome DA, Swartz M, Leone NC, et al. Oral zinc in macular degeneration. Arch Ophthalmol. 1988;106:192–8.
483. Sperduto RD, Ferris III FL, Kurinij N. Do we have a nutritional treatment for age-related cataract or macular degeneration? Arch Ophthalmol 1990;108:1403–5.
484. Trempe CL. Reply to letter by Beaumont P: Zinc and macular degeneration. Arch Ophthalmol 1993;111:1023.
485. Bergink GJ, Deutman AF, van den Broek JFCM, et al. Radiation therapy for subfoveal choroidal neovascular membranes in age-related macular degeneration; a pilot study. Graefes Arch Clin Exp Ophthalmol 1994;232:591–8.
486. Chakravarthy U, Houston RF, Archer DB. Treatment of age-related subfoveal neovascular membranes by teletherapy: a pilot study. Br J Ophthalmol 1993;77:265–73.
487. Fine AM, Elman MJ, Ebert JE, et al. Earliest symptoms caused by neovascular membranes in the macula. Arch Ophthalmol 1986;104:513–4.
488. Fine SL. Advising patients about age-related macular degeneration. Arch Ophthalmol 1993;111:1186–8.
489. Blair CJ, Ferguson Jr J. Exacerbation of senile macular degeneration following cataract extraction. Am J Ophthalmol 1979;87:77–83.
490. Feman SS, Bartlett RE, Roth AM, et al. Intraocular hemorrhage and blindness associated with systemic anticoagulation. JAMA 1972;220:1354–5.
491. Gieser DK. Visual rehabilitation: the challenge, responsibility, and reward. Ophthalmology 1992;99:1622–5.
492. Nasrallah FP, Jalkh AE, Friedman GR, et al. Visual results with low-vision aids in age-related macular degeneration. Am J Ophthalmol 1988;106:730–4.
493. Gass JDM. Stereoscopic atlas of macular diseases; diagnosis and treatment, 2nd ed. St. Louis: CV Mosby; 1977. p. 46.
494. Gass JDM, Jallow S, Davis B. Adult vitelliform macular detachment occurring in patients with basal laminar drusen. Am J Ophthalmol 1985;99:445–59.
495. Kenyon KR, Maumenee AE, Ryan SJ, et al. Diffuse drusen and associated complications. Am J Ophthalmol 1985;100:119–28.
496. Lerche W. Pigmentepithelveränderungen bei Drusen im Maculabereich. Ber Dtsch Ophthalmol Ges 1973;73:439–46.
497. Müller H. Anatomische Beiträge zur Ophthalmologie. Albrecht von Graefes Arch Ophthalmol 1856;2:1–69.
498. Coats G. The structure of the membrane of Bruch, and its relation to the formation of colloid excrescences. R Lond Ophthalmic Hosp Rep 1905;16:164–78.
499. Nakaizumi Y. The ultrastructure of Bruch's membrane. I. Human, monkey, rabbit, guinea pig, and rat eyes. Arch Ophthalmol. 1964;72:380–7.
500. Lerche W. Clinical and electron microscopic studies of degeneration in the macular region. Concilium Ophthalmologicum XXI, Mexico, 1970, Acta 1971;1:828–31.
501. Boon CJ, Klevering BJ, Hoyng CB, et al. Basal laminar drusen caused by compound heterozygous variants in the CFH gene. Am J Hum Genet 2008;82:516–23.
502. Boon CJ, van de Kar NC, Klevering BJ, et al. The spectrum of phenotypes caused by variants in the CFH gene. Mol Immunol 2009;46:1573–94.
503. Cleasby GW. Idiopathic focal subretinal neovascularization. Am J Ophthalmol 1976;81:590–6.
504. Delaney Jr WV, Torrisi PF, Hampton GR, et al. Hemorrhagic peripheral pigment epithelial disease. Arch Ophthalmol 1988;106:646–50.
505. Gass JDM. St Stereoscopic atlas of macular diseases; diagnosis and treatment, 3rd ed. Louis: CV Mosby; 1987. p. 198–201.
506. Kleiner RC, Brucker AJ, Johnston RL. The posterior uveal bleeding syndrome. Retina 1990; 10:9–17.
507. Lopez PF, Green WR. Peripapillary subretinal neovascularization; a review. Retina 1992;12: 147–71.
508. Macular Photocoagulation Study Group. Krypton laser photocoagulation for idiopathic neovascular lesions; results of a randomized clinical trial. Arch Ophthalmol 1990;108:832–7.
509. Spitznas M, Böker T. Idiopathic posterior subretinal neovascularization (IPSN) is related to myopia. Graefes Arch Clin Exp Ophthalmol 1991;229:536–8.
510. Stern RM, Zakov ZN, Zegarra H, et al. Multiple recurrent serosanguineous retinal pigment epithelial detachments in black women. Am J Ophthalmol 1985;100:560–9.
511. Thomas JW, Grossniklaus HE, Lambert HM, et al. Ultrastructural features of surgically excised idiopathic subfoveal neovascular membranes. Retina 1993;13:93–8.
512. Yannuzzi LA, Sorenson J, Spaide RF, et al. Idiopathic polypoidal choroidal vasculopathy (IPCV). Retina 1990;10:1–8.
513. Macular Photocoagulation Study Group. Argon laser photocoagulation for idiopathic neovascularization; results of a randomized clinical trial. Arch Ophthalmol 1983;101:1358–61.
514. Bardenstein DS, Char DH, Irvine AR, et al. Extramacular disciform lesions simulating uveal tumors. Ophthalmology 1992;99:944–51.
515. Mazow ML, Ruiz RS. Eccentric disciform degeneration. Trans Am Acad Ophthalmol Otolaryngol 1973;77:OP68–73.
516. Annesley Jr WH. Peripheral exudative hemorrhagic chorioretinopathy. Trans Am Ophthalmol Soc 1980;78:321–64.
517. Kingham JD. Hemorrhagic detachment of the peripheral retinal pigment epithelium. Ann Ophthalmol 1978;10:175–8.
518. Orth DH, Flood TP. Management of breakthrough vitreous hemorrhage from presumed extramacular subretinal neovascularization. Retina 1982;2:89–93.
519. Clarkson JG, Altman RD. Angioid streaks. Surv Ophthalmol. 1982;26:235–46.
520. Federman JL, Shields JA, Tomer TL. Angioid streaks. II. Fluorescein angiographic features. Arch Ophthalmol. 1975;93:951–62.
521. Gass JDM. Stereoscopic atlas of macular diseases; diagnosis and treatment, 2nd ed. St. Louis: CV Mosby; 1977. p. 78.
522. Hagedoorn A. Angioid streaks. Arch Ophthalmol. 1939;21:935–65.
523. Paton D. The relation of angioid streaks to systemic disease. Springfield, IL: Charles C Thomas; 1972.
524. Shields JA, Federman JL, Tomer TL, et al. Angioid streaks. I. Ophthalmoscopic variations and diagnostic problems. Br J Ophthalmol 1975;59:257–66.
525. Gass JDM, Clarkson JG. Angioid streaks and disciform macular detachment in Paget's disease (osteitis deformans). Am J Ophthalmol 1973;75:576–86.
526. Klien BA. Angioid streaks; a clinical and histopathologic study. Am J Ophthalmol 1947;30: 955–68.
527. Lim JI, Lam S. A retinal pigment epithelium tear in a patient with angioid streaks. Arch Ophthalmol 1990;108:1672–4.
528. Gass JDM. Pathogenesis of disciform detachment of the neuroepithelium. VI. Disciform detachment secondary to heredodegenerative, neoplastic and traumatic lesions of the choroid. Am J Ophthalmol 1967;63:689–711.
529. Smith JL, Gass JDM, Justice Jr J. Fluorescein fundus photography of angioid streaks. Br J Ophthalmol 1964;48:517–21.
530. Green WR, Friedman-Kien A, Banfield WG. Angioid streaks in Ehlers–Danlos syndrome. Arch Ophthalmol 1966;76:197–204.
531. McLane NJ, Grizzard WS, Kousseff BG, et al. Angioid streaks associated with hereditary spherocytosis. Am J Ophthalmol 1984;97:444–9.
532. Connor Jr PJ, Juergens JL, Perry HO, et al. Pseudoxanthoma elasticum and angioid streaks: A review of 106 cases. Am J Med 1961;30:537–43.
533. Grand MG, Isserman MJ, Miller CW. Angioid streaks associated with pseudoxanthoma elasticum in a 13-year-old patient. Ophthalmology 1987;94:197–200.
534. Grönblad E. Angioid streaks–pseudoxanthoma elasticum (Vorläufige Mitteilung). Acta Ophthalmol 1929;7:329.
535. Strandberg J. Pseudoxanthoma elasticum. Zentralbl Haut Geschlechtskrankh 1929;31:689.
536. Yap E-Y, Gleaton MS, Buettner H. Visual loss associated with pseudoxanthoma elasticum. Retina 1992;12:315–9.

537. Sato N, Nakayama T, Mizutani Y, et al. Novel mutations of ABCC6 gene in Japanese patients with Angioid streaks. Biochem Biophys Res Commun 2009;380:548–53.
538. Gills Jr JP, Paton D. Mottled fundus oculi in pseudoxanthoma elasticum; a report on two siblings. Arch Ophthalmol 1965;73:792–5.
539. Krill AE, Klien BA, Archer DB. Precursors of angioid streaks. Am J Ophthalmol 1973;76:875–9.
540. Shimizu K. Mottled fundus in association with pseudoxanthoma elasticum. Jpn J Ophthalmol 1961;5:1–13.
541. Kim DD, Pulido JS, Wipplinger WA. Indocyanine green angiographic findings in pseudoxanthoma elasticum. Am J Ophthalmol 1993;116:767–9.
542. Agarwal A, Patel P, Adkins T, et al. Spectrum of pattern dystrophy in pseudoxanthoma elasticum. Arch Ophthalmol 2005;123:923–8.
543. Gass JDM. Stereoscopic atlas of macular diseases; diagnosis and treatment, 3rd ed. St. Louis: CV Mosby; 1987. p. 106.
544. McDonald HR, Schatz H, Aaberg TM. Reticular-like pigmentary patterns in pseudoxanthoma elasticum. Ophthalmology 1988;95:306–11.
545. Zürcher M, Schipper I. Punktförmige bis retikuläre Pigmentverschiebungen bei einem Patienten mit Pseudoxanthoma elasticum (Grönblad-Strandberg-Syndrom). Klin Monatsbl Augenheilkd 1990;196:30–2.
546. Meislik J, Neldner K, Reeve EB, et al. Atypical drusen in pseudoxanthoma elasticum. Can J Ophthalmol 1978;13:210–2.
547. Coleman K, Ross MH, McCabe M, et al. Disk drusen and angioid streaks in pseudoxanthoma elasticum. Am J Ophthalmol 1991;112:166–70.
548. Mansour AM. Is there an association between optic disc drusen and angioid streaks?. Graefes Arch Clin Exp Ophthalmol 1992;230:595–6.
549. Khairallah M. Congenital communication of cilioretinal and retinal arteries associated with angioid streaks. Arch Ophthalmol 1997;115:1328–9.
550. Woodcock CW. Pseudoxanthoma elasticum, angioid streaks of retina, and osteitis deformans. AMA Arch Dermatol Syph 1952;65:623.
551. Kheterpal S, Downes SM, Eagling EM. Paget's disease presenting with exophthalmos. Eye 1994;8:480–1.
552. Pandit V, Seshadri S. Paget's disease complicated by hydrocephalus and dementia. Neurol India 2008;56:216–8.
553. Moiyadi AV, Praharaj SS, Pillai VS, et al. Hydrocephalus in Paget's disease. Acta Neurochir (Wien) 2006;148:1297–300. [discussion 300.]
554. Martin BJ, Roberts MA, Turner JW. Normal pressure hydrocephalus and Paget's disease of bone. Gerontology 1985;31:397–402.
555. Clarkson JG. Paget's disease and angioid streaks: One complication less?. Br J Ophthalmol 1991;75:511.
556. Dabbs TR, Skjodt K. Prevalence of angioid streaks and other ocular complications of Paget's disease of bone. Br J Ophthalmol 1990;74:579–82.
557. Mills BG, Singer FR. Nuclear inclusions in Paget's disease of bone. Science 1976;194:201–2.
558. Smith R. Paget's disease and angioid streaks: One complication less?. Br J Ophthalmol 1990;74:577–8.
559. Terry TL. Angioid streaks and osteitis deformans. Trans Am Ophthalmol Soc 1934;32:555–73.
560. Eretto P, Krohel GB, Shihab ZM, et al. Optic neuropathy in Paget's disease. Am J Ophthalmol 1984;97:505–10.
561. Ralston SH, Langston AL, Reid IR. Pathogenesis and management of Paget's disease of bone. Lancet 2008;372:155–63.
562. Pecorella I, Ciardi A, Amadeo G, et al. Orbital osteoclastoma of apparent extraskeletal origin in a pagetic patient: a case report. Hum Pathol 2000;31:1527–31.
563. Goldberg S, Slamovits TL, Dorfman HD, et al. Sarcomatous transformation of the orbit in a patient with Paget's disease. Ophthalmology 2000;107:1464–7.
564. Condon PI, Serjeant GR. Ocular findings in hemoglobin SC disease in Jamaica. Am J Ophthalmol 1972;74:921–31.
565. Condon PI, Serjeant GR. Ocular findings in homozygous sickle cell anemia in Jamaica. Am J Ophthalmol 1972;73:533–43.
566. Condon PI, Serjeant GR. Ocular findings in elderly cases of homozygous sickle-cell disease in Jamaica. Br J Ophthalmol 1976;60:361–4.
567. Deutman AF, Kovács B. Argon laser treatment in complications of angioid streaks. Am J Ophthalmol 1979;88:12–17.
568. Geeraets WJ, Guerry D. III. Angioid streaks and sickle-cell disease. Am J Ophthalmol 1960;49:450–70.
569. Goodman G, von Sallmann L, Holland MG. Ocular manifestations of sickle-cell disease. Arch Ophthalmol 1957;58:655–82.
570. Hamilton AM, Pope FM, Condon PI, et al. Angioid streaks in Jamaican patients with homozygous sickle cell disease. Br J Ophthalmol 1981;65:341–7.
571. Jampol LM, Acheson R, Eagle Jr RC, et al. Calcification of Bruch's membrane in angioid streaks with homozygous sickle cell disease. Arch Ophthalmol 1987;105:93–8.
572. Nagpal KC, Asdourian G, Goldbaum M, et al. Angioid streaks and sickle haemoglobinopathies. Br J Ophthalmol 1976;60:31–4.
573. Paton D. Angioid streaks in sickle cell anemia; a report of two cases. Arch Ophthalmol 1959;62:852–8.
574. Shilling JS, Blach RK. Prognosis and therapy of angioid streaks. Trans Ophthalmol Soc UK 1975;95:301–6.
575. Aessopos A, Voskaridou E, Kavouklis E, et al. Angioid streaks in sickle-thalassemia. Am J Ophthalmol 1994;117:589–92.
576. Goldberg MF, Charache S, Acacio I. Ophthalmologic manifestations of sickle cell thalassemia. Arch Intern Med 1971;128:33–9.
577. Gerde LS. Angioid streaks in sickle cell trait hemoglobinopathy. Am J Ophthalmol 1974;77:462–4.
578. Daneshmend TK. Ocular findings in a case of haemoglobin H disease. Br J Ophthalmol 1979;63:842–4.
579. Aessopos A, Stamatelos G, Savvides P, et al. Angioid streaks in homozygous beta thalassemia. Am J Ophthalmol 1989;108:356–9.
580. Singerman LJ. Angioid streaks in thalassaemia major. Br J Ophthalmol 1983;267:558.
581. Kinsella FP, Mooney DJ. Angioid streaks in beta thalassaemia minor. Br J Ophthalmol 1988;72:303–4.
582. O'Donnell BF, Powell FC, O'Loughlin S, et al. Angioid streaks in β thalassaemia minor. Br J Ophthalmol 1991;75:639.
583. Aessopos A, Floudas CS, Kati M, et al. Loss of vision associated with angioid streaks in beta-thalassemia intermedia. Int J Hematol 2008;87:35–8.
584. Roberts E, Madhusudhana KC, Newsom R, et al. Blindness due to angioid streaks in congenital dyserythropoietic anaemia type I. Br J Haematol 2006;133:456.
585. Dieckert J, White M, Christmann L, et al. Angioid streaks associated with abetalipoproteinemia. Ann Ophthalmol. 1989;21:173–9.
586. Mansour AM, Shields JA, Annesley Jr WH, et al. Macular degeneration in angioid streaks. Ophthalmologica 1988;197:36–41.
587. Runge P, Muller DPR, McAllister J, et al. Oral vitamin E supplements can prevent the retinopathy of abetalipoproteinaemia. Br J Ophthalmol 1986;70:166–73.
588. Lakhanpal V, Schocket SS, Hameroff SB. Angioid streaks in pituitary tumor. South Med J 1978;71:1298–302.
589. Awan KJ. Familial polyposis and angioid streaks in the ocular fundus. Am J Ophthalmol 1977;83:123–5.
590. Kalina RE. Facial angiomatosis with angioid streaks. Association of angioid streaks with a component of the Sturge-Weber syndrome. Arch Ophthalmol 1970;84:528–31.
591. Ahluwalia HS, Lukaris A, Lane CM, et al. Angioid streaks with congenital hypertrophy of the retinal pigment epithelium: an association or a mere coincidence?. Eye (Lond) 2002;16:645–6.
592. Brancato R, Menchini U, Pece A, et al. Laser treatment of macular subretinal neovascularizations in angioid streaks. Ophthalmologica 1987;195:84–7.
593. Gelisken Ö, Hendrikse F, Deutman AF. A long-term follow-up study of laser coagulation of neovascular membranes in angioid streaks. Am J Ophthalmol 1988;105:299–303.
594. Lim JI, Bressler NM, Marsh MJ, et al. Laser treatment of choroidal neovascularization in patients with angioid streaks. Am J Ophthalmol 1993;116:414–23.
595. Meislik J, Neldner K, Reeve EB, et al. Laser treatment in maculopathy of pseudoxanthoma elasticum. Can J Ophthalmol 1978;13:210–2.
596. Pece A, Avanza P, Zorgno F, et al. Photocoagulation au laser des néovaisseaux sous-rétiniens maculaires survenant au cours des stries angioïdes. J Fr Ophthalmol 1989;12:687–9.
597. Singerman LJ, Hatem G. Laser treatment of choroidal neovascular membranes in angioid streaks. Retina 1981;1:75–83.
598. Wilkinson CP. Stimulation of subretinal neovascularization. Am J Ophthalmol 1976;81:104–6.
599. Mimoun G, Tilleul J, Leys A, et al. Intravitreal ranibizumab for choroidal neovascularization in angioid streaks. Am J Ophthalmol 2010;150(692–700):e1.
600. Ladas ID, Kotsolis AI, Ladas DS, et al. Intravitreal ranibizumab treatment of macular choroidal neovascularization secondary to angioid streaks: one-year results of a prospective study. Retina 2010;30:1185–9.
601. Sawa M, Gomi F, Tsujikawa M, et al. Long-term results of intravitreal bevacizumab injection for choroidal neovascularization secondary to angioid streaks. Am J Ophthalmol 2009;148(584–590):e2.
602. Donati MC, Virgili G, Bini A, et al. Intravitreal bevacizumab (Avastin) for choroidal neovascularization in angioid streaks: a case series. Ophthalmologica 2009;223:24–7.
603. Curtin BJ, Karlin DB. Axial length measurements and fundus changes of the myopic eye. Am J Ophthalmol 1971;71:42–53.
604. Fuchs E. Der centrale schwarze Fleck bei Myopie. Z Augenheilkd 1901;5:171–81.
605. Hampton GR, Kohen D, Bird AC. Visual prognosis of disciform degeneration in myopia. Ophthalmology 1983;90:923–6.
606. Hotchkiss ML, Fine SL. Pathologic myopia and choroidal neovascularization. Am J Ophthalmol 1981;91:177–83.
607. Levy JH, Pollock HM, Curtin BJ. The Fuchs' spot: An ophthalmoscopic and fluorescein angiographic study. Ann Ophthalmol 1977;9:1433–43.
608. Avila MP, Weiter JJ, Jalkh AE, et al. Natural history of choroidal neovascularization in degenerative myopia. Ophthalmology 1984;91:1573–81.
609. Hayasaka S, Uchida M, Setogawa T. Subretinal hemorrhages with or without choroidal neovascularization in the maculas of patients with pathologic myopia. Graefes Arch Clin Exp Ophthalmol 1990;228:277–80.
610. Klein RM, Green S. The development of lacquer cracks in pathologic myopia. Am J Ophthalmol 1988;106:282–5.
611. Pruett RC, Weiter JJ, Goldstein RB. Myopic cracks, angioid streaks, and traumatic tears in Bruch's membrane. Am J Ophthalmol 1987;103:537–43.
612. Förster R. Ophthalmologische beitrage. Berlin: T.C.F. Enslin; 1862.
613. Green WR. Retina; myopia In: Spencer WH, editor. Ophthalmic pathology; an atlas and textbook, vol. 2, 3rd ed. Philadelphia: WB Saunders; 1985. p. 913–24.
614. Grossniklaus HE, Green WR. Pathologic findings in pathologic myopia. Retina 1992;12:127–33.
615. Bonnet M, Semiglia R. Evolution spontanée du décollement de la rétine du pôle postérieur du myope fort. J Fr Ophtalmol 1991;14:618–23.
616. Wakabayashi Y, Nishimura A, Higashide T, et al. Unilateral choroidal excavation in the macula detected by spectral-domain optical coherence tomography. Acta Ophthalmol 2010;88:e87–91.
617. Jampol LM, Shankle J, Schroeder R, et al. Diagnostic and therapeutic challenges. Retina 2006;26:1072–6.
618. Celorio JM, Pruett RC. Prevalence of lattice degeneration and its relation to axial length in severe myopia. Am J Ophthalmol 1991;111:20–3.
619. Phillips CI. Aetiology of myopia. Br J Ophthalmol. 1990;74:47–8.
620. Klein RM, Curtin BJ. Lacquer crack lesions in pathologic myopia. Am J Ophthalmol 1975;79:386–92.
621. Funata M, Tokoro T. Scleral change in experimentally myopic monkeys. Graefes Arch Clin Exp Ophthalmol 1990;228:174–9.
622. Jalkh AE, Weiter JJ, Trempe CL, et al. Choroidal neovascularization in degenerative myopia: role of laser photocoagulation. Ophthalmic Surg 1987;18:721–5.

623. Blankenship GW, Ibanez-Langlois S. Treatment of myopic macular hole and detachment; intravitreal gas exchange. Ophthalmology 1987;94:333–6.
624. Curtin BJ, Whitmore WG. Long-term results of scleral reinforcement surgery. Am J Ophthalmol 1987;103:544–8.
625. Woods AC, Wahlen HE. The probable role of benign histoplasmosis in the etiology of granulomatous uveitis. Am J Ophthalmol 1960;49:205–20.
626. Ganley JP. Epidemiologic characteristics of presumed ocular histoplasmosis. Acta Ophthalmol Suppl 1973:119.
627. Gass JDM. Pathogenesis of disciform detachment of the neuroepithelium. V. Disciform macular degeneration secondary to focal choroiditis. Am J Ophthalmol 1967;63:661–87.
628. Gass JDM. Correlation of fluorescein angiography and histopathology. Doc Ophthalmol Proc Ser 1976;9:359–65.
629. Gass JDM. Stereoscopic atlas of macular diseases; diagnosis and treatment, 2nd ed. St. Louis: CV Mosby; 1977. p. 90.
630. Gass JDM, Wilkinson CP. Follow-up study of presumed ocular histoplasmosis. Trans Am Acad Ophthalmol Otolaryngol 1972;76:672–94.
631. Klintworth GK, Hollingsworth AS, Lusman PA, et al. Granulomatous choroiditis in a case of disseminated histoplasmosis; histologic demonstration of *Histoplasma capsulatum* in choroidal lesions. Arch Ophthalmol 1973;90:45–8. [correspondence 1974;91: 237.]
632. Krause AC, Hopkins WG. Ocular manifestation of histoplasmosis. Am J Ophthalmol 1951;34:564–6.
633. Lewis ML, Schiffman JC. Long-term follow-up of the second eye in ocular histoplasmosis. Int Ophthalmol Clin 1983;23:125–35.
634. Maumenee AE. Clinical entities in "uveitis": an approach to the study of intraocular inflammation. Am J Ophthalmol 1970;69:1–27.
635. Sabates FN, Lee KY, Sabates R. Early argon laser photocoagulation of presumed histoplasma maculopathy. Am J Ophthalmol 1977;84:172–86.
636. Schlaegel Jr TF. Ocular histoplasmosis. New York: Grune & Stratton; 1977. p. 47, 195.
637. Weingeist TA, Watzke RC. Ocular involvement by *Histoplasma capsulatum*. Int Ophthalmol Clin 1983;23:33–47.
638. Lewis ML, Van Newkirk MR, Gass JDM. Follow-up study of presumed ocular histoplasmosis syndrome. Ophthalmology 1980;87:390–9.
639. Baskin MA, Jampol LM, Huamonte FU, et al. Macular lesions in blacks with the presumed ocular histoplasmosis syndrome. Am J Ophthalmol 1980;89:77–83.
640. Jones DB. Presumed histoplasmic choroiditis: a possible late manifestation of a benign disease. In: Ajello L, Chick EW, Furcolow ML, editors. Histoplasmosis; proceedings of the second national conference. Springfield, IL: Charles C Thomas; 1971. p. 206–20.
641. Check IJ, Diddie KR, Jay WM, et al. Lymphocyte stimulation by yeast phase *Histoplasma capsulatum* in presumed ocular histoplasmosis syndrome. Am J Ophthalmol 1979;87:311–6.
642. Ganley JP, Nemo GJ, Comstock GW, et al. Lymphocyte transformation in presumed ocular histoplasmosis. Arch Ophthalmol 1981;99:1424–9.
643. Braley RE, Meredith TA, Aaberg TM, et al. The prevalence of HLA-B7 in presumed ocular histoplasmosis. Am J Ophthalmol 1978;85:859–61.
644. Godfrey WA, Sabates R, Cross DE. Association of presumed ocular histoplasmosis with HLA-B7. Am J Ophthalmol 1978;85:854–8.
645. Meredith TA, Smith RE, Braley RE, et al. The prevalence of HLA-B7 in presumed ocular histoplasmosis in patients with peripheral atrophic scars. Am J Ophthalmol 1978;86:325–8.
646. Meredith TA, Smith RE, Duquesnoy RJ. Association of HLA-DRw2 antigen with presumed ocular histoplasmosis. Am J Ophthalmol 1980;89:70–6.
647. Spaide RF, Skerry JE, Yannuzzi LA, et al. Lack of the HLA-DR2 specificity in multifocal choroiditis and panuveitis. Br J Ophthalmol 1990;74:536–7.
648. Rivers MB, Pulido JS, Folk JC. Ill-defined choroidal neovascularization within ocular histoplasmosis scars. Retina 1992;12:90–5.
649. Beck RW, Sergott RC, Barr CC, et al. Optic disc edema in the presumed ocular histoplasmosis syndrome. Ophthalmology 1984;91:183–5.
650. Husted RC, Shock JP. Acute presumed histoplasmosis of the optic nerve head. Br J Ophthalmol 1975;59:409–12.
651. Fountain JA, Schlaegel Jr TF. Linear streaks of the equator in the presumed ocular histoplasmosis syndrome. Arch Ophthalmol 1981;99:246–8.
652. Bopp S, Laqua H. Periphere Netzhautstreifen; lineare Depigmentierung des peripheren retinalen Pigmentepithels. Klin Monatsbl Augenheilkd 1991;198:20–4.
653. Bottoni FG, Deutman AF, Aandekerk AL. Presumed ocular histoplasmosis syndrome and linear streak lesions. Br J Ophthalmol 1989;73:528–35.
654. Gass JDM. Stereoscopic atlas of macular diseases; diagnosis and treatment, 3rd ed. St. Louis: CV Mosby; 1987. p. 534–537.
655. Spaide RF, Yannuzzi LA, Freund KB. Linear streaks in multifocal choroiditis and panuveitis. Retina 1991;11:229–31.
656. Cantrill HL, Burgess D. Peripapillary neovascular membranes in presumed ocular histoplasmosis. Am J Ophthalmol 1980;89:192–203.
657. Jost BF, Olk RJ, Burgess DB. Factors related to spontaneous visual recovery in the ocular histoplasmosis syndrome. Retina 1987;7:1–8.
658. Kleiner RC, Ratner CM, Enger C, et al. Subfoveal neovascularization in the ocular histoplasmosis syndrome; a natural history study. Retina 1988;8:225–9.
659. Elliott JH, Jackson DJ. Presumed histoplasmic maculopathy: clinical course and prognosis in nonphotocoagulated eyes. Int Ophthalmol Clin 1975;15:29–39.
660. Gutman FA. The natural course of active choroidal lesions in the presumed ocular histoplasmosis syndrome. Trans Am Ophthalmol Soc 1979;77:515–41.
661. Klein ML, Fine SL, Knox DL, et al. Follow-up study in eyes with choroidal neovascularization caused by presumed ocular histoplasmosis. Am J Ophthalmol 1977;83:830–5.
662. Watzke RC, Claussen RW. The long-term course of multifocal choroiditis (presumed ocular histoplasmosis). Am J Ophthalmol 1981;91:750–60.
663. Macular Photocoagulation Study Group Krypton laser photocoagulation for neovascular lesions of ocular histoplasmosis; results of a randomized clinical trial. Arch Ophthalmol 1987;105: 1499–507.
664. Ryan Jr SJ. De novo subretinal neovascularization in the histoplasmosis syndrome. Arch Ophthalmol 1976;94:321–7.
665. Schlaegel Jr TF. The natural history of histo spots in the disc-macular area. Int Ophthalmol Clin 1975;15:19–28.
666. Smith RE, Ganley JP, Knox DL. Presumed ocular histoplasmosis. II. Patterns of peripheral and peripapillary scarring in persons with nonmacular disease. Arch Ophthalmol 1972;87:251–7.
667. Smith RE, Knox DL, Jensen AD. Ocular histoplasmosis; significance of asymptomatic macular scars. Arch Ophthalmol 1973;89:296–300.
668. Wilkinson CP. Presumed ocular histoplasmosis. Am J Ophthalmol 1976;82:140–2.
669. Sawelson H, Goldberg RE, Annesley Jr WH, et al. Presumed ocular histoplasmosis syndrome; the fellow eye. Arch Ophthalmol 1976;94:221–4.
670. Craig EL, Suie T. *Histoplasma capsulatum* in human ocular tissue. Arch Ophthalmol 1974;91:285–9.
671. Goldstein BG, Buettner H. Histoplasmic endophthalmitis; a clinicopathologic correlation. Arch Ophthalmol 1983;101:774–7.
672. Hoefnagels KLJ, Pijpers PM. *Histoplasma capsulatum* in a human eye. Am J Ophthalmol 1967;63:715–23.
673. Jester JV, Smith RE. Subretinal neovascularization after experimental ocular histoplasmosis in a subhuman primate. Am J Ophthalmol 1985;100:252–8.
674. Morinelli EN, Dugel PU, Riffenburgh R, et al. Infectious multifocal choroiditis in patients with acquired immune deficiency syndrome. Ophthalmology 1993;100:1014–21.
675. Pulido JS, Folberg R, Carter KD, et al. *Histoplasma capsulatum* endophthalmitis after cataract extraction. Ophthalmology 1990;97:217–20.
676. Ryan SJ. Histopathological correlates of presumed ocular histoplasmosis. Int Ophthalmol Clin 1975;15:125–37.
677. Scholz R, Green WR, Kutys R, et al. *Histoplasma capsulatum* in the eye. Ophthalmology 1984;91:1100–4.
678. Schwarz J, Salfelder K, Viloria HJE. *Histoplasma capsulatum* in vessels of the choroid. Ann Ophthalmol 1977;9:633–6.
679. Specht CS, Mitchell KT, Bauman AE, et al. Ocular histoplasmosis with retinitis in a patient with acquired immune deficiency syndrome. Ophthalmology 1991;98:1356–9.
680. Gass JDM, Zimmerman LE. Histopathologic demonstration of *Histoplasma capsulatum*. Am J Ophthalmol 1978;85:725.
681. Khalil MK. Histopathology of presumed ocular histoplasmosis. Am J Ophthalmol 1982;94: 369–76.
682. Makley Jr TA, editor. Presumed histoplasma chorioretinitis: case presented at the Verhoeff Society Meeting, April 23–24, 1977.
683. Roth AM. *Histoplasma capsulatum* in the presumed ocular histoplasmosis syndrome. Am J Ophthalmol 1977;84:293–8.
684. Irvine AR, Spencer WH, Hogan MJ, et al. Presumed chronic ocular histoplasmosis syndrome: a clinical-pathologic case report. Trans Am Ophthalmol Soc 1976;74:91–106.
685. Meredith TA, Green WR, Key SN, et al. Ocular histoplasmosis: Clinicopathologic correlation of 3 cases. Surv Ophthalmol 1977;22:189–205.
686. Sheffer A, Green WR, Fine SL, et al. Presumed ocular histoplasmosis syndrome; a clinicopathologic correlation of a treated case. Arch Ophthalmol 1980;98:335–40.
687. Macy JI, Minckler DS, Smith RE. Experimental inflammatory serous detachment of the retina. Arch Ophthalmol 1980;98:2217–9.
688. Smith JL, Singer JA. Experimental ocular histoplasmosis. III. Experimentally produced retinal and choroidal lesions. Am J Ophthalmol 1964;58:413–23.
689. Smith JL, Singer JA. Experimental ocular histoplasmosis. VI. Fluorescein fundus photographs of choroiditis in the primate. Am J Ophthalmol 1964;58:1021–6.
690. Smith RE, Macy JI, Parrett C, et al. Variations in acute multifocal histoplasmic choroiditis in the primate. Invest Ophthalmol Vis Sci 1978;17:1005–18.
691. Smith RE, O'Connor GR, Halde CH, et al. Clinical course in rabbits after experimental induction of ocular histoplasmosis. Am J Ophthalmol 1973;76:284–93.
692. Wong VG. Focal choroidopathy in experimental ocular histoplasmosis. Trans Am Ophthalmol Soc 1972;70:615–30.
693. Smith RE, Ganley JP. An epidemiologic study of presumed ocular histoplasmosis. Trans Am Acad Ophthalmol Otolaryngol 1971;75:994–1005.
694. Feman SS, Tilford RH. Ocular findings in patients with histoplasmosis. JAMA 1985;253: 2534–7.
695. Davidorf FH, Anderson JD. Ocular lesions in the Earth Day histoplasmosis epidemic. Trans Am Acad Ophthalmol Otolaryngol 1974;78:OP876–OP881.
696. Ellis FD, Schlaegel Jr TF. The geographic localization of presumed histoplasmic choroiditis. Am J Ophthalmol 1973;75:953–6.
697. Feman SS, Podgorski SF, Penn MK. Blindness from presumed ocular histoplasmosis in Tennessee. Ophthalmology 1982;89:1295–8.
698. Ganley JP, Smith RE, Knox DL, et al. Presumed ocular histoplasmosis. III. Epidemiologic characteristics of people with peripheral atrophic scars. Arch Ophthalmol 1973;89:116–9.
699. Giles CL, Falls HF. Amphotericin B therapy in the treatment of presumed *Histoplasma* chorioretinitis: a further appraisal. Trans Am Ophthalmol Soc 1967;65:136–45.
700. Braunstein RA, Rosen DA, Bird AC. Ocular histoplasmosis syndrome in the United Kingdom. Br J Ophthalmol 1974;58:893–7.
701. Macular Photocoagulation Study Group. Argon laser photocoagulation for ocular histoplasmosis; results of a randomized clinical trial. Arch Ophthalmol 1983;101:1347–57.
702. Macular Photocoagulation Study Group. Persistent and recurrent neovascularization after krypton laser photocoagulation for neovascular lesions of ocular histoplasmosis. Arch Ophthalmol 1989;107:344–52.
703. Macular Photocoagulation Study Group. Laser photocoagulation for juxtafoveal choroidal neovascularization; five-year results from randomized clinical trials. Arch Ophthalmol 1994;112:500–9.
704. Klein ML, Fine SL, Patz A. Results of argon laser photocoagulation in presumed ocular histoplasmosis. Am J Ophthalmol 1978;86:211–7.

705. Maumenee AE, Ryan SJ. Photocoagulation of disciform macular lesions in the ocular histoplasmosis syndrome. Am J Ophthalmol 1973;75:13–16.
706. Okun E. Photocoagulation treatment of presumed histoplasmic choroidopathy. Trans Am Ophthalmol Soc 1972;70:467–89.
707. Patz A, Fine SL. Argon laser photocoagulation in ocular histoplasmosis syndrome. Int Ophthalmol Clin 1976;16:45–57.
708. Patz A, Ticho U, Kelley JS. Some observations on argon laser photocoagulation for the presumed histoplasmosis syndrome. Mod Probl Ophthalmol 1974;12:288–94.
709. Sabates FN, Lee KY, Ziemianski MC. A comparative study of argon and krypton laser photocoagulation in the treatment of presumed ocular histoplasmosis syndrome. Ophthalmology 1982;89:729–34.
710. Schlaegel Jr TF, Cofield DD, Clark G, et al. Photocoagulation and other therapy for histoplasmic choroiditis. Trans Am Acad Ophthalmol Otolaryngol 1968;72:355–63.
711. Watzke RC, Leaverton PE. Light coagulation in presumed histoplasmic choroiditis; a controlled clinical study. Arch Ophthalmol 1971;86:127–32.
712. Yassur Y, Gilad E, Ben-Sira I. Treatment of macular subretinal neovascularization with the red-light krypton laser in presumed ocular histoplasmosis syndrome. Am J Ophthalmol 1981;91:172–6.
713. Burgess DB. Ocular histoplasmosis syndrome. Ophthalmology 1986;93:967–8.
714. Macher A, Rodrigues MM, Kaplan W, et al. Disseminated bilateral chorioretinitis due to *Histoplasma capsulatum* in a patient with the acquired immunodeficiency syndrome. Ophthalmology 1985;92:1159–64.
715. Berger AS, Kaplan HJ. Clinical experience with the surgical removal of subfoveal neovascular membranes; short-term postoperative results. Ophthalmology 1992;99:969–76.
716. Saxe SJ, Grossniklaus HE, Lopez PF, et al. Ultrastructural features of surgically excised subretinal neovascular membranes in the ocular histoplasmosis syndrome. Arch Ophthalmol 1993;111:88–95.
717. Thomas MA, Kaplan HJ. Surgical removal of subfoveal neovascularization in the presumed ocular histoplasmosis syndrome. Am J Ophthalmol 1991;111:1–7.
718. Wind BE, Sobol WM. Surgical management of a long-standing subfoveal neovascular membrane secondary to ocular histoplasmosis. Ophthalmic Surg 1993;24:36–9.
719. Hawkins BS, Bressler NM, Bressler SB, et al. Surgical removal vs observation for subfoveal choroidal neovascularization, either associated with the ocular histoplasmosis syndrome or idiopathic: I. Ophthalmic findings from a randomized clinical trial: Submacular Surgery Trials (SST) Group H Trial: SST Report No. 9. Arch Ophthalmol 2004;122:1597–611.
720. Berger AS, Conway M, Del Priore LV, et al. Submacular surgery for subfoveal choroidal neovascular membranes in patients with presumed ocular histoplasmosis. Arch Ophthalmol 1997;115:991–6.
721. Ringwald A. [PDT (photodynamic therapy) treatment of choroidal neovascularisations (CNV) associated with presumed ocular histoplasmosis syndrome (POHS)]. Klin Monbl Augenheilkd 2010;227:507–9.
722. Rosenfeld PJ, Saperstein DA, Bressler NM, et al. Photodynamic therapy with verteporfin in ocular histoplasmosis: uncontrolled, open-label 2-year study. Ophthalmology 2004;111:1725–33.
723. Ehrlich R, Ciulla TA, Maturi R, et al. Intravitreal bevacizumab for choroidal neovascularization secondary to presumed ocular histoplasmosis syndrome. Retina 2009;29:1418–23.
724. Schadlu R, Blinder KJ, Shah GK, et al. Intravitreal bevacizumab for choroidal neovascularization in ocular histoplasmosis. Am J Ophthalmol 2008;145:875–8.
725. Bass EB, Gilson MM, Mangione CM, et al. Surgical removal vs observation for idiopathic or ocular histoplasmosis syndrome-associated subfoveal choroidal neovascularization: Vision Preference Value Scale findings from the randomized SST Group H Trial: SST Report No. 17. Arch Ophthalmol 2008;126:1626–32.
726. Feman SS, Pritchett P, Johns K, et al. Intraocular tumor from disseminated histoplasmosis. South Med J 1991;84:780–1.
727. Gass JDM. Differential diagnosis of intraocular tumors; a stereoscopic presentation. St. Louis: CV Mosby; 1974. p. 196–197.
728. Jampel HD, Schachat AP, Conway B, et al. Retinal pigment epithelial hyperplasia assuming tumor-like proportions; report of two cases. Retina 1986;6:105–12.
729. Makley Jr TA, Davidorf FH, Chambers RB, et al. Massive intraocular hemorrhage in the ocular histoplasmosis syndrome. Contemp Ophthalmic Forum 1987;5:55–65.
730. Capone Jr A, Wallace RT, Meredith TA. Symptomatic choroidal neovascularization in blacks. Arch Ophthalmol 1994;112:1091–7.
731. MacCumber MW, Dastgheib K, Bressler NM, et al. Clinicopathologic correlation of the multiple recurrent serosanguineous retinal pigment epithelial detachments syndrome. Retina 1994;14:143–52.
732. Perkovich BT, Zakov ZN, Berlin LA, et al. An update on multiple recurrent serosanguineous retinal pigment epithelial detachments in black women. Retina 1990;10:18–26.
733. Byeon SH, Lee SC, Oh HS, et al. Incidence and clinical patterns of polypoidal choroidal vasculopathy in Korean patients. Jpn J Ophthalmol 2008;52:57–62.
734. de Mello PC, Brasil OF, Maia HS, et al. Prevalence and epidemiologic features of polypoidal choroidal vasculopathy in southeastern Brazil. Eye 2007;21:1247.
735. Obata R, Yanagi Y, Kami J, et al. Polypoidal choroidal vasculopathy and retinochoroidal anastomosis in Japanese patients eligible for photodynamic therapy for exudative age-related macular degeneration. Jpn J Ophthalmol 2006;50:354–60.
736. Yuzawa M, Mori R, Kawamura A. The origins of polypoidal choroidal vasculopathy. Br J Ophthalmol 2005;89:602–7.
737. Hikichi T, Ohtsuka H, Higuchi M, et al. Causes of macular serous retinal detachments in Japanese patients 40 years and older. Retina 2009;29:395–404.
738. Ahuja RM, Downes SM, Stanga PE, et al. Polypoidal choroidal vasculopathy and central serous chorioretinopathy. Ophthalmology 2001;108:1009–10.
739. Yannuzzi LA, Freund KB, Goldbaum M, et al. Polypoidal choroidal vasculopathy masquerading as central serous chorioretinopathy. Ophthalmology 2000;107:767–77.
740. Ojima Y, Hangai M, Sakamoto A, et al. Improved visualization of polypoidal choroidal vasculopathy lesions using spectral-domain optical coherence tomography. Retina 2009;29:52–9.
741. Ozawa S, Ishikawa K, Ito Y, et al. Differences in macular morphology between polypoidal choroidal vasculopathy and exudative age-related macular degeneration detected by optical coherence tomography. Retina 2009;29:793–802.
742. Kondo N, Honda S, Kuno S, et al. Coding variant I62V in the complement factor H gene is strongly associated with polypoidal choroidal vasculopathy. Ophthalmology 2009;116:304–10.
743. Aiello PD, Trautmann JC, McPhee TJ, et al. Visual prognosis in giant cell arteritis. Ophthalmology 1993;100:550–5.
744. Kinyoun JL, Kalina RE. Visual loss from choroidal ischemia. Am J Ophthalmol 1986;101:650–6.
745. McLeod D, Oji EO, Kohner EM, et al. Fundus signs in temporal arteritis. Br J Ophthalmol 1978;62:591–4.
746. Parrish R, Gass JDM, Anderson DR. Outer retina ischemic infarction–a newly recognized complication of cataract extraction and closed vitrectomy. Part 2. An animal model. Ophthalmology 1982;89:1472–7.
747. Quillen DA, Cantore WA, Schwartz SR, et al. Choroidal nonperfusion in giant cell arteritis. Am J Ophthalmol 1993;116:171–5.
748. Slavin ML, Barondes MJ. Visual loss caused by choroidal ischemia preceding anterior ischemic optic neuropathy in giant cell arteritis. Am J Ophthalmol 1994;117:81–6.
749. Newman NM, Hoyt WF, Spencer WH. Macula-sparing monocular blackouts; clinical and pathologic investigations of intermittent choroidal vascular insufficiency in a case of periarteritis nodosa. Arch Ophthalmol 1974;91:367–70.
750. van Meurs JC. Choroidal filling patterns in sickle cell patients. Int Ophthalmol 1991;15:49–52.
751. Straatsma BR, Zimmerman LE, Gass JDM. Phycomycosis; a clinicopathologic study of fifty-one cases. Lab Invest 1962;11:963–85.
752. Gass JDM. Ocular manifestations of acute mucormycosis. Arch Ophthalmol 1961;65:226–37.
753. Gass JDM. Acute orbital mucormycosis; report of two cases. Arch Ophthalmol. 1961;65: 214–20.
754. Qingli L, Orcutt JC, Seifter LS. Orbital mucormycosis with retinal and ciliary artery occlusions. Br J Ophthalmol 1989;73:680–3.
755. McLean EB. Inadvertent injection of corticosteroid into the choroidal vasculature. Am J Ophthalmol 1975;80:835–7.
756. Thomas EL, Laborde RP. Retinal and choroidal vascular occlusion following intralesional corticosteroid injection of a chalazion. Ophthalmology 1986;93:405–7.
757. Raymond LA, Sacks JG, Choromokos E, et al. Short posterior ciliary artery insufficiency with hyperthermia (Uhthoff's symptom). Am J Ophthalmol 1980;90:619–23.
758. Rodriguez A, Rodriguez FJ, Betancourt F. Presumed occlusion of posterior ciliary arteries following central retinal vein decompression surgery. Arch Ophthalmol 1994;112:54–6.
759. Mames RN, Friedman SM, Brown GC. Distribution of the posterior ciliary arteries revealed after vascular occlusions; a case report. Retina 1992;12:367–9.
760. DeLaey JJ. Fluoro-angiographic study of the choroid in man. Doc Ophthalmol 1978;45: 78–112.
761. DeLaey JJ. Fluorescein angiography of the choroid in health and disease. Int Ophthalmol 1983;6:125–38.
762. Cohen SMZ, Fine SL, Murphy RP, et al. Transient delay in choroidal filling after krypton red laser photocoagulation for choroidal neovascular membranes. Retina 1983;3:284–90.
763. Goldbaum MH, Galinos SO, Apple D, et al. Acute choroidal ischemia as a complication of photocoagulation. Arch Ophthalmol 1976;94:1025–35.
764. Johnson R, Schatz H. Delayed choroidal vascular filling after krypton laser photocoagulation. Am J Ophthalmol 1985;99:154–8.
765. Amalric P. Le territoire chorio-rétinien de l'artère ciliaire longue postérieure. Etude clinique. Bull Soc Ophtalmol Fr 1963;63:342–51.
766. Amalric PM. Choroidal vessel occlusive syndromes–clinical aspects. Trans Am Acad Ophthalmol Otolaryngol 1973;77:OP291–OP299.
767. Buettner H, Machemer R, Charles S, et al. Experimental deprivation of choroidal blood flow; retinal morphology, early receptor potential, and electroretinography. Am J Ophthalmol 1973;75:943–52.
768. Foulds WS, Lee WR, Taylor WOG. Clinical and pathological aspects of choroidal ischaemia. Trans Ophthalmol Soc UK 1971;91:323–41.
769. Gaudric A. Les occlusions vasculaires choroïdiennes aiguës. In: Ducournau D, Gaudric A, Grange J-D, editors. La vascularisation choroïdienne. Bull Soc Ophtalmol Fr Rapport Annuel Numéro spécial 1981. p. 67–133.
770. Gaudric A, Coscas G, Bird AC. Choroidal ischemia. Am J Ophthalmol 1982;94:489–98.
771. Hayreh SS. Segmental nature of the choroidal vasculature. Br J Ophthalmol 1975;59:631–48.
772. Hayreh SS, editor. Retina, 2; 1982 p. 191–2.
773. Hayreh SS, Baines JAB. Occlusion of the posterior ciliary artery. I. Effects on choroidal circulation. Br J Ophthalmol 1972;56:719–35.
774. Spolaore R, Gaudric A, Coscas G, et al. Acute sectorial choroidal ischemia. Am J Ophthalmol 1984;98:707–16.
775. Diamond JG, Kaplan HJ. Uveitis: Effect of vitrectomy combined with lensectomy. Ophthalmology 1979;86:1320–7.
776. Gass JDM, Parrish R. Outer retinal ischemic infarction–a newly recognized complication of cataract extraction and closed vitrectomy. I. A case report. Ophthalmology 1982;89:1467–71.
777. Hollenhorst RW, Svien HJ, Benoit CF. Unilateral blindness occurring during anesthesia for neurosurgical operations. Arch Ophthalmol 1954;52:819–30.
778. Rosenblum PD, Michels RG, Stark WJ, et al. Choroidal ischemia after extracapsular cataract extraction by phacoemulsification. Retina 1981;1:263–70.
779. West J, Askin G, Clarke M, et al. Loss of vision in one eye following scoliosis surgery. Br J Ophthalmol 1990;74:243–4.
780. Lieb WE, Flaharty PM, Sergott RC, et al. Color Doppler imaging provides accurate assessment of orbital blood flow in occlusive carotid artery disease. Ophthalmology 1991;98:548–52.
781. Azar P, Smith RS, Greenberg MH. Ocular findings in disseminated intravascular coagulation. Am J Ophthalmol 1974;78:493–6.
782. Cogan DG. Ocular involvement in disseminated intravascular coagulopathy. Arch Ophthalmol 1975;93:1–8.

783. Cogan DG. Fibrin clots in the choriocapillaris and serous detachment of the retina. Ophthalmologica 1976;172:298–307.
784. Klein BA. Ischemic infarcts of the choroid (Elschnig spots); a cause of retinal separation in hypertensive disease with renal insufficiency. A clinical and histopathologic study. Am J Ophthalmol 1968;66:1069–74.
785. Morse PH. Elschnig's spots and hypertensive choroidopathy. Am J Ophthalmol 1968;66:844–52.
786. Ortiz JM, Yanoff M, Cameron JD, et al. Disseminated intravascular coagulation in infancy and in the neonate; ocular findings. Arch Ophthalmol 1982;100:1413–5.
787. Stropes LL, Luft FC. Hypertensive crisis with bilateral bullous retinal detachment. JAMA 1977;238:1948–9.
788. Beck RW, Gamel JW, Willcourt RJ, et al. Acute ischemic optic neuropathy in severe preeclampsia. Am J Ophthalmol 1980;90:342–6.
789. Chaine G, Attali P, Gaudric A, et al. Ocular fluorophotometric and angiographic findings in toxemia of pregnancy. Arch Ophthalmol 1986;104:1632–5.
790. Fastenberg DM, Fetkenhour CL, Choromokos E, et al. Choroidal vascular changes in toxemia of pregnancy. Am J Ophthalmol 1980;89:362–8.
791. Jaffe G, Schatz H. Ocular manifestations of preeclampsia. Am J Ophthalmol 1987;103:309–15.
792. Kenny GS, Cerasoli JR. Color fluorescein angiography in toxemia of pregnancy. Arch Ophthalmol 1972;87:383–8.
793. Kronenberg EW. Toxemic retinopathy of pregnancy with special consideration of retinal detachment as complication of pregnancy toxicosis. Ned Tijdschr Geneeskd 1956;100:331.
794. Mabie WC, Ober RR. Fluorescein angiography in toxaemia of pregnancy. Br J Ophthalmol 1980;64:666–71.
795. Schultz JF, O'Brien CS. Retinal changes in hypertensive toxemia of pregnancy; a report of 47 cases. Am J Ophthalmol 1938;21:767–74.
796. Hoines J, Buettner H. Ocular complications of disseminated intravascular coagulation (DIC) in abruptio placentae. Retina 1989;9:105–9.
797. Gass JDM, Slamovits TL, Fuller DG, et al. Posterior chorioretinopathy and retinal detachment after organ transplantation. Arch Ophthalmol 1992;110:1717–22.
798. Snyers B, Kestens C. Choroïdite séreuse centrale après transplantation rénal. Bull Soc Belge Ophtalmol 1990;239:87–101.
799. Diddie KR, Aronson AJ, Ernest JT. Chorioretinopathy in a case of systemic lupus erythematosus. Trans Am Ophthalmol Soc 1977;75:122–31.
800. Gold DH, Morris DA, Henkind P. Ocular findings in systemic lupus erythematosus. Br J Ophthalmol 1972;56:800–4.
801. Googe Jr JM, Brady SE, Argyle JC, et al. Choroiditis in infantile periarteritis nodosa. Arch Ophthalmol 1985;103:81–3.
802. Martin VAF. Disseminated intravascular coagulopathy. Trans Ophthalmol Soc UK 1978;98:506–7.
803. Kinyoun JL, Kalina RE, Klein ML. Choroidal involvement in systemic necrotizing vasculitis. Arch Ophthalmol 1987;105:939–42.
804. Jampol LM, Lahav M, Albert DM, et al. Ocular clinical findings and basement membrane changes in Goodpasture's syndrome. Am J Ophthalmol 1975;79:452–63.
805. Snir M, Cohen S, Ben-Sira I, et al. Retinal manifestations of thrombocytopenic purpura (TTP) following use of contraceptive treatment. Ann Ophthalmol 1985;17:109–12.
806. Benson DO, Fitzgibbons JF, Goodnight SH. The visual system in thrombotic thrombocytopenic purpura. Ann Ophthalmol 1980;12:413–7.
807. Lewellen Jr DR, Singerman LJ. Thrombotic thrombocytopenic purpura with optic disk neovascularization, vitreous hemorrhage, retinal detachment, and optic atrophy. Am J Ophthalmol 1980;89:840–4.
808. Percival SPB. The eye and Moschcowitz's disease (thrombotic thrombocytopenic purpura); a review of 182 cases. Trans Ophthalmol Soc UK 1970;90:375–82.
809. Percival SPB. Ocular findings in thrombotic thrombocytopenic purpura (Moschcowitz's disease). Br J Ophthalmol 1970;54:73–8.
810. Samples JR, Buettner H. Ocular involvement in disseminated intravascular coagulation (DIC). Ophthalmology 1983;90:914–6.
811. Stefani FH, Brandt F, Pielsticker K. Periarteritis nodosa and thrombotic thrombocytopenic purpura and serous retinal detachment in siblings. Br J Ophthalmol 1978;62:402–7.
812. Vesconi S, Langer M, Rossi E, et al. Thrombotic thrombocytopenic purpura during oral contraceptive treatment. Thromb Haemost 1978;40:563–4.
813. Wyszynski RE, Frank KE, Grossniklaus HE. Bilateral retinal detachments in thrombotic thrombocytopenic purpura. Graefes Arch Clin Exp Ophthalmol 1988;226:501–4.
814. Yamaguchi K, Abe S, Shiono T, et al. Macular choroidal occlusion in dysplasminogenemia. Retina 1991;11:423–5.
815. Patchett RB, Wilson WB, Ellis PP. Ophthalmic complications with disseminated intravascular coagulation. Br J Ophthalmol 1988;72:377–9.
816. MacCumber MW, Flower RW, Langham ME. Ischemic hypertensive choroidopathy; fluorescein angiography, indocyanine green videoangiography, and measurement of pulsatile blood flow. Arch Ophthalmol 1993;111:704–5.
817. de Venecia G, Wallow I, Houser D, et al. The eye in accelerated hypertension. I. Elschnig's spots in nonhuman primates. Arch Ophthalmol 1980;98:913–8.
818. Gass JDM. Stereoscopic atlas of macular diseases; diagnosis and treatment, 2nd ed. St. Louis: CV Mosby; 1977. p. 124.
819. Gass JDM, Pautler SE. Toxemia of pregnancy pigment epitheliopathy masquerading as a heredomacular dystrophy. Trans Am Ophthalmol Soc 1985;83:114–30.
820. Gitter KA, Houser BP, Sarin LK, et al. Toxemia of pregnancy; an angiographic interpretation of fundus changes. Arch Ophthalmol 1968;80:449–54.
821. Oliver M, Uchenik D. Bilateral exudative retinal detachment in eclampsia without hypertensive retinopathy. Am J Ophthalmol 1980;90:792–6.
822. Saito Y, Omoto T, Fukuda M. Lobular pattern of choriocapillaris in pre-eclampsia with aldosteronism. Br J Ophthalmol 1990;74:702–3.
823. Talbert LM, Blatt PM. Disseminated intravascular coagulation in obstetrics. Clin Obstet Gynecol 1979;22:889–900.
824. Burke JP, Whyte I, MacEwen CJ. Bilateral serous retinal detachments in the HELLP syndrome. Acta Ophthalmol 1989;67:322–4.
825. Kirkpatrick CA. The HELLP syndrome. Acta Clin Belg. 2010;65:91–7.
826. Keiser SD, Owens MY, Parrish MR, et al. HELLP Syndrome with and without Eclampsia. Am J Perinatol 2010 [in press]
827. Wada Y, Sakamaki Y, Kobayashi D, et al. HELLP syndrome, multiple liver infarctions, and intrauterine fetal death in a patient with systemic lupus erythematosus and antiphospholipid syndrome. Intern Med 2009;48:1555–8.
828. Karaguzel H, Guven S, Karalezli A, et al. Bilateral serous retinal detachment in a woman with HELLP syndrome and retinal detachment. J Obstet Gynaecol 2009;29:246–8.
829. Stewart MW, Brazis PW, Guier CP, et al. Purtscher-like retinopathy in a patient with HELLP syndrome. Am J Ophthalmol 2007;143:886–7.
830. Murphy MA, Ayazifar M. Permanent visual deficits secondary to the HELLP syndrome. J NeuroOphthalmol 2005;25:122–7.
831. Tranos PG, Wickremasinghe SS, Hundal KS, et al. Bilateral serous retinal detachment as a complication of HELLP syndrome. Eye (Lond) 2002;16:491–2.
832. Gonzalvo FJ, Abecia E, Pinilla I, et al. Central retinal vein occlusion and HELLP syndrome. Acta Ophthalmol Scand 2000;78:596–8.
833. Gupta LY, Mansour SE. Bilateral bullous retinal detachment as a complication of the HELLP syndrome. Can J Ophthalmol 1994;29:242–5.
834. Leff SR, Yarian DL, Masciulli L, et al. Vitreous haemorrhage as a complication of HELLP syndrome. Br J Ophthalmol 1990;74:498.
835. Bussen S, Bussen D. Influence of the vascular endothelial growth factor on the development of severe pre-eclampsia or HELLP syndrome. Arch Gynecol Obstet 2010. [in press]
836. Rowe PA, Mansfield DC, Dutton GN. Ophthalmic features of fourteen cases of Goodpasture's syndrome. Nephron 1994;68:52–6.
837. Boucher MC, el Toukhy EA, Cormier G. Bilateral serous retinal detachments associated with Goodpasture's syndrome. Can J Ophthalmol 1998;33:46–9.
838. Jampol LM, Lahov M, Albert DM, et al. Ocular clinical findings and basement membrane changes in Goodpasture's syndrome. Am J Ophthalmol 1975;79:452–63.
839. Chiquet C, Lumbroso L, Denis P, et al. Acute posterior multifocal placoid pigment epitheliopathy associated with Wegener's granulomatosis. Retina 1999;19:309–13.
840. Wang M, Khurana RN, Sadda SR. Central retinal vein occlusion in Wegener's granulomatosis without retinal vasculitis. Br J Ophthalmol 2006;90:1435–6.
841. Venkatesh P, Chawla R, Tewari HK. Hemiretinal vein occlusion in Wegener's granulomatosis. Eur J Ophthalmol 2003;13:722–5.
842. Iida T, Spaide RF, Kantor J. Retinal and choroidal arterial occlusion in Wegener's granulomatosis. Am J Ophthalmol 2002;133:151–2.
843. Kinyoun JL. APMPPE associated with Wegener's granulomatosis. Retina 2000;20:419–20.
844. Janknecht P, Mittelviefhaus H, Loffler KU. Sclerochoroidal granuloma in Wegener's granulomatosis simulating a uveal melanoma. Retina 1995;15:150–3.
845. Agostini HT, Brautigam P, Loffler KU. Subretinal tumour in a patient with a limited form of Wegener's granulomatosis. Acta Ophthalmol Scand 1995;73:460–3.
846. Tanihara H, Nakayama Y, Honda Y. Wegener's granulomatosis with rapidly progressive retinitis and anterior uveitis. Acta Ophthalmol (Copenh) 1993;71:853–5.
847. Samuelson TW, Margo CE. Protracted uveitis as the initial manifestation of Wegener's granulomatosis. Arch Ophthalmol 1990;108:478–9.
848. Greenberger MH. Central retinal artery closure in Wegener's granulomatosis. Am J Ophthalmol 1967;63:515–6.
849. Gaudric A, Sterkers M, Coscas G. Retinal detachment after choroidal ischemia. Am J Ophthalmol 1987;104:364–72.
850. Wilson CA, Royster AJ, Tiedemann JS, et al. Exudative retinal detachment after photodynamic injury. Arch Ophthalmol 1991;109:125–34.
851. Ho AC, Benson WE, Wong J. Unusual immunogammopathy maculopathy. Ophthalmology 2000;107:1099–103.
852. Brody JM, Butrus SI, Ashraf MF, et al. Multiple myeloma presenting with bilateral exudative macular detachments. Acta Ophthalmol Scand 1995;73:81–2.
853. Quhill F, Khan I, Rashid A. Bilateral serous macular detachments in Waldenstrom's macroglobulinaemia. Postgrad Med J 2009;85:382.
854. Okada K, Yamamoto S, Tsuyama Y, et al. Case of POEMS syndrome associated with bilateral macular detachment resolved by autologous peripheral blood stem cell transplantation. Jpn J Ophthalmol 2007;51:237–8.
855. Leys A, Vandenberghe P. Serous macular detachments in a patient with IgM paraproteinemia: an optical coherence tomography study. Arch Ophthalmol 2001;119:911–3.
856. Ogata N, Ida H, Takahashi K, et al. Occult retinal pigment epithelial detachment in hyperviscosity syndrome. Ophthalmic Surg Lasers 2000;31:248–52.
857. Cohen SM, Kokame GT, Gass JD. Paraproteinemias associated with serous detachments of the retinal pigment epithelium and neurosensory retina. Retina 1996;16:467–73.
858. Berta A, Beck P, Mikita J. IgM paraprotein in the subretinal fluid of a patient with recurrent retinal detachment and Waldenstrom's macroglobulinaemia. Acta Med Hung 1985;42:179–86.
859. Omoti AE, Omoti CE. Ophthalmic manifestations of multiple myeloma. West Afr J Med 2007;26:265–8.
860. Thomas EL, Olk RJ, Markman M, et al. Irreversible visual loss in Waldenstrom's macroglobulinaemia. Br J Ophthalmol 1983;67:102–6.
861. Wiaux C, Landau K, Borruat FX. Unusual cause of bilateral optic disc swelling: POEMS syndrome. Klin Monatsbl Augenheilkd 2007;224:334–6.
862. Chong DY, Comer GM, Trobe JD. Optic disc edema, cystoid macular edema, and elevated vascular endothelial growth factor in a patient with POEMS syndrome. J Neuroophthalmol 2007;27:180–3.
863. Imai H, Kusuhara S, Nakanishi Y, et al. A case of POEMS syndrome with cystoid macular edema. Am J Ophthalmol 2005;139:563–6.
864. Wong VA, Wade NK. POEMS syndrome: an unusual cause of bilateral optic disk swelling. Am J Ophthalmol 1998;126:452–4.

865. Davies EWG. Annular serous choroidal detachment. Mod Probl Ophthalmol 1979;20:2–5.
866. De Bustros S, Michels RG, Rice TA, et al. Treatment of idiopathic exudative retinal detachment. Retina 1984;4:158–62.
867. De Laey JJ, Laender R, Verbraeken H. Impairment of choroidal venous outflow: possible cause of spontaneous choroidal detachment? Mod Probl Ophthalmol 1979;20:16–22.
868. Gamringer H, Schreck E, Wollensak J. Zur Pathogenese and Therapie der Cyclitis anularis exsudativa pseudotumorosa. Klin Monatsbl Augenheilkd 1959;135:638–46.
869. Gass JDM, Jallow S. Idiopathic serous detachment of the choroid, ciliary body, and retina (uveal effusion syndrome). Ophthalmology 1982;89:1018–32.
870. Geyer O, Godel V, Lazar M. Hypotony as a late complication of extracapsular cataract extraction. Am J Ophthalmol 1983;96:112–3.
871. Pollalis S, Tragakis M. Idiopathic choroidal detachment. Mod Probl Ophthalmol 1979;20:23–9.
872. Schepens CL, Brockhurst RJ. Uveal effusion. I. Clinical picture. Arch Ophthalmol. 1963;70: 189–202.
873. Stallard HB. Annular peripheral retinal detachment. Br J Ophthalmol 1954;38:115–8.
874. Verhoeff FH, Waite JH. Separation of the choroid, with report of a spontaneous case. Trans Am Ophthalmol Soc 1925;23:120–39.
875. von Graefe A. Zur Diagnose des beginnenden intraocularen Krebses. Albrecht von Graefes Arch Ophthalmol 1858;4:218–29.
876. Wilson RS, Hanna C, Morris MD. Idiopathic chorioretinal effusion: an analysis of extracellular fluids. Ann Ophthalmol 1977;9:647–53.
877. Brockhurst RJ, Lam K-W. Uveal effusion. II. Report of a case with analysis of subretinal fluid. Arch Ophthalmol 1973;90:399–401.
878. Dawidek GMB, Kinsella FM, Pyott A, et al. Delayed ciliochoroidal detachment following intraocular lens implantation. Br J Ophthalmol 1991;75:572–4.
879. Sato S, Okubo A, Sugahara M. Biochemical study of subretinal fluid. I. Uveal effusion. Jpn J Clin Ophthalmol 1981;35:1185–7.
880. Brockhurst RJ. Vortex vein decompression for nanophthalmic uveal effusion. Arch Ophthalmol 1980;98:1987–90.
881. Singh OS, Simmons RJ, Brockhurst RJ, et al. Nanophthalmos; a perspective on identification and therapy. Ophthalmology 1982;89:1006–12.
882. Forrester JV, Lee WR, Kerr PR, et al. The uveal effusion syndrome and trans-scleral flow. Eye 1990;4:354–65.
883. Tagami N, Uyama M, Yamada K, et al. Histological observations on the sclera in uveal effusion. J Jpn Ophthalmol Soc 1993;97:268–74.
884. Ward RC, Gragoudas ES, Pon DM, et al. Abnormal scleral findings in uveal effusion syndrome. Am J Ophthalmol 1988;106:139–46.
885. Fukuchi T, Sawaguchi S, Honda T, et al. Proteoglycan abnormality in a nanophthalmos sclera. J Jpn Ophthalmol Soc 1993;97:260–7.
886. Shiono T, Shoji A, Mutoh T, et al. Abnormal sclerocytes in nanophthalmos. Graefes Arch Clin Exp Ophthalmol 1992;230:348–51.
887. Stewart III DH, Streeten BW, Brockhurst RJ, et al. Abnormal scleral collagen in nanophthalmos; an ultrastructural study. Arch Ophthalmol 1991;109:1017–25.
888. Yue BYJT, Duvall J, Goldberg MF, et al. Nanophthalmic sclera; morphologic and tissue culture studies. Ophthalmology 1986;93:534–41.
889. Yue BYJT, Kurosawa A, Duvall J, et al. Nanophthalmic sclera; fibronectin studies. Ophthalmology 1988;95:56–60.
890. Gass JDM. Uveal effusion syndrome: A new hypothesis concerning pathogenesis and technique of surgical treatment. Trans Am Ophthalmol Soc 1983;81:246–60.
891. Vine AK. Uveal effusion in Hunter's syndrome; evidence that abnormal sclera is responsible for the uveal effusion syndrome. Retina 1986;6:57–60.
892. Brockhurst RJ. Nanophthalmos with uveal effusion; a new clinical entity. Arch Ophthalmol 1975;93:1289–99.
893. Brubaker RF, Pederson JE. Ciliochoroidal detachment. Surv Ophthalmol 1983;27:281–9.
894. Calhoun Jr FP. The management of glaucoma in nanophthalmos. Trans Am Ophthalmol Soc 1975;73:97–119.
895. Ryan EA, Zwaan J, Chylack Jr LT. Nanophthalmos with uveal effusion; clinical and embryologic considerations. Ophthalmology 1982;89:1013–7.
896. Shaffer RN. Discussion of Calhoun EP Jr: The management of glaucoma in nanophthalmos. Trans Am Ophthalmol Soc 1975;73:119–20.
897. Guyton AC. Textbook of medical physiology, 6th ed. Philadelphia: WB Saunders; 1981. p. 373.
898. McGetrick JJ, Wilson DG, Dortzbach RK, et al. A search for lymphatic drainage in the monkey orbit. Arch Ophthalmo 1989;107:255–60.
899. Bill A, Phillips CI. Uveoscleral drainage of aqueous humour in human eyes. Exp Eye Res 1971;12:275–81.
900. Pederson JE, Discussion of Bellows AR, Chylack Jr LT, Hutchinson BT. Choroidal detachment: clinical manifestation, therapy and mechanism of formation. Ophthalmology 1981;88: 1114–15.
901. Trelstad RL, Silbermann NN, Brockhurst RJ. Nanophthalmic sclera; ultrastructural, histochemical, and biochemical observations. Arch Ophthalmol 1982;100:1935–8.
902. Wing GL, Schepens CL, Trempe CL, et al. Serous choroidal detachment and the thickened-choroid sign detected by ultrasonography. Am J Ophthalmol 1982;94:499–505.
903. Peyman GA, Mafee M, Schulman J. Computed tomography in choroidal detachment. Ophthalmology 1984;91:156–62.
904. Allen KM, Meyers SM, Zegarra H. Nanophthalmic uveal effusion. Retina 1988;8:145–7.
905. Casswell AG, Gregor ZJ, Bird AC. The surgical management of uveal effusion syndrome. Eye 1987;1:115–9.
906. Jin JC, Anderson DR. Laser and unsutured sclerotomy in nanophthalmos. Am J Ophthalmol 1990;109:575–80.
907. Johnson MW, Gass JDM. Surgical management of the idiopathic uveal effusion syndrome. Ophthalmology 1990;97:778–85.
908. Brockhurst RJ. Cataract surgery in nanophthalmic eyes. Arch Ophthalmol 1990;108:965–7.
909. Guerry III D, Harbison JW, Wiesinger H. Bilateral choroidal detachment and fluctuating proptosis secondary to bilateral dural arteriovenous fistulas treated with transcranial orbital decompression with resolution: Report of a case. Trans Am Ophthalmol Soc 1975;73:64–73.
910. Harbison JW, Guerry D, Wiesinger H. Dural arteriovenous fistula and spontaneous choroidal detachment: new cause of an old disease. Br J Ophthalmol 1978;62:483–90.
911. DeLuise VP, Clark III SW, Smith JLS, et al. Syphilitic retinal detachment and uveal effusion. Am J Ophthalmol 1982;94:757–61.
912. Sneed SR, Byrne SF, Mieler WF, et al. Choroidal detachment associated with malignant choroidal tumors. Ophthalmology 1991;98:963–70.
913. Scheider A, Asiyo M, Habersetzer K. Seröse Ablatio retinae unter O2-Therapie bei primärer pulmonaler Hypertonie. Fortschr Ophthalmol 1991;88:346–9.
914. Bellows AR, Chylack Jr LT, Hutchinson BT. Choroidal detachment; clinical manifestation, therapy and mechanism of formation. Ophthalmology 1981;88:1107–15.
915. Dotan S, Oliver M. Shallow anterior chamber and uveal effusion after nonperforating trauma to the eye. Am J Ophthalmol 1982;94:782–4.
916. Topilow HW, Ackerman AL. Massive exudative retinal and choroidal detachments following scleral buckling surgery. Ophthalmology 1983;90:143–7.
917. Ruiz RS, Salmonsen PC. Expulsive choroidal effusion; a complication of intraocular surgery. Arch Ophthalmol 1976;94:69–70.
918. Savir H. Expulsive choroidal effusion during cataract surgery (in a case with Fuchs' heterochromic cyclitis). Ann Ophthalmol 1979;11:113–5.
919. Weiter JJ, Brockhurst RJ, Tolentino FI. Uveal effusion following pan-retinal photocoagulation. Ann Ophthalmol 1979;11:1723–7.
920. MacKay CJ, Shek MS, Carr RE, et al. Retinal degeneration with nanophthalmos, cystic macular degeneration, and angle closure glaucoma; a new recessive syndrome. Arch Ophthalmol 1987;105:366–71.
921. Krohn J, Bjune C. Uveal effusion and angle-closure glaucoma in primary pulmonary hypertension. Am J Ophthalmol 2003;135:705–6.
922. Saran BR, Brucker AJ, Bandello F, et al. Familial primary pulmonary hypertension and associated ocular findings. Retina 2001;21:34–9.
923. Bhan A, Rennie IG, Higenbottam TW. Central retinal vein occlusion associated with primary pulmonary hypertension. Retina 2001;21:83–5.
924. Akduman L, Del Priore LV, Kaplan HJ, et al. Uveal effusion syndrome associated with primary pulmonary hypertension and vomiting. Am J Ophthalmol 1996;121:578–80.
925. Van Camp G, Renard M, Verougstraete C, et al. Ophthalmologic complications in primary pulmonary hypertension. Chest 1990;98:1543–4.
926. Yang S, Jeong J, Kim JG, et al. Progressive venous stasis retinopathy and open-angle glaucoma associated with primary pulmonary hypertension. Ophthalmic Surg Lasers Imaging 2006;37:230–3.
927. Thomas AQ, Gaddipati R, Newman JH, et al. Genetics of primary pulmonary hypertension. Clin Chest Med. 2001;22:477–91, ix.
928. Mandegar M, Fung YC, Huang W, et al. Cellular and molecular mechanisms of pulmonary vascular remodeling: role in the development of pulmonary hypertension. Microvasc Res 2004;68:75–103.
929. Launay D, Mouthon L, Hachulla E, et al. Prevalence and characteristics of moderate to severe pulmonary hypertension in systemic sclerosis with and without interstitial lung disease. J Rheumatol 2007;34:1005–11.
930. Lehrman S, Romano P, Frishman W, et al. Primary pulmonary hypertension and cor pulmonale. Cardiol Rev 2002;10:265–78.
931. Rudarakanchana N, Trembath RC, Morrell NW. New insights into the pathogenesis and treatment of primary pulmonary hypertension. Thorax 2001;56:888–90.
932. Lang G, Klepetko W. Lung transplantation for end-stage primary pulmonary hypertension. Ann Transplant 2004;9:25–32.
933. Trulock EP. Lung transplantation for primary pulmonary hypertension. Clin Chest Med 2001;22:583–93.
934. Speaker MG, Guerriero PN, Met JA, et al. A case-control study of risk factors for intraoperative suprachoroidal expulsive hemorrhage. Ophthalmology 1991;98:202–10.
935. Kuhn F, Morris R, Mester V. Choroidal detachment and expulsive choroidal hemorrhage. Ophthalmol Clin North Am 2001;14:639–50.
936. Augsburger JJ, Coats TD, Lauritzen K. Localized suprachoroidal hematomas; ophthalmoscopic features, fluorescein angiography, and clinical course. Arch Ophthalmol 1990;108:968–72.
937. Hoffman P, Pollack A, Oliver M. Limited choroidal hemorrhage associated with intracapsular cataract extraction. Arch Ophthalmol 1984;102:1761–5.
938. Morgan CM, Gragoudas ES. Limited choroidal hemorrhage mistaken for a choroidal melanoma. Ophthalmology 1987;94:41–6.
939. Williams DF, Mieler WF, Lewandowski M. Resolution of an apparent choroidal melanoma. Retina 1989;9:131–5.
940. Gressel MG, Parrish 2nd RK. Fluorouracil and suprachoroidal hemorrhage. Arch Ophthalmol 1987;105:169.
941. Ruderman JM, Harbin Jr TS, Campbell DG. Postoperative suprachoroidal hemorrhage following filtration procedures. Arch Ophthalmol 1986;104:201–5.
942. Gressel MG, Parrish 2nd RK, Heuer DK. Delayed nonexpulsive suprachoroidal hemorrhage. Arch Ophthalmol 1984;102:1757–60.

CHORIORETINAL FOLDS

Any condition causing a reduction in the area of the inner surface of the sclera (scleral thickening or scleral shrinkage) will cause the inner portion of the choroid, including Bruch's membrane, the overlying retinal pigment epithelium (RPE), and the outer retinal layers, to be thrown into a series of folds or wrinkles.[1–12] Indentation of the sclera by scleral depression or by an orbital tumor in the absence of scleral thickening or shrinkage does not produce chorioretinal folds. Choroidal thickening by congestion alone or by choroidal inflammatory or neoplastic infiltration may or may not cause chorioretinal folds.[13–15] The terms "choroidal folds," "choroidal striae," or, more accurately, "chorioretinal folds" are used to refer to those folds that produce a characteristic ophthalmoscopic, biomicroscopic, and fluorescein angiographic appearance in the fundus (Figures 4.01–4.05). Figures 4.01F, 4.02B and C; and 4.03 H illustrate diagrammatically and photomicrographically the histopathologic configuration of these folds.[5,11,16]

Acutely acquired chorioretinal folds usually produce visual dysfunction caused by distortion by the overlying retinal receptors. Most patients with long-standing idiopathic folds, however, are typically asymptomatic, have excellent visual acuity, and may show no evidence of metamorphopsia on the Amsler grid (Figure 4.01A–D). Chorioretinal folds produce alternate yellow and dark streaks, which often involve the posterior pole of the eye (Figure 4.01). These folds may have a horizontal, oblique, or vertical orientation (Figure 4.01) and are generally roughly parallel to each other. They may, however, have an irregular (Figure 4.01H) or a radiating pattern (Figure 4.04D–F). The longer the duration of the folds, the more prominent they appear. Biomicroscopy reveals that the elevated portion, or crest, of the folds appears yellow in contrast to the darker appearance of the relative narrow trough between the folds. The retina, particularly its outer layers, may or may not mirror precisely the contours of the choroidal and RPE folds. The retina in the central macula is often thrown into a stellate pattern of folds.

Characteristic changes in the background choroidal fluorescence are caused by folding of the choroid and RPE (Figures 4.01 and 4.03–4.06). Figure 4.02 depicts schematically the histopathologic changes occurring in the RPE and choroid that account for the various angiographic patterns seen in chorioretinal folds. Intensification of the choroidal fluorescence occurs along the crest of the choroidal and RPE folds and produces a series of relatively hyperfluorescent streaks that are evident as early as the arterial phase. The hyperfluorescent streaks are caused by the relative normality or slight thinness of the RPE on the crest, the greater thickness of the pool of choroidal dye beneath the crest, and the shorter course of the incident blue and reflected yellow-green light through the RPE on the crest compared to that in the trough. This pattern of fluorescence remains constant, but the degree of fluorescence gradually fades along with the background fluorescence, usually within 1 hour. The troughs of the folds appear hypofluorescent. In some cases the choroidal folds are quite broad and the troughs between them may be narrow (Figures 4.03B and E and 4.04B). This results in the angiographic finding of narrow dark lines running within a background of normal or slightly intensified background choroidal fluorescence (Figures 4.01E and 4.03B and E). Indocyanine green angiography also demonstrates the lines; however the hyperfluorescent lines appear to be broader than they appear on fluorescein angiography.[17,18]

4.01 Idiopathic chorioretinal folds.

A–C: This 49-year-old man has bilateral idiopathic folds (A). He complained of difficulty with reading. Visual acuity was 20/20 right eye, 20/25 left eye. The refractive error changed from −0. 25 to +0.75 over 5 years in each eye for distance with a +2.25 add in both eyes. There was no distortion on the Amsler grid. Stereoangiograms show hyperfluorescence corresponding with the yellow elevated folds (B and C).
D and E: Bilateral idiopathic folds. Angiography showed evidence of the folds as well as evidence of retinal pigment epithelial fibrous metaplasia and degenerative changes simulating angioid streaks (arrows, E).
F: Histopathology of chorioretinal folds (arrow). Note proliferative changes and reduplication of the basement membrane.
G: Vertically oriented folds.
H: Irregularly oriented folds.
I and J: Blurred vision occurred in this woman with bilateral idiopathic folds because of development of a choroidal neovascular membrane in the right eye (arrow, J).
K and L: Serous macular detachment occurred in the left eye of this woman. Angiography (L) demonstrated a focal leak but no definite evidence of subretinal neovascularization.

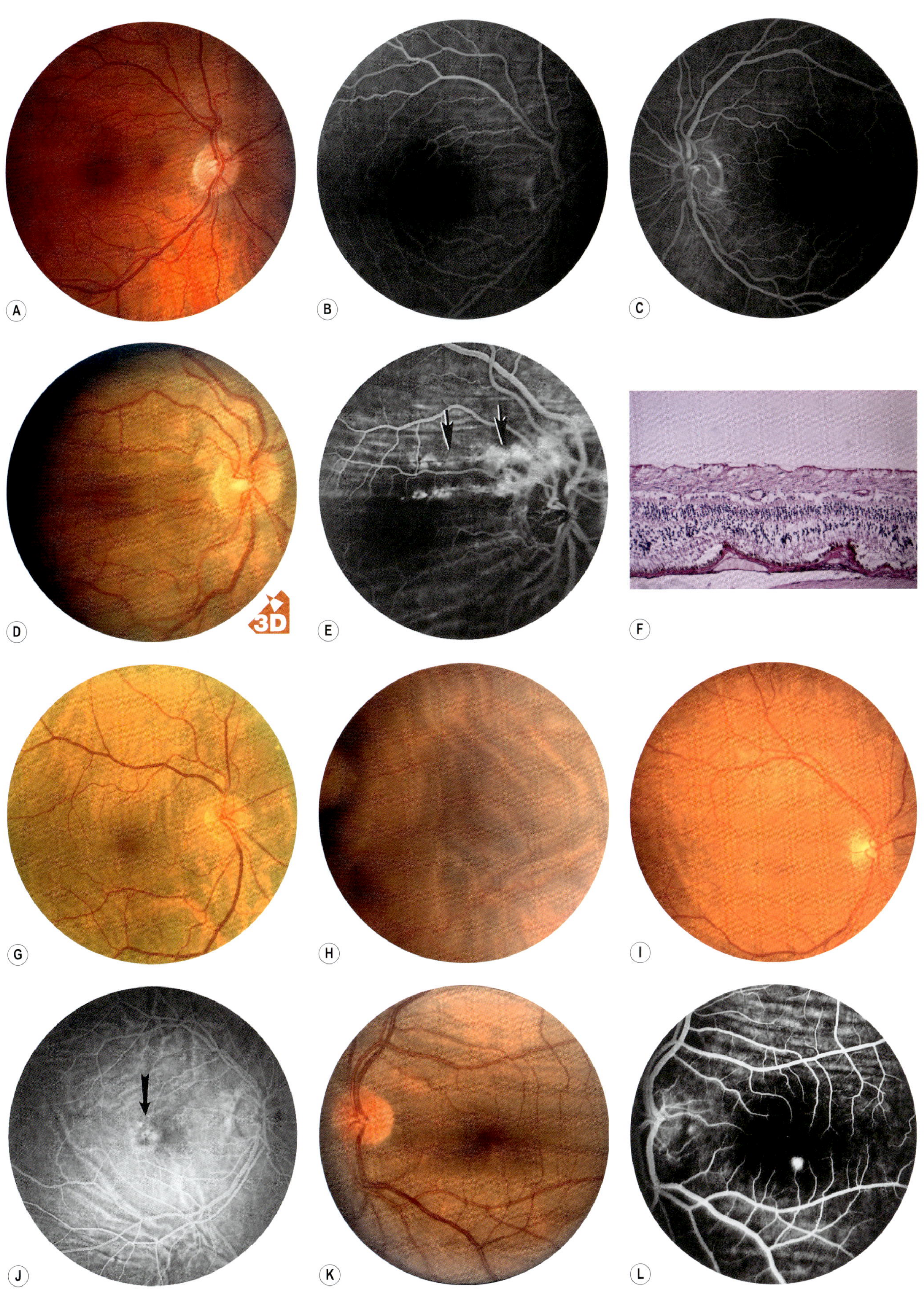
A
B
C
D
3D
E
F
G
H
I
J
K
L

Angiography is helpful in demonstrating these folds, which, if only mildly developed, may be overlooked. It is also helpful in detection of proliferative and metaplastic RPE changes (Figure 4.01E), drusen formation, focal RPE leaks, and choroidal neovascularization that may occur occasionally along these folds (Figure 4.01I and J).[19] Angiography is also useful in differentiating folds of the choroid and RPE from folds in the retina, which do not alter background fluorescence (Figure 4.06E and I). Autofluorescence imaging also demonstrates the chorioretinal folds with the color of the lines being most often opposite to the lines seen on angiography. The crests appear dark or hypoautofluorescent due to stretching of the pigment epithelium and spread of the RPE pigment while the troughs appear hyperautofluorescent due to crowding of the pigment in the pigment epithelium (Figure 4.02J and K). Autofluorescence is rapid and noninvasive and can replace fluorescein angiography. It is especially useful in monitoring folds that are expected to resolve, such as after correction of hypotony, resolution of choroidal detachments, and so forth.

Ultrasonography usually demonstrates some flattening and thickening of the posterior sclera and choroid in the area of extensive chorioretinal folding (Figure 4.04G).[20,21] Atta and Byrne studied 31 eyes with folds in 24 patients and found that over 60% had flattening of the posterior ocular wall, 40% had thickening of the retinochoroidal layer, and 25% had distended optic nerve sheaths.[20] Computed tomography of patients with idiopathic acquired folds also reveals flattening of the posterior globe and mild to moderate enlargement of the optic nerve sheaths.[21,22]

Causes of Chorioretinal Folds

Idiopathic Chorioretinal Folds

Idiopathic chorioretinal folds are most frequently encountered as an incidental finding in predominantly male patients, who are seen because of presbyopia and who have normal or near normal visual acuity. These patients typically have hyperopia that may vary from 1 to 6 D or more. When the folds occur in the macular region, they are often roughly horizontal in their course or may radiate outward from the optic disc (Figure 4.01). They may involve most of the posterior pole of the eye. Frequently, they are confined to an area either above or below the macula and optic disc. In such cases their course is often irregularly oblique. Their distribution in both eyes is

4.02 Chorioretinal folds.

Schematic diagram correlating the histopathologic and fluorescein angiographic changes caused by wrinkling of the choroid and retinal pigment epithelium (RPE). The yellow color in each diagram represents fluorescein dye in the choroid.

A: Normal relationship of the RPE to the choroid (CH) and sclera (SC).

B: Slight wrinkling of Bruch's membrane and RPE that may produce little or no change in the background choroidal fluorescence.

C: More marked folding in the choroid and RPE. The RPE on the crest of the fold is relatively thinned (left arrow) and transmits the background choroidal fluorescence better than the compressed RPE in the troughs of the folds (right arrow; Figure 4.01A–C).

D: Broad choroidal folds with relatively narrowed troughs. There is compression and heaping-up of the RPE in the trough (right arrow). The RPE over the center of the folds may be relatively normal or show some loss of pigmentation (left arrow; Figure 4.01D and E).

E: After resolution of the choroidal folds, linear lines of hyperpigmentation (arrow) may remain in the region of the previous troughs and cause dark lines angiographically.

F and G: A 58-year-old male with bilateral idiopathic folds and organ transplant retinopathy secondary to a renal transplant. Note the orange flecks in the right eye (arrows). He underwent focal laser to a leak along the ST (superotemporal) arcade.

H and I: Fluorescein angiogram a year later shows alternate light and dark lines and hypofluorescence of the two sites of laser photocoagulation in the right eye.

J and K: Increased autofluorescent lines correspond to the dark lines on the angiogram in both eyes. The pigment epithelial alterations in the peripapillary region secondary to the chronic ICSC (idiopathic central serous chorioretinopathy)/organ transplant retinopathy are seen as triradiate hypoautofluorescence around an increased autofluorescent center opposite to the colors on an angiogram.

(A–E, from Gass.[5])

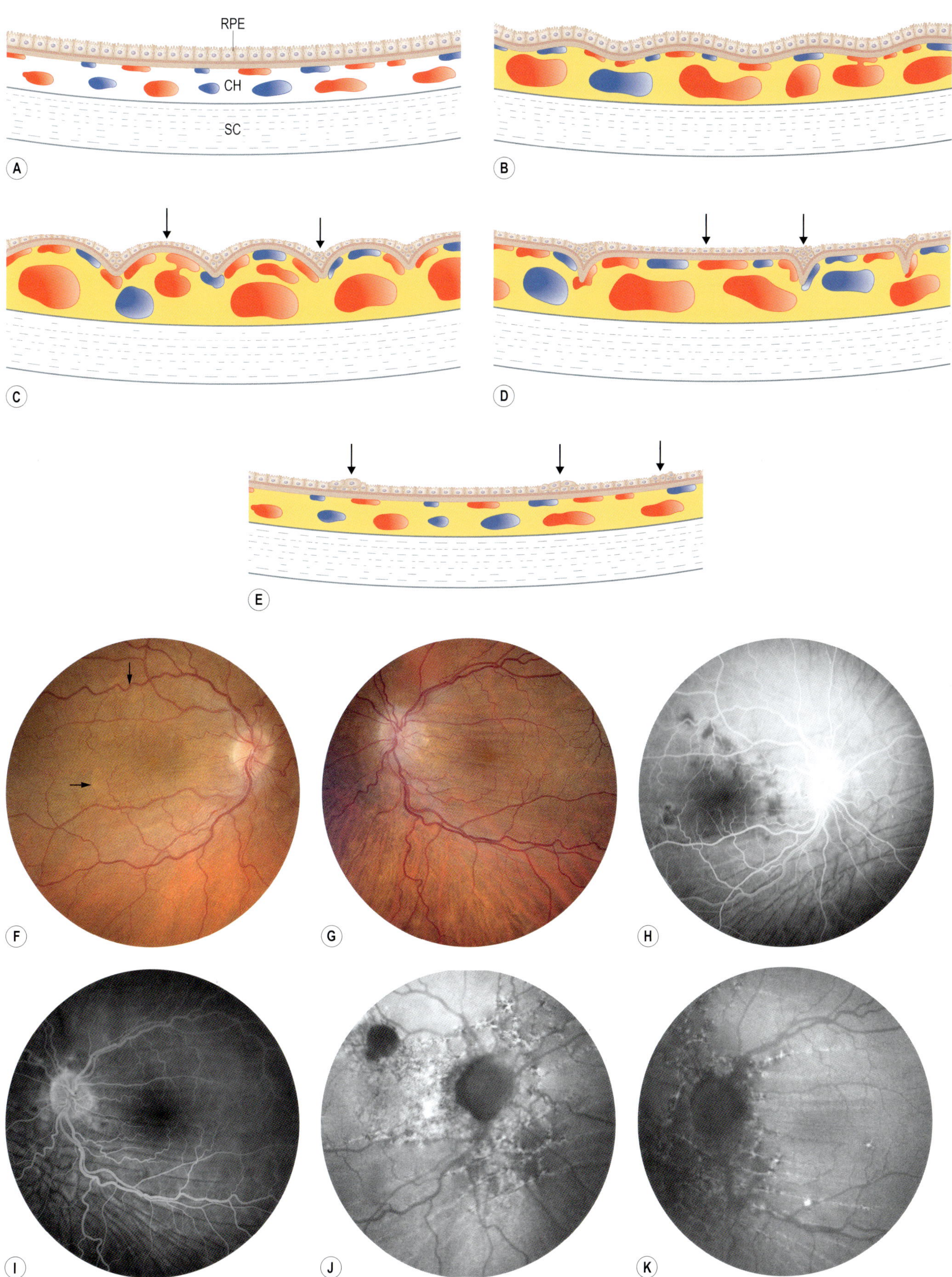

RPE
CH
SC
A
B
C
D
E
F
G
H
I
J
K

usually symmetric. They may be confined to one eye in some cases. Acquisition of folds in the second eye may occur during observation. Idiopathic central serous retinopathy occasionally occurs in these patients (Figure 4.02F–K; see Chapter 3 for discussion of associated findings in ICSC). Since in the embryonic development of the eye, the choroid should adapt itself to developing sclera in such a way that folds do not occur and since most patients with high hyperopia do not have chorioretinal folds, it is probable that these folds are acquired.[4,9,22–24] Some patients experience rather sudden change in vision, suggesting that scleral shortening may occur abruptly in some cases in the absence of any other signs of orbital inflammatory reaction.[8,24] It is likely that some inflammatory process affecting the posterior sclera, either in late prenatal life or some time during childhood in the absence of clinical signs or symptoms, causes shrinkage of the fibrous tunic of the eye.[4] This would account for the hyperopia, the flattening of the posterior sclera, and the folds that remain as a permanent residue of this inflammation.

Retrobulbar Mass Lesions

Benign and malignant orbital tumors, including Erdheim–Chester disease, lymphangioma, hemangioma, orbital pseudotumor and others, as well as orbital implants for repair of orbital wall fractures, may cause only an indentation of the globe or in some cases may cause scleral edema, choroidal congestion, and chorioretinal folds (Figure 4.03A–C and 4.04 A and B).[8,25–27] The pattern and location of these folds may or may not be helpful in defining the site of the tumor.[25] Intraconal tumors often induce hyperopia, and extraconal tumors often induce astigmatism. Broad yellow chorioretinal folds should be differentiated from the finer retinal folds that may occasionally be produced by a retrobulbar mass. These latter folds produce no changes in the angiographic picture. If the retrobulbar mass is removed or otherwise treated successfully, the chorioretinal folds usually disappear (Figure 4.03A–F).[8]

Scleral Inflammation

Thickening and inflammation of the sclera in thyroid eye disease, inflammatory pseudotumor of the orbit, and rheumatoid posterior scleritis may cause chorioretinal folds (Figure 4.03A–F).

Scleral Buckle

Thickening of the sclera in the vicinity of a scleral buckle for a rhegmatogenous retinal detachment may occasionally produce chorioretinal folds, which are usually present near the posterior slope of the buckle.

Choroidal Tumors

Choroidal tumors, particularly malignant melanomas and metastatic carcinomas, may produce folds in the choroid and retina surrounding the base of the tumor (Figure 4.03G–I).[4,11,26] These folds are produced by mechanical displacement of the surrounding choroid by the expanding tumor, as well as by vascular engorgement, choroidal edema, and scleral thickening.[11]

4.03 Secondary chorioretinal folds.

A–C: Chorioretinal folds caused by an orbital inflammatory pseudotumor in a 70-year-old woman with blurred vision and proptosis of the right eye of recent onset. Note prominent broad chorioretinal folds delineated by dark lines separating the folds (black arrows, A). Note that all the retinal folds do not correspond to the folds in the choroid. Black arrow indicates a retinal fold. Fluorescein angiography shows dark lines (arrows, B) that correspond to the troughs of the choroidal folds. Ten weeks after treatment with systemic steroids the visual acuity returned to normal. The proptosis and the chorioretinal folds disappeared (C).

D–F: Chorioretinal folds and papilledema in a middle-aged woman with severe thyroid exophthalmos. Similar changes were present in the opposite eye. Angiograms showed dark lines (arrows, E) corresponding to the troughs between relatively broad choroidal folds. There was some dilation of the capillaries on the optic nerve head. Sixteen years later (F) the proptosis, chorioretinal folds, and papilledema had resolved.

G and H: Chorioretinal folds associated with a malignant melanoma of the choroid superior to the macular region (arrow, G). In the histopathologic section of choroid (H) taken just inferior to the melanoma, note configuration of the folding of the pigment epithelium, Bruch's membrane, and the inner choroidal tissue. The crest (arrow, H) corresponded to the light lines in G. The choroid was considerably engorged in this area adjacent to the intraocular tumor. There was mild scleritis.

I–L: A 73-year-old male with limited suprachoroidal hemorrhage during cataract surgery with vertically oriented folds posterior to a temporal choroidal hemorrhage. The angiogram and autofluorescence imaging show alternate dark and light lines that are opposite in colors between the two. Chorioretinal wrinkling is seen at the retinal pigment epithelium and choroid on optical coherence tomography; note the elevation of the choroid corresponding to the choroidal hemorrhage.

(A–C, from Kroll and Norton.[8])

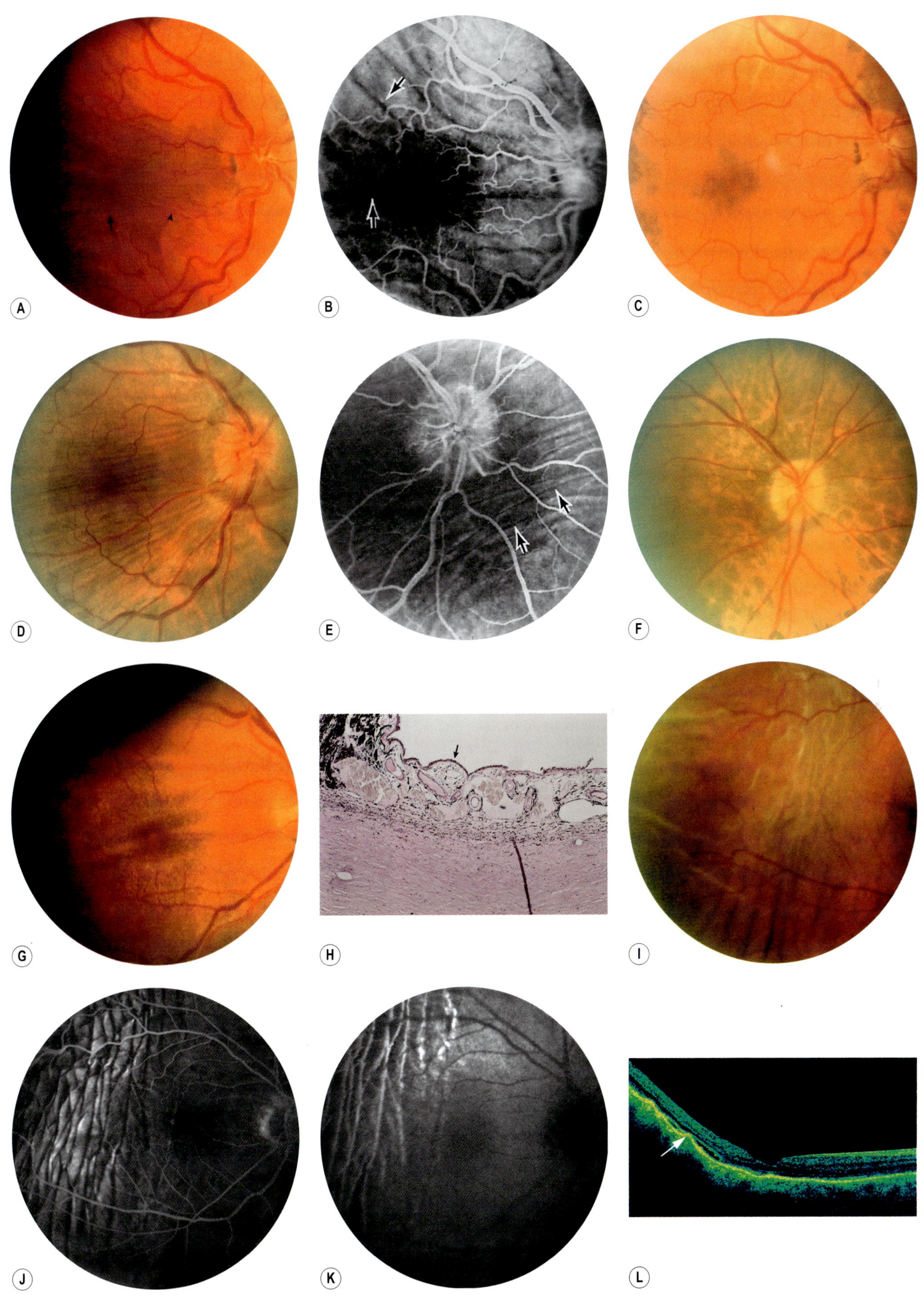
A
B
C
D
E
F
G
H
I
J
K
L

Hypotony

In some instances patients with intraocular hypotony, usually caused by a wound leak, cyclodialysis cleft, or excessive filtration after a glaucoma-filtering procedure, will develop loss of central vision secondary to marked irregular folding of the choroid, RPE, and retina.[2,5,28,29] Initially, these folds are broad and are not sharply delineated. They tend to radiate outward in a branching fashion from the optic disc temporally, whereas nasal to the disc they tend to be arranged concentrically or irregularly (Figure 4.04F and H). This difference in the pattern of the folds is probably determined partly by traction exerted nasally by the optic nerve as the eye moves.[30] There may be a broad area of swelling of the choroid surrounding the optic nerve head, which together with circumpapillary retinal folding produces a picture simulating marked papilledema. The sensory retina may be arranged into irregular folds that do not exactly parallel the choroidal and RPE folds. The sensory retina is often thrown into a series of radiating or stellate folds around the center of the fovea (Figure 4.04H). This unusual central stellate retinal wrinkling is caused by the central displacement of the normally very thick retina surrounding the very thin foveola by the thickened posterior scleral wall and engorgement of the choroid. The retinal vessels are often tortuous and sometimes engorged. Cystoid macular edema is not usually present. The primary cause of loss of visual acuity in most patients is the marked folding of the retina centrally. Shallowing of the anterior chamber caused by ciliochoroidal edema and detachment may occur. A postoperative wound leak or a cyclodialysis cleft, produced either inadvertently during an iridectomy at the time of cataract extraction or intentionally for the correction of glaucoma, were formerly the most important causes of these changes. With the development of improved techniques of wound closure and controlled trabeculectomies the incidence of hypotony maculopathy decreased dramatically during the 1980s. With the introduction of mitomycin C and 5-fluorouracil to improve the effectiveness of glaucoma-filtering procedures; however, there has been an increase in the incidence of hypotony maculopathy.[31,32] Patients with chronic hypotony caused by cyclodialysis are at risk of developing permanent anterior synechiae and intractable glaucoma after surgical closure of the cyclodialysis cleft. Early detection of the characteristic fundoscopic picture of hypotony and its causes is important because surgical correction of the cause will usually result in visual improvement. As the intraocular tension becomes normalized, the choroidal folds become flattened and may completely disappear. In cases of prolonged hypotony, however, permanent, irregularly dark, pigmented lines caused by changes in the RPE remain. These changes are often present nasally as well as in the macular area. Early in the course of hypotony, fluorescein angiography shows an irregular increase in background choroidal fluorescence corresponding to the crest of the choroidal folds and also shows some evidence of leakage of dye from the capillaries on the optic nerve head but usually not from the retinal capillaries.[5] Permanent alterations in the RPE may be demonstrable with angiography after resumption of normal intraocular pressure and marked improvement in the degree of chorioretinal wrinkling. It is not known why most eyes with the acute development of hypotony fail to develop chorioretinal folds. The maculopathy is most likely to occur in young myopic patients.[32] It is possible the sclera in young patients is more susceptible to swelling and contraction, which reduce intraocular volume and cause the redundant folds of choroid and retina to develop. The pattern of the folds cannot be explained on the basis of uveal edema alone.[29]

4.04 Secondary chorioretinal folds.

A and B: Chorioretinal folds caused by orbital infiltration by an esthesioneuroblastoma. Stereoangiograms revealed evidence of the folds in addition to many basal laminar drusen. C–E: Radial chorioretinal folds caused by contraction of a choroidal neovascular membrane (CNVM) lying beneath an exudative retinal pigment epithelium (RPE) detachment in a man with age-related macular degeneration. Angiograms showed folds and gliotic neovascular membrane (D and E). F and G: Chorioretinal wrinkling caused by hypotony in a patient following glaucoma surgery with mitomycin. Note the mild tortuosity of the retinal veins. Ultrasonography showed significant flattening of the posterior ocular wall and congested choroid. H and I: Radial, irregular, and horizontal folds in a patient with hypotony. Optical coherence tomography shows involvement of the choroid, RPE, and photoreceptors in the folds. J–L: Bilateral ischemic optic neuropathy of unknown cause in a 60-year-old woman with horizontal chorioretinal folds. Despite intensive systemic corticosteroid therapy bilateral optic atrophy occurred and visual acuity was reduced to 20/400 11 months later (I).

F and G, courtesy of Dr. Jeffrey Kammer; H and I, courtesy of Dr. Paul Sternberg, Jr.)

Choroidal Effusion

Choroidal folds are also seen posterior to choroidal elevation in patients with both serous and hemorrhagic choroidal detachments. The rapid rise in choroidal volume throws the retina and choroid posterior to this into folds that run parallel to the elevation (Figure 4.03I–K; see Chapter 3).

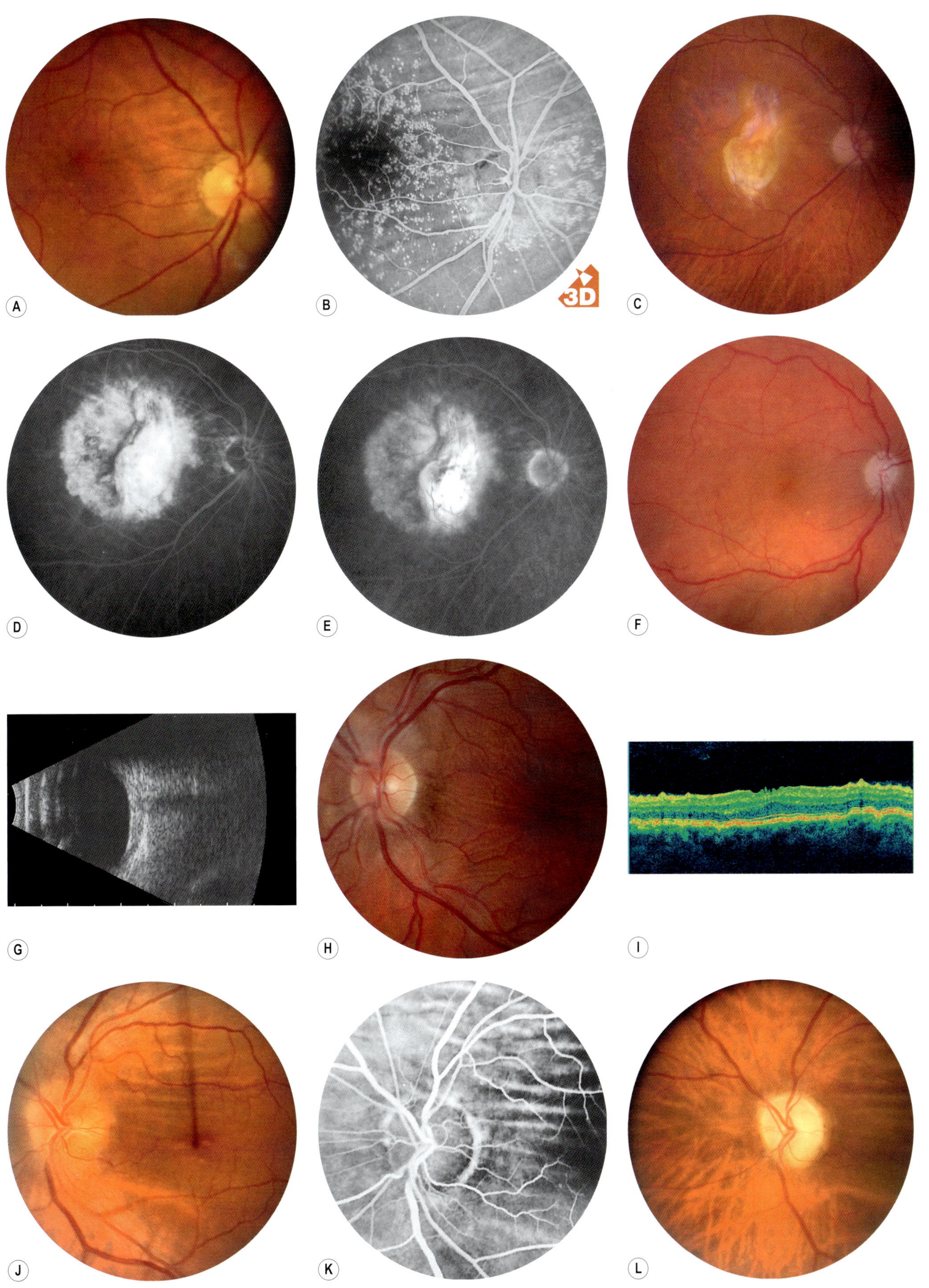
A
B
3D
C
D
E
F
G
H
I
J
K
L

Choroidal Neovascularization

Contraction of a sub-RPE choroidal neovascular complex and the underlying Bruch's membrane occurring either spontaneously or after photocoagulation may cause a radiating pattern of chorioretinal folds around the membrane (Figure 4.04C–E).[33,34] Contraction of the superficial part of a sub-RPE neovascular complex may produce a series of parallel hyperpigmented folds in the RPE overlying the neovascular complex (see discussion of occult choroidal neovascularization in age-related macular degeneration in Chapter 3). Radial chorioretinal folds are sometimes seen in association with a pigment epithelial rip following treatment with antivascular endothelial growth factor agents (Figure 4.04C–E).[35]

Vogt–Koyanagi–Harada Disease

The earliest manifestation of Harada's disease is congestion and thickening of the choroid visible as choroidal folds or striations,[13,14,36] followed by exudative retinal detachment. These striations are usually seen in the less or later involved fellow eye when the patient presents with symptoms in one eye, and can also be seen further in the disease course in areas outside the pockets of SRF (subretinal fluid). C-scan optical coherence tomography (OCT) shows these undulations on the RPE layer, which resolve once the retina flattens[13,36] (see Chapter 11).

Focal Chorioretinal Scars

Occasionally contraction of deep focal chorioretinal scars from a variety of causes at the retinal choroidal interface may cause a pattern of radiating folds. Johnson et al. observed the development of radiating folds around what they believed was a scar induced by the operating microscope.[37]

Optic Nerve Head Diseases Associated with Chorioretinal Folds

The changes in the posterior sclera responsible for shrinkage and flattening of the posterior sclera in patients with chorioretinal folds may also be responsible for reducing the diameter of the perioptic scleral ring and dura. This change may be responsible for the frequency of the "crowded disc" appearance or pseudopapilledema (Figure 4.04A and B) in these patients and for predisposing them to the development of optic disc hyaline bodies (drusen), juxtapapillary subretinal neovascularization, ischemic optic neuropathy (Figure 4.04J–L), and papilledema.[38] The small diameter of the optic disc unassociated with chorioretinal folds has been implicated in the pathogenesis of pseudopapilledema, ischemic optic neuropathy,[39,40] and hyaline bodies of the optic nerve head.[41]

Chorioretinal folds may occur in association with pseudopapilledema in patients with Alagille's syndrome (arteriohepatic dysplasia) (Figure 4.05; see Chapter 5).[7,42–47]

Chorioretinal folds often showing a horizontal course in the macula but converging on the nasal side of the optic disc have been described in association with papilledema caused by raised intracranial pressure.[48–51] The mechanism for how papilledema causes folds that extend well away from the optic disc is difficult to explain. The fact that these folds may persist after resolution of papilledema suggests that in some cases they may have been present before the development of the papilledema. Because chorioretinal folds occur with such frequency, their association with other diseases may or may not be pathogenically related.

4.05 Chorioretinal folds, pseudopapilledema, juxtapapillary chorioretinal atrophy, and streaky hypopigmentation of the retinal pigment epithelium (RPE) peripherally in arteriohepatic syndrome (Alagille's syndrome) in a father and two sons.

A–D: Note the long narrow facies of the 45-year-old father, horizontal chorioretinal folds (arrows, B and D), and streaky hypopigmentation of the RPE in the peripheral fundus (C).
E and F: The 6-year-old son. Note long facies, pseudopapilledema, and mild chorioretinal folds (arrows, F).
G–I: The 13-year-old son. Note juxtapapillary changes in the pigment epithelium, elevated nasal disc margins, and streaky depigmentation of the RPE. All three had normal visual acuity and normal electroretinograms.
J–L: Posterior embyotoxin (arrows, J and K) in a 3½-year-old child with Alagille's who died because of complications associated with hepatocellular carcinoma. Histopathologic examination revealed evidence of hypertrophy of Schwalbe's ring (arrow, K) and patchy areas of variation in the size and melanin content of the pigment epithelium (arrows, L).

(J–L, This case was presented by Dr. A.O. Jensen at the combined Verhoeff Society and European Ophthalmic Pathology Society meeting in May 1992. From Békássy et al.[43])

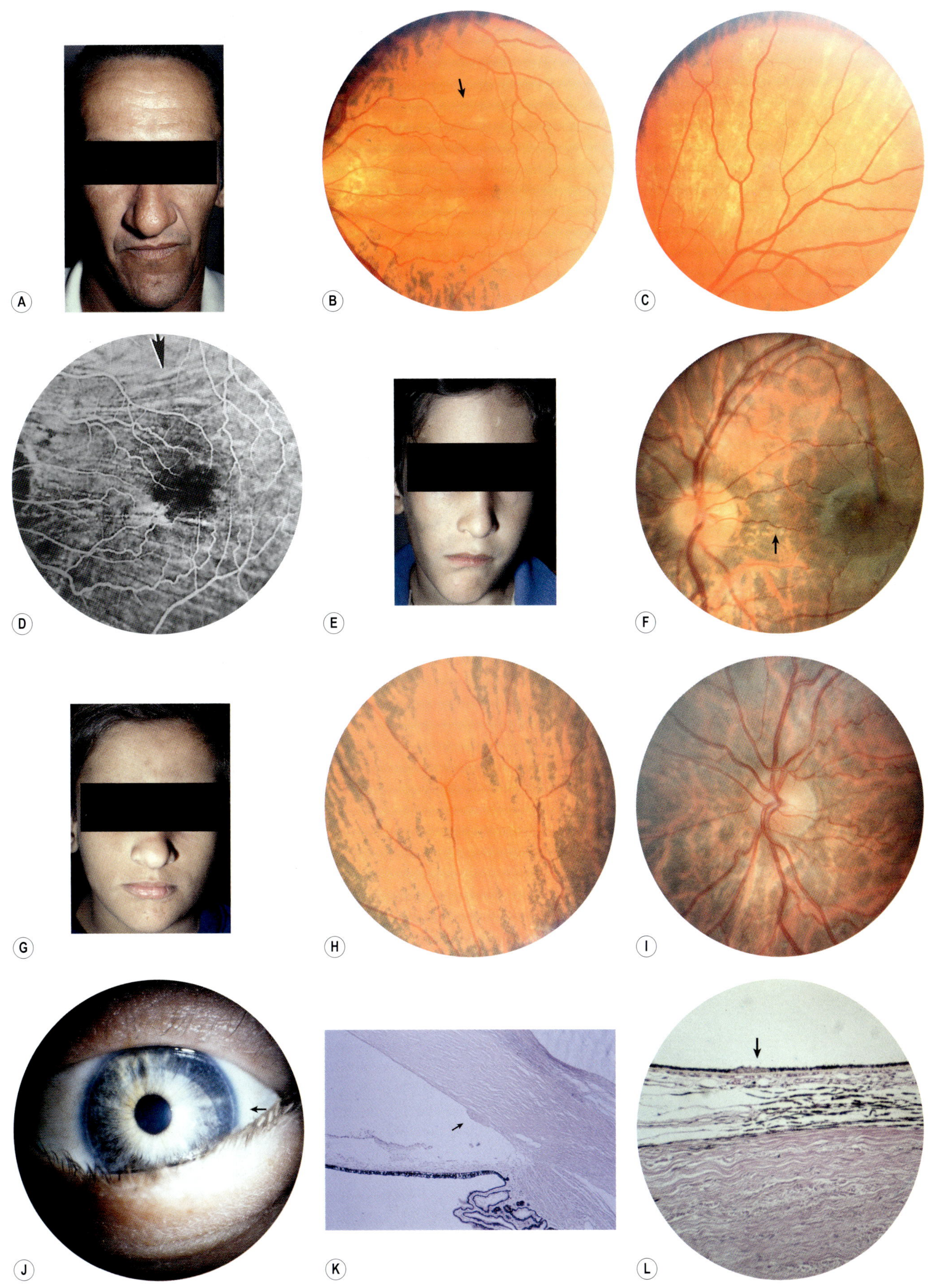
A
B
C
D
E
F
G
H
I
J
K
L

RETINAL FOLDS

Folds that involve only the neurosensory retina should be differentiated from chorioretinal folds. They may occur in a variety of circumstances and may simulate chorioretinal folds (Figure 4.06). They may be narrow and have a less striking color than chorioretinal folds. These are seen most commonly radiating away from a focal area of contraction of the inner retinal surface by an epiretinal membrane (see Chapter 7) or from an area of contraction of the outer retina in the region of a chorioretinal scar. They may occur concentrically around an acutely swollen optic nerve head, and they may be seen radiating away from the optic disc following resolution of inflammatory diseases of the nerve head and juxtapapillary choroid. A radiating pattern of retinal folds centered in the macula occurs in a variety of situations associated with uveal and scleral thickening (e.g., the uveal effusion syndrome), diffuse inflammatory cell infiltration of the choroid, scleritis, and hypotony (Figure 4.04H and I). These may or may not be associated with folds in the underlying choroid and RPE (see previous discussion of chorioretinal folds). Irregular, broad, yellowish folds involving primarily the outer layers of the neurosensory retina are often seen in bullous rhegmatogenous retinal detachments (Figure 4.06A). Prominent retinal folds extending into the macula following surgery for repair of retinal detachment may be responsible for subnormal vision. These may be caused by posterior placement of radial scleral buckles, retroretinal fibrous bands (Figure 4.06B), and folds caused by use of intravitreal gas (Figure 4.06C).[52–55] This complication is seen most commonly in patients after pars plana vitrectomy, particularly in those with subtotal retinal detachments and either internal drainage through a peripheral retinal hole or external drainage with simultaneous gas insufflation (Figure 4.06C). Figure 4.06D–F illustrates an unusual cause of transient radiating retinal folds in a patient with the acute onset of drug (chlorthalidone (Hygroton))-induced myopia.[4,56,57] Similar horizontal and radial retinal folds have occurred in the macula of patients with acutely induced myopia caused by ethoxzolamide (Cardrase), acetazolamide, acetaminophen, and hydrochlorothiazide.[58–62] In some cases, however, with acute drug-induced myopia, researchers have described no retinal changes.[63] The presence of transient radial retinal folds in these patients suggests that the drugs cause submacular edema that displaces the macula anteriorly, which might be expected to cause transient hyperopia. The greater effect of these drugs, however, is probably exerted anteriorly, where edema of the ciliary body may result in narrowing of the anterior-chamber angle, relaxation of the zonules, and increased lens curvature.

Figure 4.06G–I illustrates an unusual pattern of concentric superficial retinal folds of unknown cause occurring in both eyes of a healthy young man.

4.06 Retinal folds.

A: Outer retinal folds in a rhegmatogenous retinal detachment.
B: Prominent retinal fold caused by retroretinal fibrous band (arrows) of metaplastic retinal pigment epithelium (RPE) after scleral buckling procedure for rhegmatogenous detachment.
C: Retinal fold caused by posterior sliding of retina after vitrectomy and scleral buckling in this patient. Note two droplets of perfluorocarbon liquid under the retina temporally.
D–F: Fine retinal folds radiating outward from the macular region (D) in a 22-year-old woman who developed acute myopia while taking chlorthalidone 5 mg daily for 2 weeks, following delivery of an infant. Her uncorrected visual acuity was 20/200. With cycloplegic refraction of −4.75 in the right eye her acuity was 20/25, and with −3.75 in the left eye the acuity was 20/20. Angiography (E) was normal. The medication was stopped, and within 24 hours her uncorrected visual acuity returned to 20/15 and the retinal folds disappeared (F). Her intraocular pressure was normal before and after cessation of treatment.
G–I: An unusual concentric pattern of superficial retinal folds of unknown cause in a 20-year-old man complaining of bilateral loss of vision. His visual acuity was 6/200 in both eyes. A similar pattern of retinal folds was present in the other eye. Fluorescein angiography was normal. Neurologic examination was unremarkable. The electroretinogram was normal. Visual evoked responses were subnormal.

(C, courtesy of Dr. Baker Hubbard.)

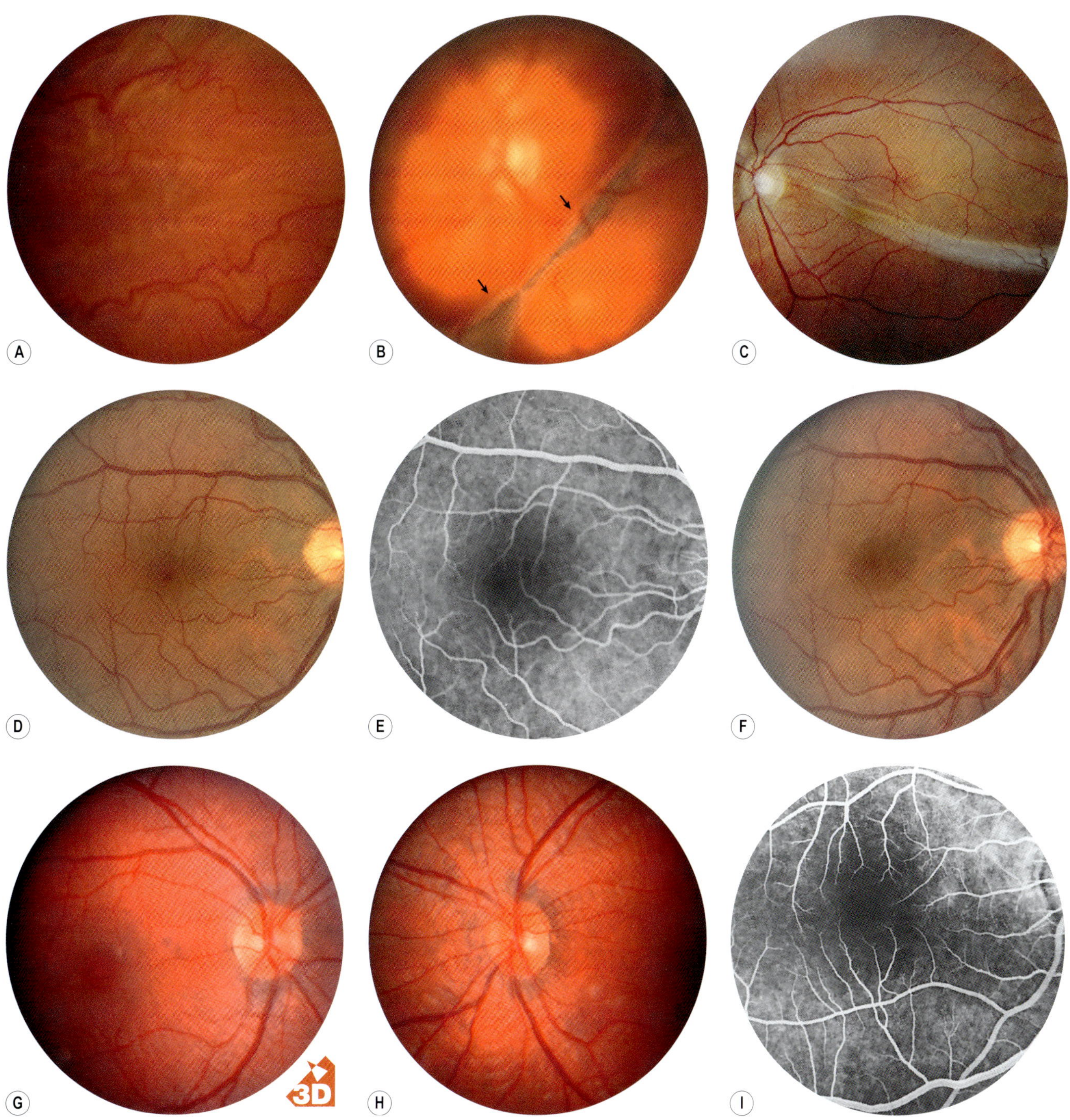
A
B
C
D
E
F
G
3D
H
I

POSTERIOR MICROPHTHALMOS

An elevated papillomacular retinal fold may occur in both eyes of patients with congenital foreshortening of the posterior ocular segment and a relatively normal anterior segment (posterior microphthalmos; Figure 4.07A–D).[64–68] The eyes are highly hyperopic (usually greater than +10.00 D), and the acuity is usually subnormal (20/30–20/400). The corneal diameter and the anterior-chamber depth are within normal limits, whereas the length of the globe from the posterior lens surface to the optic disc is shortened. Ultrasonography can measure this distance, thus confirming the clinical anomaly. Angiography reveals the absence of the retinal capillary-free zone due to crowding of the retinal elements in the fold (Figure 4.07E and F). The disorder may be inherited as an autosomal-recessive trait occurring sporadically and in siblings.[69,70] Embryologically, the retina is formed by the neuroectoderm and the mesoderm contributes to the choroid and the sclera. Since there is an anomalous paucity of the mesoderm in this condition, the normal-size neuroectoderm conforms to the shortened mesoderm thus throwing the redundant retina into a fold. Complications include uveal effusion due to the associated thickened sclera,[71] and rarely, bilateral macular holes.[72] The condition is seen worldwide and has no racial predilection.[69–77] An OCT can easily depict the fold and confirms the involvement of the neurosensory retina alone (Figure 4.07G and H).

4.07 Posterior microphthalmos.

A–F: This 22-year-old Iraqi male had poor vision in both eyes since childhood. His parents were first cousins, and he has other siblings with similar condition. His visual acuity was 20/70-2 and 20/200. He had normal corneal diameters, short axial length and high hyperopia. His refraction was +10.75 + 1.00 × 180 right eye and +12.50 + 2.00 × 170 left eye. There were typical-appearing papillomacular folds in each eye (A–D) and angiography showed an absent foveal avascular zone (E, F).

G and **H**: OCT shows the fold to involve the neurosensory retina alone sparing the pigment epithelial and photoreceptor layers.

(A–H, courtesy of Dr. William F. Mieler and Dr. Felix Y. Chau.)

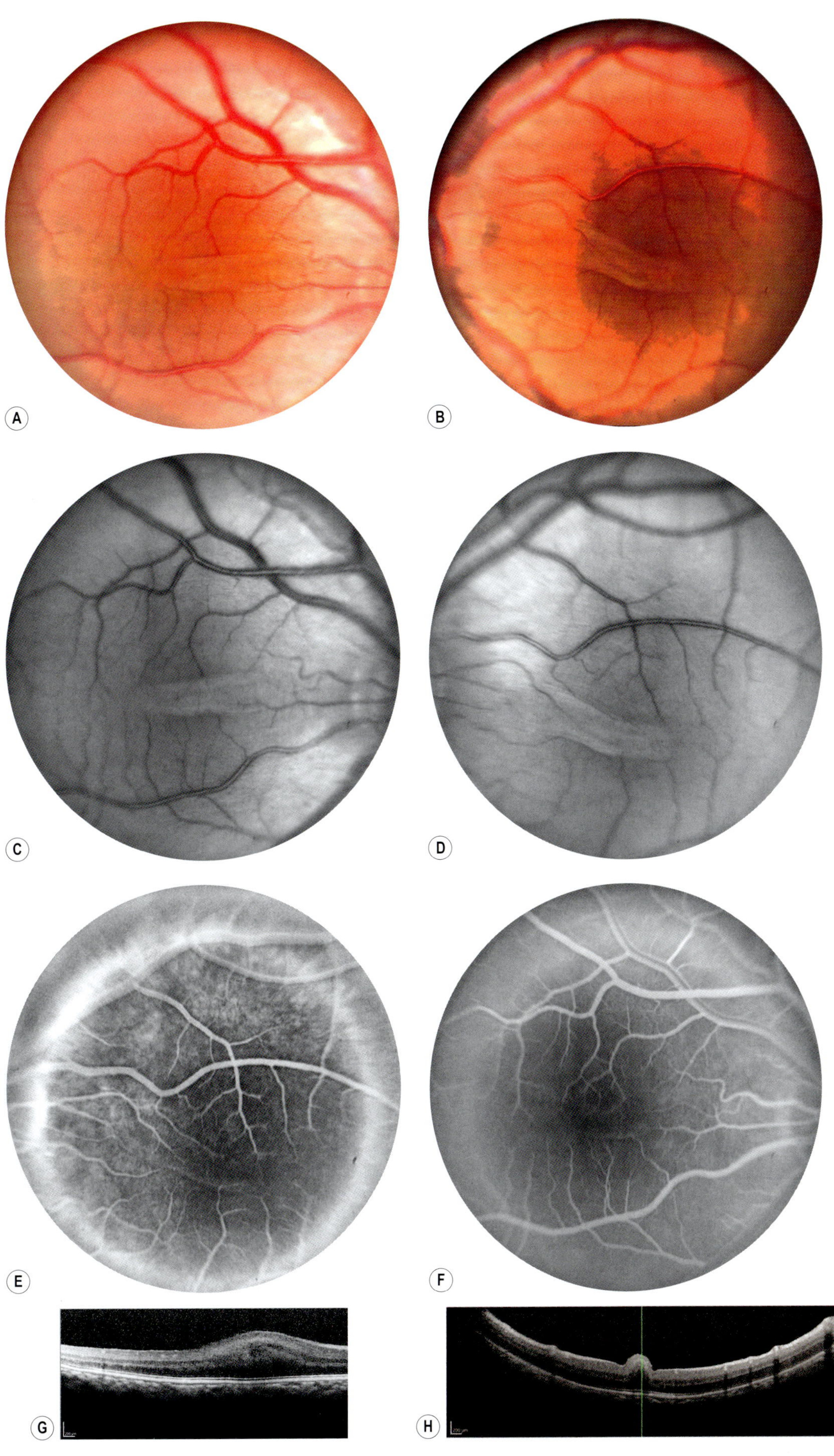
A
B
C
D
E
F
G
H

OUTER RETINAL CORRUGATIONS IN JUVENILE X-LINKED RETINOSCHISIS

These "flying seagull"-appearing corrugations are seen in some cases of X-linked juvenile retinoschisis[78–80] (Figure 4.08A, C, and D). They are seen most often temporal to the macula, except in one case where they were present all around the macula. Stratus OCT has demonstrated these corrugations to be in the outer retina (photoreceptors and outer plexiform layer) (Figure 4.08E and F); the newer high-definition OCT should be able to delineate these folds better. The corrugations can change in orientation and even disappear (Figure 4.08G), hence are speculated to be caused by tautness of the adjacent retina to changes in the height of the macular schisis.

NONACCIDENTAL AND ACCIDENTAL TRAUMA

Perimacular retinal folds are seen in nonaccidental trauma (shaken-baby syndrome) and some cases of severe accidental trauma, which result in extensive retinal hemorrhages, intracranial bleeds, and severe raised intracranial pressures.[81–84] Though initially attributed solely to nonaccidental trauma, these folds are seen at the periphery of a dome-shaped retinoschisis that involves the macula. The severe rise in intracranial pressure transmits the pressure through the perineural sheaths resulting in shearing of the retinal vessels in all layers, causing bleeding and extravasation of fluid to separate the retinal layers[84] (see Chapter 8).

4.08 Outer retinal corrugations.

A–C: Sibling 1: 17-year-old male with rapid change in vision in both eyes from 20/25 to 20/50 right eye and 20/70 left eye over 3 months. Both eyes show macular schisis with fine radiating retinal folds. Temporal to the macula are "flying seagull"-like outer retinal corrugations. Fluorescein angiogram barely shows a change corresponding to the corrugations (arrows).
D: Sibling 2: 15-year-old younger brother had presented at age 11 with similar fundus appearance of foveal schisis and outer retinal corrugations.
E and F: Optical coherence tomography demonstrates the corrugations in the outer retina in sibling 1.
G: The corrugations disappeared by age 15 in sibling 2.

(A–G, From Agarwal and Rao[79])

POST MACULAR TRANSLOCATION SURGERY

Limited translocation surgery for macular degeneration and scars involves deliberate detachment of the retina by injecting subretinal balanced salt solution and imbricating the sclera to foreshorten it, followed by flattening the retina with air or gas.[85–87] This maneuver shifts the macular neurosensory retina inferiorly, displacing it to overlie a normal RPE base. Often this results in a retinal fold to accommodate the redundant retina.[85,87–89] Retinal folds are seen occasionally in complete translocations also.

Unlike folds involving the choroid and RPE, folds of the neurosensory retina are not evident angiographically (Figures 4.06E and I and 4.07E and F).

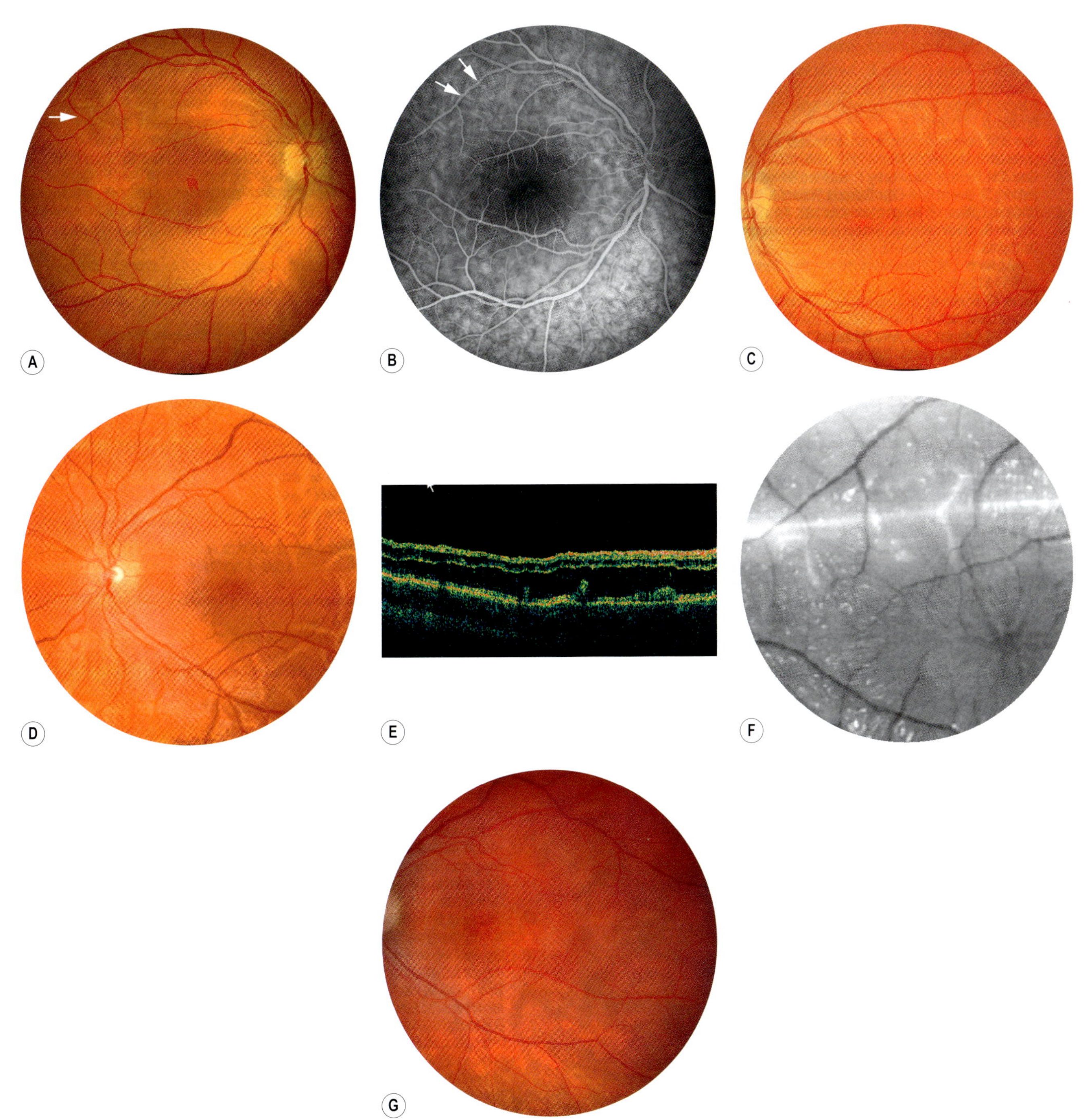
A
B
C
D
E
F
G

Some of the heredodystrophic disorders appear to affect primarily the retinal pigment epithelium (RPE) and only secondarily the retina (e.g., Best's disease). Others, such as retinitis pigmentosa, appear to affect both layers equally; still others affect primarily the sensory retina (e.g., cone dystrophies and the sphingolipidoses). Some affect primarily central vision, whereas others may affect most of the visual field. Several heredodystrophic diseases that may prove to affect primarily the RPE and retina are frequently associated with drusen and disciform detachment (dominantly inherited exudative drusen; basal laminar drusen; North Carolina dystrophy and macular staphyloma).

BEST'S DISEASE

Best's disease (vitelliform macular dystrophy) is an autosomal-dominantly inherited disorder with variable penetrance and expressivity.[1–27] Linkage analysis has mapped the gene for Best's disease for pedigrees in Sweden and Iowa to chromosome 11q13.[28–30] The gene responsible for BVMD was cloned by Petrukhin and colleagues in 1998 and named the *Bestrophin1* (*BEST1*) gene.[31] It consisits of 11 exons and 585 amino acids and spans 15 kilobases of genomic DNA. The gene is expressed predominantly in the RPE cells and the bestrophin protein is located mainly on the basolateral plasma membrane of the RPE and to a small extent within the RPE cells. The protein is believed to function as an intracellular Ca^{2+}-dependent Cl^- channel and an HCO_3^- channel.[32–35] Disruption of the ion conductance across the RPE by abnormal bestrophin1 is likely responsible for the absence of light peak response in the electro-oculogram (EOG) in both patients and unaffected carriers of Best's disease.[14,19,26,36,37] The disease appears to affect primarily the RPE.

Previtelliform or Carrier Stage

Although vitelliform lesions have been observed as early as the first week of life, the fundi of most patients probably are normal during the first few months or years of life (Figures 5.01A and 5.02A). Many carriers never manifest a change in the fundus.

5.01 Best's disease.

A–C: Changes occurring over a 21-year period in this 27-year-old man with Best's disease. His fundi were considered as normal at age 4 years (A). At age 7 years, he had developed a typical vitelliform lesion in both macular areas (B). Visual acuity was 20/30 and J-1 in both eyes. At age 27 his visual acuity was 20/30 right eye and 20/25 left eye (C).

D–F: The brother of the patient illustrated in A–C was 10 years old when his fundi showed partly scrambled vitelliform lesions (D). His visual acuity in the right eye was 20/15. At age 12 years, he returned complaining of blurred vision in his right eye. Note the submacular hemorrhage (E). Angiogram showed evidence of a choroidal neovascular membrane. At age 30 years his visual acuity was 20/50 right eye and 20/20 left eye. Note the white subretinal scar in F.

G and **H**: A 19-year-old boy with Best's disease who complained of blurred vision in both eyes. His electro-oculographic findings were 1.00 in both eyes. Four months later the vitelliform lesions and surrounding retinal detachment (G) had disappeared (H). Visual acuity was 20/20.

I and **J**: This 13-year-old female had bilaterally symmetric vitelliform macular lesions and a visual acuity of 20/15. Angiograms showed minimal fluorescence of both eye lesions (probably pseudofluorescence corresponding to the vitelliform lesion) (J).

K and **L**: A vitelliform lesion was present in both eyes of this 9-year-old boy (K), and in the right eye (L) of his 73-year-old grandfather who had a scar in the left macula.

(G and H courtesy of Dr. Mark J. Daily; K and L courtesy of Dr. Michael W. Hines.)

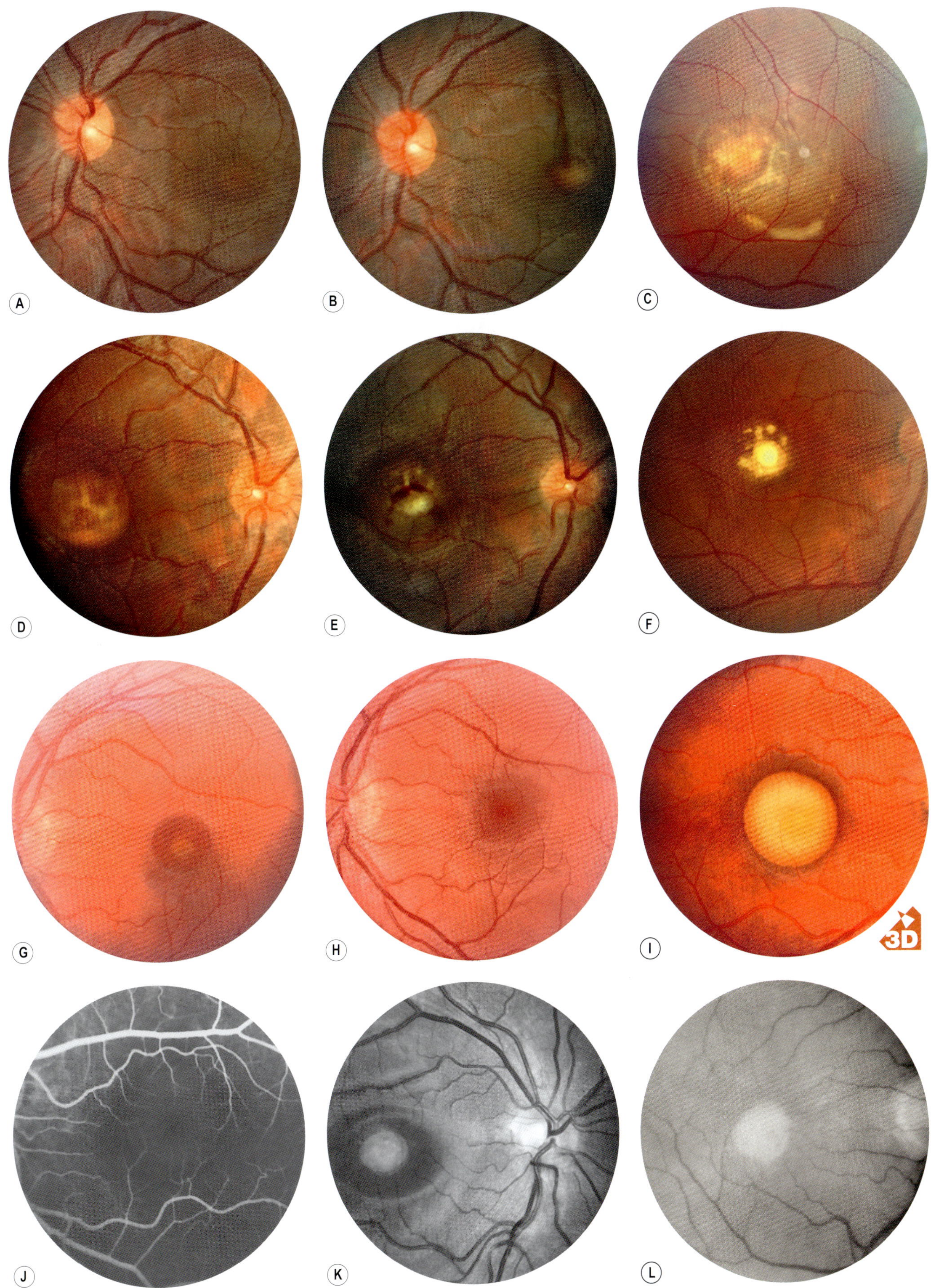
A
B
C
D
E
F
G
H
I
3D
J
K
L

Vitelliform Stage

In infancy or in early childhood patients may develop a sharply circumscribed subretinal lesion that has been likened to the yolk of a sunny-side-up fried egg (Figures 5.01B and I, 5.02A, and 5.03G). Visual acuity at this stage of the disease is usually normal. Biomicroscopy and stereophotography reveal a discrete lesion beneath the retina that is ½–2 disc diameters in size, yellowish, and usually round or oval. Early in the disease, little or no elevation of the retina occurs. Subsequently the lesion appears elevated as the yellow material increases in amount, and is found in the outer photoreceptor zone, subretinal space, and within the RPE layer.[32,38] The color and pattern of the RPE surrounding the lesion are usually normal. Variations in size and stage of development of the lesion may be present in the eyes of the same patient (Figure 5.03A and B). The lesion initially may be evident only in one eye. In some patients the fellow eye may remain near normal with 20/20 acuity throughout life.[39] The vitelliform lesion may occasionally disappear spontaneously (Figure 5.01G and H). The lesions may be eccentrically located and may be multiple (Figure 5.04).[40] In a few patients they may be unusually large and geographic in shape (Figure 5.04G–I). Some patients may show a finely mottled pattern of yellowish change in the RPE throughout the fundus (Figure 5.03F). Each of the affected family members illustrated in Figure 5.04A–F had several small, focal, yellow lesions scattered in the fundus of each eye. These yellow punctate lesions may be the only manifestation of the disease in some family members.[12]

5.02 Best's Disease-correlation of clinical appearance to schematic diagram

A: Schematic diagram of probable histopathologic changes in Best's disease. Previtelliform stage (see Fig. 5.01A). Sunny-side-up vitelliform stage (see Fig. 5.01G). RPE cells (arrows) are distended with yellow pigment. Vitelliruptive stage (see Figs. 5.01D and 5.03D). Disruption of RPE with yellow pigment beneath the retina and atrophy of the receptor elements. Serous detachment of the retina may occur over the vitelliform (see Figs. 5.01G and 5.04A and B), the atrophic or neovascular stage (see Fig. 5-03E). Atrophic stage. Choroidal neovascularization and cicatricial stage (see Fig. 5.03F).

B and C: This 36 year old male with 20/80 and 20/200 vision respectively had a pseudo hypopyon appearing vitelliform lesion on the right and an atrophic lesion on the left.

D to G: This young woman was noted to have bilateral maculopathy at age 7. Photographs done at age 10 shows multifocal vitelliform deposits in both macula (D and E). Eleven years later, at age 21, there was an increase in the yellow material with a partial scrambled egg appearance in both eyes (F and G). Her visual acuity at age 24 was best corrected to 20/40 right eye and 20/25 left eye. EOG revealed an Arden ratio of 1.26 on the right and 1.40 on the left.

Courtesy: B and C, Dr. Paul Sternberg, D -G, Dr. Edward Cherney.

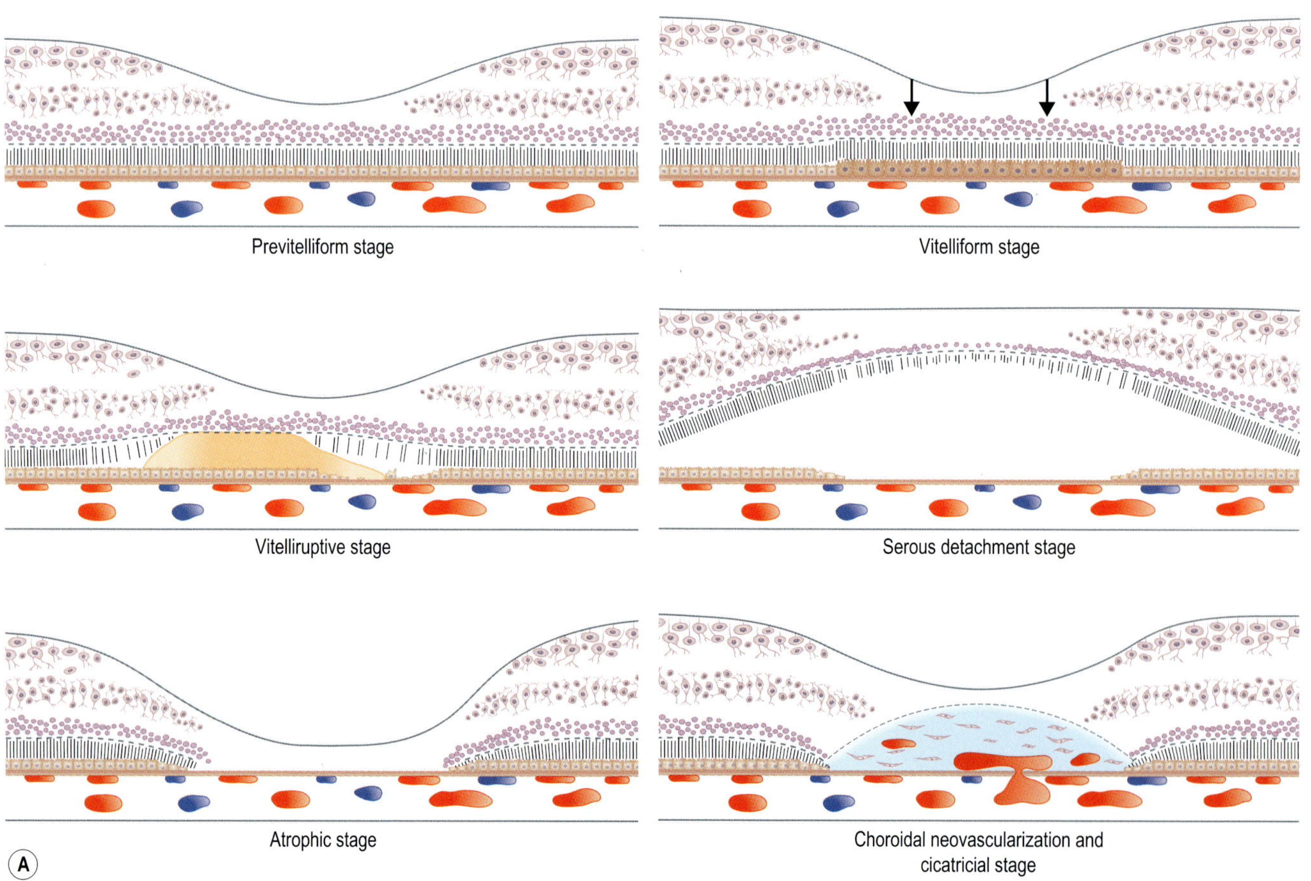

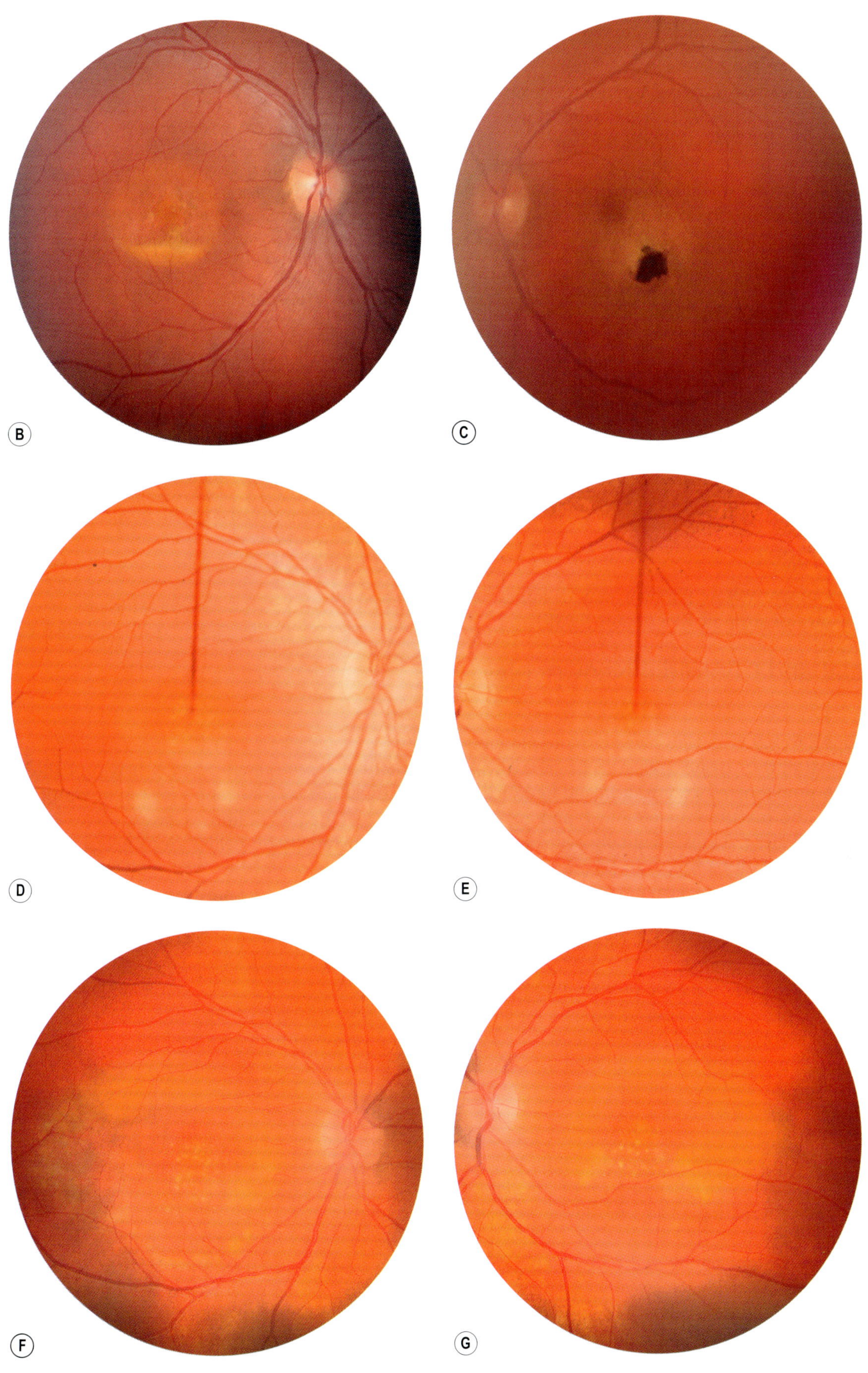
B
C
D
E
F
G

Pseudohypopyon Stage

Usually by the time the patient reaches puberty the yellowish lesion shows evidence of disruption (Figures 5.01D and 5.03A and D). It appears that the yellow material is partly taken up by the RPE cells and the heavier material gravitates inferiorly in the subretinal space. Some shifting of this material may occur when the patient's head is tilted for 60–90 minutes.[11] There is thinning of the RPE and occasionally some clumping of pigment in the superior portion of these lesions.

Scrambled-Egg Stage

With further disruption of the vitelliform lesion, multiple irregular yellowish subretinal deposits produce a picture likened to a scrambled egg. Multifocal yellow deposits may occasionally be arranged in a more orderly ring distribution near the periphery of these lesions (Figure 5.04G). The visual acuity is often decreased to the level of 20/30 to 20/40 in the presence of extensive scrambling of the vitelliform lesion.

Atrophic Stage

Eventually all of the yellow pigment may disappear and leave an oval area of atrophic RPE (Figure 5.03F).

Cicatricial and Choroidal Neovascular Stage

Many patients develop evidence of one or more plaques of white subretinal fibrous tissue, and in some cases there is evidence of choroidal neovascularization and hemorrhagic detachment of the macula (Figures 5.01E and 5.03B, C, and J).[6,12] These latter patients eventually develop a white or partly pigmented disciform scar (Figures 5.01F and 5.03F). The central vision is generally 20/100 or less at this stage of the disease. Serous detachment of the retina may occur at any stage of the development of vitelliform lesions (Figures 5.01G, 5.03A, B, and D, and 5.04A and B).

In the vitelliform stage the early phases of angiography demonstrate complete obstruction of the choroidal fluorescence by the lesion (Figure 5.01J).[12,18] There is no generalized obscuration of the choroidal fluorescence such as occurs in Stargardt's disease. During the later stages of angiography, the vitelliform lesion may appear nonfluorescent or may appear to fluoresce slightly. Possible explanations for this apparent fluorescence include reflected vitreous fluorescence from the surface of the lesion, improperly matched exciting and barrier filters, and autofluorescence of the yellow lesion. As the yellow pigment gravitates inferiorly, angiography in the area vacated by the yellow material reveals evidence of early fluorescence secondary to depigmentation and late staining of the altered RPE (Figure 5.03E). Often there is a narrow zone of hypofluorescence surrounding the atrophic lesion. Angiography permits detection of choroidal neovascularization and shows evidence of staining of fibrous tissue present in the subretinal space (Figure 5.03C). It is probable that occult choroidal neovascularization is present within some of the subretinal plaques of fibrous tissue.

Peripheral visual fields, electroretinographic findings, and dark adaptation in these patients are normal. Color vision in the late stages of the disease may be mildly disturbed. The EOG is markedly abnormal with the light to dark ratio usually being below 1.55.[8,14,19] EOGs of carriers of the disease usually yield a subnormal result. Patients who are both homozygous and heterozygous for the *Best1* gene show low Arden ratio, thus making this feature most characteristic of the condition. Vitreous fluorophotometry shows no evidence of breakdown in the outer blood–retinal barrier with few exceptions in patients with advanced macular degeneration.[15] The disease is inherited as an autosomal-dominant trait. Best's disease usually occurs in Caucasian patients but may occur occasionally in Africans and Asians (Figure 5.03A–C).[41]

Visual prognosis is good for at least the first six decades of life.[5] Most patients retain reading vision in at least one eye throughout life. The progression of visual loss is slow and occurs for the most part beyond the age of 40 years.[16] Acute and permanent loss of central vision may occur in association with bleeding from subretinal new vessels (Figure 5.01E). A macular hole may occasionally occur in patients with Best's disease as well as in patients with adult-onset foveomacular dystrophy or pattern dystrophy.[39,41,42]

5.03 Best's disease.

A–C: This 13-year-old black girl, one of three siblings with Best's disease, showed a partially scrambled vitelliform lesion in the right eye and a small disciform scar and serous macular detachment in the left eye (A and B). Visual acuity in the right eye was 20/20 and in the left eye was 20/40. Arteriovenous phase angiogram showed evidence of choroidal neovascular membrane (arrow, C).

D and E: This 14-year-old boy had the vitelliruptive stage of Best's disease. Note loss of yellow material in the superior portion of the lesion and layering of this material inferiorly. Angiography (H) showed evidence of fluorescence superiorly but not inferiorly in the region of the yellowish material inferiorly. Later angiograms showed definite evidence of leakage of dye in the superior half of this lesion.

F: The 37-year-old mother of the patient illustrated in D had a visual acuity of 20/300. Note the elevated fibrous scar beneath the retina and atrophy of surrounding retinal pigment epithelium (RPE). There is a fine mottled pattern of yellow discoloration of the RPE throughout the posterior pole. Angiography revealed staining of the subretinal scar.

G–L: This 8-year-old girl was noted to have vitelliform lesions in both maculas at age 4. An "egg yolk"-like lesion in the right macula (G) is brilliantly autofluorescent (H) and fills the subretinal space without overlying inner retinal damage (I). The left eye has a scrambled-egg appearance (J) with a fibrotic scar that is irregularly hyperautofluorescent (K). The fibrous scar is associated with subretinal fluid, implying subretinal neovascularization (L).

(G–L courtesy of Dr. Franco Recchia.)

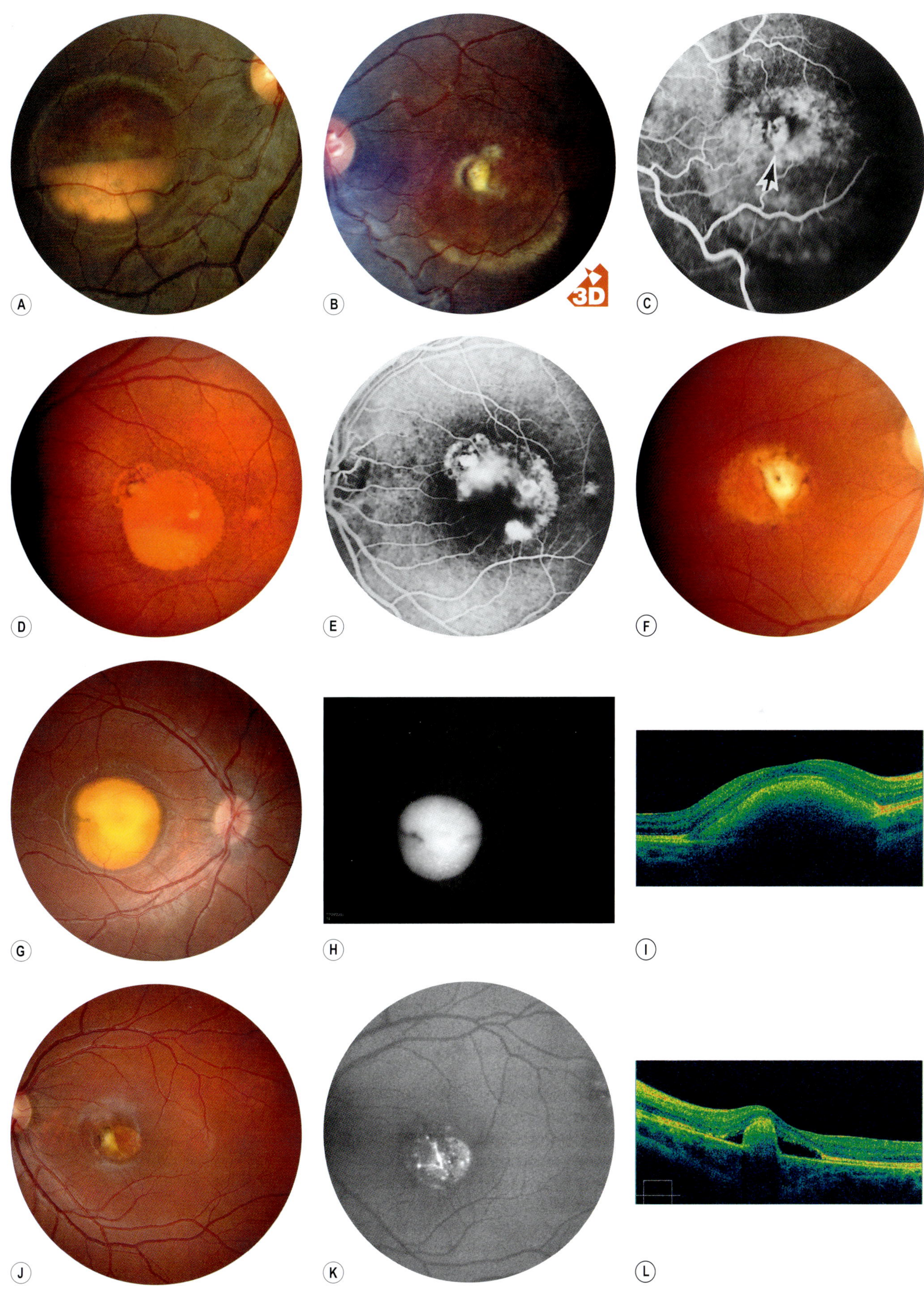
A
B
3D
C
D
E
F
G
H
I
J
K
L

The histopathology of the vitelliform or pseudohypopyon stage of the disease is unknown.[1,13,27,43] One histopathologic report concerned a relatively early scrambled-egg phase of the disease.[1] One report concerned one eye with mild pigment macular changes in a 69-year-old man with advanced degeneration in the fellow eye.[43] Findings in these reports were consistent in their demonstration of a generalized RPE abnormality that was associated with an abnormal accumulation of lipofuscin granules in the RPE and within macrophages in the subretinal space. None of these studies, however, showed the extensive lipofuscin storage characteristic of Stargardt's disease, a finding in keeping with the absence of a dark choroid angiographically outside the area of the vitelliform lesion in patients with Best's disease.

Other histopathologic findings in Best's disease included a periodic acid–Schiff (PAS)-positive, acid mucopolysaccharide-negative, electron-dense, finely granular material in the inner segments of the degenerating photoreceptors and Müller cells recently identified predominantly as A2E[44]; an abnormal fibrillar material beneath the RPE cells in the region of photoreceptor cell loss, and normal choriocapillaris.[13] Breaks in Bruch's membrane and choroidal neovascularization have been demonstrated.[1,13] One group of authors concluded that the sensory retinal changes were probably primary and the RPE changes secondary.[13] These studies, together with the in vivo demonstration of autofluorescence of vitelliform lesions in Best's disease by Miller,[7,32,38,45] suggest that the yellow pigment may at least in part be caused by lipofuscin. There is no fluorescein angiographic evidence in this disease, however, for a diffuse marked lipofuscin storage disease such as occurs in Stargardt's disease (see pp. 278–284). Histopathologic examination of a 86-year-old homozygous for *BEST1* gene showed accumulation of lipofuscin, a large component of it made up of A2E, within the RPE cells. Other RPE granules were melanoliposomes. Extraction of the granules in this eye and another 81-year-old's eye heterozygous for the gene showed the lipofuscin to be mostly made up of A2E similar to that found in diseases caused by the *ABCR* transport gene abnormality.[44]

The vitelliform stage of Best's disease should be differentiated from other diseases that cause solitary yellowish macular lesions; for example, dominantly inherited, adult-onset vitelliform foveomacular dystrophy (pattern dystrophy) (see Figure 5.06–5.08), basal laminar drusen (Figure 3.29), acute exudative vitelliform maculopathy (Figures 11.30 and 11.31), and fundus flavimaculatus (Stargardt's disease) with large central flecks. The early age of development of the yellow lesion and the progressive vitellirupti-form changes are essential findings to differentiate patients with Best's disease from those with adult-onset vitelliform foveomacular dystrophy (pattern dystrophy), because the latter disease may be associated with subnormal EOGs in one-third of cases and because both are dominantly inherited. Four other yellow lesions that may simulate Best's disease include focal serous RPE detachments containing dehemoglobinized blood pigment, some cases of central serous retinopathy with subretinal fibrin, resolving subretinal hematomas, and unusually large acute solar maculopathy lesions.[46] To be confident that one is dealing with Best's vitelliform dystrophy rather than some other type of dystrophy, the following are required: (1) the presence of one of the recognized polymorphous lesions typical of Best's disease; (2) dominant mode of inheritance; (3) moderate to severely subnormal EOG findings; and (4) onset and natural course of the disease typical for Best's disease.[21] Without this documentation the diagnosis of Best's disease is open to question.[2,42,46,47] Gene testing for the *BEST1* gene with the presence of the above features confirms the diagnosis. Future identification of specific gene defects and the nature of the vitelliform material will help elucidate the pathogenic relationship of the various disorders that demonstrate similar yellow lesions in the macula.[28,48]

5.04 Multiple vitelliform lesions in Best's disease.

A–E: This 25-year-old physician complained of mild visual blurring. Visual acuity in the right eye was 20/20 and in the left eye was 20/15. Note the multiple slightly elevated lesions scattered throughout the posterior pole of both eyes (A and B). Clinically, these lesions resemble somewhat a serous detachment of the retinal pigment epithelium (RPE). Note the ill-defined borders of the yellowish material in the large central lesions. Late angiogram (C) in the left eye revealed no evidence of staining of the large central lesion. The slight fluorescence of the paracentral lesions was probably caused by pseudofluorescence. The patient's electro-oculographic findings were definitely abnormal (1.1 right eye and 1.3 left eye). Several months after these photographs, he became asymptomatic and remained so for approximately 1 year, when the symptoms returned for approximately 6 months. He again became relatively asymptomatic. Photograph of the left fundus taken 21 months after A and B shows that the central lesion has largely resolved (D). The other lesions appear smaller, more discrete, and yellow in appearance. Similar findings were present in the right eye. His visual acuity at this time was 20/30 in the right eye and 20/15 in the left eye. Angiography (E) showed evidence of some thinning of the RPE inferior to the foveal area. The paracentral lesions appeared nonfluorescent.
F: The left fundus of the 15-year-old sister of the patient illustrated in A–E. Note the multiple, small, discrete, yellowish lesions scattered in the posterior pole (arrows). Another brother and the father had similar punctate yellow spots in the fundi. All three had a markedly subnormal electro-oculogram. The fundi and electro-oculographic findings of another sibling and the mother were normal.
G–I: Large multifocal vitelliform lesions in a 46-year-old woman who gave a 2-year history of blurred vision. Her mother had failing vision in late adulthood, and a maternal cousin had macular degeneration. Note the partly disrupted lesion in the right macula (G) and the large nondisrupted lesions in the left macula (H). Twenty months later the central macular lesion had enlarged (I). Visual acuity was 3/200 in the right eye and 20/40 + 3 in the left eye. Her electro-oculographic findings were definitely abnormal. Her electro-retinographic findings were normal. Angiography revealed the intact vitelliform lesions to be nonfluorescent.

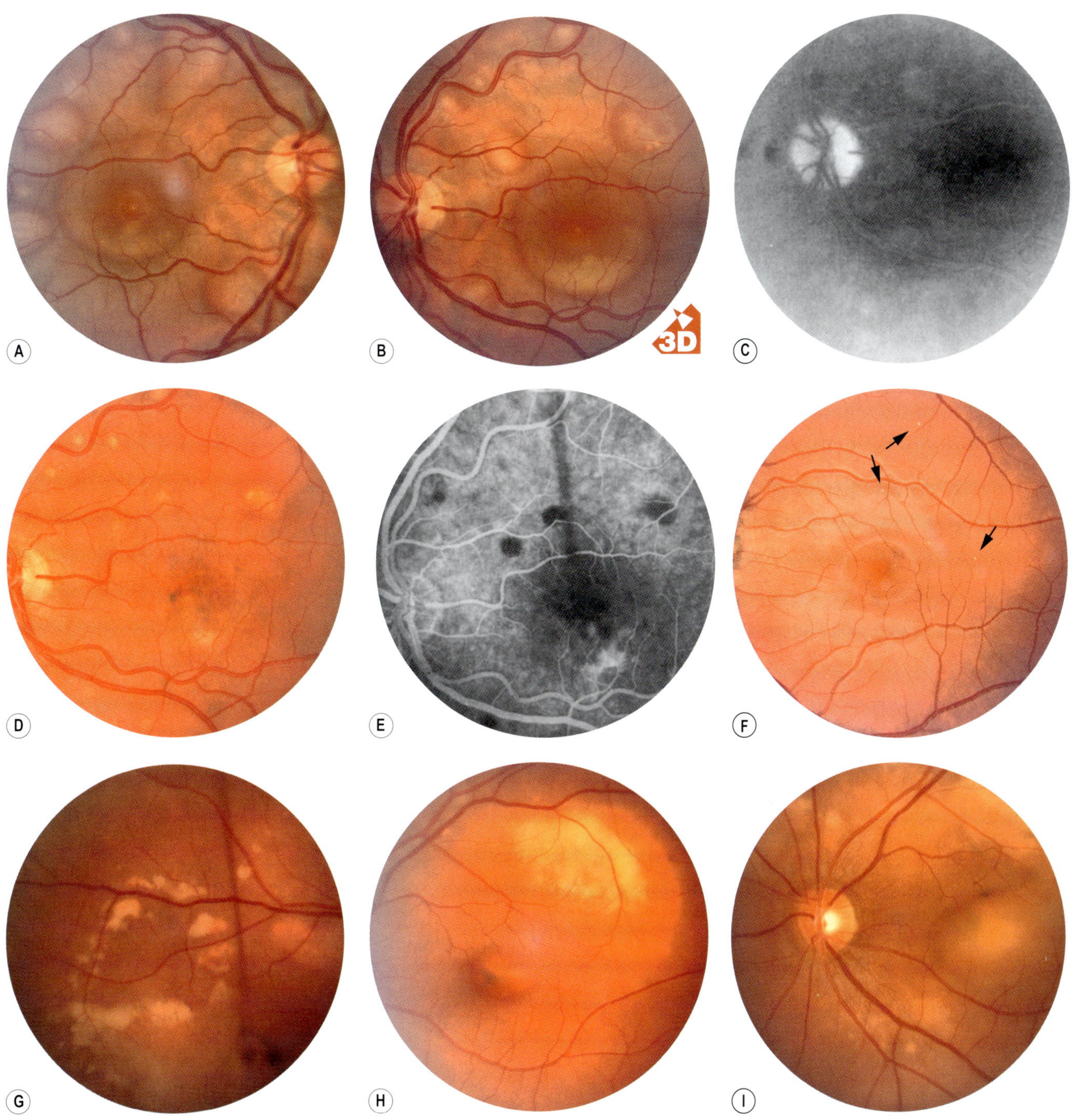
A
B
3D
C
D
E
F
G
H
I

Multifocal vitelliform lesions may occur in patients with Best's disease (Figure 5.04).[12,40] Most patients with multifocal vitelliform lesions, however, have no other evidence of Best's disease (see next section). The lesions may vary in size. Some may be several disc diameters or larger in size and often have some irregularity to their contour (Figure 5.04G–I). These larger lesions frequently demonstrate partial resolution or disruption. Multiple round flecks of yellow pigment may be arranged in a circular or oval distribution near the periphery of the partly disrupted lesions (Figure 5.04G).

Best1 gene has also been implicated in autosomal-dominant vitreoretinochoroidopathy (ADVIRC), autosomal-dominant microcornea rod–cone degeneration syndrome (ADMRCS), and autosomal-recessive bestrophinopathy (ARB), all with extraretinal features implicating the gene that may be involved in ocular development.[32]

AUTOSOMAL-DOMINANT VITREORETINOCHOROIDOPATHY

ADVIRC is a hereditary pigmentary dystrophy described in 1982 by Kaufman and associates.[49] It has an autosomal-dominant inheritance pattern and is characterized by peripheral pigmentary retinopathy for 360° with a discrete posterior boundary near the equator (Figure 5.05C–E) associated with punctate whitish opacities in the superficial retina along with vitreous cells and fibrillary condensation. Frequently, peripheral retinal arteriolar narrowing and occlusion, evidence of retinal neovascularization, choroidal atrophy, and presenile cataracts are present. Evidence of blood–retinal barrier breakdown is seen by cystoid macular edema.[32,49,50]

These patients usually do not have symptoms of night blindness. The electroretinogram (ERG) is normal or only slightly reduced. The EOG is variably affected, with Arden ratio ranging from normal to subnormal. There have been a few cases with late cone dystrophy.[51] The gene defect has been localized to the *BEST1* gene with missense mutations and exon skipping on the long arm of chromosome 11.[32,52,53]

5.05 Autosomal-dominant vitreoretinochoroidopathy.

A–H: A 47-year-old woman of Huguenot ancestry presented with progressive visual blurring and glare for a year. There was no family history of visual problems and she was otherwise healthy. Visual acuity was 20/25 in the right eye and 20/40 in the left eye. Mild bilateral posterior subcapsular cataracts were present in both eyes. The posterior poles were normal in both eyes (A and B). Mid peripheral fundus had retinal pigment epithelium (RPE) migration in the form of bone spicules that were tightly located and symmetrical between the two eyes (C–E). Fluorescein angiogram was normal in the posterior pole; the periphery showed diffuse transmission hyperfluorescence interspersed with blockage from pigment spicules.

AUTOSOMAL-DOMINANT MICROCORNEA ROD–CONE DYSTROPHY, CATARACT WITH STAPHYLOMA

A subgroup of patients who have all or some features of ADVIRC may also have microcornea and shallow anterior chamber with evidence of subacute or acute angle closure glaucoma. Some of these patients show posterior staphyloma and some of them are myopic.[54] The inheritance pattern is autosomal-dominant, and the gene again has been ascribed to the *BEST1* mutation.[32,52] The EOG is abnormal in all patients with ADMRCS syndrome. A full-field ERG may show subnormal photopic and scotopic responses. With time, these patients show progressive ERG changes with severe rod and cone photoreceptor dysfunction, unlike patients with ADVIRC who are relatively stable. The ADMRCS syndrome is generally more severe than ADVIRC. However, there are family members who have overlapping findings of the two conditions.[32]

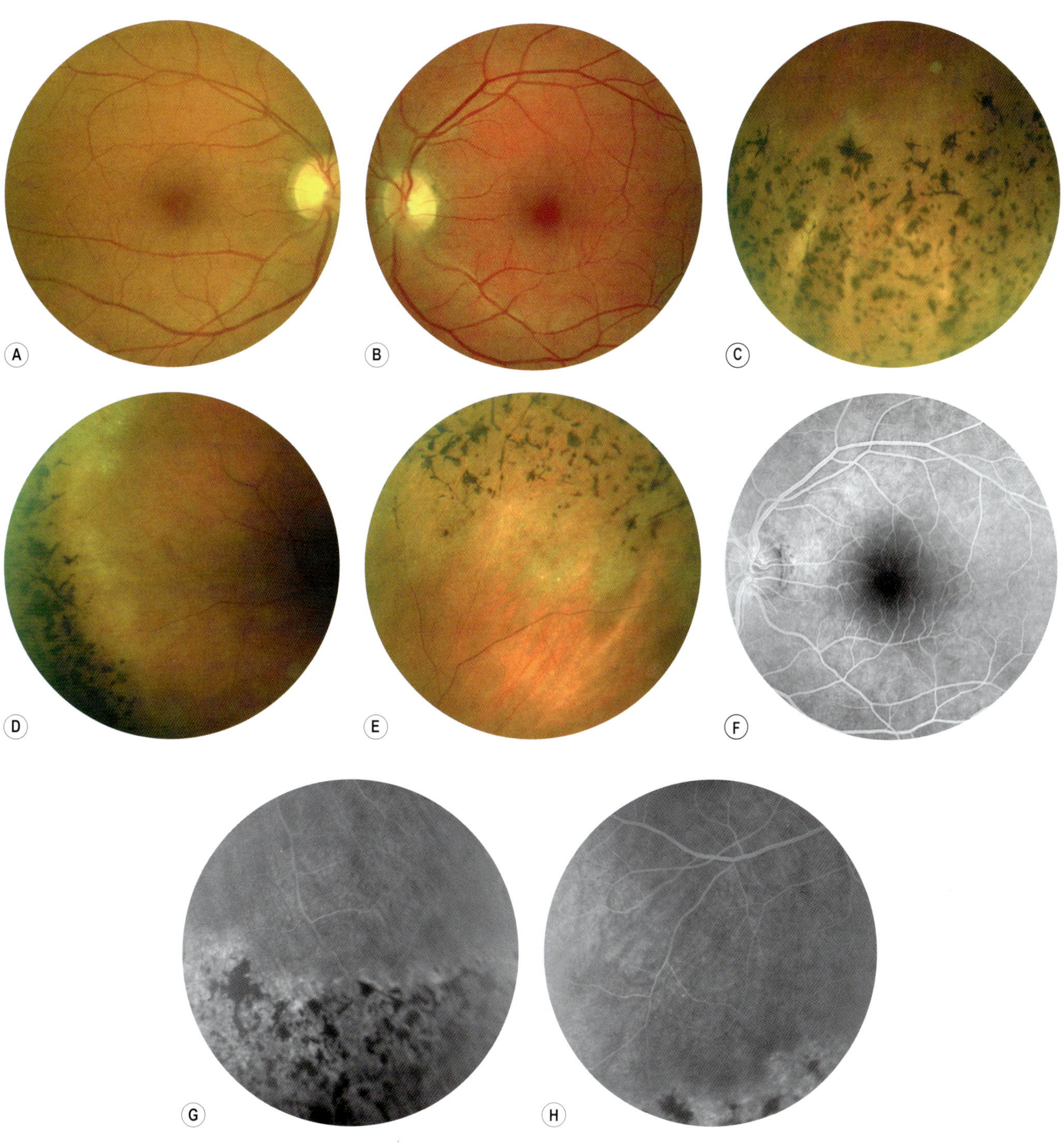
A
B
C
D
E
F
G
H

AUTOSOMAL-RECESSIVE BESTROPHINOPATHY

This condition was described by Burgess et al. in 2008.[55] It usually starts with central visual loss at an age of onset ranging from 4 to 40 years, and the mean age of onset is approximately 25 years. The visual acuity often deteriorates to less than 20/60 in both eyes within a few years. Patients are generally hyperopic and show shallow anterior chambers and may present with subacute or acute angle closure glaucoma. Fundus examination shows irregular RPE alterations with whitish subretinal deposits that are seen throughout the retina, preferentially in the macula and midperiphery (Figure 5.05I–L). Retinal edema with neurosensory retinal detachment and subretinal fluid may be observed in the macula occasionally; this can be confirmed by optical coherence tomography (OCT). Patients may not show the vitelliform lesions that are characteristic of Best's disease. The macular lesions may evolve into atrophic scars causing a further decline in vision.[55] The EOG is severely reduced or absent to light rise. The focal pattern ERG in the macula is markedly abnormal, indicating severe macular dysfunction. The full-field ERG shows reduced and delayed rod and cone responses indicating panretinal photoreceptor dysfunction. On angiography, there is widespread patchy hyperfluorescence due to RPE atrophy and retinal edema. These areas correspond to areas of increased fundus autofluorescence (Figure 5.05L), suggesting lipofuscin accumulation in the pigment epithelium. The areas of RPE loss show decreased fundus autofluorescence. High-resolution OCT of the macula shows photoreceptor detachment from the pigment epithelium, disruption of the photoreceptor layer but persevered inner retinal layers (Figure 5.05M).[32,55] Those patients who are heterozygous to the mutation are entirely normal clinically and electrophysiologically.

All the three conditions described above are caused by mutations in the *BEST1* gene, the same gene that causes Best's vitelliform macular dystrophy. Whereas Best's, ADVIRC, and ADMRCS syndromes are autosomal-dominant, ARB occurs in the presence of homozygous or compound hetereozygous *BEST1* mutation.

Nearly all mutations identified in Best's vitelliform macular dystrophy and adult-onset foveal macular vitelliform dystrophy, a type of pattern dystrophy, are missense mutations. Those mutations causing ADVIRC and the MRCS syndrome are splice mutations,[32,53,55] leading to in-frame deletions or duplications. The null phenotype of ARB is caused by homozygous or compound heterozygous nonsense or missense *BEST1* mutation.[32,56] The variable expressivity and penetrance probably account for the wide variation in the phenotype of these conditions. It is likely they are also dependent on other genetic or environmental modifiers to manifest all features of the condition.

5.05 Continued

Autosomal-recessive bestrophinopathy.

I–M: Fundus photograph of a 30-year-old female, who carried two homozygous nonsense mutations in the *BEST1* gene. The visual acuity was 20/32 (0,63) in the right eye. A faint round yellowish lesion was present in the central macula. This lesion was surrounded by some yellow-white ill-defined spots. In addition, faintly atrophic hypopigmented areas could be noted around the retinal vascular arcades (I). Fluorescein angiography revealed diffuse patchy hyperfluorescence throughout the fundus, compatible with mild diffuse atrophy of the RPE. Around the fovea similar hyperfluorescent changes were present, together with staining of a small subretinal scar inferior of the fovea (J and K).

Fundus autofluorescence imaging showed slight autofluorescence changes centrally in the macula. The brightly autofluorescent dots corresponded to (but outnumbered) the yellow-white spots seen on ophthalmoscopy. These lesions therefore seemed to reflect increased amounts of retinal lipofuscin. Around and beyond the retinal vascular arcades, small irregular spotted areas of increased and decreased autofluorescence were noted (L).

Spectral-domain optical coherence tomography image, scanned horizontally through the macula, revealed hyperreflective material – possibly shed photoreceptor outer segments between the slightly elevated retina and the RPE (M).

(A–H courtesy of Dr. Ranjit Dhaliwal; I–M courtesy of Dr. Camiel Boon.)

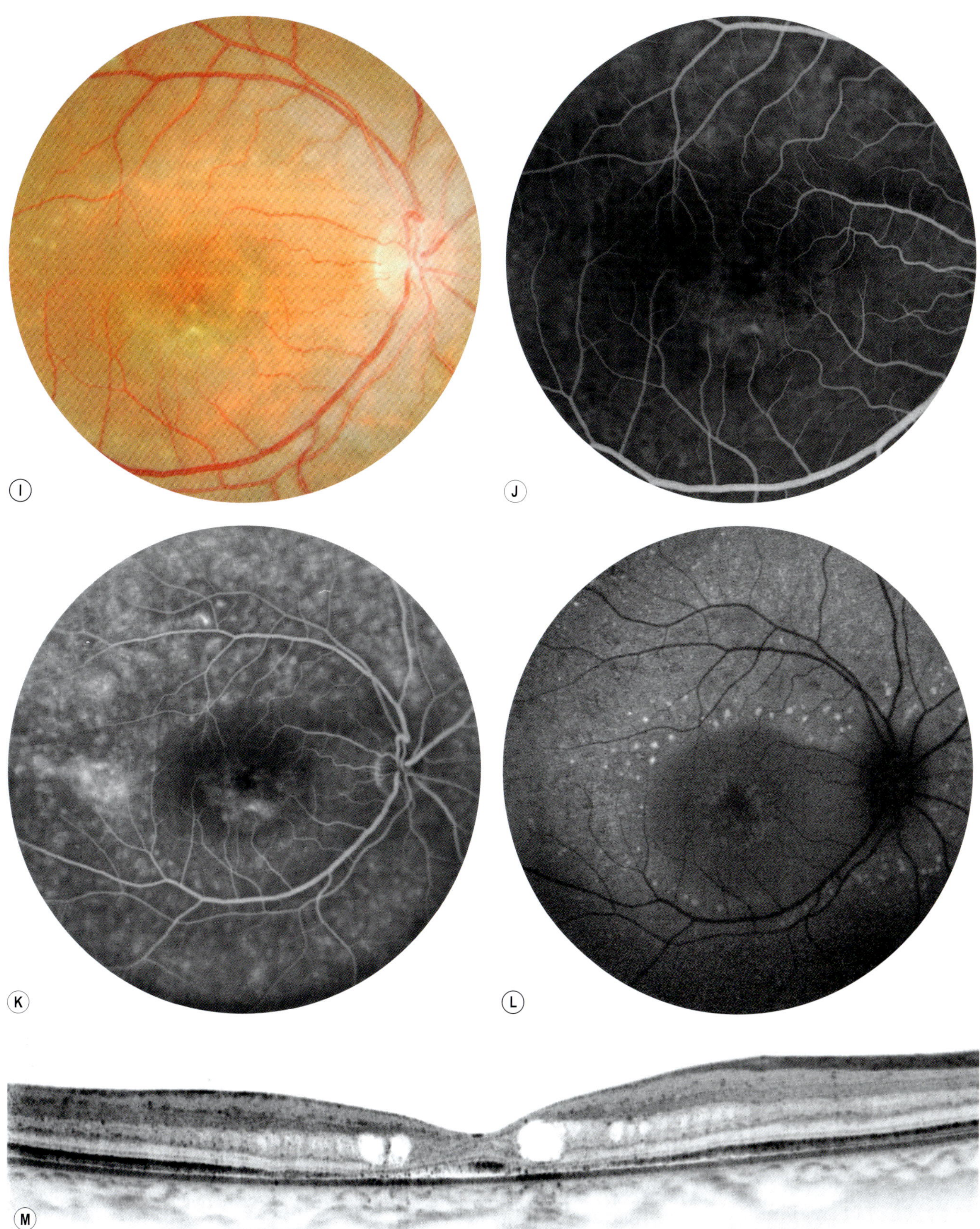
I
J
K
L
M

MULTIFOCAL VITELLIFORM LESIONS IN PATIENTS WITHOUT EVIDENCE OF BEST'S DISEASE

Multifocal vitelliform lesions with the same features as those occurring in Best's disease, in Dr. Gass' experience, occur most frequently in patients with normal EOG findings and a normal family history (Figures 5.06 and 5.07). Fluorescein angiography typically demonstrates nonfluorescence of the yellow lesions (Figures 5.06C and L, and 5.07H). Occasionally, however, the yellow lesions demonstrate early hyperfluorescence (Figure 5.07J). As in the case of Best's disease, the yellow lesions may disappear (Figure 5.07A–D). The frequency of normal EOG findings and a negative family history in patients with multifocal vitelliform lesions suggest that most of these patients do not have either Best's disease or pattern dystrophy. The absence of a family history alone does not entirely exclude these diagnoses, since many affected persons with Best's disease and pattern dystrophy are asymptomatic. This condition should be differentiated from acute exudative multifocal vitelliform maculopathy, an acute-onset inflammatory disorder of so far unknown cause,[57–59] ARB,[32,55] and paraneoplastic vitelliform maculopathy.[60,61] Deutman[17] reported a patient with loss of central vision for many years associated with peripheral and macular vitelliform lesions together with electroretinographic changes compatible with a rod–cone dystrophy. It is possible Deutman's patient had autosomal recessive bestrophinopathy.

5.06 Multifocal vitelliform lesions in adult patients with a normal family history.

A–C: This 39-year-old healthy black man with a 4-month history of metamorphopsia had a visual acuity of 20/30 in the right eye and 20/25 in the left eye. The partly disrupted paramacular lesion in the right eye (A) was partly hypofluorescent (C). The yellow lesions were nonfluorescent. His electro-oculographic findings were normal (1.88 in the right eye and 1.87 in the left eye).
D–F: This 34-year-old man complained of hazy vision in the left eye of 5 months' duration. Visual acuity in both eyes was 20/20. He had multiple vitelliform lesions in both eyes. A large vitelliform lesion involved the left macula (composite photograph, D). A fluid level was evident biomicroscopically in a lesion nasal to the left optic disc (arrow, D) and angiographically in the large macular lesion (stereoangiograms, E and F). His family history was negative. His electro-oculogram Arden ratio was 1.6 bilaterally.
G–L: This 54-year-old man noted blurred vision in the right eye. His family history was negative. Visual acuity was 20/40 in the right eye and 20/40 in the left eye. There were multiple vitelliform lesions in both eyes (G and H). His electro-oculographic findings were subnormal (1.5 in the right eye and 1.4 in the left eye). His electroretinographic findings were normal. His color vision was severely abnormal. Seven years later the lesions in the right eye were partly disrupted (I) and he had acquired a central vitelliform lesion in the left macula (J). Visual acuity was 20/20 in the right eye and 20/40 in the left eye. Angiography revealed that the disrupted lesions in both eyes were hyperfluorescent (K and L). The nondisrupted lesions in the left eye were nonfluorescent (L). The multiple large "sunny-side-up" lesions present in the sixth decade of life and the absence of a history of affected family members are atypical for Best's disease.

(G–L courtesy of Dr. Stephen J. Ryan, Jr.)

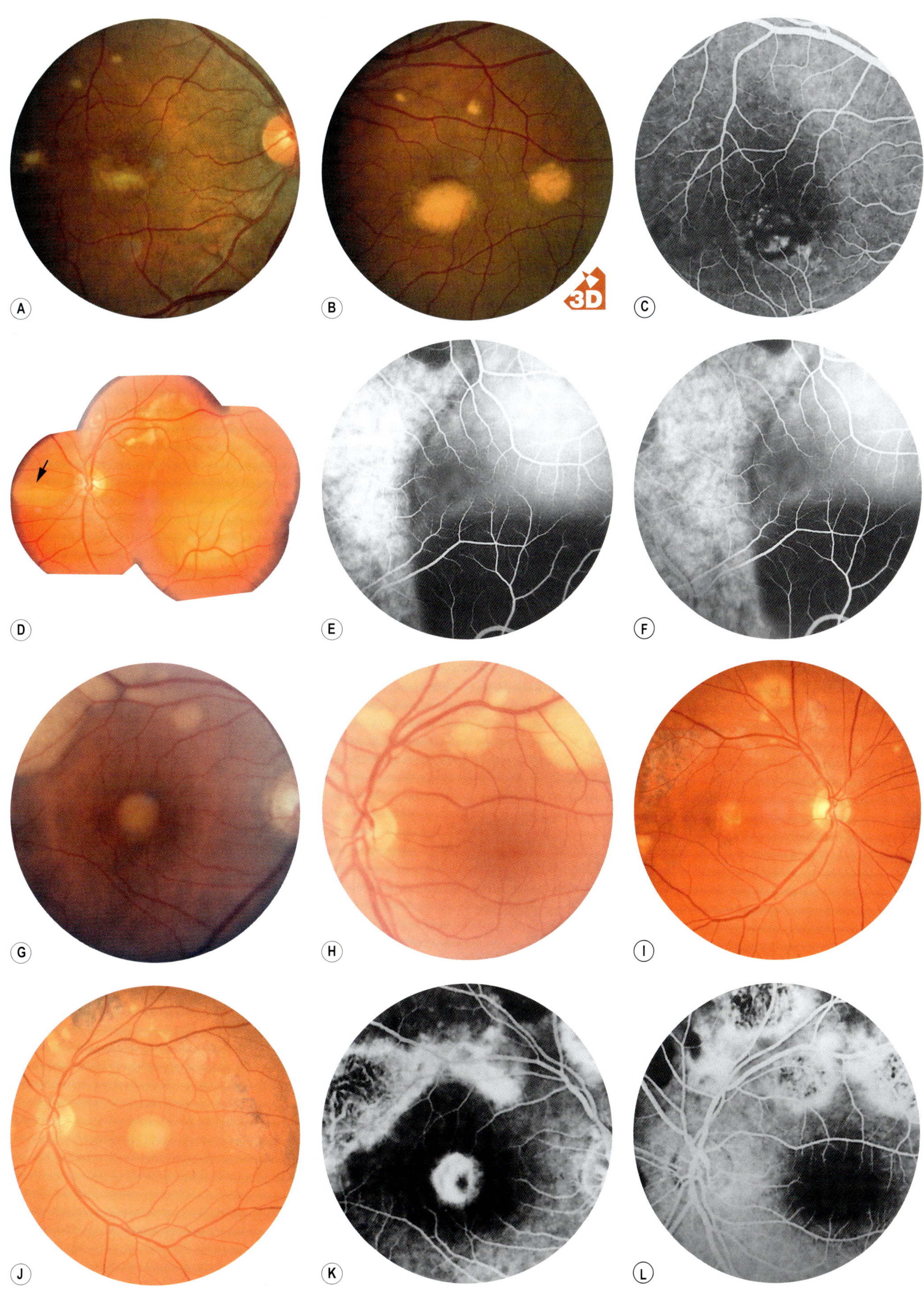
A
B
3D
C
D
E
F
G
H
I
J
K
L

AUTOSOMAL-DOMINANT PATTERN DYSTROPHIES OF THE RPE

Autosomal-dominant pattern dystrophies are characterized by the development, usually in midlife, of mild disturbances of central vision associated with a variety of patterns of deposits of yellow, orange, or gray pigment in the macular area.[21,47,62–100] The prognosis for retention of good central vision in at least one eye until late adulthood is good. The EOG may be slightly or moderately subnormal. The ERG is typically normal. These dystrophies are usually inherited as an autosomal-dominant trait. Mutations of the peripherin/*RDS* and slow gene (Pro 210 ARG) and codon 167 of the *RDS* gene were first demonstrated in family members of patients with dominantly inherited pattern dystrophy.[101–105] Since then several other mutations of the peripherin/*RDS* gene have been found in families and sporadic cases of pattern dystrophy.[98–100] Of importance are the various phenotypes, often within families seen with the same genetic mutation.[34,106–110] In addition to the association with different phenotypes of pattern dystrophy, peripherin/*RDS* gene mutations are associated with central areolar choroidal dystrophy, autosomal-dominant retinitis pigmentosa, autosomal-dominant cone and cone–rod dystrophy, retinitis punctate albescens, and digenic retinitis pigmentosa.[109,111–114] One family demonstrated phenotypic variation, including retinitis pigmentosa and fundus flavimaculatus.[104] The peripherin/*RDS* gene localizes to chromosome 6p21.2, spans 26 kilobases of genomic DNA, and contains three exons. The gene product of peripherin/*RDS* is an integral membrane protein peripherin/*RDS* within rods and cones, and plays an important role in the photoreceptor outer-segment morphogenesis by managing disc formation, alignment, and shedding.

Based on the pattern of pigment distribution, pattern dystrophies have been subdivided into at least five principal groups. A few patients will show different patterns in the two eyes. A patient may show progression from one pattern to another over a period of years. Some pedigrees will show any combination or all four of the patterns of fundus change described in the succeeding sections.[98,115,116] For these reasons it is probable that these are closely related, if not expressions of the same disorder.

5.07 Multifocal vitelliform lesions in adult patients with normal family history and normal or subnormal electro-oculographic findings.

A–E: This 40-year-old man presented to his local physician in 1973 because of difficulty with dark adaptation. His visual acuity was 20/20 in both eyes. Yellow lesions were noted in both fundi. His electro-oculographic findings were normal. Two years later his acuity was reduced to 20/25 right eye and 20/80 left eye. There were multiple geographic yellow-orange lesions in the paracentral region of both eyes and a scar in the left macula (A and B). Two years later the fundi were unchanged (C). By 1984, all of the yellow-orange deposits had disappeared, leaving in their stead geographic atrophy of the retinal pigment epithelium (D and E). His visual acuity was 20/25 right eye and 20/200 left eye. His findings were unchanged in January 1995.
F–H: This 44-year-old woman presented because of a 1-year history of visual loss. Her visual acuity was 20/40 bilaterally. There were multifocal yellow lesions in the macula and juxtapapillary area bilaterally (F and G). Angiographically these were nonfluorescent centrally and were surrounded by a ring of hyperfluorescence (H). Electroretinogram, electro-oculogram, dark adaptation, and color vision were normal. Sixteen months later her findings were unchanged.
I–L: This healthy 20-year-old man noted a central scotoma in both eyes. Multiple yellow lesions were scattered in the macula and juxtapapillary region of both eyes (I). These lesions showed early hyperfluorescence and late staining (J). Two months later he had developed evidence of subretinal fluid around each of the yellow lesions (K). His electro-oculogram was low normal in both eyes. Eighteen months later the lesions had disappeared (L) and his visual acuity was 20/15 in both eyes.

(F–H courtesy of Dr. Richard E. Goldberg; I–L courtesy of Dr. Robert N. Johnson and Patrick J. Caskey.)

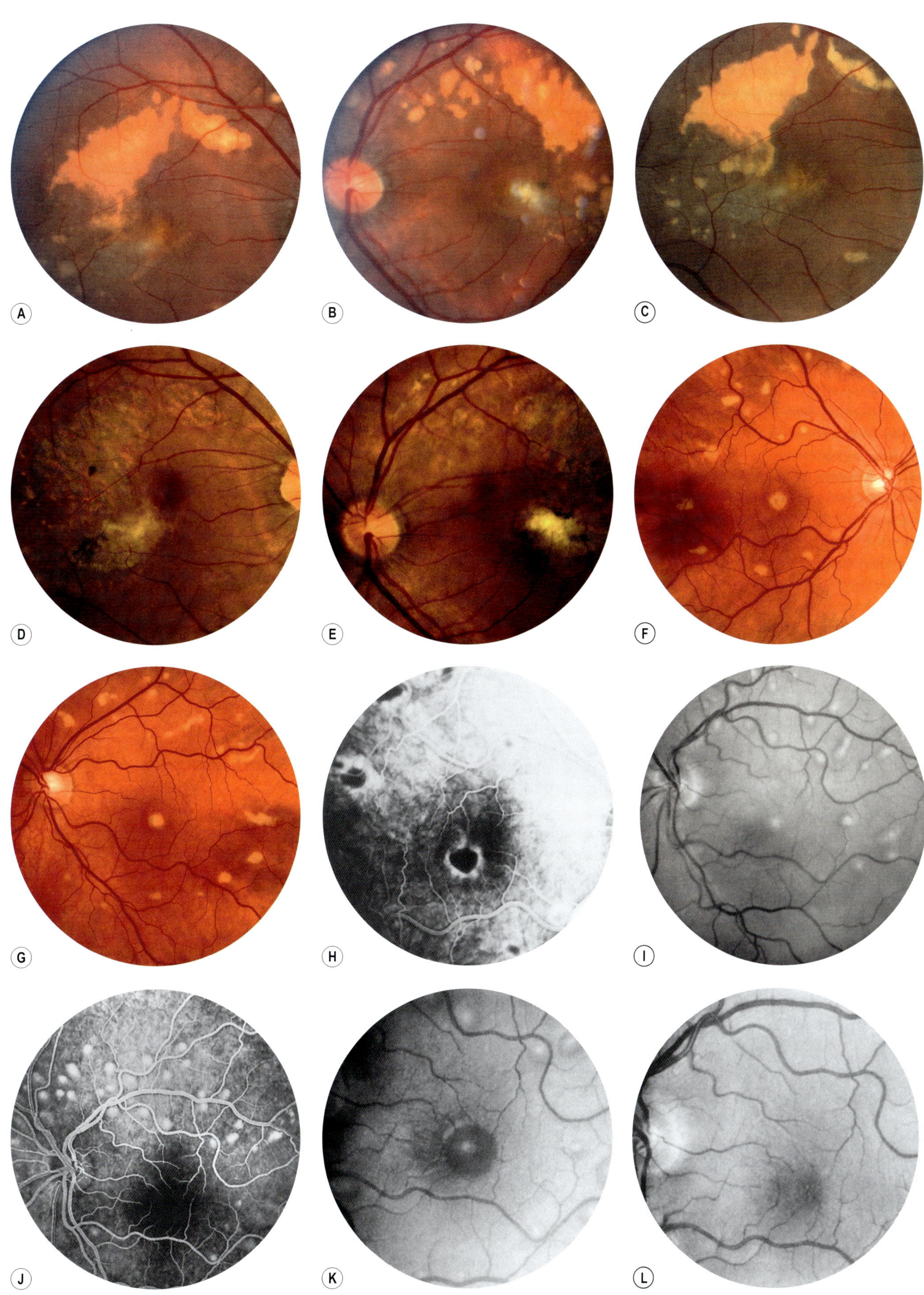
A
B
C
D
E
F
G
H
I
J
K
L

Group 1: Adult-Onset Foveomacular Vitelliform Dystrophy

Patients with adult-onset foveomacular vitelliform dystrophy share the following clinical features: (1) visually asymptomatic or mild visual blurring and metamorphopsia in one or both eyes, usually with the onset between ages 30 and 50 years; (2) symmetric, solitary, usually 1/3–1 disc diameter-size, round or oval, slightly elevated, yellow subretinal lesions, often with a central pigmented spot in each eye (Figures 5.08–5.10); and (3) small yellow flecks that may or may not be present in the paracentral region.[62–64,66,68,70–72,78,80,81,83–86,91,96] The symptoms of blurring and metamorphopsia are often unilateral despite the frequent presence of bilaterally symmetric lesions. The symptoms may improve spontaneously. Initially, the yellow lesion may be present in only one eye. Although most of the foveal lesions are approximately 1/3 disc diameter in size, occasionally they may be larger and misdiagnosed as the "sunny-side-up" stage of Best's vitelliform macular dystrophy or as bilateral serous detachment of the RPE (Figure 5.09). The yellow foveal lesions often develop a central gray or orange clump of pigment that biomicroscopically may show evidence of the pigment extending into the posterior retinal layers (Figures 5.08A and B, 5.09D, and 5.10A and B). Later the foveal lesions may fade and leave an irregular oval or round area of depigmentation of the RPE (Figure 5.08E). Some patients eventually develop additional paracentral yellow deposits, often in a triradiate pattern (Figure 5.08D–F). Fluorescein angiography during the early stages of the disease shows either a nonfluorescent lesion (Figure 5.09C) or, more typically, a small irregular ring of hyperfluorescence surrounding a central nonfluorescent spot (halo) (Figures 5.08C and I and 5.09F). Some of the extrafoveal small yellow lesions show discrete staining, such as drusen (Figure 5.10C), and others, similar to the foveal lesions, are either nonfluorescent or have a halo of fluorescence surrounding them. The yellow and gray components of the lesions are brightly autofluorescent and the depigmented RPE in late lesions are hypoautofluorescent (Figure 5.11K and L).

5.08 Adult-onset foveomacular vitelliform pattern dystrophy.

A–C: This 30-year-old white woman developed metamorphopsia and a positive scotoma in the right eye 6 weeks before examination. The symptoms had improved by the time of examination. Visual acuity in the right eye was 20/25-1 and J-1 and in the left eye was 20/50 and J-1. Symmetric, slightly elevated, oval, discrete, one-third disc diameter size, yellow lesions with a central pigment clump were present in the foveolar areas (A and B). There were several small yellow deposits in the paracentral area of the left eye (arrows). Her electro-oculographic findings were subnormal (1.4 in both eyes). Angiography showed a fluorescent ring centered in the fovea of each eye (C). Yellow lesions in the midperiphery fluoresced (arrows).

D: Right eye of the 54-year-old mother of the patient illustrated in A–C. She noted mild distortion of vision in her left eye 10 years previously. Visual acuity in the right eye was 20/40 and J-2 and in the left eye was 20/30 and J-2. In the center of the fovea is an irregular, round area of depigmentation surrounded by multiple yellowish deposits. A few deposits (arrow) are present in the extramacular area. Her electro-oculographic findings were subnormal (1.22 in the right eye and 1.40 in the left eye). The angiographic pattern was similar to that in C.

E and F: The 70-year-old maternal grandmother of the patient illustrated in A–C had noted mild difficulty with reading in her left eye for the first time 30 years previously. This remained unchanged since that time. She was asymptomatic in her right eye. Her visual acuity in both eyes was 20/40. Note the central area of depigmentation of the retinal pigment epithelium (arrow, E) and faintly visible peripheral flecks. Angiography showed a reticular pattern of irregular hyperfluorescence (F). Her electro-oculographic findings were subnormal (1.0 in both eyes).

G–L: Central yellow lesions resembling inanimate and animate objects, e.g., spaceship (G), chicken (H and I), sunfish (J), airplane (K), and hobbyhorse (L). Note the yellow paracentral flecks.

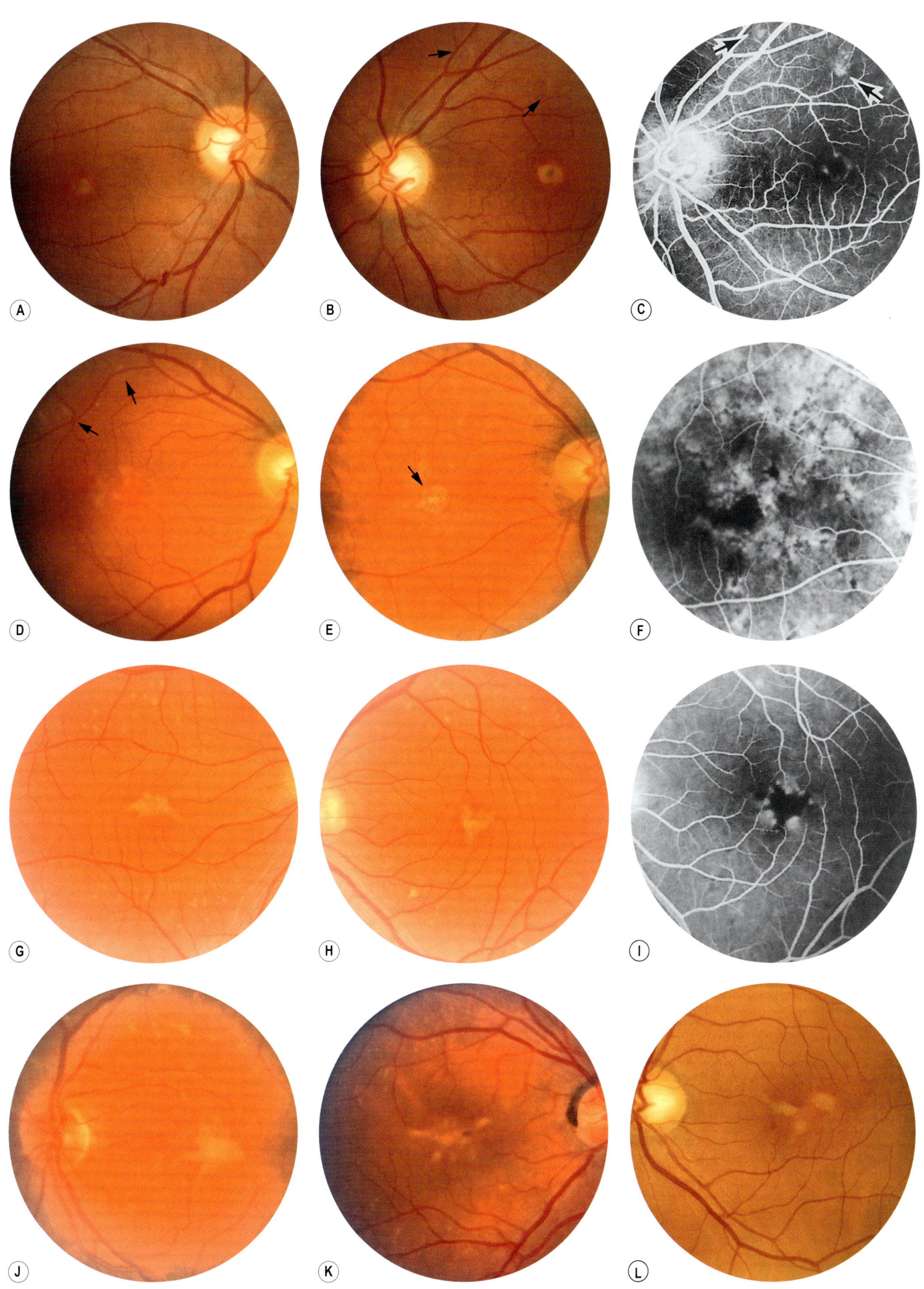
A
B
C
D
E
F
G
H
I
J
K
L

This form of pattern dystrophy was observed in females in three successive generations in one family (Figure 5.08A–F) at the Bascom Palmer Eye Institute. This family was originally reported in 1974 by this author (Gass) as having a peculiar foveomacular dystrophy, later referred to as adult-onset vitelliform foveomacular dystrophy.[83,84] Recently a mutation of the peripherin RDS gene has been demonstrated in two of these patients.[103] The mothers of two unrelated patients with adult-onset foveomacular vitelliform lesions showed evidence of butterfly dystrophy (Figure 5.12A–G).

5.09 Large vitelliform lesions associated with adult-onset vitelliform foveomacular pattern dystrophy.

A–F: This 51-year-old woman's visual acuity was 20/80 bilaterally. She had discrete slightly elevated, yellowish lesions in the center of both maculae (A and B). Angiography revealed the lesions to be nonfluorescent (C). Same patient 3 years later (D and E). Note the pigment in the center of the lesion. Visual acuity was 20/60. The angiogram now showed an irregular hyperfluorescent ring centered in the fovea (F). Similar changes took place in the left macula during this same period of time. The patient gave no family history of macular degeneration. Her electro-oculographic findings were normal.

G–L: This 68-year-old woman's visual acuity was 20/50 bilaterally. Note the large vitelliform lesions (G and H). Her electro-oculographic findings were normal (2.8 in the right eye and 3.5 in the left eye). The lesion in the left eye was nonfluorescent initially (I). Later phases (J and K, stereo, and L), however, suggested possible underlying choroidal neovascularization.

(A–F from Gass.[83])

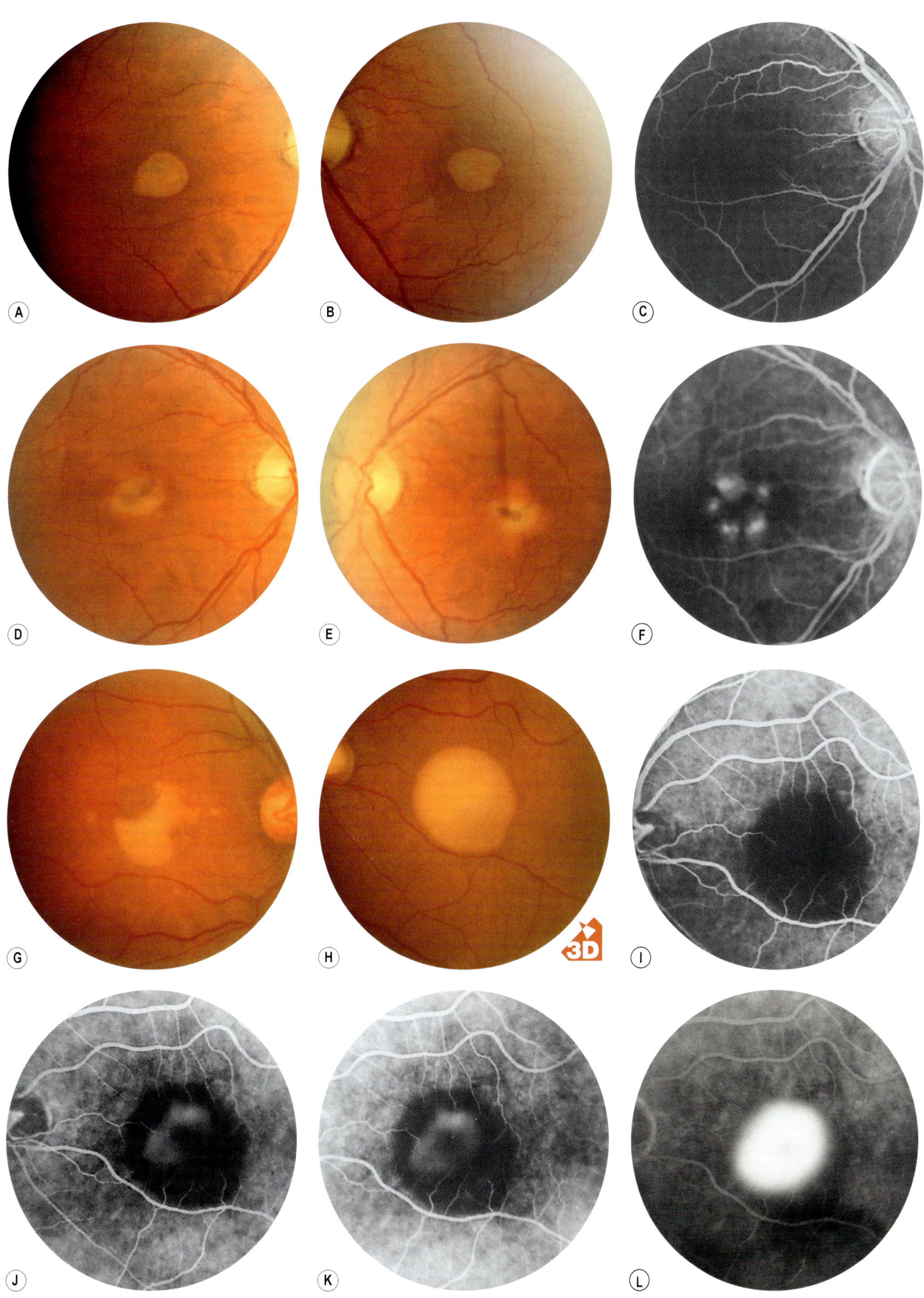
A
B
C
D
E
F
G
H
3D
I
J
K
L

Unlike those in Best's vitelliform macular dystrophy, the vitelliform lesions in patients with pattern dystrophy usually first appear in the fourth decade or beyond, are generally smaller, and do not show disruption and layering of the yellow pigment in the dependent portion of the lesions. In some families there is an overlap in the features of Best's disease and pattern dystrophy.[117]

Group 2: Butterfly-Shaped Pigment Dystrophy

When the gray or yellow pigment is arranged in a well-organized triradiate pattern confined to the center of the macula in a symmetric fashion, it has been likened to the shape of a butterfly (Figure 5.12A–C).[73,82,90] A zone of depigmentation occurs around the pigment figure. The optic disc and vessels are normal. Some patients have a reticular pigmentary pattern of drusen in the periphery. The early phases of angiography show hyperfluorescence that outlines the nonfluorescent pigment figures in the macula (Figure 5.12C). The shapes of the central yellow lesions in pattern dystrophies vary considerably and may simulate a variety of inanimate or animate objects (Figure 5.08G–L).

5.10 Clinicopathologic findings in adult-onset vitelliform foveomacular pattern dystrophy.

A–F: This 66-year-old woman had a 4-month history of gradual decrease of vision in both eyes. Her visual acuity was 20/30 and J-1 in the right eye and 20/40 and J-2 in the left eye. Note the central foveal yellowish lesions with central black dots and the scattered, small, yellowish lesions in the paracentral area (A and B). Angiography revealed a fluorescent ring in the central macular area and hyperfluorescence of the small paracentral lesions (C.) One year later the patient's vision had deteriorated slightly secondary to cataracts. The fundi were unchanged. The patient died soon after of carcinoma of the liver and the eyes were obtained for pathologic examination. Histopathologic findings in the right macula (D) showed focal loss of retinal receptor elements and pigment migration into the retina in the foveal area (arrow 1), clumping of cells laden with pigment and chorioretinal adhesion in the foveal area (arrow 2), a paracentral zone of thinning of the retinal pigment epithelium (arrows 3 and 4), and focal drusen (arrow 5). High-power view of the foveolar area (E) showed clumps of pigment-laden cells and calcific body (arrow). Note preservation of the choriocapillaris and slight thickening of the intercapillary pillars. High-power view of typical drusen (F) corresponding with one of the small yellow paracentral lesions.

G–J: Small partly faded central lesion (G and H) in the 57-year-old daughter of an 81-year-old mother with bilateral butterfly pattern of yellow flecks (I and J). The daughter's visual acuity was 20/40 in the right eye and 20/50 in the left eye and the mother's was 20/70 in both eyes.

(A–F from Gass.[83])

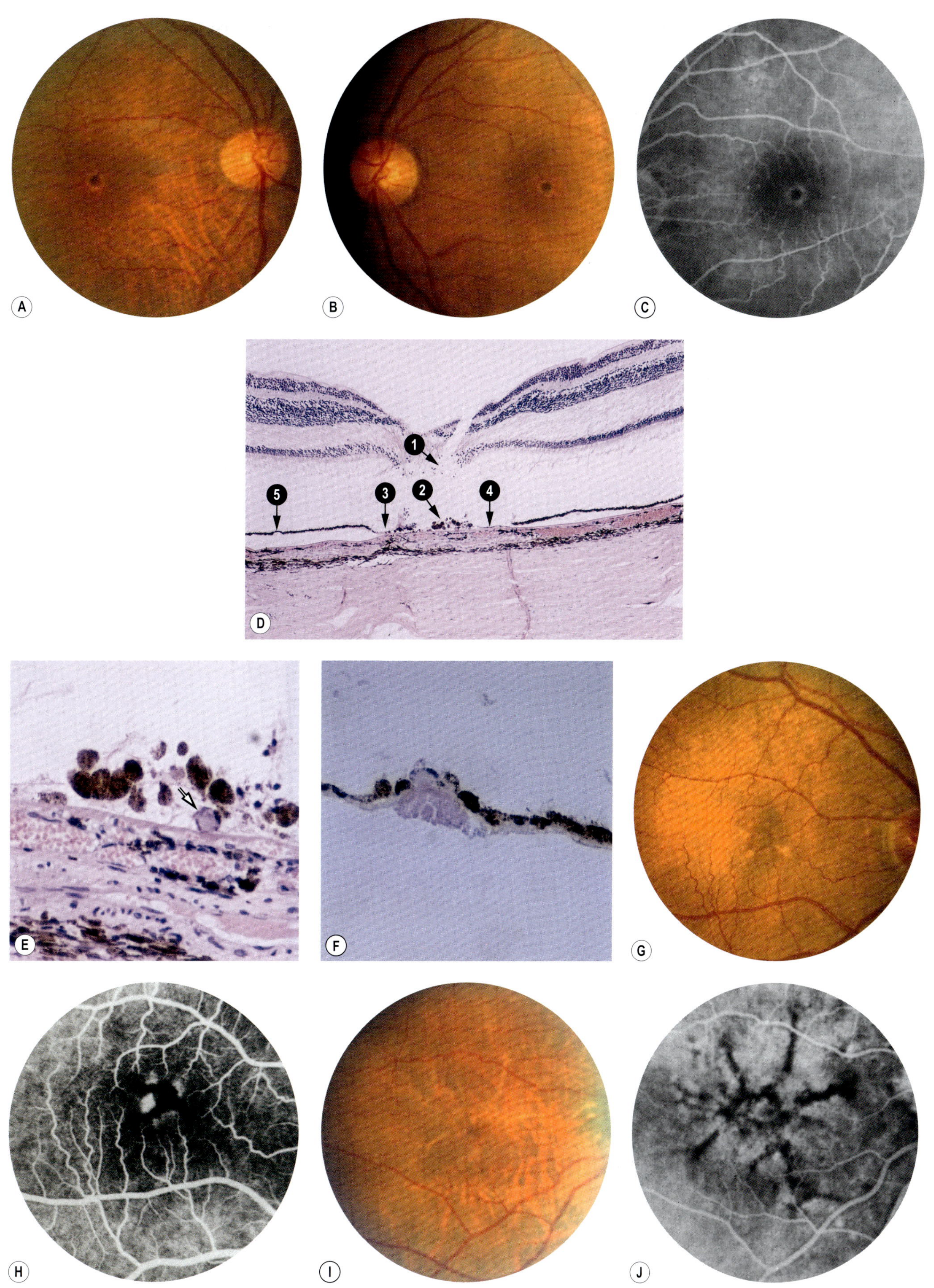
A
B
C
1
5
3
2
4
D
E
F
G
H
I
J

Group 3: Reticular Dystrophy of the RPE

In patients with reticular dystrophy the pattern of yellow pigment extends into the periphery of the macula in a highly organized pattern that has been likened to coarse, knotted fishnet or chicken wire (Figure 5.12J–L).[67,74,77,88,89,94] Its development usually begins in the foveal area. The network gradually extends four or five disc diameters from the macula in all directions. The net meshes are usually less than one disc diameter in size. The midperiphery and the periphery of the fundus are unaffected early in the disease. The network may be more apparent angiographically than ophthalmoscopically (Figure 5.12H). It usually fades with age and may be replaced by extensive atrophic changes in the RPE in later life. A similar but coarser pigmentary network has been reported by Mesker and associates.[74] Patients with reticular dystrophy may show an autosomal-recessive as well as autosomal-dominant inheritance.

5.11 Variations in pattern dystrophy.

A–C: Family with adult vitelliform foveomacular dystrophy. The 28-year-old son (A) had mild blurring of vision in the right eye and bilateral, small, focal vitelliform lesions in the macula. Visual acuity was 20/20 in the right eye and 20/15 in the left eye. Electro-oculographic ratios were 1.6 in both eyes. The 51-year-old mother had bilateral butterfly dystrophy (B and C). Her visual acuity was 20/25 in the right eye and 20/30 in the left eye. The 81-year-old maternal grandfather had bilateral geographic atrophy of the RPE and less than 20/200 vision.

D and E: Fundus pulverulentus type of pattern dystrophy in a 73-year-old man with mild visual loss of 3 years' duration. Visual acuity was 20/25. He had prominent reticular pigmentary changes in the periphery.

F–H: Reticular dystrophy in a young girl with visual acuity of 20/20 in both eyes. Her electro-oculogram and electroretinogram were normal. Two siblings had similar findings.

I–L: This 10-year-old male complained of difficulty seeing the blackboard. His visual acuity was 20/15 and 20/20 uncorrected. Both retinas show symmetrical appearance of honeycomb or chicken wire-like reticular pattern dystrophy (I and J). The hyperpigmented retinal pigment epithelium showed increased autofluorescence (K). The fovea had a normal contour with intact inner segment–outer segment junction (L, right eye).

(F–H, courtesy of Dr. Lee S. Anderson; I–L, courtesy of Dr. Scott Brodie.)

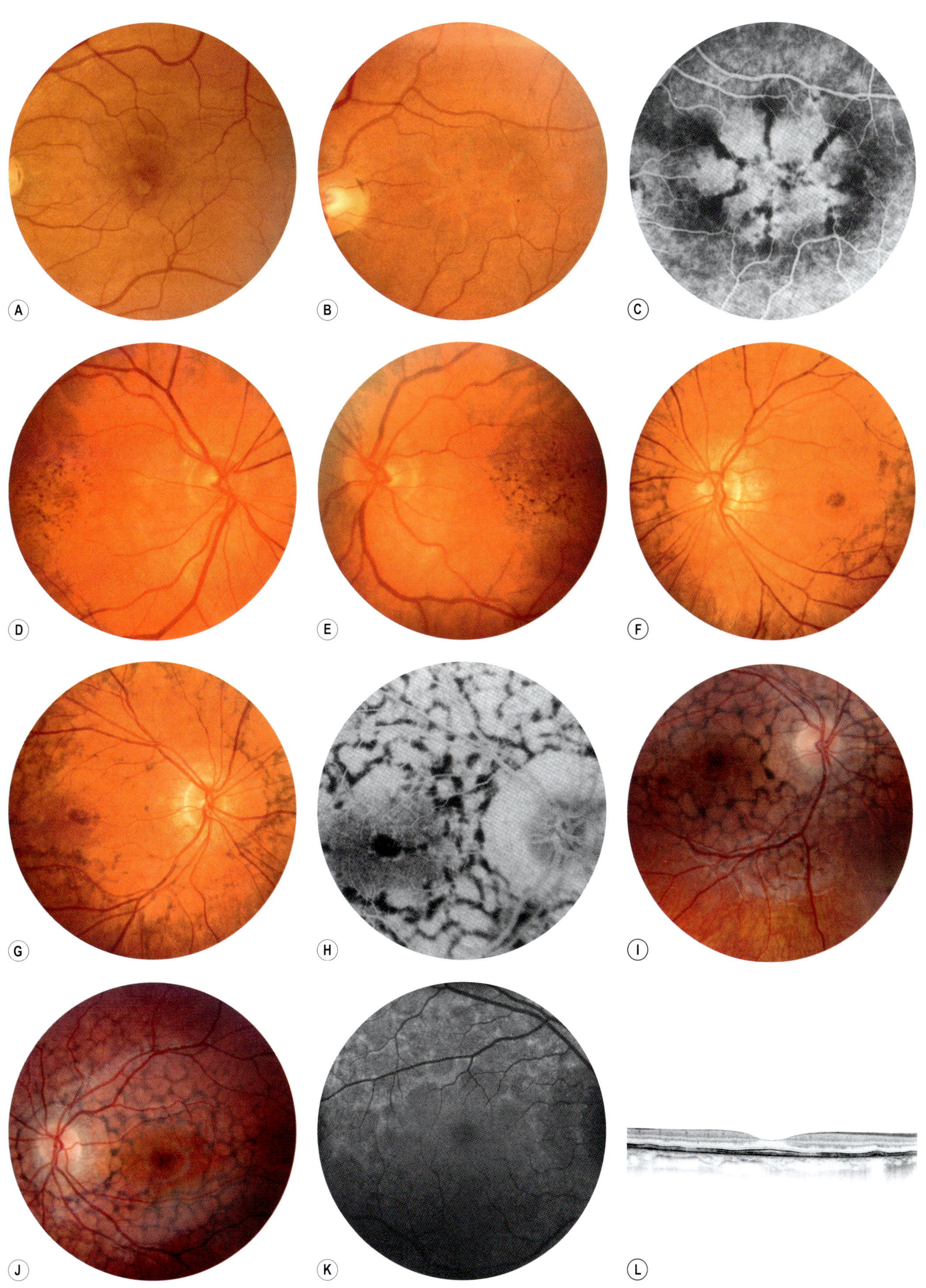
A
B
C
D
E
F
G
H
I
J
K
L

Group 4: Multifocal Pattern Dystrophy Simulating Fundus Flavimaculatus

Some patients develop multiple irregular or triradiate yellow lesions centrally or eccentrically, and in some cases these are widely scattered and partly interconnected in a triradiate fashion that may simulate that in fundus flavimaculatus (Stargardt's disease) (Figure 5.13A–H).[118–120] These patients, who do not show fluorescein angiographic evidence of a dark choroid suggesting lipofuscin storage, have been recently reported as examples of dominantly inherited fundus flavimaculatus (see p. 284). Unlike most patients with fundus flavimaculatus, these patients have good visual acuity and a more favorable visual prognosis. However, some of these patients with an exaggerated phenotype can show progressive loss of the yellow material and RPE/photoreceptor thinning and atrophy resulting in islands of, or confluent, geographic atrophy (Figure 5.13). Choroidal neovascular membranes can rarely occur (Figure 5.13). Histopathologic and electron microscopic studies of the eye of a patient with this type of pattern dystrophy have demonstrated that the flecks are not caused by abnormal lipofuscin storage (Figure 5.13G and H).[120]

Group 5: Coarse Pigment Mottling in the Macula (Fundus Pulverulentus)

Patients with fundus pulverulentus typically display mild visual loss associated with a prominent, coarse, punctiform mottling of the pigment epithelium in the central macular area (Figure 5.12D–G).[65,72,76] This pattern is most often seen in patients with pseudoxanthoma elasticum in the author's experience.[116]

Although it is convenient to subdivide patients with pattern dystrophy into these five groups, it is important to realize that the fundus findings in some patients do not fall precisely into one group. Some may show one pattern in one eye and another pattern in the fellow eye. Others may show one or more eccentric triradiate yellow or darkly pigmented lesions. Some may have one or more lesions in only one eye early in their course. The fundus findings in patients with pattern dystrophy and an asymmetric distribution of triradiate pigment figures must be differentiated from similar findings that may develop in some patients with recurrent idiopathic central serous chorioretinopathy/organ transplant retinopathy, and in patients with Elschnig spots caused by hypertensive choroidopathy, e.g., in a patient with toxemia of pregnancy. (See Chapter 3, Figures 3.57 and 3.58.)

The visual prognosis is good in all subgroups of dominantly inherited pattern dystrophy.[85,121] Late geographic atrophy (Figure 5.11I and K) and choroidal neovascularization may occur in any of the subgroups and are responsible for visual loss. Choroidal neovascularization occurs only infrequently.[102] Gass observed it most frequently in patients with the solitary vitelliform, butterfly pattern, and the exaggerated pattern simulating fundus flavimaculatus (Figures 5.11A–H and 5.12I–L). Some, if not most, of the reports of subretinal neovascularization in fundus flavimaculatus probably concern patients with pattern dystrophy.[122] Absence of a dark choroid angiographically and good visual function suggest pattern dystrophy rather than fundus flavimaculatus.[118,120] An occasional cause of loss of vision in these patients is the development of a macular hole.[123] Gass has observed the development of a macular hole in both eyes of a patient who some years previously presented with adult-onset foveomacular dystrophy.

5.12 Pattern dystrophy simulating fundus flavimaculatus.

A–C: This 53-year-old woman had 20/20 visual acuity bilaterally. Her electroretinographic and electro-oculographic findings were normal. There was no family history for eye disease. Angiograms of both eyes (B and C) showed multifocal stellate hypofluorescent lesions surrounded by hyperfluorescence and no evidence of diffuse dampening of the background fluorescence.

D–H: Clinicopathologic findings in a 51-year-old man with normal visual acuity and a fundus picture simulating fundus flavimaculatus. Note the peripheral flecks and the normal appearance of the central macular area (D–F). Light and electron microscopy revealed subtle and focal distension and minor variations in pigmentation of the retinal pigment epithelium (RPE). Occasional cells showed distended, relatively nonpigmented, dome-shaped apices extending above the adjacent RPE (G and H). The RPE did not stain with periodic acid–Schiff or for acid mucopolysaccharides. Electron microscopy showed that those RPE cells with distended cytoplasm contained tubulovesicular membranous material (H).

I–L: A 55-year-old woman from Trinidad with mixed heritage of African, East Indian, and French presented with decreased vision in her left eye to 20/100. Both fundi showed extensive fundus flavimaculatus type of pattern dystrophy extending beyond the arcades and loss of the vitelliform material in much of the lesions. Both maculas showed geographic atrophy and the left, a choroidal neovascularization in addition (I). A fluorescein angiogram confirmed the subfoveal choroidal neovascular membrane in the center of the geographic atrophy, with increasing fluorescence in the late frames (J and K). Note the absence of a dark choroid and halo of hyperfluorescence around central blockage from pigment, typical of fundus flavimaculatus type of pattern dystrophy. The right eye had a similar appearance without the choroidal neovascular membrane. She received intravitreal injections of bevacizumab every month for 4 months followed by every 2 months for a total of 8 injections. Her vision in the left eye improved to 20/40 and continued to remain stable at last follow-up 3 years later. An autofluorescence imaging shows increased autofluorescence of the yellow flecks and decreased autofluorescence of the atrophic flecks (L).

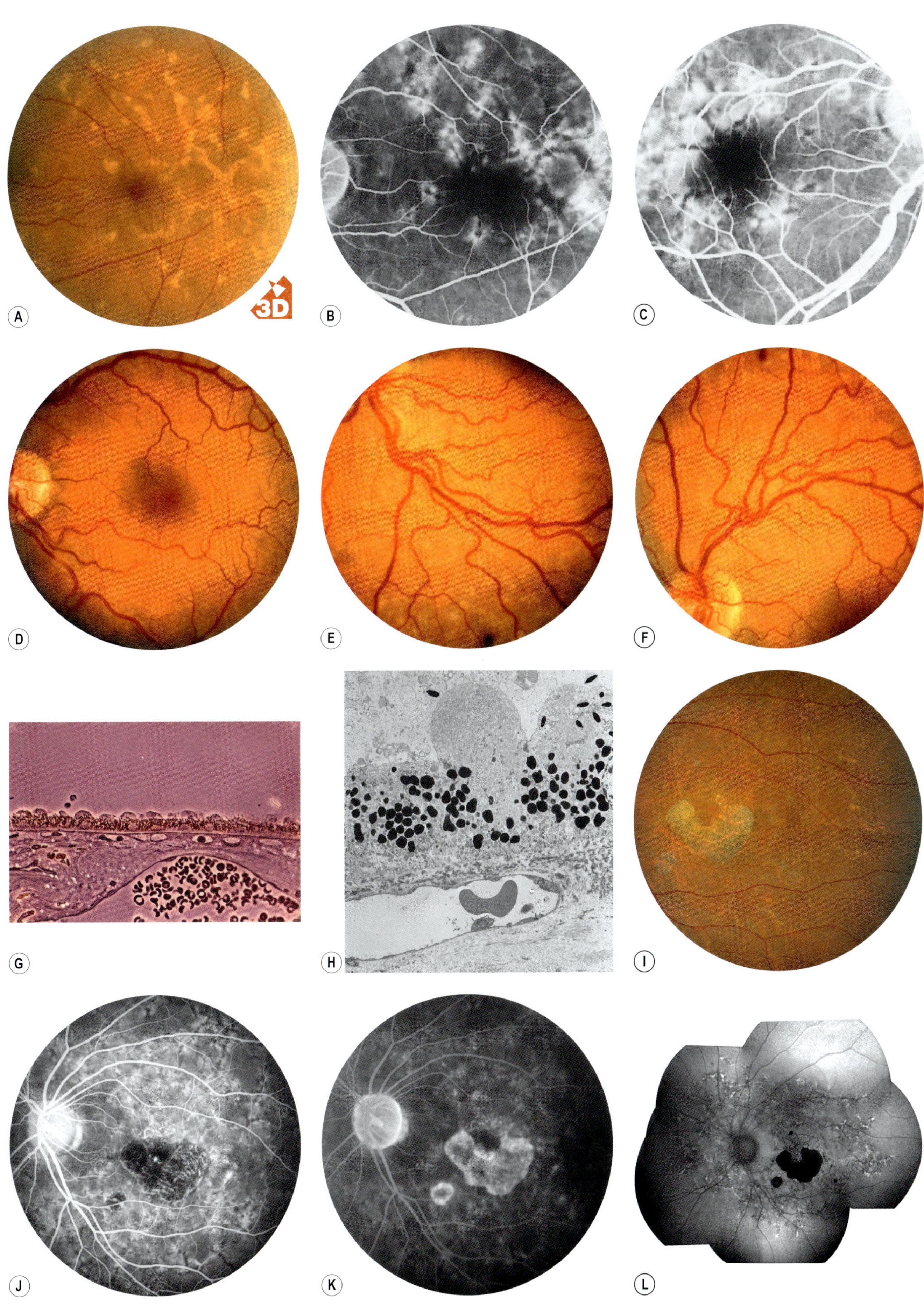
A
3D
B
C
D
E
F
G
H
I
J
K
L

Histopathologic examination of two eyes of a patient with a solitary yellow foveal lesion bilaterally (Figure 5.10A–F) showed focal loss of the retinal receptor elements and atrophy and partial loss of the RPE in the foveal area of both eyes.[83] The central pigmented spots seen biomicroscopically were caused by a clump of large pigment-laden cells and extracellular melanin pigment lying between the retina and Bruch's membrane with some extension into the outer retinal layers. In a ring-like zone surrounding this central pigment clump was a thick layer of slightly granular, eosinophilic, PAS-positive material lying between the thinned atrophic RPE and Bruch's membrane. Fluorescent microscopy showed no unusual amount of lipofuscin present within the RPE cells in this lesion. Bruch's membrane, the choriocapillaris, and the large choroidal blood vessels underlying the lesion were within normal limits. The paracentral yellow spots seen ophthalmoscopically proved to be typical drusen histopathologically (Figure 5.10F).

Histopathologic examination of the eyes of two other patients with almost identical lesions revealed similar findings.[71,124] In one case, however, the eye showed evidence of a high concentration of lipofuscin, which may be responsible for the central yellow lesion.[71] A report of the histopathologic and ultrastructural findings in two eyes of a 51-year-old man with a pattern of flecks suggesting fundus flavimaculatus and normal macula and visual acuity found no evidence of lipofuscin storage or acid mucopolysaccharide accumulation in the RPE – these are characteristic findings in fundus flavimaculatus (Figure 5.13D–H).[120] Elevated aggregates of enlarged RPE cells with apices distended by accumulated lipid membranes with a tubulovesicular appearance were responsible for the flecks (Figure 5.13G and H). The findings in this patient suggest that the yellow flecks in the pattern dystrophies, although they clinically appear similar to those in Stargardt's disease and fundus flavimaculatus, are not caused by focal lipofuscin storage in the RPE. The same may prove true in the case of vitelliform lesions in Best's disease. Unlike patients with Stargardt's disease, patients with Best's disease and adult-onset vitelliform foveomacular dystrophy do not show the angiographic feature of obstruction of the normal background choroidal fluorescence (silent choroid) that is caused by diffuse heavy deposition of lipofuscin material in the RPE.

5.13 Complications of pattern dystrophy.

Choroidal neovascular membrane (CNVM).

A–H: This 75-year-old woman had a history of solitary vitelliform lesions in both eyes and presented with a choroidal neovascular membrane in her left eye and a visual decline to 20/100 (A, B). She underwent photodynamic therapy to the left eye, which resulted in a disciform scar. Fifteen months later the vision in the right eye dropped to 20/40 with increase in the size of the vitelliform lesion and reorganization of the central pigment (C). An angiogram showed staining of the yellow material (D and E). Four months later her vision dropped to 20/100; she now showed evidence of a CNVM with subretinal fluid and blood (F). An angiogram showed a classic CNVM with lacy appearance early and late leakage (G and H). The right eye also underwent photodynamic therapy with limited success.

Geographic atrophy.

I–L: This 65-year-old male presented with a vision of 20/70 in the right and 20/20 in the left eye. There was a small island of geographic atrophy corresponding to the loss of the yellow pigment in the foveal lesion (I and J). Autofluorescence shows decreased autofluorescence consistent with loss of retinal pigment epithelium (K). The left vitelliform lesion showed hyperautofluorescence (L).

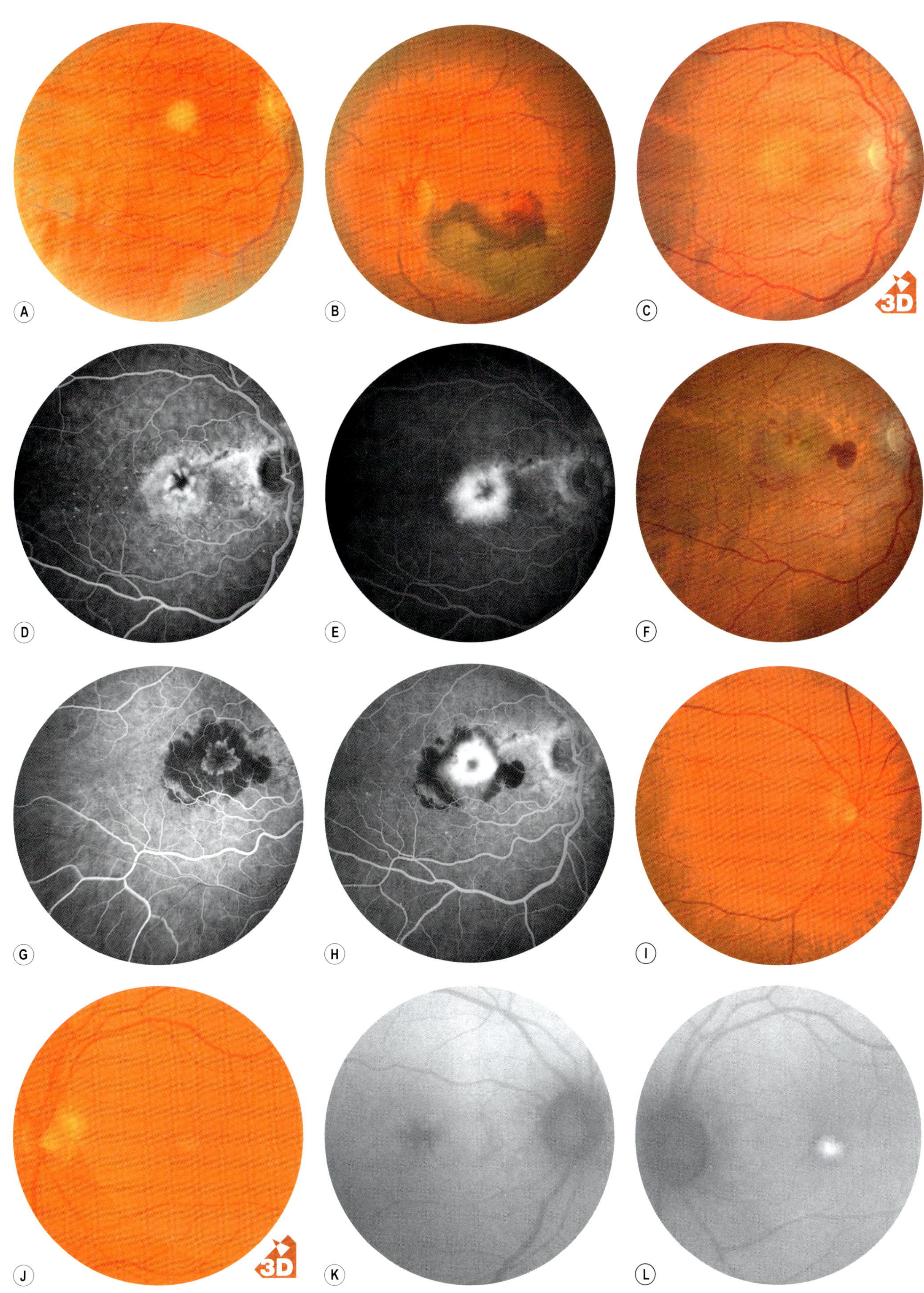
A
B
C
3D
D
E
F
G
H
I
J
3D
K
L

KJELLIN'S SYNDROME (HEREDITARY SPASTIC PARAPLEGIA)

Kjellin's syndrome is an autosomal-recessive syndrome characterized by slowly progressive spastic paraparesis and dementia.[142,143] Some of these patients may show evidence of pattern dystrophy of the retina, most often the fundus flavimaculatus type (Figure 5.15). The flecks seem to be stationary or very slowly progressive with no change noted over 5 years in a patient followed by the author (Figure 5.15A, B, K, and L). The fluorescein angiogram shows central blockage from the yellow material with halo of hyperfluorescence surrounding this, quite typical of the appearance in isolated pattern dystrophy.[144] Autofluorescence study shows brilliant fluorescence of the material in the macula (Figure 5.15H and I)[144]; in addition the pigment epithelium shows widespread reticular type of hyperautofluorescence outside the macula (Figure 5.15 H and I), the significance of which is still unknown. The OCT suggests accumulation of the material within and just anterior to the RPE (Figure 5.15J1 and J2). The flecks and the RPE changes are not associated with significant visual morbidity, suggesting very slow breakdown of the cells that may be contributing towards the accumulation of the yellow material.

Vitelliform lesions similar to pattern dystrophy have been seen in a variety of maternally inherited mitochondrial diseases, including maternally inherited diabetes and deafness (MIDD), mitochondrial myopathy, encephalopathy, lactic acidosis, and stroke-like episodes (MELAS), myoclonic epilepsy, red ragged fibers (MERRF), and more widespread pigmentary changes in Kearns–Sayre, neurogenic muscle weakness, ataxia retinitis pigmentosa (NARP), and Danon disease (see later sections).

5.15 Kjellin's syndrome (hereditary spastic paraplegia) and pattern dystrophy.

A to **L**: This 44-year-old male developed progressive ataxia, spastic paraplegia over the previous 10 years. His visual acuity was correctable to 20/20 with refraction when first examined in 2003. Both eyes showed yellow triradiate flecks, some with brown pigment within them, distributed over the posterior pole (A and B). Fluorescein angiogram showed central nonfluorescence with a halo of hyperfluorescence typical of pattern dystrophy (C–E). In 2008, autofluorescence imaging showed central increased autofluorescence corresponding to the brown pigmentation. In addition there were lattice-like autofluorescent changes in the nasal retina extending up to the equator, that corresponded to mild pigmentary changes seen on fundus photography (F–I). Optical coherence tomography revealed these lesions as thickening of the retinal pigment epithelium (J1 and J2). His lesions and vision have remained unchanged over more than 7 years (K and L), suggesting the condition is almost nonprogressive.

(A-D, Also, Yannuzzi, Lawrence J., The Retinal Atlas, Saunders 2010, 978-0-7020-3320-9, p.112).

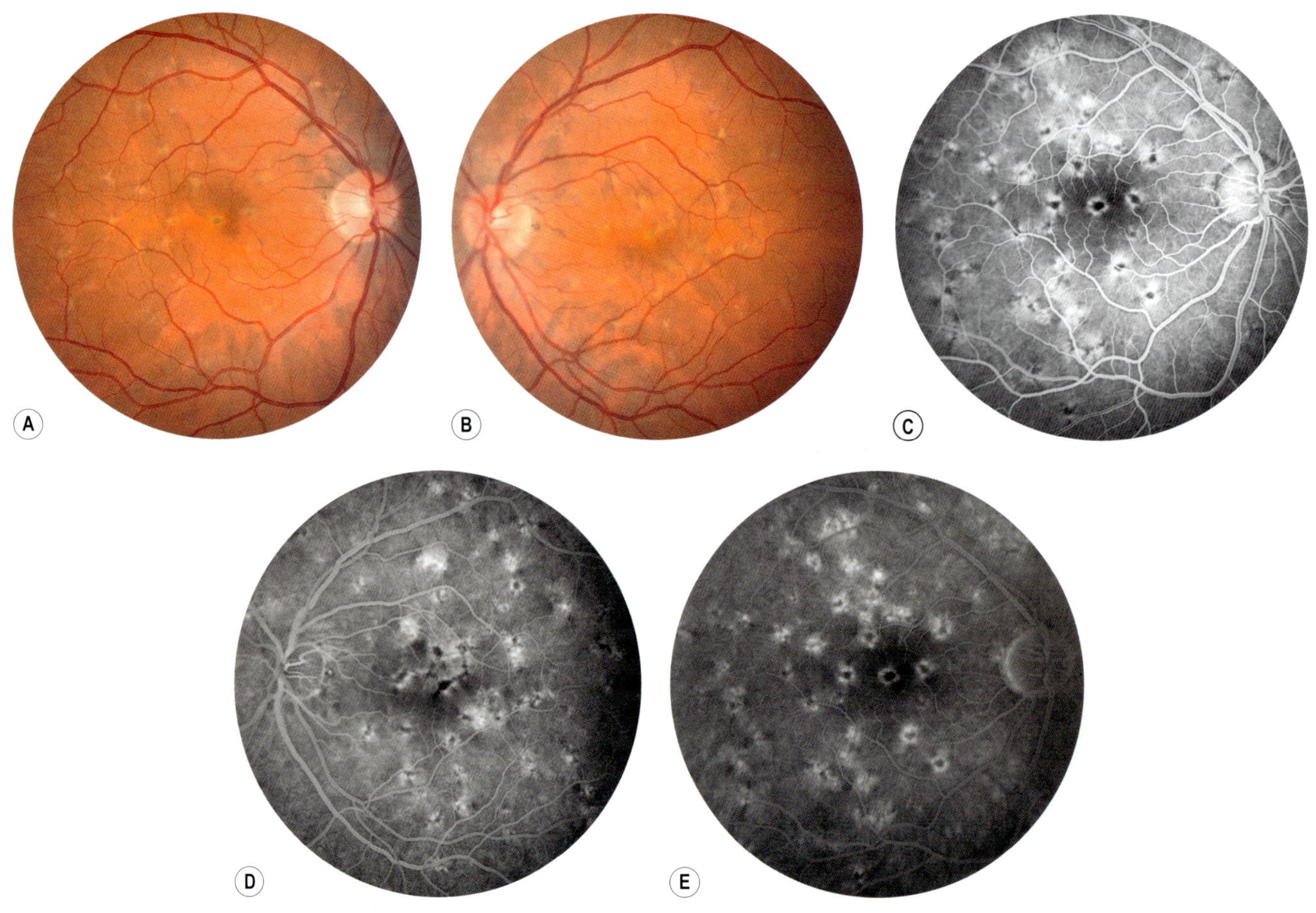

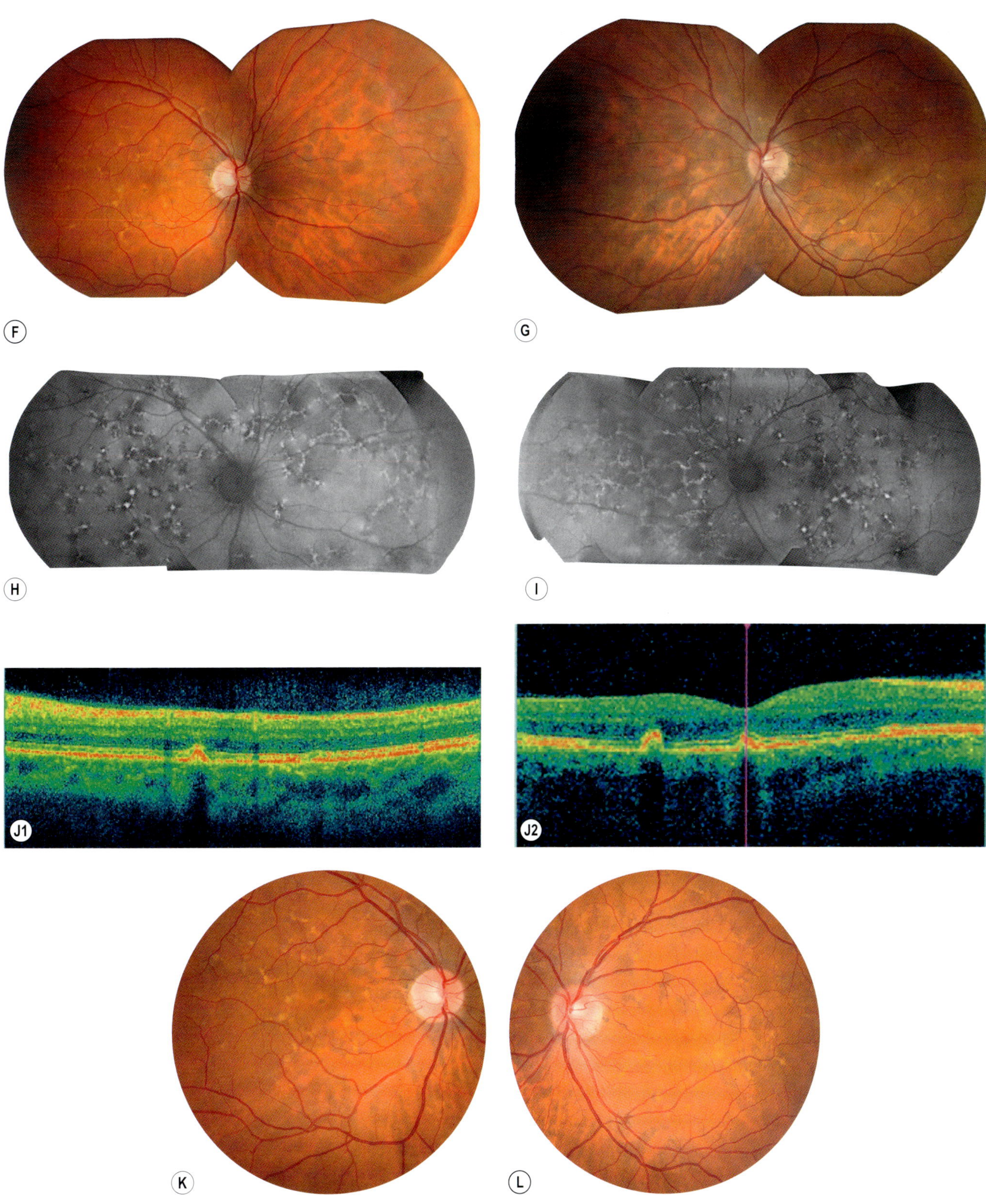
F
G
H
I
J1
J2
K
L

MACULAR PATTERN DYSTROPHY IN MIDD, MELAS, AND MERRF

Mitochondrial DNA is inherited from the mother. Mitochondrial defects affect high-energy-utilizing organs such as the central nervous system, eye, inner ear, skeletal, and cardiac muscle. A point mutation A3243G in the mitochondrial DNA causes both MIDD and MELAS. The exact reason why the same mutation causes a different phenotype is not completely understood, though there can be an overlap of findings in some patients with MIDD and MELAS to a variable extent.[145] Affected individuals can fall anywhere in the wide spectrum of clinical features. The disease can vary greatly in severity and features within a family. The degree of heteroplasmy (cells contain both mutated and normal mitochondrial DNA) likely determines the phenotypic variability between the three syndromes and in individuals within the same family.

A3243G mitochondrial mutation in individuals is seen with a wide range of mitochondrial encephalomyopathies, including MELAS or MELAS/MERRF overlap syndrome. It has been postulated that mitochondrial dysfunction causes a reduction in adenosine triphosphate, which in turn leads to an ion imbalance that results in death of hair cell and stria vascularis in the inner ear. Postmortem histopathologic examination of the temporal bone of a woman with MIDD due to the A3243G mutation has identified diffuse outer hair cell loss, severe degeneration of the stria vascularis, as well as a reduction in spiral ganglion cells. Similar histopathologic findings have been reported in association with the A3243G mutation in MELAS, though marked loss of neurons and gliosis in the ventral cochlear nuclei were also noted.[146]

Macular pattern dystrophy seen in this disease spectrum has a variable phenotype (Figures 5.16 and 5.17).[146–152] The manifestations can be: grade I: several punctate pigment dots in the macula; grade II: a butterfly or reticular pattern that on fluorescein angiography shows the typical hyperfluorescent halo around an area of decreased fluorescence; grade III: in some eyes multifocal or a continuous perifoveal atrophy of the RPE. The flecks show increased autofluorescence (Figure 5.17E) (resembling the pattern seen in fundus flavimaculatus) while the areas of RPE atrophy show decreased autofluorescence (Figure 5.17J and L).

5.16 Progression of pattern dystrophy in maternally inherited diabetes and deafness (MIDD), mitochondrial myopathy, encephalopathy, lactic acidosis, and stroke-like episodes (MELAS), and myoclonic epilepsy, red ragged fibers (MERRF).

A–F: The patient is a 51-year-old female who first presented in 2001 with a 5-year history of blurred vision which she described as words disappearing while reading. Visual acuity was 20/20 both eyes. She was found to be mutation-positive for the mitochondrial DNA A3243G mutation. Past medical history included a 31-year history of insulin-dependent diabetes, a 6-year history of decreased hearing and tinnitus, difficulty with balance, peripheral neuropathy, cardiomyopathy, weakness, and fatigue. Her mother had diabetes and deafness. The patient's 51-year-old sister had no diabetes, hearing loss or eye problems and denied other medical problems; she did not have mutation testing. The patient's 29-year-old son had no history of any systemic problems other than an appendectomy in the past. His fundus revealed myopic nerves with normal fundus autofluorescence. The patient's 27-year-old daughter also had a normal fundus exam and autofluorescence but did have a history of migraine and fatigue. Both children were found to be positive for the A3243G mutation. Her fundus exam revealed circumferential perifoveal islands of atrophy with surrounding pigment clumping (A and B). There was mild NPDR in both eyes. Angiography showed window defects in the area of the atrophy, hyperfluorescent microaneurysms and blocking defect by the subretinal pigment clumps (C and D). Fundus autofluorescence demonstrated decreased autofluorescence in areas of atrophy with surrounding speckled areas of increased and decreased autofluorescence in an area that was larger than would be expected by fundus exam alone (E and F).

G and **H**: This patient first presented in 1996 at the age of 43 with a pigmentary macular abnormality in both eyes which was diagnosed as a pattern dystrophy. Vision was 20/20 in both eyes. Past medical history was significant for hearing loss and tinnitus from the age of 25; there was no history of diabetes. In 2000 at 47 years of age she had a mild cerebrovascular accident and later developed seizures. Due to the development of additional medical problems mitochondrial DNA testing was performed. The patient was found to have the A3243G mutation. The family history was positive for a mother with diabetes. The fundus revealed mild mottling of the retinal pigment epithelium with mild pigment clumping in the periphery of both eyes; no atrophy was present (G and H).

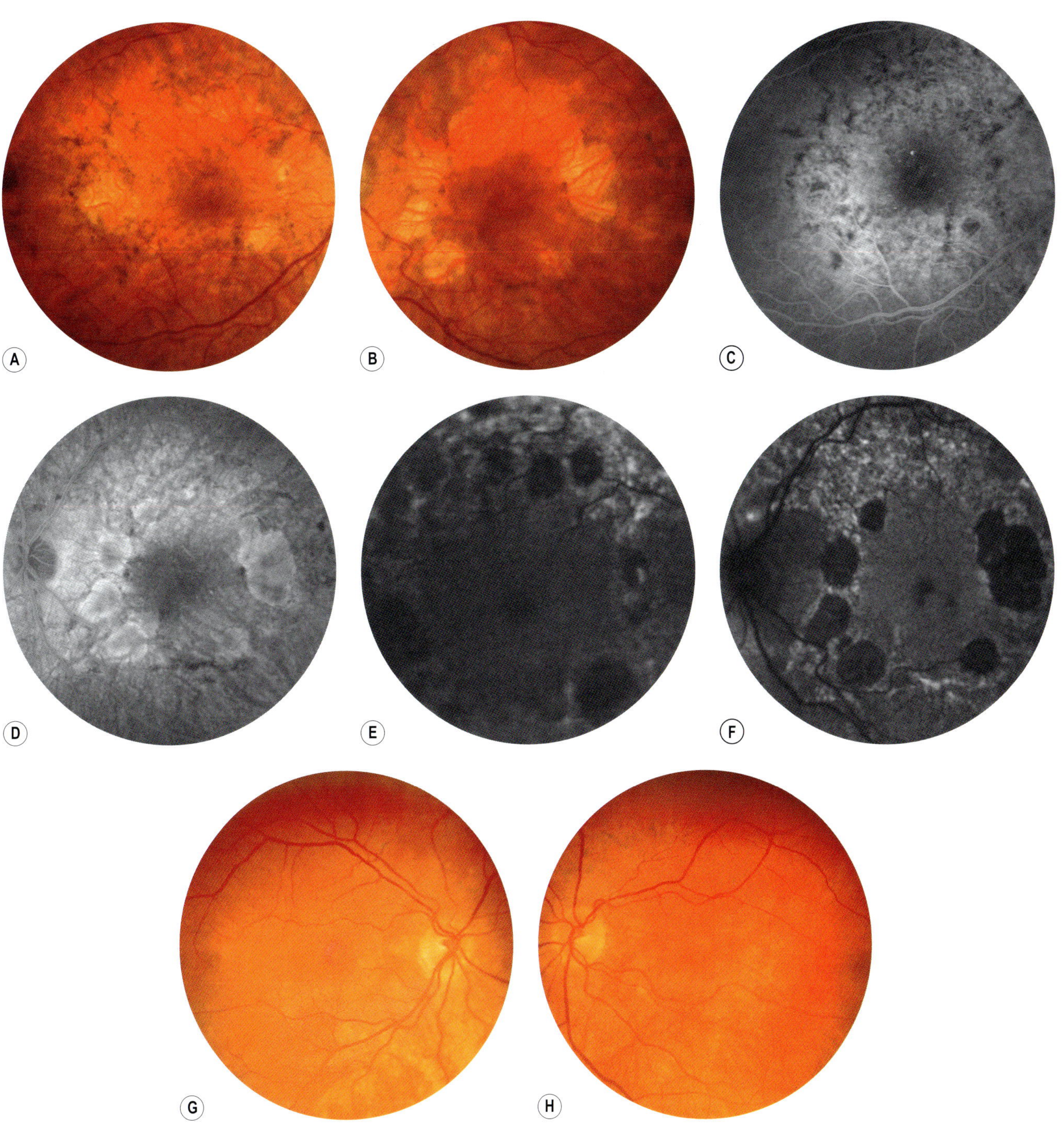
A
B
C
D
E
F
G
H

Rath et al.[148] classified MIDD A3243G mutation-associated macular dystrophy into:

- Type 1: continuous or discontinuous perifoveal geographic atrophy
- Type 2: pattern dystrophy with flecks and variable RPE atrophy.

It appears that the phenotype changes with age, with increasing geographic atrophy over time.[149]

5.16 Continued

I–P: This patient first presented in 1994 at the age of 43 with a history of paracentral scotomas and difficulty adjusting to changes in lighting. Visual acuity was 20/20 in both eyes. Medical history was significant for diabetes of 4 years duration, insulin-dependent for 2 months. Hearing loss began to develop in 1996. Fundus photos in 1994 revealed circumferential perifoveal areas of geographic atrophy (I and J). There was significant progression of the macular atrophy with visual acuity of 20/30 in both eyes in 2001 (K and L). Fundus autofluorescence in 2007 reveals decreased autofluorescence in areas of atrophy with surrounding areas of speckled autofluorescence in an area larger than would be expected based on clinical exam. Fundus autofluorescence of the patient's mother (O and P), whose fundus appeared normal, showed subtle mottling of the autofluorescence in a circumferential pattern perifoveally. Interestingly, the patient's mother's blood tested negative for the A3243G mitochondrial DNA mutation; no muscle biopsy was performed. It is known that the ability to detect the mutation in the peripheral blood decreases as a person ages; it is also possible this was a new mutation in the patient herself but, less likely given the fundus autofluorescence abnormalities in the mother. The mother also had a history of adult-onset diabetes without hearing loss.

(Courtesy of Dr. Pamela Rath and Dr. Alan Bird; A, from Bellmann et al.[1245]; B, F, H–L, from Rath et al.[148])

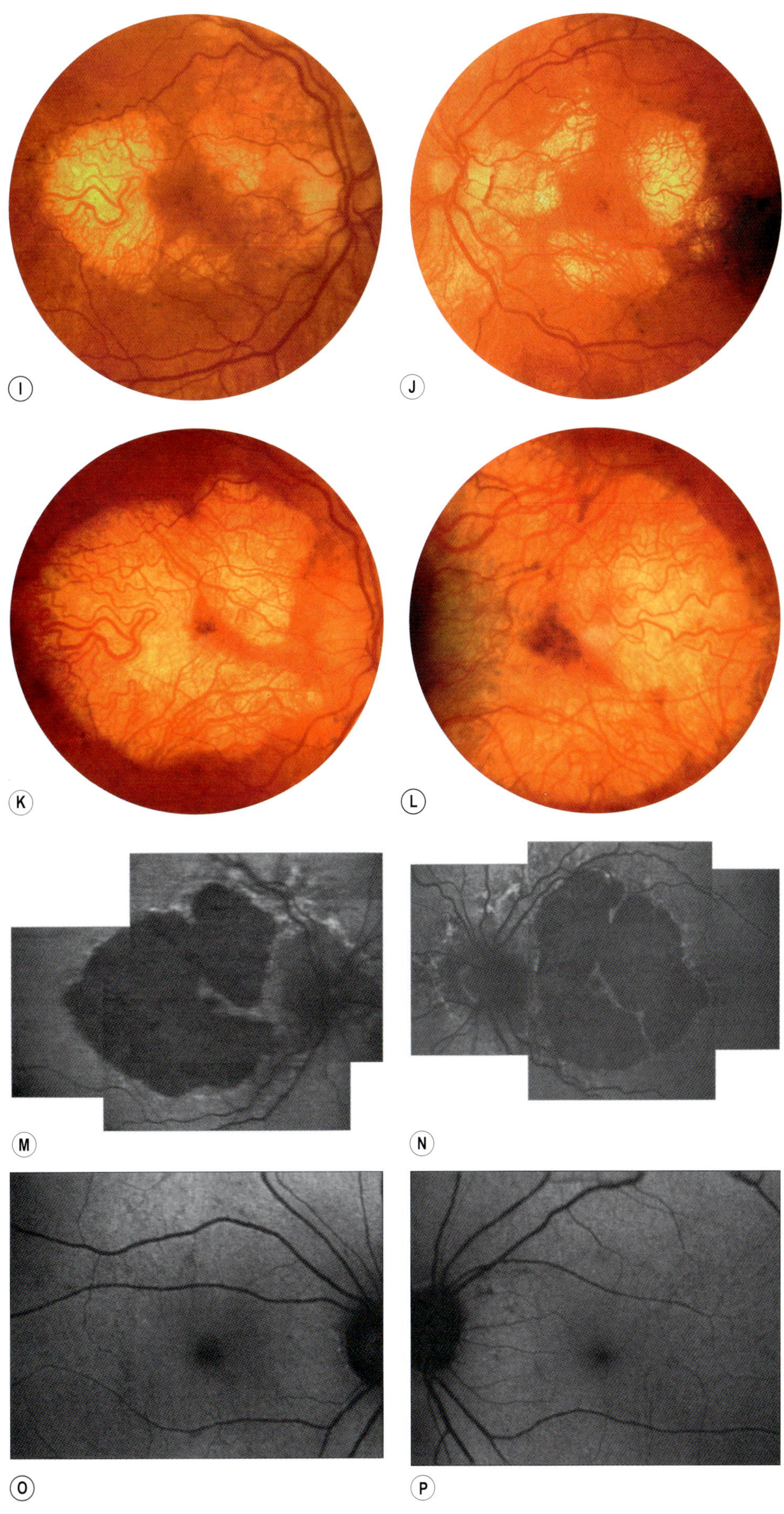
I
J
K
L
M
N
O
P

5.17 Pattern dystrophy in maternally inherited diabetes and deafness (MIDD).

A–F: Evolution of retinal lesions in a patient who was 47 years of age at first examination (A–C), and after 3 years of follow-up (D–F). She carried the mitochondrial m.3243A > G mutation, and was previously diagnosed with sensorineural hearing loss and diabetes mellitus. During follow-up, her visual acuity remained stable (20/40), although she experienced subjective central visual loss. Initially, this patient showed macular and peripapillary pigmentary alterations. In the fovea, a vitelliform lesion (A) with increased autofluorescence and some satellite lesions (B) were observed. The lesion was hypofluorescent on angiography, due to blockage of the choroidal fluorescence and was surrounded by a hyperfluorescent mildly atrophic zone (C1). Hyperreflective material was seen between the neurosensory retina and retinal pigment epithelium (C2). Three years later, the vitelliform material had disappeared leaving a zone of chorioretinal atrophy that began to encroach on the fovea (D). This chorioretinal atrophy corresponded to markedly decreased autofluorescence. Some satellite lesions faded, whereas other lesions became more prominent in size and intensity of autofluorescence (E). A hyperfluorescent well-demarcated window defect was seen on angiography (F1). On optical coherence tomography, irregular attenuation of the photoreceptor–retinal pigment epithelial layers was seen in the atrophic area of the previous vitelliform lesion. The outer retinal structures in the fovea also appeared abnormal, but still relatively preserved (F2).

G–L: Retinal phenotype of a 55-year-old patient, who was asymptomatic and had a visual acuity of 20/20 in both eyes. A few years previously, diabetes mellitus was diagnosed, but no deafness. After the retinal phenotype was diagnosed, MIDD was confirmed by the finding of the m.3243A > G mitochondrial mutation. Ophthalmoscopy revealed a broad horseshoe-shaped zone of chorioretinal atrophy that encircled the fovea of the right eye (G). A less severe appearance with foveal sparing was seen in the left eye (H). The "foveal island" of normal autofluorescence was surrounded by a large zone of absent autofluorescence due to chorioretinal atrophy. Outside this atrophic area, speckled variable autofluorescence was noted (I and J). The angiogram of the left eye shows irregular transmission hyperfluorescence except where blocked by pigment (K). Four years later, the chorioretinal atrophy has expanded with gradual narrowing of the preserved foveal area (L).

(Courtesy of Dr. Camiel Boon.)

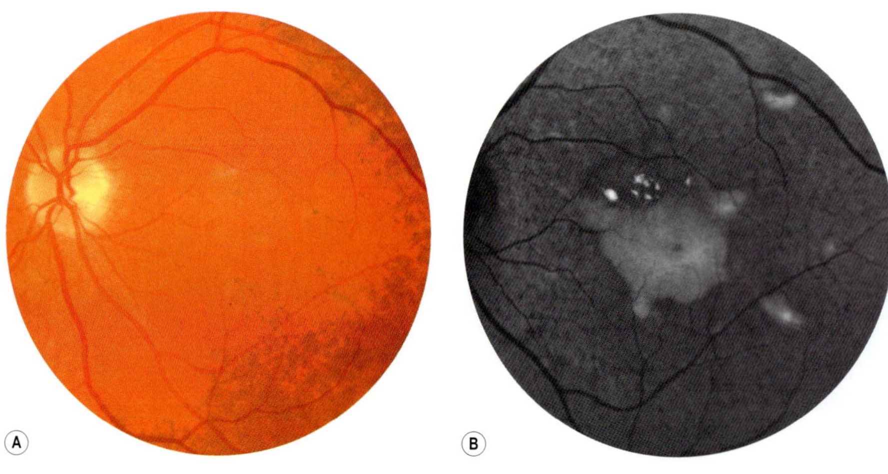

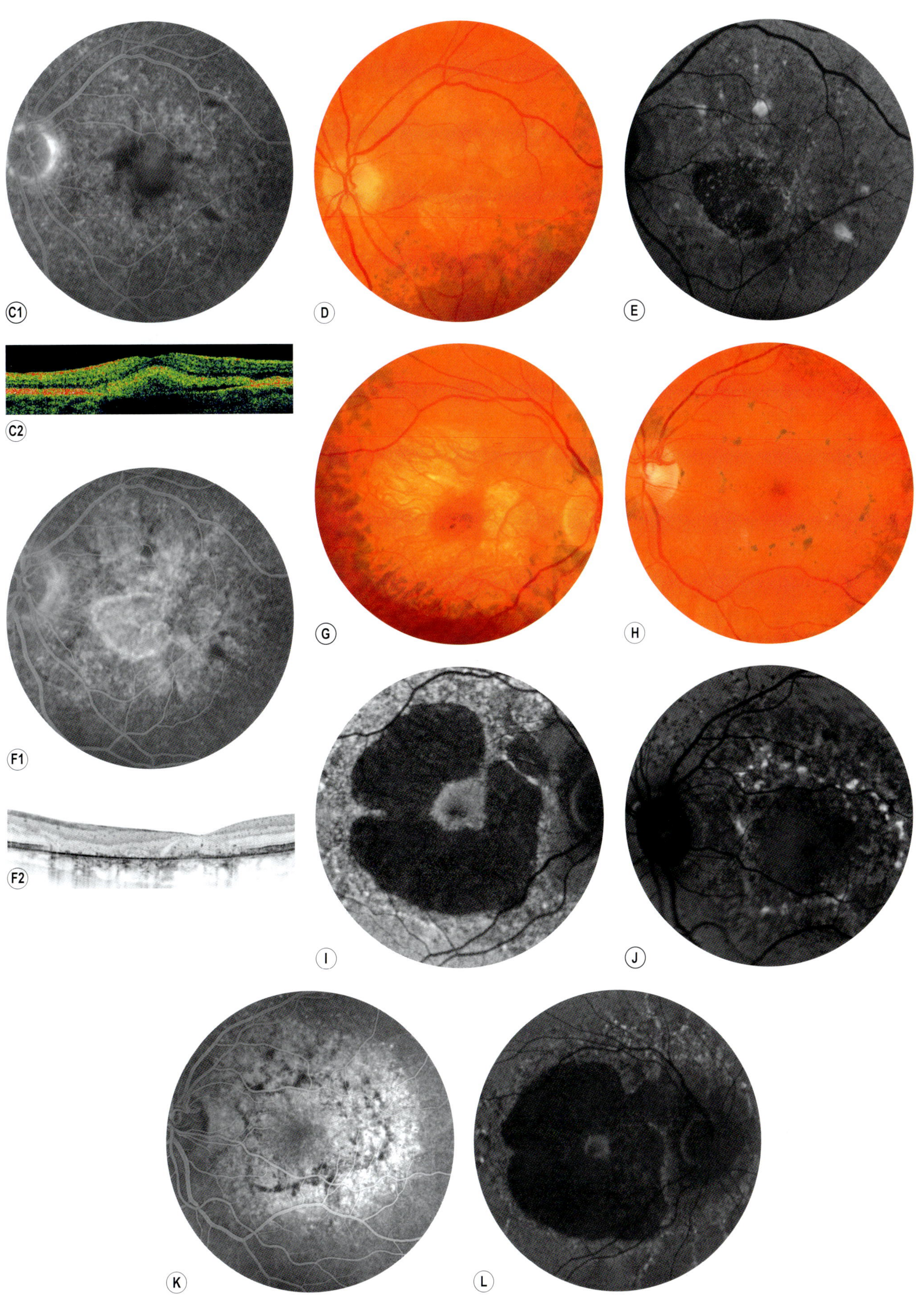
C1
D
E
C2
G
H
F1
F2
I
J
K
L

STARGARDT'S DISEASE (FUNDUS FLAVIMACULATUS)

In 1909 Stargardt described an apparently autosomal-recessive disorder in seven patients from two families, with visual loss beginning in the first two decades of life, often with a normal fundus, and later associated with macular atrophy and yellowish deep retinal flecks.[153] Rosehr examined two of Stargardt's original patients 50 years later and found that they had good peripheral function.[154] In 1965 Franceschetti described similar patients but with flecks that extended into the peripheral fundus.[155,156] Histopathologic and histochemical studies in recent years have demonstrated evidence that these patients have a diffuse lipofuscin storage disease affecting the RPE.[157–162] Stargardt's disease and fundus flavimaculatus are names now used interchangeably in the literature for what the author believes are a heterogeneous group of disorders. Most authors do not restrict the diagnosis of Stargardt's disease and fundus flavimaculatus to patients with fluorescein angiographic evidence of lipofuscin storage in the RPE, although most agree that the majority of patients show evidence of it. This author prefers to restrict the diagnosis of Stargardt's disease and fundus flavimaculatus to describe different stages of the same disease in patients who, early in life, develop a vermillion or darkly colored fundus caused by excessive storage of lipofuscin within the RPE that prevents visualization of choroidal details ("dark" choroid).[155–157,160,162–178]

Patients with Stargardt's disease, usually during childhood or early adulthood, develop visual loss that may be unassociated with any evidence of flecks or RPE atrophy initially (Figures 5.18A and B and 5.19A and B) but soon afterward is associated with atrophic macular changes and the appearance of peculiar yellowish RPE flecks (Figure 5.18C, F, H, and I). They appear somewhat similar to, but should be differentiated from, drusen. These flecks are variable in size, shape, and distribution. Unlike drusen, they are less often discretely round, oval, and dome-shaped. When located in the midperiphery, they are often arranged in a triradiate or reticular pattern that has been likened to a forked fishtail. As they begin to fade, their color changes from yellow to gray, partly due to loss of RPE substance, and they may appear larger and less discrete. Fluorescein angiography is important in differentiating the flecks in Stargardt's disease (fundus flavimaculatus) from drusen. Whereas drusen show a pattern of hyperfluorescence corresponding precisely with their size, the yellow flecks in fundus flavimaculatus either appear nonfluorescent when the lipofuscin is intracellular or show an irregular pattern of fluorescence with disruption or atrophy of RPE cells (Figures 5.18G and 5.19H).[179]

5.18 Stargardt's disease.

A–C: In 1979 this 15-year-old white man had a paracentral scotoma. His visual acuity was 20/20. Except for a deep orange-red (vermillion) color, the fundi were normal (A). Angiography (B) demonstrated a "silent" choroid and a ring of faint hyperfluorescence. In 1991 his visual acuity was 20/200 and multiple flecks (C) were evident.

D–G: This 16-year-old female with unexplained visual loss and 20/200 vision in both eyes was suspected of having a brain tumor. The fundi appear normal (D). Neurologic examination and skull roentgenograms were normal. Angiography (E) revealed a faint ring of hyperfluorescence in the central macular area and no evidence of obstruction of the choroidal fluorescence. One year later (F) there were definite atrophic changes in the retinal pigment epithelium as well as multiple small flecks in the macular areas. Angiography (G) showed greater hyperfluorescence centrally and evidence of obstruction of the choroidal fluorescence elsewhere.

H–L: Forty-year-old male followed for the past 7 years with 20/20 vision in each eye. Extensive yellow pisciform flecks in the posterior pole of both eyes with islands of geographic atrophy sparing the fovea (H and I). The yellow flecks towards the periphery are hyperautofluorescent; those that have lost the yellow material towards the center are hypoautofluorescent; the islands of RPE loss are nonautofluorescent (J and K). Optical coherence tomography localises the flecks to the retinal pigment epithelium (L).

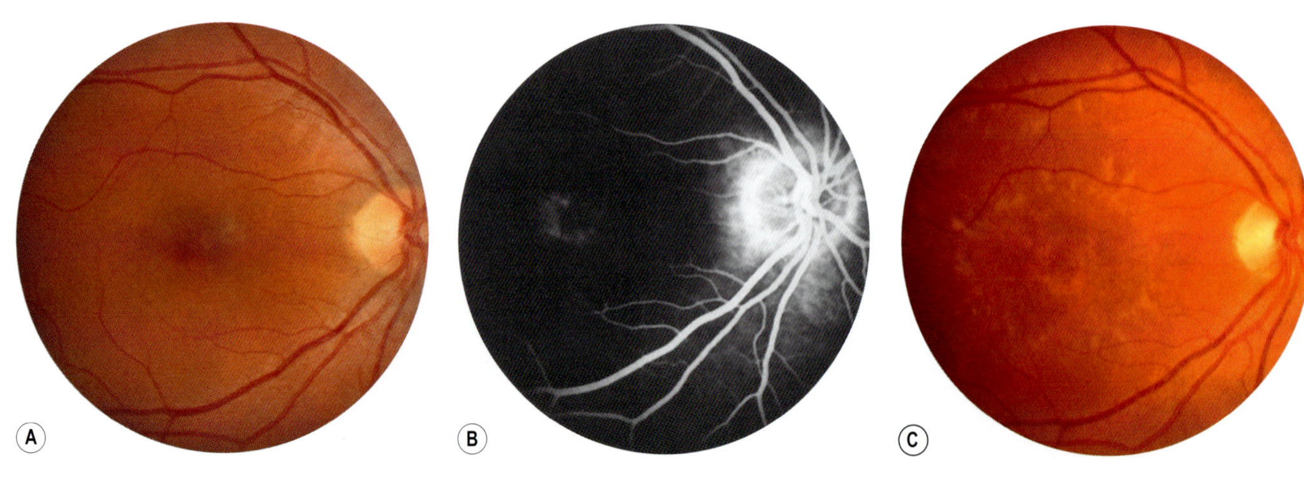

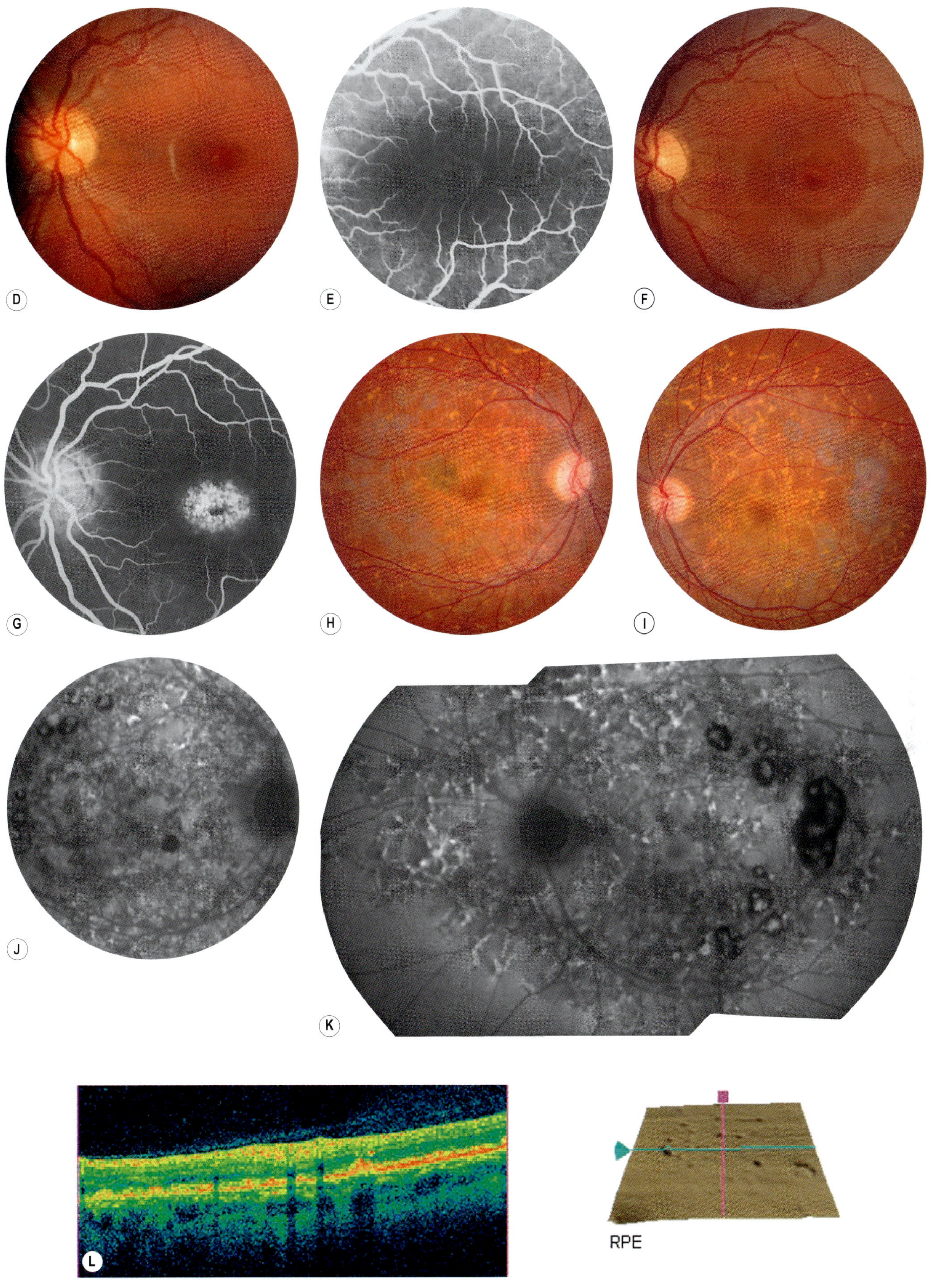
D
E
F
G
H
I
J
K
L
RPE

Most patients with this disease experience loss of central vision first in childhood or young adulthood. Some, however, first become symptomatic in midlife or beyond. Loss of central vision may be accompanied by symptomatic as well as electrophysiologic evidence of significant cone dysfunction.[165,180] Likewise some patients, particularly those who develop widespread flecks extending into the periphery, may develop evidence of rod as well as cone dysfunction.[171] On the basis of the fundus and fluorescein angiographic findings at the time of presentation, patients with Stargardt's disease can be subdivided into the following groups.

Group 1: Vermillion Fundi and Hidden Choroidal Fluorescence

Some patients with subnormal visual acuity have relatively normal-appearing fundi except for the easy-to-overlook heavily pigmented RPE that in most white patients imparts a vermillion color and that obscures most of the details of the choroid from view (Figures 5.18A and B and 5.19A and B). Angiographically the retinal vessels are displayed prominently on a dark background of minimal choroidal fluorescence. In some cases the retinal capillaries appear to be more dilated than normal.

Group 2: Atrophic Maculopathy with or without Flecks

In some patients the loss of pigment in the macula may be so minimal that only with angiography can this be demonstrated with certainty (Figure 5.18E). These patients and those in group 1 may be misdiagnosed either as having functional complaints or as having a lesion involving the optic pathways. Particularly in young children, the flecks may not be present or may be quite small and limited in number (Figure 5.18F). Likewise the vermillion fundus and dark choroid angiographically may not be present in early life (Figure 5.18D and E).[181] On subsequent follow-up, flecks as well as evidence of diffuse lipofuscin storage in the RPE occur (Figure 5.18F and G). The flecks may be confined to the macula or may extend into the midperiphery of the fundi. The degree and pattern of atrophy of the RPE in the central macular area vary and do not always correlate with the degree of visual loss. The RPE may show only mild loss of its normal color, a beaten-metal appearance, or marked geographic atrophy. A diffuse oval or bull's-eye pattern of atrophy occurs commonly (Figures 5.18H and I and 5.19J–L). The lipofuscin within the flecks accounts for the increased autofluorescence, which may be surrounded by regions of decreased autofluorescence from the adjacent atrophic RPE. The autofluorescence pattern can resemble chronic idiopathic central serous chorioretinopathy, mitochondrial myopathies, and flecks of pattern dystrophy. Patients with fundus flavimaculatus show a ring of decreased autofluorescence around the disc and in the fovea, unlike those with mitochondrial myopathies where this pattern is absent (Figure 5.18J and K). Patients with the bull's-eye change may initially be seen with normal visual acuity and a ring scotoma. A few such patients retain 20/20 visual acuity until 40 years of age or beyond (Figure 5.20G–L). Varying degrees of atrophy of the RPE surround and extend between the flecks. This is always more evident angiographically than biomicroscopically (Figure 5.19H). If the number of flecks and amount of RPE atrophy are great, the angiographic dark choroid sign typical of Stargardt's disease may not be evident in the posterior fundus, although it is often preserved in the peripapillary area. The optic disc and retinal vessels in patients in groups 1 and 2 are normal.

Patients with widespread flecks may develop in one or occasionally both eyes an eccentric well-defined zone of reactive RPE changes that includes hypertrophy, hyperplasia, fibrous metaplasia, and atrophy (Figure 5.19D). Patients with many flecks occasionally develop subretinal neovascularization and disciform detachment of the macula.[122,166,168]

5.19 Stargardt's disease with peripheral flecks (fundus flavimaculatus).

A–G: Dominantly or pseudodominantly inherited Stargardt's disease (fundus flavimaculatus). A 7-year-old girl whose visual acuity was 20/50 had vermillion fundi and angiographic evidence of obstruction of the choroidal fluorescence (A and B). She later developed a picture of fundus flavimaculatus. Her brother had a vermillion but otherwise normal fundus bilaterally when he was 8 years old (C). Five years later he developed flecks in the macula and mid peripheral fundus as well as atrophy of the retinal pigment epithlium (RPE) in the macula. Within a few weeks of being examined, the brother was struck in the right eye with a dodgeball. He noted no change in the vision but 2 months later he had evidence of a 2.5-disc diameter alteration in the RPE inferior to the right macula (arrows, D). One month later there was evidence of subretinal neovascularization, including a small amount of subretinal blood and fibrous metaplasia and hyperplasia of the RPE. In his left eye temporal to the macula he had a peculiar paracentral area of geographic atrophy of the RPE similar to that depicted in the patient illustrated in J–L. Another 12-year-old brother and their 30-year-old mother (E) had mild visual loss associated with widespread flecks and central RPE atrophy. There was no history of previously affected generations.

F–H: In this young woman note the unusual two areas of geographic atrophy of the RPE located just temporal to the macula of the left eye (arrows).

I–L: This African American male had a visual acuity of 20/20 in the right and 20/30– in the left eye. Triradiate yellow flecks along with small islands of geographic atrophy were seen in the macula of both eyes (I and J). The older central lesions showed decreased autofluorescence suggesting loss of the yellow material and atrophy of the RPE, while the more peripheral flecks showed increased autofluorescence from the lipofuscin within the RPE. The areas of geographic atrophy showed no autofluorescence (K and L).

(A–E, courtesy of Dr. Gary E. Fish; I-L, courtesy of Dr. James Otey.)

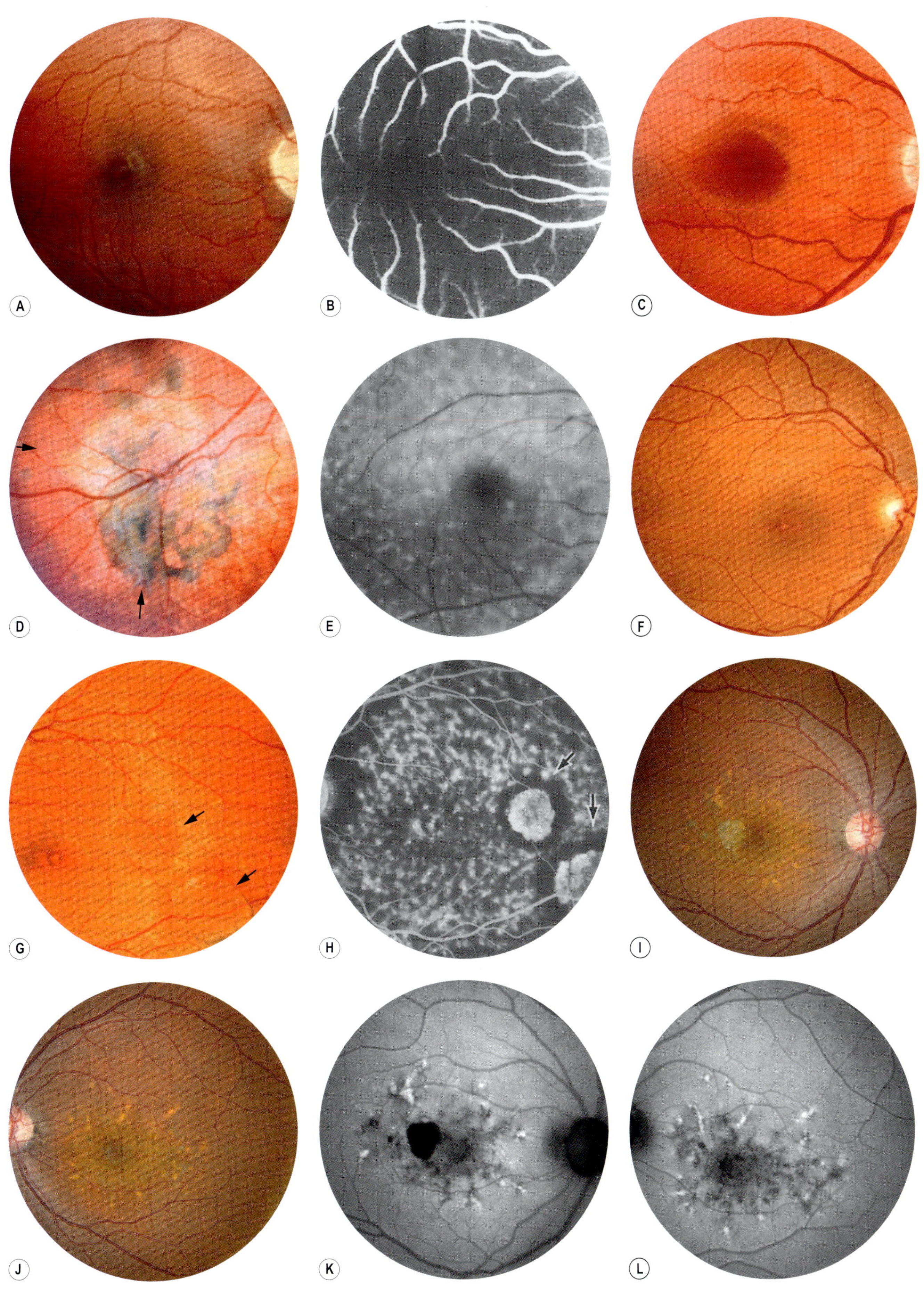
A
B
C
D
E
F
G
H
I
J
K
L

Color vision testing usually shows a mild red–green dyschromatopsia. Many patients show a prolongation in rod dark adaptation and selective prolongation of the later segment of rod recovery.[162,167,182] Electroretinographic findings are usually normal or slightly disturbed. The EOG is subnormal in some cases. Some patients may develop photophobia, loss of color vision, and electroretinographic evidence of a cone dystrophy.

Group 3: Atrophic Maculopathy with Late Signs and Symptoms of Retinitis Pigmentosa

Patients in group 3 are similar to those in group 2 but in addition show signs and symptoms of retinitis pigmentosa, including nyctalopia, diffuse loss of pigment from the RPE, narrowing of the retinal vessels, and abnormalities of both the scotopic and photopic ERG.[165]

Group 4: Flecks not Associated with Macular Atrophy

Patients may have paracentral and central flecks associated with minimal biomicroscopic and angiographic evidence of atrophy of the RPE between the flecks. Visual acuity may be normal if the center of the fovea is not involved by a fleck. Most patients with a large fleck in the foveola have subnormal acuity. Fluorescein angiography shows a dark choroid, obstruction of the background fluorescence by the flecks with minimal hyperfluorescence in a small area immediately surrounding the flecks. In the absence of information concerning other family members, and in eyes showing borderline evidence of a dark choroid, it may be difficult or impossible to differentiate some patients in group 4 from patients with dominantly inherited pattern dystrophy.[183,184]

Whereas the fundus findings and the degree and rate of visual loss are usually symmetric, the atrophic changes and visual loss in some patients may be more advanced in one eye. In general, the onset, rate, and severity of visual loss are similar in family members, but notable exceptions to this rule occur. In an appraisal of visual loss with age by both life-table analysis and cross-sectional procedures in 95 patients with Stargardt's disease, Fishman and associates found the probability of maintaining a visual acuity of 20/40 or better in at least one eye was 52% by age 19 years, 32% by age 29 years, and 22% by age 39 years.[185] The visual acuity after reaching a level of 20/40 tended to decrease rapidly and stabilize at 20/200. Low-vision correction in these patients is highly successful.[186–188]

There is considerable evidence that Stargardt's disease and fundus flavimaculatus are the same disease and that the latter probably represents a more advanced and widespread stage of lipofuscin storage and RPE damage (Figure 5.14A–F). The age of onset of visual loss and the severity of visual loss are generally greater in patients with widespread flecks (fundus flavimaculatus).[164] The electro-oculographic and electroretinographic findings are more likely to be subnormal in patients who either have or are destined to develop widespread flecks in the fundi and other signs and symptoms of a more widespread tapetoretinal dystrophy.[164,169,171] The electrophysiologic studies therefore are probably of some prognostic value, particularly in younger patients who have only minimal flecks.

5.20 Extensive flecks of fundus flavimaculatus.

A–F: This 30-year-old male had extensive involvement of the fundus in both eyes extending almost to the equator (A–D). Note the decreased autofluorescence in most of the lesions except the very anterior ones that show increased autofluorescence, signifying progressive atrophy of the retinal pigment epithelium cells and loss of their lipofuscin content (E and F). His visual acuity was count fingers in the right and 20/30 in the left eye.

Evolution of flecks in fundus flavimaculatus and normal vision.

G–L: This 21-year-old young male was asymptomatic in 2004 and the flecks were discovered on a routine examination for glasses. He had a vermillion fundus without visible choroidal vessels in the posterior pole and yellow flecks, some with central pigmentation in the superior macula and superior to the disc (G and H). The red-free images better delineate the flecks.

I and J: Five years later there was a significant increase in the flecks now distributed all over the posterior pole and nasal to the disc in both eyes (K and L). His visual acuity was still 20/20 in each eye.

(A–F, courtesy of Dr. Franco Recchia and Dr. Brad Kehler.)

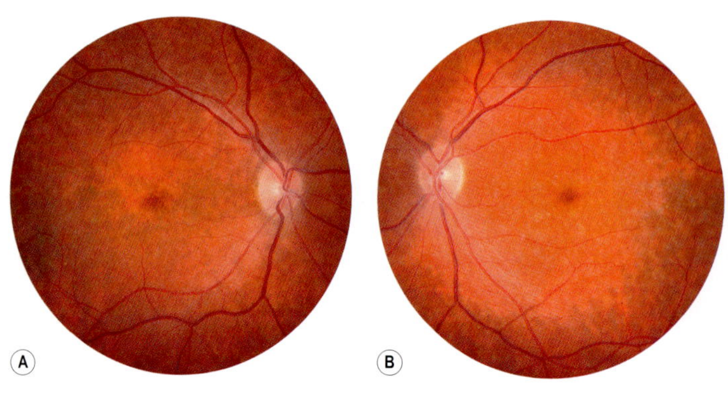

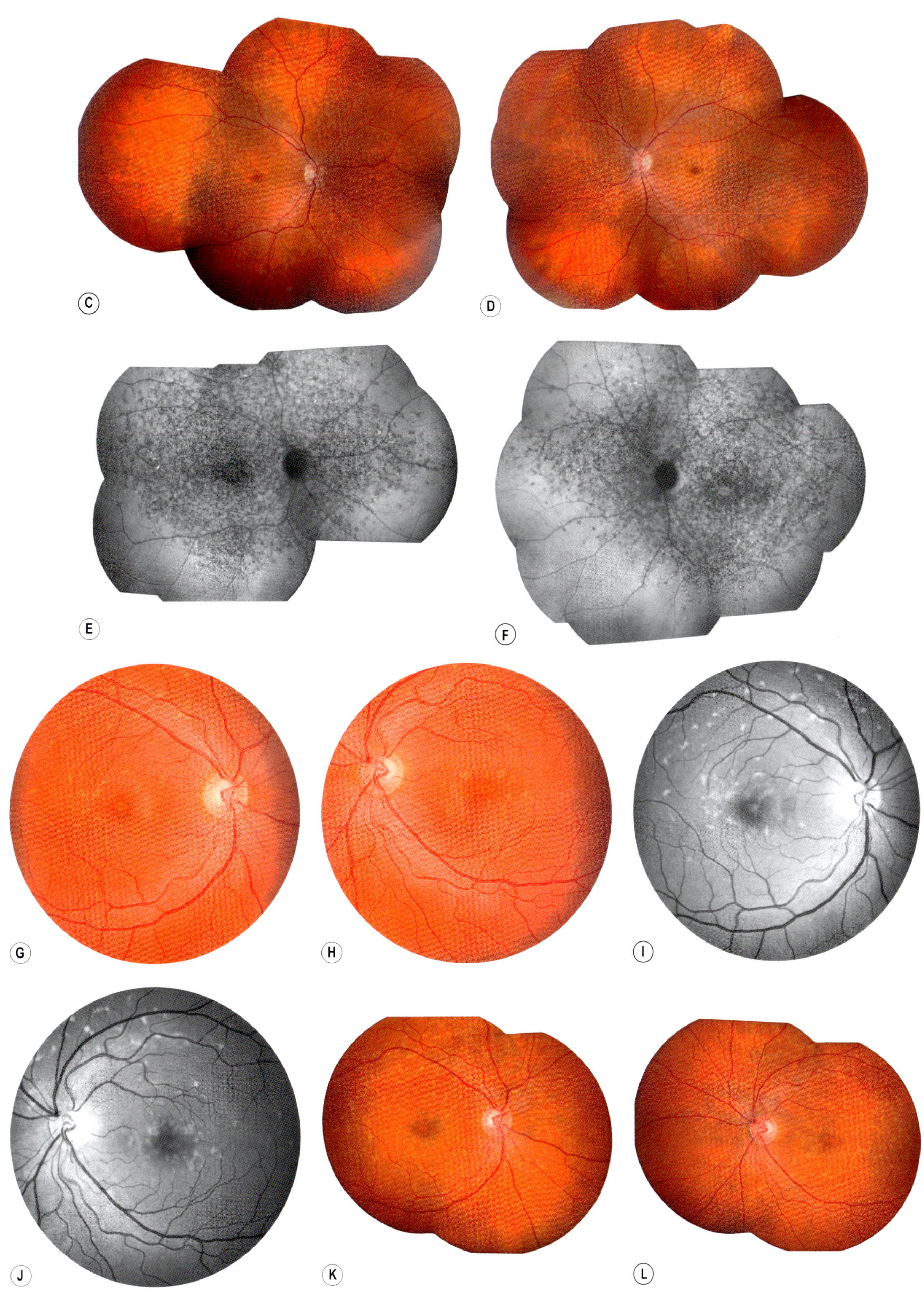
C
D
E
F
G
H
I
J
K
L

AUTOSOMAL-DOMINANT CENTRAL AREOLAR CHORIORETINAL DYSTROPHY UNASSOCIATED WITH DRUSEN OR FLECKS

This dystrophy is characterized by the development of fine, mottled depigmentation in the macular region, usually in late childhood or early adulthood in the absence of any symptoms (Figure 5.22A, B, G, and H). Visual acuity, visual fields, ERG, and dark adaptation are normal early in the course. Multifocal ERG shows abnormal central function and late stages may sometimes show more widespread cone and rod dysfunction.[195,196] The EOG may be subnormal. Fluorescein angiography is helpful in detecting the earliest pigmentary changes of the macular region that may eventually have a bull's-eye configuration (Figure 5.22B, I, and J). Associated with the gradual development of symmetric, sharply outlined, bull's-eye oval or round areas of geographic atrophy of the RPE in the macula in the absence of any flecks or drusen there is slow, mild deterioration of visual acuity during the fourth and fifth decades of life (Figure 5.22C, F, G, and H). The findings can be staged from 1 to 4 (Figure 5.23). Families with earlier age of onset of visual acuity changes (Figure 5.22G–J) are known.[197] The area of geographic depigmentation of the RPE enlarges concentrically but usually does not exceed three to four disc diameters. In some patients geographic atrophy of the RPE in the peripapillary region accompanies the macular changes. As the patient lives beyond the fifth decade, the reddish orange color of the large choroidal vessels within the area of RPE atrophy is replaced by a yellow-white color (Figure 5.22F, K, and L). Serous and hemorrhagic disciform detachment occurs rarely, if at all. Visual acuity in the range of 20/100–20/200 may be retained even during the seventh and eighth decades of life. The optic disc, retinal vessels, and RPE outside the macular area are usually normal in appearance.

5.22 Autosomal-dominant central areolar choroidal and retinal pigment epithelium (RPE) dystrophy unassociated with drusen or flecks.

A and **B**: A 19-year-old boy with visual acuity of 20/15 had minimal changes in the RPE centrally. Angiography (B) revealed definite evidence of pigment loss in the macula.
C–E: The 46-year-old father of patient in A had visual acuity of 20/70. He had a central scotoma corresponding to discrete areas of RPE atrophy bilaterally (C). Arteriovenous-stage angiogram showed delay in perfusion of the large and small choroidal vessels centrally (D). Approximately 20 minutes after injection, the angiogram showed choroidal staining that was most marked in the periphery of the central lesion (E).
F: The 74-year-old paternal grandfather of the patient in A. Note whitening of the large choroidal vessel walls. His acuity was 20/100. The patient illustrated in A had two affected siblings. The patients illustrated in A and C had moderately abnormal electro-oculographic findings. Their electroretinographic findings were normal. Several members of this family also have von Hippel–Lindau disease.
G–J: This healthy 18-year-old woman had 20/15 visual acuity in both eyes. There was mottled depigmentation of the pigment epithelium and mottled hyperfluorescence in the macular area bilaterally. Her electro-oculogram, electroretinogram, and 100-hue color vision test results were normal. Three siblings had macular degeneration.
K and **L**: The 46-year-old mother of the patient in G–I noted visual loss beginning at age 24 years. Her visual acuity was 10/200 bilaterally. The rod and cone electroretinogram and electro-oculogram findings were moderately abnormal. This patient's mother, two maternal aunts, two maternal uncles, and maternal grandmother had macular degeneration.

Initially, a relative (but later an absolute) central scotoma corresponding to the area of RPE atrophy can be demonstrated. Peripheral fields are normal. Fluorescein angiography demonstrates varying degrees of loss of the choriocapillaris within the area of RPE atrophy that correlates well with the degree of loss of visual function.[198] There usually is minimal evidence of atrophy of the large choroidal vessels throughout the course of the disease.

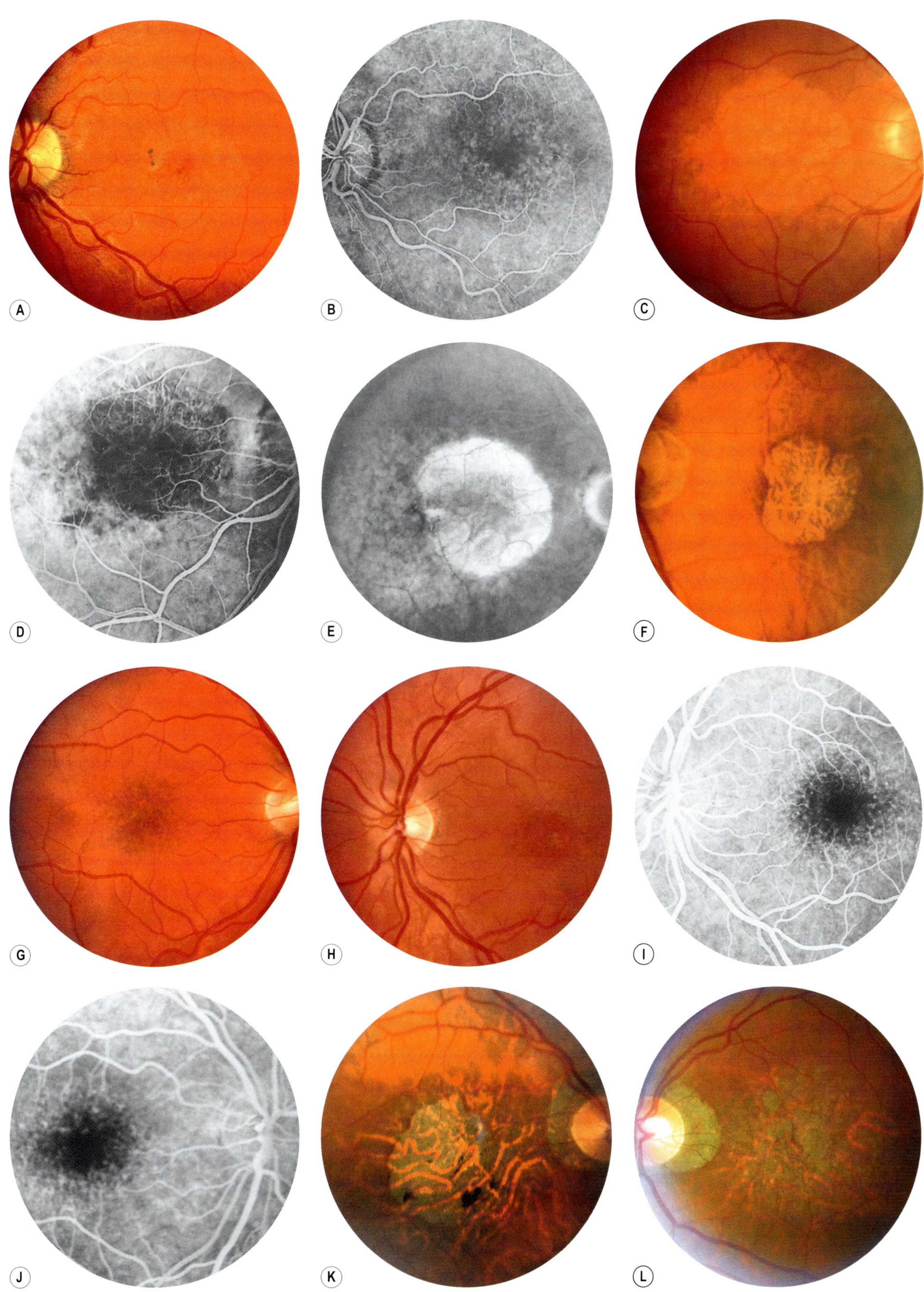
A
B
C
D
E
F
G
H
I
J
K
L

Dominantly inherited central areolar chorioretinal dystrophy unassociated with flecks occurs infrequently and has been confused in the literature with a variety of other more prevalent diseases associated with geographic atrophy of the RPE. Central areolar or geographic atrophy of the RPE and choroid is a nonspecific change that may occur in association with other diseases, including: (1) familial macular dystrophies associated with macular coloboma; (2) central areolar RPE dystrophy[199] that may be the same disease as (1); (3) dominant macular drusen associated with senile macular degeneration and disciform detachment (see Figure 3.46); (4) basal laminar drusen; (5) autosomal-recessive macular dystrophy associated with Stargardt's disease or fundus flavimaculatus (Figures 5.13 and 5.14); (6) central areolar atrophy in the cone and rod–cone dystrophies (Figure 5.16); (7) central areolar atrophy secondary to myopic degeneration (see Figure 3.34); and (8) central areolar choroidal and RPE atrophy secondary to serous or hemorrhagic disciform detachment of the RPE and retina from a variety of causes, such as idiopathic central serous chorioretinopathy or choroiditis.[200] Autosomal-dominant central areolar choroidal dystrophy may also be confused with other disorders that cause a bull's-eye pattern of pigment epithelial atrophy (see benign concentric annular macular dystrophy, p. 300, and chloroquine and hydroxychloroquine toxicity).

In 1953 Sorsby and Crick described five pedigrees of patients with "central areolar choroidal sclerosis." Only one or possibly two families had evidence of dominant inheritance.[201] Several patients showed evidence of flecks or drusen and may have had either Stargardt's disease or senile macular degeneration. Histopathologic examination of one patient showed evidence of choroidal and RPE atrophy but no evidence of sclerosis of the choroidal vessels.[202]

A family of three successive generations of patients with central areolar macular dystrophy seen in Miami also have autosomally dominantly inherited von Hippel–Lindau disease (Figure 5.22A–F). Mansour reported three brothers, each affected with central areolar choroidal dystrophy and pseudochondroplastic spondyloepiphyseal dysplasia, both of which are heterogeneous disorders with autosomal transmission.[197] The association of two rare diseases having an autosomal-dominant inheritance (germ cell mosaicism in one parent) or autosomal-recessive inheritance resulting from parental or grandparental consanguinity (new syndrome) is more likely to be a true association than a simple coincidence.[197] Mutation in the peripherin/*RDS* gene on chromosome 6 is the most common cause of autosomal-dominant central areolar choroidal dystrophy, though the disease is genetically heterogeneous.[113,203–205] Five different mutations have so far been found, the commonest being arginine 195 leucine mutation.[204,206]

5.23 Stages of central areolar choroidal dystrophy.

A–C: Stage 1 central areolar choroidal dystrophy (CACD) in a 39-year-old asymptomatic patient with a visual acuity of 20/20. She carried a p.Arg142Trp missense mutation in the *PRPH2* gene. The fundus photograph shows parafoveal zones of hypopigmentation (A), which correspond to areas of increased autofluorescence (B). Spectral-domain optical coherence tomography (OCT) horizontally through these zones just below the fovea shows disorganization and thickening of the outermost neuroretinal layers, at the level of the photoreceptor outer segments (C).
D–F: Stage 2 CACD, in a 60-year-old patient with a visual acuity of 20/20 (p.Arg142Trp *PRPH2* mutation). She complained of mild micropsia. A mildly atrophic hypopigmented oval area was seen in the macula (D). The lesion was faintly hyperfluorescent on fluorescein angiography. Fundus autofluorescence showed an oval lesion with granular areas of decreased autofluorescence and a few spots of increased autofluorescence (E). In early stage 2 CACD, speckled areas of increased autofluorescence predominate. A horizontal spectral-domain OCT scan through this lesion showed an accumulation of hyperreflective material under the fovea, between the neurosensory retina and retinal pigment epithelium. This hyperreflective material may correspond to clumping of altered photoreceptor outer segments. Outside this area was disruption of photoreceptor layer with some hyperreflective spots that may correspond to clumps of abnormal photoreceptor outer-segment material (F).
G–I: Stage 3 CACD, in a 47-year-old patient who also carried a p.Arg142Trp mutation in the *PRPH2* gene. The visual acuity was 20/25, and the patient reported a mild decrease in visual acuity. An area of well-demarcated chorioretinal atrophy was seen just outside the foveal center (G). On fundus autofluorescence, this atrophic area showed an absence of autofluorescence. Outside this, the more mildly affected area showed granular zones of altered autofluorescence (H). On a horizontal spectral-domain OCT scan, this area of chorioretinal atrophy corresponded to a thinning of the outer neuroretinal layers, marked attenuation of the photoreceptor layer, as well as an attenuated retinal pigment epithelium layer. Outside this area, these structures were more mildly disorganized and attenuated (I).
J–L: Stage 4 CACD, in a 49-year-old patient with a visual acuity of 20/200 (p.Arg142Trp mutation in *PRPH2*). Ophthalmoscopy showed a well-circumscribed area of profound chorioretinal atrophy that involved the fovea, with some pigment clumping (J). This atrophy again corresponded to an absence of fundus autofluorescence. Some residual increased autofluorescence was seen at the border of the lesion (K). On fluorescein angiography, the choroidal vessels were visible through the retinal pigment epithelial window defect. The border of the lesion showed some staining (L).

(Courtesy of Dr. Camiel Boon.)

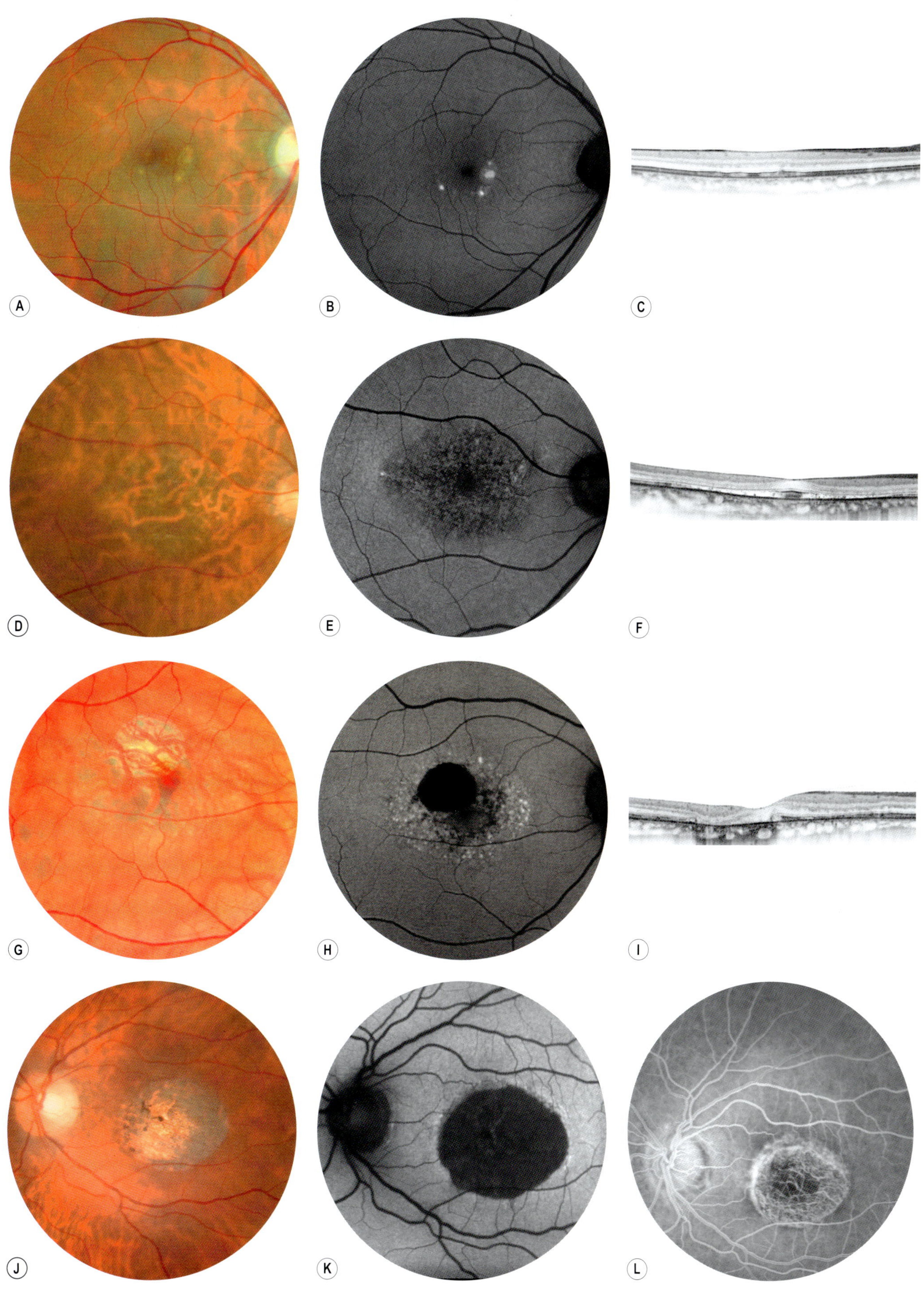

A
B
C
D
E
F
G
H
I
J
K
L

BASAL LAMINAR DRUSEN ASSOCIATED WITH TYPE II MESANGIOCAPILLARY (MEMBRANOPROLIFERATIVE) GLOMERULONEPHRITIS

Mesangiocapillary glomerulonephritis (MCGN, MPGN) is a renal disorder characterized by proliferation of mesangial cells and alterations in the basement membrane of the glomerulus.[207–214] MCGN has been classified on the basis of the localization and composition of the glomerular deposits: type I with subendothelial electron-dense deposits along the glomerular basement membrane with presence of complement and immunoglobulin within the glomerulus, type II with electron-dense ribbon like deposits of C3 in the lamina densa of the glomerular basement membrane without the presence of immunoglobulin (also called dense deposit disease), and type III with deposits like those of both types I and II, and both subepithelial and subendothelial location. Other associated features of the disease include chronic hypocomplementemia, partial lipodystrophy, and a higher incidence of diabetes. Type I is twice as common as type II and is less severe. Type II usually begins in childhood or early adulthood and tends to be a progressive unremitting disease, often recurring even after renal transplantation. MPGN comprises approximately 4–7% of patients with idiopathic nephrotic syndrome. Basal laminar drusen and larger more typical drusen occur frequently in the macular region of patients with type II MCGN (Figure 5.24A–F).[207–213] The number of deposits increases in number and size with age and duration of the disorder.[215] Although most patients are visually asymptomatic, some may develop choroidal neovascularization at an early age.[210,212] The fundus findings occur more frequently in those patients with type II MCGN who have in addition partial lipodystrophy.[207] Those patients who have undergone renal transplant may develop signs of organ transplant retinopathy with exudative retinal detachment, retinal pigment epithelial mottling, or serous pigment epithelial detachments[215,216] which may alter the fundus appearance. Light and electron microscopic study in one patient with drusen revealed diffuse and focal deposits in the basement membrane of the RPE similar to those found in the glomerulus.[207] The nature of these deposits was not determined.

A variety of mutations in the complement factor H (CFH) gene are seen in a minority of patients with MPGN II. Homozygous or compound heterozygous *CFH* mutations result in lack of plasma CFH, causing uncontrolled alternate complement pathway activation resulting in ubiquitous C3 deposition in the Bruch's membrane and glomerulus.[217–219]

5.24 Cuticular and calcified drusen in patients with type II membranoproliferative glomerulonephritis (MPGN).

A–D: A 50-year-old man, who had a history of renal transplant at ages 36 and 39 years because of type II MPGN, complained of blurred vision of 2 months' duration. Visual acuity in right eye was 20/200, left eye 20/20. Note variability of the size of the drusen, some of which appear calcified. Angiography revealed cuticular drusen (C and D).

E and F: A 19-year-old man with childhood onset diabetes and nephrotic syndrome associated with type II MPGN. Visual acuity in the right eye was 20/20 and of the left eye was 20/25. Note clusters of tiny basal laminar drusen (arrows) and mild background diabetic retinopathy.

Radial basal laminar drusen (malattia levantinese).

G–L: An 84-year-old Caucasian male from Tennessee carried a diagnosis of age-related macular degeneration from age 40 onwards. His visual acuity was 20/400 in each eye. He had moderate cataracts. Nodular drusen were distributed in the macula and nasal to the disc. The fovea showed extracellular pigment and atrophy. The temporal drusen were smaller and arranged in a radial fashion. He also had evidence of an old superotemporal branch retinal vein occlusion (G and H). His 48-year-old daughter accompanied him and was examined. Her visual acuity was 20/50 in the right and 20/60 in the left eye. Both foveas showed central fibrosis surrounded by several small drusen that had a radial arrangement temporally and were also seen nasal to the disc (I and J). The radial arrangement is more distinct on the red-free images (K); the angiogram of the right eye shows late staining of the central fibrosis (L). They had no relatives in Switzerland but the family could be traced back to the UK.

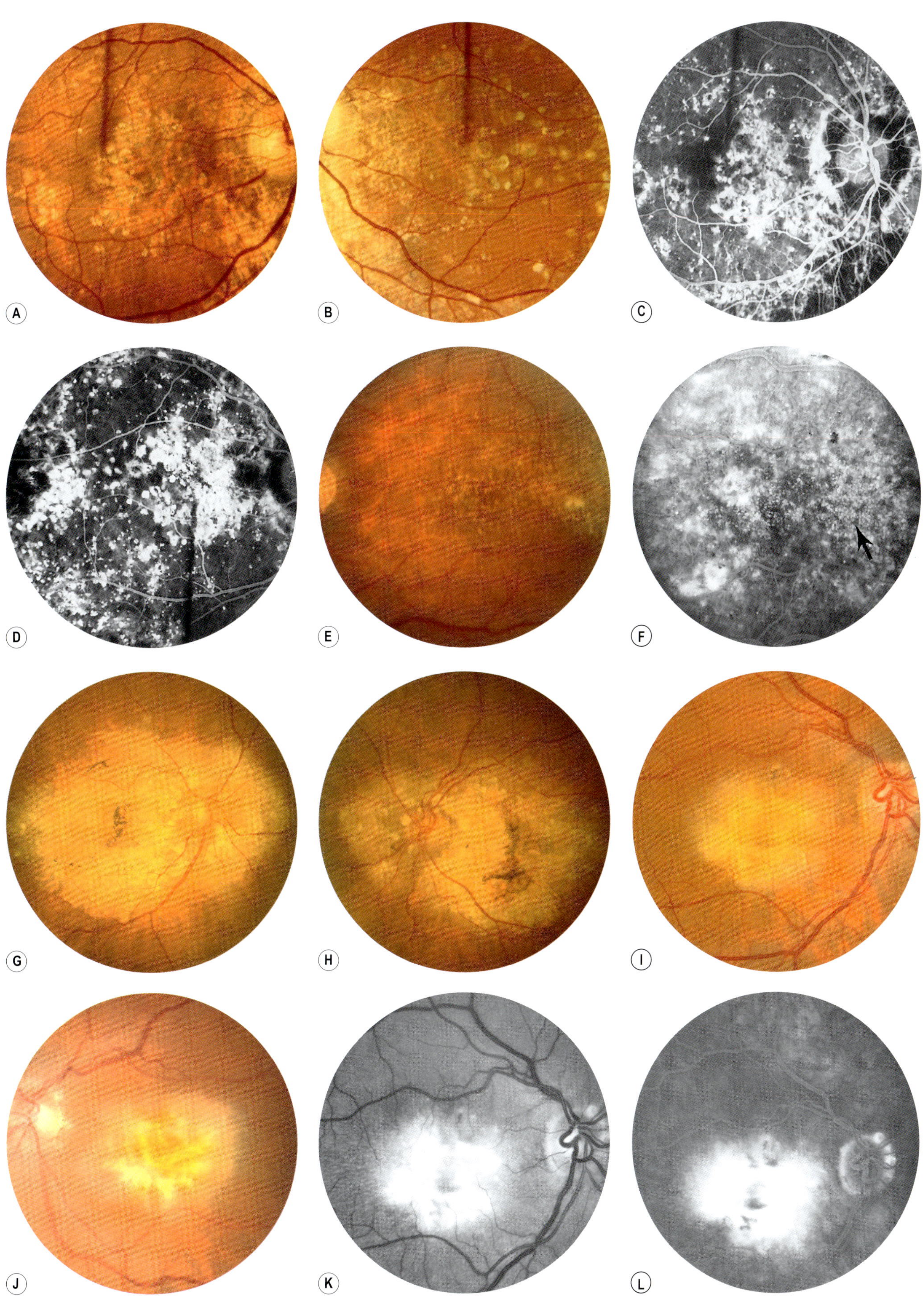
A
B
C
D
E
F
G
H
I
J
K
L

DOMINANTLY INHERITED RADIAL BASAL LAMINAR DRUSEN (MALATTIA LEVANTINESE, DOYNE'S HONEYCOMB MACULAR DYSTROPHY)

A dominantly inherited disorder characterized by a radial pattern of innumerable, small, elongated basal laminar drusen was initially reported in a family from the Levantine valley in Switzerland.[220–224] It was later found that the condition is the same as the dominantly inherited honeycomb retinal dystrophy described by Doyne in 1899.[225] Typically the radiating pattern is most prominent in the temporal macular area and is often accompanied by larger nodular, and at times papillary, drusen and variable amounts of irregular subretinal fibrous metaplasia and hyperplasia of the RPE (Figure 5.24G–J). This subretinal scar tissue may or may not be vascularized. The visual acuity is often excellent in spite of the fibrous metaplastic changes. The radial drusen demonstrate early discrete fluorescence similar to that of basal laminar drusen (Figure 5.25B, C, F, and I). On indocyanine green angiography the lesions mask the fluorescence early, and the central drusen stains late with hypofluorescence of its edge.[226] High-resolution OCT shows conical deposits between the RPE and the Bruch's membrane, and late stages secondary disruption of the outer nuclear layer.[227,228] Choroidal neovascularization is known to occur and responds to surgical removal, photodynamic therapy, and antivascular endothelial growth factor antibodies.[229,230] Streicher and Krcméry[231] and Dusek and associates[232] have reported a dominantly inherited pedigree of patients with radial basal laminar drusen. Even though the typical appearance is of nodular drusen that fill the macula and often the area nasal to the disc, phenotypic heterogeneity is seen in some families, showing less extensive drusen or predominant fibrous change rather than drusen (Figure 5.26E and F).[225,233] Mutation in the *EFEMP1* gene (Arg345Trp) is responsible for the condition.[234–236] There has been a family diagnosed clinically as malattia levantinese, without the Arg345Trp mutation, suggesting other gene defects may also cause this phenotype.[233] Light and electron microscopic findings in one patient demonstrated evidence that these drusen are caused by thickening of the basement membrane of the RPE (see Figure 3.29J and K).[232] Dr. Gass has seen one member of a family with North Carolina dystrophy who had a small zone of radial drusen (see next section). It is of interest that only one of the half-dozen patients with prominent radial basal laminar drusen examined in Miami had a family history of macular degeneration (Figure 5.25D–F).[221]

5.25 Radial basal laminar drusen (malattia levantinese).

A–C: A 31-year-old man complained of metamorphopsia of 4 months' duration. His family history was negative. Visual acuity in the right eye was 20/15 and in the left eye was 20/40. A radial pattern of drusen and subretinal scarring were present in both eyes (A). Angiograms in both eyes revealed a similar radial pattern of drusen that fluoresced during the early arteriovenous phase (B and C). There was evidence of subretinal neovascularization in the left eye (B).
D–F: Radial drusen in a 43-year-old woman with a 10-year history of poor dark adaptation and a 1-year history of blurred vision. Her brother had similar visual complaints and her mother and maternal grandmother were legally blind because of macular degeneration. The patient's visual acuity was 20/30 right eye and 20/70 left eye. Note the prominent nodulation and evidence of calcification of the central drusen in D.
G-I: Radial pattern of drusen in a 43-year-old woman whose family history was negative. Visual acuity was 20/40 in the right eye and counting fingers in the left eye. Note hyperplastic retinal pigment epithelium (RPE) scars in both eyes.
J and **K**: Histopathology J and K, electron micrographic findings of large multinodular and papillary basal laminar drusen (arrows) in patient with dominantly inherited radial drusen. Note the papillary thickening of the basal lamina (BL) of the RPE in K. Compare with the prominently elevated drusen in G. Note loss of retinal receptors and subretinal fibrous metaplasia in J.

(J and K, from Dusek et al.[232])

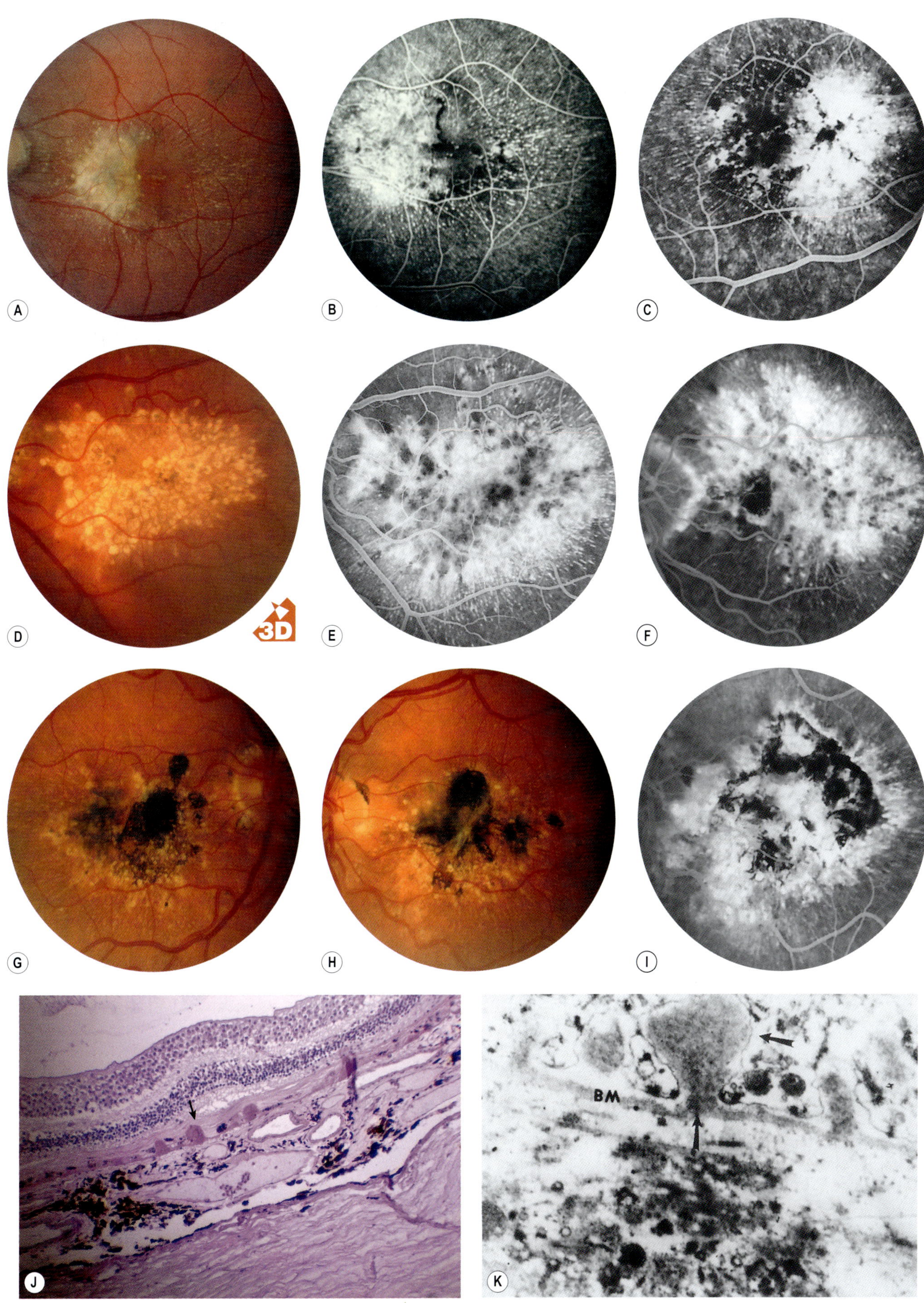
A
B
C
D
3D
E
F
G
H
I
BM
J
K

5.26 Malattia levantinese – variable phenotype.

A and B: Right and left eye of a patient with malattia levantinese showing symmetric appearance of lesions comprised of nodular drusen, pigment clumping, and the radial arrangement of the drusen temporally.
C–L: Two affected sisters among four siblings with extreme variable phenotype. The 64-year-old younger sister became symptomatic around age 40 with a visual acuity of 20/200 in each eye. Central macular atrophy surrounded by nodular cuticular drusen that extend nasal to the disc with radial temporal distribution seen in both eyes (C and D). The nodular drusen are highly autofluorescent and the central atrophic area is hypoautofluorescent(E and F). Spectralis OCT demonstrates nodular and confluent RPE accumulations corresponding to the drusen in both eyes (G to J). Her 66-year-old sister had a visual acuity of 20/40 in each eye and showed a much milder phenotype (K and L), comprising of small drusen, arranged in a radial pattern in the left eye, resembling cuticular drusen of North Carolina macular dystrophy (see Figure 5.27 A and B). Their maternal uncle carried a diagnosis of Doyne's honeycomb dystrophy; their mother was relatively asymptomatic by history till she died at age 80. A daughter and son of the two sisters examined at age 32 and 34 were unaffected.

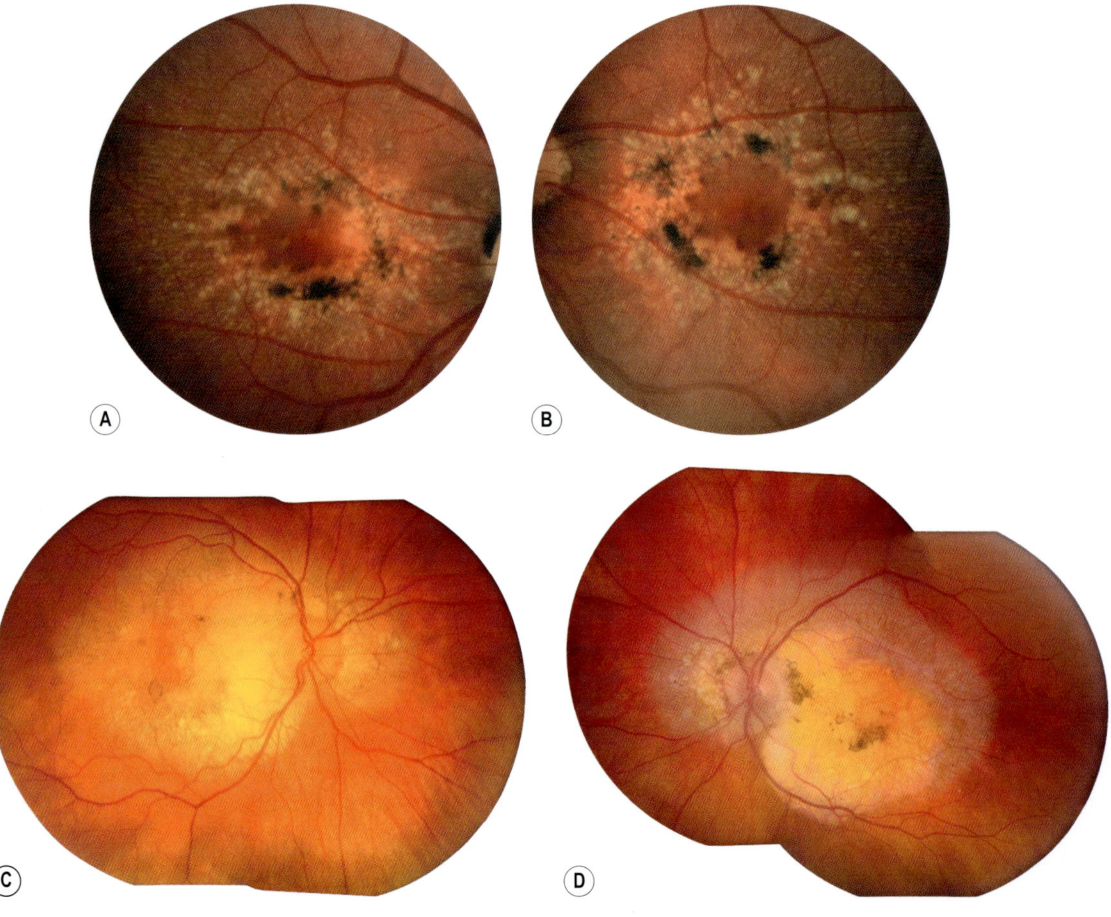

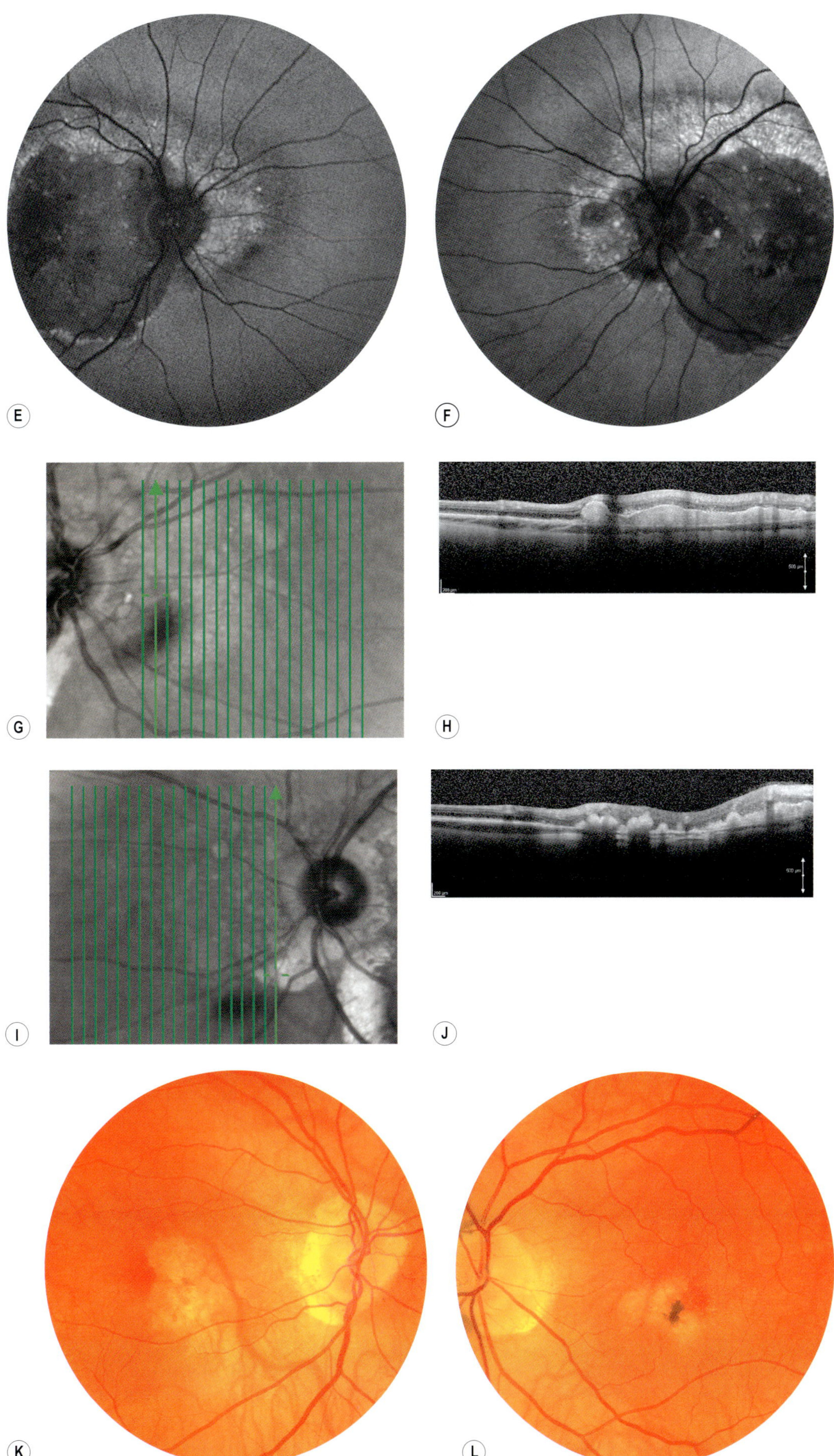
E
F
G
H
I
J
K
L

NORTH CAROLINA MACULAR DYSTROPHY AND OTHER HEREDITARY MACULAR STAPHYLOMATA (COLOBOMATA)

North Carolina macular dystrophy is an autosomal-dominantly inherited disorder with complete penetrance. Its onset is in infancy and perhaps prenatally, its course is generally stable, and its phenotype is highly variable and includes drusenlike changes, disciform lesions with choroidal neovascularization, macular staphylomata, and peripheral drusen. Electroretinography, electro-oculography, and color vision are normal. Lefler et al.[237] and Frank et al.[238] reported a large pedigree from western North Carolina consisting of 545 family members in seven generations with a dominantly inherited macular dystrophy that they characterized as progressive, usually commencing in infancy and reaching its maximum severity in the early teenage years. Scattered lesions that they believed were drusen and pigmentary changes in the macula with normal visual acuity were the earliest fundoscopic changes (stage 1) (Figures 5.27A and B, 5.28B, E–L). As the vision declined to the 20/50 range, there was an increase in the number as well as the confluence of the drusenlike changes (stage 2). In many patients the fundus changes did not progress beyond the drusen stage and visual acuity may have remained normal. Other family members showed a progressive decrease in the acuity to the 20/200 level concomitant with the development in some cases of almost total atrophy of the choroid, RPE, and retina in the macular area (stage 3). Although Lefler's and Frank's photographs appeared to show evidence of staphylomatous outpouching in association with these severe changes, they did not mention that change. Neither did they describe peripheral drusenlike changes or evidence of choroidal neovascularization and disciform detachment, although one of the patients depicted in their report as well as one of our patients showed evidence of this complication.[239] The retinal vessels, peripheral fields, color vision, ERG, and EOG were normal. The general medical examination was typically normal except for a transport type of aminoaciduria that segregated independently of the foveal dystrophy, but which was also dominantly inherited. Small et al.[240] studied 15 of the original Lefler's and Frank's patients over 10 years and noted stable vision and fundus appearance in all but one eye of one patient, thus confirming the relatively nonprogressive nature of the condition. Additionally, they noted peripheral yellow drusenlike changes in some of them.

Gass has seen members of three families from western North Carolina who demonstrated all of the clinical features reported by Lefler and associates and Frank and associates (Figure 5.27). The yellow spots in the macula appeared biomicroscopically to be caused by focal areas of depigmentation of the RPE in the absence of nodular elevation, as observed in more typical drusen (Figure 5.27A, B, F, and L). In one patient there was a radial pattern of drusen in the paracentral region (Figure 5.27A). All of the drusen as well as the central spots showed prompt fluorescence (Figure 5.27C). In one family the mother showed evidence of disciform macular scarring in one eye (Figure 5.27D). In the other family the grandmother and her sister showed large, deep, circumscribed, staphylomatous or colobomatous areas of marked atrophy of the choroid and retina, absence of high myopia, and remarkably good visual acuity (Figure 5.27G, H, J, and K).[239] The son and the grandchildren showed varying degrees of drusenlike changes in the macula. Unlike the cases reported by the previous authors, some of our patients have shown drusen in the peripheral fundus. The radial pattern (Figures 5.03B and F and 5.28G and H) has also been seen in Small's group of patients.[240] Patients with drusen are largely asymptomatic unless they develop choroidal neovascularization. Often the parents are completely asymptomatic and have been incidentally discovered when the child developed symptoms (Figure 5.28).

5.27 North Carolina macular dystrophy.

A–C: Note the cluster of peculiar, yellowish-white lesions at the level of the retinal pigment epithelium (RPE) in the macular region of both eyes (A and B) of this 18-year-old woman who had no ocular symptoms and had 20/20 visual acuity. Angiography revealed a pattern of hyperfluorescence that was apparent in the arterial phase (C) and did not change in pattern during the course of angiography. Note the faintly visible radial pattern of the lesions in the temporal macular area. The central confluent areas of depigmentation of the RPE may or may not be caused by drusenlike deposits. The radial distribution of the lesions temporally suggests that they may be basal laminar drusen.

D and **E**: The mother of the patient illustrated in A–C had subnormal vision all her life. The vision had not changed for at least 25 years. Her visual acuity in the right eye was 20/40, and the left eye was 20/200. Note the irregular white subretinal scar in addition to several drusen in the right macula (D) and atrophy of the RPE with clumping of the pigment in the left macula (E). Both the mother and daughter had many small drusenlike deposits in the periphery of both eyes. Both patients were from western North Carolina.

F: This asymptomatic 7-year-old girl from North Carolina had normal visual acuity. She had drusenlike changes similar to that in A and B bilaterally.

G–I: Excavated atrophic chorioretinal lesions in a 57-year-old woman whose vision was apparently subnormal all her life. She had noted mild progression of her visual symptoms in recent years. There was an overhanging lip of retina that partly surrounded these lesions. Visual acuity in the right eye was 20/50 and in the left eye was 20/70. Angiography revealed the presence of only a few small choroidal blood vessels in the area of the macular lesions (I).

J and **K**: The 62-year-old sister of the patient illustrated in G and H. Note the lip of retinal tissue (arrows, J) overhanging the large staphylomatous lesions. Her visual acuity in the right eye was 20/80 and in the left eye was 20/100.

L: The 20-year-old grandson of the patient illustrated in G and H. Note the multiple drusen in the macula. His visual acuity was 20/15. Similar lesions were found in this patient's father. All of these patients had multiple drusen in the periphery of the fundus. The family was originally from western North Carolina.

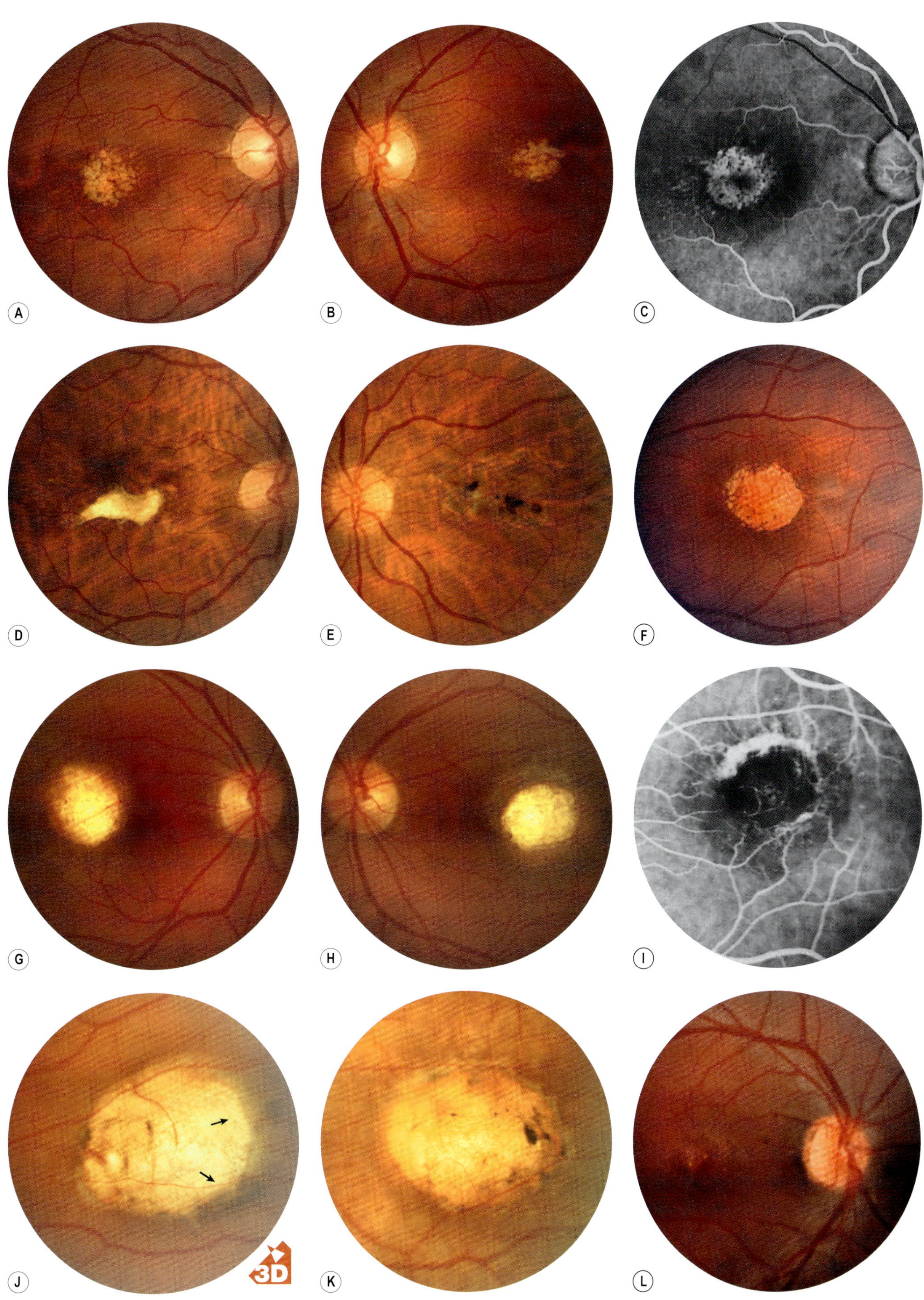
A
B
C
D
E
F
G
H
I
J
K
L
3D

The North Carolina Macular dystrophy gene (*MCDR1*) is mapped to the 6q14-q16.2 region, though the disease causing gene is yet to be identified. Though initially described in inhabitants of North Carolina with their descendancy traced to three Irish brothers, the phenotype has been found in Caucasian patients outside North Carolina and the USA,[241–243] in African American (Figure 5.29), Belize,[244] and Korean patients.[245] A black family in Chicago where three generations are affected is described in Figure 5.29.

The presumably congenital staphylomatous macular lesions (referred to by some as macular colobomas, more recently as macular caldera by Goldberg et al.[246]), similar to that illustrated in this large pedigree, may occur in families that may show other features including Leber's congenital blindness,[247–249] progressive cone–rod dystrophy,[248] and skeletal abnormalities.[248,250–258] Pedigrees with fundus findings similar to North Carolina dystrophy include those of Leveille and associates[259] in a black family, Fetkenhour and associates,[199] and Miller and Bresnick.[260] Small and associates[262] have recently established that the cases reported from North Carolina[237,238] and those by Hermsen and Judisch[261] and Fetkenhour and associates[199] are descendants of three Irish brothers who settled in the North Carolina mountains in the 1830s.

Gass has seen a 38-year-old mother and her 16-year-old son, both with moderate loss of central vision and large macular staphylomata unassociated with high myopia (Figure 5.30A–F). ERG, EOG, and color vision testing were normal in the mother. The son had a markedly abnormal rod ERG. They had no known relatives from North Carolina. Satorre and colleagues reported a Spanish family with autosomal-dominant bilateral macular colobomata.[263] Gass has seen one patient with cone dystrophy and congenital macular staphyloma (see Figure 5.32E and F).[264] Heckenlively et al. reported macular colobomas in families with Leber's congenital amaurosis and progressive cone–rod dystrophy.[248] Dr. Gass has seen another young woman who, over a period of 13 years, developed progressive macular degeneration that was accompanied by the development of a large macular staphyloma in one eye (Figure 5.30G–J). Her family history was negative.

North Carolina-Like Dominant Macular Dystrophy

Three other families with autosomal-dominant drusen and early-onset macular dystrophy resembling North Carolina macular dystrophy have been described recently with loci different from 6q14-q16.2. One is a four-generation British family localized to chromosome 5, region p13.1-p15.33, *MCDR3*[265]; second, an English family with associated progressive sensorineural deafness to chromosome 14q[266]; and the third, a North American family mapped to 6q14 between loci for cone–rod dystrophy 7 (*CORD7*) and North Carolina macular dystrophy (*MCDR1*).[267]

5.28 North Carolina macular dystrophy (NCMD): stability of lesions.

A–F: This 16-year-old female noted central metamorphopsia and distortion in her right eye for 2 months which gradually improved over the next month. Her vision was 20/25– on the right and 20/20 on the left. A hyperpigmented raised central lesion surrounded by a ring of mottled retinal pigment epithelium (RPE) with a few punctate drusen within it was seen on the right (A). Small and intermediate punctate drusen distributed within the fovea was seen on the left (B). Findings suggest a spontaneously regressed type 2 choroidal neovascular membrane in a patient with NCMD. Autofluorescence imaging showed a ring of increased autofluorescence surrounded by a ring of decreased autofluorescence corresponding to the ring of mottled RPE (C). Optical coherence tomography (OCT) showed no activity on the right, and the drusen could not be picked up by OCT (D1 and D2). Her 40-year-old asymptomatic mother with a corrected visual acuity of 20/20, showed similar small compact drusen within the fovea in both eyes (E and F).
G–L: A 13-year-old female was found to have compact small drusen with temporal radial arrangement in both eyes typical of NCMD, on a routine examination for glasses (G and H). Four years later the lesions are unchanged, demonstrating stability and very slow progression (I and J). Autofluorescence was nonspecific with some lesions showing punctate hypoautofluorescence shown. Her 45-year-old father was asymptomatic and had small compact drusen in the fovea (K and L); a brother was known to have similar changes when examined elsewhere.

(G-J, Also, Yannuzzi, Lawrence J., The Retinal Atlas, Saunders 2010, 978-0-7020-3320-9, p.74.)

Chorioretinal Coloboma

Patients with typical inferotemporal chorioretinal colobomas that extend into the macula may occasionally develop loss of central vision because of choroidal neovascularization developing at the margin of the coloboma (Figure 3.31K and L).[268–272]

Parametric linkage analysis originally localized the SFD gene to chromosome 22q13-qter.[288] Subsequently, five different missense mutations and a splice site mutation have been identified in *TIMP3* (tissue inhibitor of metalloproteinases 3).[288–294] In the UK, all SFD families carry the same Ser181Cys *TIMP3* mutation and it has been suggested that all cases relate to one single ancestor. *TIMP3* encodes an RPE-expressed member of a group of zinc-binding endopeptidases involved in retinal extracellular matrix remodeling. Most recently a susceptibility locus near *TIMP3* has been found to be associated with age-related macular degeneration, suggesting overlap of some disease mechanisms between the two conditions.[295]

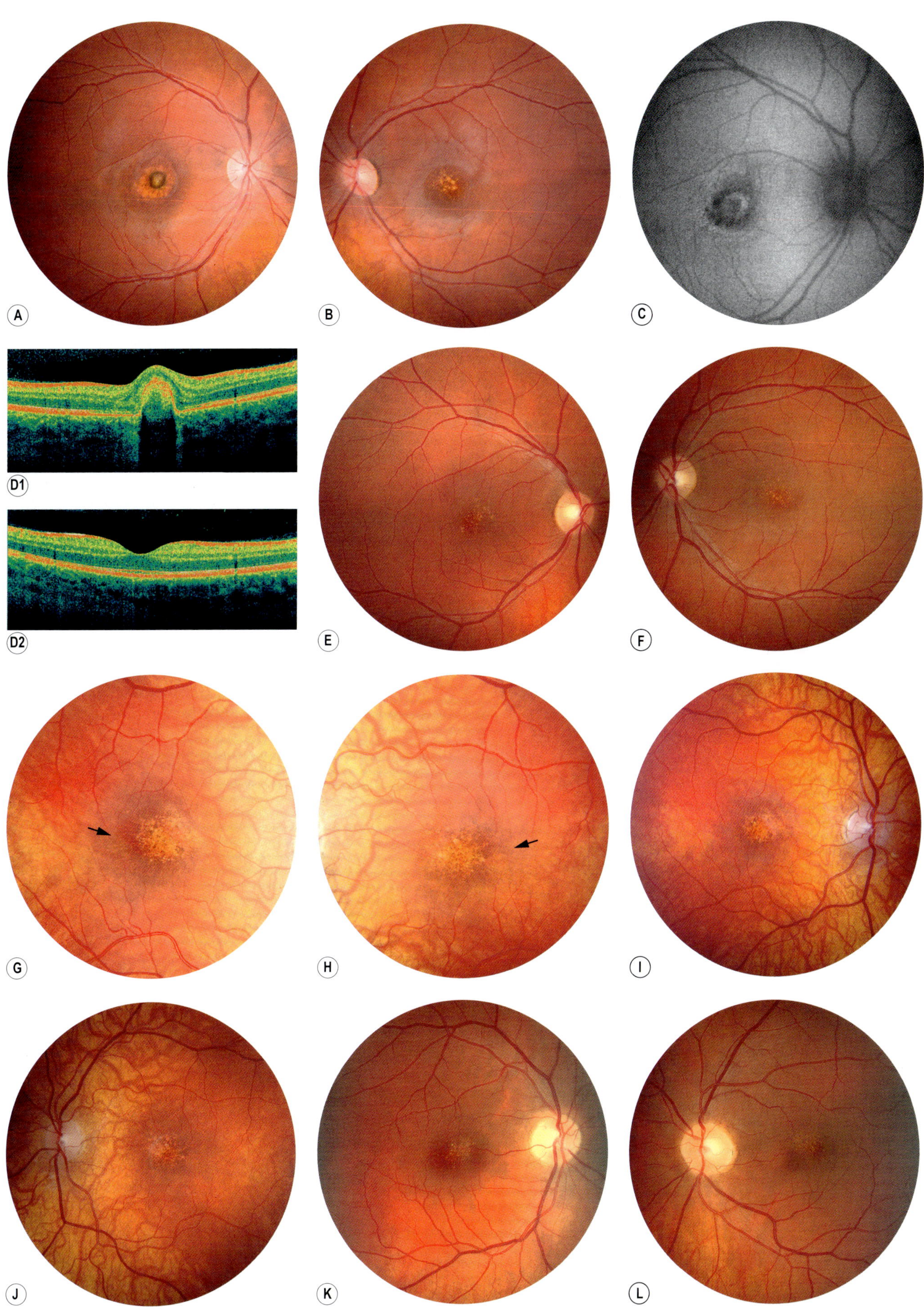
A
B
C
D1
D2
E
F
G
H
I
J
K
L

"BENIGN" CONCENTRIC ANNULAR MACULAR DYSTROPHY

In 1974 Deutman described benign, concentric, annular macular dystrophy in patients who develop a paracentral ring scotoma associated with a bull's-eye pattern of perifoveal atrophy of the RPE and variable degrees of hyperpigmentation of the central macular region.[296–299] Slight narrowing of the retinal vessels may be present. The optic discs are normal. The visual acuity is either normal or near normal. The ERG may be normal or slightly abnormal. The EOG may be subnormal. There may be a mild to moderate color vision defect. The disease is inherited as an autosomal-dominant trait. Although initially termed "benign," a recent 10-year follow-up of the pedigree described by Deutman revealed evidence of progression of benign, concentric, annular macular dystrophy into a more generalized tapetoretinal dystrophy involving both rod and cone function.[298] A progressive decrease in visual acuity, nyctalopia, and dyschromatopsia were found in some members of the pedigree as well as an increase in the pigmentary maculopathy and peripheral bone corpuscular changes. Electrophysiology confirmed equal involvement of the rod and cone systems. This progression of the phenotype is indicative of retinitis pigmentosa with bull's-eye appearance, since rod dysfunction and nyctalopia may be seen early. Photophobia and early loss of central vision, features of cone–rod degeneration, are not typical findings.[300] Benign concentric annular macular dystrophy maps to 6p12.3-q16 in the vicinity of the interphotoreceptor matrix proteoglycan1 (*IMPG1*) gene.[300] The disease is autosomal-dominantly inherited. Miyake et al. described a bull's-eye maculopathy and a negative ERG (b-wave smaller than a-wave) in four unrelated males with initially normal vision, progressive decrease in visual acuity, preserved cone ERG, and mild to moderate deficiency in color vision.[301] They believed that these patients had a disease similar to benign concentric annular dystrophy, although none of their patients had evidence of dominant inheritance. EOG is almost always subnormal or abnormal and deteriorates with age. Dark adaptation also decreases with time. Visual fields may be normal early on and show a ringlike zone of decreased sensitivity around a small central island. Blue-yellow color vision may be deficient.

The differential diagnosis of concentric, annular, macular dystrophy includes cone dystrophy, rod cone dystrophy, lipofuscinosis, chloroquine retinopathy, bull's-eye maculopathy associated with Stargardt's disease (fundus flavimaculatus), sporadic progressive loss of visual acuity secondary to bull's-eye macular atrophy without cone dystrophy, fenestrated sheen macular dystrophy, parafoveal atrophy of the RPE secondary to drusen, and autosomal-dominant central areolar chorioretinal dystrophy unassociated with flecks (Figure 5.22G–J).

5.29 North Carolina macular dystrophy in an African American family.

A–D: This African American male had 20/25 vision in both eyes and belonged to a family examined over four generations with autosomally inherited macular dystrophy in Chicago. He had confluent and nonconfluent drusen confined to the fovea in both eyes (A and B). The lesions show window defects on angiography (C and D). His mother and maternal grandfather were examined in 1979 with bilateral macular lesions and were then given a diagnosis of central areolar choroidal atrophy.
E–H: The son of the above patient had bilateral staphylomatous lesions (E and F) with central atrophy showing loss of choriocapillaris on the angiogram (G and H), surrounded by subretinal fibrosis.
I and **J**: An older maternal cousin was examined in New York who also had a similar staphylomatous lesion (I) with a visual acuity of 20/60 that showed loss of autofluorescence with a ring of hyperautofluorescence at the edge of the lesion (J). Several other members of this family have been examined at various times between 1979 and 2009 and found to have either the drusen or the staphylomatous phenotype. The inheritance has been in an autosomal-dominant pattern.

(Courtesy of Dr. Daniel Kiernan, Dr. Seenu Hariprasad, and Dr. William F. Mieler. E and F, Also, Yannuzzi, Lawrence J., The Retinal Atlas, Saunders 2010, 978-0-7020-3320-9, p.73)

JUVENILE HEREDITARY DISCIFORM MACULAR DEGENERATION

Disciform macular detachment occurs infrequently in children. When it occurs unilaterally in the absence of abnormalities in the opposite eye, it is usually attributed to an inflammatory lesion such as *Toxocara canis*, diffuse unilateral subacute neuroretinitis, and toxoplasmosis, or to a posttraumatic choroidal rupture. Occasionally, a child with rubella retinopathy (see Figure 7.27), pars planitis (see Figure 7.75), and multifocal choroiditis and panuveitis (the pseudo-presumed ocular histoplasmosis syndrome) may develop a disciform macular detachment. Some patients with Best's vitelliform macular dystrophy may develop choroidal neovascularization and the various stages of serous and hemorrhagic disciform detachment (see Figures 5.01E and 5.03C). Choroidal neovascularization has occurred in two sibling children with juxtafoveolar retinal telangiectasis.[273] In general, however, disciform macular detachment in children secondary to hereditary disease apparently occurs rarely. At the 1979 International Fluorescein Angiographic Meeting at Bath, Drs. Alan Bird and Steven Ryan briefly presented two families with multiple children with bilateral disciform macular lesions of unclassified type. In Miami we have observed bilateral disciform detachment of unknown causes in several children without a family history of macular degeneration, and in two sisters. The findings by Bird and Ryan suggest that the clinician should be cautious in making a diagnosis of bilateral disciform detachment secondary to an inflammatory cause without carefully examining other family members.

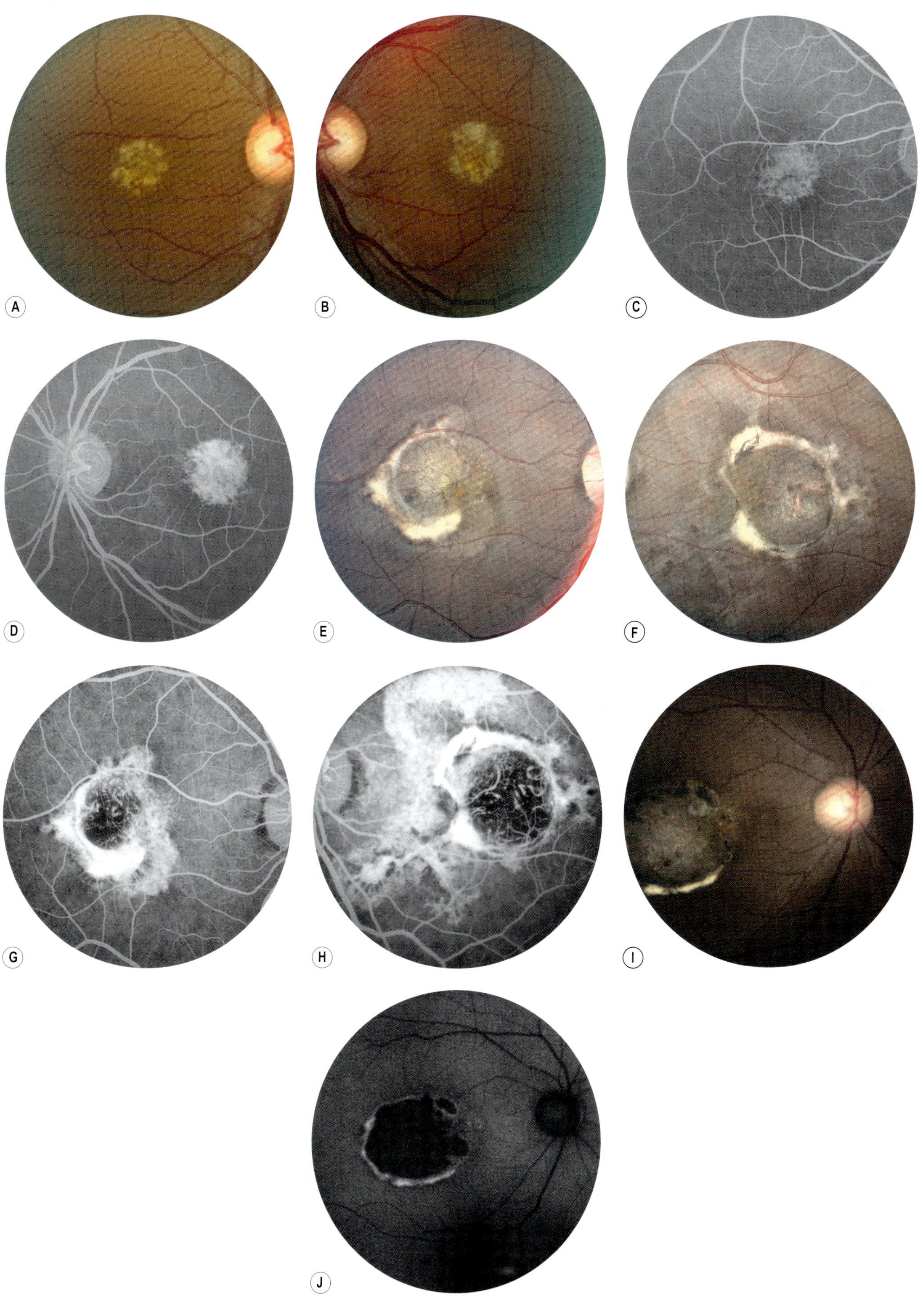
A
B
C
D
E
F
G
H
I
J

5.30 Familial bilateral macular staphylomata.

A–F: This 28-year-old mother (A–C) and her 16-year-old boy (D–F) had minimal eye complaints. She noted trouble with her near vision for 4 years. Her visual acuity was 20/200 in the right eye and 20/50 in the left eye. His visual acuity was 20/200 and J-1 in the right eye and 20/100 and J-1 in the left eye. Both had normal color vision and electro-oculographic findings. The mother's electroretinogram was normal. The son had markedly subnormal rod responses. The cone responses were normal. There was no other family history of eye disease. The family was from Indiana and had no known relatives in North Carolina.

Nonfamilial progressive macular dystrophy and unilateral macular staphyloma.

G–J: This 43-year-old woman gave a 13-year history of decreased vision in the right eye and a recent history of visual change in the left eye. Compare fundus photos made in 1975 (G and H), with those made in 1987 (I and J). Note in the right eye the change from geographic atrophy of retinal pigment epithelium (G) to a large staphyloma (arrows, I), and the development of multiple areas of geographic atrophy in the left eye (J). Her visual acuity was 20/400 right eye and 20/25 left eye at the last examination. Her family history was negative. She missed most of the HRR color plates with each eye. No electrophysiologic information was obtained.

Chorioretinal coloboma associated with choroidal neovascularization.

K and **L**: This 35-year-old man developed metamorphopsia caused by a localized serous detachment that was associated with a focal area of staining (arrow, L) at the superior rim of the staphyloma (arrows, K). The macular detachment resolved after laser photocoagulation but subsequently recurred along with further evidence of choroidal neovascularization.

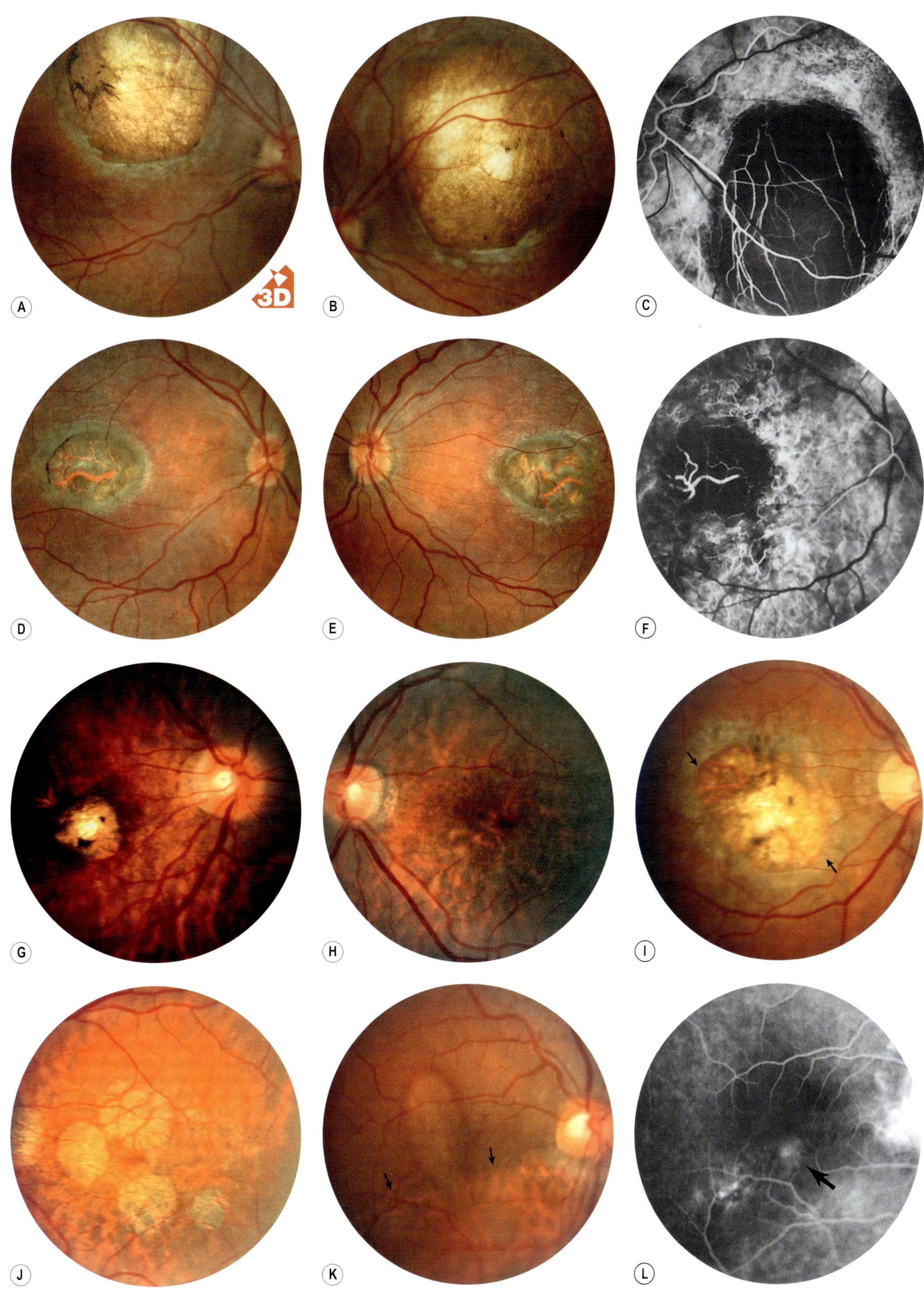
A
3D
B
C
D
E
F
G
H
I
J
K
L

PSEUDOINFLAMMATORY SORSBY'S FUNDUS DYSTROPHY (SFD)

In 1949 Sorsby and associates[274] described five families with dominantly inherited macular dystrophy that was characterized by the development, usually during the fifth decade of life, of choroidal neovascularization, subretinal hemorrhage, and changes suggestive of disciform degeneration (Figure 5.31A–F). Progressive atrophy of the peripheral choroid and RPE occurs later in life and in some cases causes loss of ambulatory vision. Unfortunately the loss of peripheral function has generally been overlooked, as indicated by the name pseudoinflammatory macular dystrophy. This name was chosen because the extensive macular and paramacular changes have suggested to some a postinflammatory change. The term "pseudoinflammatory" is perhaps unfortunate for other reasons: (1) many of the patients have a disciform scar that is indistinguishable from that seen in a host of diseases, including senile macular degeneration and angioid streaks; (2) the fact that the scar extends away from the macula is a nonspecific change that may occur in patients with senile macular degeneration and angioid streaks; and (3) some patients with typical dominantly inherited macular drusen may develop disciform detachment in the fourth decade or earlier. Ashton and Sorsby[275] studied the eyes of two sisters with this condition and noted histopathologic changes similar to those of senile macular degeneration and angioid streaks in patients with pseudoxanthoma elasticum. At least three of the original families reported by Sorsby and associates showed some evidence of drusen deposits at the level of Bruch's membrane. One of his families (Kempster pedigree) had peripheral retinal dysfunction (progressive loss of night vision for up to 25 years before loss of central vision), a deposit of yellow subretinal material throughout the fundus, a tritan color defect, and loss of vision occurring because of choroidal neovascularization by the fifth decade of life. Some patients lost central vision because of geographic atrophy.[276] The yellow material tended to become less apparent with age. Light and electron microscopic examination of the eyes of a 63-year-old descendant of the Kempster family demonstrated a thick deposit within Bruch's membrane that stained positive for lipids, gross loss of the outer retina and RPE, and atrophy of the choriocapillaris.[277] Although no yellow change in the fundus was apparent just prior to death the thickened layer of material between the basement membrane of the RPE and the inner collagenous zone of Bruch's membrane may be the homolog of the yellow material seen clinically earlier in life. These changes were not noted in the histopathologic study of the eyes of one of two sisters described by Ashton and Sorsby.[275]

Dreyer and Hidayat described the clinical and histopathologic findings in a family with dominantly inherited early-onset peripheral and central visual loss with marked EOG changes.[278] The histopathologic changes were similar to those seen by Capon et al.,[276] except no thick sub-RPE deposit was described. Hoskin et al. noted a confluent yellow deposit confined to the macula and angioid streaks in another of Sorsby's pedigrees (Ewbank).[279] The yellow material in both families was associated with some delay in the appearance of fluorescence angiographically that was interpreted as evidence of delayed choriocapillary perfusion.

It is of interest that in a follow-up report of the original five families of Sorsby and associates, two patients were found with a typical fundoscopic picture of angioid streaks and multiple fine drusenlike deposits that appear identical to the peau d'orange change occurring in patients with pseudoxanthoma elasticum.[279] There was no mention in the report as to the presence or absence of the skin lesion. Forsius and associates[280] have reported a Finnish pedigree with a recessively inherited pseudoinflammatory dystrophy characterized by colloid bodies deep within the retina that they likened to those occurring in retinitis punctata albescens (RPA), angioid streaks, and widespread areas of choroidal atrophy and pigment derangement as the disease progressed. A four-generation pedigree characterized by submacular neovascularization in the third to fourth decade, yellow punctate deposits at the level of the pigment epithelium, myopia, nyctalopia beginning in childhood, mid peripheral equatorial pigment clumping and migration, and electrophysiologic abnormalities was reported from Oklahoma.[281] Hamilton et al. reported a seven-generation pedigree with loss of central vision between the second and fourth decades.[282] White to yellow fundus spots, atypical for drusen, accompanied a disciform degeneration in many patients.[282] Some had atrophic maculopathy and others showed no spots. Atrophy of retina and RPE spread to the periphery. Wu et al. studied two brothers of family with dominant

5.31 Sorsby's fundus dystrophy.

A–G: A 55-year-old woman was diagnosed with macular degeneration 10 years previously when she received laser to bleeding in her right eye. Her mother and maternal grandmother were diagnosed with macular degeneration in their 50s and 60s. Her visual acuity was 20/150 in each eye. In addition to partly atrophic and partly fibrotic scars in both maculas the patient had multiple/large choroidal neovascular membranes with subretinal blood and fluid. There were extensive pseudodrusenlike changes extending up to, and anterior to, the equator in both eyes (A–D). Fluorescein angiogram showed early hyperfluorescence of the drusen and leakage corresponding to the choroidal neovascular membranes (E and F). Her Goldmann visual fields were moderately constricted. Given the early age of onset and strong family history she underwent genetic testing and was positive for *TIMP3* mutation. She received intravitreal anti-vascular endothelial growth factor antibodies.

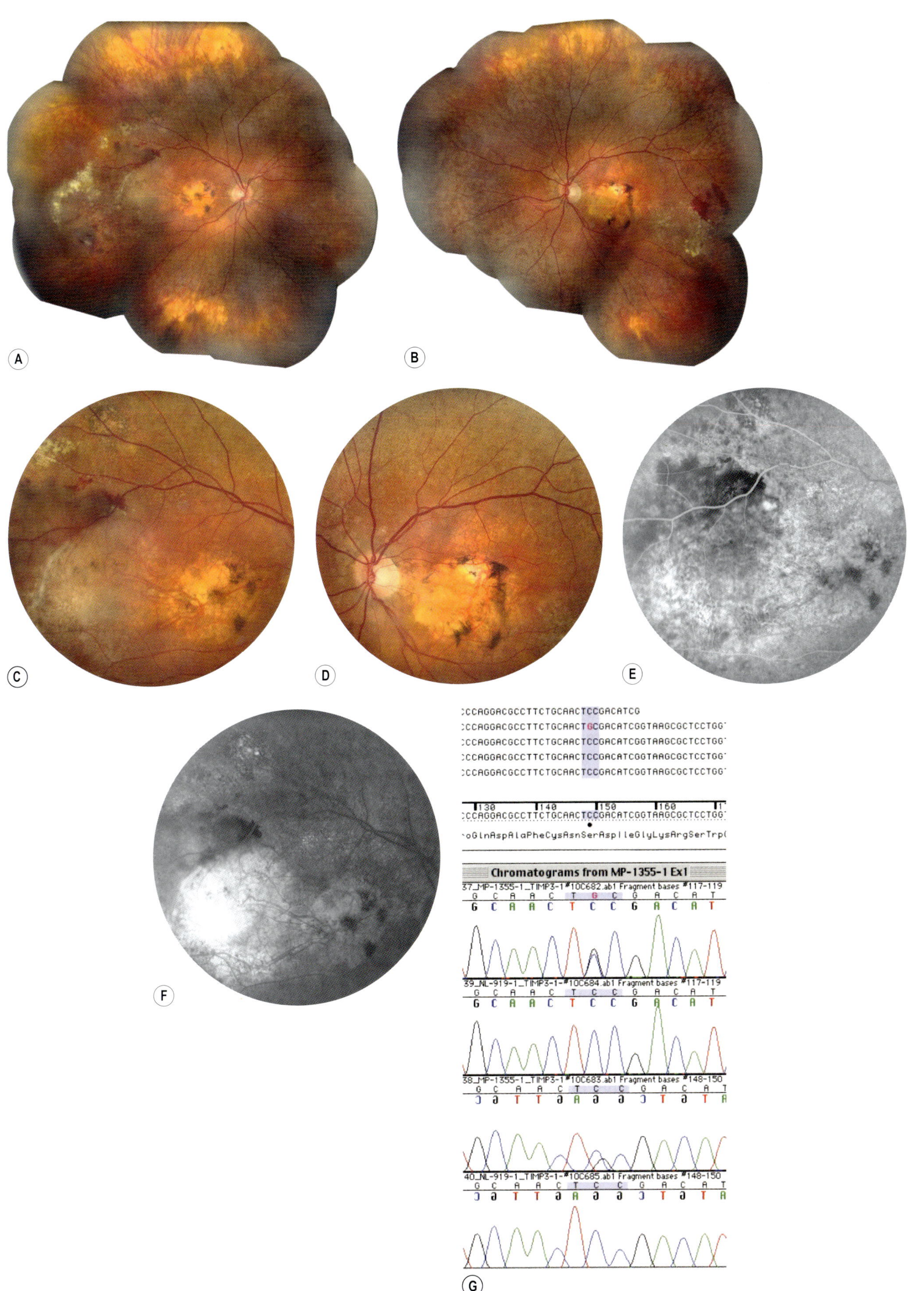
A
B
C
D
E
F
CCCAGGACGCCTTCTGCAACTCCGACATCG
CCCAGGACGCCTTCTGCAACTGCGACATCGGTAAGCGCTCCTGG
CCCAGGACGCCTTCTGCAACTCCGACATCGGTAAGCGCTCCTGG
CCCAGGACGCCTTCTGCAACTCCGACATCGGTAAGCGCTCCTGG
CCCAGGACGCCTTCTGCAACTCCGACATCGGTAAGCGCTCCTGG
130 140 150 160
CCCAGGACGCCTTCTGCAACTCCGACATCGGTAAGCGCTCCTGG
oGlnAspAlaPheCysAsnSerAspIleGlyLysArgSerTrp
Chromatograms from MP-1355-1 Ex1
37_MP-1355-1_TIMP3-1#10C682.ab1 Fragment bases #117-119
G C A A C T G C G A C A T
G C A A C T C C G A C A T
39_NL-919-1_TIMP3-1-#10C684.ab1 Fragment bases #117-119
38_MP-1355-1_TIMP3-1#10C683.ab1 Fragment bases #148-150
40_NL-919-1_TIMP3-1-#10C685.ab1 Fragment bases #148-150
G

is not possible in patients with normal vision or a more benign congenital color vision deficiency. Three genes have been implicated so far. About one-quarter of the patients are associated with *CNGA3* mutation, about 45–50% with *CNGB3* mutation, and the third gene responsible, *GNAT2*, is found in less than 2% of patients.[312]

Incomplete Achromatopsia (Atypical Achromatopsia)

These patients have a mild ability to discern color though abnormal, and have somewhat better visual acuity as compared to the complete achromats. The condition is also inherited as an autosomal-recessive inheritance where mid- and long-wavelength cones are probably present to a small extent. Mutations in *CNGA3* have been found in patients with incomplete achromatopsia. The photophobia is more severe than the loss of vision. These patients often wear more than one pair of sunglasses due to extreme photophobia. Red contact lenses help alleviate some of the photophobia.

Cone Monochromatism

Two of the three cone systems (S small, M medium, and L long) are absent or nearly absent in these patients. The more common forms of cone monochromatism are those that have either the red or the green cones, as compared to blue monochromats.

X-Linked Blue Cone Monochromatism

Patients with X-linked blue cone monochromatism are males having subnormal visual acuity, pendular nystagmus, photophobia, myopia, minimal fundus changes, and psychophysical and electrophysiologic evidence of both normal rod and blue cone functions. Neither red cone nor green cone function can be demonstrated psychophysically. Mutations in the L- and M-opsin gene array that result in the lack of functional L- and M-pigments, and thus inactivate the corresponding cones, have been identified in the majority of cases with blue cone monochromatism.[313,314] Provisional assignment of the gene locus for blue cone monochromasy is in the vicinity of Xq28.[315]

Congenital Color Blindness

Deuteranomaly results when a normal middle-wavelength (M) cone pigment is replaced by one that has a peak sensitivity at a longer wavelength (L). Protanomaly results when the normal long-wavelength pigment is replaced by one that has a peak sensitivity at a shorter midrange wavelength. Protanopia is caused by lack of a red cone pigment and deuteranopia by lack of green cone pigment. Visual acuity and the ocular fundi are normal. They are also inherited as an X-linked disorder and the gene defect is at Xq28. Congenital tritanopia, if it exists, is rare.[316]

5.32 Cone dystrophy.

A and **B**: This 51-year-old woman complained of visual distortion and day blindness. She denied color vision abnormalities and had normal responses to color vision testing. Family history was negative. Visual acuity was 20/20. Her electroretinographic cone responses were subnormal, and the rod responses were normal.
C and **D**: Cone dystrophy in a 29-year-old man complaining of loss of vision and day blindness. Note the bull's-eye pattern of retinal pigment epithelium (RPE) atrophy in both eyes. His electro-retinogram showed no cone responses and normal rod function. His electro-oculogram was normal.
E and **F**: Cone dystrophy or dysgenesis in a 32-year-old man who has had subnormal visual acuity and color blindness since childhood when he was diagnosed as having a "hole in the retina." His visual acuity had decreased from 20/80 to 20/200 during the past 2 years. He had bilaterally symmetric staphylomatous foveal lesions. Note slight narrowing of the retinal vessels. His cone electro-retinogram was moderately abnormal. The rod electroretinogram and electro-oculogram were normal. Farnsworth-Munsell 100-hue testing showed a tritan axis.
G: The 28-year-old color-blind sister of patient shown in E. There was a faint perifoveolar ring of RPE atrophy bilaterally. Results of electro-retinography, electro-oculography, and color vision testing were identical to those of her brother.
H: This 32-year-old man noted day blindness at 22 years of age and later progressive loss of central and color vision. His visual acuity was 20/40. His fundi were unremarkable. His electroretinographic and electro-oculographic findings were normal. His sister and mother had similar complaints.
I: Mother of patient illustrated in H.

Cone dystrophy with Mizuo-Nakamura phenomenon

J–L: Late-onset X-linked recessive cone dystrophy with tapeto-like sheen and Mizuo–Nakamura phenomenon. Note iridescent RPE changes (J and K) that partly disappeared after dark adaptation (L).

(J–L from Heckenlively and Weleber, [335])

Goldmann–Favre Syndrome

There is increasing evidence to suggest that Goldmann–Favre syndrome may be a genetically determined retinal receptor dysgenesis primarily affecting the cone system in which an overabundance of S-cones partly replaces the other cone types. (See p. 368, ch 5.)

PROGRESSIVE CONE DYSTROPHY

The term "cone dystrophy" is used to describe those patients with a heritable dystrophy in which predominantly the cone system is affected.[254,317–346] It includes some patients in whom no evidence of rod dysfunction develops as well as those in whom rod deficiency later develops but cone deficiency predominates.[347] Both types may be seen in the same pedigree. Most cases are sporadic, but when they are familial, most are autosomal-dominant[318,319,324,327,331,342,343] or X-linked cone

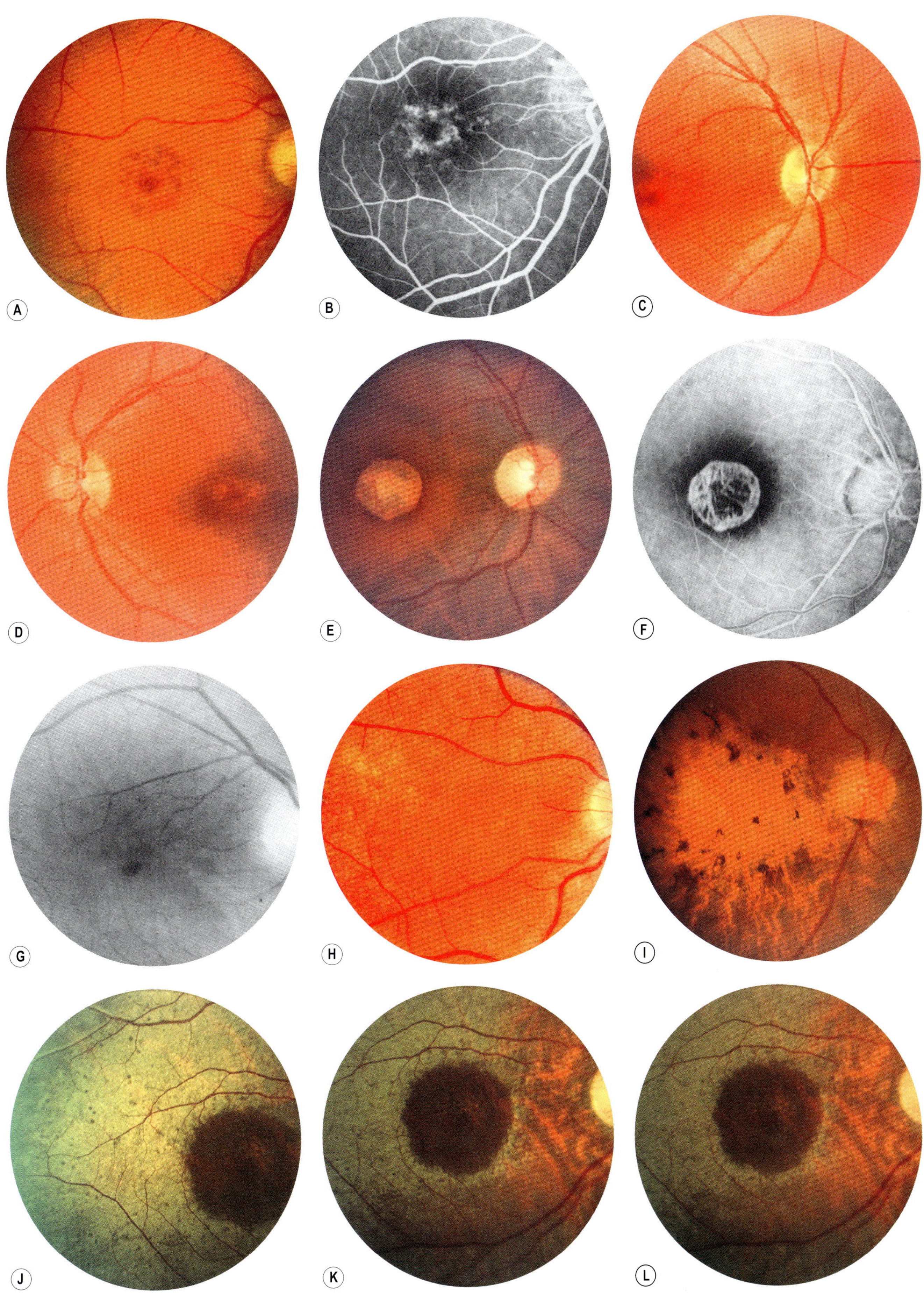
A
B
C
D
E
F
G
H
I
J
K
L

dystrophy. In X-linked cone dystrophy, pseudoprotanomaly and abnormal foveal densitometry findings have been identified in female carriers.[332] In other families fundus changes and abnormalities in color vision, ERG, and visual evoked potential were found in female carriers.[320,333] The age of onset, severity, and rate of progression vary from family to family and within the same family. The age of onset varies from childhood to midlife or beyond. The clinical features, all of which or only some of which may be present, initially include: (1) onset of progressive visual loss; (2) impairment of color vision even with minimal acuity loss; (3) impaired visual function in brightly illuminated situations and better vision in twilight or dim illumination and day blindness (hemeralopia); (4) normal or near-normal fundi initially and, later, RPE atrophy in the macula often progressing to a bull's-eye pattern; (5) temporal pallor of the optic disc in some patients; (6) fluorescein angiographic evidence of depigmentation of the RPE in the macula (often antedating visible alterations in the fundi); (7) central scotoma with normal peripheral fields; and (8) reduced or nondetectable photopic as well as abnormal flicker response ERG. Some patients may demonstrate a supernormal scotopic ERG.[339,346] Early selective involvement of the blue cone system may occur in some families with autosomal-dominant inheritance.[318,319,324,342] Visual acuity varies from 20/20 early to 20/200 or less later. The macula may be normal (Figure 5.32H), or it may show a variety of changes, including mottling and clumping of the pigment epithelium, a bull's-eye pattern of depigmentation, focal chorioretinal atrophy, and a macular staphyloma (Figure 5.32E and F).[260] The bull's-eye pattern of RPE atrophy and a corresponding zone of hyperfluorescence surrounding a central nonfluorescent spot similar to that seen in chloroquine retinopathy are the most commonly described biomicroscopic and angiographic changes in these patients (Figures 5.31G and H, 5.32A, C, and D). Occasionally temporal pallor of the optic disc may be the only fundus change. Autofluorescence testing can show increased autofluorescence in a ring around the fovea surrounding an area of central hypoautofluorescence that corresponds to the bull's-eye atrophy (Figure 5.31I and J).[348] An acquired fixation nystagmus may be present. A few patients with predominantly the peripheral portion of the cone system affected may have normal color vision performance in the presence of a subnormal photopic ERG (Figure 5.32A).

Some of these patients may present with complaints of progressive day blindness yet have normal visual acuity.[322,324,329] Conversely, if the central portion of the cone system is primarily affected, patients may have subnormal visual acuity, abnormal color vision, and a normal photopic ERG. As the disease progresses, they will develop abnormal photopic ERG findings. Many patients eventually develop some electroretinographic evidence of abnormal rod function.[349] This varies in severity. When severe, it is associated with varying degrees of optic disc pallor, narrowing of the retinal vessels, and peripheral field loss. Often there is no or only minimal evidence of pigment migration. The EOG may be normal or abnormal. Patients with cone dystrophy and fundi resembling retinitis pigmentosa rarely complain of night blindness. Despite an extinguished ERG, they may show either a normal or mildly abnormal dark adaptation curve. This discrepancy is seen also in chloroquine retinopathy. The earliest histological changes seen are distortion and kinking of the foveal receptor segments followed by loss of nucleus and the rest of the cell bodies. Histopathologic and ultrastructural findings in an eye removed after development of ERG changes of rod involvement showed changes in the peripheral retina similar to that of mild retinitis pigmentosa.[350] The differential diagnosis of a bull's-eye maculopathy has been discussed elsewhere (see p. 300).

The progression of cone dystrophy is usually more rapid in patients with early onset of visual symptoms. Visual loss is usually, but not always, symmetric. The acuity usually does not decrease much below 20/200.

Some patients with cone dystrophy will show, in addition to reduced or missing potentials at light-adapted conditions and reduced photopic flicker frequencies, a supernormal dark-adapted b-wave amplitude (supernormal rod ERG).[339,341,346] Some patients showing this latter ERG finding have a congenital stationary cone dysgenesis, whereas others demonstrate evidence of a progressive cone dystrophy. Most show pigmentary changes in the macula that in some patients has a bull's-eye pattern. Mutations in *KCNV2* which encodes a subunit of a voltage-gated potassium channel in both rods and cones has been found recently.[351]

An X-linked form of cone dystrophy may have a golden sheen that disappears on dark adaptation; this is known as the Mizuo-Nakamura phenomenon (Figure 5.32J–L). Female carriers can have a wide spectrum of findings, some appearing relatively normal to those having bull's-eye change in the macula. X-linked cone dystrophy has been mapped to three loci on the X chromosome.

Autosomal-dominant cone dystrophy or cone–rod dystrophy has been associated with several mutations that include mutations of the peripherin/*RDS* gene, the *CRX* gene, the retinal guanylate cyclase gene (*RET-GC1*), the guanylyl cyclase-activating protein 1 (*GCAP1*) gene, *AIPL1*, *GUCY2D*, *PITPNM3*, *PROM1*, *RIMS1*, *SEMA4A*, and *UNC11* gene.[352,353] Peripherin *RDS* is present on both rod and cone segments. *CRX* codes for a photoreceptor-specific domain transcription factor. The *RET-GC1* and *GCAP1* gene are involved in cyclic guanosine monophosphate (cGMP) production. Different mutations within the same gene and mutations of several genes result in variable severity of the cone dystrophy.[98]

Late-Onset Sporadic Cone Dystrophy

Patients with late-onset sporadic cone dystrophy, who are often older than 50 years of age at the onset, develop slowly progressive loss of central or paracentral vision usually in the absence of any fundoscopic abnormalities.[317,330,354] Visual acuity is often normal or near normal at presentation. Detection of color vision dysfunction is an important clue to early diagnosis because initially full-field ERG findings may be normal.[353] These patients are often subjected to extensive neurologic investigations. The differential diagnosis in patients, particularly if they present with asymmetric paracentral field defects, or with a history of rapid onset of visual loss that may be associated with photopsia, includes acute zonal occult outer retinopathy (see Chapter 11) and occult macular dystrophy. Drug toxicity has been implicated in acute cone degeneration.[319]

A subgroup of patients with Stargardt's disease (atrophic maculopathy, flecks, and a dark choroid on fluorescein angiography) present with hemeralopia and ERG changes typical for a cone dystrophy. The disorder is recessively inherited in these patients with few exceptions.

The retinal dystrophy associated with autosomal-dominant cerebellar ataxia may affect primarily the cone system (spinocerebellar ataxia 7: SCA 7, see later section). Two of the four patients described with this association showed, in addition to the typical ERG findings of a cone dystrophy, a supernormal dark-adapted b-wave.[337]

Some patients with cone and cone–rod dystrophies may exhibit a bright tapeto-like retinal reflex.[335,340,355] Heckinlively and Weleber reported a late-onset cone dystrophy with X-linked recessive inheritance in patients with a greenish-golden iridescent RPE change in the posterior pole (Figure 5.32J–L).[335] These patients demonstrated the Mizuo–Nakamura phenomenon and were prone to development of rhegmatogenous retinal detachment (see Oguchi's disease, Figure 5.37). In a family with dominant cone dystrophy, Noble et al. observed a scintillating golden reflex, identical to that seen in female carriers of X-linked retinitis pigmentosa in the son and a diffuse golden-gray sheen similar to that of Oguchi's disease in his mother.[355] A golden sheen and pigment disturbance may also occur in families with progressive visual loss, normal ERG findings, and absence of the Mizuo–Nakamura phenomenon.[356]

Analysis of genomic DNA isolated from affected members of a family of X-linked cone degeneration revealed a 6.5-kilobase deletion in the red cone pigment gene.[323] Reduced levels of alpha-l-fucosidase activity in leukocytes was found in two patients with sporadic cone dystrophy.[336] Screening of 24 patients with several forms of cone dystrophy failed to find this abnormality.[321] Antibodies against human retinal proteins have been identified in the serum of some patients with cone dystrophy.[334]

Heavily tinted glasses or miotics may be helpful in alleviating photophobia in patients with cone dystrophy.

FENESTRATED SHEEN MACULAR DYSTROPHY

Fenestrated sheen macular dystrophy is an autosomal-dominant macular disorder characterized in young patients by tiny red fenestrations occurring in a central macular zone of a golden sheen (Figure 5.33A–C).[357–361] Multifocal areas of hypopigmentation of the RPE become manifest in the paracentral area in young adulthood, and this may progress to an annular zone of depigmentation by the fourth decade. Fluorescein angiography shows window defects corresponding to the RPE changes and not related to the red fenestrations. The visual acuity may be mildly affected in late adulthood and ranges from 20/20 to 20/30. Mild changes in the ERG and EOG and color vision abnormalities may develop. The sheen reflex that appears to lie between the level of the RPE and retinal vessels persists, but the central fenestrations disappear as more changes in the RPE occur. Daily and Mets suggested that this disorder may be related to a defect or abnormality in macular xanthophyll.[360] This disease should be added to the list of bull's-eye maculopathies.

DOMINANTLY INHERITED MÜLLER CELL SHEEN DYSTROPHY (FAMILIAL INTERNAL LIMITING MEMBRANE RETINAL DYSTROPHY)

Dominantly inherited Müller cell sheen dystrophy is a rare, previously unreported disorder characterized biomicroscopically by prominent glistening light reflections emanating from the inner retinal surface that appears to be thickened, yet translucent, and thrown into a pattern of railroad track-like folds (Figure 5.33D–L).[362] These changes are most prominent but are not limited to the posterior fundus. This dominantly inherited disorder is apparently associated with minimal visual morbidity prior to midlife, when patients may experience visual loss in one or both eyes as the result of biomicroscopic and angiographic evidence of widespread intraretinal edema (Figure 5.33D–H). In addition to typical cystoid macular edema, there is a pattern of superficial microcystic changes that extend throughout the posterior fundus. Vitrectomy in three eyes of two members of the same family has failed to improve the visual function (Figure 5.33D–I). One family member developed monocular loss of central vision that was attributed to vitreomacular traction. Pars plana vitrectomy failed to change either the visual function or the appearance of the fundus (Figure 5.33D–H). Histopathologically, these fundus changes are caused by thickening and undulation of the internal limiting membrane of the retina, superficial retinal schisis, and cystic spaces in the inner nuclear layer. All of these changes suggest a primary defect in the Müller cells (Figure 5.33J–L).

5.33 Fenestrated sheen macular dystrophy.

A–C: A 32-year-old man with presumed dominantly inherited fenestrated sheen macular dystrophy. He complained of recent loss of vision. His acuity, which had previously been 20/20, was 20/40. His family history was negative. His color vision and electroretinographic findings were normal. The small, dark, fenestrated areas within the glistening sheen in the central macular area are barely visible in the photographs. Angiography showed mottled hyperfluorescence centrally but no evidence of abnormal staining.

Dominantly inherited Müller cell sheen retinal dystrophy (familial internal limiting membrane dystrophy).

D–H: This 53-year-old man, his sister, his mother, and a maternal second cousin had a long-standing history of a peculiar fundus glistening reflex change that, in the patient and his cousin, was associated with some visual loss. The patient had laser treatment for recurrent idiopathic central serous chorioretinopathy in January 1994. His symptoms failed to respond to laser treatment. There were marked glistening reflexes and some distortion of the retinal vessels in both eyes. There was clinical and angiographic evidence of macular edema in the right eye (D and E). This edema was attributed to vitreomacular traction and a pars plana vitrectomy was done in September 1994. This resulted in minimal change in the fundus appearance and visual function. In December 1994 his visual acuity was 20/200 right eye and 20/25 left eye. He missed all of the HRR plates with the right eye and got nearly all of them with the left eye. Biomicroscopically the inner retinal surface was thrown into folds that gave a railroad track-like reflex running throughout much of the posterior fundus of the right eye and to a lesser degree in the left eye (F). In the right eye there was cystoid macular edema and a fine pattern of superficial retinal cysts that extended throughout the macular area. Fluorescein angiography showed some improvement in the dye leakage from the retinal capillaries (G and H). Angiography of the left eye was normal except for evidence of focal scars related to central serous chorioretinopathy. His past medical history was positive for diabetes and carpal tunnel syndrome.

I: Note the same but less prominent fundus changes in his sister, who had normal visual acuity.

J–L: The eyes of the mother, who had a history of right hemianopia, optic disc cupping, and normal intraocular pressures, were obtained at autopsy. Gross examination of her eyes revealed prominent light reflexes on the surface of the retina. Histopathologic examination revealed thickening and undulation of the internal limiting membrane of the retina (arrows, J–L), multiple superficial schisis cavities separating the internal limiting membrane from the nerve fiber layer, ganglion cell atrophy, and cystic spaces in the inner nuclear layer. Stains for elastic tissue, amyloid, and mucopolysaccharides were negative.

(A–C, from Daily and Mets, [1246])

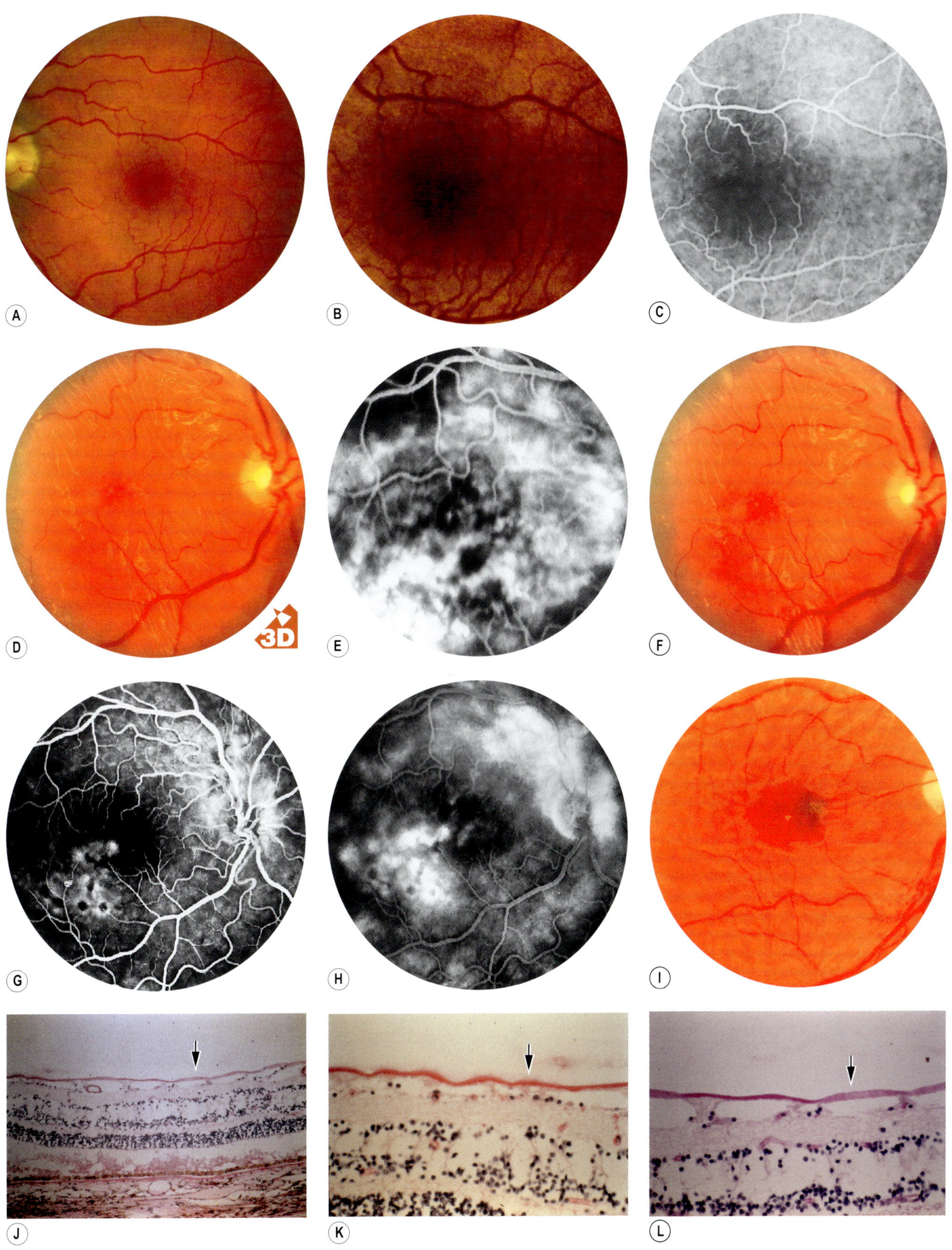
A
B
C
D
3D
E
F
G
H
I
J
K
L

ASTEROID MACULAR DYSTROPHY

Figure 5.34 (A–C), depicts the ophthalmoscopic and angiographic findings in a young woman with a striking seven-point dark stellate figure centered in the fovea of both eyes.[363] Her visual acuity was 20/20. Her family history was normal. No family members were available for examination. It is probable, however, that this is a foveomacular dystrophy or dysgenesis with a good visual prognosis.

SJÖGREN–LARSSON SYNDROME

Sjögren–Larsson syndrome, an autosomal-recessive neurocutaneous syndrome, is characterized by the following clinical features: (1) congenital ichthyosis; (2) congenital low-grade stationary mental deficiency; (3) symmetric spastic paresis with maximum involvement of the legs; (4) convulsions; (5) dental and osseous dysplasia; (6) defective sweating; (7) hypertelorism; (8) reduced life expectancy; and (9) ophthalmoscopic changes in the macula, characterized by the presence of white glistening flecks and yellowish pigmentary changes that may simulate Best's vitelliform dystrophy (Figure 5.34D and E).[364–367] These macular changes are present in a majority of patients and considered pathognomonic. The glistening dots are believed to be located in the inner retina (ganglion cells and inner plexiform layer), may appear by age 1–2 years, and increase with age. Photophobia is often present. On fluorescein angiography the foveal and perifoveal areas show hyperfluorescence. The crystals do not block fluorescence, and are hyperautofluorescent.[368] In addition to the crystals in inner retina, microcystoid spaces may be seen on OCT, a feature somewhat similar to idiopathic juxtafoveal telangiectasia type 2.[369] Macular pigment levels were found to be reduced by macular pigment reflectometer and autofluorescent testing by van der Veen et al.[370] ERG and EOG done in a few of these patients are usually normal.[368,369,371,372] Patients with this syndrome are specifically deficient in the fatty aldehyde dehydrogenase component of the fatty alcohol oxidoreductase that catalyzes the oxidation of medium- and long-chain fatty aldehydes to corresponding fatty acids. This deficiency may be detected in the skin fibroblasts of patients and in carriers of the disorder.[365]

5.34 Asteroid macular dystrophy.

A–C: This 38-year-old black woman complained of mild visual changes. Family history and past medical history were normal. Visual acuity was 20/20. Note the peculiar stellate lesion, consisting of seven fine irregular dark lines radiating from the center of the fovea in each eye. Angiography revealed no evidence of alterations of the retinal pigment epithelium (RPE).

Sjögren–Larssen syndrome.

D and **E**: Note the yellowish deposit and fine crystalline deposits in the macula (D) in this 31-month-old black boy with mental and motor retardation, ichthyosis, generalized weakness, and spasticity (E). There was some narrowing of the retinal arterioles.

Aicardi's syndrome.

F–H: Two-year-old girl with microphthalmos and orbital cyst, right side; coloboma of the iris, left eye; absence of the corpus callosum; hydrocephalus secondary to aqueductal stenosis; and psychomotor and mental retardation. The atrophic patches in the choroid and RPE were detected at birth and were initially interpreted as possible chorioretinal scars caused by cytomegalic inclusion disease.

Flecked retina in Alport's syndrome.

I–L: This 30-year-old man, with hearing loss, anterior lenticonus (D), and nephritis, had multiple flecks in the macular regions of both eyes (E and F). Angiography (G) revealed no changes corresponding with the flecks implying the flecks to be in inner retina rather than at the RPE level. His visual acuity was 20/25. His electroretinogram and electro-oculogram were normal.

(D and G, courtesy of Dr. Randy Campo; H and I. from Gilbert et al.[364]),

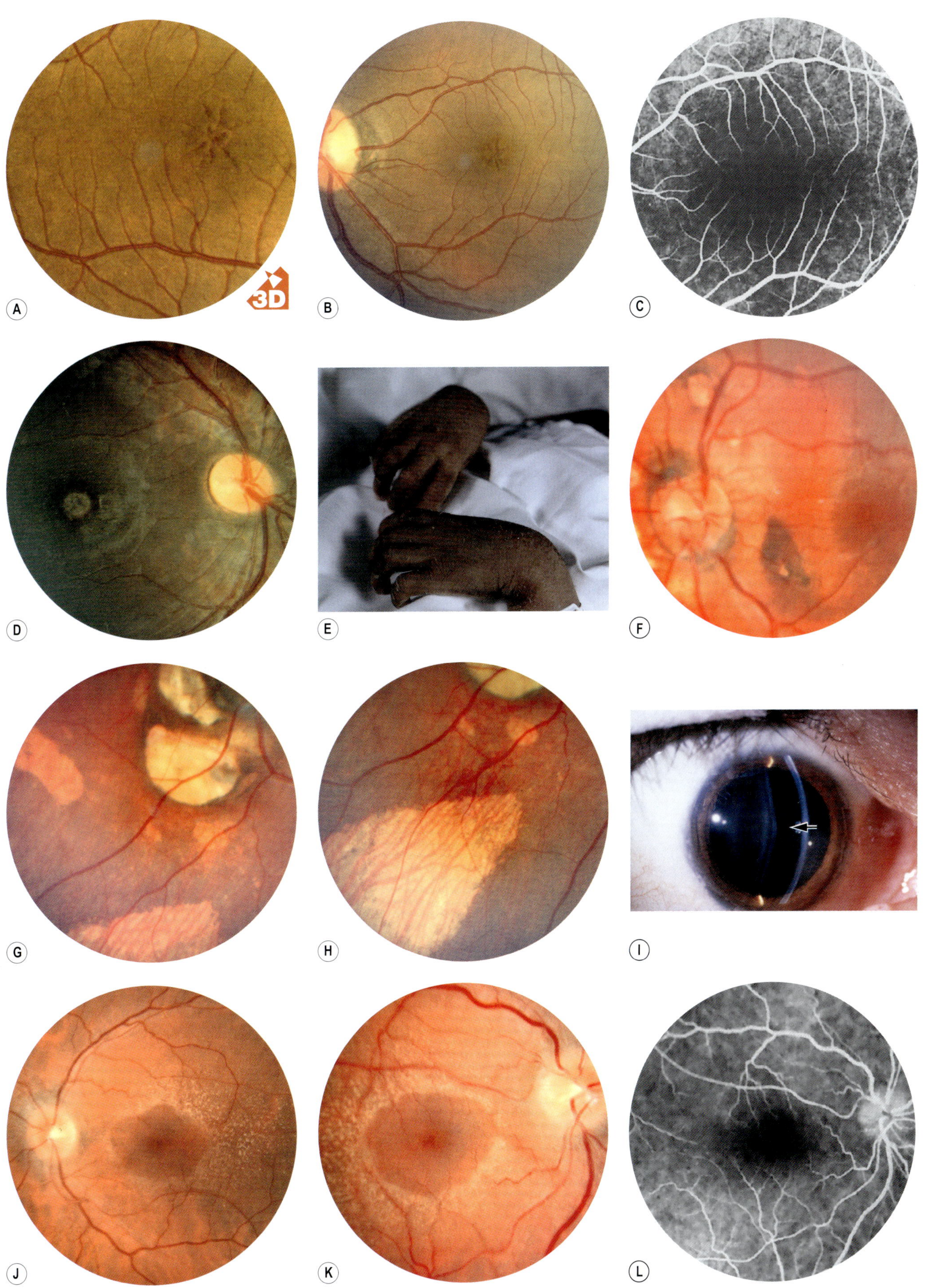
A
3D
B
C
D
E
F
G
H
I
J
K
L

AICARDI'S SYNDROME

The cardinal features of Aicardi's syndrome are infantile spasms, agenesis of the corpus callosum, and a characteristic chorioretinopathy that may occur in association with other ocular abnormalities, including microphthalmia, colobomas of the optic nerve and choroid, scleral ectasia, persistent pupillary membrane, and glial tissue extending from the optic disc.[373–384] Other associated findings are mental retardation, generalized seizures, hypotonia, cerebral malformations including microcephaly, polymicrogyria, periventricular and intracortical gray-matter heterotopias, interventricular cysts, choroid plexus papillomas and cysts, asymmetry of cerebral hemispheres, cortical atrophy, pineal gland cysts, vermian anomalies, and cerebellar hypoplasia.[383,385–389] Costovertebral defects such as scoliosis, hemivertebrae, block vertebrae, fused vertebrae, and missing or bifurcated ribs and craniosyostosis are common findings.[386,390] Characteristic fundus lesions are well-defined, circular, white lacunae with minimal pigmentation at their borders varying in size from one-tenth disc diameter to twice the normal size of the optic disc (Figure 5.34F–H). They are usually bilateral and are often symmetrically distributed. In general the lesions are clustered around the optic disc and decrease in size and number as they extend into the periphery of the fundus. Electroretinography may be normal or minimally disturbed. Histopathologically these lesions have been shown to correspond to areas of depigmentation and deficiency in the RPE as well as gross choroidal atrophy.[375,377,391] It is probable that the chorioretinal lesions represent a dysgenesis and not a progressive dystrophic disorder since new lesions do not occur. Progressive pigmentation of the lesions has been documented.[392] Aicardi's syndrome occurs only in females, and no familial cases have been reported except for one report of discordance in monozygotic twins.[393] It has been reported rarely in Klinefelter's 47,XXY males,[394,395] except for one report in a 46,XY male.[396] No study so far has been able to demonstrate a defect in the X chromosome, hence it appears that the change occurs after fertilization. Attempts to find the mutation in the Xp22 and the Xq28 regions have been unsuccessful.[390,397]

ALPORT'S DISEASE

Alport syndrome is associated with genetic abnormality involving the *COL4A3*, *COL4A4*, and *COL4A5* genes that encode the production of type IV collagen. This protein is common to the basement membrane of the glomerulus, cochlea, retina, lens capsule, and cornea. The glomerular basement membrane is irregularly thickened and splinted and stretched. The immunohistochemical stain shows absence of A5 chain. Carrier females may have variable inactivation of the X chromosome in different tissues and may manifest some of the features.[398,399] These patients present with hematuria, deafness, and progressive renal dysfunction. The condition was first described by Cecil Alport in 1927. The frequency is 1:5000. It accounts for 2.1% of end-stage renal disease in pediatric patients: 85% of affected patients are male. Affected males are more likely to be deaf and develop renal failure than females.

It is associated with the following ocular findings: microspherophakia; lenticonus (Figure 5.35E and F); anterior or posterior subcapsular cataracts; posterior polymorphous corneal dystrophy; multiple, small (20–50 μm in diameter), punctate, yellow-white lesions in the superficial pericentral retina in the macula (Figures 5.34J, K and 5.35A and C, G and H); and confluent and clustered, punctate, yellow-white lesions located deep to the retinal vessels in the midperiphery of the fundi.[400–414] The macular lesions may be present in early childhood but probably become more apparent with age and are seen in 35% of patients.[407] They are not associated with angiographic or electrophysiologic changes other than that which may occur as a result of hypertension and renal failure.[404,406,408,410,414] There may be spotty areas of window defects in the RPE associated with the peripheral lesions.[405] The nature of these lesions is unknown. These patients are known to develop giant macular holes likely due to defective Müller cell basement membrane (Figure 5.35A–D).[415] The anterior lenticonus is pathognomonic for Alport syndrome. Posterior polymorphous corneal dystrophy due to defect in the Descemet's membrane occurs infrequently. Drusen in Bruch's membrane, degeneration of the RPE in the macular area, and serous retinal detachments occurring in the terminal stage of renal insufficiency have also been reported in these patients.

5.35 Macular hole in Alport's syndrome.

A and **B**: A 34-year-old male who had a history of renal transplant and hearing loss. He showed several flecks at the posterior pole, characteristic for Alport's syndrome. He subsequently developed a traumatic cataract requiring cataract surgery with intraocular lens placement. Following this, he was found to have several small holes in the macula that became confluent into a solitary giant hole.
C and **D**: Left eye of another patient with inner retinal flecks that eventually developed a large macular hole.
E–I: A 22-year-old Indian male had progressive decrease in vision in both eyes associated with worsening renal insufficiency and deafness. His parents and sister were asymptomatic. His visual acuity was 20/50 and 20/60. Bilateral anterior lenticonus with localized cataract due to microbreaks in capsule was present (E and F). Bilateral symmetrical macular flecks were seen in the superficial retina, likely at the level of the internal limiting membrane, suggesting abnormalities of the footplates of Müller cells (G and H). Optical coherence tomography demonstrates the flecks to be at the internal limiting membrane and just beneath it. Visual acuity returned to 20/20 in both eyes following cataract surgery.

(A–D, courtesy of Dr. David Weinberg. Also, Yannuzzi, Lawrence J., The Retinal Atlas, Saunders 2010, 978-0-7020-3320-9, p.122.)

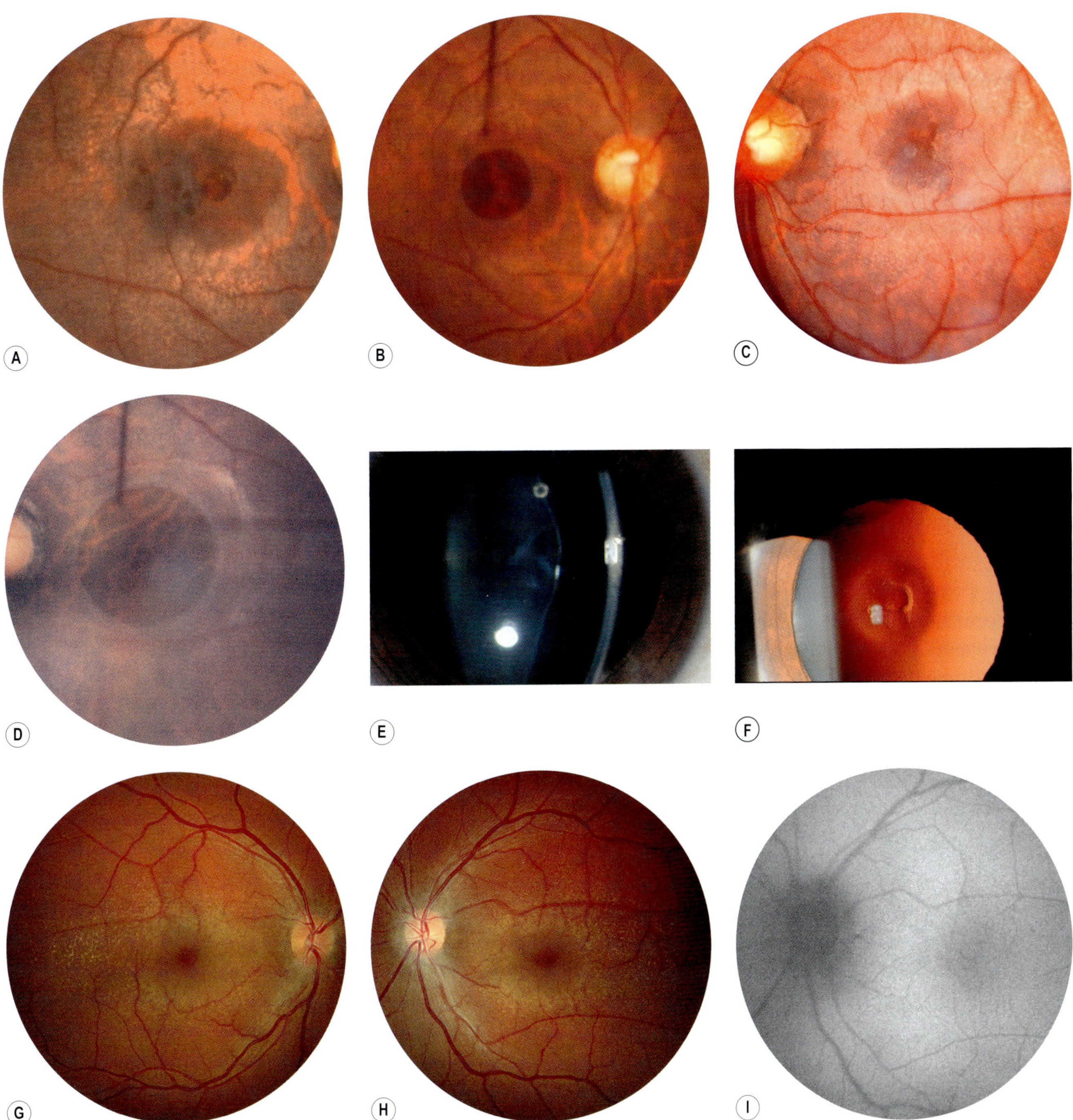
A
B
C
D
E
F
G
H
I

Because these patients have abnormalities affecting basement membranes elsewhere, particularly that of the renal glomeruli, it is possible that the mid peripheral lesions may represent nodular thickening of the basement membrane of the RPE (basal laminar drusen; see chapter 3), and that the superficial lesions in the macula are related to abnormalities of the basement membrane of the Müller cells or retinal astrocytes. Gehrs et al. have suggested that the retinal flecks may consist of an abnormal subtype alpha 5 of type IV collagen, which is a major structural component of the glomerulus basement membrane.[404] The gene encoding for this protein has been localized to the same locus (*COL45A*) at Xq22, where genetic linkage studies have placed the defect in patients with X-linked Alport syndrome.[416] Mutations in collagen type IV genes have been described to be responsible for X-linked (*COL4A5*), autosomal-recessive, and autosomal-dominant Alport syndrome (*COL4A3/COL4A4*). A related disorder, benign familial hematuria, is an autosomal-dominant disorder; about 40% of these cases cosegregate with the *COL4A3/COL4A4* loci, the same site for autosomal-dominant Alport syndrome. It is likely that some cases of benign familial hematuria may represent the carrier state for autosomal-recessive Alport syndrome. Collagen type IV nephropathy is an entity in itself, and phenotypic manifestations of *COL4A3/COL4A4* mutations may range from monosymptomatic hematuria (benign familial hematuria) to severe renal failure (Alport syndrome), depending on the gene dosage.[417]

RETINAL DYSTROPHY IN DUCHENNE AND BECKER MUSCULAR DYSTROPHY

Duchenne muscular dystrophy is a lethal X-linked recessive disorder characterized by progressive proximal muscular weakness, loss of ambulation, and early death. Ninety-five percent of patients are wheelchair-bound by age 12 years and the mortality rate is 95% by age 20 years. The dystrophin gene for the disorder is mapped to Xp21. Dystrophin, the gene product of Duchenne muscular dystrophy, is a 427-kDa submembranous cytoskeletal protein and many dystrophin-associated proteins, such as utrophin, dystroglycans, sarcoglycans, syntrophins and dystrobrevins, have been identified. Dystrophin and dystrophin-associated proteins are very important proteins for skeletal, cardiac, and smooth muscles and also for the peripheral and central nervous system, including the retina. Dystrophin and beta-dystroglycan localize at the retinal photoreceptor terminal; their deficiency results in abnormal neurotransmission between photoreceptor cells and ON bipolar cells. Dystrophin has seven isoforms in variable tissues, and the retina contains full-length dystrophin (Dp427), Dp260, and Dp71. Dp71 localizes in the inner limiting membrane and around the blood vessels, and Dp260 is expressed in the outer plexiform layer.

5.36 Fleck retina in ring 17 chromosome.

A–D: This 34-year-old man had short stature, microcephaly, café-au-lait spots, mild mental deficiency, yellow flecks throughout the postequatorial fundi (A and B), and ring 17 chromosome (D). He had no visual complaints. His visual acuity was 20/30 bilaterally. There were a few cortical flecks in both lenses. Fluorescein angiography revealed a salt-and-pepper pattern of mottled hyperfluorescence and nonfluorescence corresponding with the flecks (C). His chromosome diagnosis was 46,XY,r(17) (p13q25), that of a male with ring 17 chromosome. His family history was negative.

Benign fleck retina.

E and **F**: This asymptomatic young Australian Aborigine woman had normal visual acuity, color vision, and electroretinographic findings. There were widespread polymorphous flecks at the level of the pigment epithelium throughout the peripheral fundi. The family history was negative. No other family members were available for examination. Note similarity to Figure 5.38D.

It is generally assumed that dystrophin functions to stabilize muscle fibers with dystrophin-associated proteins by linking the sarcolemma to the basement membrane in muscles, but its function in the retina is unknown so far. Patients with Duchenne muscular dystrophy have subnormal scotopic ERG amplitudes in the form of electronegative b-waves; the extent is likely determined by the presence of, and location of, the gene deletion.[418–421] Focal hyperpigmentation of the macula may be seen, but color vision, photopic ERGs, visual acuity, and extraocular muscle function remain normal, distinguishing Duchenne muscular dystrophy from other X-linked disorders with electronegative ERGs.[422]

OCCULT MACULAR DYSTROPHY

Occult Hereditary Macular Dystrophy

Miyake et al.[423] described three patients in two generations with progressive central visual loss, normal fundus and fluorescein angiographic findings, mild or moderate color vision defects, normal full-field ERG, and severely affected macular ERG.[423,424] It is an autosomal-dominant disorder with age of presentation between 20 and 45 years, though an 11- and a 16-year-old patient have been described.[425] Since the original description, the spectrum of visual loss and progression has widened. The presenting visual acuity is from 20/20 to 20/200. Color vision is variably affected. Some patients may show no progression of visual loss or change in their central scotoma, while the majority show worsening central vision.[426–428] Multifocal ERG and more recently OCT have been useful in confirming the findings.[426,427,429–431] All patients show foveal cone involvement; some show variable involvement of foveal rods. The characterisitic multifocal ERG finding is decreased amplitudes in the central ring or hexagons, with amplitudes

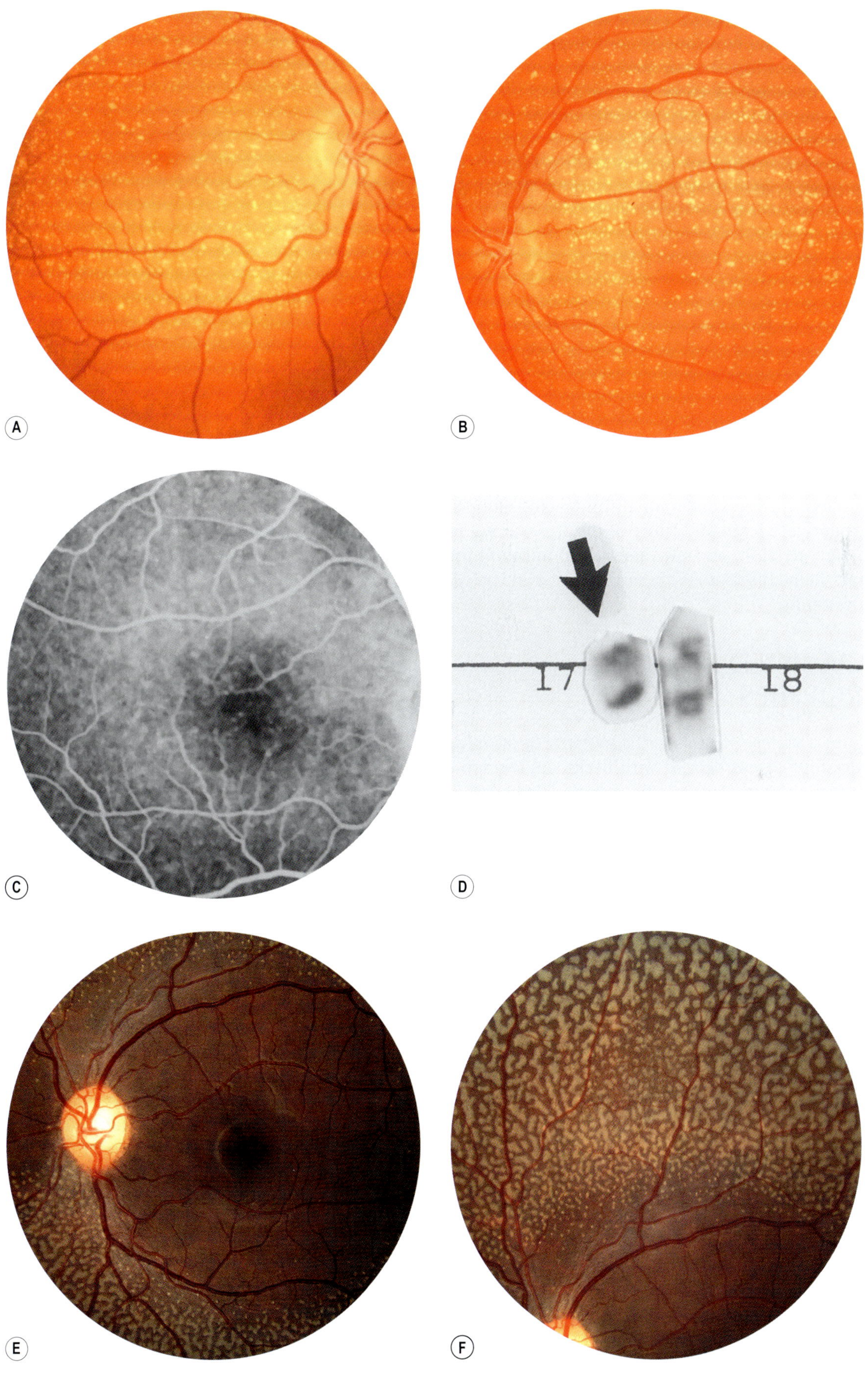
A
B
17
18
C
D
E
F

returning to the control values as one moves eccentrically towards the peripheral hexagons.[426,427,431] Implicit times, in addition, have been found to be delayed in some studies, suggesting involvement of more anterior retinal elements than cones alone. OCT shows variable thinning of the outer nuclear layer in most eyes, though some eyes with poor cone function have normal outer nuclear thickness, suggesting functional rather than structural loss.[429,432] Though the early reports were from Japan, case series have been described in Italy, the rest of Europe, and the USA.[430,431,433] No specific gene defect has so far been implicated.

Sporadic Occult Macular Dystrophy

A clinical and electrophysiologic appearance identical to the hereditary form of occult macular dystrophy has been seen in patients with no family history suggesting the disorder may have multiple etiologies or has variable penetrance.[433] Patients with autoimmune antibodies to enolase or other retinal elements can present with central scotoma, cone dysfunction, and normal fundus and fluorescein appearance.[434] A careful history of the age at onset of symptoms, progression, and any associated autoimmune disease may help differentiate these patients from occult macular dystrophy.

UNCLASSIFIED MACULAR DYSTROPHIES

Patients with a variety of nonspecific patterns of atrophic macular dystrophy unassociated with flecks, angiographic evidence of lipofuscin storage, or other electrophysiologic or systemic manifestations are occasionally encountered.[435] In such patients the author prefers to label their macular dystrophy as "unclassified" rather than Stargardt's disease.

FLECKED RETINA ASSOCIATED WITH CAFÉ-AU-LAIT SPOTS, MICROCEPHALY, EPILEPSY, SHORT STATURE, AND RING 17 CHROMOSOME

A ring chromosome is a type of deletion that results from breakage and loss in the terminal ends of each arm of a chromosome, followed by union of the broken ends (Figure 5.36D). Patients with ring 17 chromosome may have mental deficiency, seizures, short stature, microcephaly, and café-au-lait spots and demonstrate a striking pattern of yellow flecks at the level of the RPE throughout the posterior fundus (Figure 5.36A and B).[436–438] None of these patients has cutaneous neurofibromas, Lisch iris nodules, or a family history of neurofibromatosis. Their chromosome diagnosis is 46,XY,r(17) (p13q25). Although the *NF-1* gene has been mapped to chromosome 17, it is unlikely that these patients have *NF-1*. The fluorescein angiographic findings in one case suggest that the flecks are associated with irregular depigmentation or thinning of the RPE as well as focal obstruction of the background fluorescence by some of the flecks (Figure 5.36C).[437] Charles et al.[436] found some evidence of blockage of choroidal fluorescence by the flecks, which were believed to be at the level of the pigment epithelium. Although the flecks resemble drusen, their poor correlation with foci of discrete hyperfluorescence suggests they have a different morphology.

BENIGN FAMILIAL FLECK RETINA

Sabel Aish and Dajani[440] and later, McAllister et al.[439] and Audo et al.,[441] reported a beautiful pattern of somewhat polymorphous white flecks scattered widely throughout the fundi unassociated with any visual deficit or electrophysiologic deficits (Figure 5.36E–L). The flecks appear round posteriorly but become more polygonal towards the equator and periphery (Figure 5.36K and L). There is a suggestion the shape follows the choroidal venous lobular pattern especially beyond the arcades (Figure 5.36H and I). The flecks are hyperautofluorescent, suggesting accumulation of fluorphores within the RPE.[441] No progressive changes in the flecks, the RPE, or photoreceptor function have been described to date and the condition remains benign. The pattern of flecks appears similar to that reported by Miyake and Harada[442] in three patients in two families with congenital stationary night blindness. Two of their patients had absent scotopic ERG responses, subnormal EOG responses, and delayed dark adaptation.

5.36 Continued

G–L: This 42-year-old Hispanic woman was seen for intermittent blurred vision in both eyes. She was hospitalized for acute myeloid leukemia and had received prednisone, cytarabin, daunorubicin, vincristine, methotrexate, and radiation. Her vision was 20/20 in both eyes with normal color vision. Both fundi had symmetrical appearance of flecks that were smaller in the posterior pole resembling those of fundus flavimaculatus and larger towards the midperiphery and extended anterior to the equator. There was no known family history; she succumbed to her illness and the eyes could not be obtained for histology. The fundus appearance was typical of familial benign fleck retina and not secondary to leukemia or the effects of her medications.

(E and F, from McAllister et al.[439] G–L, courtesy of Dr. Michael Ober. K and L, Also, Yannuzzi, Lawrence J. The Retinal Atlas, Saunders 2010, 978-0-7020-3320-9, p.128.)

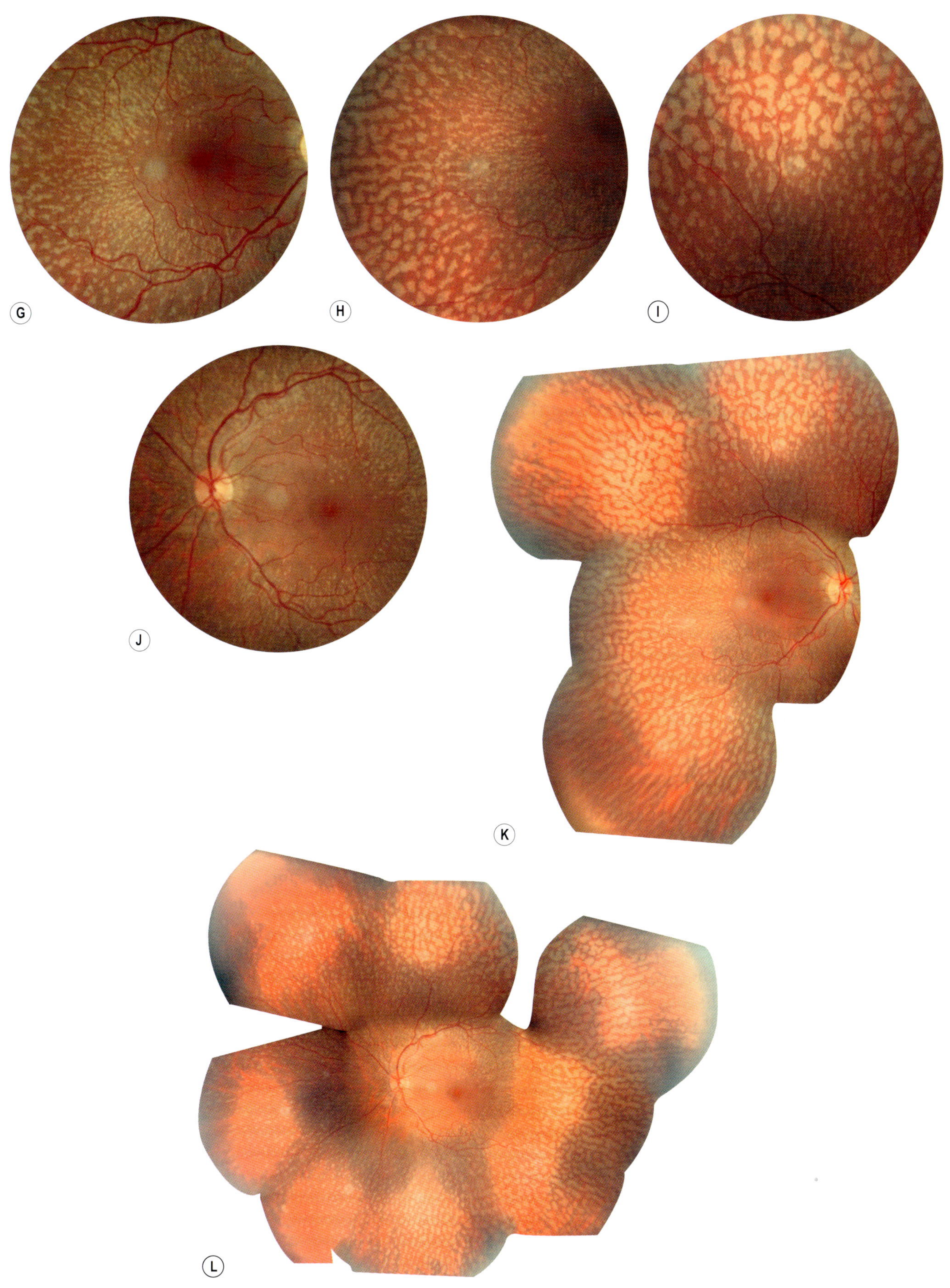
G
H
I
J
K
L

Oguchi's Disease

Oguchi's disease is one form of congenital stationary night blindness in patients with normal visual acuity, visual fields, and color vision.[453,458–462] Ophthalmoscopy in the light-adapted state reveals either a greenish-white or a golden-yellow color to the fundus (Figure 5.37A and B). It may be confined to the posterior pole or to the periphery, or it may involve both. The density of these RPE changes obscures the details of the choroidal vasculature. The retinal vessels stand out in bold relief, and the color of the arteries and veins may be similar. The fundus achieves a normal color in from 30 minutes to several hours after dark adaptation (Mizuo phenomenon) (Figure 5.37F).[459,461] Fluorescein angiography yields normal results (Figure 5.37E). Dark adaptation shows a delayed secondary adaptation (type I) or, rarely, absence of secondary adaptation (type II). The ERG shows subnormal rod responses that usually persist after prolonged adaptation. Oguchi's disease is similar to fundus albipunctate dystrophy in that there is reversibility of the psychophysical function following prolonged dark adaptation, but it is different from X-linked congenital stationary night blindness associated with myopia, in which this adaptation does not occur. Histopathologic studies have revealed abnormally large cones in an area that extends 20° temporal from the optic disc and an additional layer of granular pigment between the photoreceptors and the true RPE.[460] Yamanaka[462] failed to find evidence of a distinct layer between the RPE and the receptors. De Jong et al. in four patients with X-linked retinoschisis postulated that the Mizuo–Nakamura phenomenon may be caused by an excess of extracellular potassium in the retina as a result of a decreased potassium-scavenging capacity of retinal Müller cells.[463]

This disease is inherited as an autosomal-recessive trait and mutations have been identified mostly in the arrestin gene and occasionally in the rhodopsin kinase gene.[464,465]

A golden sheen confined to the macular area and the Mizuo phenomenon may occur in some patients with progressive, late-onset X-linked cone dystrophy (Figure 5.32J–L) and X-linked retinoschisis.[463]

Nonprogressive Albipunctate Dystrophy (Fundus Albipunctatus)

Patients with nonprogressive albipunctate dystrophy complain of night blindness. Visual acuity, visual fields, and color vision are normal. Fundoscopic examination reveals a large number of discrete, small, punctate, white spots at the level of the RPE (Figure 5.38).[466–469] These lesions have their maximum density in the postequatorial region, but the center of the macula is usually spared (Figure 5.38). The spots generally increase in number over the years[469] but some spots can disappear over time in older people.[470–472] The disc and retinal vessels are normal. The ERG is usually normal, but when it is abnormal, it usually improves toward normal levels after prolonged adaptation. The EOG may be subnormal but becomes normal after prolonged dark adaptation. The dark adaptation thresholds are markedly elevated but return to normal absolute threshold levels if the test is continued for several hours or longer.[450] Overnight patching of the eyes prior to electrophysiological tests is a useful way to achieve prolonged dark adaptation. Fluorescein angiography reveals a mottled pattern of fluorescence throughout the midperiphery of the fundus. In general there is no correlation between the areas of hyperfluorescence and the white spots. Angiography may demonstrate changes in the RPE in the macular area, and occasionally a few patients may lose central vision because of a cone dystrophy or atrophic maculopathy (Figure 5.38B and C).[472,473] The flecks are not hyperautofluorescent suggesting that these changes may not be at the pigment epithelial level but rather in the outer part of the photoreceptor layer. High-definition OCT confirms that the flecks correspond to dome-shaped opacifications at the photoreceptor outer-segment layer and continuous with the RPE cells.[474] The disease demonstrates an autosomal-recessive inheritance with the gene defect in 11-*cis* retinol dehydrogenase (RDH5), the enzyme found in the RPE cells responsible for the production of 11-*cis* retinal, which is transported to the rods and cones to act as the chromophore in rhodopsin and cone opsins.[475,476] A total of 19 different mutations have been found thus far in patients with fundus albipunctatus.

5.37 Oguchi's disease.

A–F: This 46-year-old black woman had normal visual acuity. Note the golden color of the fundus in the light-adapted state (A–D). Her electro-oculographic findings were normal. The electroretinogram showed depression of the b-wave and reduced rod function. Angiography (E) was normal. Fundus photographs (F) of the right eye following 1 hour of dark adaptation. Note the color of the retinal pigment epithelium is normal.

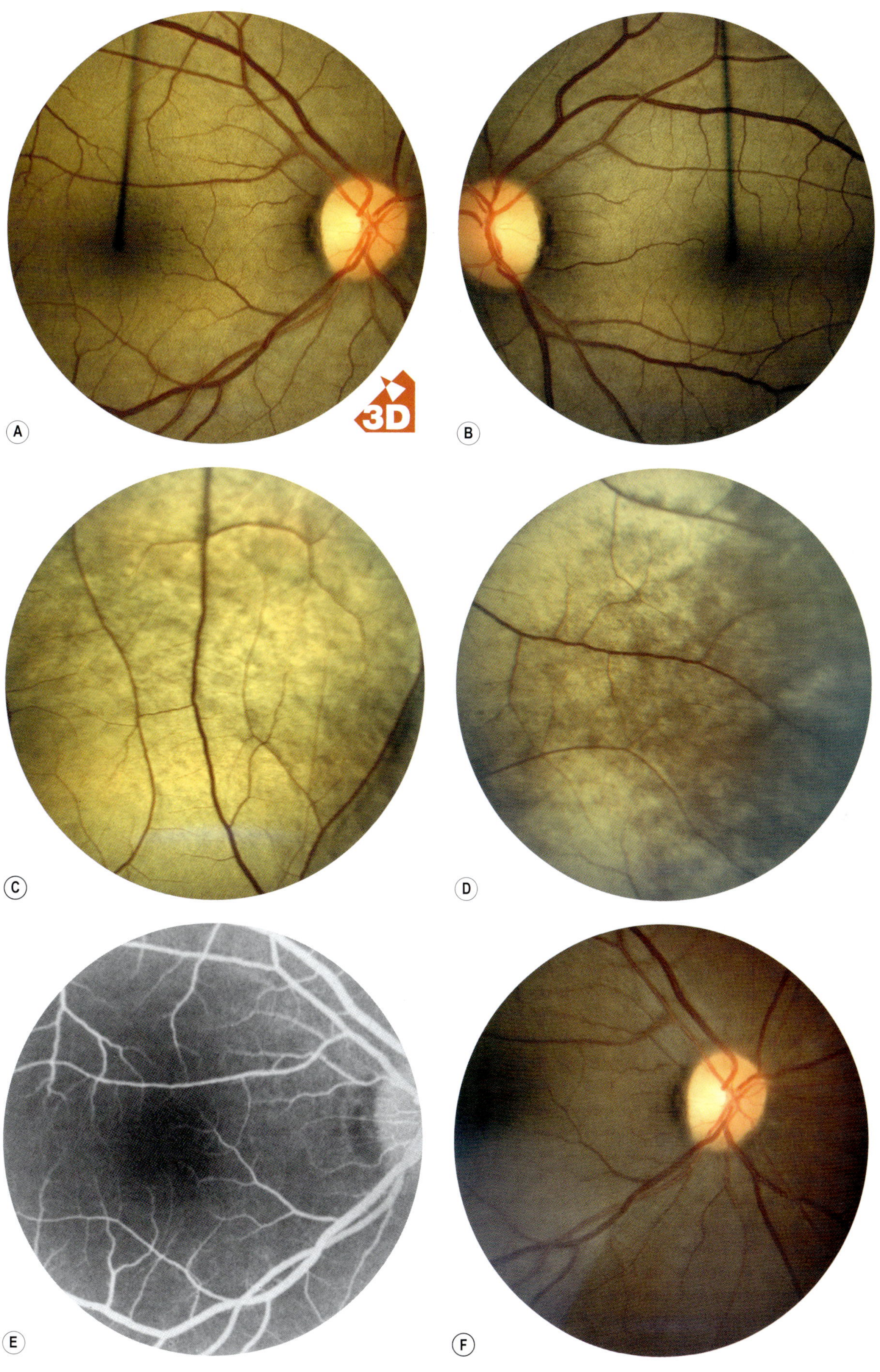
A
3D
B
C
D
E
F

This typically nonprogressive form of the disease is more common than its counterpart, RPA[477–479] (see Figure 5.38B–D) and Bothnia (Figure 5.44) and Newfoundland rod–cone dystrophy (Figure 5.45). Differentiation of these two diseases in younger patients may be difficult.[267] Occasionally both forms of the disease may occur in the same family.[477,480] RPA shows progressive nyctalopia, bone corpuscular pigment change, and vascular narrowing beginning by the third decade. Some patients, especially from Japan (38–43%), have a macular or cone dystrophy in addition to the flecks of fundus albipunctatus, all of whom have mutations in the *RDH5* gene of fundus albipunctatus.[472,481–484] Most, but not all, patients with macular involvement were older; whether this is a function of longer duration of disorder or a common Japanese ancestor in these various families remains to be determined.[472] This macular change associated with decreased cone ERG amplitudes resembles the macular change seen in patients with Bothnia dystrophy; however the gene defects in the two conditions are different (see section on Bothnia dystrophy, below). It is conceivable the metabolic derangements caused by the two mutations have some similarity or overlap, given that they are both involved in the metabolism of 11-*cis* retinol.

Fundus albipunctatus should be differentiated from acquired nyctalopia associated with vitamin A deficiency (Figure 9.12A–F)[468] as well as crystalline retinal dystrophy (see Figure 5.46), oxalosis (see Figure 5.67), cystinosis (see Figure 5.64), canthaxanthine retinopathy (see Figure 9.10), basal laminar drusen (see Figure 3.31 and 3.32), and Alport's syndrome (Figure 5.35). Pedigrees with larger "scale" or "silkworm-shaped" flecks with[442] or without[439,440] similar electrophysiologic findings may represent variants of albipunctate dystrophy (Figure 5.38D). Hayashi et al. found compound heterozygous mutations p.V177G and p.L310delinsEV in the *RDH5* gene in a 3-year-old proband with night blindness and fundus changes similar to benign fleck retina.[485] His asymptomatic parents and one of the grandparents each carried one of the mutations, explaining the autosomal-recessive inheritance.

5.38 Fundus albipunctatus.

A and **B**: This 14-year-old female had normal vision, normal electroretinogram, and an abnormal electro-oculogram. The central and peripheral visual fields were normal. Dark adaptation studies revealed absence of rod vision. Small punctate opacities extended almost to the ora serrata (A and B). Two brothers, 15 and 17 years of age, had similar findings. All the patients were night-blind. A 12-year-old sister had normal eyes. Angiography revealed a mottled pattern of hyperfluorescence indicative of depigmentation of the retinal pigment epithelium (RPE) everywhere except in the macular area. Some of the punctate spots obscured choroidal fluorescence, whereas others did not.

C: Fundus albipunctatus in a 33-year-old man with bilateral macular dystrophy. His visual acuity was 20/40 in both eyes. His electro-oculographic findings were normal. His electroretinogram showed moderately abnormal rod and normal cone function. After 50 minutes of dark adaptation the electroretinogram was normal. His Farnsworth-Munsell 100-hue test revealed a blue-yellow defect. Angiography showed evidence of RPE atrophy in the macula.

Hereditary stationary night blindness with polymorphous flecked retina.

D: Large white flecks confined to the peripheral fundi of an 11-year-old girl with familial stationary night blindness. Note similarity to Figure 5.36E–L.

E to **K**: The parents of this now 33 year old woman, (second of 3 siblings) noted a visual behavior in the dark different from her older sister when she was 3-5 years of age. Her vision was 20/20 in each eye at age 33, fundus showed symmetric appearance of several punctate white dots distributed up to the periphery and a bull's eye maculopathy (E to I). The visual function with stationary night blindness and fundus appearance was unchanged 6 years later (J and K).

(D, from Miyake and Harada.[442])

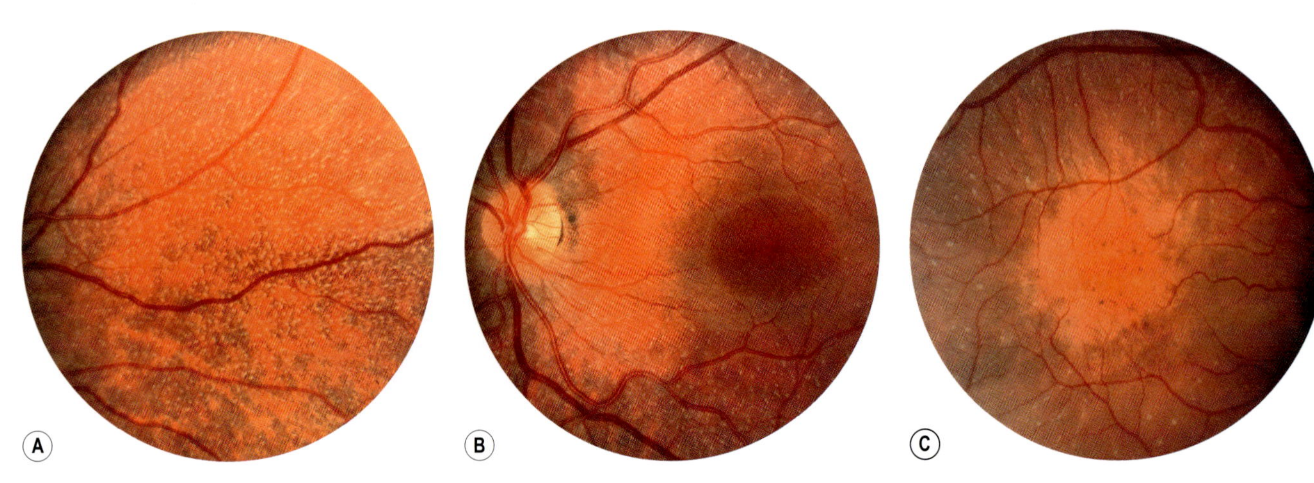

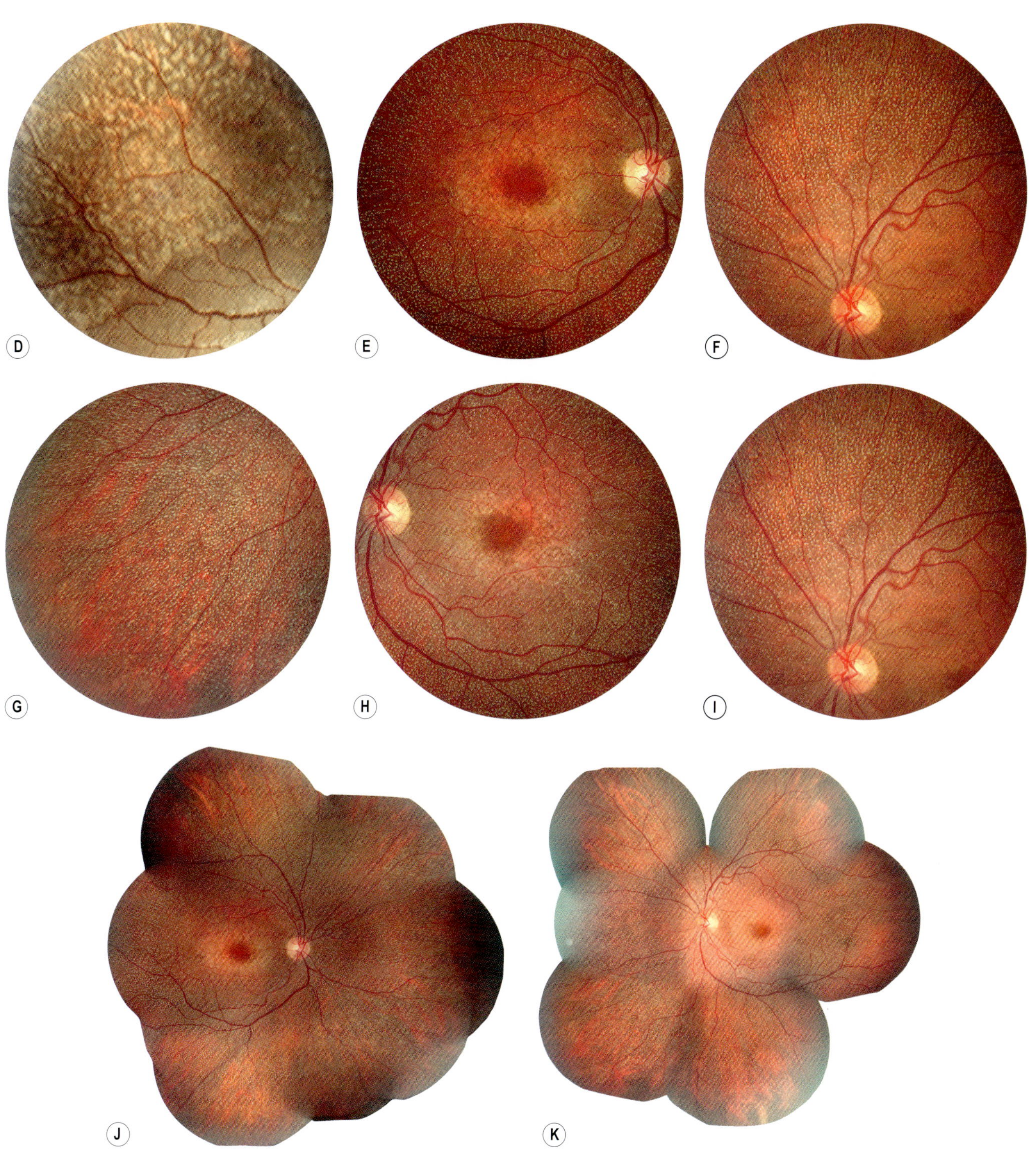
D
E
F
G
H
I
J
K

Kandori's Flecked Retina

Kandori's flecked retina[449,486] is an apparently rare, atypical type of congenital nonprogressive night blindness; it was described in four patients with sharply defined, dirty yellow, irregular relatively large flecks or patches of RPE atrophy distributed in the equatorial region between the macula and the equator. The macula was uninvolved. The retinal vessels and optic nerve were normal. Dark adaptation was delayed but returned to normal in 30–40 minutes. Visual acuity, visual fields, EOG, ERG, and visual evoked potentials were normal. Fluorescein angiography showed evidence of focal depigmentation of the RPE corresponding with the peripheral lesions. None of the four patients was from the same family. The flecks in these patients appear similar to, if not identical to, congenital grouped albinotic RPE spots. This is believed to be a congenital anomaly of the RPE that is usually unassociated with night blindness (see Figure 12.05).

RETINITIS PIGMENTOSA (ROD–CONE DYSTROPHIES)

Retinitis pigmentosa, tapetoretinal dystrophy, and primary pigmentary retinal dystrophy are names used interchangeably to refer to a large spectrum of disorders of variable age of onset, rate of progression, severity, and mode of inheritance. These can be subdivided into two broad categories: typical and atypical.

Typical Retinitis Pigmentosa

"Typical retinitis pigmentosa" is used to refer to those patients with a hereditary dystrophy characterized by the onset of night blindness in childhood or young adulthood, progressive contraction of the peripheral visual field beginning as a mid zonal ring scotoma with preservation of central vision, and frequently profound visual loss or blindness in middle or later life (Figures 5.39–5.41).[487–533] Early in the course of the disease the most common presenting complaints are headache (53%) and photopsias (35%).[534] Photopsias are spontaneous impulses exhibited by dying or disintegrating photoreceptors. Patients describe them as tiny blinking or shimmering lights or gold sparkles. A total of 10–15% of patients may not be aware of symptoms until central vision is affected. They experience variability in their visual function and may note worsening of vision during stress. There is a high incidence of relative myopia.[492] The earliest fundoscopic changes consist of gray-green discoloration of the RPE giving a tapetal-like reflex, depigmentation of the RPE, mild narrowing of the peripheral retinal blood vessels, and migration of pigment into the overlying retina in a bone spicule pattern in a mid peripheral annular zone of both eyes. This annular zone progressively enlarges in an anterior and posterior direction and is associated with further attenuation of the retinal blood vessels, waxy pallor of the optic disc, and the development of a glistening reflex and crinkling of the inner retinal surface secondary to an epiretinal membrane. The pallor of the optic disc is due to astroglial proliferation on the surface of the optic disc. Retinal arterial and venular narrowing is a secondary phenomenon from retinal autoregulation. Loss of photoreceptors, the highest metabolically active cells in the retina, results in diffusion of nutrients from the choroidal capillary circulation into the inner retina reducing the metabolic demand on the inner retina and consecutively narrowing the retinal arteries and veins. Posterior polar cataract and fine vitreous opacities or cells often develop.[492] This adds to visual loss. Classically, the macula has been described as being relatively normal and visual acuity is excellent until the later stages of the disease. Recent investigation has revealed that 50% or more of patients at the time of initial presentation will have

5.39 Retinitis pigmentosa.

A–D: Cystoid macular edema in an 8-year-old boy with nyctalopia. Note the narrowing of the retinal arterioles (A). Visual acuity was 20/30. His electroretinogram was extinguished. The periphery of the fundus (B) showed mild bone corpuscular pigmentary changes. Early angiography (C) revealed evidence of generalized depigmentation of the retinal pigment epithelium. Note the nonfluorescent cross in the foveolar area. This is probably caused by central compression of the retinal xanthophyllic pigment by the large central retinal cysts. One-hour angiogram (D) revealed minimal evidence of fluorescein staining in the macula.

E and **F**: Widespread retinal edema and cystoid macular edema in a 42-year-old woman with night blindness, moderate number of vitreous cells, and minimal intraretinal pigment migration. Her electroretinogram was severely abnormal but not extinguished. Her sister had similar findings.

G–I: This 37-year-old man with an 8-year history of nyctalopia developed evidence of retinal telangiectasis inferiorly in the right eye in 1984 (H and I). Note narrowing of the retinal vessels (G). Because of progressive exudation he was treated with transscleral cryopexy in 1990.

J–L: Development of peripheral retinal telangiectasis and subretinal exudation occurred in the right eye of this patient during observation for typical retinitis pigmentosa, 2 + vitreous cells, and cystoid macular edema. The retinal telangiectasis was not present at the time of initial examination at age 14 but developed at age 18 years (K). There was extensive leakage of fluorescein from retinal vessels in macular and paramacular retina. The exudation seen in K cleared spontaneously over a period of 3 years (L). In spite of chronic cystoid macular edema she maintained 20/40 visual acuity during the 18 years of observation. She experienced gradual loss of peripheral vision. Her electroretinogram was extinguished at the time of initial examination.

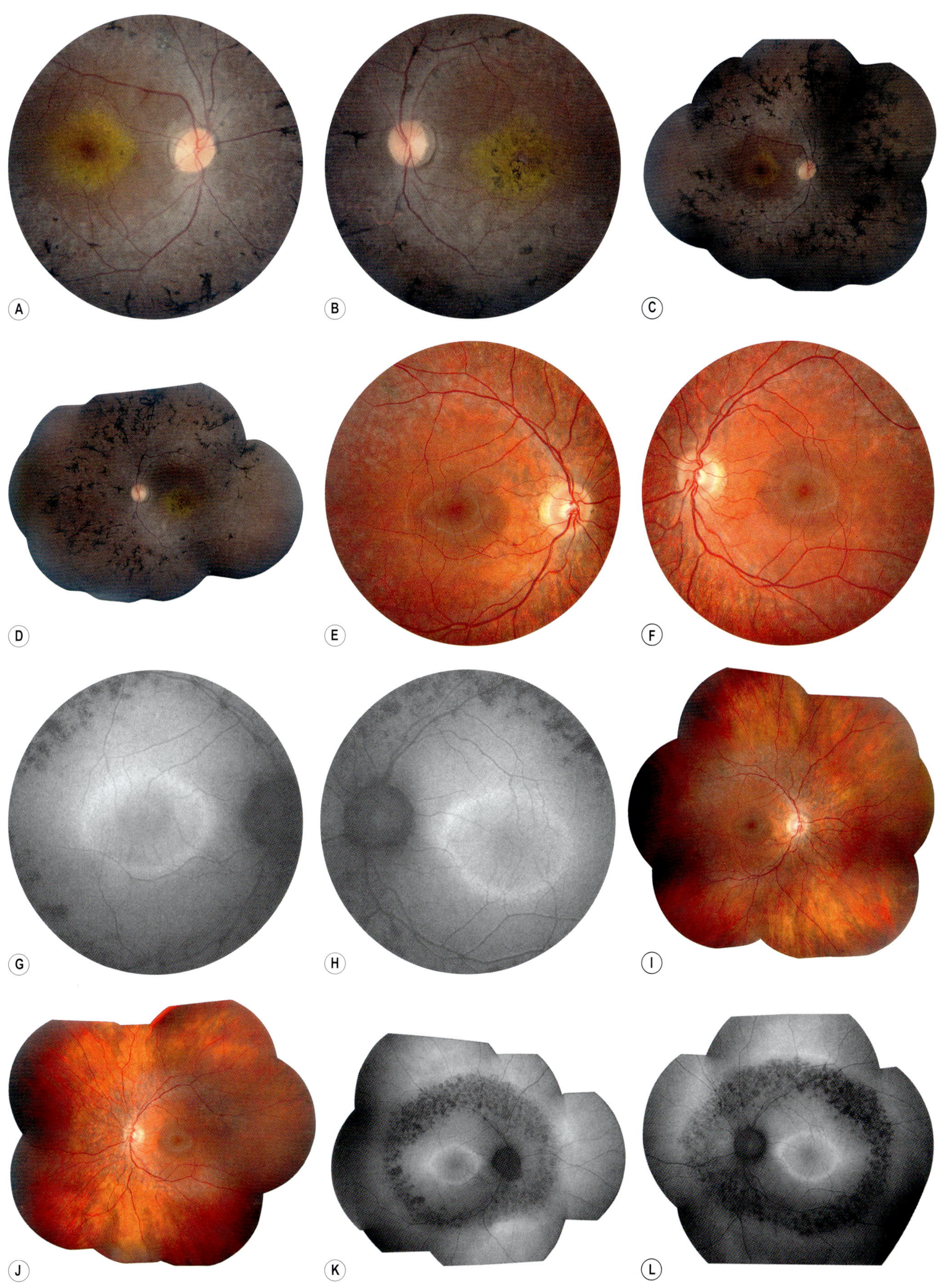
A
B
C
D
E
F
G
H
I
J
K
L

biomicroscopic and angiographic evidence of macular changes, including cystoid macular edema (Figure 5.42A–D),[491,498,499,514,517,519,520,528,535–538] epiretinal membrane,[509,514,517,539] and atrophic changes in the RPE. Some degree of epiretinal membrane change in the macula is evident in most patients with retinitis pigmentosa.[509] Cystoid macular edema is visible biomicroscopically in fewer than 10% of patients, in the author's experience. The high incidence of 70% in 58 patients studied retrospectively by Fetkenhour and associates[520] probably reflects the fact that patients with central visual loss are more likely to be referred for photographic studies. Those with cystoid macular edema often have more cells than usual in the vitreous. Although the incidence of cystoid macular edema probably is higher in younger patients showing minimal pigment migration into the retina, it may occur in all age groups and in patients with typical pigmentary changes. In most patients with subtle macular edema that is evident only angiographically in the paracentral area, visual acuity is good. By the time cysts become visible biomicroscopically, the patients are complaining of loss of central vision and the acuity is usually 20/40 or less. Some patients with chronic macular edema may retain good visual acuity for many years (Figure 5.42A–D). Most patients with macular edema have 1+ or 2+ vitreous cells. Loss of Snellen acuity in some patients is associated with atrophic RPE changes in the macula. This appears to occur more often in black patients than white patients.[538]

5.40 Retinitis pigmentosa with Coats'-type response.

A and **B**: This 40-year-old woman from Iraq complained of difficulty seeing at night for more than 5 years. Her visual acuity was 20/20 in each eye. Visual fields were narrowed to central 20° in each eye. Both optic nerves were pale, the vessels were diffusely narrowed, the retinal pigment epithelium was atrophic everywhere except the macula and bone spicule pigment migration spared the macula, typical of retinitis pigmentosa (A and B).

C and **D**: This 37-year-old man with an 8-year history of nyctalopia developed evidence of retinal telangiectasis inferiorly in the right eye in 1984 (C and D). Note narrowing of the retinal vessels. Because of progressive exudation he was treated with transscleral cryopexy in 1990.

E and **F**: Development of peripheral retinal telangiectasis and subretinal exudation occurred in the right eye of this patient during observation for typical retinitis pigmentosa, 2 + vitreous cells, and cystoid macular edema. The retinal telangiectasis was not present at the time of initial examination at age 14 but developed at age 18 years (E). There was extensive leakage of fluorescein from retinal vessels in macular and paramacular retina. The exudation seen in E cleared spontaneously over a period of 3 years (F). In spite of chronic cystoid macular edema she maintained 20/40 visual acuity during the 18 years of observation. She experienced gradual loss of peripheral vision. Her electroretinogram was extinguished at the time of initial examination.

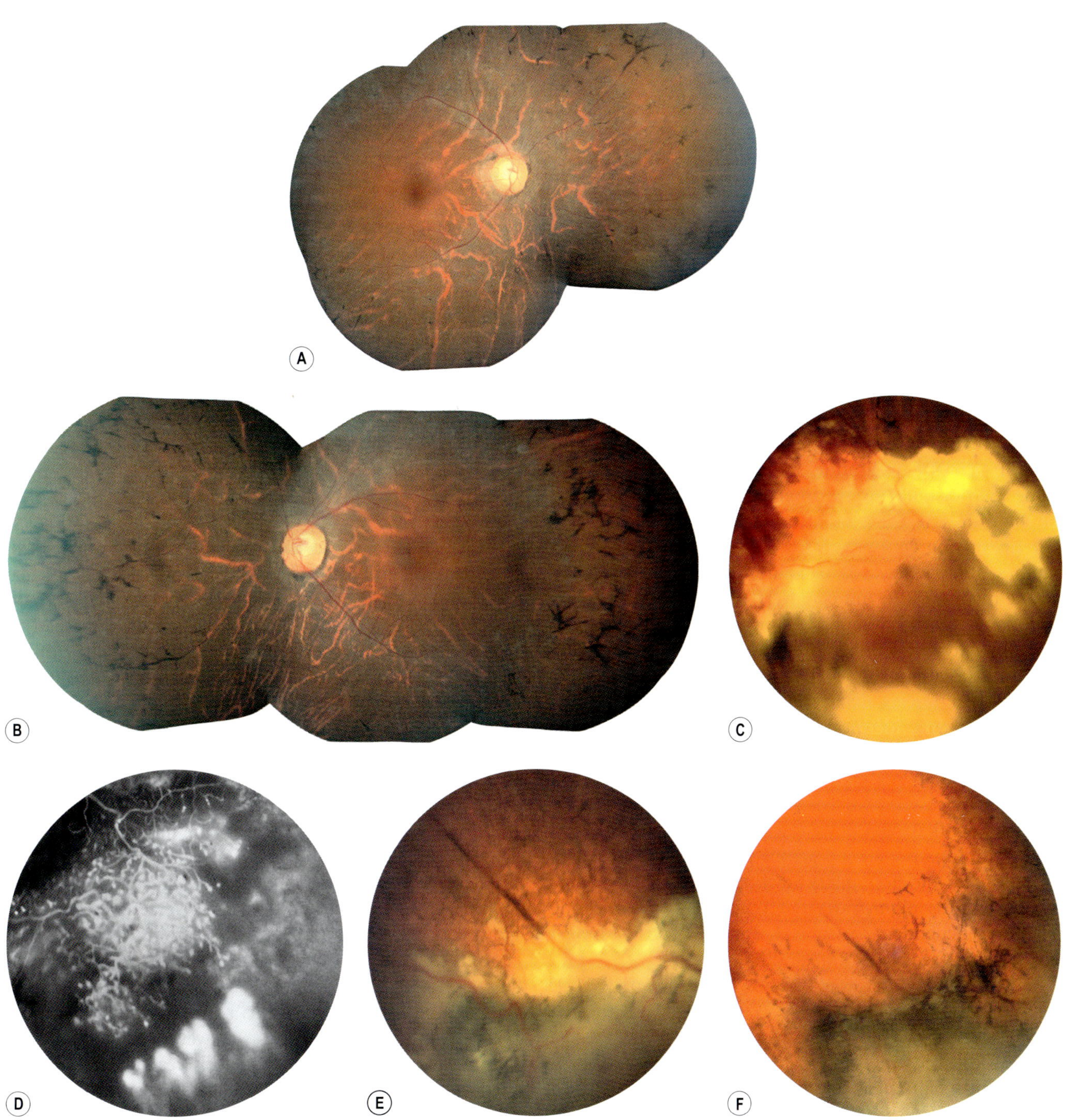
A
B
C
D
E
F

Several subtypes of retinitis pigmentosa due to various gene defects can show a variable appearance of the RPE change. A type of retinitis pigmentosa with RPE preservation is seen in patients with Crumbs homolog 1 (*CRB1*) or *CRUMB* gene defect (See Figure 5.43G and H). Some patients show very little migration of pigment epithelial cells, called retinitis pigmentosa sine pigmenti. Those patients with autosomal-recessive retinitis pigmentosa have earlier onset of symptoms and findings. Women, who are X-linked carriers, can show a variable amount of involvement. Sometimes involvement is sectoral and occasionally it is extensive. Irregular lyonization of cells is responsible for the varying degrees of symptoms in female carriers of X-linked recessive retinitis pigmentosa. Pericentral retinitis pigmentosa patients have most of the findings related to the mid peripheral fundus around the arcades. Sectoral retinitis pigmentosa was first described in 1937. These patients generally have fine shiny crystals in addition to the sectoral consideration of the photoreceptor loss. Several of the patients can progress from cone to cone–rod degeneration.

Associated findings in typical retinitis pigmentosa include congenital deafness (Usher's syndrome) that may or may not be associated with other evidence of central nervous system abnormalities,[529,554–556] vitiligo,[508,526,533,554,557] and calcific nodular drusen within the optic nerve head.[494,497,525,558]

Calcified bodies on the optic nerve head in patients with retinitis pigmentosa have been attributed to hyaline bodies (drusen) by some[495,558] and to astrocytic hamartomas by others.[494,497,525] The evidence in favor of the former is more convincing.

Retinitis pigmentosa may be inherited in any one of the three classic modes. There is a general tendency for earlier and more severe involvement in those showing X-linked recessive and autosomal-recessive modes of inheritance.[316,347,349,351,456,504,516,559] There are notable exceptions to the general rule that the disease in families with dominant inheritance is milder.[560] Patients with X-linked disease are usually almost blind by the age of 30–40 years, whereas many affected patients with autosomal-recessive disease or no family history of disease retain central vision until they are 45–60 years old.[516,531] An alteration in sperm axoneme is present in patients with X-linked retinitis pigmentosa.[561,562] Almost 100% of the female carriers of X-linked retinitis pigmentosa can be identified on the basis of either or both fundus and ERG changes.[563] The fundus changes include tapeto-like reflex in the macula, isolated regions of peripheral retinal degeneration, and occasionally widespread retinal degeneration.[563]

Some authors have subdivided patients with dominantly inherited retinitis pigmentosa into two primary subgroups: one having diffuse pigmentation, concentric visual field loss, and no recordable ERG, the other with regionalized pigmentation, sectoral field loss, and some recordable ERG.[515,521,560,564–567] The cumulative probability of maintaining a visual acuity of 20/40 or better over each decade of life decreased rapidly in the former type and remained above 90% through the fifth decade in the latter type. Patients with dominant disease can retain central vision beyond the age of 60 years.

A number of distinct mutations in the rhodopsin gene have been identified in different families with autosomal-dominant retinitis pigmentosa.[523,524,564,567–578] There is evidence that some cases of dominant retinitis pigmentosa are the result of mutations in the retinal degeneration slow (*RDS*) gene on chromosome 6.[579] Rosenfeld et al. reported a rhodopsin gene defect in one family with autosomal-recessive retinitis pigmentosa.[580] Distinct mutations have not been identified in patients with X-linked retinitis pigmentosa.[554,581] Jacobson et al. found discernible differences in the pattern of retinal dysfunction in patients with different rhodopsin mutations.[567]

A natural course study of retinitis pigmentosa unassociated with systemic disease showed significant decline of full-field ERG amplitudes over a 3-year period in 77% of patients with detectable levels at baseline.[531] Patients lost an average of 16–18.5% of remaining ERG amplitudes per year and 4.6% of remaining visual field per year.

Most patients with retinitis pigmentosa have myopia except for those with early-onset autosomal-dominant retinitis pigmentosa with nanophthalmos,[582] Leber's congenital amaurosis,[583] and preserved para-arterial RPE (Figure 5.43G and H).[584]

Autoimmune responses have been detected in many degenerative ocular diseases, including retinitis pigmentosa, but their role in the pathogenesis of retinitis pigmentosa is unknown.[585–588]

5.41 Retinitis pigmentosa and central serous chorioretinopathy.

A–C: Recurrent episodes of idiopathic central serous retinopathy associated with multiple serous detachments of the retinal pigment epithelium (RPE: arrows, A and C) in both eyes occurred in this 30-year-old woman with retinitis pigmentosa sine pigmenti and an extinguished electroretinogram.

Late onset retinitis pigmentosa.

D–F: Long-standing "late-onset" retinitis pigmentosa occurred in this 66-year-old woman who was asymptomatic until 3 months prior to these pictures. Her family history was negative. Her visual acuity was 20/25 right eye and 20/80 left eye. She had marked concentric constriction of the visual fields bilaterally. Angiography revealed relative preservation of the RPE centrally and mild intraretinal staining in the central macular area of both eyes (E and F).

G–J: Histopathology of retinitis pigmentosa. Macular area (G) showing extensive atrophy of the receptor cell layer that is thinned to one cell thickness (arrows), and mild degeneration of the RPE and slight attenuation of the choriocapillaris. Mid peripheral fundus (H and I) showing extensive gliosis and atrophy of the retina, intraretinal migration of RPE around sclerosed retinal blood vessels, atrophy of the RPE and choriocapillaris (lower arrow), and cellular epiretinal membrane (upper arrow, I). High-power view showing vitreous cell filled with melanin pigment (J).

(A–C: from Lewis[502].)

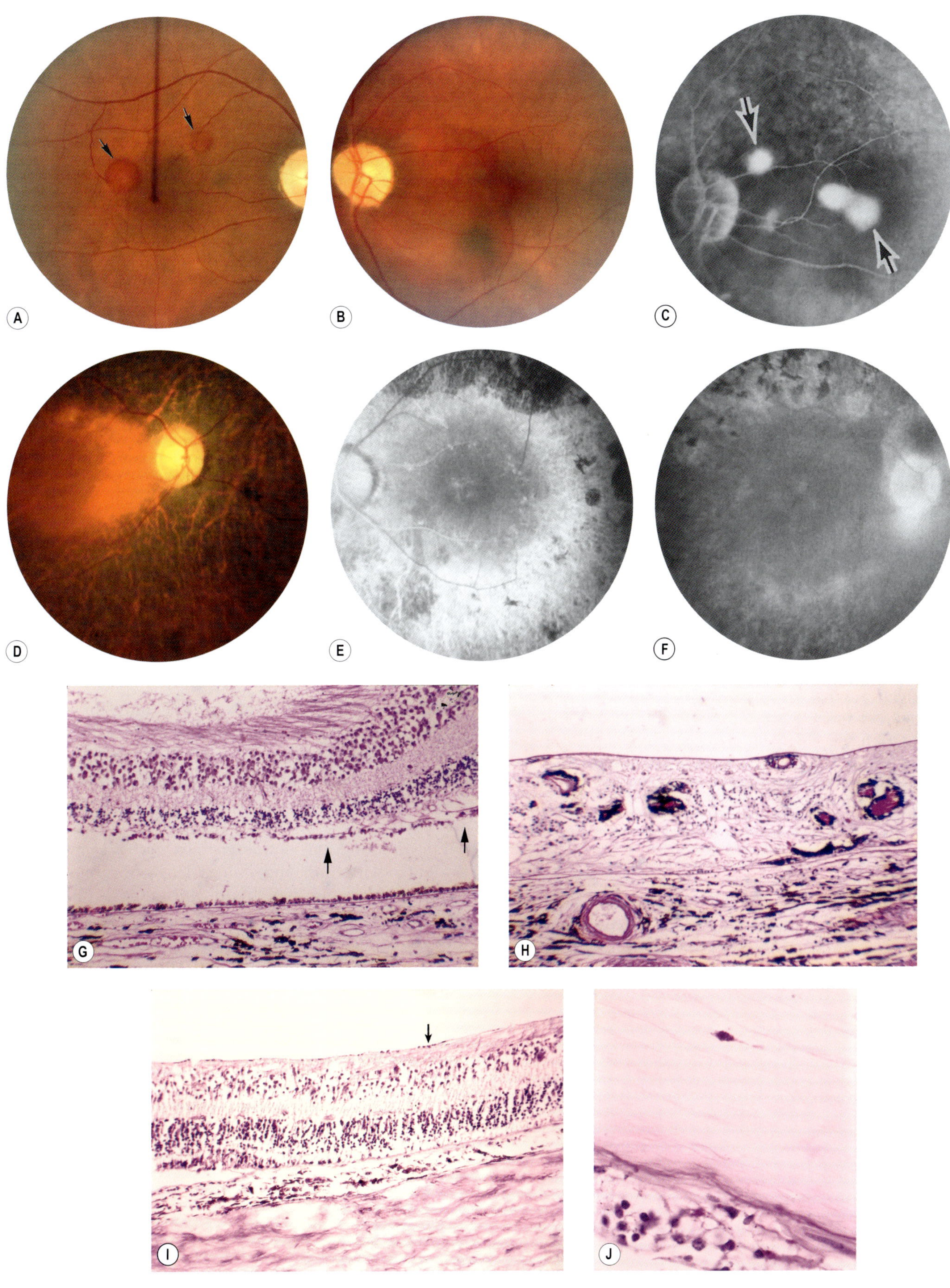
A
B
C
D
E
F
G
H
I
J

There is no proven effective treatment to slow the loss of visual function in patients with retinitis pigmentosa. A randomized trial of vitamin A (15 000 IU/day) and vitamin E (400 IU/day) supplementation for retinitis pigmentosa showed a beneficial effect of vitamin A in regard to inhibiting decline of ERG amplitudes, but it failed to demonstrate any benefit in slowing the course of loss of visual field.[589–592] The results of the trial suggest an adverse effect of vitamin E on the course of retinitis pigmentosa. Use of oral acetazolamide and methazolamide and topical dorzolamide for the treatment of chronic cystoid macular edema in patients with retinitis pigmentosa has been beneficial in some cases.[518,593] In some cases acuity improves without demonstrable improvement in the degree of angiographic fluorescein leakage. The mechanism seems to be via stimulation of the pump function of the RPE. Results of a scatter pattern of grid laser treatment for cystoid macular edema in a small series of patients with retinitis pigmentosa are unimpressive, and risks of this treatment in patients with only a limited peripheral field are high.[594,595] There is some hope for the therapeutic value of transplantation of retinal tissues and gene therapy for retinitis pigmentosa and macular degenerative disorders. Transscleral transplantation of RPE into the subretinal space of animals has retarded photoreceptor degeneration in the vicinity of the transplant. Transfer of corrective genes into the subretinal space by the use of viral vectors is another possible strategy for therapy.[596] Tissue growth factors appear to inhibit or slow the rate of hereditary retinal degeneration in animals.[522] Although studies of patients with diabetes and retinitis pigmentosa have shown a protective effect of the latter in regard to the development of diabetic proliferative retinopathy, optic disc and retinal neovascularization does occasionally occur.[597–599] When retinal neovascularization occurs in diabetics with retinitis pigmentosa, it usually develops in the periphery at the junction of perfused and nonperfused retina. There is a negative association of rhegmatogenous retinal detachment in patients with retinitis pigmentosa.[600] Recent studies with implantable chips that function as retinal receptors are in progress. Rapid and extensive expanse in genotyping and genetherapy processes is likely to result in novel therapeutic approaches for these patients in the near future.

Electroretinography, dark-adaptation studies, and automated light- and dark-adapted perimetry are useful in the diagnosis, classification, and follow-up of patients with retinitis pigmentosa.[601]

Usher Syndrome

Usher syndrome is an autosomal-recessive disorder of deafness, often congenital, combined with features typical of retinitis pigmentosa (Figure 5.42G to J). Cystic or atrophic macular changes are seen earlier in patients with Usher's than typical retinitis pigmentosa, and are more prevalent in type I (62%) than type II (32%), most likely due to the more severe and earlier involvement in the former.[602] Though von Graefe first described the condition in 1858, Charles Usher, a British ophthalmologist, noticed the hereditary nature of the disorder.

Usher syndrome can be divided into three major groups. The two most frequent forms are types I and II. In type I there is profound congenital sensorineural deafness resulting in prelingual deafness and speech impairment. Vestibular symptoms and childhood-onset retinopathy accompany the deafness. Type II is characterized by partial or profound, but nonprogressive, deafness, absence of vestibular symptoms and milder, later-onset retinopathy. The least common is type III, in which there is progressive deafness starting late in the second to fourth decade of life, onset of retinopathy in adult life, and hypermetropic astigmatism.[603] Type III resembles type II except for progressive worsening of hearing.

Approximately 3–6% of persons have profound prelingual deafness of type I Usher syndrome. Type II Usher is more common and accounts for about two-thirds of patients. Type III constitutes less than 20%. The ERG is nondetectable in all groups early on in life. Occasionally, a type II Usher can have cerebellar atrophy resulting in ataxia. Type III has been associated with psychotic symptoms and magnetic resonance imaging (MRI) changes associated with this.[604,605] The disorder is genetically and clinically heterogeneous and at least nine genetic loci have been identified. Usher type I has six different gene loci, mapping to 14q32, 11q13, 11p15, 10q, 21q21 and chromosome 10. Usher type II has been mapped to 1q41, 3p, and 5q, and others have been postulated.[606]

5.42 Retinitis pigmentosa: response of cystoid macular edema (CME) to acetazolamide.

A–F: This 35-year-old African American male had a best-corrected visual acuity of 20/80 and 20/70. In addition to the peripheral pigmentary retinopathy, a large central cyst surrounded by a few small cysts were present in both maculas (A and B). Optical coherence tomography documented the cystoid macular edema in each eye (C and D). He was treated with oral acetazolamide 250 mg three times a day, which he tolerated well. Eight weeks later his vision had improved to 20/40 and 20/30 respectively; the cysts had decreased significantly in both eyes (E and F). Acetazolamide was continued at the same dose for 2 more months and slowly tapered off over the next 3 months. The CME recurred once he came off the acetazolamide and he was kept on maintenance dose of it from then onwards. The cyst in the right eye persisted, but the left eye remained resolved.

Usher's syndrome.

G–J: A 68-year-old older brother has been followed for Usher's syndrome for more than 20 years. His visual acuity has remained at hand motions for the past 20 years. Both eyes had extensive retinal atrophy, including the macula with bone corpuscles retinal pigment epithelium (RPE) migration (G and H). His 64-year-old younger brother had 20/400 vision in each eye. The optic nerves were pale bilaterally; vessels were narrowed with extensive pigment migration in each eye (I and J). The macula had some preservation of RPE that accounted for the 20/400 vision.

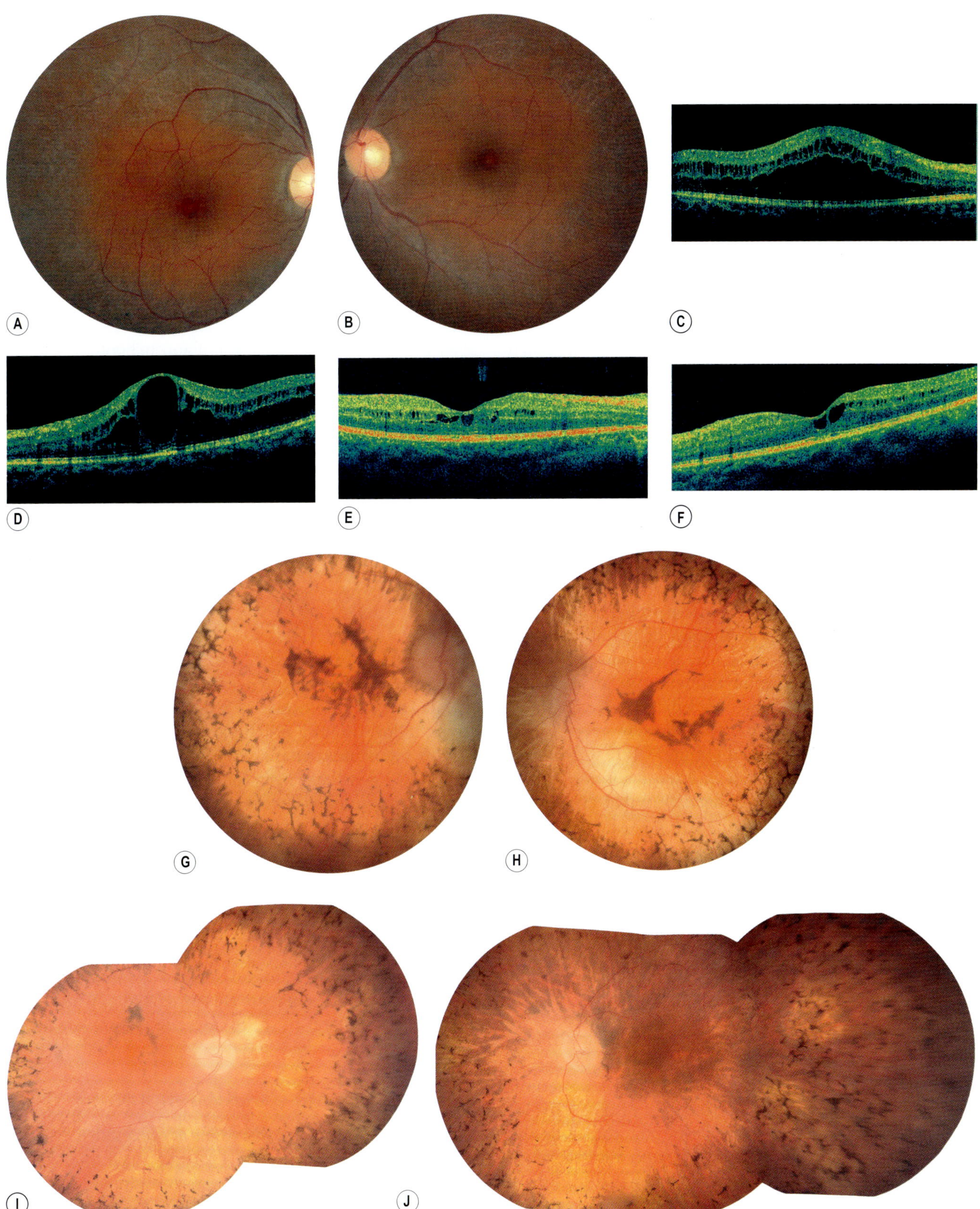
A
B
C
D
E
F
G
H
I
J

Cochlear implants can be placed in profoundly deaf children and this has helped their speech. Usher syndrome can be mistaken for rubella retinopathy due to the deafness and pigmentary changes. However, an ERG will be useful in confirming the diagnosis of Usher's. Other syndromes that can be associated with deafness and pigmentary retinopathy include infantile Refsum disease, adult Refsum disease, Cocayne syndrome, Bardet–Biedl syndrome, Alstrom disease, Flynn–Aird syndrome, Friedreich's ataxia, and Kearns–Sayre syndrome.

Typical Pigmentary Retinal Dystrophy with Coats' Syndrome

Some patients with typical sporadic or familial retinitis pigmentosa, usually during adulthood, may develop yellowish subretinal exudation derived primarily from the peripheral retinal vessels and present with a Coats' syndrome picture (Figure 5.40C–F and G–L).[487,488,493,500,503,507,511,513,607–609] The exudative detachment may be confined to the peripheral fundus, or it may be massive and extend into the posterior pole. Total retinal detachment may occasionally occur.[609] Focal areas of irregular telangiectatic dilation of the retinal blood vessels, and occasionally angiomatous proliferation of retinal capillaries, occur usually in the peripheral fundus on a background of the typical findings of retinitis pigmentosa. Fluorescein angiography may show widespread evidence of capillary leakage in the retina in areas outside as well as within the area of exudative retinal detachment. Cystoid macular edema is usually present. The exudation may be self-limited (Figure 5.40E and F), or it may be progressive and result in extensive loss of vision. These patients require photocoagulation and cryotherapy to control the exudation (Figure 5.40J–L). This exudative response may also be the cause of massive segmental retinal gliosis in these patients.[610] Histopathologic findings in one case revealed evidence of communication of choroidal blood vessels with the overlying exudative retinal mass.[513] It is uncertain whether this communication is of primary importance in causing retinal exudation or occurs only secondarily after a long-standing exudative retinal detachment.

Angiographic evidence of retinal vascular leakage, either confined to the macular area or involving the entire fundus, has been frequently observed in retinitis pigmentosa,[490,491,511] as well as a variety of other atypical tapetoretinal dystrophies, cone dystrophy, rod–cone dystrophy, Stargardt's macular dystrophy, and familial exudative vitreoretinopathy. It is probable that massive yellowish exudative detachment in patients with retinitis pigmentosa represents an unusually severe alteration in the retinal vascular permeability that can probably occur in any of the inheritance patterns of retinitis pigmentosa. The frequency of bilaterality, adult onset, and absence of sex predilection suggest strongly that this exudative response in patients with retinitis pigmentosa is unrelated to congenital retinal telangiectasia, the most frequent cause of Coats' syndrome. Dr. Gass has observed it developing in one patient during follow-up for a unilateral localized area of pseudoretinitis pigmentosa change caused by trauma. Mutations in the *CRB1* gene have been found in 65% of patients with Coats'-type retinitis pigmentosa. The condition has been seen in patients as young as 4 years and in patients with Usher syndrome type II.[611,612]

5.43 Retinitis pigmentosa with unusual peripheral retinal changes.

A–C: Retinitis punctata albescens in a 32-year-old man with nyctalopia, progressive loss of peripheral vision, and multiple, discrete, round, white flecks at the level of the retinal pigment epithelium (RPE) in the pericentral area (A). These flecks were more numerous and smaller in the mid peripheral area where there were more advanced atrophic changes in the RPE and retina. Note the narrowing of the retinal vessels (B). Angiography revealed widespread depigmentation of the RPE that was more marked peripherally (C).

D–F: Peculiar perivascular and geographic distribution of subretinal white lesions (F–H) in a woman with nyctalopia and evidence of a tapetoretinal degeneration.

G and **H**: Periarterial sparing of the pigment epithelium and an Oguchi-like metallic reflex in the periphery of a healthy 8-year-old boy with nyctalopia, onset of progressive visual loss at age 5 years, and an extinguished electroretinogram. His visual acuity was 20/200 bilaterally. There was no nystagmus. He had three normal siblings. There was no history of consanguinity.

I–L: Three-dimensional lacelike network of white retinal capillaries (J–L) in a 34-year-old woman with a lifelong history of nyctalopia, severe loss of peripheral visual field, and an extinguished electroretinogram. She had a sister with the same ocular disorder. Her visual acuity was 20/60 in the right eye and 20/50 left eye. Her electroretinogram was extinguished bilaterally.

ATYPICAL FORMS OF RETINITIS PIGMENTOSA

"Atypical pigmentary retinal dystrophy" is a term applied to retinal dystrophies that are closely related to typical retinitis pigmentosa and in some cases are incomplete forms of the disease.

Leigh Syndrome (NARP Syndrome)

Leigh syndrome is a hereditary neurodegenerative disorder of infancy or childhood, and is characterized by developmental delay, psychomotor regression, signs of brainstem dysfunction, lactic acidosis, and symmetrical necrotizing lesions in the basal ganglia on the brainstem. The clinical course is variable with most cases of a poor outcome with progressive neurological deterioration leading to death within months or years. The definitive diagnosis depends on MRI changes, described as hyperintense lesions of the putamen and the brainstem.

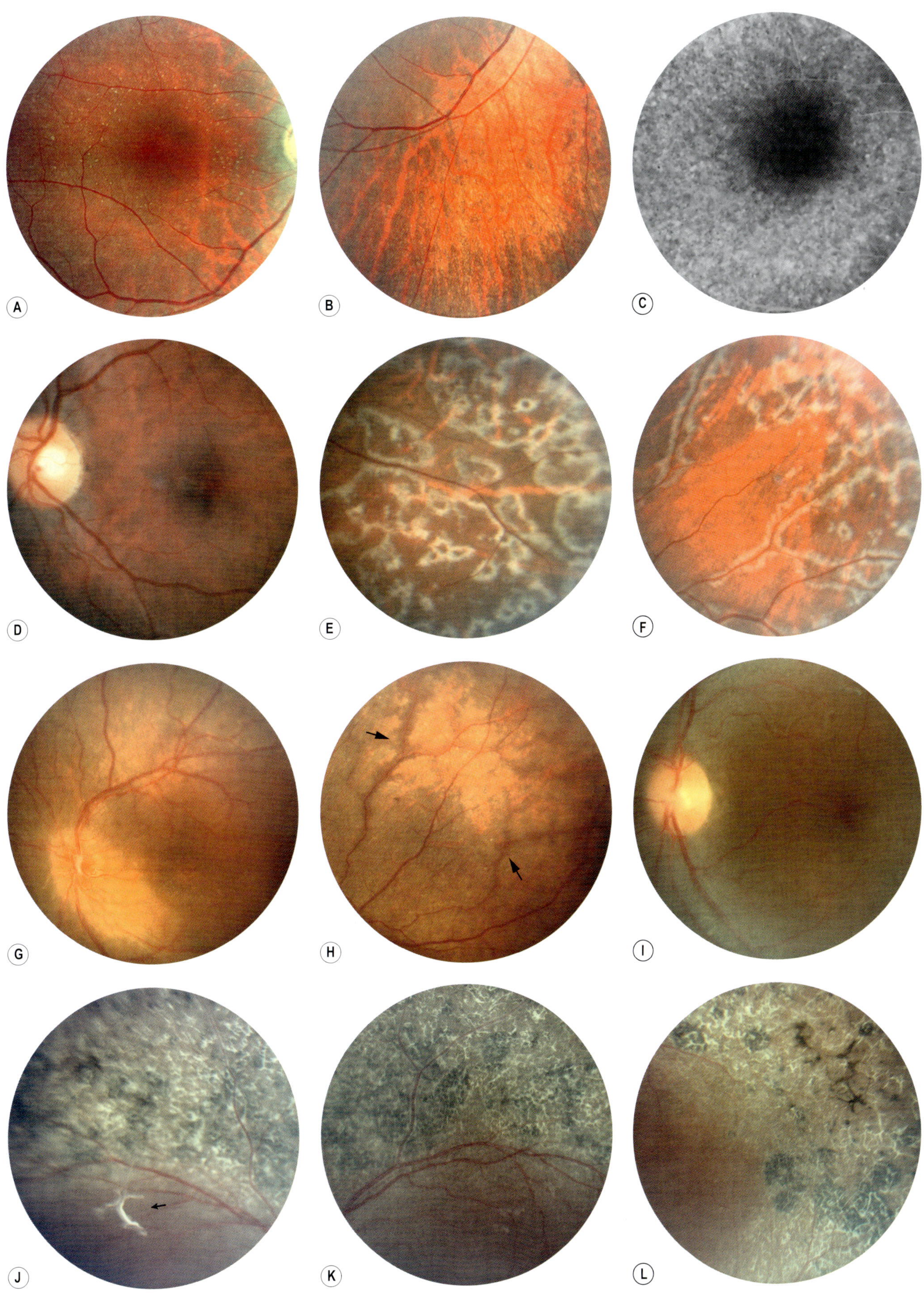
A
B
C
D
E
F
G
H
I
J
K
L

NARP syndrome is typically caused by defects of the mitochondrial enzymes including pyruvate dehydrogenase and complexes 1, 2, and 4 of the respiratory chain. In most cases, the deficiencies are due to mutations in the nuclear genes and coding subunits of the complexes PDHA1, and SDHA, proteins implicated with assembly of complexes such as SURF1 and LRPPRC. In addition, mitochondrial DNA mutations are important causes of Leigh syndrome. A T8993C mitochondrial DNA mutation is a cause of Leigh syndrome.[613–615]

The clinical picture is variable, and some patients have a milder phenotype. These patients who do not fulfill all the criteria for Leigh syndrome, are classified as Leigh-like syndrome, and they have a better prognosis but a lower biochemical and molecular diagnostic yield than patients with Leigh syndrome. The phenotypic variation in the mitochondrial DNA mutation is due to heteroplasmy or variable affection of the mitochondrial DNA mutations.[616] The *MT-ATP6* gene encoding to subunit 6 of the adenosine triphosphate synthase complex 5 is the commonest DNA gene mutation seen in cases with NARP. The *T8993* gene mutation is the commonest mutation seen.[614]

Some patients are known to improve significantly after 16–18 years of age.[617] This may be due to the decrease in the mutational load with age that has been observed in some patients. The ocular changes that have been seen in these patients can be variable, bull's-eye maculopathy has been discovered in an infant with Leigh's disease noted at the age of 8 months. In addition, the retinal arterioles are diffusely narrowed with consecutive pallor of the optic disc,[618] consistent with diffuse loss of photoreceptors. Optic atrophy, nystagmus, strabismus, ophthalmoplegia along with developmental delay, hypotonia, seizures, and psychomotor regressions are all features of Leigh's disease. Leigh's disease should be considered in the differential diagnosis of neurologically impaired infants presenting with a bull's-eye maculopathy.

5.44 Bothnia dystrophy.

A: A 15-year-old male with night blindness since early childhood, with 20/20 vision in both eyes. Visual fields were full bilaterally, rod responses were undetectable, mixed rod and cone responses were poor, and the cone response was subnormal. Left eye shows uniform white dots resembling flecks of fundus albipunctatus (A). The severely diminished scotopic and photopic amplitudes differentiate it from fundus albipunctatus.
B and **C**: This 16-year-old female with a visual acuity of 20/30 both eyes had a relative ring scotoma and suffered night blindness since early childhood. Her rod and mixed rod and cone responses were undetectable and the cone responses were subnormal. The right fundus shows diffuse glistening punctuate white dots interspersed with hyperpigmented dots (B and C).
D and **E**: This 26-year-old female with history of night blindness since early childhood and progressive loss of central vision had a visual acuity of 20/200 both eyes. She shows an older phenotype of Bothnia dystrophy with diffusely altered pigmentation of her fundus (D) and peripheral islands of geographic atrophy resembling gyrate atrophy (E). Her visual fields showed relative central and paracentral scotomas. The rod and mixed responses were undetectable and the cone responses were low.
F and **G**: A 36-year-old woman with distinct punctate white dots in the macula and diffusely mottled pigment epithelium outside the macula (F and G). Her vision was 20/100 right eye and count fingers left eye. She had bilateral central scotomas and undetectable rod and cone responses.
H: A 42-year-old female with 20/200 vision in both eyes, undetectable rod and cone electroretinograms with white dots all over the fundus and foveal atrophy (H).

(Courtesy of Dr. Ola Sandgren and Dr. Marie Burstedt.)

Retinitis Pigmentosa Sine Pigmenti

Patients with otherwise typical retinitis pigmentosa may show minimal or no evidence of pigment migration into the retina (Figure 5.39E–J).[619,620] Pearlman and associates[620] have presented evidence to suggest that the absence of pigment migration represents an initial stage of typical retinitis pigmentosa and is manifested by shorter duration of symptoms, less severe night blindness, and less impairment of the electroretinographic b-wave. Because some patients may initially be seen with visual loss secondary to cystoid macular edema or with field defects simulating arcuate scotomata, these patients may be misdiagnosed as having a neurologic disease or glaucoma. The ophthalmoscopic findings of waxy pallor of the optic disc, a glistening reflex secondary to epiretinal membrane change, a greenish or gray tapeto-like reflex from the altered RPE, and slight narrowing of the retinal arterioles should alert the clinician to inquire concerning symptoms of night blindness and to obtain electrophysiologic studies. Fluorescein angiography is helpful in detecting zones of depigmentation of the RPE not readily apparent ophthalmoscopically. Histopathologically, the changes are similar but less severe than those in typical retinitis pigmentosa. There is evidence of pigment migration into the retina but in amounts insufficient to be detected ophthalmoscopically.

Preserved Para-arterial RPE in Retinitis Pigmentosa

Heckenlively reported five patients with retinitis pigmentosa, probable autosomal-recessive inheritance, hypermetropia, and preservation of the RPE beneath the retinal arteries in areas of otherwise severe pigment epithelial and retinal atrophy (Figure 5.43G and H).[584,621] Mutations in the *CRB1* gene have been reported in a variety of autosomal-recessive retinal dystrophies, including retinitis pigmentosa with preserved para-arteriolar RPE,[622] retinitis pigmentosa with Coats'-like exudative vasculopathy, early-onset RPE with preserved para-arterial RPE (PPRPE), and Leber's congenital amaurosis.[623] It appears that loss of function of members of the *CRB/CRB* complex in *Drosophila* and vertebrate retina results in typical architectural disorganization and light-induced degeneration. The alterations occur at the RPE photoreceptor level and also at the Müller cells.

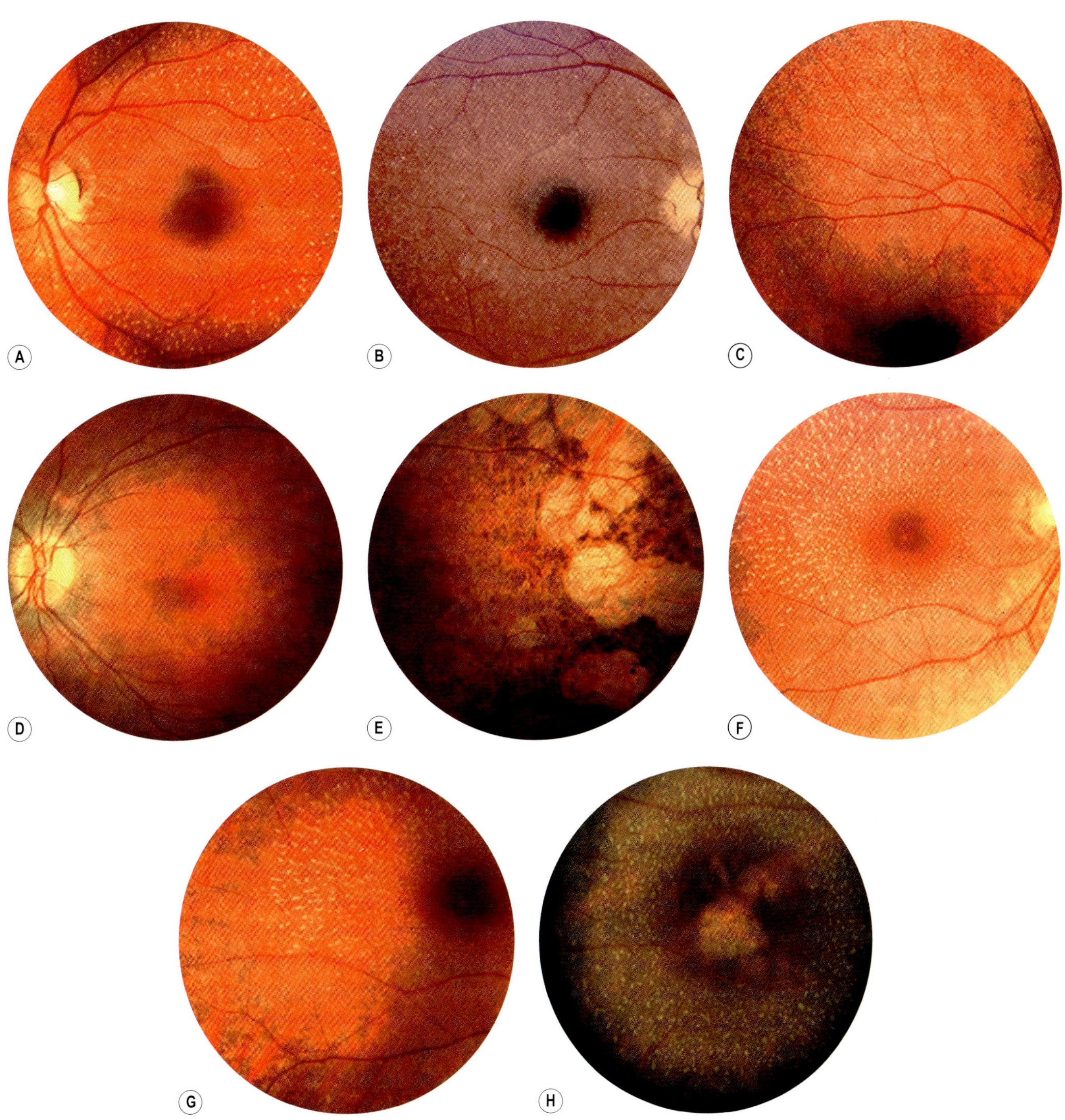
A
B
C
D
E
F
G
H

Retinitis Punctata Albescens (RPA)

RPA is mostly an autosomal-recessive condition (rarely dominant)[624] with multiple small gray or white dots that resemble the flecks of fundus albipunctatus. Confinement of the flecks to the region just outside the macula (not reaching the periphery), progressive night blindness, narrowing of retinal vessels, loss of peripheral field, and appearance of pigment spicules differentiate it from fundus albipunctatus (Figure 5.43A–C).[467,599,625–627] Intermediate forms of these disorders exist.

RPA is mostly associated with mutations in *RLBP1*,[480,628–633] and occasionally in *RHO*, *RDS*, and *RDH5* genes.[624,634] There is a wide genetic heterogeneity amongst a reasonable phenotypic uniformity in this condition. Various mutations in the *RLBP1* gene have been found, and in some cases none of the known mutations is positive.[630] Bothnia dystrophy and NFRCD closely resemble RPA in many features and the gene affected is *RLBP1*[635–639]; however the mutations are different from those known for RPA.

The differential diagnosis includes basal laminar drusen, fundus flavimaculatus, abetalipoproteinemia, oxalosis, cystinosis, talc emboli, Alport's syndrome, canthaxanthine retinopathy, and fundus xerophthalmicus. Other types of flecks and peculiar color changes of the peripheral retina occasionally occur in patients with retinitis pigmentosa (Figure 5.43D–L).

Bothnia Dystrophy

The onset is in early childhood with symptoms of night blindness when the retina appears normal. Punctate white dots of RPA appear in teenage and young adults (Figure 5.44A). Macular pigment deposits (Figure 5.44B, C) followed by macular atrophic changes occur next (Figure 5.44D, H). This is followed by paracentral and mid peripheral round chorioretinal atrophic lesions resembling gyrate atrophy (Figure 5.44E) and narrowing of retinal vessels. Widespread pigment epithelial migration in the form of bone spicules occurs occasionally. Visual acuity progressively declines with age, leading to legal blindness by the fourth decade of life. Those whose vision never develops beyond 20/80 show nystagmus. Premature cataract has not been a feature. Fluorescein angiography shows mottled transmission defects from RPE atrophy.[640]

Visual fields are normal in young patients; gradually increasing central scotomas develop in the teens or in young adults, eventually leaving only peripheral islands of visual field. Color vision is affected early and worsens with age. Dark adaptation studies show abnormalities of both rod and cone function that progressively worsen. Electroretinography shows decreased amplitudes and increased implicit times for rod and rod–cone function early, and progressive cone dysfunction later on. Individuals heterozygous for the mutation show near-normal ERG amplitudes and implicit times. EOG is subnormal in all patients.[640–642]

It is a unique autosomal-recessive rod–cone retinal dystrophy first described in the Bothnia Occidentalis region of Västerbotten county of northern Sweden, with a high prevalence of 1 per 4500 population. The disorder is caused by a mutation in the *RLBP1* gene mapped to chromosome 15q26, encoding the human cellular retinaldehyde-binding protein (CRALBP). Patients affected by Bothnia dystrophy are homozygous for a C-to-T transition in exon 7 of the *RLBP1* gene, leading to an arginine to tryptophan substitution at position 234 of the protein (R234W). CRALBP is located in the RPE, Müller cells, ciliary body pigment epithelium, outer epithelium of the iris, cornea, the optic nerve, and pineal gland. In the RPE it functions as the carrier protein for endogenous retinoids such as 11-*cis*-retinol involved in the visual cycle. Defect in the *RLBP1* gene leads to defective binding of 11-*cis* retinaldehyde, thus preventing its regeneration, and subsequently loss of rod function.[637] He et al. found R234W displays fivefold increased resistance to light-induced photoisomerization relative to wild-type CRALBP, caused by unanticipated domino-like structural rearrangements causing Bothnia-type retinal dystrophy by the impaired release of 11-*cis*-retinal from R234W.[635]

Other mutations in the *RLBP1* gene have been described: R150Q in exon 5 in three patients from India and in patients from Saudi Arabia, three additional mutations in a small family of European ancestry and two splice junction mutations, one of which causes NFRCD. Most of these patients present with white flecks, peripheral degenerative changes, and maculopathy and resemble the phenotype of Bothnia dystrophy, except NFRCD, which has an earlier onset and more rapid progression and so far has not developed the macular areolar atrophy.[638,639,641]

5.45 Newfoundland rod–cone degeneration (NFRCD).

A and **B**: This 47-year-old male was investigated for hyperreflexia and abnormal gait in 1993. In 2000, gait disturbance worsened and a retinal degeneration was noted. Cerebellar and cerebral atrophy was found on magnetic resonance imaging in 2001, and by 2007, the spasticity confined him to a wheelchair. He was found to have punctate white dots all over the fundus (early stage) with some patches of retinal pigment epithelium/choriocapillary atrophy (A and B). One sister had similar history and findings and two other siblings and parents were unaffected. His rod electroretinogram was flat and cone responses were diminished.

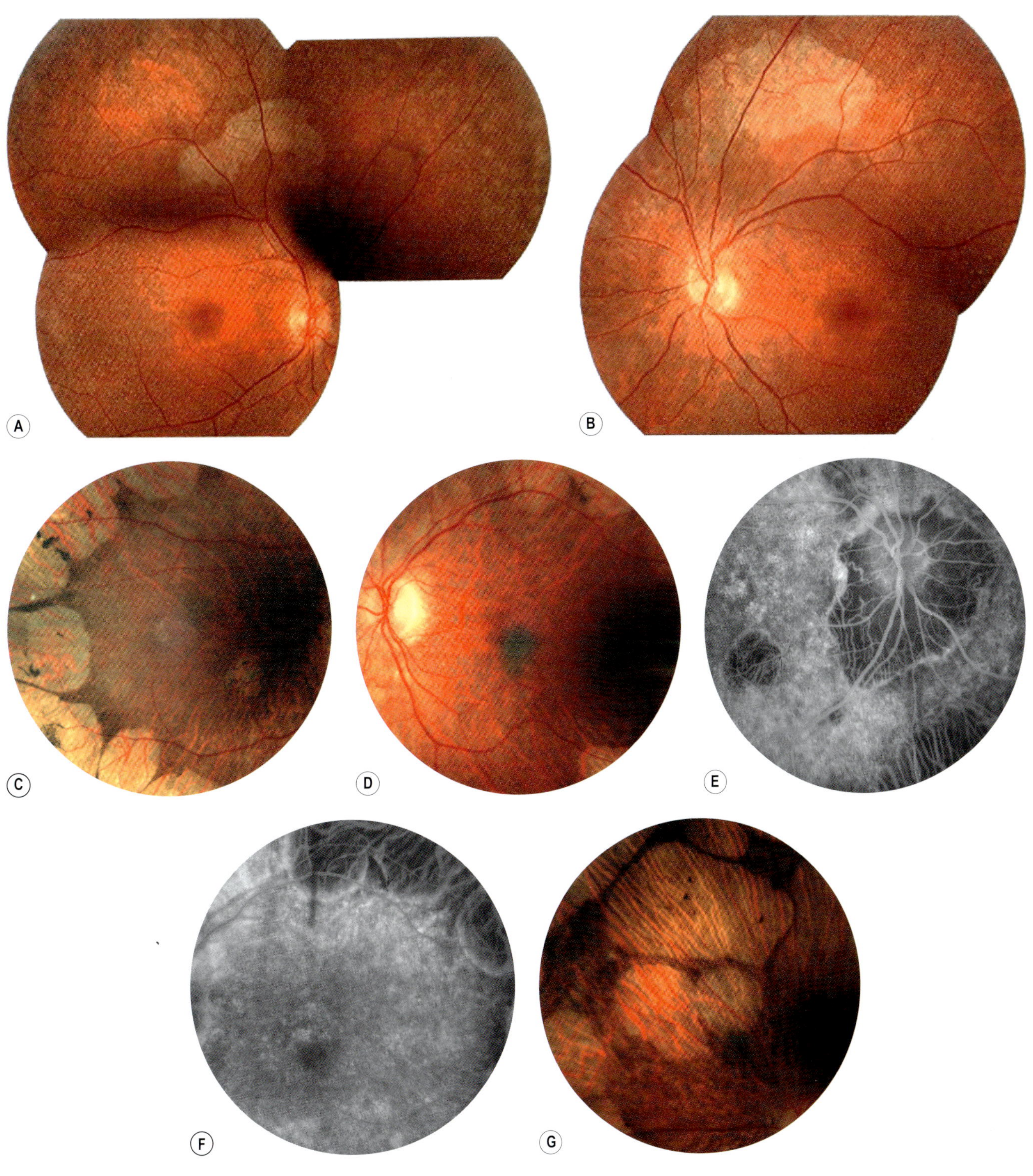
A
B
C
D
E
F
G

Newfoundland Rod–Cone Dystrophy

Symptoms begin in infancy with night blindness, followed by progressive loss of peripheral, central, and color vision in childhood, resulting in severe visual loss by the second to fourth decade of life. Several white dots similar to fundus punctata albescens/fundus albipunctatus and Bothnia dystrophy may be seen in the posterior pole and midperiphery in some patients. In contrast to Bothnia dystrophy, where macular involvement occurs early, the macula in NFRCD is normal or exhibits a "beaten-bronze" atrophy. A perimacular ring of white stippling similar to that in RPA is observed in young patients, and a scallop-bordered geographic atrophy of the mid peripheral RPE develops over time (Figure 5.45A and B).[638] This is similar in appearance to early gyrate atrophy, choroideremia, and Bothnia dystrophy; however, plasma ornithine levels are normal. Cataracts have not been documented, myopia is not seen consistently, and glaucoma has not been identified. Bone spicule pigmentation is not seen, optic discs are either normal or show trace pallor until late stage, and only mild attenuation of retinal vessels is seen in advanced disease (Figure 5.45G–K).[638]

The ERG rod responses are selectively reduced early, and the ERG rod and cone responses are both extinguished in advanced disease. The early visual field defect is a ring scotoma close to fixation rather than in the mid peripheral field seen in classic retinitis pigmentosa (Figure 5.45L). Central visual acuity may be as good as 20/20–20/60, although the central field may be less than 5°. The rate at which the ring scotoma widens and becomes a complete central scotoma is an indicator of the rate of progression of the disease. Color vision defects are initially mild red/green with or without blue/yellow defects, but this progresses rapidly to eventual loss of color perception. There are however exceptions where patients in their 30s or 40s have only mild to moderate color vision defects.[638]

The area in Newfoundland in which the majority of affected patients reside is within a 10-mile (16-km) radius. Most inhabitants here migrated from southwestern England in the mid 18th century, and the population has remained fairly isolated till recently. A single common ancestor has not been identified. Two *RLBP1* splice junction mutations are responsible for NFRCD, whereas missense mutations of *RLBP1* are responsible for RPA, Bothnia dystrophy, and autosomal-recessive RP.[629,637,638,640]

5.45 Continued

C–L: This patient with NFRCD had confluent peripheral and mid peripheral lacunar atrophy in both eyes (midstage, C and D). Angiogram showing "moth-eaten" retinal pigment epithelium in the macula and loss of choriocapillaris in the areas of lacunar atrophy. Composite images show the extent and distribution of the atrophy in the midperiphery in both eyes (G–I). Five years later, the lacunar atrophy appears stable without progression into the macula in both eyes (J and K). Visual field defects correspond to the lacunar atrophy with ring scotomas early in the disease, but only remaining temporal field when the disease is advanced and extends to the macula (L).

(Courtesy of Dr. James Whelan.)

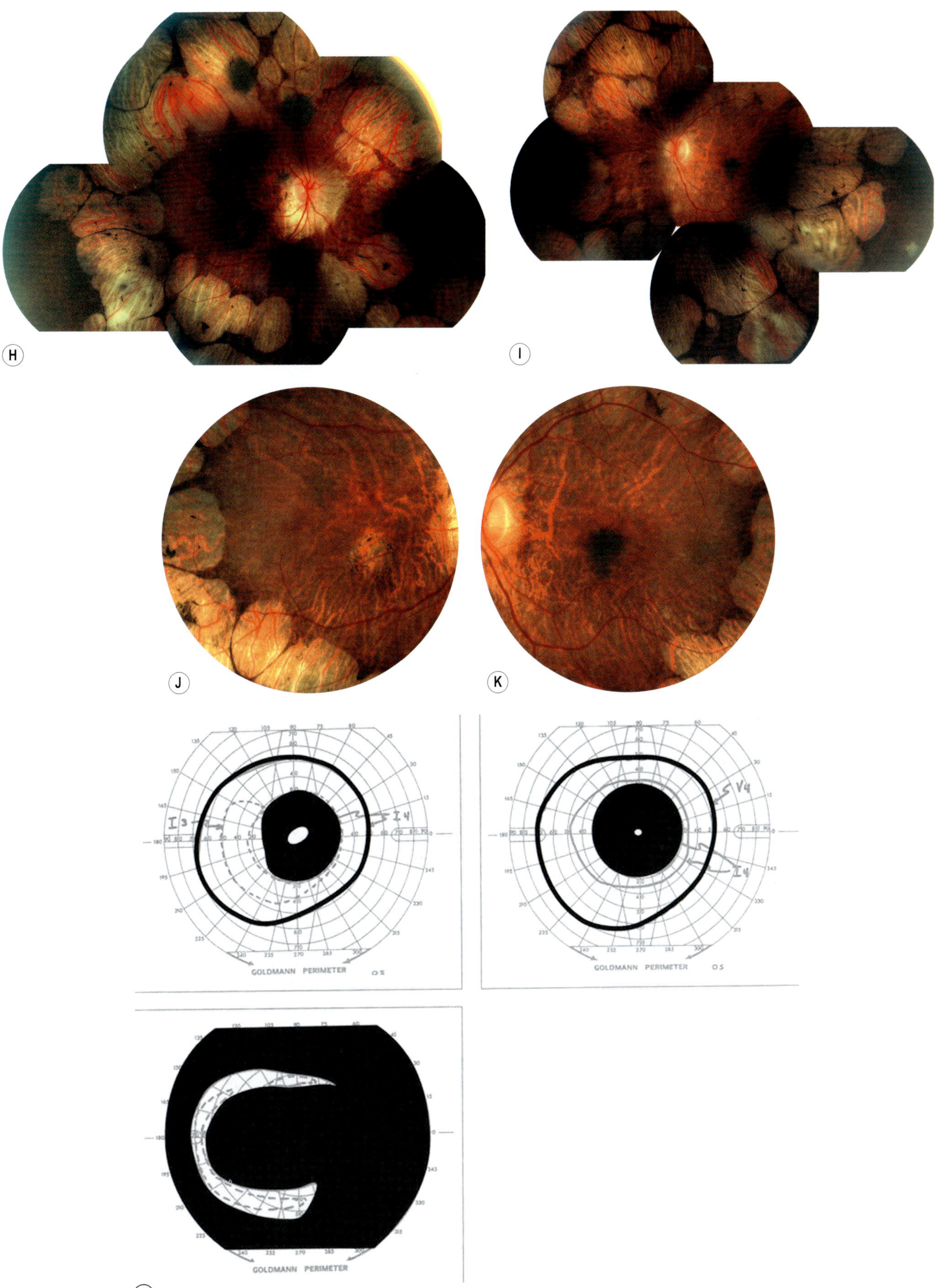
H
I
J
K
I3
I4
GOLDMANN PERIMETER
OS
V4
I4
GOLDMANN PERIMETER
OS
GOLDMANN PERIMETER
L

Bietti's Crystalline Tapetoretinal Dystrophy

Patients with Bietti's crystalline tapetoretinal dystrophy, usually males, are initially seen in middle age because of slowly progressive loss of vision frequently unassociated with nyctalopia.[643–653] In the early stages of the disease fundoscopic examination reveals a striking fundoscopic picture characterized by the presence of glittering crystals scattered throughout the posterior fundus (Figure 5.46A, B, H, and I). These are located in all layers of the retina and can be confirmed on OCT.[654–657]

There are often multiple areas of geographic atrophy of the RPE in the posterior fundus (Figures 5.46 and 5.47). Autofluorescence imaging shows decreased autofluorescence corresponding to the areas of RPE loss, punctate increased autofluorescence corresponding to pigment dots, possibly RPE hyperplasia, and very little hyperautofluorescence of the crystals.[655] The crystals are less apparent in the areas of pigment epithelial atrophy. The optic disc and retinal vessels are typically normal. There may or may not be marginal crystalline dystrophy of the cornea characterized by the presence of sparkling yellow or white, round, polygonal, or needlelike crystals located in the anterior stroma of the perilimbal region.[644,646,650,653] These crystals may become more prominent late in the disease[653] and biopsy of the limbal conjunctiva and cornea has shown these crystals to be complex lipid inclusions within fibroblasts.[658] The electroretinographic and electro-oculographic findings are usually subnormal. Fluorescein angiography reveals atrophy of the choriocapillaris in the zones of pigment epithelial atrophy. These zones progressively enlarge, become confluent, and extend into the periphery of the fundus. The rate of progression and severity of the disease are variable. Figure 5.46 (H–L) illustrates a black woman who had rapid progression of the disease. Most cases have been reported in patients of Italian or oriental extraction, in particular Chinese and Japanese.[654,659–663]

5.46 Bietti's crystalline tapetoretinal dystrophy.

A–D: Atypical pigmentary retinal dystrophy associated with widespread subretinal crystalline deposits in a 54-year-old man of Italian descent who had recently noted paracentral scotomas in both eyes. His visual acuity was normal. Note the relative paucity of crystalline deposits in those areas of geographic atrophy of the retinal pigment epithelium (RPE) (A and B). Visual field defects corresponded with the areas of RPE depigmentation. The corneas and conjunctivae were normal. His electro-oculogram was normal. Electroretinography showed subnormal rod and cone responses in both eyes. His past medical history was unremarkable. He had normal levels of serum ornithine and urine oxalates. There was no family history of consanguinity or visual loss.

E and **G**: This 34-year-old Lebanese man noted slow loss of central vision for several years. His family history was negative. His visual acuity was 20/70 right eye and 20/50 left eye. He had many retinal crystals in the posterior fundi (E) and subtle crystals in the corneas. There was evidence of early geographic atrophy of the RPE in the right eye (E–G). Note evidence of nonperfusion of the choriocapillaris paracentrally (arrows) and depigmentation of the RPE throughout the macula (F and G). An electroretinogram revealed mild decrease in cone amplitudes.

H–L: This 15-year-old female had many variably sized crystalline deposits throughout the postequatorial fundi (H and I). Three and one-half years later, she had severe visual loss, atrophy of the pigment epithelium, loss of the crystalline material, and sheathing of the choroidal vessels (J). Note the extensive loss of the choriocapillaris evident in the angiograms (K and L).

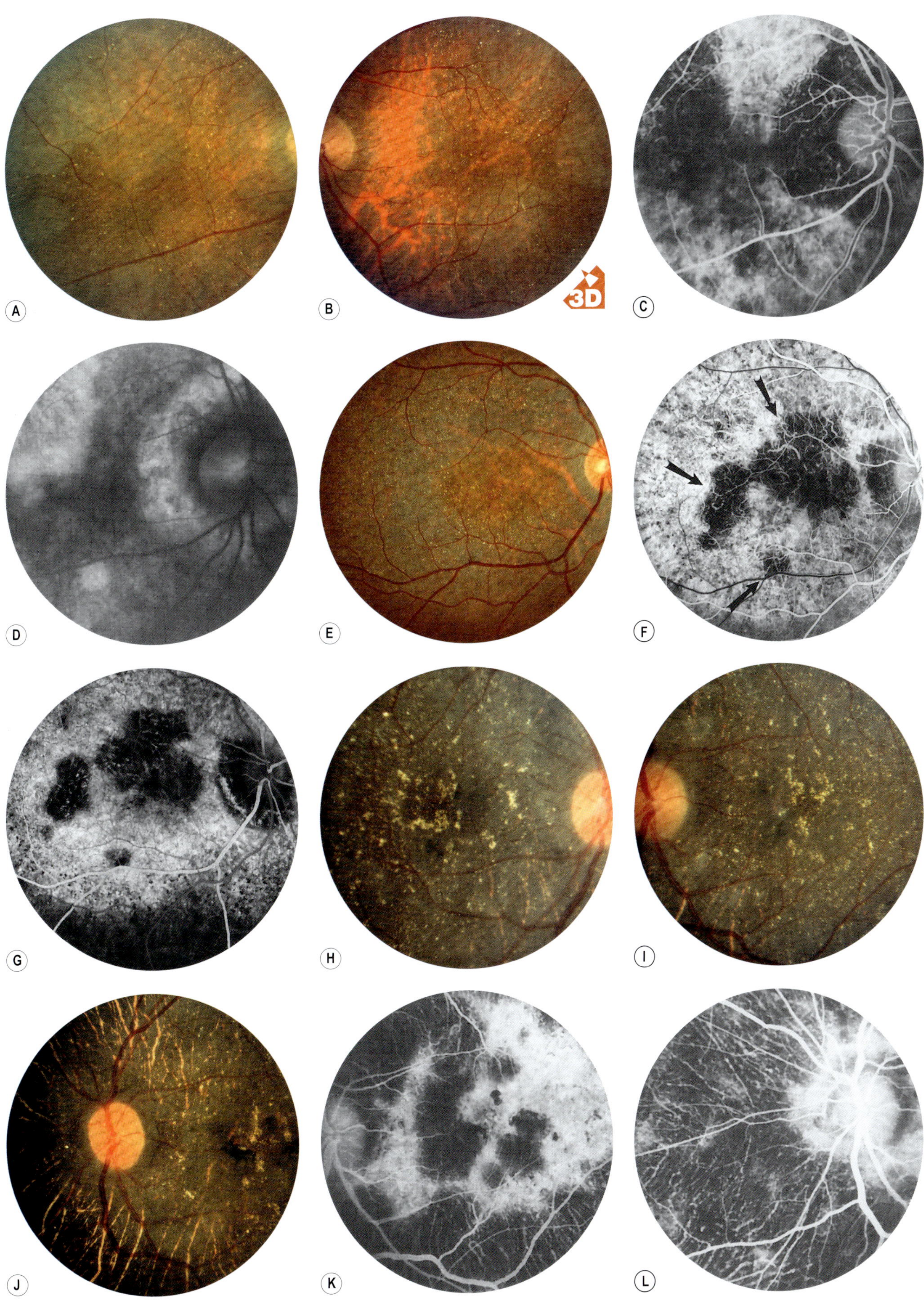
A
B
3D
C
D
E
F
G
H
I
J
K
L

The hereditary pattern is autosomal-recessive and the causative gene is *CYP4V2,* which belongs to the cytochrome P450 hemithiolate protein superfamily and is responsible for oxidizing various substrates in the metabolic pathway. Several mutations in the *CYP4V2* gene have been described.[662–665] Cultured cells and peripheral lymphocytes from patients with Bietti's crystalline tapetoretinal dystrophy are found to have abnormally high triglycerides and cholesterol storage, and reduced metabolism of labeled fatty acid precursors, suggesting that Bietti's crystalline dystrophy may result from abnormality of lipid metabolism.[654,658,664]The nature of the crystals within the retina is unknown, but is presumed to be similar or related to the inclusions in the corneal and dermal fibroblasts and peripheral blood lymphocytes.

5.47 Bietti's crystalline dystrophy.

A–D: This 47-year-old woman of German descent complained of night blindness for more than 10 years. Her visual acuity was 20/40 on the right and 20/100 on the left. Diffuse atrophy of the retinal pigment epithelium (RPE) and choriocapillaris was seen in the posterior pole with shiny yellow white crystals all over in both eyes. Fluorescein angiography showed diffuse chorioretinal atrophy with patch preservation of RPE and choriocapillaris (B–D).
E–I: A 50-year-old Hispanic woman with complaints of photophobia and nycatalopia had a visual decline to 20/40 and 20/100. Color vision was diminished to 2/12 on the right and 0/12 on the left by Ishihara testing. Both eyes showed central RPE/choriocapillary atrophy with shiny crystals throughout the fundus (E and F). Choriocapillary and RPE loss were seen on angiography (G–I).

(Courtesy of Dr. Brian Berger.)

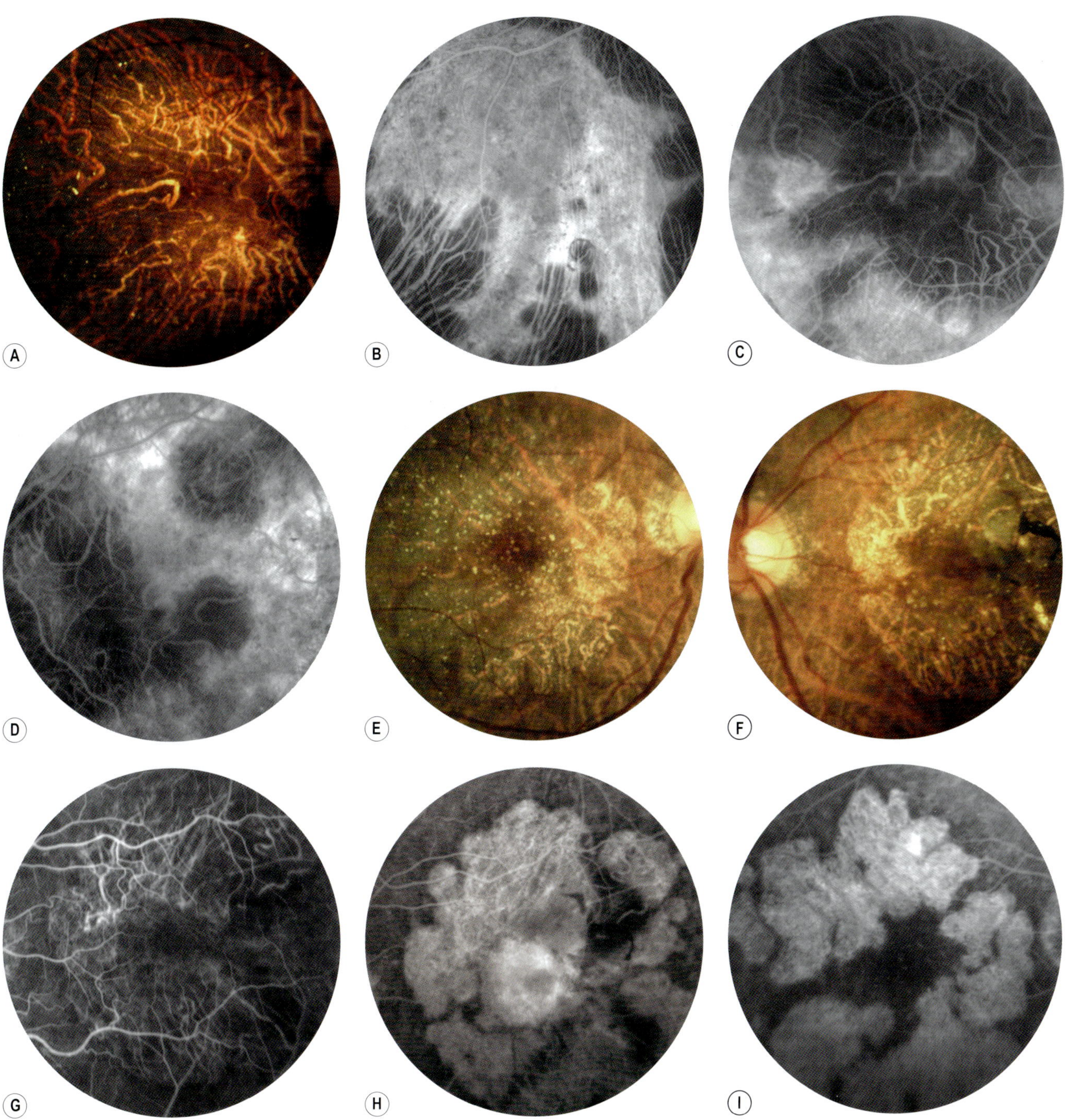
A
B
C
D
E
F
G
H
I

Leber's Amaurosis (Infantile Tapetoretinal Dystrophy, Retinal Neuroepithelial Dysgenesis)

Leber used the name "congenital amaurosis" to describe an autosomal-recessively inherited disorder characterized by blindness or very low vision at birth, failure to fix, nystagmus, sluggish pupillary reaction, occasional photophobia, a positive oculodigital sign, and hyperopia in patients who later developed evidence of retinitis pigmentosa.[256,583,666–682]Patients with Leber's amaurosis are usually hyperopic, unlike patients with retinitis pigmentosa, who are typically myopic. Because there is accumulating evidence that many patients with congenital amaurosis have a retinal dysgenesis associated with minimal evidence of progressive visual loss, it is useful to group these patients, who are otherwise normal, apart from those with congenital blindness associated with a host of systemic disorders, including psychomotor retardation, mental retardation, hydrocephaly, deafness, epilepsy, cardiomyopathy, myopathy, dyscephaly, dwarfism, and other skeletal anomalies.[512,683–685] It is possible that some of these latter patients may have an infantile-onset progressive tapetoretinal dystrophy.

At birth the fundi of most patients with Leber's amaurosis are normal. Some patients, however, may show dysplastic fundus changes, including pseudopapilledema (Figure 5.48A), optic disc pallor (Figure 5.48D),[686] optic disc hypoplasia (Figure 5.48D),[677] macular coloboma,[248,256,674] and chorioretinal coloboma (Figure 5.48E and F). A variety of pigment epithelial and retinal changes develop in early childhood and continue into adulthood. These include salt-and-pepper pigmentation,[670] yellowish flecks,[669,675,677,679,681] "marbleized" fundus with mosaic pattern (Figure 5.48C and I),[687] periarteriolar distribution of well-demarcated yellow lesions located external to the retinal vessels,[669,675,681] nummular pigmented lesions (Figure 5.48C),[688,689] retinitis pigmentosa,[674] choroideremia,[675] gyrate atrophy,[670] macular colobomata,[248,256,683] and bull's-eye maculopathy.[677,690] A variety of progressive chorioretinal degenerative changes associated with narrowing of the retinal vessels and optic atrophy eventually develop (Figure 5.48B and C). Only occasionally does the typical bone spicule pattern of retinitis pigmentosa occur. Cataract and keratoconus are late complications.

The ERG is extinguished in approximately 75% of patients and is markedly abnormal in the remainder. For infants with unexplained visual loss, an ERG is essential in differentiating Leber's amaurosis from other causes of congenital blindness.[676] Fluorescein angiography may show evidence of RPE atrophy not appreciated ophthalmoscopically as well as evidence of papilledema.

LCA is usually inherited as an autosomal recessive trait, although dominant inheritance has also been reported. Mutations in 10 retinal genes have so far been shown to cause LCA, namely *AIPL1, CRB1, CRX, GUCY2D, RDH, RPE65, RPGRIP1, TULP1, IMPDH1* and, more recently, *CEP290*. Because of the increasing number of LCA-causing genes, it is difficult to classify patients with LCA on a molecular basis and consequently to evaluate phenotype–genotype correlations. Gene therapy trials are underway in RPE65 involved patients. Long-term follow-up studies of patients with Leber's amaurosis reveal that, although there is a progression of the fundus changes throughout life, the visual function remains relatively stable in most patients.[683,691] Loss of function is most likely to occur in those with macular colobomas, and those who in later life develop keratoconus and cataracts. Most patients with Leber's congenital amaurosis have the capability of normal cognitive function, but most perform poorly on standard IQ tests.[692]

In childhood, histopathologic changes consist primarily of failure of development or loss of the rods and cones (Figure 5.48J).[672] These changes are followed by progressive degenerative changes involving all of the retinal layers and RPE similar to that seen in retinitis pigmentosa (Figure 5.48K).[668]

5.48 Leber's congenital amaurosis.

A: This 2-year-old girl had only light perception in both eyes. Note the anomaly of the optic disc. The electroretinogram was extinguished. Her refractive error was + 4.50.
B and C: This 8-year-old boy had hand movements vision in the right eye and 20/70 in the left eye. Note the extensive geographic areas of atrophy of the retinal pigment epithelium (RPE) posteriorly and the round clumping of pigment in the periphery of the fundus. His electroretinogram was extinguished.
D: Optic disc hypoplasia, and marked narrowing of the retinal vessels in this boy with nystagmus, night blindness, and an extinguished electroretinogram.
E and F: This 14-year-old boy had poor vision since birth, nyctalopia, marked narrowing of the retinal vessels, pigmentary mottling in the macula (E), marked constriction of the visual fields, an extinguished electroretinogram, and an inferior colobomata of the choroid and retina bilaterally (F). His visual acuity was 20/40 right eye and 20/50 left eye. A first cousin had poor vision of uncertain cause. At age 25 years his findings were similar but his visual acuity was 20/200 bilaterally.
G–I: Coats' syndrome in the left eye of this woman with nystagmus and marked loss of vision since birth. She had marked narrowing of the retinal vessels and extensive degeneration of the RPE with punctate RPE hyperplasia (H and I) in both eyes. In the left eye inferiorly there was extensive yellowish exudative detachment of the retina and retinal telangiectasis (G and H). Arrows in G and H indicate optic disc.
J: Histopathology of the eye of a 12-year-old boy with Leber's amaurosis and xeroderma pigmentosa. Note monolayer of retinal receptors and absence of cone outer segments (arrow) in the macula, which was otherwise unremarkable. The mid peripheral retina showed disruption of the normal retinal architecture by gliosis.
K: Histopathology of the eye of another patient with Leber's amaurosis who developed spontaneous rupture of the cornea that had severe keratoconus. Note in this section of the peripheral retina the marked degeneration and gliosis, the migration of RPE (left arrow) into the retina, and the focal areas of subretinal RPE hyperplasia beneath the retina (right arrow).

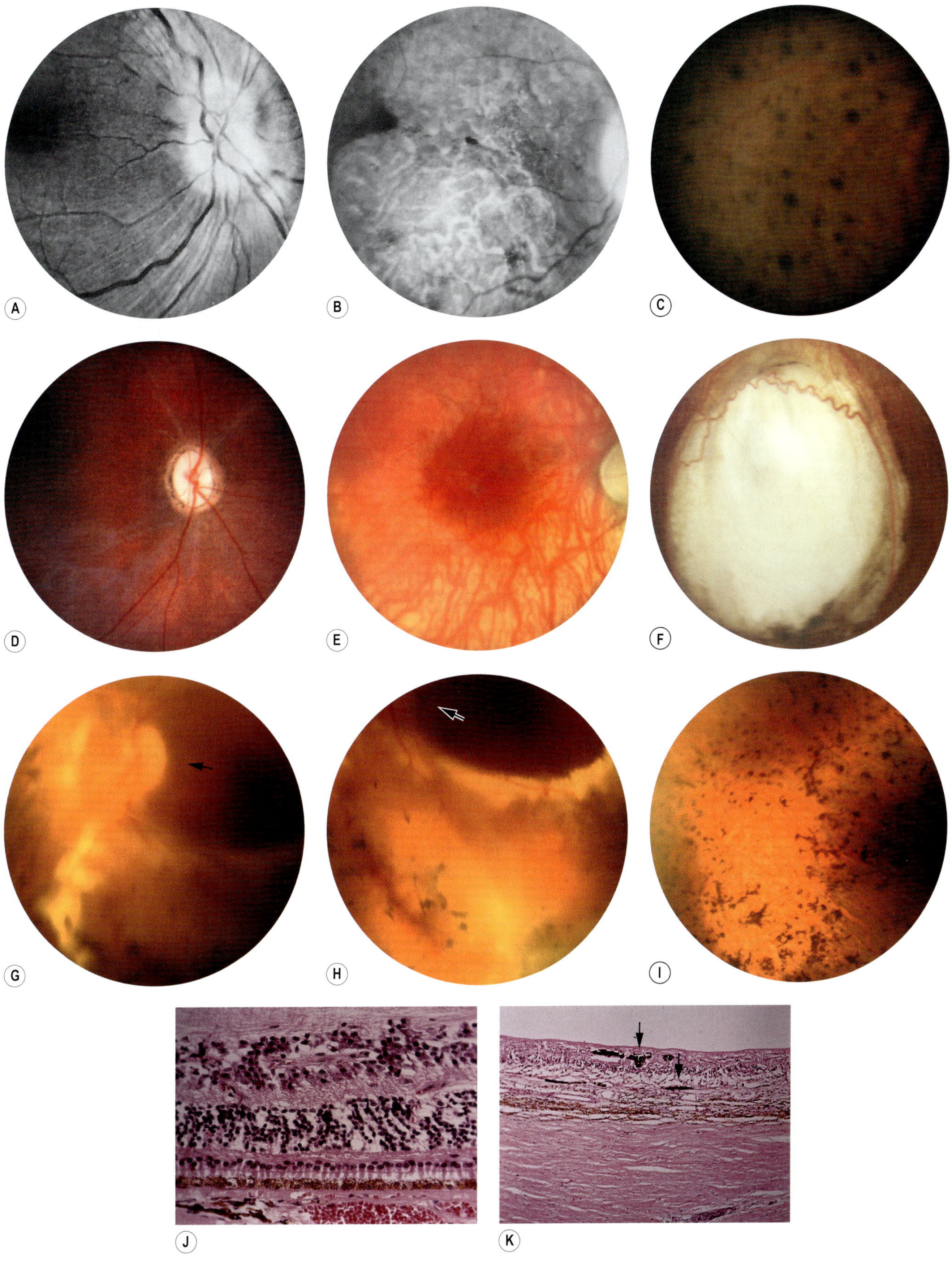
A
B
C
D
E
F
G
H
I
J
K

The natural course of most patients with Leber's congenital amaurosis suggests that it is a retinal dysgenesis and not a progressive tapetoretinal degeneration. The progressive fundoscopic and histopathologic changes observed in these patients can all be explained on the basis of reactive changes occurring in the retina and pigment epithelium in response to the widespread absence at birth of the retinal receptor cells. These reactive changes include degeneration, proliferation, and intraretinal migration of the pigment epithelium; narrowing of the retinal blood vessels; proliferation of retinal glial cells; and transsynaptic degeneration of the ganglion cells.

The differential diagnosis of Leber's congenital amaurosis includes cortical blindness, achromatopsia, congenital stationary night blindness, infantile-onset retinitis pigmentosa, and infantile ceroid lipofuscinoses. Electroretinography is important in establishing whether the retina is affected, and to what degree it is affected. Although the ERG may be severely abnormal or extinguished in Leber's amaurosis, it is not affected in cortical blindness, and only mildly or moderately affected in congenital stationary night blindness. It may be severely affected early in infantile-onset tapetoretinal dystrophies. Absence of searching nystagmus, relatively good visual acuity, and absence of high hyperopia in these latter patients are features atypical for Leber's amaurosis.[512,583]

Neonatal Retinal Dysgenesis and Dystrophies Associated with Systemic Diseases

Several well-defined single-gene defects and other less well-defined disorders occur in which retinal dysfunction is one aspect of a generalized disease affecting other organ systems. These include Zellweger's cerebrohepatorenal syndrome (see p. 397), Saldino–Mainzer syndrome, Senior–Loken syndrome (see p. 390), Joubert syndrome (see p. 398), and Arima's syndrome (see p. 398). Unlike Leber's congenital amaurosis, hyperopia is not characteristic of these disorders. Russell-Eggitt et al. have reported seven members of four families with neonatal nystagmus, poor vision, photophobia, severely abnormal or extinguished ERG responses, cardiomyopathy, and short obese habitus.[685] Six had a life-threatening episode of cardiac failure and two died. Examination of muscle obtained at autopsy was unremarkable. Mrak et al. reported a congenital myopathy associated with congenital features of Leber's amaurosis, hypotonia, delayed motor development, and histologic evidence of broadened or smeared A bands.[684]

5.49 Slowly progressive dominantly inherited dystrophy in a family with nystagmus, myopia, microcornea, S-shaped lower-lid deformity, variable degrees of visual acuity loss, field loss, retinal degeneration, optic disc pallor, and electroretinographic abnormalities.

A–C: Ten-year-old black girl with lid deformity, optic disc pallor, and juxtapapillary and peripheral retinal pigment epithelium and retinal atrophy. Her electroretinographic study was normal.
D and E: Brother, 28 years old, of patient in A. Electroretinography revealed severely abnormal rod and cone function.
F: Father, 51 years old, of patient in A. His electroretinogram was nonrecordable.
G: Paternal aunt, 56 years old, of patient in A. Electroretinography revealed moderately abnormal rod and cone functions.
H and I: Eight-year-old grandson of patient in G.

Stationary or Slowly Progressive Dominantly Inherited Tapetoretinal Dystrophy

Three successive generations of a black family seen at the Bascom Palmer Eye Institute demonstrated an early-onset, slowly progressive, atypical tapetoretinal dystrophy of variable severity associated with S-shaped deformity of the upper eyelid, microcornea, and angle closure glaucoma (Figure 5.49).[693] Some of the family members showed only mild RPE and retinal degenerative changes without visual loss. Others had more severe loss of central as well as peripheral vision. This family shares some features with a dominantly inherited RPE dystrophy with variable expressivity and complete penetrance characterized by myopia, nystagmus, and an RPE dystrophy of varying severity reported by Noble and associates.[694] In some patients the fundus changes were mild and confined to the macula. The severity of the changes was not related to the extent of involvement or to the degree of myopia. Visual acuity varied from near normal to 20/200 or worse. The pendular nystagmus was not related to the visual function. Electroretinographic changes were present in all patients but varied from mild to severe. These families might be considered as having a dominant, less severe form of Leber's amaurosis.

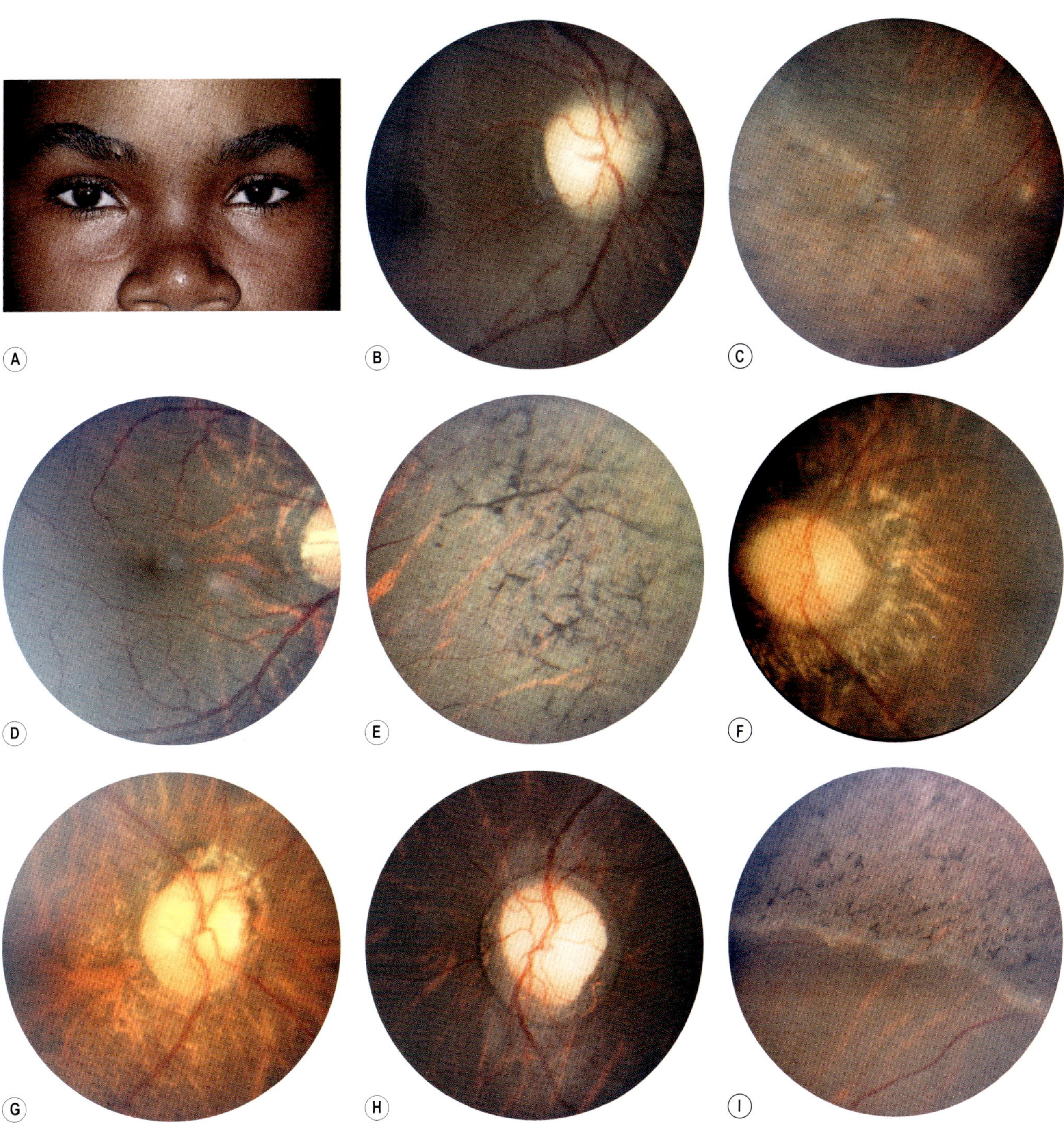
A
B
C
D
E
F
G
H
I

Late-Onset Retinal Macular Degeneration (LORMD)

Patients with Scottish ancestry were first described with this autosomal-dominant condition.[695] They are asymptomatic and have normal fundus till their fifth decade. Symptoms of night blindness begin in the fifth to sixth decade and progress rapidly over a few years. Early retinal changes include "drusenlike" yellow spots throughout the fundus that represent sub-RPE deposits (Figure 5.50C). Soon islands of RPE atrophy ensue, leaving intervening spaces of RPE that have scalloped edges (Figure 5.50D, E, J–L). The photoreceptor function rapidly worsens over an average of 5 years to leave the patient with severely constricted visual fields; central vision is lost later with further geographic atrophy of the macular RPE. There may be patchy involvement with preservation of the RPE in some parts of the fundus (Figure 5.50D, E, K, and L). Early in the course of the disease dark adaptation is affected. The retinal appearance resembles gyrate atrophy; however in patients with gyrate atrophy, the islands of geographic atrophy begin in the periphery and slowly progress towards the posterior pole, whereas those in LORMD are present early in the posterior retina, and ornithine and other amino acids are normal.

Some patients with abnormally long and anterior-attached lens zonules have been described.[696] Histology, electron microscopy, and immunohistochemistry show deposition of material made up of components similar to deposits in age-related macular degeneration and SFD under the RPE.[695,697–700] In addition there is accumulation of esterified (stains with oil red O) and unesterified cholesterol similar to contents of atheromatous plaques. The gene defect has been localized to *CTRP5*.

5.50 Late-onset retinal macular degeneration (LORMD).

A–H: This 62-year-old woman of German descent complained of difficulty with night vision for the past 5 years. Her optometrist noted retinal changes that were not seen 5 years before when he had last examined her. She was amblyopic in her right eye since early childhood and read 20/200 right eye and 20/50 left eye. Several nummular atrophic patches that became larger towards the periphery were seen in the posterior pole (A and B) and temporal fundus (D and E). The nasal retina showed fine drusen. Window defects were seen on angiography and the lesions were hypoautofluorescent. Visual fields showed peripheral constriction and electroretinogram revealed severely depressed rod and cone amplitudes in both eyes. Her father was known to have developed poor vision in his later life; she had two living siblings with no visual dysfunction. Two sons aged 32 and 34 were also asymptomatic.

I–L: This 60-year-old Hispanic male complained of nyctalopia and reduced central vision for 5 years. Several of his cousins had poor vision; no history was available about his own siblings. His vision was 20/100 and 20/80. Round patches of retinal pigment epithelium (RPE)/choriocapillaris atrophy were seen around the fovea and diffusely in the inferior fundus of both eyes (I–L). Patchy pigment migration and clumping were seen; there were intervening scalloped areas of RPE preservation typical of LORMD (J).

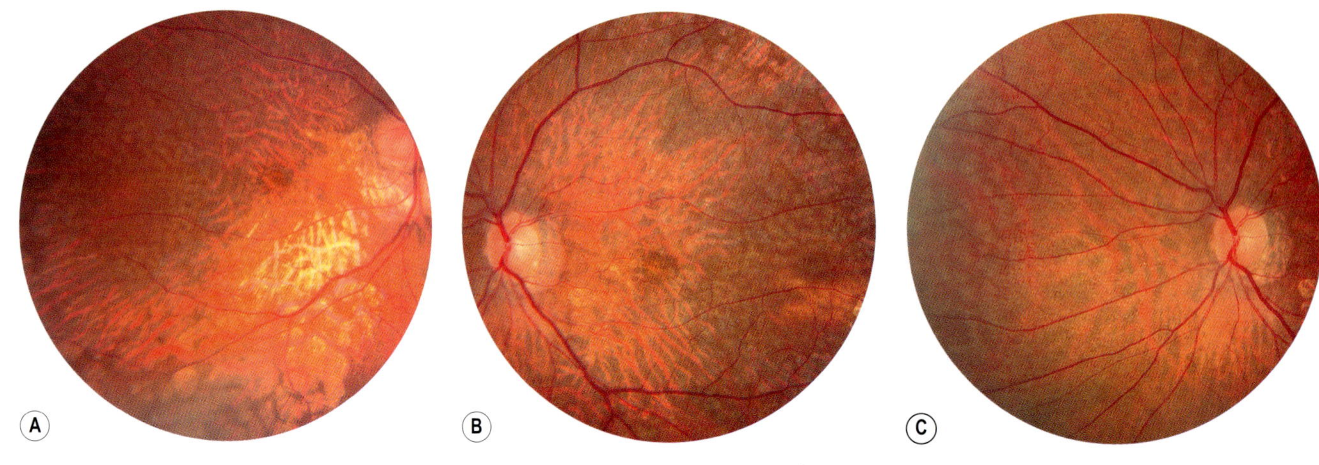

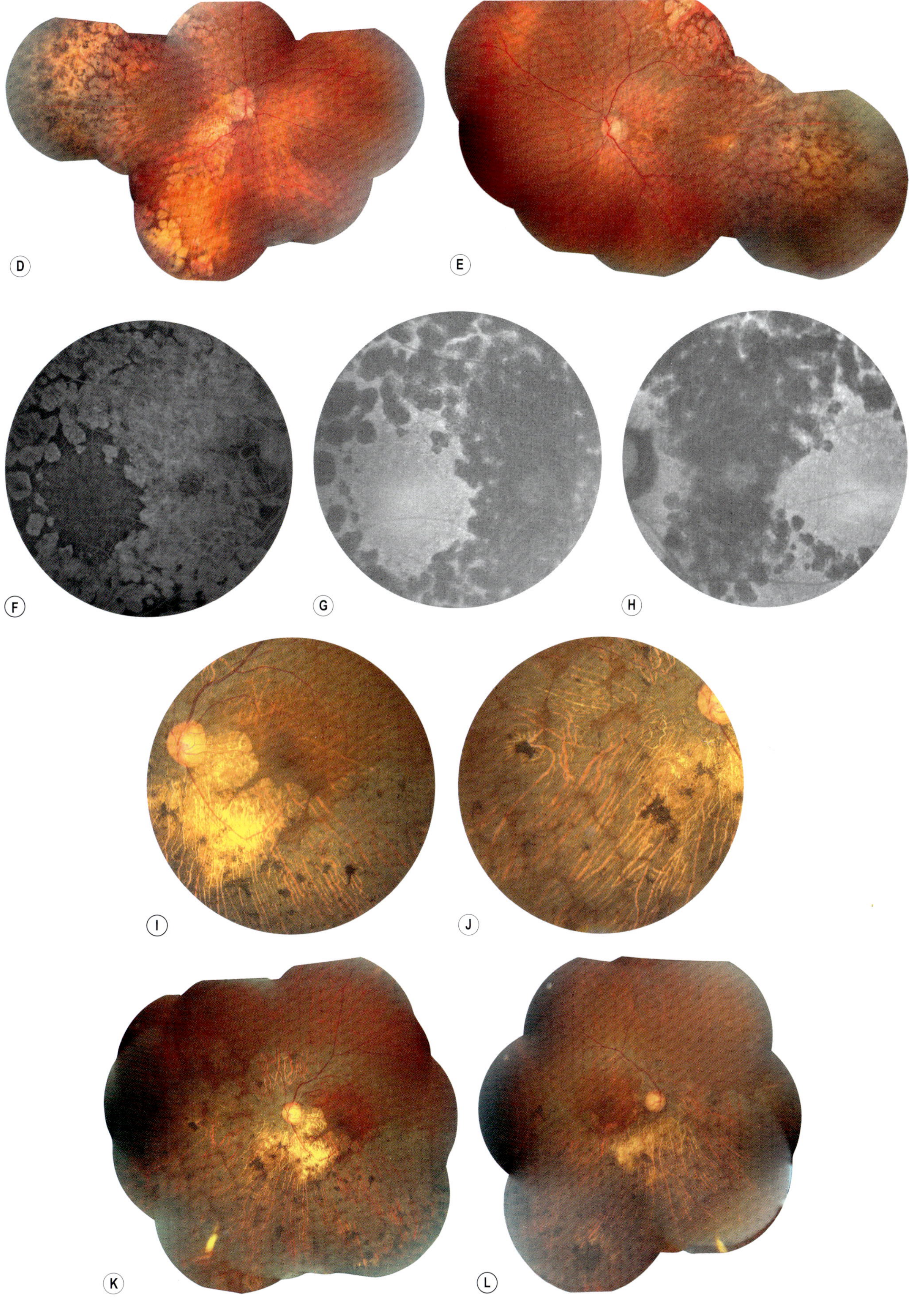
D
E
F
G
H
I
J
K
L

Extensive Macular Atrophy with Pseudo Drusenlike Appearance

Hamel et al. described 18 patients with an onset before age 50 of a rapidly increasing atrophic macular lesion that involves the entire posterior pole up to the arcades, resembling geographic atrophy of age-related macular degeneration (Figure 5.51).[701] This vertically oriented atrophic macular lesion is surrounded by numerous drusenlike deposits (resembling reticular pseudodrusen) found throughout the posterior pole and the midperiphery in all cases (Figure 5.51A–C). All patients also had paving-stone degeneration in the far inferior periphery. No patient developed choroidal neovascularization and the disorder is not familial.

5.51 Macular atrophy with pseudodrusen.

A–F: This 54-year-old white woman had a family history of blindness in the elderly. Onset of symptoms started at age 50 with night blindness, marked photophobia, and difficulty in reading and face recognition at distance. Her visual acuity was right eye: 20/40 with −3.25 sph −1.25 × 170° and left eye: 20/400 with −4.00 sph −1.25 × 180°. Intraocular pressure was 13 mmHg right eye and 12 mmHg left eye. On Goldmann perimetry she had bilateral absolute central scotomas (E, F), and dark adaptation was delayed. Bilateral large macular atrophy with the largest diameter in the vertical axis, and numerous pseudodrusen were seen in the midperiphery (A, B). Optical coherence tomography showed the atrophy of the outer layers of the retina (D). Pseudodrusen were not autofluorescent (C) and were not visible on angiography or on optical coherence tomography.

(Courtesy of Dr. Christian Hamel.[701])

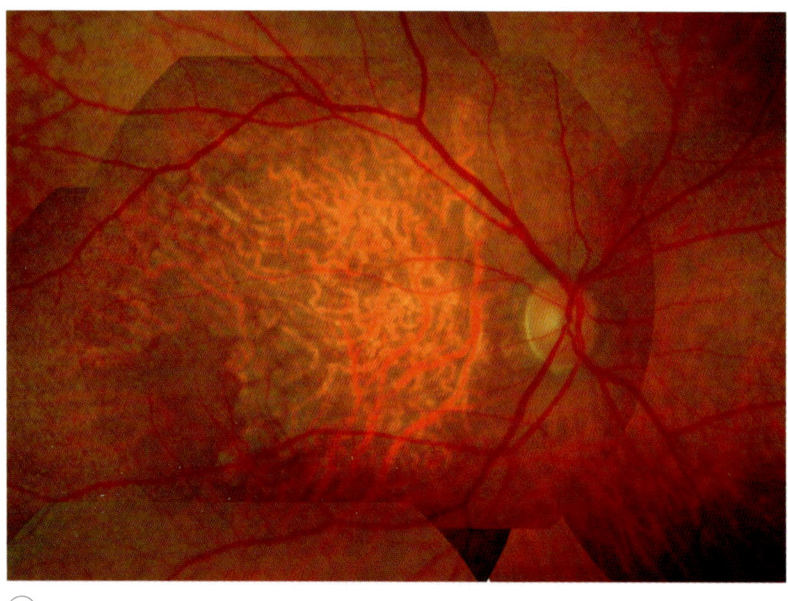

A

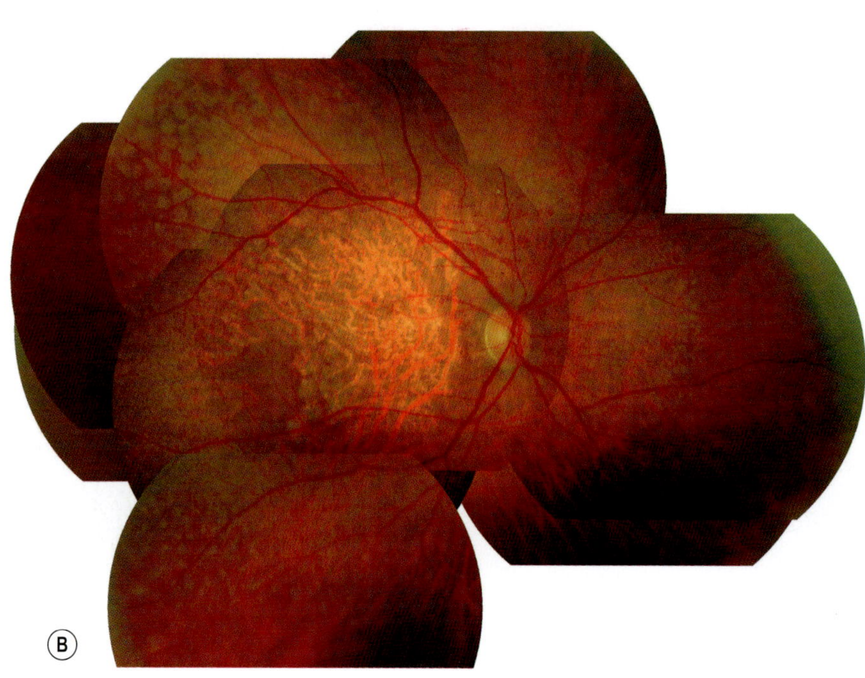

B

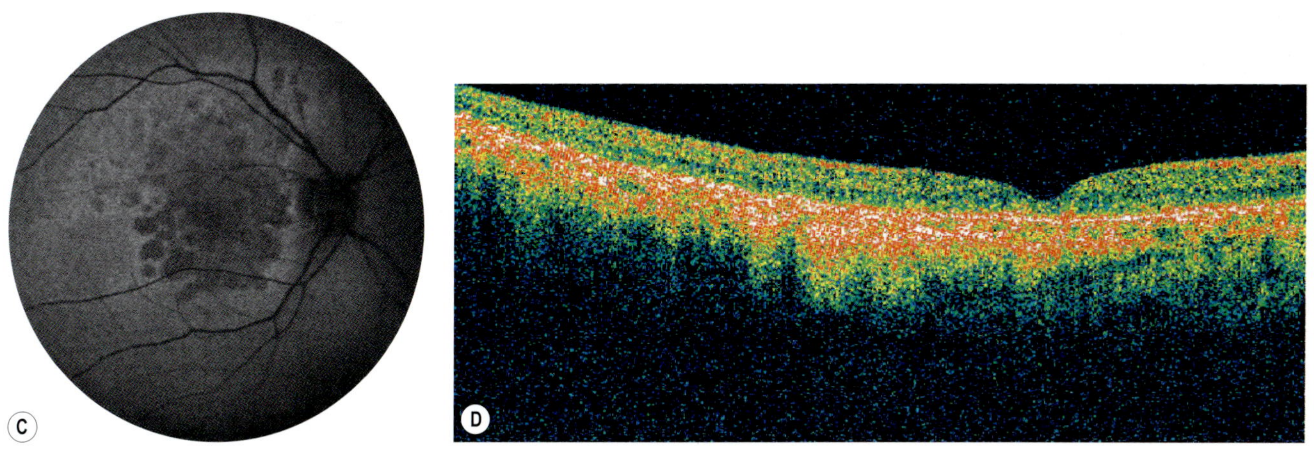
C
D

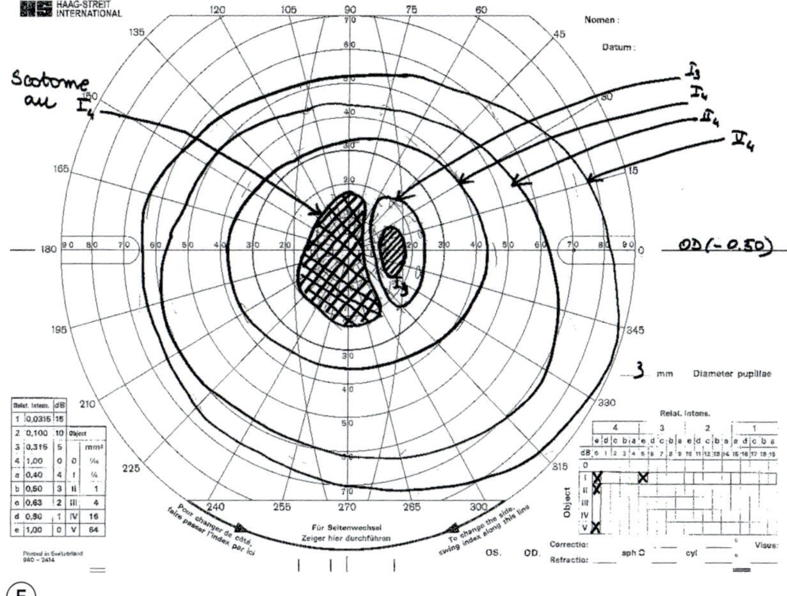
HAAG-STREIT INTERNATIONAL
Nomen:
Datum:
Scotome au I4
I3
I4
II4
V4
OD (-0.50)
3 mm Diameter pupillae
Relat. Intens.
Object
Pour changer de côté, faire passer l'index par ici
Für Seitenwechsel Zeiger hier durchführen
To change the side, swing index along this line
OS.
OD.
Correctio:
Refractio:
Visus:
E

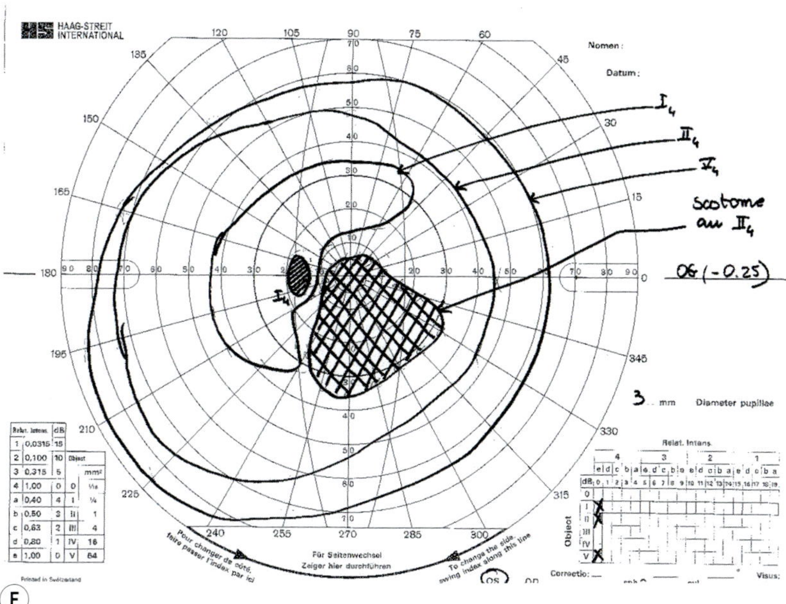
HAAG-STREIT INTERNATIONAL
Nomen:
Datum:
I4
II4
V4
Scotome au II4
I4
OG (-0.25)
3 mm Diameter pupillae
Relat. Intens.
Object
Pour changer de côté, faire passer l'index par ici
Für Seitenwechsel Zeiger hier durchführen
To change the side, swing index along this line
OS
Correctio:
Visus:
F

West Indies Crinkled Retinal Pigment Epitheliopathy

Recently, a novel retinal dystrophy (Figure 5.52) was reported by Cohen et al. (presented at the Macula society annual meeting, February, 2010). All reported patients were black or from black ancestry, and originated in Martinique, a French West Indies island. The disease affected a whole family of an 86-year-old mother and her four children. Two other patients were diagnosed with the condition, one related (cousin) to this family, and one unrelated, but originating from the same geographic area.

The main fundus feature is the presence of a white reticular net located at the level of the RPE, dense in the macular area, but also present in the midperiphery, resembling crackled dry mud (Figure 5.52A–C). Some pigment may be observed within the reticular pattern either in the macula or the periphery. Autofluorescence pattern is variable, with hypoautofluorescence of the white lines (Figure 5.52D). Fluorescein angiography reveals a hyperfluorescent network pattern in the early frames, with late staining (Figure 5.52E–H). Indocyanine green angiography also displays the reticular pattern on late frames (Figure 5.52I). On OCT the RPE appears rippled, giving the crinkled appearance (Figure 5.52J). The etiopathogenesis of the disorder is unclear, be it an acquired or a dystrophic condition. Two patients developed subretinal hemorrhages related to possible polypoidal choroidal vasculopathy. Two patients also had disciform macular scarring which may have been secondary to hemorrhages and/or choroidal neovascularization. Electrophysiology and genetic testing are ongoing.

5.52 West Indies crinkled retinal pigment epitheliopathy.

A and **B**: Composite of right and left eye of a patient with crinkled corrugations of the retinal pigment epithelium appearing as a white reticular net more densely packed in the macular area but extending to the midperiphery, resembling a crackled dry land. Mild pigmentation of the corrugations in the fovea and periphery.

C–I: Left eye of a second patient showing the distinct crinkling (C). The autofluorescence is variable,; most of the wrinkles correspond to hypoautofluorescence suggesting displacement of retinal pigment epithelium (RPE) pigment away from the wrinkles (similar to that seen in chorioretinal folds) (D). Fluorescein angiography revealed the wrinkle to be hyperfluorescent, again suggesting relative lack of pigment within the RPE (E) with late staining (F). Right eye of the same patient showed evidence of choroidal neovascularization with subretinal hemorrhage (G and H). Indocyanine green angiography showed a reticular pattern on late frames, but less distinctly (I). Optical coherence tomography showed that the RPE was thrown into ripples, giving the crinkled appearance (J). Electrophysiology and genetic testing is ongoing.

(Courtesy of Drs. SY Cohen, A Jean-Charles, and H Merle.)

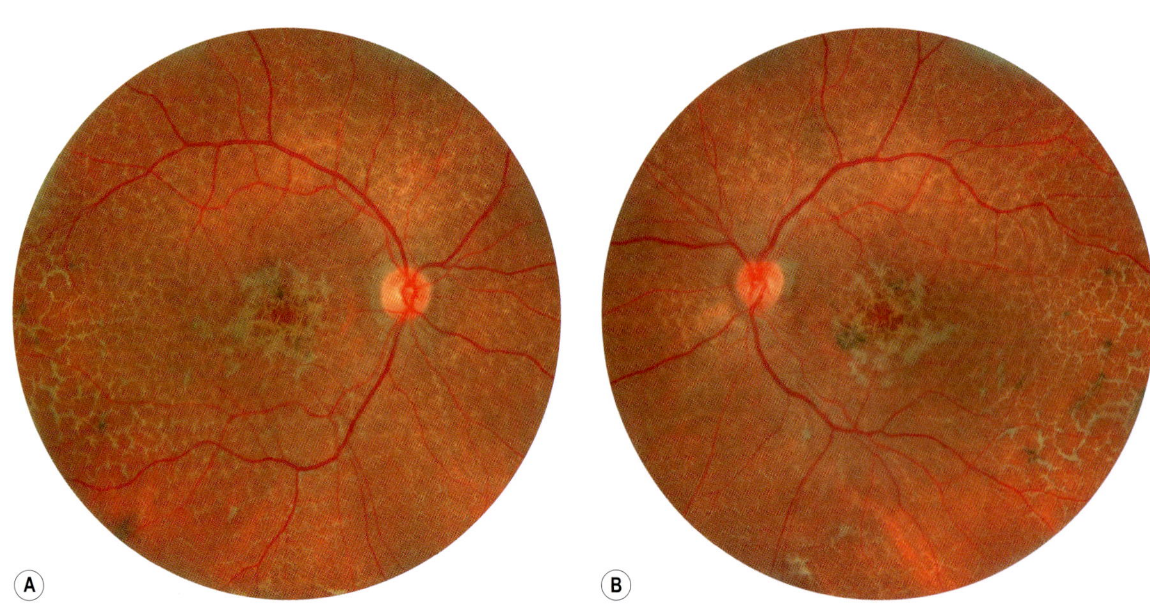

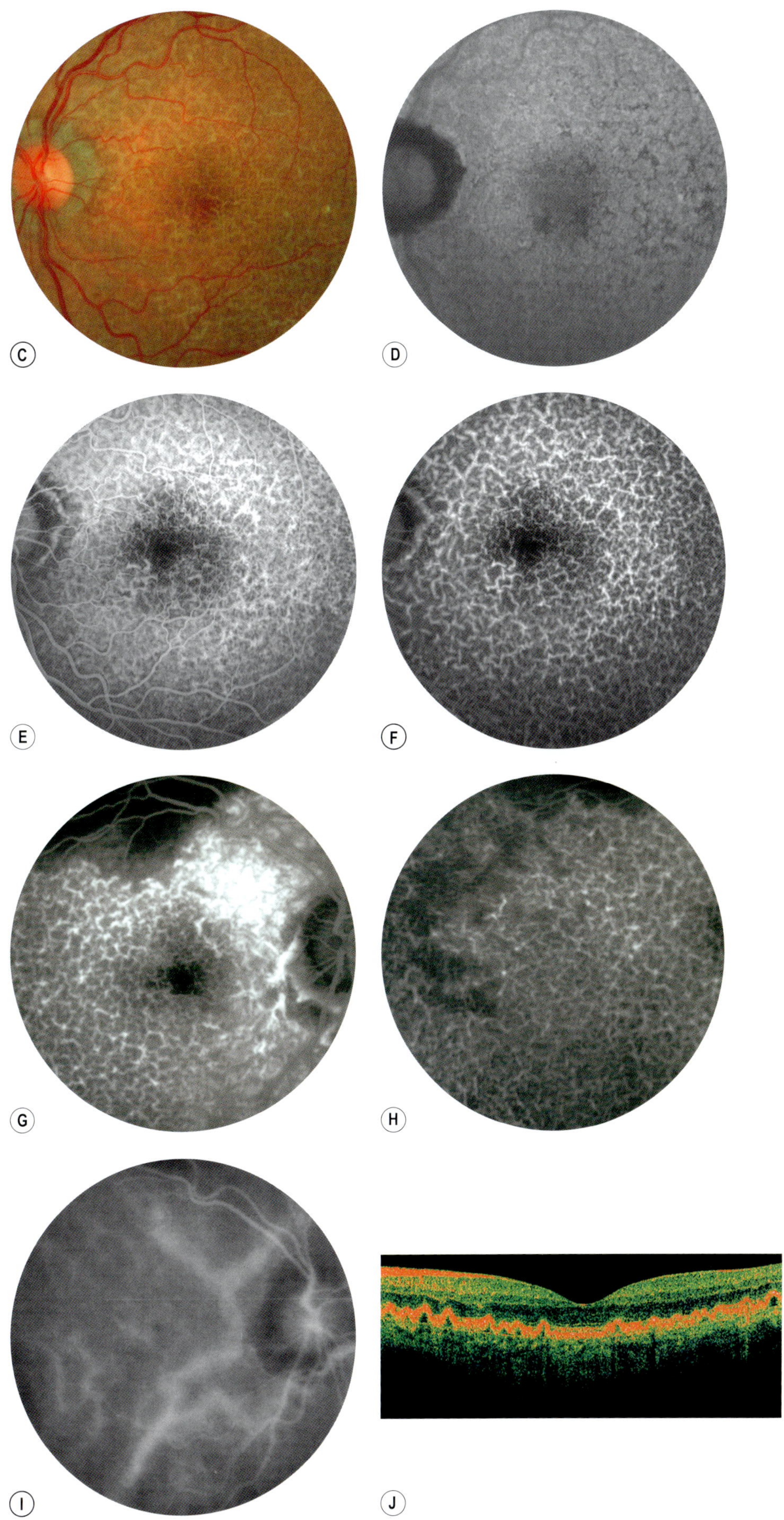
C
D
E
F
G
H
I
J

CHOROIDEREMIA

Choroideremia is a X-linked recessive chorioretinal dystrophy.[702–712] It probably is the same disorder reported previously by some authors as X-linked choroidal sclerosis.[713] Affected males usually note the onset of night blindness between 10 and 30 years of age. Some years later they become aware of loss of peripheral fields. Central vision is affected only in middle or later life. Mottled depigmentation of the RPE may be the only finding initially. Large patches of RPE and choroidal atrophy, however, develop in the midperiphery of the fundus and spread gradually in anterior and posterior directions. Eventually the patient is left with only a small island of relatively normal choroid and RPE in the macular area (Figure 5.53I and J, and 5.54F and L). Choroidal neovascularization may rarely occur.[709] Narrowing of the retinal vessels and optic atrophy accompany the later stages of the disease. Fluorescein angiography during the late stages of the disease demonstrates slowing of the retinal and choroidal circulation, marked loss of the RPE, and choroidal vasculature, but relative preservation of the RPE and the choroidal vessels, including the choriocapillaris in the central macular area (Figure 5.53E). Angiography usually demonstrates the presence of many choroidal vessels that may be difficult to see ophthalmoscopically. Some patients show severe impairment of the photopic functions in dark adaptation. Color vision is essentially normal. The ERG is abnormal early and becomes extinguished usually by midlife.

The female carrier demonstrates normal visual acuity, visual fields, dark adaptation studies, and electroretinographic findings and, with few exceptions, shows characteristic RPE mottling and depigmentation that is most marked in the midperiphery (Figure 5.53B and C, G and H, 5.54E and K). The pigment granules in carriers have been described as being irregularly square in appearance. The pigmentary changes are not associated with abnormalities of either the optic nerve head or retinal vessels. The fundi resemble those seen in rubella retinopathy (see Figure 7.27) and toxic retinopathy caused by thioridazine (see Figure 9.02A) but are different from the streaky iridescent changes in the fundi of some carriers of X-linked retinitis pigmentosa.

It is important to identify these carriers because their sons will have a 50% chance of having choroideremia and their daughters a 50% chance of being carriers of the disease. Some female carriers are known to manifest clinical features of choroideremia, especially later in life due to irregular inactivation of the X chromosome (lyonization).

No known systemic association has been described in patients with choroideremia, except for one male with polydactyly, which was caused by an autosomal-dominant inheritance of polydactyly on his paternal side. He had normal growth, normal mentation, and no evidence of hypogonadism.[714]

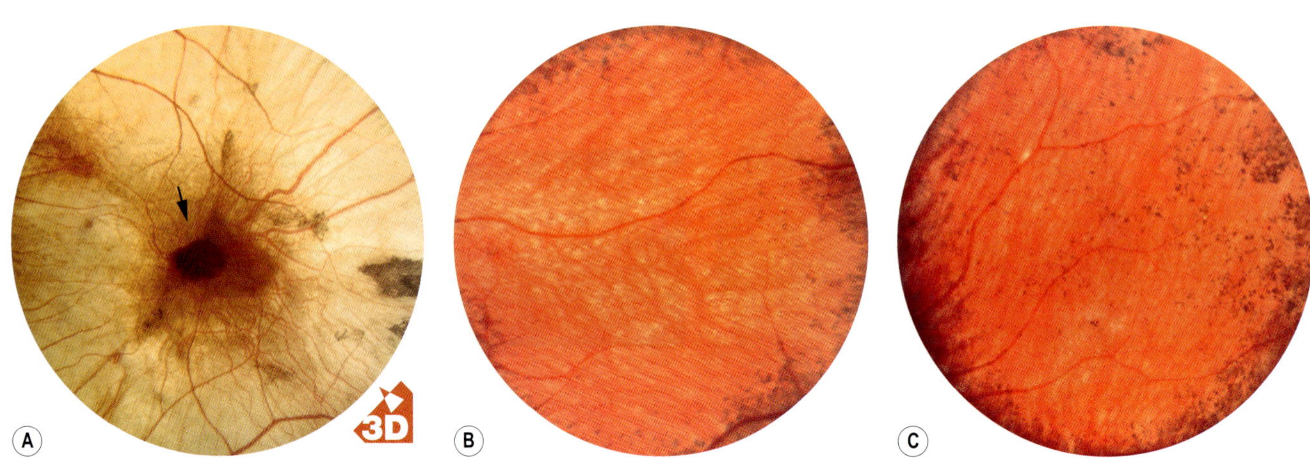

5.53 Choroideremia.

A: A 33-year-old man with visual acuity of 20/40 in the right eye and 20/200 in the left eye had extensive atrophy of the choroid and retinal pigment epithelium (RPE) in both eyes. There was preservation of some of the RPE centrally (arrow, A). The retinal vessels were narrowed.

B and C: Carrier state of choroideremia with widespread mottling of the RPE throughout the fundus of a 9-year-old girl with normal visual acuity. Her father had choroideremia. Her electro-oculographic and electroretinographic findings were normal.

D and E: Choroideremia in a 34-year-old man. Visual acuity was 20/25 in the right eye and 20/20 in the left eye. His electroretinogram was extinguished. His brother was similarly affected. Two sisters had pigmentary changes in the fundi but normal visual function.

F–J: This 34-year-old woman complained of mild metamorphopsia in her right eye. Visual acuity was 20/25 in the right eye and 20/20 in the left eye. She gave a history of "retinitis pigmentosa" associated with long-standing nyctalopia in her father. Both eyes had stippled pigmentation resembling "cracked clay" (F–H). Her visual fields were full, and electroretinogram was normal in both eyes. A diagnosis of carrier state of choroideremia was made and father asked to be evaluated. Father had diffuse loss of pigment in the fundus with preservation of the RPE in the fovea, narrowed retinal arteries, severely constricted visual fields and a visual acuity of 20/60 in each eye (I and J). The findings were typical of choroideremia.

(L-J, Also, Yannuzzi, Lawrence J., The Retinal Atlas, Saunders 2010, 978-0-7020-3320-9, p.148.)

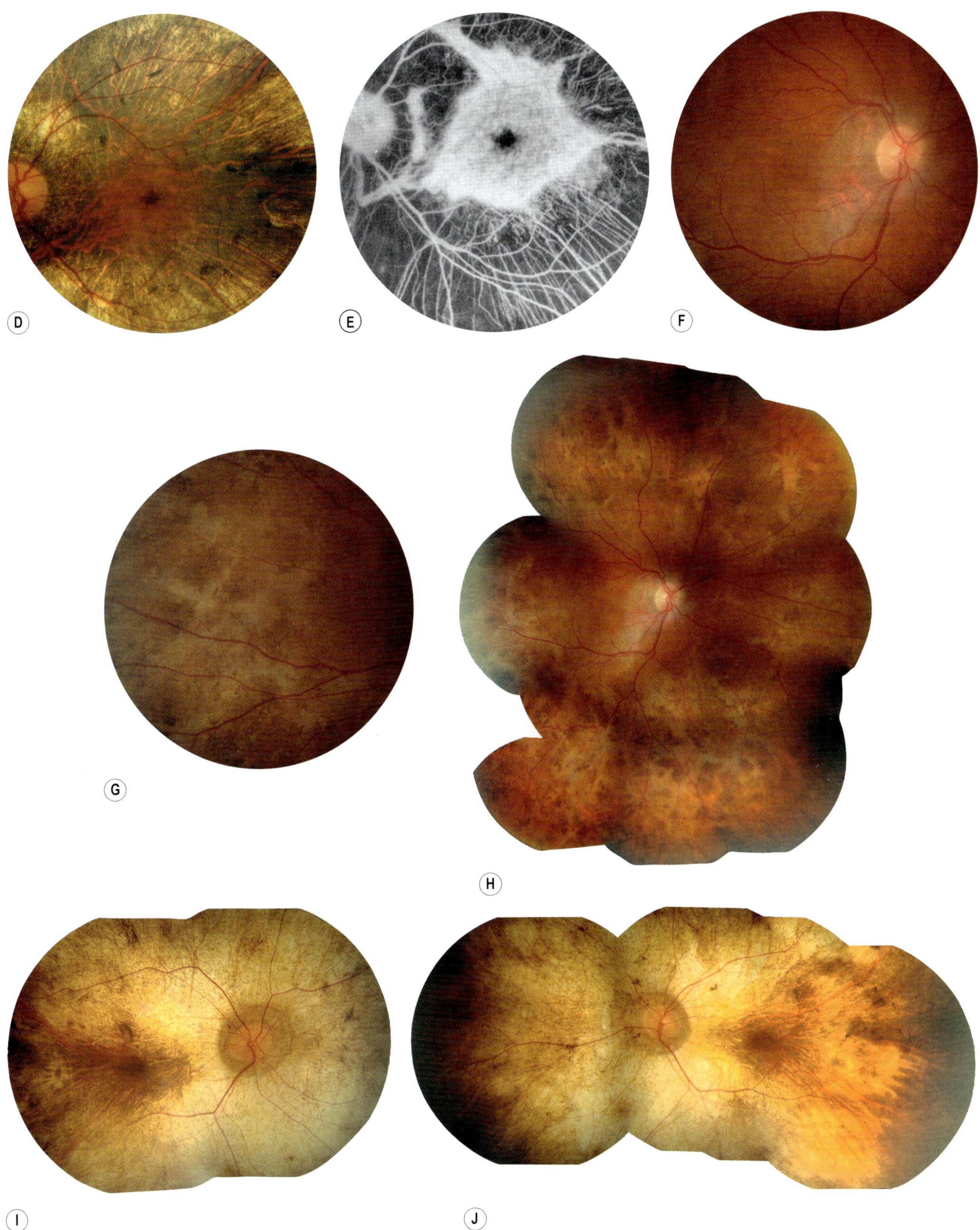
D
E
F
G
H
I
J

Choroideremia is caused by mutations in the *CHM* gene localized to the long arm of X-chromosome (Xq21.2). The mutation affects the production of Rab escort protein isoform 1 (REP-1), previously known as component A of Rab geranylgeranyltransferase (GGTase), the enzyme that plays a key role in the activation of Rab proteins that are responsible for the regulation of exocytic and endocytic cellular pathways. They control the protein trafficking of secretory and endocytic pathways. A reduction in particular of activated Rab27a by preferential binding by REP-1 is implicated in choroideremia.[715–718] Several types of mutation in the *CHM* gene, including point deletions, large basepair deletions, splice site substitutions, and translocations, have been associated with the clinical findings of choroideremia. Though these patients lack REP-1 in all other cells too, the retina and choroid are the only structures affected in choroideremia; it is believed that REP-2, that resembles REP-1 to about 75% is enough to activate Rab proteins in cells outside the retina and choroid.[719]

DNA analysis of chorionic villi obtained during pregnancy permits prenatal exclusion of choroideremia.[720]

Histopathologic examination during the late stages of the disease reveals atrophy of the choroid, RPE, and overlying retina with relative sparing of the macula and periphery.[704,705,707,710,712,721] Ultrastructurally, the curvilinear trilaminar structures within macrophages in the RPE and outer retina are similar to those seen in abetalipoproteinemia.[710]

5.54 Choroideremia.

A–L: A 15-year-old boy was found to have mild visual field constriction on a routine Humphrey field test done at an optometrist's office. His visual acuity was 20/20 in each eye. There was diffuse loss of pigment in the fundus in each eye sparing the central macula. Small pigment clumps were seen here and there in the fundus (A–C). His 8-year-old half-brother was also asymptomatic and had fine pigment stippling in the fovea and moderate loss of pigment in the midperiphery and anterior fundus in each eye (D). Their 40-year-old mother was asymptomatic with 20/20 vision and an almost normal fundus appearance (E). Their 75-year-old maternal grandfather had lost his right eye to advanced glaucoma, and the left fundus showed complete absence of pigment, narrowed retinal vessels and a visual acuity of 20/400. The fundus 3 years later showed further loss of retinal pigment in both half-brothers (G–J), normal pigmentation in their carrier mother (K), and complete absence of retinal pigment in their grandfather (L).

(G and H, Also, Yannuzzi, Lawrence J., The Retinal Atlas, Saunders 2010, 978-0-7020-3320-9, p.147.)

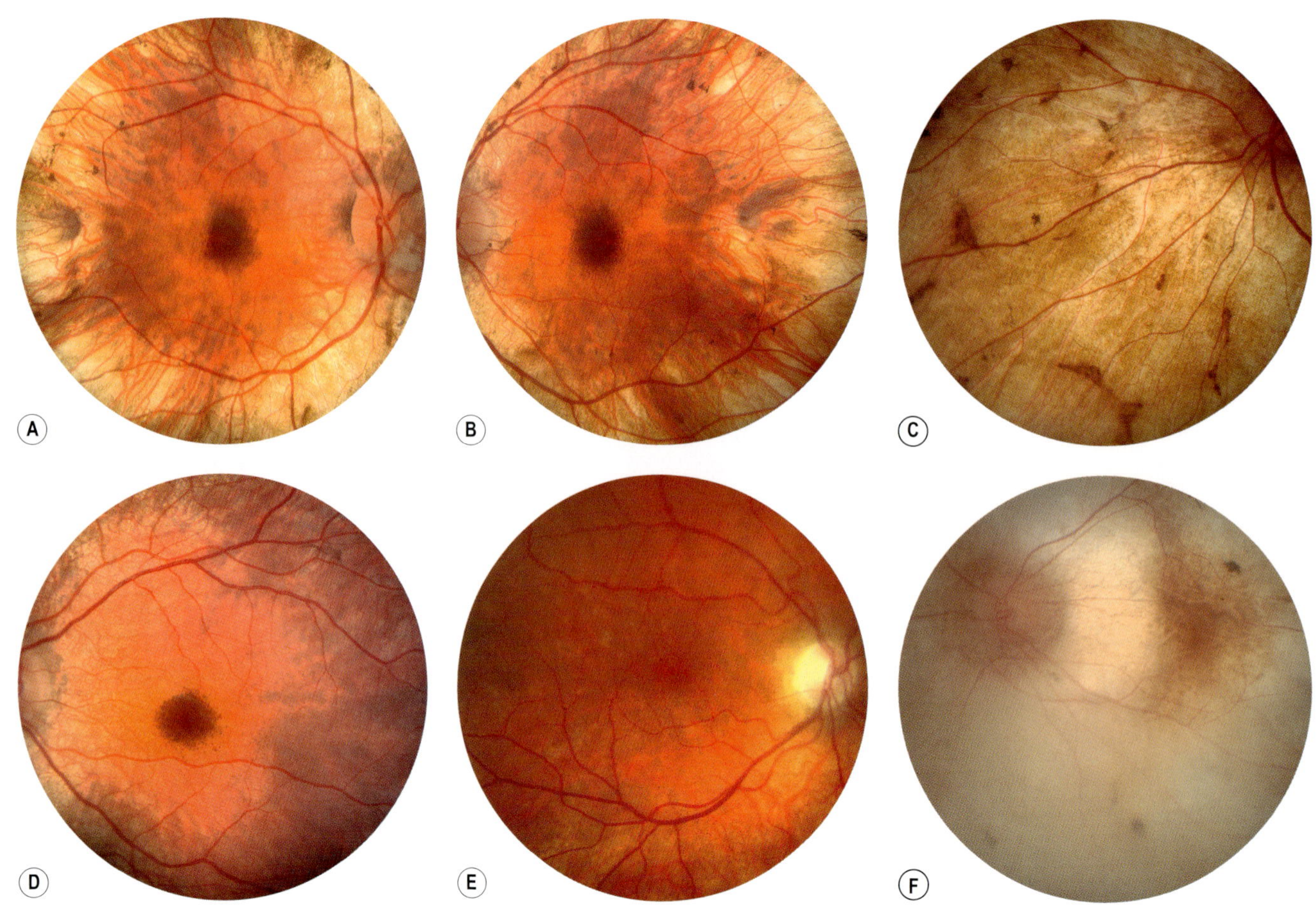

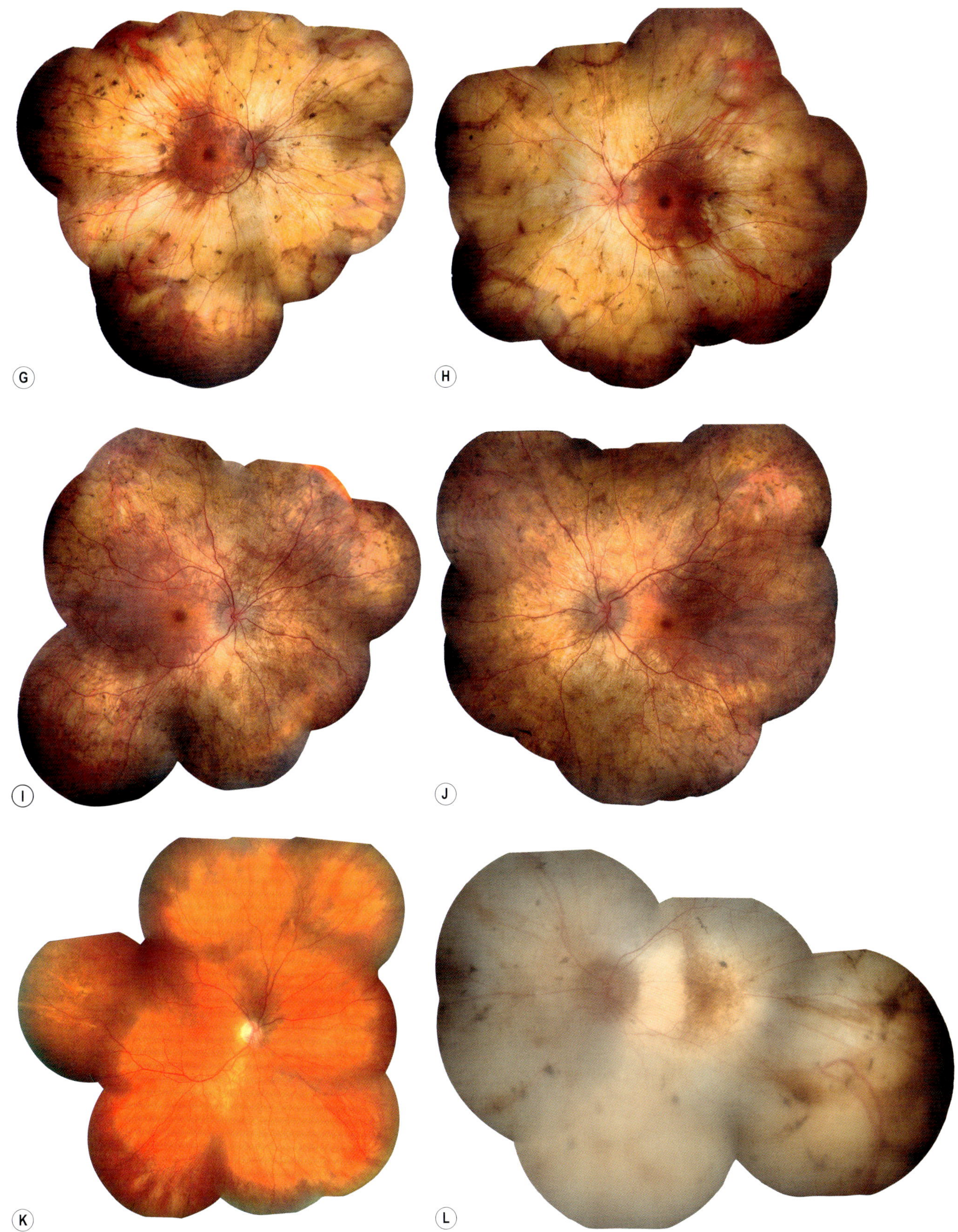
G
H
I
J
K
L

CONE–ROD DYSTROPHIES (INVERSE PIGMENTARY RETINAL DYSTROPHY)

Loss of central and color vision and development of nyctalopia, usually early in life, are the hallmarks of cone–rod dystrophy.[248,347,507,725–731] The onset of symptoms may not begin until adulthood (Figure 5.56A). Initially some patients may manifest only clinical and electrophysiologic evidence of cone dystrophy (see p. 306). In the beginning the RPE in the macular area may be normal (Figure 5.56F and G). Later, mottling of the pigment in the macula along with slight narrowing of the retinal vessels occur. The pigmentary changes progress and may or may not be associated with bone spicules in the periphery. A bull's-eye-like pattern of pigmentary derangement frequently develops centrally followed later by temporal pallor and capillary telangiectasis of the optic disc (Figure 5.56A, B, E, and H).[507] The ERG, however, usually reveals markedly abnormal or absent cone responses and reduced rod responses. It may become extinguished. The EOG is flat. These patients show severe abnormalities of color vision. There may be some value to subclassification of these patients into groups depending upon the relative severity of the reduction of cone versus rod ERG amplitudes.[732,733] Vitreous fluorophotometry is less likely to be abnormal in these patients than those with typical retinitis pigmentosa.[729]

Cone–rod dystrophies are a heterogeneous group of inherited disorders. They may be inherited by all three main modes. The four major causative genes in the pathogenesis of cone–rod dystrophies are *ABCA4* (which causes Stargardt disease and also 30–60% of autosomal-recessive cone–rod dystrophies), *CRX* and *GUCY2D* (which are responsible for many reported cases of autosomal-dominant cone–rod dystrophies and cone dystrophies), and *RPGR* (which causes about two-thirds of X-linked retinitis pigmentosa and also an undetermined percentage of X-linked cone–rod dystrophies).[734] It occasionally is associated with neurologic disease (Figure 5.56F–I). Rabb et al. reported the clinicopathologic findings in a patient with cone–rod dystrophy.[735] They can also be part of a syndrome such as Bardet–Biedl and SCA 7. A similar disease in baboons and Rdy cats has been studied by light and electron microscopy.[725–727,736] Deletion mapping of a cone–rod dystrophy resulted in assignment to 18q211.[737]

5.56 Cone–rod dystrophy.

A–C: Sporadic late onset of cone–rod dystrophy in this 31-year-old man with a 27-year history of nyctalopia and a 1-year history of visual loss. Visual acuity, which at the age of 28 was 20/20, was now 20/400 in the right eye (A) and 20/20 in the left eye (B). His electroretinographic findings revealed severely abnormal rod and cone responses.

D and **E**: Early-onset cone–rod dystrophy in a 12-year-old boy with peripheral bone corpuscular changes in the retina and a nonrecordable electroretinogram. His visual acuity was 20/200. A brother had similar findings. Note bull's-eye pattern of retinal pigment epithelium (RPE) atrophy.

F–I: Cone dystrophy, probably progressing to a cone–rod dystrophy, in a 17-year-old female with progressive spinocerebellar degeneration and spastic quadriplegia. She noted progressive loss of vision beginning at age 14 years. Her visual acuity was 20/200. An electroretinogram showed markedly abnormal cone function and normal rod function. Her fundi (F) and angiography (G) were within normal limits. At 22 years of age, her vision had decreased further and there was narrowing of the retinal vessels and widespread RPE changes (H). Angiography (I) revealed a bull's-eye pattern of hyperfluorescence in the macula of both eyes and evidence of diffuse atrophy of the RPE.

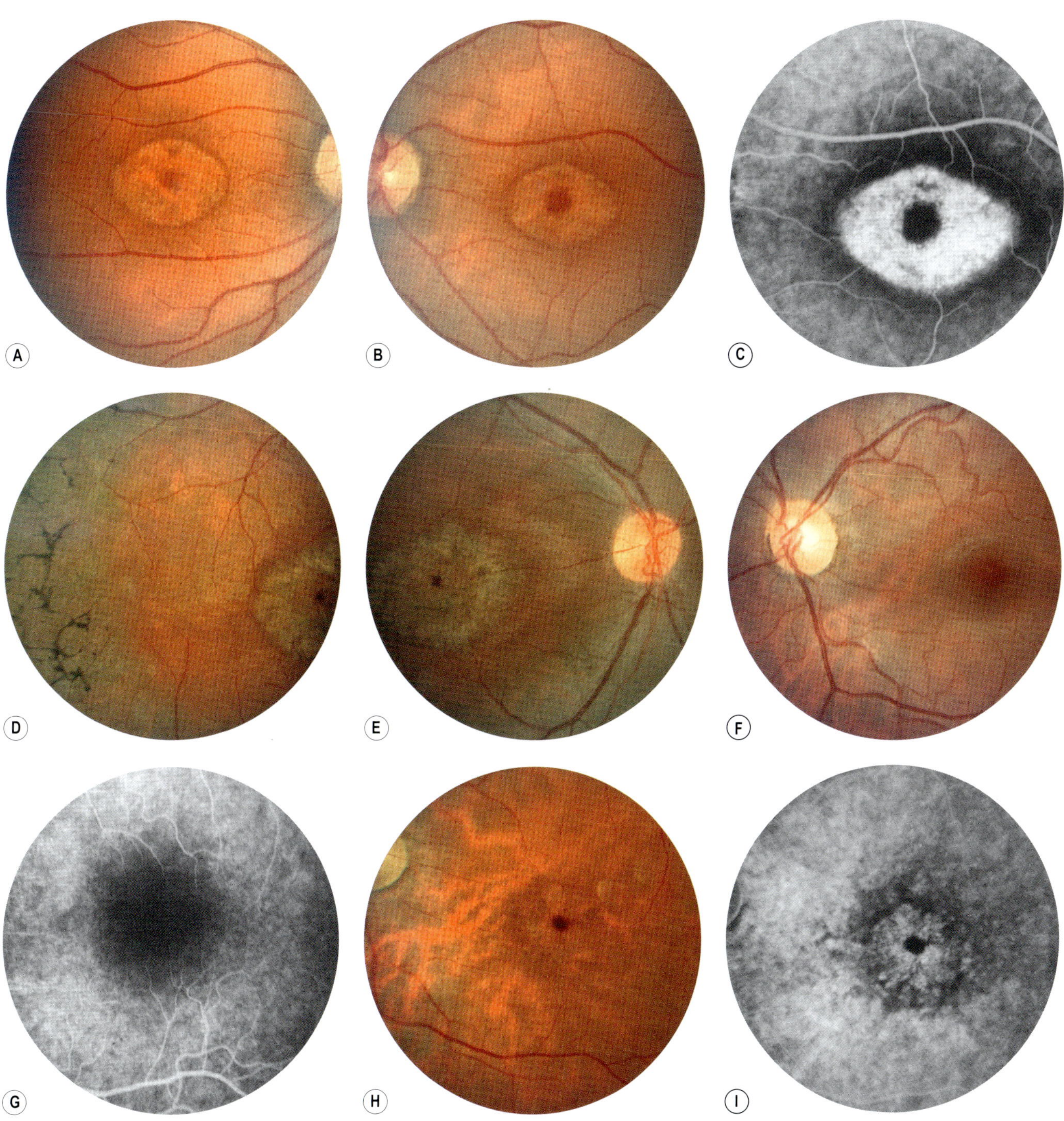
A
B
C
D
E
F
G
H
I

Goldmann–Favre Syndrome (Enhanced S-Cone Syndrome)

Goldmann–Favre syndrome (hyaloideotapetoretinal degeneration) is an autosomal-recessive disease characterized by night blindness, atypical peripheral pigmentary dystrophy, central and peripheral retinoschisis, complicated cataract at an early age, optically empty vitreous with an occasional vitreous band, and a markedly abnormal, often nonrecordable, ERG.[738–744] In addition to narrowing of the retinal vessels and waxy pallor of the disc, the macula appears diffusely thickened by prominent superficially located macrocysts that fail to stain on fluorescein angiographic study (Figure 5.57C, E, and F). Giant macular schisis and cyst formation can be confirmed on OCT testing (Figure 5.57J–L). There have been reports of benefit with oral acetazolamide in decreasing the macular thickness in patients with enhanced S-cone syndrome.

Cases of night blindness and peripheral retinoschisis without macular schisis occur.[745] Histopathologic examination of a peripheral biopsy specimen in one case showed nonspecific degeneration of the sensory retinal layers, thickened retinal vessel basement membranes, areas of retinal vascular occlusion, preretinal glial membranes, and choroidal vascular changes.[744] Some patients with Goldmann–Favre syndrome demonstrate relatively enhanced S-cone function electrophysiologically identical to that found in the enhanced S-cone syndrome.[746–750] These latter patients have night blindness, maculopathy (often cystoid), degenerative changes with partly pigmented yellow flecks in the region of the major vascular arcades, relatively mild visual field loss, slow progression, and a characteristic ERG.[750] The dark-adapted ERG shows no response to low-intensity stimuli that normally activate the rods but large, slow responses to high-intensity stimuli. The large, slow waveforms persist without change under light adaptation and show a striking mismatch to photopically balanced short- and long-wavelength stimuli, with sensitivity much greater to short than to long wavelengths. It is possible that patients with Goldmann–Favre syndrome and those with enhanced S-cone syndrome, some of whom do not have macular schisis, are not distinct entities but are simply two identifiable phenotypes of clinical expression of a retinal degenerative disease with a single pattern of retinal dysfunction. Patients with both syndromes have been observed in the same family.[748] There is evidence that patients with the enhanced S-cone syndrome have a retinal dysgenesis that probably occurs during the early development of the retina and results in many more S-cones that form in the place of many L/M-cones and rods.[746] Many of the clinical and functional characteristics of enhanced S-cone syndrome, e.g., the negative waveform, reduced oscillatory potentials, retinoschisis, and vitreous changes, may be consequences of this early abnormality in the complex development sequence of the retina.[746] Both patients illustrated in Figure 5.57 (A–F) reported in previous editions of this atlas as examples of Goldmann–Favre syndrome were recalled and both have enhanced S-cone syndrome.

Mutations in *NR2E3* which encodes a photoreceptor nuclear receptor are responsible for enhanced S-cone syndrome, Goldmann–Favre syndrome, and clumped pigmentary retinopathy.[751–757]

5.57 Goldmann–Favre syndrome (enhanced S-cone syndrome).

A–C: This 19-year-old boy's visual acuity in the right eye was 20/50 and J-1 and in the left eye was 10/200. He had a mid zonal scotoma. There were extensive schisis and large cystoid changes of the entire macular region (A). There was a broad mid zonal area of atrophy of the retinal pigment epithelium associated with some migration of pigment and narrowing of the retinal vessels (B). There was no peripheral retinoschisis. Fluorescein angiography (C) was within normal limits. There was no leakage of dye in the late stages of angiography. His electroretinogram showed absent photopic responses and markedly abnormal scotopic responses. His color vision was normal (Farnsworth D-15).

D–F: Goldmann–Favre disease in a 12-year-old boy complaining of mild loss of vision. His family history was negative. Visual acuity was 20/40 in the right eye and 20/100 in the left eye. He had retinal thickening and cystic changes throughout the macular areas (D). There were ill-defined subretinal white flecks (arrows, D and E) in the perimacular area. Angiography revealed focal areas of hyperfluorescence corresponding with the flecks (arrow, E and F). There was no evidence of intraretinal staining. An electroretinogram showed severely abnormal rod and cone function. The electro-oculographic findings were markedly abnormal. Eight years later the fundi were unchanged. Visual acuity was 20/400 and J-3 in the right eye and 20/300 and J-2 in the left eye.

G–L: This present 30-year-old male was examined by Dr. Gass at age 19 with a history of running into bushes when the child got out of the car in the dark for the previous 10 years. At that time he carried a diagnosis of juvenile macular schisis in both eyes. He was found to have a disciform scar in the macula of the right eye and extensive schisis in the macula of the left eye rephotographed at age 30 (G and H). He also had pigmented nummular lesions (arrow) sourrounding the arcades in each eye (I and J). The retinal vessels were of reasonable caliber and no bone spicule pigment migration was visible in either eye. A diagnosis of Goldmann–Favre (enhanced S-cone dystrophy) disease was made by Dr. Gass. Optical coherence tomography shows a scar from involuted choroidal neovascular membrane in the right eye with collapsed schisis and extensive schisis of the left macula extending up to the arcades (K and L).

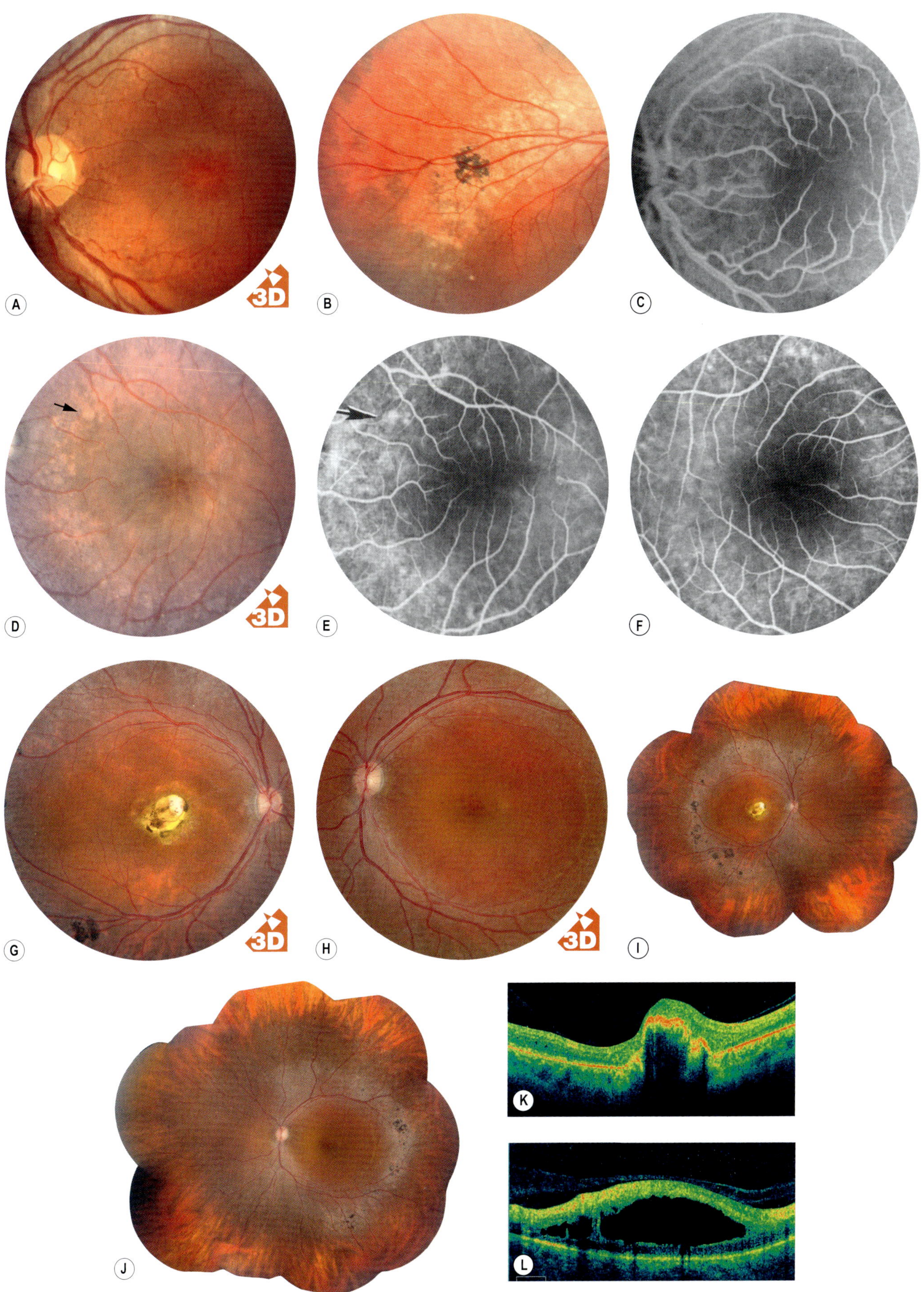
A
3D
B
C
D
3D
E
F
G
3D
H
3D
I
J
K
L

Familial Foveal Retinoschisis

Foveal retinoschisis, which is characterized by a delicate network of radiating cystic changes in the superficial retina and confined generally to the foveal area, is the hallmark of X-linked juvenile retinoschisis and should be differentiated from macular schisis, which is composed of a more coarse pattern of larger cystoid spaces that may extend throughout most of the macular area and is the hallmark of Goldmann–Favre syndrome. With rare exceptions,[758,759] familial foveal retinoschisis is found only in males.[758,760–776] The macula is involved in all cases, and many patients demonstrate evidence of widespread changes in the retina and RPE.

X-Linked Juvenile Retinoschisis

A constant diagnostic feature of X-linked juvenile retinoschisis, which is present at birth or soon afterward in all affected males, is a characteristic macular lesion referred to as "foveal schisis" (Figure 5.58A, C, G, J, and L and 5.59A–C, E–G). Only 50% of patients will have evidence of peripheral retinoschisis or related findings, mostly in the inferotemporal quadrant (Figure 5.58A, B, J, and K). There may be large oval or round holes in the inner retinal layers creating "vitreous veils" (Figure 5.58B). Retinal blood vessels may or may not accompany the inner retinal layer. Unsupported retinal vessels may course into the vitreous cavity. Semitranslucent gray-white arborescent scrolls, a dendriform pattern of occluded retinal vessels (Figure 5.58H), silver-gray glistening patches on the retinal surface, perivascular cuffing, chorioretinal scars, vitreous detachment, intraretinal gray-white spots (Figure 5.58G), intraretinal blood cysts, and evidence of recent or old vitreous hemorrhage are other findings that may be present. Nasal dragging of the retina may be present in infancy and is presumed to be related to temporal dehiscence of the nerve fiber layer.[777] Retinal and optic disc neovascularization may occur.[776,778] Usually these patients are initially seen during the early school years, either because of reading difficulty or because of symptoms of vitreous hemorrhage. An occasional patient may be seen early in life because of a massive area of schisis that partly or completely obstructs the pupillary space.

5.58 X-linked juvenile retinoschisis.

A and B: Typical radiating inner retinal cysts associated with foveal schisis in a boy with peripheral retinoschisis and large holes in the inner retinal layers.
C and D: Foveomacular schisis in a 24-year-old man who first noted decreased vision at age 5 years. Visual acuity was 20/30. Angiography showed minimal changes in the retinal pigment epithelium.
E and F: Cystic changes simulating foveal retinoschisis in a 7-year-old boy with a rhegmatogenous retinal detachment. These disappeared after a scleral buckling procedure.
G–I: Foveal and peripheral retinoschisis in a 14-year-old boy with widespread intraretinal gray-white spots and sheathed and occluded peripheral retinal vessels. There were large holes in the inner retinal layers temporally in the right eye.
J–L: Twenty-two-year follow-up of X-linked juvenile retinoschisis in a patient who was age 15 years with visual acuity of 20/60 bilaterally when first seen with foveomacular schisis (J and K). Visual acuity at last examination was 20/200 right eye and 20/80 left eye. There was minimal change in the fundi (L).

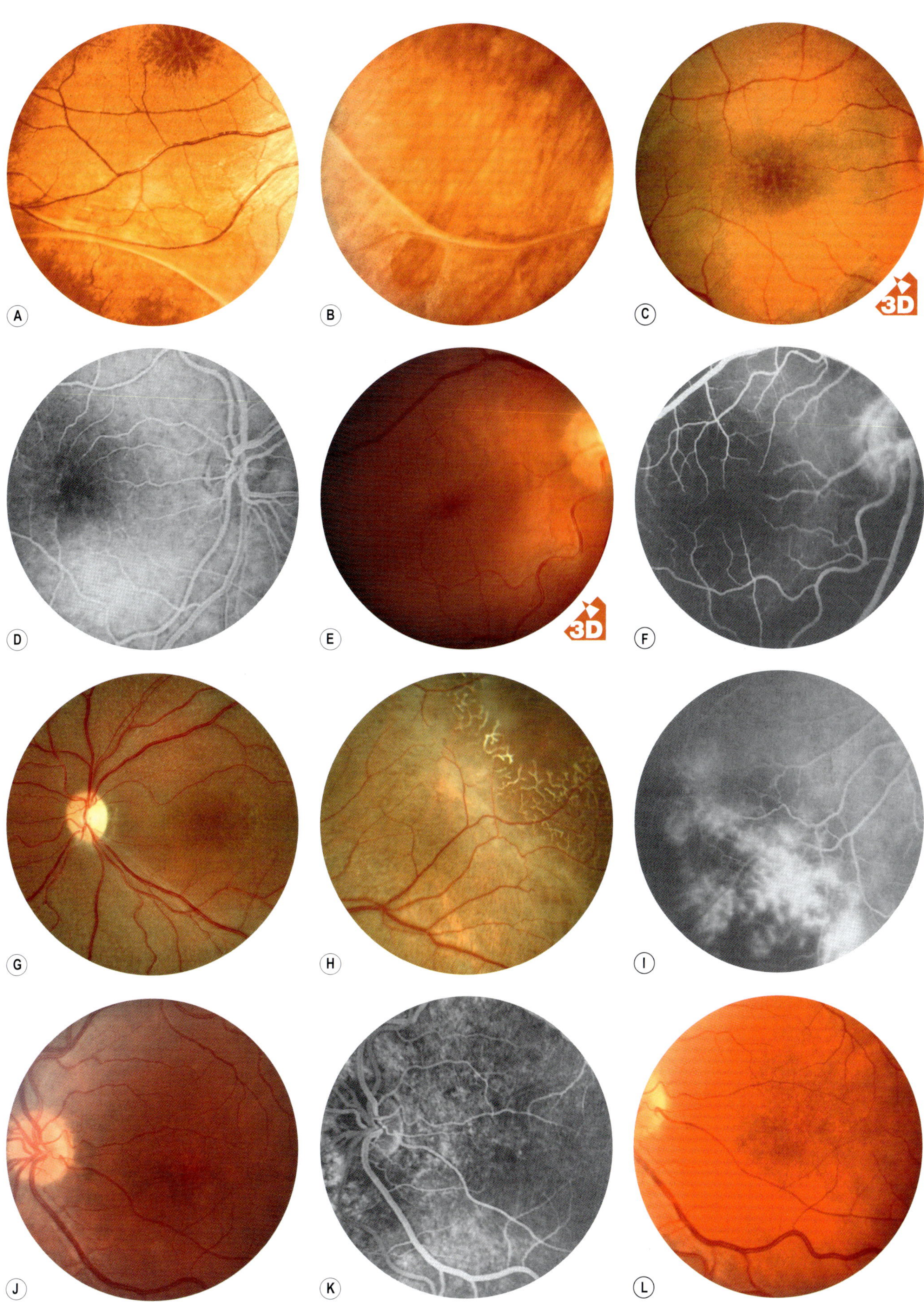
A
B
C
3D
D
E
3D
F
G
H
I
J
K
L

Biomicroscopically, foveal schisis presents a characteristic picture of small superficially located cysts arranged in a stellate pattern and radial striae centered in the foveal area (Figures 5.58A, C, G, J, and L and 5.59C, E, F, and G). The central cysts often have a fusiform shape. Additional cysts become evident more peripherally. This is associated with some elevation of the inner portion of the retina. A peculiar sheen develops on the retinal surface. This occasionally may present a golden tapetal reflex and the Mizuo–Nakamura phenomenon.[779] Eventually the cyst walls may coalesce and form a large central schisis cavity. This is followed in some cases in adulthood by disappearance of the cystic changes, alterations in the underlying RPE, and finally development of a nonspecific atrophic macular lesion. Some patients demonstrate corrugations of the outer retina either in the temporal macula, or more extensively throughout the fundus. These corrugations appear to be at the photoreceptor and outer plexiform layers and are known to change in orientation and shape over time, and sometimes may disappear altogether. Two brothers are shown in Figure 5.59. The younger sibling, who became symptomatic first, lost the corrugations over 5 years (Figure 5.59B and K). Whether the change in height and tautness of the schisis cavity impart forces to the temporal retinal to cause these corrugations is a hypothesis.[779a]

Some patients show progressive narrowing of the retinal vessels and develop peripheral changes of pigmentary retinal dystrophy. In childhood the RPE may be normal (Figure 5.58C and D) or may be diffusely or irregularly depigmented (Figure 5.58J and K). Rhegmatogenous detachment infrequently occurs, and spontaneous reattachment may occur. Rupture of a superficial retinal neovascular tuft within the area of schisis may cause either vitreous hemorrhage or bleeding into a peripheral retinal cyst.[773] Most vitreous hemorrhages resolve spontaneously. Anomalous vascular looping or branching on the optic disc is common.

Most of the changes occurring in X-linked juvenile retinoschisis occur during the first two decades of life.[780] Visual acuity often stabilizes at 20/50–20/100. The peripheral visual field is affected only when peripheral schisis is present.

On fluorescein angiography the posterior fundus is frequently normal (Figure 5.58D). In some patients there may be diffuse mottled hyperfluorescence indicative of extensive pigmentary changes present throughout the retina (Figure 5.32J and K). Patients with evidence of peripheral schisis may show leakage of dye from the retinal vessels within the area of schisis, as well as adjacent areas (Figure 5.58I). Evidence of nonperfusion of segments of the retina may be present. OCT demonstrates the cavities with vertical pillars separating them from each other (Figure 5.59H1 and H2). Dark adaptation is usually normal or minimally affected. Electroretinography typically shows abnormal b-wave and normal a-wave amplitudes, prolonged b-wave latencies and implicit times, reduced oscillatory potential generated by either rods or cones, and reduced 30-Hz flicker response.[781,782] The findings are probably partly dependent upon the severity of the retinoschisis and the age of the patient. Electro-oculographic studies are usually normal in young patients.They may be subnormal in patients with severe involvement of the RPE.

5.59 X-linked juvenile retinoschisis and outer retinal corrugations.

This 12-year-old male (sibling A) had a best-corrected visual acuity of 20/60 in each eye. There were cystic changes in the fovea in both eyes, more prominent on the right (A) than the left. In addition corrugations of the outer retina were likened to "flying seagulls" temporal to the schisis cavity in his left eye (B). His mother's eye examination was normal. His vision gradually worsened over 5 years to the 20/200 level. Five years later his brother older by 2 years (sibling B) noted a rapid change in vision and could not be corrected with his contact lenses beyond 20/40. He had foveal schisis in both eyes associated with similar outer retinal corrugations, in his right eye (C and E). The schisis cavity was not detected by fluorescein angiography, while the corrugations were mildly fluorescent (D, arrow). Over the next year the corrugations changed in shape in his right eye and appeared in the left eye (arrows, F and G). Optical coherence tomography (OCT) of both maculas showed schisis cavity in multiple layers (H1 and H2). OCT through the corrugations showed them to be in the outer retina with processes of the photoreceptors and external limiting membrane (arrows, I1 and I2). Sibling A now had lost the retinal corrugations in his left eye, the schisis was more widespread in both eyes (J and K), and the OCT showed schisis cavity on the left was larger (L).[779a]

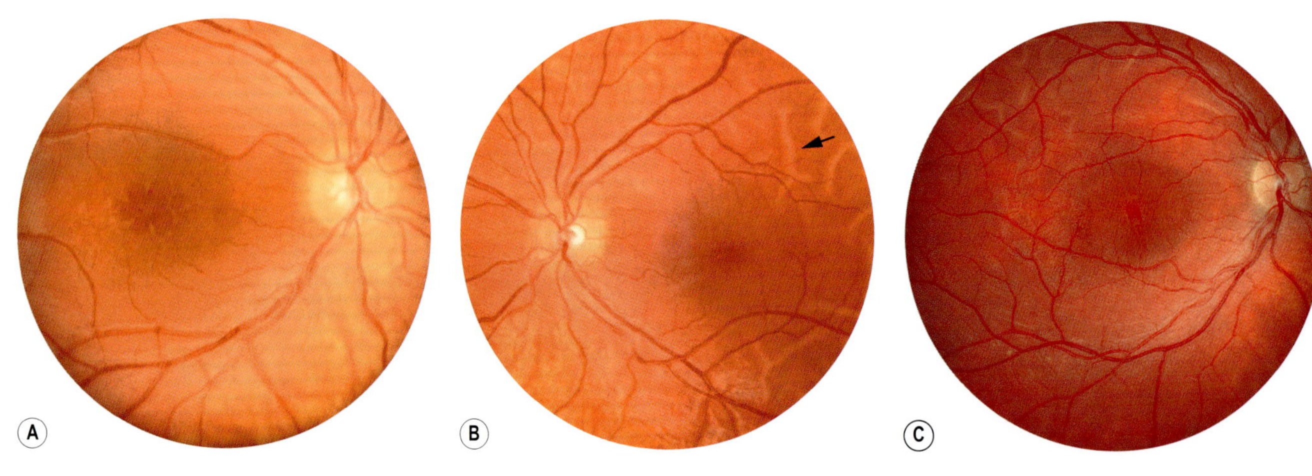

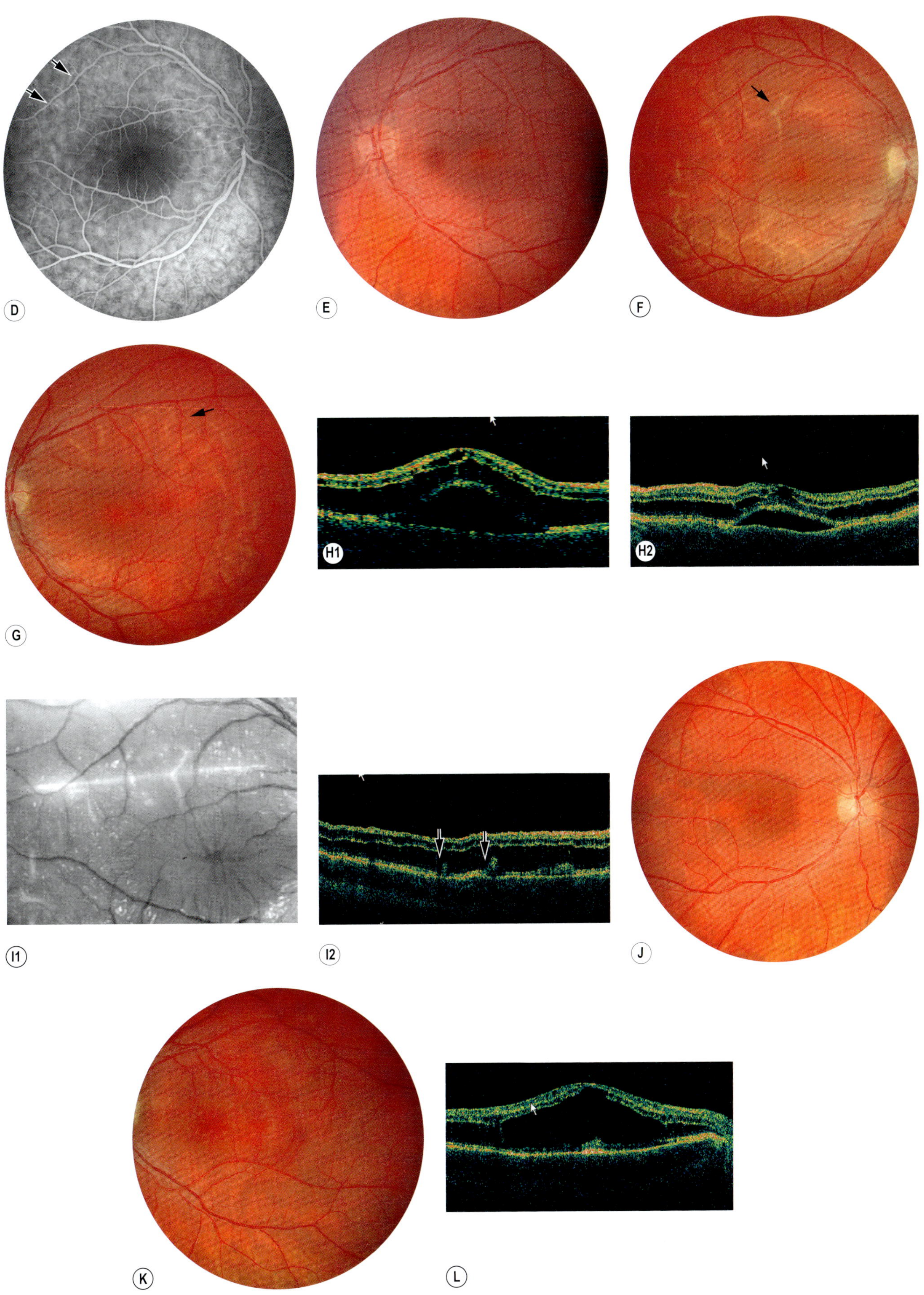
D
E
F
G
H1
H2
I1
I2
J
K
L

Histopathologically, the splitting in juvenile retinoschisis occurs in the nerve fiber layer and ganglion cell layers.[760,762,783] The internal limiting membrane of the retina is thinned over the area of schisis. The inner layer may or may not contain retinal blood vessels. To date no histopathology is available concerning the typical early stages of foveal schisis. The histopathologic findings and ERG abnormalities affecting the b-wave implicate the Müller cells at the primary cell involved in this disorder.[760,783] (See p. 506 for the histopathologic findings of infantile cystoid maculopathy that macroscopically resemble foveal retinoschisis.) Unlike senile schisis, where retinal splitting occurs predominantly in the outer plexiform layer and adjacent nuclear layers, the superficial juvenile retinoschisis cavities do not contain acid mucopolysaccharides.

Progression of visual loss is usually slow and may be associated with minimal changes in the appearance of the fundi (Figure 5.58J and L). Peripheral schisis usually does not progress, and in some cases spontaneous reapposition of the inner and outer layers occurs.

There are no fundus changes in the female carriers.[767] Arden et al. reported identification of obligate heterozygous X-linked juvenile retinoschisis: all patients demonstrated a lack of rod–cone interaction electroretinographically.[781] Linked DNA probes have been used for carrier detection and diagnosis of X-linked juvenile retinoschisis.[772]

Mutations including deletions, missense mutations, and null mutations in the Retinoschisin gene *XRLS1* are responsible for the condition.

Foveal schisis may be simulated by focal contraction of the internal limiting membrane caused by contracted prefoveolar vitreous cortex following an aborted macular hole (see Figure 12.14J–L), by changes occurring in the inner retina in patients with a rhegmatogenous retinal detachment (Figure 5.32E and F), and by infantile cystoid maculopathy (see p. 506).

Bullous peripheral retinoschisis affecting the macula is seen mainly in infants and children and there is a marked tendency for spontaneous resolution. Prophylactic treatment to prevent spread of the schisis or to reattach the inner retina is generally unnecessary and may lead to severe complications.[784]

Non X-Linked Foveal Retinoschisis

Typical foveal schisis has been reported in females with peripheral schisis,[785] and in families showing evidence of autosomal-dominant inheritance (Figure 5.60).[759,786] The pattern of the foveal cystic changes is variable (Figure 5.60A, B, G, and H); some resemble cystoid edema in patients with retinitis pigmentosa whereas others have more vertically oriented columns of tissue between lucent spaces (Figure 5.61). Lewis and associates have reported typical foveal schisis in three daughters of a nonconsanguineous marriage.[758] Yamaguchi and Hara have reported a family of probable autosomal-recessively inherited peripheral retinoschisis without foveal schisis.[788]

5.60 Non X-linked foveomacular schisis.

A–C: Foveomacular schisis in a 19-year-old woman with visual acuity 20/20 right eye, and 20/40 left eye. Angiography was normal (C). Her family history was negative. Her electroretinographic study was normal.

D–I: Familial foveomacular schisis in a brother and sister. Macular lesions were first noted in the sister at age 6 years. At age 15 years her acuity in the right eye was 20/30 bilaterally. She had mild epiretinal membrane changes and cystic foveal changes bilaterally that were associated with a yellowish change at the level of the retinal pigment epithelium (RPE) in the right eye (D and E). A few vitreous cells were present. There were no pars plana exudates. Fluorescein angiography in the left eye was normal (F). An electroretinogram was normal. The brother presented at age 21 years complaining of gradual visual loss for 5 years. He denied nyctalopia or hemeralopia. His visual acuity was 20/60 bilaterally. There were minimal vitreous cells present bilaterally, mild epiretinal membrane changes, and a large central cyst surrounded by smaller cysts in the center of the macula bilaterally (G and H). There was no peripheral retinoschisis. Angiography revealed a focal window defect hyperfluorescence centrally in both eyes (I). The retinal vessels and RPE appeared normal. An electroretinogram revealed some reduction of rod and cone amplitudes.

J–L: This 63-year-old woman had bilateral foveomacular schisis (J and K) and peripheral retinal schisis. Angiography was unremarkable (L). Her family history was negative.

Localized or Segmental Forms of Retinitis Pigmentosa

Autosomal-Dominant Peripheral Annular Pigment Dystrophy (Autosomal-Dominant Vitreoretinochoroidopathy, see ADVIRC p. 248 in Chapter 5)

Autosomal-dominant peripheral annular pigment dystrophy is characterized by coarse hyperpigmentation and hypopigmentation for 360°, with a sharp posterior border at approximately the equator, superficial and deep punctate yellowish-white opacities, retinal vascular attenuation, transudation and neovascularization, cystoid macular edema, choroidal atrophy, vitreous degeneration, and cataract formation[788–791]. It is a relative stable disease and, unlike retinitis pigmentosa, is associated with minimal nyctalopia and visual field loss. ERG responses are normal in younger patients and moderately abnormal in older patients. Histopathologically the findings show some similarities to that in retinitis pigmentosa. Unusual findings include multifocal areas of loss of retinal receptors and extensive preretinal membrane formation with cellular debris and layers of Müller cells. There is no histopathologic evidence to suggest a primary involvement of either the vitreous or choroid in the pathogenesis of this disorder.

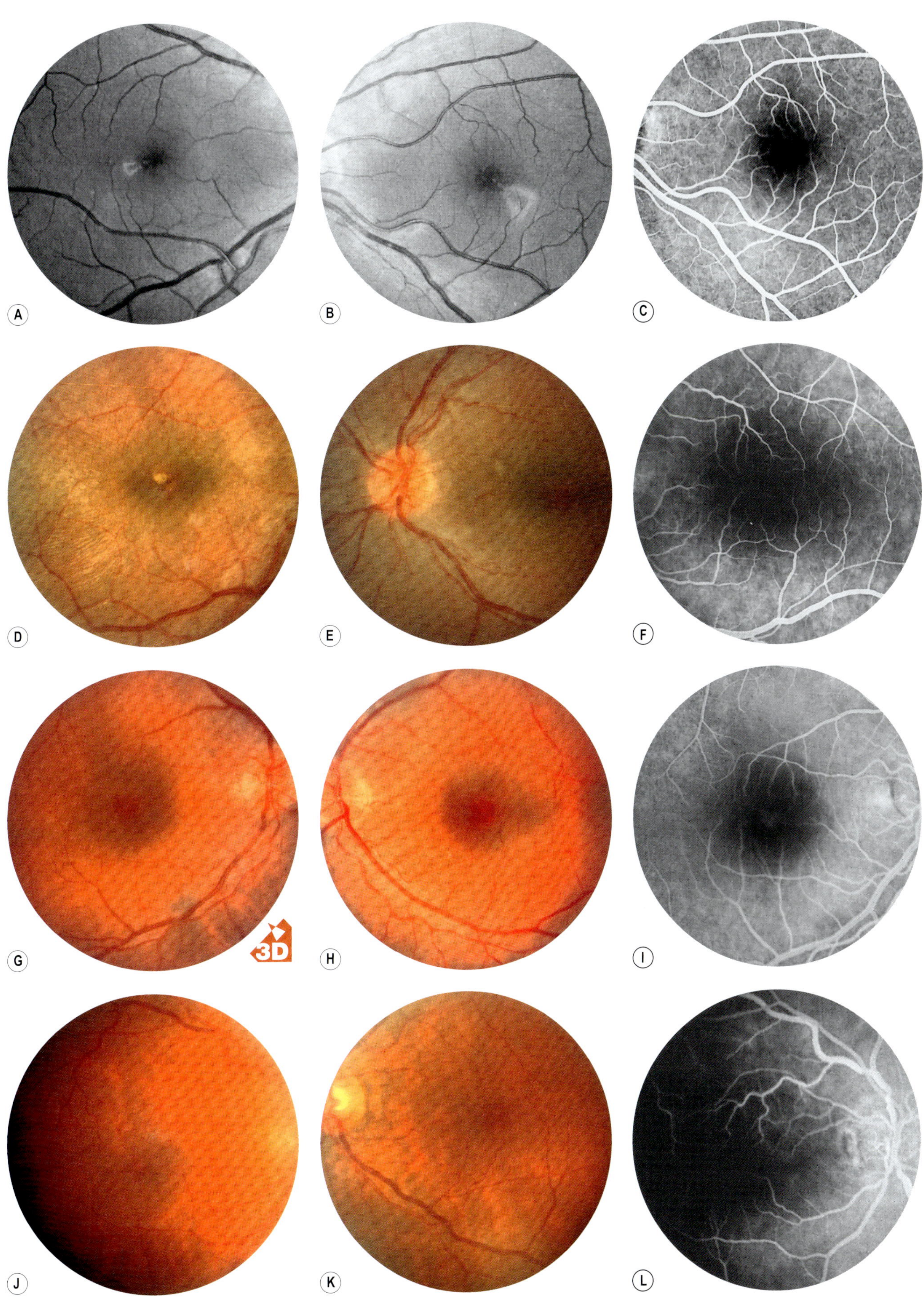
A
B
C
D
E
F
G
3D
H
I
J
K
L

Posterior Annular (Pericentral, Circinate, Peripapillary) Pigmentary Retinal Dystrophy

A variety of names has been given to the development of a ring of pigmentary atrophy with or without intraretinal pigment migration in a ringlike zone immediately surrounding the posterior pole (Figure 5.62A–F).[792–797] These patients usually have normal visual acuity. The ERG typically is subnormal and may be extinguished. When this condition is not associated with pigment migration into the retina, it has been called circinate choroidal sclerosis.[798] Progression in most patients appears to be slow.[793,797] Its mode of inheritance is probably most often autosomal-recessive.

Paravenous Retinochoroidal Atrophy

Patients with paravenous retinochoroidal atrophy, many of whom are asymptomatic and have normal visual function, show a striking pattern of sharply outlined zones of atrophy of the RPE that follow the course of the major retinal veins (Figure 5.62G).[799–809] These may extend posteriorly and be confluent with zones of atrophy surrounding the optic disc. There is often migration of pigment into the retina to surround the retinal veins. The condition is bilaterally symmetric. In most patients the optic nerve and the caliber of the retinal vessels are normal. Some cases have shown evidence of narrowing of the retinal vessels, optic disc pallor, and changes in the RPE in the macula and subnormal acuity. One boy seen in Miami had eccentrically located macular staphylomata (Figure 5.62G). Chen et al. described bilateral macular colobomata associated with pigmented paravenous atrophy.[810] Fluorescein angiography outlines the areas of RPE atrophy and in some cases may demonstrate evidence of atrophy of the choriocapillaris. Autofluorescence imaging shows decreased autofluorescence corresponding to the area of atrophy surrounded by a zone of normal or isofluorescence, outside which there is a ring of increased autofluorescence.[811,812] This appearance is seen in a variety of dystrophies associated with photoreceptor loss, including cone dystrophy, sector retinitis pigmentosa, and cone–rod dystrophy. The increased fundus autofluorescence, and therefore, excessive lipofuscin accumulation in RPE cells, may result from an abnormally high turnover of photoreceptor outer segments or impaired RPE lysosomal degradation of normal or altered phagocytosed molecular substrates. This arc of increased fundus autofluorescence in different retinal dystrophies migrates with time as the area of involvement spreads.

Paravenous retinochoroidal atrophy may occur in siblings and in successive generations.[800,802,813] Some cases of paravenous atrophy are probably acquired as the result of inflammatory disease.[814–816] Gass has seen one patient who presented initially with a widespread perivenous distribution of acute chorioretinitis that over a period of several years progressed to severe typical serpiginous choroiditis. The occurrence of paravenous atrophy bilaterally in one of two monozygotic twins is evidence that in some patients it may have a cause unrelated to genetic makeup. Males are affected more than females, in about a 4:1 ratio.[817,818] Some cases are familial, most are sporadic; no definite inheritance pattern has been established.[819–821] Mutations within the *CRB1* gene have been found by various groups; other conditions associated with *CRB1* mutations include some cases of Leber's congenital amaurosis, early-onset retinitis pigmentosa (PPRPE, RP12), and retinitis pigmentosa associated with Coats'-like vasculopathy. It appears that loss of *CRB1* leads to displaced photoreceptors and focal degeneration of all neural layers attributable to loss of adhesion between photoreceptors and Müller cells.

Electrophysiologic tests are usually normal or only mildly affected but in some instances may be markedly subnormal.[808,809] Most cases fail to show progression. In some cases, however, the disease may progress and result in significant visual loss. In a study of 15 patients over time, the mean change in remaining visual field and ERG amplitudes was much slower than in patients with typical retinitis pigmentosa.[817]

Differential diagnosis includes angioid streaks, helicoid peripapillary chorioretinal degeneration, radial lattice retinal degeneration, and chorioretinitis.

Sector Pigmentary Retinal Dystrophy

In some patients the ophthalmoscopic evidence of pigmentary retinal dystrophy that may or may not be associated with bone spicule pigmentary migration may be confined to one sector of the fundus, most frequently the inferonasal quadrant (Figure 5.62H and I).[822–830] The disease is usually discovered in adult patients who may have mild symptoms of night blindness. They usually show slow progression of the disease, which rarely reaches the disabling stage. The visual acuity is usually normal. Retinal arterioles in the area of pigmentary changes are narrowed. The field defect usually corresponds with the area of RPE atrophy. Absolute visual thresholds, however, may be elevated throughout the retina.[828,831] Occasionally chronic angle closure glaucoma, macular holes, and exudative vasculopathy have been associated with it.[832–835]

5.61 Non-X-linked macular schisis.

A–F: This 60-year-old woman had best-corrected vision of 20/25 vision in each eye. Careful examination of the fovea showed faint yellow stippling of the temporal fovea in each eye that did not capture well on the photographs. Optical coherence tomography showed only mild thickening and cysts in the temporal macula of both eyes. The intervening pillars were obliquely oriented in the macula and vertically oriented in the temporal retina (A–D). There was no family history suggestive of retinoschisis. She was treated with oral acetazolamide for more than 3 months with only mild changes in the height of the schisis cavity in both eyes (E and F). She maintained a vision of 20/25 and the acetazolamide was stopped.

(Courtesy of Dr. Edward Cherney.)

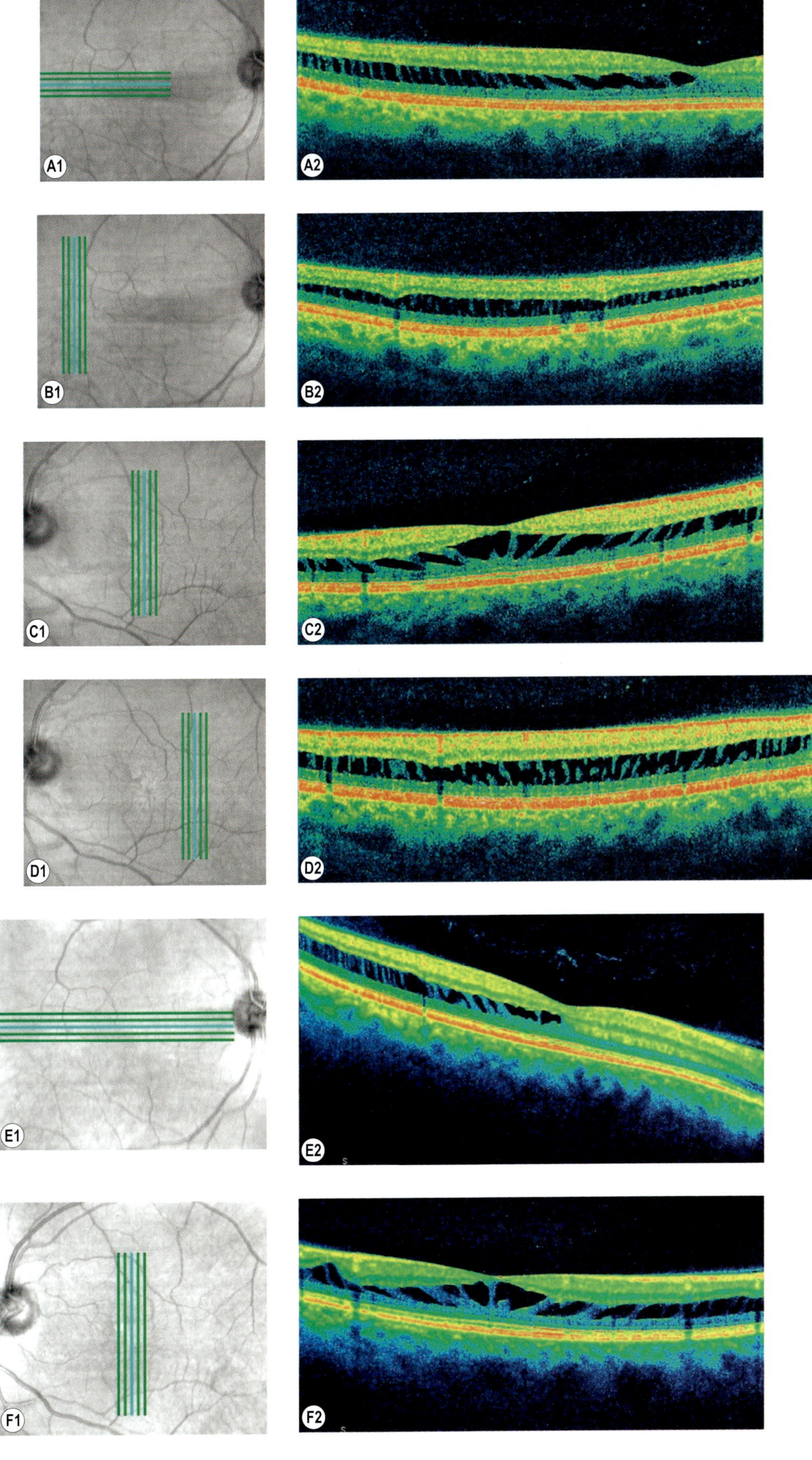
A1
A2
B1
B2
C1
C2
D1
D2
E1
E2
F1
F2

Juvenile nephronophthisis and sectoral retinitis pigmentosa have been associated in one instance.[836] Histopathologic and metabolic abnormalities involving the normal-appearing retina have also been demonstrated.[826,829] In patients showing minimal ophthalmoscopic evidence of RPE changes in the affected area, the field defects may simulate a nerve fiber bundle defect or bitemporal hemianopia and lead to the mistaken diagnosis of glaucoma or an intracranial lesion.[837] Electroretinography may show evidence of rod, cone, or combined dysfunction.[825] Fluorescein angiography is helpful in detecting the sector areas of atrophy of the RPE that may be overlooked ophthalmoscopically. Most cases are sporadic, but autosomal-recessive and dominant inheritance occurs.[829–830,838–839] Rod opsin mutations are responsible for autosomal-dominant inheritance of segmental retinitis pigmentosa in some families.[830,838,839] These latter patients demonstrate abnormal dark adaptation kinetics with marked prolongation of the later phase of rod adaptation.[839]

Patients with sector pigmentary retinal dystrophy should be clearly differentiated from patients with segmental areas of bone spicule pigmentation related to long-standing serous detachment, such as occurs particularly in some patients with a severe form of idiopathic central serous chorioretinopathy (see Figure 3.06) and in patients with acute zonal occult outer retinopathy (see Figure 11.18). In such cases the distribution of pigmentary changes is usually asymmetric. Although sector pigmentary retinal dystrophy may occasionally occur unilaterally, pigmentary changes when confined to one eye are much more likely to be the result of trauma (see Figures 8.02D–F and 8.03L); previous long-standing retinal detachment related to a retinal hole, choroidal hemangioma (see Figure 14.16) or choroidal nevus; or previous occlusion of a large choroidal artery.

Unilateral Retinitis Pigmentosa

The diagnosis of unilateral retinitis pigmentosa should be made only when: (1) there is functional electroretinographic and ophthalmoscopic evidence suggesting a primary pigmentary degeneration in one eye; (2) the visual function, ERG, and appearance of the other eye are normal; (3) follow-up has been at least 5 years in order to rule out delayed involvement of the second eye; and (4) inflammatory, traumatic, or other causes in the affected eye have been excluded.[841–843] Patients with these criteria rarely have other affected family members, and their fundus changes probably are caused by some acquired disease rather than by a primary genetically determined dystrophy (Figure 5.62J and K).[842,843] Female carriers of X-linked retinitis pigmentosa can develop unilateral symptomatic retinitis pigmentosa when the process of lyonization inactivates the normal X chromosome. Inflammation, trauma, and combined choroidal and retinal vascular occlusion are probably responsible for most cases. In the southeastern USA diffuse unilateral subacute neuroretinitis is the commonest cause of a unilateral retinitis pigmentosa-like syndrome (see Figure 10.28). Patients with acute zonal occult outer retinopathy and multifocal choroiditis and panuveitis may also present with unilateral fundus changes typical of retinitis pigmentosa (see Figures 11.18 and 11.19).

5.62 Localized forms of pigmentary retinal dystrophy.

A–D: Annular pigmentary retinal dystrophy in a 63-year-old man complaining of nyctalopia of 18 months' duration. His family history was negative. Visual acuity was 20/20 in the right eye and 20/200 in the left eye. Color vision testing was markedly abnormal. His electroretinographic studies showed moderately abnormal rod and cone dysfunction. Note the ring of retinal pigment epithelium atrophy surrounding the macula (A–C). Angiography in the left eye (D) showed evidence of a faint bull's-eye pattern of hyperfluorescence centrally (arrows). There has been only minimal change in the fundi and visual function during the 8 years of follow-up.

E and **F**: Identical twin females developed mild visual loss associated with foveomacular schisis in their teenage years. The schisis disappeared in their 20s, and they developed an incomplete segmental annular dystrophy of the pigment epithelium and retina in their 30s (E and F). Their visual acuity was 20/20 bilaterally. Electroretinography was within normal limits.

G: Paravenous retinochoroidal atrophy and macular staphylomata in a 14-year-old Latin boy whose visual acuity was 20/25 in the right eye and 20/200 in the left eye. His electroretinogram showed severely abnormal rod and cone function. His family history was negative. A similar picture was present in both eyes. This was observed at age 4 years and photographs during the past 5 years have revealed only minor changes in the fundus appearance.

H and **I**: Segmental retinitis pigmentosa involving the nasal half of the fundi (H) in a 47-year-old man with a bitemporal hemianopsia. A paternal aunt had retinitis pigmentosa. Visual acuity was 20/20, The temporal halves of the fundi were normal (I). His cone and rod electroretinographic findings were moderately abnormal.

J–L: Unilateral retinitis pigmentosa-like fundus in a 34-year-old woman who was asymptomatic before presenting with acute loss of central vision in the right eye caused by a subretinal neovascular membrane in the right eye (arrow, J). In addition to the typical findings of pseudoxanthoma elasticum with angioid streaks and peau d'orange changes in both eyes, she had marked narrowing of the retinal vessels and extensive 360° bone–corpuscular changes that were confined to the left eye (L). An electroretinogram was normal in the right eye and severely abnormal in the left eye. Visual acuity was 20/30 right eye and 20/20 left eye.

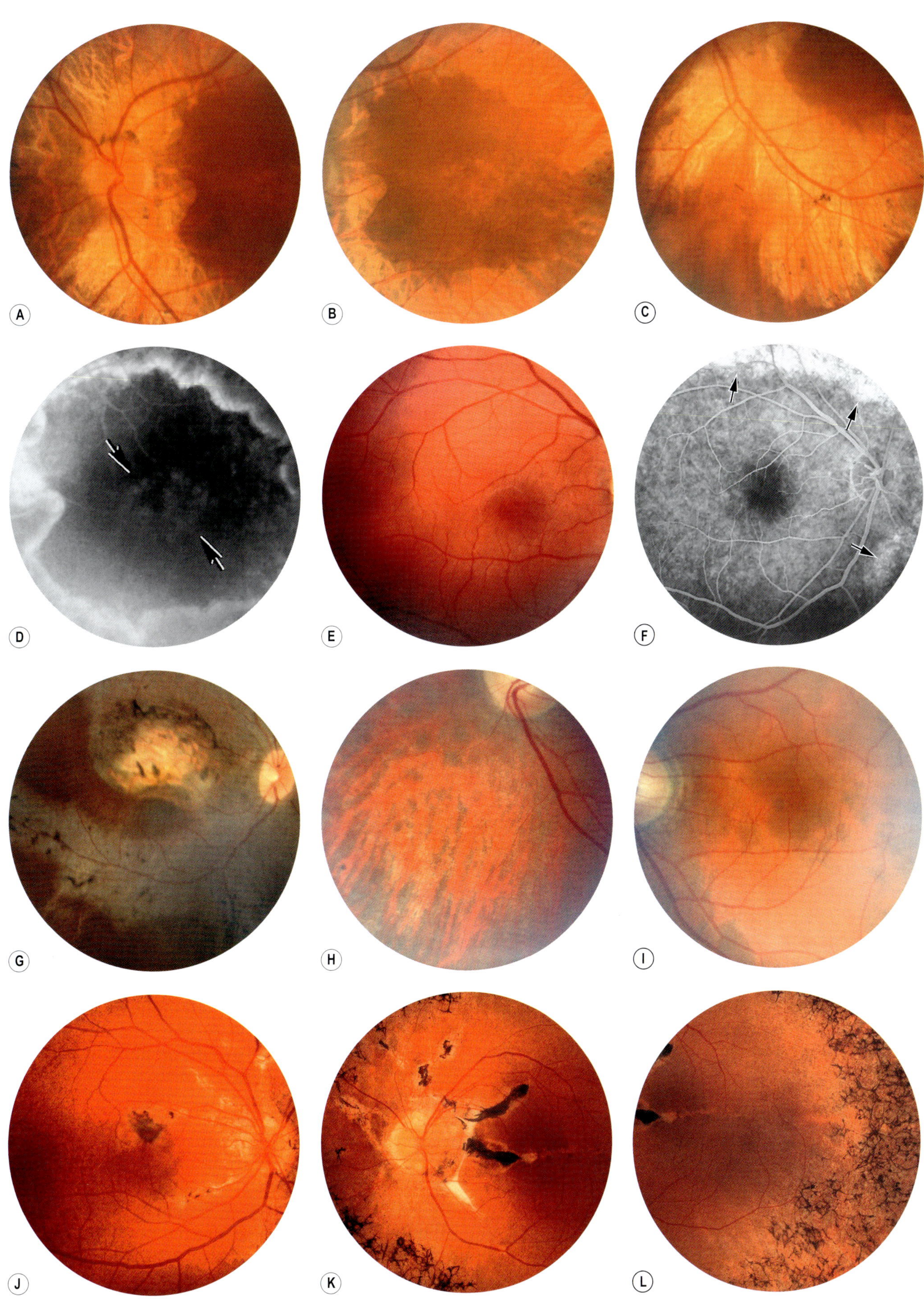

ATYPICAL PIGMENTARY RETINAL DYSTROPHIES ASSOCIATED WITH METABOLIC AND NEUROLOGIC DISORDERS

Gyrate Atrophy of the Choroid

Gyrate atrophy of the choroid is a rare recessively inherited chorioretinal dystrophy and inborn error of metabolism caused by a generalized deficiency of the mitochondrial matrix enzyme ornithine aminotransferase. Myopia and night blindness are the first clinical symptoms and the disease appears in childhood. It is manifest early in life as garland-shaped, sharply defined zones of chorioretinal atrophy involving the midperiphery of the fundus (Figure 5.63A and B).[843–865] These lesions spread peripherally and posteriorly. The macula is usually involved later in life. Focal areas of atrophy are variable in size and fuse to form large atrophic areas with festooned edges (Figure 5.63). The mechanism for the chorioretinal atrophy remains unknown; adverse effects of creatinine or deficiency of pyrroline-5-carboxilate on retinal function may be a cause.[866] Small glittering crystals may be visible on the fine velvet-like RPE in areas unaffected by choroidal atrophy. Some pallor of the optic disc, vitreous opacities, narrowing of the retinal vessels, and cataracts occur during the later stages of the disease. Optic disc drusen and cystoid macular edema may occasionally occur.[844,868] The late fundus picture may simulate that of advanced choroideremia (Figure 5.63I and J) or LORMD. Most patients have a high degree of myopia and manifest varying degrees of night blindness. Progressive peripheral field loss accompanies the fundus changes.[846] Color vision is normal until later life. The EOG is markedly abnormal. The scotopic ERG is usually extinguished. Both rod and cone amplitudes may be severely reduced in early childhood at a time when the fundus changes may be minimal.[857] Dark adaptation reveals progressive loss of rod function. Takki[844,845] and McCollough and Marliss[850–852] have demonstrated abnormal levels of ornithine in the plasma, urine, cerebrospinal fluid, and aqueous humor in these patients. The enzyme ornithine ketoacid transaminase is deficient in these patients.[862]

At least 50 different mutations have been found in the *OAT* gene mapped to 10q26.[868] Nearly half the patients that are known are of Finnish origin. In addition to the eye changes, other systemic findings include: (1) minor decreases in intelligence; (2) changes in the electroencephalogram (EEG); (3) minor weakness of muscle; (4) changes in staining of type II muscle fibers; (5) tubular inclusions in muscle cells on electron microscopy; (6) fine, sparse, straight hair with microstructural changes; and (7) lengthening and enlargement of mitochondria in liver cells.[869–871] The central nervous system involvement in patients with gyrate atrophy and hyperornithinemia involves degenerative changes in the white matter in approximately 50% of patients with gyrate atrophy and 70% of patients have premature atrophic changes, a striking increase in the Virchow's spaces. About half the patients show abnormal background activity on EEG. The EEG and MRI findings do not correlate with each other.

There are two clinical subtypes of gyrate atrophy based on the presence or absence of an in vivo response to vitamin B_6, which is the cofactor of the enzyme ornithine aminotransferase. Vitamin B_6 responsiveness is defined as a 50% reduction in serum ornithine levels. Patients with B_6 responsiveness generally have a milder disease than those who are not responsive. Somatic cell hybridization studies have demonstrated absence of complementation among B_6 responders and nonresponders, which indicates that these two forms of gyrate atrophy probably represent different allelic mutants of the same gene.[872,873] Use of arginine-restricted diet has also been shown to slow progression of the vision loss in patients with gyrate atrophy due to lower plasma ornithine levels. Carriers of gyrate atrophy have no clinical signs but may have slight elevation of blood ornithine levels, clear ornithine more slowly on loading test, and demonstrate only 50% enzyme activity on cell culture. Mutations of the ornithine aminotransferase gene show a high degree of heterogeneity, reflecting the heterogeneity of the disease.[854,874,877]

Histopathologic examination of eyes of a patient with vitamin B_6-responsive gyrate atrophy has shown abrupt transition between normal retina and near-total atrophy of the retina, pigment epithelium, and choroid corresponding with the gyrate areas of atrophy seen clinically.[876] Mitochondrial abnormalities may be evident in the corneal epithelium, nonpigmented ciliary epithelium, and to a lesser extent in the photoreceptors.[876]

5.63 Gyrate atrophy of the choroid.

A–C: Gyrate atrophy in a 25-year-old woman whose visual acuity was 20/100 right eye and 20/80 left eye. The rod and cone electroretinogram was extinguished. Her serum ornithine level was 753 μmol/L.

D–L: A 43-year-old mother complained of nyctalopia for 2 years. She carried a diagnosis of Retinitis pigmentosa for 30 years. Her visual acuity was 20/20 both eyes. Wide-field photographs show peripheral pigment change in a reticular or fishnet-like pattern with normal-caliber vessels (D–G). Her angiogram showed hypofluorescence corresponding to the pigment with adjacent areas of hyperfluorescence (H). Her two affected sons with progressive gait disturbance showed peripheral nummular chorioretinal atrophy that was symmetric between the two eyes and between each other typical of gyrate atrophy (I and J). The atrophic patches were hypoautofluorescent with intervening areas of increased autofluorescence (K) in her and her sons. Optical coherence tomography showed preservation of retinal pigment epithelium and photoreceptors in the intervening areas but loss corresponding to the atrophic zones (L). The angiogram showed loss of choriocapillaris in those areas.

(D–L, courtesy of Dr. David Sarraf.)

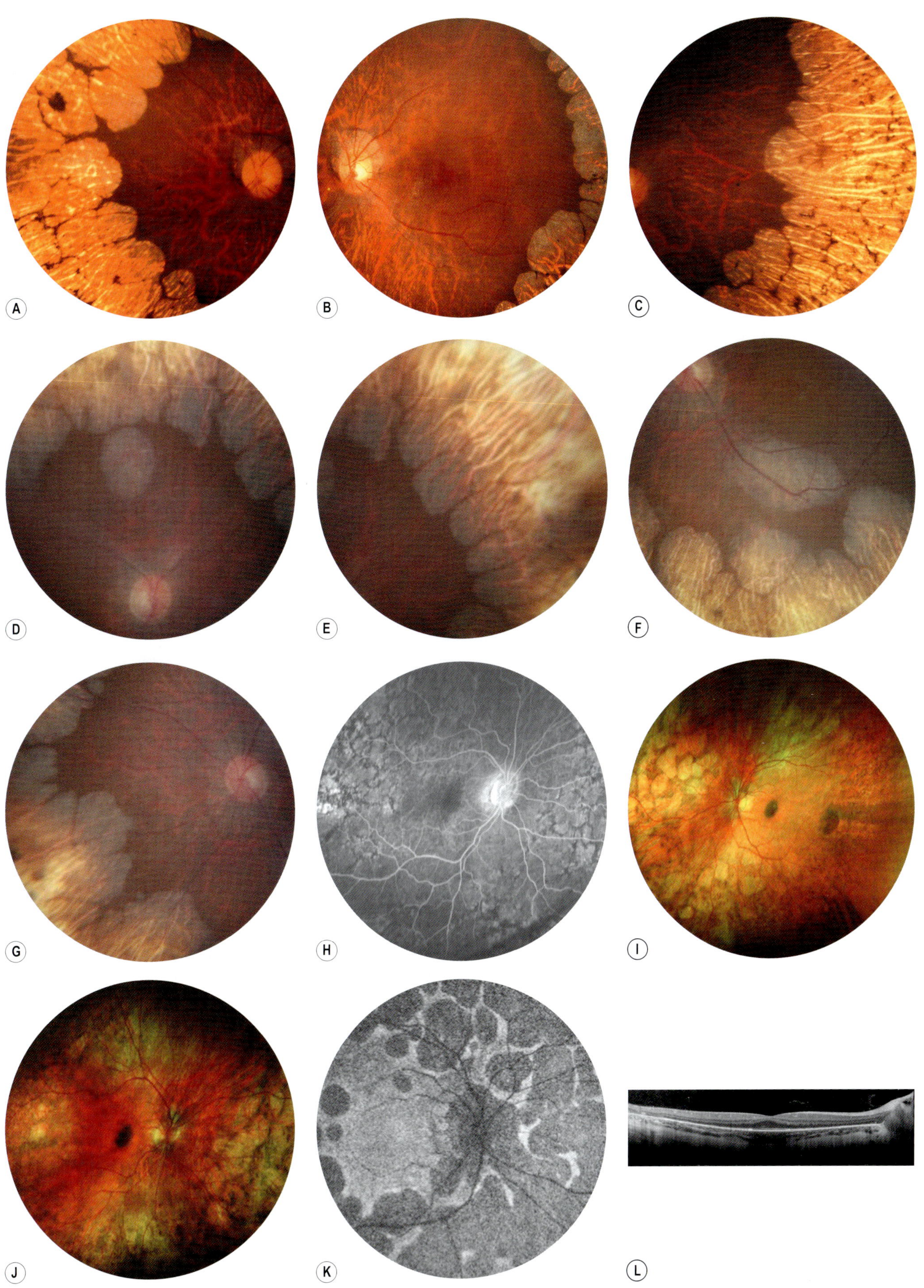
A
B
C
D
E
F
G
H
I
J
K
L

The differential diagnosis of gyrate atrophy includes choroideremia and generalized choroidal sclerosis.[724] Peripheral confluent zones of old inactive chorioretinitis secondary to congenital or secondary syphilis or other inflammatory disease if discovered in young patients might be confused with gyrate atrophy. Similar multiple geographic zones of atrophy also occur after spontaneous resolution of large zones of sub-RPE large-cell lymphoma. (See Chapter 13, p. 1150.) NFRCD, Bothnia dystrophy, and LORMD are other conditions that have large areas of geographic atrophy in the midperiphery that progress over time.

Blood ornithine levels have been successfully lowered through the therapeutic use of vitamin B_6,[843,860,877] pyridoxal phosphate,[878] and a low-arginine diet.[847,855] The results of therapeutic trials to date are inconclusive as to whether treatment is of benefit in retarding progression of the disease.[843,847,849,859,860,863,867,878]

5.64 Cystinosis.

A and **B**: There was a peculiar yellow crystalline material at the level of the choroid and retinal pigment epithelium in a 7-year-old girl with renal insufficiency diagnosed as cystine storage disease.

C: A 14-year-old female with cystinosis developed a urinary tract infection at 6 months of age. She was diagnosed as having Fanconi's syndrome. At 6 years she developed photophobia and multiple corneal crystals were noted. At 7 years, bright refractile deposits were noted in the choroid. Visual acuity was normal. She died at 14 years of age from complications of immunosuppressant therapy following renal transplantation. Histopathologic examination of the eyes revealed square, rectangular, and sliverlike crystals in the choroid. These crystals were also found in the cornea, iris, ciliary body, sclera, episclera, and optic nerve sheath.

(A, from Fellers et al.[883], C, from Winter.[890])

Hooft's Syndrome

Hooft's syndrome is an autosomal-recessive disorder of tryptophan metabolism, characterized by atypical pigmentary retinal dystrophy, extinguished ERG, panhypolipidemia, hypoglycemia, mental and growth retardation, erythematous skin rash involving the face and extremities, whitish discoloration of the nails, dry hair, tooth decay, and a progressive course leading to death by 2 years of age.[879,880] The fundus may show a dusty-gray appearance with pigmented spots or gray or yellow patches. The macula has been described as appearing to be "covered by a kind of snail's slime."[880] This is a variant of the Bassen–Kornzweig syndrome but without steatorrhea and acanthocytosis.

Cystinosis

Nephropathic cystinosis is an autosomal-recessively inherited storage disorder in which nonprotein cystine accumulates within cellular lysosomes caused by a defect in lysosomal cystine transport. Early in life these patients experience growth retardation, renal tubular and glomerular dysfunction, anemia, and hyperthyroidism. Renal transplantation is usually necessary by 10 years of age. Ocular manifestations usually develop in the first year of life and include photophobia; progressive accumulation of corneal, conjunctival, and iris crystals; and yellowish mottling of the pigment epithelium in the macula and more marked mottled RPE degenerative changes in the peripheral fundi (Figure 5.64A and B).[881-890] Corneal crystal deposition begins in the superficial peripheral corneal stroma and subsequently involves the central and deeper corneal stroma. Fine crystals may be visible in the retina in some patients.[883,885,887] With longer survival made possible by renal transplantation, additional ocular complications have occurred.[883] These include incapacitating photophobia, blepharospasm, posterior synechiae, thickened iris stroma, crystal deposition on the anterior lens surface, tritan color vision abnormalities, elevated dark adaptation thresholds, reduction in rod and cone amplitudes electroretinographically, and impairment in visual function. There is some evidence that cystinosis in the French Canadian population may be associated with milder complications of the disease.[887] Histopathologic and ultrastructural examinations have shown evidence of intracellular crystals within the RPE and choroid but not in the retina (Figure 5.64C). It is probable that accumulation of cystine crystals within the RPE is responsible for the characteristic fundus pictures seen in these patients,[888] although Winter found the crystals only in the choroid[889] (Figure 5.64C).

Cellular cystine accumulation, which is the putative cause of the ocular damage, can be reduced by over 90% with the free thiol cysteamine, both in vitro and in vivo. This treatment apparently stabilizes renal function but does not reverse existing renal damage. Likewise, it does not reverse the corneal deposition of crystals and probably does not reverse the retinal dysfunction.[883] Studies are needed to determine whether cysteamine therapy, which is usually discontinued after successful renal transplantation, is of benefit in retarding progressive ocular changes. Cysteamine eye drops have been used to reverse corneal crystal deposition.[884]

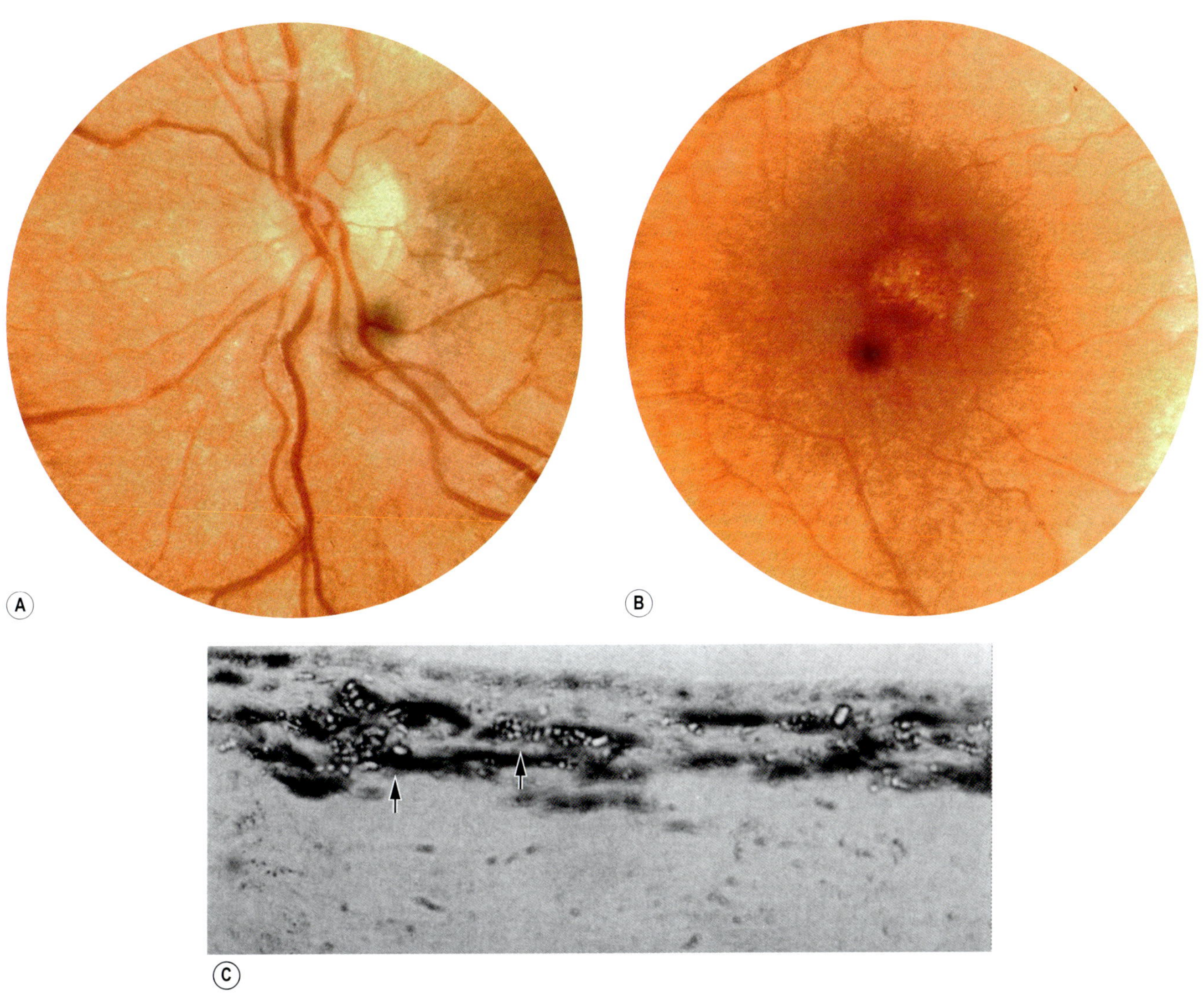
A
B
C

Albinism

Albinism is a group of disorders associated with an inborn error of amino acid metabolism affecting the production of melanin. Associated defects that may occur include nystagmus; strabismus; large refractive errors, particularly myopic and astigmatic errors; macular dysplasia (hypoplasia); deafness; mental retardation; reticuloendothelial incompetence; and coagulation defects.[891–908] Macular dysplasia is characterized by loss of the foveal depression and reflex and absence of or ill-defined capillary-free zone (Figure 5.65C, E, F, and H). Some patients, however, demonstrate a capillary-free zone by fluorescein angiography.[909] Prominent retinal blood vessels may course directly through, rather than arching around, the dysplastic macula (Figure 5.65E).[892]

Oculocutaneous Albinism

Oculocutaneous albinism may be inherited as either an autosomal-recessive or a dominant trait (Figure 5.65A–F).[898,910,911] Most patients with ophthalmic symptoms have the recessive form of the disease. Patients whose hair bulbs lack tyrosinase have platinum blonde hair, pink skin, severe photophobia, nystagmus, subnormal acuity, diaphanous, light-colored irides that transilluminate diffusely (Figure 5.65B), absence of pigmentation of the fundi, and macular dysplasia. Patients with tyrosinase in the hair bulbs usually have more ocular pigmentation and less visual symptoms and disability. Three subtypes of tyrosine-negative oculocutaneous albinism include: (1) tyrosinase-negative albinism; (2) platinum albinism; and (3) the yellow mutant type. Eight subtypes of tyrosinase-positive oculocutaneous albinism include: (1) minimal pigment oculocutaneous albinism; (2) tyrosinase-positive albinism; (3) brown albinism; (4) minimal pigment albinism; (5) Hermansky–Pudlak syndrome; (6) Chédiak–Higashi syndrome; (7) rufous albinism; and (8) autosomal-dominant albinism.[910,912–914] Other features of Chédiak–Higashi syndrome include: reticuloendothelial incompetence associated with susceptibility to infection and lymphomatous disease, lymphadenopathy, hepatosplenomegaly, mental retardation, cytoplasmic inclusions in leukocytes, and death in childhood (Figure 5.65K and L).[891] Features accompanying oculocutaneous albinism in Hermansky–Pudlak syndrome include: blood-clotting defect (caused by defective glutathione peroxidase activity) and Cross's syndrome (microphthalmos, cloudy vascularized corneas, skeletal anomalies, athetosis, and mental retardation).[905]

Ocular Albinism

Patients with a defect in melanogenesis that is largely confined to the eye fall into three major categories: (1) the Nettleship–Falls X-linked type (the most common of the three categories)[898–904,908–910,915,916]; (2) the Forsius–Eriksson X-linked type (Åland Island disease), accompanied by an atypical protanomalous defect (Figure 5.65G–I)[917]; and (3) the autosomal-recessive type. All have impaired visual acuity, translucent irides, congenital nystagmus, photophobia, hypopigmentation of the fundi, and macular dysplasia. Some of the female carriers of the Nettleship–Falls type show patchy areas of iris transillumination and a coarsely mottled or irregular streaky change in the RPE peripherally (Figure 5.65J). The affected patients and obligate carriers have abnormal giant melanosomes in the skin.[895,897,908] The pigmentary mosaicism in carriers is not found in the Forsius–Eriksson type.

In a variant of X-linked ocular albinism in black males there may be a lack of iris transillumination defects and characteristic fundus hypopigmentation.[894] The visual acuity is better than in typical X-linked ocular albinism and diagnosis may require skin biopsy. The carriers, in addition to having the typical fundus changes, may have a striking alternating spokewheel-like pattern of the iris stromal hypo- and hyperpigmentation.[915]

Histopathologic examination has revealed evidence of foveomacular dysplasia, including absence of the foveal pit in patients with oculocutaneous as well as ocular albinism.[895,897,902,916] The ganglion cell layer is present throughout the macula, and the cones resemble those seen in the normal parafoveal area.

Variable results have been reported in regard to ERG findings in patients with albinism. Whereas some have suggested that increased a-wave amplitudes and shorter latencies of both a- and b-waves are characteristic of patients with ocular as well as oculocutaneous albinism, others have reported that most of these patients have normal ERG findings.[918,919] Patients with ocular albinism should be distinguished from patients with isolated foveomacular dysplasia and those with dysplasia associated with aniridia.[920–922] Flash visual evoked potentials and ERG may be helpful in this regard.[918,919]

5.65 Albinism.

A–C: Oculocutaneous albinism in a 16-year-old girl with full transillumination of the irides. She had nystagmus. Visual acuity was 5/200. Her paternal grandfather and his brothers had albinism. There was no well-defined capillary-free zone or foveolar depression biomicroscopically (C).
D–F: Oculocutaneous albinism, optic nerve hypoplasia, and flecked retina in a 27-year-old Latin man with nystagmus, poor vision, and mild hyperopic astigmatism all of his life. The mother and paternal grandfather were blond but had good vision.
G–I: X-linked ocular albinism in a 19-year-old man with nystagmus and 20/70 acuity. He had dark hair, brown irides that showed some transillumination defects, and albinotic fundi with foveal dysplasia.
J: Streaky and mottled retinal pigment epithelium in an asymptomatic female carrier of X-linked ocular albinism.
K: Oculocutaneous albinism in Chédiak–Higashi disease.
L: Stippling of white cells in Chédiak–Higashi syndrome.

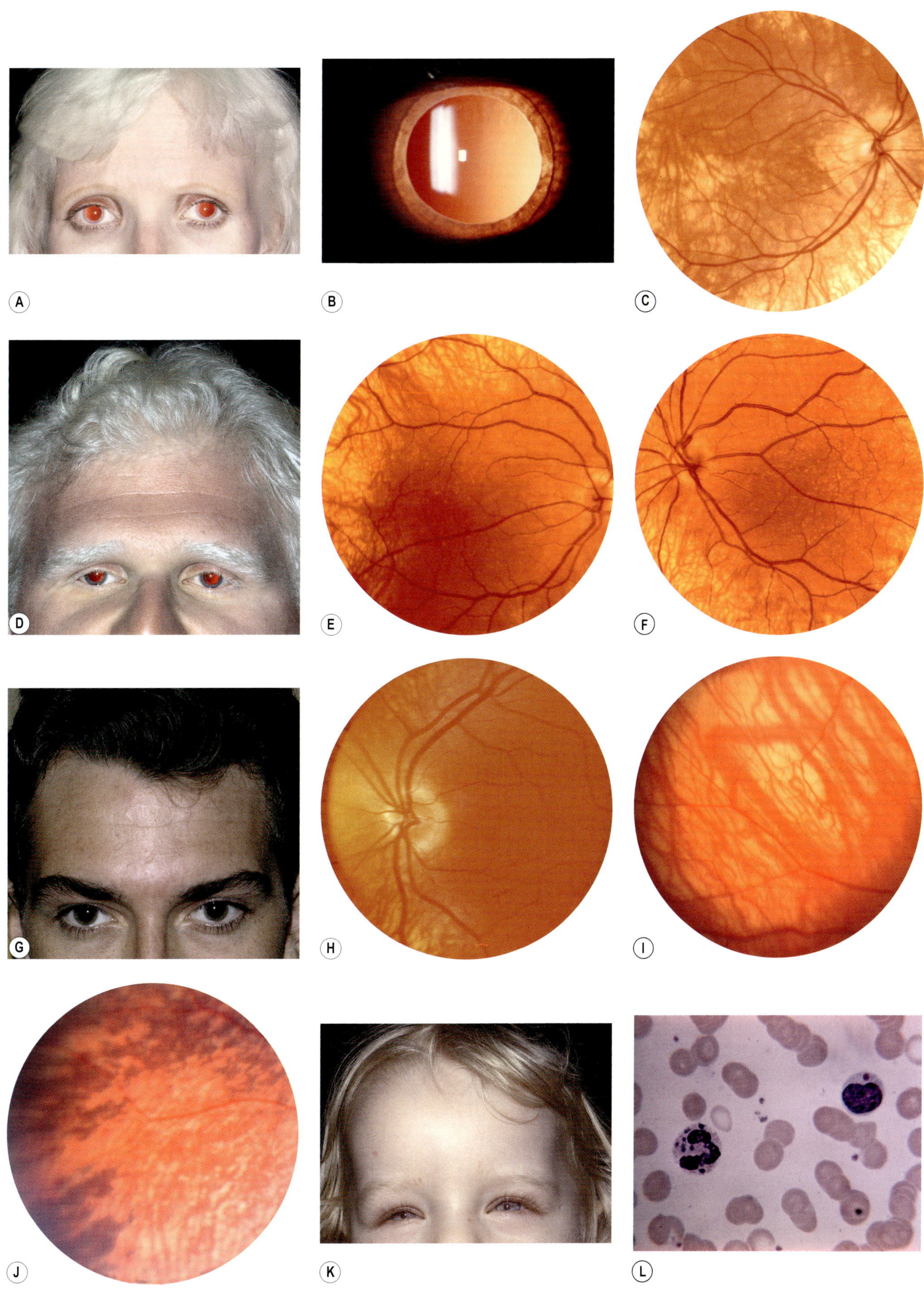
A
B
C
D
E
F
G
H
I
J
K
L

Partial Ocular Albinism

Congenital heterochromia of the iris and fundus may occur alone (Figure 5.66D–J) or may be associated with localized congenital depigmentation of the skin and hair, for example, Waardenburg's syndrome (Figure 5.66A–C).[900,906,914]

Primary Hereditary Hyperoxaluria

Primary hereditary hyperoxaluria is a rare inborn error of glyoxalate metabolism characterized by calcium oxalate nephrolithiasis, chronic renal failure, and systemic deposition of oxalate crystals in many tissues, including the heart, bone, testes, central nervous system, thyroid, media of arteries, adipose tissue, lymph nodes, muscles, skin, and eye.[923–930] Approximately 30% of patients will demonstrate retinopathy.[931] There are two types of hereditary oxaluria. Type I hyperoxaluria results from deficiency of the cytoplasmic enzyme hepatic peroxisomal alanine:glycolate aminotransferase.[932,933] These patients have increased urinary excretion of oxalate and glycolate. Type II hyperoxaluria is caused by a deficiency of D-glyceric dehydrogenase, which causes an increased synthesis of oxalate. Only patients with type I are symptomatic and develop eye signs. These include crystalline flecks widely scattered throughout all layers of the retina and RPE (Figure 5.67). Irregular dense clumps of RPE hyperplasia and hypertrophy, and fibrous metaplasia, ranging in size from small ringlets to large several disc diameter-size geographic plaques, occur in the macular area.[927,930,931] Optic atrophy as well as choroidal neovascularization may occur. Visual acuity loss is greater in those patients with optic atrophy.[931,934]

In type I primary hyperoxaluria, the calcium oxalate crystals early in life may be deposited primarily in the RPE at the posterior pole.[935] In older children, however, the crystals clinically and histopathologically are found in great numbers in the retina with a tendency for periarterial distribution.[927] Hypertrophy and hyperplasia of the RPE are prominent in the macular area (Figure 5.67A and B).[927,935] In a 46-year-old man with a clinically milder and later-onset familial hyperoxaluria, ophthalmoscopically and histopathologically the crystals were located primarily in the outer plexiform and nuclear layers of the retina and not in the pigment epithelium and inner retinal layers.[936] Histopathologically, oxalate crystals may be found in the other ocular and body tissues, including the kidneys.[927]

Similar retinopathy has been described in acquired oxalosis following methoxyflurane anesthesia that produced acute renal failure (see Figure 9.09G–K).[937,938] A similar retinopathy has been produced in rabbits by injecting calcium oxalate subcutaneously.[938] The differential diagnosis includes the fleck retina syndromes, Bietti's crystalline dystrophy, cystinosis, gyrate atrophy, Sjögren–Larsson syndrome, tamoxifen retinopathy, Alport's syndrome, and talc embolization. The progressive RPE changes that may occur in association with oxalate crystals may simulate any of the disorders associated with atypical retinitis pigmentosa.

5.66 Partial albinism.

A–C: Partial albinism in Waardenburg's syndrome in this 13-year-old black girl with partial deafness, white forelock, synophrys, lateral displacement of the medial canthus, and heterochromia of the irides and fundi. Her visual acuity in the right eye was 20/25 and in the left eye was 20/40. She did not have poliosis of the eyelashes and brow or congenital vitiligo of the skin. The left iris (A) and fundus (C) were hypopigmented.
D–G: This 20-year-old Latin male with visual acuity of 20/20 bilaterally had heterochromia of the irides and fundi (D and E), some loss of hearing in the right ear, pectus excavatum (F), and a few café-au-lait spots (G). His parents were cousins. The family history was negative for ocular abnormalities.
H–J: Heterochromia of the iris (H) and fundi (I) in a 6-year-old black boy with 20/20 visual acuity in both eyes.

(D–I, from Thompson and Curtin.[914],)

Inborn Error of Vitamin B_{12} Metabolism

There are at least three autosomal-recessive inborn errors of intracellular cobalamin that may cause methylmalonic aciduria with homocystinuria. The cobalamin C form may be caused by deficiency of a cytoplasmic hydroxycobalamin reductase that results in faulty synthesis of the two active forms of cobalamin and absence of adenosylcobalamin and methylcobalamin. Absence of these latter two cofactors results in methylmalonic acidemia and aciduria, accumulation of homocysteine and its derivatives, and decreased methionine. Early in life, patients with the cobalamin C type of methylmalonic aciduria and homocystinuria develop failure to thrive, developmental delay, seizures, megaloblastic anemia, and a progressive maculopathy.[939–944] Reported ocular findings include pigment epithelial mottling in the macula with progression to a bull's-eye appearance,[943] peripheral salt-and-pepper pigment changes,[942] and optic disc pallor.[943] Most patients develop nystagmus early in life, but its onset may be delayed in some patients. Visual acuity is reduced to 20/200 or worse in most patients. Pupillary response may be sluggish. Eyelid clonus may be evident.[940] The electroretinographic amplitudes are reduced early. The cones may be more affected than the rods.[942]

Histopathologic and ultrastructural examination of the eyes of a 22-month-old child revealed depigmentation of the RPE and loss of receptor cells in the macula, reduced numbers of the small ganglion cells in the papillomacular bundle area, thickening of the posterior sclera associated with accumulation of acidic and weakly sulfated mucopolysaccharide, and diffuse storage of material in clear or granular cytoplasm in most of the ocular tissues.[944]

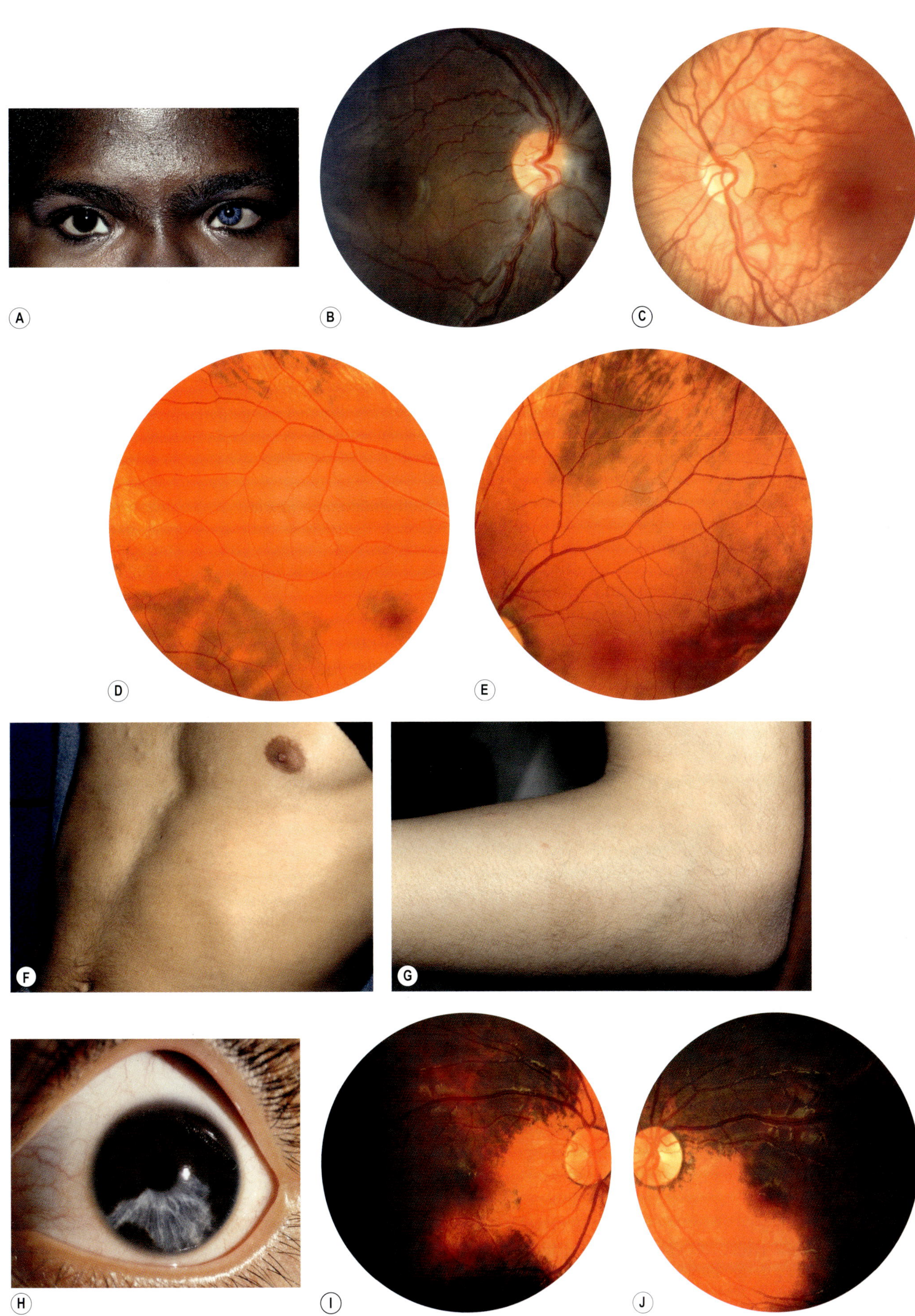
A
B
C
D
E
F
G
H
I
J

Methylmalonic Acid Urea Cobalamin-C Type

Methylmalonic acid urea with homocysteinuria cobalamin-C type is the commonest inborn error of vitamin B_{12} metabolism. It is an autosomal-recessive disorder caused by mutation in the *MMACHC* gene. Early- and late-onset subgroups are distinguished based on their age of onset.[945,946] Patients who present within the first year of life are affected more severely than those with later onset. The early-onset group of patients presents with failure to thrive, lethargy, and feeding difficulties. These children show neurological deterioration, multisystem pathology, pancytopenia, megaloblastic anemia, cognitive disabilities, and progressive retinopathy. The late-onset group presents with gait abnormalities, extrapyramidal symptoms, psychiatric disturbances, dementia, mild to moderate cognitive disability, but no retinopathy. Early recognition of the condition and treatment with hydroxycobalamin, vitamin supplementation, carnitine and B_{10} help to modify the severity of the disease.

The ocular findings have shown progressive macular changes which initially appear to be a bull's-eye maculopathy, which continues to progress with central atrophy and hyperpigmentation (Figure 5.67G and H). Coarse pigmentary retinopathy with bone spicule formation is seen over time (Figure 5.67I).[945–948] Consecutive optic atrophy occurs subsequently. Those patients with late-onset disease show reasonably good ocular function, including rod and cone-mediated ERG responses. No significant ocular pathology has been noted. Subtle ERG or EOG changes may not be functionally significant.[945,946]

Vitamin A and E Deficiency

Combined deficiency of vitamins A and E may cause nyctalopia and progressive retinal degeneration in humans.[949] Berger et al. reported these same changes in a patient with an 18-year history of avitaminosis E associated with an autosomal-recessive form of intrahepatic cholestasis with malabsorption of predominantly vitamin E.[950] They suggest that the vitamin E deficiency may be the major cause of the retinal degeneration previously attributed to combined deficiency of vitamins A and E.

RETINAL CILIOPATHIES

Disruption of the function of proteins associated with photoreceptor cilia results in a wide variety of phenotypes ranging from isolated retinal degeneration to more widespread phenotypes. Systemic associations include neurosensory hearing loss, developmental delay, situs inversus, infertility, disorders of limb and digit development, obesity, and kidney, liver, and respiratory disease. The retinal ciliopathies include retinitis pigmentosa, macular degeneration, cone dystrophy, cone–rod dystrophy, Leber's congenital amaurosis, retinal degenerations associated with Usher syndrome, primary ciliary dyskinesia, Senior–Loken syndrome, Joubert syndrome, Bardet–Biedl syndrome, Laurence–Moon syndrome, McKusick–Kaufman syndrome, and Biemond syndrome. Mutations for these disorders have been found in retinitis pigmentosa-1 (*RP1*), retinitis pigmentosa GTPase regulator (*RPGR*), retinitis pigmentosa GTPase regulator-interacting protein (RPGR-IP), and in the Usher, Bardet–Biedl, and nephronophthisis genes. Systemic disorders associated with retinal degenerations that may also involve ciliary abnormalities include: Alstrom, Edwards–Sethi, Ellis–van Creveld, Jeune, Meckel–Gruber, orofaciodigital type 9, and Gurrieri syndromes. Understanding these conditions as "ciliopathies" may help the clinician to recognize associations between seemingly unrelated diseases and have a high degree of suspicion that a systemic feature may be present.[951]

5.67 Primary hyperoxaluria.

A and **B**: This 14-year-old female was referred for evaluation of black macular lesions. At 9 years of age her visual acuity was 20/20. At 13 years, she had a renal transplant because of shrunken calcified kidneys. Her visual acuity at the time of these photographs was 20/50. Many yellow crystals were scattered throughout the retina at all levels. Note their predilection for periarterial distribution. Irregular geographic black subretinal lesions with lacunae and some fibrous tissue were present in the macular areas. She subsequently died, and the histopathologic findings were similar to those found in secondary oxalosis (see Figure 9.09).
C–F: Primary familial hyperoxaluria in a 33-year-old Iranian woman who developed nephrolithiasis at 20 years of age. Renal dialysis was necessary at age 30 years. At that time she had peripheral neuropathy, hyperuricemia, pericarditis, and migratory arthritis. One brother had a renal transplant. Four other relatives had renal stones. Visual acuity was 20/25 in the right eye and 20/30 in the left eye. The fundi showed widespread retinal crystals and grade 3 hypertensive retinopathy (C and D). Angiography revealed marked loss of the peripheral retinal vessels (F) and extensive retinal vascular changes (E).

Methylmalonic aciduria

G to **I**: This 18 year old male with CF vision at 3 feet in each eye, was born at full term by emergency C-section for fetal distress. At age 6 weeks, he was found to feed poorly, was lethargic, irritable, had emesis and poor muscle tone. Methylmalonic acid was found in his urine, fundus was normal at that time. Vitamin B12 shots were given with reduction in MMA. Methylmalonic aciduria, cobalamin C type (cbl-C) was diagnosed. At 9 months of age he had nystagmus, a "bulls eye maculopathy" was noted bilaterally and ERG was non recordable. He received orientation and mobility training, learnt Braille in kindergarten, has average IQ, graduated high school with peers and attends community college. He skis in the blind program and aspires to become a sports radio and TV statistician. Both macula show central chorioretinal atrophy surrounded by hyperpigmented RPE (G and H). The rest of the fundus shows diffuse pigmentary alteration with coarse RPE clumps and bone spicules (I). There was mild waxy pallor of the optic discs in both eyes.

(A and B, from Meredith et al.[927], © 1984, American Medical Association. All rights reserved. C–F, courtesy of Dr. Richard A. Lewis G to I, courtesy of Dr. Alan Kimura.)

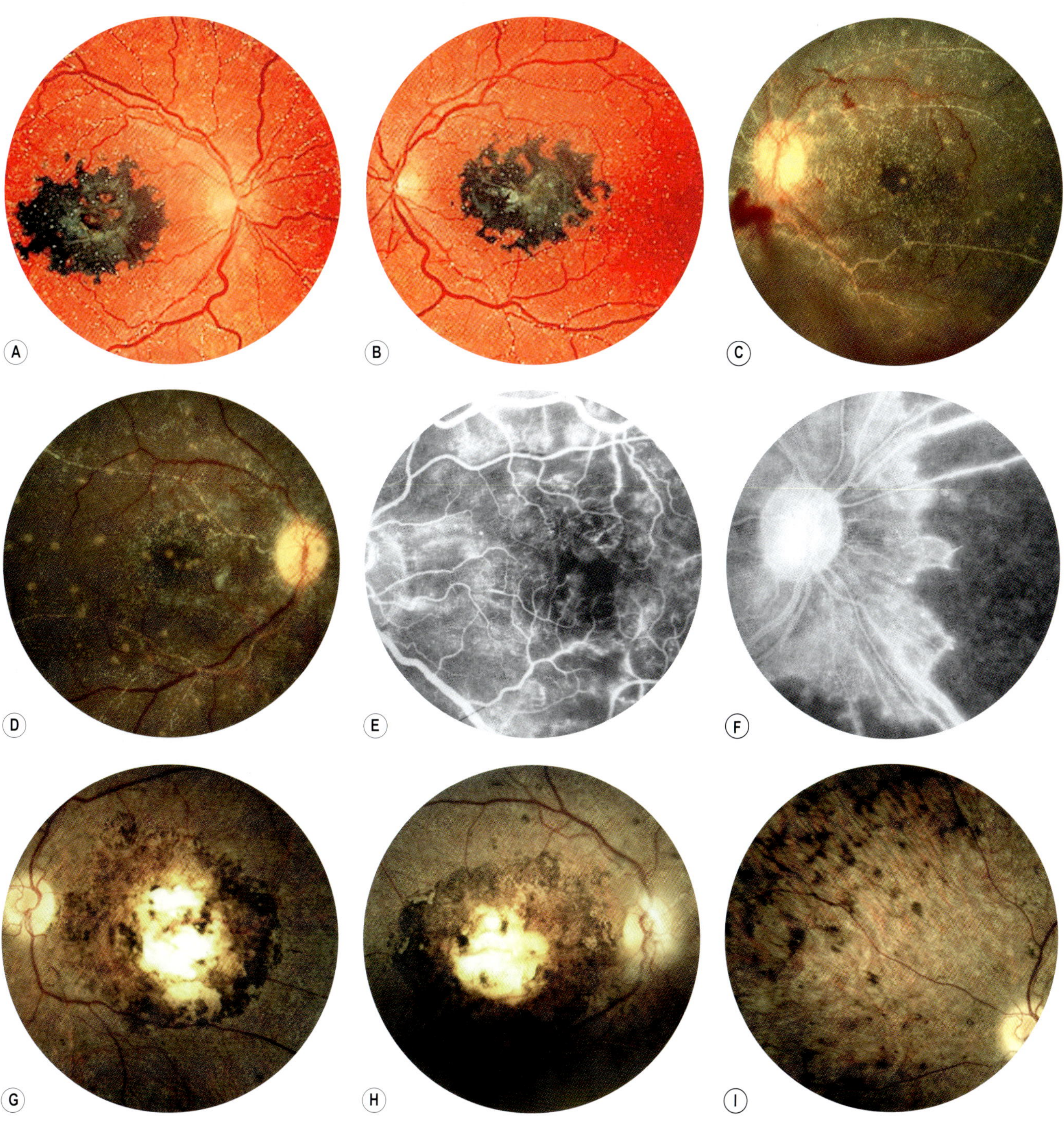
A
B
C
D
E
F
G
H
I

BARDET–BIEDL SYNDROME

Bardet–Biedl syndrome is characterized by: (1) pigmentary retinal dystrophy; (2) mental retardation; (3) congenital obesity (usually a Fröhlich type); (4) hypogenitalism (more frequently in males); and (5) polydactyly or syndactyly (Figure 5.68).[952–960] In any one patient, the syndrome may be incomplete. Other defects include deafness, nystagmus, strabismus, shortness of stature, genu valgum, pes plana, congenital heart disease, cystic kidney dysplasia, and atrophic pyelonephritis. It occurs more commonly in males. The fundus often shows the typical changes of retinitis pigmentosa and may in addition show evidence of a bull's-eye maculopathy (Figure 5.68A).[958] Retinal wrinkling caused by an epiretinal membrane may be present.[958,961]

Fluorescein angiography shows evidence of hyperfluorescence in areas of RPE atrophy and frequently shows leakage of dye from the capillaries on the optic nerve head and paramacular area without evidence of cystoid macular edema (Figure 5.68B–D).[958,962] The ERG is markedly abnormal or extinguished. Patients with no measurable peripheral visual field may show a variety of different patterns of central visual dysfunction: an island of only cone function centered in a bull's-eye lesion, patches of rod function surrounding geographic atrophy, or a central island of excellent rod sensitivity but severely impaired cone function.[963] The EOG is markedly abnormal.[956] Whereas most patients retain central vision through their early school years, many develop macular changes and 20/200 visual acuity or less during the second decade of life.[955] Approximately 50% are legally blind beyond 20 years of age. Most patients eventually become virtually blind. The disease is inherited as an autosomal-recessive trait. Premature death is often caused by renal failure secondary to low-grade vesicourethral reflux, urinary tract infection, and hypertensive vascular disease.[958] There is an increased incidence of diabetes mellitus in these patients.[964]

LAURENCE–MOON SYNDROME

Patients with Laurence-Moon syndrome are similar to those with Bardet–Biedl syndrome except polydactyly and obesity are not present, and these patients develop spastic paraparesis.[961,965,966] Further, these patients show extensive choroidal atrophy approaching that seen in choroideremia. Some patients may show features of both syndromes.[961] A hypothalamic hamartoma was found in one patient.[967]

ALSTRÖM SYNDROME

Patients with Alström syndrome (Alstrom-Hallgren syndrome) manifest a tapetoretinal degeneration (infantile retinal dystrophy) in association with obesity, diabetes mellitus, acanthosis nigricans, polycystic ovaries, hypogonadism, cardiomyopathy, and neurosensory deafness.[968–973] Other features occasionally presented include mental deficiency, baldness, hepatic dysfunction, and hypertriglyceridemia.[970,974] Renal dysfunction is variable, age-related, and probably the most frequent cause of death.[975] They present with nystagmus and photophobia, with severe cone dysfunction in infancy, progressive loss of rod function, and usually an extinguished ERG by 5 years of age and no light perception by age 20.[973,976] These patients may be initially misdiagnosed as achromotopsia, Bardet–Biedl, Leber's congenital amaurosis, or cone–rod dystrophy. Infantile cardiomyopathy and/or weight above the 90th percentile associated with severe early-onset cone–rod dystrophy should alert one towards the diagnosis.[977] The condition is recessively inherited and the defective gene *ALMS1* maps to chromosome 2p13. The *ALMS1* gene encodes a protein found primarily in the centrosomes and basal bodies of ciliated cells, suggesting a function in cilia formation, maintenance, and function.[976]

5.68 Bardet–Biedl syndrome.

A–D: This 12-year-old girl with mental retardation, Fröhlich-type obesity, polydactyly, night blindness, and a negative family history had visual acuity of 20/300. There were many vitreous cells. Her electroretinogram showed severely abnormal rod and cone function. Note the narrowing of the retinal arterioles (A). Fluorescein angiography (B–D) showed evidence of diffuse mild pigmentary changes and leakage of dye from the retinal capillaries along the major arcades.
E and **F**: Fröhlich-type obesity and polydactyly (arrow) in another patient with the same syndrome.

JUVENILE FAMILIAL NEPHROPHTHISIS ASSOCIATED WITH TAPETORETINAL DEGENERATION (SENIOR–LOKEN SYNDROME)

Some patients with autosomal-recessively inherited juvenile familial nephrophthisis or cystic disease of the renal medulla may have an associated tapetoretinal degeneration.[978–986] The earliest signs of the renal disorder are polydipsia, polyuria, and nocturia secondary to impaired urinary concentrating ability. The renal disease is insidious; there is little warning before development of uremia or anemia. Results of urinalysis are essentially normal. The retinal degeneration resembles Leber's amaurosis, pigmentary retinal degeneration, and RPA. Usher's syndrome, segmental retinitis pigmentosa, and Coats' syndrome have been reported in these patients.[985]

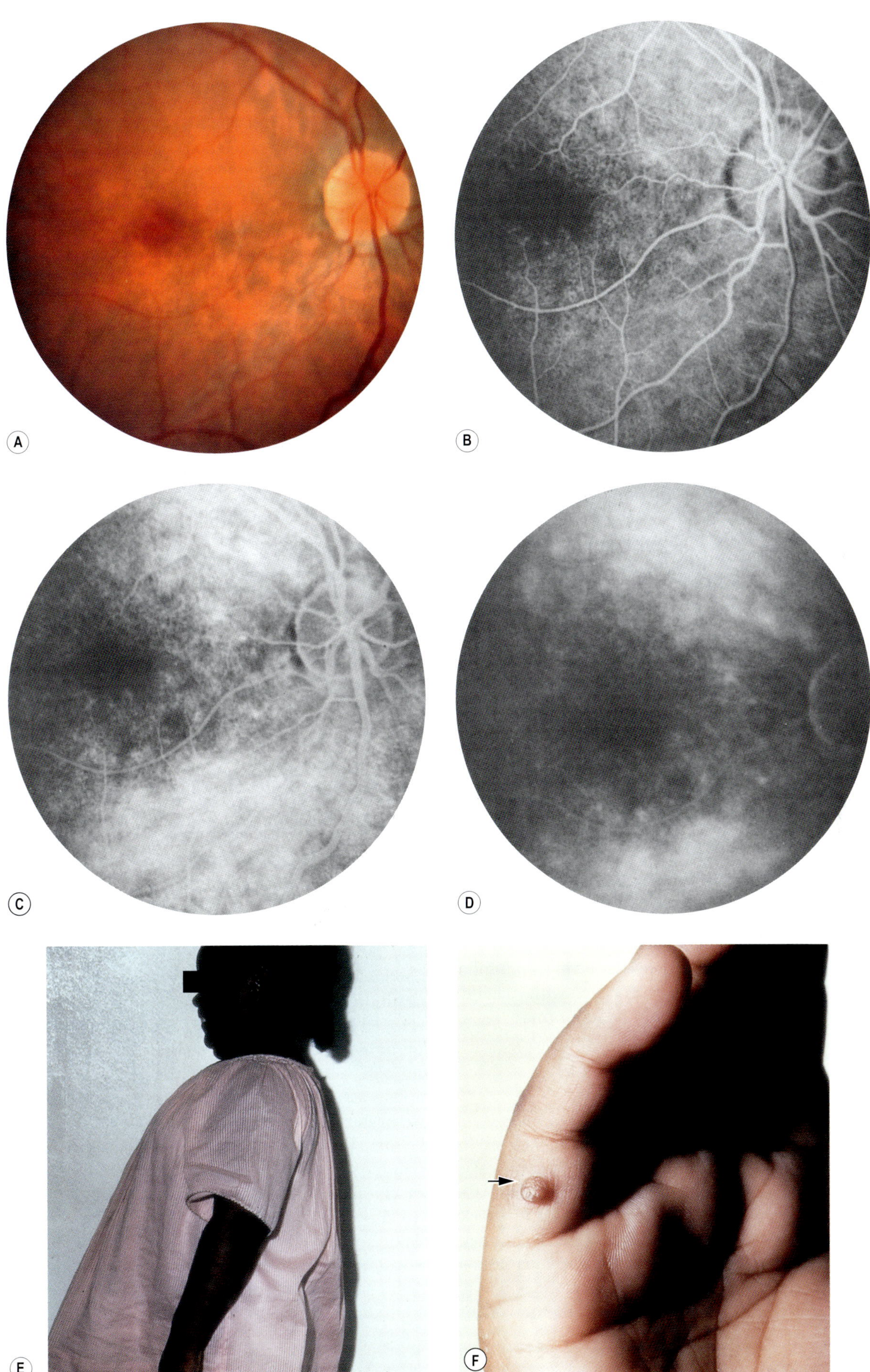
A
B
C
D
E
F

JEUNE SYNDROME

This is an autosomal-recessive disorder characterized by skeletal abnormalities (short-limbed structure, short ribs), long thorax with respiratory insufficiency that may lead to infantile death, brachydactyly, metaphyseal irregularity, polydactyly, progressive renal disease, occasional ocular abnormalities, including reduced visual acuity, photophobia, nystagmus, strabismus, and abnormal ERG.[987,988] Histopathologic examination and electron microscopy show mildly altered RPE, marked loss of retinal receptor cells with relative sparing of cones, and moderate loss of peripheral ganglion cells.[989]

ARTERIOHEPATIC DYSPLASIA (ALAGILLE'S SYNDROME)

Alagille's syndrome is an autosomal-dominantly inherited syndrome characterized by intrahepatic biliary hypoplasia, neonatal jaundice, pruritus, cardiovascular anomalies (particularly pulmonary artery stenosis), vertebral anomalies, growth retardation, hypogonadism, and a characteristic facies (deep-set eyes, mild hypertelorism, overhanging forehead, straight nose, and small pointed chin), and hoarse voice (see Figure 4.05).[990–998] Associated ocular anomalies that are apparent in at least 50% of cases include posterior embryotoxon (Axenfeld's anomaly),[995] pigmentary retinal degeneration, pseudopapilledema, chorioretinal folds (see Figure 4.05),[992,996] band keratopathy, ectopic pupil, esotropia, high myopia, and tortuous retinal blood vessels. Posterior embryotoxon and the peripheral retinal pigmentary changes are the most consistent findings and may be helpful in differentiating this benign form of neonatal jaundice from other more serious causes of neonatal jaundice. The disorder is of variable penetrance and is benign in most patients. Some, however, may have severe cardiovascular and renal complications as well as progressive neurovascular deterioration caused by vitamin A and E deficiency.[991,997] The "cholestasis" facies, although occurring frequently in this disorder, may be seen in patients with congenital intrahepatic cholestatic liver disease unassociated with Alagille's syndrome.[998] The ERG and EOG may be subnormal.

INCONTINENTIA PIGMENTI ACHROMIANS

Incontinentia pigmenti achromians (hypomelanosis of Ito) is characterized by linear and whorled, "marble-cake" streaks of cutaneous depigmentation on the trunk and extremities (along the lines of Blaschko) similar to streaks of hyperpigmentation seen in patients with incontinentia pigmenti, and anomalies of the central nervous system, including psychomotor retardation and seizures, eyes, hair, teeth, nails, musculoskeletal system, and internal organs (Figure 5.69).[999–1007] The name "incontinentia pigmenti acromians" should not link this condition with incontinentia pigmenti, which occurs only in females (transmitted by X-linked inheritance and lethal in males); they are in no way related, except for the superficial resemblance of the skin changes. Incontinentia pigmenti achromians occurs in both sexes with a female-to-male ratio of 2.5:1 and genetically is not well defined.[1001–1002,1006] Evidence documenting single-gene transmission is unconvincing and recurrence risks in the same family are negligible in most cases. Karyotyping of blood lymphocytes, skin fibroblasts, and/or keratinocytes of 115 individuals reported in the literature as reviewed by Sybert[1008] revealed abnormal chromosome constitutions in 60. Three patients were 46,XX/46,XY chimeras, and two were 46,XX/46,XX chimeras. Most patients were mosaic for aneuploidy or unbalanced translocations, with two or more chromosomally distinct cell lines either within the same tissue or between tissues. The common alterations were mosaic trisomy 18, diploidy/triploidy, mosaicism for sex chromosome aneuploidy, microdeletion of the proximal region of 15q, and tetrasomy 12p.[985,1003,1004,1006–1008] Features frequently seen in incontinentia pigmenti such as vesicobullous and verrucous phases predating the skin pigment changes and severe retinal vascular anomalies leading to blindness (see Figure 6.69) are not seen.

5.69 Incontinentia pigmenti achromians.

A–E: A 7-year-old Latin boy was seen because of progressive cataract in the left eye, mild visual loss in the right eye, and left exotropia. He was the product of a 37-week gestation and a breech delivery. Congenital anomalies included right hemiatrophy of the body, including the tongue (D) and palate, cryptorchism, and foot deformities; retinal pigment epithelium (RPE) abnormalities were noted in the fundi at 1 month and myopia at 1 ½ years. Abnormal dentition (E), alopecia areata, deafness, and streaks of cutaneous hypopigmentation (hypomelanosis of Ito) (C) occurred before 5 years of age. Visual acuity in the right eye (− 6.00 D) was 20/50 and in the left eye (− 4.50 D) was hand movements. There were bilateral cortical cataracts, worse in the left eye. The right fundus showed an anomalous optic disc, coarse streaks, and changes in the RPE (A and B). Electroretinographic findings showed reduced rod and cone amplitudes.

Hypomelanosis of Ito associated with medulloblastoma.

F–L: This 19-year-old female was operated for a medulloblastoma and was found to have a congenital ankle deformity and whorls of skin pigmentation along the lines of Blaschko. A trisomy of chromosome 3 was found on genetic testing, a defect so far not known to be associated with medulloblastoma. She had punctate areas of RPE hypopigmentation more visible in the right than the left macula (F and G), that were hypoautofluorescent (H and I) and appeared as transmission defects on angiography (J). Her visual acuity was normal in both eyes. The streaks of hypopigmentation were present on her back (K), forearm (L), and face. There was no family history of medical disorders.

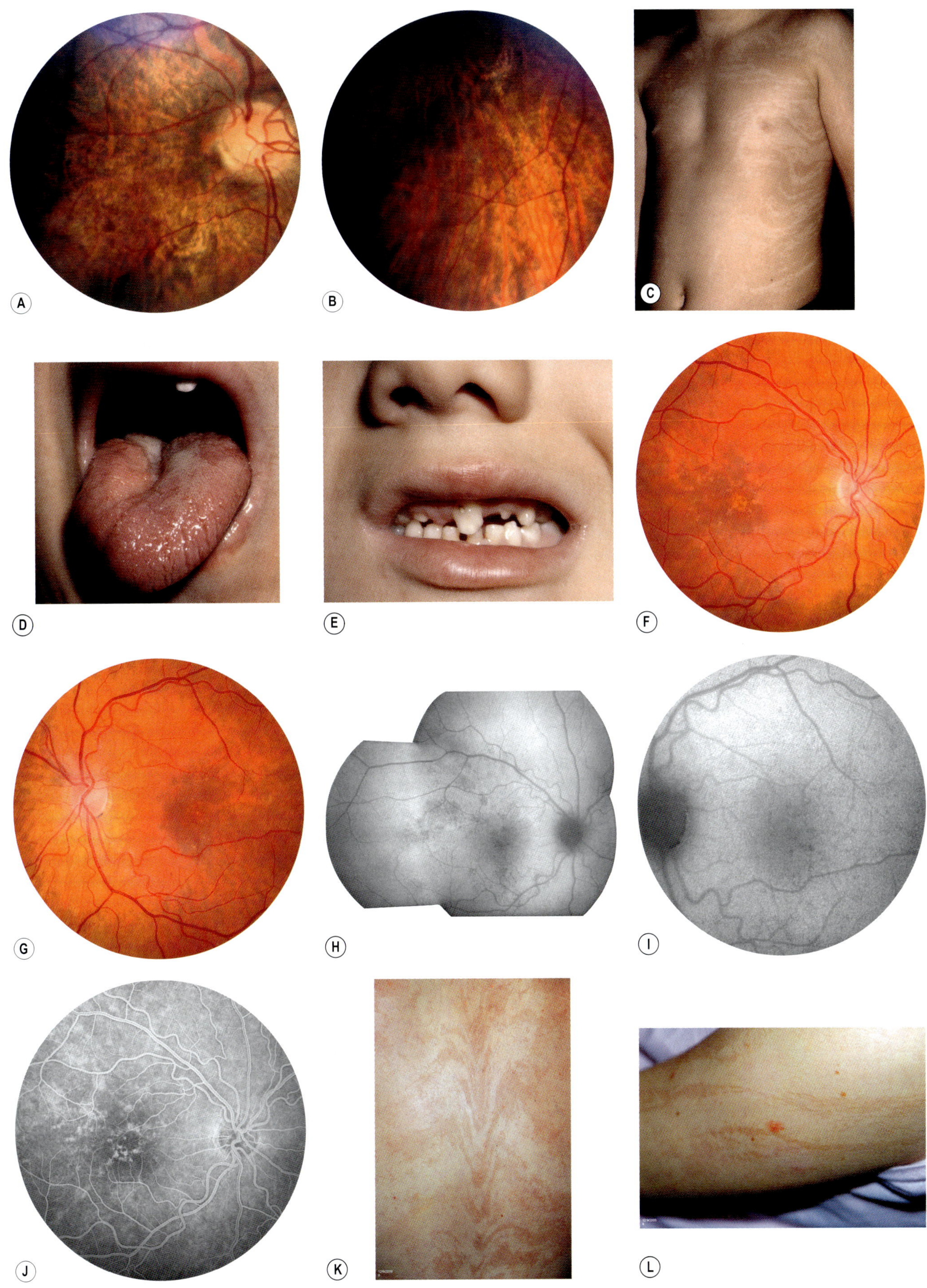
A
B
C
D
E
F
G
H
I
J
K
L

A variety of ocular anomalies, including strabismus, epicanthal folds, coloboma, myopia, microphthalmos, corneal asymmetry, atrophic irides, irregular pupil, heterochromia of the iris, cataract, and retinal detachment, have been reported.[1006,1009–1012] Streaks of hypopigmentation of the RPE and optic disc anomalies occurred in a 7-year-old boy with incontinentia pigmenti achromians seen at the Bascom Palmer Eye Institute (Figure 5.69A–E).[1005] He also had bilateral congenital cataracts, myopia, and dental anomalies. Other cases with ocular changes limited to pigmentation of the fundus alone without visual compromise have been described.[1013] We have seen an 18-year-old female with medulloblastoma, dysmorphic facies including epicanthic folds, broad nasal bridge, congenital ankle deformity, and bilateral large great and second toes with extensive whorls of skin pigmentation following the lines of Blaschko, especially on the face, back, and arms (Figure 5.69F–L). She was visually asymptomatic and her fundus showed patchy depigmentation of the RPE (Figure 5.69F–J). She was found to carry a partial duplication of the long arm of chromosome 3 (46,XX, dup (3) (q23q27).

Overall, it appears that the skin changes of hypomelanosis of Ito are associated with a variety of chromosomal anomalies rather than a specific gene defect; hence it may best be addressed as a feature rather than a disorder, as suggested by Sybert.[1008]

HEIMLER'S SYNDROME

Heimler et al. in 1991 described two siblings with sensorineural deafness that began in early childhood, associated with Beau's lines (horizontal ridges) and leukonychia (white dots) on their finger- and toenails with hypoplastic enamel in their permanent teeth – more so the molars, with relative sparing of the incisors (Figure 5.70G and H).[1014] The primary dentition is normal in all cases. The condition is believed to be autosomal-recessive; subsequently there have been three reports in two siblings, one sporadic case, and a set of monozygotic twins.[1015] The original patient described by Heimler was recently examined at age 26 and found to have visual acuity of 20/40 in each eye, symmetric widespread gray white changes at the pigment epithelial level throughout the posterior pole, and cystoid macular edema in both eyes (Figure 5.70A, B, E, and F). The pigment epithelial changes correspond to punctate decreased and increased autofluorescence (Figure 5.70C and D). ERG showed mild decrease in scotopic and photopic function.

5.70 Heimler syndrome.

A–H: This 26-year-old woman was described by Dr. Heimler in 1991 when she was 6 years of age with dental and nail anomalies (G and H). An ocular examination was not performed at that time. Both eyes now had graying of the posterior pole at the level of the retinal pigment epithelium, extending up to the equator (A and B). Visual acuity was 20/40 in each eye. Optical coherence tomography showed cysts/schisis cavity in the macula (E and F). Autofluorescence imaging revealed punctate hyper- and hypoautofluorescent changes in both eyes that were symmetrical (C and D). Electroretinogram showed mildly subnormal amplitudes for cones and within the normal range for rods.

(A–H, Courtesy of Dr. Irene Barbazatto and Dr. Lawrence Yannuzzi.)

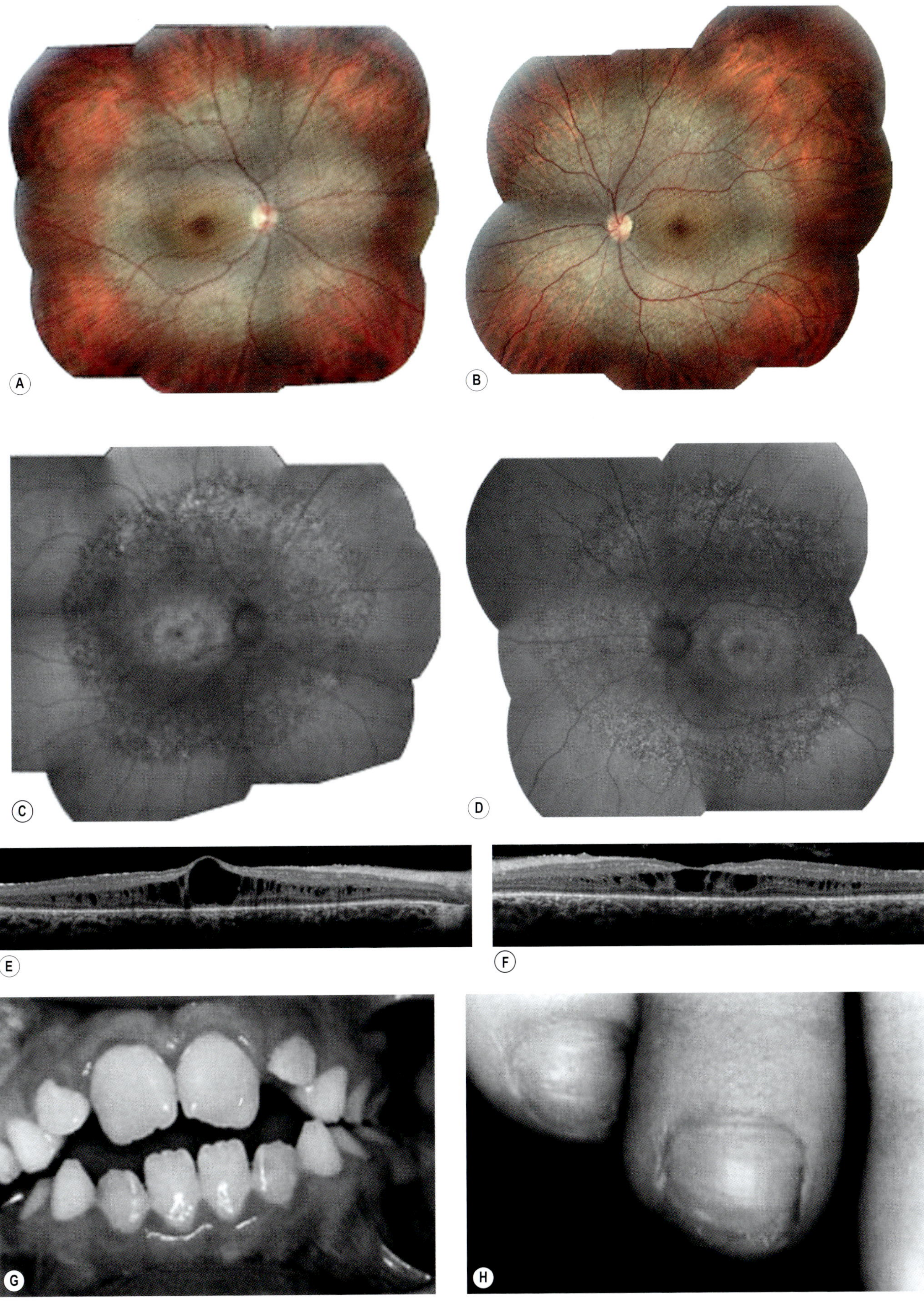
A
B
C
D
E
F
G
H

COCKAYNE'S SYNDROME

Cockayne's syndrome is an autosomal-recessive form of dwarfism associated with premature aging, characteristic "birdlike" facies, microcephaly, sunken eyes, beak nose, prognathism, disproportionately large hands and feet, flexion contractures of the limbs, kyphosis, hearing loss, intention tremor, nystagmus, ataxia, muscle rigidity, incontinence, mental retardation, hyperpigmentation and photosensitivity of the skin, "salt-and-pepper" retinopathy with waxy optic atrophy, and narrowed retinal vessels.[1016–1019] Vision is generally poor. Electroretinographic findings are normal or minimally abnormal. A French family of four brothers whose parents were first cousins showed hypermetropia and bilateral maculopathies with decreased cone amplitudes in all four. No retinal vascular or pigmentary changes were seen. Their mother had unilateral peripapillary pigmentary retinopathy on the left side and the father was normal.[1020]

On the basis of a neuropathologic finding it has been regarded as a leukodystrophy and a subgroup of the Pelizaeus–Merzbacher disease. The basic defect is unknown. Histopathology shows evidence of loss of nerve fiber and ganglion cells as well as loss of photoreceptor cells, irregular hypopigmentation, hyperpigmentation, and migration of pigment cells into the retina and subretinal space.[1018]

HEREDITARY MICROCEPHALY AND RETINAL DEGENERATION

Although the association of chorioretinal degeneration, electroretinographic abnormalities, and microcephaly has been reported most often in families with autosomal-recessive inheritance, it may occur in families with autosomal-dominant inheritance.[1021]

OSTEOPETROSIS AND CHORIORETINAL DEGENERATION

Osteopetrosis is a group of hereditary metabolic diseases characterized by increased bone mass caused by defective bone resorption. It is subdivided into juvenile- and adult-onset types. Infantile malignant osteopetrosis is an autosomal-recessive disorder present at birth and is lethal during childhood unless treated. Osteoclast dysfunction causes abnormal bone resorption, thickened cortical bone skeletal defects, and frequent bone fractures. Hematological abnormalities due to bone expansion into the marrow space with extramedullary hematopoiesis are present. Hearing and visual loss may occur as the result of encroachment on the auditory and optic foramen, optic atrophy, or progressive retinal degeneration.[1022–1026] Retinal degeneration may be evident on ophthalmoscopic examination as depigmentation and atrophy of the pigment epithelium in the macula,[1022] or electroretinographically in patients whose fundi are within normal limits.[1022,1023] Thorough neuroradiologic and imaging studies and electroretinography are important in these children when they present with poor visual function, optic disc pallor, and otherwise normal fundi before proceeding with surgery to decompress the optic foramen. The optic foramen may show only minimal narrowing, and most of the visual loss may be on the basis of the progressive retinal degeneration.[1022]

Allogenic hematopoietic stem cell transplantation done early in the course has resulted in survival and increased life expectancy in these children.[1026] Mutations in the *Tcirg1* (Atp6V0a3), locus which encodes the a3 subunit of the vaculolar-type proton-transporting ATPase, an enzyme involved in the development of visual function, is known to cause half the cases of severe autosomal-recessive osteopetrosis.[1025,1026]

PERIOXISOMAL DISEASES

Malfunction of the peroxisome, a subcellular organelle, results in several childhood ophthalmological disorders. These disorders have been divided into three groups: (1) defective biogenesis of the peroxisome (Zellweger syndrome, neonatal adrenoleukodystrophy, and infantile Refsum's disease); (2) multiple enzyme deficiencies (rhizomelic chondrodysplasia punctata); and (3) a single-enzyme deficiency (X-linked adrenoleukodystrophy, primary hyperoxaluria type 1).

Zellweger syndrome, the most lethal of the three peroxisomal biogenesis disorders, causes infantile hypotonia, seizures, and death within the first year. Ophthalmic manifestations include corneal opacification, cataract, glaucoma, pigmentary retinopathy, and optic atrophy. Neonatal adrenoleukodystrophy and infantile Refsum's disease appear to be genetically distinct, but clinically, biochemically, and pathologically similar to Zellweger syndrome, although milder. Rhizomelic chondrodysplasia punctata, a peroxisomal disorder which results from at least two peroxisomal enzyme deficiencies, presents at birth with skeletal abnormalities and patients rarely survive past 1 year of age. The most prominent ocular manifestation consists of bilateral cataracts. X-linked (childhood) adrenoleukodystrophy results from a deficiency of a single peroxisomal enzyme, and presents in the latter part of the first decade with behavioral, cognitive, and visual deterioration. The vision loss results from demyelination of the entire visual pathway, but the outer retina is spared. Primary hyperoxaluria type 1 manifests as parafoveal subretinal pigment proliferation. Classical Refsum's disease is also a peroxisomal disorder.

Cerebrohepatorenal Syndrome (Zellweger's Syndrome)

Zellweger's syndrome is a multisystem congenital disorder characterized by severe central nervous system involvement (hypotonia, seizures, and psychomotor retardation), hepatic interstitial fibrosis (jaundice, hepatomegaly, hypoprothrombinemia, and gastrointestinal bleeding), multiple renal cortical cysts, calcified stippling of the bony epiphysis, characteristic facies (high forehead, micrognathia, flat supraorbital ridges, and high arched palate), and in some patients evidence of a tapetoretinal degeneration.[1027–1029] Most of these patients die within the first year of life. Histopathologic examination reveals changes similar to retinitis pigmentosa.[1028] Ultrastructural examination shows bileaflet inclusions of the RPE. These patients have an excessive amount of very-long-chain fatty acids in the ocular tissue. These histopathologic and biochemical findings are similar to those in neonatal adrenoleukodystrophy, a metabolic neurodegenerative disorder characterized by generalized visceral dysfunction, central nervous system white-matter degeneration, and adrenal hypofunction.[1031]

ADRENOLEUKODYSTROPHIES

The adrenoleukodystrophies are a group of rare disorders that include a childhood-onset X-linked variant (Schilder's disease), adrenoleukomyelonephropathy, and neonatal adrenoleukodystrophy. Patients with all three disorders demonstrate central nervous system demyelinization, adrenal cortical atrophy and/or lamellar inclusions, and increased serum levels of long-chain fatty acids.[1031] Features of neonatal adrenoleukodystrophy include: onset of hypotonia and seizures in the neonatal period, visual loss, optic atrophy, cataract, pigmentary retinopathy (50%), autosomal-recessive mode of inheritance, long-chain fatty acid in multiple organs, and diminution in size and number of hepatocellular peroxisomes.[1031] The mean age of death is 3 years. Histopathologic and ultrastructural changes in the eye include loss of the ganglion cell and nerve fiber layers, optic atrophy, atrophy of the retinal receptors, cystoid macular edema, pigment cell migration into the retina, cataracts, and characteristic bileaflet inclusions in retinal macrophages, pigment epithelial cells, photoreceptor cells, and vitreous macrophages.[1030,1031]

Zellweger's syndrome is similar to neonatal adrenoleukodystrophy but is associated with renal cysts but no adrenal cortical atrophy (see Zellweger's syndrome). The features of childhood adrenoleukodystrophy include: onset at 4–8 years of life of progressive dementia, gait disturbances, visual loss, primary adrenal insufficiency leading to skin pigmentation and symptoms of hypoadrenalism, X-linked recessive mode of inheritance, morphologically normal hepatic peroxisomes, and death in adolescence.[1033] Visual loss is primarily caused by central nervous system demyelinization, but ganglion cell degeneration may also be operative. Pigmentary macular changes occur in some patients.[1033] Adrenoleukomyeloneuropathy is associated with late-onset (range 20–30 years) hypogonadism, spastic quadriparesis, and X-linked inheritance.[1033]

REFSUM'S SYNDROME (HEREDOPATHIA ATACTICA POLYNEURITIFORMIS)

Refsum's syndrome is a familial disease characterized by night blindness, atypical pigmentary retinal dystrophy, chronic polyneuropathy, cerebellar ataxia, and elevated cerebrospinal fluid protein without pleocytosis.[1034–1038] This disease begins insidiously in either infancy or early childhood. The average delay in diagnosis of Refsum's disease is approximately 10 years after the diagnosis of retinitis pigmentosa.[1034] Cataracts, ichthyosis, skeletal anomalies, and electrocardiographic evidence of conduction defects frequently appear. Some patients develop hearing loss. The pupils may be small and nonreactive. Oculomotor apraxia may be seen. The ERG amplitudes decrease as the disease progresses. Death is caused by heart failure or respiratory paralysis.

This is a recessively inherited disorder of lipid metabolism with mutations in the gene encoding a peroxisomal enzyme phytanoyl-coenzyme A alpha-hydroxylase, which results in the inability to alpha-oxidize phytanic acid.[1037,1039,1040] As a result phytanic acid, which is not an endogenous product but is supplied with food mainly as phytanic acid or its precursor, phytol, accumulates in the urine, plasma (normal, $< 1\ \mu mol/l$), and body tissues and nerves. Two hypotheses have been postulated: (1) phytanic acid methyl groups may act to destabilize the myelin lipid layer in axons; or (2) the phytanic acid may replace long-chain fatty acids in phospholipids and triglycerides, resulting in decreased function of the affected tissues. In the eye, abundant fat-staining substances have been found within the RPE; this may eventually lead to photoreceptor cell death. Esterification of vitamin A with phytanic acid may also lead to the demise of photoreceptors. Treatment with a diet low in phytol and phytanic acid reduces plasma phytanic acid levels and causes some improvement in neurologic signs[1034] and may retard the progression of retinal degeneration.[1034,1041] Plasmapheresis can help lower serum phytanic acid levels in severe metabolic aberrations.[1042–1045] Early diagnosis, however, is important to prevent development of the neurologic complications.[1034]

CEREBRO-OCULOHEPATORENAL SYNDROME (ARIMA'S SYNDROME)

Arima's syndrome consists of characteristic facies (blepharoptosis and telecanthus), nystagmus, Leber's amaurosis, hypotonia, profound psychomotor retardation, agenesis of cerebellar vermis, infantile polycystic kidneys, progressive chronic renal insufficiency, and liver disease.[1046] Its features are similar to those of Joubert's syndrome, which in addition includes infantile episodic respiratory abnormalities that may be life-threatening.[1046,1047]

5.71 Spinocerebellar atrophy (SCA7).

A–G: This 36-year-old male complained of decreased vision in both eyes for 10 years. He had a 5-year history of gait, limb, and speech ataxia. His vision was 20/100 in each eye with bilateral central scotomas (C). Both foveas were thinned out with reddish coloration (A–B). A foveolar window defect was seen on a fluorescein (D and E) and no changes on an indocyanine green angiogram (F). Electroretinogram showed diminished rod and cone function. Foveal photoreceptors were lost on optical coherence tomography (G). His gene testing showed 48 CAG repeats on the *ATXN7* gene consistent with SCA7.

CHORIORETINOPATHY AND PITUITARY DYSFUNCTION

The syndrome of chorioretinopathy and pituitary dysfunction is characterized by severe congenital or early-onset atypical pigmentary retinal dystrophy; hypothalamic–pituitary dysfunction manifested by growth retardation; sexual infantilism; hair abnormalities, including long lashes, sparse, fine scalp hair, long bushy eyebrows (trichomegaly), and failure to develop postpubertal hair patterns; and perhaps, to a lesser degree, hypothyroidism.[1048–1051] Less consistent features include low birth weight, abnormal pregnancy, and mental retardation. Patients may show an extinguished ERG, widespread areas of thinning, and coarse clumping of the RPE.

RETINITIS PIGMENTOSA AND AUTOIMMUNE POLYENDOCRINOPATHY

During childhood or early adulthood, patients with type I autosomal-recessive autoimmune polyendocrinopathy develop hypoparathyroidism, mucocutaneous moniliasis, Addison's disease, and keratoconjunctivitis.[1052–1054] This syndrome may also include chronic hepatitis, malabsorption, pernicious anemia, alopecia, and primary hypogonadism. A few patients may develop typical retinitis pigmentosa.[1053] I have seen one such patient and the medical records of another. Neither had evidence of malabsorption, and both had normal serum vitamin A levels. The occasional association of retinitis pigmentosa with type I polyendocrinopathy may be related to the proximity of the gene locus for these two disorders, which in the case of the polyendocrinopathy, has been assigned to chromosome 21.[1054] Wood and coworkers observed the development of an asymmetric fundus picture of retinitis pigmentosa in a young man with type I autoimmune polyendocrinopathy.[1055] They demonstrated markedly elevated titers against the retina and optic nerve and hypothesized that the eye findings were autoimmune and part of the syndrome.

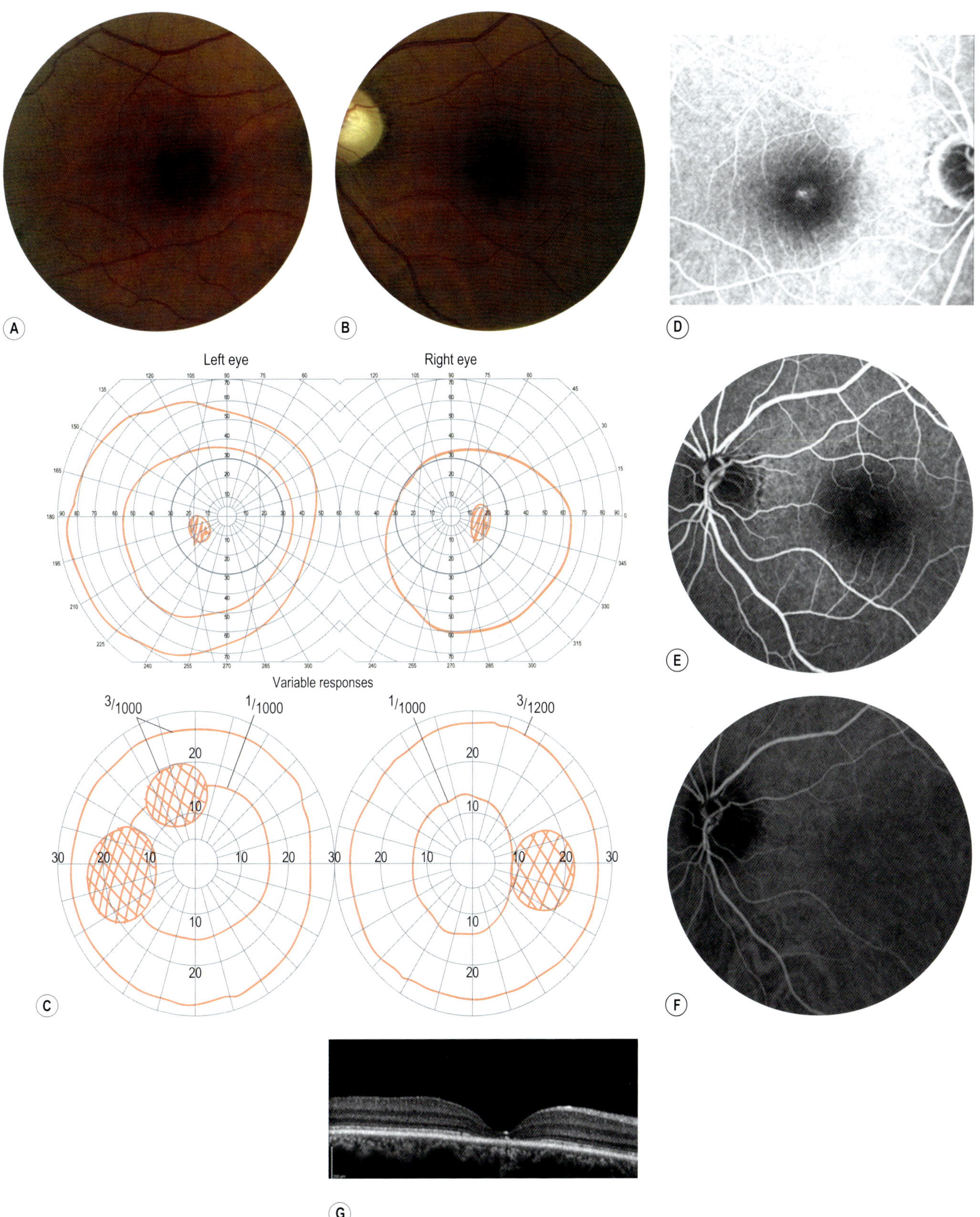
A
B
D
Left eye
Right eye
Variable responses
3/1000
1/1000
1/1000
3/1200
C
E
F
G

ATYPICAL TAPETORETINAL DYSTROPHY ASSOCIATED WITH OLIVOPONTOCEREBELLAR ATROPHY, KONIGSMARK TYPE III, HARDING TYPE II

Atypical tapetoretinal dystrophy associated with cerebellar ataxia is an autosomal-dominantly inherited disease characterized by loss of central vision that is caused by atrophic changes of the retina and RPE, which are initially confined to the macula but which gradually spread to involve the peripheral fundus (Figure 5.56F–I).[1056–1065] Patients with infantile-onset disease typically have pigmentary changes and exhibit a rapidly progressive course that often leads to early death.[1066] Later onset in childhood is less severe, and adult-onset disease is accompanied by relatively mild and slowly progressive cerebellar degeneration and circumscribed macular lesions.[1066] Some patients may have pyramidal, extrapyramidal, and brainstem dysfunction. Findings in some patients may include dystonia, nystagmus, internuclear ophthalmoplegia, progressive ophthalmoplegia, ptosis, and disturbances in esophageal, bladder, and bowel function. Electrophysiologic testing may be normal early but severely abnormal in the later stages of the disease. Some patients have progressive external ophthalmoplegia. Histopathologic and ultrastructural findings in the infantile type III olivopontocerebellar atrophy and degeneration show retinal degeneration affecting primarily the retinal receptor layer with maximal involvement being in the macular area, striking variability in pigmentation of the RPE, osmiophilic multimembranous and complex lipofuscin inclusions in conjunctiva, keratocytes, lens epithelium, iris and ciliary body fibrocytes, outer retinal cells, and pigment epithelial cells.[1057,1062,1067,1068] These inclusions are similar to those seen in the neuronal ceroid lipofuscinoses (NCL). Unlike in the latter patients, however, there are no curvilinear inclusions.

Olivopontocerebellar degeneration type III should be suspected in infants presenting with a neurodegenerative and retinal degenerative picture. These patients should be differentiated from those with the infantile form of NCL, infantile phytanic acid storage disease, abetalipoproteinemia, and recessive neonatal adrenoleukodystrophy. Detection of evidence of the disease in a parent and clinical evidence of ataxia are important findings to differentiate this from the other disorders. Conjunctival biopsy is helpful to confirm the diagnosis but does not differentiate it from the lipofuscinoses. Family members with normal fundi and visual acuity may show ERG changes.[1067]

5.71 Continued

H–M: This 28-year-old African American woman had a family history of decreased vision in mother, a sister, and a brother. Her mother carried a diagnosis of multiple sclerosis. One other sister had normal vision. She was a type 2 diabetic for 5 years. She complained of decreased vision in both eyes and said her vision was better at night. She was a −8.50 myope with significant astigmatism of +3.25 on the right and +5.25 on the left. Vision was 20/200 in each eye. Her fundus was normal (H and I) and HVF showed central scotoma in both eyes. No specific diagnosis could be made and when re-examined 2 years later her fundus was still unremarkable with 20/400 vision in both eyes. Three years later the macula developed bull's-eye-type change in both foveas, more prominent on the right than the left (J), which continued to evolve over the next 2 years. The foveal change was hypoautofluorescent (K) and showed a window defect on angiography (L). Optical coherence tomography through the fovea confirmed loss of foveal cones and thinning of inner retina (M). Over the 8 years she was followed her ataxia progressed and she became wheelchair-bound. She and her mother tested positive for CAG repeats on 3p12-13, confirming the diagnosis of SCA7.

(A–G, courtesy of Dr. Jose Pulido; H–M, courtesy of Dr. Joel Miller.)

Spinocerebellar Ataxia 7

SCA 7 is an autosomal-dominant neourodegenerative disease with progressive retinal and cerebellar degeneration. Clinical features in patients with SCA 7 consist of early blue-yellow color blindness, progressive visual impairment with central vision becoming compromised first. The fundus may look normal in the early stages of the disease, then develops a subtle reddish change with thinning (Figure 5.71A and B) that can be discerned only on high-resolution OCT imaging. Progressive RPE hypopigmentation ensues that manifests as window defects on angiography (Figure 5.71D). The OCT at this stage shows complete loss of foveal photoreceptors (Figure 5.71G). These changes are usually accompanied by progressive limb ataxia, dysarthria, slowing of saccades, and ophthalmoplegia. Patients become wheelchair-bound over time. Gene ataxin is expressed in the brain and eye. The repeat expression of CAG gene causes cytotoxic gain of function of the protein and aggregation, resulting in structural changes to the involved tissue. The repeats are unstable between generations, and this results in anticipation in the children of these patients. The higher the number of repeats, the more severe the disease manifestation.[1069–1071]

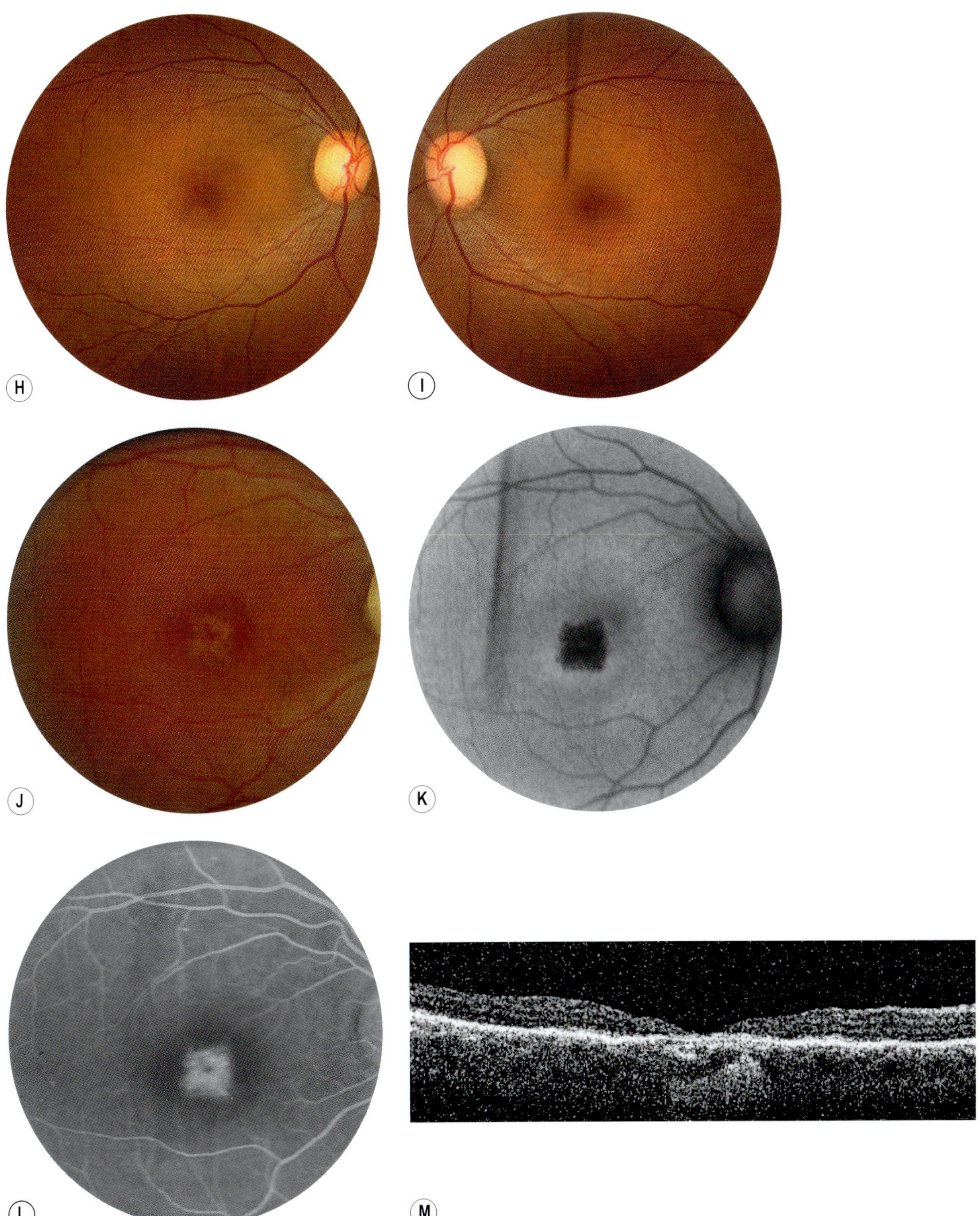
H
I
J
K
L
M

PANTOTHENATE KINASE-ASSOCIATED NEURODEGENERATION (HALLERVORDEN–SPATZ SYNDROME)

Pantothenate kinase-associated neurodegeneration, formely known as Hallervorden–Spatz syndrome, is characterized by the early onset of an extrapyramidal motor disorder (dystonic posturing, muscular rigidity, choreoathetoid movements, ataxia, hyperreflexia, and spasticity), dementia, iron accumulation in the brain, and a relentlessly progressive course leading to death in early adulthood.[1073–1077] Approximately one-fourth of these patients will demonstrate retinal degeneration that initially may show only mottling of the RPE but subsequently may show evidence of a flecked retina and later bone spicule formation and a bull's-eye annular maculopathy.[1078] There is some evidence to suggest that those patients with the retinal findings have an earlier onset of the disease and a much more rapid course, with death occurring in late childhood. Some patients have an associated acanthocytosis and normal beta-lipoprotein levels.[1074] Pupillary abnormalities resmbling Adie's pupil, poor convergence reflex, patchy loss of pupillary ruff, and sector iris atrophy are seen in some patients, likely due to proximal degeneration of the fibers destined to the iris due to iron deposition in the midbrain in or near the substantia nigra.[1078] Patients with a variant of Hallervorden–Spatz syndrome have hypoprebetalipoproteinemia, acanthocytosis, retinitis pigmentosa, and pallidal degeneration (HARP syndrome).[1079] Computed tomography of the brain may show basal ganglia opacities and T2-weighted MRI shows characteristic abnormalities of the globus pallidus described as "eye of the tiger" sign (much darker with a central bright spot).[1077,1078,1080] Neuropathologic criteria for diagnosis include: (1) symmetric, partially destructive lesions of the globus pallidus; (2) widely disseminated rounded or oval nonnucleated structures ("spheroids"), identifiable as swollen axons, especially numerous in the globus pallidus and pars reticulata; and (3) accumulation of pigment, much of it containing iron, in the affected regions. Histopathologic examination of the eye shows absence of the photoreceptor cells, attenuation of the plexiform and outer nuclear layers, normal inner retinal layers, and degenerative changes with accumulation of melanofuscin in the RPE.[1074,1076,1081] There are accumulations of RPE cells as well as extracellular pigment around equatorial blood vessels.[1074,1081] The disease is inherited autosomal-recessively secondary to mutations in the gene encoding pantothenate kinase 2 (PANK2) located on chromosome 20p13, involved in the biosynthesis of coenzyme A.[1082–1087] Deficiency of PANK2 enzyme results in accumulation of cysteine in the globus pallidus, causing neuronal death. The exact mechanism leading to iron accumulation in the area is not understood.[1088] Two forms, classic or early-onset, with a more severe phenotype and progression, and an atypical form, adult-onset slowly progressive parkinsonism, are known.[1082]

5.72 Kearns–Sayre syndrome.

A–C: This 16-year-old female with atypical pigmentary retinal dystrophy, external ophthalmoplegia (A), complete heart block, amenorrhea, and retarded growth had Stokes–Adams attacks that were relieved by a cardiac pacemaker. Her visual acuity was 20/25. There was concentric contraction of the visual fields to color test objects. Diffuse pigment abnormalities that were not prominent ophthalmoscopically were readily apparent angiographically.
D–H: This 36-year-old black man with heart block complained of ptosis of both eyelids of several years' duration (D). Note the plaque of hyperplastic retinal pigment epithelium (RPE) nasally (E) and mottling of the RPE in the macula (F). Angiography shows coarse pattern of hyperfluorescence (G and H).

MITOCHONDRIAL ENCEPHALOMYOPATHIES

The mitochondrial encephalomyopathies are a group of clinically heterogeneous disorders that share common biochemical and morphologic abnormalities in the mitochondria. This group includes the Kearns–Sayre syndrome, MELAS syndrome,[1089] and MERRF syndrome,[149,1090–1092]. A patient who shows features of two or three of these disorders is referred to by some as having a mitochondrial encephalomyopathy overlap syndrome.[1097] A number of DNA mutations have been localized in patients with these disorders.[1098–1100] Interestingly, in some instances a specific gene mutation can account for more than one phenotype. Two patients with the overlap syndrome demonstrated identical mitochondrial DNA mutations at nucleotide position 3243 (MELAS mutation).[1097]

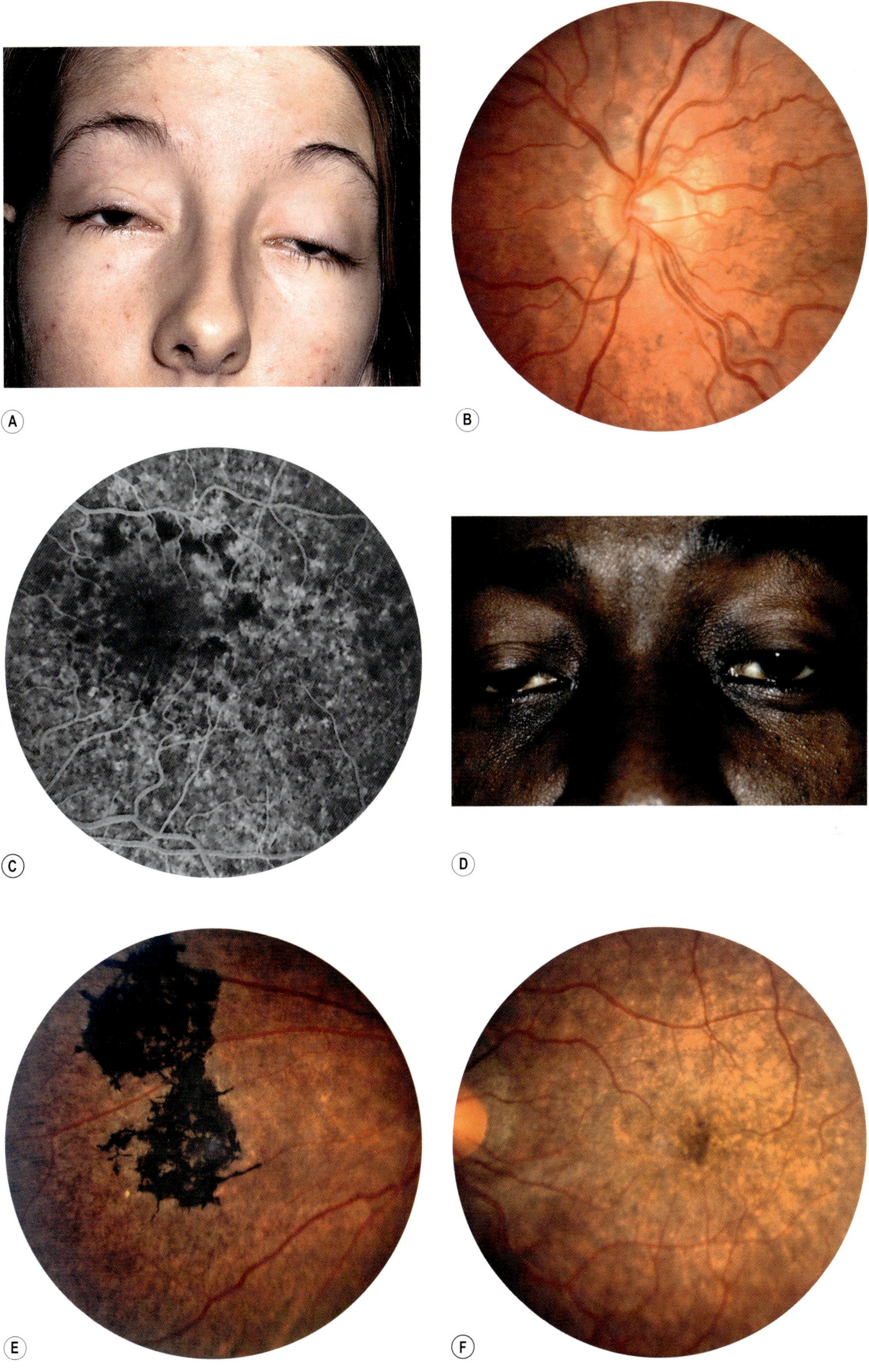
A
B
C
D
E
F

Kearns–Sayre Syndrome

Kearns–Sayre syndrome is a rare sporadic multisystem mitochondrial disorder affecting the central nervous system, muscles, and endocrine organs. Clinical features include atypical pigmentary retinal dystrophy (Figure 5.72), myopathic external ophthalmoplegia with the onset of ptosis in early childhood, and heart block.[1101] Other features that may be present include widespread muscular dystrophy, deafness, vestibular dysfunction, elevated spinal fluid protein, dwarfism, hypogonadism, cerebellar and corticospinal dysfunction, endocrine dysfunction, nephropathy, and corneal opacity.[1101–1108] "Ragged-red" myopathy and spongiform degeneration of the central nervous system are characteristic histopathologic findings.[1104] These patients usually have excellent visual function. There may be some loss of central vision in later life. Less than 50% experience nyctalopia. Diplopia is uncommon. The characteristic fundus finding is the presence of widespread salt-and-pepper RPE mottling that is most striking in the macula and depigmentation of the RPE in the peripapillary area (Figure 5.72B, E, F, I, and J). There is rarely evidence of pigment migration into the overlying retina. The retinal vessels are of normal caliber, and the optic disc is normal. Later in life some patients may develop a picture more closely simulating retinitis pigmentosa and in a few cases demonstrate severe chorioretinal atrophy simulating choroideremia.[1109] The EOG may be normal or subnormal. The ERG may be subnormal or extinguished. A patient with findings typical of adult vitelliform pattern dystrophy has been described recently – a feature similar to that seen in patients with MELAS/MIDD, signifying changes affecting the RPE.[1110] Early in life the histopathologic changes in the eye may be confined to an irregular area of hypopigmentation and hyperpigmentation of the RPE, macrophages in the subretinal space, mild loss of rod and cone cells (Figure 5.72K), and dystrophic changes in the extraocular muscles that are characteristic yet nonspecific (Figure 5.72L).[1106,1111–1113] Later there may be loss of the RPE and receptor cells that is most marked in the macular area (Figure 5.72K). Ultrastructural study reveals enlarged mitochondria in the basal part of the RPE, the photoreceptor ellipsoid, outer plexiform layer, and nonpigmented ciliary epithelium.[1113,1114] Macrophages containing phagocytosed lamellar discs were present in the subretinal space. The clinical and histopathologic findings suggest that the primary disease affects the RPE and that the posterior fundus is affected more than the peripheral fundus. The use of systemic corticosteroids in these patients may precipitate hyperglycemic acidotic coma and death.[1102] A similar syndrome but with progressive optic atrophy and absence of tapetoretinal dystrophy may occur.[1115]

MIDD/MELAS

See earlier section under pattern dystrophies.

5.72 Continued

I–L: This 14-year-old boy with Kearns–Sayre syndrome developed ptosis and restricted eye movements at 9 years of age. He had mild reduction in visual acuity and subnormal electroretinographic findings. There were mottled pigmentary changes in the macular area (I and J) that were relatively inapparent in this blond fundus. He developed syncopal attacks and heart block 5 months before death following complications of an upper respiratory infection. His eyes were obtained at autopsy. Histopathologic examination revealed evidence of hyperpigmentation and depigmentation of the RPE (K). In some areas there was evidence of some loss of the retinal receptor elements. The retina and choroid were otherwise unremarkable. There were marked degenerative changes involving the extraocular muscles (L). Similar alterations were noted in the muscles of the lower extremities, shoulder girdle, and diaphragm.

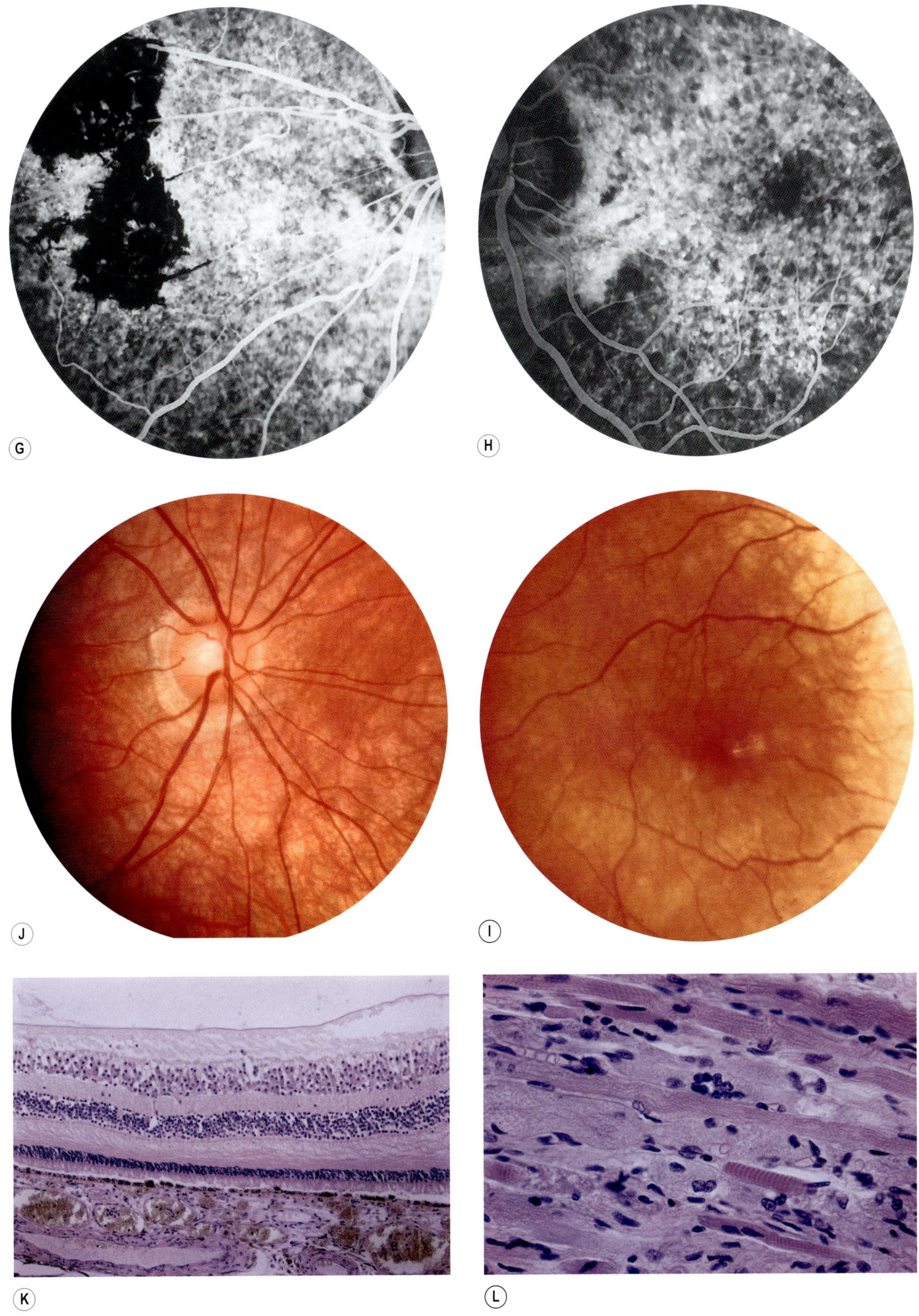
G
H
J
I
K
L

DANON DISEASE

Danon disease is a rare X-linked disorder characterized by cardiomyopathy, skeletal myopathy, and mental retardation.[1096,1116,1117] The skeletal myopathy is generally mild and the mental retardation variable and nonprogressive, but cardiomyopathy is progressive and determines the outcome. Mutations in the *LAMP2* gene on Xq24 have been shown to be responsible for the disease, the cellular pathogenesis being caused by a deficiency of lysosome-associated membrane protein-2 (LAMP2). Lysosomal storage occurs in this disorder, with elevated muscle glycogen in spite of normal α-glucosidase activity. Cytoplasmic vacuoles containing autophagic material and glycogen are seen in skeletal and cardiac muscle cells. An animal model, the lamp2-deficient mouse, shows reduced weight and increased mortality, with accumulation of autophagic vacuoles in many tissues, including skeletal and heart muscle, liver, pancreas, spleen, and kidney. In hepatocytes, the autophagic degradation of long-lived proteins is severely impaired, cardiac myocytes are ultrastructurally abnormal, and heart contractility is severely reduced.[1096] The affected males present early in age (2–5 years) with fatigue and show evidence of progressive hypertrophic cardiomyopathy and secondary arrhythmias, the commonest being Wolff–Parkinson–White. Unless a cardiac transplant is done, death can occur suddenly from an arrhythmia or due to progressive heart failure from a heavy heart and thickened ventricular wall and interventricular septum. Women present later in life, in the fourth decade or later (Figure 5.73H–J), with signs of dilated cardiomyopathy.[1096] The less severe disease in women is likely from irregular lyonization of the X chromosome.

Male patients have moderate decrease in vision in the 20/40–20/60 range and may complain of nyctalopia while women may have normal or near-normal acuity. The retina of affected men shows diffuse loss of RPE and choroidal pigment resembling the fundi of choroideremia (Figure 5.73A–C, F, and G), though may not be as severe. Women show annular mid peripheral and peripheral fine pigment mottling (Figure 5.73H–J) resembling salt-and-pepper fundus of rubella and the carrier state of choroideremia. Fluorescein angiogram delineates the pigment mottling better (Figure 5.73D and E). Electoretinogram in affected males is subnormal and mildly affected in women. Lens changes in the form of stellate dots or fine flecks may be present.[1094,1095,1116] Macular changes have been mentioned in one case but no images are available. Tying the ocular findings with the cardiac history is important to make the diagnosis, which in turn can save the patient's life with a timely heart transplant.

5.73 Danon disease.

A–G: This 35-year-old visually asymptomatic male was found to have 20/20 vision with hypopigmented patches of the retinal pigment epithelium in both eyes (A–C). Angiogram revealed punctate blocked fluorescence from pigment (D and E). Three years later the fundus appearance was unchanged in both eyes (F and G). His ocular examination was prompted by his medical findings of cardiomyopathy requiring heart transplant.

H–J: Visually asymptomatic sister of a patient with cardiomyopathy and arrhythmia showed fine mottling of pigment more prominent outside the posterior pole. Electroretinogram amplitudes were normal but implicit times were prolonged.

(A–G, courtesy of Dr. Susan Malinowski; H–J, courtesy of Dr. Naresh Mandava.)

BASSEN–KORNZWEIG SYNDROME

Bassen–Kornzweig syndrome is characterized by atypical pigmentary retinal dystrophy (retinitis pigmentosa albescens in some cases), night blindness, spinal cerebellar ataxia (Friedreich's type), celiac syndrome, acanthocytosis, low serum levels of cholesterol, triglycerides, and fat-soluble vitamins, extinguished ERG, and abetalipoproteinemia.[950,1118–1126] Abnormalities of extraocular movements, including ptosis, strabismus, nystagmus, and progressive ophthalmoplegia, have been noted.[1125]

Bassen–Kornzweig syndrome is recessively inherited, with mutations in the gene encoding the large subunit of microsomal triglyceride transfer protein (MTP) on 4q22-24. MTP acts as a chaperone that facilitates the transfer of lipids on to apoB.[1127] ApoB-100 is an essential component of very-low-density lipoproteins and low-density lipoproteins (LDLs). ApoB-48 is secreted from the intestine and is needed for the assembly and secretion of chylomicrons by the intestine.[867] The patient can assimilate fat into the intestinal mucosa, but a defect exists in its removal from this site because of the deficiency of plasma chylomicrons. The liver and the retina become depleted of vitamin A. The role of vitamin A deprivation in causing the retinal degeneration in this syndrome is supported by observations that large doses of vitamin A have produced return of dark adaptation thresholds and electroretinographic responses.[1123] Large-dose vitamin E supplementation combined with low-fat diet and soluble vitamin supplementation appeared to prevent the retinopathy in one small uncontrolled study.[1128] Studies have shown prevention of the neurological and retinal degeneration to a large extent if water-soluble vitamin A, E, and sometimes K supplementation is begun before age 2.[867,1119–1122] Some progression may still occur, and reversal of changes does not occur.

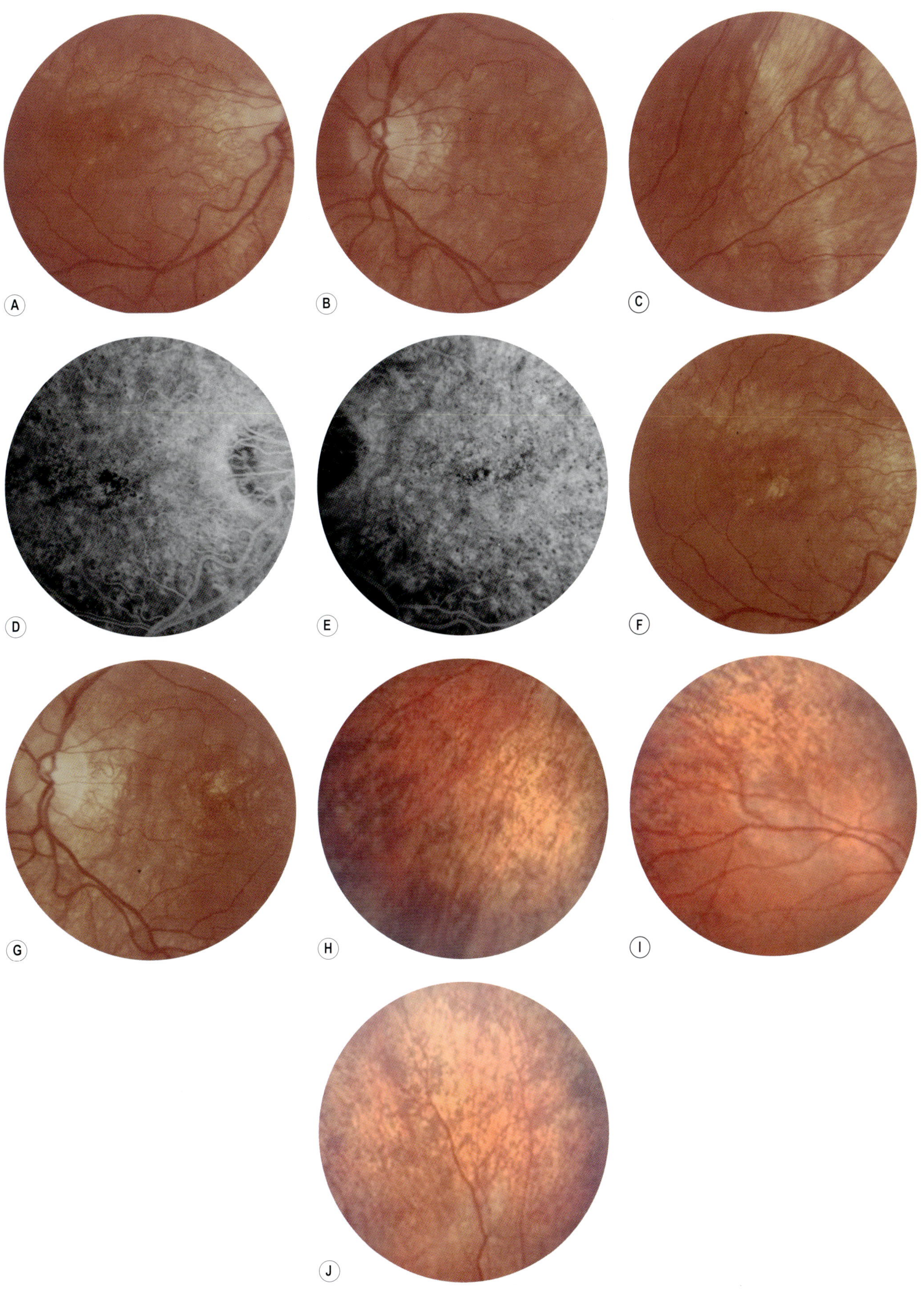
A
B
C
D
E
F
G
H
I
J

The pigmentary retinal degeneration in these patients is often associated with waxy pallor of the optic disc, attenuation of the retinal vessels, peripheral ring scotoma, and RPE atrophic changes associated with clump or spot pigmentation rather than bone corpuscular pigmentation. The retinal degenerative changes were milder in two brothers with the syndrome seen at the Bascom Palmer Eye Institute (Figure 5.74). One of these brothers has maintained excellent visual function while being given 25 000 units of water-soluble vitamin A for 20 years (Figure 5.74E and F). He recently noted progression of nyctalopia to the point that he had to give up driving. His serum vitamin A levels were low. After treatment with 50 000 units of vitamin A, the serum levels of vitamin A returned to normal and he experienced marked improvement of the nyctalopia and some improvement in the ERG.

Histopathologically, there is widespread loss of photoreceptors and abnormal PAS-positive granules in the RPE.[949,1124] Electron microscopically the RPE contains abnormal amounts of lipofuscin and lamellar inclusions.[949]

FAMILIAL HYPOBETALIPOPROTEINEMIA

Familial hypobetalipoproteinemia is a distinct entity from the Bassen–Kornzweig syndrome.[1126,1129] It is a dominantly inherited disorder characterized by low total plasma cholesterol levels and low levels of LDLs. Hepatic vitamin A transport is normal but vitamin E transport is severely affected due to lack of LDL. Patients may be asymptomatic or may have a variety of neurologic defects ranging from psychomotor retardation to polyneuropathy, mostly attributed to lack of vitamin E. An atypical form of pigmentary degeneration may occur in homozygous patients. A patient with heterozygous hypobetalipoproteinemia developed night blindness at age 51 years and ophthalmoscopic evidence of severe progressive retinal degeneration before she died at age 75 years.[1129] Histopathologic examination of her eyes revealed absent photoreceptors and massive deposition of basal linear deposit and minimal migration of pigment epithelium into the retina. Vitamin E supplementation, along with A and K, can limit the neurological and retinal degeneration if begun early and maintained lifelong.[867]

NEUROLIPIDOSES

The term "neurolipidoses" is used to describe the neuronal storage diseases. These can be divided into two broad types: (1) the sphingolipidoses; and (2) the nonglycolipid neuronal storage diseases, or ceroid lipofuscinoses.

5.74 Bassen–Kornzweig syndrome.

A–D: This 22-year-old man with high myopia and his brother had mild pigmentary retinal dystrophy, abetalipoproteinemia, progressive spinocerebellar degeneration, tremor, acanthocytosis, and celiac syndrome. Their parents were first cousins. His visual acuity was 20/40 in both eyes when he was initially examined. His fundi showed paracentral and patchy peripheral zones of depigmentation of the retinal pigment epithelium (RPE) and minimal narrowing of the retinal vessels (A–D). An electroretinogram revealed slightly abnormal rod and cone function. His acuity was unchanged until age 32 years. At age 46 years his visual acuity had declined to 8/200 right eye and 5/200 left eye. He had bull's-eye maculopathy. There was no nyctalopia and moderate constriction of the peripheral visual fields. The peripheral fundi were blond and free of pigmentary migration.
E and **F**: His 19-year-old brother showed similar but less severe pigmentary changes in addition to a prominent angioid streak (arrow, E) and a blond fundus peripherally. A large, flat, scalloped, hypopigmented lesion in the periphery of one eye was probably hypertrophy of the RPE (F). His visual acuity was 20/25 in the right eye and 20/40 in the left eye. His electroretinogram in the right eye was normal and in the left eye showed moderately abnormal rod and cone responses. He took vitamin A, 25 000 units daily. There was minimal change in his visual function and fundi when examined at age 43 years. During the following 2 years, however, he developed moderately severe nyctalopia that responded favorably to 50 000 units of vitamin A daily.

(E and F, courtesy of Dr. John T Flynn.)

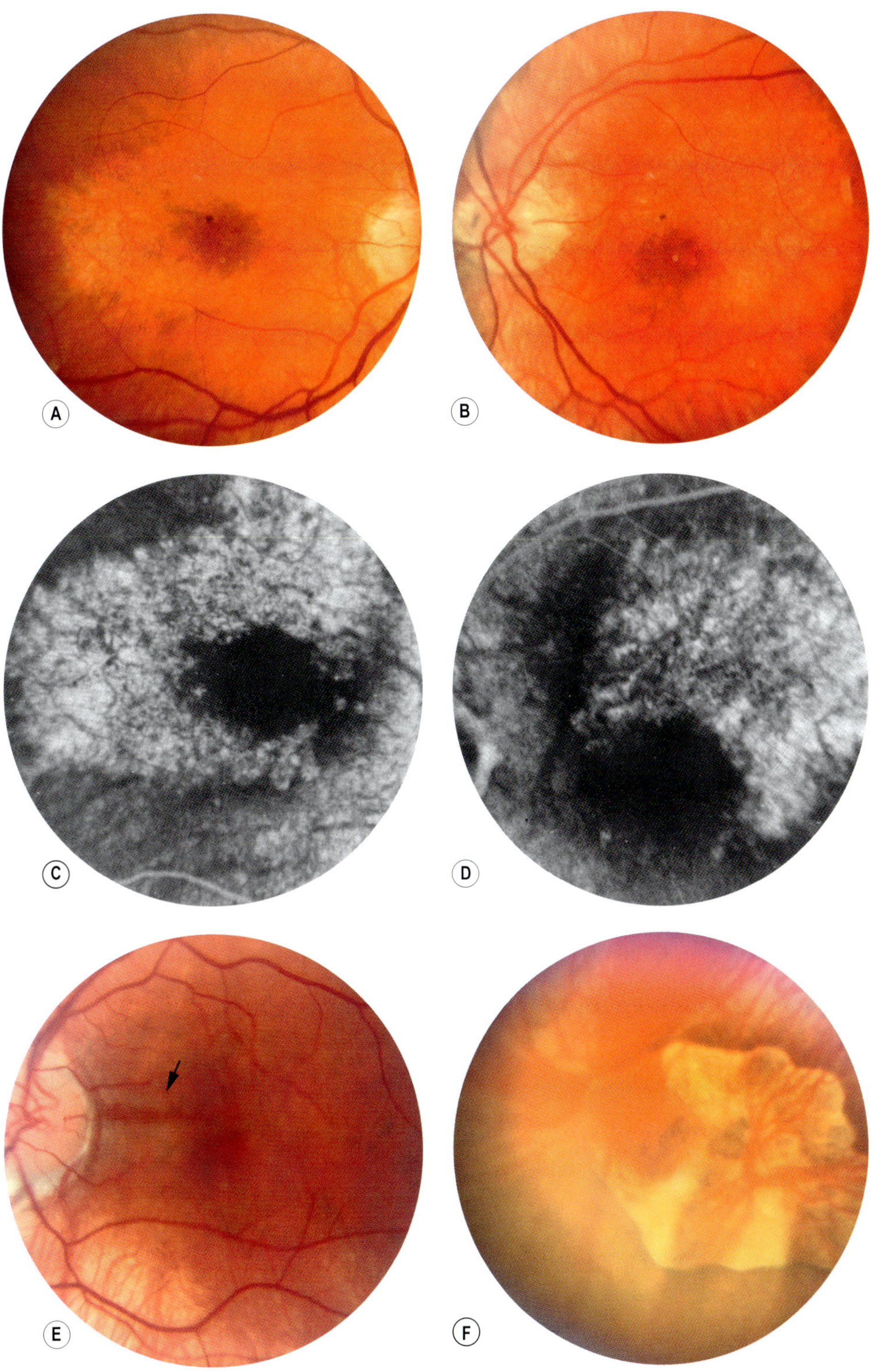
A
B
C
D
E
F

Sphingolipidoses

The sphingolipidoses are lysosomal metabolic disorders involving conjugated derivatives of ceramide with phospholipid or sugars.[1130] Specific catabolic enzyme deficiencies are responsible for abnormal accumulation of normal cell constituents. Demonstration of the enzyme deficiency makes it possible to detect heterozygotes (carriers) so that prenatal counseling can be provided.[1131] In some of the sphingolipidoses, abnormal accumulation of lipids within the retinal ganglion cells causes opacification of these cells and results ophthalmologically in the so-called cherry-red spot macular lesion (Figure 5.75A–C). The sphingolipidoses that may be associated with a cherry-red spot include the following types.

Gangliosidosis

The β-hexosaminidase system consists of two major isoenzymes, β-hexosaminidase A (α − β) and β-hexosaminidase B (β − β) as well as one minor isoenzyme, β-hexosaminidase S (α–α). These isoenzymes are formed by the different combinations of the two subunits, α and β. The α subunit is encoded in the *HEX A* gene located on chromosome 15q 23-24 and the β subunit is encoded in the *HEX B* gene located on chromosome 5q 13.9. A defect of the β subunit leads to total absence of both β-hexosaminidase A and B, and gives rise to Sandhoff disease, while a defect of the α subunit results in Tay–Sachs disease due to the absence of α-hexosaminidase A and S. Storage in Tay–Sachs disease is mainly in the central nervous system, whereas in Sandhoff's disease storage is abundant in the liver, pancreas, kidney, and other tissues. These two diseases present an identical ophthalmic and neurological clinical picture[1132–1136] but organomegaly and skeletal abnormalities are seen in addition in Sandhoff's disease.

GM_2 Gangliosidosis, Type I

Tay–Sachs Disease

Although patients appear normal at birth, by approximately 6 months they manifest blindness, irritability, and psychomotor deterioration that results in death by 2–4 years of age. Nystagmus, cherry-red spot, and poor vision are prominent early (Figure 5.75A). The cherry-red spot may fade or disappear shortly before death due to loss of ganglion cells; it is accompanied by progressive optic atrophy. Occasionally corneal clouding and endothelial changes can be seen.[1137,1138] In Tay–Sachs disease there is a selective deficiency of the A component of hexosaminidase, whereas in Sandhoff's disease there is almost total absence of both the A and B components of hexosaminidase. The pathogenesis of Tay–Sachs disease is attributable to the accumulation of GM2 trihexosylceramide due to defective β hexosaminidase A enzyme, caused by mutation in the alpha subunit of the hexominidase A gene on chromosome 15q(1). GM2 trihexosylceramide accumulates predominantly in retinal ganglion cells whereby retina becomes turbid with milky-white coloration and the cherry-red spot. Gangliosides are most plentiful in the gray matter with most of the clinical and pathologic manifestations occurring in the nervous system. The commonest form is the infantile form, as described earlier, with death by age 4. A juvenile form with later onset and slower progression is also known. The mildest form of the disease is the adult subtype, also called late-onset Tay–Sachs disease. Manifestations include ataxia, dysarthria, muscle weakness, and dementia. In this form, no cherry-red spot is seen, as the amount of accumulated ganglioside is smaller. The last variant is the chronic form, with patients surviving well into adulthood. There are approximately 78 described mutations, although the majority of patients have the infantile form. The diagnosis is confirmed by assaying the activity of individual β hexosaminidase isoenzymes in serum and cultured cells of patients. Tay–Sachs is most common among Ashkenazi Jewish children.

Substrate reduction therapy that uses small molecules to slow the rate of glycolipid biosynthesis shows efficacy in mouse models of Tay–Sachs. Enzyme replacement therapy and gene substitution hold promise for the future.

GM_2 Gangliosidosis, Type II

Sandhoff's Disease

The clinical presentation is similar to Tay–Sachs with similar neurological and ophthalmic features, including seizures. An infantile and a late-onset form are seen clinically based on the amount of accumulated gangliosides. Hepatosplenomegaly is present. The disease is autosomal-recessive and has been seen worldwide and is not particular to Ashkenazi Jews.[1139,1140]

5.75 Sphingolipidoses.

A: Cherry-red spot in an infant with Tay–Sachs disease.
B: Histopathology of retina in Tay–Sachs disease showed marked loss and disruption of the ganglion cell layer. Special stains for fat showed fat within the remaining ganglion cells as well as within the inner retinal layers.
C: Electron micrograph showed lysosomal bodies distended with laminated sphingolipids within a ganglion cell (× 20000).
D–F: Granular white macula halo lesion (E) associated with Niemann–Pick disease type B in a 6-year-old girl with normal intelligence, hepatosplenomegaly (D), and normal visual acuity. Note lipid-laden macrophages in bone marrow (F).
G–I: Granular white macular halo (G) first detected at age 21 years in a 43-year-old patient with peripheral polyneuropathy, 20/20 visual acuity bilaterally, associated with sea-blue histiocytosis (H). Electron microscopy revealed striking collection of heterogeneous material stored in cells of various types (I). It was most prominent in endoneural fibroblasts. The appearance of the stored material was most like that seen in Niemann–Pick disease. The patient's older sister had similar findings. Both patients were otherwise healthy.

(C, from Yanoff and Fine[1171]; D–F, from Harzer et al.[1144], © 1978, American Medical Association. All rights reserved. G–I, courtesy of Dr. Gordon Harris. D, Also, Yannuzzi, Lawrence J., The Retinal Atlas, Saunders 2010, 978-0-7020-3320-9, p.105)

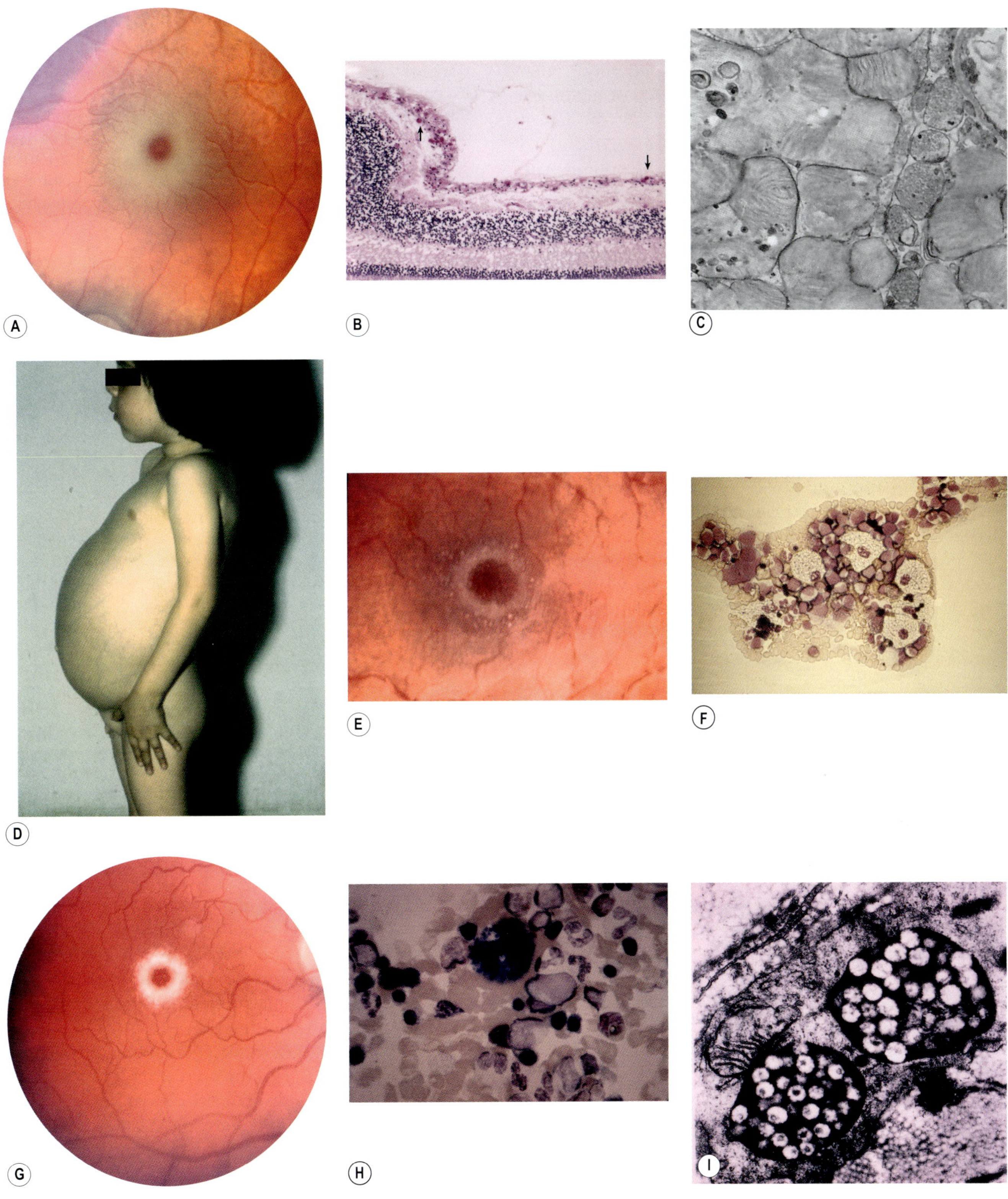
A
B
C
D
E
F
G
H
I

Niemann–Pick Disease

Niemann–Pick disease, an autosomal-recessive disorder, has been subdivided into five types differing in their clinical manifestation, age of onset, severity of neurologic involvement, and genetic background.[1141–1147] All have in common a deficiency of sphingomyelinase enzyme or isoenzyme. Macular changes have been noted only in types A–C.

Type A (infantile form) of Niemann–Pick disease is the most common and most severe form. It is of particular interest to ophthalmologists because of the occurrence of cherry-red spot in at least 50% of cases, mild corneal clouding, and brown granular discoloration of the anterior lens cortex or capsule. These children have a clinical course similar to that of Tay–Sachs disease. The visual loss, however, is delayed because of preservation of the ganglion cells. This results in a less well-defined white opacification that extends farther into the periphery and persists in Niemann–Pick type A disease. Fifty percent of reported patients with this autosomal-recessive disease have been Ashkenazi Jews. Hepatosplenomegaly, progressive neurodegenerative features followed by death in infancy, ensues.

Type B is a nonneuropathic form of Niemann–Pick disease that occurs in patients with normal vision, hepatosplenomegaly, hyperlipidemia, interstitial lung disease, and variable survival to adulthood (Figure 5.75D–F). A brownish-red foveola surrounded by a granular gray halo, less prominent than the typical cherry-red spot, may occur in some patients (Figure 5.44E).[1141–1143,1148–1150] Cogan et al. coined the term "macular halo syndrome" to describe this ringlike perifoveolar distribution of crystalloid opacities.[1141] The macula has multiple layers of ganglion cells and the foveola is devoid of ganglion cells. Lipid storage in the multilayered ganglion cells results in the grayish-white macular halo. This finding is present in several of the lipid storage disorders, including Tay–Sachs, Sandhoff's, GM2 gangliosidosis, galactosialoidosis, and α neuraminidase deficiency.[1151]

Figure 5.75G depicts a macular halo that occurred in two siblings who were in good health until middle life when they developed moderately severe peripheral polyneuropathy associated with sea-blue histiocytosis, absence of foam cells typical of Niemann–Pick disease, marked depletion of sphingomyelinase activity in leukocytes and cultured skin fibroblasts, and electron microscopic evidence of a striking collection of heterogeneous material stored in cells of various types in a biopsy of the sural nerve. Storage of material was most prominent in endoneural fibroblasts in the form of electron-dense inclusions with some suggestion of lamellar structure; dense inclusions containing numerous vesicular or vacuolar structures, often with fine electron-dense floccular material centrally; structures with a concentrically arranged laminated appearance; structures having the appearance of myelin debris; and some multilaminated structures bearing a resemblance to zebra bodies. Although the appearance of the stored material most closely resembled that seen in Niemann–Pick disease, the clinical picture and bone marrow biopsy findings were unlike any of the various forms of Niemann–Pick disease.

Type C Niemann–Pick disease occurs in non-Jewish patients and is a milder, chronic form of the disease that is characterized by normal early development but later progressive psychomotor deterioration and death between age 5 and 15 years. There is moderate visceral and central nervous system involvement. Some patients have vertical ophthalmoplegia. The cherry-red spot is less prominent and granular in appearance, similar to that in type B. Visual acuity is usually within normal limits. Histopathologic and ultrastructural studies of eyes with type C Niemann–Pick disease have shown variable degrees of lipid storage in the ocular tissues.[1152,1153]

5.76 Gaucher's disease.

A–D: This 54-year-old woman with the adult form of Gaucher's disease had a splenectomy at 10 years of age. Except for bilateral hip replacement for degenerative joint disease, her general health was good. She had prominent yellow pinguecula at the nasal and temporal limbus of both eyes. Visual acuity was 20/20 in the right eye and 20/30 in the left eye. Note the variably sized white deposits, some of which are anterior to the retinal vessels scattered throughout the fundus. Relatively few small lesions were present in the macular area (arrow, D).

E and **F**: Similar white lesions in this 6-year-old boy with the infantile form of Gaucher's disease. Histopathologically, the lesions were caused by clusters of foamy macrophages (asterisk) on the inner retinal surface.

Galactosialidosis.

G and **H**: Cherry-red spot in a 21-year-old woman with the cherry-red spot–myoclonus syndrome. She had a slowly progressive neurologic disease characterized by reduced visual acuity, nystagmus, dysarthria, and myoclonic spasms. A sister was similarly affected. Angiography was normal except for slight blurring of details of macular capillaries (H).

I: Histopathologic findings in the macular area of a 22-year-old woman with bilateral cherry-red spots, generalized tremor, muscular weakness, convulsions, and mental deterioration. The eyes were obtained at autopsy following death from bronchopneumonia. Note that the ganglion cells in the macular region are enlarged and contain an eosinophilic granular intracytoplasmic material with eccentric displacement of the nuclei. Special stains revealed periodic acid–Schiff-positive, diastase-resistant material in the cytoplasm of the ganglion cells. The material in the ganglion cells stained positively with oil red O, Luxol fast blue, and Sudan black. Stains for acid mucopolysaccharides, with and without hyaluronidase and iron stains, were negative.

(E and F, from Ueno et al.[1166]; I, from Font.[1202])

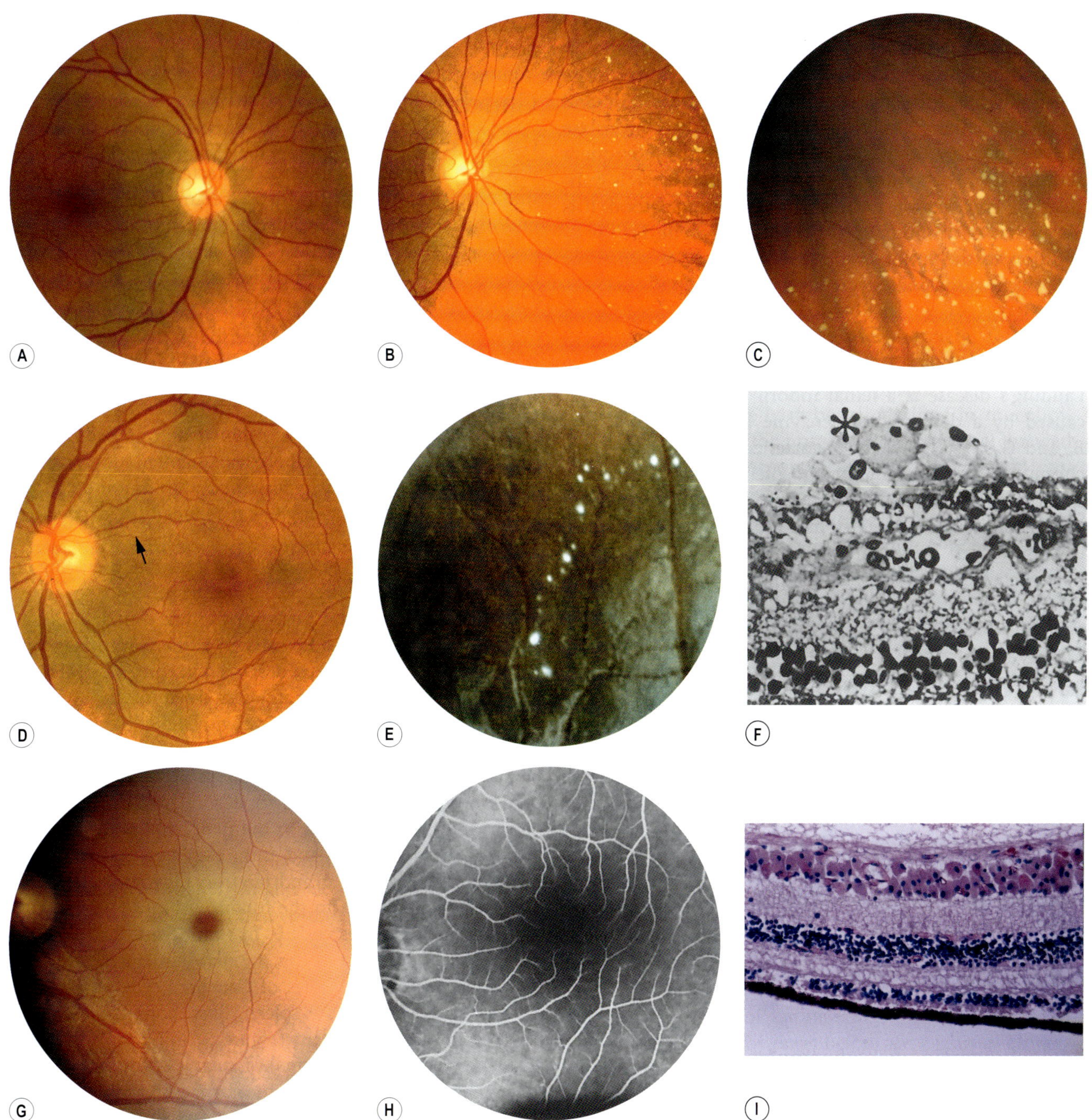
A
B
C
D
E
F
G
H
I

Mucolipidosis I (Sialidosis, Type II)

Patients with mucolipidosis I have facies resembling those in Hurler's syndrome, skeletal abnormalities, and often low beta-galactosidase activity. Myoclonus is less prominent. Many of the patients are mentally retarded, and some have corneal and lens opacities and are deaf. Almost all have cherry-red spots. Many patients are Japanese.

Mucolipidosis Type II (ML II Alpha/Beta, I-Cell Disease)

Clinical findings present at birth include Hurler-like facies, bulbous nose, and thick doughy skin. Linear growth stops at age 1 year. Progressive joint stiffness, dysostosis multiplex, recurrent respiratory infections, and congestive heart failure lead to death by 5–8 years of age. Corneal clouding and glaucoma may occur. A characteristic histological feature is the presence of enlarged lysosomes filled with undigested compounds in patient fibroblasts, also called inclusion or I-cells. The affected gene is *GNPTAB* 12q23.3.

Mucolipidosis Type III A (ML III Alpha/Beta, Pseudo-Hurler Polydystrophy)

Patients with mucolipidosis type III develop the onset during the first few years of life of joint stiffening, mild facial coarseness, stature below third percentile for age, kyphoscoliosis, and X-ray evidence of dysostosis multiplex similar to that seen in the mucopolysaccharidoses with the arms and hands most prominently affected.[1191] They have a milder form of ML II alpha/beta. The disease stabilizes after 18 years of age and patients may live up to the eighth decade. Patients may, however, have aortic insufficiency. As a result of an enzymatic defect there is an excess intracellular storage of acid mucopolysaccharides and glycolipids that are apparent ultrastructurally as fibrillogranular inclusion bodies and membranous lamellar vacuoles, respectively. Corneal clouding and hyperopic astigmatism are constant ocular features. Retinal haziness, surface wrinkling retinopathy, and optic disc edema may be present. They may have a relatively mild retinal dystrophy.[1191,1203] The affected gene is *GNPTAB* 12q23.3.

Mucolipidosis IIIC (MLIII Variant, ML III Gamma)

The affected gene is *GNPTG* 16p13.3. It has a milder phenotype of the pseudo-Hurler type.

Mucolipidosis Type IV

Patients with type IV mucolipidosis manifest delayed development, psychomotor retardation, and generalized hypotonia soon after birth.[1203] Skeletal anomalies, hepatosplenomegaly, and coarse facial features are typically absent. Strabismus, corneal clouding, optic disc pallor, narrowed retinal vasculature, pigmentary retinopathy, and extinguished ERG may develop during early life. Light and electron microscopy have demonstrated loss of retinal photoreceptors, pigment migration into the retina, and fine granular material consistent with mucopolysaccharides and concentric lamellar bodies, presumably representing phospholipids, in macrophages, plasma cells, ciliary epithelial cells, Schwann cells, retinal ganglion cells, and vascular endothelium.[1189] ERG changes in isolated cases include severely reduced rod and cone-mediated responses and an electronegative scotopic response.[1207] Patients (both girls) with a mild phenotype consisting of corneal clouding alone without neurological or skeletal changes have been reported.[1206,1207] ML IV is caused by mutations in *MCOLN1*, which codes for mucolipin-1, a 580-amino-acid protein that is a member of the transient receptor potential family.[7–9] Thus far, most of the patients have been Ashkenazi Jews (80%), and the mutations in them seem to differ from the mutations seen in affected non-Ashkenazi Jews.[1208]

5.77 Lipofuscinosis.

A and **B**: This 5-year-old white girl complained of the recent onset of poor vision. Her visual acuity in the right eye was 20/30 and in the left eye was 20/40. Note the bull's-eye pattern of retinal pigment epithelium (RPE) atrophy and the slightly narrowed retinal vessels in the left macula in A and the coarse mottling of the RPE in the peripheral fundus in B. One year previously the patient had been asymptomatic. Her visual acuity was 20/20, and the fundi appeared within normal limits. At 7 years of age the patient's visual acuity was reduced to counting fingers in the right eye and hand movements in the left eye. At 8 years of age she developed grand mal seizures and nystagmus. At that time she had light perception with poor projection in both eyes.

C and **D**: This 8-year-old brother of the patient illustrated in A and B had first noted visual disturbances 1 year previously. Visual acuity at that time was 20/50. Visual acuity at the time these photographs were made was finger counting in both eyes. Note the pallor of the optic disc, marked attenuation of the retinal vessels, and coarse clumping of pigment in the peripheral fundus. Over the subsequent 3 years he developed further visual loss, generalized seizures, nystagmus, dysarthria, and mild dementia.

E and **F**: Histopathology of the macular region of a child who died of juvenile lipofuscinosis. Note the marked atrophy involving all of the retinal layers in the foveal area (E) and the peripheral macular area (F) of the same eye. Note loss of ganglion cells and marked degenerative changes involving the outer nuclear layer and receptor elements. There were pigment-laden cells present in the outer layers of the retina.

GALACTOSIALIDOSIS (GOLDBERG–COTLIER SYNDROME)

Galactosialidosis is a lysosomal storage disease characterized by decreased alpha-neuraminidase and beta-galactosidase caused by a decrease in a protective protein/cathepsin A, an intralysosomal protein that protects these enzymes from premature proteolytic processing.[1209–1212] Three types of galactosialidosis are recognized clinically.

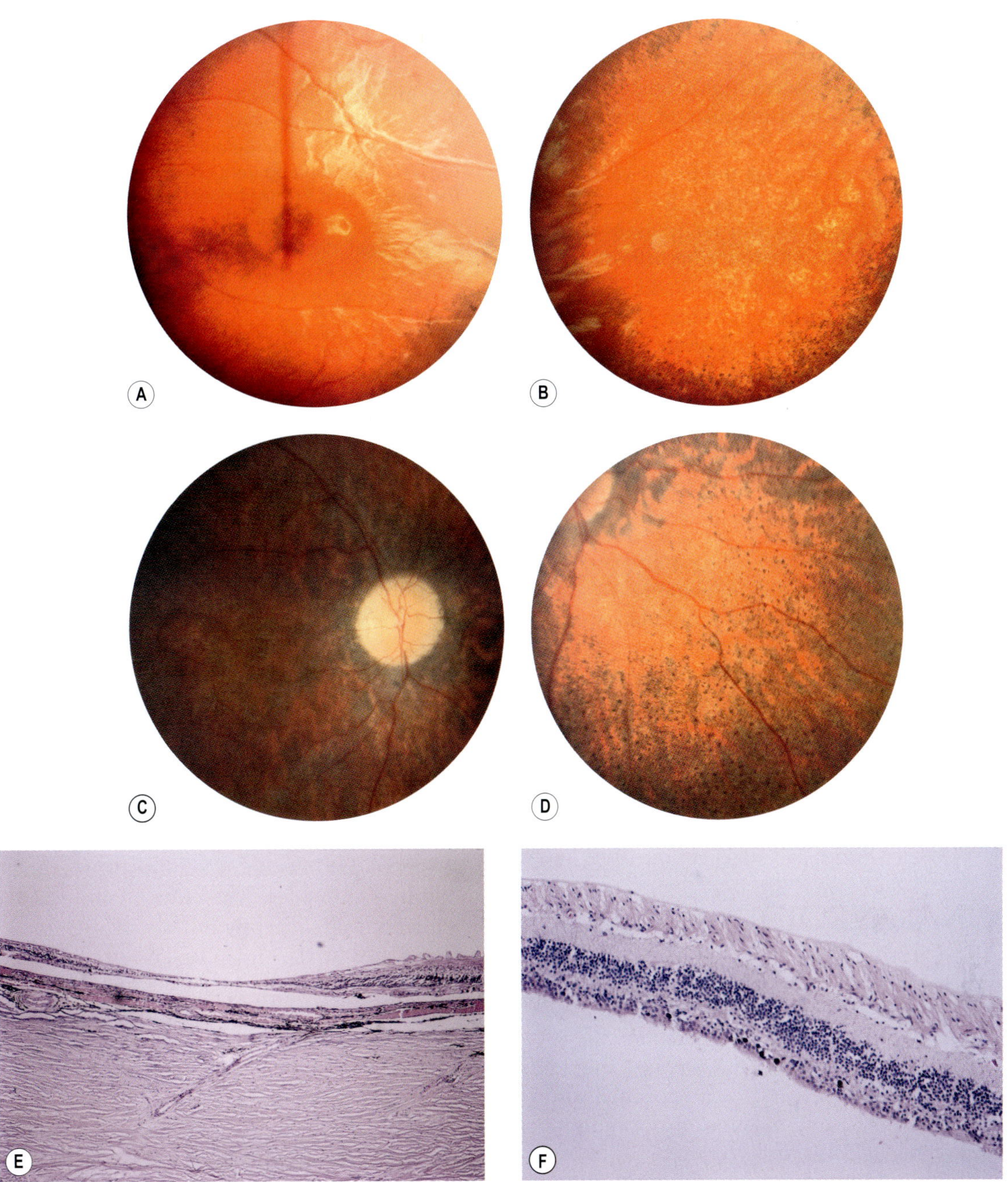
A
B
C
D
E
F

1. Early infantile form: presents neonatally with Hurler-like facies, dysostosis multiplex, progressive neurological changes, progressive visceromegaly, and early death. Ocular abnormalities are common and fetal hydrops occurs in one-third of cases.[1213,1214]
2. Late infantile form: presents in the first 2 years of life with visceromegaly, valvular heart disease, with or without cardiomyopathy, growth retardation, dysostosis multiplex, mild neurological compromise, ocular changes, and angiokeratomata. The disease progresses slowly: cardiac management is of primary concern.[1215]
3. Juvenile/adult form: found exclusively in Japanese presents anywhere from 3 years of age to adulthood. Neurological, cardiac, and ophthalmological features are prominent with cherry-red spot, myoclonus, and ataxia. Corneal clouding, decreased vision, coarse facies, and arrhythmias can also occur.[1209,1211,1212] The cherry-red spot may fade and be relatively inapparent in older patients.

Histopathologic and ultrastructural examination of the eyes of a 13-year-old boy with late infantile form revealed loss of retinal ganglion cells, abnormal accumulation of lipid and proteinaceous material in residual ganglion cells, optic atrophy, and intracytoplasmic inclusion bodies in retinal and amacrine cells.[1211] Conjunctival biopsy in two siblings with the adult form showed several types of intracytoplasmic inclusions in the fibroblasts, lymphatic capillary endothelial cells, Schwann cells, and epithelial cells. Membrane-bound vesicles with fibrillogranular content, dense granular inclusions, and oil droplets were also seen.[1216]

NEURONAL CEROID LIPOFUSCINOSES

Batten in 1903 described two siblings with progressive macular dystrophy and cerebral degeneration, the juvenile form of NCL. The name "Batten's disease" should be reserved for this form of NCL. NCL is a lysosomal storage disease that involves the accumulation of insoluble fluorescent lipoproteins believed to be ceroid and lipofuscin, pigments normally associated with aging.[1217–1231] The term "neuronal" is misleading, since many different cell types, including smooth muscle, glands, Schwann cells, and vascular endothelium, contain the storage product.[1217] Psychomotor retardation, seizures, visual loss, and premature death characterize the clinical features of this group of neurodegenerative disorders. These patients can be divided into four principal groups on the basis of the age of onset as well as ultrastructural findings related to the deposition of this autofluorescent pigment in neurons and other body tissues. The mode of inheritance in these disorders is autosomal-recessive and genes *CLN1–CLN8* have been identified.[1232–1234]

5.78 Long-chain fatty acid dehydrogenase deficiency (LCHAD).

A–I: An almost 5-year-old was examined with a visual acuity of 20/40 in each eye and fine pigment mottling through out the fundus (A–C). Photographs were repeated at age 11 and 13 (D–G) with no apparent change in the retinal appearance. The patient had LCHAD deficiency. She was maintained on a low-fat carbohydrate-rich diet and showed no progressive chorioretinal degeneration. Optical coherence tomography showed choroidal shadowing from the increased foveal retinal pigment epithelium pigment (H and I).

(Courtesy of Dr. Michael Goldbaum.)

Infantile Group (*CLN1*, Haltia–Santavuori Type)

Infantile-group patients manifest microcephaly, severe neurologic and visual symptoms usually before 2 years of age. Infantile-onset NCL is caused by mutations in a palmitoyl-protein thioesterase 1 gene, *CLN1*, located at1p32.

Late Infantile Group (*CLN2*, Jansky–Bielchowsky Type)

The onset of severe neurologic disease, including ataxia, seizures, loss of speech, and regression of developmental milestones, begins between 2 and 4 years of age and usually precedes the visual symptoms. These patients typically have a rapid progression of the disease, resulting in coma and death within a few years. Late infantile NCL is caused by mutations in a pepstatin-resistant peptidase 1 gene, *CLN2*, located at 11p15. Up to 85% of these patients also have an approximately 1-kb deletion in the *CLN3* gene located at 16p12, which codes a hydrophobic protein of unknown function. *CLN5* at 13q31-32, *CLN6* at 15q21-23, and *CLN7* and *CLN8* at 8p23 are associated with certain variants of late infantile NCL.

The Juvenile Group (*CLN3*, Spielmeyer–Sjögren Type)

Juvenile group patients, resulting from the mutation of *CLN3* gene at 16p12, who constitute the major subgroup of these disorders, typically are seen initially in childhood at a peak age of 6–7 years because of visual symptoms, which are often advanced. Mental disturbances, such as loss of recent memory, tantrums, speech disturbances, and inability to learn, may be present at the time of presentation but are often overlooked. Fundoscopic examination may reveal very mild changes in the RPE. Soon they develop signs of a bull's-eye type of macular atrophy, followed by progressive alterations in the RPE throughout the

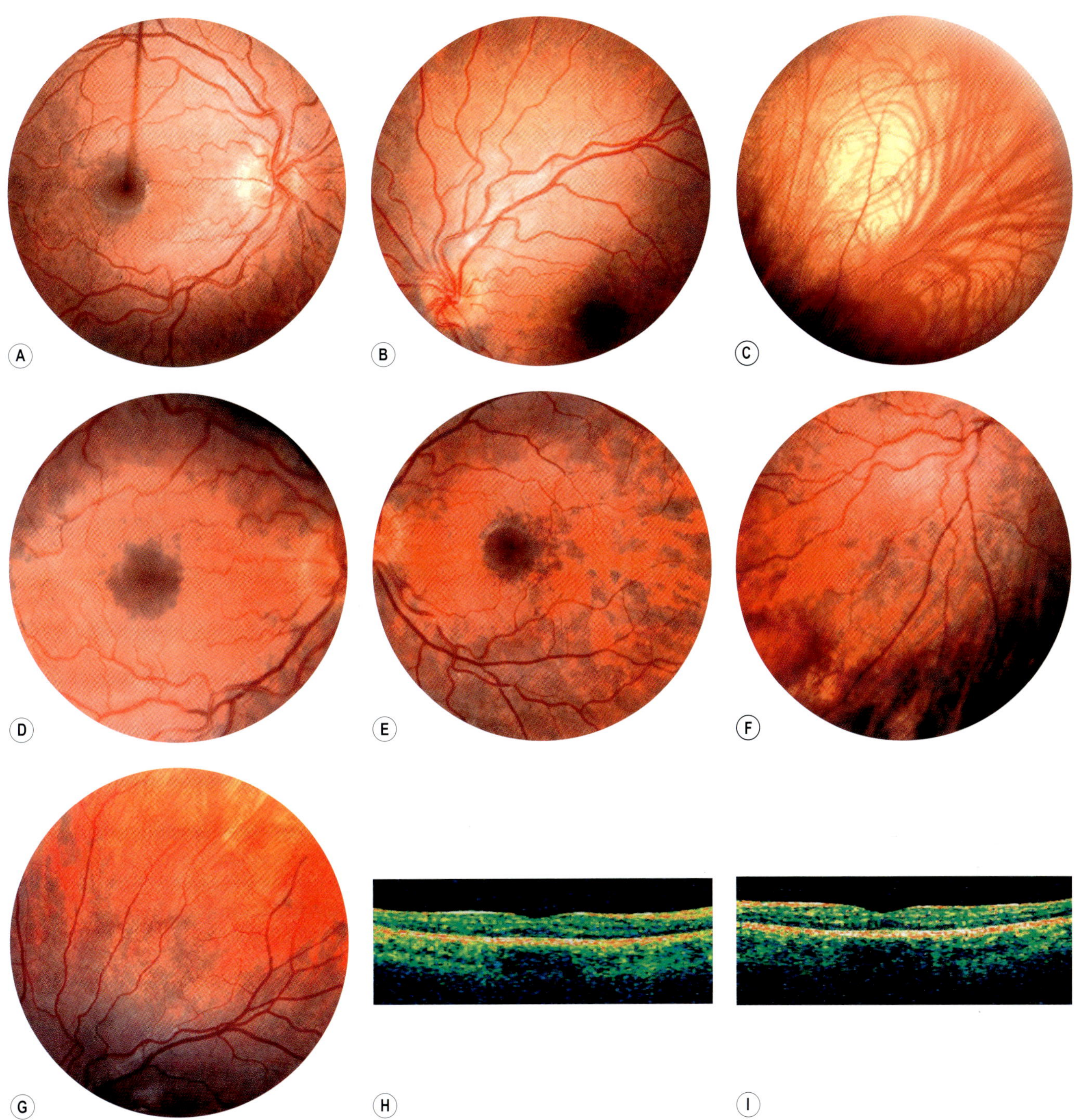
A
B
C
D
E
F
G
H
I

fundus together with narrowing of the retinal vessels and optic atrophy (Figure 5.77A–D).[1235] Fluorescein angiography is helpful in detecting the early signs of the disease. Electroencephalography and electroretinography are useful in making a correct diagnosis before the onset of definite neurologic symptoms.[1232,1236,1237] Diagnostic findings in the juvenile type include vacuolated lymphocytes in the peripheral blood; rectal biopsy ultrastructurally shows fingerprint forms intracellularly in neuronal tissue. These patients experience progressive neurologic symptoms, including seizures, with a peak incidence of 1–2 years after the onset of symptoms, tremors, ataxia, dementia, and paralysis, resulting in death usually by 20 years of age.

Histopathologic examination reveals extensive loss of the rod and cone cells, outer nuclear layer, and outer plexiform layer; accumulation of a PAS-positive lipid substance in the ganglion cell layer; narrowing of small retinal vessels; and gliosis of the nerve fiber layer (Figure 5.77E and F).[1220–1223,1227,1238] Of note is the absence of autofluorescent inclusions in the photoreceptors, suggesting that photoreceptors may be rescued if a therapy for Batten disease can be developed.[1238] Changes are more marked posteriorly than anteriorly. There is extensive RPE atrophy and migration of pigment into the overlying retina. Electron microscopy reveals curvilinear bodies and fingerprint profiles in the ganglion cells.[1221,1227,1231] The differences in retinal pathology of the three childhood forms of the neuronal ceroid lipofuscinoses are of a quantitative rather than a qualitative nature.[1222]

Kuf's Disease (Adult Neuronal Ceroid Lipofuscinosis)

Kuf's disease is the rarest form (1.3–10%) of the neuronal ceroid lipofuscinoses and is autosomal-dominant in inheritance. Cerebellar, extrapyramidal, and motor signs predominate. Visual failure is infrequent. Mild central visual and color deficiency and impaired smooth pursuit have been noted.[1239] Seizures are rare, and the patients are often demented. Two clinical phenotypes, type A, with progressive myoclonic epilepsy, and type B, with progressive dementia, extrapyramidal symptoms, suprabulbar and cerebellar dysfunction, are known. The underlying molecular defect in Kuf's disease (*CLN4*) is still not known.[1233,1234] Electron microscopic examination of the peripheral blood lymphocytes for characteristic "finger profiles," single membrane-bound intracytoplasmic vacuoles, and osmiophilic granular bodies is a sensitive means of detecting patients with any of the four forms as well as the carriers.[1219]

Long-Chain 3-Hydroxy-Acyl-Coenzyme A Dehydrogenase (LCHAD) Deficiency

Fatty acids are metabolized within the mitochondria by beta-oxidation by the LCHAD enzyme. Deficiency of LCHAD results in hypoketotic hypoglycemia, hepatic steatosis, cardiomyopathy, and rhabdomyolysis. In addition, peripheral neuropathy and retinopathy occur. Deficiency of LCHAD is a severe disease that usually results in death during the first 2 years of life unless the natural course can be modified by a low-fat, high-carbohydrate diet. Death is usually due to hepatic or cardiorespiratory failure. Children who have been diagnosed early and have been maintained on a low-fat, high-carbohydrate diet show ocular findings.

The ocular findings in a large cohort were classified into four stages.[1240] In stage I, the retina appears normal at birth. Soon after pigment dispersion occurs at the retinal pigment epithelial level (stage II) (Figure 5.78A–C). Patchy chorioretinal atrophy, progressive occlusion of choroidal vessels and choriocapillaris in the posterior pole follows, resulting in deterioration of central vision, often with relative sparing of the peripheral fundus (Figure 5.78F and G) (stage III). Central scotomas and posterior staphyloma develop in stage IV. Developmental cataracts, which are flaky opacities around the nucleus, progressive myopia, and deterioration of visual fields and color vision are the findings of LCHAD deficiency. ERG abnormalities and chorioretinopathy precede the development of myopia and posterior staphyloma.[1240,1241]

Fluorescein angiography in the second stage onwards shows poor choroidal filling and progressive loss of choriocapillaris. Subsequently, dropout of choriocapillary lobules occurs with large areas of chorioretinal atrophy. In late stages, the large choroidal vessels are preserved mostly temporal to the macula. Color vision and dark adaptation are affected by stages II–III. It is possible that derangement of the RPE and choriocapillaris is the primary defect in this condition, and the photoreceptors' function is lost secondarily. The fundus changes in stage III onward resemble central areolar choroidal sclerosis, progressive bifocal chorioretinal dystrophy, choroideremia, and pathological myopia. In the early stages, it resembles a carrier state of choroideremia or rubella retinopathy with fine pigment mottling (Figure 10.50). Both night blindness and difficulty with central vision eventually occur.

The condition is inherited in an autosomal-recessive fashion with a G1528C mutation in the gene of the LCHAD enzyme.[1240–1242] The treatment is early recognition and management with a low-fat and a high-carbohydrate diet, and survival up to age 31-plus has been noted.[1243]

References

1. Weingeist TA, Kobrin JL, Watzke RC. Histopathology of Best's macular dystrophy. Arch Ophthalmol 1982;100:1108–14.
2. Pece A, Gaspari G, Avanza P, et al. Best's multiple vitelliform degeneration. Int Ophthalmol 1992;16:459–64.
3. Noble KG, Scher BM, Carr RE. Polymorphous presentations and vitelliform macular dystrophy: Subretinal neovascularisation and central choroidal atrophy. Br J Ophthalmol 1978;62:561–70.
4. Morse PH, MacLean AL. Fluorescein fundus studies in hereditary vitelliruptive macular degeneration. Am J Ophthalmol 1968;66:485–94.
5. Mohler CW, Fine SL. Long-term evaluation of patients with Best's vitelliform dystrophy. Ophthalmology 1981;88:688–92.
6. Miller SA, Bresnick GH, Chandra SR. Choroidal neovascular membrane in Best's vitelliform macular dystrophy. Am J Ophthalmol 1976;82:252–5.
7. Miller SA. Fluorescence in Best's vitelliform dystrophy, lipofuscin, and fundus flavimaculatus. Br J Ophthalmol 1978;62:256–60.
8. Massof RW, Fleischman JA, Fine SL, et al. Flicker fusion thresholds in Best macular dystrophy. Arch Ophthalmol 1977;95:991–4.
9. Maloney WF, Robertson DM, Duboff SM. Hereditary vitelliform macular degeneration; variable fundus findings within a single pedigree. Arch Ophthalmol 1977;95:979–83.
10. Krill AE, Morse PA, Potts AM, et al. Hereditary vitelliruptive macular degeneration. Am J Ophthalmol 1966;61:1405–15.
11. Kraushar MF, Margolis S, Morse PH, et al. Pseudohypopyon in Best's vitelliform macular dystrophy. Am J Ophthalmol 1982;94:30–7.
12. Gass JDM. Stereoscopic atlas of macular diseases; diagnosis and treatment, 2nd ed. St. Louis: CV Mosby; 1977. p. 162.
13. Frangieh GT, Green WR, Fine SL. A histopathologic study of Best's macular dystrophy. Arch Ophthalmol 1982;100:1115–21.
14. François J, De Rouck A. Fernandez-Sasso D. L'électrooculographie dans les dégénérescences vitelliformes de la macula. Bull Soc Belge Ophtalmol 1966;143:547–52.
15. Fishman GA, Ward LM, Rusin MM. Vitreous fluorophotometry in patients with Best's macular dystrophy. Retina 1990;10:102–4.
16. Fishman GA, Baca W, Alexander KR, et al. Visual acuity in patients with Best vitelliform macular dystrophy. Ophthalmology 1993;100:1665–70.
17. Deutman AF. The hereditary dystrophies of the posterior pole of the eye. Assen: Van Gorcum; 1971. p. 198.
18. Curry Jr HF, Moorman LT. Fluorescein photography of vitelliform macular degeneration. Arch Ophthalmol 1968;79:705–9.
19. Cross HE, Bard L. Electro-oculography in Best's macular dystrophy. Am J Ophthalmol 1974;77:46–50.
20. Cavender JC. Best's macular dystrophy. Arch Ophthalmol 1982;100:1067.
21. Birndorf LA, Dawson WW. A normal electrooculogram in a patient with a typical vitelliform macular lesion. Invest Ophthalmol 1973;12:830–3.
22. Best F. Über eine hereditäre Maculaaffektion; Beitrag zur Vererbungslehre. Z Augenheilkd 1905;13:199–212.
23. Berkley WL, Bussey FR. Heredodegeneration of the macula. Am J Ophthalmol 1949;32:361–5.
24. Benson WE, Kolker AE, Enoch JM, et al. Best's vitelliform macular dystrophy. Am J Ophthalmol 1975;79:59–66.
25. Barricks ME. Vitelliform lesions developing in normal fundi. Am J Ophthalmol 1977;83:324–7.
26. Bard LA, Cross HE. Genetic counseling of families with Best macular dystrophy. Am Acad Ophthalmol Otolaryngol 1975;79:OP865–OP873.
27. Anderson SR, editor. Ocular pathology in hereditary (vitelliform) macular degeneration. In: European ophthalmic pathology society meeting, May 28, 1970, Ghent, Belgium.
28. Forsman K, Graff C, Nordstrom S, et al. The gene for Best's macular dystrophy is located at 11q13 in a Swedish family. Clin Genet 1992;42:156–9.
29. Nichols BE, Bascom R, Litt M, et al. Refining the locus for Best vitelliform macular dystrophy and mutation analysis of the candidate gene ROM1. Am J Hum Genet 1994;54:95–103.
30. Stone EM, Nichols BE, Streb LM, et al. Genetic linkage of vitelliform macular degeneration (Best's disease) to chromosome 11q13. Nat Genet 1992;1:246–50.
31. Petrukhin K, Koisti MJ, Bakall B, et al. Identification of the gene responsible for Best macular dystrophy. Nat Genet 1998;19:241–7.
32. Boon CJ, Klevering BJ, Leroy BP, et al. The spectrum of ocular phenotypes caused by mutations in the BEST1 gene. Prog Retin Eye Res 2009;28:187–205.
33. Yu K, Qu Z, Cui Y, et al. Chloride channel activity of bestrophin mutants associated with mild or late-onset macular degeneration. Invest Ophthalmol Vis Sci 2007;48:4694–705.
34. Boon CJ, Klevering BJ, den Hollander AI, et al. Clinical and genetic heterogeneity in multifocal vitelliform dystrophy. Arch Ophthalmol 2007;125:1100–6.
35. Bakall B, Marknell T, Ingvast S, et al. The mutation spectrum of the bestrophin protein – functional implications. Hum Genet 1999;104:383–9.
36. Hartzell HC, Qu Z, Yu K, et al. Molecular physiology of bestrophins: multifunctional membrane proteins linked to best disease and other retinopathies. Physiol Rev 2008;88:639–72.
37. Hartzell C, Qu Z, Putzier I, et al. Looking chloride channels straight in the eye: bestrophins, lipofuscinosis, and retinal degeneration. Physiology (Bethesda) 2005;20:292–302.
38. Spaide RF, Noble K, Morgan A, et al. Vitelliform macular dystrophy. Ophthalmology 2006;113:1392–400.
39. Schachat AP, de la Cruz A, Green WR, et al. Macular hole and retinal detachment in Best's disease. Retina 1985;5:22–5.
40. Miller SA. Multifocal Best's vitelliform dystrophy. Arch Ophthalmol 1977;95:984–90.
41. Thu T, Chan WM, Dung D, et al. A large macular hole in a young patient with Best's disease. Clin Experiment Ophthalmol 2003 Dec;31:539–40.
42. Mehta M, Katsumi O, Tetsuka S, et al. Best's macular dystrophy with a macular hole. Acta Ophthalmol 1991;69:131–4.
43. O'Gorman S, Flaherty WA, Fishman GA, et al. Histopathologic findings in Best's vitelliform macular dystrophy. Arch Ophthalmol 1988;106:1261–8.
44. Bakall B, Radu RA, Stanton JB, et al. Enhanced accumulation of A2E in individuals homozygous or heterozygous for mutations in BEST1 (VMD2). Exp Eye Res 2007;85:34–43.
45. Spaide R. Autofluorescence from the outer retina and subretinal space: hypothesis and review. Retina 2008;28:5–35.
46. Gross JG, Freeman WR. Posttraumatic yellow maculopathy. Retina 1990;10:37–41.
47. Fletcher RC, Jampol LM, Rimm W. An unusual presentation of Best's disease. Br J Ophthalmol 1977;61:719–21.
48. Yoder FE, Cros HE, Chase GA, et al. Linkage studies of Best's macular dystrophy. Clin Genet 1988;34:26–30.
49. Kaufman SJ, Goldberg MF, Orth DH, et al. Autosomal-dominant vitreoretinochoroidopathy. Arch Ophthalmol 1982;100:272–8.
50. Blair NP, Goldberg MF, Fishman GA, et al. Autosomal-dominant vitreoretinochoroidopathy (ADVIRC). Br J Ophthalmol 1984;68:2–9.
51. Oh KT, Vallar C. Central cone dysfunction in autosomal-dominant vitreoretino choroidopathy (ADVIRC). Am J Ophthalmol 2006;141:940–3.
52. Yardley J, Leroy BP, Hart-Holden N, et al. Mutations of VMD2 splicing regulators cause nanophthalmos and autosomal-dominant vitreoretinochoroidopathy (ADVIRC). Invest Ophthalmol Vis Sci 2004;45:3683–9.
53. Burgess R, MacLaren RE, Davidson AE, et al. ADVIRC is caused by distinct mutations in BEST1 that alter pre-mRNA splicing. J Med Genet 2009;46:620–5.
54. Reddy MA, Francis PJ, Berry V, et al. A clinical and molecular genetic study of a rare dominantly inherited syndrome (MRCS) comprising of microcornea, rod–cone dystrophy, cataract, and posterior staphyloma. Br J Ophthalmol 2003;87:197–202.
55. Burgess R, Millar ID, Leroy BP, et al. Biallelic mutation of BEST1 causes a distinct retinopathy in humans. Am J Hum Genet 2008;82:19–31.
56. Gerth C, Zawadzki RJ, Werner JS, et al. Detailed analysis of retinal function and morphology in a patient with autosomal-recessive bestrophinopathy (ARB). Doc Ophthalmol 2009;118:239–46.
57. Vaclavik V, Ooi KG, Bird AC, et al. Autofluorescence findings in acute exudative polymorphous vitelliform maculopathy. Arch Ophthalmol 2007;125:274–7.
58. Chan CK, Gass JD, Lin SG. Acute exudative polymorphous vitelliform maculopathy syndrome. Retina 2003;23:453–62.
59. Gass JD, Chuang EL, Granek H. Acute exudative polymorphous vitelliform maculopathy. Trans Am Ophthalmol Soc 1988;86:354–66.
60. Eksandh L, Adamus G, Mosgrove L, et al. Autoantibodies against bestrophin in a patient with vitelliform paraneoplastic retinopathy and a metastatic choroidal malignant melanoma. Arch Ophthalmol 2008;126:432–5.
61. Nieuwendijk TJ, Hooymans JM. Paraneoplastic vitelliform retinopathy associated with metastatic choroidal melanoma. Eye (Lond) 2007;21:1436–7.
62. Wiznia RA, Perina B, Noble KG. Vitelliform macular dystrophy of late onset. Br J Ophthalmol 1981;65:866–8.
63. Watzke RC, Folk JC, Lang RM. Pattern dystrophy of the retinal pigment epithelium. Ophthalmology 1982;89:1400–6.
64. Vine AK, Schatz H. Adult-onset foveomacular pigment epithelial dystrophy. Am J Ophthalmol 1980;89:680–91.
65. Slezak H, Hommer K. Fundus pulverulentus. Albrecht von Graefes Arch Klin Exp Ophthalmol 1969;178:177–82.
66. Skalka HW. Vitelliform macular lesions. Br J Ophthalmol 1981;65:180–3.
67. Sjögren H. Dystrophia reticularis laminae pigmentosae retinae: an earlier not described hereditary eye disease. Acta Ophthalmol 1950;28:279–95.
68. Singerman LJ, Berkow JW, Patz A. Dominant slowly progressive macular dystrophy. Am J Ophthalmol 1977;83:680–92.
69. Shiono T, Ishikawa A, Hara S, et al. Pattern dystrophy of the retinal pigment epithelium. Retina 1990;10:251–4.
70. Sabates R, Pruett RC, Hirose T. Pseudovitelliform macular degeneration. Retina 1982;2:197–205.
71. Patrinely JR, Lewis RA, Font RL. Foveomacular vitelliform dystrophy, adult type; a clinicopathologic study including electron microscopic observations. Ophthalmology 1985;92:1712–8.
72. O'Donnell FE, Schatz H, Reid P, et al. Autosomal-dominant dystrophy of the retinal pigment epithelium. Arch Ophthalmol 1979;97:680–3.
73. Mejia JR, Gieser RG. Sporadic butterfly macular dystrophy. Ann Ophthalmol 1981;13:1253–4.
74. Mesker RP, Oosterhuis JA, Delleman JW. A retinal lesion resembling Sjögren's dystrophia reticularis laminae pigmentosae retinae . In: Winkelman JE, Crone RA, editors. Perspectives in ophthalmology, vol. II. Amsterdam: Excerpta Medica; 1970. p. 40–5.
75. Marmor MF. "Vitelliform" lesions in adults. Ann Ophthalmol 1979;11:1705–12.
76. Marmor MF, Byers B. Pattern dystrophy of the pigment epithelium. Am J Ophthalmol 1977;84:32–44.
77. Kingham JD, Fenzl RE, Willerson D, et al. Reticular dystrophy of the retinal pigment epithelium; a clinical and electrophysiologic study of three generations. Arch Ophthalmol 1978;96:1177–84.
78. Kingham JD, Lochen GP. Vitelliform macular degeneration. Am J Ophthalmol 1977;84:526–31. [correspondence 1979;88:955.]
79. Hsieh RC, Fine BS, Lyons JS. Patterned dystrophies of the retinal pigment epithelium. Arch Ophthalmol 1977;95:429–35.
80. Hodes BL, Feiner LA, Sherman SH, et al. Progression of pseudovitelliform macular dystrophy. Arch Ophthalmol 1984;102:381–3.
81. Hittner HM, Ferrell RE, Borda RP, et al. Atypical vitelliform macular dystrophy in a 5-generation family. Br J Ophthalmol 1984;68:199–207.
82. Gutman I, Walsh JB, Henkind P. Vitelliform macular dystrophy and butterfly-shaped epithelial dystrophy: a continuum? Br J Ophthalmol 1982;66:170–3.
83. Gass JDM. A clinicopathologic study of a peculiar foveomacular dystrophy. Trans Am Ophthalmol Soc 1974;72:139–56.

84. Gass JDM. Stereoscopic atlas of macular diseases; diagnosis and treatment, 2nd ed. St. Louis: CV Mosby; 1977. p. 170.
85. Gass JDM. Dominantly inherited adult form of vitelliform foveomacular dystrophy. In: Fine SL, Owens SL, editors. Management of retinal vascular and macular disorders. Baltimore: Williams & Wilkins; 1983. p. 182–6.
86. Girard P, Setbon G, Forest A, et al. Dystrophies en réseau de l'épithélium pigmentaire (dystrophies macroréticulaires et en aile de papillon). J Fr Ophtalmol 1980;3:101–8.
87. Fishman GA, Trimble S, Rabb MF, et al. Pseudovitelliform macular degeneration. Arch Ophthalmol 1977;95:73–6.
88. Fishman GA, Woolf MB, Goldberg MF, et al. Reticular tapeto-retinal dystrophy as a possible late stage of Sjögren's reticular dystrophy. Br J Ophthalmol 1976;60:35–40.
89. Deutman AF. Rümke AML. Reticular dystrophy of the retinal pigment epithelium; dystrophia reticularis laminae pigmentosa retinae of H. Sjogren. Arch Ophthalmol 1969;82:4–9.
90. Deutman AF, van Blommestein JDA, Henkes HE, et al. Butterfly-shaped pigment dystrophy of the fovea. Arch Ophthalmol 1970;83:558–69.
91. Epstein GA, Rabb MF. Adult vitelliform macular degeneration: Diagnosis and natural history. Br J Ophthalmol 1980;64:733–40.
92. de Jong PTVM, Delleman JW. Pigment epithelial pattern dystrophy; four different manifestations in a family. Arch Ophthalmol 1982;100:1416–21.
93. Cortin P, Archer D, Maumenee IH, et al. A patterned macular dystrophy with yellow plaques and atrophic changes. Br J Ophthalmol 1980;64:127–34.
94. Chopdar A. Reticular dystrophy of retina. Br J Ophthalmol 1976;60:342–4.
95. Burgess D. Subretinal neovascularization in a pattern dystrophy of the retinal pigment epithelium. Retina 1981;1:151–5.
96. Bloom LH, Swanson DE, Bird AC. Adult vitelliform macular degeneration. Br J Ophthalmol 1981;65:800–1.
97. Ayazi S, Fagan R. Pattern dystrophy of the pigment epithelium. Retina 1981;1:287–9.
98. Renner AB, Fiebig BS, Weber BH, et al. Phenotypic variability and long-term follow-up of patients with known and novel PRPH2/RDS gene mutations. Am J Ophthalmol 2009;147:518–30, e1.
99. Zhuk SA, Edwards AO. Peripherin/RDS and VMD2 mutations in macular dystrophies with adult-onset vitelliform lesion. Mol Vis 2006;12:811–5.
100. Wells J, Wroblewski J, Keen J, et al. Mutations in the human retinal degeneration slow (RDS) gene can cause either retinitis pigmentosa or macular dystrophy. Nat Genet 1993;3:213–8.
101. Nichols BE, Sheffield VC, Vandenburgh K, et al. Butterfly-shaped pigment dystrophy of the fovea caused by a point mutation in condon 167 of the RDS gene. Nat Genet 1993;3:191–2.
102. Feist RM, White Jr MF, Skalka H, et al. Choroidal neovascularization in a patient with adult foveomacular dystrophy and a mutation in the retinal degeneration slow gene (Pro 210 Arg). Am J Ophthalmol 1994;118:259–60.
103. Gorin MB, Jackson KE, Ferrell RE, et al. A peripherin/retinal degeneration slow mutation (Pro-210-Arg) associated with macular and peripheral retinal degeneration. Ophthalmology 1994;102:246–55.
104. Weleber RG, Carr RE, Murphey WH, et al. Phenotypic variation including retinitis pigmentosa, pattern dystrophy, and fundus flavimaculatus in a single family with a deletion of codon 153 or 154 of the peripherin/RDS gene. Arch Ophthalmol 1993;111:1531–42.
105. Wells J, Wroblewski J, Keen J, et al. Mutations in the human retinal degeneration slow (RDS) gene can cause either retinitis pigmentosa or macular dystrophy. Nat Genet 1993;3:213–8.
106. Gamundi MJ, Hernan I, Muntanyola M, et al. High prevalence of mutations in peripherin/RDS in autosomal-dominant macular dystrophies in a Spanish population. Mol Vis 2007;13:1031–7.
107. Testa F, Marini V, Rossi S, et al. A novel mutation in the RDS gene in an Italian family with pattern dystrophy. Br J Ophthalmol 2005;89:1066–8.
108. Francis PJ, Schultz DW, Gregory AM, et al. Genetic and phenotypic heterogeneity in pattern dystrophy. Br J Ophthalmol 2005;89:1115–9.
109. Yang Z, Li Y, Jiang L, et al. A novel RDS/peripherin gene mutation associated with diverse macular phenotypes. Ophthalmic Genet 2004;25:133–45.
110. van Lith-Verhoeven JJ, van den Helm B, Deutman AF, et al. A peculiar autosomal-dominant macular dystrophy caused by an asparagine deletion at codon 169 in the peripherin/RDS gene. Arch Ophthalmol 2003;121:1452–7.
111. Boon CJ, den Hollander AI, Hoyng CB, et al. The spectrum of retinal dystrophies caused by mutations in the peripherin/RDS gene. Prog Retin Eye Res 2008;27:213–35.
112. Conley S, Nour M, Fliesler SJ, et al. Late-onset cone photoreceptor degeneration induced by R172W mutation in Rds and partial rescue by gene supplementation. Invest Ophthalmol Vis Sci 2007;48:5397–407.
113. Keilhauer CN, Meigen T, Stohr H, et al. Late-onset central areolar choroidal dystrophy caused by a heterozygous frame-shift mutation affecting codon 307 of the peripherin/RDS gene. Ophthalmic Genet 2006;27:139–44.
114. Yang Z, Lin W, Moshfeghi DM, et al. A novel mutation in the RDS/Peripherin gene causes adult-onset foveomacular dystrophy. Am J Ophthalmol 2003;135:213–8.
115. Wabbels B, Preising MN, Kretschmann U, et al. Genotype–phenotype correlation and longitudinal course in ten families with Best vitelliform macular dystrophy. Graefes Arch Clin Exp Ophthalmol 2006;244:1453–66.
116. Agarwal A, Patel P, Adkins T, et al. Spectrum of pattern dystrophy in pseudoxanthoma elasticum. Arch Ophthalmol 2005;123:923–8.
117. Giuffrè G. Autosomal-dominant pattern dystrophy of the retinal pigment epithelium; intrafamilial variability. Retina 1988;8:169–73.
118. Aaberg TM, Han DP. Evaluation of phenotypic similarities between Stargardt flavimaculatus and retinal pigment epithelial pattern dystrophies. Trans Am Ophthalmol Soc 1987;85:101–19.
119. Lopez PF, Aaberg TM. Phenotypic similarities between Stargardt's flavimaculatus and pattern dystrophies. Aust NZ J Ophthalmol 1992;20:163–71.
120. McDonnell PJ, Kivlin JD, Maumenee IH, et al. Fundus flavimaculatus without maculopathy; a clinicopathologic study. Ophthalmology 1986;93:116–9.
121. Lim JI, Enger C, Fine SL. Foveomacular dystrophy. Am J Ophthalmol 1994;117:1–6.
122. Bottoni F, Fatigati G, Carlevaro G, et al. Fundus flavimaculatus and subretinal neovascularization. Graefes Arch Clin Exp Ophthalmol 1992;230:498–500.
123. Noble KG, Chang S. Adult vitelliform macular degeneration progressing to full-thickness macular hole. Arch Ophthalmol 1991;109:325.
124. Jaffe GJ, Schatz H. Histopathologic features of adult-onset foveomacular pigment epithelial dystrophy. Arch Ophthalmol 1988;106:958–60.
125. Finger RP, Charbel Issa P, Ladewig MS, et al. Pseudoxanthoma elasticum: genetics, clinical manifestations and therapeutic approaches. Surv Ophthalmol 2009;54:272–85.
126. Li Volti S, Avitabile T, Li Volti G, et al. Optic disc drusen, angioid streaks, and mottled fundus in various combinations in a Sicilian family. Graefes Arch Clin Exp Ophthalmol 2002;240:771–6.
127. McDonald HR, Schatz H, Aaberg TM. Reticular-like pigmentary patterns in pseudoxanthoma elasticum. Ophthalmology 1988;95:306–11.
128. Leonardy NJ, Harbin RL, Sternberg Jr P. Pattern dystrophy of the retinal pigment epithelium in a patient with McArdle's disease. Am J Ophthalmol 1988;106:741–2.
129. Babel J, Tsacopoulos M. Les lesions rétiniennes de la dystrophie myotonique; étude clinique. Ann Oculist 1970;203:1049–65.
130. Betten MG, Bilchik RC, Smith ME. Pigmentary retinopathy of myotonic dystrophy. Am J Ophthalmol 1971;72:720–3.
131. Burian HM, Burns CA. Ocular changes in myotonic dystrophy. Am J Ophthalmol 1967;63:22–34.
132. Burns CA. Ocular histopathology of myotonic dystrophy; a clinicopathologic case report. Am J Ophthalmol 1969;68:416–22.
133. Deutman AF. Genetically determined retinal and choroidal disease. Trans Ophthalmol Soc UK 1974;94:1014–32.
134. Dumont P, Malthieu D, Turut P, et al. Dystrophie reticulee de la macula et maladie de Steinert. Bull Soc Ophthalmol Fr 1989;89:277–82.
135. Godtfredsen E, Jensen SF. Dystrophia myotonica and retinal dystrophy. Acta Ophthalmol 1969;47:565–9.
136. Hayasaka S, Kiyosawa M, Katsumata S, et al. Ciliary and retinal changes in myotonic dystrophy. Arch Ophthalmol 1984;102:88–93.
137. Manschot WA. Histological findings in a case of dystrophia myotonica. Ophthalmologica 1968;155:294–6.
138. Meyer E, Navon D, Auslender L, et al. Myotonic dystrophy: Pathological study of the eyes. Ophthalmologica 1980;181:215–20.
139. Kimizuka Y, Kiyosawa M, Tamai M, et al. Retinal changes in myotonic dystrophy; clinical and follow-up evaluation. Retina 1993;13:129–35.
140. Raby O, Bonsch M. Hypotonie oculaire et lésions rétiniennes dans la maladie de Steinert: aspects angiographiques. J Fr Ophtalmol 1986;9:543–53.
141. ter Brugggen JP, van Meel GJ, Paridaens ADA, et al. Foveal photopigment kinetics-abnormality: an early sign in myotonic dystrophy? Br J Ophthalmol 1992;76:594–7.
142. Farmer SG, Longstreth Jr WT, Kalina RE, et al. Fleck retina in Kjellin's syndrome. Am J Ophthalmol 1985;99:45–50.
143. Kjellin K. Familial spastic paraplegia with amyotrophy, oligophrenia, and central retinal degeneration. AMA Arch Neurol 1959;1:133–40.
144. Frisch IB, Haag P, Steffen H, et al. Kjellin's syndrome: fundus autofluorescence, angiographic, and electrophysiologic findings. Ophthalmology 2002;109:1484–91.
145. Takeshima T, Nakashima K. MIDD and MELAS: a clinical spectrum. Intern Med 2005;44:276–7.
146. Michaelides M, Jenkins SA, Bamiou DE, et al. Macular dystrophy associated with the A3243G mitochondrial DNA mutation. Distinct retinal and associated features, disease variability, and characterization of asymptomatic family members. Arch Ophthalmol 2008;126:320–8.
147. Sivaprasad S, Kung BT, Robson AG, et al. A new phenotype of macular dystrophy associated with a mitochondrial A3243G mutation. Clin Experiment Ophthalmol 2008;36:92–3.
148. Rath PP, Jenkins S, Michaelides M, et al. Characterisation of the macular dystrophy in patients with the A3243G mitochondrial DNA point mutation with fundus autofluorescence. Br J Ophthalmol 2008;92:623–9.
149. Ambonville C, Meas T, Lecleire-Collet A, et al. Macular pattern dystrophy in MIDD: long-term follow-up. Diabetes Metab 2008;34:389–91.
150. Isashiki Y, Nakagawa M, Ohba N, et al. Retinal manifestations in mitochondrial diseases associated with mitochondrial DNA mutation. Acta Ophthalmol Scand 1998;76:6–13.
151. Harrison TJ, Boles RG, Johnson DR, et al. Macular pattern retinal dystrophy, adult-onset diabetes, and deafness: a family study of A3243G mitochondrial heteroplasmy. Am J Ophthalmol 1997;124:217–21.
152. Rummelt V, Folberg R, Ionasescu V, et al. Ocular pathology of MELAS syndrome with mitochondrial DNA nucleotide 3243 point mutation. Ophthalmology 1993;100:1757–66.
153. Stargardt K. Über familiäre, progressive Degeneration in der Maculagegend des Auges. Albrecht von Graefes Arch Ophthalmol 1909;71:534–50.
154. Rosehr K. Über den weiteren Verlauf der von Stargardt und Behr beschriebenen familiären Degeneration der Makula. Klin Monatsbl Augenheilkd 1954;124:171–9.
155. Franceschetti A. Über tapeto-retinale Degenerationen im Kindesalter Dritter Fortbildungskurs der Deutschen Ophthalmologischen Gesellschaft, Hamburg, 1962. In: Sautter H, editor. Entwicklung und Fortschritt in der Augenheilkunde. Stuttgart: Enke; 1963. p. 107.
156. Franceschetti A. A special form of tapetoretinal degeneration: fundus flavimaculatus. Trans Am Acad Ophthalmol Otolaryngol 1965;69:1048–53.
157. Steinmetz RL, Garner A, Maguire JI, et al. Histopathology of incipient fundus flavimaculatus. Ophthalmology 1991;98:953–6.
158. Newell FW, Krill AE, Farkas TG. Drusen and fundus flavimaculatus: clinical, functional, and histologic characteristics. Trans Am Acad Ophthalmol Otolaryngol 1972;76:88–100.
159. Lopez PF, Maumenee IH, de la Cruz Z, et al. Autosomal-dominant fundus flavimaculatus; clinicopathologic correlation. Ophthalmology 1990;97:798–809.
160. Eagle Jr RC, Lucier AC, Bernardino Jr VB, et al. Retinal pigment epithelial abnormalities in fundus flavimaculatus; a light and electron microscopic study. Ophthalmology 1980;87:1189–200.
161. Birnbach CD, Järveläinen M, Possin DE, et al. Histopathologic and immunocytochemistry of the neurosensory retina in fundus flavimaculatus. Ophthalmology 1994;101:1211–9.
162. Klien BA, Krill AE. Fundus flavimaculatus; clinical, functional and histopathologic observations. Am J Ophthalmol 1967;64:3–23.

163. Uliss AE, Moore AT, Bird AC. The dark choroid in posterior retinal dystrophies. Ophthalmology 1987;94:1423–7.
164. Moloney JBM, Mooney DJ, O'Connor MA. Retinal function in Stargardt's disease and fundus flavimaculatus. Am J Ophthalmol 1983;96:57–65.
165. Leys A, van de Sompel W. Dark choroid in cone–rod dystrophy. Eur J Ophthalmol 1992;2:39–40.
166. Leveille AS, Morse PH, Burch JV. Fundus flavimaculatus and subretinal neovascularization. Ann Ophthalmol 1982;14:331–4.
167. Krill AE, Klien BA. Flecked retina syndrome. Arch Ophthalmol 1965;74:496–508.
168. Klein R, Lewis RA, Meyers SM, et al. Subretinal neovascularization associated with fundus flavimaculatus. Arch Ophthalmol 1978;96:2054–7.
169. Itabashi R, Katsumi O, Mehta MC, et al. Stargardt's disease/fundus flavimaculatus: Psychophysical and electrophysiologic results. Graefes Arch Clin Exp Ophthalmol 1993;231:555–62.
170. Irvine AR, Wergeland Jr FL. Stargardt's hereditary progressive macular degeneration. Br J Ophthalmol 1972;56:817–26.
171. Hadden OB. Gass JDM. Fundus flavimaculatus and Stargardt's disease. Am J Ophthalmol 1976;82:527–39.
172. Gelisken O, De Laey JJ. A clinical review of Stargardt's disease and/or fundus flavimaculatus with follow-up. Int Ophthalmol 1985;8:225–36.
173. Fishman GA. Fundus flavimaculatus; a clinical classification. Arch Ophthalmol 1976;94:2061–7.
174. Fish G, Grey R, Sehmi KS, et al. The dark choroid in posterior retinal dystrophies. Br J Ophthalmol 1981;65:359–63.
175. Ernest JT, Krill AE. Fluorescein studies in fundus flavimaculatus and drusen. Am J Ophthalmol 1966;62:1–6.
176. Doka DS, Fishman GA, Anderson RJ. Refractive errors in patients with fundus flavimaculatus. Br J Ophthalmol 1982;66:227–9.
177. Deutman AF. The hereditary dystrophies of the posterior pole of the eye. Assen: Van Gorcum; 1971. p. 100.
178. Bonnin P, Passot M, Triolaire-Cotten M-T. Le signe du silence choroïdien dans les dégénérescences tapéto-rétiniennes posterieures. Doc Ophthalmol Proc Ser 1976;9:461–3.
179. Anmarkrud N. Fundus fluorescein angiography in fundus flavimaculatus and Stargardt's disease. Acta Ophthalmol 1979;57:172–82.
180. Iijima H, Gohdo T, Hosaka O. Fundus flavimaculatus with severely reduced cone electroretinogram. Jpn J Ophthalmol 1992;36:249–56.
181. Gass JDM. Stereoscopic atlas of macular diseases; diagnosis and treatment, 3rd ed. St. Louis: CV Mosby; 1987. p. 256-57.
182. Fishman GA, Farbman JS, Alexander KR. Delayed rod dark adaptation in patients with Stargardt's disease. Ophthalmology 1991;98:957–62.
183. Stone EM, Nichols BE, Kimura AE, et al. Clinical features of a Stargardt-like dominant progressive macular dystrophy with genetic linkage to chromosome 6q. Arch Ophthalmol 1994;112:765–72.
184. Zhang K, Bither PP, Park R, et al. A dominant Stargardt's macular dystrophy locus maps to chromosome 13q34. Arch Ophthalmol 1994;112:759–64.
185. Fishman GA, Farber M, Patel BS, et al. Visual acuity loss in patients with Stargardt's macular dystrophy. Ophthalmology 1987;94:809–14.
186. Fonda G, Gardner LR. Characteristics and low vision corrections in Stargardt's disease: educational and vocational achievements enhanced by low vision corrections. Ophthalmology 1985;92:1084–91.
187. McMahon TT, Maino JH, Farber MD. Treatment of low vision in fundus flavimaculatus. Arch Ophthalmol 1985;103:1325–8.
188. Szlyk JP, Fishman GA, Severing K, et al. Evaluation of driving performance in patients with juvenile macular dystrophies. Arch Ophthalmol 1993;111:207–12.
189. Maumenee IH, Maumenee AE, editors. Fundus flavimaculatus; clinical, genetic, and pathologic observations, Blutzirkulation in der Uvea, in der Netzhaut und im Sehnerven (Physiologie und Pathologie). 5th Congress of the European Society of Ophthalmology, April 5–9, 1976. Hamburg: Stuttgart, Enke; 1978. p. 80–2.
190. Del Buey MA, Huerva V, Minguez E, et al. Posttraumatic reaction in a case of fundus flavimaculatus with atrophic macular degeneration. Ann Ophthalmol 1993;25:219–21.
191. Cibis GW, Morey M, Harris DJ. Dominantly inherited macular dystrophy with flecks (Stargardt). Arch Ophthalmol 1980;98:1785–9.
192. Kaplan J, Gerber S, Larget-Piet D, et al. A gene for Stargardt's disease (fundus flavimaculatus) maps to the short arm of chromosome 1. Nat Genet 1993;5:308–11. [erratum, 1994;6:214.]
193. Mansour AM. Long-term follow-up of dominant macular dystrophy with flecks (Stargardt). Ophthalmologica 1992;205:138–43.
194. Gass JDM, Weleber RG, Johnson DR. Non-Hodgkin's lymphoma causing fundus picture simulating fundus flavimaculatus. Retina 1987;7:209–14.
195. Lotery AJ, Silvestri G, Collins AD. Electrophysiology findings in a large family with central areolar choroidal dystrophy. Doc Ophthalmol 1998;97:103–19.
196. Hartley KL, Blodi BA, VerHoeve JN. Use of the multifocal electroretinogram in the evaluation of a patient with central areolar choroidal dystrophy. Am J Ophthalmol 2002;133:852–4.
197. Mansour AM. Central areolar choroidal dystrophy in a family with pseudoachondroplastic spondyloepiphyseal dysplasia. Ophthalmic Paediatr Genet 1988;9:57–65.
198. Gass JDM. Stereoscopic atlas of macular diseases; diagnosis and treatment, 2nd ed. St. Louis: CV Mosby; 1977. p. 156.
199. Fetkenhour CL, Gurney N, Dobbie JG, et al. Central areolar pigment epithelial dystrophy. Am J Ophthalmol 1976;81:745–53.
200. Noble KG. Central areolar choroidal dystrophy. Am J Ophthalmol 1977;84:310–8.
201. Sorsby A, Crick RP. Central areolar choroidal sclerosis. Br J Ophthalmol 1953;37:129–39.
202. Ashton N. Central areolar choroidal sclerosis; a histo-pathological study. Br J Ophthalmol 1953;37:140–7.
203. Ouechtati F, Belhadj Tahar O, Mhenni A, et al. Central areolar choroidal dystrophy associated with inherited drusen in a multigeneration Tunisian family: exclusion of the PRPH2 gene and the 17p13 locus. J Hum Genet 2009;54:589–94.
204. Boon CJ, Klevering BJ, Cremers FP, et al. Central areolar choroidal dystrophy. Ophthalmology 2009;116:771–82, e1.
205. Klevering BJ, Blankenagel A, Maugeri A, et al. Phenotypic spectrum of autosomal-recessive cone–rod dystrophies caused by mutations in the ABCA4 (ABCR) gene. Invest Ophthalmol Vis Sci 2002;43:1980–5.
206. Keilhauer CN, Meigen T, Weber BH. Clinical findings in a multigeneration family with autosomal-dominant central areolar choroidal dystrophy associated with an Arg195Leu mutation in the peripherin/RDS gene. Arch Ophthalmol 2006;124:1020–7.
207. Duvall-Young J, MacDonald MK, McKechnie NM. Fundus changes in (type II) mesangiocapillary glomerulonephritis simulating drusen: a histopathological report. Br J Ophthalmol 1989;73: 297–302.
208. Duvall-Young J, Short CD, Raines MF, et al. Fundus changes in mesangiocapillary glomerulonephritis findings. Br J Ophthalmol 1989;73:900–6.
209. Kim DD, Mieler WF, Wolf MD. Posterior segment changes in membranoproliferative glomerulonephritis. Am J Ophthalmol 1992;114:593–9.
210. Leys A, Michielsen B, Leys M, et al. Subretinal neovascular membranes associated with chronic membranoproliferative glomerulonephritis type II. Graefes Arch Clin Exp Ophthalmol 1990;228:499–504.
211. Leys A, Vanrenterghem Y, Van Damme B. Fundus changes in membranoproliferative glomerulonephritis type II: A fluorescein angiographic study of 23 patients. Graefes Arch Clin Exp Ophthalmol 1991;229:406–10.
212. Leys A, Vanrenterghem Y, Van Damme B, et al. Sequential observation of fundus changes in patients with long standing membranoproliferative glomerulonephritis type II (MPGN type II). Eur J Ophthalmol 1991;1:17–22.
213. Raines MF, Duvall-Young J, Short CD. Fundus changes in mesangiocapillary glomerulonephritis type II: Vitreous fluorophotometry. Br J Ophthalmol 1989;73:907–10.
214. Ulbig MRW, Riordan-Eva P, Holz FG, et al. Membranoproliferative glomerulonephritis type II associated with central serous retinopathy. Am J Ophthalmol 1993;116:410–3.
215. McAvoy CE, Silvestri G. Retinal changes associated with type 2 glomerulonephritis. Eye 2005;19:985–9.
216. Awan MA, Grierson DJ, Walker S. Bilateral macular sub-retinal fluid and retinal pigment epithelial detachment associated with type 2 membrano-proliferative glomerulonephritis. Clin Exp Optom 2008;91:476–9.
217. Boon CJ, van de Kar NC, Klevering BJ, et al. The spectrum of phenotypes caused by variants in the CFH gene. Mol Immunol 2009;46:1573–94.
218. Mandal MN, Ayyagari R. Complement factor H: spatial and temporal expression and localization in the eye. Invest Ophthalmol Vis Sci 2006;47:4091–7.
219. Xing C, Sivakumaran TA, Wang JJ, et al. Complement factor H polymorphisms, renal phenotypes and age-related macular degeneration: the Blue Mountains Eye Study. Genes Immun 2008;9:231–9.
220. Forni S, Babel J. Etude clinique et histologique de la malattia leventinese; affection appartenant au groupe de dégénérescences hyalines du pôle postérieur. Ophthalmologica 1962;143: 313–22.
221. Gass JDM. Stereoscopic atlas of macular diseases; diagnosis and treatment, 3rd ed. St. Louis: CV Mosby; 1987. p. 96–97.
222. Haimovici R, Wroblewski J, Piguet B, et al. Symptomatic abnormalities of dark adaptation in patients with EFEMP1 retinal dystrophy (Malattia Leventinese/Doyne honeycomb retinal dystrophy). Eye 2002;16:7–15.
223. Miyanaga Y, Mizutani T, Yamanishi R. A pedigree of Doyne's honeycomb macular degeneration. Jpn J Clin Ophthalmol 1977;31:431–5.
224. Piguet B, Haimovici R, Bird AC. Dominantly inherited drusen represent more than one disorder: a historical review. Eye 1995;9:34–41.
225. Evans K, Gregory CY, Wijesuriya SD, et al. Assessment of the phenotypic range seen in Doyne honeycomb retinal dystrophy. Arch Ophthalmol 1997;115:904–10.
226. Souied EH, Leveziel N, Querques G, et al. Indocyanine green angiography features of malattia leventinese. Br J Ophthalmol 2006;90:296–300.
227. Gerth C, Zawadzki RJ, Werner JS, et al. Retinal microstructure in patients with EFEMP1 retinal dystrophy evaluated by Fourier domain OCT. Eye 2009;23:480–3.
228. Souied EH, Leveziel N, Letien V, et al. Optical coherent tomography features of malattia leventinese. Am J Ophthalmol 2006;141:404–7.
229. Pager CK, Sarin LK, Federman JL, et al. Malattia leventinese presenting with subretinal neovascular membrane and hemorrhage. Am J Ophthalmol 2001;131:517–8.
230. Dantas MA, Slakter JS, Negrao S, et al. Photodynamic therapy with verteporfin in mallatia leventinese. Ophthalmology 2002;109:296–301.
231. Streicher T, Krcméry K. Das fluoreszenzangiographische Bild der hereditären Drusen. Klin Monatsbl Augenheilkd 1976;169:22–30.
232. Dusek J, Streicher T, Schmidt K. Hereditäre Drusen der Bruchschen Membran. II. Untersuchung von Semidünnschnitten und elektronenmikroskopischen Ergebnissen. Klin Monatsbl Augenheilkd 1982;181:79–83.
233. Toto L, Parodi MB, Baralle F, et al. Genetic heterogeneity in Malattia Leventinese. Clin Genet 2002;62:399–403.
234. Stone EM, Lotery AJ, Munier FL, et al. A single EFEMP1 mutation associated with both malattia leventinese and Doyne honeycomb retinal dystrophy. Nat Genet 1999;22:199–202.
235. Fu L, Garland D, Yang Z, et al. The R345W mutation in EFEMP1 is pathogenic and causes AMD-like deposits in mice. Hum Mol Genet 2007;16:2411–22.
236. Matsumoto M, Traboulsi EI. Dominant radial drusen and Arg345Trp EFEMP1 mutation. Am J Ophthalmol 2001;131:810–2.
237. Lefler WH, Wadsworth JAC, Sidbury Jr JB. Hereditary macular degeneration and amino-aciduria. Am J Ophthalmol 1971;71:224–30.
238. Frank HR, Landers III MB, Williams RJ, et al. A new dominant progressive foveal dystrophy. Am J Ophthalmol 1974;78:903–16.

239. Gass JDM. Stereoscopic atlas of macular diseases; diagnosis and treatment, 2nd ed. St. Louis: CV Mosby; 1977. p. 74.
240. Small KW, Killian J, McLean WC. North Carolina's dominant progressive foveal dystrophy: how progressive is it? Br J Ophthalmol 1991;75:401–6.
241. Rohrschneider K, Blankenagel A, Kruse FE, et al. Macular function testing in a German pedigree with North Carolina macular dystrophy. Retina 1998;18:453–9.
242. Reichel MB, Kelsell RE, Fan J, et al. Phenotype of a British North Carolina macular dystrophy family linked to chromosome 6q. Br J Ophthalmol 1998;82:1162–8.
243. Small KW, Puech B, Mullen L, et al. North Carolina macular dystrophy phenotype in France maps to the MCDR1 locus. Mol Vis 1997;3:1.
244. Rabb MF, Mullen L, Yelchits S, et al. A North Carolina macular dystrophy phenotype in a Belizean family maps to the MCDR1 locus. Am J Ophthalmol 1998;125:502–8.
245. Kim SJ, Woo SJ, Yu HG. A Korean family with an early-onset autosomal-dominant macular dystrophy resembling North Carolina macular dystrophy. Korean J Ophthalmol 2006;20:220–4.
246. Khurana RN, Sun X, Pearson E, et al. A reappraisal of the clinical spectrum of North Carolina macular dystrophy. Ophthalmology 2009;116:1976–83.
247. Freedman J, Gombos GM. Bilateral macular coloboma, keratoconus, and retinitis pigmentosa. Ann Ophthalmol 1971;3:664–8.
248. Heckenlively JR, Foxman SG, Parelhoff ES. Retinal dystrophy and macular coloboma. Doc Ophthalmol 1988;68:257–71.
249. Murayama K, Adachi-Usami E. Bilateral macular colobomas in Leber's congenital amaurosis. Doc Ophthalmol 1989;72:118–88.
250. Car A. Mikrozephalie and beiderseitiges Kolobom im Bereiche der Makula. Z Augenheilkd 1925;57:618–30.
251. Clarke E. Coloboma at the macula (both eyes). Br J Ophthalmol 1927;11:97–9.
252. Clausen W. Typisches, beiderseitiges hereditäres Makula-Kolobom. Klin Monatsbl Augenheilkd 1921;67:116.
253. Clausen W. Zur Frage der Vererbung der Makulakolobom. Klin Monatsbl Augenheilkd 1928;81:385.
254. Goodman G, Ripps H, Siegel IM. Cone dysfunction syndromes. Arch Ophthalmol 1963;70:214–31.
255. Klein R, Bresnick G. An inherited central retinal pigment epithelial dystrophy. Birth Defects 1982;18:281–96.
256. Margolis S, Scher BM, Carr RE. Macular colobomas in Leber's congenital amaurosis. Am J Ophthalmol 1977;83:27–31.
257. Phillips CI, Griffiths DL. Macular coloboma and skeletal abnormality. Br J Ophthalmol 1969;53:346–9.
258. Sorsby A. Congenital coloboma of the macula: together with an account of the familial occurrence of bilateral macular coloboma in association with apical dystrophy of hands and feet. Br J Ophthalmol 1935;19:65–90.
259. Leveille AS, Morse PH, Kiernan JP. Autosomal-dominant central pigment epithelial and choroidal degeneration. Ophthalmology 1982;89:1407–13.
260. Miller SA, Bresnick G. Familial bilateral macular colobomata. Br J Ophthalmol 1978;62:261–4.
261. Hermsen VM, Judisch GF. Central areolar pigment epithelial dystrophy. Ophthalmologica 1984;189:69–72.
262. Small KW, Hermsen V, Gurney N, et al. North Carolina macular dystrophy and central areolar pigment epithelial dystrophy; one family, one disease. Arch Ophthalmol 1992;110:515–8.
263. Satorre J, López JM, Martínez J, et al. Dominant macular colobomata. J Pediatr Ophthalmol Strabismus 1990;27:148–52.
264. Gass JDM. Stereoscopic atlas of macular diseases; diagnosis and treatment, 3rd ed. St Louis: CV Mosby; 1987. p. 98-9, 264–65.
265. Michaelides M, Johnson S, Tekriwal AK, et al. An early-onset autosomal-dominant macular dystrophy (MCDR3) resembling North Carolina macular dystrophy maps to chromosome 5. Invest Ophthalmol Vis Sci 2003;44:2178–83.
266. Francis PJ, Johnson S, Edmunds B, et al. Genetic linkage analysis of a novel syndrome comprising North Carolina-like macular dystrophy and progressive sensorineural hearing loss. Br J Ophthalmol 2003;87:893–8.
267. Kniazeva M, Traboulsi EI, Yu Z, et al. A new locus for dominant drusen and macular degeneration maps to chromosome 6q14. Am J Ophthalmol 2000;130:197–202.
268. Brodsky MC, Ford RE, Bradford JD. Subretinal neovascular membrane in an infant with a retinochoroidal coloboma. Arch Ophthalmol 1991;109:1650–1.
269. Leff SR, Britton Jr WA, Brown GC, et al. Retinochoroidal coloboma associated with subretinal neovascularization. Retina 1985;5:154–6.
270. Maberley AL, Gottner MJ, Antworth MV. Subretinal neovascularization associated with retinochoroidal colobomas. Can J Ophthalmol 1989;24:172–4.
271. Rouland J-F, Hochart G, Constantinides G. Colobome chorio-rétinien et membrane néovasculaire. Bull Soc Ophtalmol Fr 1990;90:643–4.
272. Steahly LP. Laser treatment of a subretinal neovascular membrane associated with a retinochoroidal coloboma. Retina 1986;6:154–6.
273. Gass JDM, Blodi BA. Idiopathic juxtafoveolar retinal telangiectasis; update of classification and follow-up study. Ophthalmology 1993;100:1536–46.
274. Sorsby A, Joll Mason ME, Gardener N. A fundus dystrophy with unusual features (late onset and dominant inheritance of a central retinal lesion showing oedema, haemorrhage and exudates developing into generalised choroidal atrophy with massive pigment proliferation). Br J Ophthalmol 1949;33:67–97.
275. Ashton N, Sorsby A. Fundus dystrophy with unusual features; a histological study. Br J Ophthalmol 1951;35:751–64.
276. Capon MRC, Polkinghorne PJ, Fitzke FW, et al. Sorsby's pseudoinflammatory macular dystrophy – Sorsby's fundus dystrophies. Eye 1988;2:114–22.
277. Capon MRC, Marshall J, Krafft JI, et al. Sorsby's fundus dystrophy; a light and electron microscopic study. Ophthalmology 1989;96:1769–77.
278. Dreyer RF, Hidayat AA. Pseudoinflammatory macular dystrophy. Am J Ophthalmol 1988;106:154–61.
279. Hoskin A, Sehmi K, Bird AC. Sorsby's pseudoinflammatory macular dystrophy. Br J Ophthalmol 1981;65:859–65.
280. Forsius HR, Eriksson AW, Suvanto EA, et al. Pseudoinflammatory fundus dystrophy with autosomal-recessive inheritance. Am J Ophthalmol 1982;94:634–49.
281. Balyeat RM, Kingsley RM. Dominant macular subretinal neovascularization with peripheral retinal degeneration. Ophthalmology 1987;94:1140–7.
282. Hamilton WK, Ewing CC, Ives IJ, et al. Sorsby's fundus dystrophy. Ophthalmology 1989;96:1755–62.
283. Wu G, Pruett RC, Baldinger J, et al. Hereditary hemorrhagic macular dystrophy. Am J Ophthalmol 1991;111:294–301.
284. Steinmetz RL, Polkinghorne PC, Fitzke FW, et al. Abnormal dark adaptation and rhodopsin kinetics in Sorsby's fundus dystrophy. Invest Ophthalmol Vis Sci 1992;33:1633–6.
285. Carr RE, Noble KG, Nasaduke I. Hereditary hemorrhagic macular dystrophy. Am J Ophthalmol 1978;85:318–28.
286. Deutman AF. The hereditary dystrophies of the posterior pole of the eye. Assen, The Netherlands: Van Gorcum; 1971. p. 400.
287. Polkinghorne PJ, Capon MRC, Berninger T, et al. Sorsby's fundus dystrophy; a clinical study. Ophthalmology 1989;96:1763–8.
288. Weber BHF, Vogt G, Pruett RC, et al. Mutations in the tissue inhibitor of metalloproteinases-3 (TIMP3) in patients with Sorsby's fundus dystrophy. Nat Genet 1994;8:352–6.
289. Majid MA, Smith VA, Newby AC, et al. Matrix bound SFD mutant TIMP-3 is more stable than wild type TIMP-3. Br J Ophthalmol 2007;91:1073–6.
290. Majid MA, Smith VA, Matthews FJ, et al. Tissue inhibitor of metalloproteinase-3 differentially binds to components of Bruch's membrane. Br J Ophthalmol 2006;90:1310–5.
291. Li Z, Clarke MP, Barker MD, et al. TIMP3 mutation in Sorsby's fundus dystrophy: molecular insights. Expert Rev Mol Med 2005;7:1–15.
292. Clarke M, Mitchell KW, Goodship J, et al. Clinical features of a novel TIMP-3 mutation causing Sorsby's fundus dystrophy: implications for disease mechanism. Br J Ophthalmol 2001;85:1429–31.
293. Chong NH, Alexander RA, Gin T, et al. TIMP-3, collagen, and elastin immunohistochemistry and histopathology of Sorsby's fundus dystrophy. Invest Ophthalmol Vis Sci 2000;41:898–902.
294. Wijesuriya SD, Evans K, Jay MR, et al. Sorsby's fundus dystrophy in the British Isles: demonstration of a striking founder effect by microsatellite-generated haplotypes. Genome Res 1996;6:92–101.
295. Chen W, Stambolian D, Edwards AO, et al. Genetic variants near TIMP3 and high-density lipoprotein-associated loci influence susceptibility to age-related macular degeneration. Proc Natl Acad Sci U S A 2010;107:7401–6.
296. Coppeto J, Ayazi S. Annular macular dystrophy. Am J Ophthalmol 1982;93:279–84.
297. Deutman AF. Benign concentric annular macular dystrophy. Am J Ophthalmol 1974;78:384–96.
298. van den Biesen PR, Deutman AF. Pinckers AJLG. Evolution of benign concentric annular macular dystrophy. Am J Ophthalmol 1985;100:73–8.
299. Weise EE, Yannuzzi LA. Ring maculopathies mimicking chloroquine retinopathy. Am J Ophthalmol 1974;78:204–10.
300. van Lith-Verhoeven JJ, Hoyng CB, van den Helm B, et al. The benign concentric annular macular dystrophy locus maps to 6p12.3-q16. Invest Ophthalmol Vis Sci 2004;45:30–5.
301. Miyake Y, Shiroyama N, Horiguchi M, et al. Bull's-eye maculopathy and negative electroretinogram. Retina 1989;9:210–5.
302. Babel J. Les choroïdopathies géographiques et hélicoïdales. Etude clinique et angiographique; essai de classification. J Fr Ophthalmol 1983;6:981–93.
303. Brazitikos PD, Safran AB. Helicoid peripapillary chorioretinal degeneration. Am J Ophthalmol 1990;109:290–4.
304. Franceschetti A. A curious affection of the fundus oculi: helicoid peripapillar chorioretinal degeneration. Its relation to pigmentary paravenous chorioretinal degeneration. Doc Ophthalmol Proc Ser 1962;16:81–110.
305. Rubino A. Su una particolare anomalia bilaterale e simmetrica dello strato pigmentato retinico. Boll Oculist 1940;19:318–22.
306. Sveinsson K. Choroiditis areata. Acta Ophthalmol 1939;17:73–80.
307. Sveinsson K. Helicoidal peripapillary chorioretinal degeneration. Acta Ophthalmol 1979;57: 69–75.
308. Fossdal R, Jonasson F, Kristjansdottir GT, et al. A novel TEAD1 mutation is the causative allele in Sveinsson's chorioretinal atrophy (helicoid peripapillary chorioretinal degeneration). Hum Mol Genet 2004;13:975–81.
309. Fossdal R, Magnusson L, Weber JL, et al. Mapping the locus of atrophia areata, a helicoid peripapillary chorioretinal degeneration with autosomal-dominant inheritance, to chromosome 11p15. Hum Mol Genet 1995;4:479–83.
310. Falls HF, Wolter JR, Alpern M. Typical total monochromacy; a histological and psychophysical study. Arch Ophthalmol 1965;74:610–6.
311. Glickstein M, Heath GG. Receptors in the monochromat eye. Vision Res 1975;15:633–6.
312. Wiszniewski W, Lewis RA, Lupski JR. Achromatopsia: the CNGB3 p.T383fsX mutation results from a founder effect and is responsible for the visual phenotype in the original report of uniparental disomy 14. Hum Genet 2007;121:433–9.
313. Michaelides M, Holder GE, Hunt DM, et al. A detailed study of the phenotype of an autosomal-dominant cone–rod dystrophy (CORD7) associated with mutation in the gene for RIM1. Br J Ophthalmol 2005;89:198–206.
314. Michaelides M, Holder GE, Bradshaw K, et al. Cone–rod dystrophy, intrafamilial variability, and incomplete penetrance associated with the R172W mutation in the peripherin/RDS gene. Ophthalmology 2005;112:1592–8.
315. Lewis RA, Holcomb JD, Bromley WC, et al. Mapping X-linked ophthalmic diseases. III. Provisional assignment of the locus for blue cone monochromacy to Xq28. Arch Ophthalmol 1987;105:1055–9.
316. Krill AE, Smith VC, Pokorny J. Further studies supporting the identity of congenital tritanopia and hereditary dominant optic atrophy. Invest Ophthalmol 1971;10:457–65.

317. Zervas JP, Smith JL. Neuro-ophthalmic presentation of cone dysfunction sydromes in the adult. J Clin Neuro-Ophthalmol 1987;7:202–18.
318. Went LN, van Schooneveld MJ, Oosterhuis JA. Late onset dominant cone dystrophy with early blue cone involvement. J Med Genet 1992;29:295–8.
319. van Schooneveld MJ, Went LN, Oosterhuis JA. Dominant cone dystrophy starting with blue cone involvement. Br J Ophthalmol 1991;75:332–6.
320. van Everdingen JAM, Went LN, Keunen JEE, et al. X-linked progressive cone dystrophy with specific attention to carrier detection. J Med Genet 1992;29:291–4.
321. Stoumbos VD, Weleber RG, Kennaway NG. Normal α-l-fucosidase and other lysosomal enzyme activities in progressive cone dystrophy. Am J Ophthalmol 1988;106:11–16.
322. Siegel IM, Smith BF. Acquired cone dysfunction. Arch Ophthalmol 1967;77:8–13.
323. Reichel E, Bruck AM, Sandberg MA, et al. An electroretinographic and molecular genetic study of X-linked cone degeneration. Am J Ophthalmol 1989;108:540–7.
324. Pinckers A. Dominant cone dystrophy starting with blue cone involvement. Br J Ophthalmol 1992;76:127.
325. Pinckers A, Deutman AF. Peripheral cone disease. Ophthalmologica 1977;174:145–50.
326. Pinckers A, Deutman AF. X-linked cone dystrophy; an overlooked diagnosis? Int Ophthalmol 1987;10:241–3.
327. Pearlman JT, Owen WG, Brounley DW. Cone dystrophy with dominant inheritance. Am J Ophthalmol 1974;77:293–303.
328. Ohba N. Progressive cone dystrophy: Four cases of unusual form. Jpn J Ophthalmol 1974;18:50–69.
329. Noble KG, Siegle IM, Carr RE. Progressive peripheral cone dystrophy. Am J Ophthalmol 1988;106:557–60.
330. Krill AE, Deutman AF, Fishman M. The cone degenerations. Doc Ophthalmol 1973;35:1–80.
331. Krill AE, Deutman AF. Dominant macular degenerations: the cone dystrophies. Am J Ophthalmol 1972;73:352–69.
332. Keunen JEE, van Everdingen JAM, Went LN, et al. Color matching and foveal densitometry in patients and carriers of an X-linked progressive cone dystrophy. Arch Ophthalmol 1990;108:1713–9.
333. Jacobson DM, Thompson HS, Bartley JA. X-linked progressive cone dystrophy; clinical characteristics of affected males and female carriers. Ophthalmology 1989;96:885–95.
334. Isashiki Y, Ohba N, Nakagawa M, et al. Antibodies against human retinal proteins in serum from patients with cone dystrophy. Jpn J Ophthalmol 1992;36:323–30.
335. Heckenlively JR, Weleber RG. X-linked recessive cone dystrophy with tapetal-like sheen; a newly recognized entity with Mizuo–Nakamura phenomenon. Arch Ophthalmol 1986;104:1322–8.
336. Hayasaka S, Nakazawa M, Okabe H, et al. Progressive cone dystrophy associated with low αa-l-fucosidase activity in serum and leukocytes. Am J Ophthalmol 1985;99:681–5.
337. Hamilton SR, Chatrian G-E, Mills RP, et al. Cone dysfunction in a subgroup of patients with autosomal-dominant cerebellar ataxia. Arch Ophthalmol 1990;108:551–6.
338. Grey RHB, Blach RK, Barnard WM. Bull's eye maculopathy with early cone degeneration. Br J Ophthalmol 1977;61:702–18.
339. Gouras P, Eggers HM, MacKay CJ. Cone dystrophy, nyctalopia, and supernormal rod responses; a new retinal degeneration. Arch Ophthalmol 1983;101:718–24.
340. François J, De Rouck A, Verriest G, et al. Progressive generalized cone dysfunction. Ophthalmologica 1974;169:255–84.
341. Foerster MH, Kellner U, Wessing A. Cone dystrophy and supernormal dark-adapted b-waves in the electroretinogram. Graefes Arch Clin Exp Ophthalmol 1990;228:116–9.
342. Bresnick GH, Smith VC, Pokorny J. Autosomal-dominantly inherited macular dystrophy with preferential short-wavelength sensitive cone involvement. Am J Ophthalmol 1989;108: 265–76.
343. Berson EL, Gouras P, Gunkel RD. Progressive cone degeneration, dominantly inherited. Arch Ophthalmol 1968;80:77–83.
344. Babel J, Stangos N. Progressive degeneration of the photopic system. Am J Ophthalmol 1973;75:511–25.
345. Babel J, Stangos N. Dégénérescence progressive du système photopique. Ophthalmologica 1972;165:392–5.
346. Alexander KR, Fishman GA. Supernormal scotopic ERG in cone dystrophy. Br J Ophthalmol 1984;68:69–78.
347. Berson EL, Gouras P, Gunkel RD. Progressive cone–rod degeneration. Arch Ophthalmol 1968;80:68–76.
348. Wang NK, Fine HF, Chang S, et al. Cellular origin of fundus autofluorescence in patients and mice with a defective NR2E3 gene. Br J Ophthalmol 2009;93:1234–40.
349. Forsius H, Erkkilä H, Eriksson AW. Rod–cone dystrophy of the retina; continuation of a family study described in 1923. Acta Ophthalmol 1990;68:2–10.
350. Buchanan TAS, Gardeiner TA, de Jesus V, et al. Retinal ultrastructural findings in cone degeneration. Am J Ophthalmol 1988;106:405–13.
351. Robson AG, Webster AR, Michaelides M, et al. "Cone dystrophy with supernormal rod electroretinogram": a comprehensive genotype/phenotype study including fundus autofluorescence and extensive electrophysiology. Retina 2010;30:51–62.
352. Small KW, Silva-Garcia R, Udar N, et al. New mutation, P575L, in the GUCY2D gene in a family with autosomal-dominant progressive cone degeneration. Arch Ophthalmol 2008;126:397–403.
353. Langwinska-Wosko E, Szulborski K, Broniek-Kowalik K. Late onset cone dystrophy. Doc Ophthalmol 2010;120:215–8.
354. Rowe SE, Trobe JD, Sieving PA. Idiopathic photoreceptor dysfunction causes unexplained visual acuity loss in later adulthood. Ophthalmology 1990;97:1632–7.
355. Noble KG, Margolis S, Carr RE. The golden tapetal sheen reflex in retinal disease. Am J Ophthalmol 1989;107:211–7.
356. Noble KG, Sherman J. Central pigmentary sheen dystrophy. Am J Ophthalmol 1989;108:255–9.
357. Slagsvold JE. Fenestrated sheen macular dystrophy. A new autosomal-dominant maculopathy. Acta Ophthalmol (Copenh) 1981;59:683–8.
358. O'Donnell FE, Welch RB. Fenestrated sheen macular dystrophy. Arch Ophthalmol 1980;98:575.
359. O'Donnell Jr FE, Welch RB. Fenestrated sheen macular dystrophy. A new autosomal-dominant maculopathy. Arch Ophthalmol 1979;97:1292–6.
360. Daily MJ, Mets MB. Fenestrated sheen macular dystrophy. Arch Ophthalmol 1984;102: 855–6.
361. Sneed SR, Sieving PA. Fenestrated sheen macular dystrophy. Am J Ophthalmol 1991;112: 1–7.
362. Timothy D. Polk, J. Donald M. Gass, W. Richard Green, et al. Familial Internal Limiting Membrane Dystrophy A New Sheen Retinal Dystrophy. Arch Ophthalmol 1997;115:878–885.
363. Gass JDM. Stereoscopic atlas of macular diseases; diagnosis and treatment, 3rd ed. St. Louis: CV Mosby; 1987. p. 266.
364. Gilbert Jr WR, Smith JL, Nyhan WL. The Sjögren–Larsson syndrome. Arch Ophthalmol. 1968;80:308–16.
365. Kelson TL, Craft DA, Rizzo WB. Carrier detection for Sjogren–Larsson syndrome. J Inherit Metab Dis 1992;15:105–11.
366. Nilsson SEG, Jagel S. Lipofuscin and melanin content of the retinal pigment epithelium in a case of Sjögren–Larsson syndrome. Br J Ophthalmol 1987;71:224–6.
367. Sjögren T, Larsson T. Oligophrenia in combination with congenital ichthyosis and spastic disorders; a clinical and genetic study. Acta Psychiatr Neurol Scand Suppl 1957;113:32–44.
368. Mirshahi A, Piri N. Fundus autofluorescence changes in two cases of Sjogren–Larsson syndrome. Int Ophthalmol 2008 Oct 2.
369. Fuijkschot J, Cruysberg JR, Willemsen MA, et al. Subclinical changes in the juvenile crystalline macular dystrophy in Sjogren–Larsson syndrome detected by optical coherence tomography. Ophthalmology 2008;115:870–5.
370. van der Veen RL, Fuijkschot J, Willemsen MA, et al. Patients with Sjogren–Larsson syndrome lack macular pigment. Ophthalmology 2010;117:966–71.
371. Willemsen MA, Cruysberg JR, Rotteveel JJ, et al. Juvenile macular dystrophy associated with deficient activity of fatty aldehyde dehydrogenase in Sjogren–Larsson syndrome. Am J Ophthalmol 2000;130:782–9.
372. Aslam SA, Sheth HG. Ocular features of Sjogren–Larsson syndrome. Clin Experiment Ophthalmol 2007;35:98–9.
373. Aicardi J, Lefebvre J, Lerique-Koechlin A. A new syndrome: spasm in flexion, callosal agenesis, ocular abnormalities. Electroenceph Clin Neurophysiol 1965;19:609–10.
374. Aicardi J, Chevrie J-J, Rousselie E. Le syndrome spasmes en flexion, agenesie calleuse, anomalies chorio-retiniennes. Arch Fr Pediatr 1969;26:1103–20.
375. Del Pero RA, Mets MB, Tripathi RC, et al. Anomalies of retinal architecture in Aicardi syndrome. Arch Ophthalmol 1986;104:1659–64.
376. Déodati F, Bec P, Carrière J-P, et al. Manifestations ophtalmologiques du syndrome d'Aicardi. Bull Soc Ophtalmol Fr 1973;73:161–4.
377. Font RL, Marines HM, Cartwright Jr J, et al. Aicardi syndrome; a clinicopathologic case report including electron microscopic observations. Ophthalmology 1991;98:1727–31.
378. Gloor P, Pulido JS, Judisch GF. Magnetic resonance imaging and fundus findings in a patient with Aicardi's syndrome. Arch Ophthalmol 1989;107:922–3.
379. Hoyt CS, Billson F, Ouvrier R, et al. Ocular features of Aicardi's syndrome. Arch Ophthalmol 1978;96:291–5.
380. Limnaios EE, Panayiotopoulos CP, Theodosiadis G, et al. Ophthalmologic features of Aicardi's syndrome: report of two cases. Br J Ophthalmol 1979;63:713–7.
381. Tillmann W, von Bernuth H. Das Aicardi-Syndrom. Klin Monatsbl Augenheilkd 1975;167: 496–9.
382. Weleber RG, Lovrien EW, Isom JB. Aicardi's syndrome; case report, clinical features, and electrophysiologic studies. Arch Ophthalmol 1978;96:285–90.
383. Carney SH, Brodsky MC, Good WV, et al. Aicardi syndrome: more than meets the eye. Surv Ophthalmol 1993;37:419–24.
384. Singhi PD, Gupta A, Agarwal A. Aicardi syndrome. Indian Pediatr 1991;28:1513–6.
385. Frye RE, Polling JS, Ma LC. Choroid plexus papilloma expansion over 7 years in Aicardi syndrome. J Child Neurol 2007;22:484–7.
386. Mutlu FM, Akin R, Uysal Y, et al. Aicardi syndrome: an unusual case associated with pineal gland cyst and ventricular septal defect. J Child Neurol 2006;21:1082–4.
387. Lee SW, Kim KS, Cho SM, et al. An atypical case of Aicardi syndrome with favorable outcome. Korean J Ophthalmol 2004;18:79–83.
388. Nielsen KB, Anvret M, Flodmark O, et al. Aicardi syndrome: early neuroradiological manifestations and results of DNA studies in one patient. Am J Med Genet 1991;38:65–8.
389. Lorenz B, Hasenfratz G, Laub MC, et al. Retrobulbar cysts in Aicardi's syndrome. Ophthalmic Paediatr Genet 1991;12:105–10.
390. Jensen AA, Christiansen SP. Aicardi syndrome with Pierre Robin sequence. J AAPOS 2004;8:187–9.
391. McMahon RG, Bell RA, Moore GRW, et al. Aicardi's syndrome; a clinicopathologic study. Arch Ophthalmol 1984;102:250–3.
392. Ospina LH, Nayak H, McCormick AQ. Progressive pigmentation of chorioretinal lesions in Aicardi syndrome. Arch Ophthalmol 2004;122:790.
393. Costa T, Greer W, Rysiecki G, et al. Monozygotic twins discordant for Aicardi syndrome. J Med Genet 1997;34:688–91.
394. Anderson C, Pahk P, Blaha GR, et al. Preferential hyperacuity perimetry to detect hydroxychloroquine retinal toxicity. Retina 2009;29:1188–92.
395. Aggarwal KC, Aggarwal A, Prasad MS, et al. Aicardi's syndrome in a male child: an unusual presentation. Indian Pediatr 2000;37:542–5.
396. Chappelow AV, Reid J, Parikh S, et al. Aicardi syndrome in a genotypic male. Ophthalmic Genet 2008;29:181–3.
397. Yilmaz S, Fontaine H, Brochet K, et al. Screening of subtle copy number changes in Aicardi syndrome patients with a high resolution X chromosome array-CGH. Eur J Med Genet 2007;50:386–91.
398. Vetrie D, Flinter F, Bobrow M, et al. X inactivation patterns in females with Alport's syndrome: a means of selecting against a deleterious gene? J Med Genet 1992;29:663–6.

399. Jais JP, Knebelmann B, Giatras I, et al. X-linked Alport syndrome: natural history and genotype–phenotype correlations in girls and women belonging to 195 families: a "European Community Alport Syndrome Concerted Action" study. J Am Soc Nephrol 2003;14:2603–10.
400. Alport AC. Hereditary familial congenital haemorrhagic nephritis. Br Med J 1927;1:504–6.
401. Arnott EJ, Crawfurd MDA, Toghill PJ. Anterior lenticonus and Alport's syndrome. Br J Ophthalmol 1966;50:390–403.
402. Davies PD. Pigment dispersion in a case of Alport's syndrome. Br J Ophthalmol 1970;54:557–61.
403. Gelisken O, Ozçetin H, Erturk H. Alport's syndrome and flecked retinopathy. Bull Soc Belge Ophthalmol 1987;220:75–9.
404. Gehrs KM, Pollock SC, Zilkha G. Clinical features and pathogenesis of Alport retinopathy. Retina 1995;15:305–11.
405. Govan JAA. Ocular manifestations of Alport's syndrome: a hereditary disorder of basement membranes? Br J Ophthalmol 1983;67:493–503.
406. Jacobs M, Jeffrey B, Kriss A, et al. Ophthalmologic assessment of young patients with Alport syndrome. Ophthalmology 1992;99:1039–44.
407. Kanamori M, Hayasaka S, Furuse N, et al. Macular flecks in a 5-year-old boy with Alport's syndrome. Graefes Arch Clin Exp Ophthalmol 1988;226:227–9.
408. Perrin D, Jungers P, Grunfeld JP, et al. Perimacular changes in Alport's syndrome. Clin Nephrol 1980;13:163–7.
409. Peterson WS, Albert DM. Fundus changes in the hereditary nephropathies. Trans Am Acad Ophthalmol Otolaryngol 1974;78:OP762–OP770.
410. Polak BCP, Hogewind BL. Macular lesions in Alport's disease. Am J Ophthalmol 1977;84:532–5.
411. Sabates R, Krachmer JH, Weingeist TA. Ocular findings in Alport's syndrome. Ophthalmologica 1983;186:204–10.
412. Sohar E. A heredo-familial syndrome characterized by renal disease, inner ear deafness and ocular changes. Harefuah 1954;47:161–2.
413. Teekhasaenee C, Nimmanit S, Wutthiphan S, et al. Posterior polymorphous dystrophy and Alport syndrome. Ophthalmology 1991;98:1207–15.
414. Zylbermann R. Silverstone B-Z, Brandes E, et al. Retinal lesions in Alport's syndrome. J Pediatr Ophthalmol Strabismus 1980;17:255–60.
415. Rahman W, Banerjee S. Giant macular hole in Alport syndrome. Can J Ophthalmol 2007;42:314–5.
416. Myers JC, Jones TA, Pohjolainen E-R, et al. Molecular cloning of α5(IV) collagen and assignment of the gene to the region of the X-chromosome containing the Alport syndrome locus. Am J Hum Gen 1990;46:1024–33.
417. Tazon Vega B, Badenas C, Ars E, et al. Autosomal-recessive Alport's syndrome and benign familial hematuria are collagen type IV diseases. Am J Kidney Dis 2003;42:952–9.
418. Pascual Pascual SI, Molano J, Pascual-Castroviejo I. Electroretinogram in Duchenne/Becker muscular dystrophy. Pediatr Neurol 1998;18:315–20.
419. Jensen H, Warburg M, Sjo O, et al. Duchenne muscular dystrophy: negative electroretinograms and normal dark adaptation. Reappraisal of assignment of X linked incomplete congenital stationary night blindness. J Med Genet 1995;32:348–51.
420. Tremblay F, De Becker I, Dooley JM, et al. Duchenne muscular dystrophy: negative scotopic bright-flash electroretinogram but not congenital stationary night blindness. Can J Ophthalmol 1994;29:274–9.
421. Sigesmund DA, Weleber RG, Pillers DA, et al. Characterization of the ocular phenotype of Duchenne and Becker muscular dystrophy. Ophthalmology 1994;101:856–65.
422. Sigesmund DA, Weleber RG, Pillers DAM, et al. Characterization of the ocular phenotype of Duchenne and Becker muscular dystrophy. Ophthalmology 1994;101:856–65.
423. Miyake Y, Ichikawa K, Shiose Y, et al. Hereditary macular dystrophy without visible fundus abnormality. Am J Ophthalmol 1989;108:292–9.
424. Deutman AF. The hereditary dystrophies of the posterior pole of the eye. Assen: Van Gorcum; 1971. p. 172–98.
425. Kondo M, Ueno S, Piao CH, et al. Occult macular dystrophy in an 11-year-old boy. Br J Ophthalmol 2004;88:1602–3.
426. Piao CH, Kondo M, Tanikawa A, et al. Multifocal electroretinogram in occult macular dystrophy. Invest Ophthalmol Vis Sci 2000;41:513–7.
427. Fujii S, Escano MF, Ishibashi K, et al. Multifocal electroretinography in patients with occult macular dystrophy. Br J Ophthalmol 1999;83:879–80.
428. Miyake Y, Horiguchi M, Tomita N, et al. Occult macular dystrophy. Am J Ophthalmol 1996;122:644–53.
429. Koizumi H, Maguire JI, Spaide RF. Spectral domain optical coherence tomographic findings of occult macular dystrophy. Ophthalmic Surg Lasers Imaging 2009;40:174–6.
430. Brockhurst RJ, Sandberg MA. Optical coherence tomography findings in occult macular dystrophy. Am J Ophthalmol 2007;143:516–8.
431. Wildberger H, Niemeyer G, Junghardt A. Multifocal electroretinogram (mfERG) in a family with occult macular dystrophy (OMD). Klin Monatsbl Augenheilkd 2003;220:111–5.
432. Kiernan DF, Mieler WF, Hariprasad SM. Spectral-domain optical coherence tomography: a comparison of modern high-resolution retinal imaging systems. Am J Ophthalmol 2010 Jan;149:18–31.
433. Lyons JS. Non-familial occult macular dystrophy. Doc Ophthalmol 2005;111:49–56.
434. Weleber RG, Watzke RC, Shults WT, et al. Clinical and electrophysiologic characterization of paraneoplastic and autoimmune retinopathies associated with antienolase antibodies. Am J Ophthalmol 2005;139:780–94.
435. Hoyng C, Pinckers A, Deutman A. Juvenile atrophy of pigment epithelium and choriocapillaris. Graefes Arch Clin Exp Ophthalmol 1992;230:230–2.
436. Charles SJ, Moore AT, Davison BCC, et al. Flecked retina associated with ring 17 chromosome. Br J Ophthalmol 1991;75:125–7.
437. Gass JDM, Taney BS. Flecked retina associated with café au lait spots, microcephaly, epilepsy, short stature, and ring 17 chromosome. Arch Ophthalmol 1994;112:738–9.
438. Ono K, Suzuki Y, Fujii I, et al. A case of ring chromosome E 17:46,r(17)(p13-q25). Jpn J Hum Genet 1974;19:235–42.
439. McAllister IL, Isaacs TW, Wade MS. Benign fleck retina. Br J Ophthalmol 1996;20:267–9.
440. Sabel Aish SF, Dajani B. Benign familial fleck retina. Br J Ophthalmol 1980;64:652–9.
441. Audo I, Tsang SH, Fu AD, et al. Autofluorescence imaging in a case of benign familial fleck retina. Arch Ophthalmol 2007;125:714–5.
442. Miyake Y, Harada K. Familial fleck retina with night blindness. Ann Ophthalmol 1982;14:836–41.
443. Noble KG, Carr RE, Siegel IM. Autosomal-dominant congenital stationary night blindness and normal fundus with an electronegative electroretinogram. Am J Ophthalmol 1990;109:44–8.
444. Miyake Y, Yagasaki K, Horiguchi M, et al. Congenital stationary night blindness with negative electroretinogram; a new classification. Arch Ophthalmol 1986;104:1013–20.
445. Miyake Y, Kawase Y. Reduced amplitude of oscillatory potentials in female carriers of X-linked recessive congenital stationary night blindness. Am J Ophthalmol 1984;98:208–15.
446. Merin S, Rowe H, Auerbach E, et al. Syndrome of congenital high myopia with nyctalopia; report of findings in 25 families. Am J Ophthalmol 1970;70:541–7.
447. Kubota Y. Seven cases of congenital hemeralopia. Acta Soc Ophthalmol Jpn 1972;76:179–83.
448. Krill AE. Congenital stationary night blindness. In: Krill AE, Archer DB, editors. Krill's hereditary retinal and choroidal diseases, vol. 2. Clinical characteristics. New York: Harper & Row; 1977. p. 391–420.
449. Kandori F, Tamai A, Kurimoto S, et al. Fleck retina. Am J Ophthalmol 1972;73:673–85.
450. Carr RE. Congenital stationary nightblindness. Trans Am Ophthalmol Soc 1974;72:448–87.
451. Heckenlively JR, Martin DA, Rosenbaum AL. Loss of electroretinographic oscillatory potentials, optic atrophy, and dysplasia in congenital stationary night blindness. Am J Ophthalmol 1983;96:526–34.
452. Ruttum MS, Lewandowski MF, Bateman JB. Affected females in X-linked congenital stationary night blindness. Ophthalmology 1992;99:747–52.
453. Oguchi C. Über die eigenartige Hemeralopie mit diffuser weissgraulicher Verfärbung des Augenhintergrundes. Albrecht von Graefes Arch Ophthalmol 1912;81:109–17.
454. Aldred MA, Dry KL, Sharp DM, et al. Linkage analysis in X-linked congenital stationary night blindness. Genomics 1992;14:99–104.
455. Bech-Hansen NT, Moore BJ, Pearce WG. Mapping of locus for X-linked congenital stationary night blindness (CSNB1) proximal to DXS7. Genomics 1992;12:409–11.
456. Keith CG, Denton MJ, Chen J-D. Clinical variability in a family with X-linked retinal dystrophy and the locus at the RP3 site. Ophthalmic Paediat Genet 1991;12:91–8.
457. Weleber RG, Tongue AC. Congenital stationary night blindness presenting as Leber's congenital amaurosis. Arch Ophthalmol 1987;105:360–5.
458. Wilder H. Oguchi's disease. Am J Ophthalmol 1953;36:718–9.
459. Mizuo A. On new discovery in dark adaptation in Oguchi's disease. Acta Soc Ophthalmol Jpn 1913;17:1148.
460. Kuwabara Y, Ishihara K, Akiya S. Histopathological and electron microscopic studies on the retina of Oguchi's disease. Acta Soc Ophthalmol Jpn 1963;67:1323–51.
461. Carr RE, Gouras P. Oguchi's disease. Arch Ophthalmol 1965;73:646–56.
462. Yamanaka M. Histologic study of Oguchi's disease; its relationship to pigmentary degeneration of the retina. Am J Ophthalmol 1969;68:19–26.
463. de Jong PT, Zrenner E, van Meel GJ, et al. Mizuo phenomenon in X-linked retinoschisis. Pathogenesis of the Mizuo phenomenon. Arch Ophthalmol 1991;109:1104–8.
464. Nakamura M, Yamamoto S, Okada M, et al. Novel mutations in the arrestin gene and associated clinical features in Japanese patients with Oguchi's disease. Ophthalmology 2004;111:1410–4.
465. Yoshii M, Murakami A, Akeo K, et al. Visual function and gene analysis in a family with Oguchi's disease. Ophthalmic Res 1998;30:394–401.
466. Carr RE, Margolis S, Siegel IM. Fluorescein angiography and vitamin A and oxalate levels in fundus albipunctatus. Am J Ophthalmol 1976;82:549–58.
467. Lauber H. Die sogenannte Retinitis punctata albescens. Klin Monatsbl Augenheilkd 1910;48:133–48.
468. Levy NS, Toskes PP. Fundus albipunctatus and vitamin A deficiency. Am J Ophthalmol 1974;78:926–9.
469. Marmor MF. Long-term follow-up of the physiologic abnormalities and fundus changes in fundus albipunctatus. Ophthalmology 1990;97:380–4.
470. Sekiya K, Nakazawa M, Ohguro H, et al. Long-term fundus changes due to Fundus albipunctatus associated with mutations in the RDH5 gene. Arch Ophthalmol 2003;121:1057–9.
471. Yamamoto H, Yakushijin K, Kusuhara S, et al. A novel RDH5 gene mutation in a patient with fundus albipunctatus presenting with macular atrophy and fading white dots. Am J Ophthalmol 2003;136:572–4.
472. Nakamura M, Hotta Y, Tanikawa A, et al. A high association with cone dystrophy in Fundus albipunctatus caused by mutations of the RDH5 gene. Invest Ophthalmol Vis Sci 2000;41:3925–32.
473. Miyake Y, Shiroyama N, Sugita S, et al. Fundus albipunctatus associated with cone dystrophy. Br J Ophthalmol 1992;76:375–9.
474. Querques G, Carrillo P, Querques L, et al. High-definition optical coherence tomographic visualization of photoreceptor layer and retinal flecks in fundus albipunctatus associated with cone dystrophy. Arch Ophthalmol 2009;127:703–6.
475. Yamamoto H, Simon A, Eriksson U, et al. Mutations in the gene encoding 11-cis retinol dehydrogenase cause delayed dark adaptation and fundus albipunctatus. Nat Genet 1999;22:188–91.
476. Dryja TP. Molecular genetics of Oguchi disease, fundus albipunctatus, and other forms of stationary night blindness: LVII Edward Jackson Memorial Lecture. Am J Ophthalmol 2000;130:547–63.
477. Brew GA. Retinitis punctata albescens. Trans Ophthalmol Soc Aust 1949;9:154–66.
478. Katajakunnas M, Mäntyjärvi M. Retinitis punctata albescens; a family study. Acta Ophthalmol 1989;67:703–9.
479. Smith BF, Ripps H, Goodman G. Retinitis punctata albescens; a functional and diagnostic evaluation. Arch Ophthalmol 1959;61:93–101.
480. Katsanis N, Shroyer NF, Lewis RA, et al. Fundus albipunctatus and retinitis punctata albescens in a pedigree with an R150Q mutation in RLBP1. Clin Genet 2001;59:424–9.

481. Niwa Y, Kondo M, Ueno S, et al. Cone and rod dysfunction in fundus albipunctatus with RDH5 mutation: an electrophysiological study. Invest Ophthalmol Vis Sci 2005;46: 1480–5.
482. Nakamura M, l in J, Miyake Y. Young monozygotic twin sisters with fundus albipunctatus and cone dystrophy. Arch Ophthalmol 2004;122:1203–7.
483. Hotta K, Nakamura M, Kondo M, et al. Macular dystrophy in a Japanese family with fundus albipunctatus. Am J Ophthalmol 2003;135:917–9.
484. Nakamura M, Miyake Y. Macular dystrophy in a 9-year-old boy with fundus albipunctatus. Am J Ophthalmol 2002;133:278–80.
485. Hayashi T, Goto-Omoto S, Takeuchi T, et al. Compound heterozygous RDH5 mutations in familial fleck retina with night blindness. Acta Ophthalmol Scand 2006;84:254–8.
486. Kandori F. Very rare case of congenital nonprogressive nightblindness with fleck retina. J Clin Ophthalmol (Tokyo) 1959;13:384–6.
487. Zamorani G. Una rara associazione di retinite di Coats con retinite pigmentosa. Ital Oftalmol 1956;9:429–43.
488. Witschel H. Retinopathia pigmentosa and "Morbus Coats." Klin Monatsbl Augenheilkd 1974;164:405–11.
489. Tso MOM. Pathology and pathogenesis of drusen of the optic nervehead. Ophthalmology 1981;88:1066–80.
490. Spalton DJ, Rahi AHS, Bird AC. Immunological studies in retinitis pigmentosa associated with retinal vascular leakage. Br J Ophthalmol 1978;62:183–7.
491. Spalton DJ, Bird AC, Cleary PE. Retinitis pigmentosa and retinal oedema. Br J Ophthalmol 1978;62:174–82.
492. Sieving PA, Fishman GA. Refractive errors of retinitis pigmentosa patients. Br J Ophthalmol 1978;62:163–7.
493. Schmidt D, Faulborn J. Retinopathia pigmentosa mit Coats-Syndrom. Klin Monatsbl Augenheilkd 1970;157:643–52.
494. Robertson DM. Hamartomas of the optic disk with retinitis pigmentosa. Am J Ophthalmol 1972;74:526–31.
495. Puck A, Tso MOM, Fishman GA. Drusen of the optic nerve associated with retinitis pigmentosa. Arch Ophthalmol 1985;103:231–4.
496. Pruett RC. Retinitis pigmentosa; a biomicroscopical study of vitreous abnormalities. Arch Ophthalmol 1975;93:603–8.
497. Pillai S, Limaye SR, Saimovici L-B. Optic disc hamartoma associated with retinitis pigmentosa. Retina 1983;3:24–6.
498. Merin S. Macular cysts as an early sign of tapeto-retinal degeneration. J Pediatr Ophthalmol 1970;7:225–8.
499. Metge P, Chovet M, Ebagosti A, et al. Oedème maculaire cystoïde dans la rétinopathie pigmentaire. Bull Soc Ophtalmol Fr 1974;74:119–23.
500. Morgan III WE, Crawford JB. Retinitis pigmentosa and Coats' disease. Arch Ophthalmol 1968;79:146–9.
501. Marmor MF. Visual loss in retinitis pigmentosa. Am J Ophthalmol 1980;89:692–8.
502. Lewis ML. Coexisting central serous choroidopathy and retinitis pigmentosa. South Med J 1980;73:77–80.
503. Lanier JD, McCrary III JA, Justice J. Autosomal-recessive retinitis pigmentosa and Coats disease; a presumed familial incidence. Arch Ophthalmol 1976;94:1737–42.
504. Jay B, Bird A. X-linked retinitis pigmentosa. Trans Am Acad Ophthalmol Otolaryngol 1973;77:OP641–OP651.
505. Hyvärinen L, Maumenee AE, Kelley J, et al. Fluorescein angiographic findings in retinitis pigmentosa. Am J Ophthalmol 1971;71:17–26.
506. Heckenlively JR, Yoser SL, Friedman LH, et al. Clinical findings and common symptoms in retinitis pigmentosa. Am J Ophthalmol 1988;105:504–11.
507. Heckenlively JR, Martin DA, Rosales TO. Telangiectasia and optic atrophy in cone–rod degenerations. Arch Ophthalmol 1981;99:1983–91.
508. Haye C. Guyot-Sionnest, Coulon G. Association de rétinite pigmentaire et de vitiligo. Bull Soc Ophtalmol Fr 1973;73:1155–8.
509. Hansen RI, Friedman AH, Gartner S, et al. The association of retinitis pigmentosa with preretinal macular gliosis. Br J Ophthalmol 1977;61:597–600.
510. Haim M. Prevalence of retinitis pigmentosa and allied disorders in Denmark. III. Hereditary pattern. Acta Ophthalmol 1992;70:615–24.
511. Grizzard WS, Deutman AF, Pinckers AJLG. Retinal dystrophies associated with peripheral retinal vasculopathy. Br J Ophthalmol 1978;62:188–94.
512. Foxman SG, Heckenlively JR, Bateman JB, et al. Classification of congenital and early onset retinitis pigmentosa. Arch Ophthalmol 1985;103:1502–6.
513. Fogle JA, Welch RB, Green WR. Retinitis pigmentosa and exudative vasculopathy. Arch Ophthalmol 1978;96:696–702.
514. Fishman GA, Maggiano JM, Fishman M. Foveal lesions seen in retinitis pigmentosa. Arch Ophthalmol 1977;95:1993–6.
515. Fishman GA, Alexander KR, Anderson RJ. Autosomal-dominant retinitis pigmentosa; a method of classification. Arch Ophthalmol 1985;103:366–74.
516. Fishman GA, Farber MD, Derlacki DJ. X-linked retinitis pigmentosa; profile of clinical findings. Arch Ophthalmol 1988;106:369–75.
517. Fishman GA, Fishman M, Maggiano J. Macular lesions associated with retinitis pigmentosa. Arch Ophthalmol 1977;95:798–803.
518. Fishman GA, Gilbert LD, Fiscella RG, et al. Acetazolamide for treatment of chronic macular edema in retinitis pigmentosa. Arch Ophthalmol 1989;107:1445–52.
519. Ffytche TJ. Cystoid maculopathy in retinitis pigmentosa. Trans Ophthalmol Soc UK 1972;92: 265–83.
520. Fetkenhour CL, Choromokos E, Weinstein J, et al. Cystoid macular edema in retinitis pigmentosa. Trans Am Acad Ophthalmol Otolaryngol 1977;83:OP515–OP521.
521. Farber MD, Fishman GA, Weiss RA. Autosomal-dominantly inherited retinitis pigmentosa; visual acuity loss by subtype. Arch Ophthalmol 1985;103:524–8.
522. Faktorovich EG, Steinberg RH, Yasumura D, et al. Photoreceptor degeneration in inherited retinal dystrophy delayed by basic fibroblast growth factor. Nature 1990;347:83–6.
523. Dryja TP. Rhodopsin and autosomal-dominant retinitis pigmentosa. Eye 1992;6:1–10.
524. Dryja TP, McGee TL, Hahn LB, et al. Mutations within the rhodopsin gene in patients with autosomal-dominant retinitis pigmentosa. N Engl J Med 1990;323:1302–7.
525. De Bustros S, Miller NR, Finkelstein D, et al. Bilateral astrocytic hamartomas of the optic nerve heads in retinitis pigmentosa. Retina 1983;3:21–3.
526. Cowan Jr CL, Grimes PE, Chakrabarti S, et al. Retinitis pigmentosa associated with hearing loss, thyroid disease, vitiligo, and alopecia areata; retinitis pigmentosa and vitiligo. Retina 1982;2:84–8.
527. Cogan DG. Symposium: primary chorioretinal aberrations with night blindness. Pathology. Trans Am Acad Ophthalmol Otolaryngol 1950;54:629–61.
528. Bonnet M, Pingault C. Oedème maculaire cystoïde et rétinopathie pigmentaire. Bull Soc Ophthalmol Fr 1973;73:715–8.
529. Bloom TD, Fishman GA, Mafee MF. Usher's syndrome; CNS defects determined by computed tomography. Retina 1983;3:108–13.
530. Bird AC. X-linked retinitis pigmentosa. Br J Ophthalmol 1975;59:177–99.
531. Berson EL, Sandberg MA, Rosner B, et al. Natural course of retinitis pigmentosa over a three-year interval. Am J Ophthalmol 1985;99:240–51.
532. Ayesh I, Sanders MD, Friedmann AI. Retinitis pigmentosa and Coats's disease. Br J Ophthalmol 1976;60:775–7.
533. Albert DM, Nordlund JJ, Lerner AB. Ocular abnormalities occurring with vitiligo. Ophthalmology 1979;86:1145–58.
534. Newsome DA. Retinal fluorescein leakage in retinitis pigmentosa. Am J Ophthalmol 1986;101:354–60.
535. Shahidi M, Fishman G, Ogura Y, et al. Foveal thickening in retinitis pigmentosa patients with cystoid macular edema. Retina 1994;14:243–7.
536. Gass JDM. Stereoscopic atlas of macular diseases; a fundoscopic and angiographic presentation. St. Louis: CV Mosby; 1970. p. 151.
537. François J, de Laey JJ, Verbraeken H. L'oedeme kystoide de la macula. Bull Soc Belge Ophtalmol 1972;161:708–21.
538. Fishman GA, Lam BL, Anderson RJ. Racial differences in the prevalence of atrophic-appearing macular lesions between black and white patients with retinitis pigmentosa. Am J Ophthalmol 1994;118:33–8.
539. Gartner S, Henkind P. Pathology of retinitis pigmentosa. Ophthalmology 1982;89:1425–32.
540. Piermarocchi S, Segato T, Midena E. Retinal fluorescein leakage in retinitis pigmentosa. Am J Ophthalmol 1986;102:674.
541. Spallone A. Retinal fluorescein leakage in retinitis pigmentosa. Am J Ophthalmol 1986; 102:408.
542. Tucker GS, Jacobson SG. Morphological findings in retinitis pigmentosa with early diffuse rod dysfunction. Retina 1988;8:30–41.
543. Szamier RB, Berson EL. Retinal histopathology of a carrier of X-chromosome-linked retinitis pigmentosa. Ophthalmology 1985;92:271–8.
544. Rodrigues MM, Wiggert B, Hackett J, et al. Dominantly inherited retinitis pigmentosa; ultrastructure and biochemical analysis. Ophthalmology 1985;92:1165–72.
545. Kolb H, Gouras P. Electron microscopic observations of human retinitis pigmentosa, dominantly inherited. Invest Ophthalmol 1974;13:487–98.
546. Berson EL, Adamian M. Ultrastructural findings in an autopsy eye from a patient with Usher's syndrome type II. Am J Ophthalmol 1992;114:748–57.
547. Henkind P, Gartner S. The relationship between retinal pigment epithelium and the choriocapillaris. Trans Ophthalmol Soc UK 1983;103:444–7.
548. Reppucci V, Henkind P. Retinal pigment epithelial damage and secondary choriocapillary atrophy. ARVO Abstracts. Invest Ophthalmol Vis Sci 1983;24:283.
549. Stone JL, Barlow WE, Humayun MS, et al. Morphometric analysis of macular photoreceptors and ganglion cells in retinas with retinitis pigmentosa. Arch Ophthalmol 1992;110:1634–9.
550. Albert DM, Pruett RC, Craft JL. Transmission electron microscopic observations of vitreous abnormalities in retinitis pigmentosa. Am J Ophthalmol 1986;101:665–72.
551. Gouras P. Transmission electron microscopic observations of vitreous abnormalities in retinitis pigmentosa. Am J Ophthalmol 1987;103:345.
552. Newsome DA, Michels RG. Detection of lymphocytes in the vitreous gel of patients with retinitis pigmentosa. Am J Ophthalmol 1988;105:596–602.
553. Ogura Y, Cunha-Vaz JG, Zeimer RC. Evaluation of vitreous body integrity in retinitis pigmentosa by vitreous fluorophotometry. Arch Ophthalmol 1987;105:517–9.
554. Kimberling W, Smith RJ. Gene mapping of the Usher syndromes. Otolaryngol Clin North Am 1992;25:923–34.
555. Piazza L, Fishman GA, Farber M, et al. Visual acuity loss in patients with Usher's syndrome. Arch Ophthalmol 1986;104:1336–9.
556. Piazza L, Fishman GA, Kaplan RD, et al. Magnetic resonance imaging of central nervous system defects in Usher's syndrome. Retina 1987;7:241–5.
557. McDonald JM, Newsome DA, Rintelmann WF. Sensorineural hearing loss in patients with typical retinitis pigmentosa. Am J Ophthalmol 1988;105:125–31.
558. Novack RL, Foos RY. Drusen of the optic disk in retinitis pigmentosa. Am J Ophthalmol 1987;103:44–7.
559. Jacobson SG, Roman AJ, Cideciyan AV, et al. X-linked retinitis pigmentosa: Functional phenotype of an RP2 genotype. Invest Ophthalmol Vis Sci 1992;33:3481–92.
560. Jay M, Bird AC, Moore AN, et al. Nine generations of a family with autosomal-dominant retinitis pigmentosa and evidence of variable expressivity from census records. J Med Genet 1992;29:906–10.
561. Hunter DG, Fishman GA, Kretzer FL. Abnormal axonemes in X-linked retinitis pigmentosa. Arch Ophthalmol 1988;106:362–8.
562. Hunter DG, Fishman GA, Mehta RS, et al. Abnormal sperm and photoreceptor axonemes in Usher's syndrome. Arch Ophthalmol 1986;104:385–9.

717. Seabra MC, Brown MS, Goldstein JL. Retinal degeneration in choroideremia: deficiency of rab geranylgeranyl transferase. Science 1993;259:377–81.
718. Seabra MC, Brown MS, Slaughter CA, et al. Purification of component A of Rab geranylgeranyl transferase: possible identity with the choroideremia gene product. Cell 1992;70:1049–57.
719. MacDonald IM, Mah DY, Ho YK, et al. A practical diagnostic test for choroideremia. Ophthalmology 1998;105:1637–40.
720. van den Hurk JA, van Zandvoort PM, Brunsmann F, et al. Prenatal exclusion of choroideremia. Am J Med Genet 1992;44:822–3.
721. Cameron JD, Fine BS, Shapiro I. Histopathologic observations in choroideremia with emphasis on vascular changes of the uveal tract. Ophthalmology 1987;94:187–96.
722. Bonilha VL, Trzupek KM, Li Y, et al. Choroideremia: analysis of the retina from a female symptomatic carrier. Ophthalmic Genet 2008;29:99–110.
723. Krill AE. Diffuse choroidal atrophies. In: Krill AE, Archer DB, editors. Krill's hereditary retinal and choroidal diseases, vol. 2. Clinical characteristics. New York: Harper & Row; 1977. p. 979–1041.
724. Hayasaka S, Shoji K, Kanno C-I, et al. Differential diagnosis of diffuse choroidal atrophies; diffuse choriocapillaris atrophy, choroideremia, and gyrate atrophy of the choroid and retina. Retina 1985;5:30–7.
725. Vainisi SJ, Beck BB, Apple DJ. Retinal degeneration in a baboon. Am J Ophthalmol 1974;78:279–84.
726. Tso MOM, Santos-Anderson RM, Vainisi SJ. Heredofamilial retinal dystrophy in Guinea baboons. I. A histopathologic study. Arch Ophthalmol 1983;101:1597–603.
727. Santos-Anderson RM, Tso MOM, Vainisi SJ. Heredofamilial retinal dystrophy in Guinea baboons. II. Electron microscopic observations. Arch Ophthalmol 1983;101:1762–70.
728. Miyake Y, Ichikawa K, Tokuda H, et al. The clinical properties in progressive cone–rod dystrophy. Jpn J Clin Ophthalmol 1982;36:323–9.
729. Miyake Y, Goto S, Ota I, et al. Vitreous fluorophotometry in patients with cone–rod dystrophy. Br J Ophthalmol 1984;68:489–93.
730. Hittner HM, Murphree AL, Garcia CA, et al. Dominant cone–rod dystrophy. Doc Ophthalmol 1975;39:29–52.
731. Fishman GA. Progressive human cone–rod dysfunction (dystrophy). Trans Am Acad Ophthalmol Otolaryngol 1976;81:OP716–OP724.
732. Szlyk JP, Fishman GA, Alexander KR, et al. Clinical subtypes of cone–rod dystrophy. Arch Ophthalmol 1993;111:781–8.
733. Yagasaki K, Jacobson SG. Cone–rod dystrophy; phenotypic diversity by retinal function testing. Arch Ophthalmol 1989;107:701–8.
734. Hamel CP. Cone rod dystrophies. Orphanet J Rare Dis 2007;2:7.
735. Rabb MF, Tso MOM, Fishman GA. Cone–rod dystrophy; a clinical and histopathologic report. Ophthalmology 1986;93:1443–51.
736. Leon A, Curtis R. Autosomal-dominant rod–cone dysplasia in the Rdy cat. 1. Light and electron microscopic findings. Exp Eye Res 1990;51:361–81.
737. Warburg M, Sjo O, Tranebjaerg L, et al. Deletion mapping of a retinal cone–rod dystrophy; assignment to 18q211. Am J Med Genet 1991;39:288–93.
738. Favre M. A propos de deux cas de dégénérescence hyaloïdéorétinienne. Ophthalmologica 1958;135:604–9.
739. Fishman GA, Jampol LM, Goldberg MF. Diagnostic features of the Favre-Goldmann syndrome. Br J Ophthalmol 1976;60:345–53.
740. Gass JDM. Stereoscopic atlas of macular diseases; diagnosis and treatment, 3rd ed. St. Louis: CV Mosby; 1987. p. 290–91.
741. Goldmann H. Présentation du rapport sur la biomicroscopie du corps vitré et du fond de l'oeil. Bull Mem Soc Fr Ophthalmol 1957;70:265–72.
742. Nasr YG, Cherfan GM, Michels RG, et al. Goldmann–Favre maculopathy. Retina 1990;10: 178–80.
743. Noble KG, Carr RE, Siegel IM. Familial foveal retinoschisis associated with a rod–cone dystrophy. Am J Ophthalmol 1978;85:551–7.
744. Peyman GA, Fishman GA, Sanders DR, et al. Histopathology of Goldmann–Favre syndrome obtained by full-thickness eye-wall biopsy. Ann Ophthalmol 1977;9:479–84.
745. Hirose T, Schepens CL, Brockhurst RJ, et al. Congenital retinoschisis with night blindness in two girls. Ann Ophthalmol 1980;12:848–56.
746. Hood DC, Cideciyan AV, Roman AJ, et al. Enhanced S cone syndrome: evidence for an abnormally large number of S cones. Vision Res 1995;35:1473–81.
747. Jacobson SG, Marmor MF, Kemp CM, et al. SWS (blue) cone hypersensitivity in a newly identified retinal degeneration. Invest Ophthalmol Vis Sci 1990;31:827–38.
748. Jacobson SG, Román AJ, Román MI, et al. Relatively enhanced S cone function in the Goldmann–Favre syndrome. Am J Ophthalmol 1991;111:446–53.
749. Kellner U, Foerster MH. Netzhautdegeneration mit Blauzapfenhypersensitivität. Fortschr Ophthalmol 1991;88:637–41.
750. Marmor MF, Jacobson SG, Foerster MH, et al. Diagnostic clinical findings of a new syndrome with night blindness, maculopathy, and enhanced S cone sensitivity. Am J Ophthalmol 1990;110:124–34.
751. Schorderet DF, Escher P. NR2E3 mutations in enhanced S-cone sensitivity syndrome (ESCS), Goldmann–Favre syndrome (GFS), clumped pigmentary retinal degeneration (CPRD), and retinitis pigmentosa (RP). Hum Mutat 2009;30:1475–85.
752. Pachydaki SI, Klaver CC, Barbazetto IA, et al. Phenotypic features of patients with NR2E3 mutations. Arch Ophthalmol 2009;127:71–5.
753. Escher P, Gouras P, Roduit R, et al. Mutations in NR2E3 can cause dominant or recessive retinal degenerations in the same family. Hum Mutat 2009;30:342–51.
754. Chavala SH, Sari A, Lewis H, et al. An Arg311Gln NR2E3 mutation in a family with classic Goldmann–Favre syndrome. Br J Ophthalmol 2005;89:1065–6.
755. Wright AF, Reddick AC, Schwartz SB, et al. Mutation analysis of NR2E3 and NRL genes in Enhanced S Cone Syndrome. Hum Mutat 2004;24:439.
756. Sharon D, Sandberg MA, Caruso RC, et al. Shared mutations in NR2E3 in enhanced S-cone syndrome, Goldmann–Favre syndrome, and many cases of clumped pigmentary retinal degeneration. Arch Ophthalmol 2003;121:1316–23.
757. Haider NB, Jacobson SG, Cideciyan AV, et al. Mutation of a nuclear receptor gene, NR2E3, causes enhanced S cone syndrome, a disorder of retinal cell fate. Nat Genet 2000;24:127–31.
758. Lewis RA, Lee GB, Martonyi CL, et al. Familial foveal retinoschisis. Arch Ophthalmol 1977;95:1190–6.
759. Yassur Y, Nissenkorn I, Ben-Sira I, et al. Autosomal-dominant inheritance of retinoschisis. Am J Ophthalmol 1982;94:338–43.
760. Yanoff M, Rahn EK, Zimmerman LE. Histopathology of juvenile retinoschisis. Arch Ophthalmol 1968;79:49–53.
761. Tasman W. Macular changes in congenital retinoschisis. Mod Probl Ophthalmol 1975;15:40–7.
762. Manschot WA. Pathology of hereditary juvenile retinoschisis. Arch Ophthalmol 1972;88:131–8.
763. Krause U, Vainio-Mattila B, Eriksson A, et al. Fluorescein angiographic studies on X-chromosomal retinoschisis. Acta Ophthalmol 1970;48:794–807.
764. Harris GS, Yeung JW-S. Maculopathy of sex-linked juvenile retinoschisis. Can J Ophthalmol 1976;11:1–10.
765. Green Jr JL, Jampol LM. Vascular opacification and leakage in X-linked (juvenile) retinoschisis. Br J Ophthalmol 1979;63:368–73.
766. Gieser EP, Falls HF. Hereditary retinoschisis. Am J Ophthalmol 1961;51:1193–200.
767. Forsius H, Krause U, Helve J, et al. Visual acuity in 183 cases of X-chromosomal retinoschisis. Can J Ophthalmol 1973;8:385–93.
768. Forsius H, Vainio-Mattila B, Eriksson A. X-linked hereditary retinoschisis. Br J Ophthalmol 1962;46:678–81.
769. Ewing CC, Cullen AP. Fluorescein angiography in X-chromosomal maculopathy with retinoschisis (juvenile hereditary retinoschisis). Can J Ophthalmol 1972;7:19–28.
770. Ewing CC, Ives EJ. Juvenile hereditary retinoschisis. Trans Ophthalmol Soc UK 1969;89:29–39.
771. Deutman AF. The hereditary dystrophies of the posterior pole of the eye. Assen: Van Gorcum; 1971. p. 48.
772. Dahl N, Pettersson U. Use of linked DNA probes for carrier detection and diagnosis of X-linked juvenile retinoschisis. Arch Ophthalmol 1988;106:1414–6.
773. Conway BP, Welch RB. X-chromosome-linked juvenile retinoschisis with hemorrhagic retinal cyst. Am J Ophthalmol 1977;83:853–5.
774. Constantaras AA, Dobbie JG, Choromokos EA, et al. Juvenile sex-linked recessive retinoschisis in a black family. Am J Ophthalmol 1972;74:1166–78.
775. Burns RP, Lovrien EW, Cibis AB. Juvenile sex-linked retinoschisis: clinical and genetic studies. Trans Am Acad Ophthalmol Otolaryngol 1971;75:1011–21.
776. Arkfeld DF, Brockhurst RJ. Vascularized vitreous membranes in congenital retinoschisis. Retina 1987;7:20–3.
777. Tasman W, Greven C, Moreno R. Nasal retinal dragging in X-linked retinoschisis. Graefes Arch Clin Exp Ophthalmol 1991;229:319–22.
778. Pearson R, Jagger J. Sex linked juvenile retinoschisis with optic disc and peripheral retinal neovascularisation. Br J Ophthalmol 1989;73:311–3.
779. de Jong PTVM, Zrenner E, van Meel GJ, et al. Mizuo phenomenon in X-linked retinoschisis. Arch Ophthalmol 1991;109:1104–8.
[779a] Agarwal A, Rao US. Outer retinal corrugations in x-linked juvenile retinoschisis. Arch Ophthalmol 2007;125(2):278–9.
780. Kellner U, Brümmer S, Foerster MH, et al. X-linked congenital retinoschisis. Graefes Arch Clin Exp Ophthalmol 1990;228:432–7.
781. Arden GB, Gorin MB, Polkinghorne PJ, et al. Detection of the carrier state of X-linked retinoschisis. Am J Ophthalmol 1988;105:590–5.
782. Peachey NS, Fishman GA, Derlacki DJ, et al. Psychophysical and electroretinographic findings in X-linked juvenile retinoschisis. Arch Ophthalmol 1987;105:513–6.
783. Condon GP, Brownstein S, Wang N-S, et al. Congenital hereditary (juvenile X-linked) retinoschisis; histopathologic and ultrastructural findings in three eyes. Arch Ophthalmol 1986;104:576–83.
784. Turut P, François P, Castier P, et al. Analysis of results in the treatment of peripheral retinoschisis in sex-linked congenital retinoschisis. Graefes Arch Clin Exp Ophthalmol 1989;227:328–31.
785. Han DP, Sieving PA, Johnson MW, et al. Foveal retinoschisis associated with senile retinoschisis in a woman. Am J Ophthalmol 1988;106:107–9.
786. Shimazaki J, Matsuhashi M. Familial retinoschisis in female patients. Doc Ophthalmol 1987;65:393–400.
787. Yamaguchi K, Hara S. Autosomal juvenile retinoschisis without foveal retinoschisis. Br J Ophthalmol 1989;73:470–3.
788. Blair NP, Goldberg MF, Fishman GA, et al. Autosomal-dominant vitreoretinochoroidopathy (ADVIRC). Br J Ophthalmol 1884;68:2–9.
789. Goldberg MF, Lee F-L, Tso MOM, et al. Histopathologic study of autosomal-dominant vitreoretinochoroidopathy; peripheral annular pigmentary dystrophy of the retina. Ophthalmology 1989;96:1736–46.
790. Kaufman SJ, Goldberg MF, Orth DH, et al. Autosomal-dominant vitreoretinochoroidopathy. Arch Ophthalmol 1982;100:272–8.
791. Traboulsi EI, Payne JW. Autosomal-dominant vitreoretinochoroidopathy; report of the third family. Arch Ophthalmol 1993;111:194–6.
792. Bridges CDB, Alvarez RA. Selective loss of 11-cis vitamin A in an eye with hereditary chorioretinal degeneration similar to sector retinitis pigmentosa. Retina 1982;2:256–60.
793. Gass J. Stereoscopic atlas of macular diseases; diagnosis and treatment, 3rd ed. St. Louis: CV Mosby; 1987. p. 294.
794. Noble KG. Peripapillary (pericentral) pigmentary retinal degeneration. Am J Ophthalmol 1989;108:686–90.
795. Noble KG, Carr RE. Peripapillary pigmentary retinal degeneration. Am J Ophthalmol 1978;86:65–75.
796. O'Connor PR, John ME, Lawwill T, et al. Atypical retinitis pigmentosa. Ann Ophthalmol 1974;6:824–6.
797. Traboulsi EI, O'Neil JF, Maumenee IH. Autosomal-recessive pericentral pigmentary retinopathy. Am J Ophthalmol 1988;106:551–6.

798. Schocket SS, Ballin N. Circinate choroidal sclerosis. Trans Am Acad Ophthalmol Otolaryngol 1970;74:527–33.
799. Watanabe I, Miyake Y, Asano T, et al. Pigmented paravenous retinochoroidal atrophy. Jpn Rev Clin Ophthalmol 1972;66:1156–9.
800. Traboulsi EI, Maumenee IH. Hereditary pigmented paravenous chorioretinal atrophy. Arch Ophthalmol 1986;104:1636–40.
801. Takei Y, Harada M, Mizuno K. Pigmented paravenous retinochoroidal atrophy. Jpn J Ophthalmol 1977;21:311–7.
802. Skalka HW. Hereditary pigmented paravenous retinochoroidal atrophy. Am J Ophthalmol 1979;87:286–91.
803. Pearlman JT, Kamin DF, Kopelow SM, et al. Pigmented paravenous retinochoroidal atrophy. Am J Ophthalmol 1975;80:630–5.
804. Noble KG, Carr RE. Pigmented paravenous chorioretinal atrophy. Am J Ophthalmol 1983;96:338–44.
805. Miller SA, Stevens TS, Myers F, et al. Pigmented paravenous retinochoroidal atrophy. Ann Ophthalmol 1978;10:867–71.
806. Hirose T, Miyake Y. Pigmentary paravenous chorioretinal degeneration: fundus appearance and retinal functions. Ann Ophthalmol 1979;11:709–18.
807. Chisholm IA, Dudgeon J. Pigmented paravenous retino-choroidal atrophy; helicoid retino-choroidal atrophy. Br J Ophthalmol 1973;57:584–7.
808. Amalric P, Pigmentierte Schum U. paravenöse Netz- und Aderhautatrophie. Klin Monatsbl Augenheilkd 1968;153:770–5.
809. Rothberg DS, Cibis GW, Trese M. Paravenous pigmentary retinochoroidal atrophy. Ann Ophthalmol 1984;16:643–6.
810. Chen M-S, Yang C-H, Huang J-S. Bilateral macular coloboma and pigmented paravenous retinochoroidal atrophy. Br J Ophthalmol 1992;76:250–1.
811. Fleckenstein M, Charbel Issa P, Fuchs HA, et al. Discrete arcs of increased fundus autofluorescence in retinal dystrophies and functional correlate on microperimetry. Eye 2009;23:567–75.
812. Fleckenstein M, Charbel Issa P, Helb HM, et al. Correlation of lines of increased autofluorescence in macular dystrophy and pigmented paravenous retinochoroidal atrophy by optical coherence tomography. Arch Ophthalmol 2008;126:1461–3.
813. Noble KG. Hereditary pigmented paravenous chorioretinal atrophy. Am J Ophthalmol 1989;108:365–9.
814. Limaye SR, Mahmood MA. Retinal microangiopathy in pigmented paravenous chorioretinal atrophy. Br J Ophthalmol 1987;71:757–61.
815. Small KW, Anderson Jr WB. Pigmented paravenous retinochoroidal atrophy; discordant expression in monozygotic twins. Arch Ophthalmol 1991;109:1408–10.
816. Yamaguchi K, Hara S, Tanifuji Y, et al. Inflammatory pigmented paravenous retinochoroidal atrophy. Br J Ophthalmol 1989;73:463–7.
817. Choi JY, Sandberg MA, Berson EL. Natural course of ocular function in pigmented paravenous retinochoroidal atrophy. Am J Ophthalmol 2006;141:763–5.
818. Kukner AS, Yilmaz T, Celebi S, et al. Pigmented paravenous retinochoroidal atrophy. A literature review supported by seven cases. Ophthalmologica 2003;217:436–40.
819. Obata R, Yanagi Y, Iriyama A, et al. A familial case of pigmented paravenous retinochoroidal atrophy with asymmetrical fundus manifestations. Graefes Arch Clin Exp Ophthalmol 2006;244:874–7.
820. Bozkurt N, Bavbek T, Kazokoglu H. Hereditary pigmented paravenous chorioretinal atrophy. Ophthalmic Genet 1998;19:99–104.
821. Traboulsi EI, Maumenee IH. Hereditary pigmented paravenous chorioretinal atrophy. Arch Ophthalmol 1986;104:1636–40.
822. Bietti G. Su alcune forme atipiche o rare di degenerazione retinica (degenerazioni tappeto-retiniche e quadri morbosi similari). Boll Oculist 1937;16:1159–244.
823. Bisantis C. La retinopathie pigmentaire en secteur de G.B. Bietti; contribution á la connaissance de ses divers aspects cliniques. Ann Oculist 1971;204:907–54.
824. Franceschetti A, François J, Babel J. Chorioretinal heredodegenerations. Springfield, IL: Charles C Thomas; 1974. p. 254.
825. François J, de Rouck A, Golan A. ERG in sectorial pigmentary retinopathy. Doc Ophthalmol Proc Ser 1977;13:239–44.
826. Hollyfield JG, Frederick JM, Tabor GA, et al. Metabolic studies on retinal tissue from a donor with a dominantly inherited chorioretinal degeneration resembling sectoral retinitis pigmentosa. Ophthalmology 1984;91:191–6.
827. Krill AE, Archer D, Martin D. Sector retinitis pigmentosa. Am J Ophthalmol. 1970; 69:977–87.
828. Massof RW, Finkelstein D. Vision threshold profiles in sector retinitis pigmentosa. Arch Ophthalmol 1979;97:1899–904.
829. Rayborn ME, Moorhead LC, Hollyfield JG. A dominantly inherited chorioretinal degeneration resembling sectoral retinitis pigmentosa. Ophthalmology 1982;89:1441–54.
830. Sullivan LJ, Makris GS, Dickinson P, et al. A new codon 15 rhodopsin gene mutation in autosomal-dominant retinitis pigmentosa is associated with sectorial disease. Arch Ophthalmol 1993;111:1512–7.
831. Fulton AB, Hansen RM. The relationship of rhodopsin and scotopic retinal sensitivity in sector retinitis pigmentosa. Am J Ophthalmol 1988;105:132–40.
832. Omphroy CA. Sector retinitis pigmentosa and chronic angle-closure glaucoma: a new association. Ophthalmologica 1984;189:12–20.
833. Osman SA, Aylin Y, Arikan G, et al. Photodynamic treatment of a secondary vasoproliferative tumour associated with sector retinitis pigmentosa and Usher syndrome type I. Clin Experiment Ophthalmol 2007;35:191–3.
834. Meyerle CB, Fisher YL, Spaide RF. Autofluorescence and visual field loss in sector retinitis pigmentosa. Retina 2006;26:248–50.
835. Saperstein DA. Sector retinitis pigmentosa with bitemporal visual field defects and macular hole. Retina 2001;21:73–4.
836. Godel V, Iaina A, Nemet P, et al. Sector retinitis pigmentosa in juvenile nephronophthisis. Br J Ophthalmol 1980;64:124–6.
837. Heidemann DG, Beck RW. Retinitis pigmentosa: A mimic of neurologic disease. Surv Ophthalmol. 1987;32:45–51.
838. Heckenlively JR, Rodriguez JA, Daiger SP. Autosomal-dominant sectorial retinitis pigmentosa; two families with transversion mutation in codon 23 of rhodopsin. Arch Ophthalmol 1991;109:84–91.
839. Moore AT, Fitzke FW, Kemp CM, et al. Abnormal dark adaptation kinetics in autosomal-dominant sector retinitis pigmentosa due to rod opsin mutation. Br J Ophthalmol 1992;76:465–9.
840. Carr RE, Siegel IM. Unilateral retinitis pigmentosa. Arch Ophthalmol 1973;90:21–6.
841. François J, Verriest G. Rétinopathie pigmentaire unilatérale. Ophthalmologica 1952;124:65–88.
842. Henkes HE. Does unilateral retinitis pigmentosa really exist? An ERG and EOG study of the fellow eye. In: Burian HM, Jacobson JH, editors. Clinical electroretinography: proceedings of the Third International Symposium held in October, 1964. Oxford: Pergamon Press; 1966. p. 327–50.
843. Weleber RG, Kennaway NG. Clinical trial of vitamin B6 for gyrate atrophy of the choroid and retina. Ophthalmology 1981;88:316–24.
844. Takki K. Gyrate atrophy of the choroid and retina associated with hyperornithinaemia. Br J Ophthalmol 1974;58:3–23.
845. Takki K, Simell O. Genetic aspects in gyrate atrophy of the choroid and retina with hyperornithinaemia. Br J Ophthalmol 1974;58:907–16.
846. Takki KK, Milton RC. The natural history of gyrate atrophy of the choroid and retina. Ophthalmology 1981;88:292–301.
847. Valle D, Walser M, Brusilow S, et al. Gyrate atrophy of the choroid and retina; biochemical considerations and experience with arginine-restricted diet. Ophthalmology 1981;88:325–30.
848. Vannas-Sulonen K. Progression of gyrate atrophy of the choroid and retina; a long-term follow-up by fluorescein angiography. Acta Ophthalmol 1987;65:101–9.
849. Sipilä I, Rapola J, Simell O, et al. Supplementary creatine as a treatment for gyrate atrophy of the choroid and retina. N Engl J Med 1981;304:867–70.
850. McCulloch C, Marliss EB. Gyrate atrophy of the choroid and retina: clinical, ophthalmologic, and biochemical considerations. Trans Am Ophthalmol Soc 1975;73:153–71.
851. McCulloch C, Marliss EB. Gyrate atrophy of the choroid and retina with hyperornithinemia. Am J Ophthalmol 1975;80:1047–57.
852. McCulloch JC, Arshinoff SA, Marliss EB, et al. Hyperornithinemia and gyrate atrophy of the choroid and retina. Ophthalmology 1978;85:918–28.
853. Mehta MC, Katsumi O, Shih VE, et al. Gyrate atrophy of the choroid and retina in a five-year-old girl. Acta Ophthalmol 1991;69:810–4.
854. Mashima Y, Murakami A, Weleber RG, et al. Nonsense-codon mutations of the ornithine aminotransferase gene with decreased levels of mutant mRNA in gyrate atrophy. Am J Hum Genet 1992;51:81–91.
855. Kaiser-Kupfer MI, de Monasterio F, Valle D, et al. Visual results of a long-term trial of a low-arginine diet in gyrate atrophy of choroid and retina. Ophthalmology 1981;88:307–10.
856. Kaiser-Kupfer MI, Kuwabara T, Askanas V, et al. Systemic manifestations of gyrate atrophy of the choroid and retina. Ophthalmology 1981;88:302–6.
857. Kaiser-Kupfer MI, Ludwig IH, de Monasterio F, et al. Gyrate atrophy of the choroid and retina; early findings. Ophthalmology 1985;92:394–401.
858. Kuwabara T, Ishikawa Y, Kaiser-Kupfer MI. Experimental model of gyrate atrophy in animals. Ophthalmology 1981;88:331–4.
859. Hayasaka S, Mizuno K, Yabata K, et al. Atypical gyrate atrophy of the choroid and retina associated with iminoglycinuria. Arch Ophthalmol 1982;100:423–5.
860. Hayasaka S, Saito T, Nakajima H, et al. Gyrate atrophy with hyperornithinaemia: different types of responsiveness to vitamin B6. Br J Ophthalmol 1981;65:478–83.
861. Enoch JM, O'Donnell J, Williams RA, et al. Retinal boundaries and visual function in gyrate atrophy. Arch Ophthalmol 1984;102:1314–6.
862. Deutman AF, Sengers RCA, Trybels JMF. Gyrate atrophy of the choroid and retina with reticular pigmentary dystrophy and ornithine-ketoacid-transaminase deficiency. Int Ophthalmol 1978;1:49–56.
863. Berson EL, Shih VE, Sullivan PL. Ocular findings in patients with gyrate atrophy on pyridoxine and low-protein, low-arginine diets. Ophthalmology 1981;88:311–5.
864. Bargum R. Differential diagnosis of normoornithinaemic gyrate atrophy of the choroid and retina. Acta Ophthalmol 1986;64:369–73.
865. Bakker HD, Abeling NG, van Schooneveld MJ, et al. A far advanced case of gyrate atrophy in a 12-year-old girl. J Inherit Metab Dis 1991;14:379–81.
866. Weleber RG, Kurz DE, Trzupek KM. Treatment of retinal and choroidal degenerations and dystrophies: current status and prospects for gene-based therapy. Ophthalmol Clin North Am 2003;16:583–93. vii
867. Feldman RB, Mayo SS, Robertson DM, et al. Epiretinal membranes and cystoid macular edema in gyrate atrophy of the choroid and retina. Retina 1989;9:139–42.
868. Brody LC, Mitchell GA, Obie C, et al. Ornithine delta-aminotransferase mutations in gyrate atrophy. Allelic heterogeneity and functional consequences. J Biol Chem 1992;267:3302–7.
869. Fleury M, Barbier R, Ziegler F, et al. Myopathy with tubular aggregates and gyrate atrophy of the choroid and retina due to hyperornithinaemia. J Neurol Neurosurg Psychiatry 2007;78:656–7.
870. Valtonen M, Nanto-Salonen K, Jaaskelainen S, et al. Central nervous system involvement in gyrate atrophy of the choroid and retina with hyperornithinaemia. J Inherit Metab Dis 1999;22:855–66.
871. Kaiser-Kupfer MI, Kuwabara T, Askanas V, et al. Systemic manifestations of gyrate atrophy of the choroid and retina. Ophthalmology 1981;88:302–6.
872. Wilson DJ, Weleber RG, Green WR. Ocular clinicopathologic study of gyrate atrophy. Am J Ophthalmol 1991;111:24–33.
873. Wirtz MK, Kennaway NG, Weleber RG. Heterogeneity and complementation analysis of fibroblasts from vitamin B6 responsive and non-responsive patients with gyrate atrophy of the choroid and retina. J Inherit Metab Dis 1985;8:71–4.
874. Akaki Y, Hotta Y, Mashima Y, et al. A deletion in the ornithine aminotransferase gene in gyrate atrophy. J Biol Chem 1992;267:12950–4.

876. Brody LC, Mitchell GA, Obie C, et al. Ornithine delta-aminotransferase mutations in gyrate atrophy; allelic heterogeneity and functional consequences. J Biol Chem 1992;267:3302–7.
876. Mito T, Shiono T, Ishiguru S, et al. Immunocytochemical localization of ornithine aminotransferase in human ocular tissues. Arch Ophthalmol 1989;107:1372–4.
877. Kaiser-Kupfer MI, Caruso RC, Valle D. Gyrate atrophy of the choroid and retina; long-term reduction of ornithine slows retinal degeneration. Arch Ophthalmol 1991;109:1539–48.
878. Vannas-Sulonen K, Simell O, Sipilä I. Gyrate atrophy of the choroid and retina; the ocular disease progresses in juvenile patients despite normal or near normal plasma ornithine concentration. Ophthalmology 1987;94:1428–33.
879. François J. Ocular manifestations in certain congenital errors of metabolism. In: Symposium on surgical and medical management of congenital anomalies of the eye; transactions of the New Orleans Academy of Ophthalmology, St. Louis, 1968. p. 157–98.
880. Hooft C, DeLaey P, Herpol J, et al. Familial hypolipidaemia and retarded development without steatorrhoea; another inborn error of metabolism? Helv Paediatr Acta 1962;17:1–23.
881. Dufier JL, Dhermy P, Gubler MC, et al. Ocular changes in long-term evolution of infantile cystinosis. Ophthalmic Paediatr Genet 1987;8:131–7.
882. Fellers FX, Cogan DG, Donaldson DD. Cystinosis with extensive choroidal involvement. Arch Ophthalmol 1965;74:868–969.
883. Kaiser-Kupfer MI, Caruso RC, Minkler DS, et al. Long-term ocular manifestations in nephropathic cystinosis. Arch Ophthalmol 1986;104:706–11.
884. Kaiser-Kupfer MI, Gazzo MA, Datiles MB, et al. A randomized placebo-controlled trial of cysteamine eye drops in nephropathic cystinosis. Arch Ophthalmol 1990;108:689–93.
885. Okami T, Nakajima M, Higashino H, et al. Ocular manifestations in a case of infantile cystinosis. Acta Soc Ophthalmol Jpn 1992;96:1341–6.
886. Read J, Goldberg MF, Fishman G, et al. Nephropathic cystinosis. Am J Ophthalmol 1973;76:791–6.
887. Richler M, Milot J, Quigley M, et al. Ocular manifestations of nephropathic cystinosis; the French-Canadian experience in a genetically homogeneous population. Arch Ophthalmol 1991;109:359–62.
888. Sanderson PO, Kuwabara T, Stark WJ, et al. Cystinosis; a clinical, histopathologic, and ultrastructural study. Arch Ophthalmol 1974;91:270–4.
889. Winter FC, editor. Case report presented at the Verhoeff Society meeting, Washington, DC: 1975.
890. Wong VG, Lietman PS, Seegmiller JE. Alterations of pigment epithelium in cystinosis. Arch Ophthalmol 1967;77:361–9.
891. Spencer WH, Hogan MJ. Ocular manifestations of Chédiak-Higashi syndrome; report of a case with histopathologic examination of ocular tissues. Am J Ophthalmol 1960;50:1197–203.
892. Spedick MJ, Beauchamp GR. Retinal vascular and optic nerve abnormalities in albinism. J Pediatr Ophthalmol Strabismus 1986;23:58–63.
893. Simon JW, Kandel GL, Krohel GB, et al. Albinotic characteristics in congenital nystagmus. Am J Ophthalmol 1984;97:320–7.
894. O'Donnell Jr FE, Green WR, Fleischman JA, et al. X-linked ocular albinism in blacks; ocular albinism cum pigmento. Arch Ophthalmol 1978;96:1189–92.
895. O'Donnell Jr FE, Hambrick Jr GW, Green WR, et al. X-linked ocular albinism; an oculocutaneous macromelanosomal disorder. Arch Ophthalmol 1976;94:1883–92.
896. O'Donnell Jr FE, King RA, Green WR, et al. Autosomal-recessively inherited ocular albinism; a new form of ocular albinism affecting females as severely as males. Arch Ophthalmol 1978;96:1621–5.
897. Nettleship E. On some hereditary diseases of the eye. Trans Ophthalmol Soc UK 1909;29: LVII–CXCVIII.
898. Naumann GOH, Lerche W, Schroeder W. Foveola-Aplasie bei Tyrosinase-positivem oculocutanen Albinismus; Klinisch-pathologische Befunde. Graefes Arch Klin Exp Ophthalmol 1976;200: 39–50.
899. Jay B, Carroll W. Albinism; recent advances. Trans Ophthalmol Soc UK 1980;100:467–71.
900. Goldberg MF. Waardenburg's syndrome with fundus and other anomalies. Arch Ophthalmol 1966;76:797–810.
901. Gillespie FD. Ocular albinism with report of a family with female carriers. Arch Ophthalmol 1961;66:774–7.
902. Fulton AB, Albert DM, Craft JL. Human albinism; light and electron microscopy study. Arch Ophthalmol 1978;96:305–10.
903. Falls HF. Sex-linked ocular albinism displaying typical fundus changes in the female heterozygote. Am J Ophthalmol 1951;34:41–50.
904. Epstein RL. Inborn metabolic disorders and the eye. In: Peyman GA, Sanders DR, Goldberg MF, editors. Principles and practice of ophthalmology. Philadelphia: WB Saunders; 1980. p. 1755–7.
905. Cross HE, McKusick VA, Breen W. A new oculocerebral syndrome with hypopigmentation. J Pediatr 1967;70:398–406.
906. Bard LA. Heterogeneity in Waardenburg's syndrome; report of a family with ocular albinism. Arch Ophthalmol 1978;96:1193–8.
907. Bergsma DR, Kaiser-Kupfer M. A new form of albinism. Am J Ophthalmol 1974;77:837–44.
908. Garner A, Jay BS. Macromelanosomes in X-linked ocular albinism. Histopathology 1980;4: 243–54.
909. Gregor Z. The perifoveal vasculature in albinism. Br J Ophthalmol 1978;62:554–7.
910. King RA, Lewis RA, Townsend D, et al. Brown oculocutaneous albinism; clinical, ophthalmological, and biochemical characterization. Ophthalmology 1985;92:1496–505.
911. Witkop Jr CJ, Quevedo Jr WC, Fitzpatrick TB, et al. Albinism. In: Scriver CR, Beaudet AC, Sly WS, editors. The metabolic basis of inherited disease (6th ed.). New York: McGraw-Hill; 1989. p. 2905–51.
912. Summers CG, King RA. Ophthalmic features of minimal pigment oculocutaneous albinism. Ophthalmology 1994;101:906–14.
913. Summers CG, Knobloch WH, Witkop Jr CJ, et al. Hermansky–Pudlak syndrome; ophthalmic findings. Ophthalmology 1988;95:545–54.
914. Thompson WS, Curtin VT. Congenital bilateral heterochromia of the choroid and iris. Arch Ophthalmol 1994;112:1247–8.
915. Maguire AM, Maumenee IH. Iris pigment mosaicism in carriers of X-linked ocular albinism cum pigmento. Am J Ophthalmol 1989;107:298–9.
916. Mietz H, Green WR, Wolff SM, et al. Foveal hypoplasia in complete oculocutaneous albinism; a histopathologic study. Retina 1992;12:254–60.
917. Weleber RG, Pillers D-AM, Powell BR, et al. Åland Island eye disease (Forsius–Eriksson syndrome) associated with contiguous deletion syndrome at Xp21; similarity to incomplete congenital stationary night blindness. Arch Ophthalmol 1989;107:1170–9.
918. Russell-Eggitt I, Kriss A, Taylor DSI. Albinism in childhood: a flash VEP and ERG study. Br J Ophthalmol 1990;74:136–40.
919. Wack MA, Peachey NS, Fishman GA. Electroretinographic findings in human oculocutaneous albinism. Ophthalmology 1989;96:1778–85.
920. Curran RE, Robb RM. Isolated foveal hypoplasia. Arch Ophthalmol 1976;94:48–50.
921. O'Donnell Jr FE, Pappas HR. Autosomal-dominant foveal hypoplasia and presenile cataracts; a new syndrome. Arch Ophthalmol 1982;100:279–81.
922. Oliver MD, Dotan SA, Chemke J, et al. Isolated foveal hypoplasia. Br J Ophthalmol 1987;71: 926–30.
923. Besio R, Meerhoff E, Laza J, et al. Oxalosis. Am J Ophthalmol 1983;95:397–8.
924. Fielder AR, Garner A, Chambers TL. Ophthalmic manifestations of primary oxalosis. Br J Ophthalmol 1980;64:782–8.
925. Franceschetti A, François J, Babel J. Chorioretinal heredodegenerations. Springfield, IL: Charles C Thomas; 1974. p. 907.
926. Gottlieb RP, Ritter JA. "Flecked retina" – an association with primary hyperoxaluria. J Pediatr 1977;90:939–42.
927. Meredith TA, Wright JD, Gammon JA, et al. Ocular involvement in primary hyperoxaluria. Arch Ophthalmol 1984;102:584–7.
928. Timm G. Das Krankheitsbild der Retinopathia oxalogenica. Klin Monatsbl Augenheilkd 1976;168:537–43.
929. Toussaint D, Vereerstraeten P, Goffin P, et al. Hyperoxalurie primaire: Étude clinique, histologique et cristallographique des lésions oculaires. Arch Ophthalmol (Paris) 1976;36:97–112.
930. Zak TA, Buncic R. Primary hereditary oxalosis retinopathy. Arch Ophthalmol 1983;101:78–80.
931. Small KW, Letson R, Scheinman J. Ocular findings in primary hyperoxaluria. Arch Ophthalmol 1990;108:89–93.
932. Danpure CJ, Jennings PR. Peroxisomal alanine:glycolate aminotransferase deficiency in primary hyperoxyluria type I. FEBS Lett 1986;201:20–4.
933. Small KW. Enzyme deficiency for type 1 primary hyperoxaluria. Arch Ophthalmol 1992; 110:13.
934. Small KW, Pollock S, Scheinman J. Optic atrophy in primary oxalosis. Am J Ophthalmol 1988;106:96–7.
935. Small KW, Scheinman J, Klintworth GK. A clinicopathological study of ocular involvement in primary hyperoxaluria type I. Br J Ophthalmol 1992;76:54–7.
936. Sakamoto T, Maeda K, Sueishi K, et al. Ocular histopathologic findings in a 46-year-old man with primary hyperoxaluria. Arch Ophthalmol 1991;109:384–7.
937. Albert DM, Bullock JD, Lahav M, et al. Flecked retina secondary to oxalate crystals from methoxyflurane anesthesia: clinical and experimental studies. Trans Am Acad Ophthalmol Otolaryngol 1975;79:OP817–OP826.
938. Bullock JD, Albert DM. Flecked retina; appearance secondary to oxalate crystals from methoxyflurane anesthesia. Arch Ophthalmol 1975;93:26–31.
939. Carmel R, Bedros AA, Mace JW, et al. Congenital methylmalonic aciduria–homocystinuria with megaloblastic anemia: observations on response to hydroxocobalamin and on the effect of homocysteine and methionine on the deoxyuridine suppression test. Blood 1980;55:570–9.
940. Cogan DG, Schulman J, Porter RJ, et al. Epileptiform ocular movements with methylmalonic aciduria and homocystinuria. Am J Ophthalmol 1980;90:251–3.
941. Fenton WA, Rosenberg LE. Inherited disorders of cobalamine transport and metabolism. In: Scriver CR, Beaudet AC, Sly WS, editors. The metabolic basis of inherited disease, 6th ed. New York: McGraw-Hill; 1989. p. 2065.
942. Mitchell GA, Watkins D, Melançon SB, et al. Clinical heterogeneity in cobalamin C variant of combined homocystinuria and methylmalonic aciduria. J Pediatr 1986;108:410–5.
943. Robb RM, Dowton SB, Fulton AB, et al. Retinal degeneration in vitamin B12 disorder associated with methylmalonic aciduria and sulfur amino acid abnormalities. Am J Ophthalmol 1984;97:691–6.
944. Traboulsi EI, Silva JC, Geraghty MT, et al. Ocular histopathologic characteristics of cobalamin C type vitamin B12 defect with methylmalonic aciduria and homocystinuria. Am J Ophthalmol 1992;113:269–80.
945. Gerth C, Morel CF, Feigenbaum A, et al. Ocular phenotype in patients with methylmalonic aciduria and homocystinuria, cobalamin C type. J AAPOS 2008;12:591–6.
946. Ricci D, Pane M, Deodato F, et al. Assessment of visual function in children with methylmalonic aciduria and homocystinuria. Neuropediatrics 2005;36:181–5.
947. Tsina EK, Marsden DL, Hansen RM, et al. Maculopathy and retinal degeneration in cobalamin C methylmalonic aciduria and homocystinuria. Arch Ophthalmol 2005;123:1143–6.
948. Francis PJ, Calver DM, Barnfield P, et al. An infant with methylmalonic aciduria and homocystinuria (cblC) presenting with retinal haemorrhages and subdural haematoma mimicking non-accidental injury. Eur J Pediatr 2004;163:420–1.
949. Cogan DG, Rodrigues M, Chu FC, et al. Ocular abnormalities in abetalipoproteinemia; a clinicopathologic correlation. Ophthalmology 1984;91:991–8.
950. Berger AS, Nychsen L, Rosenblum JL. Retinopathy in human vitamin E deficiency. Am J Ophthalmol 1991;111:774–5.
951. Adams NA, Awadein A, Toma HS. The retinal ciliopathies. Ophthalmic Genet 2007;28:113–25.
952. Stiggelbout W. The Bardet–Biedl syndrome, including Hutchinson–Laurence–Moon syndrome. In: Vinkin PJ, Bruyn GW, editors. Handbook of clinical neurology, vol. 13. Neuroretinal degenerations. New York: American Elsevier; 1972. p. 380–412.
953. Jacobson SG, Borruat F-X, Apáthy PP. Patterns of rod and cone dysfunction in Bardet–Biedl syndrome. Am J Ophthalmol 1990;109:676–88.

954. Gershoni-Baruch R, Nachlieli T, Leibo R. Cystic kidney dysplasia and polydactyly in 3 sibs with Bardet–Biedl syndrome. Am J Med Genet 1992;44:269–73.
955. Fulton AB, Hansen RM, Glynn RJ. Natural course of visual functions in the Bardet–Biedl syndrome. Arch Ophthalmol 1993;111:1500–6.
956. Fishman G. Hereditary retinal and choroidal diseases: electroretinogram and electro-oculogram findings. In: Peyman GA, Sanders DR, Goldberg MF, editors. Principles and practice of ophthalmology. Philadelphia: WB Saunders; 1980. p. 876.
957. De Marchi S, Cecchin E, Bartoli E. Bardet–Biedl syndrome and cystinuria. Ren Fail 1992;14:587–90.
958. Campo RV, Aaberg TM. Ocular and systemic manifestations of the Bardet–Biedl syndrome. Am J Ophthalmol 1982;94:750–6.
959. Biedl A. Ein Geschwisterpaar mit adiposo-genitaler Dystrophie. Dtsch Med Wochenschr 1922;48:1630.
960. Bardet G. Sur un syndrome d'obésité congénitale avec polydactylie et rétinite pigmentaire. (Contribution à l'étude des formes clinique de l'obésité hypophysaire). Thesis. Paris, 1920.
961. Ackerman J, Brody PE, Kanarek I, et al. Macular wrinkling and atypical retinitis pigmentosa in Laurence–Moon–Biedl–Bardet syndrome. Ann Ophthalmol 1980;12:632–4.
962. Gass JDM. Stereoscopic atlas of macular diseases; diagnosis and treatment, 2nd ed. St. Louis: CV Mosby; 1977. p. 196.
963. Sachdev MS, Verma L, Garg SP. Bilateral disc oedema in retinitis pigmentosa – an unusual sign. Jpn J Ophthalmol 1987;31:621–6.
964. Escallon F, Traboulsi EI, Infante R. A family with the Bardet–Biedl syndrome and diabetes mellitus. Arch Ophthalmol 1989;107:855–7.
965. Laurence JZ, Moon RC. Four cases of "retinitis pigmentosa," occurring in the same family, and accompanied by general imperfections of development. Ophthalmic Rev 1866;2:32–41.
966. Rizzo III JF, Berson EL, Lessell S. Retinal and neurologic findings in the Laurence–Moon–Bardet–Biedl phenotype. Ophthalmology 1986;93:1452–6.
967. Diaz LL, Grech KF, Prados MD. Hypothalamic hamartoma associated with Lawrence–Moon–Biedl syndrome; case report and review of the literature. Pediatr Neurosurg 1991-1992:30–3. 17 1991-1992:30–3.
968. Alström CH, Hallgren B, Nilsson LB, et al. Retinal degeneration combined with obesity, diabetes mellitus and neurogenous deafness; a specific syndrome (not hitherto described) distinct from the Laurence–Moon–Bardet–Biedl syndrome. A clinical, endocrinological and genetic examination based on a large pedigree. Acta Psychiatr Neurol Scand Suppl 1959;129:1–35.
969. Charles SJ, Moore AT, Yates JR. Alström's syndrome: further evidence of autosomal-recessive inheritance and endocrinological dysfunction. J Med Genet 1990;27:590–2.
970. Connolly MB, Jan JE, Couch RM. Hepatic dysfunction in Alström disease. Am J Med Genet 1991;40:421–4.
971. Johnson J. Diabetes, neurogenous deafness, and retinal degeneration. Br Med J 1961;2:646.
972. Sebag J, Albert DM, Craft JL. The Alström syndrome: ophthalmic histopathology and retinal ultrastructure. Br J Ophthalmol 1984;68:494–501.
973. Tremblay F, LaRoche RG, Shea SE, et al. Longitudinal study of the early electroretinographic changes in Alström's syndrome. Am J Ophthalmol 1993;115:657–65.
974. Boor R, Herwig J, Schrezenmeir J. Familial insulin resistant diabetes associated with acanthosis nigricans, polycystic ovaries, hypogonadism, pigmentary retinopathy, labyrinthine deafness, and mental retardation. Am J Med Genet 1993;45:649–53.
975. Millay RH, Weleber RG, Heckenlively JR. Ophthalmologic and systemic manifestations of Alström's disease. Am J Ophthalmol 1986;102:482–90.
976. Malm E, Ponjavic V, Nishina PM, et al. Full-field electroretinography and marked variability in clinical phenotype of Alstrom syndrome. Arch Ophthalmol 2008;126:51–7.
977. Russell-Eggitt IM, Clayton PT, Coffey R, et al. Alstrom syndrome. Report of 22 cases and literature review. Ophthalmology 1998;105:1274–80.
978. Abraham FA, Yanko L, Licht A, et al. Electrophysiologic study of the visual system in familial juvenile nephronophthisis and tapetoretinal dystrophy. Am J Ophthalmol 1974;78:591–7.
979. Avasthi PS, Erickson DG, Gardner KD. Hereditary renal-retinal dysplasia and the medullary cystic disease–nephronophthisis complex. Ann Intern Med 1976;84:157–61.
980. Lauweryns B, Leys A, Van Haesendonck E, et al. Senior–Løken syndrome with marbleized fundus and unusual skeletal abnormalities; a case report. Graefes Arch Clin Exp Ophthalmol 1993;231:242–8.
981. Løken AC, Hanssen O, Halvorsen S, et al. Hereditary renal dysplasia and blindness. Acta Paediatr 1961;50:177–84.
982. Meier DA, Hess JW. Familiar nephropathy with retinitis pigmentosa; a new oculorenal syndrome in adults. Am J Med 1965;39:58–69.
983. Polak BCP, Hogewind BL, Van Lith FHM. Tapetoretinal degeneration associated with recessively inherited medullary cystic disease. Am J Ophthalmol 1977;84:645–51.
984. Proesmans W, van Damme B, Macken J. Nephronophthisis and tapetoretinal degeneration associated with liver fibrosis. Clin Nephrol 1975;3:160–4.
985. Schuman JS, Lieberman KV, Friedman AH. Senior–Loken syndrome (familial renal-retinal dystrophy) and Coats' disease. Am J Ophthalmol 1985;100:822–7.
986. Senior B, Friedmann AI, Braudo JL. Juvenile familial nephropathy with tapetoretinal degeneration; a new oculorenal dystrophy. Am J Ophthalmol 1961;52:625–33.
987. Bard LA, Bard PA, Owens GW, et al. Retinal involvement in thoracic-pelvic-phalangeal syndrome. Arch Ophthalmol 1978;96:278–81.
988. Wilson DJ, Weleber RG, Beals RK. Retinal dystrophy in Jeune's syndrome. Arch Ophthalmol 1987;105:651–7.
989. Allen Jr AW, Moon JB, Hovland KR, et al. Ocular findings in thoracic-pelvic-phalangeal dystrophy. Arch Ophthalmol 1979;97:489–92.
990. Alagille D, Odièvre M, Gautier M, et al. Hepatic ductular hypoplasia associated with characteristic facies, vertebral malformations, retarded physical, mental and sexual development, and cardiac murmur. J Pediatr 1975;86:63–71.
991. Alvarez F, Landrieu P, Laget P. Nervous and ocular disorders in children with cholestasis and vitamin A and E deficiencies. Hepatology 1983;3:410–4.
992. Gass JDM. Stereoscopic atlas of macular diseases; diagnosis and treatment, 3rd ed. St. Louis: CV Mosby; 1987. p. 230.
993. Johnson BL. Ocular pathologic features of arteriohepatic dysplasia (Alagille's syndrome). Am J Ophthalmol 1990;110:504–12.
994. Raymond WR, Kearney JJ, Parmley VC. Ocular findings in arteriohepatic dysplasia (Alagille's syndrome). Arch Ophthalmol 1989;107:1077.
995. Riely CA, Cotlier E, Jensen PS, et al. Arteriohepatic dysplasia: a benign syndrome of intrahepatic cholestasis with multiple organ involvement. Ann Intern Med 1979;91:520–7.
996. Romanchuk KG, Judisch GF, LaBrecque DR. Ocular findings in arteriohepatic dysplasia (Alagille's syndrome). Can J Ophthalmol 1981;16:94–9.
997. Shulman SA, Hyams JS, Gunta R. Arteriohepatic dysplasia (Alagille syndrome): extreme variability among affected family members. Am J Med Genet 1984;19:325–32.
998. Sokol RJ, Heubi JE, Balistreri WF. Intrahepatic "cholestasis facies": is it specific for Alagille syndrome? J Pediatr 1983;103:205–8.
999. Amon M, Menapace R, Kirnbauer R. Ocular symptomatology in familial hypomelanosis Ito; incontinentia pigmenti achromians. Ophthalmologica 1990;200:1–6.
1000. Grazia R, Tullini A, Rossi PG. Hypomelanosis of Ito with trisomy 18 mosaicism. Am J Med Genet 1993;45:120–1.
1001. Ito M. Incontinentia pigmenti achromians: a singular case of nevus depigmentosus systematicus bilateralis. Tohoku J Exp Med 1952;55(Suppl. I):57–9.
1002. Ross DL, Liwnicz BH, Chun RW, et al. Hypomelanosis of Ito (incontinentia pigmenti achromians) – a clinicopathologic study: macrocephaly and gray matter heterotopias. Neurology 1982;32:1013–6.
1003. Rott H-D, Lang GE, Huk W, et al. Hypomelanosis of Ito (incontinentia pigmenti achromians): Ophthalmological evidence for somatic mosaicism. Ophthalmic Paediatr Genet 1990;11:273–9.
1004. Steichen-Gersdorf E, Trawöger R, Duba HC. Hypomelanosis of Ito in a girl with plexus papilloma and translocation (X;17). Hum Genet 1993;90:611–3.
1005. Takematsu H, Sato S, Igarashi M, et al. Incontinentia pigmenti achromians (Ito). Arch Dermatol 1983;119:391–5.
1006. Turleau C, Taillard F, Doussau de Bazignan M. Hypomelanosis of Ito (incontinentia pigmenti achromians) and mosaicism for a microdeletion of 15q1. Hum Genet 1986;74:185–7.
1007. Weaver Jr RG, Martin T, Zanolli MD. The ocular changes of incontinentia pigmenti achromians (hypomelanosis of Ito). J Pediatr Ophthalmol Strabismus 1991;28:160–3.
1008. Sybert VP. Hypomelanosis of Ito: a description, not a diagnosis. J Invest Dermatol 1994;103(Suppl):141S–3S.
1009. Weaver Jr RG, Martin T, Zanolli MD. The ocular changes of incontinentia pigmenti achromians (hypomelanosis of Ito). J Pediatr Ophthalmol Strabismus 1991;28:160–3.
1010. Flaherty MP, Padilla CD, Sillence DO. Axenfeld anomaly in association with hypomelanosis of Ito. Ophthalmic Paediatr Genet 1991;12:23–30.
1011. Rott HD, Lang GE, Huk W, et al. Hypomelanosis of Ito (incontinentia pigmenti achromians). Ophthalmological evidence for somatic mosaicism. Ophthalmic Paediatr Genet 1990;11:273–9.
1012. Amon M, Menapace R, Kirnbauer R. Ocular symptomatology in familial hypomelanosis Ito. Incontinentia pigmenti achromians. Ophthalmologica 1990;200:1–6.
1013. Ikeda T, Sato K, Miyaura T. Fundus and fluorescein documentation of hypomelanosis of Ito. Arch Ophthalmol 1999 Jul;117(7):976–7.
1014. Heimler A, Fox JE, Hershey JE, et al. Sensorineural hearing loss, enamel hypoplasia, and nail abnormalities in sibs. Am J Med Genet 1991;39:192–5.
1015. Ong KR, Visram S, McKaig S, et al. Sensorineural deafness, enamel abnormalities and nail abnormalities: a case report of Heimler syndrome in identical twin girls. Eur J Med Genet 2006;49:187–93.
1016. Cockayne EA. Dwarfism with retinal atrophy and deafness. Arch Dis Child 1936;11:1–8.
1017. Cockayne EA. Dwarfism with retinal atrophy and deafness. Arch Dis Child 1946;21:52–4.
1018. Levin PS, Green WR, Victor DI, et al. Histopathology of the eye in Cockayne's syndrome. Arch Ophthalmol 1983;101:1093–7.
1019. Pearce WG. Ocular and genetic features of Cockayne's syndrome. Can J Ophthalmol 1972;7:435–44.
1020. Hamdani M, El Kettani A, Rais L, et al. [Cockayne's syndrome with unusual retinal involvement (report of one family).] J Fr Ophtalmol 2000;23:52–6.
1021. Manning FJ, Bruce AM, Berson EL. Electroretinograms in microcephaly with chorioretinal degeneration. Am J Ophthalmol 1990;109:457–63.
1022. Hoyt CS, Billson FA. Visual loss in osteopetrosis. Am J Dis Child 1979;133:955–8.
1023. Keith CG. Retinal atrophy in osteopetrosis. Arch Ophthalmol 1968;79:234–41.
1024. Ruben JB, Morris RJ, Judisch GF. Chorioretinal degeneration in infantile malignant osteopetrosis. Am J Ophthalmol 1990;110:1–5.
1025. Driessen GJ, Gerritsen EJ, Fischer A, et al. Long-term outcome of haematopoietic stem cell transplantation in autosomal-recessive osteopetrosis: an EBMT report. Bone Marrow Transplant 2003;32:657–63.
1026. Kawamura N, Tabata H, Sun-Wada GH, et al. Optic nerve compression and retinal degeneration in Tcirg1 mutant mice lacking the vacuolar-type H-ATPase a3 subunit. PLoS One 2010:58.
1027. Cohen SMZ, Brown III FR, Martyn L. Ocular histopathologic and biochemical studies of the cerebrohepatorenal syndrome (Zellweger's syndrome) and its relationship to neonatal adrenoleukodystrophy. Am J Ophthalmol 1983;96:488–501.
1028. Garner A, Fielder AR, Primavesi R, et al. Tapetoretinal degeneration in the cerebro-hepato-renal (Zellweger's) syndrome. Br J Ophthalmol 1982;66:422–31.
1029. Stanescu B, Dralands L. Cerebro-hepato-renal (Zellweger's) syndrome; ocular involvement. Arch Ophthalmol 1972;87:590–2.
1030. Cohen SMZ, Green WR, de la Cruz ZC, et al. Ocular histopathologic studies in neonatal and childhood adrenoleukodystrophy. Am J Ophthalmol 1983;95:82–96.
1031. Glascow BJ, Brown HH, Hannah JB, et al. Ocular pathologic findings in neonatal adrenoleukodystrophy. Ophthalmology 1987;94:1054–60.
1032. Traboulsi EI, Maumenee IH. Ophthalmologic manifestations of X-linked childhood adrenoleukodystrophy. Ophthalmology 1987;94:47–52.

1033. Rosen NL, Lechtenberg R, Wisniewski K. Adrenoleukomyeoneuropathy with onset in early childhood. Ann Neurol 1985;17:311–2.
1034. Claridge KG, Gibberd FB, Sidey MC. The presentation and ophthalmic aspects of Refsum disease in a series of 23 patients. Eye 1992;6:371–5.
1035. Refsum S. Heredopathia atactica polyneuritiformis; a familial syndrome not hitherto described. A contribution to the clinical study of the hereditary diseases of the nervous system. Acta Psychiatr Neurol Suppl 1946;38:1–303.
1036. Refsum S. Heredopathia atactica polyneuritiformis phytanic acid storage disease (Refsum's disease) with particular reference to ophthalmological disturbances. Metab Ophthalmol 1977;1:73–9.
1037. Steinberg D. Refsum disease. In: Scriver CR, Beaudet AL, Sly WS, editors. The metabolic basis of inherited disease, 6th ed. New York: McGraw-Hill; 1989. p. 1533–50.
1038. Weleber RG, Tongue AC, Kennaway NG. Ophthalmic manifestations of infantile phytanic acid storage disease. Arch Ophthalmol 1984;102:1317–21.
1039. Jansen GA, Hogenhout EM, Ferdinandusse S, et al. Human phytanoyl-CoA hydroxylase: resolution of the gene structure and the molecular basis of Refsum's disease. Hum Mol Genet 2000;9:1195–200.
1040. Jansen GA, Wanders RJ, Watkins PA, et al. Phytanoyl-coenzyme A hydroxylase deficiency – the enzyme defect in Refsum's disease. N Engl J Med 1997;337:133–4.
1041. Hansen E, Bachen NI, Flage T. Refsum's disease; eye manifestations in a patient treated with low phytol low phytanic acid diet. Acta Ophthalmol 1979;57:899–913.
1042. Marroun I, Delevaux I, Andre M, et al. Refsum's disease with severe neuropathy: efficiency of the diet and plasmapheresis. Rev Med Interne 2005;26:523–5.
1043. Lou JS, Snyder R, Griggs RC. Refsum's disease: long term treatment preserves sensory nerve action potentials and motor function. J Neurol Neurosurg Psychiatry 1997;62:671–2.
1044. Millaire A, Warembourg A, Leys D, et al. Refsum's disease. Apropos of 2 cases disclosed by myocardiopathy. Ann Cardiol Angeiol (Paris) 1990;39:173–8.
1045. Hungerbuhler JP, Meier C, Rousselle L, et al. Refsum's disease: management by diet and plasmapheresis. Eur Neurol 1985;24:153–9.
1046. Matsuzaka T, Sakuragawa N, Nakayama H. Cerebro-oculo-hepato-renal syndrome (Arima's syndrome): a distinct clinicopathological entity. J Child Neurol 1986;1:338–46.
1047. Lambert SR, Kriss A, Gresty M. Joubert syndrome. Arch Ophthalmol 1989;107:709–13.
1048. Cant JS. Ectodermal dysplasia. J Pediatr Ophthalmol 1967;4:13–17.
1049. Corby DG, Lowe Jr RS, Haskins RC, et al. Trichomegaly, pigmentary degeneration of the retina, and growth retardation; a new syndrome originating in utero. Am J Dis Child 1971;121:344–5.
1050. Judisch GF, Lowry RB, Hanson JW, et al. Chorioretinopathy and pituitary dysfunction; the CPD syndrome. Arch Ophthalmol 1981;99:253–6.
1051. Oliver GL, McFarlane DC. Congenital trichomegaly with associated pigmentary degeneration of the retina, dwarfism, and mental retardation. Arch Ophthalmol 1965;74:169–71.
1052. Gass JDM. The syndrome of keratoconjunctivitis, superficial moniliasis, idiopathic hypoparathyroidism and Addison's disease. Am J Ophthalmol 1962;54:660–74.
1053. McMahon F, Cookson DU, Kabler JD, et al. Idiopathic hypoparathyroidism and idiopathic adrenal cortical insufficiency occurring with cystic fibrosis of the pancreas. Ann Intern Med 1959;51:371.
1054. Aaltonen J, Bjorses P, Sandkuliji L. An autosomal locus causing autoimmune disease: autoimmune polyglandular disease type I assigned to chromosome 21. Nature Genetics 1994;8:83–7.
1055. Wood LW, Jampol LM, Daily MJ. Retinal and optic nerve manifestations of autoimmune polyendocrinopathy-candidiasis-ectodermal dystrophy. Arch Ophthalmol 1991;109:1065.
1056. Carpenter S, Schumacher GA. Familial infantile cerebellar atrophy associated with retinal degeneration. Arch Neurol 1966;14:82–94.
1057. de Jong PTVM, de Jong JGY, de Jong-Ten Doeschate JMM, et al. Olivopontocerebellar atrophy with visual disturbances; an ophthalmologic investigation into four generations. Ophthalmology 1980;87:793–804.
1058. Duinkerke-Eerola KU, Cruysberg JRM, Deutman AF. Atrophic maculopathy associated with hereditary ataxia. Am J Ophthalmol 1980;90:597–603.
1059. Harding AE. The hereditary ataxias and related disorders. New York: Churchill Livingstone; 1984. p. 129.
1060. Havener WH. Cerebellar-macular abiotrophy. Arch Ophthalmol 1951;45:40–3.
1061. Konigsmark BW, Weiner LP. The olivopontocerebellar atrophies; a review. Medicine 1970;49:227–41.
1062. Ryan Jr SJ, Knox DL, Green WR, et al. Olivopontocerebellar degeneration; clinicopathologic correlation of the associated retinopathy. Arch Ophthalmol 1975;93:169–72.
1063. Ryan SJ, Smith RE. Retinopathy associated with hereditary olivopontocerebellar degeneration. Am J Ophthalmol 1971;71:838–43.
1064. Weiner LP, Konigsmark BW, Stoll Jr J, et al. Hereditary olivopontocerebellar atrophy with retinal degeneration; report of a family through six generations. Arch Neurol 1967;16:364–76.
1065. Woodworth JA, Beckett RS, Netsky MG. A composite of hereditary ataxias; a familial disorder with features of olivopontocerebellar atrophy, Leber's optic atrophy, and Friedreich's ataxia. Arch Intern Med 1959;104:594–606.
1066. Drack AV, Traboulsi EI, Maumanee IH. Progression of retinopathy in olivopontocerebellar atrophy with retinal degeneration. Arch Ophthalmol 1992;110:712–3.
1067. To KW, Adamian M, Jakobiec FA, et al. Olivopontocerebellar atrophy with retinal degeneration; an electroretinographic and histopathologic investigation. Ophthalmology 1993;100:15–23.
1068. Traboulsi EI, Maumenee IH, Green WR. Olivopontocerebellar atrophy with retinal degeneration; a clinical and ocular histopathologic study. Arch Ophthalmol 1988;106:801–6.
1069. Hugosson T, Granse L, Ponjavic V, et al. Macular dysfunction and morphology in spinocerebellar ataxia type 7 (SCA 7). Ophthalmic Genet 2009;30:1–6.
1070. Tsai HF, Liu CS, Leu TM, et al. Analysis of trinucleotide repeats in different SCA loci in spinocerebellar ataxia patients and in normal population of Taiwan. Acta Neurol Scand 2004;109:355–60.
1071. Modi G, Modi M, Martinus I, et al. The clinical and genetic characteristics of spinocerebellar ataxia type 7 (SCA 7) in three Black South African families. Acta Neurol Scand 2000;101:177–82.
1072. Puertas-Bordallo D, De-Domingo-Baron B, Lozano-Vazquez M, et al. Alstròm Hallgren syndrome. Arch Soc Esp Oftalmol 2007;82:649–52.
1073. Hallervorden J, Spatz H. Eigenartige Erkrankung im extrapyramidalen System mit besonderer Beteiligung des Globus pallidus und der Substantia nigra: ein Beitrag zu den Beziehungen zwischen diesen beiden zentren. Z Ges Neurol Psychiatr 1922;79:254–302.
1074. Luckenbach MW, Green WR, Miller NR. Ocular clinicopathologic correlation of Hallervorden–Spatz syndrome with acanthocytosis and pigmentary retinopathy. Am J Ophthalmol 1983;95:369–82.
1075. Newell FW, Johnson II RO, Huttenlocher PR. Pigmentary degeneration of the retina in the Hallervorden–Spatz syndrome. Am J Ophthalmol 1979;88:467–71.
1076. Roth AM, Hepler RS, Mukoyama M. Pigmentary retinal dystrophy in Hallervorden–Spatz disease: Clinicopathological report of a case. Surv Ophthalmol 1971;16:24–35.
1077. Van Kirk MP, Larsen PD, O'Conner PS. New computed tomography scan finding in Hallervorden–Spatz syndrome. J Clin Neuro-Ophthalmol 1986;6:86–90.
1078. Egan RA, Weleber RG, Hogarth P, et al. Neuro-ophthalmologic and electroretinographic findings in pantothenate kinase-associated neurodegeneration (formerly Hallervorden–Spatz syndrome). Am J Ophthalmol 2005;140:267–74.
1079. Higgins JJ, Patterson MC, Papadopoulos NM. Hypoprebetalipoproteinemia acanthocytosis, retinitis pigmentosa, and pallidal degeneration (HARP syndrome). Neurology 1992;42:194–8.
1080. Angelini L, Nardocci N, Rumi V. Hallervorden–Spatz disease; clinical and MRI study of 11 cases diagnosed in life. J Neurol 1992;239:417–25.
1081. Tripathi RC, Tripathi BJ, Bauserman SC, et al. Clinicopathologic correlation and pathogenesis of ocular and central nervous system manifestations in Hallervorden–Spatz syndrome. Acta Neuropathol 1992;83:113–9.
1082. Seo JH, Song SK, Lee PH. A novel PANK2 mutation in a patient with atypical pantothenate-kinase-associated neurodegeneration presenting with adult-onset parkinsonism. J Clin Neurol 2009;5:192–4.
1083. Cangul H, Ozdemir O, Yakut T, et al. Pantothenate kinase-associated neurodegeneration (PKAN): molecular confirmation of a Turkish patient with a rare frameshift mutation in the coding region of the PANK2 gene. Turk J Pediatr 2009;51:161–5.
1084. Bozi M, Matarin M, Theocharis I, et al. A patient with pantothenate kinase-associated neurodegeneration and supranuclear gaze palsy. Clin Neurol Neurosurg 2009;111:688–90.
1085. Westaway SK, Robinson SW, Hayflick SJ, et al. Gene symbol: PANK2. Disease: pantothenate kinase-associated neurodegeneration (PKAN). Hum Genet 2006;119:679.
1086. Koyama M, Yagishita A. Pantothenate kinase-associated neurodegeneration with increased lentiform nuclei cerebral blood flow. AJNR Am J Neuroradiol 2006;27:212–3.
1087. Antonini A, Goldwurm S, Benti R, et al. Genetic, clinical, and imaging characterization of one patient with late-onset, slowly progressive, pantothenate kinase-associated neurodegeneration. Mov Disord 2006;21:417–8.
1088. Doi H, Koyano S, Miyatake S, et al. Siblings with the adult-onset slowly progressive type of pantothenate kinase-associated neurodegeneration and a novel mutation, Ile346Ser, in PANK2: clinical features and (99m)Tc-ECD brain perfusion SPECT findings. J Neurol Sci 2010 Mar 15;290:172–6.
1089. Pavlakis SG, Phillips PCD, Mauro S. Mitochondrial myopathy encephalopathy, lactic acidosis, and strokelike episodes: a distinctive clinical syndrome. Ann Neurol 1984;16:481–8.
1090. Fukuhara N. Myoclonus epilepsy and mitochondrial myopathy. In: Cerri C, Scarlato G, editors. Mitochondrial pathology in muscle diseases; proceedings of the satellite symposium of the Vth International Congress on Neuromuscular Diseases, Sanremo, Italy, September 19, 1982. Padua: Piccin Editore; 1983. p. 87.
1091. Barboni P, Savini G, Plazzi G, et al. Ocular findings in mitochondrial neurogastrointestinal encephalomyopathy: a case report. Graefes Arch Clin Exp Ophthalmol 2004;242:878–80.
1092. Latkany P, Ciulla TA, Cacchillo PF, et al. Mitochondrial maculopathy: geographic atrophy of the macula in the MELAS associated A to G 3243 mitochondrial DNA point mutation. Am J Ophthalmol 1999;128:112–4.
1093. van der Kooi AJ, van Langen IM, Aronica E, et al. Extension of the clinical spectrum of Danon disease. Neurology 2008;70:1358–9.
1094. Schorderet DF, Cottet S, Lobrinus JA, et al. Retinopathy in Danon disease. Arch Ophthalmol 2007;125:231–6.
1095. Prall FR, Drack A, Taylor M, et al. Ophthalmic manifestations of Danon disease. Ophthalmology 2006;113:1010–3.
1096. Balmer C, Ballhausen D, Bosshard NU, et al. Familial X-linked cardiomyopathy (Danon disease): diagnostic confirmation by mutation analysis of the LAMP2gene. Eur J Pediatr 2005;164:509–14.
1097. Chang TS, Johns DR, Walker D. Ocular clinicopathologic study of the mitochondrial encephalomyopathy overlap syndromes. Arch Ophthalmol 1993;111:1254–62.
1098. Oritz RG, Newman NJ, Shoffner JM. Variable retinal and neurologic manifestations in patients harboring the mitochondrial DNA 8993 mutation. Arch Ophthalmol 1993;111:1525–30.
1099. Rummelt V, Folberg R, Ionasescu V. Ocular pathology of MELAS syndrome with mitochondrial DNA nucleotide 3243 point mutation. Ophthalmology 1993;100:1757–66.
1100. Ota Y, Miyake Y, Awaya S. Early retinal involvement in mitochondrial myopathy with mitochondrial DNA deletion. Retina 1994;14:270–6.
1101. Kearns TP, Sayre GP. Retinitis pigmentosa, external ophthalmoplegia, and complete heart block. Arch Ophthalmol 1958;60:280–9.
1102. Bachynski BN, Flynn JT, Rodrigues MM. Hyperglycemic acidotic coma and death in Kearns–Sayre syndrome. Ophthalmology 1986;93:391–6.
1103. Bosche J, Hammerstein W, Neuen-Jacob E, et al. Variation in retinal changes and muscle pathology in mitochondriopathies. Graefes Arch Clin Exp Ophthalmol 1989;227:578–83.
1104. Daroff RB, Solitare GB, Pincus JH, et al. Spongiform encephalopathy with chronic progressive external ophthalmoplegia; central ophthalmoplegia mimicking ocular myopathy. Neurology 1966;16:161–9.
1105. Gross-Jendroska M, Schatz H, McDonald HR, et al. Kearns–Sayre syndrome: a case report and review. Eur J Ophthalmol 1992;2:15–20.
1106. Kearns TP. External ophthalmoplegia, pigmentary degeneration of the retina, and cardiomyopathy: a newly recognized syndrome. Trans Am Ophthalmol Soc 1965;63:559–625.

1107. Leveille AS, Newell FW. Autosomal-dominant Kearns–Sayre syndrome. Ophthalmology 1980;87:99–108.
1108. Zeviani M, Moraes CT, DiMauro S. Deletions of mitochondrial DNA in Kearns–Sayre syndrome. Neurology 1988;38:1339–46.
1109. Herzberg NH, van Schooneveld MJ, Bleeker-Wagemakers EM. Kearns–Sayre syndrome with a phenocopy of choroideremia instead of pigmentary retinopathy. Neurology 1993;43:218–21.
1110. Ascaso FJ, Lopez-Gallardo E, Del Prado E, et al. Macular lesion resembling adult-onset vitelliform macular dystrophy in Kearns–Sayre syndrome with multiple mtDNA deletions. Clin Experiment Ophthalmol 2010;38:812–6.
1111. Gass JDM. Stereoscopic atlas of macular diseases; diagnosis and treatment, 2nd ed. St. Louis: CV Mosby; 1977. p. 198.
1112. McKechnie NM, King M, Lee WR. Retinal pathology in the Kearns–Sayre syndrome. Br J Ophthalmol 1985;69:63–75.
1113. Newell FW, Polascik MA. Mitochondrial disease and retinal pigmentary degeneration. In: Shimizu K, Oosterhuis J, editors. XXIII Concilium Ophthalmologicum, Kyoto 1978, Acta. Amsterdam: Excerpta Medica; International Congress series No. 450; 1979. p. 615–17.
1114. Eagle Jr RC, Hedges TR, Yanoff N. The atypical pigmentary retinopathy of Kearns–Sayre syndrome; a light and electron microscopic study. Ophthalmology 1982;89:1433–40.
1115. Treft RL, Sanborn GE, Carey J. Dominant optic atrophy, deafness, ptosis, ophthalmoplegia, dystaxia, and myopathy; a new syndrome. Ophthalmology 1984;91:908–15.
1116. Maron BJ, Roberts WC, Arad M, et al. Clinical outcome and phenotypic expression in LAMP2 cardiomyopathy. JAMA 2009;301:1253–9.
1117. Nadeau A, Therrien C, Karpati G, et al. Danon disease due to a novel splice mutation in the LAMP2 gene. Muscle Nerve 2008 Mar;37(3):338–42.
1118. Bassen FA, Kornzweig AL. Malformation of the erythrocytes in a case of atypical retinitis pigmentosa. Blood 1950;5:381–7.
1119. Berson EL. Nutrition and retinal degenerations; vitamin A, taurine, ornithine, and phytanic acid. Retina 1982;2:236–55.
1120. Bishara S, Merin S, Cooper M. Combined vitamin A and E therapy prevents retinal electrophysiological deterioration in abetalipoproteinaemia. Br J Ophthalmol 1982;66:767–70.
1121. Gouras P, Carr RE, Gunkel RD. Retinitis pigmentosa in abetalipoproteinemia: effects of vitamin A. Invest Ophthalmol 1971;10:784–93.
1122. Kornzweig AL. Bassen–Kornzweig syndrome – present status. Metab Ophthalmol 1976;1:51–3.
1123. Sperling MA, Hiles DA, Kennerdell JS. Electroretinographic responses following vitamin A therapy in a-beta-lipoproteinemia. Am J Ophthalmol 1972;73:342–51.
1124. Von Sallmann L, Gelderman AH, Laster L. Ocular histopathologic changes in a case of a-beta-lipoproteinemia (Bassen–Kornzweig syndrome). Doc Ophthalmol 1969;26:451–60.
1125. Yee RD, Cogan DG, Zee DS. Ophthalmoplegia and dissociated nystagmus in abetalipoproteinemia. Arch Ophthalmol 1976;94:571–5.
1126. Yee RD, Herbert PN, Bergsma DR, et al. Atypical retinitis pigmentosa in familial hypobetalipoproteinemia. Am J Ophthalmol 1976;82:64–71.
1127. Zamel R, Khan R, Pollex RL, et al. Abetalipoproteinemia: two case reports and literature review. Orphanet J Rare Dis 2008;3:19.
1128. Runge P, Müller DPR, McAllister J. Oral vitamin E supplements can prevent the retinopathy of abetalipoproteinaemia. Br J Ophthalmol 1986;70:166–73.
1129. Brosnahan DM, Kennedy SM, Converse CA. Pathology of hereditary retinal degeneration associated with hypobetalipoproteinemia. Ophthalmology 1994;101:38–45.
1130. Brady RO, Kanfer JN, Shapiro D. Metabolism of glucocerebrosides. II. Evidence of an enzymatic deficiency in Gaucher's disease. Biochem Biophys Res Commun 1965;18:221–5.
1131. Cogan DG, Kuwabara T. The sphingolipidoses and the eye. Arch Ophthalmol 1968;79:437–51.
1132. Brownstein S, Carpenter S, Polomeno RC, et al. Sandhoff's disease (GM2 gangliosidosis type 2); histopathology and ultrastructure of the eye. Arch Ophthalmol 1980;98:1089–97.
1133. Cogan DG, Kuwabara T, Kolodny E, et al. Gangliosidoses and the fetal retina. Ophthalmology 1984;91:508–12.
1134. Kivlin JD, Sanborn GE, Myers GG. The cherry-red spot in Tay–Sachs and other storage diseases. Ann Neurol 1985;17:356–60.
1135. Sandhoff K, Andreae U, Jatzkewitz H. Deficient hexozaminidase activity in an exceptional case of Tay–Sachs disease with additional storage of kidney globoside in visceral organs. Life Sci 1968;7:283–8.
1136. Tay W. Symmetrical changes in the region of the yellow spot in each eye of an infant. Trans Ophthalmol Soc UK 1881;1:55–7.
1137. Ghosh M, Hunter WS, Wedge C. Corneal changes in Tay–Sachs disease. Can J Ophthalmol 1990;25:190–2.
1138. Sorcinelli R, Sitzia A, Loi M. Cherry-red spot, optic atrophy and corneal cloudings in a patient suffering from GM1 gangliosidosis type I. Metab Pediatr Syst Ophthalmol 1987;10:62–3.
1139. Yun YM, Lee SN. A case refort of Sandhoff disease. Korean J Ophthalmol 2005;19:68–72.
1140. Brownstein S, Carpenter S, Polomeno RC, et al. Sandhoff's disease (GM2 gangliosidosis type 2). Histopathology and ultrastructure of the eye. Arch Ophthalmol 1980;98:1089–97.
1141. Cogan DG, Chu FC, Barranger J, et al. Macula halo syndrome. Trans Am Ophthalmol Soc 1982;80:184–92.
1142. Cogan DG, Kuwabara T, Kolodny EH. A variant of Tay–Sachs disease. Concilium Ophthalmologicum XXII, Paris, 1974. Acta 1976;1:700–1.
1143. Harzer K, Ruprecht KW, Seuffer-Schulze DS, et al. Morbus Niemann–Pick Typ B – enzymatisch gesichert – mit unerwarteter retinaler Beteiligung. Albrecht von Graefes Arch Klin Exp Ophthalmol 1978;206:79–88.
1144. Libert J, Toussaint D, Guiselings R. Ocular findings in Neimann–Pick disease. Am J Ophthalmol 1975;80:991–1002.
1145. Niemann A. In unbekanntes Krankheitsbild. Jahrb Kinderheilkd 1914;79:1–10.
1146. Pick L. Über die lipoidzellige Splenohepatomegalie Typus Niemann–Pick als Stoffwechselerkrankung. Med Klin 1927;23:1483–8.
1147. Walton DS, Robb RM, Crocker AC. Ocular manifestations of group A Niemann–Pick disease. Am J Ophthalmol 1978;85:174–80.
1148. Cogan DG, Federman DD. Retinal involvement with reticuloendotheliosis of unclassified type. Arch Ophthalmol 1964;71:489–91.
1149. Lipson MH, O'Donnell J, Callahan JW. Ocular involvement in Niemann–Pick disease type B. J Pediatr 1986;108:582–4.
1150. Matthews JD, Weiter JJ, Kolodny EH. Macular halos associated with Niemann–Pick type B disease. Ophthalmology 1986;93:933–7.
1151. McGovern MM, Wasserstein MP, Aron A, et al. Ocular manifestations of Niemann–Pick disease type B. Ophthalmology 2004;111:1424–7.
1152. Emery JM, Green WR, Huff DS, et al. Niemann–Pick disease (type C); histopathology and ultrastructure. Am J Ophthalmol 1972;74:1144–54.
1153. Palmer M, Green WR, Maumenee IH. Niemann–Pick disease-type c; ocular histopathologic and electron microscopic studies. Arch Ophthalmol 1985;103:817–22.
1154. Mihaylova V, Hantke J, Sinigerska I, et al. Highly variable neural involvement in sphingomyelinase-deficient Niemann–Pick disease caused by an ancestral Gypsy mutation. Brain 2007;130:1050–61.
1155. Emery JM, Green WR, Wyllie RG, et al. G_{M1}-gangliosidosis; ocular and pathological manifestations. Arch Ophthalmol 1971;85:177–87.
1156. O'Brien JS, Stern MB, Landing BH. Generalized gangliosidosis; another inborn error of ganglioside metabolism? Am J Dis Child 1965;109:338–46.
1157. Cogan DG, Kuwabara T, Moser H, et al. Retinopathy in a case of Farber's lipogranulomatosis. Arch Ophthalmol 1966;75:752–7.
1158. Farber S. A lipid metabolic disorder – disseminated "lipogranulomatosis" – a syndrome with similarity to, and important difference from, Niemann–Pick and Hand–Schüller–Christian disease. Am J Dis Child 1952;84:499–500.
1159. Zarbin MA, Green WR, Moser HW, et al. Farber's disease; light and electron microscopic study of the eye. Arch Ophthalmol 1985;103:73–80.
1160. Libert J, Van Hoof F, Toussaint D. Ocular findings in metachromatic leukodystrophy; an electron microscopic and enzyme study in different clinical and genetic variants. Arch Ophthalmol 1979;97:1495–504.
1161. Quigley HA, Green WR. Clinical and ultrastructural ocular histopathologic studies of adult-onset metachromatic leukodystrophy. Am J Ophthalmol 1976;82:472–9.
1162. Grabowski GA. Phenotype, diagnosis, and treatment of Gaucher's disease. Lancet 2008;372:1263–71.
1163. Cogan DG, Chu FC, Gittinger J, et al. Fundal abnormalities of Gaucher's disease. Arch Ophthalmol 1980;98:2202–3.
1164. Ueno H, Ueno S, Kajitani T. Clinical and histopathological studies of a case with juvenile form of Gaucher's disease. Jpn J Ophthalmol 1977;21:98–108.
1165. Ueno H, Ueno S, Matsuo N, et al. Electron microscopic study of Gaucher cells in the eye. Jpn J Ophthalmol 1980;24:75–81.
1166. Wang TJ, Chen MS, Shih YF, et al. Fundus abnormalities in a patient with type I Gaucher's disease with 12-year follow-up. Am J Ophthalmol 2005;139:359–62.
1167. East T, Savin LH. A case of Gaucher's disease with biopsy of the typical pingueculae. Br J Ophthalmol 1940;24:611–3.
1168. Petrohelos M, Tricoulis D, Kotsiras I, et al. Ocular manifestations of Gaucher's disease. Am J Ophthalmol 1975;80:1006–10.
1169. Sasaki T, Tsukahara S. New ocular findings in Gaucher's disease: report of two brothers. Ophthalmologica 1985;191:206–9.
1170. Yanoff M, Fine BS. Ocular pathology; a text and atlas, 2nd ed. Philadelphia: Harper & Row; 1982. p. 552.
1171. Abraham FA, Yatziv S, Russell A, et al. Electrophysiological and psychophysical findings in Hunter syndrome. Arch Ophthalmol 1974;91:181–6.
1172. Del Monte MA, Maumenee IH, Green WR, et al. Histopathology of Sanfilippo's syndrome. Arch Ophthalmol 1983;101:1255–62.
1173. Epstein RL. Inborn metabolic disorders and the eye. In: Peyman GA, Sanders DR, Goldberg MF, editors. Principles and practice of ophthalmology. Philadelphia: WB Saunders; 1980. p. 1729.
1174. Matalon R, Dorfman A. Hurler's syndrome, an α-l-iduronidase deficiency. Biochem Biophys Res Commun 1972;47:959–64.
1175. Sanfilippo SJ, Yunis J, Worthen HG. An unusual storage disease resembling the Hunter–Hurler syndrome. Am J Dis Child 1962;104:553.
1176. Scheie HG, Hambrick Jr GW, Barness LA. A newly recognized forme fruste of Hurler's disease (gargoylism). Am J Ophthalmol 1962;53:753–69.
1177. Usui T, Shirakashi M, Takagi M. Macular edema-like change and pseudo-papilledema in a case of Scheie syndrome. J Clin Neuro-Ophthalmol 1991;11:183–5.
1178. Pitz S, Ogun O, Bajbouj M, et al. Ocular changes in patients with mucopolysaccharidosis I receiving enzyme replacement therapy: a 4-year experience. Arch Ophthalmol 2007;125: 1353–6.
1179. Goldberg MF, Duke JR. Ocular histopathology in Hunter's syndrome; systemic mucopolysaccharidosis type II. Arch Ophthalmol 1967;77:503–12.
1180. Koliopoulos J, Bartsokas C, Kenyon K. Ocular manifestations of the mucopolysaccharidoses. Bull Soc Hellén Ophtalmol 1977;45:70–84.
1181. Lindsay S, Reilly WA, Gotham TH, et al. Gargoylism II. Study of pathologic lesions and clinical review of twelve cases. Am J Dis Child 1948;76:239–306.
1182. McDonnell JM, Green WR, Maumenee IH. Ocular histopathology of systemic mucopolysaccharidosis, Type II-A (Hunter syndrome, severe). Ophthalmology 1985;92:1772–9.
1183. Topping TM, Kenyon KR, Goldberg MF, et al. Ultrastructural ocular pathology of Hunter's syndrome; systemic mucopolysaccharidosis type II. Arch Ophthalmol 1971;86:164–77.
1184. Ashworth JL, Biswas S, Wraith E, et al. The ocular features of the mucopolysaccharidoses. Eye (Lond) 2006;20:553–63.
1185. Ashworth JL, Biswas S, Wraith E, et al. Mucopolysaccharidoses and the eye. Surv Ophthalmol 2006;51:1–17.
1186. Sato S, Maeda N, Watanabe H, et al. Multiple iridociliary cysts in patients with mucopolysaccharidoses. Br J Ophthalmol 2002;86:933–4.

1187. Dolman CL. Diagnosis of neurometabolic disorders by examination of skin biopsies and lymphocytes. Semin Diagn Pathol 1984;1:82–97.
1188. Summers CG, Purple RL, Krivit W. Ocular changes in the mucopolysaccharidoses after bone marrow transplantation; a preliminary report. Ophthalmology 1989;96:977–85.
1189. Riedel KG, Zwaan J, Kenyon KR. Ocular abnormalities in mucolipidoses IV. Am J Ophthalmol 1985;99:125–36.
1190. Spranger JW, Wiedemann HR. The genetic mucolipidoses; diagnosis and differential diagnosis. Humangenetik 1970;9:113–39.
1191. Traboulsi EI, Maumenee IH. Ophthalmologic findings in mucolipidosis III (pseudo-Hurler polydystrophy). Am J Ophthalmol 1986;102:592–7.
1192. Dierks T, Schlotawa L, Frese MA, et al. Molecular basis of multiple sulfatase deficiency, mucolipidosis II/III and Niemann–Pick C1 disease – Lysosomal storage disorders caused by defects of non-lysosomal proteins. Biochim Biophys Acta 2009;1793:710–25.
1193. Cathey SS, Kudo M, Tiede S, et al. Molecular order in mucolipidosis II and III nomenclature. Am J Med Genet A 2008;146A:512–3.
1194. Spranger J, Mucolipidosis I. Birth Defects 1975;11:279–82.
1195. Kirkham TH, Coupland SG, Guitton D. Sialidosis: the cherry-red spot–myoclonus syndrome. Can J Ophthalmol 1980;15:35–9.
1196. Rapin I, Goldfischer S, Katzman R. The cherry-red spot–myoclonus syndrome. Ann Neurol 1978;3:234–42.
1197. Sogg RL, Steinman L, Rathjen B. Cherry-red spot-myoclonus syndrome. Ophthalmology 1979;86:1861–73.
1198. Spranger J, Cantz M. Mucolipidosis I the cherry-red-spot–myoclonus syndrome and neuraminidase deficiency. Birth Defects 1978;14:105–12.
1199. Goldberg MF. Macular cherry-red spot and corneal haze in sialidosis (mucolipidosis type 1). Arch Ophthalmol 2008;126:1778.
1200. Heroman JW, Rychwalski P, Barr CC. Cherry red spot in sialidosis (mucolipidosis type I). Arch Ophthalmol 2008;126:270–1.
1201. Font RL, editor. Case presented at the joint meeting of the verhoeff and european ophthalmic pathology societies, April 25–28, 1971, London.
1202. Gass J. Stereoscopic atlas of macular diseases; diagnosis and treatment, 2nd ed. St. Louis: CV Mosby; 1977. p. 327.
1203. Pourjavan S, Fryns JP, Van Hove JL, et al. Ophthalmological findings in a patient with mucolipidosis III (pseudo-Hurler polydystrophy). A case report. Bull Soc Belge Ophtalmol 2002;286:19–24.
1204. Berman ER, Livni N, Shapira E. Congenital corneal clouding with abnormal systemic storage bodies; a new variant of mucolipidosis. J Pediatr 1974;84:519–26.
1205. Pradhan SM, Atchaneeyasakul LO, Appukuttan B, et al. Electronegative electroretinogram in mucolipidosis IV. Arch Ophthalmol 2002;120:45–50.
1206. Dobrovolny R, Liskova P, Ledvinova J, et al. Mucolipidosis IV: report of a case with ocular restricted phenotype caused by leaky splice mutation. Am J Ophthalmol 2007;143:663–71.
1207. Casteels I, Taylor DS, Lake BD, et al. Mucolipidosis type IV. Presentation of a mild variant. Ophthalmic Paediatr Genet 1992;13:205–10.
1208. Bach G. Mucolipidosis type IV. Mol Genet Metab 2001;73:197–203.
1209. Goldberg MF, Cotlier E, Fichenscher LG. Macular cherry-red spot, corneal clouding and β-galactosidase deficiency. Arch Intern Med 1971;128:387–98.
1210. Tsuji S, Yamada T, Tsutsumi A, et al. Neuraminidase deficiency and accumulation of sialic acid in lymphocytes in adult type sialidosis with partial beta-galactosidase deficiency. Ann Neurol 1982;11:541–3.
1211. Usui T, Sawaguchi S, Abe H. Late-infantile type galactosialidosis; histopathology of the retina and optic nerve. Arch Ophthalmol 1991;109:542–6.
1212. Patel MS, Callahan JW, Zhang S, et al. Early-infantile galactosialidosis: prenatal presentation and postnatal follow-up. Am J Med Genet 1999;85:38–47.
1213. Landau D, Meisner I, Zeigler M, et al. Hydrops fetalis in four siblings caused by galactosialidosis. Isr J Med Sci 1995;31:321–2.
1214. Carvalho S, Martins M, Fortuna A, et al. Galactosialidosis presenting as nonimmune fetal hydrops: a case report. Prenat Diagn 2009;29:895–6.
1215. Hisahara S, Fujita T, Yoshizawa K, et al. Two siblings of galactosialidosis with marked progression of cardiac involvement during 10 years. Rinsho Shinkeigaku 1996;36:562–5.
1216. Usui T, Abe H, Takagi M, et al. Electroretinogram and visual evoked potential in two siblings with adult form galactosialidosis. Metab Pediatr Syst Ophthalmol 1993;16:19–22.
1217. Bateman JB, Philippart M. Ocular features of the Hagberg-Santavuori syndrome. Am J Ophthalmol 1986;102:262–71.
1218. Batten FE. Cerebral degeneration with symmetrical changes in the maculae in two members of a family. Trans Ophthalmol Soc UK 1903;23:386–90.
1219. Brod RD, Packer AJ, Van Dyk HJL. Diagnosis of neuronal ceroid lipofuscinosis by ultrastructural examination of peripheral blood lymphocytes. Arch Ophthalmol 1987;105:1388–93.
1220. De Venecia G, Shapiro M. Neuronal ceroid lipofuscinosis; a retinal trypsin digest study. Ophthalmology 1984;91:1406–10.
1221. Goebel HH, Fix JD, Zeman W. The fine structure of the retina in neuronal ceroid-lipofuscinosis. Am J Ophthalmol 1974;77:25–39.
1222. Goebel HH, Klein H, Santavuori P, et al. Ultrastructural studies of the retina in infantile neuronal ceroid-lipofuscinosis. Retina 1988;8:59–67.
1223. Goebel HH, Zeman W, Damaske E. An ultrastructural study of the retina in the Jansky–Bielschowsky type of neuronal ceroid-lipofuscinosis. Am J Ophthalmol 1977;83:70–9.
1224. Gottlob I, Leipert KP, Kohlschütter A, et al. Electrophysiological findings of neuronal ceroid lipofuscinosis in heterozygotes. Graefes Arch Clin Exp Ophthalmol 1988;226:516–21.
1225. Hittner HM, Zeller RS. Ceroid-lipofuscinosis (Batten disease); fluorescein angiography, electrophysiology, histopathology, ultrastructure, and a review of amaurotic familial idiocy. Arch Ophthalmol 1975;93:178–83.
1226. Raitta C, Santavuori P. Ophthalmological findings in infantile type of so-called neuronal ceroid lipofuscinosis. Acta Ophthalmol 1973;51:755–63.
1227. Schochet Jr SS, Font RL, Morris III HH. Jansky–Bielschowsky form of neuronal ceroid-lipofuscinosis; ocular pathology of the Batten–Vogt syndrome. Arch Ophthalmol 1980;98:1083–8.
1228. Spalton DJ, Taylor DSI, Sanders MD. Juvenile Batten's disease: an ophthalmological assessment of 26 patients. Br J Ophthalmol 1980;64:726–32.
1229. Traboulsi EI, Green WR, Luckenbach MW, et al. Neuronal ceroid lipofuscinosis; ocular histopathologic and electron microscopic studies in the late infantile, juvenile, and adult forms. Graefes Arch Clin Exp Ophthalmol 1987;225:391–402.
1230. Zeman W. Batten disease: ocular features, differential diagnosis and diagnosis by enzyme analysis. Birth Defects 1976;12:441–53.
1231. Zeman W. Studies in the neuronal ceroid-lipofuscinosis. J Neuropathol Exp Neurol 1974;33:1–12.
1232. Collins J, Holder GE, Herbert H, et al. Batten disease: features to facilitate early diagnosis. Br J Ophthalmol 2006;90:1119–24.
1233. Mole SE. The genetic spectrum of human neuronal ceroid-lipofuscinoses. Brain Pathol 2004;14:70–6.
1234. Mole SE, Williams RE, Goebel HH. Correlations between genotype, ultrastructural morphology and clinical phenotype in the neuronal ceroid lipofuscinoses. Neurogenetics 2005;6:107–26.
1235. Hainsworth DP, Liu GT, Hamm CW, et al. Fundoscopic and angiographic appearance in the neuronal ceroid lipofuscinoses. Retina 2009;29:657–68.
1236. Weleber RG, Gupta N, Trzupek KM, et al. Electroretinographic and clinicopathologic correlations of retinal dysfunction in infantile neuronal ceroid lipofuscinosis (infantile Batten disease). Mol Genet Metab 2004;83:128–37.
1237. Eksandh LB, Ponjavic VB, Munroe PB, et al. Full-field ERG in patients with Batten/Spielmeyer-Vogt disease caused by mutations in the CLN3 gene. Ophthalmic Genet 2000;21:69–77.
1238. Bensaoula T, Shibuya H, Katz ML, et al. Histopathologic and immunocytochemical analysis of the retina and ocular tissues in Batten disease. Ophthalmology 2000;107:1746–53.
1239. Ivan CS, Saint-Hilaire MH, Christensen TG, et al. Adult-onset neuronal ceroid lipofuscinosis type B in an African-American. Mov Disord 2005;20:752–4.
1240. Tyni T, Kivela T, Lappi M, et al. Ophthalmologic findings in long-chain 3-hydroxyacyl-CoA dehydrogenase deficiency caused by the G1528C mutation: a new type of hereditary metabolic chorioretinopathy. Ophthalmology 1998;105:810–24.
1241. Fahnehjelm KT, Holmstrom G, Ying L, et al. Ocular characteristics in 10 children with long-chain 3-hydroxyacyl-CoA dehydrogenase deficiency: a cross-sectional study with long-term follow-up. Acta Ophthalmol 2008;86:329–37.
1242. Tyni T, Paetau A, Strauss AW, et al. Mitochondrial fatty acid beta-oxidation in the human eye and brain: implications for the retinopathy of long-chain 3-hydroxyacyl-CoA dehydrogenase deficiency. Pediatr Res 2004;56:744–50.
1243. Lund AM, Skovby F, Vestergaard H, et al. Clinical and biochemical monitoring of patients with fatty acid oxidation disorders. J Inherit Metab Dis 2010;33:495–500.
1244. Bellmann C, Neveu MM, Scholl HP, et al. Localized retinal electrophysiological and fundus autofluorescence imaging abnormalities in maternal inherited diabetes and deafness. Invest Ophthalmol Vis Sci 2004;45:2355–60.
1245. Daily MJ, Mets MB. Fenestrated sheen macular dystrophy. Arch Ophthalmol 1984;102:855–6.

CHAPTER 6

Macular Dysfunction Caused by Retinal Vascular Diseases

Diseases affecting primarily the retinal arteries, capillaries, and veins or any combination of the three may be the underlying cause of central vision loss. Angiography provides information concerning alterations in retinal blood flow, the normal retinal vascular pattern, and retinal vascular permeability. In addition, in the sensory retina, which normally has very little extracellular space, stereo angiography provides a means of pictorially defining expansions of the extracellular space produced by extracellular fluid accompanying alterations in vascular permeability and cellular destruction. Optical coherence tomography (OCT) has enhanced the ability to define these lesions in a vertical cross-section and three-dimensional layout. For a more detailed discussion of the basic pathophysiologic and histopathologic changes occurring in retinal vascular disorders and their correlation with fluorescein angiographic and biomicroscopic changes, the reader should see Chapter 2.

RETINAL VASCULAR ANOMALIES

A variety of minor anomalies of the retinal vascular tree occur commonly and are unassociated with visual morbidity. Some of the vascular anomalies, however, may cause visual loss.

Hereditary Retinal Artery Tortuosity

Recurrent macular hemorrhages occurring in family members with congenital arteriolar tortuosity constitute a recognized syndrome (Figure 6.01A–C).[1–6] Visual loss in these patients may occur spontaneously or following relatively minor trauma (see the discussion on Valsalva maculopathy, p. 730 in Chapter 8). Retinal arteriolar tortuosity may increase with age, particularly during adolescence.[7,8] The tortuosity affects primarily the second- and third-order retinal arterioles in the macular area and the veins are spared. Fluorescein angiography has failed to disclose any primary alterations in the retinal vascular tree that would account for the predilection for hemorrhages. The pathogenesis is unknown. Despite recurrent bleeding, vision usually returns to normal. Retinal bleeding during scleral buckling procedure has been reported.[9] There is no evidence that a systemic hemorrhagic diathesis is present in patients with this disease, which is inherited as an autosomal-dominant trait. Families with increased nail bed capillary tortuosities, carotid aneurysm, and microscopic hematuria have been described.[10–12] Congenital retinal arteriolar tortuosity must be differentiated from other diseases associated with acquired retinal vascular tortuosity, including polycythemia, leukemia, dysproteinemia, sickle-cell disease, familial dysautonomia, mucopolysaccharidosis VI, and Fabry's disease. Pulsatile three-dimensional arteriolar tortuosity, previously reported in patients with coarctation of the aorta, rarely occurs now because of early surgical intervention.[13]

6.01 Retinal vascular anomalies.

A–C: Congenital retinal arterial tortuosity and spontaneous macular hemorrhage in a 26-year-old man who developed loss of central vision in the right eye while weight-lifting. He had had a similar episode in both eyes previously. Each time the hemorrhages cleared and he regained 20/20 acuity. He was of Eastern European descent and had two paternal first cousins with the same ocular problem.
D–F: Congenital retinal arterial loop in an asymptomatic boy.
G–I: Congenital retinal arterial malformation in a young asymptomatic woman with 20/20 visual acuity.
J–L: Congenital venous loop in an asymptomatic young woman.

(A–C, courtesy of Dr. Donald J. D'Amico.)

Spontaneous retinal hemorrhages may occur in multiple family members in the absence of related systemic disease or retinal arterial tortuosity.[7]

Inherited Retinal Venous Beading

Meredith described five affected members in two generations with sausagelike beading of the major retinal veins and conjunctival venules, focal retinal infarctions, altered retinal vascular permeability, and in some cases abnormalities of arteriolar and venular distribution.[14] Large venules crossed the horizontal raphe in some cases. Three members had retinal and/or optic disc neovascularization and vitreous hemorrhage. Some members had renal disease (Alport's disease) and decreased leukocyte counts. Stewart and Gitter reported four affected members of two generations with retinal venous beading but no conjunctival vessel tortuosity.[15] The affected members had low to normal neutrophil leukocyte counts that differed significantly from unaffected members.

Retinal Venous Tortuosity in Infants

Neonates born to mothers who smoke during pregnancy have a higher incidence of venous dilation and tortuosity, arteriolar straightening and narrowing, and intraretinal hemorrhages. This is likely the result of a combination of higher hematocrit and higher peripheral vascular resistance in these babies. All vascular changes correct by age 6 months.[16] Infants with congenital heart diseases show a higher incidence of retinal vascular tortuosity (46%), more so those with cyanotic heart disease, low hematocrit, and low oxygen saturation.[17]

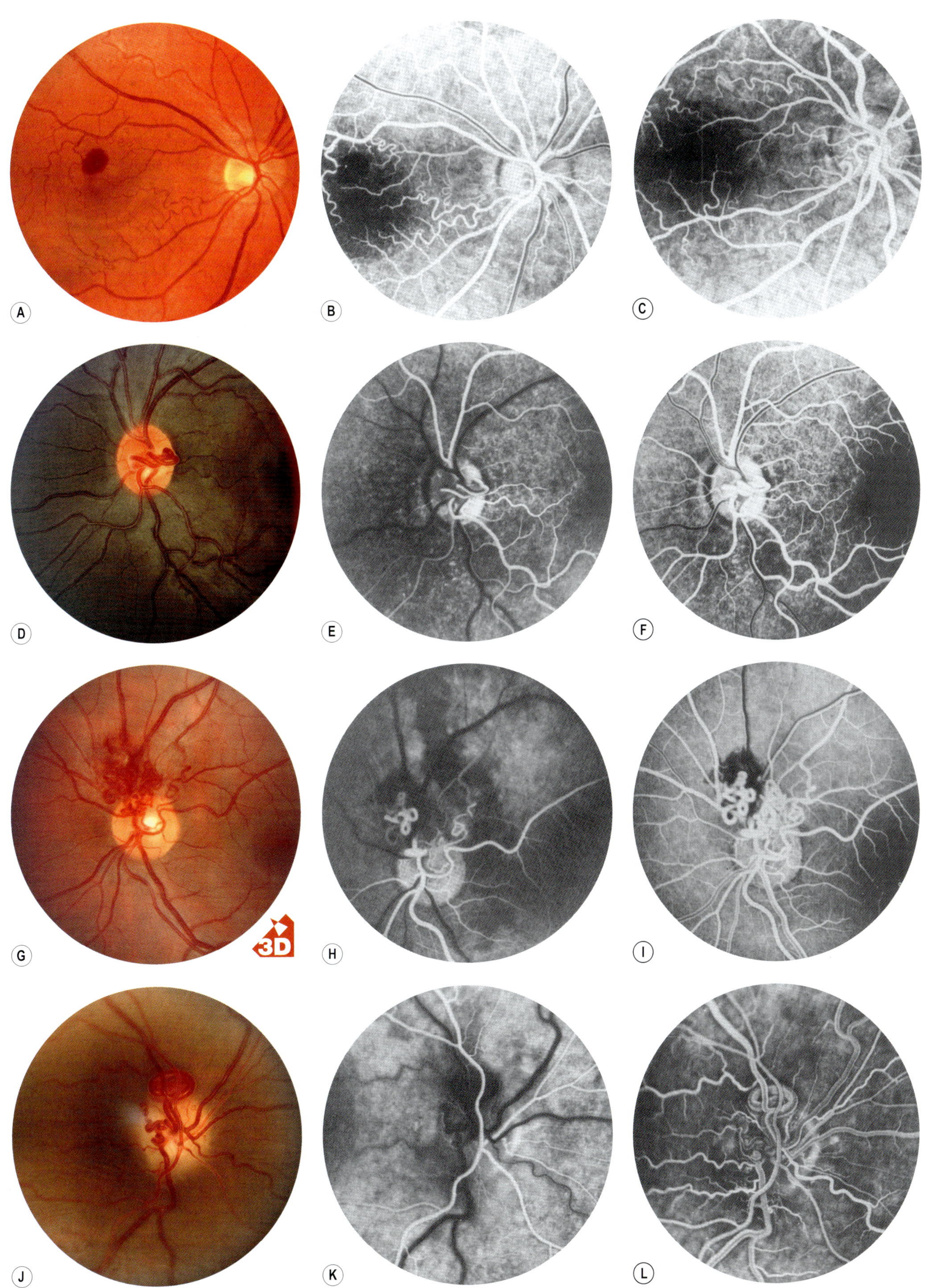
A
B
C
D
E
F
G
3D
H
I
J
K
L

Congenital Prepapillary Vascular Loops

Dilated loops involving either the veins or the arteries may occur in and around the optic nerve head (Figure 6.01 D–L).[18–29] Loops involving the retinal arteries are more common than those involving veins (4:1).[21] Retinal arterial loops may arise on or near the optic disc from a major branch retinal artery, the central retinal artery, or a cilioretinal artery (Figure 6.01D–F). They extend anteriorly into the vitreous, are composed of one or more twists, and usually supply one of the retinal quadrants. The loops often exhibit movement within the vitreous and cast a shadow on the surrounding fundus. They may pulsate. They occasionally occur bilaterally, may be familial, and may be partly surrounded by glial or fibrous sheaths.[22,24] Retinal circulation time in the affected quadrant may be slightly increased. There is a high incidence of cilioretinal arteries in these eyes, and they often supply much of the retinal circulation.[21,26] A small percentage of these patients may lose vision secondary to occlusion of the arterial loop (Figure 6.02A–G),[18,19,21,23,26,27] vitreous hemorrhage,[20,21,27] amaurosis fugax,[21] and hyphema.[21] Thrombosis or twisting of the loop probably causes the obstruction (Figure 6.02A–G). Histologically the artery comprising the loop is of normal structure.[28] The pathogenesis of the vitreous hemorrhage occurring in and around these loops is uncertain but probably is caused by rupture of small vessels near the base of the loop caused by its movement.

6.02 Prepapillary loop with branch retinal artery occlusion.

A–G: This 17-year-old female developed a sudden temporal field defect in her left eye. She had a history of sickle-cell trait but was otherwise normal. Her visual acuity was 20/25 in each eye. A prepapillary loop emanated from the disc along with retinal opacification in the upper nasal quadrant secondary of a branch retinal artery to occlusion within the loop. The retinal color recovered in 4 weeks but the visual field defect remained. Thrombotic occlusion of the communication from the loop to the superonasal branch retinal artery was noted (arrow).

Congenital macrovessel

H–J: A 34-year-old male presented with a 3-year history of type 2 diabetes. Visual acuity was 20/15 in both eyes. Dilated fundus examination of the right eye showed a large macrovessel coursing the macula. The macrovessel was a vein and the angiogram showed it draining into the superotemporal vein after crossing the horizontal raphe and lateral to the fovea and dipping back inferior to the fovea and recrossing nasal to the fovea.

(A–G, courtesy of Dr. Franco Recchia; H–J, from Jager et al.,[1361] reprinted with permission from *Retina*. H, Also, Yannuzzi, Lawrence J., The Retinal Atlas, Saunders 2010, 978-0-7020-3320-9, p.384.)

Congenital prepapillary venous loops (Figure 6.01J–L) and macroretinal vessels should be differentiated from acquired dilated venous collateral channels caused by retinal venous obstruction (see Figure 6.81J and K) and meningioma of the optic nerve (see Figure 15.16).

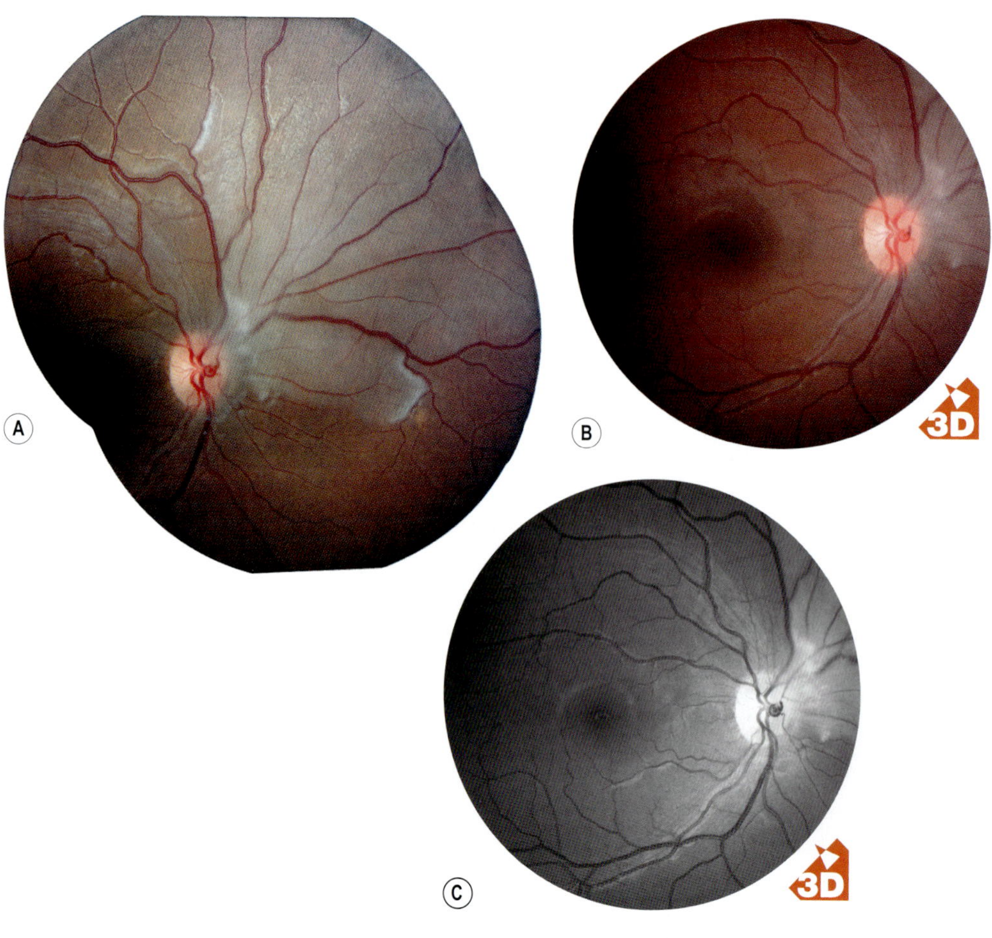

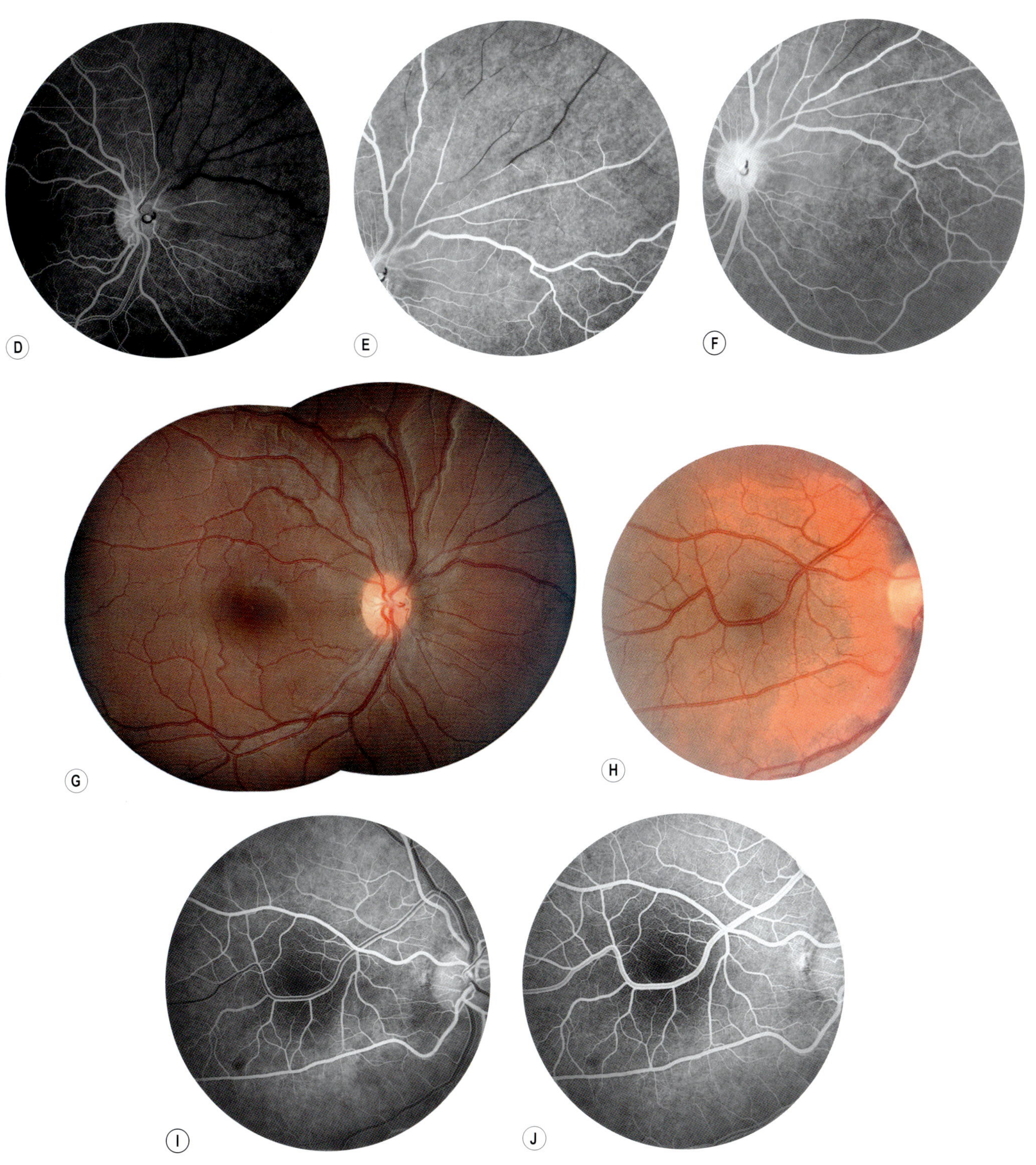
D
E
F
G
H
I
J

Congenital Retinal Macrovessels and Arteriovenous Communications

A large aberrant retinal vessel, more often a vein than artery, may extend from the optic disc into the central macular area, where it typically sends tributaries across the horizontal raphe (Figures 6.02H–J and 6.03A–I).[30,31] In some patients, both an artery and a vein are affected. Visual function is usually normal. Fluorescein angiography typically shows no permeability alterations but may show small areas of capillary nonperfusion and focal capillary dilations (Figure 6.03C and D). In some cases the capillary bed separating the dilated artery and vein may be normal (Figure 6.02H–J). In others there is a direct arteriovenous anastomosis (Figure 6.03E–G).[32] Changes in blood flow or permeability within these communications may precipitate loss of visual function (Figure 6.03A and B, and E–G) and are reported following bungee jumping. These malformations typically occur unilaterally in single or multiple sites. There is a predilection for involvement of the papillomacular bundle area and the superotemporal quadrant.[33] Both sexes are affected. Detection of the anomaly usually occurs on routine examination. Retinal macrovessels may occasionally be associated with similar vascular anomalies affecting the conjunctiva and mouth (Figure 6.03J–L). Macrovessels are isolated findings and should be differentiated from large-caliber retinal vessels (artery or vein) associated with anomalies such as Coats' disease, retinal capillary hemangioma, familial exudative vitreoretinopathy (FEVR), incontinentia pigmenti, and other peripheral vascular occlusive diseases.

Retinal arteriovenous anomalies have been subdivided into groups, depending on the severity of the anomaly.[33,34] Archer's group 1 comprises patients with retinal macrovessels with interposition of an arteriolar or abnormal capillary plexus between the major communicating artery and vein. These well-compensated arteriovenous communications rarely extend to involve the papillary vasculature and are rarely associated with cerebrovascular malformations.

6.03 Congenital retinal macrovessels.

A and **B**: Macular hemorrhage occurring in a 50-year-old man who on awakening noted a central scotoma caused by a retinal hemorrhage associated with a congenital macroartery and vein. His visual acuity was 20/40.
C and **D**: Microaneurysms (arrows) associated with congenital macroartery and vein. There was minimal staining of the microaneurysms.
E–G: Blurred vision occurred in this healthy boy with macrovessels associated with angiographic evidence of arteriovenous shunting (arrow, F), and hypoperfusion of the juxtafoveal retinal capillary network (G).
H–L: Congenital retinal macroveins (arrows, H and I) associated with macrovessels of the conjunctiva (J) and the dorsal (K) and ventral side (L) of the tongue in an apparently healthy 51-year-old man. Computed tomography of the brain revealed multiple venous anomalies.

(C and D, courtesy of Dr. J. S. Cohen.)

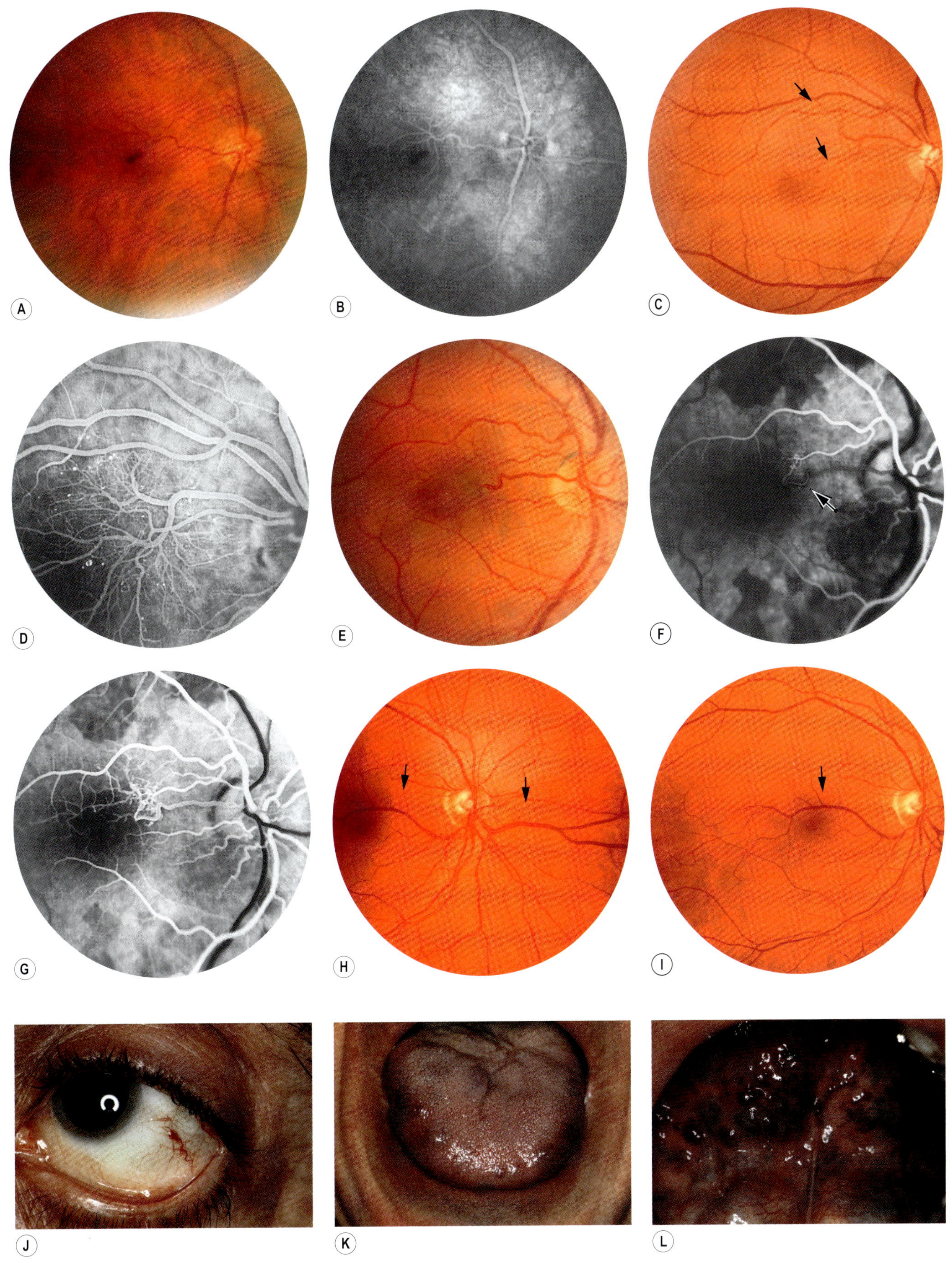
A
B
C
D
E
F
G
H
I
J
K
L

In group 3 patients (Figure 6.05) there are many anastomosing channels of large caliber that are so intertwined and convoluted that separation into their arterial and venous components may be difficult. Visual acuity is usually poor. Ophthalmoscopically and angiographically, the retina may show perivascular sheathing, exudation, and pigmentary degeneration. Some eyes may be blind from birth. Patients with severe retinal involvement are the most likely to have periorbital or cerebral involvement (Wyburn–Mason syndrome).[31,33,34,37,40,44,49,52,54,55]

Complications of these vascular anomalies include intraretinal hemorrhage, aneurysm formation with intraretinal exudation, retinal artery occlusion, Valsalva retinopathy,[56] central and peripheral retinal vein occlusions, neovascular glaucoma, vitreous hemorrhage, arterial macroaneurysm,[57] and macular hole (Figure 6.04B, E, G, and I).[36,51,58–60] Severe visual loss caused by occlusion of the malformation occurs infrequently (Figure 6.04D and E). Slow visual loss may occur because of mechanical compression of the optic nerve.[44] Spontaneous regression of the lesions may occur occasionally.[49,61] The histopathology of arteriovenous communications identical to those seen in humans has been described in rhesus monkeys (Figure 6.04J–L).[38,45] Anomalous arteriovenous communications should be distinguished from those acquired secondary to peripheral vascular occlusive disease (see Figure 6.81J and K).[62]

Photocoagulation treatment may occasionally be warranted in those patients who develop exudative maculopathy.[51]

For a discussion of congenital retinal telangiectasis and retinal vascular hamartomas, see p. 514 in Chapter 6 and Chapter 13, respectively.

6.05 Retinal arteriovenous malformation.

A and **B**: Ths 16-year-old female was seen for intractable headaches and migraine with aura. Her vision was 20/15 in each eye. She had several anomalous vessels emanating from the disc and peripapillary area. Some of the larger-caliber vessels appeared to communicate with the choroidal circulation as they dipped into the substance of the retina while the others were part of a network of vessels seen on the disc and superficial peripapillary retina. She had had an inflammatory workup, which showed minimally elevated angiotensin-converting enzyme. Magnetic resonance imaging (MRI) of the head did not reveal other anomalous foci. She was treated medically for headaches and migraine.

C–F: This 28-year-old male with count-fingers vision in the right and 20/20 vision in the left eye complained of several episodes of headache for the past 2 years. He had a previous MRI that showed arteriovenous malformations in his brain. A large arteriovenous malformation simulating a bag of worms was seen in the right fundus involving the vessels on the disc and in the macula associated with dilated and tortuous retinal arteries and veins extending up to the periphery. One large vessel that dipped into the retina communicating with the choroid showed whitening of its wall (C and F). Fluorescein angiogram showed rapid filling of the malformation, making it difficult to determine if the majority of the vessels filled from the choroid or from the retinal side – they likely filled simultaneously from the choroid and retina (D and E). He was treated symptomatically for the migrainous headache.

Retinal capillary hamartoma.

G–K: This 34-year-old male noted metamorphopsia in his right eye for a few months. A 2 × 2 disc diameter subtle elevation (arrows) was noted in his right eye just temporal to the fovea associated with cystoid swelling of the temporal fovea (G). An angiogram revealed deep dilated plexus of vessels with several bulbous dilatations in the inner retina (I and J). The anomalous capillary plexus leaked with fluid accumulation into cystoid spaces (K). The malformation appears to be an isolated hamartoma of the retinal capillaries without an astrocytic component. There was no evidence of hamartomas elsewhere in the eye or body, thus ruling out tuberous sclerosis.

(A and B, courtesy of Dr. Patrick Lavin; G–K, courtesy of Dr. David Weinberg.)

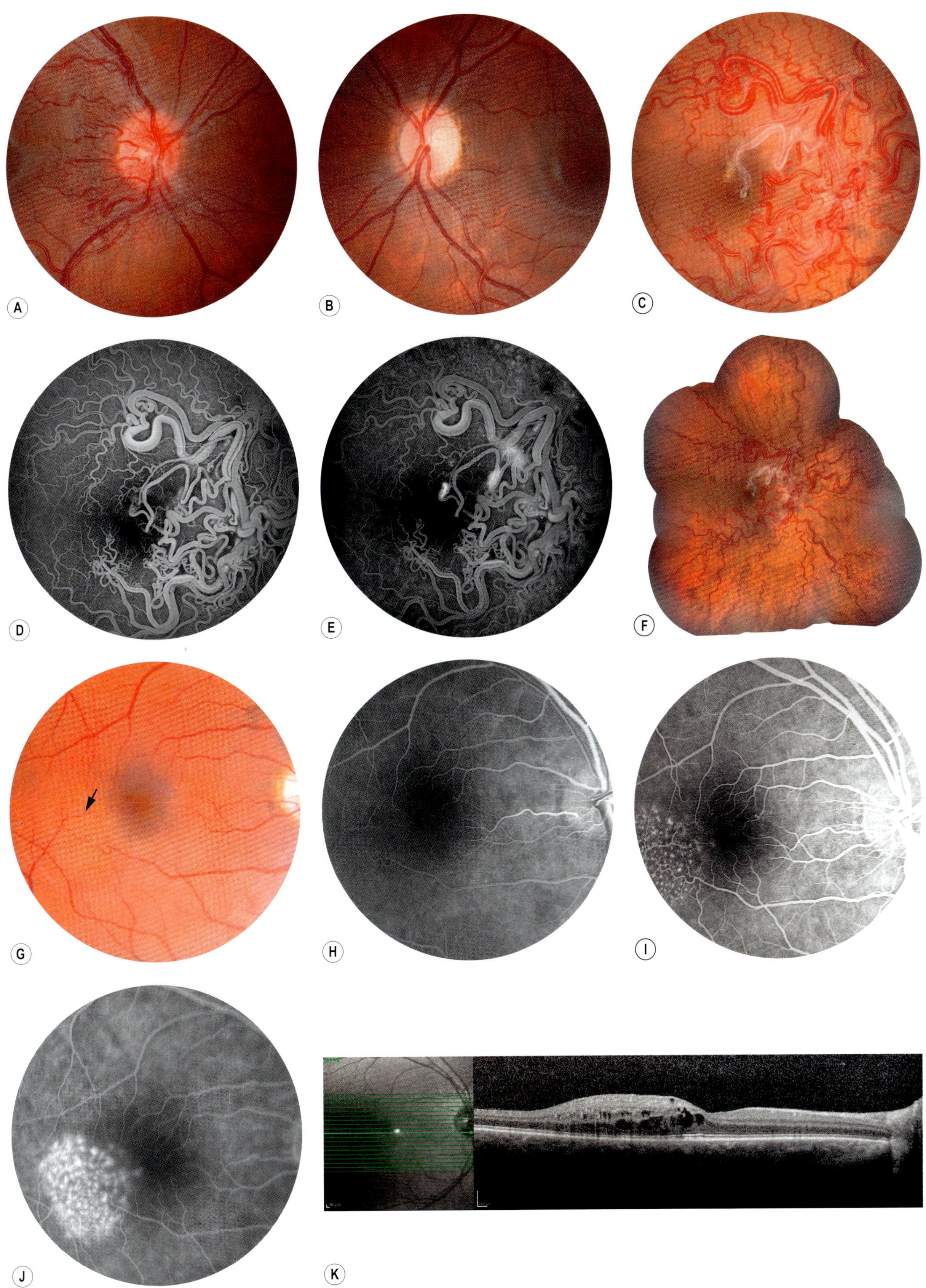
A
B
C
D
E
F
G
H
I
J
K

Anomalous Foveal Avascular Zone

Controversy exists about the development of the foveal avascular zone (FAZ); one school believes the future FAZ is initially vascularized, and by a process similar to apoptosis the capillaries are lost to form a capillary-free zone. Absence of the FAZ and multilayered foveola seen in retinopathy of prematurity (ROP) is explained by this theory.[63] The other school studied seven retinal whole mounts aged between 26 and 41 weeks' gestation and found a blood vessel-free zone in all retinas, including at the 26-week gestational age.[64] This ring was open temporally at age 26 weeks and closed by 37 weeks' gestation to form a complete circle. It is believed that the superior and inferior blood vessels grow faster than the horizontal raphe and the nasal vessels grow faster than the temporal ones, resulting in the open temporal ring till about the 37-week gestational age. The diameter of the FAZ gradually decreased in size from 500 μm at 35 weeks to 300–350 μm at 40 weeks. After birth, the accelerated retinal growth stretches the foveal pit, making it wider and shallower; this remodeling of the FAZ continues to occur even up to 15 months to eventually yield an FAZ that is 500–750 μm in size.

It is likely various factors influence formation of the foveal vascular zone during development: astrocytes, macular pigment, ganglion cells, vasoendothelial growth factor (VEGF) levels and their alteration in hypoxia, to consider a few.[65–68] Whatever the insult that allows blood vessels to invade the future foveal pit during development (Figure 6.06), this in turn likely prevents normal foveal pit formation, resulting in a multilayered foveal center (Figure 6.06E, F, K, and L). Hypoplastic fovea with small or absent FAZ associated with multilayered foveal pit on OCT is a feature of albinism, chiasmal misrouting,[69] ROP, and aniridia. It is likely we will discover more developmental vasculopathies and other disorders that harbor a multilayered foveal center.

6.06 Absent foveal avascular zone (FAZ) and foveal pit.

A–F: This 40-year-old male had a history of "jumping eyes" with subnormal vision since childhood. When his son was evaluated for nystagmus at age 6 months, he was sent in for a retina consultation to help find a diagnosis for the infant. He was best corrected to 20/60 in each eye with a moderately high myopic refractive error. He was not albinotic. The fundus had a blonde coloration with orange color at the posterior pole. A fluorescein angiogram showed no specific abnormality. Due to the myopia and light fundus background, a good perfusion of the fovea vascular pattern was not obtainable. Scanning through the entire macula, a foveal depression could not be found on optical coherence tomography (E and F), suggesting arrested foveal development as the cause of the subnormal vision and nystagmus.

G–L: This 16-year-old girl could only be corrected to 20/25 all through her refractive evaluations for the previous 10 years. Her color vision was full bilaterally and she had no nystagmus. The right eye had an anomalous architecture of the retinal arteries with two branches each supplying the superior and inferior posterior pole (G). The left eye's architecture appeared within the normal variation (H). Careful examination of the fovea and its angiogram revealed possible small foveal avascular zone. Optical coherence tomography through the fovea could not localize the foveal pit in either eye (K and L), confirming the arrested foveolar development as a plausible cause of the subnormal vision.

(G–L, courtesy of Dr. Janice C. Law.)

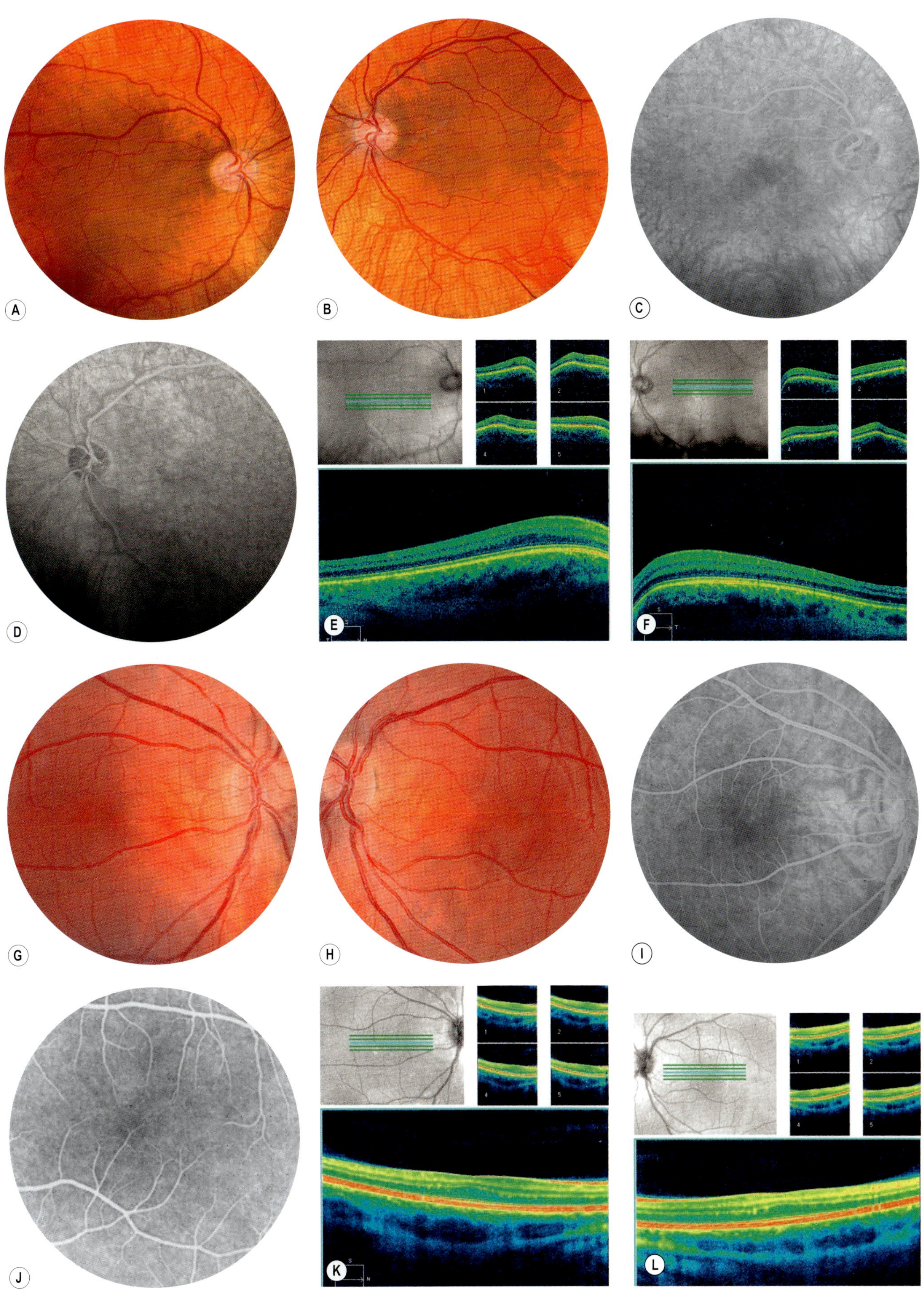
A
B
C
D
E
F
G
H
I
J
K
L

OBSTRUCTIVE RETINAL ARTERIAL DISEASES

Pathophysiologically, diseases may cause obstruction of the retinal arterial blood flow, primarily through one or a combination of the following processes: (1) embolism; (2) vascular narrowing; (3) thrombosis; (4) arterial spasm; (5) vascular narrowing caused by extravascular disease; and (6) reduction in blood flow caused by carotid or ophthalmic artery obstruction, lowered systemic blood pressure, or elevated intraocular pressure.

Embolic Obstruction

Obstruction of the retinal circulation may be caused by emboli derived from within the human body (endogenous emboli) or from without (exogenous emboli).

Endogenous Embolization From the Major Arteries and Heart

Emboli derived from ulcerated atheromatous plaques in the carotid artery, occurring either spontaneously or during manipulation of the carotid artery during arteriography or surgery, are probably the most common cause of major retinal arterial occlusions (Figures 6.07–6.10).[70–84] Other important sources of emboli are diseased or anomalous heart valves. Embolization from the heart may occur spontaneously or during open-heart surgery or coronary artery angioplasty.[85–88] Patients with embolic occlusion usually experience sudden monocular loss of vision. This loss may be antedated by episodes of transient loss of monocular vision lasting 1–2 minutes (amaurosis fugax) in 20–25% of cases, and transient ischemic attacks in approximately 5–10% of cases.[89] The average age of onset of symptoms is approximately 60 years. Fewer than 10% of occlusions occur in persons under 30 years of age.[85,90] Occlusion is more common in men than in women. In all, 50–75% of patients over 40 years of age with retinal artery occlusion will have clinical evidence of carotid artery disease.[91,92] In younger patients the emboli are usually derived from heart valves damaged by rheumatic fever, congenital anomalies of the heart valves and great vessels, or prolapse of the mitral valve (Barlow's syndrome) (Figure 6.07E–I).[85,93,94] Most patients with central retinal artery occlusion (CRAO) will have a small area of preservation of light perception caused by the presence of small cilioretinal arteries (Figure 6.08D and K, arrow).[95] In patients with no light perception, the physician should look for evidence of abnormalities of choroidal and optic nerve head circulation.[96,97]

6.07 Central retinal artery obstruction.

A–D: Central retinal artery obstruction occurred 1 week after replacement of an aortic and mitral valve for rheumatic heart disease in a 55-year-old man whose visual acuity consisted of light perception only. Note the cherry-red spot and "boxcar" formation of blood in the retinal vessels (A). Angiography shows marked retinal artery obstruction and retrograde filling of proximal retinal veins via the optic disc collateral circulation (B–D).
E and **F**: Central retinal artery obstruction in a 19-year-old woman. Angiography shows fluorescein leakage from perifoveal arterioles.
G–I: Central retinal artery obstruction and retinal hemorrhages in a 29-year-old man with rheumatic mitral valvular disease and subacute bacterial endocarditis. Note the cherry-red spot, "boxcar" formation, and angiographic evidence of marked increase in retinal circulation time.
J–L: Patchy retinal ischemia and delayed perfusion of both the retinal and choroidal circulation caused by ophthalmic artery obstruction in a 73-year-old hypertensive man with ultrasonographic evidence of thyroid ophthalmopathy. He experienced sudden almost complete loss of vision in the right eye several weeks before these photographs. He noted partial return of peripheral vision soon afterward. Angiography showed that dye appeared in the choroid at 21 seconds and in the central retinal artery at 25 seconds (K and L).

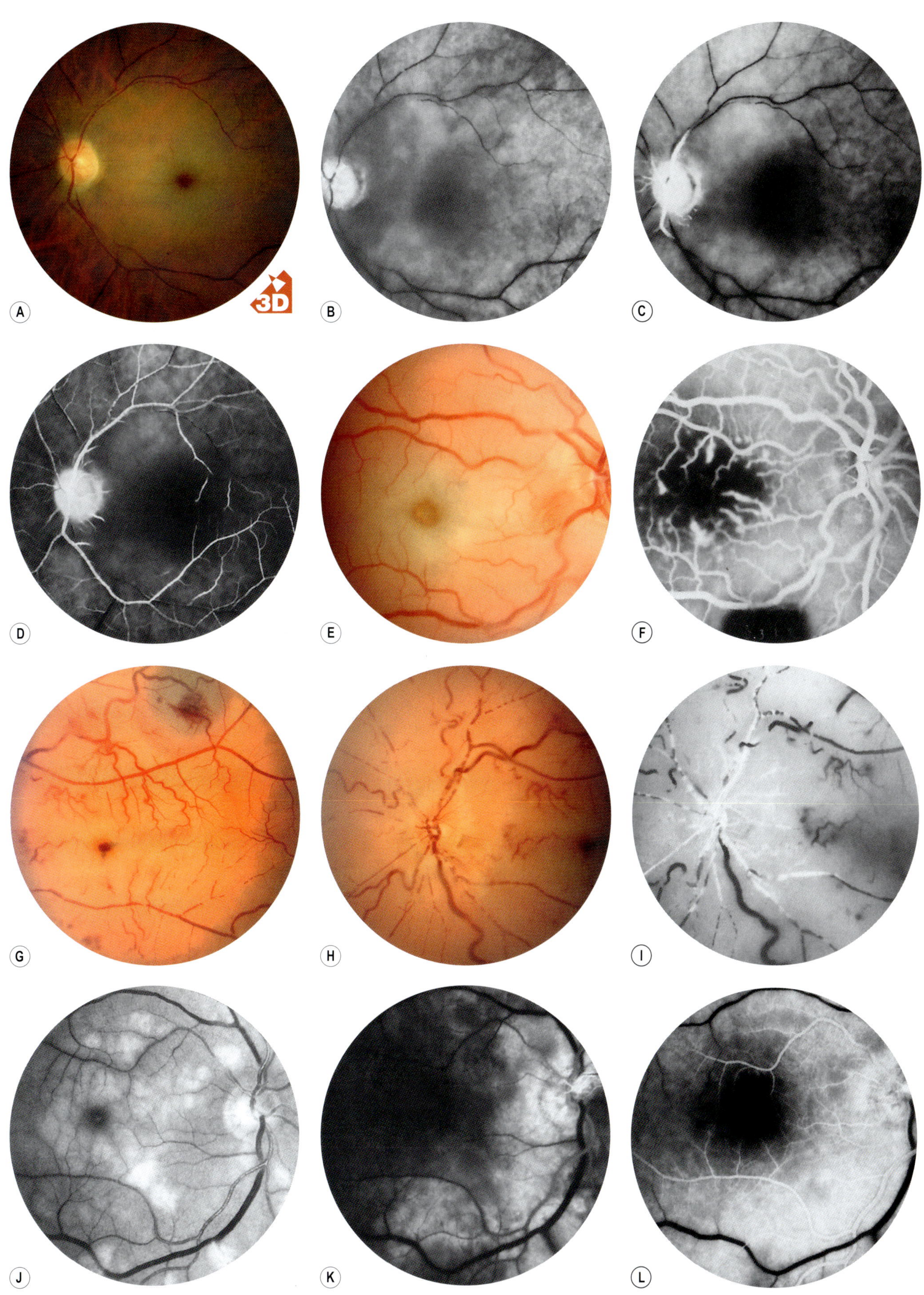
3D
A
B
C
D
E
F
G
H
I
J
K
L

If retinal artery obstruction is incomplete and of short duration, only a slight gray haze may result, and little or no permanent damage to the retina may occur (Figure 6.09G and H).[71,98] If the block is more complete, progressive whitening and swelling of the inner half of the retina develop (Figure 6.07A and E). These physical changes are caused by denaturation and breakdown of the normally transparent intracellular protein, an increase in the intracellular water, and, finally, complete cellular necrosis (Figure 6.10I).[99,100] Acute ischemic whitening of the retina is a more accurate descriptive term for this change than retinal edema, which is best reserved for retinal thickening secondary to the accumulation of serous fluid escaping from retinal capillaries into the extracellular space, producing multiple cystoid changes in the outer retinal layers.[101] Acute ischemic retinopathy may be localized (cotton-wool patch), as in small arteriolar obstruction, or more diffuse, as in obstruction of the central retinal artery or one of its major branches. Intensified retinal whitening along the peripheral edge of ischemic areas that cut across nerve fiber layers is related to the damming effect of the orthograde and retrograde axoplasmic flow.[102]

Patients with visual loss caused by acute retinal artery obstruction usually seek treatment in the first week after obstruction and show a variety of clinical pictures, depending on the portion of the retinal arterial tree involved. In central retinal artery obstruction, widespread ischemic whitening of the retina occurs, except in the foveolar area (cherry-red spot), whose blood supply is derived from the choriocapillaris (Figures 6.07A and 6.08G), and except in some patients in whom focal peripapillary areas are supplied by a cilioretinal artery. Absence of the cherry-red spot in patients with CRAO should suggest the presence of choroidal vascular ischemia as well.[103] In some patients, particularly those with chronic systemic hypertension, transient obstruction of the central retinal artery may produce a peculiar picture of multiple gray patches of retinal whitening simulating that seen in Purtscher's retinopathy (Figures 6.07J–L; see Figures 6.23H, and 6.25J). This pattern is probably the result of regional variations in arterial perfusion that occur normally or that are the result of formation of collateral pathways of retinal capillary flow caused by focal narrowing of the origin of the first-order arterioles in hypertensive patients. The visual prognosis in patients showing this pattern of retinal whitening is relatively good.[104]

Branch artery obstruction may be overlooked or mistaken for other disease processes, particularly if the patient has a central scotoma caused by obstruction of a cilioretinal artery or other small arterioles supplying most of the macular area.[97,105–107] Varying degrees of arterial narrowing occur. Segmentation of the blood column indicates marked slowing of arterial flow (Figure 6.07A, H, and I). Often one or more emboli are visible in the arterial tree, either as a large embolus at a bifurcation of the central retinal artery on the optic nerve head (Figures 6.09 G and H and 6.10K and L) or as one or more emboli lodged at distal bifurcations (Figure 6.09D).

6.08 Central retinal artery occlusion (CRAO) with neovascularization of disc.

A–F: This 68-year-old hypertensive diabetic woman with a history of end-stage renal disease presented with light perception vision in her right eye. The posterior pole was opacified and the blood column in all the retinal arterioles and some of the veins were fragmented (A). A tiny corkscrew vessel was present on the optic disc. A small zone of retina adjacent to the superotemporal edge of the disc appeared to be perfused by a cilioretinal artery. The left eye had scattered microaneurysms and dot hemorrhages from diabetes (B). Four weeks later she was found to have a vitreous hemorrhage, bleeding from the corkscrew-shaped vessel seen previously on the disc (C and D). An angiogram showed almost no perfusion of the retina except for a small zone from a cilioretinal artery (E and F). It is likely the ischemia secondary to the CRAO enhanced the pre-existing diabetic ischemia to cause the new vessel to bleed.
G–J: The right fundus of this male patient who presented with severe headache and sudden loss of vision in his right eye shows opacification of the retina with a cherry-red spot and boxcarring of the blood column in the retinal arterioles (G). An angiogram shows poor perfusion through the central retinal artery (H). Carotid angiogram shows dissection of the right internal carotid artery resulting in the CRAO (I and J). A few weeks later, the optic nerve turned pale. The boxcarring of the retinal arterioles continued with regaining of the orange color of the retina. The vision remained at light perception.
K and L: This 75-year-old male with hypercholesterolemia, hypertension, and previous history of bilateral carotid endarterectomies shows a retinal embolus in the superotemporal arteriole and opacification of the posterior pole secondary to a CRAO. There is a small patch of unopacified orange retina temporal to the disc from perfusion through a cilioretinal artery (arrow). Note three cotton-wool spots that likely predate the CRAO. Optical coherence tomography showed thickening and opacification of the inner retina and shadowing of the photoreceptor layer (L).

(G–J, courtesy of Dr. Robert Mittra. G and J, Also, Yannuzzi, Lawrence J., The Retinal Atlas, Saunders 2010, 978-0-7020-3320-9, p.387.)

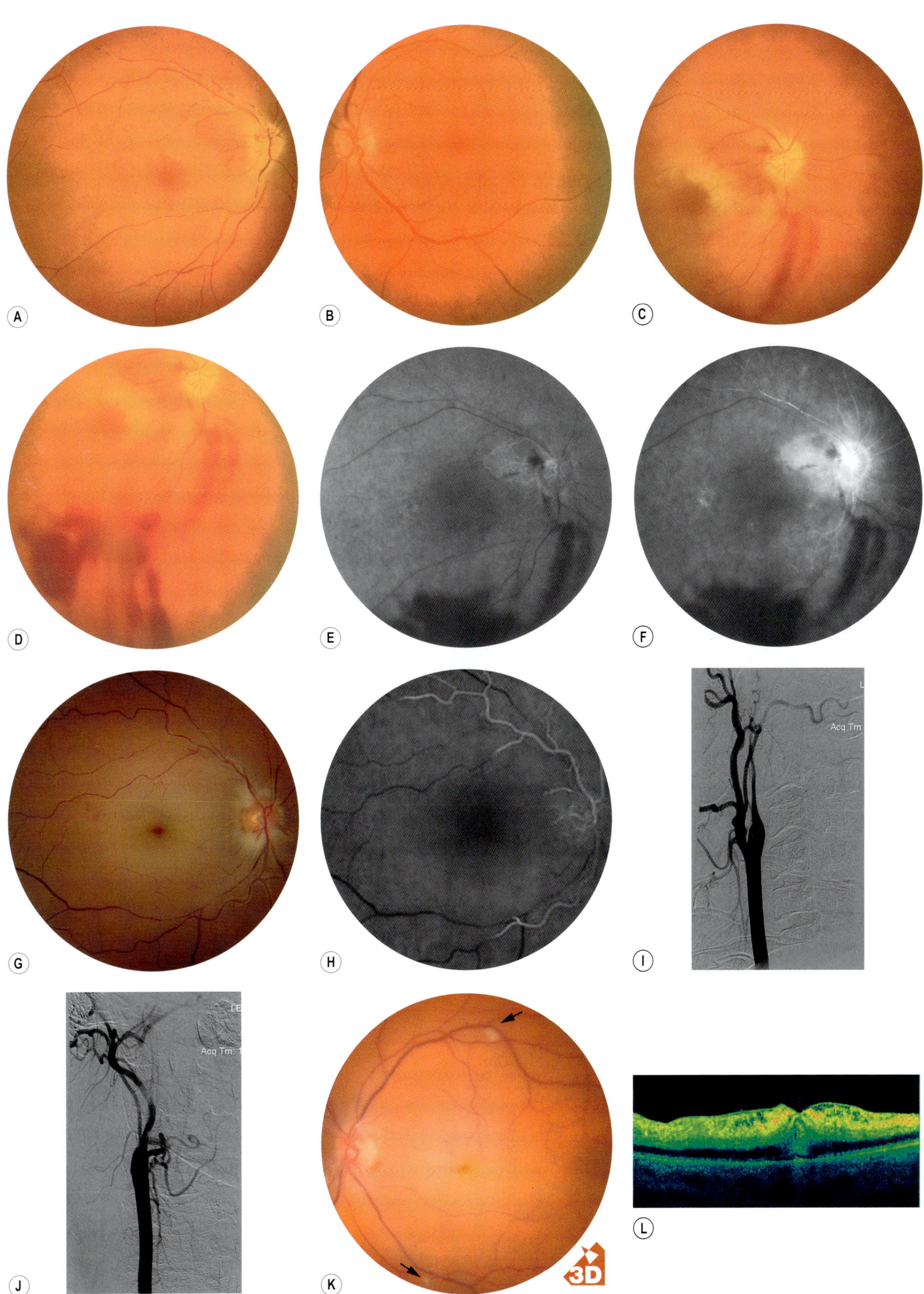
A
B
C
D
E
F
G
H
Acq Tm:
I
Acq Tm:
J
K
3D
L

Three major types of emboli occur. Platelet fibrin emboli are dull, gray-white, often elongated plugs that are subject to fragmentation and movement into more distal arterioles (Figure 6.09J and K). They may be either single or multiple and are most often lodged at a bifurcation. Cholesterol emboli are often multiple, yellow or copper-colored iridescent globules that are most often seen in the peripheral radicles on the temporal side of the fundus (Figures 6.09D and 6.10C).[78,108,109] They are often unassociated with obstruction of blood flow. When causing obstruction, cholesterol emboli are usually located near the optic nerve head. Calcific emboli are usually single, solid, white, nonrefractile, ovoid or angulated emboli derived from the aortic or mitral valve (Figure 6.10A, B, K, and L).[110] They are usually near the optic nerve head and, unlike cholesterol emboli, which often disappear in a few days, they may remain visible permanently. Occult calcified emboli may be detected ultrasonographically at the level of the lamina cribrosa in patients with CRAO and in some patients who present with ischemic optic neuropathy.[111] The narrowest site of central retinal artery is where the artery perforates the dural sheath and enters the optic nerve; any of the three types of emboli can lodge here and not be visible.[112] Occasionally a stream of emboli may be present, many behind the lamina cribrosa, hence not visible. Cholesterol emboli arise primarily from atheromatous disease affecting the proximal carotid artery. Calcific emboli arise primarily from the aortic valve and less often the aorta and carotid artery.

Focal areas of periarterial sheathing and focal accumulation of serum lipids within the artery wall at the site of embolic damage to the endothelium may be evident rather than the emboli themselves (Figure 6.09J).

Because both platelet fibrin and cholesterol emboli are soft and consequently become rapidly fragmented and cast into the distal radicles of the retinal circulation, fluorescein angiography often fails to demonstrate complete obstruction of either a branch or the central retinal artery by the time the patient reports for examination (Figure 6.09J and K).[101,113–115] Likewise, the rapid development of collateral flow around an embolus obstructing the central retinal artery behind the level of the lamina cribrosa may restore intraocular blood flow to nearly normal levels soon after the occlusion. The best scenario for improvement in vision is with occlusion at the entry of the central retinal artery into the optic nerve, since several pial and intraneural collaterals vessels can contribute to filling the central retinal artery distal to its occlusion.[112] In most cases, however, fluorescein angiography reveals a delayed appearance time and an increased retinal circulation time in the area of the occluded segment (Figure 6.09B). In complete occlusion of the central retinal artery, no dye enters the eye by the artery, but dye filling the optic nerve capillaries by way of the ciliary artery circulation may pass through collateral channels and fill the proximal branches of both the central retinal vein and artery (Figure 6.07A–D). In complete branch artery obstruction the arterial tree may be perfused in a retrograde fashion by neighboring collateral vessels.[101] In most instances an embolus lodged in an arterial bifurcation either on the optic nerve head or in the periphery is only partly successful in impeding the flow of fluorescein into the artery distal to the site of obstruction. In some instances the dye seeps by the embolus, and in others it bypasses the embolus by way of collateral flow.[101,116,117] A significant reduction in flow is usually demonstrated angiographically in either case (Figure 6.07A–D). Retinal flow remains depressed even after dissolution of the embolus because of the collapse of the capillary bed by the ischemic and swollen retinal tissue. Fragmented emboli may completely plug the paramacular arterioles. The dye column entering the partly blocked area may show a pattern of laminar flow. In other cases there may be alternating nonfluorescent zones caused by packets of erythrocytes and hyperfluorescent zones caused by stagnant plasma (Figure 6.07D and H). Focal fluorescein leakage may occur at the site of the obstructing emboli and less often at sites where emboli have previously

6.09 Branch retinal artery obstruction.

A–C: Branch retinal artery obstruction of unknown cause in a 36-year-old man. Note the obscuration of the proximal part of the obstructed retinal artery that suggests the possibility of a focal area of retinitis and late staining at the site of obstruction.

D–F: This 61-year-old man developed sudden onset of central scotoma in his right eye secondary to embolic obstruction of a cilioretinal artery. Note the bright plaques in the cilioretinal artery and the superior branch of the central retinal artery (arrows, D). After 16 seconds there was delayed perfusion of the retina in the region of distribution of the cilioretinal artery (E). Several months later the scotoma persisted, but the retinal whitening had cleared (F). This patient had angiographic evidence of obstruction of his right carotid artery.

G–I: Transient embolic obstruction (arrow, G) of the inferior retinal artery. Note ischemic whitening of the retina inferiorly. The patient had an altitudinal field defect superiorly. Visual acuity was 20/20. Nineteen months later the retina had regained its transparency, and the patient had no field defect. He later developed loss of the inferior field of vision caused by embolization of the superior branches of the central retinal artery (arrow, H and I). Note that perivascular cuffing persists at the site of the previous embolus in the inferior artery (H).

J and **K**: Focal atheroma (arrows) of a retinal arterial bifurcation following resolution of an impacted cholesterol embolus. Note the slight narrowing of the arterial wall indicated in the angiogram (arrow, K).

L: Arterioarterial anastomosis in a 62-year-old woman distal to a previous atheromatous embolus in the main trunk of the arteriole. She had another tiny plaque at the foveal end of the arteriole not seen in fig. This patient had suffered a central retinal artery occlusion on the right side and subsequently developed another branch retinal artery occlusion in this eye with loss of a significant part of her visual field. She had a diseased aortic valve and an arrhythmia.

(D and E, from Gass.[101];)

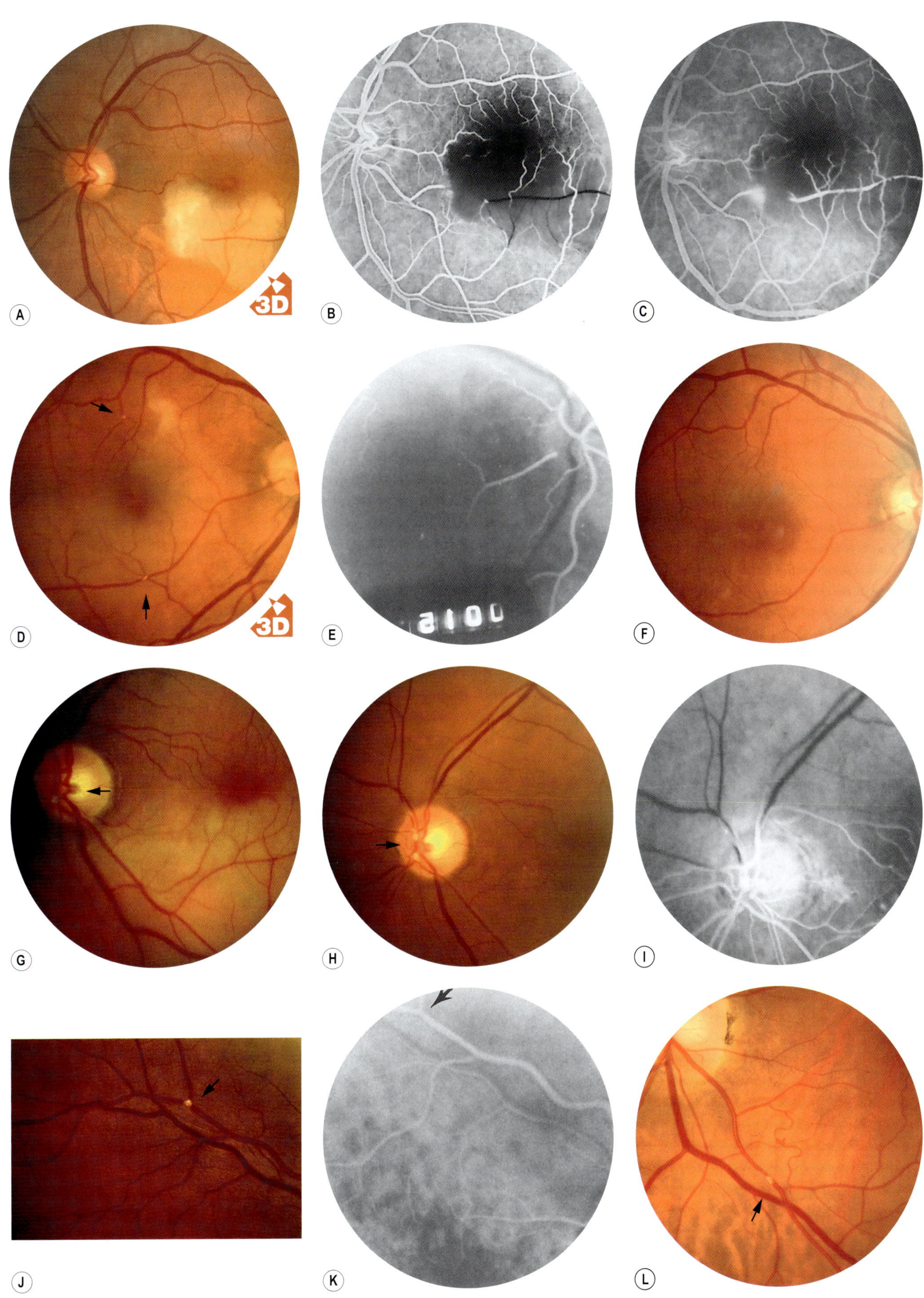

impacted on the arterial wall (Figures 6.07F and 6.09).[118] Failure of fluorescein to leak from the blood vessels distal to the site of arterial obstruction, even when circulation has been partly restored, testifies to the resistance of the retinal vessel endothelium to the effects of ischemia. In rare instances massive embolization of the retinal circulation may cause marked damage to the endothelium of the major retinal artery segments and produce striking periarterial dye leakage. Small emboli frequently observed in the arterial tree beyond the site of obstruction and elsewhere in the fundus usually show little or no tendency to alter the flow of fluorescein. No staining occurs at the site of these nonobstructing emboli. Very few patients with endogenous retinal arterial embolization show angiographic evidence of embolic occlusion of the choroidal circulation.

Some patients with branch artery occlusion may subsequently develop another branch artery occlusion or central retinal artery obstruction (Figure 6.09G–I). Patients with recurrent episodes of multiple branch retinal artery occlusions are more likely to have a nonembolic cause for the obstruction. (See discussion of recurrent branch retinal artery occlusion (Susac syndrome), p. 474 in Chapter 6.)

Electroretinography in eyes with central retinal artery obstruction reveals loss of the oscillatory potential and transient depression of the b-wave with either a normal or supernormal a-wave. The electro-oculogram is diminished or absent.

The intraocular pressure may be subnormal in both the affected and the opposite eye in some patients with both branch artery and CRAO.[77] Relative hypotony in the affected eye suggests the presence of ciliary as well as retinal arterial obstruction. The reported incidence of neovascular glaucoma after CRAO varies from under 2.5% to 15% or more.[77,119–126]Some authors suggest that it occurs most often in patients with chronic ocular ischemia associated with severe carotid or ophthalmic artery disease,[127] whereas others have not found this association.[91,122] Glaucoma usually develops within 2–3 months, often earlier than occurs with central retinal vein occlusion likely due to the rapid onset of retinal ischemia. Even rarer is the development of neovascularization of the disc and subsequent vitreous hemorrhage (Figure 6.08D).

During the first few days after retinal artery occlusion, light microscopy reveals swelling of the inner half of the retina. The swelling is caused by intracellular edema and cellular dissolution (Figure 6.10I).[100] Histologic examination 3 or 4 weeks later reveals marked loss of the inner retinal layers and preservation of the outer retinal layers (Figure 6.10J).

The white inner retinal lesions caused by arterial obstruction should be differentiated from white lesions caused by: (1) retinitis (e.g., toxoplasmosis, acute multifocal inner retinitis[128]; see Behçet's disease, Fig. 11. 40 and 11.41); (2) inflammatory disease of the choroid and retinal pigment epithelium (RPE) (e.g., acute posterior multifocal placoid pigment epitheliopathy); (3) outer retinal whitening from choroidal ischemia caused by prolonged elevation of the intraocular pressure (see Figure 3.63); (4) retinal contusion (commotio retinae, Berlin's edema); (5) neoplasia (e.g., reticulum cell sarcoma); and (6) opaque subretinal fibrin (e.g., idiopathic central serous chorioretinopathy; Figures 3.03J and 3.04J and L). Emboli may be simulated by atheromatous plaques developing within the arterial wall at a focal site of retinal artery endothelial defect, e.g., patients who are prone to develop arterial macroaneurysms (see p. 494 in Chapter 6) or focal arterial wall damage caused by previous impact of an embolus, an immune complex, or inflammatory reaction, e.g., in patients with bilateral idiopathic recurrent branch retinal artery occlusion (see Figures 6.19–6.21); acute retinal necrosis caused by herpes zoster virus (see Chapter 10); toxoplasmosis (see Kyrieleis plaques, and Figure 10.22F–H); chronic uveitis[129]; or neoplasia (see Figure 13.31H).

Inner retinal infarction occurs experimentally after complete occlusion of the central retinal artery lasting beyond approximately $1^1/_2$ hours.[130] Only occasionally does the patient who develops an acute retinal arterial obstruction report for therapy within the first few hours. Treatment, therefore, is infrequently beneficial. Nevertheless, in some patients with incomplete arterial obstruction, obstruction due to spasm, or obstruction of short duration, the ischemic damage associated with the retinal whitening may be reversible (Figure 6.09G and H). Even the presence of biomicroscopic evidence of slow blood flow (rouleaux formation) does not exclude the possibility of visual recovery.[131]

6.10 Embolic retinal artery obstruction.

A: Calcified embolus from the aortic valve is lodged in a bifurcation of the retinal artery.
B: Histopathology of a calcified embolus (arrow).
C: Histopathology of a retinal artery embolus containing cholesterol crystals (arrow).
D–F: Obstruction of the central retinal artery (left arrow, D and arrow, E) and ciliary arteries (right arrows, D and arrows, F) caused by chondrosarcoma that metastasized from the hip in a 27-year-old man. His symptoms were acute onset of headache, left hemiplegia, and loss of vision in the right eye. E and F show a high magnification of tumor obstructing the central retinal artery and ciliary arteries, respectively.
G: Multiple cotton-wool patches in a patient with fat embolism associated with multiple bone fractures.
H: Fat embolus (arrow, I) in a retinal capillary.
I: Histopathology of acute retinal artery obstruction. Note the swelling of the inner half of the retina.
J: Histopathology showing atrophy of the inner half of the retina months after retinal artery occlusion.
K and L: Large calcific embolus in the main trunk of the inferior retinal artery coming off the disc, resulting in opacification of the inferior half of the retina in this man with a diseased aortic valve.

(B, courtesy of Dr. Andrew P. Ferry; C, courtesy of Dr. Louis Karp; D–F, from Burde et al.[103]; G, courtesy of Dr. Elaine L. Chuang; I, from Hogan and Zimmerman[170]; L, reprinted with permission from Fekrat S, Moshfeghi D, Elliott D (eds) Curbside consultation in retina. Thorofare, NJ: Slack, 2010, p. 38.)

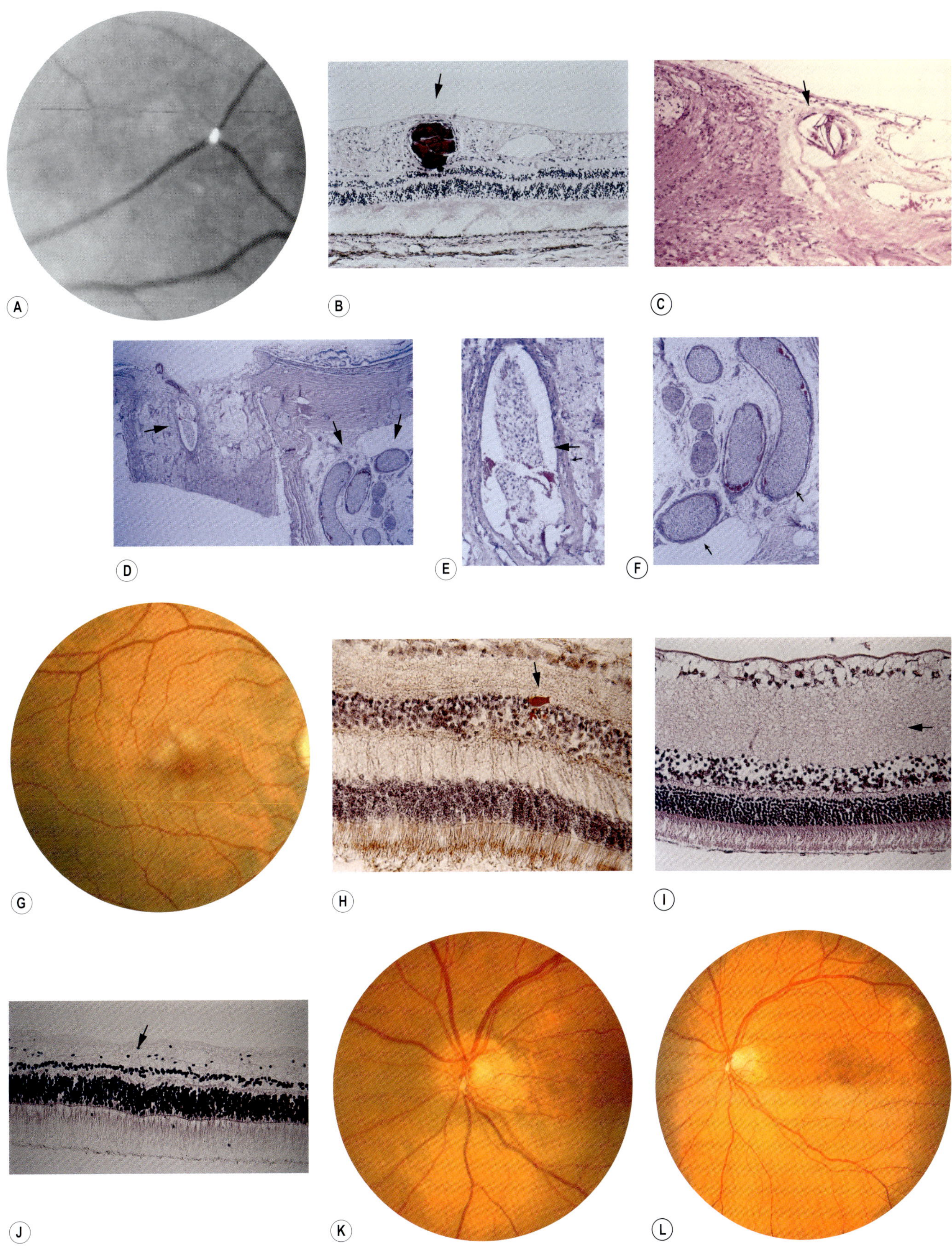
A
B
C
D
E
F
G
H
I
J
K
L

Therefore, in any patient with a history of occlusion of 24 hours or less, therapy consisting of paracentesis, intermittent massage, breathing of 95% oxygen and 5% carbon dioxide, and administration of acetazolamide may be helpful.[131,132] Other modes of therapy that have been employed include the intravenous administration of vasodilators such as papaverine, perfusion of the ocular circulation by cannulation of the supraorbital artery, hyperbaric oxygen, surgical removal of the embolus, and Nd-YAG laser disruption of the embolus.[79,133–135] Experimental use of recombinant tissue plasminogen activator to lyse retinal arterial thrombi was first reported with retinal artery occlusion.[136–138] Most recent, has been the interest in intra-arterial thrombolysis by cannulating the ophthalmic artery via the femoral artery and injecting tissue plasminogen activator. This treatment has a role if it can be performed within 4 hours of occlusion. When arrangements for intra-arterial cannulation are not possible, intravenous use of tissue plasminogen activator in the correct settings to manage any complications can be tried if the patient arrives within 4 hours of visual loss.[139–141] Even without therapy some patients will experience a remarkable visual recovery.[131,142,143]

In the absence of ophthalmoscopic evidence of emboli in patients over 65 years of age, a sedimentation rate should be obtained along with an exhaustive review of systems to exclude the possibility of cranial arteritis as the cause of the occlusion. Auscultation of the heart and carotid arteries and comparison of the pulsation of the carotid arteries with the ophthalmic artery pressures, either by ophthalmodynamometry or by finger pressure, are useful measures for determining the source of the emboli. Transesophageal echocardiography in addition to transthoracic echocardiography is necessary for detecting mitral valve prolapse or other cardiac abnormalities such as patent foramen ovale, endocardial vegetations, and noninfectious masses.[83,144,145]All patients should have a medical evaluation. In patients who are reasonable surgical candidates and who have no other explanation for the emboli, the evaluation should include at least digital subtraction carotid arteriography, which may demonstrate evidence of carotid stenosis and/or atheromatous plaques ipsilaterally in approximately 50% of cases.[146,147]

Normal retinal transparency usually returns 2–3 weeks after acute retinal artery obstruction, but the retinal flow through the involved area is only partly restored. This probably is primarily caused by collapse of the capillary bed accompanying the postnecrotic atrophy of the retina. In most cases following central artery obstruction and in many cases following branch artery obstruction, optic atrophy and some narrowing of the retinal arterial tree occur. In others with less ischemic retinal damage the retina may return to a relatively normal appearance. Some with persistent low-grade chronic retinal ischemia may show multiple peripheral retinal hemorrhages (venous stasis retinopathy) identical to that seen in patients with carotid artery obstruction.[148,149] Although visual recovery is generally poor, as many as 35% of patients after central retinal artery obstruction regain 20/100 or better visual acuity.[142] Only 1–5% of patients with CRAO will develop rubeosis and glaucoma, usually within 1–3 months.[95] These latter patients are likely to have significant obstruction of the carotid artery on the ipsilateral side. Relatively few patients with embolic retinal artery obstruction in one eye develop a similar process in the second eye. Some authors have found that the life expectancy for patients with retinal artery obstruction is reduced,[150–152] whereas others have not.[91] Although there is an increased incidence of stroke, most patients die of atherosclerotic heart disease.

It is clinically relevant to classify CRAO into:

1. nonarteretic CRAO: most often due to embolism
2. arteretic CRAO: secondary to giant cell arteritis, almost all associated with ischemic optic neuropathy
3. transient CRAO: recovers almost complete vision within a few hours of occlusion.

6.11 Carotid maneuvering during internal carotid aneurysm embolization causing retinal embolization.

A–J: This 42-year-old woman underwent onyx embolization for an internal carotid aneurysm on the left side. Soon after the procedure she complained of a "film with spotty holes" with her left eye. Her vision was 20/20 on the right and 20/50 on the left with a relative afferent pupillary defect. She had numerous white intraarteriolar refractile emboli and patchy areas of retinal whitening, more so in the temporal periphery of the left eye (A–C, G). Angiogram revealed patchy choroidal and retinal arteriolar filling with late wedge-shaped hyperfluorescence of the temporal retina simulating Amalric's triangles. The triangular areas of hyperfluorescence were secondary to choroidal ischemia from occlusion of large choroidal vessels. Her vision spontaneously improved to 20/25. Three months later she still had refractile emboli within her retinal arterioles (H–J), the peripheral retinal vessels were sheathed, and the previous areas of choroidal infarcts showed pigmentation (I and J). The emboli are believed to be cholesterol emboli originating in the carotid bulb due to manipulation of the hardware such as the guidewire and catheter, and not the onyx used for embolizing the intracranial aneurysm (which would be black in color).

(Courtesy of Dr. Karen Joos and Dr. Franco Recchia.)

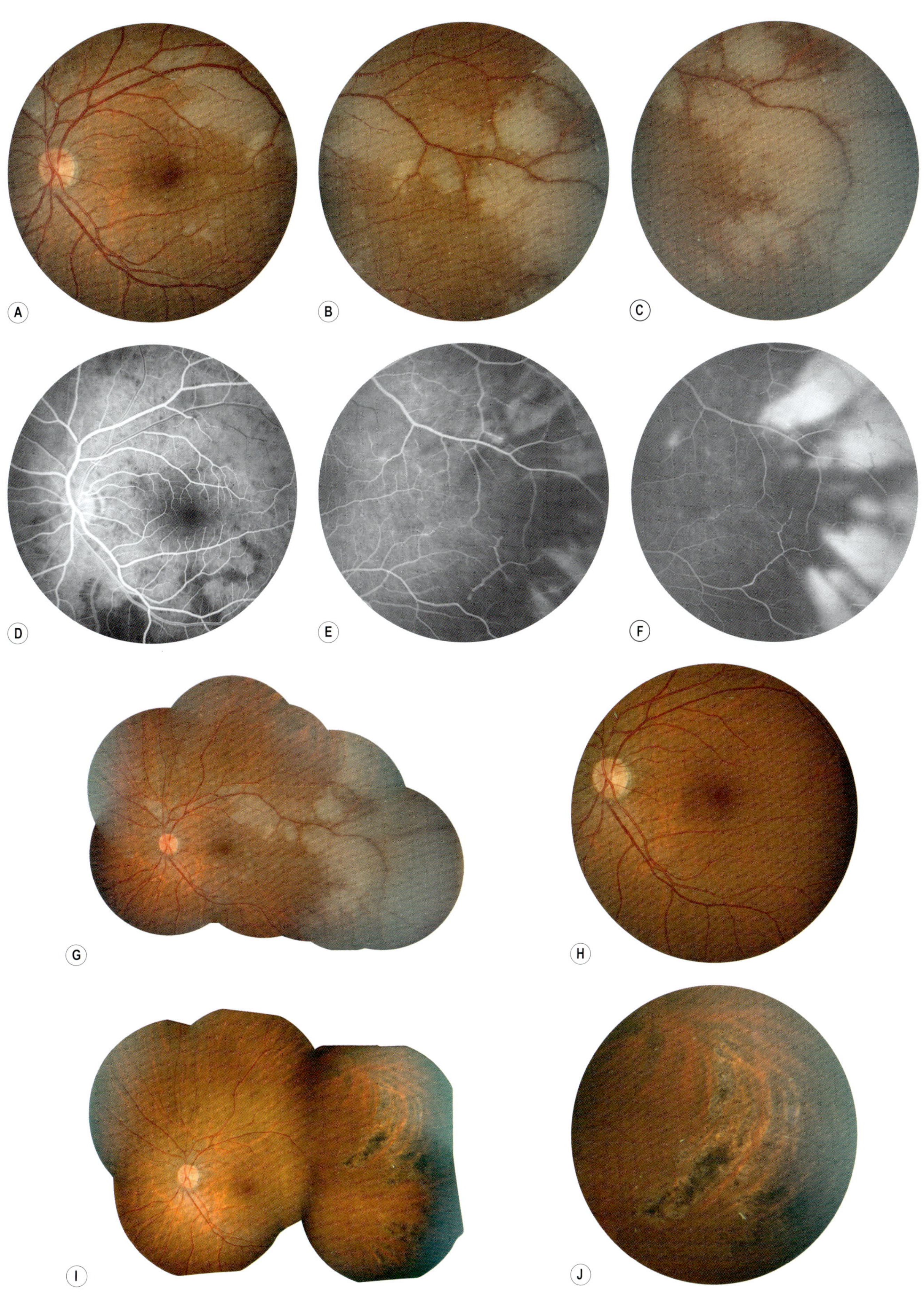
A
B
C
D
E
F
G
H
I
J

Systemic risk factors and retinal artery occlusion

In 33 patients with CRAO seen over 11 years, 64% (21 patients) showed additional vascular risk factors after the event; hyperlipidemia was seen in 36%, new diagnosis or poor control of hypertension in 21%, 27% had >50% carotid stenosis, 18% (6 patients) needed carotid endarterectomy, and two developed a vascular event, with coronary artery syndrome in one and a stroke in the other.[153] Hayreh et al. have reported in 439 patients (499 eyes) with CRAO and branch retinal artery occlusion a significantly higher prevalence of hypertension, smoking, diabetes mellitus, ischemic heart disease, and cerebrovascular disease compared to a comparable US population. They also report a 71% incidence of carotid plaques in patients with CRAO and 66% in branch retinal artery occlusion, abnormal echocardiogram in 52% of CRAO and 42% of branch retinal artery occlusion.[123] Hence patients who present with a central or branch retinal artery occlusion should be (re)assessed for the associated risk factors and necessary corrections undertaken.

Atheromatous Retinal Arterial Embolization Following Use of Onyx to Embolize Internal Carotid Aneurysm

Onyx is a liquid embolic agent used for occluding intracranial, renal, and peripheral aneurysms and arteriovenous malformations (AVMs). It comes in ready-to-use vials containing ethylene-vinylalcohol copolymer, dimethylsulfoxide, and tantalum. The polymer is dissolved in dimethylsulfoxide, and micronized tantalum powder, which is radiopaque, is added. Concentrations of 6, 6.5, and 8% are variably used. The higher the concentration, the more viscous is the agent. After injecting heparin, a microcatheter is threaded to the nidus of the aneurysm and dimethylsulfoxide is first injected to fill the dead space in the catheter, followed by the selected onyx concentration. The aneurysm is filled to its neck under fluoroscopic guidance. This material forms an acrylic cast occluding the aneurysm completely.[153,154]

During the procedure, manipulation of the guidewire/catheter and other hardware near the carotid bulb can dislodge a stream of cholesterol plaques that can embolize the retinal and choroidal vessels. Two such cases are illustrated in Figures 6.11 and 6.12G–J. The overwhelming feature seems to be the multiple emboli affecting the retinal and/or the choroidal circulation. Since these two cases, attention is being paid by the interventional neuroradiologists to minimize manipulation of the guidewire and other hardware at the carotid root. Other complications include bleeding at the site of the AVM, bleeding at the percutaneous entry site, and anesthetic complications resulting in oxygen desaturation from dimethylsulfoxide, though small and transient most of the time.[155]

6.12 Fat embolism.

A–B: This 15-year-old boy broke his collarbone while playing soccer. He noted a superior visual field loss the next morning. His visual acuity was 20/25 and the superior half of the macula was perfused via a cilioretinal artery while the rest of his retina was opacified from occlusion of his central retinal artery (A). Autofluorescence imaging showed altered fluorescence from the opacified retina (B). A transesophageal echo revealed a persistent foramen ovale, which led to the paradoxical fat embolus from the fractured clavicle.

Branch retinal artery occlusion in protein S deficiency.

C–F: This 40-year-old woman of African American ancestry woke up with a superior field loss in her right eye. In addition to the compact cuticular drusen in the fovea bilaterally, there was a right inferotemporal branch retinal artery occlusion (C). Angiogram revealed minimal perfusion of the involved arteriole and staining of the endothelium at the site of the thrombosis (D–F). She was otherwise healthy and had no known cardiac or vascular disease. There was no family history of strokes or other vascular diseases. Evaluation of her heart and carotids yielded no cause for the occlusion. A laboratory workup revealed protein S deficiency. She was placed on aspirin therapy and has had no further episodes. Her vision remains at 20/20 in each eye.

Choroidal vascular emboli during onyx embolization of internal carotid aneurysm.

G–J: This 51-year-old woman underwent onyx embolization of her right superior hypophyseal aneurysm. A few hours after the procedure she noticed a "veil" over her right eye with fluctuating vision. Her vision was 20/25 on the right and 20/20 on the left with a relative afferent pupillary defect on the right side. There was faint whitening of the inferior half of her right retina (G). No retinal arteriolar emboli were seen. Angiogram revealed delayed choroidal and retinal filling in the inferior half (H–J) secondary to choroidal embolic infarct and partial inferotemporal retinal trunk occlusion. Her vision eventually improved to 20/20 and subjectively the scotoma faded to become almost imperceivable.

(A and B, courtesy of Dr. Richard Spaide; A, Also, Yannuzzi, Lawrence J., The Retinal Atlas, Saunders 2010, 978-0-7020-3320-9, p.481. G–J, Dr. Karen Joos and Dr. Franco Recchia.)

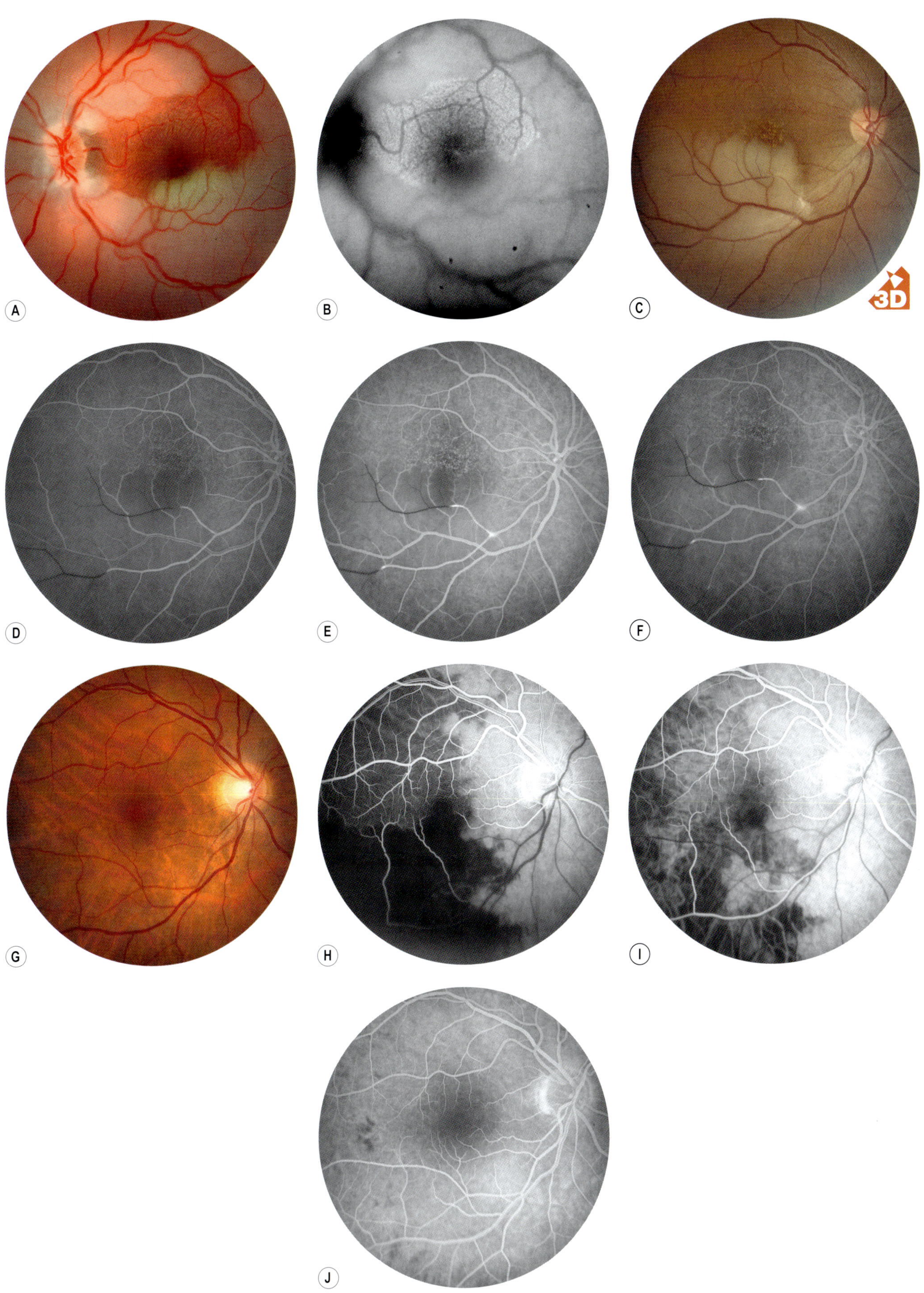
A
B
C
3D
D
E
F
G
H
I
J

Other Causes of Endogenous Embolization

Atrial Myxoma

Emboli from atrial myxomas, benign polypoid tumors of endocardial origin arising in the left atrium, should be suspected in patients who have symptoms of retinal artery occlusion, usually involving the left eye, and repetitive neurologic symptoms suggestive of ipsilateral ischemia affecting the distribution of the middle cerebral artery.[156–162] Signs and symptoms suggesting pulmonary hypertension and bacterial endocarditis also may be present.[163] The tumor is more common in middle-aged women and 75% originate in the left atrium. Tumor embolization of the ciliary arteries (swelling of the optic discs and choroidal lesions) has been shown clinically and histopathologically.[160] The relatively large size and friable nature of the embolus or emboli as compared to a cholesterol or fibrin platelet embolus is likely the reason for multiple, large-caliber vessels such as the ophthalmic, choroidal, and cerebral involvement.[164,165] Embolization of the ciliary and retinal vessels with tumor emboli from extracardiac sources has been observed (Figure 6.10D–F).[76,103,166]

6.13 Purtscher's-like retinopathy.

A–C: Bilateral retinopathy associated with acute pancreatitis in an alcoholic patient complaining of bilateral loss of central vision. Angiogram (C) shows evidence of focal retinal arteriolar occlusions in the perifoveal area.

D–F: Retinopathy associated with acute pancreatitis (D) in a 32-year-old alcoholic patient who subsequently became comatose and died. Histopathologic examination of the eye revealed necrosis and swelling of the inner two-thirds of the retina (E) and thrombotic arteriolar occlusion (arrow, F).

G–K: Purtscher's-like retinopathy in a 24-year-old woman who noted severe visual loss in both eyes on awaking after a cesarean section done because of toxemia of pregnancy (G and H). Her visual acuity was 20/200 bilaterally. Angiography showed evidence of capillary nonperfusion corresponding with the white lesions (I and J). She recovered 20/25 visual acuity in both eyes within several months but showed evidence of optic atrophy (K).

L: Purtscher's-like retinopathy occurred in both eyes of this 39-year-old woman with hypereosinophilia, skin rash, chest pain, arthritis, and eosinophilic fasciitis. Visual acuity was 20/40 in both eyes.

(A–C, courtesy of Dr. Raul E. Valenzuela; D–F, from Kincaid et al.[185]; G–K, from Blodi et al.[201]; L, courtesy of Dr. Arun Patel.)

Fat Embolization

Following liberation of neutral fat into the circulation at the time of long-bone fracture or, less often, after injury to fatty tissues, patients may experience sudden cardiopulmonary and neurologic deterioration. This usually occurs after a latent period of 12–36 hours. The pathogenesis is poorly understood but apparently is the result of release of free fatty acids, a toxic vasculitis, platelet fibrin thrombosis, and obstruction of small vascular radicles by macroaggregates of fat. Approximately 50% of patients with fat embolism syndrome may show retinal abnormalities, including cotton-wool patches, small blot hemorrhages, and, rarely, obstruction of major branches of the central retinal artery (Figure 6.12A and B) or a fundus picture of Purtscher's retinopathy (see discussion to follow).[167–171] Young people presenting with retinal artery occlusion following a fracture should alert the physician for presence of a patent foramen ovale, the incidence of which is approximately 29% in the general population (Figure 6.12A and B).

Embolization Caused by Intravascular Aggregation of Blood Elements

The spontaneous aggregation of thrombocytes, leukocytes (Purtscher's), or erythrocytes (sickle-cell; see later) may be the cause of embolic occlusion of the retinal vasculature in certain disease states.

Disseminated Intravascular Coagulopathy

Disseminated intravascular coagulopathy, or pathologic aggregation of thrombocytes, may cause vascular occlusion in many of the body organs. This occlusion is much more likely to affect the choroidal arterioles and choriocapillaris than the retinal circulation (see Chapter 3). Thromboembolization of the retinal circulation is probably responsible for arterial occlusions that may affect the brain, heart, lungs, and kidneys of patients with idiopathic persistently elevated blood eosinophilic count (Churg–Strauss syndrome; see Chapter 11).[172,173]

Protein S Deficiency

Protein C and protein S are vitamin K-dependent proteins. Protein S is a cofactor for protein C. Protein C is activated to protein Ca, which inactivates factor Va and VIIIa, thus acting as an anticoagulant, and proteolytically inactivates the inhibitor to tissue plasminogen activator, thus increasing fibrinolytic activity. Deficiency of protein C and S can increase thrombus formation in both venous and arterial circulation. The deficiencies can be congenital (autosomal-dominant) or acquired. Homozygous deficiency results in life-threatening thrombotic disease in the neonatal period, whereas heterozygous deficiency may result in symptoms in early adulthood or later. Acquired deficiency occurs due to poor hepatic synthesis of proteins.[174] The thrombus occurs at the site of the occlusion and has been reported in the central and branch retinal artery (Figure 6.12C and D), cerebral, common carotid, brachiocephalic, and as a cause of anterior ischemic optic neuropathy.[175–180] Recurrent branch arterial occlusions may occur in some patients, simulating Susac syndrome.[181] The absence of arterial wall staining on fluorescein angiography (see Figure 6.21C and E) helps differentiate Susac sydrome from this. Any artery or vein can be affected. Other factors such as pregnancy, trauma, childbirth, or surgery can sometimes precipitate thrombosis in these patients. Treatment involves anticoagulation with heparin and warfarin.

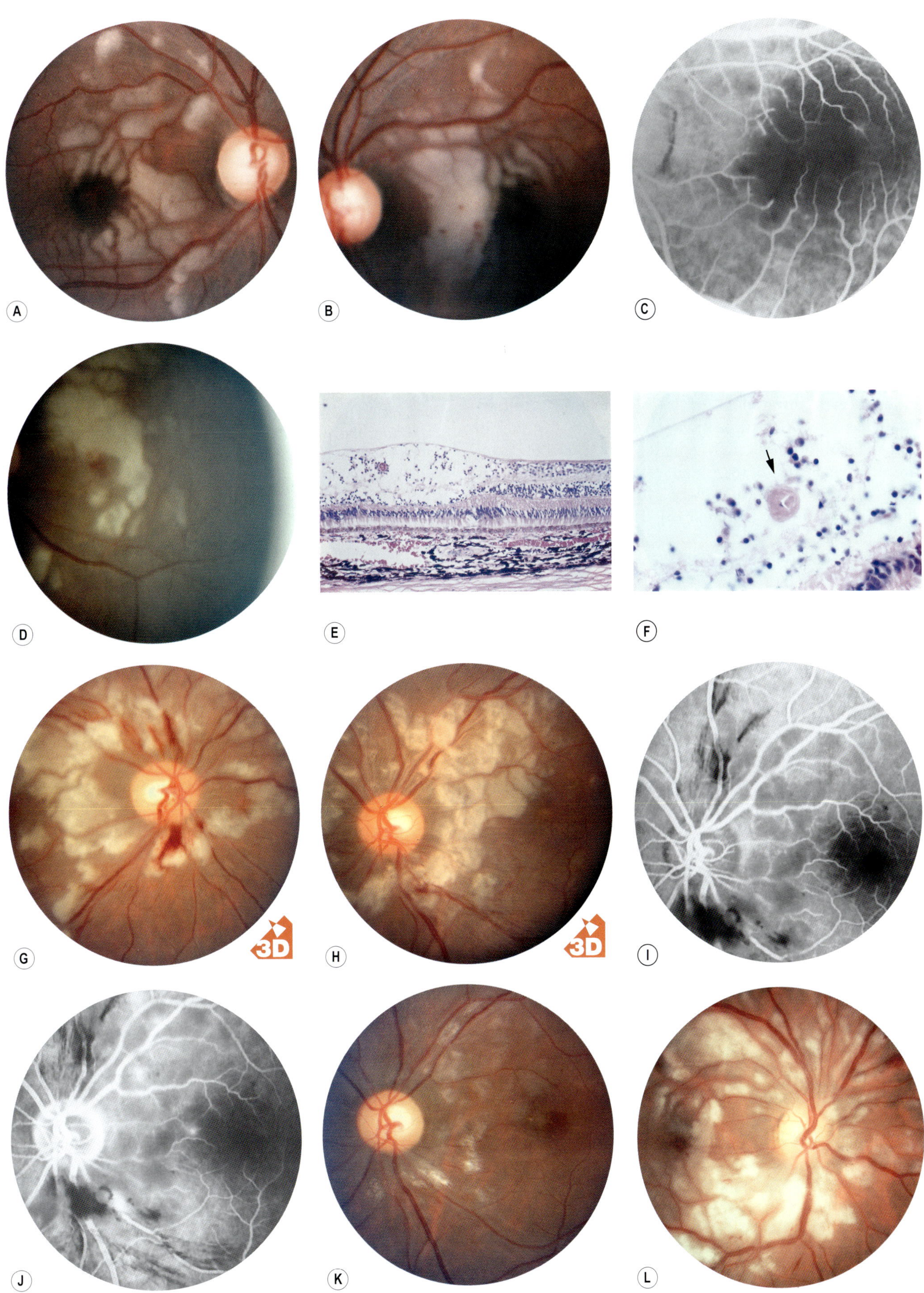
A
B
C
D
E
F
G
3D
H
3D
I
J
K
L

Leukoembolization (Purtscher's and Purtscher's-Like Retinopathy)

Intravascular aggregation of leukocytes in response to unusual activation of complement C5a has been incriminated as the possible cause of retinal arterial embolization that produces the ophthalmoscopic picture of Purtscher's retinopathy. This response occurs after trauma (see Figure 8.06) and in patients with acute pancreatitis (Figure 6.13A–F).[182–189] Similar findings have been reported in patients with collagen vascular diseases (Figure 6.14)[190–192]; in patients receiving hemodialysis[193]; in patients with chronic renal failure[194] or hemolytic–uremic syndrome[195]; during plasmapheresis for thrombotic thrombocytopenic purpura[196] and thrombotic thrombocytopenic purpura per se,[197–199] Still's disease[12–19] and[200] (Figure 6.15A–E), in normotensive obstetric patients after a precipitous delivery induced with intravenous oxytocin (Pitocin),[201] following delivery by cesarean section (Figure 6.13G–K); and in patients with amniotic fluid embolism,[201–203] HELLP syndrome (see Figure 3.58),[204] fat embolism,[205,206] cardiac aneurysm,[207] ophthalmic artery obstruction,[104] hypereosinophilia syndrome (Figure 6.15F–H), post bone marrow transplant, cytotoxic drug therapy[208,209] and retrobulbar anesthesia (see Figure 8.12J).[210–212] The frequent association of central nervous system symptoms in patients whose ophthalmoscopic picture resembles Purtscher's retinopathy suggests that leukoembolization may affect the cerebral vessels as well.

Purtscher described multiple, superficial, white retinal patches, superficial retinal hemorrhages, and papillitis occurring in five patients with severe head trauma[186,187] (see Figure 8.06). The pathogenesis of the fundus changes is not completely understood. The white lesions were attributed to lymphatic extravasations secondary to a sudden increase in intrathoracic pressure, fat embolism, reflux shock waves through the venous system, air embolism,[213] and, later, granulocytic aggregation.[184]

Chronic alcoholics hospitalized for treatment of acute pancreatitis, with or without signs of central nervous system involvement, may suddenly lose vision in both eyes secondary to a fundoscopic picture identical to that of Purtscher's retinopathy (Figure 6.13A–F).[183,184,188,214] Shapiro and Jacob studied blood samples of 12 consecutive alcoholic patients admitted for acute pancreatitis and were able to demonstrate marked granulocyte aggregation, reflecting the presence of activated complement C5a in eight patients. This lends some support to the concept that leukoembolization may be responsible for the fundus picture.[188]

Complement, platelet, and neutrophil activation and endothelial dysfunction and inflammation characterize pre-eclampsia.[215] These likely exert an effect similar to the mechanism of pancreatitis causing leukocyte and platelet aggregation and vascular thrombosis in Purtscher's-like retinopathy occurring around childbirth.

Most patients with collagen vascular disease have normal fundi. Some patients, usually those who have hypertension, may develop retinal or choroidal changes (see pp. 488–490 in Chapter 6, and p. 188 in Chapter 3).[192,216] A few patients, particularly those with an exacerbation of disseminated lupus erythematosus, lupuslike syndrome associated with autoantibodies to Sjögren's syndrome A antigen, dermatomyositis, Still's disease and scleroderma, may develop acute loss of vision in one or both eyes with a fundoscopic picture suggesting multifocal embolic retinal arterial occlusions simulating those seen in Purtscher's retinopathy (Figures 6.16 and 6.14).[190,217–229] These patients often have central nervous system symptoms as well. The occlusive process may be confined to the posterior pole or may involve extensively the peripheral fundus (Figures 6.16 and 6.14A–F).[222,227,230–236] The retinal arterioles and arteries may be partly filled with a milky white material. Those with involvement of the periphery may develop severe retinal neovascular proliferation and vitreous hemorrhage. The presence of antiphospholipid antibodies in patients with systemic lupus erythematosus also plays an important role in retinal vascular thrombosis. (See unusual causes for retinal artery and arteriolar thrombosis in subsequent sections.)

6.14 Purtscher's-like retinopathy associated with collagen vascular diseases.

A–F: Ischemic retinopathy in a 26-year-old normotensive black woman with lupus erythematosus who noted acute bilateral loss of vision, lethargy, mental confusion, and hallucinations (A). Visual acuity was 3/200. Both eyes showed a similar appearance. Her blood pressure was 120/78. Angiography showed multiple branch retinal arteriolar occlusions and dye leakage from the retinal veins (B and C). Three years later visual acuity was 20/300 in the right eye and 20/200 in the left eye. Note in D and E the optic atrophy, large areas of retinal vascular nonperfusion, and optic disc new vessels (arrows, E). After panphotocoagulation, there were atrophy and occlusion of the disc new vessels (F).

G–K: Ischemic retinopathy associated with severe scleroderma and systemic hypertension in a 54-year-old woman who developed blurred vision in both eyes. Visual acuity was 20/200 in each eye. Note the multiple cotton-wool patches and incomplete macular star (G). The nonfluorescent areas (H and I) correspond to cotton-wool patches and dye leakage from the first-order arterioles (arrow, I) and capillaries adjacent to the cotton-wool patches. The patient developed pulmonary edema, became semicomatose, and died soon after these photographs were made. Histopathologic examination revealed multiple cytoid bodies (K) and retinal arteriolar occlusions as well as some areas of fibrinoid necrosis of choroidal arteries and the choriocapillaris (arrow, J).

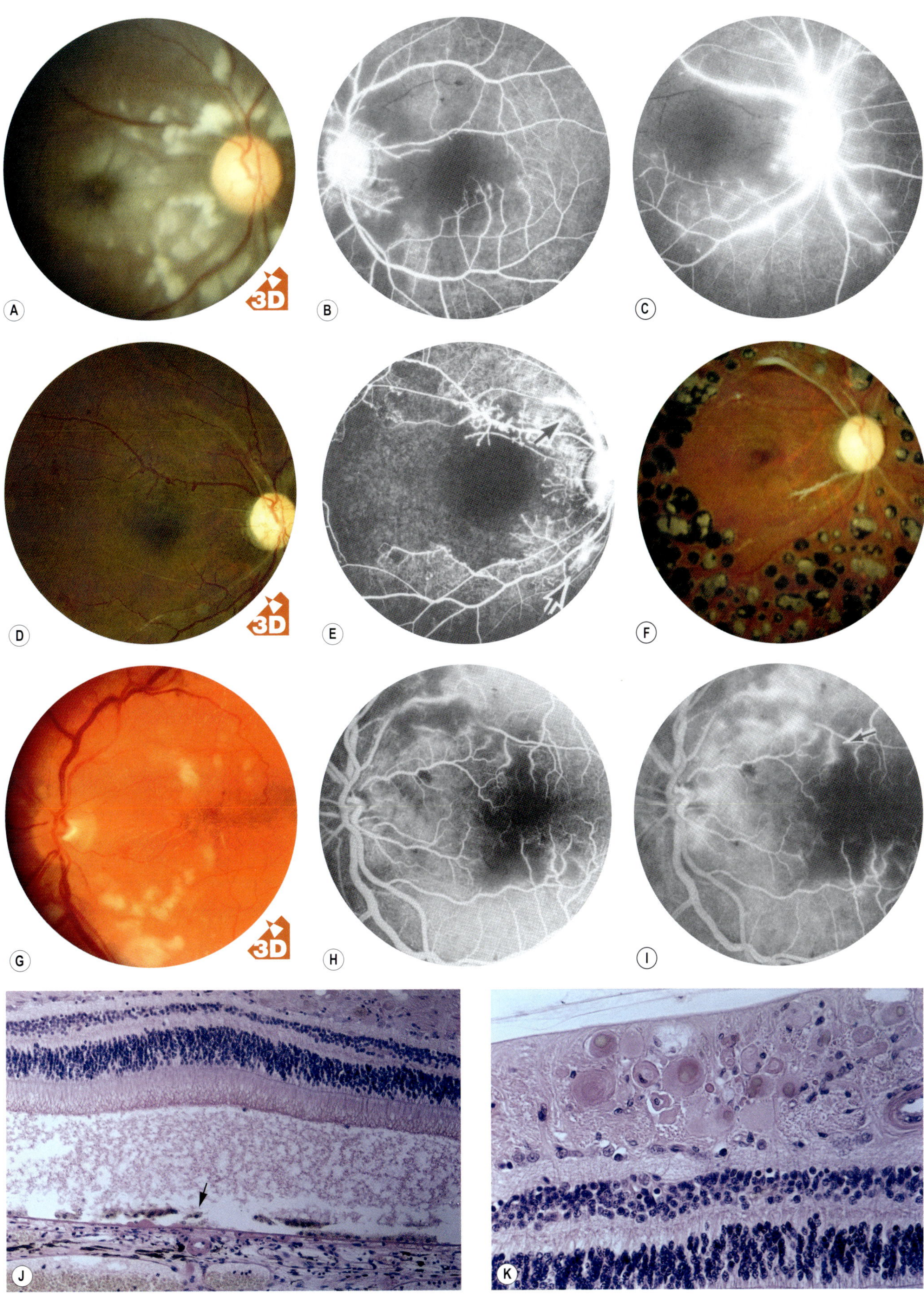
A
B
C
D
E
F
G
H
I
J
K
3D
3D
3D

The retinal whitening is referred to as a Purtscher "flecken" and it typically has a clear zone between its edge and an adjacent retinal arteriole (Figure 6.13A, L). Fluorescein angiography in all of these patients who have an ophthalmoscopic picture simulating Purtscher's retinopathy is similar. It reveals multiple focal areas of retinal arteriolar and arterial obstruction, adjacent areas of capillary nonperfusion, and extensive leakage from the vessels in the areas of infarction (Figures 6.13 and 6.14). This latter feature is uncommonly seen in branch arterial occlusion caused by emboli from the heart and great vessels. Resolution of the white peripapillary and macular ischemic areas may require several months. Varying degrees of narrowing and sheathing of the retinal arteries, optic atrophy, and retinal neovascularization may occur (Figure 6.14D–F). In some patients with collagen vascular disease, evidence of occlusive arterial disease may be confined to the peripheral fundus and be associated with evidence of vasculitis and venous stasis.[237]

Histopathology of an eye studied 23 days after onset of Purtscher's retinopathy in a patient secondary to pancreatitis, showed material occluding retinal and choroidal arterioles to be positive for fibrin. Focal areas of retinal edema, cystoid degeneration, and loss of inner retinal architecture with a sharp demarcation from an area of normal retina was noted.[238]

Further research is required to determine the role of complement activation and leukocytic aggregation and embolization in all of these disorders resembling Purtscher's retinopathy. By the time many of these patients consult the physician, the level of complement C5a may have returned to nearly normal. If elevation of complement proves to be important, then the use of systemic corticosteroids has some rationale.[184]

Erythrocytic Aggregation

Although the role of erythrocytic aggregation in the pathogenesis of retinal vascular occlusion is uncertain in diseases such as diabetes mellitus and Eales' disease, there is good evidence that it is important in the case of sickle-cell disease.[239] Increased deformity of the erythrocytes caused by hypoxia in the peripheral fundus is probably responsible for occluding the small retinal arterioles, capillary nonperfusion, and reactive proliferation of new vessels into the vitreous (for further discussion, see p. 556 in Chapter 6).

6.15 Purtscher-like retinopathy associated with thrombotic thrombocytopenic purpura.

A–E: Right and left fundus appearance in a 27-year-old male who presented with acute blurry vision in both eyes for 3 days. His acuity was 20/40 on the right and 20/300 on the left. There were several cotton-wool spots and small retinal infarcts in both posterior poles (A and B). Angiogram showed occluded retinal arterioles and late staining of the vessel walls and breakdown of the blood–retinal barrier in both eyes (C–E). He had had a rash, fever, sore throat, myalgia, chest pain, shortness of breath, paresthesia, and weakness for the past month. His sedimentation rate was 93 mm/h, C-reactive protein 234 mg/dl, white count 27 cells/μl, hemoglobin 8.7 g/dl, and liver function tests were abnormal. He also had a pleural and pericardial effusion and hepatosplenomegaly. He was diagnosed with adult-onset Still's disease and required plasma exchange, antimetabolites such as cytoxan, vincristine, and intravenous immunoglobulin after no response to ibuprofen and pulse steroids.

Purtscher-like retinopathy associated with hypereosinophilia syndrome.

F–H: This 25-year-old African American patient developed decrease in vision in both eyes associated with cough, rash, and muscle soreness. His white count was elevated to 51 000/mm^3 with 60% eosinophils. Both retinas showed several retinal infarcts and cotton-wool spots simulating Purtscher's retinopathy (F). The small retinal vessels showed leakage on angiography (G). Bone marrow biopsy showed several eosinophils with "spectacle-like nuclei" (H). Three days later he developed pleural and pericardial effusions, cardiomyopathy, uncontrolled hypertension, seizures, right middle cerebral and bilateral occipital infarcts.

(A–E, courtesy of Dr. Kourous Rezaei; A and B, Also, Yannuzzi, Lawrence J., The Retinal Atlas, Saunders 2010, 978-0-7020-3320-9, p.294. F–H, courtesy of Dr. Joseph Maguire.)

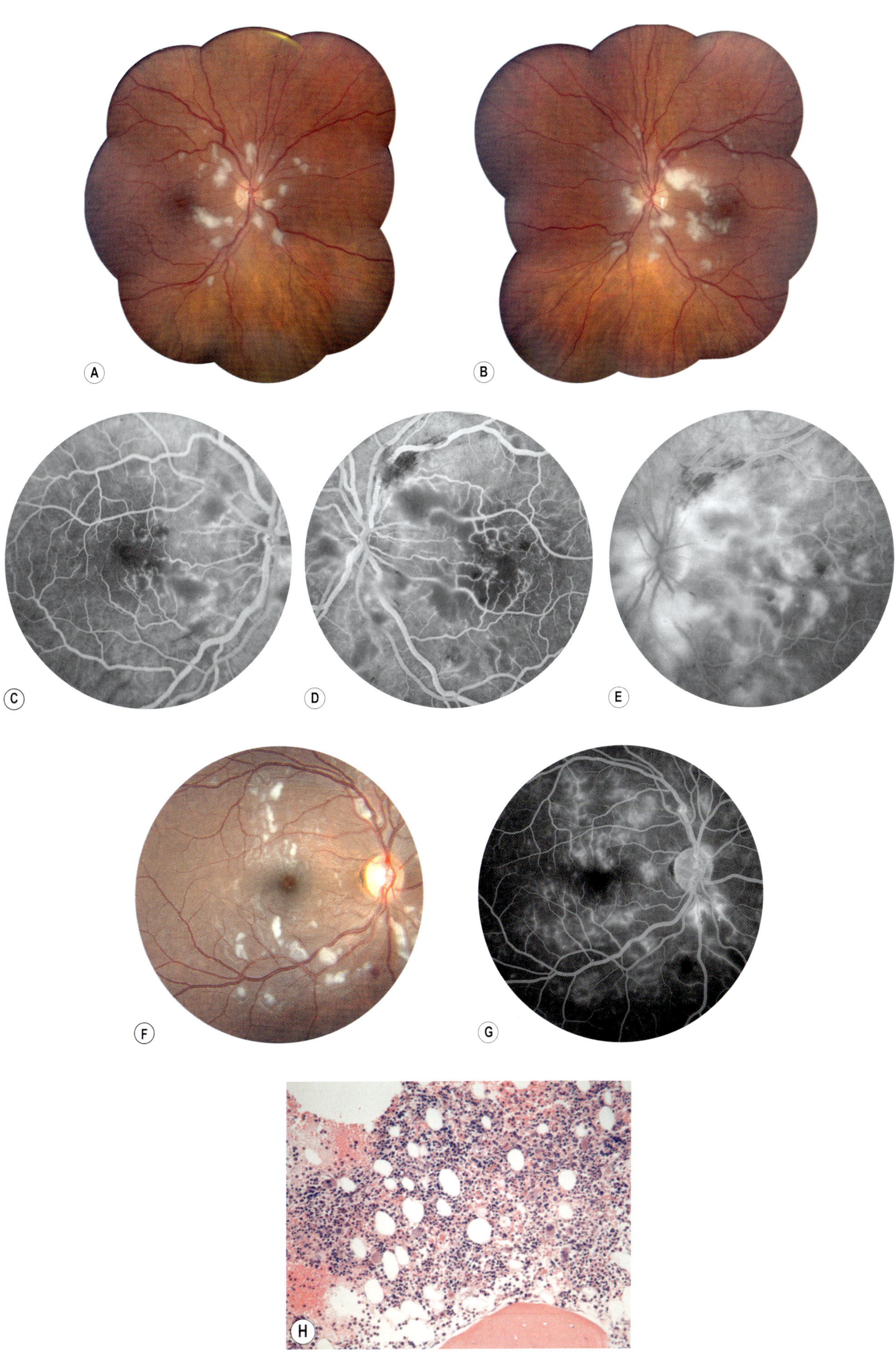
A
B
C
D
E
F
G
H

Exogenous Embolization

Talc Retinopathy

Drug users may prepare a suspension for injection by dissolving crushed tablets, most often methylphenidate (Ritalin), in boiling water. The suspension may be inadequately filtered and injected intravenously, causing showers of insoluble fillers, principally talc and cornstarch, to embolize the pulmonary vasculature. Large-caliber collateral vessels are created around areas of occluded pulmonary vasculature after repeated embolization. The trapped particles also produce pulmonary granulomatosis and pulmonary hypertension; particles that are 7 μm or smaller can traverse the intact pulmonary bed. Together with larger particles that pass through the pulmonary collateral vessels, they may be deposited as multiple, tiny, glistening, irregularly shaped particles in the retinal vasculature, particularly in the macular area (Figure 6.17A, B, and D).[240–245] In most patients they produce no symptoms. In some patients deposits of this material in the peripheral retina may cause areas of retinal capillary nonperfusion and retinal neovascularization at the junction of perfused and nonperfused retina similar to that in sickle-cell disease.[242,245,246] Angiography may show no evidence of obstruction or may show small areas of capillary nonperfusion, microaneurysmal changes, and widening and irregularities of the FAZ. Some such patients may have subnormal acuity. Optic disc neovascularization, vitreous hemorrhage, and traction retinal detachment have occurred.[245,247] Only those patients with long-term drug use develop fundoscopic changes. The retinopathy has been produced experimentally in primates.[241,248,249] In patients with a patent foramen ovale, that is prevalent in 29% of population, larger particles can occlude branch retinal arteries (Figure 6.17C).[250] Biopsy of the pulmonary nodules showed material consistent with talc that was birefringent under polarizing microscope (Figure 6.17F and G). Other foreign materials may occasionally lodge in the retinal vessels of drug addicts.[251,252] In those with retinal artery occlusion after use of cocaine, heroin, and methamphetamine, the mechanism of the retinal artery occlusion may be pharmacologic rather than embolic.[252,253] (See Chapter 9). Very tiny talc particles in a chronic methamphetamine snorter using for more than 15 years has been reported. The mechanism may be from absorption of the particles into the nasal mucosal vessels eventually reaching the lungs and the retina.[254]

6.16 Central retinal artery and vein occlusion associated with thrombotic thrombocytopenic purpura (TTP) and Still's disease.

A–J: A previously healthy 50-year-old woman developed rash, fever, abdominal pain, and weakness over 1 week and was diagnosed as having adult-onset Still's disease. She developed encephalopathy and secondary TTP, after which she noted bilateral loss of vision to counting fingers at 6 feet (2 meters). She had symmetric-appearing extensive retinal opacification and blot hemorrhages consistent with a combined central retinal artery occlusion/central retinal vein occlusion picture (A and B). Angiography revealed very poor perfusion of both retinal arteries (C–F). Her vision continued to decline and dropped to hand motions and light perception. Intravitreal triamcinolone (4 mg) did not help her retinal changes, and she developed neovascularization of the iris on the right side requiring intravitreal bevacizumab and panretinal photocoagulation. Both eyes ended with extreme atrophy of the retina and sclerosed vessels with no light perception vision (G–J).

(From Schwartz et al.,[1362] with permission.)

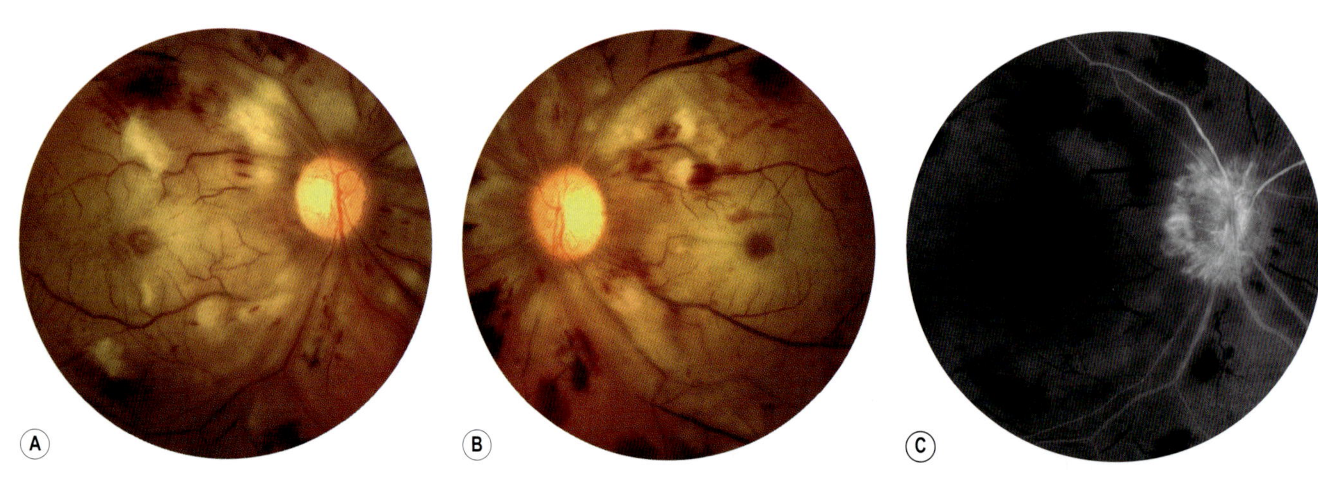

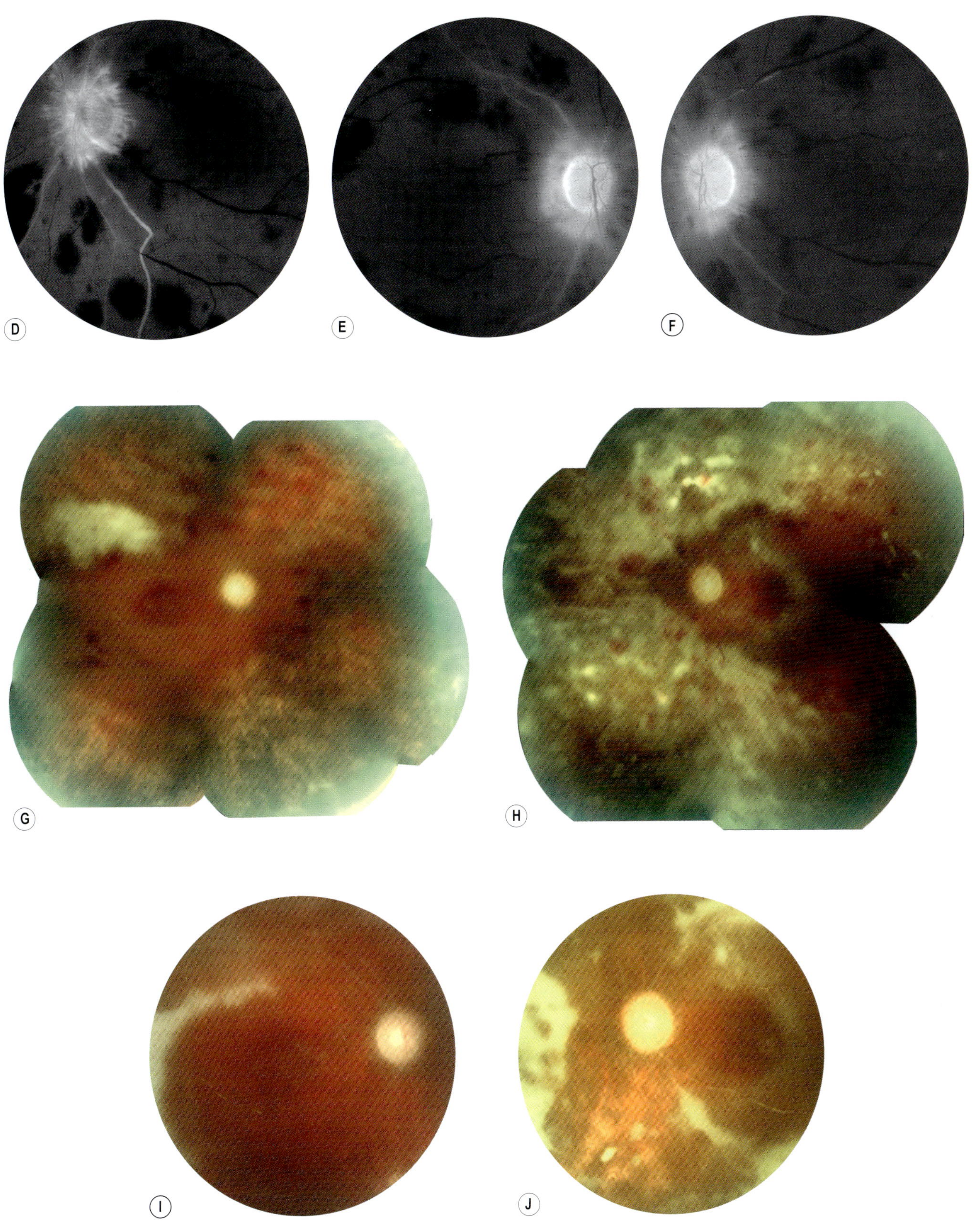
D
E
F
G
H
I
J

Retinal Emboli From Artificial Cardiac Valves

Cloth particles derived from cloth-covered artificial cardiac valves may cause loss of central vision secondary to retinal arterial embolization.[255]

Retinal Arterial Embolization Following Corticosteroid Suspension Injection

Injection of corticosteroid suspensions such as methylprednisolone acetate (Depo-Medrol) into the nasal mucosa, lips, face, scalp, tonsillar fossa, and orbit, as well as directly into periocular lesions (chalazion, hemangioma), may pass in a retrograde fashion into the ophthalmic, central retinal, and short ciliary arteries and produce visual loss caused by infarction of either the retina[82,256–265] or the optic nerve.[264,266–269] Both eyes may occasionally be affected.[260] The presence of the drug in both the retinal and choroidal circulation may be evident over widespread areas in the fundus (Figures 6.17I and J and 6.18A–C). In some cases the patient may regain normal visual acuity.[256,269] A similar picture has been produced experimentally in dogs.[270]

Other causes of exogenous embolization include retrobulbar injection of silicone and fat (Figure 6.18F–I),[2205,271] surgical embolization of intracranial arteries with polyvinyl alcohol,[272] platelet transfusion,[273] fragments of artificial heart valves and arterial implants, and air.[274] A picture suggesting multifocal retinal artery occlusions after local anesthesia for blepharoplasty was attributed to tissue substance released into the lacrimal artery.[275]

6.17 Exogenous embolization of the central retinal artery.

A and B: Intra-arterial talc emboli in a patient who chronically injected methylphenidate (Ritalin) intravenously.
C–G: This 24-year-old woman was asked to be evaluated for positive fungal blood cultures during a hospital admission for osteomyelitis. She was visually asymptomatic and found to have a branch retinal artery occlusion on the right and several intra-arteriolar white particles (C and D). She admitted to having used recreational drugs intravenously for several years. A transesophageal echo revealed a patent foramen ovale, which allowed larger talc particles into her left circulation that resulted in the retinal emboli. A computed tomography angiogram of her chest revealed a diffuse nodular pattern and focal nodules (E, arrows). Lung biopsy showed foreign-body giant-cell reaction to polarizable material consistent with talc (F and G).
H: Retinal arterial embolization after intranasal injection of methylprednisolone acetate in a 24-year-old woman who complained of "champagne bubbles," numbness of the upper lip, and transient blindness of the ipsilateral eye. Visual acuity returned to 20/20 30 minutes after injection.
I and J: Retinal (arrows) and widespread choroidal arteriolar embolization in a 35-year-old patient who experienced a positive scotoma, orbital pain, diplopia, and visual loss immediately after injection of methylprednisolone acetate into the ipsilateral nasal turbinates. Visual acuity initially was 20/80 but returned to 20/20. One day later most of the retinal emboli were no longer present. Note the intrachoroidal emboli were less apparent (J).

(A and B, courtesy of Dr. Mark J. Daily; C–G, from Tarantola et al.,[250]; H–J, from Byers.[256];

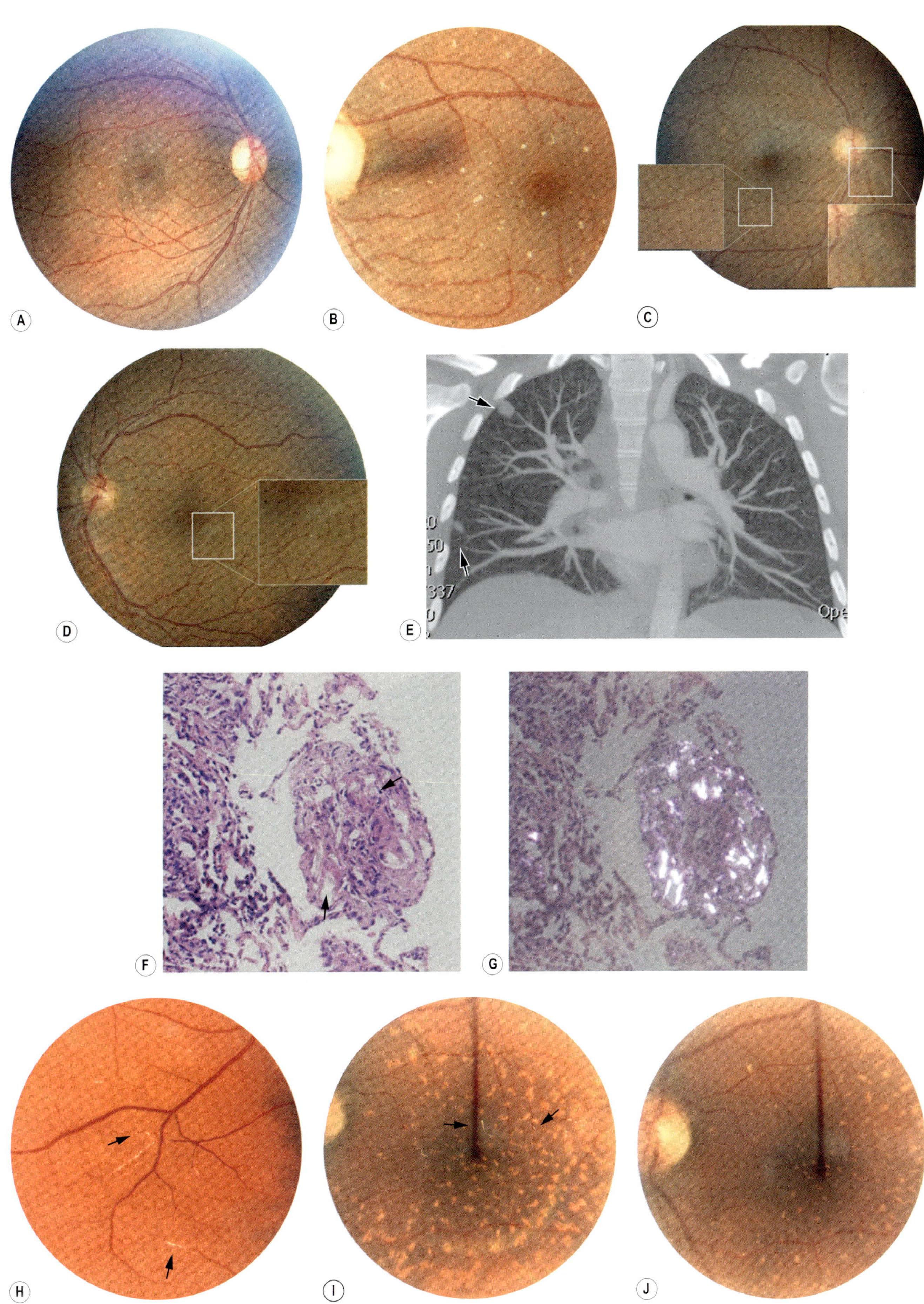
A
B
C
D
E
F
G
H
I
J

Obliterative Retinal Arterial Diseases

Arteriosclerosis and Atherosclerosis

Focal narrowing of the major arteries supplying the retina caused by arteriosclerosis and atherosclerosis with thrombosis may cause the typical picture of CRAO or, less often, branch retinal artery occlusion. It is probable that this mechanism for occlusion occurs less commonly than embolization, particularly in cases of branch artery occlusion. Systemic atherosclerosis may affect the ophthalmic artery and the central retinal artery up to the level of the lamina cribrosa, but rarely does it affect the more anterior portions of the central retinal artery. The reason for this is uncertain but may be related to the absence of the internal elastic lamina in the retinal arteries, which have a complete muscular coat out as far as the equator.[276] Although primary atherosclerosis of the retinal arterial tree is rare, the formation of secondary, often nonobstructive atheromatous plaques at focal sites of retinal arterial wall damage may develop in association with a variety of disorders, including arterial macroaneurysms, usually in patients with hypertension (see p. 494 in Chapter 6), toxoplasmosis retinitis (see Kyrieleis plaques, figure 10.22F-H), bilateral idiopathic recurrent branch retinal artery occlusion (see p. 474 in Chapter 6), acute retinal necrosis caused by herpes zoster (see Chapter 10) large-cell lymphoma (see figure 13.31 H), and chronic uveitis.[129]

Unusual Causes of Retinal Artery and Arteriolar Thrombosis

Occlusion of the central retinal artery, presumably caused by thrombosis, may occur occasionally in association with systemic diseases including essential thrombocythemia,[277] thrombotic thrombocytopenic purpura,[196,278] homocystinuria,[279] mild hyperhomocysteinemia in heterozygotes,[280] antiphospholipid antibody syndrome (Snedden's syndrome),[191,227,281–284]protein S deficiency,[179,180] (Figure 6.16C–F) protein C deficiency,[181] and Lyme disease.[285] Multifocal arteriolar occlusions associated with bone marrow transplantation may simulate Purtscher's retinopathy.[286–290] It is uncertain whether these arteriolar occlusions occur primarily as a complication of irradiation or some other mechanism such as leukoembolization. The administration of fibrinolytic agents, such as tranexamic acid, to reduce the chances of bleeding may occasionally promote spontaneous thrombosis and branch retinal artery occlusion.[291]

6.18 Exogenous embolization of the central retinal artery.

A–E: A 23-year-old girl received 1 ml of methyl prednisone acetate to a progressive hemangioma at the tip of her nose. She lost consciousness 15–20 seconds after the injection. On regaining consciousness she complained of visual loss in both eyes, to no light perception. Both retinas showed several intra-arterial embolic material and areas of retinal and choroidal whitening (A and B). Paracentesis of the anterior chamber in both eyes improved vision to count fingers bilaterally. The emboli had broken down 48 hours later and the vision had improved to 20/200 (C). Her vision gradually improved to 20/60 on the right and 20/30 on the left over 10 days when the retinal opacification had faded and all the emboli had disappeared (D and E) and eventually to 20/30 on the right and 20/20 on the left by 1 year.
F–I: Ischemic retinopathy and choroidopathy caused by embolization of silicone injected into the lid. The patient experienced sudden loss of vision immediately after the injection. Note the multiple blotchy retinal hemorrhages (G). Angiography revealed multifocal filling defects in the choroid (H) and focal retinal arteriolar leakage (I).

(A–E, courtesy of Dr. Vishali Gupta and Dr. Amod Gupta.)

Arteritis and Arteriolitis

A variety of inflammatory disorders, some infectious and some of unknown etiology, may cause acute obstruction of either or both the ophthalmic and retinal arterial circulation, e.g., cat-scratch disease, (see p. 812 in Chapter 10), herpes zoster (see pp. 898–900), mucormycosis (see p. 844 in Chapter 10), toxoplasmosis (see pp. 848–852 in Chapter 10),[292] giant cell arteritis[231] (see figure 6.23G-I), hypereosinophilic syndrome,[172] eosinophilic fasciitis (Figure 6.13L and 6.15F–H), Churg–Strauss syndrome (allergic angiitis and granulomatosis, Figure 11.51),[173,293] Kawasaki disease,[294] idiopathic multifocal retinitis (see p. 86 in Chapter 11), and acute multiple sclerosis (MS).[295] Although the retinal occlusive disease seen in these patients, as well as in patients with collagen vascular disease, has been attributed by some authors to arteritis, the arterial obstruction may be caused by other mechanisms, including hypertensive arteriolar narrowing, immune complex vascular damage, thromboembolization or leukocytic aggregation, and embolization (see discussion under leukoembolization, p. 464 in Chapter 6).[192,219,220,228,296]

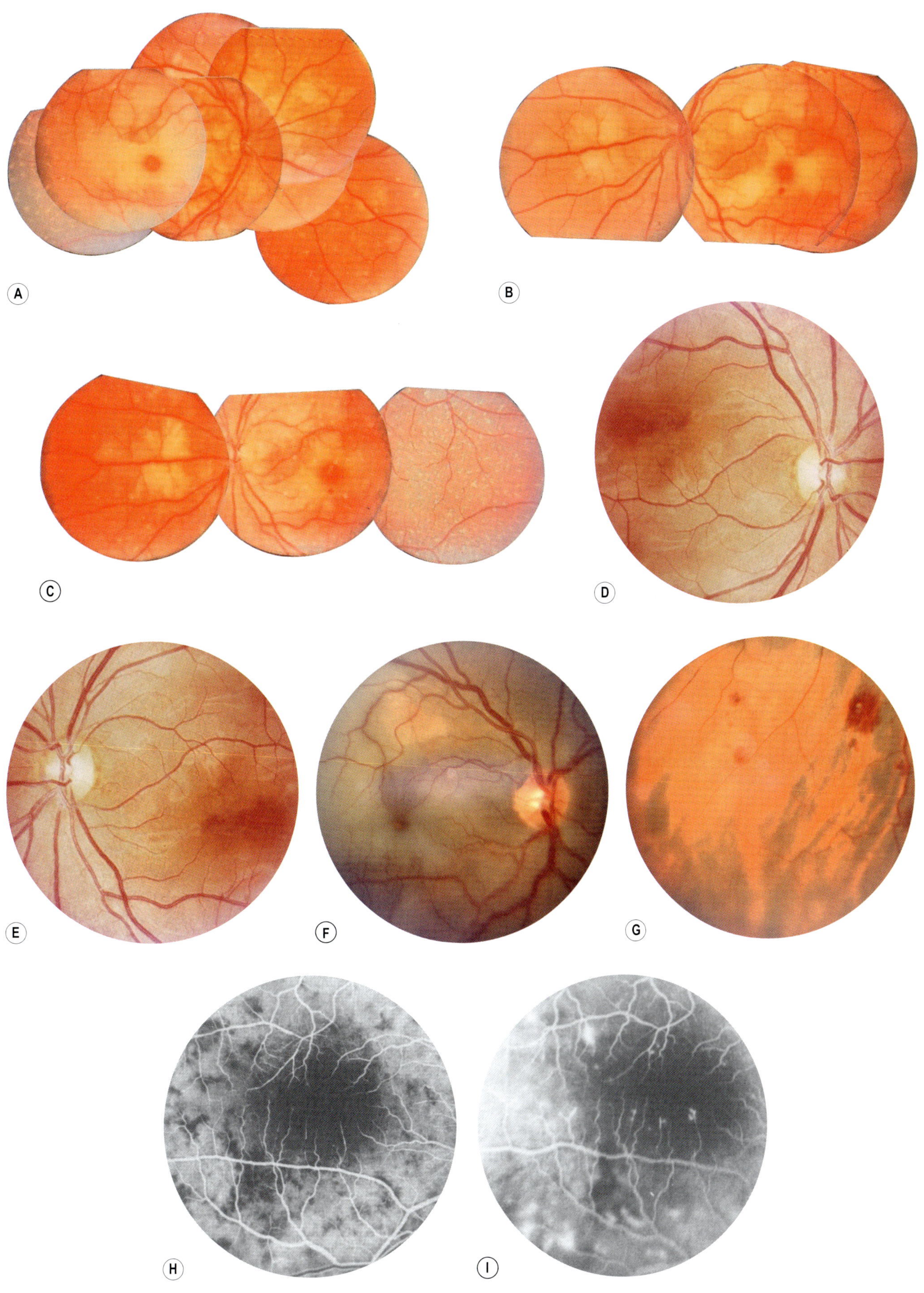
A
B
C
D
E
F
G
H
I

Idiopathic Recurrent Branch Retinal Arterial Occlusion (Susac Syndrome)

Apparently healthy individuals may develop, in one or both eyes, visual loss caused by recurrent episodes of multiple branch retinal arterial and arteriolar occlusions that often spare central vision (Figures 6.19–6.21).[182,297–302] The scotomata may be accompanied by photopsia, typically characterized as irregular shimmering, geometric lines or shapes of light just preceding a new scotoma and confined to the area destined to become scotomatous (45%); vestibuloauditory symptoms (50%); other transient focal neurologic symptoms, often affecting the face and upper extremities (30%) (Figure 6.19A–F); and a history of migraine (40%), defined as recurrent episodes of scintillating scotoma (with or without headache) or severe one-sided headache with nausea.[301] Memory and cognition disturbances with confusion and bizarre behavior with mood and personality changes may accompany, precede, or antecede the other symptoms. The disease affects 20–40-year-olds of both sexes with a slight preponderance in females.

It is considered to be an autoimmune endotheliopathy involving the arterioles of the brain, eye, and cochlea and is also referred to as retinocochleocerebral vasculopathy. The focal retinal arterial obstruction is unassociated with visible emboli, may occur in the midportion of an artery and at arterial bifurcations, and is frequently associated with focal periarterial whitening and fluorescein angiographic evidence of segmental arterial staining near the site of the obstruction and elsewhere in the fundus (Figure 6.19A–F).[299,303] Sheathing and multiple periarterial yellow-white plaques often develop along the obstructed arterial segment and may remain permanently (Figure 6.19G, H, K, and L). Egan et al. named these Gass plaques (Figure 6.19 K).[304–306] In some cases only a ghost remnant of the completely occluded arterial segment remains (Figure 6.21A and G). These patients are subject to recurrent retinal artery occlusive events that, in some cases, may extend over a period of 10 years or more.[301] Retinal, optic disc, and iris neovascularization may develop in 25% of eyes and requires photocoagulation or in some cases vitrectomy (Figure 6.19I and J).[299,301,307,308] These patients are frequently subjected to multiple extensive unrewarding medical evaluations. Standard screening tests for blood dyscrasia, dysproteinemias, and coagulopathies, including those for antiphospholipid antibodies and natural anticoagulant deficient states; imaging tests of the carotid arteries, heart, and brain; and screening tests (excluding magnetic resonance imaging: MRI) for systemic vasculitis are typically negative. Johnson et al. found multiple lesions compatible with focal brain infarcts in one of three patients studied with MRI.[301] The angiographic and ophthalmoscopic findings suggest that focal retinal arteritis and arteriolitis, perhaps caused by precipitation of immune complexes along the arterial wall, are responsible for the occlusions. The occasional association with serologic evidence of cytomegalic infection and protein S and protein C deficiency disease in these patients may be coincidental.[179,181,298]

6.19 Idiopathic, bilateral, recurrent, branch retinal arterial occlusion (Susac syndrome).

A–F: This 26-year-old woman noted tinnitus and multiple negative and scintillating scotomata in the left eye associated with multiple branch retinal arteriolar occlusions (A). Angiography revealed multiple focal areas of retinal artery and arteriolar staining and occlusion (B and C). She subsequently developed similar occlusions in the right eye (arrows, D–F) and had multiple other episodes of branch arterial occlusion over a 3-year period. Medical evaluation was negative. When last seen 5 years after the onset of symptoms, her visual acuity was 20/20 in both eyes.

G–J: This 48-year-old man had multiple branch retinal artery occlusions in both eyes over a 9-year period. Despite multiple extensive medical evaluations, no cause was found. Note the ghosting and sheathing of the retinal arteries, periarterial plaques, and focal area of retinal neovascularization (arrows, I and J). When last seen 13 years after the onset of symptoms, visual acuity was 20/20.

K and L: Periarterial plaque associated with bilateral, recurrent branch retinal artery occlusions of unknown cause in a 51-year-old man. The plaques became less prominent over a 4-year period (arrows).

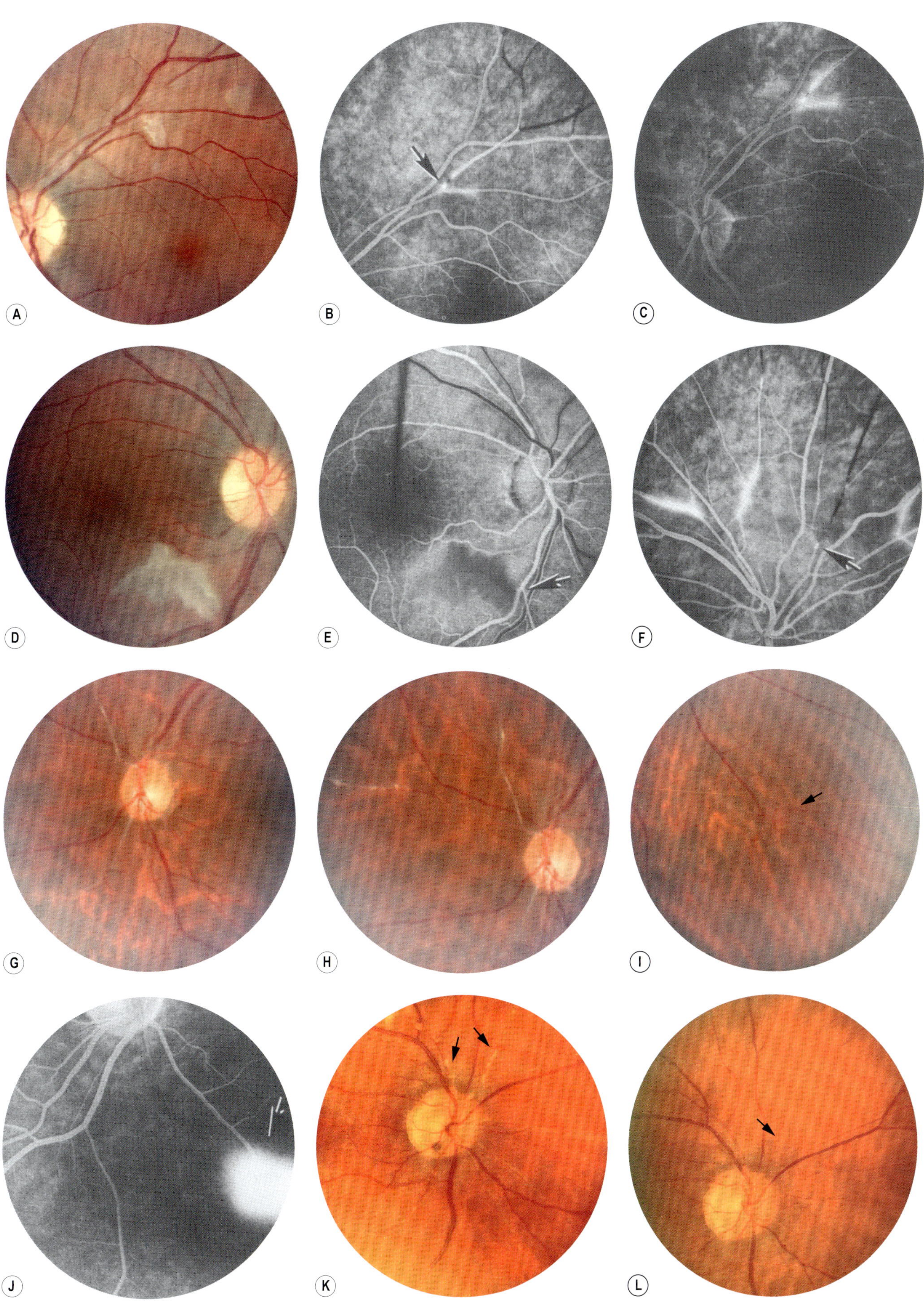
A
B
C
D
E
F
G
H
I
J
K
L

Most patients with idiopathic recurrent branch retinal artery occlusion are part of the triad of the syndrome of multiple branch retinal arterial occlusions, hearing loss, and encephalopathy (Susac sydrome). The triad sometimes is not apparent for a few years and the diagnosis may be delayed.[309] The encephalopathy usually develops subacutely and often includes psychiatric features, personality change, and bizarre and paranoid behavior.[310] The hearing loss is usually bilateral, asymmetric, and is often associated with tinnitus, vertigo, and ataxia. Low and medium frequencies are affected, localizing the lesion to the apical portion of the cochlea. MRI of the inner ear fails to show microinfarcts in the inner ear. MRI typically shows numerous infarcts in white and gray matter, more often in the periventricular region and the central part of the corpus callosum, and may show leptomeningeal involvement.[309–311] The lesions in the corpus callosum are small, multifocal, and enhance in the early stages of the diseases (Figure 6.21J). They are responsible for the behavioral manifestations. The lesions are hyperintense on T2 fluid-attenuated inversion recovery (FLAIR). Diffuse tensor imaging may be able to detect white-matter abnormalities in the early phase of the disease. The clinical findings and MRI changes are often attributed to MS[301,312] or acute disseminated encephalomyelitis. The key differentiating features on MRI are central corpus callosum involvement in Susac's but peripheral in MS and acute disseminated encephalomyelitis, leptomeningeal involvement is limited to Susac, and basal ganglial lesions are seen more often in Susac and are rare in MS.[310] The cerebrospinal fluid examination usually reveals minimal pleocytosis. The clinical course in these patients with encephalopathy, hearing loss, and multiple branch retinal artery occlusion can be self-limited, ranging from 1 to 2 years, with a good prognosis.[312] However, in some patients, the disorder may be progressive and result in severe visual loss and death (Figure 6.11G–L).

Pathogenesis of the disease is poorly understood. Endothelial deposition of C4d demonstration histologically (Magro CM, unpublished data), serum anti endothelial antibodies at a titre of 1:960, and indirect immunofluorescence demonstration of IgG_1 subclass antibodies[311] suggest the disorder to be autoimmune in nature. Elevated levels of factor VIII and von Willebrand factor antigen may be the result of endothelial damage.[305] Response to steroids and immunosuppressives also lends strength to the autoimmune hypothesis.

6.20 Idiopathic recurrent branch retinal artery occlusion associated with cerebrovascular involvement.

A–F: In February 1986 this 48-year-old woman with a long history of migraine headaches experienced a sudden onset of a paracentral scotoma in the right eye associated with a small branch retinal artery occlusion. In the asymptomatic fellow eye she had evidence of a branch retinal artery obstruction (arrow, A) and multiple focal areas of retinal arterial wall permeability changes (C and D). Several days after initial examination she developed dizziness and difficulty swallowing and talking. The diagnosis was "brainstem migraine." Over the next 2 years she experienced multiple branch retinal arterial occlusions (E, February 1986; F, August 1986). Extensive medical and neurologic investigations including assay for protein C, protein S, and lupus anticoagulant were normal. Over the next 5 years she had no further ocular or neurologic symptoms. Her visual acuity when last seen corrected to 20/15 bilaterally.

G–L: In December 1984 this 71-year-old man presented with a 3-month history of progressive loss of vision in the left eye and a 5-day history of headaches and loss of vision in the right eye. His past medical history was unremarkable except for well-controlled systemic hypertension. His visual acuity was 20/25 right eye and hand movements left eye. There were multiple branch retinal arteriolar occlusions, extensive atheromatous retinal arterial changes, and scattered retinal hemorrhages in both eyes (G–I). The left optic disc was pale. Fluorescein angiography revealed evidence of extensive retinal artery and arteriolar occlusion (J). The patient was hospitalized, and medical and neurologic evaluations, including temporal artery biopsy, cerebral arteriograms, and computerized scans of the brain, were negative. In January 1985 he developed new paracentral branch retinal artery occlusions in the right eye (K). In April 1985 he developed bilateral vitreous hemorrhage and proliferative retinopathy (L). His family noted that he had a change in personality. In June 1985 he developed signs of a right-sided stroke, and progressive mental deterioration; he died after cardiac arrest in September 1985.

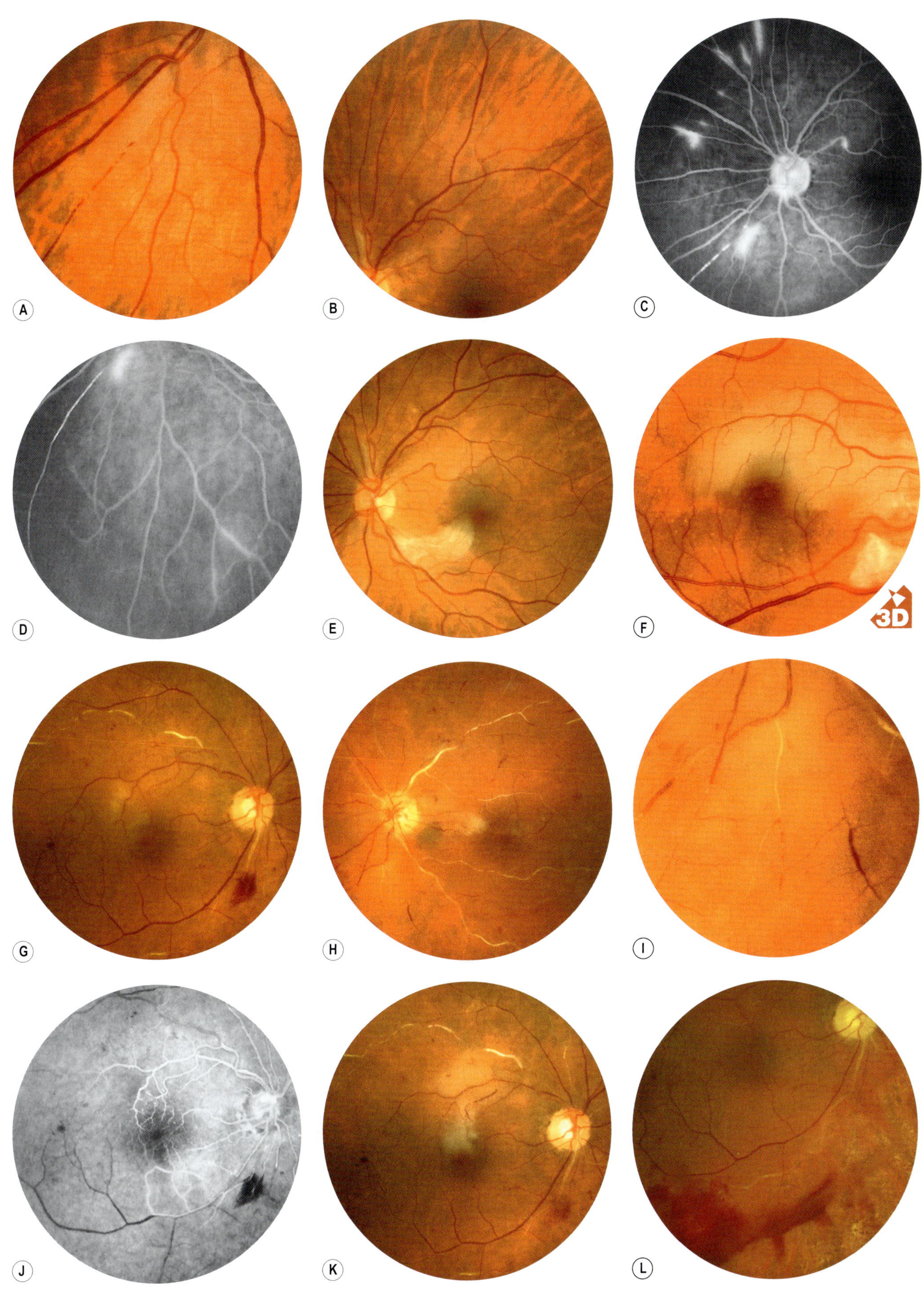
A
B
C
D
E
F
3D
G
H
I
J
K
L

A specific treatment is yet to be confirmed since the disease etiopathogenesis is not completely understood. Treatment has evolved over the years and currently is a combination of systemic corticosteroids, immunosuppressives, and immunomodulating drugs. For an acute severe presentation, intravenous immunoglobulin (IVIG, 2 g/kg divided over five doses) every other day along with a high dose of systemic steroids is begun. IVIG is given every month for the first year or so and then maintained at 2-monthly intervals indefinitely till the disease shows no flareups over a few years. Systemic steroid is maintained at a moderate dose for the first few months then at a low dose for a few years. Mycophenolate mofetil has been substituted as a steroid-sparing agent in some patients. Cyclophosphamide has also been used as a long-term immunosuppressant in place of IVIG. Most recently rituximab, a monoclonal antibody, is being tried.[309,313,314] Some patients have a self-limiting disease that quietens in 1–2 years and do not require long-term maintenance therapy.

Young patients with branch retinal artery occlusion associated with idiopathic multifocal retinitis and neuroretinitis (cat-scratch disease) may simulate idiopathic recurrent branch retinal artery occlusion (see Chapter 10, Figure 10.04).

X-Ray Irradiation

Exposure of the retina to X-ray irradiation may cause retinal arteriolar narrowing, cotton-wool patches, capillary telangiectasia, and retinal arterial occlusion (see pp. 554–556).[315–317]

6.21 Susac's syndrome.

A–H: This 25-year-old woman presented with diplopia and ataxia in 1999. She was diagnosed with multiple sclerosis when magnetic resonance imaging (MRI) showed white-matter changes, and was treated with intravenous methyl prednisolone and placed on interferon-1-alpha. Two years later she developed a visual field defect in her right eye and hearing loss, when she received intravenous methyl prednisolone. Her visual loss improved but hearing remained impaired. A year later she noted a new field loss in her left eye when she was evaluated at Vanderbilt and diagnosed as having Susac's syndrome. She had a fresh superotemporal branch retinal artery occlusion on the left with retinal whitening and evidence of old occlusion on the right (A and B). Angiogram showed typical finding of Susac syndrome with fusiform staining of the involved vessel wall (C) and other uninvolved vessels (E) and previously occluded vessels on the right (D). The retinal whitening faded somewhat by 2 weeks; over the course of several previous and further episodes her optic nerves became pale (G and H). She had patchy field loss, though her central vision remained at 20/25 in each eye. She was treated with intravenous immunoglobulin (IVIG) and systemic steroids and maintained on monthly IVIG injections. She continues to remain stable.
I–L: This 34-year-old woman in 1995, soon after the birth of her second child, was evaluated by her psychiatrist for personality changes and diagnosed with anxiety and depression. Over the next 10 years she developed episodic hearing loss, and visual field loss that was attributed to "multiple sclerosis." In the meanwhile her cognition was impaired and she had become a "slow thinker." She was treated with intravenous methyl prednisolone and started on interferon-1-alpha. In 2007 she presented to Vanderbilt with bilateral visual field defects attributable to fresh branch retinal artery occlusions (I). She was diagnosed as having Susac's syndrome and started on IVIG, oral steroids, and methotrexate. An MRI of her brain showed several callosal (J), periventricular, cortical, cerebellar, and pontine hyperintense lesions on T2 fluid-attenuated inversion recovery (FLAIR) imaging. She developed a superotemporal artery occlusion in the right eye a few months later when she self-decreased her oral prednisone (K). Note the narrowing at the site of previous occlusion in the inferotemporal arteriole (arrow). An angiogram showed the typical fusiform staining of the affected and unaffected vessel walls (L, arrow heads). She also shows evidence of past occlusions in the inferonasal arteriole. She has remained without further retinal occlusions over the next 3 years and is on maintenance IVIG and a very low dose of prednisone.

(J, courtesy of Dr. Siddharama Pawate.)

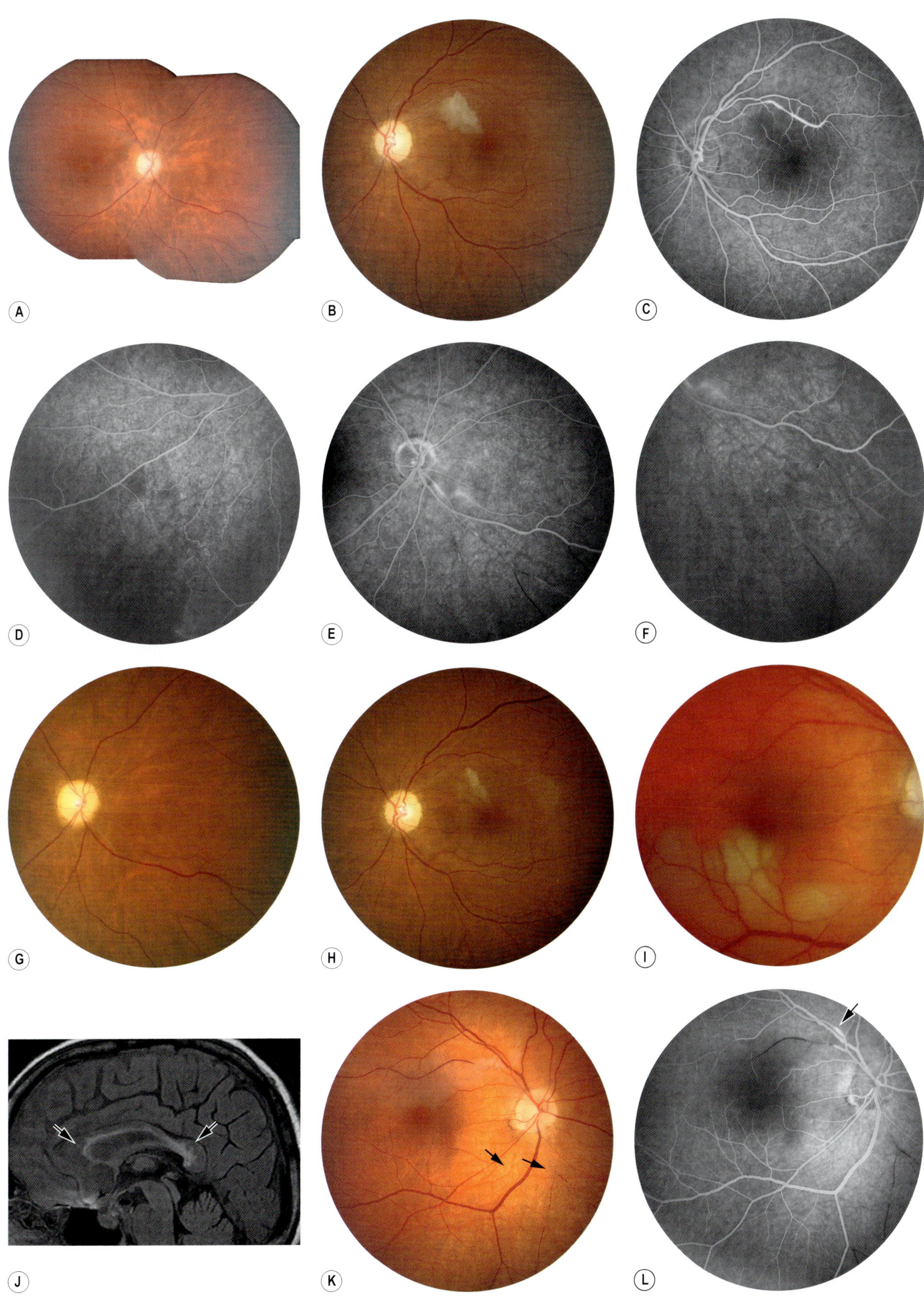
A
B
C
D
E
F
G
H
I
J
K
L

Retinal Arterial Obstruction Caused by Spasm

Some degree of reflex spasm probably plays a role in retinal arterial obstruction from many causes. The ocular fundi of patients with amaurosis fugax have been observed numerous times during an attack.[318,319] The characteristic picture described is pallor of the optic disc and marked narrowing of the retinal arteries. With restoration of circulation, vision promptly returns. In some cases this spasm may be associated with recognizable causes, such as ocular migraine, collagen vascular disease, sickle-cell disease (see Figure 6.60A–H), inhalation of cocaine (Figure 9.13) and amphetamines, and administration of propranolol.[182,216,253,320–322] It is probable that some cases of ischemic infarction resulting from retinal artery occlusion are caused by prolonged spasm of the central retinal artery. In the review by Brown and associates of a series of 27 patients under the age of 30 years who had retinal artery occlusion, the only associated finding was migraine headaches.[85,90] Wolter and Burchfield[322] reported a 12-year history of recurrent episodes of total vision loss in one eye associated with a cherry-red spot and complete recovery of vision in a 20-year-old man with ocular migraine. It is of interest that the photographs in their case show narrowing of the retinal veins rather than the arteries. This same phenomenon was noted in another patient by Dr. Mark Daily (Figure 6.22H and I).

6.22 Episodic vasospastic central retinal artery occlusion.

A–G: This young black woman with lupus erythematosus and sickle-cell hemoglobin C disease experienced episodes of blindness, each lasting 1–3 minutes, in the right eye several times daily. During an episode the retinal arteries were narrowed (A). Angiography revealed total obstruction of the central retinal artery and slow filling of both retinal veins and arteries via optic disc collateral vessels (B, 12 seconds; C, 27 seconds; D, 40 seconds; E, 85 seconds after injection of the dye). As vision returned to normal, dilation of the retinal arteries and veins occurred (F) and angiography revealed normal retinal perfusion (G). Her signs and symptoms failed to respond to blood transfusions but did so after systemic corticosteroid treatment.
H and **I**: Focal constriction of retinal veins (E) occurring during an episode of ocular migraine. Compare H with asymptomatic state in I.

(A, E, F, and G from Shaw et al.[216]; H and I, courtesy of Dr. Mark J. Daily.)

Retinal Migraine

Retinal migraine is a rare cause of transient monocular visual loss, first described by Galezowski in 1882. It is usually characterized by episodes of partial or complete reversible monocular visual loss ipsilateral to the headache and lasting less than an hour. Sometimes it can result in irreversible visual loss.[182,323] The 2004 International Headache Society criteria for the diagnosis of retinal migraine are as follows[324]:

A. At least two attacks fulfilling criteria B and C
B. Fully reversible monocular positive and/or negative visual phenomena confirmed by examination during an attack or by the patient's drawing of a monocular field defect during an attack
C. Headache fulfilling criteria - migraine without aura begins during the visual symptoms or follows them within 60 minutes
D. Normal ophthalmological examinations between attacks
E. Not attributed to another disorder.

The condition is more common in young women in their second and third decades. The field defect may not always be from the retina; the optic nerve or the choroid may be the site of spasm, hence "monocular migraine" may be a better term.[325,326] When examined during an episode these patients may have an afferent pupillary defect, constricted retinal arterioles, pallor of the optic disc, retinal whitening, and occasionally retinal venous constriction.[325,327,328] The documentation of a visual field defect that completely reverses in association with headache on the side of the visual loss is necessary to make the diagnosis. Treatment with propranolol can prevent future episodes and should be begun in a confirmed case.[324,327] These patients should be differentiated from patients with recurrent branch retinal artery occlusion of Susac syndrome,[329] amaurosis fugax from carotid embolic disease, retinal artery occlusions from collagen vascular disease such as lupus and antiphospholipid syndrome, protein C and S deficiency, and in older patients from giant cell arteritis, polyarteritis nodosa, and eosinophilic vasculitis.

Retinal Arterial Obstruction Caused by Diseases of Surrounding Structures

Acute closure of the retinal arterial circulation may be caused by diseases primarily affecting the surrounding tissues, including inflammatory diseases such as retinal toxoplasmosis (Figure 10.22A–C), neuroretinitis,[330] Bartonella associated multifocal retinitis and neuroretinitis[128] (see Figure 10.04), and orbital cellulitis; external pressure on the ophthalmic, central retinal, and cilioretinal arteries such as in orbital hemorrhage,[331] cavernous sinus thrombosis,[332] intersheath perioptic hemorrhage,[194] papilledema,[333,334]ischemic optic neuropathy, optic disc drusen,[335] central retinal vein occlusion,[336] and neoplastic diseases of the orbit, optic nerve, and retina[337]; carcinomatosis of the meninges of the brain and optic nerve[338]; and surgical manipulation such as retrobulbar procedures.[339,340]

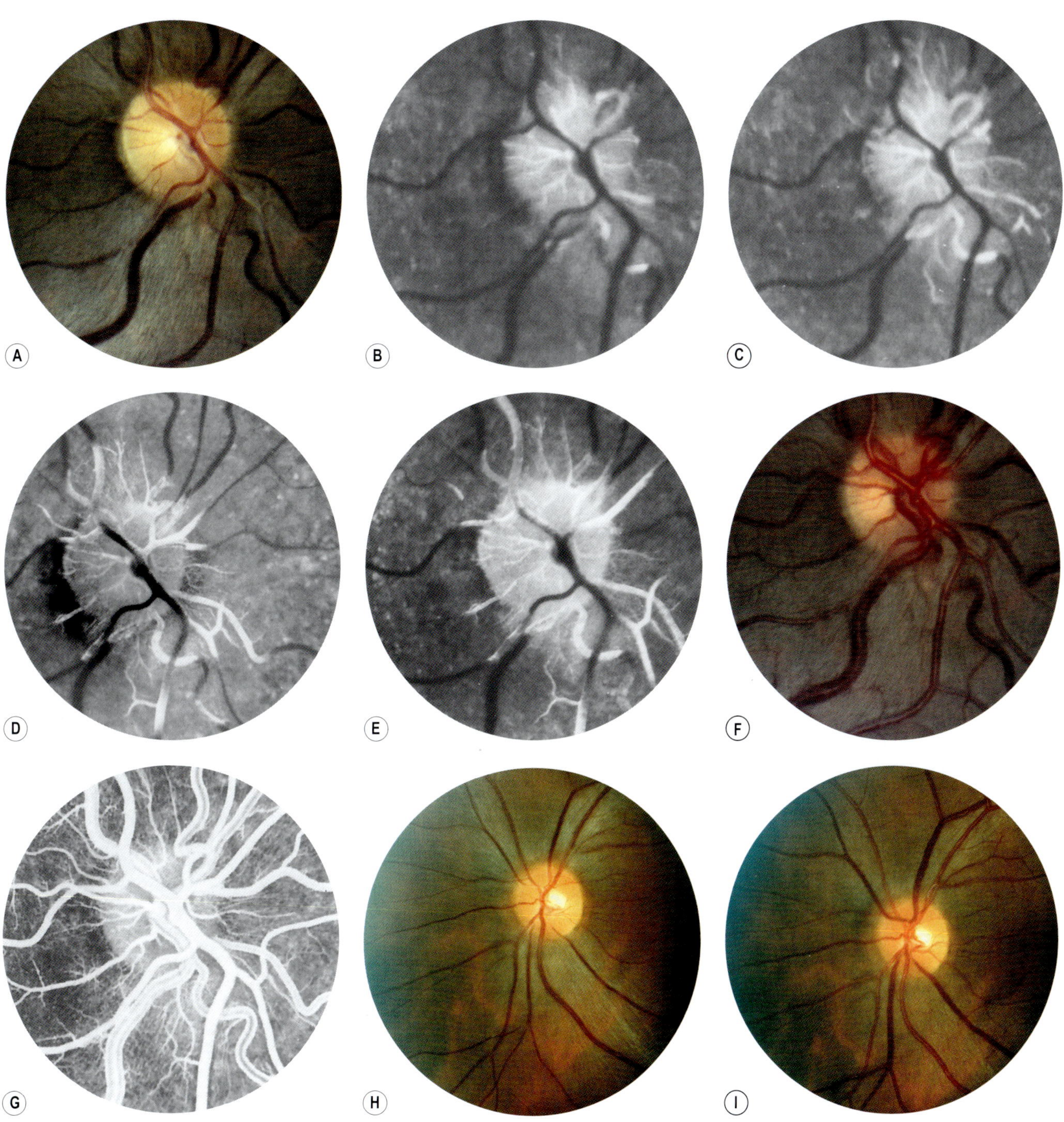
A
B
C
D
E
F
G
H
I

Branch retinal or cilioretinal artery occlusion may accompany central retinal vein obstruction in the same eye.[341,342] In some cases both may be the result of primary disease affecting the optic nerve head. In other patients, particularly those with cilioretinal artery obstruction, the central retinal vein obstruction may be the cause of decreased perfusion within the cilioretinal artery that normally has a lower perfusion pressure than the central retinal artery.[342]

Retinal Arterial Hypoperfusion Caused by Systemic Hypotension and Ocular Hypertension

Reduction of retinal blood flow in patients during systemic hypotensive episodes rarely produces evidence of retinal ischemia unless it occurs in patients with pre-existing disease causing reduced retinal flow.[343] Marked elevation of intraocular pressure may cause symptomatic optic nerve or retinal ischemia, particularly when it occurs in patients with other diseases, such as sickle-cell disease. Compression of the eye and orbital tissues during general anesthesia in the face-down position may occlude the ciliary and central retinal arterial blood supply to the eye.[344,345] (See Figure 3.54K and L.) This can also cause posterior ischemic optic neuropathy.

Retinal Arterial Hypoperfusion Caused by Carotid and Ophthalmic Artery Obstruction

Reduction of retinal arterial blood flow may be caused by obstruction of either or both the ipsilateral carotid and ophthalmic arteries.[104,346] Whereas this obstruction is usually caused by slow progressive narrowing associated with atheromatous disease, it may have a variety of other causes, including giant-cell arteritis,[347] spontaneous dissection,[348] fibromuscular dysplasia (FMD),[349] surgical complication,[350] Takayasu's disease,[351–353] and cavernous sinus thrombosis.[332] Rapid obstruction such as may occur in cranial arteritis (Figure 6.23G–L), mucormycosis, or herpes zoster causes acute visual loss and ischemic retinal infarction.[354] This is often accompanied by signs of ciliary artery obstruction, pallor of the optic disc, and hypotony (Figure 6.23J and K)[85,90,133,346,347,355–357] In a few patients multifocal areas of ischemia simulating Purtscher's retinopathy may occur (Figure 6.16H).[104] If obstruction of the major arteries occurs more slowly from atheromatous disease or chronic inflammation of the large arteries (Takayasu's disease), reduction in blood flow to the eye may or may not be sufficient to cause visual complaints (Figure 6.23A–C). A variety of fundus pictures may occur: (1) minimal or no ophthalmoscopic changes in patients complaining of transient loss of vision in one eye (amaurosis fugax)[318]; (2) few widely scattered blot and dot retinal hemorrhages and mild dilation of the retinal veins (venous stasis retinopathy), usually in patients with minimal visual complaints (Figure 6.23A–C)[358–362]; (3) dilation of the retinal arterial tree, dilation of the retina veins, and cotton-wool ischemic patches (Figure 6.23H); (4) retinal capillary changes, including microaneurysms, cystoid macular edema (CME), and angiographic evidence of areas of capillary nonperfusion that may be confined to the area along the horizontal raphe (Figure 6.23A–C)[363,364]; (5) larger areas of peripheral capillary nonperfusion, retinal neovascularization, and hemorrhage; (6) any degree of branch or central retinal vein or arterial obstruction (Figure 6.23H); (7) ischemic optic neuropathy (Figure 6.23I); and (8) any of the above associated with panuveitis, neovascular glaucoma, and a rapidly progressing cataract (ischemic ocular syndrome).[365,366]

6.23 Carotid and ophthalmic artery obstruction.

A–C: Blotchy peripheral retinal hemorrhages and retinal capillary changes (arrows, A) in a 57-year-old man with a 4-month history of frequent 8–10-minute episodes of "fogging" of vision of the right eye. There was no other history of transient ischemic attacks. He had xanthelasma for 12 years. Visual acuity was 20/20. Ophthalmodynamometry was 35/20 in the right eye and 110/40 in the left eye. Angiography showed increased retinal circulation time, microaneurysms, and dilation of retinal capillaries (C). The left fundus was normal.

D–F: Loss of peripheral vision, hypotony, and a 360° serous detachment of the ciliary body and choroid developed in a 72-year-old aphakic man 8 weeks after medical evaluation detected ipsilateral carotid artery obstruction. Ciliochoroidal detachment nasally extended almost to the optic disc (D and E, arrows). Note the round retinal hemorrhages that were present throughout the midperiphery of the eye. There was ophthalmodynamometric evidence of marked reduction in the ophthalmic artery pressure.

G–I: This elderly woman noted the sudden loss of vision in the left eye. Her vision and the fundus of the right eye were normal (G). Visual acuity in the left eye was 20/200. Note in the left fundus the patchy dense whitening of the inner juxtapapillary retina (H) and the diffuse whitening of the retina superiorly. On the following day she awoke with no light perception in the right eye. The right optic disc showed swelling and pallor (I) typical of ischemic optic neuropathy associated with giant-cell arteritis, which was demonstrated histopathologically on temporal artery biopsy. Intensive corticosteroid therapy was given. Ten months later she remained blind in the right eye and retained 20/70 in the left eye.

J and K: Unilateral blindness caused by ophthalmic artery occlusion in an elderly patient with cranial arteritis. Note the pallor of the optic disc and narrowing of the retinal vessels caused by previous obstruction of circulation in the central retinal artery; also note the segmental atrophy of the retinal pigment epithelium caused by obstruction of the short ciliary arterial circulation (J and K).

L: Histopathology of the temporal artery in a patient with cranial arteritis. Note severe narrowing of the vessel lumen by granulomatous arteritis.

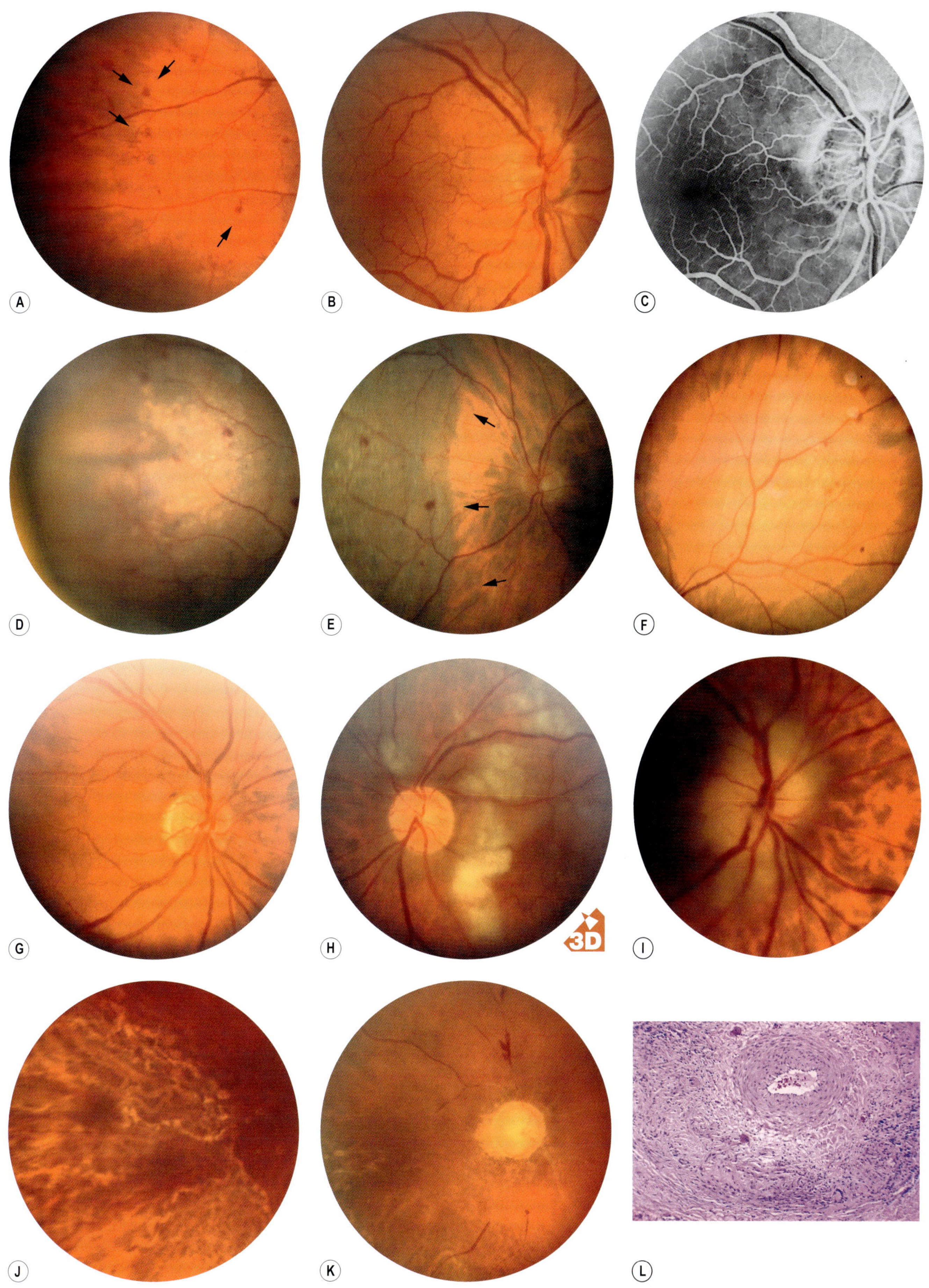
A
B
C
D
E
F
G
H
3D
I
J
K
L

Dr. Gass has seen one aphakic patient with carotid artery obstruction develop loss of vision caused by acute exudative detachment of the choroid and ciliary body (Figure 6.23D–F). The detachment resolved rapidly after carotid endarterectomy. The ophthalmologist faced with any patient who has these ocular signs or symptoms should inquire about other signs or symptoms of transient ischemic attacks and should look for other evidence of ipsilateral carotid artery obstruction, such as reduction of carotid artery pulsation, a bruit over the carotid artery and orbit, and ease of collapse of the ipsilateral central retinal artery with finger pressure on the eye compared with that of the contralateral eye. Fluorescein angiography in all such cases should show a late appearance time of the dye in the central retinal artery and choroid and a prolonged retinal circulation time. In some cases a dramatic improvement in the fundus changes may occur after carotid endarterectomy.[367]

Takayasu Retinopathy

Mikito Takayasu in 1908 described the ocular manifestations of this condition as "peculiar changes in the central retinal vessels and wreath of arertiovenous communication" around the optic disc. The retinal changes include dilatation of the retinal arteries and veins with beading (Figure 6.24I and J), microaneurysms at the capillary level and along the arterioles (very typical; Figure 6.24A–F, I–L), vascular occlusion, large zones of nonperfusion, arteriovenous shunts, retinal and optic disc neovascularization (Figure 6.24I and L), and, occasionally, vitreous hemorrhages. The arm to retina time and the arteriovenous transit times are prolonged.[368–371] Poor blood flow to the eye is the basis of the ocular findings and is seen in those patients with involvement of the common carotid arteries (Figure 6.24G and H). The left side is more commonly involved than the right. Since the intravascular hydrostatic pressure is low, these patients have very few retinal hemorrhages, and minimal leakage from the new vessels (Figure 6.24L) and microaneurysms. The poor endothelial oxygenation causes a break in the blood–retinal barrier and mild fluorescein leakage, but much less intensely than other conditions such as diabetic retinopathy. Intraocular pressure is low due to poor perfusion of the ciliary body; eventually rubeosis irides (but rarely neovascular glaucoma) and cataract develop. Traction retinal detachment and phthisis bulbi have been seen very occasionally. Those patients with renal artery stenosis without involvement of the carotids show features of hypertensive retinopathy in the form of arteriolar narrowing, retinal hemorrhages, and arteriovenous crossing changes.

Takayasu arteritis, also known as "aorta arteritis" and "pulseless disease," is a form of chronic granulomatous panarteritis with possible autoimmune origin that affects the aorta and its branches. The coronary and pulmonary arteries can sometimes be involved. Why it is more common in Asia, Mexico, and other tropical countries is not fully understood. A link to poststreptococcus autoimmune change or to tuberculosis has been postulated.[372,373] Intimal proliferation and fibrosis of the media with scarring, thrombus formation, and eventual stenosis of the affected artery occur.

A female preponderence of up to 9:1 is seen in Asia, and affects young adults who present with clinical features based on the vessels involved. Those with involvement of the branches of the aortic arch present with amaurosis fugax, dizziness, and syncope. Renal artery stenosis leads to hypertension and its manifestations.

Takayasu arteritis is classified based on vessel involvment using radiological imaging into six groups[374]:

- Type I: branches of aortic arch
- Type IIa: ascending aorta, aortic arch, and its branches
- Type IIb: descending thoracic aorta with or without ascending aorta, arch, and its branches

6.24 Takayasu retinopathy.

A–H: A 28-year-old East Indian woman had a 6-month history of diminution of vision in both eyes accompanied by giddiness, which recovered on lowering her head. Her visual acuity was 20/200 in each eye and intraocular pressure 6 and 7 mmHg respectively. There were no iris new vessels and pupils were sluggish. Multiple microaneurysms were seen in both eyes, which were significantly more common anterior to the equator, and several on the larger arterioles (arrows A and B). There was remarkable delay in dye appearance in both the choroidal and retinal circulation. Several microaneurysms as well as dilated capillary bed filled on angiography. The late frames showed diffuse vessel wall staining of all retinal vessels (C to F). Her physical exam was significant for absent radial and brachial pulses. She underwent computed tomography; angiogram of the arch of the aorta and its branches was suggestive of type 4 Takaysu arteritis involving the ascending arch and descending aorta, left pulmonary artery, bilateral common carotid artery, brachiocephalic trunk, bilateral subclavian and axillary arteries (G and H). She was treated with oral steroids.

I–L: This 17-year-old Indian female was seen for episodic headaches and frequent blackouts. Her vision at initial evaluation was 20/30 both eyes, but subsequently declined over a year to count fingers in both eyes. Both eyes showed several microaneurysms, many of them on the arterioles (arrow), dilated and sausage-shaped veins (I and J). There were no retinal hemorrhages due to slow flow in the vessels. The left eye also had a large NVD (I). An angiogram picks up the numerous microaneurysms (K), and late frames show breakdown in the blood–retinal barrier due to endothelial hypoxia. Note the NVD does not leak early due to the very slow blood flow throughout the retina (L). Her blood pressure was unrecordable in the upper limbs and measured 160/80 mmHg in both lower limbs. Her carotid, radial, brachialis, and subclavian pulses were absent bilaterally, but the femoral, popliteal, posterior tibial, and dorsalis pedis were present. On an aortogram the right subclavian artery was absent, only stumps of the left common carotid and subclavian were seen, and there were rich collaterals between the intercostals and axillary vessels. She had type 2 Takayasu arteritis.

(A–L, courtesy of Dr. Amod Gupta; I–L, courtesy of Dr. Vishali Gupta and Dr. Amod Gupta.)

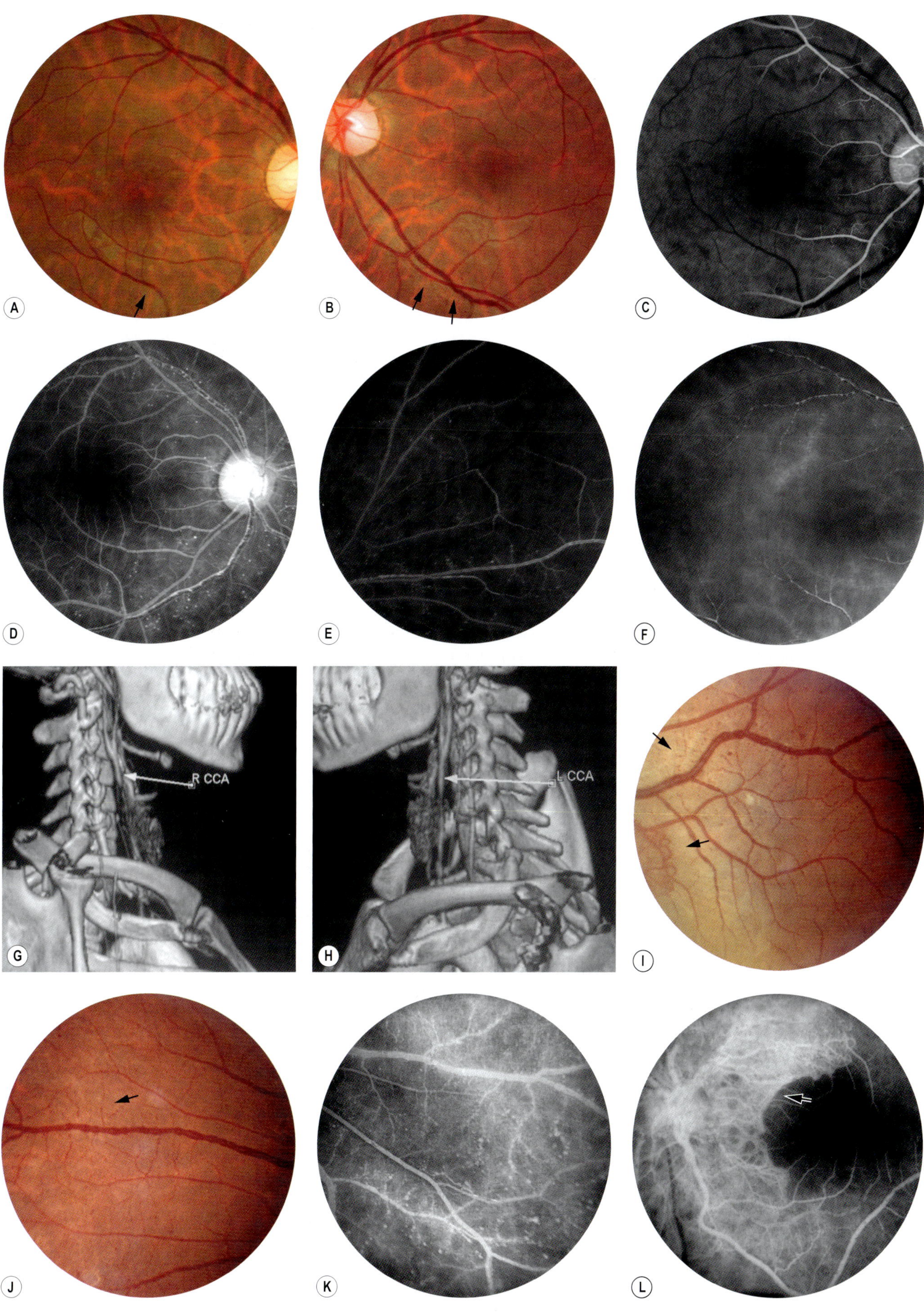
A
B
C
D
E
F
R CCA
G
L CCA
H
I
J
K
L

- Type III: descending thoracic aorta and abdominal aorta
- Type IV: abdominal aorta only
- Type V: aortic arch, descending thoracic aorta, and abdominal aorta.

Therapy depends on the stage of the disease. If the patient is seen early in the course of arteritis without significant occlusion, systemic steroids and immunosuppressives alone are indicated. Once occlusion or significant stenosis occurs, angioplasty and bypass grafts are needed in addition to the immunosuppressives.[369,373,375–379] Medical management of hypertension, nephrectomy, and autotransplantation of the kidney may be necessary. Antituberculous drugs in those patients with highly positive Mantoux test is indicated.[372]

Fibromuscular Dysplasia

FMD is a nonatheromatous, noninflammatory vascular disorder that commonly affects the renal and internal carotid arteries. It is known to cause choroidal hypoperfusion central retinal artery, and cilioretinal artery occlusion, though extremely rarely.[380–382] Retinal hypoperfusion, and its various manifestations, leading to retinal neovascularization and traction retinal detachment, similar to Takayasu retinopathy, has been described in one patient.[349] A fatal stroke and multiple retinal hemorrhages have been seen in an 11-month-old infant.[381] When a young patient without cardiovascular risk factors presents with a CRAO, one should rule out FMD. These patients may have recurrent strokes, transient ischemic attacks, syncope, headache, tinnitus, and cranial nerve palsies.[383] Unlike atherosclerosis that affects the proximal or origin of the caroid artery, FMD affects the middle or distal part and has a typical appearance on carotid Doppler/angiogram with the "pulled screw" configuration, focal tubular narrowing, or localized outpouching of the artery.[349] These configurations occur specifically in the three types of FMD (1) pulled screw or multiple constrictions in the medial type; (2) focal tubular narrowing in the intimal type; and (3) outpouching in the adventitial type. Aneurysms and involvement of other medium-sized arteries can also occur. Genetic risk factors are being investigated, as the disease is known to occur in first-degree relatives.

Retinal Hypoperfusion Caused by Cardiac Anomalies

Young patients with congenital cyanotic heart disease commonly develop some dilation and tortuosity of the major retinal vessels often associated with polycythemia.[81,384]Frank central retinal vein occlusion, atypical rubeosis iridis can be seen rarely.[385,386] Patients with pulmonary hypertension and a reversed bidirectional shunt through an intracardiac defect (Eisenmenger's syndrome) may develop retinal microvascular changes similar to that in patients with carotid artery obstruction.[387] Paradoxical embolus due to a right-to-left shunt can cause retinal artery occlusion.[388]

6.25 Hypertensive retinopathy.

A–C: This 32-year-old woman had a visual acuity of 20/80 secondary to severe hypertensive retinopathy. Note the macular star, cotton-wool patches, and hemorrhages. Early arteriovenous-stage angiograms showed narrowing of the first- and second-order arterioles (arrows) supplying the macula (B) and patchy staining of the retina corresponding to areas of dilated capillaries (C). Note the absence of fluorescein staining in the macula.

D–F: Foveal hemorrhage (D) caused by hypertensive microvascular changes evident in the angiogram (E). Note the white punctate flecks on the surface of the oval superficial retinal blood and the larger area of subretinal blood. Several months later the blood cleared (F) and the visual acuity returned to normal.

G–I: Ischemic optic neuropathy and branch retinal arterial occlusion in a patient with severe chronic hypertension. Note the sharp demarcation line (arrows, G) separating the ischemic retinal whitening from the nonischemic peripheral retina in the areas of distribution of the obstructed artery. The peripheral retina retained its transparency because of previously established collateral arterial channels (arrows) that became more apparent several months later in H and I.

J–L: Purtscher's-like retinopathy in this 58-year-old man caused by central retinal artery obstruction in a patient with hypertension. He noted blurred central vision in the left eye that progressed over a period of 24 hours to include the entire visual field. His visual acuity was 1/200. Note the severe retinal whitening in the papillomacular bundle area and patchy retinal whitening in the macular area. Angiography revealed delay in perfusion of the retinal circulation. Echography revealed distension of the left optic nerve sheath with fluid. Carotid artery studies were negative. His serum triglyceride was 944.

Retinal Arterial Hypoperfusion Caused by Occlusion of Retinal Venous Outflow

If severe and rapid obstruction of the central venous outflow occurs before collateral channels of venous outflow begin to function, severe ischemic whitening of the retina, in addition to widespread retinal hemorrhages, occurs, producing the ophthalmoscopic picture of combined central retinal arterial and venous occlusion.[338,389] Obstruction of the central retinal vein may cause selective obstruction of a cilioretinal artery because of relatively low perfusion pressure of the cilioretinal arteries).[336,342,390,391]

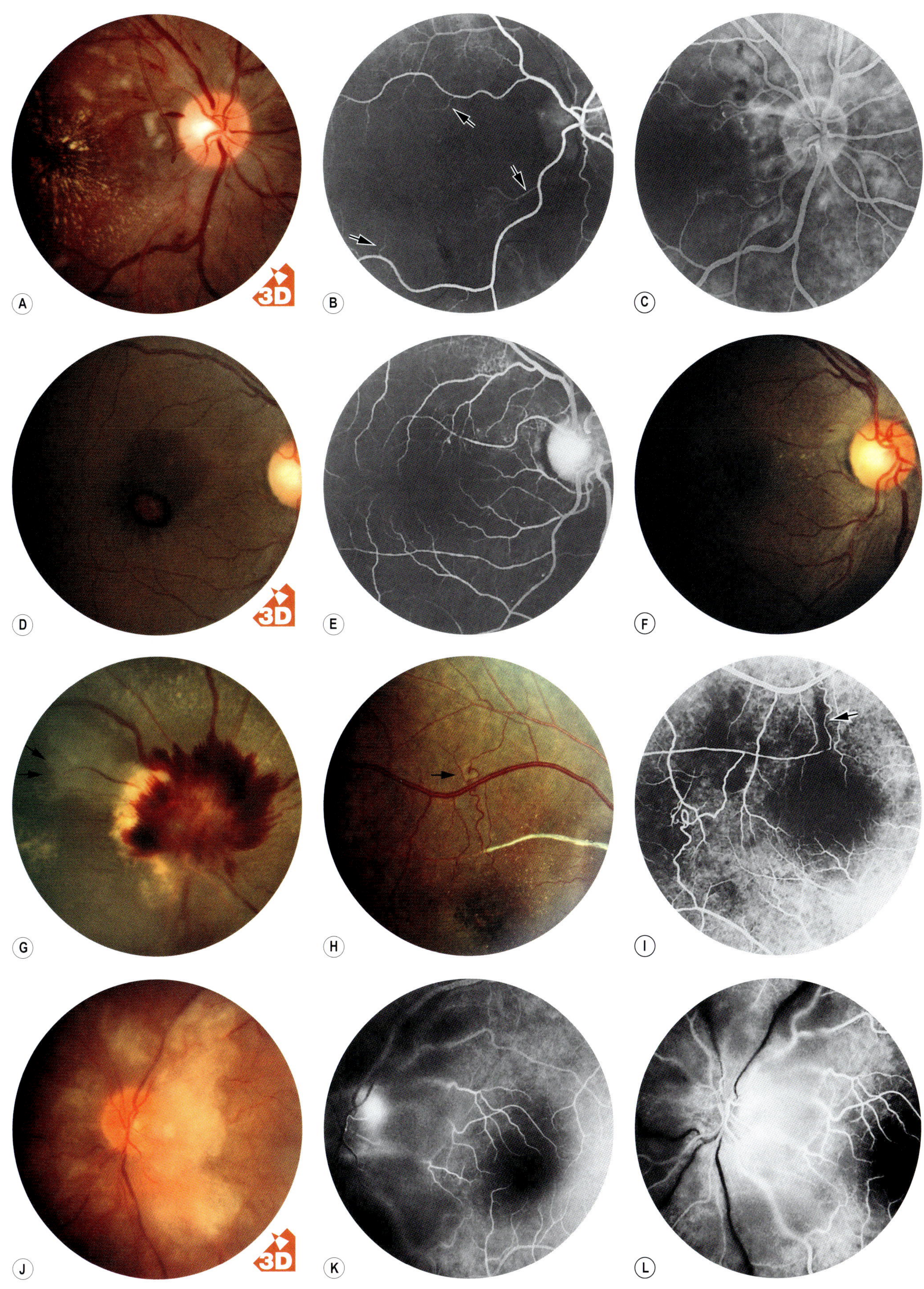
A
3D
B
C
D
3D
E
F
G
H
I
J
3D
K
L

Angiographic changes in the microvasculature, even in the presence of grade IV hypertensive retinopathy, are primarily outside the central macular area. Following medical control of malignant hypertension, angiographic evidence of permanent remodeling of the retinal capillary bed (microaneurysms, capillary telangiectasis, small areas of capillary nonperfusion, and permeability alterations) is most prominent in the juxtapapillary area and along the course of the major retinal vessels posteriorly (Figures 6.25D–F, and 6.26H and I).[414] Hemorrhagic detachments of the internal limiting membrane of the retina in the macula may arise from these permanent microvascular alterations (Figures 6.25D–F, and 6.26G–J). There is probably an increased incidence of epiretinal membrane formation in the macular region in patients who have severe hypertensive vascular changes (Figure 6.26H and L). These patients are susceptible to all of the complications of arteriolar sclerosis mentioned previously in patients with less severe hypertension.

During exacerbation of collagen vascular diseases patients may develop cotton-wool patches that may occur in the absence of significant elevation of systemic blood pressure.[192,219,221,296,402,408,415–418] Although in some cases the cause of the arteriolar obstruction is identical to that produced by severe hypertension, in other cases it may occur by a different mechanism such as thrombosis from a hypercoagulable state associated with a lupus anticoagulant[191,227,283,284] (see discussion of leukocytic aggregation and embolization, pp. 464, 565 and Figures 6.13, 6.14 and 6.62). These patients also may show evidence of occlusive vascular disease affecting the choroidal vasculature (see pp. 40, 84, 464).

6.27 Hypertensive retinopathy, optic neuropathy, and choroidopathy.

A–D: A 19-year-old African American woman with history of systemic lupus erythematosus, chronic renal failure, and hypertension presented with vision of 20/160 on the right and counting fingers on the left. Both eyes had swollen optic discs, with exudation of fluid and lipid along with retinal hemorrhages and cotton-wool spots secondary to hypertensive retinopathy and optic neuropathy (A and B). She was hospitalized and the blood pressure was brought under control. Two weeks later her vision had improved to 20/80 and 20/300; the optic disc edema had improved significantly, more on the right than the left (C and D). She returned to the hospital for uncontrolled hypertension a few weeks later but ocular exam was not sought.

Hypertensive retinopathy and choroidopathy.

E and **F**: Hypertensive retinopathy, choroidopathy, and exudative retinal detachment in this patient showing peripapillary nerve fiber hemorrhages, cotton-wool spots, choroidal infarcts (Elschnig's spots), and inferior dependent subretinal fluid in both eyes (E and F, arrows).

(A–D, courtesy of Dr. William F Mieler. A and B, Also, Yannuzzi, Lawrence J., The Retinal Atlas, Saunders 2010, 978-0-7020-3320-9, p. 488.)

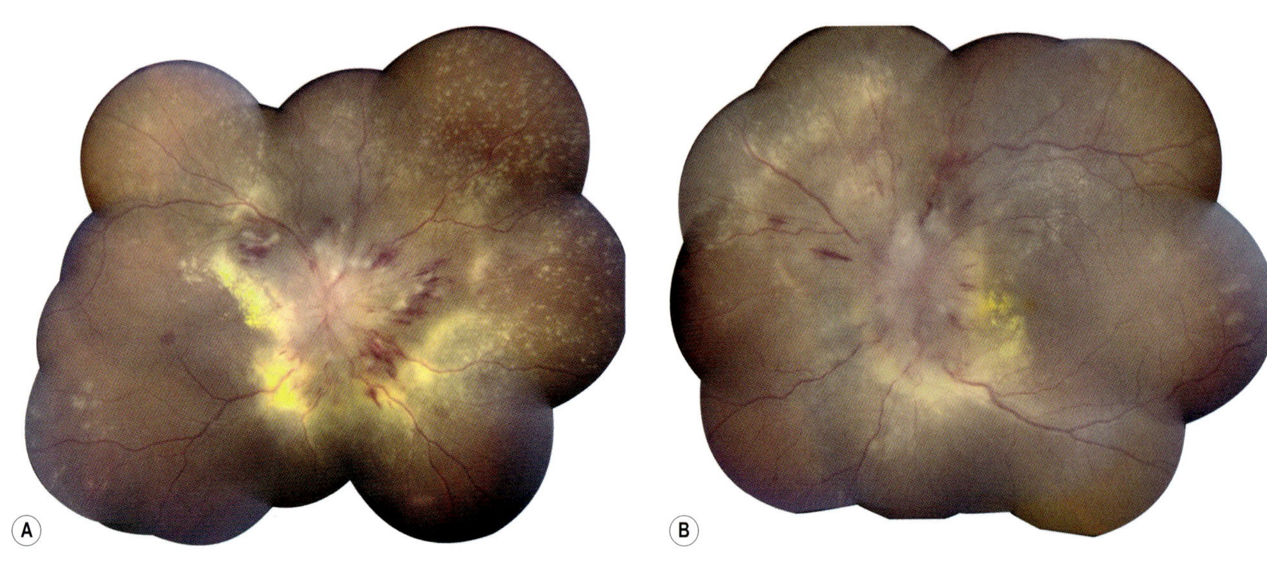

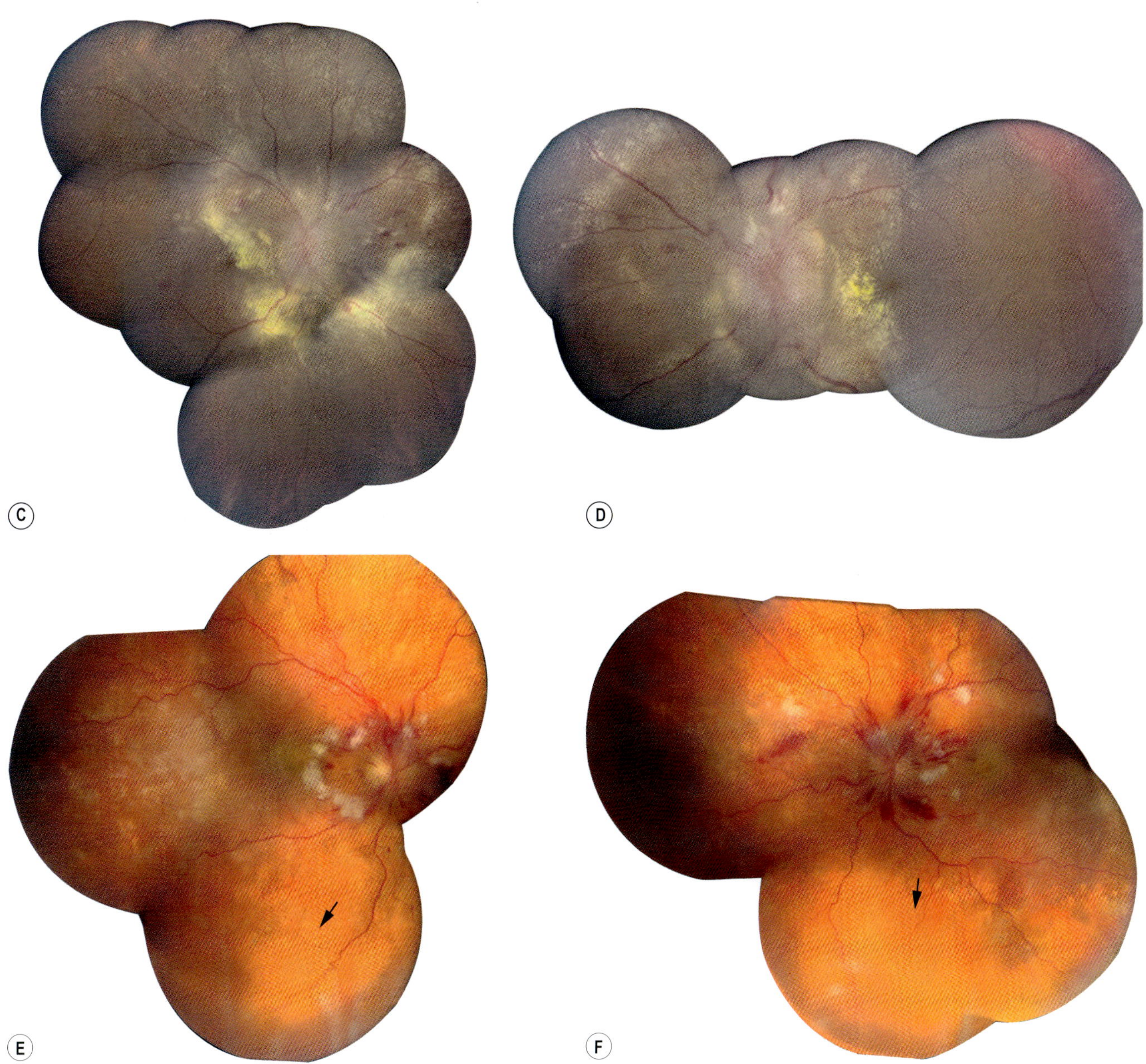
C
D
E
F

All of the retinal, choroidal, and optic nerve head changes seen in humans with accelerated hypertension have been reproduced in the rhesus monkey using a modified Goldblatt procedure.[399,400,419–422] Hayreh and others described a peculiar focal intraretinal periarteriolar transudate that frequently develops during the first few weeks after the onset of experimentally induced malignant hypertension.[419] Unlike cotton-wool spots, these pinhead-sized, dull-white, deep retinal lesions that are associated with punctate foci of fluorescein leaks are specific for malignant hypertension (Figure 6.28). They probably represent focal ischemic damage to the RPE.

6.28 Hypertensive choroidopathy with exudative retinal detachment.

A–L: This short-statured male had received a kidney transplant for end-stage renal disease resulting from a posterior urethral valve. He had developed secondary hyperparathyroidism and renal osteodystrophy due to noncompliance with phosphate binders. Vision was counting fingers at 1–2 foot (30–60 cm) in both eyes. Both retinas had small yellow distinct-appearing spots all over the posterior pole with overlying macular detachments and large inferior detachments with shifting fluid (A–D). Angiography showed initial hyperfluorescence of the lesions that leaked dye late, which pooled in the subretinal space (E and F). Optical coherence tomography confirmed loculated subretinal fibrosis in both maculas (G and H). He was hospitalized, his blood pressure was brought under control from 190/130 mmHg, and anemia and hypokalemia were treated. One week later his vision improved to 20/50 on the right and 20/200 on the left and 2.5 weeks later to 20/25 and 20/30. The exudative retinal detachments resolved, leaving residual chronic Elschnig's spots with distinct edges (I–L).

(Courtesy of Dr. Mark Hatfield.)

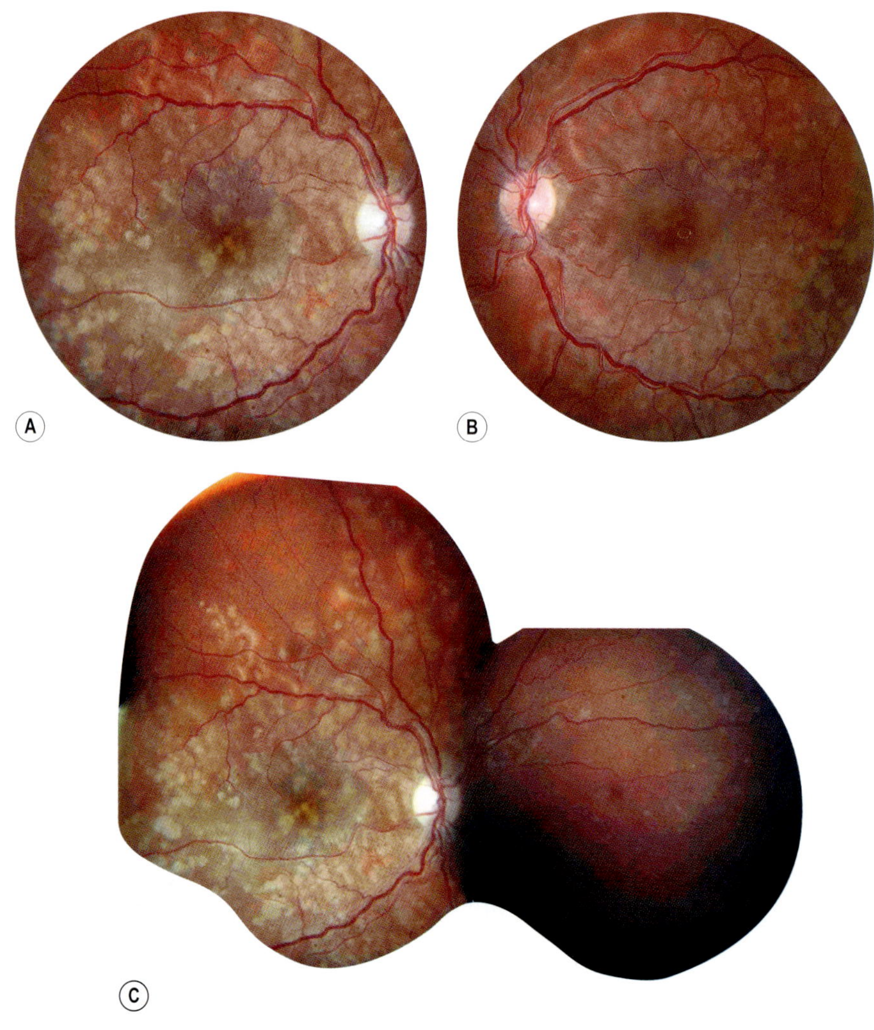

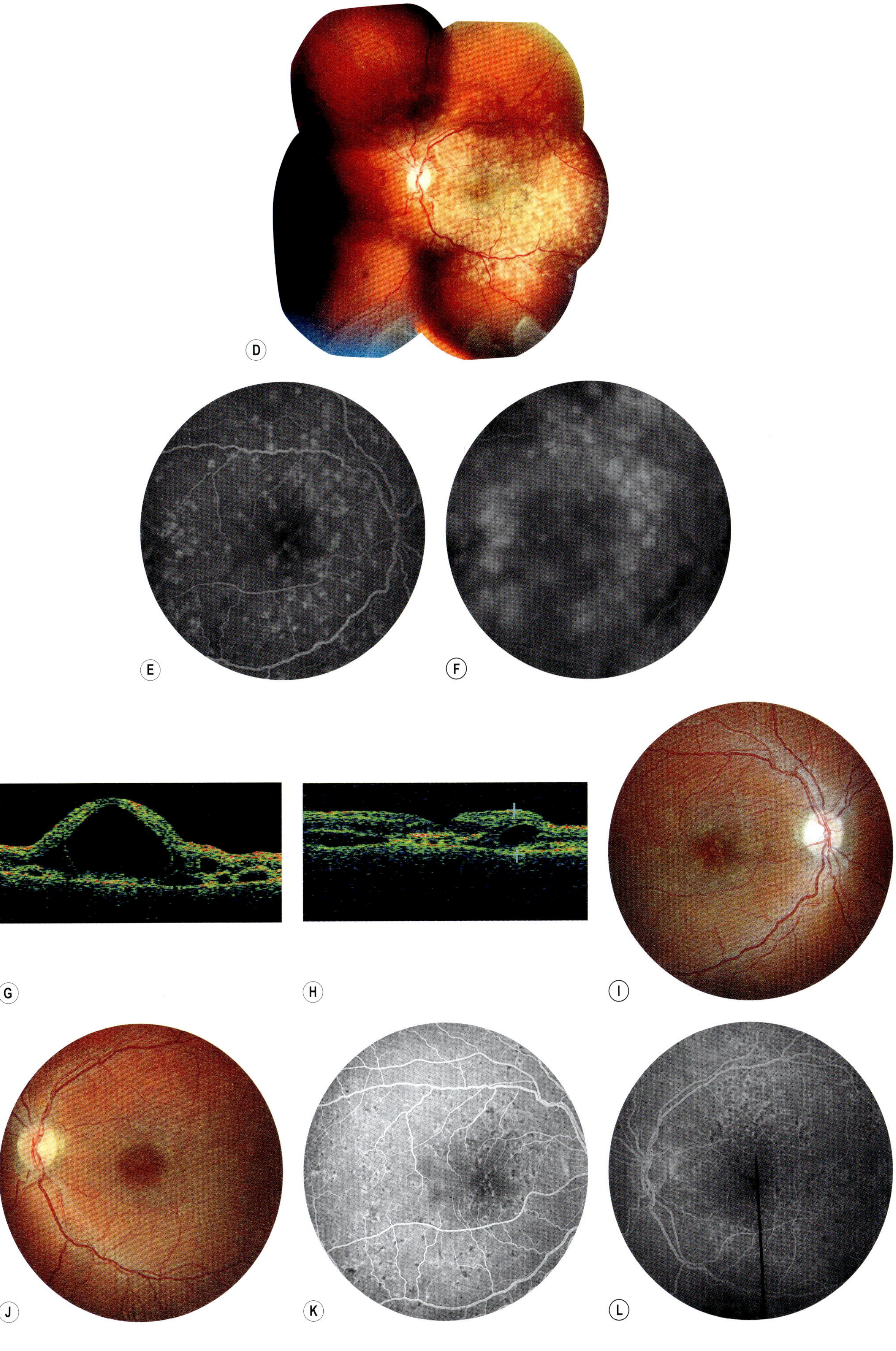
D
E
F
G
H
I
J
K
L

ACQUIRED RETINAL ARTERIAL MACROANEURYSMS

Patients who develop acquired retinal arterial macroaneurysms are usually in their sixth to seventh decade of life when they seek treatment because of visual loss caused by exudation or bleeding from the aneurysm. Typically a solitary round or fusiform aneurysm arises on one of the four major branch retinal arteries, usually within the third-order branches (Figures 6.29 and 6.30).[423–440] The aneurysm occasionally develops on a cilioretinal artery or on the optic nerve head.[441–444] It occurs more frequently in women.[435,445,446] The superotemporal artery is most commonly affected. The aneurysm often occurs at the site of an arterial bifurcation or an arteriovenous crossing. In some cases it may pulsate.[445,447] Pulsation is not a reliable indicator for high risk of hemorrhage.[445] The author has seen one pulsating macroaneurysm spontaneously disappear. The right eye is affected more commonly than the left eye. Aneurysms may be present in both eyes in approximately 10% of cases. A total of 50–75% of patients with acquired arterial macroaneurysms have a history of systemic hypertension and/or ophthalmoscopic evidence of retinal arteriolar sclerosis. Some association with systemic sarcoidosis has been noted, though the relationship is not understood. Visual loss is most frequently caused by leakage of proteinaceous and lipid-rich exudates, often along with some blood from the aneurysm, into the surrounding retina. This leakage produces an area of circinate retinopathy that includes the macular area (Figures 6.29A, F, and G, and 6.30D). Serous detachments of the macula (Figure 6.30D) and bleeding beneath the retina, the internal limiting membrane, posterior hyaloid and into the vitreous are other causes of vision loss (Figures 6.29J, 6.30H and K, and 6.31).[448] Bleeding may occasionally be precipitated by a Valsalva maneuver.[425] In cases associated with bleeding, the blood is often present in front of and posterior to the retina and may partly or totally obscure the aneurysm from view (Figure 6.30H). Full-thickness macular holes can occur as a complication. High pressure under the internal limiting membrane resulting in foveolar necrosis or secondary vitreofoveal traction as a sequela to the hematoma may play a role in the pathgenesis of the hole.[449–452]

6.29 Acquired retinal artery macroaneurysm.

A–F: Circinate maculopathy caused by retinal arterial macroaneurysm in a 49-year-old hypertensive woman with a visual acuity of 20/40. Note the focal atheromatous cuff (arrow, A) just proximal to the aneurysm. There was minimal evidence of obstruction of arterial flow either by the aneurysm (left arrow, B) or by the atheromatous cuff (right arrow). The late angiogram (C) showed minimal staining of the retina surrounding the aneurysm (arrow). Argon laser treatment (D) was applied to the aneurysm and surrounding retina. Five months later (E) visual acuity was 20/20. Note the atheroma lesion in the small retinal artery (arrow) is still visible. Several years later she had developed a new macroaneurysm and exudation nasally in the same eye (F). Note the atheroma (arrow, F) in the arterial wall distal to the aneurysm.

G–I: Vitreous hemorrhage and circinate maculopathy caused by an acquired retinal arterial macroaneurysm (arrow, G). Angiography (H) confirmed the presence of the aneurysm (arrow). Sixteen months later, following partial spontaneous resolution of vitreous blood and retinal exudate (I), visual acuity was 20/30. Note that there was no longer any exudate in the foveolar area (arrow).

J–L: Serous and hemorrhagic detachment of the internal limiting membrane of the retina was caused by a macroaneurysm (arrows) in this patient. Note the blood in the inferior part of the detachment as well as another boat-shaped area of subhyaloid blood inferiorly. Angiography (K and L) demonstrated dye leaking from the aneurysm.

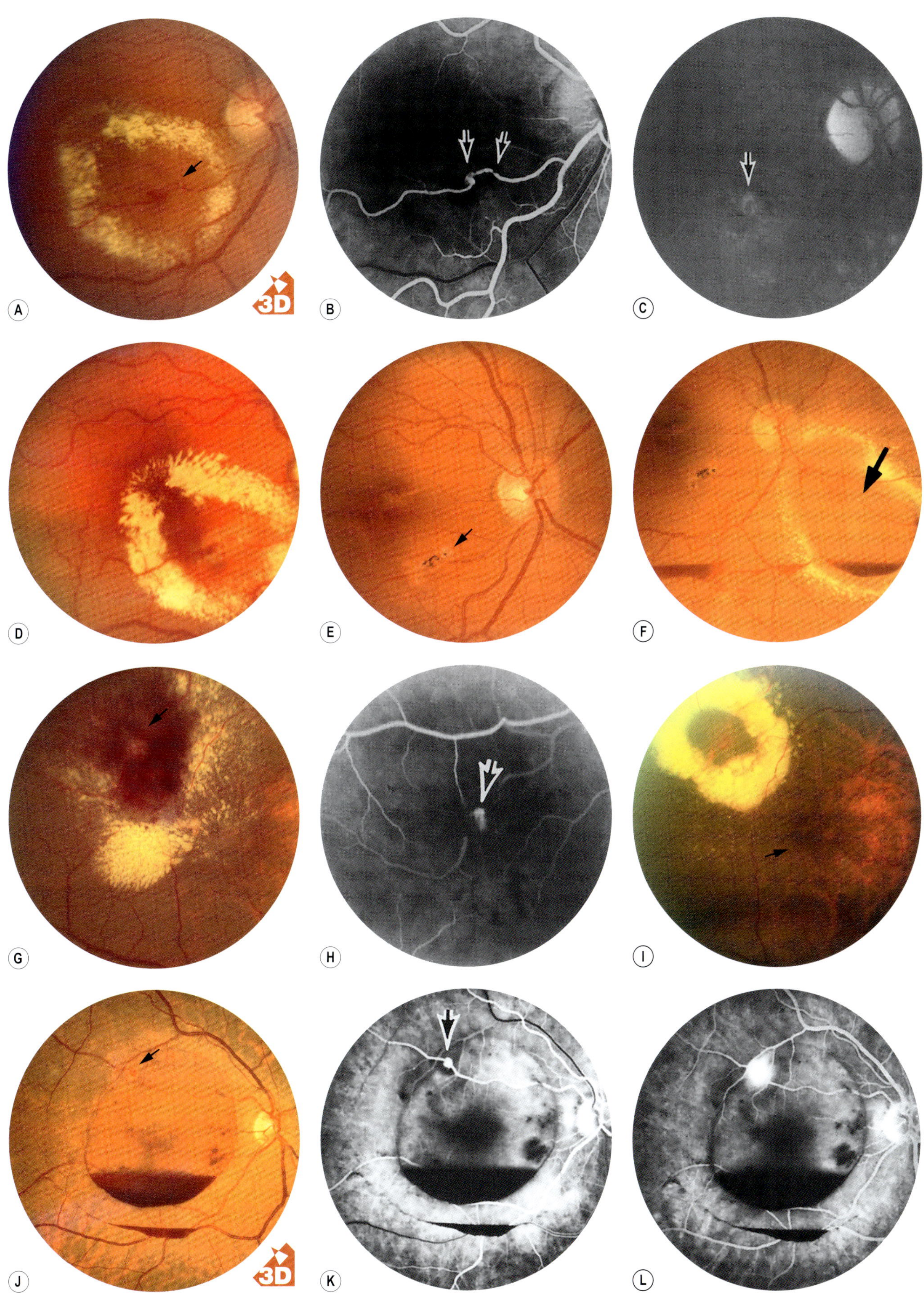
A
B
C
D
E
F
G
H
I
J
K
L
3D
3D

Subretinal neovascularization, though rare, has been reported.[453] Occasionally multiple aneurysms occur along the same artery (Figure 6.30G) or elsewhere in the eye. Approximately 10% of patients have one or more focal yellow arterial wall plaques either proximal to or, less often, distal to the aneurysm (Figure 6.29A and F). These lesions, which often incompletely surround the blood column and do not interfere with blood flow, are probably localized deposits of serum fat (atheromata) occurring at the site of defects in the arterial wall. These represent potential sites for future development of an aneurysm. Previously these atheromata have been misinterpreted as emboli.[429,433,446,453] Patients with these plaques show no clinical evidence to suggest embolic disease. Evidence of branch arterial occlusion distal to the aneurysm may be present (Figure 6.30D and E).

Branch retinal vein occlusions occasionally may occur within the same or opposite eye.[446] The arterial macroaneurysm may be within the area of the branch vein obstruction or remote to it. This association of these two disorders is not unexpected since hypertension is a risk factor for the development of both. Fluorescein angiography may fail to demonstrate the aneurysm when it is partly obscured by blood or exudate (Figure 6.30I). Angiography may show evidence of complete (Figure 6.30E), partial (Figure 6.29B), or no obstruction of the artery at the site of the aneurysm.[446] In some cases a few microvascular abnormalities may be present in the vicinity of the aneurysm. These include widening of the periarterial capillary-free zone around the aneurysm, capillary dilation, small areas of capillary nonperfusion, microaneurysms, and intra-arterial collateral vessels. Leakage of fluorescein occurs primarily from the site of the aneurysm and to a much lesser degree from the microvascular abnormalities immediately surrounding the aneurysm.

6.30 Acquired retinal arterial macroaneurysm.

A–C: Macroaneurysm (arrow, A) causing subretinal and retinal hemorrhage, as well as macular detachment. Note the evidence of staining angiographically (arrow, B). Visual acuity was 15/200. Eleven months later there was spontaneous resolution of the exudate and blood (C). The aneurysm (arrow) appeared shrunken and scarred. Visual acuity was 20/30.

D and **E**: Serous macular detachment (small arrows) caused by an acquired macroaneurysm (large arrow). Note obstruction of the dye flow at the site of the aneurysm (arrow, E).

F and **G**: Acquisition of a macroaneurysm (right arrow, G) and circinate exudation in a 67-year-old hypertensive woman. Note the small arterial aneurysm (left arrow, G) at the site of a previous retinal hemorrhage (F). G was made 5 years after F.

H and **I**: Hemorrhagic retinal detachment and vitreous hemorrhage that simulated a melanoma was caused by rupture of an acquired retinal arterial macroaneurysm (arrows, H and I). Note the failure of the aneurysm, which was totally obscured by blood, to obstruct the flow of fluorescein. The subretinal blood cleared spontaneously, and visual acuity was 20/30 3 years later.

J: Subretinal hemorrhage caused by arterial macroaneurysm, and cystoid macular edema caused by old inferotemporal branch retinal vein obstruction in a hypertensive patient.

K and **L**, Subretinal and subinternal limiting membrane hemorrhage with fluid level caused by arterial macroaneurysm (arrows).

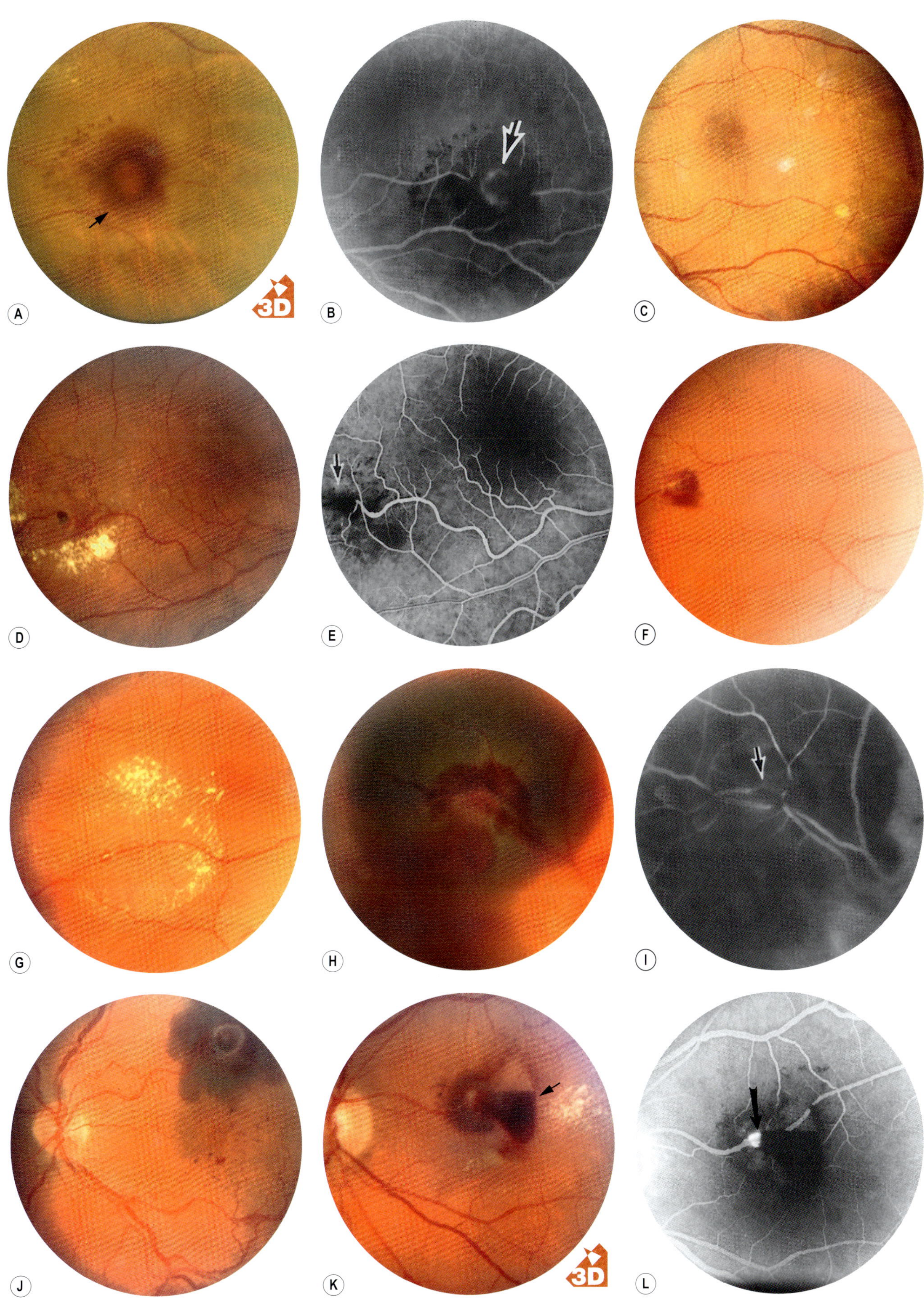
3D
A
B
C
D
E
F
G
H
I
J
K
3D
L

Histopathologically macroaneurysms show evidence of a linear break in the artery wall surrounded by a thick laminated layer of fibrin platelet clot and varying amounts of blood, exudate, lipid-laden macrophages, hemosiderin, and fibroglial reaction (Figure 6.31C–E).[427,429,430,436] Similar miliary aneurysms may occur in the central nervous system on vessels that are 100–300 μm.[397] These are more commonly found in hypertensive individuals than in normal individuals. Although the pathogenesis of these aneurysms in the eye and central nervous system is uncertain, they probably occur at sites of focal arterial wall developmental and aging defects, which particularly in a patient with hypertension are more likely to decompensate (Figure 6.29A). The presence of focal atheromata either adjacent to or in other parts of the retinal arterial tree is evidence of the presence of other focal defects in the arterial wall, which in some cases may lead to future development of additional aneurysms. Because of the association of hypertension, these patients probably are at higher than normal risk for stroke and cardiovascular disease.[445]

Evidence suggests that, following a period of exudation and hemorrhage, the defect in the arterial wall may close spontaneously through a process of thrombosis and sclerosis (Figures 6.29G–I and 6.30A and C).[429] In some cases the retinal artery may be almost completely restored to its normal caliber. Additional aneurysms may arise elsewhere (Figures 6.29F and 6.30F and G). The visual prognosis is excellent in most cases. Patients with chronic yellowish exudation in the macula and those with evidence of bleeding into the subfoveal area are the most likely to lose some vision permanently. Large hemorrhagic detachments of the retina in these patients are often mistaken for subretinal hematomas caused by age-related macular degeneration, and occasionally for a choroidal melanoma (Figures 6.30H and I and 6.31A–C).[429,430,435] The eccentric location of the hematoma centered beneath a major retinal artery is an important clue to the correct diagnosis when the aneurysm is obscured by intraretinal or preretinal blood. When associated with circinate yellowish exudation, a macroaneurysm may be misdiagnosed as retinal telangiectasis, branch retinal vein occlusion, diabetes, and irradiation retinopathy. There is usually no difficulty in differentiating patients with acquired arterial macroaneurysms from older patients with congenital retinal telangiectasis. These latter patients, most of whom are males, usually have multiple arterial aneurysms, larger areas of capillary dropout, and more extensive telangiectatic changes involving both the capillaries and the veins (see p. 514). A peculiar disorder characterized by multiple Y-shaped macroaneurysms occurring at the bifurcation of the major retinal arteries of both eyes causing exudative neuroretinopathy is of uncertain etiology (idiopathic retinal vasculitis, aneurysms, and neuroretinopathy: IRVAN) (see Figures 6.52 and 6.53).

Since spontaneous healing of macroaneurysms is part of the natural course of this disorder, treatment is not always indicated. The primary indication for photocoagulation is the persistence or progressive accumulation of yellowish exudate in the central macular area (Figure 6.29A–E).[428,429,432,433,435,437,445,455–457] Moderately heavy argon green or dye yellow laser photocoagulation using large-spot-size (500 μm), long-duration (0.5-second) applications directed to the aneurysm is successful in expediting the healing of the defect (Figure 6.29A–E). This treatment may cause a transient obstruction of the artery and occasionally may cause bleeding from the aneurysm. Since the site of the leakage is the aneurysm, the use of indirect treatment confined to the area surrounding the aneurysm has little rationale. Surgical drainage of the subretinal hematoma is technically possible but has not been demonstrated to produce visual results better than achieved by either laser treatment or by the natural course of the disease.[458–460] It does expediate the visual recovery. The same can be said for the technique of using the Q-switched Nd:YAG laser to release subinternal limiting membrane hematomas into the vitreous[439,461] or pneumatic displacement of the hematoma.

6.31 Histopathology of retinal arterial macroaneurysm.

A–C: An arterial macroaneurysm caused hemorrhagic detachment of the macula (A) that was misdiagnosed as a melanoma. Rupture of the aneurysm (arrow, B) caused extension of blood into the subretinal space (hematoxylin and eosin stain). A periodic acid–Schiff section (C) taken adjacent to B showed whorls of fibrinous exudate and blood that caused swelling of the retina and largely closed the flaplike opening (arrow) in the arterial wall. Note also the patency of the aneurysm.

D and **E**: Arterial microaneurysm causing intraretinal and subretinal hemorrhage. Note the thick fibrin platelet wall (arrow D) surrounding the large defect in the internal elastic lamina (arrow E) shown in the elastic stain.

(A–C, from Perry et al.[436], ; D and E, courtesy of Fichte et al.[427])

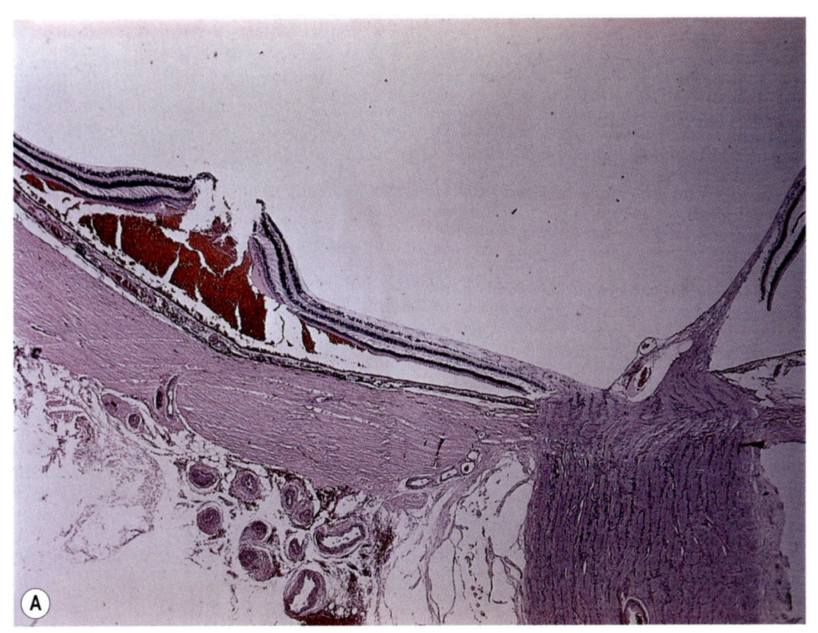
A

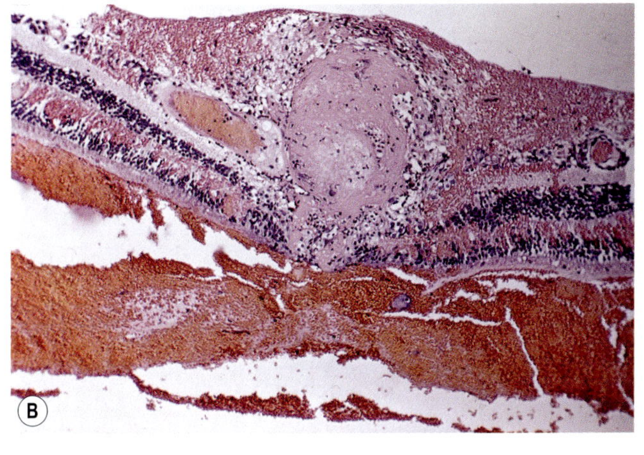
B

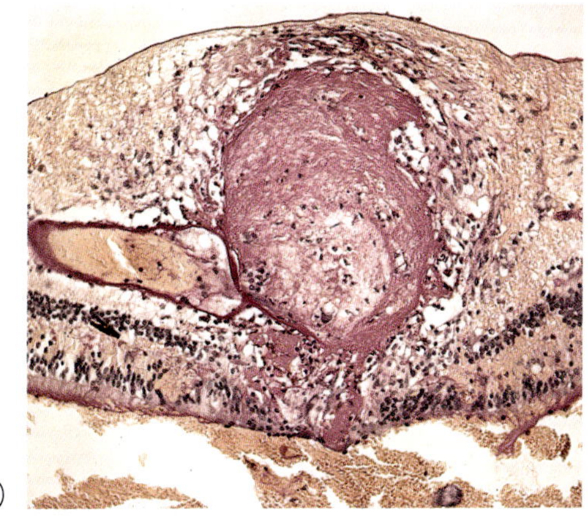
C

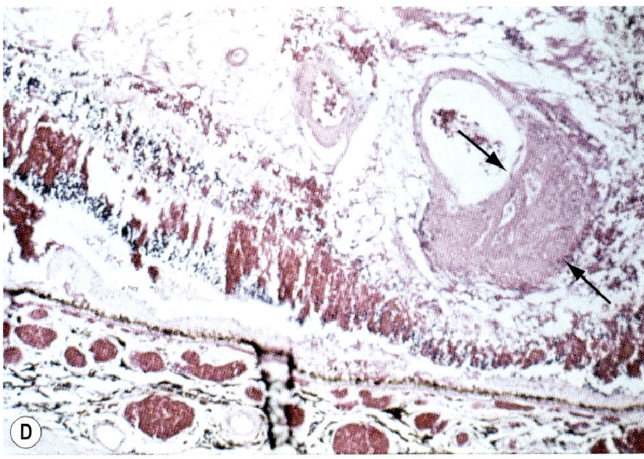
D

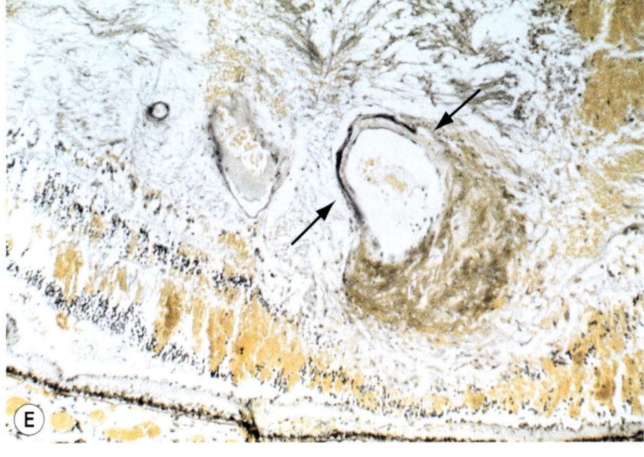
E

RETINAL CAPILLARY DISEASES

The retina normally contains very little extracellular fluid. Some diseases primarily affect the structure and permeability of the retinal capillary bed. These alterations often result in leakage of exudate and, in some cases, escape of blood cells into the retinal tissue. The content of exudate depends on the severity of the capillary endothelial damage. Intravenous fluorescein is helpful in detecting the structural and permeability alterations in the retinal capillary bed and the degree to which the extracellular space of the retina is expanded (see Chapter 2).

Cystoid Macular Edema After Cataract Extraction

Approximately 50–70% of the patients who have an uneventful intracapsular cataract extraction will develop fluorescein angiographic evidence of leakage of fluorescein from the parafoveal retinal capillaries (Figure 6.32).[462–474] More than 90% of these patients will show no biomicroscopic evidence of CME, and they will not have any significant decrease in their visual acuity. The incidence of this subclinical CME is so high that it may be considered as a normal physiologic response to intracapsular cataract extraction. Approximately 5–15% of all patients will develop loss of visual acuity secondary to clinically significant CME after uneventful intracapsular cataract extraction.[464,465] These patients will demonstrate the typical biomicroscopic and fluorescein angiographic changes caused by a polycystic pattern of expansion of the extracellular space by serous exudation (Figures 6.32–6.34). These changes are described in detail in Chapter 2. The incidence is much lower after extracapsular cataract extraction and phacoemulsification surgery. Clinically significant CME usually occurs within 4–12 weeks postoperatively, but in some instances its onset may be delayed for months or many years after surgery.[475] It infrequently occurs before the third postoperative week.[476] Blurred vision is the usual complaint. Visual acuity is generally reduced to the range of 20/30–20/70. A few patients may complain of mild irritation of the eye and show some circumlimbal conjunctival injection. The anterior hyaloid face is ruptured in approximately 50% of patients after intracapsular cataract extraction[464] or the posterior capsule is dehisced with or without anterior vitrectomy in eyes undergoing phacoemulsification. Some inflammatory cells may be present in the posterior vitreous, which typically shows evidence of extensive liquefaction. Vitreous attachment to the macula usually cannot be demonstrated. Mild and rarely severe degrees of papilledema may be present. Usually there is no ophthalmoscopically visible change in the structure of the capillary bed. An occasional small intraretinal hemorrhage or microaneurysm may be present.[464,477] Approximately 10% of patients will show some evidence of epiretinal membrane formation, or so-called cellophane maculopathy (see Chapter 7). Over 50% of these patients will have either clinical evidence of systemic hypertension or fundoscopic evidence of focal retinal artery narrowing.[464] The eyes are typically normotensive. CME after cataract extraction appears to be more common and more severe in patients with blue rather than brown irides. It occurs as a complication of cataract extraction less frequently in blacks than in whites and occurs infrequently after extracapsular cataract extraction in children.[466,478–480] If lens extraction in infants is accompanied by an anterior vitrectomy, significant and persistent CME may occur.[464]

6.32 Aphakic cystoid macular edema (CME).

A–D: Note thickening of the macular region and the presence of multiple cystoid spaces (A). An early angiogram showed evidence of perifoveal dye leakage from the retinal capillary bed (B). There was some evidence of dye leakage from the optic nerve head. The dye leaked into the cystoid spaces in the outer retinal layers and spread centrally and peripherally 1 hour after injection (C and D). The dye stained the fluid in the cystoid spaces. Note the dark stellate figure centrally, the feathery margins of the intraretinal dye peripherally, and the presence of retinal vessels that appear as dark lines overlying the fluorescein.

E and **F**: CME following cataract extraction. The vitreous haze partly obscured the cystoid spaces from view (E). The arrow indicates a small yellow deposit lying deep within the retina. Mild papilledema was present. A 1-hour angiogram (F) showed a typical angiographic pattern of CME.

G–L: This African American woman who underwent uneventful phacoemulsification and placement of posterior-chamber intraocular lens bilaterally developed CME and subretinal fluid in both eyes (G–J). After minimal response to topical steroids and nonsteroidals for nearly a year, she was started on oral acetazolamide 250 mg three times a day. She responded with resolution of subretinal and intraretinal fluid in approximately 3 months. The CME recurred in a mild fashion after discontinuation of acetazolamide, but resolved on its reinstitution (K and L). She was slowly tapered off the acetazolamide after another 3 months and remained stable with 20/20 vision in each eye.

(From Gass and Norton.[463],)

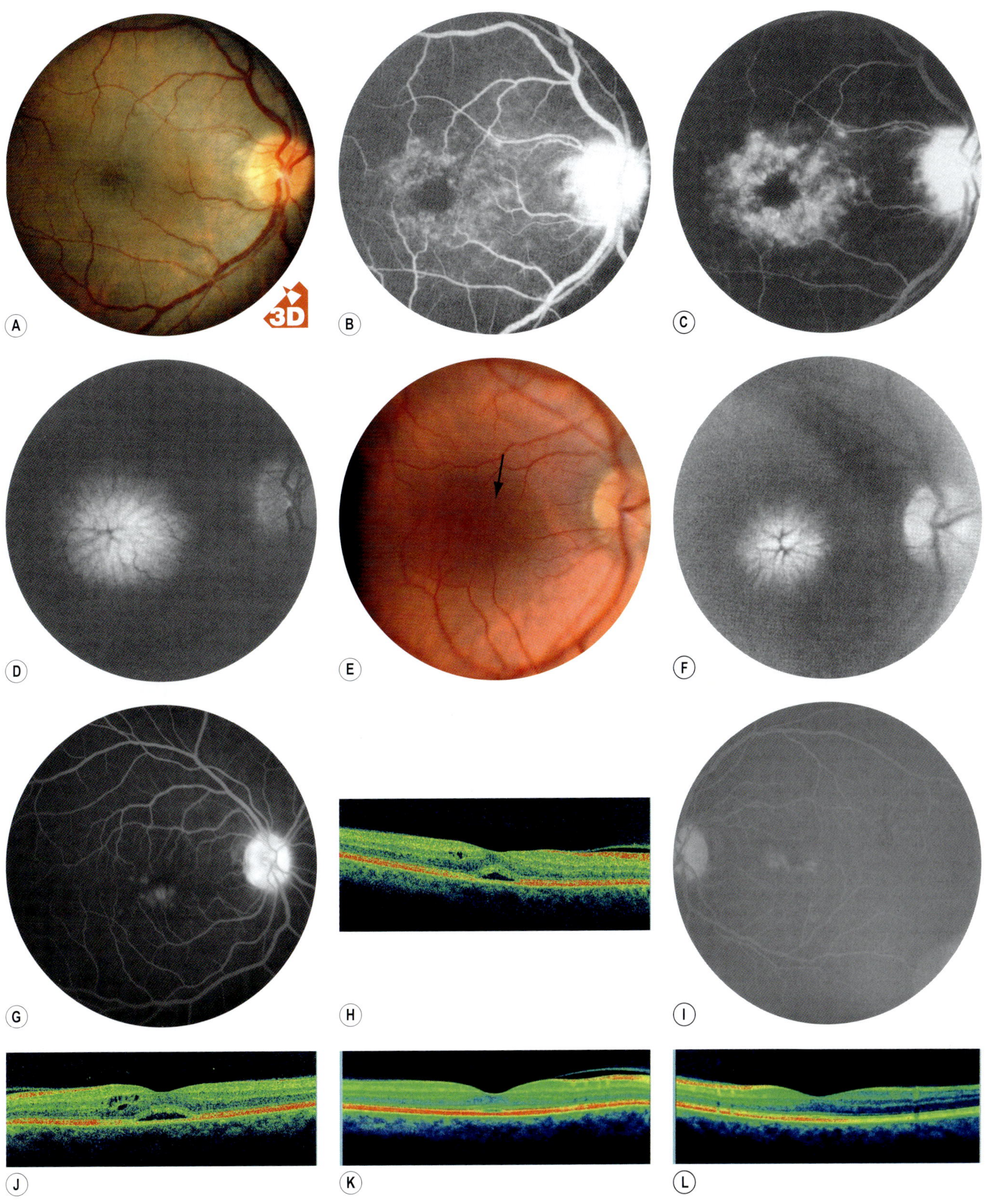
A
3D
B
C
D
E
F
G
H
I
J
K
L

Early phases of fluorescein angiography demonstrate dye leakage from the parafoveal retinal capillaries, and later phases show the characteristic picture of CME (Figure 6.32). Angiography can be helpful in the diagnosis of CME in these patients, who often have hazy ocular media that prevent detailed biomicroscopic examination of the macula. Leakage of fluorescein often occurs from the capillaries of the optic nerve head and anterior uveal tract. The aqueous humor typically stains heavily with fluorescein. CME disappears spontaneously, and visual acuity returns to 20/30 or better within 3–12 months in two-thirds of these patients after intracapsular cataract extraction and no lens implant. Other patients will show clearing of the edema and return of good vision from 1 to 5 years following the onset of CME. The incidence of permanent visual loss caused by CME after extracapsular cataract extraction and posterior-chamber intraocular lens implantation is approximately 1–1.5%. The duration of CME is usually longer and recurrences are more frequent in patients with a history of vitreous loss at the time of extraction or in those who develop incarceration of vitreous in the wound postoperatively. Angiography of the opposite phakic eye shows no evidence of abnormal retinal or iris vessel permeability, except in the rare patient who has chronic bilateral vitritis of unknown cause before cataract extraction.

Vitreous fluorophotometry in patients with aphakic CME shows evidence of increased ocular vascular permeability that parallels the severity of the CME.[481] Eyes with iris-supported implants that develop CME have a higher incidence of developing chronic CME and corneal edema.

Histopathologically, the extracellular space of the retina, particularly in the inner nuclear and outer plexiform layers, is expanded by serous fluid of low protein content (Figures 6.34 and 6.35). Small numbers of chronic inflammatory cells have been found histologically in eyes with aphakic CME.[482] Fine and Brucker's electron microscopic findings suggested that the cystic spaces in CME might be caused by accumulation of intracellular fluid within expanded Müller cell processes.[483] Gass et al., however, demonstrated that CME is caused by accumulation of serous exudate in the extracellular space, which is more in keeping with clinical, angiographic, and light microscopic findings in patients with CME.[484]

The pathogenesis of aphakic and pseudophakic CME is unknown. Direct traction on the macula by the vitreous does not appear to be an important factor. The incidence of CME is higher in patients who have had vitreous loss during cataract extraction and patients who develop a peaked pupil with vitreous adherence to the wound following delayed rupture to the anterior hyaloid face. The typical findings of inflammatory cells in the posterior vitreous of most, but not all, patients suggest the possible importance of inflammation. It may however be that these cells are the result of, rather than the cause of, the retinal capillary abnormality. Comparable inflammatory reaction in the vitreous from other intraocular surgical procedures usually does not produce macular edema. Removal of the lens is undoubtedly a key factor in this disease, but the mechanism by which it leads to retinal edema is not clear. Diffusion of prostaglandins from the anterior segment to the retina, hyperosmolarity of the vitreous secondary to a ruptured anterior hyaloid face, smoldering low-grade cyclitis, and vitreous traction acting on the peripheral retina are suggested but unproved causes of CME. The frequent findings of narrowing of the retinal arterial tree and systemic hypertension suggest that underlying retinal vascular disease is also an important factor in the pathogenesis of CME. The incidence of CME occurring following cataract extraction in patients with background diabetic retinopathy is much higher than in healthy patients.[485] In one study the incidence of clinically significant CME was 75% versus 6% of the control eyes, and the CME persisted for more than 1 year in 56% of diabetic eyes.[485] The incidence of CME occurring in the second eye following an uneventful cataract extraction may be as high as 50%.[464] It may occur soon after the subsequent opening of the posterior lens capsule. The incidence of CME after posterior-chamber lens implantation with simultaneous capsulotomy versus that after the same procedure without capsulotomy is probably slightly greater.[486,487] The incidence of CME after delayed Nd:YAG laser capsulotomy is probably less than 1–2%.[488,489]

6.33 Diagram illustrating the biomicroscopic appearance of the macula in the presence of cystoid macular edema.

The anterior bowing of the inner retinal surface in the foveal region is caused by thickening of the retina. The cystic pockets of extracellular serous fluid are seen best with retroillumination.

(From Gass and Norton.[463], © 1966, American Medical Association. All rights reserved.)

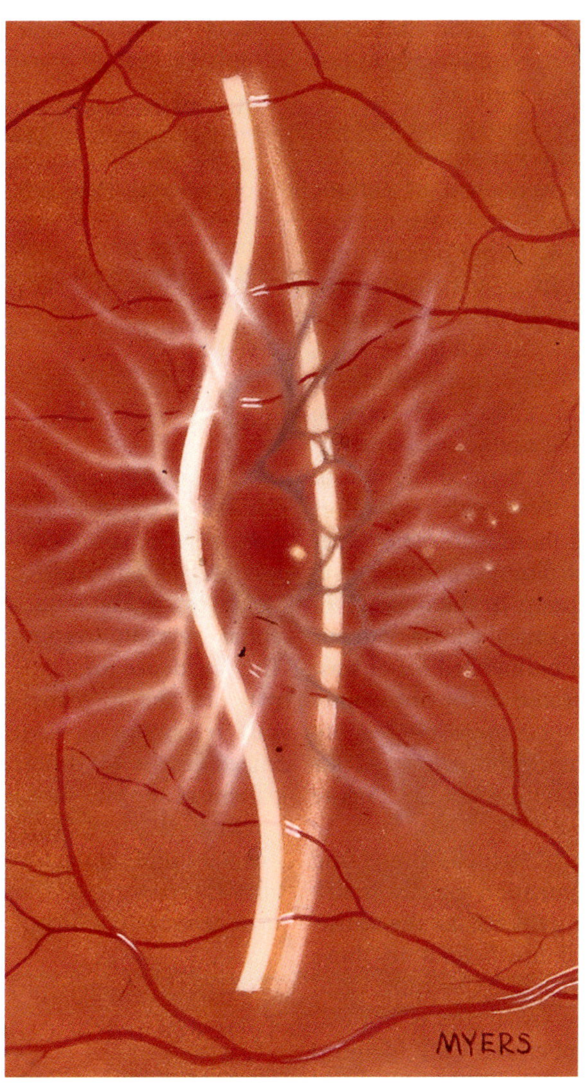
MYERS

Complications Following Cystoid Macular Edema

Although visual acuity may return to 20/30 or better after 2 or more years of CME, some patients develop permanent retinal damage secondary to the prolonged edema. The spontaneous rupture of the inner wall of a large central cystoid space to form a lamellar hole is one of the complications of CME.[522] When this occurs, it produces a characteristic biomicroscopic and a diagnostic angiographic change (Figures 6.35 and 6.36). Biomicroscopically, a round or oval, one-third disc diameter, punched-out defect occurs in the center of the macula. The RPE in the base of the hole is undisturbed. A sheen or light reflex is usually evident on the surface of the remaining retina as a slit beam is moved across the hole. Yellow deposits within the hole and a halo of marginal retinal detachment typical of a full-thickness hole are not present. Small perifoveal cystoid spaces surrounding the inner lamellar hole may be difficult to visualize. Late-phase fluorescein angiography, however, demonstrates a polycystoid pattern of dye in the perifoveolar area surrounding a round or oval, nonfluorescent zone that corresponds with the inner lamellar hole (Figure 6.36D). Following rupture of the inner cyst wall, the fluorescein can no longer concentrate in the area of the lamellar hole (Figures 6.35 and 6.36). Following resolution of the CME surrounding the lamellar hole, fluorescein angiography of the macula appears normal. Occasionally, multiple ruptures of the inner cyst walls produce a multifaceted lamellar macular hole, rather than a solitary oval or round hole.

In the aphakic patient with poor central vision and CME, failure to demonstrate the presence of central cysts during the late stages (10–60 minutes) of angiography suggests a poor prognosis caused by the presence of a lamellar hole, retinal atrophy, or a nonmacular cause for the visual loss.

Cellophane maculopathy and macular pucker caused by epiretinal membrane formation may be evident at the onset of CME, or they may occur as late complications of CME. When they occur, it is less likely that central acuity will return to normal following resolution of the CME. Occasionally, however, these membranes may peel spontaneously from the surface of the retina, and good acuity may be restored (see Figure 7.23).

Prolonged CME may occasionally produce atrophy of the outer retinal layers, and the macula may appear relatively normal except for the absence of a foveal reflex.

Infantile Cystoid Maculopathy

Infantile cystoid maculopathy that macroscopically resembled that seen in X-linked juvenile retinoschisis was observed on gross examination of the eyes of three premature infants of both sexes by Trese and Foos.[523] Cystoid changes were noted at various retinal levels. Reduced numbers of ganglion cells were found in the retina and central nervous system of all patients.

6.35 Electron microscopic findings in phakic woman with cystoid macular edema and a choroidal melanoma.

A–E: Before enucleation, angiography revealed evidence of cystoid macular edema (A and B). Epoxy resin-embedded section of the eye (C) revealed cystic expansion of the extracellular space in the inner nuclear and outer plexiform layers (×40). Electron microscopic section through the edge of one of the smaller cystoid spaces (D) showed the extracellular space filled with homogeneous material between healthy well-preserved cells. Glycogen granules (arrow) indicate prompt fixation (×15 000). There was thickening of the retinal capillary basement membrane (E, ×7200).

(From Gass et al.[484])

Cystoid Macular Edema Associated with Choroidal Melanomas

Patients with peripherally located melanomas may develop the typical biomicroscopic and angiographic appearance of CME unassociated with serous detachment of the macula (Figure 6.35).[484,524] The cause of this edema may be the chronic inflammatory cell infiltration within the choroid adjacent to the melanoma and retinal vasculitis. It is important that patients with unilateral CME have a careful examination of the peripheral fundus to exclude the presence of a melanoma.

Cystoid Macular Edema and Topical Epinephrine and Prostaglandin Inhibitor Therapy

Either aphakic or phakic patients may develop the typical biomicroscopic and angiographic appearance of CME following the use of topical epinephrine-like and antiprostaglandin drops for glaucoma.[525–529] If CME occurs and is caused by the drops, it can be reversed by discontinuing the medication.

Cystoid Macular Edema Associated with Ocular Inflammatory Diseases

CME may occur in a variety of recognized inflammatory diseases of the eye, such as pars planitis, Behçet's disease, vitiliginous chorioretinitis, sarcoidosis, idiopathic vitritis, and scleritis.

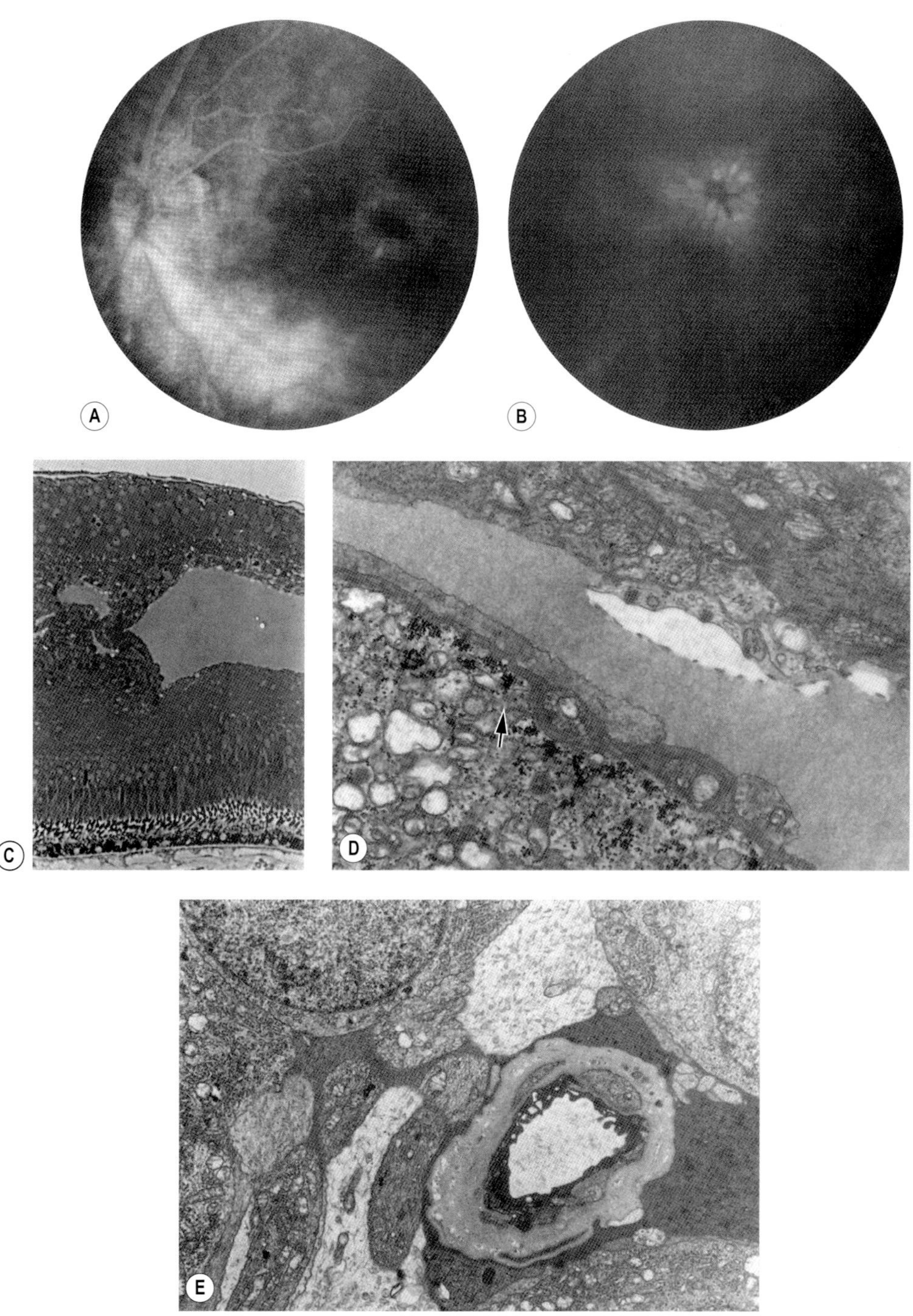
A
B
C
D
E

Cystoid Macular Edema From Other Causes

Discussions of CME associated with tapetoretinal dystrophies, carotid artery occlusion, congenital juxtafoveolar capillary telangiectasia, overlying occult choroidal neovascularization, and occurring after occult central retinal vein occlusion are found on pp. 330, 522, 570 and 588, respectively.

Idiopathic Cystoid Macular Edema

CME of uncertain cause occasionally occurs in one or both eyes of patients (Figures 6.37 and 6.38A–H). The CME may be associated with a typical pattern of fluorescein leakage, or with no evidence of fluorescein staining. Some of these patients may eventually develop evidence of a tapetoretinal dystrophy.

Pseudocystoid Macular Edema

Superficial changes in the retina occurring in patients with sex-linked juvenile retinoschisis (see Figures 5.59A, C, and E and 5.58), Goldmann–Favre syndrome (see Figure 5.57A, D, and H), infantile cystoid maculopathy, and rhegmatogenous retinal detachment, lightning maculopathy (see Figure 8.16), and following spontaneous vitreoretinal separation (see Figure 7.14J–L) may be mistaken for CME. Fluorescein angiography is helpful in this differential diagnosis. In patients with suspected CME and a negative angiogram, care must be taken to exclude the possibility of a tapetoretinal dystrophy (see Figure 5.42) and nicotinic acid maculopathy (Figure 6.38I–L).

6.36 Lamellar macular hole developing in a patient with prolonged cystoid macular edema (CME) after cataract extraction.

A–D: Note the yellow pigment centrally lying within the retina (arrow, A). Visual acuity was 20/40. A 1-hour angiogram (B) shows a typical picture of CME. Note that the dye fills the central cystoid spaces. Four years later (C), the patient has developed a circumscribed defect involving the inner layers of the retina centrally. There was biomicroscopic evidence of an epiretinal membrane and cystoid edema of the retina around the lamellar hole (C). The visual acuity was 20/70. Angiography demonstrated evidence of CME surrounding the lamellar hole (D). There was no pooling of the dye centrally because it was free to diffuse into the vitreous through the defect in the inner retinal layer. The patient died soon after the photographs in C and D were taken.
E: Histopathologic examination revealed a lamellar hole (1), epiretinal membrane (2), the slit-like areas of retinal edema in the outer plexiform layer (3), and small pockets of exudate in the inner nuclear layer. There was some loss of the receptor elements (4) in the vicinity of the lamellar macular hole where because of postmortem artifact the receptor cell layer is folded back on itself.
F and **G**: Schematic diagram showing the development of a lamellar macular hole in a patient with CME.
F: CME before rupture of the internal limiting membrane.
G: Lamellar macular hole with surrounding epiretinal membrane.

(From Gass.[522])

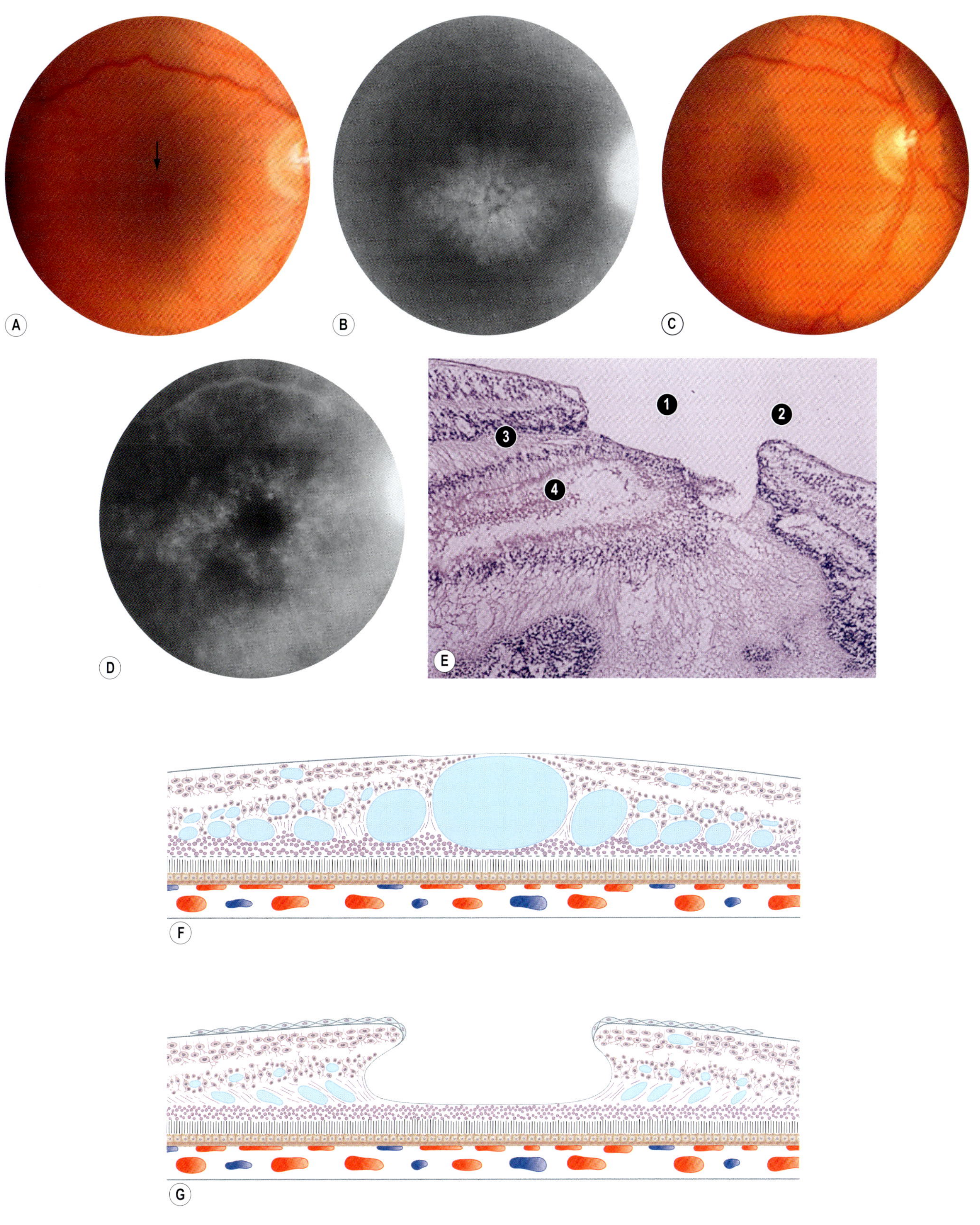
A
B
C
D
E
1
2
3
4
F
G

Nicotinic Acid Maculopathy

A small percentage of patients (probably under 1%) receiving high oral doses of nicotinic acid (1.5–5 g/day) for the treatment of hypercholesterolemia will develop bilateral blurring of vision caused by CME (Figure 6.38I–L).[530–534] Although the biomicroscopic appearance of CME is identical to that seen in patients after cataract extraction, it is unaccompanied by vitritis, other retinal vascular changes, and fluorescein angiographic evidence of retinal capillary permeability alterations (Figure 6.38K). Cystic spaces are seen in the outer plexiform and inner nuclear layer on OCT.[535,536] The reason for the absence of fluorescein leakage is speculative. Whether the permeability change in the retinal capillaries is so mild that fluorescein particles do not leak out or Müller cell edema is the cause of the cystic spaces is still debated.[537,538] Prompt recovery of normal vision and complete resolution of macular edema occur after nicotinic acid therapy is stopped (Figure 6.38L).[536,539] Reinstitution of the therapy results in recurrence of the CME.

Dominantly Inherited Cystoid Macular Edema

Deutman et al. described an autosomally dominant macular dystrophy characterized by CME, fluorescein leakage from the retinal capillaries throughout the posterior pole, normal electroretinographic findings, subnormal electro-oculographic findings, and hyperopia.[540–542] Atrophic pigment epithelial changes with a "beaten bronze" appearance may eventually develop. Histopathologic examination reveals large retinal schisis spaces in the macula, marked disorganization of the inner retinal layers, and advanced degeneration of Müller cells.[540] Treatment with oral acetazolamide has not been successful.[543] However a somatostatin analog, octreotide acetate, stabilized visual acuity and decreased fluorescein leakage in seven out of eight eyes.[544]

6.37 Idiopathic cystoid macular edema (CME).

A: Idiopathic unilateral CME in the left eye of this man who was complaining of blurred vision. There were no vitreous cells or biomicroscopic evidence of vitreomacular traction. Stereoscopic angiograms showed thickening of the retina centrally but no fluorescein staining. One month later the CME had disappeared and there was evidence of posterior vitreous detachment.

B–D: Idiopathic self-limited bilateral CME in this 37-year-old woman with a 4-month history of visual loss in both eyes. Soon after the onset of symptoms examination revealed marked bilateral CME and only a few vitreous cells. Except for multiple allergies her past medical history was negative. The CME failed to respond to long-acting prednisolone orbital injections and oral prednisone. When seen in Miami her visual acuity was 20/70 both eyes. There were no vitreous cells. Prominent CME in the absence of any other abnormalities was present bilaterally (B and C). Angiography (D) showed no staining. Her family history was negative. An electroretinogram was normal. Approximately 1 month later she had surgery for abdominal scarring caused by endometriosis. Three months later the CME had cleared spontaneously.

E–G: Idiopathic, possibly congenital, nonstaining CME in a 34-year-old woman with pendular nystagmus, poor vision all her life, and no history of nyctalopia or hemeralopia. Her visual acuity was 20/60 right eye and 20/200 left eye. Fluorescein angiography revealed evidence of slight mottled depigmentation of the RPE paracentrally (G). Color vision by Ishihara color plates was normal. An electroretinogram revealed mild decrease in cone and rod amplitudes with the b-wave much more affected than the a-wave.

H–L: This 55-year-old phakic woman complained of blurred vision in her right eye for 6 months. Biomicroscopic examination revealed cysts in the right fovea (H) that did not accumulate dye on angiography (I). There were no vitreous cells, vitreofoveal traction, or other ocular pathology. She was on no medications. Observation over 4 months did not change her ocular status. Optical coherence tomography (OCT) confirmed persistence of cysts and revealed a pre-existing posterior vitreous separation. She was treated with oral acetazolamide 250 mg three times daily, the cysts resolved, and vision returned to 20/20 (K) by 3 months. Acetazolamide was tapered over 2 months and repeat OCT 2 further months later (L) revealed no recurrence of CME.

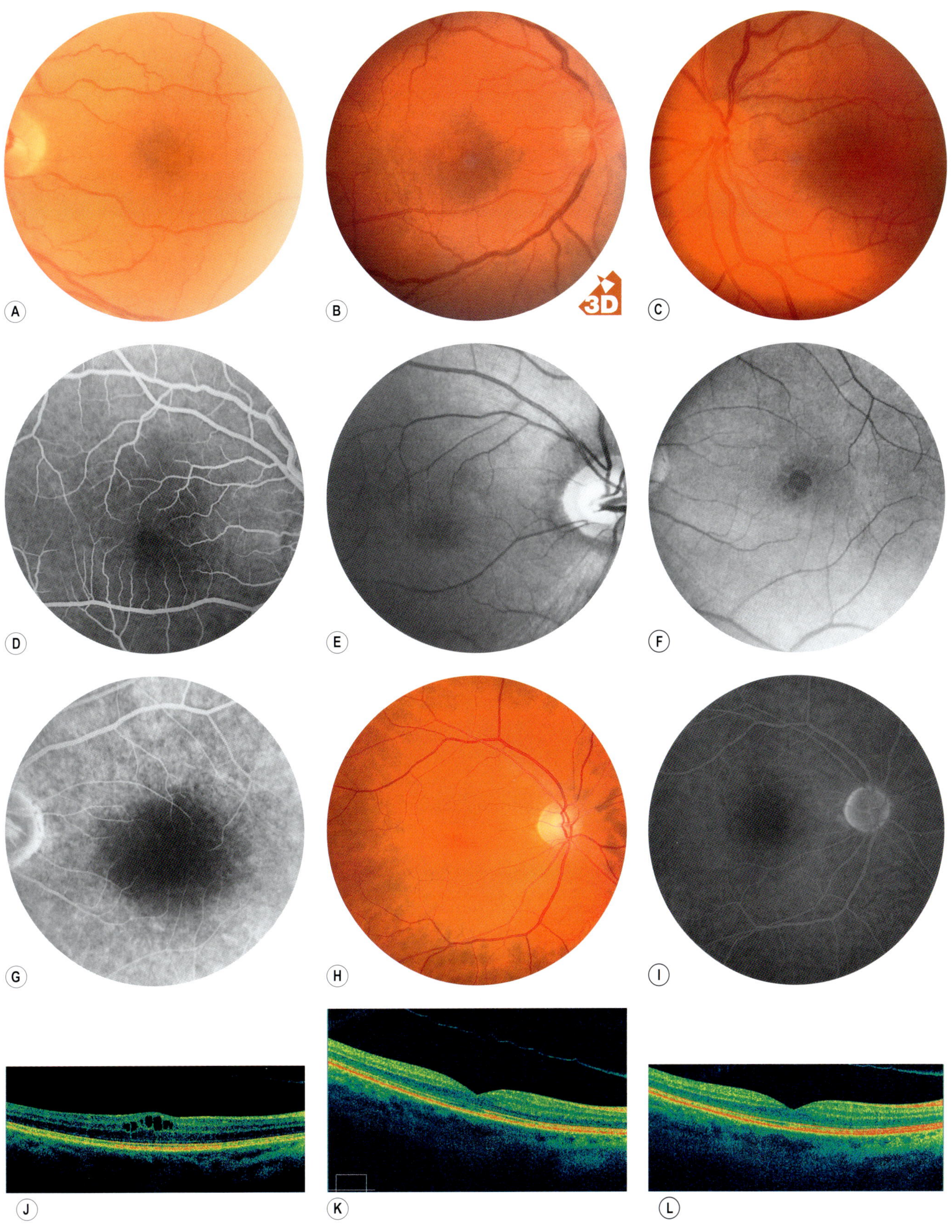
A
B
3D
C
D
E
F
G
H
I
J
K
L

6.38 Idiopathic cystoid macular edema (CME).

A–D: Idiopathic bilateral CME (A and B) occurring 1 week after a mild viral-like gastrointestinal illness, in an otherwise healthy woman, who on awakening noted marked loss of central vision bilaterally. Examination revealed 20/200 acuity, prominent CME in both eyes (A and B), and no signs of intraocular inflammation. There was a poorly defined equatorial zone of leopard-spot hyperpigmentation in both eyes (C). Angiography revealed a prominent staining pattern typical for CME (D). An electroretinogram and peripheral visual fields were normal. Within 6 weeks she was asymptomatic and her visual acuity returned to 20/25 right eye and 20/20 left eye.
E and **F**: Bilateral postpartum CME and mild vitreous cellular infiltration in a 22-year-old woman who noted blurred vision 3 days after a normal delivery of a full-term healthy infant. Visual acuity was 20/50 in the right eye and 20/25 in the left eye. Two months later the visual acuity was 20/40 in the right eye and 20/20 in the left eye. There was an epiretinal membrane in the right eye but no macular edema or vitreous cells in either eye.
G and **H**: Idiopathic unilateral CME in a 52-year-old healthy man with a 4-month history of blurred vision. His visual acuity was 20/30 in the right eye and 20/20 in the left eye. There were no vitreous cells. His past medical and family history was negative. His findings were unchanged 5.5 years later.

Nicotinic acid maculopathy.

I–L: This 50-year-old man experienced progressive loss of central vision bilaterally. He was receiving 3–5 grams of nicotinic acid a day for the treatment of hypercholesterolemia. Visual acuity in the right eye was 20/70, and in the left eye was 20/50. The fundi were normal except for typical CME (I and J). Fluorescein angiography showed no evidence of capillary permeability in the macula (K). Six months after cessation of nicotinic acid therapy, his visual acuity returned to 20/20, and the CME had resolved (L) bilaterally.

(F–I, from Gass.[530];)

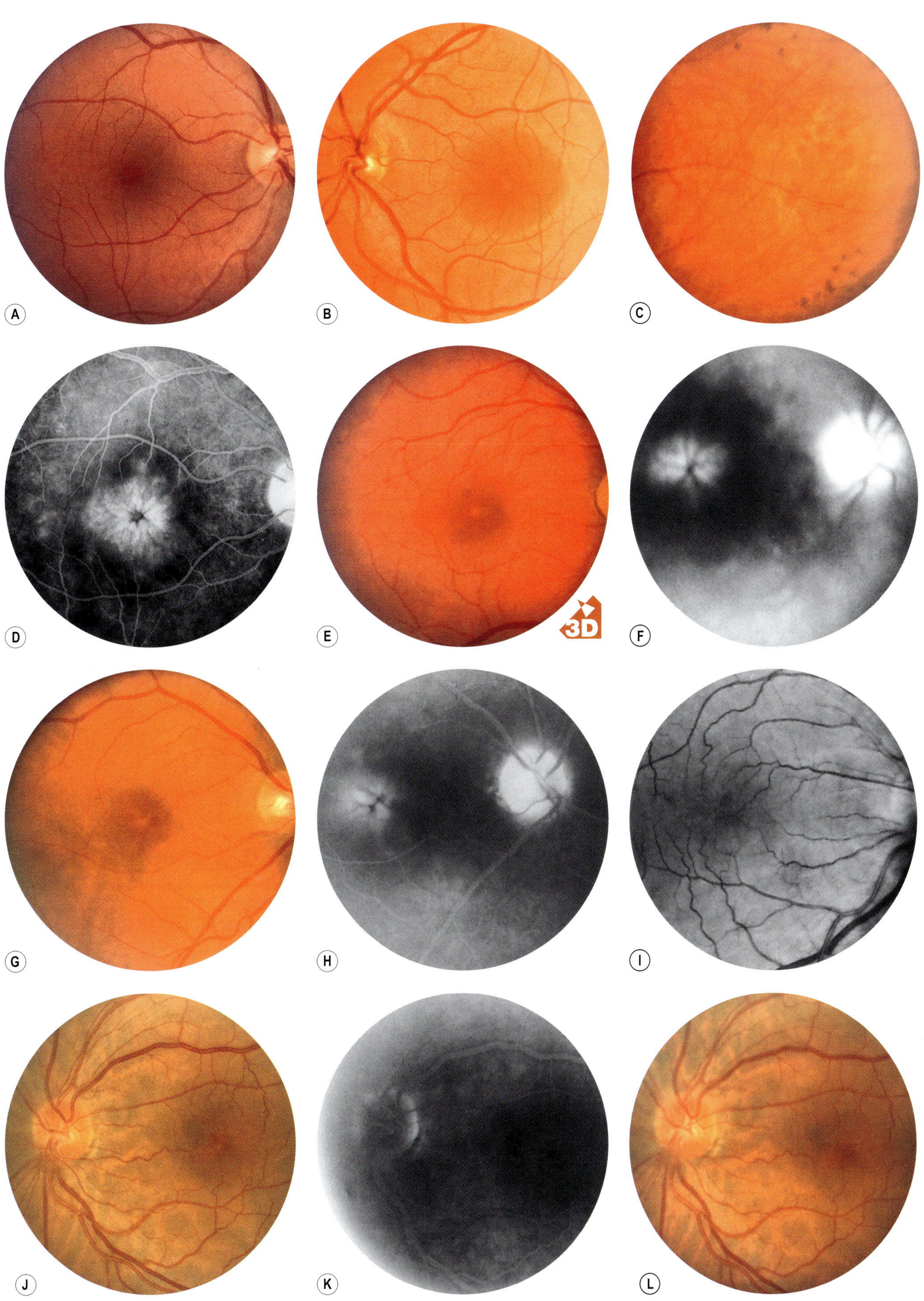
A
B
C
D
E
3D
F
G
H
I
J
K
L

PRIMARY OR CONGENITAL RETINAL TELANGIECTASIS (LEBER'S MILIARY ANEURYSMS, COATS' SYNDROME)

Retinal telangiectasis, a term originally proposed by Reese,[545] is a nonfamilial, developmental, retinal vascular anomaly characterized by irregular dilation and incompetence of the retinal vessels that typically occurs in one eye of a male patient (Figures 6.39–6.42).[546–554] Although primarily the retinal capillaries are affected, multiple focal aneurysms of the major retinal vessels, particularly the arteries, may be present. Women are occasionally affected (fewer than 10% of cases), and a few patients may show bilateral involvement. The extent of the retinal involvement and the degree of permeability alterations are variable. At one end of the spectrum are patients, usually infants or children, in whom most or all of the retinal vessels, including the arteries and veins, are telangiectatic, with massive yellow exudative and occasionally hemorrhagic retinopathy and detachment of the retina. This clinical picture is referred to as "Coats' disease," or, more correctly, "Coats' syndrome" (Figure 6.40). Congenital retinal telangiectasis is only one of the three causes of yellow exudative retinal detachment described by Coats.[548,555–558] At the other end of the spectrum are patients with the retinal telangiectasis confined to a small segment of the juxtafoveolar area. These patients constitute type I juxtafoveolar retinal telangiectasis (Figures 6.42 and 6.43). Decompensation of these localized areas of telangiectasis and visual loss often do not occur until adulthood. Approximately one-third of patients are 30 years or older before the onset of symptoms.

Patients with loss of macular function may present a variety of ophthalmoscopic pictures: (1) telangiectasis of the capillary bed, which may or may not be confined to the macular area, with minimal evidence of intraretinal exudation (Figure 6.43A, G, and H); (2) telangiectasis of the macular capillaries with extensive evidence of intraretinal exudation, including CME and circinate maculopathy (Figures 6.43E and I and 6.44A and E); (3) telangiectasis of the macular capillaries with extension of the exudate into the subretinal space; (4) exudative detachment of the macula caused by gravitation of protein- and lipid-rich exudate derived from peripheral areas of retinal telangiectasis (Figure 6.39A and J); and (5) a focal, organized, subretinal disciform mass (Figure 6.39L) or atrophic scar (Figure 6.39H) caused by chronic pooling of exudate into the macular region, often seen after laser or cryo treatment of the telangiectasis.[549] The latter two changes are most often seen in infants and children with extensive areas of peripheral retinal telangiectasis. These patients often have esotropia or an abnormal pupillary reflex caused by the massive accumulation of yellow exudate in the posterior pole (Figures 6.39A and D and 6.42). The yellow exudate is always more prominent remote from the areas of the retinal telangiectasis, which in some cases may be confined to the equatorial region (Figure 6.39A–C and J–L). As the cloudy, often greenish, subretinal exudate gravitates more posteriorly, particularly during sleep, the serous component is reabsorbed into the retinal vessels, leaving the yellowish, lipid-rich residue beneath and within the outer retinal layers (Figures 6.39A and J, 6.41G–I, and 6.42). The accumulation of this material in the macular region probably occurs during sleep. Over a period of many months the yellowish exudate in the macular area may incite the ingrowth of blood vessels and fibrous tissue into the submacular exudate (Figure 6.39A). Extension of exudation into the posterior fundus from telangiectasis confined to the periphery, particularly if it is located inferiorly, may not occur in some patients until late in life.

Fluorescein angiography is helpful in defining this structural and permeability alteration in the affected vessels and in demonstrating the extent of the extravascular leakage of serous exudate into and beneath the retina.[549] Angiography demonstrates focal aneurysmal dilation of the capillaries (Figures 6.39C, E, and I, 6.40D–F, 6.42D, E, and H, and 6.43B and C), retinal arteries, and veins (Figure 6.39C and E). The surrounding capillary bed may be dilated from slow flow and portions of the capillary

6.39 Congenital retinal telangiectasis.

A–C: Submacular scar surrounded by yellowish intraretinal and subretinal exudate in a 17-year-old boy with unilateral equatorial telangiectasis. Note the retinal vessels dipping into the subretinal scar (arrow, A) and large aneurysms and telangiectatic vessels (B) that perfused with dye (C).

D–F: Intraretinal and subretinal yellowish exudate in a 12-year-old boy with unilateral retinal telangiectasis involving the arteries, veins, and capillary bed in the paramacular area (D). Visual acuity was 20/400. Note the fusiform dilation and focal narrowing of the retinal vein (lower arrow) and aneurysmal dilation of the retinal artery (upper arrow). Arteriovenous-phase angiography demonstrated aneurysmal dilation of the first-order arteriole (arrow), the capillary bed, and the infratemporal vein (E). After photocoagulation, most of the yellowish exudate in the macula resolved (F). Visual acuity was 20/100.

G–I: Spontaneous resolution of submacular exudation in a young man who had poor vision in the left eye all of his life. The right eye was normal. Note the sheathed and partly occluded retinal vessels in the area of active exudation around the patch of retinal telangiectasis superior to the large atrophic macular scar (H and I) as well as elsewhere in the fundus (G). There were many areas of occluded retinal arterial aneurysms (arrow, H) and telangiectatic vessels throughout the periphery of the eye.

J–L: Unilateral exudative retinal detachment (Coats' syndrome) in a $2^1/_2$-year-old boy caused by peripheral retinal telangiectasis (K). The subretinal exudate resolved after xenon photocoagulation of the telangiectasis. Note the residual disciform scar in the macula 7 years after treatment. Visual acuity was limited to counting fingers at 6 foot (1.80 meters).

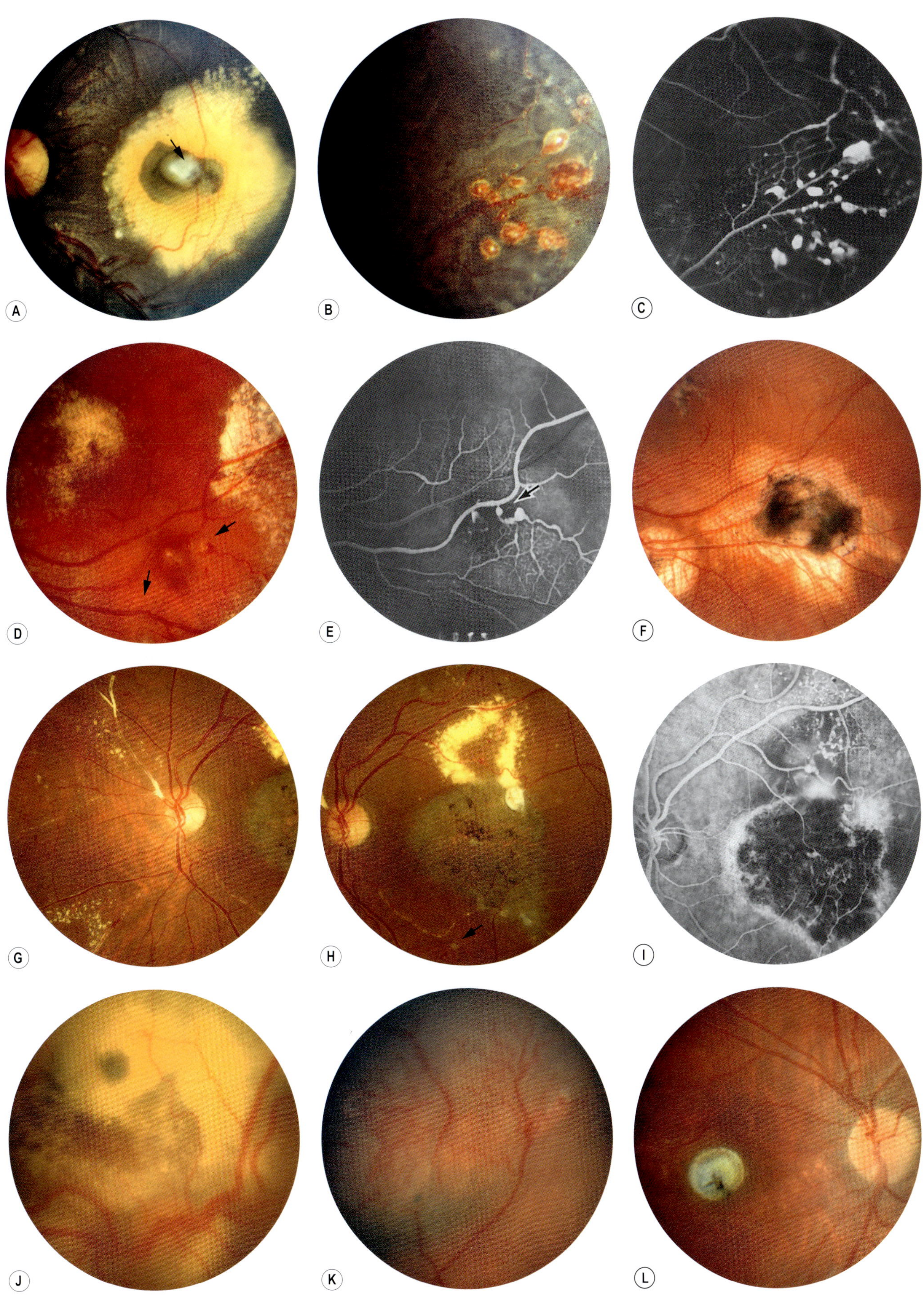
A
B
C
D
E
F
G
H
I
J
K
L

bed may show nonperfusion (Figure 6.42D). This is particularly prominent in those patients with large aneurysmal vascular anomalies in the peripheral fundus. There may be some delay in passage of dye through the telangiectatic capillary bed, particularly if there is extensive saccular aneurysmal formation. The permeability of the telangiectatic vessels is quite variable. Dye leakage is largely confined to the dilated vessels. When intraretinal serous exudation is extensive, fluorescein stains the extravascular fluid pooled in the outer layers to produce a characteristic angiographic pattern of CME (Figure 6.44F). The dye diffuses into the subretinal exudate. It may not, however, stain subretinal exudate pooled beneath the retina in an area remote from the telangiectatic vessels. The yellowish exudate beneath or within the retina will not show fluorescence. Retinal function remains intact in an area of telangiectasis if the permeability of the retinal vessels is relatively normal.

The natural course of retinal telangiectasis is variable. Patients who seek treatment early in life because of exudation are more likely to have more widespread retinal involvement and develop progressive detachment and degeneration. In some cases this may be followed by rubeosis, retinal and vitreous hemorrhage, secondary glaucoma, and loss of the eye. Acute orbital cellulitis secondary to transscleral movement of toxic products may occasionally occur (Figure 6.41J–L). This presentation closely mimics retinoblastoma. In patients with milder degrees of the disease, there may be fluctuations in the degree of vascular leakage. Spontaneous resolution of exudation may occur (Figures 6.39H and 6.43E–G). Patients with telangiectasis confined to several clock areas, usually inferiorly, may gradually develop over a period of many years an elevated, organized, exudative mass that may be mistaken for a melanoma or an exophytic capillary hemangioma. In some cases it may not be possible to differentiate this stage of the disease from exudative intraretinal and subretinal masses caused by primary retinal capillary hemangiomas or secondary fibrovascular proliferation caused by branch vein occlusion, focal inflammation, trauma, or chronic retinal detachment (see Figure 7.28). Vitreous hemorrhage secondary to localized areas of retinal or optic disc neovascularization may occasionally occur.

Primary retinal telangiectasis is rarely associated with clinical evidence of vascular anomalies elsewhere in the body. Although congenital telangiectasis of the cerebral blood vessels is occasionally found at autopsy, it rarely is associated with clinical symptoms and has not been associated with retinal involvement.[559] Gass has seen one boy with a prominent facial angioma associated with typical retinal telangiectasis.

In treating children with Coats' syndrome, photocoagulation and cryotherapy should be used whenever possible to destroy telangiectatic vessels so as to preserve visual function and prevent rubeotic glaucoma (Figure 6.39D–F and J–L). Drainage of the subretinal exudate may be required in some cases to treat highly elevated abnormal blood vessels. A more conservative approach is possible in older patients who seek treatment later in life because of peripheral localized detachment or mild loss of central vision caused by telangiectasis confined to the paracentral retina. Some patients with chronic cystoid edema caused by juxtafoveal telangiectasis may retain nearly normal visual acuity for many years (Figure 6.43A–D).[557] Those showing progressive accumulation of yellowish exudate in the central macular area should, however, be considered for laser treatment if the telangiectasis is localized outside the papillomacular bundle region (Figure 6.44A–H).[551,560–562] Recently intravitreal anti-VEGF agents have been used in conjunction with laser photocoagulation with the intention of trying to decrease the accumulation of lipid under the macula.[563,564] Intravitreal triamcinolone in addition to laser photocoagulation has also been tried with variable success. Surgery to remove the submacular lipid has been tried anecdotally.[565] Macular distortion secondary to epiretinal membrane formation and contraction may accompany retinal telangiectasis or may follow photocoagulation treatment. Gass has seen one adult patient who developed total retinal detachment and massive periretinal proliferation following cryotherapy to peripheral retinal telangiectasis in an eye with 20/20 vision discovered late in life.

The histopathology of advanced retinal telangiectasis in eyes enucleated with the incorrect clinical diagnosis of retinoblastoma reveals irregular dilation of the retinal capillaries, arteries, and veins and is often associated with a massive outpouring of periodic acid–Schiff-positive exudate into the outer retinal layers (Figure 6.41D–I).[550,558,566,567] This outpouring is associated with varying degrees of degeneration and disruption of the normal retinal architecture. Retinal detachment may or may not be present. Cholesterol clefts are seen within the subretinal exudates and lipid-laden macrophages are usually found remote from the site of the retinal telangiectasis, both beneath and in the outer layers of the overlying

6.40 Congenital retinal telangiectasis associated with systemic disease.

A–F: Bilateral peripheral and macular retinal telangiectasis in a 17-year-old man with facioscapulohumeral muscular dystrophy. Note the macular star and exudative retinopathy surrounding large arterial and venous aneurysms temporally in the right eye (A and B) and the subtle microaneurysms in the temporal macula of the left eye (C). His visual acuity was 20/200 right eye and 20/20 left eye. Angiography showed evidence of telangiectasis and large peripheral zone of capillary nonperfusion temporally in the right eye (D and E), and retinal staining in the paracentral area in the left eye (F).

G and H: Peculiar unilateral retinal telangiectasis in a patient with tuberous sclerosis.

I–L: Retinal telangiectasis and exudative retinal detachment in the contralateral eye of a patient with progressive hemifacial atrophy (Parry–Rhomberg syndrome).

(G and H, from Jost and Olk[583]; I–L, from Gass et al.[571])

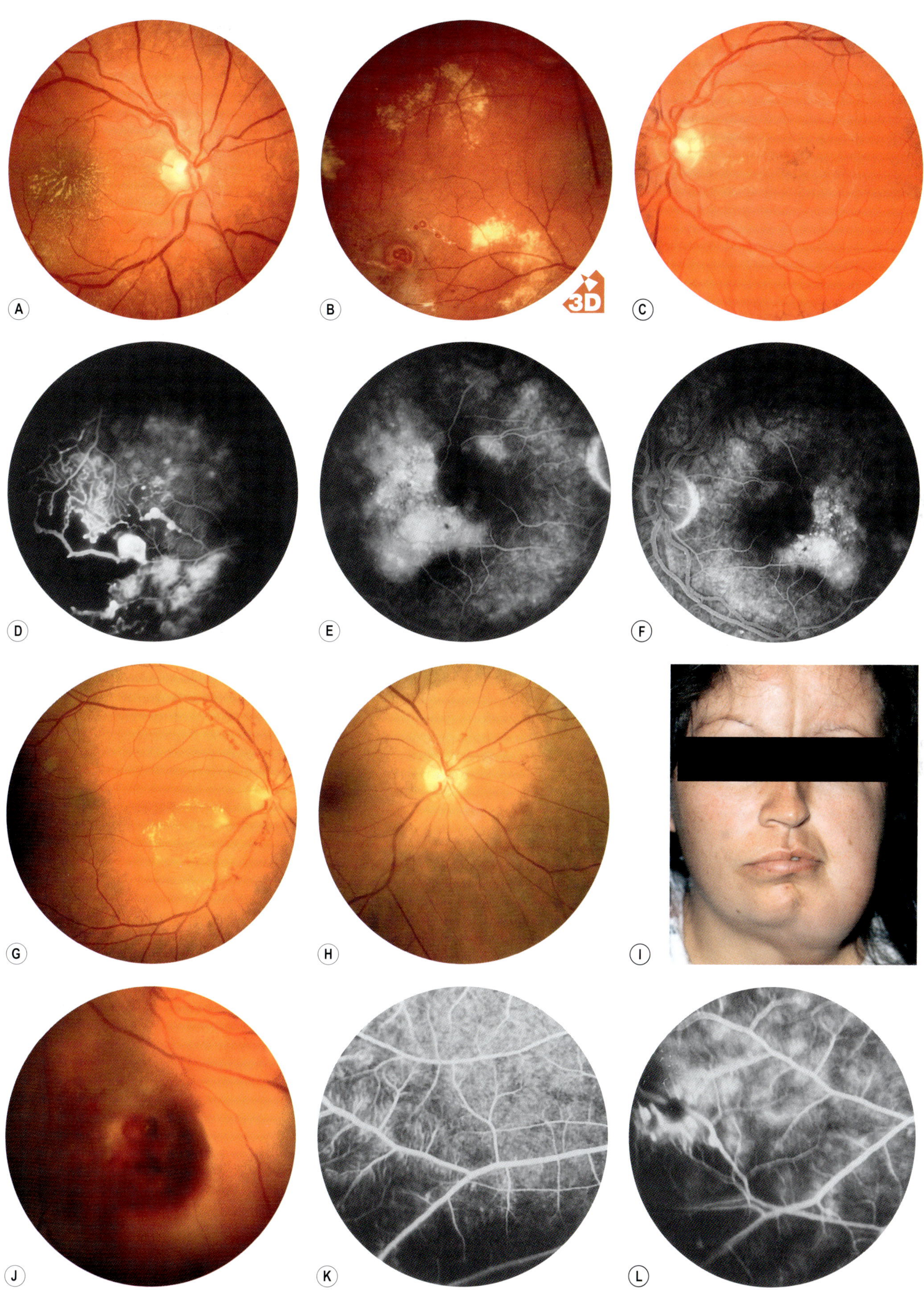
A
B
3D
C
D
E
F
G
H
I
J
K
L

retina (Figure 6.41I). Marked retinal vascular endothelial proliferation and hemorrhagic infarction of the retina may occur in some children with severe retinal telangiectasis (Figure 6.41A–F).

Shields et al., in an attempt to streamline management and understand the prognosis, have classified Coats' disease as[568]

- stage 1: telangiectasia only
- stage 2: telangiectasia and exudation
  - stage 2A: extrafoveal exudation
  - stage 2B: foveal exudation
- stage 3: exudative retinal detachment
  - stage 3A: subtotal
  - stage 3B: total
- stage 4: total detachment with secondary glaucoma
- stage 5: advanced end-stage disease.

This staging has prognostic significance, with patients presenting in stage 1 with almost no visual loss, and stage 2B with some amount of visual loss that can be treated with laser photocoagulation. Stage 3 had worse visual prognosis, although some could be treated, while eyes with stage 4 and 5 disease had to be enucleated.

In a recent finding, both a mother who had Coats' disease and her son with Norrie's disease had a missense mutation for the *NDP* gene on chromosome Xp11.2. The same investigators also analyzed retinas of nine enucleated eyes from males with Coats' disease and found a somatic mutation of the retinal tissue in one of the nine cases.[569] They speculated that Coats' disease might be the result of a somatic mutation in the *NDP* gene, which results in deficiency of the protein norrin. Coats' disease may occur as a postfertilization change in the X chromosome in a recessive fashion, similar to Aicardi syndrome. However, given that Aicardi's is an X-linked dominant condition, the mutation is lethal for males. No study so far has been able to demonstrate a defect in the X chromosome in Coats' or Aicardi syndrome.[570]

6.41 Congenital retinal telangiectasis.

A–F: Exudative and hemorrhagic retinopathy and detachment caused by widespread severe retinal telangiectasis in one eye of a 3-year-old boy who had a white pupillary reflex. Vision in this eye was no light perception. The other eye was normal. Because of the possibility of retinoblastoma, the eye was enucleated. Histopathologic examination of the eye revealed prominent intraretinal exudation and blood (arrows, E), telangiectatic retinal vessels (arrow, D), and vascular endothelial proliferation (E and F).

G–I: The eye of this child was enucleated because of suspected retinoblastoma. Clinically, the patient probably had a fundus picture similar to that in Figure 6.27 J and K. Gross examination of the eye revealed a peripheral mass (arrows, G) and intraretinal and subretinal exudation extending posteriorly to the macular area. Photomicrographs revealed dilated retinal vessels (arrow, H), massive intraretinal and subretinal exudation with cholesterol clefts, lipid-laden macrophages, hemosiderin, and retinal degeneration. Lipid-laden macrophages were present within and beneath the retina far posterior to the area of retinal telangiectasis (arrows, I).

J–L: Orbital cellulitis and chemosis (J) simulating endophthalmitis and retinoblastoma in a 2-year-old infant with massive subretinal lipoproteinaceous exudation (K) (Coats' syndrome) caused by congenital retinal telangiectasis. Histopathologic examination revealed total retinal detachment and marked telangiectasis of the retinal blood vessels (arrows, L).

(A–F from Gass.[550])

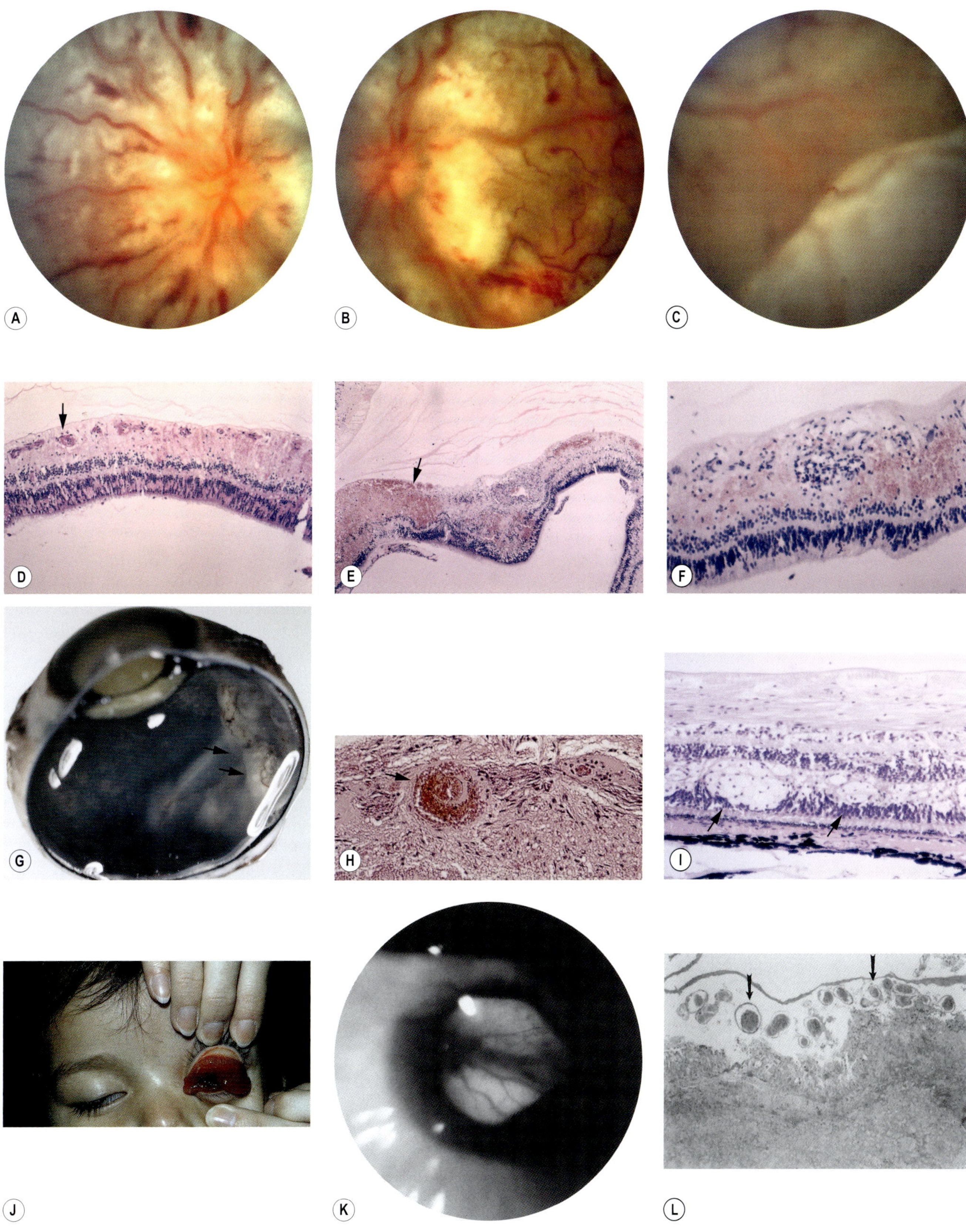
A
B
C
D
E
F
G
H
I
J
K
L

A clinical picture of retinal telangiectasis and Coats' syndrome may develop in one or both eyes of patients with progressive facial hemiatrophy (Figures 6.40I–L and 15.12),[550,571,572] in multiple family members with facioscapulohumeral muscular dystrophy (FSHD) and deafness (Figure 6.40A–F),[573–580] Alport's syndrome,[581] the epidermal nevus syndrome,[582] tuberous sclerosis (Figure 6.40G and H),[583] isolated hemihyperplasia,[584] and in patients with retinitis pigmentosa (Figure 6.42F–H).[585] In one report of retinal telangiectasis in a patient with hypogammaglobulinemia, the retinal lesion was a cavernous retinal hemangioma rather than telangiectasis.[586,587]

The differential diagnosis in young patients with exudative retinal detachment caused by congenital retinal telangiectasis includes retinoblastoma (see Figure 13.01A–F), retrolental fibroplasia, FEVR (see Figure 6.68), angiomatosis retinae, *Toxocara canis*, incontinentia pigmenti, retinitis pigmentosa (see Figure 5.40), proliferative retinopathy caused by inflammatory diseases such as pars planitis or by chronic rhegmatogenous retinal detachment (see Figure 7.28), and endophthalmitis (Figure 6.41J–L).[557] Globular, yellowish exudative detachments of the retina secondary to telangiectasis in infants and children may simulate closely those with exophytic retinoblastomas. Telangiectatic vessels may occur on the surface of the mass lesions in both cases. In retinoblastoma these dilated vessels are continuous with large vascular trunks that extend into the depth of the tumor, whereas the dilated vessels in retinal telangiectasis do not extend into the subretinal exudative mass. Fluorescein angiography may be helpful in establishing the diagnosis (Figure 13.01A and F). Ultrasonographic demonstration of calcium in the eye with retinoblastoma is also important in this regard. Patients with localized congenital telangiectasis associated with retinal arterial and venous aneurysms may be misdiagnosed as cavernous hemangioma of the retina (see Figure 13.16A–C), acquired arterial macroaneurysms (Figure 6.29), branch vein occlusion (see Figure 6.81C–H), and bilateral multiple retinal arterial aneurysms associated with neuroretinitis (see Figures 6.52 and 6.53). (See a later subsection for the differential diagnosis of type I juxtafoveolar telangiectasis.)

Facioscapulohumeral Muscular Dystrophy and Coats' Syndrome

FSHD is an autosomal-dominant disorder with a variable age of onset from childhood to old age, and severity from mild weakness to severe disability. A family history may be difficult to elicit because expression of the gene is variable and penetrance is incomplete. The characteristic clinical features include wasting of the shoulder girdle, upper deltoid, pectoralis, biceps, and triceps muscles, with relative preservation of the lower deltoid and prominence of the upper trapezius muscles. Muscle weakness can progress to the trunk and lower limbs over time and 20% can become confined to the wheelchair. Loss of tone of the abdominal musles leads to a protruding belly, and of the facial muscles to a drool and protruding tongue.[588] Leg muscle involvement can lead to tiptoe walking and foot drop, resulting in an unstable gait. Loss of vision caused by retinal telangiectasis and deafness (high-frequency hearing loss) occur in some of these patients and rarely may be the initial manifestation of FSHD (Figure 6.40A–F).[573,574,576–580,589] Early onset of symptoms and deafness herald more severe cases. Myoclonus and temporal-lobe absence attacks can occur.[588] Unlike congenital retinal telangiectasis, both eyes are affected and both sexes are affected equally. The onset of visual loss is variable and may occur in early childhood. Asymptomatic family members with minimal evidence of FSHD may show evidence of retinal telangiectasis without evidence of exudation. The patients and family members should be screened for evidence of retinal telangiectasis since early treatment with photocoagulation may prevent visual loss. A young girl's presentation with neovascular glaucoma at age 2 led to the detection of bilateral Coats' disease; further onset of seizures led to the diagnosis of FSHD.[588] Coats' syndrome has also been reported in a scapulohumeral muscular dystrophy that is probably is a variant of FSHD.[575]

Deletion in the long arm of chromosome 4 (4q35) is the locus for the gene for FSHD; however the exact gene has not been found.[588]

6.42 Coats' disease.

A–E: This 36-year-old male noted trouble with his vision on the right 3 months previously. His vision was 3/200 on the right and 2/20 on the left. In the superotemporal quadrant 3–4 disc areas of retinal telangiectasia with hemorrhages surrounded by dense circinate lipid exudates and retinal thickening were seen (A–C). Another patch was present nasally. Angiogram showed the bulbous vessels, capillary nonperfusion, surrounding dilated capillary bed, and leakage from the telangiectatic vessels (D and E). He underwent laser treatment and moved to Texas.

Coats' disease with retinal degeneration.

F–H: A 72-year-old man, followed since 1980 from age 45 for retinitis pigmentosa, initially presented with retinal and vitreous hemorrhage in the right eye, requiring pars plana vitrectomy ×3 and phacoemulsification cataract surgery. That eye turned phthisical. The left eye has had several episodes of vitreous hemorrhage and received laser treatment (F–H).

(F–H, courtesy of Dr. Laurence W. Arend.)

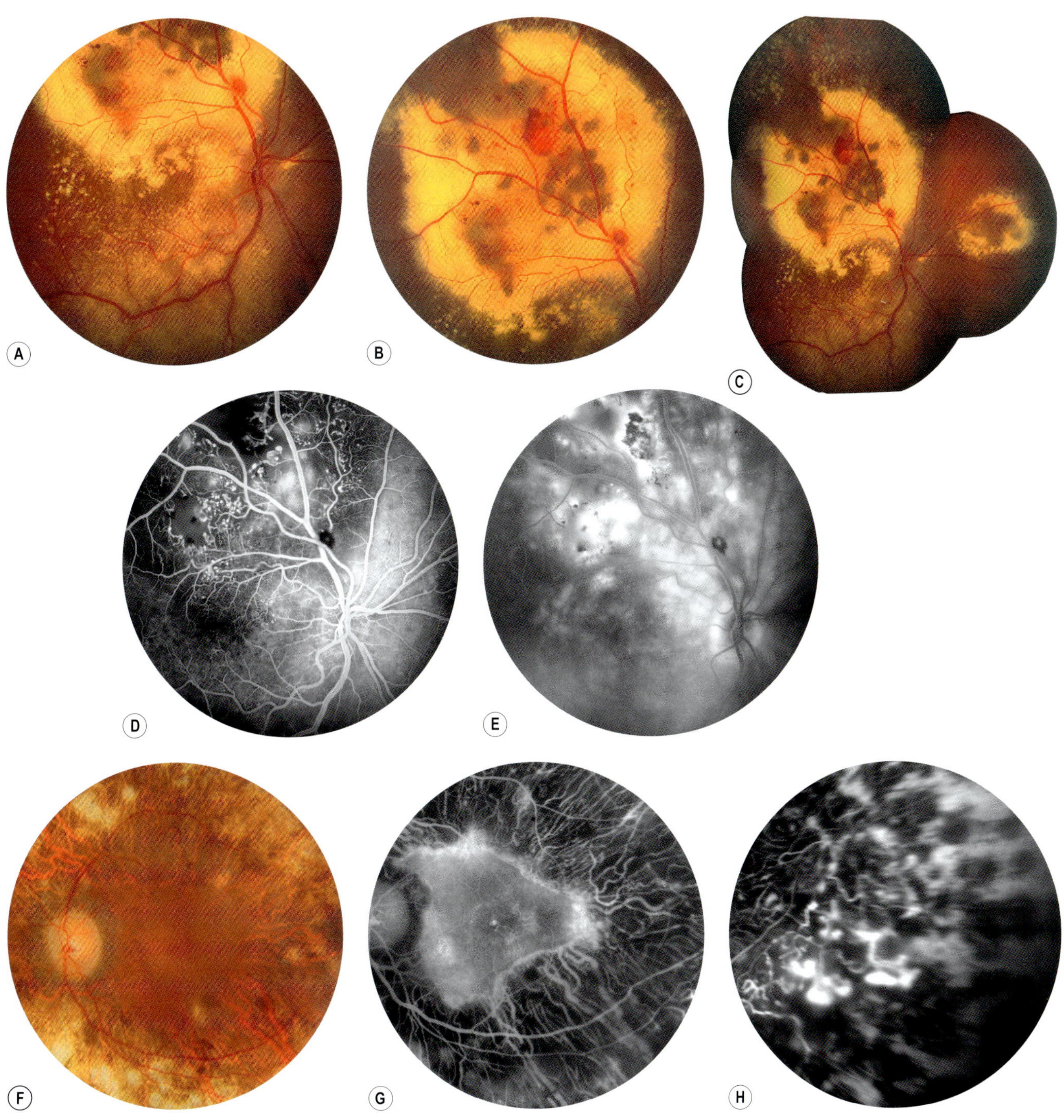
A
B
C
D
E
F
G
H

CONGENITAL AND ACQUIRED IDIOPATHIC MACULAR RETINAL TELANGIECTASIA

Adult patients may develop loss of central vision caused by exudation, diffusion abnormalities, or from ischemia and nonperfusion of ectatic and incompetent retinal capillaries that are confined to the foveal and perifoveal region, which are either congenital or of unknown cause.[547,551,556,560,590,591] These patients fall into several subgroups. Since the extent of the telangiectasia may vary and extend beyond the fovea, "macular telangiectasia" appears to be an appropriate name.

Group 1A: Unilateral Congenital Macular Telangiectasia

Patients with unilateral congenital foveal and parafoveolar telangiectasis probably suffer from a localized mild form of congenital retinal telangiectasis, a nonfamilial disorder affecting predominantly one eye of males without other evidence of systemic disease[549,551,560] (see previous discussion of congenital retinal telangiectasis and Coats' syndrome). The localized form of congenital retinal telangiectasis is typically confined to an area between 1½ and 2 disc diameters in the temporal half of the macula, where it straddles the horizontal raphe (Figures 6.43 and 6.44).[551,560] Approximately one-third of patients will have some focal telangiectasis in the extramacular area, usually temporally. Yellow, lipid-rich exudation is usually present at the outer margins of the area of telangiectasis, often in a ring configuration (Figures 6.43I, and 6.44A and E). The mean age of onset of symptoms is approximately 35 years. Polycystic macular edema and exudation are the cause of the loss of acuity, which usually ranges from 20/25 to 20/40. Telangiectatic capillaries are easily visualized with biomicroscopy and fluorescein angiography. Blunted right-angle venules, superficial retinal crystals, intraretinal pigment plaques, and subretinal neovascularization, features of group 2 juxtafoveal capillary telangiectasis, are not found in these patients. Early-phase stereoscopic fluorescein angiography shows prompt filling of the telangiectatic vessels, affecting both the superficial and the deep capillary network, and late intraretinal staining. The natural course of this disorder is variable. Some patients may retain excellent visual acuity for many years in spite of chronic waxing and waning CME (Figure 6.43A–I).[551,560] Those with yellow lipid exudate in or near the center of the macula are probably at greatest risk of developing progressive loss of visual acuity. Focal applications of laser photocoagulation of the telangiectatic vessels may be helpful in restoring and preserving central acuity (Figure 6.44A–H). Congenital telangiectasis confined to the capillary bed in the region of the macular area should be differentiated from idiopathic bilateral acquired juxtafoveal capillary telangiectasis (Figures 6.45–6.48),[551,556,560,590,591] and telangiectasis caused by branch vein obstruction (see Figure 6.79D–F), diabetic retinopathy (Figure 6.52A–C), X-ray irradiation retinopathy (Figure 6.57), Eales' disease,[586,592] sickle-cell maculopathy, tuberous sclerosis (Figure 6.40G and H), and carotid artery obstruction.[363,364,593] Group 1A patients should be clearly differentiated from patients with dilated perifoveal capillaries and evidence of vitreous cellular infiltration, whether it is caused by acquired inflammatory disease or is part of a tapetoretinal dystrophy.

6.43 Natural course of congenital juxtafoveolar retinal telangiectasis, group 1A.

A–D: This 52-year-old man noted blurred vision in the left eye. His visual acuity in the left eye was 20/30. The right eye was normal. Note the localized zone of capillary telangiectasis, which was confined to the juxtafoveolar region temporally (arrows, A). Angiography demonstrated the telangiectasis (B) and showed evidence of cystoid macular edema (C). No treatment was given. Twelve years later he had developed some lipid exudation (D) and his visual acuity was 20/40.

E–I: Spontaneous resolution of circinate maculopathy caused by juxtafoveolar retinal telangiectasis occurred in a 16-year-old boy, who when he was seen initially in 1958 had marked exudative maculopathy (E); his visual acuity was approximately 20/100. Six years later the exudate had cleared, he was asymptomatic, and his visual acuity was 20/20 (F and G). Angiography demonstrated that the telangiectasis extended into the peripheral fundus temporally (H). At age 38 years he noted decreased vision in the right eye. His visual acuity was 20/50. Note the recurrence of the lipid exudation (I).

J–L: This 57-year-old man presented with a 6-year history of blurred vision in the left eye and a 2-week history of blurred vision in the right eye. His visual acuity was 20/20, right eye, and 20/30, left eye. He had bilateral juxtafoveolar telangiectasis associated with mild cystoid edema but no lipid exudation in both eyes (J). Ten years later his visual acuity was 20/30, right eye, and 20/40, left eye. Note the temporal location of the telangiectatic capillaries and the lipid exudate (K and L).

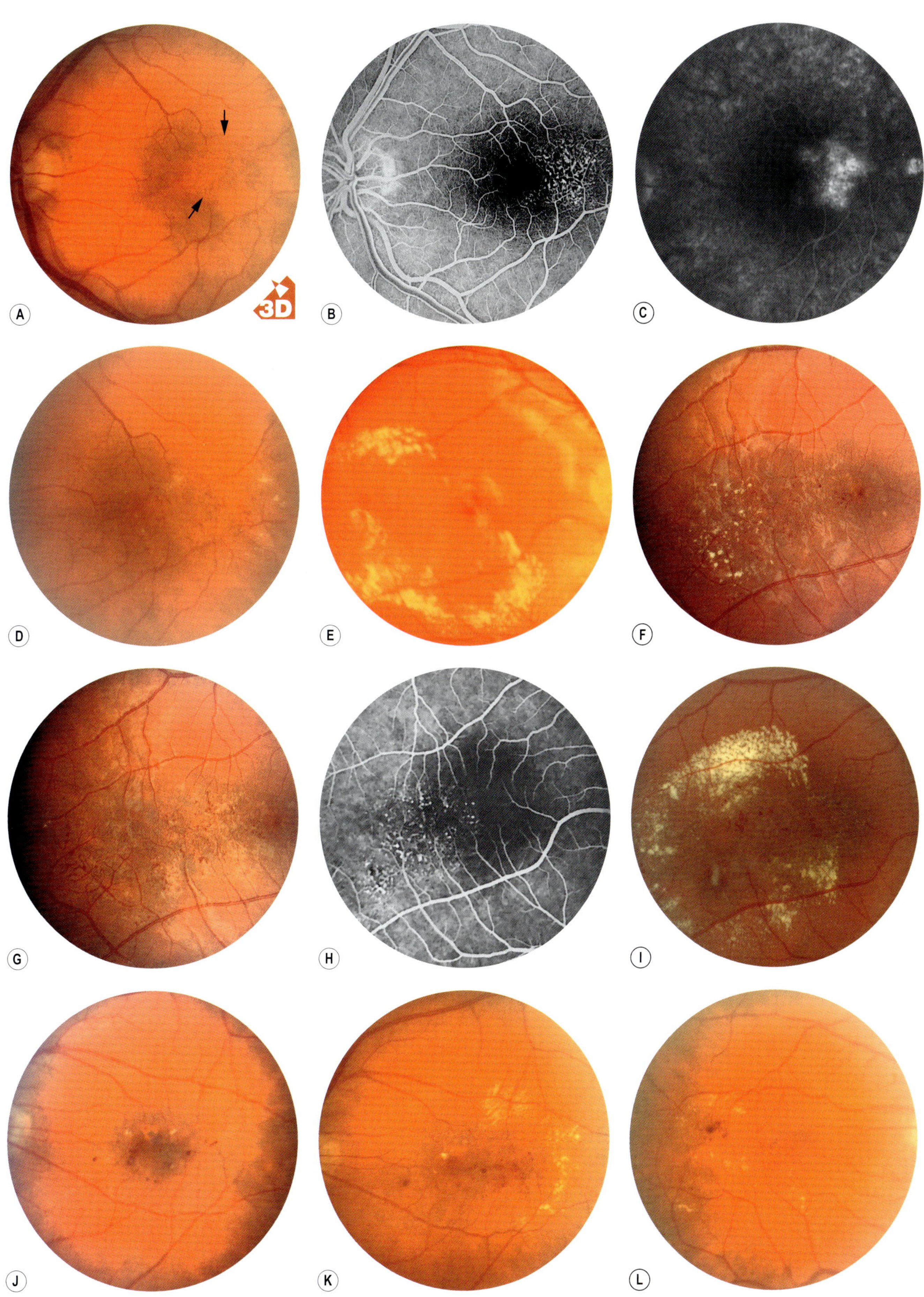
A
3D
B
C
D
E
F
G
H
I
J
K
L

Group 1B: Unilateral, Idiopathic, Focal Macular Telangiectasis

Most patients with unilateral idiopathic focal juxtafoveolar telangiectasis are middle-aged men who have mild metamorphopsia or blurring caused by exudation from a minute area of capillary telangiectasis that is usually confined to 2 hours of the clock or less at the edge of the capillary-free zone (Figure 6.44I–L).[551,560] It may or may not be associated with a small amount of yellow exudate. The visual acuity is usually 20/25 or better. Angiography shows the focal capillary telangiectasis and minimal staining. Photocoagulation is usually not advisable because of the proximity of the leakage to the capillary-free zone and the good visual prognosis without treatment. It is uncertain whether this is an acquired lesion or merely represents a minute focus of congenital telangiectasis.

6.44 Congenital juxtafoveolar retinal telangiectasis, group 1A.

A–D: Retinal telangiectasis involving the capillary bed temporal to the macula associated with a localized serous detachment of the retina, retinal edema, and circinate retinopathy in a 27-year-old man (A). Note the sheathed capillaries just temporal to the macula (arrow). The elevation of the lesion was caused primarily by thickening of the retina secondary to edema. Angiography revealed extensive telangiectatic involvement of the capillary bed temporal to the macula (B and C). There was marked leakage of dye from the capillary bed in the area surrounded by circinate retinopathy (G). Note the partial dark figure in the macula (arrow). Twelve months after xenon photocoagulation, the exudate had cleared (D) and visual acuity was 20/20.

E–H: Unilateral congenital juxtafoveolar telangiectasis in the right eye (E and F) of this 49-year-old man, whose visual acuity was 20/50. Following focal argon laser photocoagulation his visual acuity improved to 20/20 and the exudation resolved (H).

Congenital monocular focal juxtafoveolar retinal telangiectasis, group 1B.

I and **J**: This 40-year-old man noted blurred vision in the right eye caused by exudation from a focal area of capillary telangiectasis (arrows, I and J) at the edge of the capillary-free zone at 1 o'clock.

K and **L**: This healthy 28-year-old man noted metamorphopsia in the left eye caused by yellow exudation from focal retinal telangiectasis confined to a small area at the edge of the capillary-free zone.

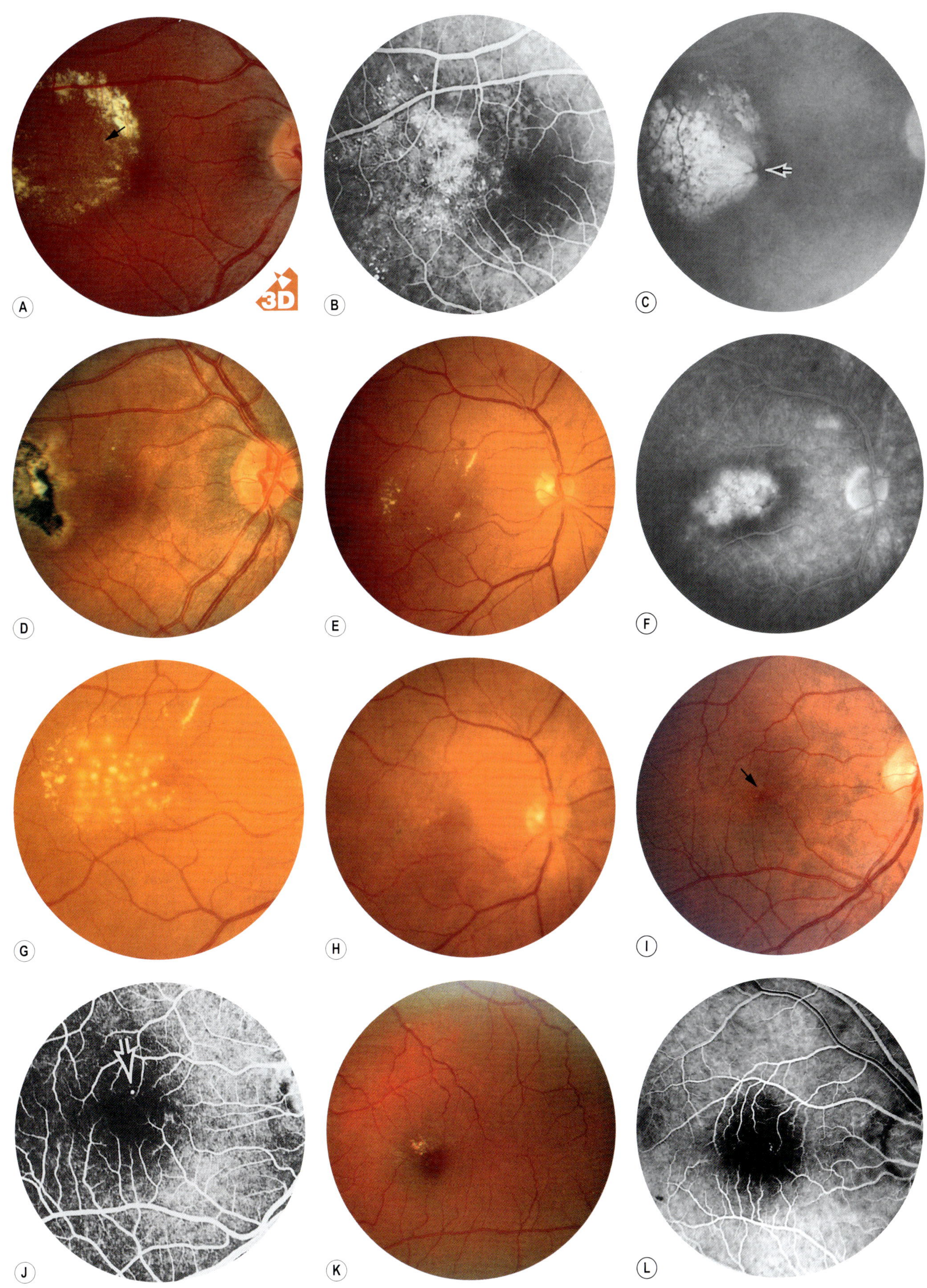
A
B
C
D
E
F
G
H
I
J
K
L
3D

OCT shows one or more cysts or lacunae in the inner or outer retina in all stages of the disease (Figure 6.47H and I). These cysts or lacunae may be the result of breakdown and loss of the Müller cell bodies in the Müller cell cone and the rest of the fovea.

Visual acuity is usually normal in stages 1 and 2. Most patients become symptomatic at stage 3, and some maintain good acuity after developing stage 4. Loss of central vision in these patients typically occurs slowly over many years and is associated with atrophy of the foveolar retina that develops in the absence of typical CME. This atrophy may produce a picture simulating a lamellar macular hole (Figure 6.46E and F).[596] Fluorescein angiography in stages 1–4 fails to show late staining extending into the center of the fovea in all but a few eyes that develop angiographic evidence of capillary ingrowth into the FAZ (Figure 6.45H and I). OCT demonstrates some degree of thinning in almost all patients and is extremely useful in confirming this observation, made by Gass. Cystoid edema, yellow exudate, and loss of the foveolar depression develop only in those patients who develop subretinal neovascularization (Figure 6.46G–L).[560] This complication may be associated with rapid loss of vision, subretinal hemorrhage, disciform scarring, and retinochoroidal anastomosis (Figure 6.46G–L).

The yellow foveal lesions in these patients may be mistaken for those seen in the adult form of vitelliform foveomacular dystrophy (see Figures 5.08 and 5.09) or Best's disease (see Figures 5.01 and 5.02). Those with stellate pigment plaques or with choroidal neovascularization may be misdiagnosed as having senile macular degeneration or chorioretinal scars secondary to focal choroiditis.

Histopathologic examination in one patient with group 2A telangiectasis reported by Green and coworkers showed focal thickening of the sensory retina in the parafoveolar region, thickening of the retinal vessel walls, evidence of capillary endothelial abnormalities, but minimal or no evidence of capillary telangiectasis (Figure 6.48).[591] In a review of histopathologic sections of the eye previously reported by Green and coworkers, Gass found evidence of retinal capillary invasion of the retinal receptor layer and minimal evidence of cystic accumulation of extracellular fluid (Figure 6.48F–H).

6.46 Bilateral acquired juxtafoveolar telangiectasis, group 2A.

A–E: This woman first noted loss of central vision at age 50 years. At that time her visual acuity was 20/25 bilaterally. There was mild loss of retinal transparency and superficial retinal crystals in the juxtafoveolar region temporally in both eyes (A). Stereoscopic angiograms revealed evidence of juxtafoveal telangiectasis in both eyes temporally and evidence of a peculiar remodeling of dilated blood vessels in the outer retina in the left eye (B–D). When she returned 13 years later, visual acuity was 20/200, right eye, and 20/30, left eye. She had developed stellate foci of intraretinal retinal pigment epithelium hyperplasia temporally in both eyes (E). Note the multiple, superficial, pale yellow crystalline deposits, and the focal atrophy of the retina centrally simulating an inner lamellar hole.

F: This woman had bilateral acquired juxtafoveolar retinal telangiectasis. Note the sharply delineated foveolar atrophy simulating a macular hole.

G–L: This 36-year-old man was being observed because of mild blurring of vision caused by acquired, bilateral, perifoveolar telangiectasis, before developing marked metamorphopsia in the right eye caused by subretinal neovascularization (G). He was asymptomatic in the left eye (H). Note the prominent superficial crystalline retinal opacities in both eyes (G and H). Six years later in the left eye he developed subretinal neovascularization (I–K) that resulted in a large disciform scar (L).

(G–L, from Gass and Oyakawa.[560],)

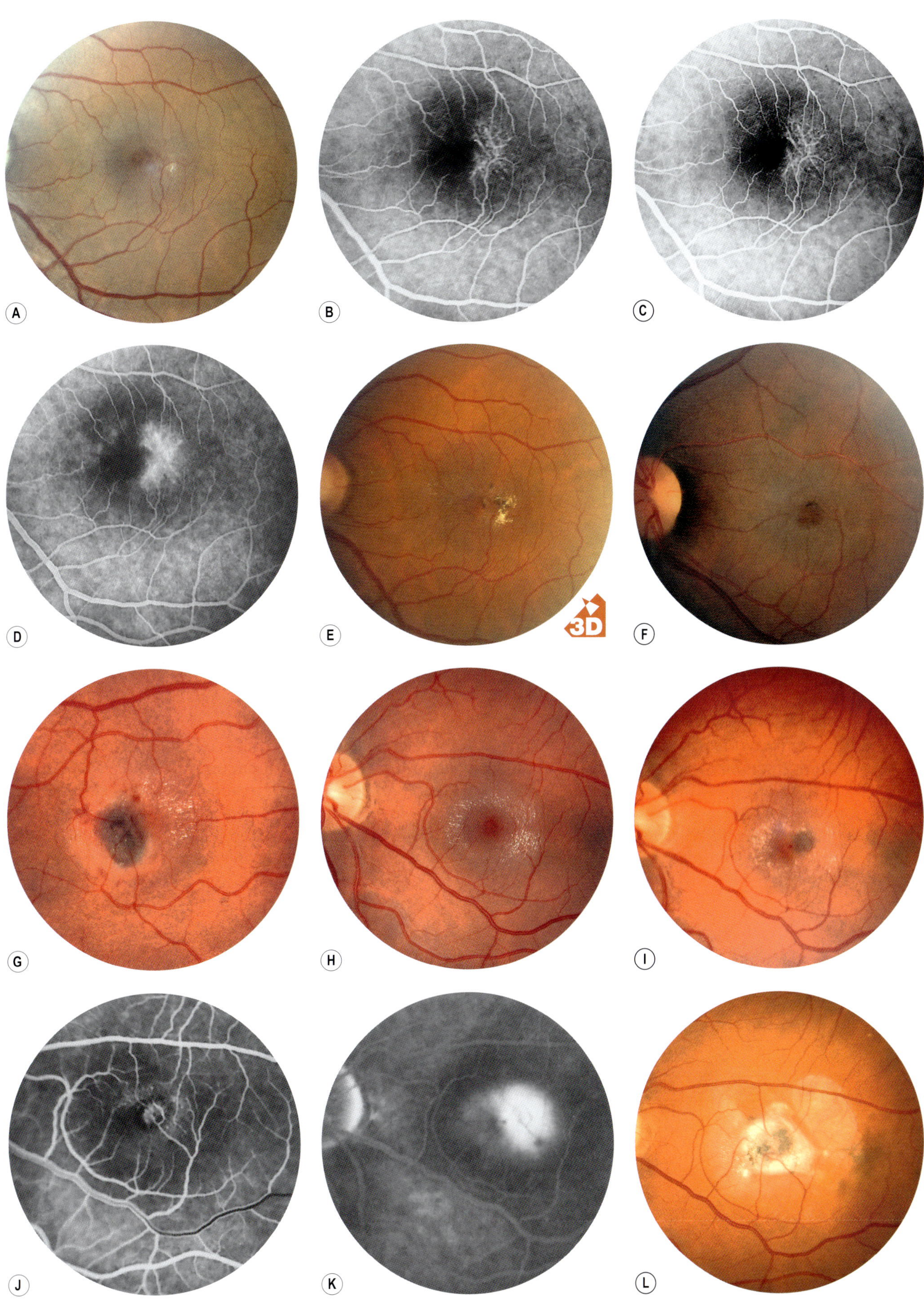
A
B
C
D
E
3D
F
G
H
I
J
K
L

How do we account for the retinal staining and the absence of evidence of migration of extracellular fluid into the central macular region to form cystoid edema in patients with group 2A juxtafoveolar telangiectasis? The following sequence of events appears to occur (Figure 6.47J). Early fluorescein staining of the thickened capillary walls, particularly those in the deeper plexus, is responsible for the early-phase angiographic appearance of "telangiectatic" vessels. The altered structure of the capillary wall is associated with decreased metabolic exchange and minimal increased endothelial permeability. These changes result in low-grade chronic nutritional damage to the retinal cells, particularly those at the level of the inner nuclear layer that includes the Müller cells. The late diffuse staining that stereoscopically appears to occur at the middle and outer retina is probably caused by staining of minimal amounts of extracellular matrix and intracellular diffusion of fluorescein into damaged retinal cells. Further changes in the outer capillary bed, which may include capillary proliferation and invasion of the outer retina and occasionally the foveolar retina, are accompanied by alteration of the pattern of venous outflow and formation of dilated right-angled venules (Figure 6.47J, stage 3). Nutritional deprivation of the retinal cells in the middle retina, particularly the Müller cells, leads to degeneration and atrophy of these cells and the connecting photoreceptor cells. This loss of photoreceptor cells is responsible for the gradual loss of visual acuity and biomicroscopic picture that may simulate a lamellar macular hole. Loss of photoreceptor cells permits RPE cells to migrate into the overlying retina, particularly along the right-angle venules, to form black stellate plaques (Figure 6.47J, stage 4). Stage 5 disease results when loss of retinal cells induces proliferative changes in the deep capillary network that may eventually gain entrance into the subsensory retinal space, where a type II pattern of subretinal neovascular growth and reactive proliferation of the RPE occurs (Figure 6.47J, stage 5). Although it is probable that this neovascularization is primarily derived from the retinal vessels, evidence of chorioretinal vascular anastomosis may eventually occur. The cause of the golden refractile structures at the inner retinal surface in the juxtafoveolar area is unknown. Their appearance suggests that they are lipid. Their location in the region of the internal limiting membrane of the retina suggests that they may be a product of degenerating Müller cells whose nuclei are located in the inner nuclear layer at the site of the altered deep retinal capillary plexus, and whose foot plates form the internal limiting membrane.[551]

6.47 Bilateral acquired juxtafoveolar telangiectasis, group 2A with good vision and lacunae.

A–I: This 67-year-old woman noted a change in her vision in her right eye in 2004 to 20/40. She saw 20/20 with her left eye. Both foveas had fine telangiectatic vessels, no pigmentation, crystals or hemorrhages (A and B). Angiogram was consistent with bitemporal hyperfluorescence and staining of tissue (C and D). Four years later her vision continues to remains at 20/40 right and 20/25 left eye. She now has a few pigment figures in the left fovea (F and G). Optical coherence tomography shws the typical lacunae seen in this condition likely from changes in the Müller cell cone (H and I).
J: Diagram of presumed anatomic changes accompanying stages 3, 4, and 5 of development of acquired juxtafoveolar telangiectasis involving the deep retinal plexus.

Stage 3, Incompetent retinal capillaries, swelling of the retina on the left side of the fovea, development of dilated right-angle venules (RaV) draining the deep capillary plexus (DCP), and early proliferation of capillaries into the outer retinal layers. Arrow indicates superficial retinal crystals.

Stage 4, Atrophy of outer retinal layers, hyperplasia of the retinal pigment epithelium (RPE), intraretinal migration of RPE cells alongside the RaV, further proliferation and remodeling of the DCP.

Stage 5, Type 2 subretinal neovascularization, subretinal bleeding, and exudation. The subretinal new vessels may or may not anastomose with the choroidal vessels.

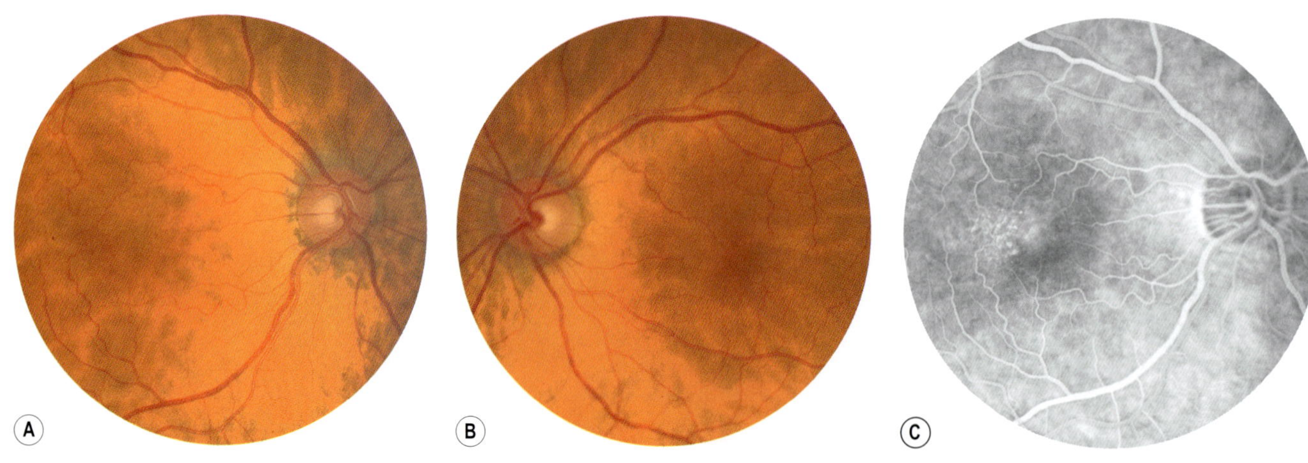

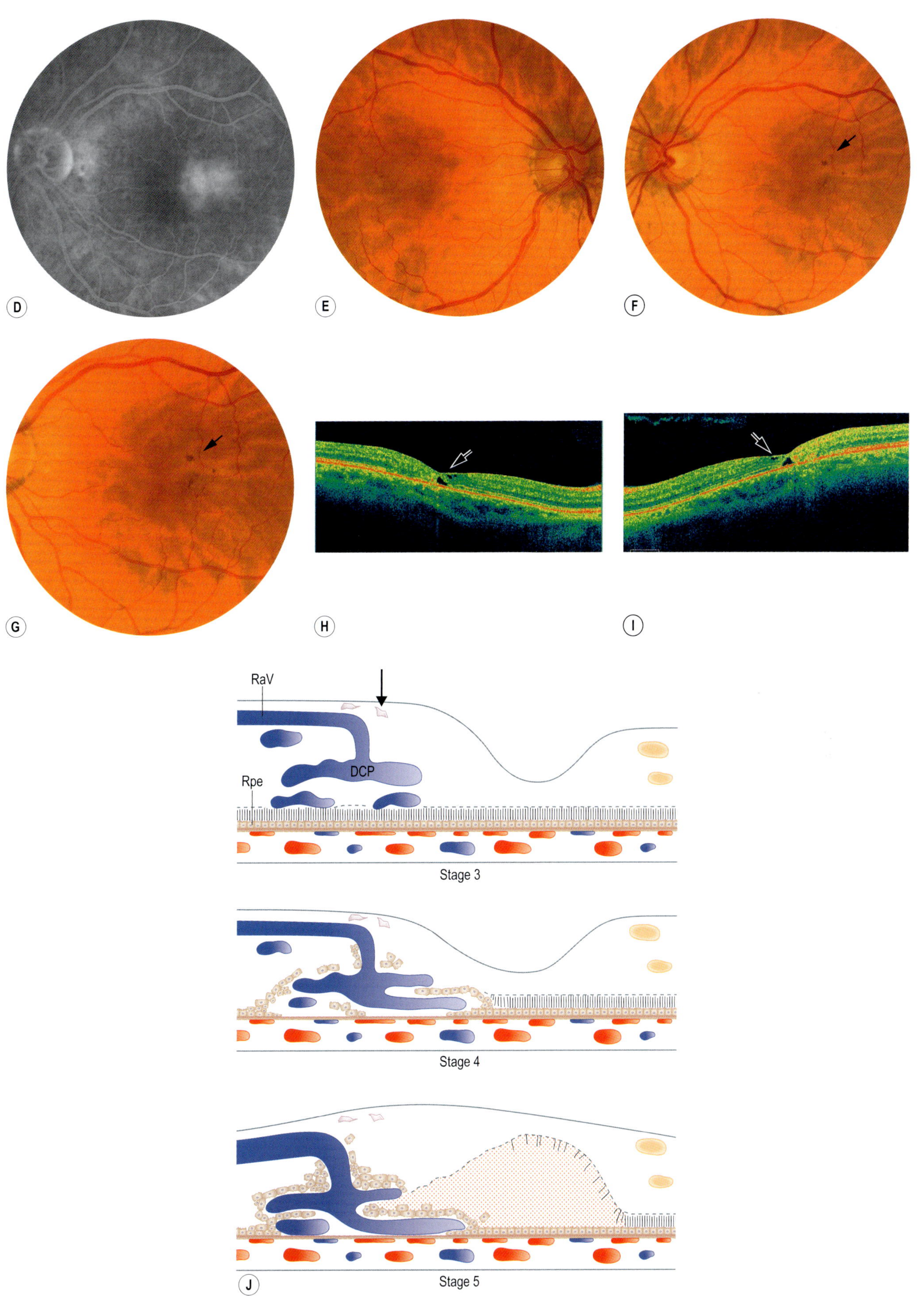
D
E
F
G
H
I
RaV
DCP
Rpe
Stage 3
Stage 4
Stage 5
J

The cause for group 2A telangiectasis, which is the most common form of idiopathic juxtafoveolar telangiectasis, is unknown. Chronic venous stasis caused by obstruction of the retinal veins as they cross the retinal arteries on both sides of the horizontal raphe may be a factor.[560] More recently, study of the FAZ using whole mounts at 26–41-week gestational age has shown that the vessels making up the temporal FAZ are the last to close in to complete the ring.[64] The temporal juxtafoveolar vessels are the earliest vessels to be affected in type 2 juxtafoveolar telangiectasis. Whether there is a relationship between these two features is interesting and needs further exploration. Although approximately 15% of these patients may have evidence of systemic diseases including systemic hypertension, borderline diabetes, coronary artery disease, and renal failure associated with Alport's disease, long-term follow-up studies have failed to link group 2A telangiectasis to systemic disease in the majority of patients.[551] Familial cases of group 2A telangiectasis occur occasionally.[560]

Patients with group 2A telangiectasis should be differentiated from cases of bilateral retinal telangiectasis with other causes, including bilateral group 1A congenital juxtafoveal telangiectasis (Figure 6.43J–L), juxtafoveal telangiectasis associated with Eales' disease (see Figure 6.62A–H), diabetes mellitus, and irradiation retinopathy.

There is limited information available concerning the results of photocoagulation treatment of group 2A telangiectasis. It is probable that photocoagulation is ineffective in restoring visual function in these patients before the development of subretinal neovascularization because loss of function is associated with retinal atrophy rather than intraretinal exudation, as in the case of group 1 telangiectasis.[586] It is also unlikely that prophylactic photocoagulation of the paracentral retinal capillaries will either slow or prevent the loss of visual acuity. In most instances the close proximity of subretinal neovascular networks to the center of the fovea precludes photocoagulation as a means of restoring or preventing loss of central vision.

Group 2B: Juvenile Occult Familial Idiopathic Juxtafoveolar Retinal Telangiectasis

Juxtafoveolar retinal telangiectasis similar to group 2A, but without evidence of right-angle venules, superficial retinal refractile deposits, or stellate pigmented plaques, has been reported in two siblings, 9 and 12 years of age.[551,597]

Group 3A: Occlusive Idiopathic Juxtafoveolar Retinal Telangiectasis

Group 3A patients experience variable degrees of loss of central vision in both eyes associated with juxtafoveolar retinal telangiectasis and progressive loss of the juxtapapillary capillary network in later life associated with a variety of systemic diseases, including polycythemia, hypoglycemia, ulcerative colitis, multiple myeloma, and chronic lymphatic leukemia (Figure 6.49A–F).[551,598] The macular changes in this group are similar to those that occasionally occur in patients with sickle-cell retinopathy, diabetic retinopathy (Figure 6.52), and X-ray radiation retinopathy (Figure 6.57B and D). The loss of central vision may be abrupt and be associated with ischemic whitening of the retina centrally, occlusion of the perifoveolar retinal capillaries, and minimal evidence of telangiectasis, which develops only later (Figure 6.51A). In others the loss of parafoveolar retinal capillaries may occur slowly and be associated with telangiectasis of the adjacent capillaries, probably as the result of development of collateral pathways of flow.

6.48 Spontaneous retinal hemorrhage in bilateral acquired juxtafoveolar telangiectasis, group 2A.

A–D: This 65-year-old asymptomatic woman with vision of 20/30 in each eye when seen for a routine exam was found to have bilateral foveal telangiectasia with fine intraretinal pigment, and a fleck of blood in the superficial retina in her left eye. An angiogram revealed the typical pattern of staining of the intraretinal tissue, but no late pooling of dye. Optical coherence tomography did not reveal intra- or subretinal thickening or fluid (D). No treatment was given and the retinal hemorrhage disappeared by 3 months. Examination 15 months later revealed no change in vision, or signs of subretinal neovascular membrane (D).

Clinicopathologic correlation of bilateral juxtafoveolar retinal telangiectasis, group 2A.

E–H: This 58-year-old woman, whose visual acuity was 20/25 in both eyes, had angiographic evidence of intraretinal fluorescein staining in the temporal juxtafoveolar region bilaterally (E). Light microscopy revealed focal thickening of the retina in the juxtafoveolar area (F). Compare the normal retina on the right side of the arrow in B with the affected retina on the left side of the arrow. The ganglion cells appear vacuolated and swollen. There is minimal evidence of focal accumulation of extracellular fluid in the inner nuclear and outer plexiform layers. Higher-power views of the affected retina showed evidence of focal invasion of the nerve fiber layer of Henle and the receptor cell layer with fine capillaries (arrows, G and H). The retinal pigment epithelium and choroid were normal.

(E and F, from Green et al.[591])

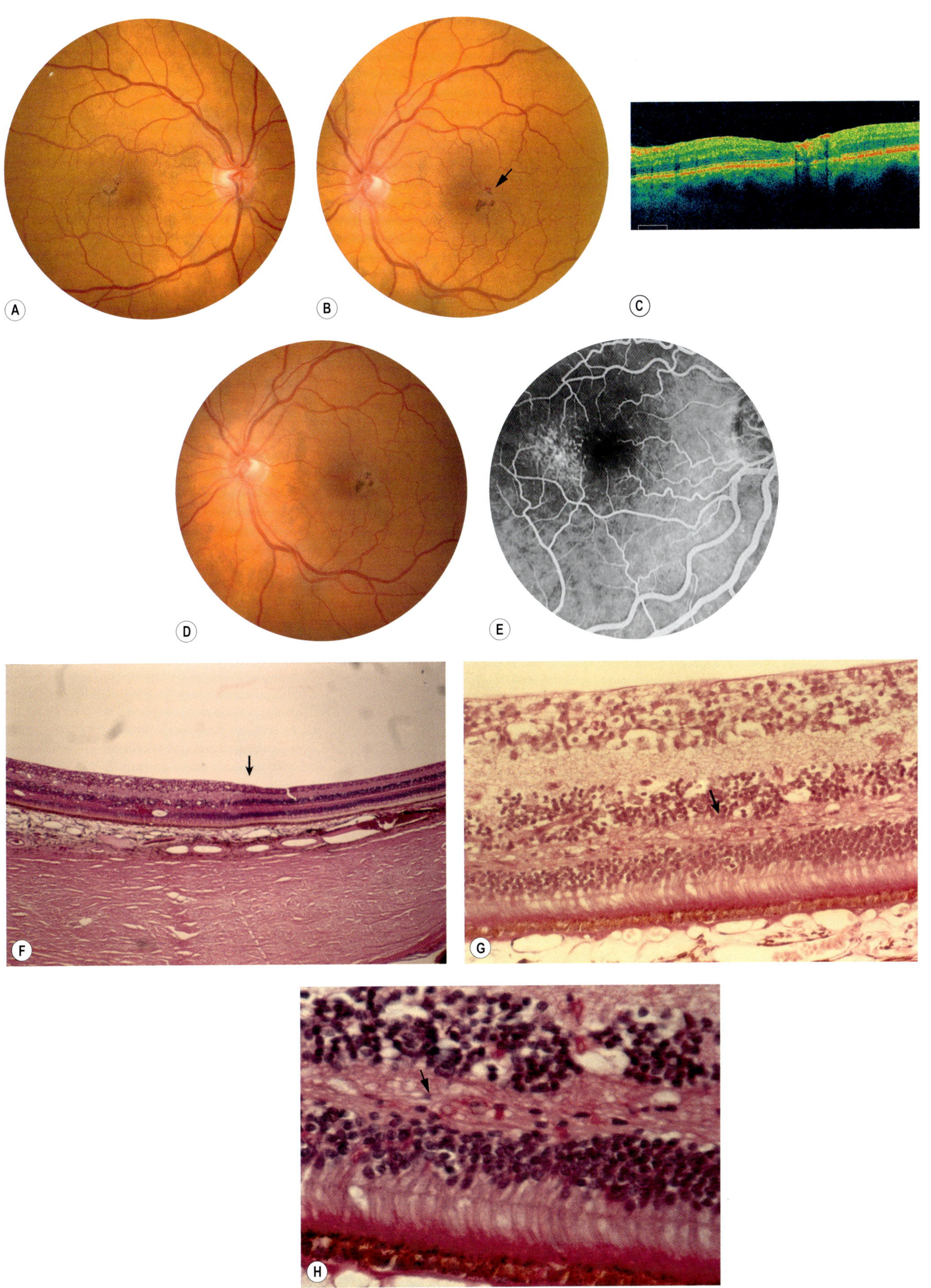
A
B
C
D
E
F
G
H

Group 3B: Occlusive Idiopathic Juxtafoveolar Retinal Telangiectasis Associated with Central Nervous System Vasculopathy

Group 3B patients have a hereditary oculocerebral syndrome characterized by the onset in middle or later life of progressive loss of central vision in both eyes caused by progressive obliteration and telangiectasis of the perifoveolar capillary network, which in some patients is associated with optic atrophy, abnormal deep tendon reflexes, and other evidence of central nervous system involvement (Figure 6.49).[550,551,560,599–603] Loss of the juxtafoveolar capillaries, marked aneurysmal dilation of the terminal capillary network, and relatively little fluorescein leakage from the affected capillary bed are features that differentiate these patients from those in groups 1 and 2. In one family the retinal telangiectasis was associated with frontoparietal-lobe pseudotumors, comprised of small blood vessel damage and fibrinoid necrosis of white matter in the absence of evidence of vasculitis.[599] Van Effenterre et al. described three sisters with similar retinal findings involving retinal telangiectasis and capillary occlusion in the peripheral retina and posterior pole, associated with poikiloderma, graying of the hair, and idiopathic nonarteriosclerotic cerebral calcifications.[603] Pathology studies revealed small-vessel hyalinosis caused by basement membrane thickening involving the digestive tract, kidney, and calcified areas in the brain. In another family with evidence of autosomal-dominant inheritance of both central and peripheral retinal obliterative vasculopathy, there was associated Raynaud's phenomena and mental changes, mainly forgetfulness, aggression, and depression.[601,603] Ehlers and Jensen[556] reported similar macular lesions in three family members of two successive generations. These patients did not have optic atrophy or neurologic disease.

CEREBRORETINAL VASCULOPATHY

Cerebroretinal vasculopathy is a rare adult-onset (fourth decade onwards) autosomal-dominant disorder involving the microvessels of the brain and retina due to frameshift mutations in the gene *TREX1*.[604] Patients present with vision loss, seizures, hemiparesis, apraxia, dysarthria, or memory loss. Progression to blindness, a neurovegetative state, and death ensues within 5–10 years. It was first described by Grand et al. in 10 family members and suspected in eight others, spanning over four generations.[599] Retinal capillary and small-vessel obliteration and telangiectasia involving the macula alone, or including the periphery, are seen.[605,606] Retinal or optic disc neovascularization occurs occasionally.[607]

Pseudotumor of the brain due to fibrinoid necrosis from ischemia can mimic a tumor in approximately half of patients, while the other half may have multiple small white-matter lesions, which may be misdiagnosed as demyelinating disease.[608–610] Migraine and Raynaud's phenomenon may be associated in some. Other organs sometimes involved include the liver with elevated enzymes, kidney, and osteonecrosis of the hip.[611,612] Three disorders that appear to be related to each other and share the same genetic locus at 3p21.1-p21.3 are: (1) hereditary vascular retinopathy; (2) cerebroretinal vasculopathy; and (3) hereditary endotheliopathy with retinopathy, nephropathy, and stroke.[612,613]

6.49 Bilateral, idiopathic, juxtafoveolar, retinal capillary occlusion and telangiectasis, group 3A.

A–C: This 59-year-old woman complained of onset of a positive scotoma of the right eye that began 6 weeks previously but increased in size 1 week previously after taking prednisone 60 mg daily for 2 weeks. She had a past history of iritis in the left eye and recurrent ulcerative colitis. Visual acuity in the right eye was 20/200 and in the left eye, 20/20. Note the irregular ischemic whitening of the retina in the central macular area of the right eye (A). There was no evidence of iridocyclitis. Angiography revealed evidence of retinal capillary arteriolar and occlusion and irregular dilation of the paracentral retinal arterioles (B and C). Nine years later she had evidence of posterior synechia and an immature cataract in the right eye. The visual function was unchanged. There was focal dilation of the retinal capillaries adjacent to the enlarged capillary-free zone centrally. The left eye was normal.

D–F: Acquired perifoveolar retinal telangiectasis and capillary occlusion in a middle-aged woman with polycythemia vera. Despite large areas of capillary nonperfusion centrally in both eyes, her visual acuity was 20/25.

Bilateral, idiopathic juxtafoveolar retinal capillary occlusion and telangiectasis associated with central nervous system involvement, group 3B.

G–J: A 47-year-old man had a 1-year history of progressive loss of vision in both eyes. Note the slight temporal pallor of both optic discs, focal obliteration of the capillaries in the central macular region, and aneurysmal dilation of some of the terminal capillaries (G and H). Angiography showed irregular widening of the capillary-free zone, aneurysmal dilation of the abnormal blood vessels, and no evidence of dye leakage (I and J).

K and **L**: This 51-year-old man with a poorly defined neurologic disease developed progressive loss of central vision in both eyes. His visual acuity was 20/70 in the right eye and 20/30 in the left eye. The macular changes and angiographic findings were identical to those of the patient depicted in G–J.

HEREDITARY HEMORRHAGIC TELANGIECTASIA (RENDU–OSLER–WEBER DISEASE)

Hemorrhagic hereditary telangiectasia is a dominantly inherited disorder characterized by telangiectasias of the capillaries and venules involving many organ systems, including the skin and mucous membranes and visceral AVMs. The affected blood vessels are friable and prone to bleeding. The most frequent signs and symptoms include epistaxis, gastrointestinal tract bleeding, and dyspnea on exertion caused by either hemorrhage or shunting

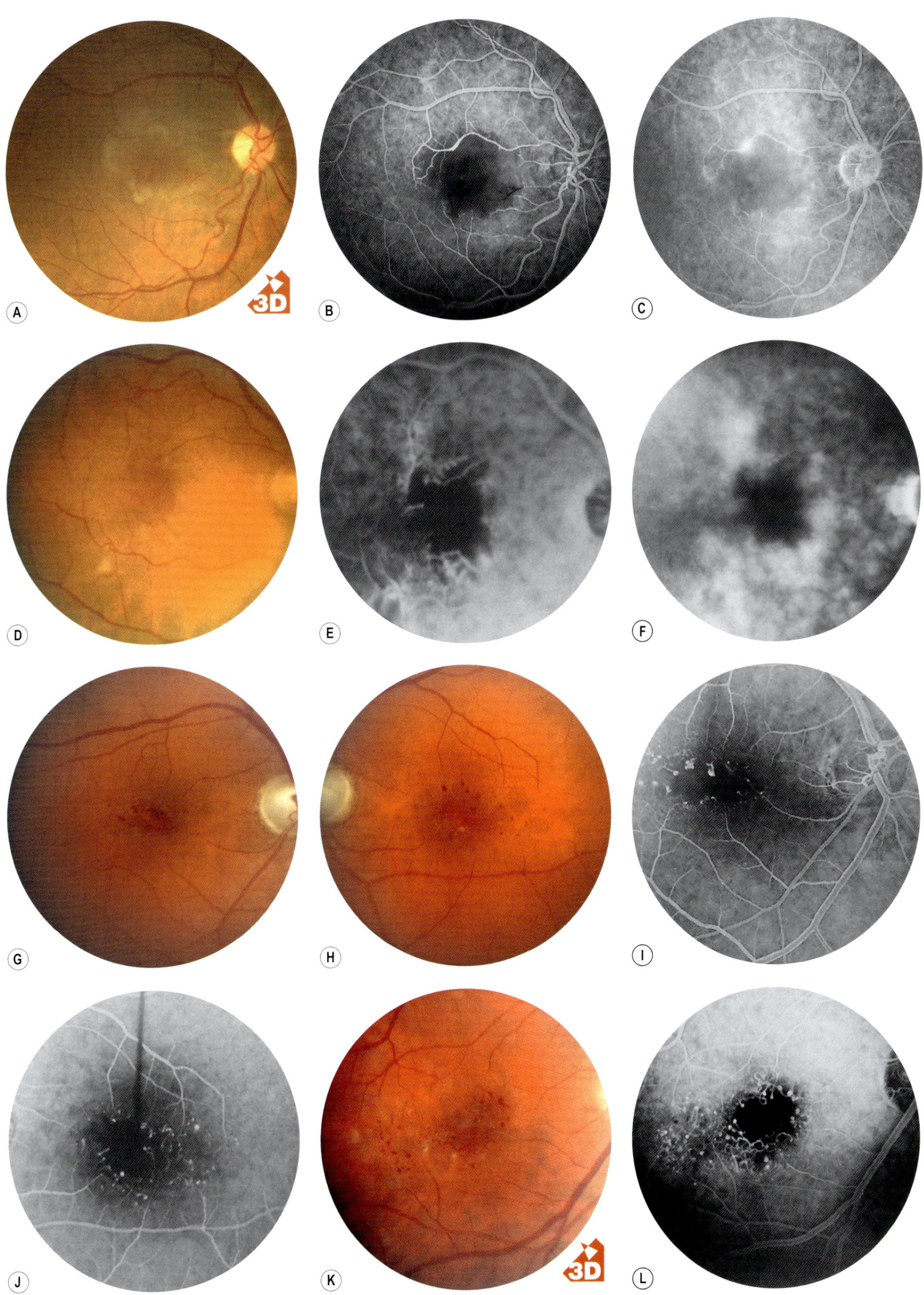
A
3D
B
C
D
E
F
G
H
I
J
K
3D
L

of blood through abnormal vessels in the nasal mucosa, gastrointestinal tract, liver, brain, and lung. Paradoxical embolization and stroke may occur when venous thrombi from the lower extremities and pelvis pass through AVMs in the lung and lodge in the brain.

Multiple spiderlike telangiectases involving the palpebral conjunctiva occur frequently and may cause bloody tearing. Involvement of the retinal blood vessels occurs infrequently.[614–618] Brant and coworkers[614] examined 20 patients with hereditary hemorrhagic telangiectasia and found retinal telangiectasis in two patients.[614] In their review of the literature they cited reports of four patients with retinal vascular malformations, primarily AVMs, in association with hereditary hemorrhagic telangiectasia. Geisthoff and coworkers examined 75 patients, of whom none had retinal telangiectasia, but 28 had conjunctival telangiectases.[619] Intraoperative choroidal hemorrhage has been reported in each eye of a 68-year-old Caucasian woman, one during vitrectomy and the other during phacoemulsification,[620] and large choroidal vessels visible on fluorescein and indocyanine green angiography in a 73-year-old with serous RPE detachments.[621]

6.50 Idiopathic retinal vasculitis, aneurysms, and neuroretinopathy.

A–L: This patient presented with several hard exudates in the posterior pole associated with aneurysmal dilations of the blood vessels on optic disc and in the surrounding area (A and B). Fluorescein angiogram confirmed the multiple aneurysms along the retinal arterioles (C and E). A mid peripheral angiogram showed peripheral nonperfusion 360° in both eyes (D–G). The patient underwent panretinal photocoagulation in both eyes. The aneurysms worsened over time (H) and he also developed flat NVE in the left eye. There was progressive sheathing and occlusion of the retinal vessels and further NVE in both eyes (I–L) over the next year.

(Courtesy of Dr. Richard Spaide.)

Two types of hereditary hemorrhagic telangiectasia, HHT-1 (more frequent pulmonary and cerebral AVMs), from mutation in the endoglin gene (*ENG*) and HHT-2 (more frequent hepatic AVMs) from mutation in activin receptor-like kinase 1 gene (*ACVRL1*, *ALK1*, chromosome 12q13) are known.[622,623]

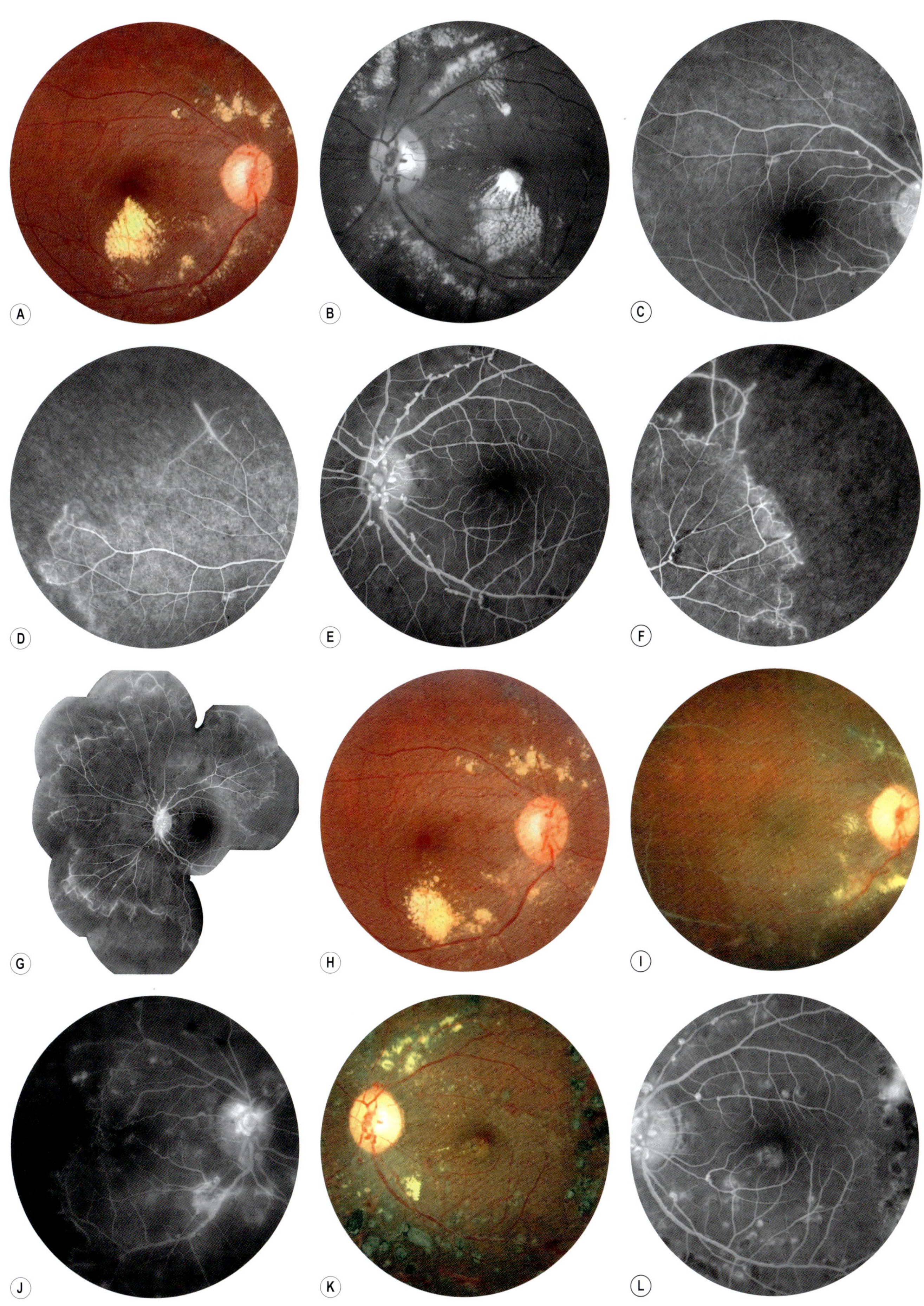
A
B
C
D
E
F
G
H
I
J
K
L

IDIOPATHIC RETINAL VASCULITIS, ANEURYSMS, AND NEURORETINOPATHY: BILATERAL NEURORETINOPATHY WITH MULTIPLE RETINAL ARTERIAL ANEURYSMS

Multiple, peculiar, saccular, and fusiform aneurysms involving all of the major retinal arteries in both eyes may be accompanied by neuroretinopathy, vitreous and anterior-chamber inflammatory cell infiltration, and angiographic evidence of arteritis in children and young adults (Figures 6.50 and 6.51).[624–630] The multiple aneurysms protruding from both sides of the retinal arteries, as well as the Y-shaped aneurysms affecting the arterial bifurcations, give the impression of a series of knots in the arterial tree (Figures 6.50 and 6.51). They may extend from the optic nerve head into the midperiphery of the fundus and may be associated with irregular dilation of the retinal veins, vascular sheathing, focal areas of capillary telangiectasis, retinal hemorrhages, peripheral zones of occlusion of the retinal circulation, retinal neovascularization, and vitreous hemorrhage. Swelling of the optic nerve head may be accompanied by retinal exudation, juxtapapillary retinal detachment, and a macular star (Figures 6.50 and 6.51).[624] Fluorescein angiography may demonstrate dye leakage from some of the arterial aneurysms, focal perivenous staining, optic nerve head staining, focal areas of retinal capillary staining, peripheral zones of capillary nonperfusion (Figures 6.50 and 6.51), and retinal neovascularization. Development of these arterial aneurysms over a 3-year period has been observed in a young woman who presented initially with symptoms related to peripheral retinal neovascularization.[625] It is uncertain whether the arterial aneurysms and the other retinal vascular alterations are caused by a congenital retinal arterial defect or are the product of an acquired inflammatory allergic vascular disease. If the latter is true, then these patients may have some pathogenetic relationship to those with Eales' disease. The value of anti-inflammatory medications including steroids and immunosuppressives and photocoagulation in the management of exudative complications is uncertain but should be tried in appropriate cases. Panretinal photocoagulation (PRP) is required for those eyes with extensive retinal nonperfusion and new-vessel formation (Figure 6.50).

6.51 Multiple retinal and optic nerve head arterial aneurysms, arteritis, and neuroretinitis (IRVAN).

A–F: A 21-year-old woman complained of progressive loss of central vision in both eyes. Note the marked tortuosity and irregular dilation of the major optic nerve head and retinal arteries that extend into the peripheral fundus (A, B, and D) and the circinate pattern of lipid-rich exudate surrounding the optic disc in both eyes. There was peripheral capillary telangiectasis in areas posterior to zones of retinal vascular obliteration (D). Angiography demonstrated tortuosity, irregular caliber, aneurysm formation, and focal areas of staining of the major arteries of the optic disc and retina (E and F).
G–J: A 7-year-old female who was healthy complained of blurred spot in the right eye. She saw 20/20 in both eyes. Fundus examination revealed aneurysms in the arterioles coming off the disc with large areas of hard exudates in both eyes. Fluorescein angiogram showed aneurysmal dilations of the retinal artery in and around the disc. Her peripheral retina was perfused normally.

(G–J, courtesy of Dr. Dharma Le.)

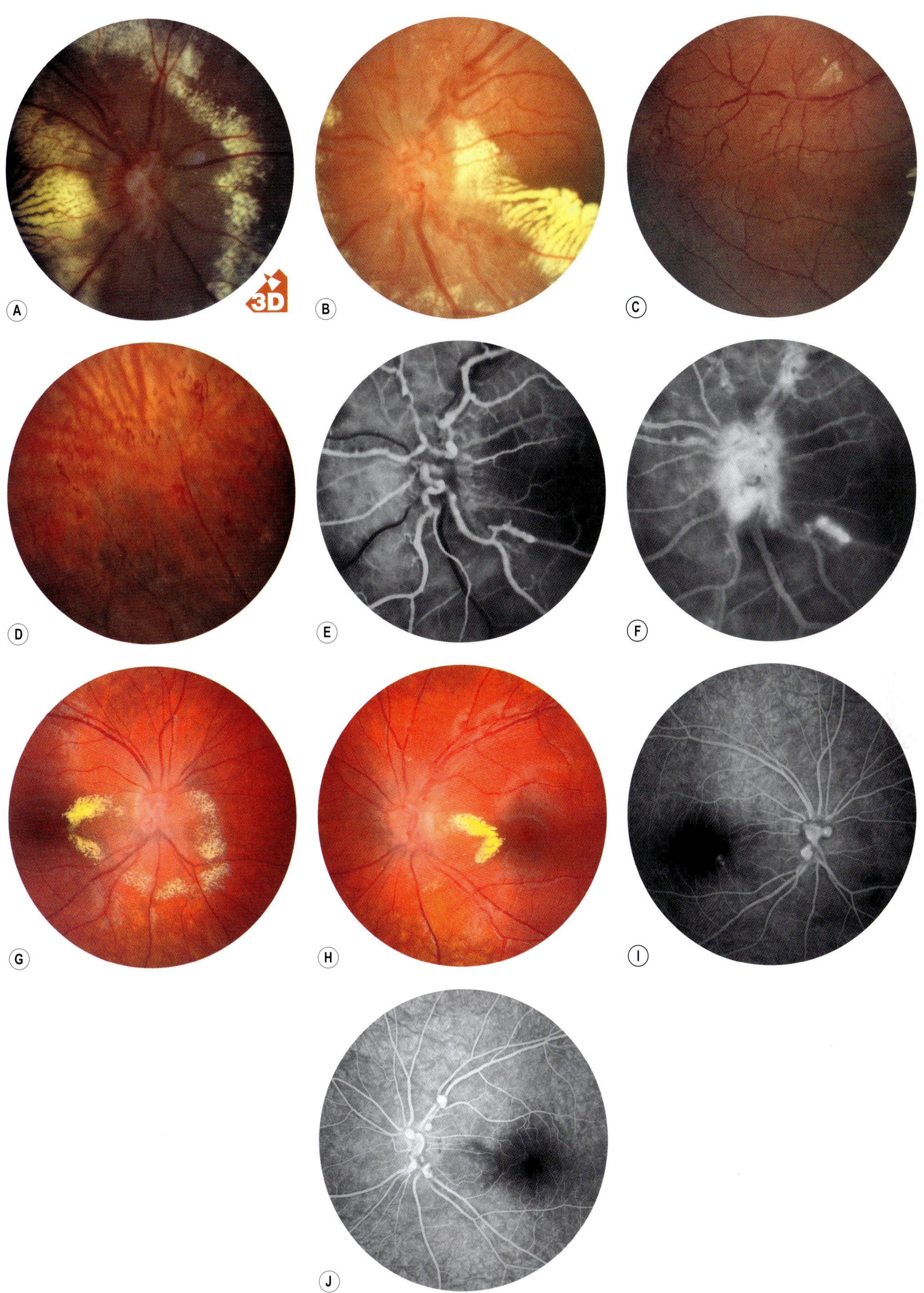

A
3D
B
C
D
E
F
G
H
I
J

DIABETIC RETINOPATHY

Diabetes mellitus is a heterogeneous disorder of carbohydrate metabolism with multiple etiologic factors that ultimately lead to hyperglycemia. There are two primary types of diabetes. Type 1 insulin-dependent diabetes mellitus (IDDM) is an autoimmune disease characterized by hyperglycemia resulting from loss of the pancreatic islet cells. Up to 90% of these patients and 3.1% of their nondiabetic relatives have demonstrable serum titers of islet cell antibodies.[631] The age of onset is before 30 years and often the disease begins in childhood. Type 2 noninsulin-dependent diabetes (NIDDM) is characterized by late-onset hyperglycemia typically occurring in obese patients who are often asymptomatic at the time of diagnosis.[632] It appears to result from deficiency in the regulation of insulin secretion and/or in its action at the cellular level in the liver and peripheral tissues. Secondary types of diabetes may be associated with pancreatic disease, excess counterinsulin hormonal disorders, and drug-induced and gestational diabetes. In all types, hyperglycemia, although of primary importance, is only one of many pathogenetic factors (aldose reductase-mediated cell damage; vasoproliferative factors produced by hypoxic retina; growth hormone and erythrocyte, platelet, and blood viscosity abnormalities) involved in this complex metabolic disorder affecting all of the major organ systems, including the eye.[633–637] Although there has been much emphasis on the importance of the alterations of the blood vessels in regard to the morbidity associated with diabetes, primary metabolic damage to the parenchymal cells is important.[638,639] For example, the development of color vision abnormalities (acquired blue-yellow defect), abnormalities in contrast sensitivity, and electroretinographic alterations in some diabetics may precede any demonstrable evidence of retinal vascular abnormalities.[640–642]

India ink injection techniques, trypsin digestion preparations, and fluorescein angiography have been important in elucidating the anatomic and physiologic changes that constitute diabetic retinopathy.[643–654] The initial changes involve the retinal capillary bed and include selective loss of pericytes, microaneurysm formation, thickening of the basement membrane, focal closure of the capillary bed, dilation of adjacent capillaries, shunt formation, and permeability alterations (Figure 6.52).[643,646,647] These changes may be followed by arteriolar closure, large zones of vascular nonperfusion, and proliferative neovascular changes within and on the inner retinal surface.[647] Microaneurysms develop as outpouchings that initially involve primarily the prevenular capillaries at sites of loss of pericytes (perithelial cells). They may arise as an isolated change or may be clustered around focal zones of capillary occlusion. Their walls may be thin by weakening or thickened by proliferation of the endothelial basement membrane. Their lumen occasionally may be packed with agglutinated erythrocytes or a thrombus. Focal zones of loss of capillary endothelial cells, thickening of the capillary basement membrane, and reduction of blood flow develop and are associated with surrounding areas of compensatory capillary dilation, capillary endothelial proliferation, and permeability alterations. This change in permeability of the dilated capillaries and microaneurysms is associated with extravasation of serous and lipoproteinaceous exudate and, in some cases, intraretinal bleeding (Figure 6.52J). Other physiologic changes accompanying diabetic retinopathy include alterations of blood flow and blood viscosity.[655–658] Autoregulation causes venous dilation when local tissue hypoxia and hypoglycemia are detected. With constant changes in the vessel caliber from fluctuating tissue glucose levels, the venous tone is eventually lost, resulting in chronic venous dilation. Hyperglycemia per se can cause dysfunction of autoregulation.

These early anatomic and physiologic changes are responsible for the ophthalmoscopic changes referred to as background and nonproliferative diabetic retinopathy. These include red dotlike microaneurysms, areas of dilated retinal capillaries, superficial flame-shaped or deeper dot and blot retinal hemorrhages, white-centered hemorrhages, yellow exudates, and focal areas of gray-whitening of the retina (cotton-wool spots) (Figure 6.52).[640,659,660]Microaneurysms are the earliest clinical sign of diabetic retinopathy (Figure 6.52 A). They may occur anywhere in the retina. In some cases they are widely distributed, whereas in others they may be concentrated in the central macular area.

Visual loss in patients with nonproliferative diabetic retinopathy occurs primarily as the result of macular exudation, particularly in patients with late-onset diabetes (Figure 6.52 A–F).[654,661–671] This may occur either as the result of focal leakage of exudate from one or more clusters of microaneurysms and dilated capillaries, each often surrounded by a ring of yellow, deep retinal exudates, or as the result of diffuse leakage from most of the retinal vasculature in the macular area. In general, the loss of central vision parallels the degree of intraretinal exudation seen biomicroscopically and angiographically. Minimal loss of acuity may be associated with mild intraretinal exudation from capillary microaneurysms that are either confined to the posterior pole or are more widely scattered. More pronounced degrees of intraretinal exudation are often associated with greater evidence

6.52 Background diabetic retinopathy.

A–F: Progression of retinopathy that occurred between September 1985 (A) and January 1987 (C–E). Argon laser treatment was given. In January 1991, visual acuity was 20/25 and there was minimal evidence of retinopathy (F).

G–I: Ischemic background retinopathy in an insulin-dependent diabetic with prominent cystoid macular edema, dilated peripheral macular retinal capillaries, and evidence of loss of the juxtafoveolar capillary network (stereo photos G and H). Angiography (I) showed loss of pericentral capillary network, and capillary nonperfusion in the area of the cotton-wool patch and in the temporal periphery of the macula.

J–L: Submacular hemorrhage (J) cause by bleeding from juxtafoveolar microvascular changes (K) cleared spontaneously (L) and the patient recovered 20/30 visual acuity.

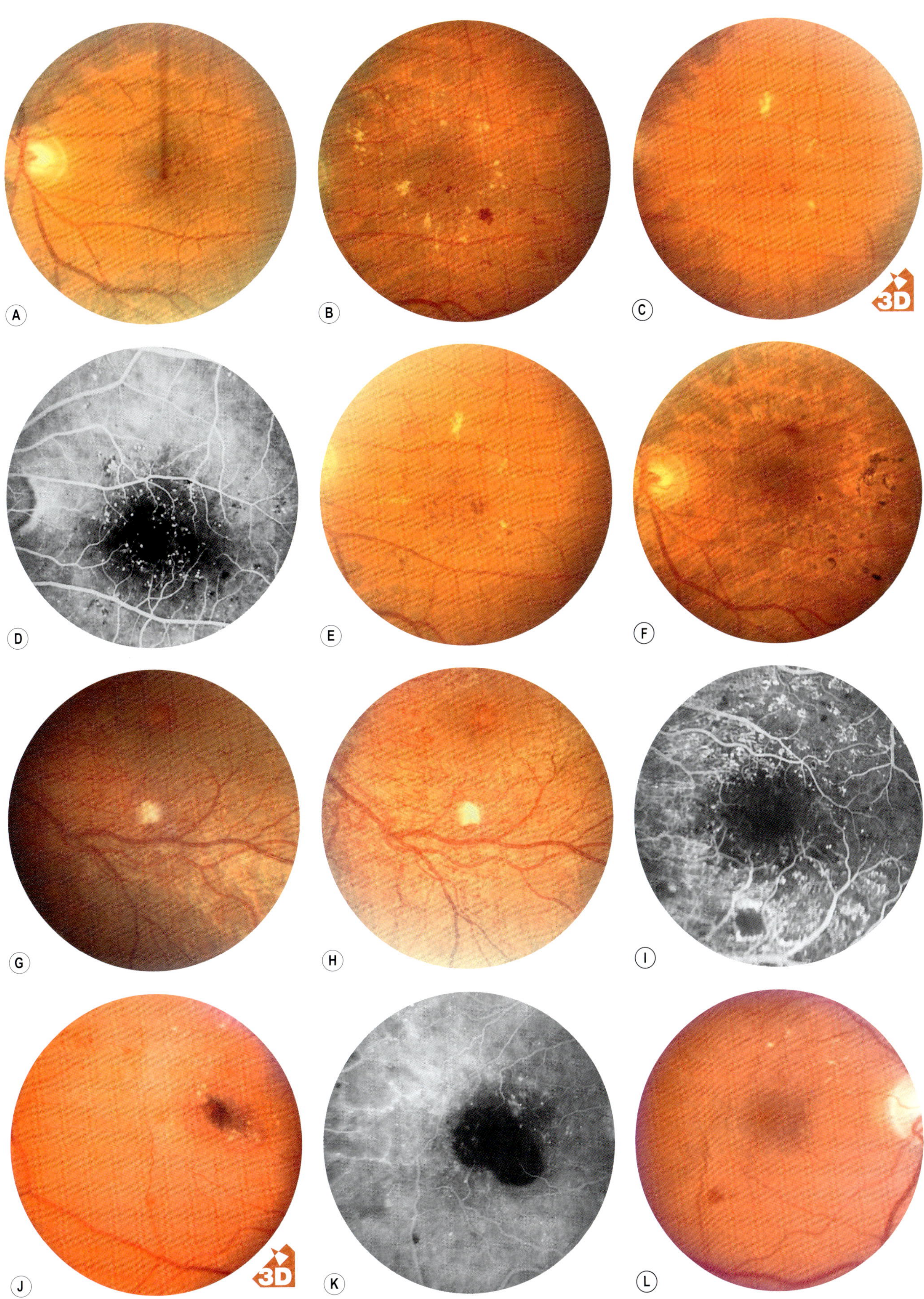
A
B
C
3D
D
E
F
G
H
I
J
3D
K
L

of dilation of both the small and large retinal blood vessels. Scattered yellow exudates, retinal hemorrhages, and occasional cotton-wool spots may be present. Cotton-wool spots in diabetic retinopathy are indicative of focal zones of relative retinal ischemia caused by either partial or, in some cases, complete closure of the capillary bed in the zone of retinal whitening (Figure 6.53).[660,672,673] They occur commonly during the early development of nonproliferative diabetic retinopathy, are not necessarily related to elevated blood pressure, and do not necessarily suggest a high risk of progression of the retinopathy. In general they persist for a longer period of time in diabetes than in hypertension. When they resolve, they may be associated with a local scotoma, nerve fiber bundle scotoma, or no scotoma.[672,674] The presence of numerous cotton-wool spots, particularly when associated with other signs of preproliferative retinopathy, may indicate rapidly progressing retinopathy.

A frequent clinical picture seen in patients with early loss of vision is that of one or more circinate zones of yellow, lipid-rich exudation, usually centered in the paramacular area and extending into the fovea (Figures 6.52B and C, and 6.53D). The yellowish deposits surround clusters of microaneurysms and cloudy intraretinal and subretinal exudate. Circinate zones may be round, oval, or irregular. They are most frequently centered in the temporal portion of the macula. The amount of lipid exudation around the retinal capillary abnormalities in these patients is related to their serum lipid levels and their diastolic blood pressure. The presence of extensive deposits of intraretinal lipid exudates may be indicative of hyperlipidemia (see Figure 6.85J–L).[675] (See discussion of hyperlipemic retinopathy, p. 610.) Transudation of serum lipids into the vitreous in such patients may occasionally simulate endophthalmitis.[676]

Some patients with diffuse retinal capillary leakage and CME angiographically may show minimal evidence of yellow exudate and loss of retinal transparency biomicroscopically.[663,677,678] The edema may wax and wane, remain stationary for long periods, or steadily progress. Occasionally the CME may occur in the absence of prominent background retinopathy and dilation of the major retinal vessels.[665,678] Other causes of central vision loss in diabetic patients include hemorrhage from the perifoveal capillary abnormalities (Figure 6.52), perifoveolar capillary occlusion (Figure 6.52), vitreofoveal traction (Figure 7.09I and J), and epiretinal membrane formation.

When the vascular occlusive phenomenon caused by diabetes begins to involve the precapillary arterioles and larger retinal arterioles, fundus changes characteristic of preproliferative retinopathy develop. These include multiple cotton-wool spots and retinal hemorrhages, dark blot hemorrhages, venous beading and loops, irregular dilated segments of the capillary bed (intraretinal microvascular abnormalities, or IRMA), and large areas of loss of retinal vascular details or "featureless" retina (Figures 6.52G and 6.54A–B). These latter areas show extensive vascular nonperfusion angiographically (Figure 6.54). This process of vascular occlusion frequently involves the peripheral retina and in some cases may initially be largely confined to the extramacular areas. In other cases capillary nonperfusion affects the central macular area early and may cause loss of visual acuity.[679] The IRMA occur near areas of vascular nonperfusion and in some cases represent dilated segments of the capillary bed or shunt vessels, whereas in other cases they are intraretinal newly developed blood vessels.[680]

The risk of developing proliferative diabetic retinopathy (PDR) is approximately 50% within 15 months in eyes with preproliferative diabetic retinopathy.[681] It is important to realize that, by the time neovascularization has commenced, many of the signs of active preproliferative retinopathy may no longer be present. Neovascularization usually begins within 45° of the optic disc and often arises on the optic disc. New vessels are subdivided on the basis of their location as follows: those arising on or within 1 disc diameter of the optic disc (NVD), and those elsewhere in the fundus (NVE). The NVD begins as fine loops or networks of vessels lying on the surface of the optic disc or bridging across the physiologic cup. They may be difficult to differentiate from dilated optic nerve vessels. Likewise, differentiating NVE from IRMA may also be difficult, particularly when the NVE do not yet show any of their characteristic features, including wheel-like network, extension across both arterial and venous branches of the underlying retinal vascular network, and accompanying fibrous

6.53 Diabetic exudative maculopathy and response to treatment.

A and B: Circinate lipid associated with foveal thickening in this patient who has had panretinal photocoagulation for proliferative diabetic retinopathy (A). Four months later a lot of the lipid exudates have disappeared (B).
C–F: Nonproliferative diabetic retinopathy and circinate maculopathy before (C and D) and after (F) argon laser photocoagulation. Note resolution of the lipid exudate (F).
G and H: Histopathology of diabetic exudative maculopathy. Note the macrophages (arrows) engulfing the lipid exudate and evidence of cystic degeneration of the retina (G).

Diabetic neuroretinopathy (papillopathy).

I–K: This young woman with childhood diabetes noted the sudden onset of visual loss in the right eye. Note the macular star, the optic disc swelling, and minimal evidence of background diabetic retinopathy (I and J). Six months later her visual acuity had improved to 20/20. Note the pallor of the optic disc (K). Three months later she experienced the same sequence of events in the left eye.

DIDMOAD (Wolfram syndrome).

L: Right pale optic disc (left, not shown) of an 18-year-old with type 1 diabetes, nephrogenic diabetes insipidus, bilateral progressive optic atrophy, and deafness. He also had hydronephrosis secondary to the diabetes insipidus and renal insufficiency. Gene testing for *WFS1* gene was positive.

(I–K, from Barr et al.[828], G-J, Also, Yannuzzi, Lawrence J., The Retinal Atlas, Saunders 2010, 978-0-7020-3320-9, p.281.)

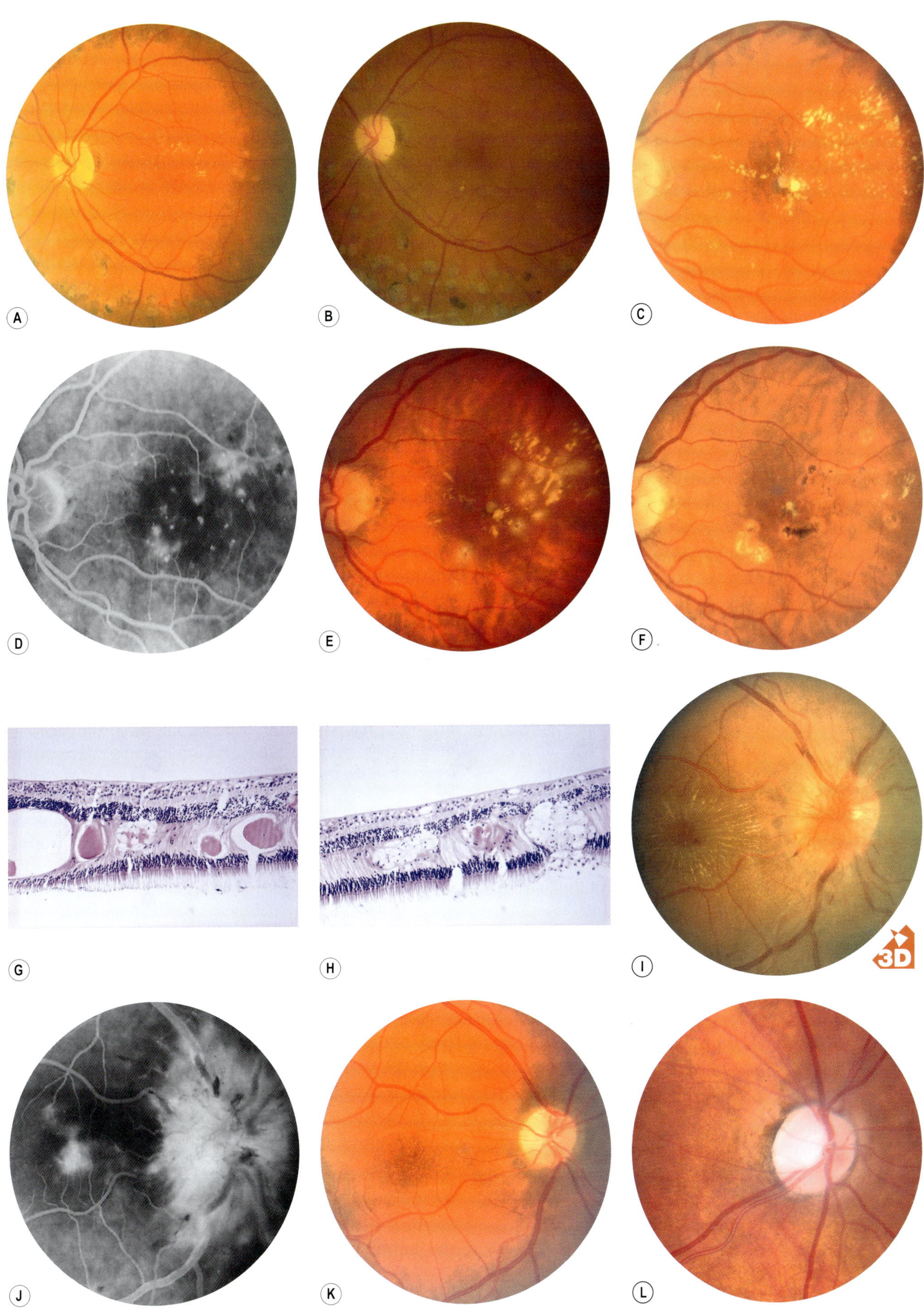
A
B
C
D
E
F
G
H
I
3D
J
K
L

proliferation. Fluorescein angiography is helpful in distinguishing new vessels, which leak diffusely, from vessels located within the optic disc and retina, which show minimal leakage. New vessels typically form networks simulating sea fans (Figure 6.55A–C), but, in some cases, particularly when they arise from the optic disc, they may grow across the retinal surface and present the appearance of mature retinal blood vessels (Figure 6.55F–H). Patients with new vessels are often asymptomatic until vitreous separation elevates the new vessels and causes intravitreal bleeding. Vitreous separation often begins along the superotemporal vessels, temporal to the macula, and above or below the optic disc.[682–684] The vitreous usually does not separate from the disc in patients with NVD. Traction on the new vessels by the partly separated vitreous may cause vitreous hemorrhage. Bleeding into the vitreous may also be caused by avulsion of retinal blood vessels (usually a vein) or a retinal tear. Displacement and distortion of the macula caused by vitreoretinal traction and epiretinal membrane contraction and tractional detachment of the macula may cause loss of visual acuity, dimness of vision, metamorphopsia, and diplopia.[645,685–687] Focal serous detachment of the macula is an infrequent complication of diabetic retinopathy unless it occurs secondary to vitreous traction with or without macular hole formation (Figure 7.08E–H).

A peculiar form of occult vitreomacular traction occurring in patients, particularly after unsuccessful scatter macular photocoagulation, may be responsible for severe macular edema and diffuse fluorescein staining of the macula.[688] Visual function in these latter patients may improve dramatically following pars plana vitrectomy (see Figures 7.05G and H, and 7.08I–K). Nasrallah et al. found that adult-onset diabetic eyes with macular edema were less likely to have posterior vitreous detachment than eyes without edema.[689] They found the reverse was true in eyes of patients with type 1 diabetes.[690]

PDR may occur in the perimacular area (Figure 6.55) but it infrequently occurs near the center of the macula.[691] What may be an aborted form of intraretinal and preretinal neovascularization may give rise to a peculiar cluster of coiled aneurysmal blood vessels in the juxtafoveolar area, particularly in insulin-dependent diabetics with evidence of macular capillary nonperfusion and following PRP (Figure 6.53).[691–693] These juxtafoveolar aneurysmal changes are associated with excellent visual acuity and good visual prognosis and may occur in both eyes. Similar abortive nodular neovascular outgrowths without an extravascular fibrous component may arise along the major vascular arcades in eyes with extensive areas of capillary nonperfusion (Figure 6.53A–C).[694] Histopathologically, they are nodules of vessels with gross hyalinization of their walls and without a fibrous component.[692] These lesions may represent aborted forms of neovascularization that develop in the absence of a vitreous scaffold.

There are significant differences in the natural courses of IDDM and NIDDM.[669,682,695,696] In childhood-onset type 1 diabetes, retinal microaneurysms and other diabetic retinopathy seldom develop before puberty.[697–700] In a population-based study of 271 insulin-dependent patients diagnosed before 30 years of age and without retinopathy at the time of initial examination, 59% of patients developed retinopathy, including 11% with proliferative retinopathy, by the time they were examined 4 years later.[701] Overall worsening of retinopathy occurred in 41% of the population, whereas improvement occurred in only 7%. The incidence of proliferative retinopathy rose with increasing duration until 13–14 years of diabetes and thereafter remained between 14% and 17%. Klein and coworkers found that 10.2% of adult-onset diabetics have retinopathy at the time of initial diagnosis.[702] During a 4-year period they found that 47% nonusers of insulin without retinopathy developed it, that 7% of those without proliferative retinopathy developed it, and that worsening of the retinopathy occurred in 34% of all of the patients.[703] For nonusers of insulin the corresponding rates were 34% for any retinopathy, 2% for developing proliferative retinopathy, and 25% for worsening retinopathy. In those initially free of retinopathy approximately 50% of those using insulin and 35% of nonusers will develop retinopathy within 4 years of diagnosis.[703] During this same period of time approximately 35% of users and 25% of nonusers will develop worsening of their retinopathy.

The most important risk factor for developing diabetic retinopathy is duration of the disease.[667,704] Retinopathy in IDDM occurs infrequently before 5 years after onset of the disease. It is present in 27% of patients with disease duration of 5–10 years, in 71% with longer than 10 years, and in over 90% after 30 years. The prevalence of background retinopathy in NIDDM 11–13 years after the onset is 23%, after 16 or more years it is 60%, and after 11 or

6.54 Accelerated proliferative diabetic retinopathy.

A–K: This 18-year-old African American girl with type 1 diabetes had very minimal NVD in the right eye and no new vessels in the left eye. Her retinal veins were dilated and she had several intraretinal microvascular abnormalities (IRMA) in both eyes (arrows) in addition to scattered cotton-wool spots (A and B). Angiogram confirmed extensive capillary nonperfusion and the presence of widespread IRMA in both eyes. Montage images of the right and left eye show extensive ischemia. Her renal function was abnormal and blood sugars were in the 600s mg/dl. In spite of panretinal photocoagulation begun in both eyes soon after these pictures, she developed bilateral extensive capillary drop-out and new vessels (F, G, I, and J). The left eye still had some perfusion of her native vessels while the right only showed dye in the residual vessels on the disc (H). Further panretinal photocoagulation did not prevent neovascular glaucoma that developed in both eyes requiring bilateral tube shunts (K). Complicated cataracts developed quickly with new vessels on the anterior surface of the lens (K) and vision dropped to no light perception, followed by tractional retinal detachment confirmed on ultrasound. She died within a year of her initial evaluation.

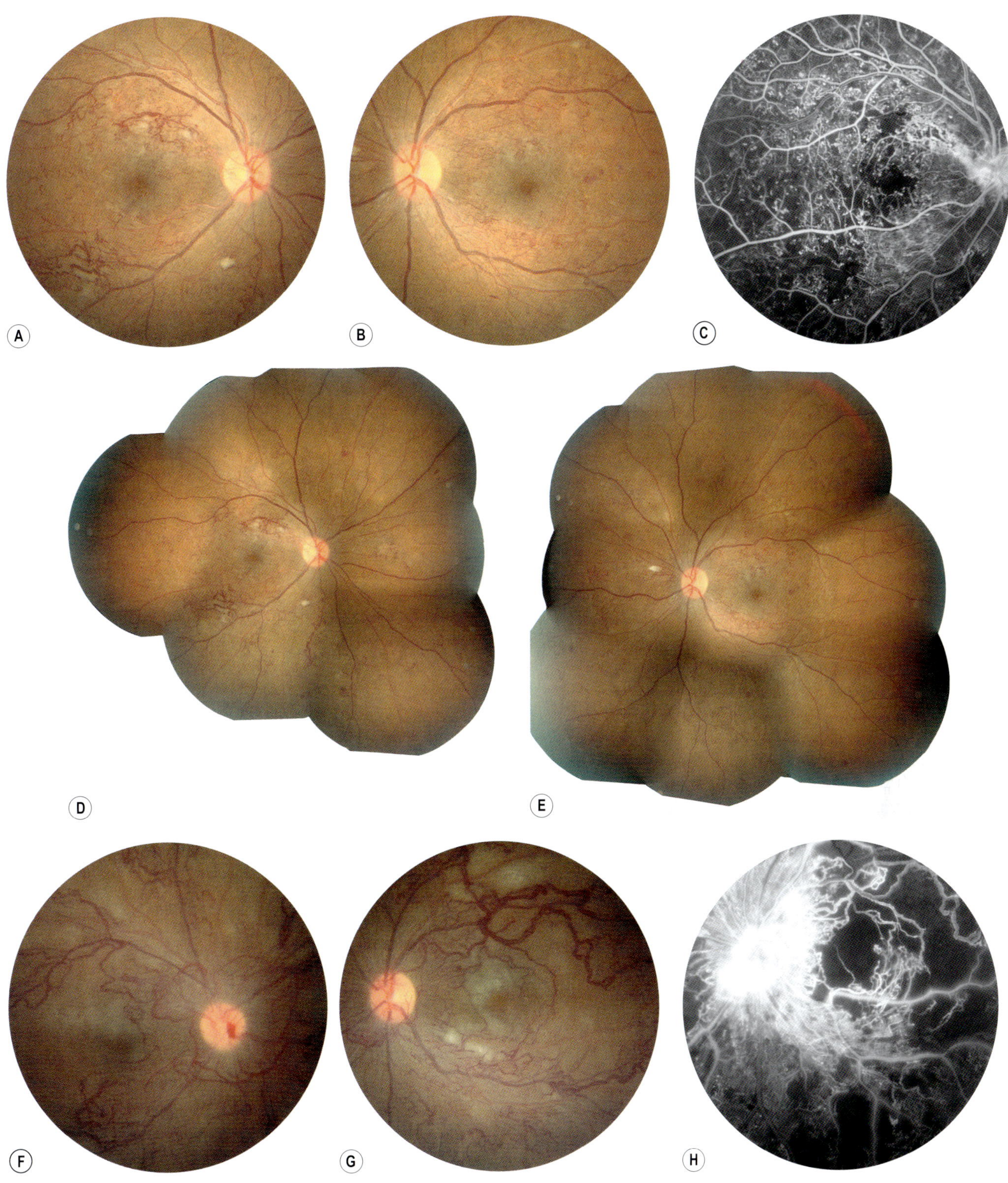
A
B
C
D
E
F
G
H

more years 3% have proliferative retinopathy.[705] Other risk factors associated with progression of diabetic retinopathy include number of microaneurysms,[706] albuminuria,[707] elevation of blood pressure,[708,709] posterior vitreous attachment,[616,684,710] increased foveal thickening,[711] blue or gray irides,[712] smoking,[709,713,714] increased testosterone levels in males with type 1 diabetes,[715] previous irradiation to the eye,[716] reduction in electroretinographic oscillatory potentials,[717] environmental and racial factors,[718] pregnancy,[719] and cataract extraction.[720–725] Carotid artery obstruction may have a favorable effect on diabetic retinopathy in some patients.[726–728]

Fluorescein angiography has provided great understanding of the microvascular changes caused by diabetes.[649,650,652–654,660,669,677,693,717,729–733] Clinicopathologic correlations have helped in interpreting and understanding these findings.[643,644,646–648,652,734,735] The development of microaneurysms and alterations in the capillary permeability are the earliest changes detectable with angiography in the diabetic retina (Figure 6.52A). The microaneurysms are predominantly on the venular side of the capillary bed. Round and occasionally fusiform microaneurysms are scattered in the macula and perimacular region and have no particular relationship to the distribution of the major retinal vessels such as occurs in hypertensive retinopathy. Focal areas of capillary closure may develop within the capillary bed affected by marked aneurysm formation. Capillary closure occurs much more frequently and to a greater extent initially in the mid peripheral fundus and generally increases towards the periphery.[654] Some enlargement of the FAZ occurs commonly in diabetes but is usually unassociated with visual loss until the FAZ approaches 1000 μm in diameter (Figure 6.52G–I).[679,729] Capillary closure occurs less frequently in the macula and rarely, if ever, in the area of the juxtapapillary radial capillary network.[654,717,730,733,736] Extensive mid peripheral and peripheral capillary closure may be relatively inapparent ophthalmoscopically, and its extent is directly correlated with the development of disc and retinal neovascularization. Dilated, tortuous, shunt capillaries may traverse large areas of capillary closure that are often more evident in the more peripheral retina. Extensive microaneurysmal changes in the capillary bed may be demonstrated angiographically in the macular region in patients who do not have significant loss of visual acuity. The permeability changes in the capillary bed and the degree of serous exudation into the extracellular space of the retina are variable and are the most important factors causing loss of macular function. In some cases, however, progressive closure of the perifoveal capillary network is the cause of loss of macular function (Figures 6.52G–I, and 6.54A–J). This closure occurs more commonly in patients with juvenile-onset diabetes.[654,669,671] There is no fluorescein angiographic evidence of choroidal vascular disease to account for the loss of central vision in diabetes. There is some indocyanine green angiographic, histopathologic, and scanning electron microscopic evidence that the choroidal vessels may be affected in diabetes.[737,738] Areas of neovascular proliferation on the surface of the retina are always accompanied by angiographic evidence of dye leakage from these vessels (Figure 6.55).

The pathogenesis of diabetic retinopathy is complicated, controversial, and beyond the scope of this book. There is overwhelming evidence that hyperglycemia is important in the pathogenesis of retinopathy, but genetic and other factors are important.[635,679,683] Release of angiogenic factors (VEGF) in the hypoperfused hypoxic retina is important in the development of proliferative retinopathy.[636,637,739–741]

Photocoagulation treatment has been advocated for treatment of exudative and PDR for many years.[632,637,646,670,681,705,742–759] In recent years randomized controlled clinical trials have established useful guidelines for use of photocoagulation and vitrectomy for the treatment of diabetic retinopathy.[659,681,743–745,760–774] Before publication of the results of the Early Treatment Diabetic Retinopathy Study (ETDRS), several randomized clinical trials reported photocoagulation to be of value in the treatment of diabetic macular edema.[743,760] Although employing somewhat different protocols and case selection, all of these studies have concluded that laser treatment is effective in reducing the rate of visual loss in eyes with macular edema but results in significant visual improvement in only a limited number of cases. The ETDRS concluded that eyes with mild to moderate nonproliferative diabetic retinopathy and clinically significant macular edema, when treated with focal argon blue-green or argon green laser to microaneurysms and a grid treatment to zones of diffuse leakage and nonperfusion, show the maximum benefit of treatment (Figures 6.52D–F, and 6.53A–F).[772] Clinically significant macular edema was defined as: (1) retinal thickening involving, or within 500 μm from, the center of the macula; (2) hard exudate(s) (with thickening of the adjacent retina) at or within 500 μm from the center of the macula; and (3) a zone of retinal thickening 1 disc area or larger in size, any part of which is within 1 disc diameter from the center of the macula.

Because of the risk involved in treating lesions closer than 500 μm to the center of the macula, it may be prudent to follow eyes with clinically significant macular edema showing such lesions when the visual acuity is normal and

6.54 Continued

L and **M**: This patient with proliferative diabetic retinopathy and subhyaloid hemorrhage underwent panretinal photocoagulation (L), following which he developed contraction of the posterior hyaloid and traction thickening of the underlying retina (M).

N and **O**: This young patient sought treatment because of vitreous hemorrhage in the right eye. She had extensive neovascularization of the optic discs and periphery of both eyes. There was angiographic evidence of extensive capillary nonperfusion in the mid peripheral and peripheral fundi. Panretinal photocoagulation in the right eye (N) resulted in closure of the optic disc new vessels but incomplete closure of the retinal new vessels (arrow, O).

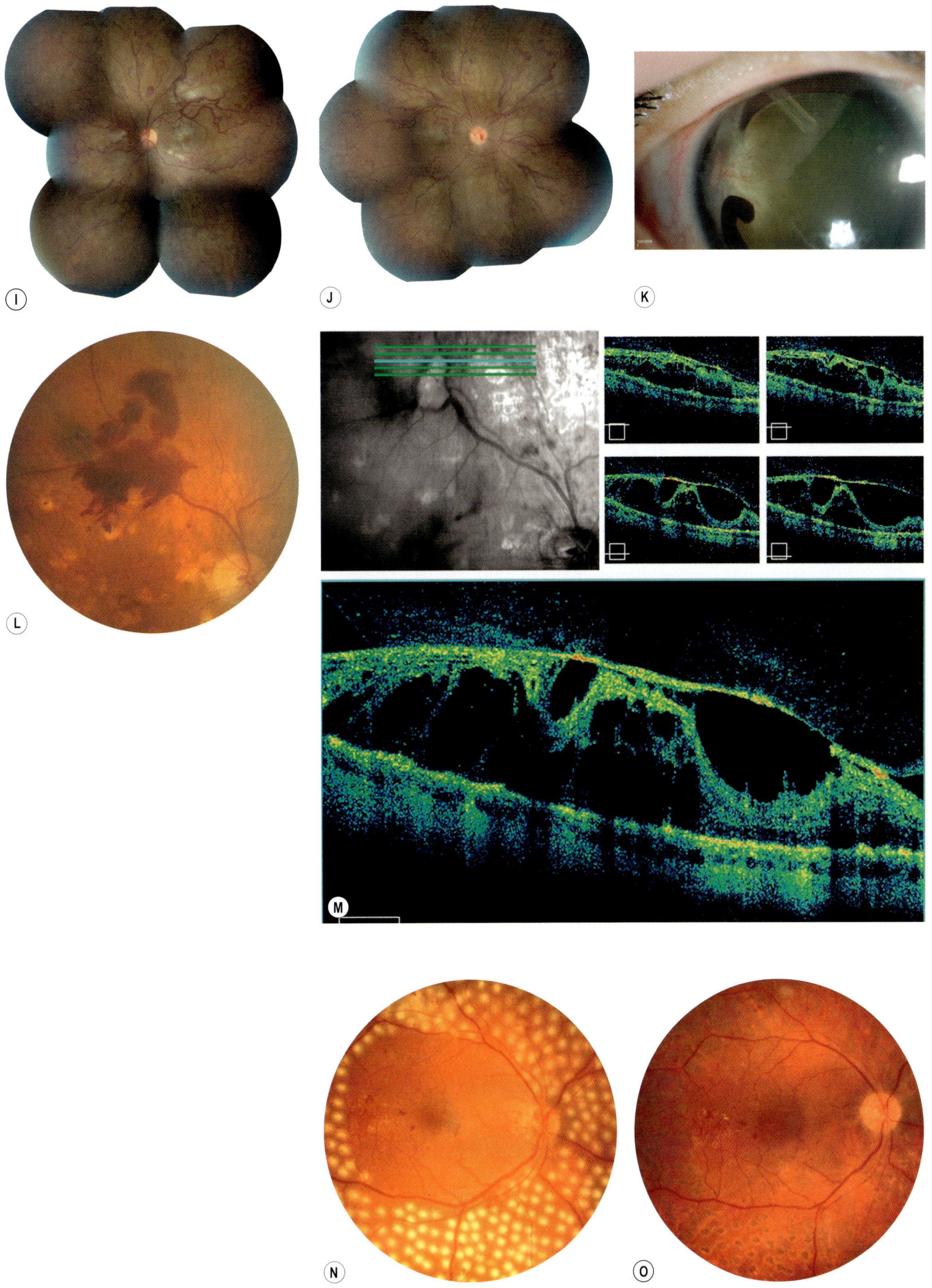
I
J
K
L
M
N
O

the center of the macula is uninvolved. There is little risk in following such eyes to determine whether the edema is worsening.[769] Olk and coworkers have used a modified grid pattern technique for treating diffuse diabetic macular edema, emphasizing treatment of diffuse leakage rather than focal leakage.[775–777] They have demonstrated that visual acuity and foveal threshold in these patients are preserved at the expense of generalized loss of threshold sensitivity across the central 10° of visual fields.[777]

In eyes with mild to moderate macular edema, PRP should not be used till the macular edema is treated. PRP treatment increases the risk of loss of visual acuity, particularly in patients with macular edema.[751,772,774,778] Reduction in the area of retina needing to be perfused following PRP redirects more blood flow to the posterior pole, thus increasing the intravascular hydrostatic force within these vessels, causing increased leakage. Treatment of the macular edema with focal and grid treatment given before scatter treatment reduces this risk.[772,774] If high-risk characteristics for PDR are also present, dividing the scatter treatment into multiple sessions beginning with the nasal quadrants, using a more peripheral pattern of scatter treatment, using smaller spot size applications, and using less intense treatment are techniques that may reduce the risk of aggravating the macular edema.[734,738,769,774,779,780]

PRP treatment should be carried out promptly in most eyes with PDR that have well-established NVD and/or vitreous or preretinal hemorrhage. When high-risk characteristics are present, scatter photocoagulation should be carried out even in the presence of fibrous proliferations and/or localized traction retinal detachment. Likewise, scatter treatment is indicated in eyes with extensive neovascularization of the anterior-chamber angle, or in eyes with preproliferative retinopathy and evidence of rapidly progressive closure of the retinal capillary, whether or not high-risk characteristics are present (Figure 6.54A–J).[772] These latter patients should be warned of the high risk of further loss of central vision caused by occlusion of the remaining vessels supplying the macula.

The prognosis for recovery of central vision is poor in patients with angiographic evidence of loss of the perifoveal capillary network; severe CME, particularly when associated with significant background retinopathy; organized yellow exudate in the macula; and severe renal disease and hypertension. Retreatment of eyes that fail to show an initial response to scatter treatment is indicated and is successful in approximately 50% of cases.[665,772,781,782] Those who fail after retreatment have an unfavorable prognosis.

The wavelength of laser light used for the treatment of the various stages of diabetic retinopathy appears to be relatively unimportant.[783–788] Although all of the clinical trials have used fluorescein angiography as part of the investigation of patients with diabetic exudative maculopathy, the decision as to whether to treat, and where to treat, depends primarily on biomicroscopic observations. For that reason some have suggested that pretreatment angiography is unnecessary.[789]

6.55 Proliferative diabetic retinopathy.

A–C: Retinal venous loop (arrow, A) and retinal neovascularization.

D–H: Severe proliferative retinopathy in the right eye of a young diabetic patient (D–F). Note the subhyaloid hemorrhage (E) and the prominent nonelevated neovascular trunks radiating from a nasal retinal vein (arrows, F–H). Angiography showed sluggish blood flow within the new vessel network (G and H).

I: Histopathology of diabetic proliferative retinopathy (arrowheads) and dilated intraretinal blood vessel (arrow).

J–L: Ring of preretinal fibrovascular tissue surrounding the macula in a patient with severe proliferative diabetic retinopathy.

The favorable effect of photocoagulation treatment on diabetic retinopathy is multifactorial. Hypotheses to explain how photocoagulation causes resolution of the neovascular and exudative complications of diabetic retinopathy include reduction of VEGF levels, improvement of the blood–outer retinal barrier by photocoagulation debridement of sick or fatigued RPE cells; release by photocoagulation-damaged RPE cells of a factor that reduces retinal capillary endothelial proliferation and causes restoration of the integrity of the blood–inner retinal barrier[713,790]; and increased oxygen tension at the inner retinal surface caused by partial photocoagulation destruction of the retinal receptor cells and RPE cells.[791–794] The increased oxygen tension occurs in spite of the partial loss of the choriocapillaris that accompanies PRP. Long-term follow-up studies after panphotocoagulation have demonstrated persistence of the treatment effect for as long as 15 years.[795,796]

Complications of laser photocoagulation treatment of diabetic retinopathy include development of subretinal neovascularization,[797–799] subfoveal fibrosis,[800–803] serous macular detachment,[804] ciliochoroidal detachment, and enlargement of photocoagulation scars.[799,802,805]

Transscleral cryotherapy is a useful adjunct to photocoagulation treatment when recurrent vitreous hemorrhage occurs without visible new vessels posteriorly. It is likely small new vessels are present very anteriorly; these can be easily destroyed by two or more rows of transconjunctival peripheral cryopexy.[806–808] This is also especially useful in those eyes that show recurrent vitreous hemorrhages after pars plana vitrectomy where no new vessels can be found. Applying two to three spots to the sclerostomy sites helps in those eyes where a vessel may be bridging the sclerostomy site on the inside.

Pars plana vitrectomy has become the standard treatment for serious visual loss caused by dense, nonclearing vitreous hemorrhage; traction retinal detachment; and macular heterotopia.[673,685,761,762,766,795,809–815] Early vitrectomy is beneficial in patients with type 1 diabetes and recent severe diabetic vitreous hemorrhage reducing visual acuity to 5/200 or less for at least 1 month.[763,764,766] In older patients with type 2 diabetes and recent severe diabetic retinal hemorrhage, it is reasonable to allow time for spontaneous clearing of the vitreous hemorrhage for 4–6 weeks before considering vitrectomy. Partial posterior vitreous

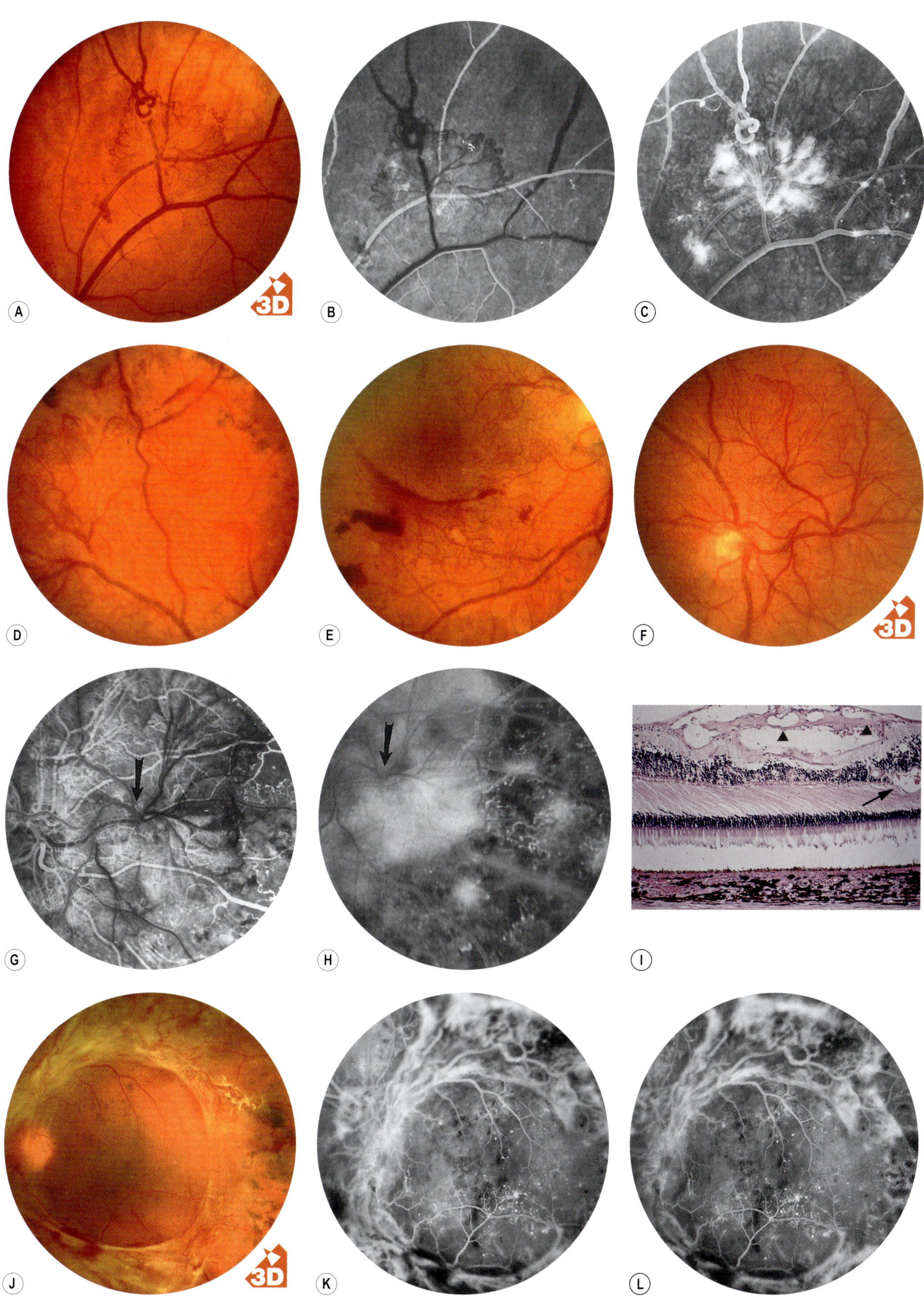
A
3D
B
C
D
E
F
3D
G
H
I
J
3D
K
L

separation that may follow a vitreous hemorrhage in some cases may help in en bloc dissection during vitrectomy. Early vitrectomy should be considered as an adjunct to photocoagulation in eyes with useful vision and advanced, active PDR with extensive new vessels that fail to show substantial regression after photocoagulation, or when additional photocoagulation is precluded by vitreous hemorrhage and when iris vessels begin to appear.[764] Although vitrectomy is of value in restoring central vision in patients who have developed macular detachment secondary to vitreous traction detachment,[816,817] it may not be indicated when the traction detachment does not extend into the macula.[818] Because of the high association of cataracts in diabetes and their frequent development soon after vitrectomy, combined vitrectomy and intraocular lens insertions are frequently done in these patients.[819] The 5-year survival rate of patients undergoing vitrectomy for complications of diabetic retinopathy is approximately 75%.[811]

Pharmacotherapies for diabetic retinopathy include treatment of macular edema using intravitreal injection of triamcinolone or sustained-release corticosteroids, and to a lesser effect intravitreal antiangiogenic agents.[820,821] Machemer first reported the use of intravitreal steroids to halt cellular proliferation in diabetes, which was not very successful.[822] Corticosteroids have antipermeability, antiangiogenic, and antifibrotic effects.[823] They help stabilize the blood–retinal barrier, downregulate inflammatory factors, and increase absorption of fluid. Triamcinolone (most recently without preservatives) at 1 and 4 mg can be used in those eyes, which fail to, or do not completely, respond to focal laser photocoagulation.[824] It is also indicated in eyes with CME without significant capillary leakage on angiography and in those eyes with diffuse leakage from all vessels in the macula. Complications include cataract formation, elevation of intraocular pressure, infectious endophthalmitis and acute toxic/inflammatory response; hence judicious use of intravitreal steroids bearing in mind the potential complications is recommended. Posurdex, a biodegradable copolymer consisting of 70% dexamethasone (350 or 700 μg) and 30% polylactic-glycolic acid, and Retisert, a sustained-release implant of fluocinolone acetonide which linearly releases fluocinolone for 3 years, have been tested. Cataract formation and elevated intraocular pressure are very common following these implants and hence have limited their use.

Antiangiogenic agents bevacizumab and ranibizumab have a role for adjunctive treatment of proliferative retinopathy in eyes that show persistent new vessels in spite of adequate PRP, in those eyes with recurrent vitreous hemorrhage following PRP or vitrectomy, preoperatively to decrease the caliber of large new vessels before pars plana vitrectomy, and in those eyes with neovascularization of the iris.[825,826] By themselves as primary treatment for proliferative retinopathy they are not beneficial in the long run due to short duration of effect. The ability of anti-VEGF agents in reducing macular edema alone by altering vascular permeability is limited and variable; response is seen only in eyes with associated significant retinal ischemia.

6.56 Diabetic intraretinal proliferative retinopathy.

A–C: Peripheral intraretinal neovascularization (arrows).
D and **E**: This 38-year-old type 1 diabetic developed several small intraretinal neovascular fronds in both eyes (D). There were a few tufts of intraretinal microvascular abnormalities (arrow) that did not leak on the angiogram while the NVE leaked profusely (E).
F–I: Focal juxtafoveolar intraretinal neovascularization with blood (arrow, F) in a patient with proliferative diabetic retinopathy (F). The preretinal neovascularization seen elsewhere disappeared after panretinal photocoagulation but the juxtafoveolar intraretinal neovascularization became more prominent (G–I).
J–L: Juxtafoveal intraretinal neovascularization (arrow) and NVE persisted following panretinal photocoagulation in this 40-year-old type 1 diabetic. She received further photocoagulation, went on to develop traction retinal detachment involving the macula, and vision dropped to 20/400. Pars plana vitrectomy with removal of traction membranes and fill-in panretinal photocoagulation restored her vision to 20/20 in spite of moderate nonperfusion of the posterior pole.

Nonretinal Ocular Changes in Diabetes

Cornea

Diabetics have a higher incidence of dry eyes and decreased tear production. In addition, corneal sensitivity is decreased. The ability of the corneal epithelium to adhere to the basement membrane is altered by impaired glucose metabolism. This includes thickening of the basement membrane of the corneal epithelium, decreased hemidesmosomal frequency, and decreased penetration of anchoring fibrils. All these contribute to frequent corneal erosion and corneal epithelial defects. This is especially noted after surgery or laser therapy where the corneal epithelium can break down easily as a sheet.

Glaucoma

Those patients with significant ischemia, especially of the peripheral retina, develop neovascularization of the iris and neovascular glaucoma due to diffusion of VEGF into the anterior chamber. Contraction of the new vessels in the iris can cause ectropion uvea and peripheral-angle closure, resulting in neovascular glaucoma. Recurrent vitreous hemorrhages can result in ghost cell glaucoma via blockage of the trabecular meshwork by enlarged macrophages that have engulfed blood pigment. Khaki-colored large cells containing Heinz bodies, which are precipitated hemoglobin, are seen in these eyes.

Lens Abnormalities

Increase and decrease in the osmolarity of the tissues surrounding the lens and the lens itself due to increase and decrease in the level of the blood sugar cause abnormal focusing resulting in fluctuating vision. The hyperglycemia per se causes changes in the basement membrane of the lens epithelium, resulting in posterior subcapsular and

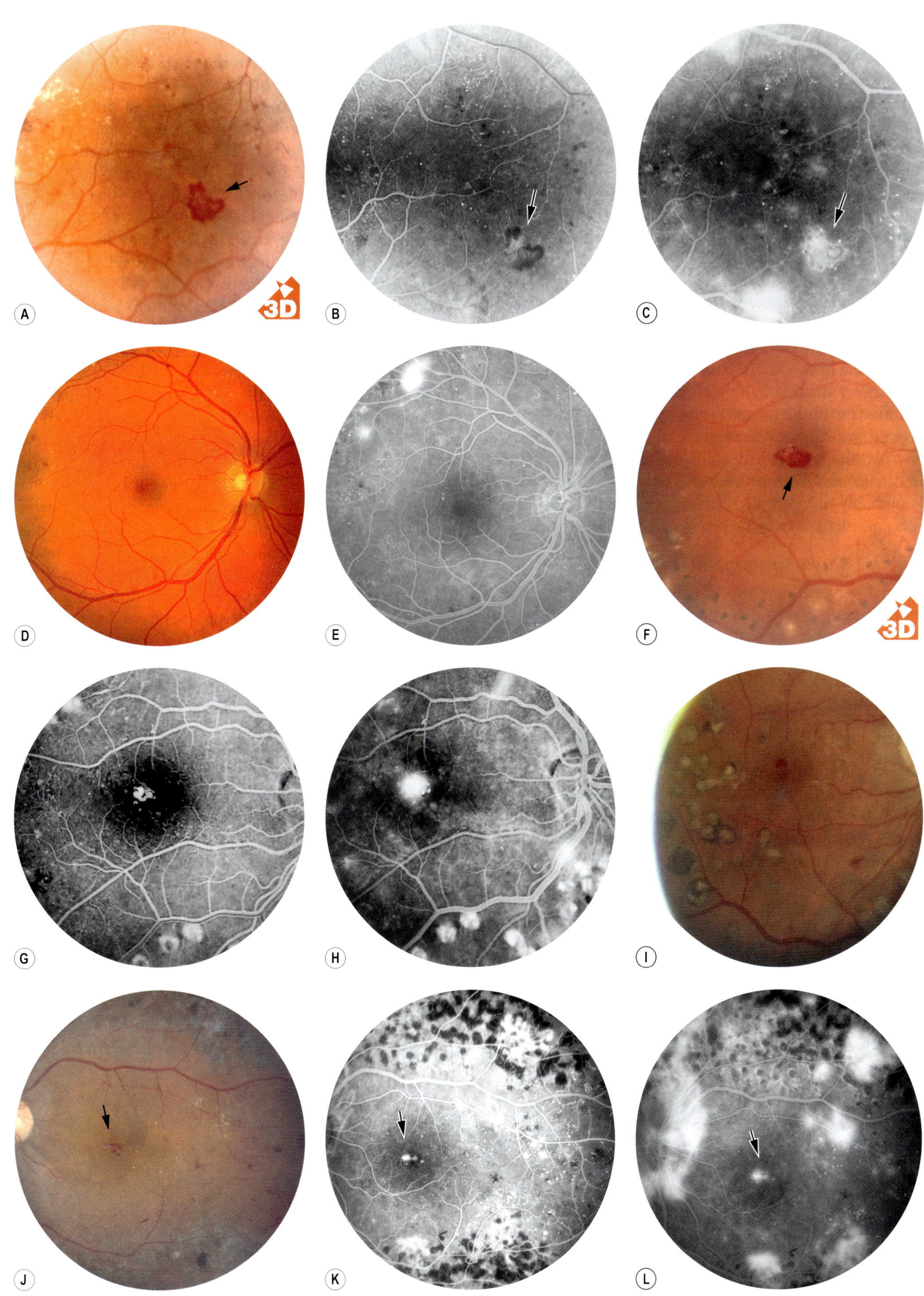
A
3D
B
C
D
E
F
3D
G
H
I
J
K
L

RADIATION RETINOPATHY

Structural and permeability alterations in the blood vessels of the retina and optic nerve that develop months or several years after X-ray irradiation of the orbital region may cause loss of visual function (Figure 6.57).[288,593,856–876] Ophthalmoscopic alterations in the retinal vasculature include the development of focal arteriolar narrowing, cotton-wool patches, microaneurysms, dilated capillary channels, perivascular sheathing, irregular loss of the retinal capillary bed, intraretinal exudation and hemorrhage, and circinate exudation (Figure 6.57). These changes are identical in all respects to diabetic retinopathy. They are usually most marked in the macular region, and loss of central acuity may be primarily a result of CME, yellowish exudative maculopathy, or loss of the perifoveal capillary network. Retinitis proliferans, optic disc new vessels, vitreous hemorrhage, retinal detachment, rubeosis, and glaucoma may eventually occur. Subretinal neovascularization that in some cases may be derived from the retinal circulation occasionally develops.[877] Fluorescein angiography highlights the structural and permeability alterations of the retinal vasculature (Figure 6.57). The latent period until the onset of retinopathy after irradiation therapy is slightly shorter in patients receiving the episcleral cobalt plaque treatment than in those receiving external-beam irradiation, and is more prolonged after irradiation of periorbital than of orbital tumors.[859,861,871] The retinopathy may appear as soon as 6 months or as late as 5 years or longer after irradiation treatment.[856,871] Retinopathy may develop after as little as 1500 rad of external-beam irradiation, but usually 3000–3500 rad is necessary to produce changes.[872] Lower doses of irradiation may produce retinopathy in patients receiving chemotherapy, e.g., 1200 cGy total-body irradiation after bone marrow transplantation, and in patients and experimental animals with diabetes mellitus.[288,856,878] High dosages of cobalt plaque therapy (mean dose of 15 000 rad delivered to the fovea) are required to produce the same changes.[861]

Visual acuity loss after irradiation may be caused also by acute irradiation optic neuropathy that is often characterized by swelling of the optic disc, peripapillary hard exudates, hemorrhages, subretinal fluid, and cotton-wool spots.[860,865,869,879–883] Fluorescein angiography in patients shows evidence of optic nerve head ischemia with superficial vascular nonperfusion accompanied usually by changes in the neighboring retinal blood vessels. Disc swelling usually lasts several weeks to months and is followed by optic atrophy. Loss of acuity in these patients is usually severe but in some cases may partly improve with resolution of the disc edema.[860] Optic disc swelling and retinal changes may be absent in patients with acute severe visual loss in one or both eyes occurring usually 1–1.5 years after irradiation of parasellar tumors.[881] These patients typically show visual field loss indicating optic nerve or chiasmal involvement. Contrast-enhanced MRI and orbital ultrasonography are invaluable in identifying the sites of radionecrosis of the optic pathway and may obviate the necessity for biopsy to exclude recurrence of the primary tumor or a radiation-induced tumor.[874,882–884] Some patients who have received irradiation treatment to the chiasmal region may experience abrupt late-onset visual loss in one or both eyes 4–35 months after receiving irradiation doses of less than 200 Gy daily and less than 6000 Gy total dosage.[874] The visual loss is permanent and no treatment is effective.

6.57 Radiation retinopathy.

A and **B**: A 37-year-old white man developed macular edema and extensive microaneurysmal formation in both eyes secondary to X-ray irradiation of a recurrent basal cell carcinoma of the nose. Visual acuity in the left eye was 20/80. Note the focal area of serous detachment of the retina surrounded by a yellowish exudate (arrows) at the superotemporal margin of the optic nerve head (A). Early angiography demonstrated multiple microaneurysms that later showed evidence of dye leakage (B). Similar changes occurred in the opposite eye.

C and **D**: Extensive cystoid macular edema (CME) with circinate retinopathy caused by X-ray irradiation therapy of a carcinoma of the antrum in a 53-year-old woman whose visual acuity was 20/50 (C). Angiography showed microaneurysms and dilation and partial loss of retinal capillaries in the temporal half of the macula. One hour after dye injection, angiography showed staining of the serous fluid in the outer layers of the retina in a typical pattern of CME. Thirty-two months after xenon photocoagulation (D) visual acuity was 20/30. There was no longer any angiographic evidence of CME.

E–H: X-ray irradiation retinopathy associated with exudative and hemorrhagic maculopathy in the right eye (E) and a subhyaloid hemorrhage in the left eye (F). Angiography showed loss of the juxtafoveal retinal capillaries bilaterally (G) and proliferative retinopathy (arrows, H) in the left eye.

Stability of radiation retinopathy over 3 years.

I–L: This 44-year-old male with radiation retinopathy maintained a vision of 20/25 and 20/20 respectively over more than 5 years of follow-up. Scattered microaneurysms and microvascular abnormalities were photographed in both eyes in 2005 (I and J). Three years later both retinas appear relatively unchanged with minimal alteration in the appearance of the microaneurysms and the microvascular changes (K and L). His vision remained unchanged in both eyes.

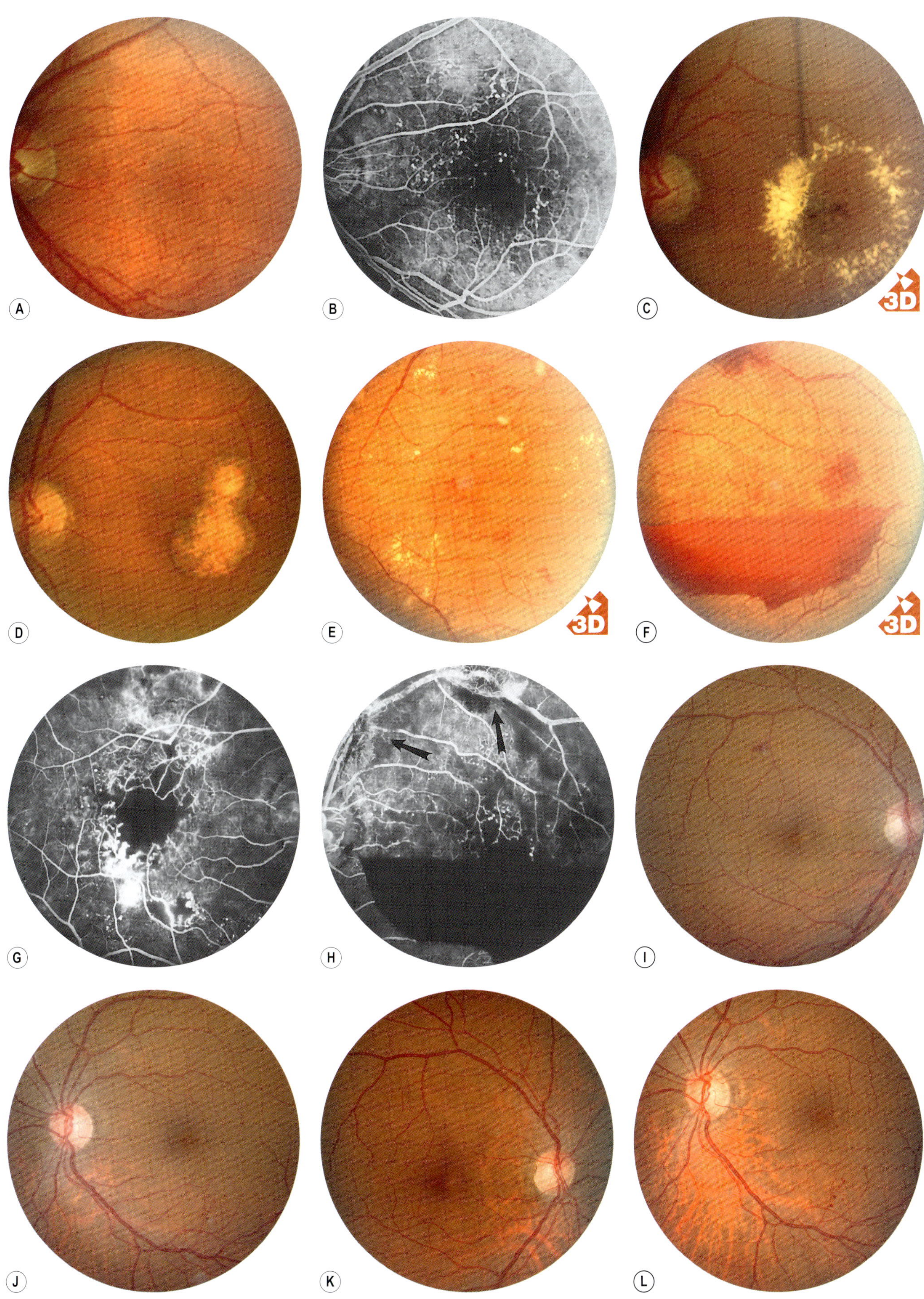
A
B
C
3D
D
E
3D
F
3D
G
H
I
J
K
L

High-dose irradiation delivered to the choroid and retina via episcleral plaques will cause postirradiation atrophic changes in the choroid and pigment epithelium in addition to the retinal vascular changes mentioned previously.[859,885–887] The size and location of the tumor and the amount of radiation delivered affect the incidence of radiation retinopathy. In a study by Paul Finger only one eye of a patient with a tumor in the anterior uvea developed radiation retinopathy[888] while 52% of the posterior choroidal melanoma patients developed radiation retinopathy. The radiation retinopathy occurred closer to the tumor, closer to the macula and the optic nerve, and more often in higher metabolic posterior retina than nasal or anterior retina.

In a similar study by Gunduz et al. of 1300 patients with posterior uveal melanoma, radiation retinopathy developed in 43.1% of patients; 5% had nonproliferative radiation retinopathy at 1 year and 42% at 5 years. Proliferative retinopathy occurred in 1% at 1 year and 8% at 5 years. Tumor margin of less than 4 mm from foveola had the highest incidence of radiation retinopathy along with radiation dose greater than 260 cGy/hour to the tumor base.[889]

In humans and experimental animals the principal histopathologic changes caused by X-ray irradiation involve loss of the retinal capillary endothelial and perithelial cells, capillary occlusion, dilation and hyalinization of thick-walled collateral channels, focal ischemic retinal infarcts, intraretinal exudation, and intraretinal and preretinal neovascularization.[860,864,878,890] Smaller vessels show thickening of the walls by fibrillar and hyaline material. Mild myointimal proliferation of both the choroidal and central retinal arteries occurs.[860,864] These changes are occasionally sufficiently severe to result in occlusion of the central retinal artery.[875] The outer retinal layers are more resistant to irradiation damage. The pathogenesis of radiation retinopathy is considered to be toxicity to the endothelial cells. The toxicity is progressive and occurs even after several years of radiation. Some eyes show no or minimal progression of the radiation retinopathy even after several years (Figure 6.57I–L).

The patients with exudative retinopathy caused by localized capillary changes outside the papillomacular bundle may be helped by photocoagulation (Figure 6.57C–F).[593] PRP may be of value in patients who develop severe proliferative retinopathy.[862] Treatment of irradiation optic neuropathy is generally unsatisfactory, although some patients may experience restoration of vision after administration of hyperbaric oxygen soon after the onset of visual loss.[880,891] Radiation maculopathy and macular edema with lipid exudates can be treated. Focal laser photocoagulation to the microaneurysms has improved vision and decreased incidence of further vision loss. Most recently, use of bevacizumab has been considered. The treatment is followed by reduction retinal hemorrhage, exudation, and edema. Visual acuities either remain stable or improve in most patients.[892–894]

6.58 Sickle-cell retinopathy.

A–C: Subretinal and preretinal macular hemorrhage in an 8-year-old black boy with sickle-cell hemoglobin C disease. Angiography showed nonperfusion of the retinal vascular bed temporal to the macula (B). Several months later the blood partly cleared, leaving an iridescent pigmented patch of hemosiderin and depigmentation of the retinal pigment epithelium (C).

D–F: Acute loss of central vision occurred in this man with sickle-cell hemoglobin C disease. Note the subinternal limiting membrane hematomas (arrows, D). A patch of fine orange hemosiderin crystals was located in the superficial retina (arrowheads, D) superior to a large sunburst pattern of pigment. There was extensive retinal capillary nonperfusion throughout the temporal fundus, including the temporal macular area (E and F). Within 4 months the hematomas disappeared and he recovered 20/25 visual acuity.

G and **H**: Peripheral salmon-patch hemorrhage before and after partial clearing of the blood.

I: "Sunburst" pigment spot with surrounding depigmentation at the site of a previous retinal hemorrhage.

J and **K**: Peripheral proliferative retinopathy at the junction of the perfused and nonperfused retina. Note early staining of the neovascular "sea fan."

L: Histopathology of a "sea fan" overlying the peripheral nonperfused retina.

(L, courtesy of Dr. W. Richard Green.)

SICKLE-CELL RETINOPATHY

Black patients with homozygous sickle-cell disease (SS), hemoglobin SC disease (SC), and sickle-cell thalassemia disease (S-thal) and hemoglobin SO Arab[895] may develop occlusive vascular disease of the peripheral retina that is associated with circumferential arteriovenous communications, retinal neovascularization ("sea fans"), and focal intraretinal and subretinal hemorrhages ("salmon-patch" hemorrhages) at the juncture of the perfused and nonperfused retina (Figure 6.58).[307,895–912] These latter hemorrhages (Figure 6.58A and D), which occur near an occluded arteriole, resolve and leave either an iridescent patch of hemosiderin (Figure 6.58C, G, and H) or, if the blood extends beneath the retina, a black patch of hyperplastic RPE ("sunburst" spots) (Figure 6.58D–F, and I) or a hyperpigmented scar.[903] These may be mistaken for focal areas of chorioretinitis. Fluorescein angiographic evidence of peripheral retinal vascular occlusion develops in 50% of children with SS and SC disease by the age of 6 years and in 90% by age 12 years.[913,914] Sanders et al. found the mean largest diameter of the FAZ in patients with SC and SS disease was 1.0 mm compared to 0.61 mm in normals.[915] There was no significant difference in the FAZ diameter within the sickle-cell group in regard to the degree of retinopathy, type of sickle-cell disease, or the visual acuity.

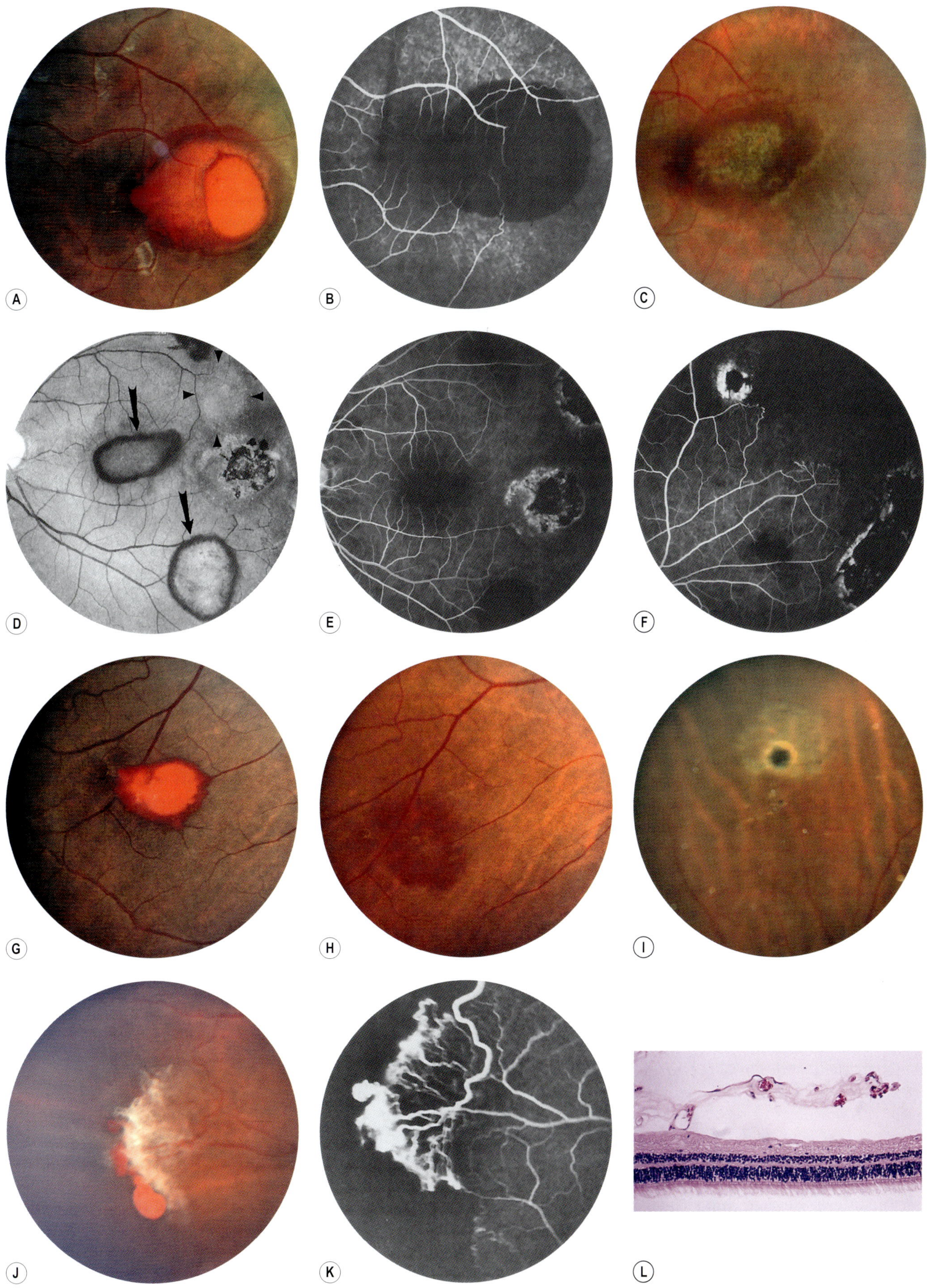
A
B
C
D
E
F
G
H
I
J
K
L

Despite the frequency of development of retinal vascular changes, they cause visual loss in 10% or fewer of patients with SC and SS disease.[916–918] Visual symptoms are most frequently caused by vitreous hemorrhage derived from the retinal neovascularization (Figures 6.58J–L and 6.59C and D), both of which are more likely to occur in males between the ages of 20 and 39 years, and in patients with SC rather than SS disease.[902,917,919] Some patients, however, initially experience acute loss of central vision caused by occlusion of one or more paracentral arterioles (Figure 6.60A–F). They have multiple patches of ischemic retinal whitening that disappear in several weeks. Angiography shows loss of localized areas of the parafoveal capillary network (Figure 6.60D–F and 6.61A–D). These paracentral occlusive vascular changes are more likely to occur in SS than in SC disease.[910,916,920,921] It is probable that many of the small microvascular changes seen in the parafoveal capillary network in asymptomatic sickle-cell disease are the result of minute arteriolar and capillary obstructions.[908,910,922–924] Evidence of juxtafoveal capillary obstruction may occur in as many as 29% of patients with sickle-cell hemoglobinopathies,[923] but has been observed much less frequently in the patients in Miami. Asdourian and coworkers[923] noted continuous remodeling of the macular and paramacular vasculature in such cases. Loss of central vision is occasionally caused by occlusion of the central retinal artery[216,925]; occlusion of the central retinal vein (see Figure 6.74A–F)[904]; macular hole formation, usually associated with retinal traction caused by proliferative retinopathy[926]; subretinal and preretinal bleeding from retinal new vessels at the junction of the perfused and nonperfused retina that in some cases may extend posteriorly into the macular area[904,927]; traction retinal detachment (Figure 6.61G and H); rhegmatogenous retinal detachment (Figure 6.59G)[928]; neovascular glaucoma[929]; retrobulbar ischemic optic neuropathy[930]; possible choroidal infarcts (Figure 6.60I–L); and, rarely, exudative retinal detachment (Figure 6.61I).[931] Macular epiretinal membranes, which occur in approximately 4% of patients with SS and SC disease, may be responsible for subnormal visual acuity.[932,933] Although angioid streaks occur in as many as 22% of patients with SS disease and less frequently in those with SC disease, rarely are they associated with central vision loss caused by choroidal neovascularization (Figure 3.32G–I and 6.59E and F).[934,935] The incidence of angioid streaks and retinitis proliferans increases with age.[936]

Other ocular findings occurring in sickle-cell disease include optic disc neovascularization,[937] hairpin neovascular loops,[938] spontaneous peripheral chorioretinal neovascularization,[939] occlusion of the posterior ciliary arteries,[940,941] pseudocapillary angiomas of the retina,[938,942] ischemic infarction of the optic nerve secondary to elevated intraocular pressure,[943–945] ischemic optic neuropathy in normotensive eyes,[946] and focal capillary stasis in the inferior conjunctival cul-de-sac and optic nerve head.[947] These latter two findings are helpful in making the clinical diagnosis of sickle-cell disease, which ultimately requires hemoglobin electrophoresis for confirmation. Goldbaum described a peculiar light reflex seen when viewed via an indirect ophthalmoscope of the thin temporal retina resulting from posterior retinal infarcts.[948] This is illustrated well on OCT (Figure 6.61E and F). Nonocular signs and symptoms, including musculoskeletal and joint pain, abdominal discomfort, cholelithiasis, and episodic anemia, that are often present in patients with SS disease are frequently minimal or absent in patients with SC disease. Ocular complications, however, are more frequent in patients with SC disease. Rare forms of sickle-cell hemoglobinopathies also may be associated with ocular complications.[895,949–951] Retinal vascular changes rarely occur in patients with sickle-cell trait unless they have additional systemic diseases that affect the retina or other retinal vascular diseases.[895] Gass has seen one such young patient who developed extreme peripheral proliferative retinopathy and recurrent vitreous hemorrhage after initially developing bilateral central retinal vein occlusion (see Figure 6.74).

6.59 Sickle-cell retinopathy.

A and **B**: A 10-year-old boy with sickle-cell (SS) disease was asymptomatic and seen with a vision of 20/20 during a screening exam. There were no retinal hemorrhages, scars, new vessels, or nonperfusion. Both temporal peripheral small vessels were prominent, suggesting dilated capillary bed and slow flow in these vessels in response to relative tissue hypoxia. The dilated capillary bed is visible on the angiograms in the temporal periphery of both eyes (A and B). **C** and **D**: This 28-year-old with Hb SC disease had a flat retinal neovascularization in the upper nasal quadrant of the left eye with nonperfusion of the retina anterior to it (Arrow C). In the superotemporal quadrant was an NVE with partial autoinvolution (Arrow D) and a pigmented chorioretinal scar at the site of a previous hemorrhage (D).

Angioid streaks in sickle-cell retinopathy.

E and **F**: This 55-year-old male with Hb SS disease had a best-corrected vision of 20/20 in each eye. Angioid streaks were seen radiating from the optic disc in both eyes (E and F). There was no evidence of pattern dystrophy, peau d'orange, comets, choroidal neovascularization or skin changes, thus eliminating pseudoxanthoma elasticum.
G and **H**: This 54-year-old male from Ghana presented with sudden loss of vision in his right eye to count fingers: 360° of peripheral retinal nonperfusion was seen associated with several autoinfarcted raised and flat neovascular tufts. There were three tears in the inferior and inferotemporal retinal periphery cuasing the retinal detachment (G). The left eye had peripheral nonperfusion to a lesser degree and autoinvoluted new vessels (H). Vision in the left eye was 20/20. He underwent a pars plana vitrectomy with silicone oil placement as the inferior vitreous was extremely adherent to the avascular retina.

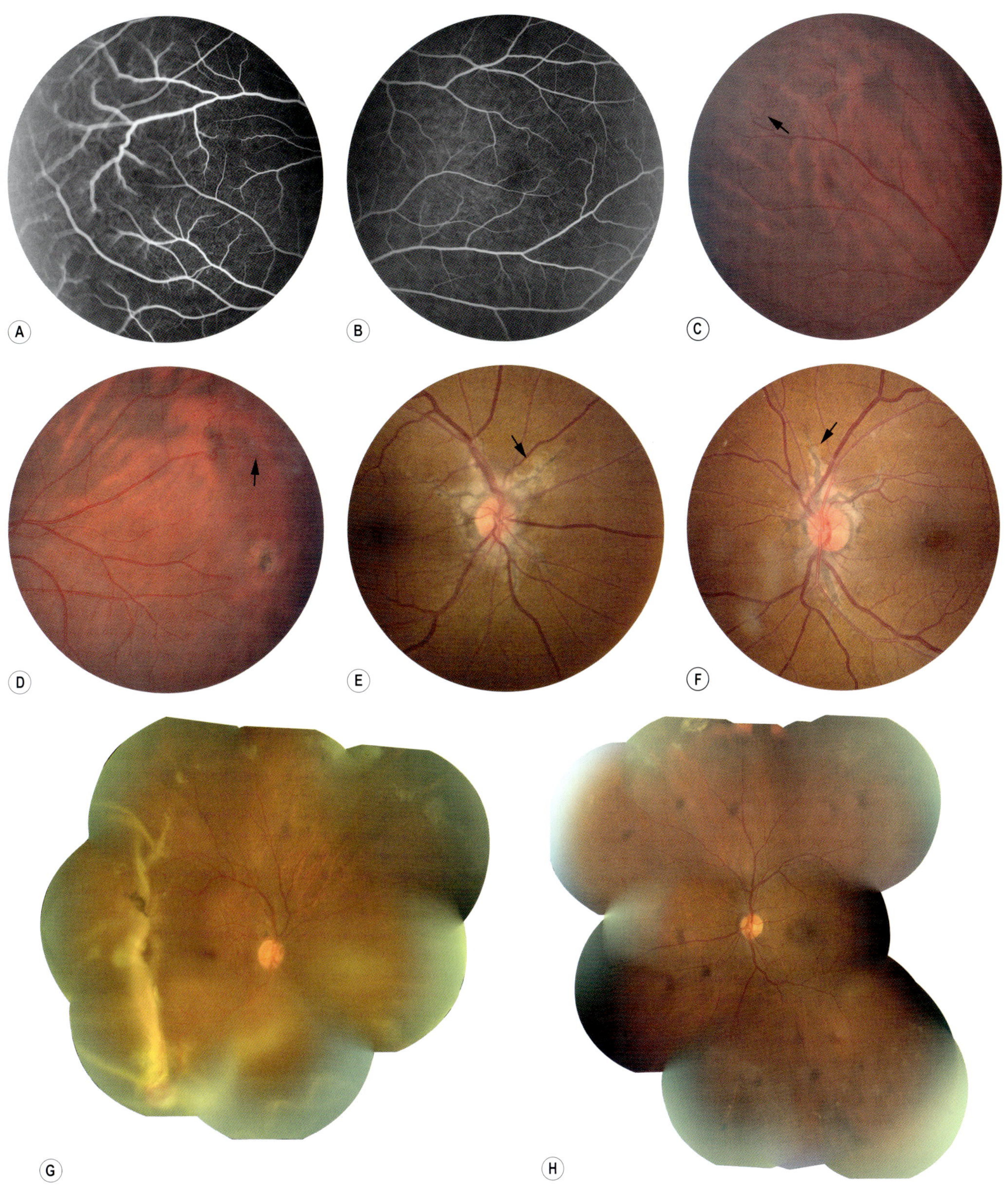
A
B
C
D
E
F
G
H

Patients with SC and SS disease prior to the development of proliferative retinopathy may demonstrate evidence of color vision abnormalities, electroretinographic changes, and abnormalities of retinal vascular autoregulation.[952–955]

There is a predilection for spontaneous regression or autoinfarction of retinal neovascularization in sickle-cell disease.[898,906,916,917,932,956] This may be more common in SS disease.[917] For this reason, treatment is probably necessary only in patients experiencing vitreous hemorrhage. In such patients, focal photocoagulation or cryotherapy applied directly to areas of neovascularization or scatter treatment in zones of retinal vascular nonperfusion are usually successful in causing regression of the new vessels.[307,896,899,900,914,937,957–962] The use of the feeder vessel technique of occluding neovascular fronds is associated with a significant incidence (94%) of posttreatment development of choriovitreal neovascularization and should be avoided in favor of scatter treatment to the peripheral zones of retinal capillary nonperfusion.[929,958,963,964] Posttreatment choriovitreal neovascularization may result in further vitreoretinal complications and permanent loss of visual function.[964,965] Other postphotocoagulation complications are the development of choroidal neovascularization,[895,964,966,967] choroidal ischemia,[941] and retinal holes.[928] Scleral buckling procedures, vitrectomy, and Nd:YAG laser vitreolysis are techniques used in these patients with rhegmatogenous and tractional retinal detachment.[968,969] Exchange transfusions, formerly done before scleral buckling procedures to reduce the chance of severe ocular ischemic complications, probably should be abandoned since the development of newer procedures for managing retinal detachment.[920,970,971]

6.60 Reversible macular infarction in sickle-cell retinopathy.

A–H: This 24-year-old woman came in for a routine exam and noted a right-eye field defect when she looked up. She saw 20/400 on the right and 20/20 on the left. Branch retinal artery occlusions were seen in the right macula and nasal retina (A and B). The far temporal periphery of the right showed vascular occlusion (C). Angiogram showed delayed filling of the involved retinal artrioles. When examined 1 and 3 weeks later the vision had improved marginally to 20/200, the retina was transparent again, and the vascular perfusion had re-established in the right macula (H). She was known to have Hb SS disease with several crises.

Choroidal ischemia in sickle-cell retinopathy.

I–L: This 42-year-old African American male was seen with poor vision in both eyes for a few years. His best-corrected visual acuity was 20/200 in each eye. Both maculas had thinning with pigmentation at the retinal pigment epithelial level (I and J). An angiogram revealed possible choriocapillaris loss in the macula, possibly from choroidal infarcts secondary to sickle-cell disease (K and L).

(A–H, courtesy of Dr. William Mieler, A and D, Also, Yannuzzi, Lawrence J., The Retinal Atlas, Saunders 2010, 978-0-7020-3320-9, p.472. I–L, courtesy of Dr. Paul Sternberg.)

The differential diagnosis includes Eales' disease, FEVR, retrolental fibroplasia, sarcoidosis, incontinentia pigmenti, branch retinal vein occlusion, talc retinopathy, chronic myelogenous leukemia, uveitis, pars planitis, radiation retinopathy, aortic arch syndromes, carotid cavernous fistula, diabetes, and collagen vascular disease.

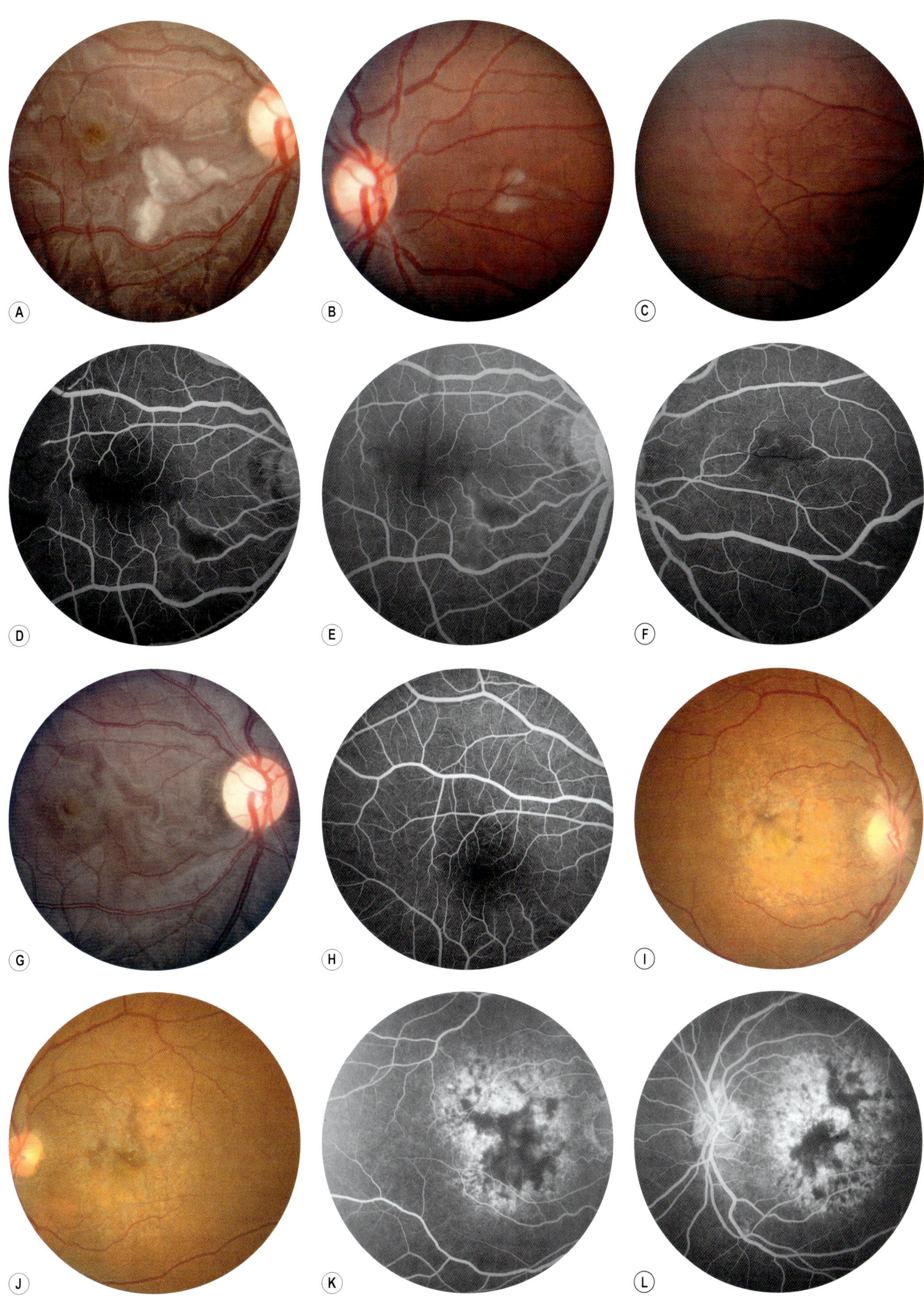
A
B
C
D
E
F
G
H
I
J
K
L

Constant remodeling of the vascular tree secondary to microinfarcts and micro-occlusions, especially in the retina temporal to the macula, has been noted (Figure 6.61A–D). Goldbaum described the retinal depression sign indicating a small retinal infarct temporal to the macula.[972] This is best seen by indirect ophthalmoscopy with a deflection of the light reflex. More recently, this has been documented by OCT findings, showing the temporal fovea to be thinner than the nasal fovea (Figure 6.61E and F).

In a study by Lima et al.,[973] conjunctival vessel alteration was not influenced by age, gender, fetal hemoglobin estimation, serum creatine albumin levels, presence of alpha-thalassemia or beta-globin gene haplotypes. However, increasing the conjunctival vessel alteration was seen in patients with hemoglobin less than 9.0 grams per 100 ml, hematocrit of less than 26.7%, and SS phenotype of sickle-cell anemia, suggesting that lower hemoglobin and lower hematocrit and SS phenotype are risk factors for conjunctival vascular anomalies. Age over 17 years was a risk for retinal vascular anomalies in sickle-cell disease patients. Treatment of acute CRAO or occlusion of larger retinal vessels can be done with immediate-exchange transfusion, improvement of the oxygen-carrying capacity, and delivery of 100% oxygen by nasal cannula or other means. The occlusion of the sickle cells is worsened by a mechanism called logjam where more sickle cells pile up behind the initial site of occlusion, increasing the area of nonperfusion, including surrounding areas for nonperfusion and occlusion. It is believed that similar stagnation of cells occurs in the choroid as occurs in the retinal circulation. The smaller choroidal vessels in the choriocapillary lobules are more prone to vaso-occlusion by the effect of sickling on choroidal circulation (Figure 6.60I–L). It is known from studies that the blood flow is slower in patients with sickle-cell disease rather than normal patients. It is also useful to monitor these patients for desferrioxamine toxicity, since many of them are on chelating agents to treat the iron overload from repeated transfusions.[973]

6.61 Sickle cell retinopathy

A–F: This 28-year-old male from west Africa gave a history of diplopia and a stroke that resulted in weakness of the left side of his body. He was hospitalized for poor mentation. When he regained consciousness he noted subnormal vision in his right eye that improved to a small extent over time. When examined 3 years later both maculas showed enlarged foveal avascular zone (B and C) associated with microvascular changes in the foveal vessels (A). The peripheral retina showed extensive nonperfusion bilaterally but no new vessels (D). The temporal foveal retina was thin compared to the nasal fovea in both eyes (E and F, arrows).

G and H: Autoinfarction of the raised new vessels resulting in gliosis and traction of the feeding arterioles in a patient with Hb SS disease.

I: This 10-year-old girl with sickle-cell disease was asymptomatic. She had an outer retinal/choroidal white lesion associated with surrounding subretinal fluid. It is likely that the yellow lesion is subretinal or outer retinal dehemoglobinized blood. The yellow patch and subretinal fluid had resolved spontaneously when she was re-examined 2 months later.

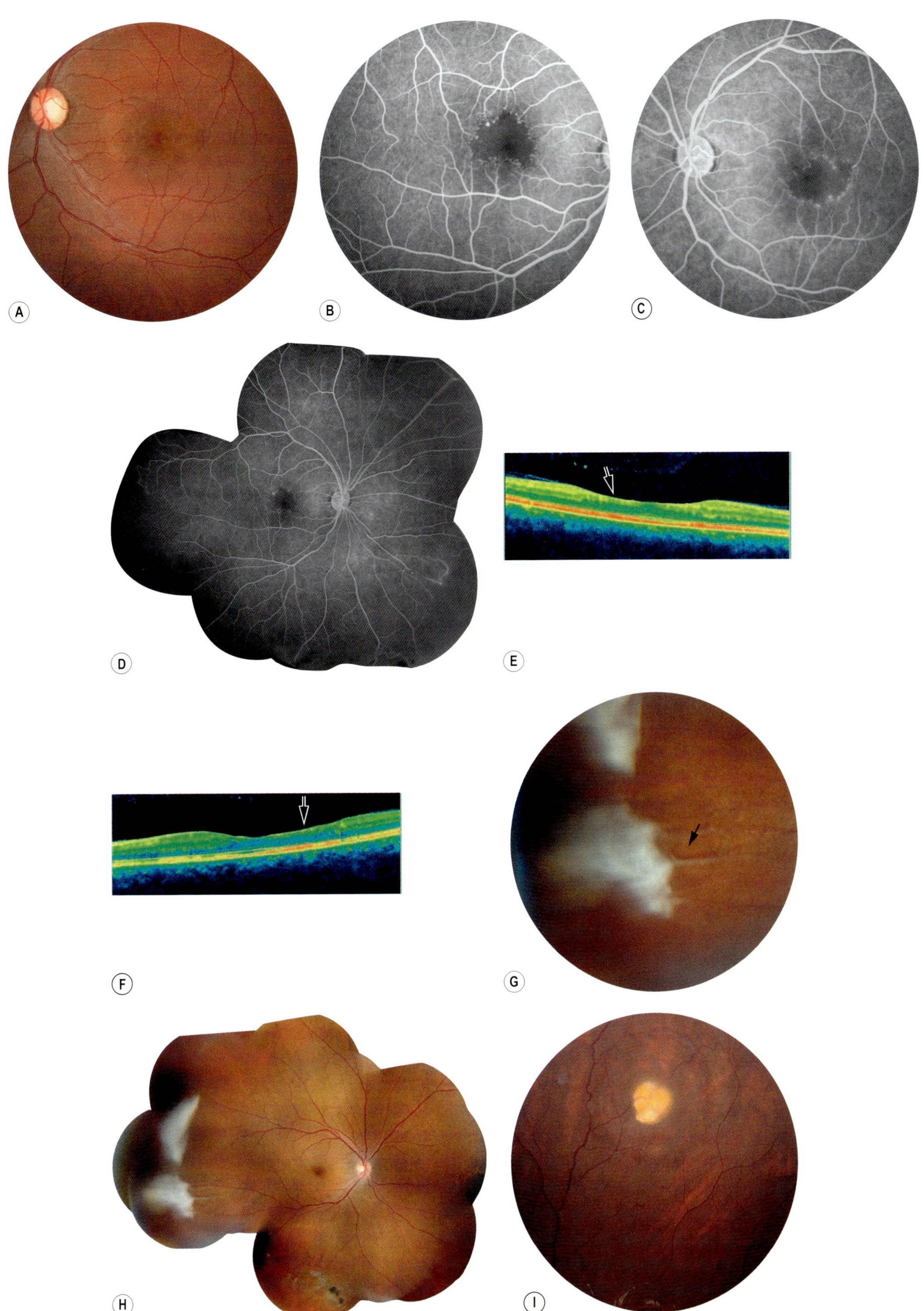
A
B
C
D
E
F
G
H
I

PRIMARY RETINAL VASCULITIS OR VASCULOPATHY (EALES' DISEASE)

Although Eales originally described the association of retinal hemorrhages with epistaxis and constipation, the term "Eales' disease" is now used to describe patients who, in the early course of this disorder of unknown cause, have active occlusive vasculopathy affecting primarily the major retinal vessels in the peripheral fundus and who later develop neovascularization occurring along the posterior edge of broad areas of peripheral retinal vascular occlusion.[308,974–982] Most of these patients are asymptomatic at the time of the active occlusive vasculopathy or "vasculitis," which may involve primarily the retinal veins, retinal arteries, or both. If seen during this active phase of the disease, because of complaints of visual field loss, photopsias, or floaters, fundoscopic examination may reveal a variety of pictures, including peripheral retinal perivenous exudation, retinal hemorrhages and exudation, or retinal periarterial exudation, arterial occlusion, and ischemic retinal whitening. Because many patients are asymptomatic during the early active vasculopathy stages of Eales' disease, we have little information concerning the relative frequency of the various fundoscopic pictures that occur early in these patients, who later present with a similar fundoscopic picture of peripheral retinal vascular occlusive disease (Figures 6.62 and 6.63). Patients with Eales' disease are typically healthy young men between the ages of 20 and 30 years who seek treatment because of floaters or vision loss secondary to vitreous hemorrhage. The hemorrhage is caused by peripheral retinal neovascularization and in some cases optic disc neovascularization (Figure 6.62J–L). Occasionally, loss of vision is caused by retinal capillary telangiectasis and CME (Figure 6.62) or macular pucker caused by an epiretinal membrane. Similar changes in the peripheral fundus are often present in both eyes. Although there is a higher than normal incidence of positive reaction to the tuberculin protein, there is no evidence that the ocular changes are directly related to active tuberculosis. In most patients examined before developing vitreous hemorrhage, there is minimal evidence of inflammation in either the vitreous or retina. One or more retinal neovascular fronds are usually found near the posterior border separating the anterior nonperfused retina from the normal retina (Figure 6.63A and B). These retinal vascular changes are usually more prominent temporally.

6.62 Eales' disease.

A–D: Recurrent vitreous hemorrhage occurred in the right eye of a 35-year-old man with 20/20 visual acuity. In both eyes he had large equatorial zones of retinal capillary nonperfusion and retinitis proliferans as well as capillary telangiectasis in the temporal macula of both eyes (arrows, A and B). In the asymptomatic left eye he had optic disc neovascularization (A). Angiography demonstrated minimal leakage of the telangiectatic capillaries in the macular areas (B) and staining of the optic disc and peripheral new vessels (C and D). Panretinal photocoagulation of the nonperfused retinal zones and later a vitrectomy were required to stop the vitreous hemorrhages.

E–H: This healthy 30-year-old man noted loss of paracentral vision in the left eye. His visual acuity was 20/15 bilaterally. Note the prominent papillary and juxtapapillary telangiectasis, irregular narrowing of the retinal arteries, and cotton-wool patches bilaterally (E and F). He had extensive obliteration of his peripheral retinal vasculature in both eyes. Angiography demonstrated extensive microvascular changes and a focal area of capillary nonperfusion (arrow, H) corresponding with a patch of ischemic whitening on the left optic disc. Soon afterward he began to experience recurrent vitreous hemorrhages with peripheral and optic disc neovascularization that required panretinal photocoagulation and vitrectomy.

I–L: This healthy young man experienced severe bilateral loss of vision associated with severe peripheral occlusive retinal vein and arterial disease that extended posteriorly and was associated with extensive proliferative retinopathy.

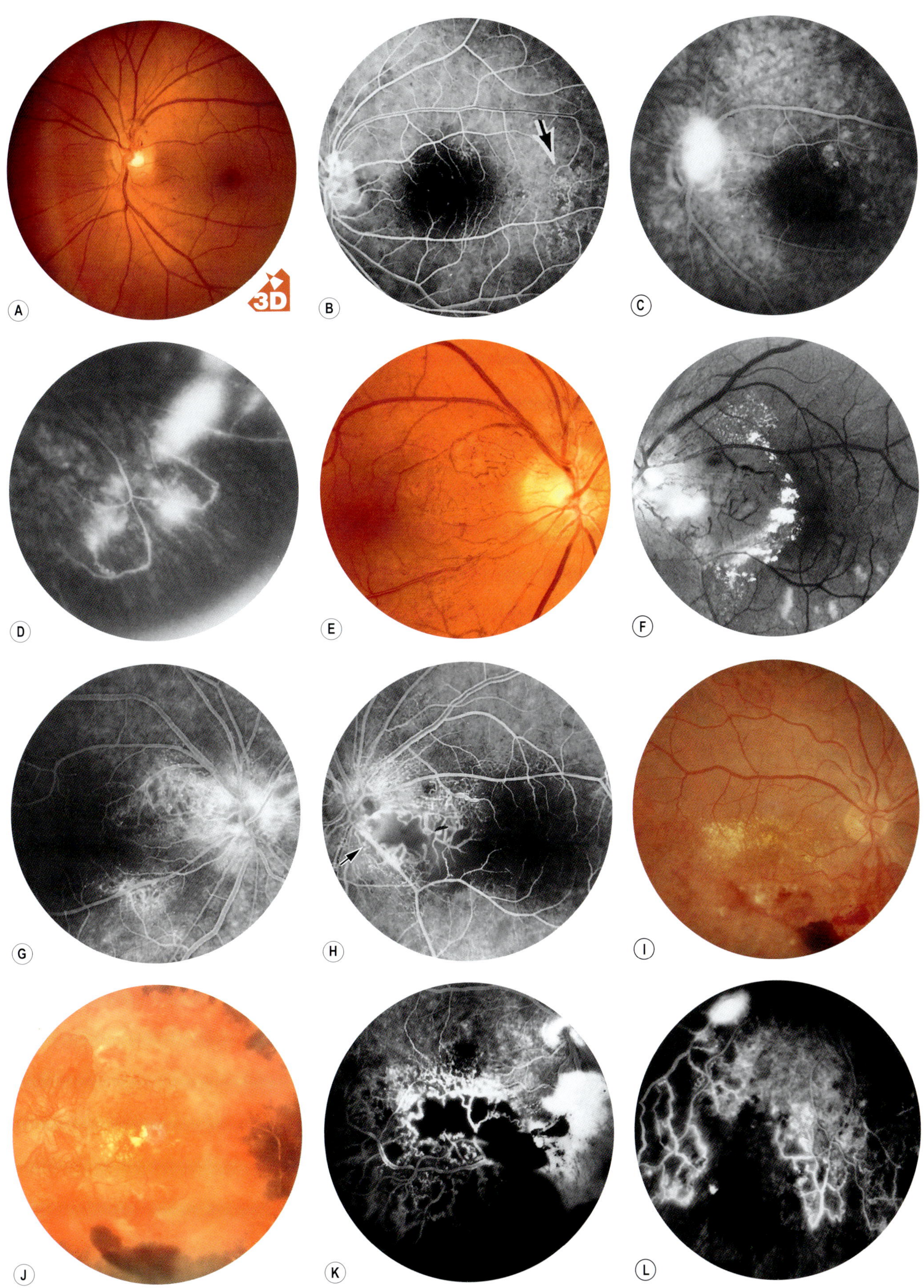
3D
A
B
C
D
E
F
G
H
I
J
K
L

Fluorescein angiography during the acute vascular occlusive phase of the disease reveals evidence of severe permeability alterations and obstruction that may affect primarily the retinal veins or the arteries. During the later stages of the disease angiography defines the zones of loss of the retinal vasculature and the remodeling of the retinal circulation, which often includes retinal neovascularization along the posterior border of the zones of perfused and nonperfused retina (Figures 6.62K and L, and 6.63C and D, J–L).

Eales' disease probably is a heterogeneous disorder that involves at least two groups of patients. In one group, who are predominantly males, the vasculopathy involves primarily the retinal veins. In the other group, with no sex predilection, the retinal arteries are primarily affected. These latter patients are probably part of the spectrum of idiopathic bilateral recurrent branch retinal arterial occlusion (see p. 482). Recent follow-up study of these patients, who typically present with visual loss caused by multiple branch retinal artery occlusions caused by focal "arteriolitis" involving the posterior fundi, reveals a high incidence of development of evidence of peripheral retinal vascular occlusive disease and proliferative retinopathy. Some of these patients may develop other evidence of focal central nervous involvement.[983] Evidence suggests a higher than normal incidence of auditory and vestibular abnormalities in these patients with bilateral recurrent branch retinal artery occlusion as well as in series of patients with Eales' disease.[984]

Laboratory investigations of patients with Eales' disease have failed to determine the cause of the vasculopathy. Elevation of the patient's serum alpha-1 acid glycoprotein levels has been demonstrated in these patients during the active phase of the disease.[985] This is a nonspecific finding that may be present in some patients with inflammatory disease, malignancies, and tissue necrosis. In a large group of patients from India with Eales' disease, Rengarajan and coworkers found two specific serum proteins, one of which was an anionic peptide, that were not present in normal control patients.[986]

6.63 Eales' disease.

A–G: This 29-year-old physician from India was evaluated for floaters in his right eye. He had no history suggestive of tuberculosis. There was a partly gliotic raised NVE in the superotemporal quadrant, anterior to which was retinal nonperfusion. There were sheathed retinal veins in the inferonasal quadrant and one chorioretinal scar (A and B). No areas of active vasculitis were found. A fluorescein angiogram defined the areas of nonperfusion and neovascularization (C and D). He underwent scatter laser to the areas of nonperfusion. A tuberculosis skin test returned strongly positive, but a chest X-ray was normal. He was followed, the new vessels regressed, and the vitreous hemorrhage cleared. A year later he was seen to develop several small retinal hemorrhages and phlebitis (arrow) in the temporal periphery of the right eye (E). Since he now showed active vasculitis with breakdown of the blood–retinal barrier on fluorescence angiogram (F), he was treated with an 18-month course of a four-drug antituberculous regimen and tapering dose of oral steroids for 2 months. The vasculitis and retinal hemorrhages cleared and his vision remained at 20/20 (G). The left eye was normal throughout.

H–L: This healthy 51-year-old male gave a 4-month history of progressive loss of vision in both eyes associated with severe occlusive retinal vascular disease affecting primarily the retinal arterial system. Recently he had developed mild vitreous hemorrhage caused by peripheral retinal neovascularization. His visual acuity was 20/400, right eye, 20/200, left eye. Note the multiple atheromatous plaques in the arterial walls (H and I), pallor of the optic discs, and the widespread dot and blot retinal hemorrhages. Medical and neurologic evaluations, including magnetic resonance imaging of the brain, were negative. Angiography revealed extensive loss of the retinal microvasculature in the macula areas and peripherally (J–L). There was marked microaneurysmal change and late staining in the area of partly perfused retina posteriorly. Both eyes subsequently required panretinal photocoagulation and vitrectomy.

(H–L, courtesy of Dr. Frank J. Culotta.)

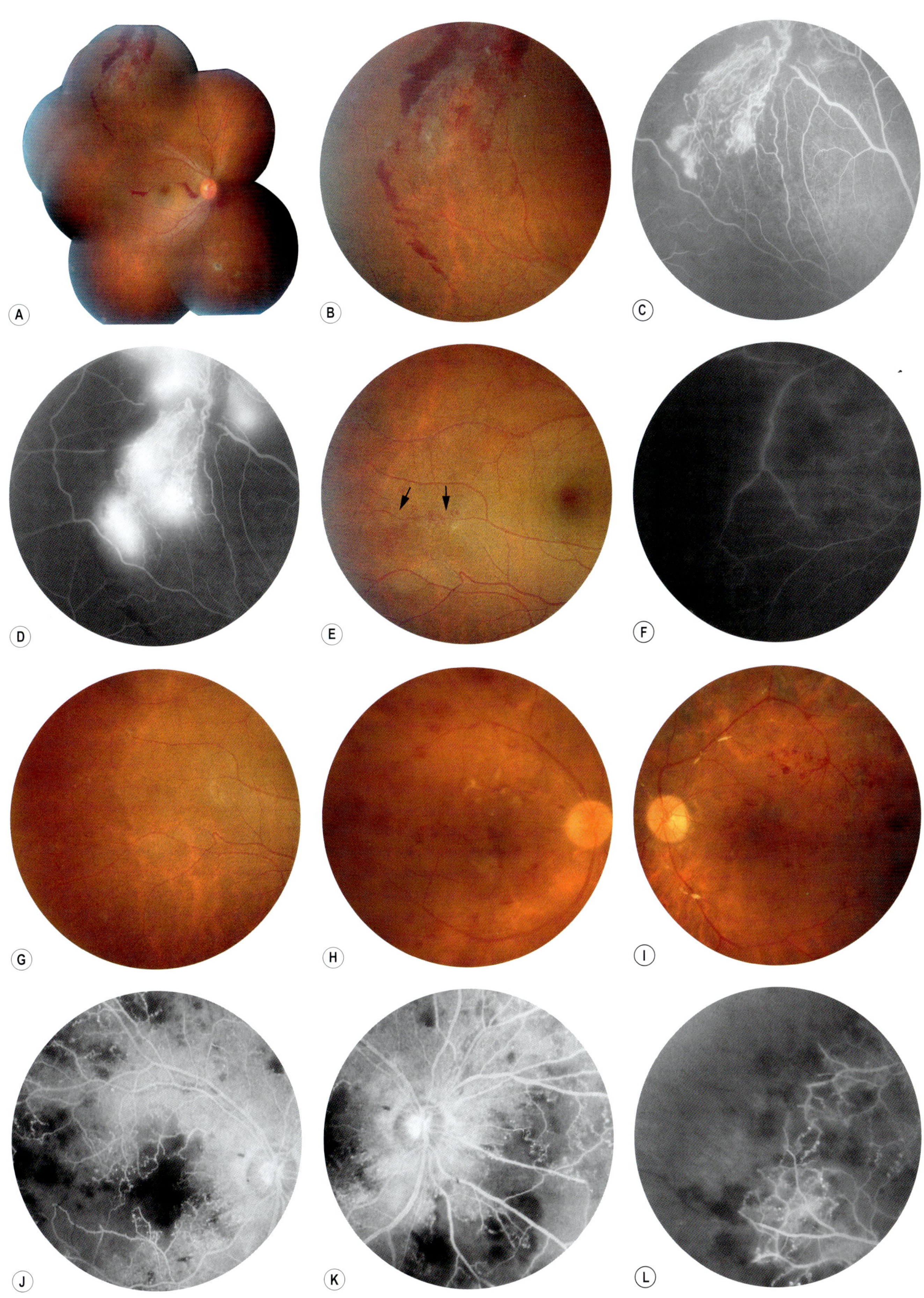
A
B
C
D
E
F
G
H
I
J
K
L

The diagnosis of Eales' disease should be reserved for patients with no evidence of other diseases that can produce the identical fundus changes. These diseases include sickle-cell disease, diabetes, collagen vascular disease (Figure 6.64A–F), incontinentia pigmenti, ROP (see p. 570), FEVR (see p. 576), MS,[295,987–994] branch retinal vein occlusion, FSHD, sarcoidosis, pars planitis, serpiginous choroiditis (see pp. 962–968), frosted retinal angiitis (see p. 950), ulcerative colitis,[995] chronic idiopathic central serous chorioretinopathy (see p. 76), and a familial syndrome that includes young women with graying of the hair, poikiloderma, and idiopathic nonarteriosclerotic cerebral calcifications.[603] (See discussion of retinal vasculitis in Chapter 11.) Patients with IRVAN syndrome have a peripheral obliterative vasculopathy that resembles Eales' disease in all ways except for the presence of arterial aneurysms (Figure 6.50 and 6.51). Whether these two conditions are causally related is yet to be determined.

The natural course of Eales' disease is variable. In some patients spontaneous occlusion of the new vessels occurs, and in others recurrent vitreous hemorrhage and progression of the occlusive vascular disease may lead to total retinal detachment.

Photocoagulation of the nonperfused peripheral retina, avoiding the large areas of retinal neovascularization, is indicated in patients experiencing vitreous hemorrhage. In some patients with vitreous traction, a vitrectomy also may be necessary. Photocoagulation may be beneficial in the few patients who develop CME or circinate maculopathy caused by paracentral telangiectasia.

6.64 Collagen vascular disease associated vasculitis.

A–F: This 18-year-old male with polyarthritis, circulating lupus anticoagulant, mild Raynaud's phenomena, proteinuria, mucous membrane lesions, and severe ischemic changes of the digits of both hands developed peripheral occlusive retinal vasculopathy affecting primarily the venous system (G–I). Ten weeks later there was extensive whitening of the occluded retinal vessels (J) and proliferative retinopathy (K and L). Biopsy of the kidney, liver, and femur revealed arteritis.

Idiopathic obliterative arteritis.

G–L: A 47-year-old Latin American male was seen for blurred vision for 25 days associated with few floaters and flashes of light. His vision was 20/20 on the right and 20/30 on the left. 1+ vitreous cells were seen on the left. Most of the retinal arterioles showed patchy periarterial whitening in both eyes associated with few cotton-wool patches. Angiogram showed occlusion of the inferotemporal arteriole on the right and inferonasal arteriole on the left. Systemic work-up for tuberculosis and collagen vascular disease was negative. He received systemic steroids; the left eye developed neovascular glaucoma and vitreous hemorrhage requiring a tube shunt and vitrectomy. His final visual acuity was 20/60 and 20/40. The working diagnosis was Eales' disease, which may or may not be the accurate term for his condition.

(A–F, from Hall et al.[1363]; G–L, courtesy of Dr. Scott Sneed.)

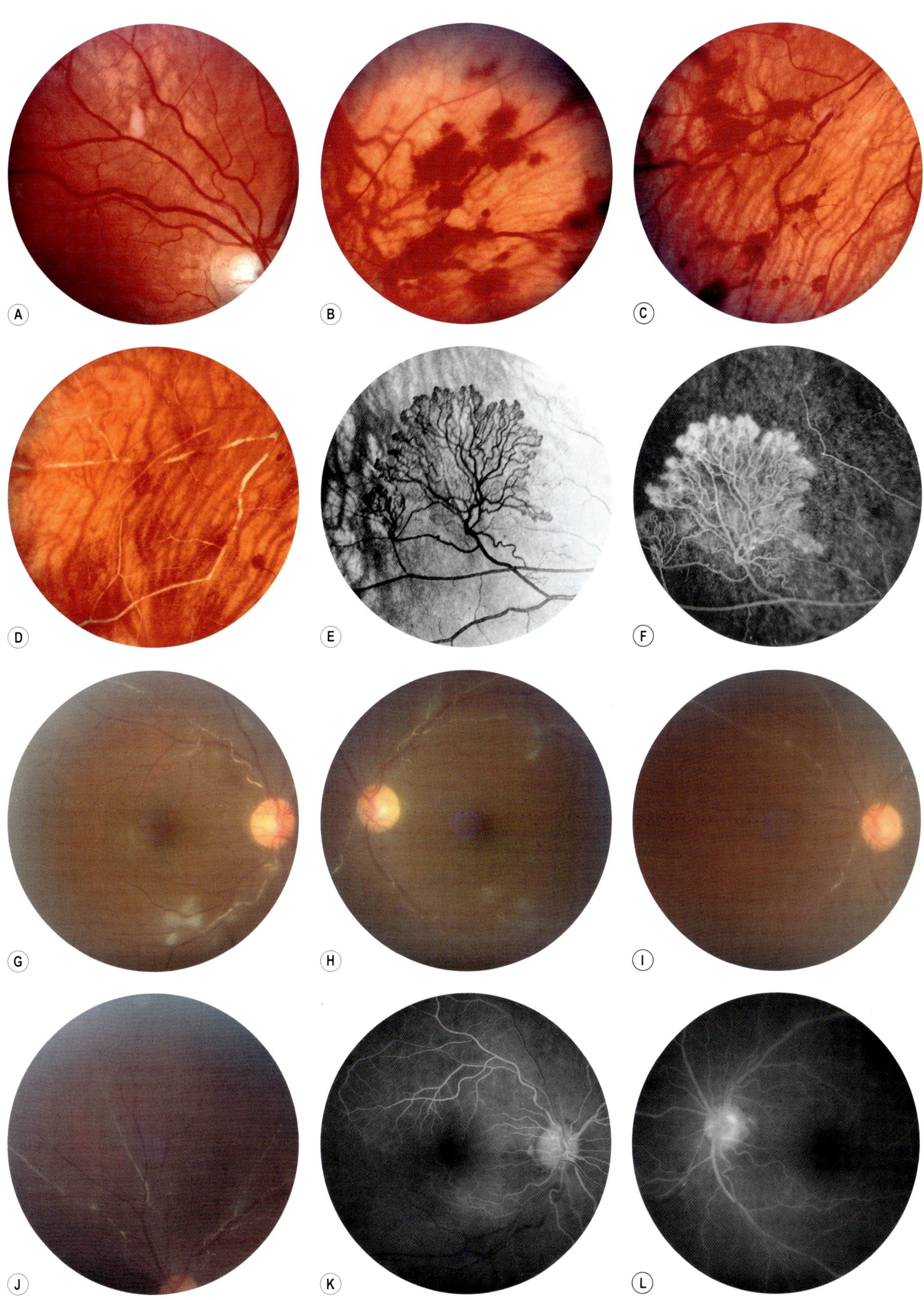
A
B
C
D
E
F
G
H
I
J
K
L

RETINOPATHY OF PREMATURITY

Premature infants with a birth weight less than 1500 grams and born at less than 32 weeks of postconceptional age are at risk of developing ROP.[996–1016] The fundamental process underlying the development of ROP is incomplete vascularization of the retina, and the ophthalmoscopic findings stem from this arrested development. During normal retinal development, vessels migrate from the optic disc to the ora serrata, beginning at approximately 16 weeks of gestation. Vasculogenesis transforms precursor cells into capillary networks. Mature vessels differentiate from these networks and extend to the nasal ora serrata by 36 weeks of gestation and to the temporal ora serrata by 39–41 weeks. The location of the interruption of normal vasculogenesis is related to the time of premature birth. The clinical appearance of the various stages of ROP is related to the location of the vascular–avascular junction.

For the purposes of defining the location and extent of the retinopathy the International Classification of ROP divides the fundus into two circular and one crescentic zones centered on the optic disc: zone I (posterior pole or inner zone) is a circular zone, the radius of which subtends an angle of 30° from the optic disc (the radius of the circle is equal to twice the distance of the foveal center from the disc edge). As a practical approach for the clinician, the approximate temporal extent of zone I can be determined by using a 25- or 28-D condensing lens. By placing the nasal edge of the optic disc at one edge of the field of view, the limit of zone I is at the temporal field of view. Zone II extends from the edge of zone I to a point tangential to the nasal ora serrata. Zone III is the residual temporal crescent of retina anterior to zone II.[1017] The extent of the disease is specified as 30° hours of the clock. The stages of abnormal retinal vascular response are as follows: stage 1 of this disease is associated with a flat circumferential white retinal demarcation line caused by proliferating primitive vascular endothelial spindle cells at the junction of the vascularized and the nonvascularized retina. Stage 2 is associated with widening and elevation of the demarcation line into a ridge of tissue anterior to the plane of the retina (Figures 6.65 and 6.66A–C). The ridge may change from white to pink as retinal vessels leave the plane of the retina to enter it. Multiple isolated polypoid neovascular tufts ("popcorn") may occur near the posterior edge of the ridge and occasionally in the posterior fundus (Figure 6.65).[1004,1018] These neovascular tufts are not considered part of the fibrovascular growth required for stage 3. Microscopically the ridge anteriorly is composed primarily of retinal astrocyte precursors that stimulate the proliferation of mature endothelial cells into a capillary network (Figure 6.65J and K).[1019,1020] Stage 3 is associated with extraretinal fibrovascular proliferation: (1) continuous with the posterior aspect of the ridge, often causing a ragged appearance of the ridge; (2) immediately posterior to the ridge but not always connected to it; or (3) extending into the vitreous perpendicular to the retinal plane. In some patients the fibrovascular proliferation begins nasally.[1021] "Plus" disease is used to designate a more severe form of each stage of ROP. When any of the stages of the peripheral retinal vascular changes are accompanied by evidence of progressive vascular incompetence, including dilation of the posterior retinal veins, tortuosity of the retinal arteries, iris vascular engorgement, pupillary rigidity, and vitreous haze, a plus sign is added to the stage.[1011,1022] This definition was further refined to be made only when sufficient vascular dilatation and tortuosity were present in at least two quadrants of the posterior fundus.[1023] Stage 4 designates a subtotal retinal detachment, either exudative or tractional. Stage 4A is used for extrafoveal detachments and 4B for detachments involving the fovea. Stage 5 is associated with a total funnel-shaped retinal detachment (Figure 6.67A–F).

6.65 Retinopathy of prematurity (ROP).

A–C: Premature infant with stage 2 ROP. Arrows indicate neovascular tufts ("popcorn") along the posterior edge of the neovascular ridge.

D–I: Stage 2 ROP in a premature infant. Note the dilated retinal veins and the multiple round neovascular tufts ("popcorn") (arrows, D–I) posterior to the neovascular ridge and on the optic disc (F).

J and **K**: Histopathology of stage 2 ROP showing the anterior zone of proliferation of primitive mesenchymal cells in the nonvascularized retina (arrow, J) and the intraretinal and preretinal neovascular tissue comprising the ridge (arrowheads, J) posterior to the avascular zone. The arrow in K indicates a neovascular tuft ("popcorn") arising from the vascularized retina posterior to the ridge.

(A–I, from Garoon et al.[1018])

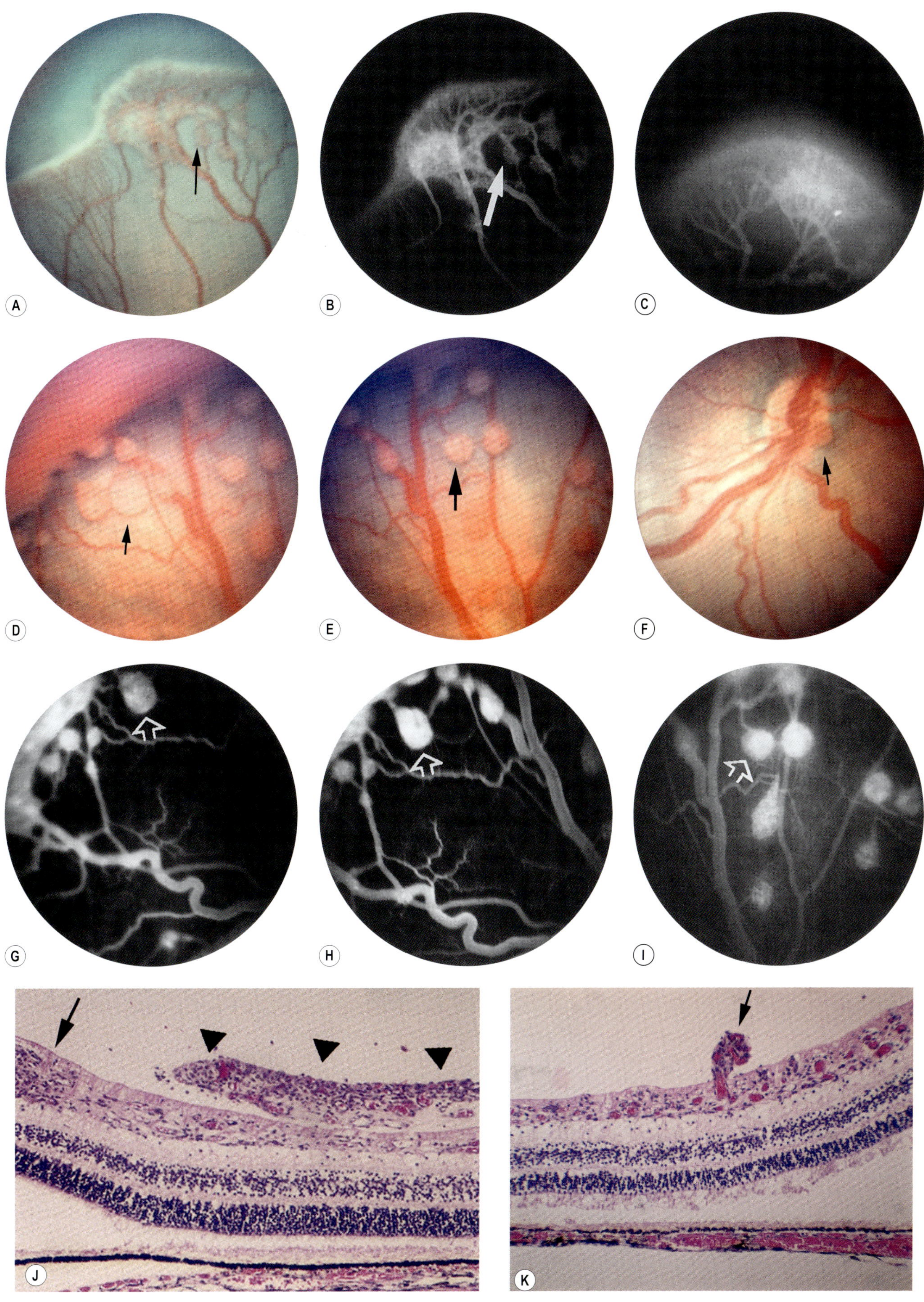
A
B
C
D
E
F
G
H
I
J
K

An uncommon, rapidly progressing, severe form of ROP is designated aggressive posterior ROP. If untreated, it usually progresses to retinal detachment, often without moving sequentially through the classic stages 1–3. The characteristic features of this type of ROP are its posterior location, anterior-segment vascular congestion, prominence of plus disease out of proportion to the peripheral retinopathy, and the ill-defined nature of the retinopathy.[1023] Most infants with ROP show partial or almost complete regression of the retinopathy without treatment. Typically, by 45 weeks of postconceptional age, the demarcation line and ridge may atrophy and disappear as retinal vascular migration into the peripheral avascular zone resumes. Nearly all patients with stage 1 and 2 ROP undergo complete resolution.[999] Less severe changes that may accompany the mild cicatricial disease (stage 3) include myopia; amblyopia; strabismus; retinal pigmentation; vitreous membranes; and equatorial folds at the junction of a vascularized and avascular retina[1008,1017,1024]; straightening of the retinal blood vessels in the temporal arcade, with decrease in the angle of insertion of the temporal arcades into the optic disc; dragging of the retina and macular displacement, usually in a temporal direction (Figures 6.66A, B, D, and H and 6.67K); and retinal neovascularization occurring near the equator (Figure 6.66I–L).[1025–1027] Amblyopia may be caused in part by arrest of the normal postnatal development of the central macula,[1008,1028,1029] occult hyperoxemic retinal necrosis,[1030] and progressive RPE and retinal atrophy.[1031,1032] Peripheral fundus changes include incomplete vascularization of the peripheral retina; abnormal, nondichotomous branching of retinal vessels; vascular arcades with circumferential interconnecting telangiectatic vessels (Figure 6.67I); retinal pigmentary changes; vitreoretinal interface changes; falciform retinal folds (Figure 6.67K; vitreous membranes with or without attachment to retina (Figure 6.67G and J); latticelike degeneration; irregular retinal breaks; posterior displacement of the vitreous base; and exudative, tractional, and rhegmatogenous retinal detachment. Pseudoexotropia usually accompanies the ectopia of the macula (Figure 6.66G).[1025]

Patients with mild to moderate degrees of cicatricial ROP may later in life develop rhegmatogenous, tractional, and exudative retinal detachment as well as pseudoangiomatous masses (Figure 6.67G).[1011,1020,1028,1033–1038] The exudative changes may resemble those seen in Coats' syndrome caused by congenital retinal telangiectasis, angiomatosis retinae, and FEVR (Figures 6.66L and 6.67I).[1039] Interestingly, patients with a history of premature birth often show a significantly smaller FAZ[63] and absence of a normal foveal contour. These changes likely represent developmental arrest of the normal centripetal migration of retinal ganglion and inner nuclear cells. They appear to be independent of refractive error or retinal ablative treatment and may be compatible with excellent visual acuity.[1040]

Other diseases that must be included in the differential diagnosis are FEVR, incontinentia pigmenti, sickle-cell retinopathy, Eales' disease, diabetic retinopathy, and the ectodermal dysplasia, ectrodactyly, and clefting syndrome.[1041]

ROP has been reported in full-term infants,[513,996,998,1042] though these diagnoses may actually represent cases of FEVR.

While improvements in maternal antenatal and neonatal care have lowered the incidence of ROP, low birth weight and gestational age remain the most important risk factors. Exposure to ambient light in the nursery has been proven not be a risk factor.[1043]

The role of oxygen supplementation in ROP pathogenesis remains complex and controversial. Growing clinical experience suggests that lower, but narrowly contained, oxygen saturations (85–92%) early in postnatal life significantly lowered the incidence and severity of ROP.[1044,1045] Newer protocols for oxygen supplementation provide for age-directed target ranges, in which saturations are targeted to 85–92% until 34 weeks' postconception, and then raised to 92–100% after 34 weeks' postconceptional age.[1046]

The majority of premature infants will develop some ROP in at least one eye, and in most infants, the disease will regress spontaneously.[1047] Screening for ROP should be initiated no sooner than 31 weeks of postconceptional age or 4–6 weeks of chronological age, whichever is later.[1048]

The median onset of stage 1 ROP is 34 weeks' postconception, and the median age of ROP requiring treatment is approximately 36 weeks' postconception.[1048] Laser photocoagulation of the avascular retinal periphery, in a near-confluent pattern of spots, has been shown to reduce the chance of unfavorable visual and structural outcomes in infants with type I ROP. Type I ROP was defined as: (1) any stage of ROP with plus disease in zone 1; (2) stage III ROP in zone 1; (3) stage II or III ROP with plus disease in zone 2. Fluorescein angiography may be of value in demonstrating peripheral retinal vascular changes associated with cicatricial ROP and may reveal areas of retinal nonperfusion requiring laser ablation.[513,1003,1049]

6.66 Retinopathy of prematurity (ROP).

A–C: Dragging of the left macula and retinal vessels temporally in a premature infant. Compare A, before dragging, with B. Note the neovascular complex (C) at the equator temporally and the absence of retinal vessels beyond the complex.
D–F: ROP causing heterotopia of the right macula (D) and a retinal fold extending from the left optic disc to the temporal periphery (E and F). Note the absence of retinal vessels in the temporal retina (F).
G–K: Late mild cicatricial stage of ROP causing temporal dragging of the right macula and pseudoexotropia (G and H) in a 12-year-old girl whose visual acuity was 20/30. Note the evidence of occlusive retinal vascular disease at the equator temporally (I and J). Angiography showed a broad zone of retinal nonperfusion temporally and staining of the abnormal vascular arcades just posterior to this zone (K).
L: Late mild cicatricial ROP causing peripheral Coats' syndrome in a 38-year-old man whose birth weight was 2 lb (0.9 kg). Note the subretinal and intraretinal lipid exudate derived from peripheral intraretinal neovascularization.

(A–C, courtesy of Dr. John T. Flynn.)

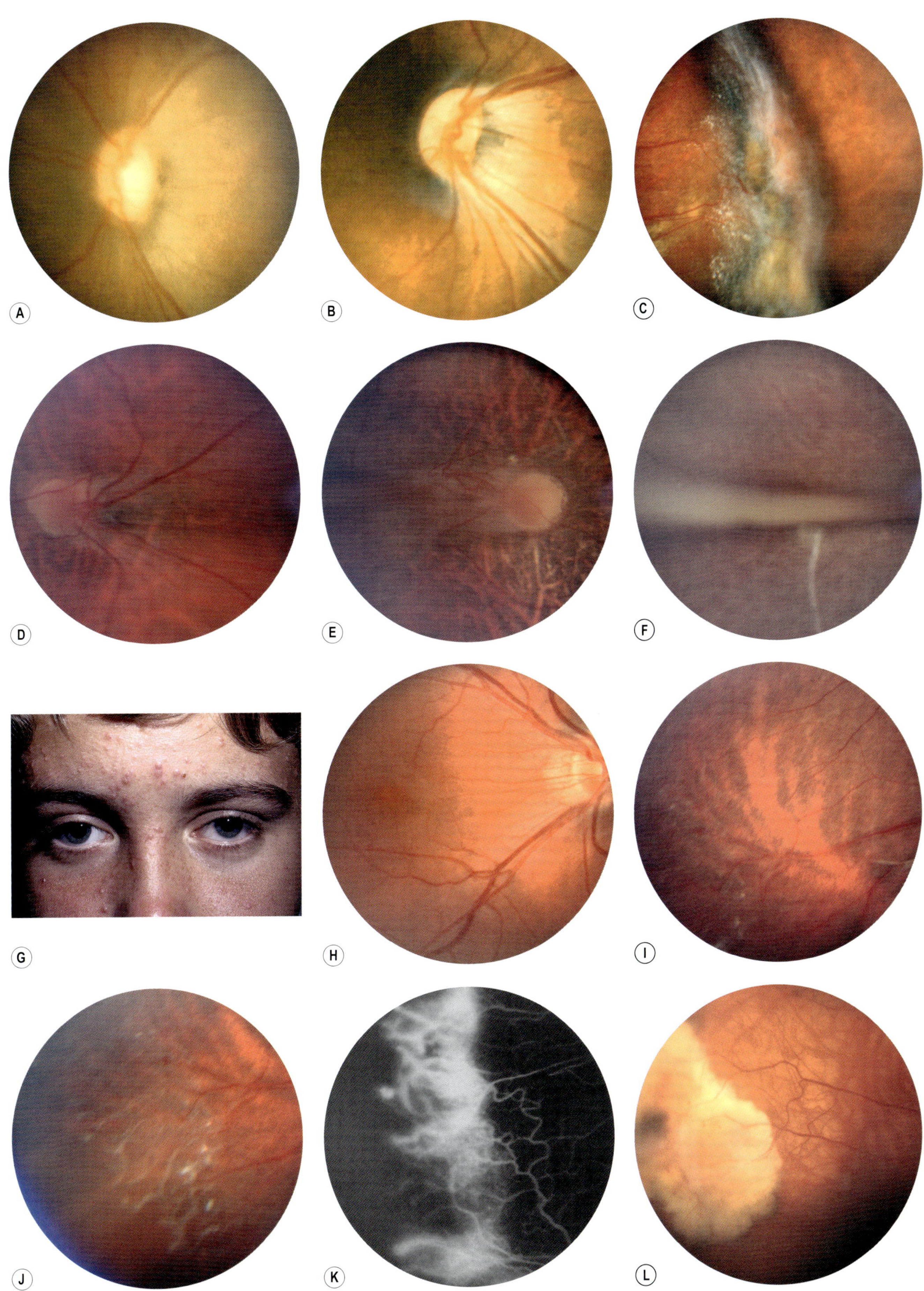
A
B
C
D
E
F
G
H
I
J
K
L

Converging lines of laboratory research and empiric clinical evidence support the rationale of targeted pharmacologic inhibition of VEGF as a treatment for advanced ROP. Intravitreal injection of bevacizumab (Avastin) has been shown to be highly effective in reducing vascular activity and eliminating retinal neovascularization, primarily in eyes with posterior disease and a guarded prognosis. It has been used successfully as rescue therapy following laser treatment, as an adjuvant to laser in eyes with impaired fundus visualization due to anterior-segment congestion, and as monotherapy.[1050]

Although retinal ablation is effective in most cases of advanced ROP, a significant number of these eyes progress to retinal detachment. Detachment is often seen associated with areas of incomplete peripheral ablation (skip areas) or in eyes with inexorably progressive, usually postequatorial disease. Contraction of neovascularization along the ridge and growth into the overlying vitreous precede tractional retinal detachment. Condensation of vitreous into sheets and strands acts as a scaffold for further extension of the fibrovascular tissue. Traction along the retinal surface and contraction of the posterior hyaloid face contribute to distortion of posterior-pole architecture. The configuration of the retinal detachment in ROP depends primarily on the location of the ridge and the orientation of vectors of vitreoretinal traction. Tractional forces are exerted by contraction of the posterior hyaloid as well as in the directional vectors intrinsic to the retina, from the ridge to the lens, transvitreally from ridge to ridge, from ridge to ciliary body, and extending from the disc stalk (Figure 6.66G–K). Some or all of the above components are present in ROP-related retinal detachments. The configuration of the detachment is determined by the relative force vector contribution of tractional component.[1051] Spontaneous reattachment of the retina in stages 4 and 5 rarely occurs.[1052]

6.67 Stages of retinopathy of prematurity (ROP).

A–F: Stages 1–5.

1. Abrupt end to the vessels, beyond which is avascular retina (A). 2. Demarcation line between vascularized and avascular retina (B). 3. Vascular growth over a ridge between vascular and avascular retina (C). 3 plus. Dilated and tortuous vessels posterior to the ridge, signifying plus disease (D). 4. Contraction of the ridge with localized traction detachment not involving the macula (E, arrow). 5. Traction retinal detachment involving the macula (F).

G and H: Coats'-like response and traction retinal detachment in an 8-year-old girl with ROP. Note the avascular retina temporally and the vascular alteration in the posterior pole on angiography (H).

I: Coats'-like response with lipid accumulation posterior to the ridge (I).

J: Contraction of the hyaloid where attached to the previous ridge. Note the extensive avascularity superiorly.

K: Adult ROP with dragging of the temporal retina into a falciform fold.

(Courtesy of Dr. Franco Recchia.)

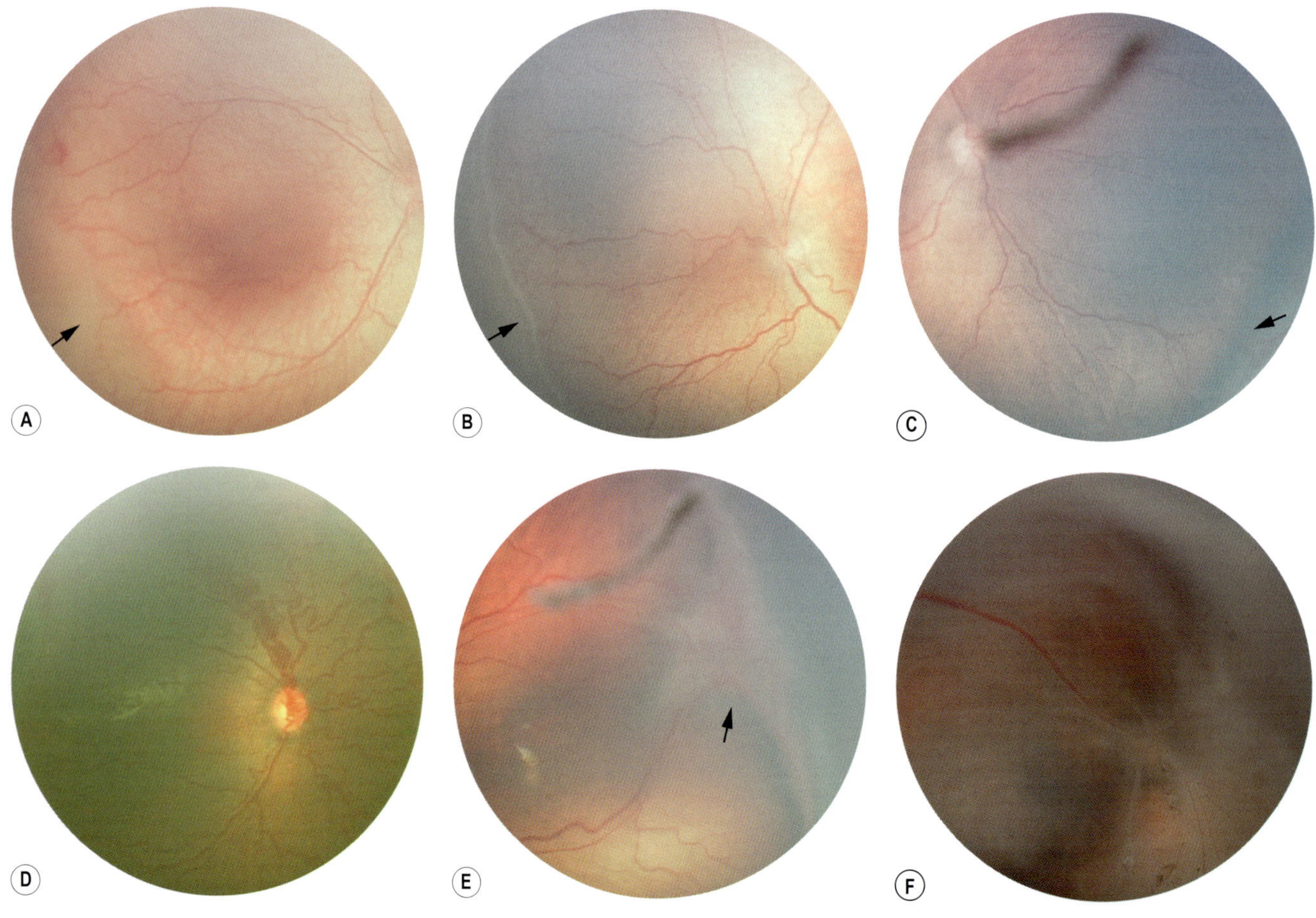

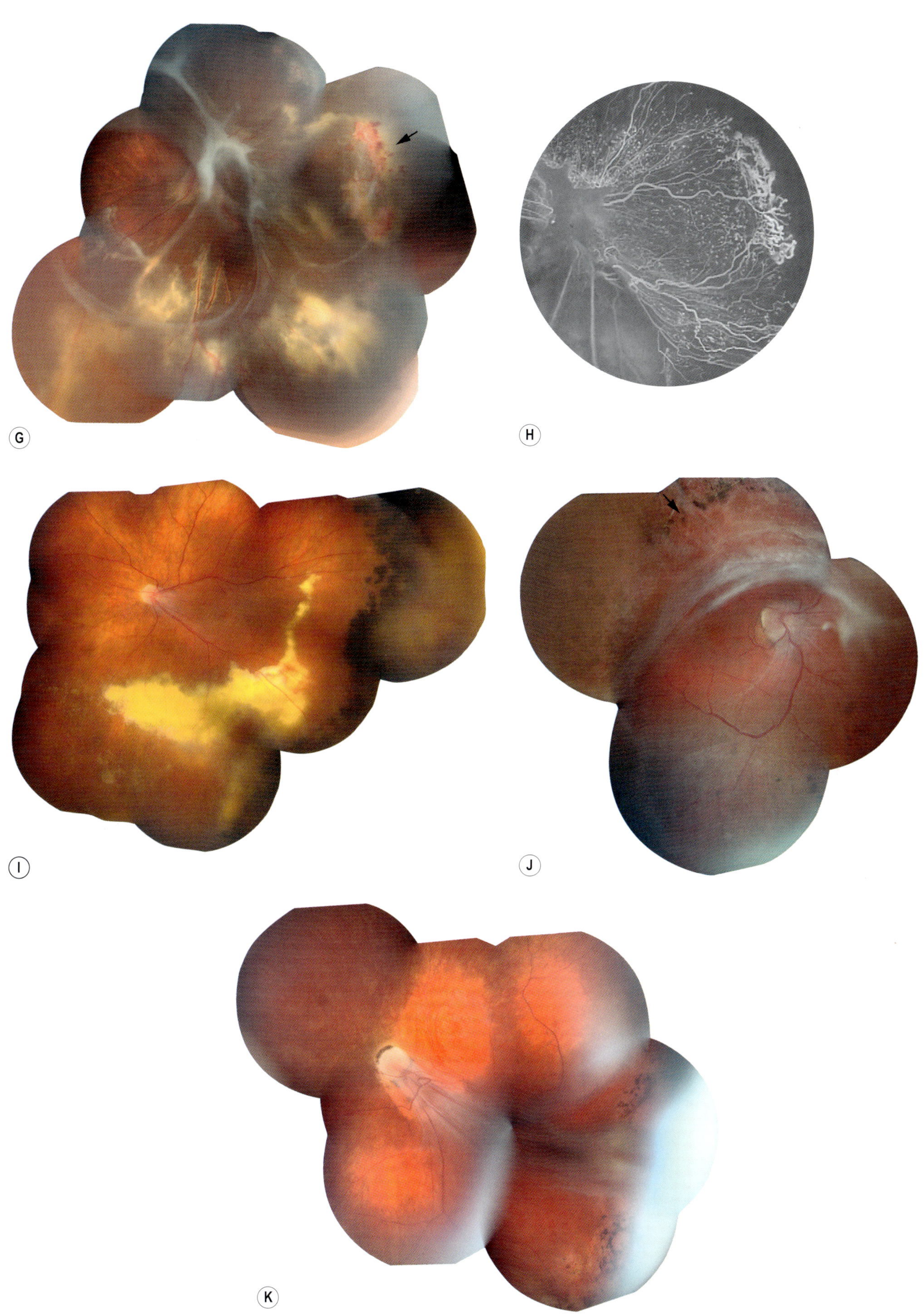
G
H
I
J
K

FAMILIAL EXUDATIVE VITREORETINOPATHY

FEVR is a hereditary ocular disorder first described by Criswick and Schepens in 1969. It can be inherited as an autosomal-dominant, recessive or X-linked trait with high penetrance and variable expressivity. It resembles ROP but occurs in patients with no history of prematurity or neonatal oxygen therapy.[1053–1068] In its earliest and mildest form, areas of peripheral retinal whitening without scleral depression, peripheral cystoid degeneration, vitreous band formation, vitreous traction, and minimal or no retinal vascular changes are present in the temporal periphery of otherwise normal eyes. Peripheral retinal avascularity, retinal neovascularization, disc neovascularization, fibrous proliferation, exudation, and localized retinal detachment in the area between the equator and ora serrata with traction and dragging of the major retinal vessels and macula in a temporal direction represent a moderately advanced stage of the disease (Figure 6.68B and C). These changes cause retinal and subretinal exudation (Coats' syndrome), vitreous traction, retinoschisis, retinal hole formation, falciform retinal folds, total retinal detachment, cataract, intraocular hemorrhage, and neovascular and angle closure glaucoma (Figure 6.68). Loss of central vision may be caused by heterotopia of the macula, retinal striae, cystoid retinal edema, epiretinal membrane, and retinal detachment.[1069] Pseudoexotropia caused by temporal dragging of the macula is frequently evident (Figure 6.68A and F). Fluorescein angiography shows areas of capillary nonperfusion anterior to the equator, dilated retinal vessels and retinal neovascularization, and dye leakage into the fibrovascular masses and from retinal capillaries elsewhere (Figure 6.68E).[1056,1070] Angiography of the temporal periphery may be helpful in diagnosing the mildest form of the disease.[1070,1071]

Three FEVR genes have been identified to date: *NDP* (MIM 300658, X-linked), *FZD4* (MIM 604579, dominant), and *LRP5* (MIM 603506, dominant and recessive).[1072–1080] Linkage analysis in one family suggests a gene locus either at Xq21.3 or at Xp11. It is of interest that the gene for Norrie disease, an X-linked disorder characterized by severe proliferative retinopathy, is also located at Xp11.[1081] The *NDP* gene codes for norrin protein that is also defective in Norrie's disease. The gene for autosomal-dominant FEVR has been mapped to the long arm of chromosome 11.[1082,1083] More than 50% of FEVR cases do not carry any of the mutations so far known; hence it is likely more genes will be identified in the future.

6.68 Familial exudative vitreoretinopathy.

A–F: This 25-year-old mother and 8-year-old child had pseudoexotropia caused by temporal dragging of the macula in both eyes (A–C, and F). Visual acuity in the mother was light perception in the right eye and 20/25 in the left eye. The retina in the right eye was totally detached by yellow exudates (B). Fibrovascular proliferative retinal changes occurred in the temporal periphery. In the left eye (C and D) there was peripheral retinal schisis with inner retinal holes (arrows, D). The son had temporal dragging of the macula, retinal proliferative changes, and exudation in the temporal periphery (E and F). His visual acuity was 20/20. Cryotherapy was successful in obliterating peripheral retinal vascular abnormalities. The visual function in both patients was unchanged 20 years later.

G–I: This 4-year-old child had fibrovascular changes in the inferotemporal and inferior periphery of the right eye (G and H) and inferior periphery of the left eye. The left eye in addition had an abnormally adherent vitreous band extending from nasal to the disc.

J and K: Histopathology of familial exudative vitreoretinopathy showing funnel-shaped exudative retinal detachment (H) and dense preretinal vitreous membranes (arrow, K) lying on the inner surface of a degenerated peripheral retina containing occluded blood vessels.

(G–I, courtesy of Dr. Franco Recchia.)

Histopathologic examination of eyes with advanced stages of the disease demonstrates total retinal detachment, peripheral retinal vascular proliferation, extensive preretinal fibrovascular membranes, intraretinal and subretinal exudation, and usually iris neovascularization and angle closure glaucoma (Figure 6.68K and L).[1054,1055,1084] Massive subretinal hemorrhage occurred in one case,[1054] and focal inflammation in the region of the peripheral fibrovascular retinal mass occurred in three eyes.[1054,1055,1084] The role of inflammation in the pathogenesis and progression of this disease is uncertain. Evidence of thrombocytopathy has been found in some, but not in other, families.[1057,1085,1086]

Unusual fibrovascular proliferation from the retina into the vitreous occurring in late intrauterine life or neonatally in FEVR is also a feature of incontinentia pigmenti (see next section), Norrie disease, a congenital X-linked recessive disorder in males who present either at birth or soon afterward with bilateral blindness and a white retrolental mass,[1081] and nonfamilial retinal vascular hypoplasia associated with persistence of the primary vitreous.[1087]

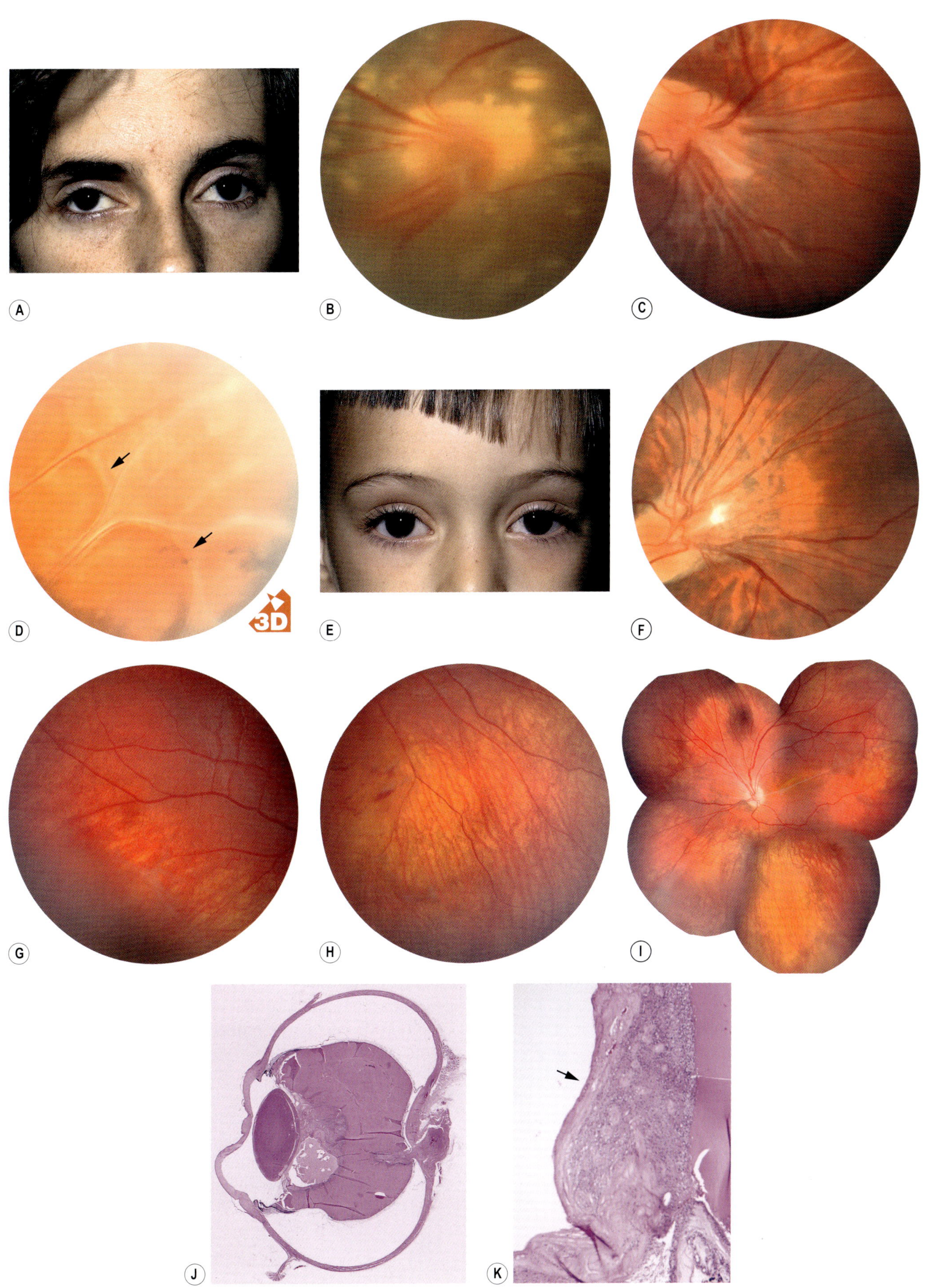
A
B
C
D
3D
E
F
G
H
I
J
K

INCONTINENTIA PIGMENTI

Incontinentia pigmenti (Bloch–Sulzberger syndrome) is an inherited generalized ectodermal dysplasia that often involves the eyes (35% of cases), hair, teeth, and central nervous system (30%) (Figures 6.69 and 6.70).[1041,1088–1110] It is usually inherited as an X-linked dominant trait that is lethal in males. Ocular and dermatologic findings of incontinentia pigmenti may occur in males with Klinefelter karyotype 47,XXY[1093] or from genetic mosaicism.[1111,1112] A less common form of the disease (Naegeli type) probably has a dominant mode of inheritance, affects both sexes, and is without ocular malformation.[1094] Incontinentia pigmenti achromians is a closely related syndrome that also occurs in both sexes (see Figure 5.69). The skin, particularly of the extremities and trunk in patients with incontinentia pigmenti, is involved at birth or soon afterward with bullous, erythematous lesions that may progress to the verrucous stage (Figure 6.69A) and may further progress to the flat pigmented lesions that are arranged in whorls and splotches (Figure 6.70I), as well as in a linear fashion around the ribcage (nevus lines of Blaschko) (Figure 6.69B, C, E, and J). The pigmentation may fade and disappear in later years. Alopecia, nail changes, and dental hypoplasia are frequent (Figures 6.69D and 6.70H). Central nervous system disorders include seizures, spastic paralysis, mental retardation, and occasionally rapidly progressing neonatal cerebral ischemia.[1095] Ocular abnormalities that are frequently unilateral or asymmetric include strabismus, cataract, myopia, nystagmus, blue sclera, corneal opacities, conjunctival pigmentation, diffuse mottled pigmentary change in the fundus[1113] (Figure 6.69F), patches of chorioretinal atrophy, retinal vascular anomalies, peripheral retinal nonperfusion, preretinal neovascularization, infantile retinal detachment, optic atrophy, retinal dysplasia, foveal hypoplasia, pseudoglioma (Figure 6.69C), and phthisis bulbi. Progression from only mild retinal involvement neonatally to total retinal detachment and blindness may occur within 3 or 4 months after birth.[1090] Abnormalities of the peripheral retinal vasculature near the temporal equator include vascular dilation, arteriovenous anastomosis, preretinal fibrous proliferation, vascular proliferation, exudation, and absence of the retinal vessels peripheral to these changes (Figures 6.69H and I and 6.70A–G, J–L).[1097–1099,1102,1103,1109,1114] Spontaneous reattachment of the retina can occur at times (Figure 6.70F).[1112] These changes simulate those in ROP, FEVR, sickle-cell disease, and Eales' disease. Abnormalities of the retinal vessels in the posterior fundus occur less frequently[1097]; abnormal vasculature of the FAZ,[1115,1116] dragging of the retinal vessels and heterotopia of the macula and retinal folds may occur (Figure 6.69J–L). Whereas there is a predilection for the retinal vascular changes to involve the periphery, the posterior pole may be affected by similar findings.[1090,1093,1097,9] Patchy variegated and whorl-like pigmentary changes in the fundus, similar to those of the skin, may occur (Figure 6.69F).[1092,1100]

The pathogenesis of the fundus changes is uncertain; the similarity of the pathology to ROP suggests a congenital defect in the development of the retinal vasculature. On the other hand, the retinal vascular and fibroproliferative changes may be secondary to a primary abnormality of the RPE.[1105,1109] Nishimura and associates[1102] observed the progressive development of avascular areas in the peripheral retina of a full-term newborn during the first month and a half of life (Figure 6.69H and I). This was much more severe in one eye than in the other and was accompanied by ischemia, a cherry-red spot, and optic atrophy in the more severely affected eye. They believed that proliferative retinopathy was caused by progressive postnatal vascular obstruction and postulated that the circulatory impairment may also involve the choroid, optic nerve, and other tissues in the body. A similar case of extreme retinal avascularity with vasculature limited to approximately 1.5 disc diameters on either side of the optic disc has been noted in the left eye of a 26-day-old infant by Meallet et al.[1117] and in a newborn by Chao et al.[1118] Some authors have demonstrated what they interpreted as a favorable effect of photocoagulation and cryotherapy in the treatment of proliferative retinopathy (Figure 6.69H and I).[1102,1103,1109,1119] Other authors have reported less favorable results.[1120]

6.69 Incontinentia pigmenti.

A: Bullous and verrucous lesions on the foot of a female infant with incontinentia pigmenti.

B: Linear arrangement of pigmented skin lesions around the rib cage (nevus lines of Blaschko).

C and D: Pseudoglioma in the right eye and pigmented skin lesion in the armpit of this 10-year-old girl who had dental hypoplasia (D).

E–G: Blotchy pigmentation of the legs and fundi in a young girl with optic disc anomalies, peculiar radiating lines or folds, and subretinal lesions in the macular areas (G).

H and I: Angiogram (H) showing peripheral retinal vascular proliferation and shunts at the posterior edge of the zone of retinal vascular nonperfusion before photocoagulation. Composite fundus photograph (I) shows same area after photocoagulation.

J–L: Infant girl with typical pigmented lesions around the trunk (J), dragging of the macula (arrow, K and L), and a retinal fold. Cryotherapy was used to treat proliferative retinal vascular changes (not shown) in the peripheral fundus. She was delivered after a full-term pregnancy and did not receive supplemental oxygen after delivery.

(F and G, from McCrary and Smith[1100], H and I, from Nishimura et al.[1102])

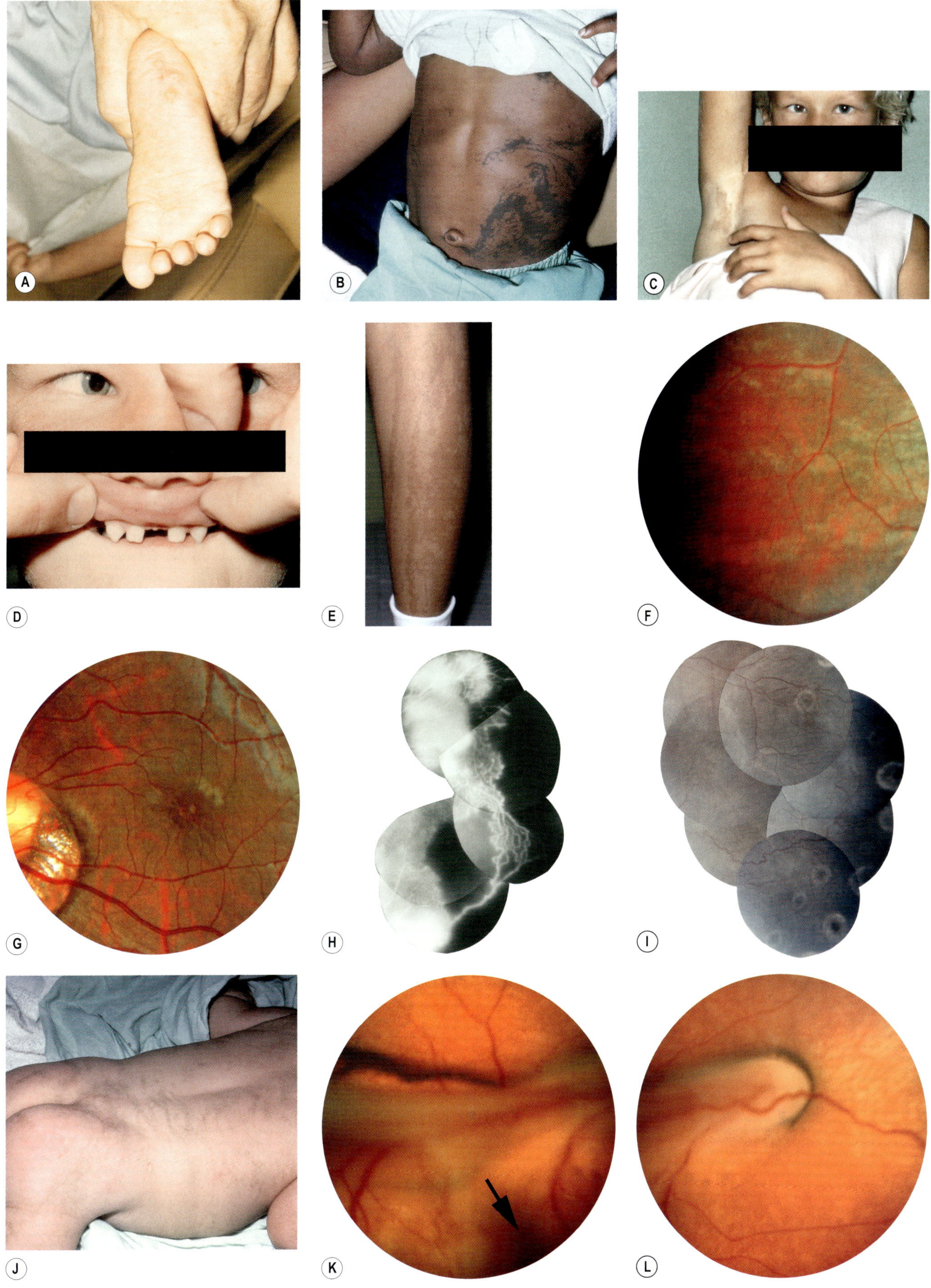
A
B
C
D
E
F
G
H
I
J
K
L

Mutations in the inhibitor of kappa light polypeptide gene enhancer in B cells, kinase gamma, *IKBKG* (GenBank NM_003639.3; MIM# 300248), also called nuclear factor kappaB (NF-κB) essential modulator (*NEMO/IKKgamma*) at the Xq28 location, is responsible for incontinentia pigmenti in about 80% of patients.[1121] Mutation in this gene leads to activation of eotaxin, an eosinophil chemokine. Accumulation of eosinophils in tissue, and in or around blood vessels, results in skin vesicles and vaso-occlusive findings in the eye and brain.[1113] The mutation may occur de novo or may be transmitted in an X-linked dominant fashion.

6.70 Incontinentia pigmenti.

A–I: This 40-year-old youngest of five siblings with no family history of eye or systemic disease was found to have anomalous vessels in the right eye (A). She was a moderate myope with corrected vision to 20/20 in each eye. The temporal and inferotemporal retina showed peripheral nonperfusion with pigmentary changes suggesting spontaneous reattachment of a detached retina (B–D). Angiogram confirmed peripheral avascularity (E and F). The left fundus had a normal vascular pattern. She had small vitiliginous patches on her skin similar to her father. Nail (H) and skin changes of incontinentia pigmenti were seen over her forearms and thighs (I). She gave a history of having blisters over her body and scalp as a neonate. Two older brothers and sisters and mother were unaffected, indicating the possibility of de novo mutation in her.

J–L: This 52-year-old white female presented with vitreous hemorrhage in the left eye. She had a past history of vitreous hemorrhage in the right eye requiring laser photocoagulation approximately 6 years previously. The posterior pole was normal. The temporal periphery showed laser scars with sheathing of the retinal vessels and absent vessels anterior to the laser scar. Far periphery of the left eye showed peripheral nonperfusion and ghost-like proliferative vessels, some intraretinally and some growing into vitreous at the junction of the perfused and nonperfused retina (J and K). Fluorescein angiogram of the periphery showed dilated collaterals and capillary bed corresponding to the ghost-like vessels seen on the color photographs (L). The retinal vessels were short in other areas of the periphery. She had skin lesions typical of incontinentia pigmenti with whorl-like defects.

(J–L, courtesy of Dr. William Mieler.)

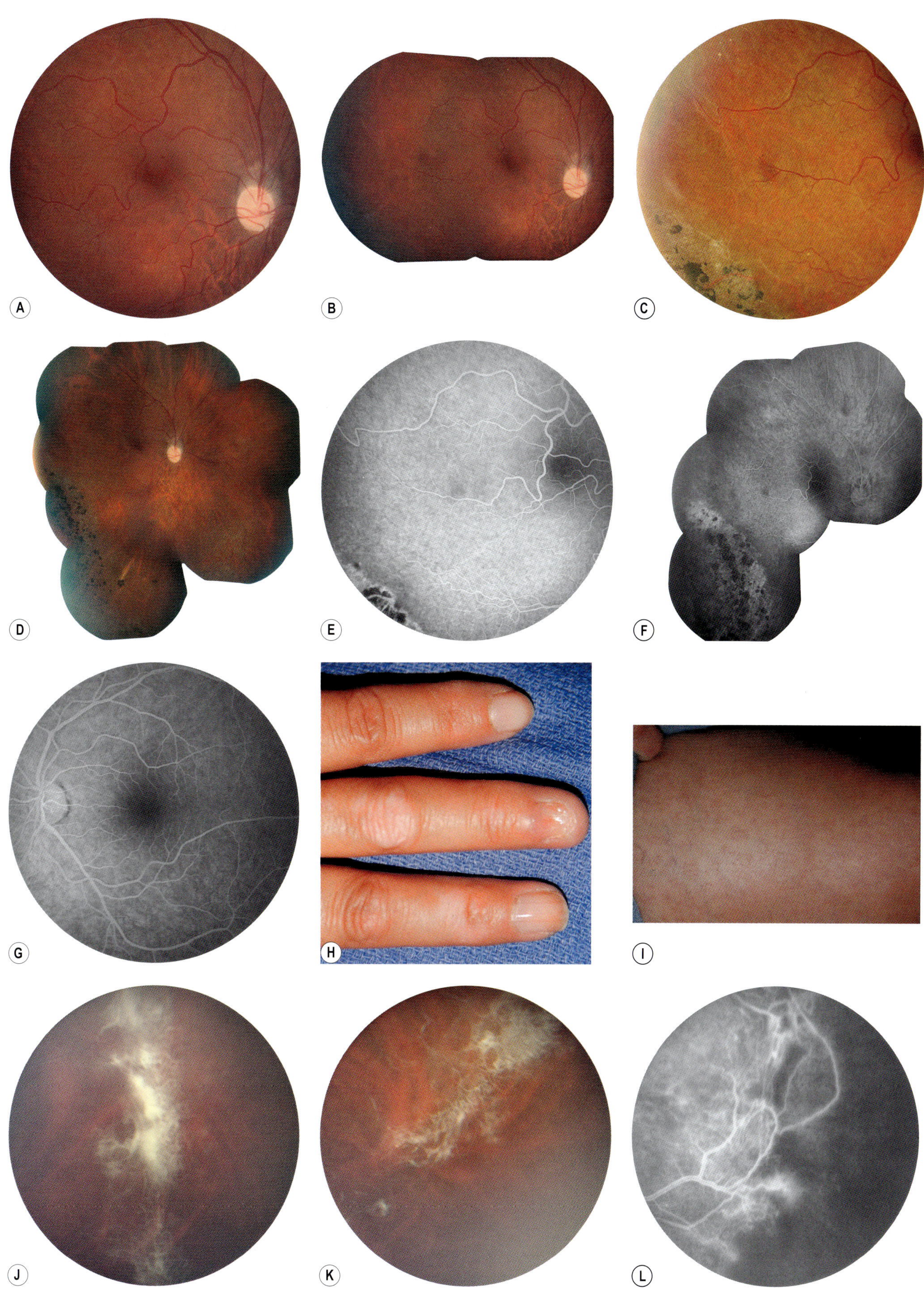
A
B
C
D
E
F
G
H
I
J
K
L

Dystroglycanopathies (Muscle–Eye–Brain Disease)

Dystroglycanopathies are a group of genetic disorders that involve both central (brain and eye) and peripheral nervous system (skeletal muscle) caused by underglycosylation of alpha-dystroglycan with O-linked carbohydrates. Alpha-dystroglycan is a 156-kDa peripheral transmembrane protein that undergoes multiple glycosylation steps to interact with extracellular matrix proteins such as laminin, neurexin, and perlecan.[1122] So far, mutations in six different genes – *POMT1, POMT2, POMGnT1, Fukutin (FKTN), FKRP*, and *LARGE* – have been recognized.[1123] There is considerable phenotypic variation in the clinical syndromes with a wide spectrum of clinical findings in each – Walker–Warburg syndrme, muscle-eye-brain disease, Fukuyama congenital muscular dystrophy, congenital muscular dystrophy types 1D and 1C, and limb girdle muscular dystrophy variants, LGMD2I, LGMD2L, and LGMD2N.[1124]

The clinical findings of hypotonia, muscle weakness, contractures, seizures, hyporeflexia, and mental retardation coupled with elevated serum creatine kinase activity guide the diagnosis of dystroglycanopathy. The group of disorders is characterized by variable involvement and severity of cerebral cobblestone lissencephaly (agyria, pachygyria, or polymicrogyria), cerebellar, pons or brainstem hypoplasia, absent corpus callosum, hydrocephaly, muscular dystrophy, eye involvement including myopia, retinal detachment, abnormal retinal vasculature, anterior-chamber abnormalities, microphthalmia, and persistent hyaloid system.[1122,1125–1128]

6.71 Muscle–eye–brain (MEB) disease.

A–F: This 2-month-old presented with poor fixation in both eyes and was found to have microphthalmia and retinal detachment in the right eye and abnormal foveal reflex in the left eye. She was born at full term by cesarean section, and was noted to have hip dysplasia. There were no skin lesions. Computed tomography scan showed enlarged lateral ventricles and thin corpus callosum. The right retina was dysplastic with peripheral avascularity in the superior quadrant and exudative retinal detachment (A and B). The left retina was also hypoplastic but attached (C). A fluorescein angiogram of the right eye confirmed the peripheral nonperfusion on the right and anomalous vascular pattern in the left (D–F). Further delay in milestones, hypotonia, floppy muscles, and elevated creatine kinase (CK) levels prompted testing for MEB disease that returned positive for heterozygous mutation in *POMGnT1* gene. The exudative retinal detachment in the right eye settled over 2 years, leaving a fold in the posterior pole in her right eye. The left eye underwent peripheral scatter ablation to areas of nonperfusion. Both retinas remained unchanged at age 4.

(Courtesy of Dr. Franco Recchia.)

Muscle–eye–brain (*POMGnT1*) has more ocular involvement involving both anterior and posterior segments, including microphthalmos, glaucoma, myopia, coloboma, secondary cataracts, retinal hypoplasia resulting in peripheral avascularity similar to ROP (Figure 6.71D and E), exudative (Figure 6.71A and B) or secondary tractional retinal detachment and optic nerve hypoplasia.[1125,1126,1129–1132]

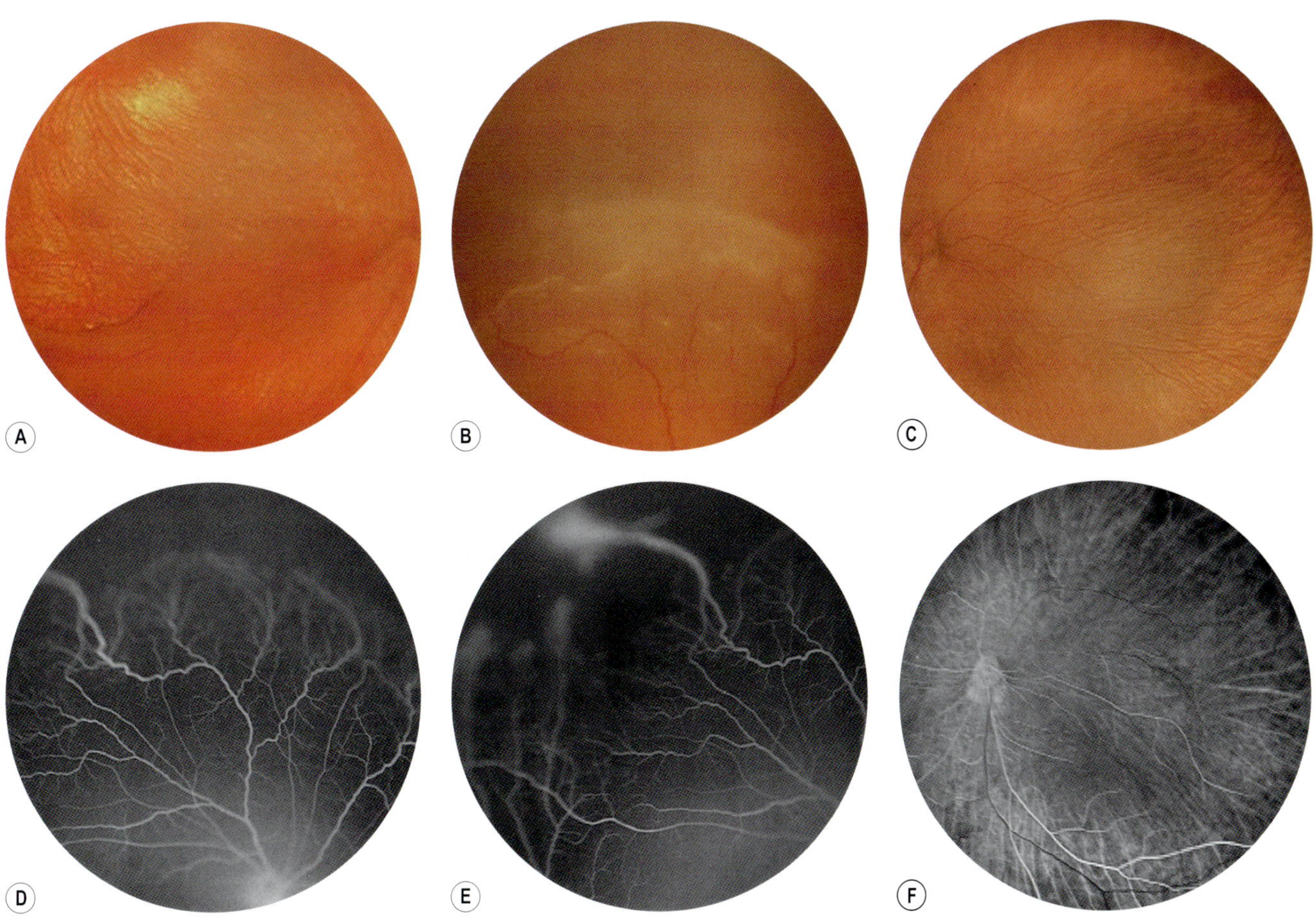
A
B
C
D
E
F

DYSKERATOSIS CONGENITA

Dyskeratosis congenita is a multisystem disorder that is caused by defects in telomere maintenance. Telomeres are complex DNA protein structures that protect chromosome ends from degradation and inappropriate recombination. Telomeres shorten with each cell division, and when they become critically short a DNA damage response is activated, causing cell cycle arrest and cell death. Shelterin, a complex of six proteins, binds to telomeric DNA and protects it. Telomerase enzyme synthesizes telomeric repeat sequences on to telomere ends. It is inherited as an autosomal-dominant, X-linked recessive, or sporadically by de novo gene mutations. In the X-linked form, mutation occurs at the Xq28 locus, resulting in dysfunction of dyskerin, a protein in the telomerase complex.[1133] The dominant form is caused by mutations in the other components of the enzyme telomerase, such as the telomerase RNA, TERC, and a reverse transcriptase TERT.[1134]

Poor telomere function affects cells with high turnover such as the epithelium, bone marrow, skin, and nails, resulting in multisystem manifestation. The disease was first described with a triad affecting nails, skin pigmentation, and mucosal leukoplakia more than 100 years ago. Bone marrow failure, premature aging, pulmonary fibrosis, and malignancy are serious manifestations. Pancytopenia, short, ridged fingernails, and patchy skin hypopigmentation are hallmarks of this condition. Ocular findings may include epiphora due to tear duct obstruction, dilated conjunctival blood vessels, corneal limbal stem cell failure, corneal vasculopathy, dry eyes, conjunctivitis, blepharitis, loss of eyelashes, microphthalmia, strabismus, and cataract.[1135] Retinal changes are rare but can include retinal hemorrhages, nerve fiber layer infarction, narrowing of the retinal vessels, preretinal fibrosis, and optic atrophy. Retinal vasculopathy in the form of aneurysm formation with leakage resembling Coats' disease is seen.[1136] Occasionally, progressive peripheral vaso-occlusive retinopathy occurs (Figure 6.72).[1137]

Other systemic features that have been recognized include premature graying of hair, premature tooth loss, enteropathy with malabsorption, immune deficiency, esophageal stricture, cardiomyopathy, liver cirrhosis, osteoporosis, and avascular necrosis of the bone, urinary tract abnormalities, testicular atrophy, mental retardation, intracranial calcifications, and cerebellar hypoplasia with ataxia. They have a predisposition to develop malignancies such as secondary acute myeloid leukemia, myelodysplasia, head and neck cancers, and esophageal cancers. More than one cancer may occur in an individual.[1138,1139] All features are not present in childhood; many develop over time.

The Nobel Prize in medicine was awarded to Elizabeth H. Blackburn, Carol W. Greider, and Jack W. Szostak in 2009 for the discovery of how chromosomes are protected by telomeres and the enzyme telomerase.

6.72 Dyskeratosis congenita.

A–L: A 20-year-old male was the proband with 20/20 vision in the right eye and 20/200 in the left eye. He was known to have interstitial lung disease, and had a biopsy of his lung, liver, and bone marrow. His father's diagnosis was established 10 years previously and a sister had died in her early 20s from renal failure. His platelet count was 19000 cells/μl, total white count 2500 cells/μl, hemoglobin 13.1 g/dl, with elevated liver enzymes and bilirubin. Blood urea nitrogen and creatinine were normal. The right fundus was normal; telangiectatic changes were seen in the left macula (A and B). In addition to dilated and leaking capillaries and aneurysms in the left macula, angiogram showed peripheral nonperfusion which was worse on the left compared to the right, and mild foveal capillary leakage on the right (C–G). The left fovea was thickened on optical coherence tomography. His 47-year-old father had 20/20 vision in both eyes, and showed mild foveal telangiectasia (I and J) that leaked very minimally on the angiogram (K and L). He had pulmonary fibrosis and peripheral edema. Another sister and two nieces of the proband were also positive, in addition to the proband and his father, for the *TERC* gene mutation. The family clearly depicts genetic anticipation; the father was less severely affected compared to the son (proband) and a daughter who died in her early 20s.

(From Johnson et al.,[1137] with permission. A, B, E, and G, Also, Yannuzzi, Lawrence J., The Retinal Atlas, Saunders 2010, 978-0-7020-3320-9, p.45.)

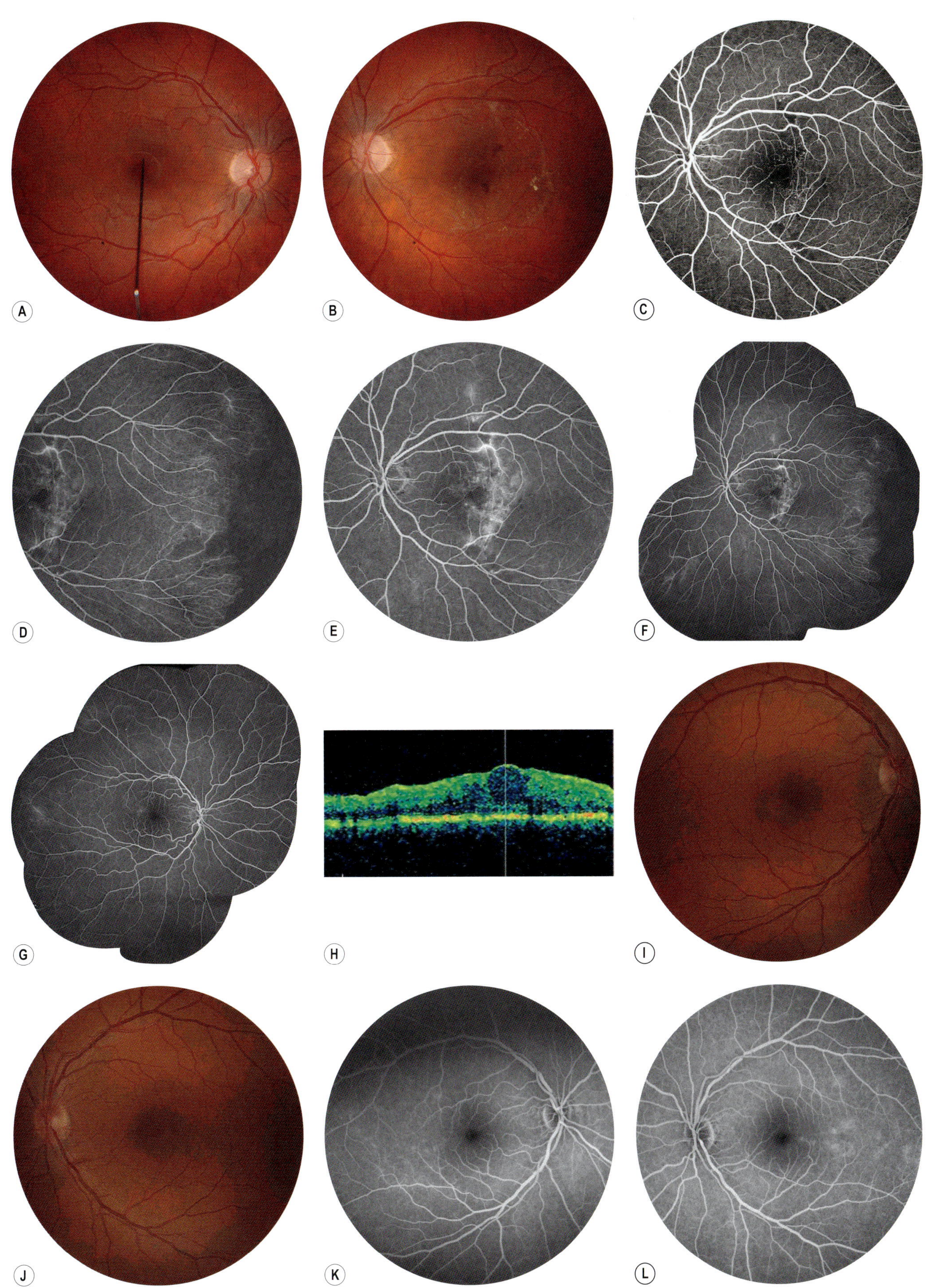
A
B
C
D
E
F
G
H
I
J
K
L

RETINAL VENOUS OBSTRUCTIVE DISEASES

In the end-artery vascular system found in the retina, obstruction of a retinal vein causes elevation of the venous and intracapillary pressure and a slowing of arterial blood flow in the area drained by the vein. The visual defects and retinal damage produced by venous obstruction depend primarily on the rapidity of its development, the degree of obstruction, and the availability of collateral pathways of venous outflow. If the degree of obstruction is mild, capillary endothelial damage is minimal and leakage of serous exudation and extravasation of erythrocytes into the retina may be unassociated with significant ischemic damage to the retina (Figures 6.73A and 6.74A–D). Complete resolution of the fundus changes and return of retinal function may occur following venous recanalization and the establishment of collateral venous channels.[1140] With moderate venous obstruction, the degree of retinal hemorrhage, exudation, and ischemia is greater. Following restoration of normal venous pressure, the retina may remain edematous secondary to prolonged or permanent damage to the retinal capillary endothelium (secondary retinal telangiectasis). If the degree of venous obstruction is great, hemorrhagic infarction of the retina causes extensive loss of the retinal capillary bed and postischemic cystoid degenerative and atrophic changes that remain after restoration of normal venous pressure (Figures 6.73B–D and 6.74G–L). The presence of retinal arterial insufficiency enhances the likelihood of venous obstruction and increases the retinal damage caused by the venous obstruction. There is little clinical or experimental evidence, however, to support the view that some degree of arterial insufficiency is necessary for venous obstruction to produce retinal hemorrhages.[336,1141–1149] There is color Doppler imaging evidence to suggest that diffuse small-vessel disease and reduced blood velocity may be important in the pathogenesis of central retinal vein obstruction in some patients.[1150,1151]

6.73 Histopathology of retinal vein obstruction.

A: Mild venous obstruction with intraretinal extravasation of erythrocytes and maintenance of relatively normal retinal architecture in a hypertensive patient with evidence of arteriolar sclerosis (arrow).
B: Severe venous obstruction with hemorrhagic infarction of the inner retina.
C: Cystic degeneration of the retina many months after severe venous obstruction.
D: Cystic degeneration of the retina and macular hole formation after severe central retinal vein occlusion.
E: Macular schisis, exudative retinopathy, retinal degeneration, and epiretinal membrane and pucker secondary to severe central retinal vein occlusion and rubeotic glaucoma. Note the lipid-laden macrophages (arrow) in Henle's layer.

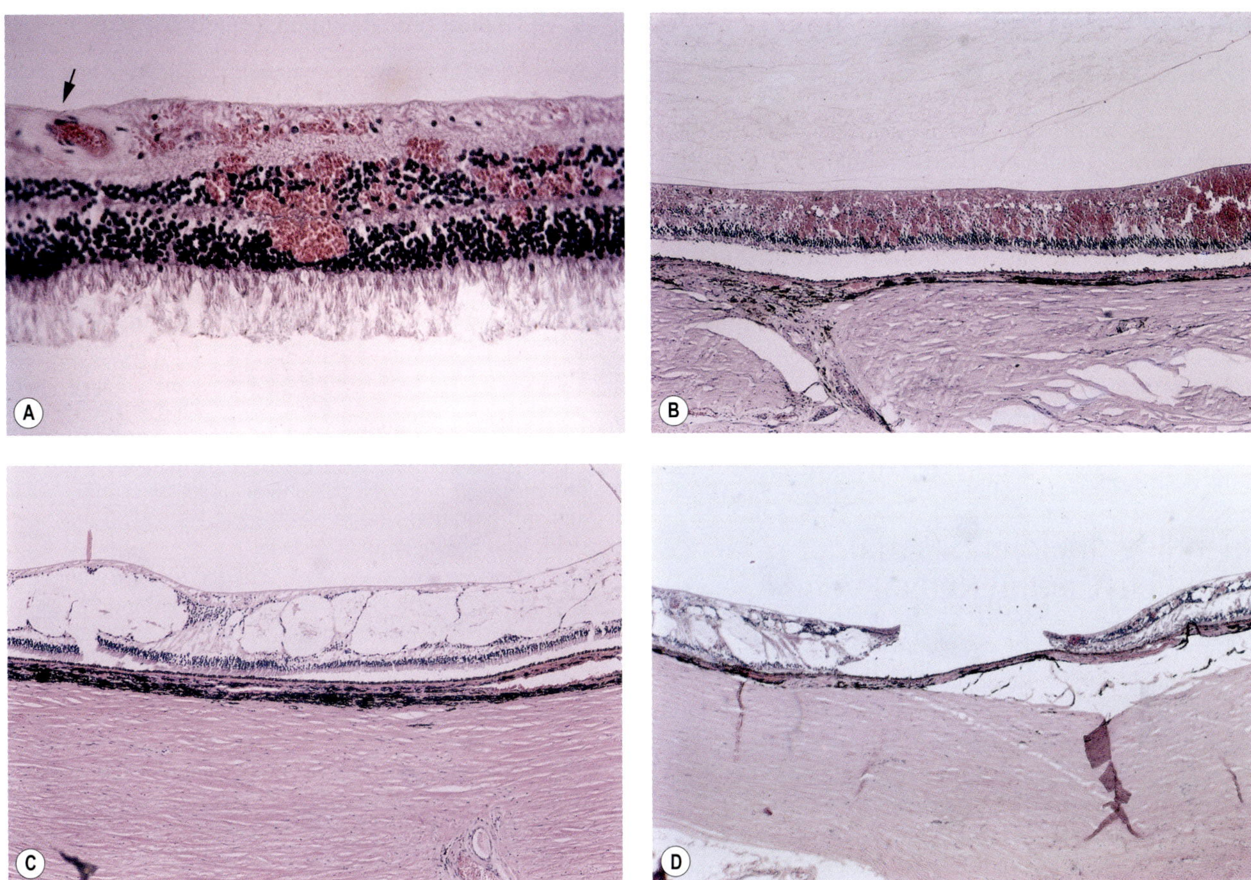
A
B
C
D

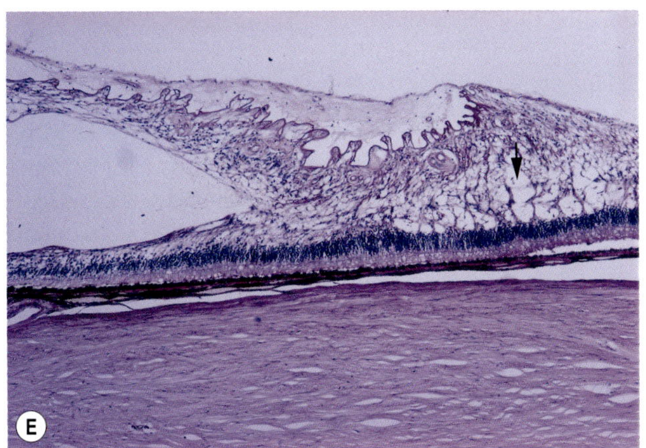
E

CENTRAL RETINAL VENOUS OBSTRUCTION

Various terms have been used to describe the severity of retinopathy associated with central retinal venous obstruction (Figures 6.73 and 6.74).[1152–1166] None is completely satisfactory. The clinical terms used to describe the ocular fundus reflect the degree of obstruction of the entire venous outflow from the retina (central retinal vein plus collateral vessels) and not just the central retinal vein alone. A patient may have complete anatomic obstruction of the central retinal vein at the level of the lamina cribrosa, with well-developed collateral venous channels, and manifest only minimal fundoscopic changes of venous occlusion.

Impending, Incipient, Partial, or Incomplete Central Retinal Vein Obstruction

These terms are used synonymously to describe the fundi of patients who are either asymptomatic or who may complain of mild, often transient episodes of blurring of vision. Their fundi demonstrate mild venous dilation, a few widely scattered retinal hemorrhages (Figure 6.74D), and a mild increase in retinal circulation time angiographically.[1152,1166] The term "venous stasis retinopathy" to describe these patients probably should be avoided, since it was originally used in the literature to describe focal retinal hemorrhages scattered in the peripheral fundi in patients with reduced retinal artery pressure caused by carotid artery obstruction.[360,1167]

Nonischemic Central Retinal Vein Obstruction (Perfused Central Retinal Vein Occlusion)

Mild to moderate loss of acuity, usually 20/200 or better; widespread retinal hemorrhages; angiographic evidence of mild to moderate cystoid retinal and optic disc edema; minimal or no areas of capillary nonperfusion; and an increase in retinal circulation time characterize these patients (Figures 6.74B, C, and G–I, and 6.75A–C). Blood levels are often seen within the large retinal cysts in the foveolar area.[1168] Some cotton-wool patches, particularly in hypertensive patients, may be present. Transient retinal vessel wall sheathing may occur.[1169] The intraocular pressure in the affected eye is often lower than in the fellow eye.[1170]

Severe (Ischemic) Central Retinal Vein Obstruction (Nonperfused Central Retinal Vein Occlusion)

Patients with severe central retinal vein obstruction typically have severe visual loss, usually less than 20/200; an afferent pupillary defect; widespread confluent retinal hemorrhages; marked swelling and obscuration of the optic disc margins; multiple focal zones of ischemic whitening; cotton-wool patches; diffuse loss of retinal transparency; marked increase in the central retinal vein pressure as determined by an inability to collapse the retinal vein with digital pressure; angiographic evidence of marked increase in retinal circulation time; evidence of large zones of capillary nonperfusion; severe capillary permeability alterations; and severe alterations in the electroretinogram (Figure 6.74K and L).[1171] The term "combined central retinal artery and vein obstruction" may be warranted in patients with severe visual loss and extensive ischemic whitening of the retina as well as scattered retinal hemorrhages. These patients are more likely to have evidence of ophthalmic or carotid artery insufficiency. Patients initially exhibiting one of the lesser degrees of obstruction may subsequently develop a more severe form of obstruction.[1166,1172] A timed fluorescein angiographic study, preferably using a wide-angle fundus camera, can document the degree of obstruction, the severity of the capillary permeability alterations, and after partial resolution of the intraretinal hemorrhages the extent of the retinal capillary nonperfusion (Figure 6.74K and L). It is important to include views of the peripheral fundus and the posterior pole, since capillary nonperfusion is most likely to occur in these areas. In the presence of

6.74 Central retinal vein obstruction.

A–F: Moderately severe central retinal vein obstruction in the left eye (B) of a 42-year-old black woman with sickle-cell trait. Visual acuity was 20/20 in the right eye (A) and was finger counting in the left eye (B). Both optic discs were slightly pale. Angiography demonstrated evidence of prolonged retinal circulation time and diffuse dye leakage from the retinal capillaries, venules, and veins (C). Two years later the patient returned because of blurred vision secondary to impending central retinal vein obstruction in the right eye (D). Note the dilated venous collateral vessel on the optic disc (arrow). The left fundus was normal (E). Visual acuity was 20/25 in the right eye and 20/20 in the left eye. Two months later the retinal hemorrhages had cleared (F); however, a few microaneurysms remained. Visual acuity was 20/20 bilaterally and has remained so for 7 years, despite recurrent vitreous hemorrhages secondary to peripheral areas of retinitis proliferans and retinal vessel nonperfusion identical to that seen in sickle-cell hemoglobin C disease.

G–J: Moderately severe nonischemic central retinal vein occlusion and optic disc edema (G). Angiography revealed an increased retinal circulation time and intraretinal staining (H and I). Note following spontaneous resolution of the obstruction the venous collateral vessel (arrow, J) on the optic disc and the retinal pigment epithelium atrophy centrally caused by dissection of intraretinal blood into the subretinal space during the acute phase of the disorder.

K and L: Severe central retinal vein obstruction. Note the pallor of the optic disc, cotton-wool patches, diffuse ischemic whitening of the retina, and multiple retinal hemorrhages (K). Angiography revealed massive drop-out of the retinal capillary bed (L).

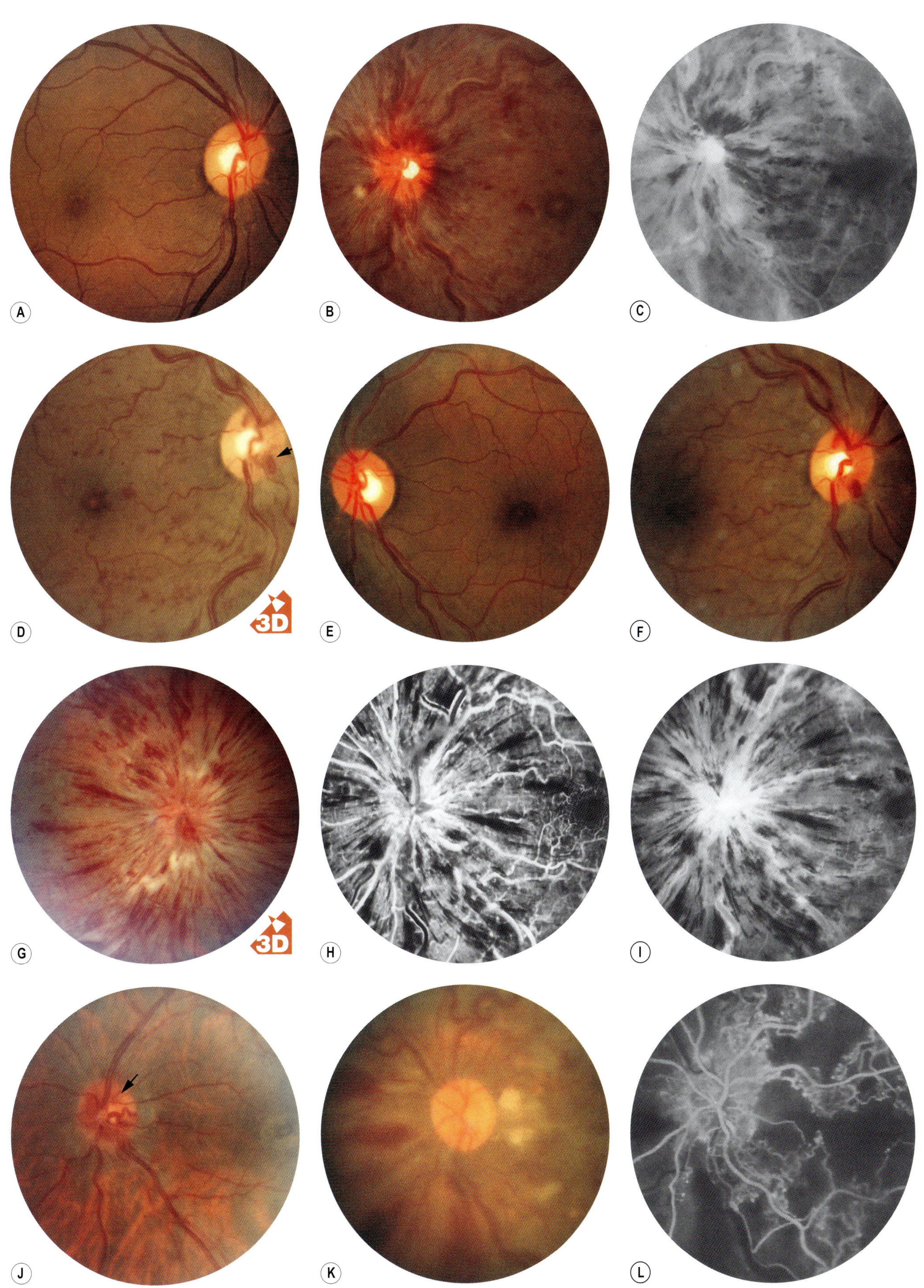
A
B
C
D
3D
E
F
G
3D
H
I
J
K
L

widespread confluent hemorrhages, it may not be possible to determine angiographically the extent of capillary closure.[1173] Late staining along the large retinal veins is a characteristic finding in moderate and severe degrees of central retinal vein obstruction (Figure 6.74I). The clinical findings of visual acuity of less than 20/200, an afferent pupillary defect, marked intraretinal hemorrhage with loss of retinal transparency, and inability to collapse the central retinal vein with finger pressure are adequate to make an accurate diagnosis of an ischemic-type central retinal vein occlusion.[1174–1176] Ancillary tests including fluorescein angiography and electroretinography are rarely necessary.[1161,1171,1177,1178]

Unusual changes that may accompany central retinal vein obstruction include shallowing of the anterior chamber,[1179] angle closure glaucoma,[1180] malignant glaucoma following a glaucoma filtering procedure,[1181] exudative retinal detachment,[1182,1183] and cilioretinal artery occlusion.[336] Very rarely, ongoing vascular remodeling can occur for years after a central retinal vein occlusion, resulting in telangiectasis and formation of collaterals leading to a Coats'-type response (Figure 6.76).

The natural course of this disorder is variable and in large measure correlates with the degree of obstruction evident initially, the location of the occlusion in the course of the vein, and the length of occluded segment of the vein.[1164,1184–1186] Some patients with mild to moderate obstruction may show complete recovery of vision and restoration of the fundus to normal within a matter of months (Figure 6.74A–F) from restoration of the flow within the vein. Others show slower resolution of the retinal changes and incomplete visual recovery. Some develop evidence of prominent venous and collateral channels on the optic nerve head that shunt blood through the choroidal circulation and thus decompress the congested vasculature (Figures 6.74D).[1140] Progression from the nonischemic to the ischemic form of central retinal vein obstruction occurs in approximately 10–20% of older patients and 5–10% of patients less than 65 years of age.[1157] After resolution of all retinal hemorrhages and venous engorgement, varying degrees of permanent retinal capillary dilation, capillary loss, and permeability alteration may remain in the macular area (Figures 6.74J).

Permanent macular changes include CME with or without evidence of cystic degeneration (Figure 6.75C, E and F), an inner lamellar macular hole, a full-thickness macular hole, epiretinal membrane change, RPE atrophy, and proliferation caused by dissection of blood beneath the retina during the acute phase of the disease (Figure 6.74J), and traction detachment of the macula.

6.75 Central retinal vein obstruction.

A–C: Chronic cystoid macular edema (B and C) remaining as the only sign of a previous central retinal vein occlusion (A) that occurred 12 months previously.

D–F: In 1965 this patient had a moderately severe central retinal vein obstruction in the left eye (D). All of the retinal hemorrhages cleared but his visual acuity remained at 10/200 because of chronic cystoid macular degeneration and edema until 1971 (E). In the late angiogram was a large irregularly shaped central cyst indicative of permanent damage to the foveal retina (not shown). At that time six applications of xenon photocoagulation were placed in the area of the retinal arteries supplying the macular area. Six months later the cystoid macular edema had resolved, but there was no improvement in visual acuity (F).

G and **H**: Occult central retinal vein occlusion occurred during the course of follow-up of this patient at yearly intervals because of idiopathic central serous retinopathy in the right eye. Note the development of numerous small venous collaterals on the optic disc of the left eye that occurred over a 1-year interval in the absence of any symptoms or other evidence of venous obstruction.

I–K: This 48-year-old African American otherwise healthy woman presented with headache and visual blurring of her left eye. Petalloid-shaped deep outer plexiform layer hemorrhage and some white-centered hemorrhages prompted a head computed tomography to rule out subarachnoid hemorrhage and blood dyscrasias causing anemia (I). Angiogram revealed good retinal perfusion. Other than being on oral contraceptives, no other risk factor was detected. She progressed to a central retinal vein occlusion with dilated and tortuous retinal veins, increase in number and extent of retinal hemorrhages and cotton-wool spots, and a decline in vision to 20/200 2 weeks later. Within 12 weeks she developed iris neovascularization requiring panretinal photocoagulation. The iris vessels regressed and her intraocular pressure remained under 21 mmHg with topical medications. Her vision remained at 20/200.

For uncertain reasons, proliferative retinopathy occurs less frequently after central than after branch retinal vein occlusion.[1161,1187,1188] Probably fewer than 20% of patients with central retinal vein occlusion will develop evidence of iris neovascularization and hemorrhagic glaucoma. This severe complication is most likely to develop within 3–4 months in those patients who have the severe ischemic forms of the disorder.[1189,1190] The risk of developing neovascularization is less in patients with a posterior vitreous separation.[1191] The risk of developing a central retinal vein occlusion in the second eye is approximately 10–15% and is more likely to occur if the patient is diabetic or has some other associated systemic disorder such as polycythemia or macroglobulinemia.[1192]

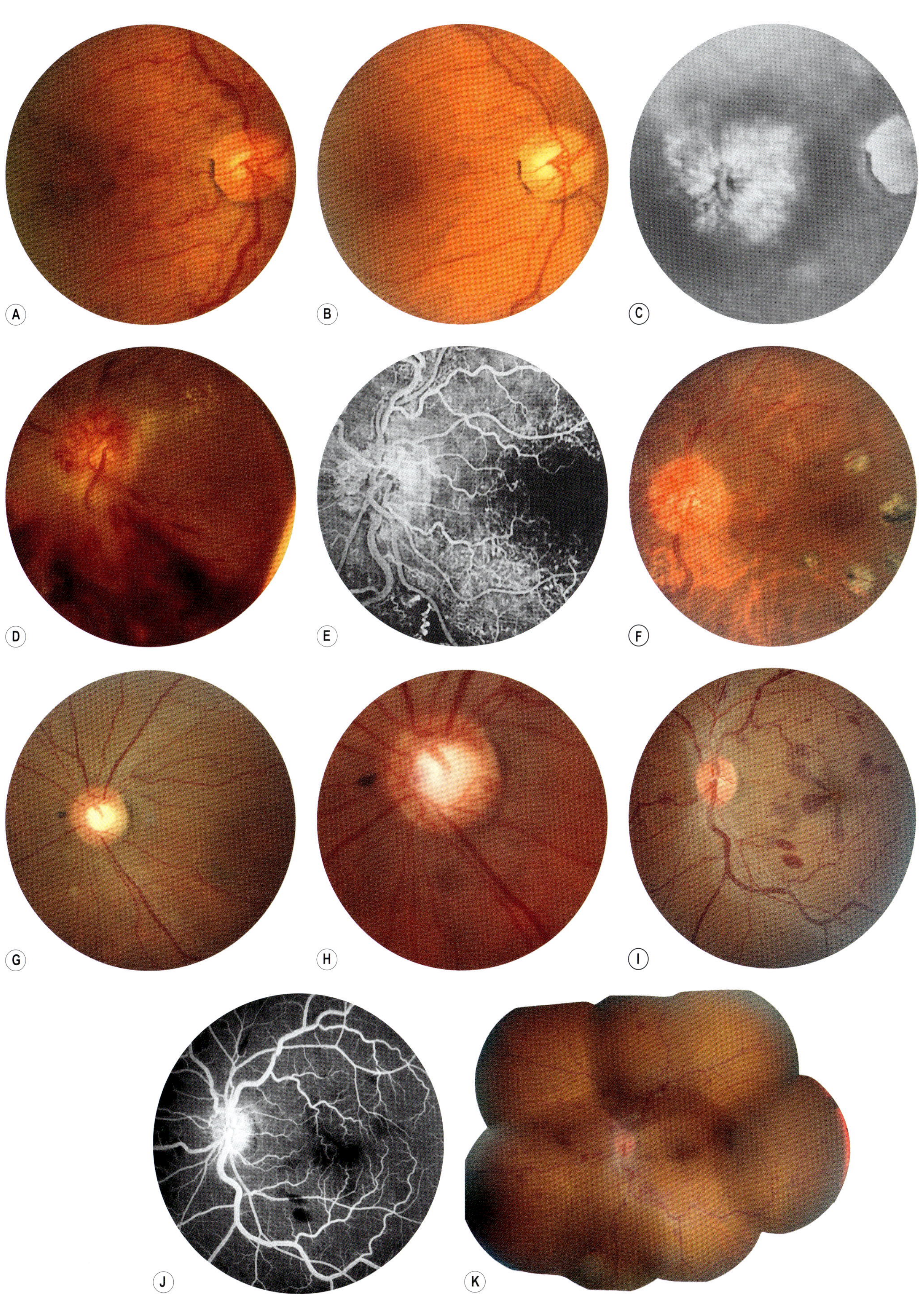
A
B
C
D
E
F
G
H
I
J
K

The visual prognosis in patients below the age of 50 years is better than in older patients (Figure 6.74A–F).[1185,1186,1193,1194] Fewer of the younger patients show the severe acute phase of obstruction, and a high percentage of younger patients with all stages of the disease show greater degrees of visual recovery.[1164] The term "papillophlebitis" is used by some authors to describe the incipient and mild to moderate degrees of central retinal vein occlusion in younger patients, particularly in patients with prominent optic disc swelling and with retinal hemorrhages largely confined to the posterior fundus.[1195,1196] Some patients with papillophlebitis may manifest evidence of partial obstruction of the central or branch retinal artery and optic disc ischemia as well (Figure 6.77A–E, and H).[336,1197] In younger patients venous obstruction is probably caused primarily by disorders producing optic nerve and disc swelling with secondary venous compression, rather than a primary venous thrombosis occurring at the level of the lamina cribrosa, as is usually the case in older patients (Figures 6.76 and 6.77F–J). In most patients with papillophlebitis there is no associated systemic disease and there are no inflammatory cells in the vitreous near the optic nerve head. In a few patients it may be associated with other disorders including pregnancy, use of birth control medications, optic neuritis, and ulcerative colitis.[1195,1198,1199] Although young, otherwise healthy adults with central retinal vein obstruction have a more favorable prognosis than older patients, as many as one-third of those referred to retinal specialists may have a final visual acuity of 20/200 or worse.[1200]

6.76 Sequelae of central retinal vein occlusion with Coats'-like response.

A–L: This 37-year-old African American man noted a sudden loss of vision in his left eye associated with severe headache that lasted only minutes. He was found to have sectoral deep retinal whitening associated with several blot retinal hemorrhages (A). Angiogram revealed some delay in the arm to retina/choroid time (18 seconds) (B and C). His vision was 20/25 when seen, which was 7 days after his symptoms began. An orbital anomalous circulation was suspected in this otherwise healthy man. Blood work, orbital and head magnetic resonance imaging revealed no abnormalities. The whitening and hemorrhages had improved 8 days later (D). His blood pressure was mildly elevated and he was started on medications. Six weeks later he returned with no new symptoms and a vision of 20/20 in both eyes. He now had venous tortuosity, and several retinal hemorrhages in all four quadrants consistent with a central retinal vein occlusion (E–G). His central vision dropped to 20/40 over the next month secondary to cystoid macular edema. Coagulation studies and cardiac workup revealed no abnormalities; he was monitored. A year later his vision had improved to 20/25, most of the hemorrhages had resolved (H and I), and the cysts in the fovea had decreased. He was found to have peripheral lipid in the inferonasal and temporal periphery 3 years later that gradually increased. An angiogram revealed dilated capillary bed in the adjoining areas and microaneurysm formation (K and L) simulating Coats' response. Given the 20/20 vision and the peripheral location of the exudates, he was monitored and gradually the lipid decreased over the next 3 years.

Experimental production of the clinical picture of a central retinal vein occlusion in animals is difficult because of the availability of collateral pathways of venous outflow near the optic nerve head.[1141,1144,1145] Histopathologic studies in humans have demonstrated a thrombosis occurring at the level of, or posterior to, the lamina cribrosa.[1201] It is likely the thrombus is a secondary event due to sludging proximal to the site of occlusion. The greater likelihood of associated central retinal arterial disease in older patients may explain why they have a poorer visual prognosis than young patients.

Although some patients have factors predisposing them to central retinal vein occlusion, such as glaucoma, diabetes mellitus, hypertension, polycythemia, sickle-cell trait (Figure 6.74A–F), Reye's syndrome, moyamoya syndrome, homocysteinemia, dysproteinemias, carotid artery insufficiency, carotid cavernous fistula, and use of oral contraceptives, amphetamine, cocaine, phenylpropanolamine, and tranexamic acid, most have no recognizable cause for developing venous thrombosis.[253,280,361,1154,1202–1220] Mansour et al. followed 78 patients for 2 years or more and found no increased risk of mortality or morbidity.[1221] Retinal venous obstruction occasionally may occur following accidental trauma, surgical trauma, such as repair of a blowout fracture or scleral buckling procedure, ischemic optic neuropathy, papillitis, papilledema, cilioretinal and branch retinal artery occlusion, congenital anomalies of the optic disc, drusen of the optic nerve head, and pregnancy.[1195,1198,1222–1225] Other factors incriminated in venous thrombosis include abnormal blood viscosity,[1226–1228] elevated erythrocyte aggregation,[1229]and lipoprotein and platelet abnormalities.[1230–1232] Although patients with glaucoma are at increased risk of venous obstruction,[1214] optic disc size and optic cup disc ratio in fellow eyes of patients with venous obstruction are no different than that seen in normal eyes.[1208,1233–1236] Likewise, congenitally tilted optic nerve heads do not appear to be a risk factor for central retinal vein occlusion.[1237] Although some have found evidence to suggest a seasonal variation in the onset of central retinal vein obstruction, others have not.[1238,1239]

There is no convincing evidence of medical treatment favorably altering the natural course of central retinal vein occlusion. Pilot studies have suggested that oral troxerutin, an inhibitor of platelet and erythrocyte aggregation, and hemodilution treatment to lower blood viscosity may be of some benefit.[1228,1240,1241] Intravenous administration of streptokinase appeared to reduce the morbidity but has never gained favor because of the risk of intravitreal hemorrhage.[1242] The value of systemic steroids in the treatment of young patients with central retinal vein obstruction with the presumption that it is caused by a "papillophlebitis" is uncertain, since most young patients have a favorable course without treatment.

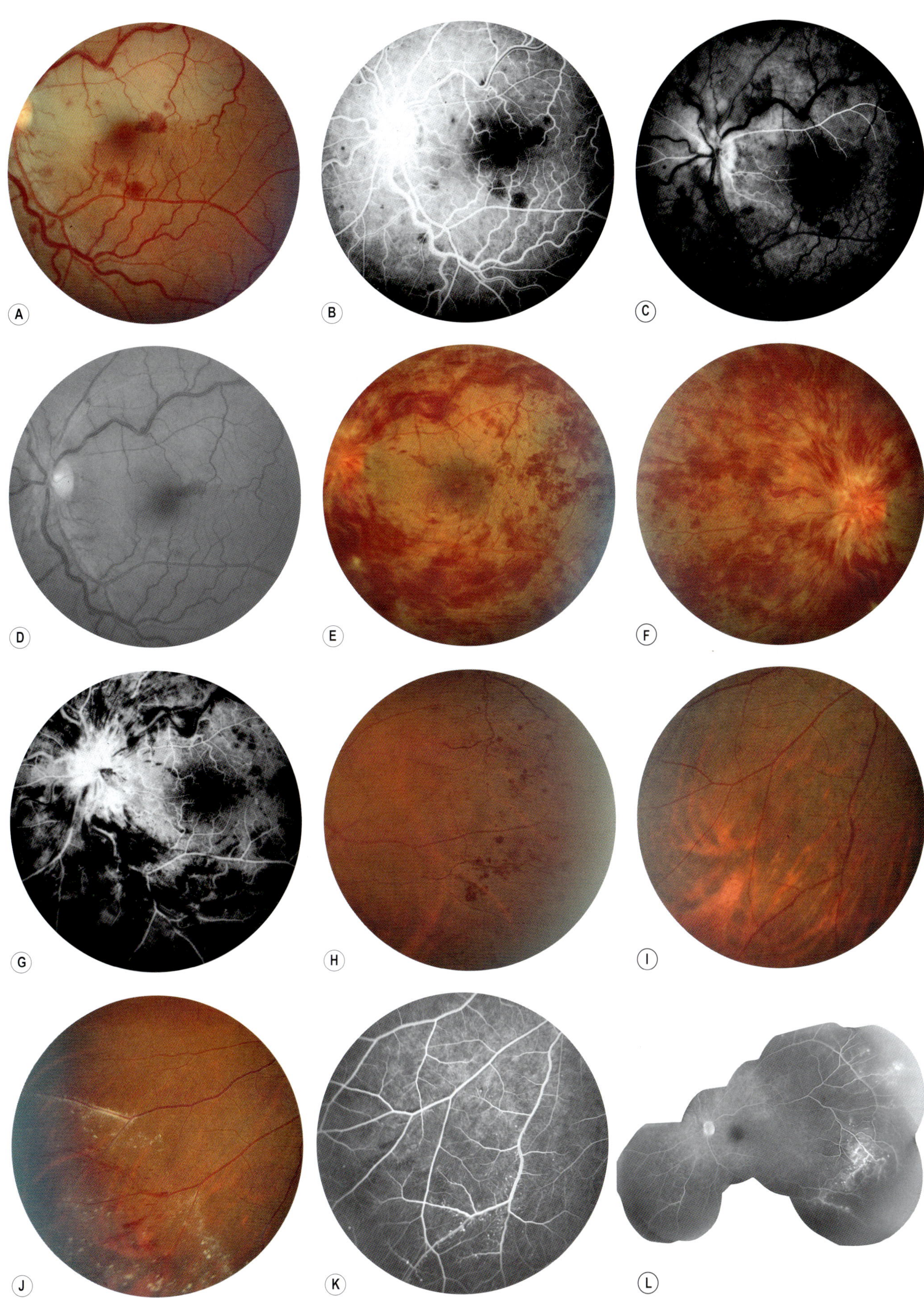
A
B
C
D
E
F
G
H
I
J
K
L

The results of the Central Vein Occlusion Study concerning the value of early prophylactic PRP treatment in patients with ischemic-type central retinal vein occlusion in preventing iris neovascularization demonstrated that prophylactic treatment does not totally prevent iris and angle neovascularization, and that prompt regression of iris and angle neovascularization in response to PRP is more likely to occur in eyes that have not been treated previously.[1243] They identified four risk factors for developing iris and angle neovascularization: (1) extent of nonperfusion on fluorescein angiography; (2) large amounts of retinal hemorrhage; (3) short duration of central retinal vein occlusion; and (4) male sex. If adequate fluorescein angiography cannot be done because of hazy media or because of extensive intraretinal hemorrhage, eyes should be followed as if they had an ischemic vein occlusion.[1243,1244] The study found no apparent benefit in performing PRP before development of iris and angle neovascularization, provided frequent follow-up examinations can be performed. Since 20% of early treated patients later developed iris and angle neovascularization, frequent follow-up is necessary following PRP. The study group recommended careful observation of all patients with recent central retinal vein occlusion with frequent (approximately monthly) follow-up examinations for 6–8 months (including undilated slit-lamp examination of the iris and gonioscopy) and prompt PRP of eyes in which iris and angle neovascularization develops. It is important to follow patients with nonischemic central retinal vein occlusion since the study found that, within 4 months, 10% of cases of nonischemic patients progressed to ischemic central retinal vein occlusion.[1244]

The use of scatter treatment for CME caused by central retinal vein occlusion was evaluated by the Central Retinal Vein Occlusion Study, which found the treatment ineffective in preserving or improving central visual acuity.[1245–1247] The SCORE study found that use of 1 mg and 4 mg of triamcinolone to improve visual loss from macular edema in patients with central retinal vein occlusion was better than observation alone. The 1-mg dose had a better safety profile than the 4-mg dose.[1248] More recently, intravitreal injection of ranibizumab and dexamethasone implants have been shown to be better than observation alone; however these studies have been short-term studies lasting up to 6 months only.[1249–1251]

Surgical incision in the area of the sclera at the junction of the sclera and optic nerve dura has been suggested as a means of relieving obstruction of the central retinal vein.[1252] Radial optic neurotomy by introducing the microvitrectomy blade into the optic nerve and dehiscing the lamina cribrosa and the compartment behind it does not have a strong rationale to be effective. Those eyes that have improved following this procedure have done so by the development of collateral vessels between the retinal venous and choroidal venous circulation. There is experimental and clinical evidence that production of retinochoroidal anastomosis, using photocoagulation distal to the site of branch venous thrombosis, may be efficacious in relieving outflow obstruction (Figure 6.81).[1162,1253,1254]

6.77 Idiopathic central retinal vein obstruction associated with optic disc edema ("papillophlebitis").

A–E: Optic nerve head swelling associated with partial obstruction of the central retinal artery and vein caused acute visual loss in the left eye of this healthy 31-year-old man. Note the venous dilation, optic disc, and peripapillary retinal hemorrhages, and ischemic whitening of the retina centrally (A). Angiography revealed early retinal artery filling at 21 seconds (B, arrow), and no venous perfusion at 35 seconds (C). Echography of the optic nerve and orbit was negative. Two weeks later there were more peripapillary hemorrhages and some vitreous hemorrhage, but less retinal ischemia (D). One year later there was mild optic atrophy (E). His visual acuity was 20/70. The right eye was normal.

F–J: This mildly hypertensive 40-year-old man presented with vision change in his right eye to 20/25. Peripapillary hemorrhages, cotton-wool spots, dilated and tortuous veins were seen in the right eye (F). The left eye was normal; note an absent optic disc cup (G). Extensive workup done elsewhere, including coagulation profile, collagen vascular, carotid workup and magnetic resonance imaging of his head revealed no other abnormality. The retinal findings resolved over 4 months (I); approximately 8 weeks after the onset in his right eye he noted a change in his left eye. His vision was still 20/20 but he had peripapillary nerve fiber whitening and hemorrhages, dilated and tortuous retinal veins and hemorrhages in all four quadrants (H). The retinal findings resolved over the following 3 months and his final visual acuity was 20/15– in each eye. The left optic disc had mild residual pallor (J).

K: Combined central retinal vein obstruction and branch retinal artery obstruction associated with a swollen optic disc in an otherwise healthy 31-year-old woman whose visual acuity was 20/20 bilaterally. The left eye was normal. Angiography revealed evidence of central retinal vein and branch artery obstruction and staining of the right optic disc. Echography of the optic nerves and orbit was normal. Her past medical history was positive only for the use of birth control pills. Two years later her visual acuity was unchanged. The fundi were unremarkable except for segmental optic atrophy in the right eye.

L: Acute loss of vision caused by large premacular hematoma that was associated with swollen optic disc and central retinal vein obstruction in a 41-year-old man. There were scattered superficial and deep retinal hemorrhages as well as extension of blood into the vitreous near the optic disc. Angiography showed evidence of increased retinal circulation time and probable location of a large hematoma in the subhyaloid space.

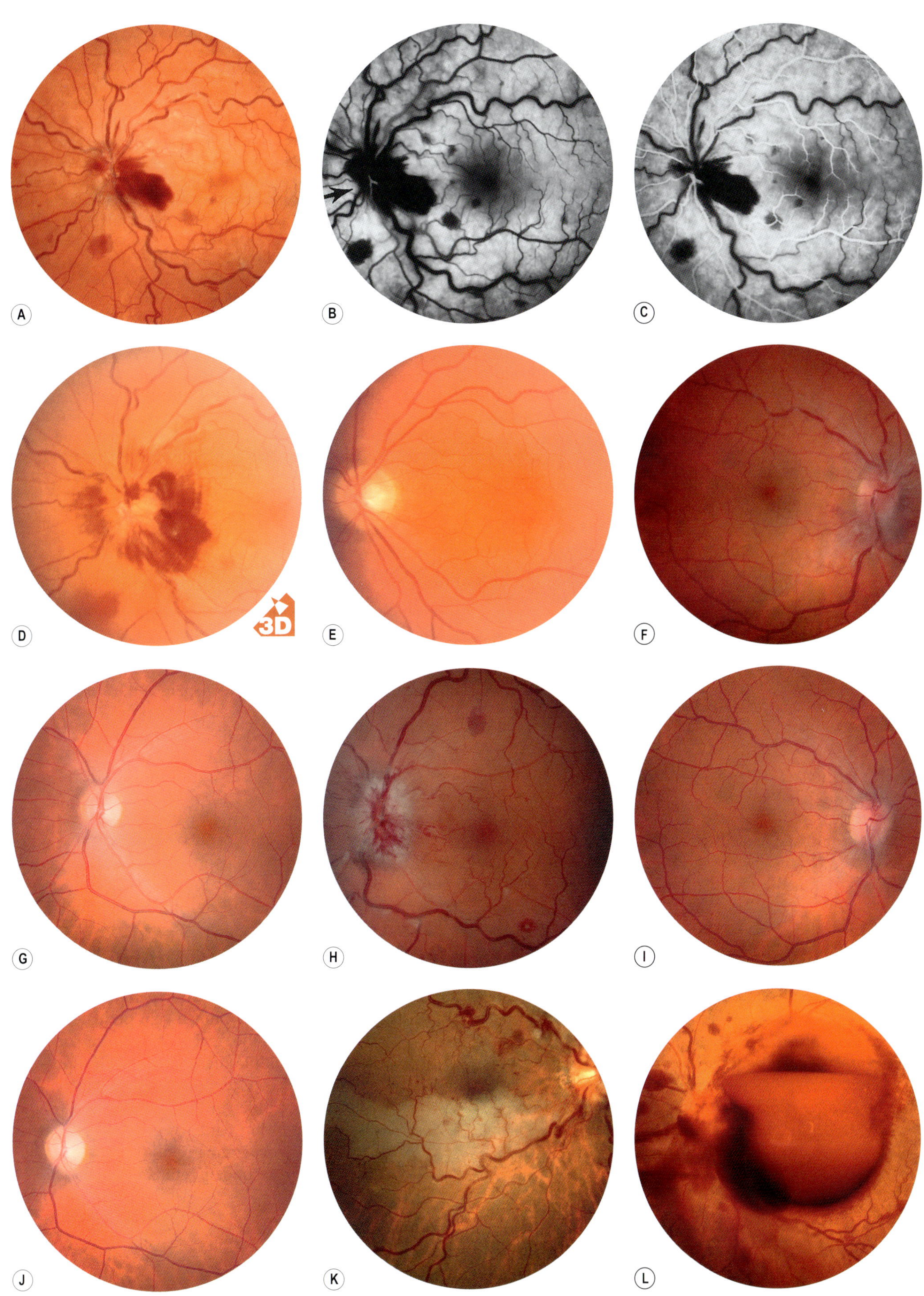
A
B
C
D
3D
E
F
G
H
I
J
K
L

Fluorescein angiography during the acute hemorrhagic phase of the disease may show nothing more than a large nonfluorescent area where the blood obscures both the retinal and choroidal circulation (Figure 6.78A–C). Late photographs are important in detecting evidence of intraretinal extravasation of dye, which may extend beyond the area of hemorrhage. A focal area of dye leakage may occur either at or just proximal to the site of the arteriovenous crossing (Figure 6.78). It occasionally occurs at a focal area of venous wall decompensation before the development of the venous obstruction. Angiography may demonstrate either complete or incomplete venous obstruction at the arteriovenous crossing and usually shows minimal interference with arterial flow.[1194] Collateral channels bridging the site of the arteriovenous crossing and draining into adjacent quadrants usually become evident angiographically as the retinal hemorrhages begin to clear (Figure 6.78E and F). These collateral channels typically do not show evidence of dye leakage during the early stages of venous obstruction. After resolution of the hemorrhages and restoration of relatively normal intracapillary pressure, angiography often demonstrates residual damage to the structure and permeability of the retinal vascular bed (Figure 6.78E, F, H, and I, 6.79 H and I). During the early stages after branch venous occlusion, fluorescein angiography demonstrates increased retinal circulation time, evidence of capillary leakage, and perivenous staining in the obstructed zone. Within a matter of weeks or several months after partial clearing of the subretinal blood, angiography in patients with relatively mild venous obstruction typically shows varying degrees of mild capillary telangiectasis, dilation of the collateral venous channels, and staining of the retina, including the typical pattern of CME in some patients with persistent subnormal visual acuity. In patients with more severe acute venous obstruction and retinal ischemia, large areas of capillary nonperfusion, which in some cases may include the macula, are evident angiographically and may be accompanied by retinal and/or optic disc neovascularization. Initial reports described a poor visual prognosis in those patients with persistent macular edema with angiographic evidence of segmental nonperfusion of the perifoveolar capillary network.[1261,1270] Finkelstein, however, found that the prognosis for spontaneous visual acuity improvement was better in those patients with angiographic evidence of juxtafoveal capillary nonperfusion.[1288]

6.79 Branch retinal vein obstruction (BRVO).

A–C: This 55-year-old otherwise healthy woman was seen because of blurred vision in the right eye associated with small retinal hemorrhages in the inferior half of the macula and a focal area of whitening (A) at an inferotemporal retinal artery and vein crossing site where angiography revealed a focal area of staining (arrow, B). The foveal capillaries showed leakage with dye accumulation in a cystoid pattern (C). All systemic investigations were normal and she was normotensive. The venous endothelial damage at the site of an arteriovenous crossing may be responsible for the BRVO.
D: Serous detachment of the macula (arrows) caused by BRVO.
E–I: This 54-year-old hypertensive woman presented with sudden superior field change in her right eye from a localized BRVO (E) and a vision of 20/40. Within a week her vision dropped to 20/200 when the cystoid macular edema (CME) increased in size (F). She received an intravitreal injection of 4 mg Triesence, which promptly resolved the CME (G) and vision returned to 20/30. By 9 months she developed a small NVE (H and I, arrow) in spite of limited nonperfusion requiring scatter laser to the affected quadrant.
J and K: This 60-year-old asymptomatic woman with a foveal-sparing superior BRVO (J) progressed with increase in hemorrhages, venous tortuosity, and development of CME over 2 months (K). Note the collaterals on the optic disc.

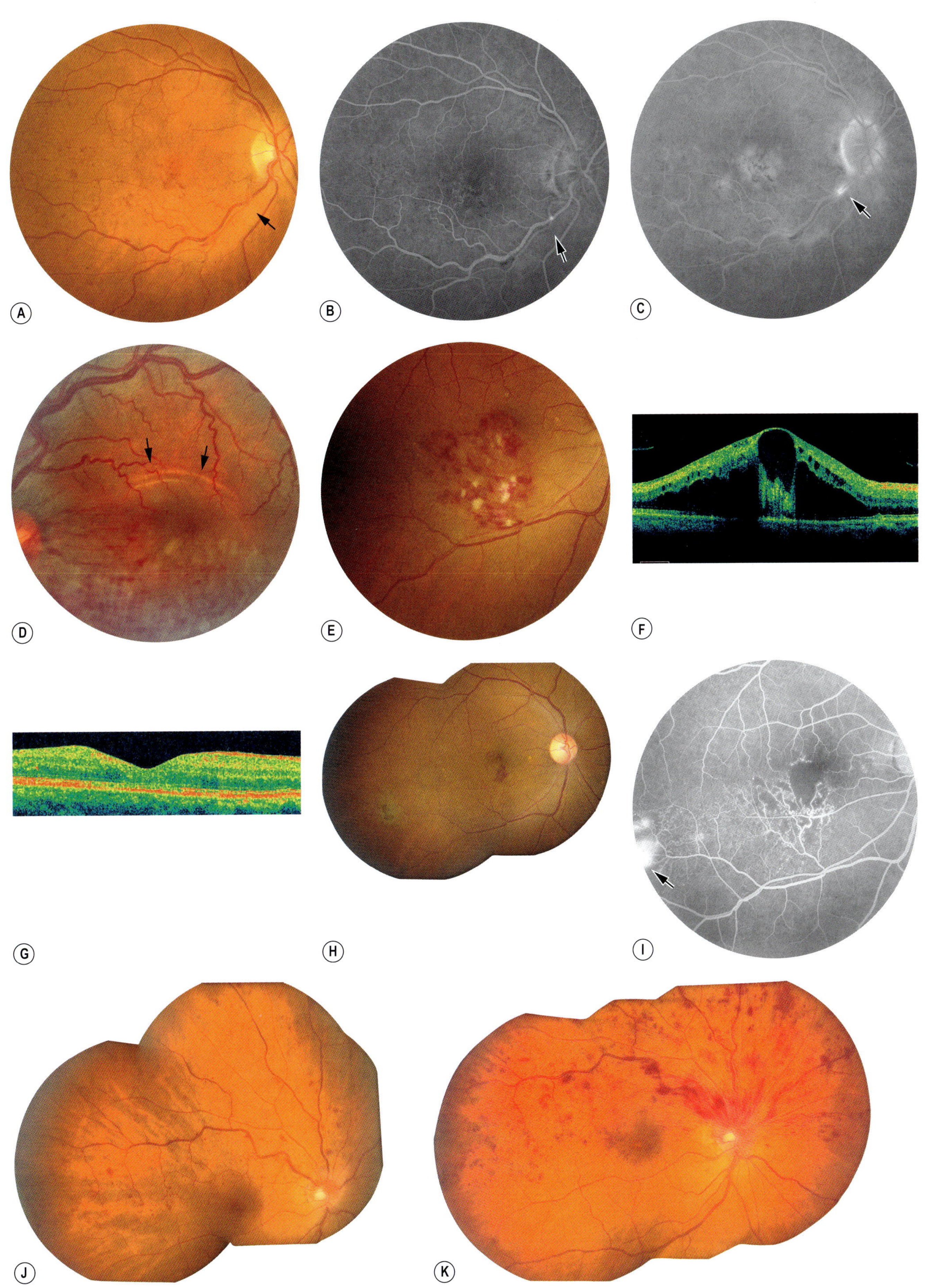
A
B
C
D
E
F
G
H
I
J
K

The development of retinal and optic disc new vessels is one of the major complications of branch vein obstruction.[1270,1289,1290] New vessels are most likely to occur in patients who initially have multiple cotton-wool patches, diffuse ischemic whitening, and extensive hemorrhages in the retina, and who later show multiple zones of retinal capillary nonperfusion. The new vessels often occur at the junction between the perfused and nonperfused retina. Occasionally, however, they may develop remote from the zone of retina affected by the venous obstruction (Figure 6.80H and I).[1289] Retinal and optic disc neovascularization is less likely to develop in eyes after posterior vitreous detachment.[1291–1293] Retinal neovascularization probably develops in fewer than 25% of patients with branch vein obstruction, and probably 50% or fewer of these ever develop a vitreous hemorrhage.[1256] Sheathing of the retinal arteries and veins in an area of venous occlusion may occur in some cases.[1169] Other complications of branch vein occlusion affecting the macula include distortion secondary to epiretinal membranes, lamellar and full-thickness macular holes, traction retinal holes and detachment,[1293–1296] hemorrhagic detachment of the internal limiting membrane of the retina,[1297] and rhegmatogenous retinal detachment.[1267,1280,1294,1296–1298] Disorders occasionally associated with branch retinal vein occlusion include optic disc drusen,[1299] sarcoidosis,[1300] toxoplasmosis, serpiginous choroiditis, idiopathic multifocal retinitis and neuroretinitis, acute intermittent porphyria,[1301] hyperlipidemia and hypercholesterolemia,[1231] and beta-thromboglobulin and platelet factor 4 abnormalities.[1232]

Varicosities and decompensation of venous collaterals, usually along the horizontal raphe, may be a delayed cause of loss of visual acuity many months or years after resolution of branch retinal vein occlusion (Figure 6.80).[1263] This complication typically occurs in patients with a large zone of capillary nonperfusion in the area of previous vein occlusion and is associated with the development of a ring of yellow exudate surrounding the foveal side of the leaking collateral vessels (Figure 6.80). On occasion, acute bleeding from the collateral vessels into the subretinal space may cause visual loss (Figure 6.80A and B).

Histopathologic examination of eyes with branch retinal vein occlusion has demonstrated a fresh or canalized thrombus at the site of obstruction and varying degrees of sclerosis of the wall of the corresponding retinal artery at the site of the obstruction.[1272,1302] Inner ischemic retinal atrophy, retinal neovascularization, IRMA, and CME and degeneration are found in the area of the venous occlusion.

Many of the ophthalmoscopic and angiographic changes seen in humans with branch retinal vein obstruction have been reproduced experimentally.[1142,1143,1146–1148,1303–1306] However, chronic CME and retinitis proliferans, which are of visual significance in humans, have not been reproduced.

6.80 Venous collateral varicosities causing late-onset visual loss after branch retinal vein obstruction.

A and **B**: Sudden loss of central vision caused by bleeding from parafoveolar venous collateral varicosities in the left eye of a 32-year-old black patient with severe cupping of the optic disc and normal intraocular pressures. There was angiographic evidence of occult superior hemiretinal vein obstruction. His visual acuity was 20/20, right eye, and 20/25, left eye. Note the central nodule of altered intraretinal and subretinal blood and the multiple patches of subretinal blood (arrows, A) beneath the dilated venous collaterals seen best in the angiogram (B).
C–E: Circinate pattern of macular exudation caused by leaking collateral venous channels (arrows, D) in a patient who had evidence of a previous inferotemporal branch retinal vein occlusion. Note the late filling of the aneurysm involving the collateral vessel (E).
F–I: Two years before these photographs this patient developed a superotemporal vein obstruction in the left eye. One year later his visual acuity was 20/20. Yet 1 year later it declined to 20/200. Note the circinate maculopathy surrounding aneurysmal dilation of a venous collateral (arrow, F) temporal to the left macula and the delay in perfusion and incomplete filling of the aneurysm (arrow, G). Argon laser photocoagulation (arrow, H) resulted in disappearance of the aneurysm and circinate exudate (I). There was minimal improvement in visual acuity because of subfoveal fibrosis. Arrow (I) indicates site of aneurysm.
J and **K**: Prominent venous collateral vessels simulating a congenital arteriovenous malformation in a hypertensive patient following a superotemporal branch retinal vein occlusion.

Photocoagulation treatment for the edematous and neovascular complications of branch retinal vein occlusion has been investigated by numerous authors.[1260,1264,1270,1307–1315] A randomized controlled clinical trial has demonstrated that a scatter pattern of argon laser applied to the area of capillary leakage within the macular area and outside the FAZ was of value in preserving central vision in patients with persistent macular edema and visual acuity of 20/40 or worse (Figure 6.78A–F).[1255,1309] Because of the relatively low frequency of development of neovascularization, peripheral scatter photocoagulation was recommended as a means of reducing the risk of vitreous hemorrhage only in those patients who demonstrated neovascularization. There is no evidence that photocoagulation during the acute stage of branch vein occlusion is of value. Laser treatment is of benefit for patients with delayed loss of vision caused by decompensation of venous collateral vessels (Figure 6.80).

Experimentally recombinant tissue plasminogen activator is effective in lysing laser-induced branch retinal venous occlusions in rabbits.[1316] Surgical separation of the retinal vein and artery where they cross is technically possible and has been tried in animals and humans with branch retinal vein obstruction, but its value in improving venous perfusion is uncertain.[1317]

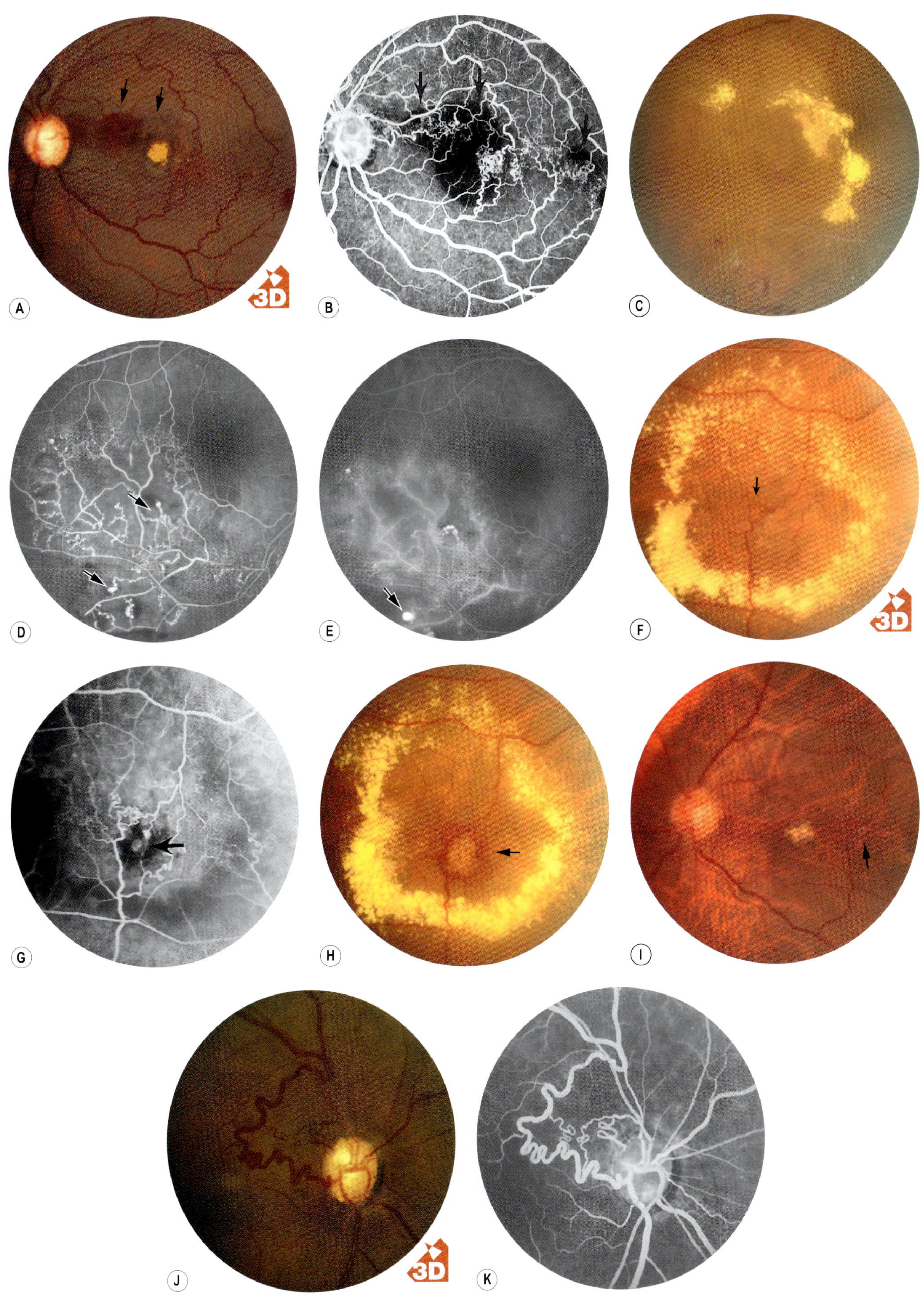
A
B
C
D
E
F
G
H
I
J
K
3D
3D
3D

Widespread retinal hemorrhages that may simulate those caused by central retinal vein occlusion may occur because of decreased blood flow to the eye (carotid artery obstruction[1318]; venous stasis retinopathy); marked reduction in intraocular pressure (ocular decompression retinopathy after filtering procedures)[1319]; capillary permeability abnormalities caused by anemia, leukemia, and septic retinopathy; reduction of blood flow associated with hyperviscosity (macroglobulinemia); and transient rise in central retinal vein pressure associated with compression injuries of the chest and by mechanisms that are not well understood in patients with subarachnoid hemorrhage (Terson's syndrome) and cocaine inhalation (see Chapter 9).

More recently, treatment of macular edema secondary to branch retinal vein occlusion has involved the use of intravitreal triamcinolone acetonide, anti-VEGF agents such as ranibizumab and bevacizumab, and long-acting dexamethasone implants.[1320–1325] The belief that these agents decrease vascular permeability is the underlying hypothesis of the treatment. The response is variable in patients; in many the edema recurs once the treatment is discontinued unless the eye develops adequate collaterals: this is the only certain mechanism for resolution of edema. It is reasonable to consider any of these treatments till one can either demonstrate development of good collateral vessels, or not, in which case no treatment is likely to improve vision and edema.

Hemiretinal Vein Occlusion

Retinal vein occlusion may involve half of the fundus and may be caused by obstruction of one of the dual trunks of the central retinal vein (Figure 6.79 J and K), an anomaly that occurs in approximately 20% of individuals.[1326–1329] The obstruction probably occurs at the level of the lamina cribrosa and pathogenetically is more closely related to occlusion of the central rather than the branch retinal veins.

6.81 Laser treatment for retinal vein obstruction.

A–F: Small branch retinal vein obstruction causing exudative maculopathy (A–D). The visual acuity was 20/80. Five years following argon laser photocoagulation (E), there was minimal exudation (F) and visual acuity was 20/20.

G and **H**: This patient developed optic disc and retinal neovascularization (arrows, G) and a macular scar following an inferotemporal branch vein occlusion. Angiography showed marked loss of the retinal capillary bed in the area of retinal vascular sheathing inferior to the macula. A scatter pattern of argon laser treatment was applied to the area of capillary nonperfusion. Twelve months later the disc and retinal neovascularization had resolved (H).

I–L: Laser retinochoroidal anastomosis in the treatment of central retinal vein occlusion in this patient, who experienced progressive decrease in vision (I). Several months following intense 0.1-second, 50-μm laser applications to create a retinochoroidal venous anastomosis inferiorly (arrow, J), the retinal hemorrhages had cleared. The laminar flow pattern in the angiograms indicates retrograde flow of venous blood toward the anastomotic site (arrows, K and L).

(I–L, from McAllister and Constable.[1162],)

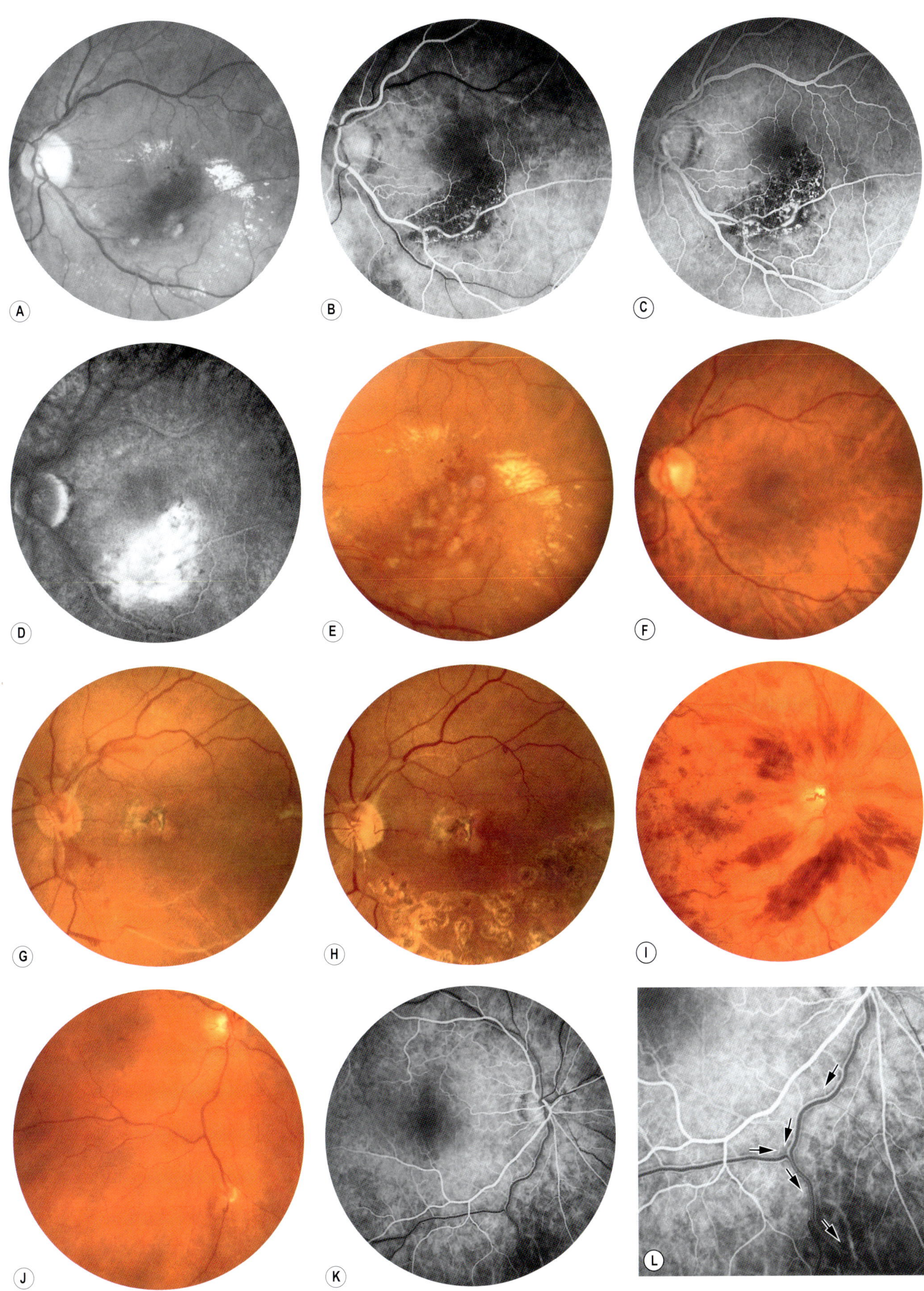
A
B
C
D
E
F
G
H
I
J
K
L

RETINAL VASCULAR CHANGES CAUSED BY HEMATOLOGIC DISORDERS

Changes in the composition of the cellular and extracellular components of blood may alter its viscosity, flow characteristics, coagulability, and transport system for oxygen, carbon dioxide, and other metabolites, which in turn may cause alterations in the retinal blood vessel caliber, length, color, and permeability. Some of these blood alterations have been discussed previously, such as sickle-cell disease, thrombocytopenia, disseminated intravascular coagulopathy, and complement-activated leukocytic aggregation. Alterations associated with leukemias are presented in Chapter 13.

Retinopathy Associated with Anemia

Patients with moderately severe or severe anemia may exhibit fundoscopic changes, including flame-shaped, white-centered, and subinternal limiting membrane hemorrhages; cotton-wool spots; retinal venous dilation and tortuosity; retinal exudation; pallor of the fundus with increased choroidal markings; and optic disc swelling (Figures 6.82A, B, F, J, and K, 6.83 A-E and 6.84 B-F). In some cases intraretinal hemorrhage may be associated with proliferative retinal vascular changes that may simulate a retinal vascular hematoma (Figure 6.82F and G).[1330]

Retinopathy is more likely to be present in cases of rapid development of anemia and in older patients with anemia.[1331,1332] Unless one of the hemorrhages involves the central macular area, the patient usually has no visual symptoms. In some cases of severe blood loss, retinal and optic nerve ischemia may be associated with profound visual loss.[1333–1335]

A small subset of patients with anemia may present as idiopathic intracranial hypertension with bilateral papilledema, peripapillary hemorrhages, retinal cotton-wool spots, and preretinal hemorrhages.[1336–1338] Cerebrospinal fluid pressures are normal and so is the MRI; these patients may have severe iron-deficiency anemia. As soon as the anemia is treated, their signs and symptoms of papilledema, retinal hemorrhages, and cotton-wool spots resolve. Anemia should be considered in those patients who do not fit the usual profile of idiopathic intracranial hypertension of excess weight and who are otherwise negative for other causes of isolated papilledema. Anemia associated with kidney disease and diabetic nephropathy may aggravate the retinopathy. The relative hypoxia causes multiple-organ tissue injury. There have been cases of anemic retinopathy with microaneurysms and dot-blot hemorrhages, all of which reversed as soon as the anemia was corrected.[1339] There have been reports of branch retinal artery occlusion in patients with iron-deficiency anemia.

6.82 Anemic chorioretinopathy.

A–D: This 19-year-old woman noted a scotoma in the left eye while in the hospital for treatment of severe anemia and idiopathic thrombocytopenic purpura. Her hemoglobin was 2.9 g/dl and hematocrit was 9%. Note the superficial retinal hemorrhages in both eyes, the prominent choroidal vascular markings, the light color of the fundus, and the retinal vessel tortuosity (A and B), all of which disappeared after blood transfusion and splenectomy (C and D).

E–I: This 3-year-old child with Klippel–Trenaunay–Weber syndrome developed severe hemolytic anemia, thrombocytopenia, hepatosplenomegaly, hypertension, and chronic renal failure. Her hemoglobin was 5.1 g/dl and her hematocrit was 15%. Superonasally in the right eye (E and F), and in the left macular area (G), she had two focal areas of intraretinal hemorrhage, retinal thickening, and mildly dilated capillaries surrounded by yellowish exudation. The appearance of the fundi was similar to that illustrated in photographs made at age 20 months (E–G). She appeared to have good visual acuity in the right eye, whose macula was unaffected by the retinal vascular changes. When seen at age 20 months the fundus changes were interpreted as retinal vascular malformations.[1290] The author believes that the retinal changes were more likely acquired as a complication of anemia, thrombocytopenia, and hypertension. Note the telangiectasis of the leg and foot (H and I).

J–L: This 26-year-old Latin man with anemia (hemoglobin 6.3 g/100 ml) related to treatment for acquired immunodeficiency syndrome (AIDS) developed bilateral blurred vision caused by subinternal limiting membrane hemorrhages in the macula bilaterally. Note the widespread white-centered superficial retinal hemorrhages (J and K). Three months later, after correction of his anemia, the hemorrhages were gone but he had developed cytomegalovirus retinopathy in the inferior macula area of the left eye (L).

(I, from Brod et al.[1330])

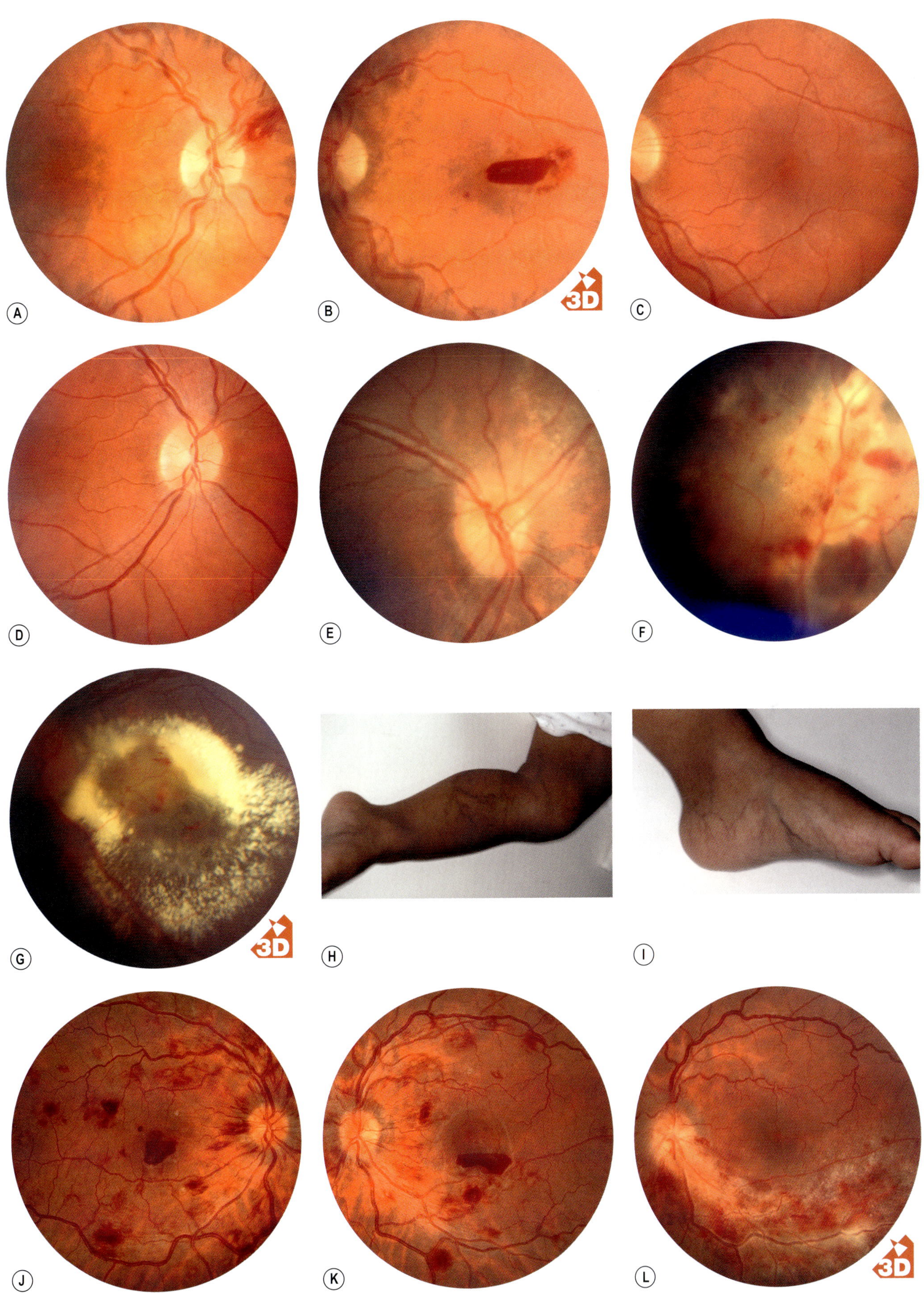
A
B
3D
C
D
E
F
G
3D
H
I
J
K
L
3D

Anemic retinopathy is often characterized by blot hemorrhages that look like an ink dot made up of multiple little clumps of red blood cells (Figure 6.83, E). It is believed that the low oxygen-carrying capacity causes damage to the endothelium and the blood cells seep out through the damaged endothelium and hence the hemorrhages are more like an ink blot rather than nerve fiber layer or more dense. Along with the blot hemorrhages, the veins are dilated due to autoregulation and as a compensatory mechanism to decrease the flow through the retina to extract as much oxygen as possible by the retinal cells.

The cause of anemia, as well as accompanying hematologic abnormalities such as thrombocytopenia, leukemia, and macroglobulinemia, may be more important than the level of hemoglobin in the production of retinal hemorrhages.[1331,1332,1340–1343] Thrombocytopenia, thrombasthenia, and other platelet abnormalities in the absence of anemia may be the underlying cause of retinal hemorrhages[1343,1344] and retinal edema (Figure 6.84G–I).

6.83 Anemic retinopathy.

A–D: This 45-year-old woman was post unknown donor peripheral stem cell transplant for acute myeloid leukemia who had developed graft-versus-host disease (GvHD). Her vision was 20/40 in each eye. She had both nerve fiber and deep ink blot-type retinal hemorrhages (arrow), some with white centers (arrow), secondary to anemia related to her blood dyscrasia (A–D). The retinal hemorrhages resolved once her anemia improved.

E: This 58-year-old patient had advanced glaucoma and had undergone repeat keratoplasties in this eye. She was found to have several target-shaped (arrow) deep retinal hemorrhages typical of anemia during her postoperative visit. She had anemia of chronic disease with a hemoglobin of 8.4 g/100 ml that improved to 11 g/100 ml with treatment.

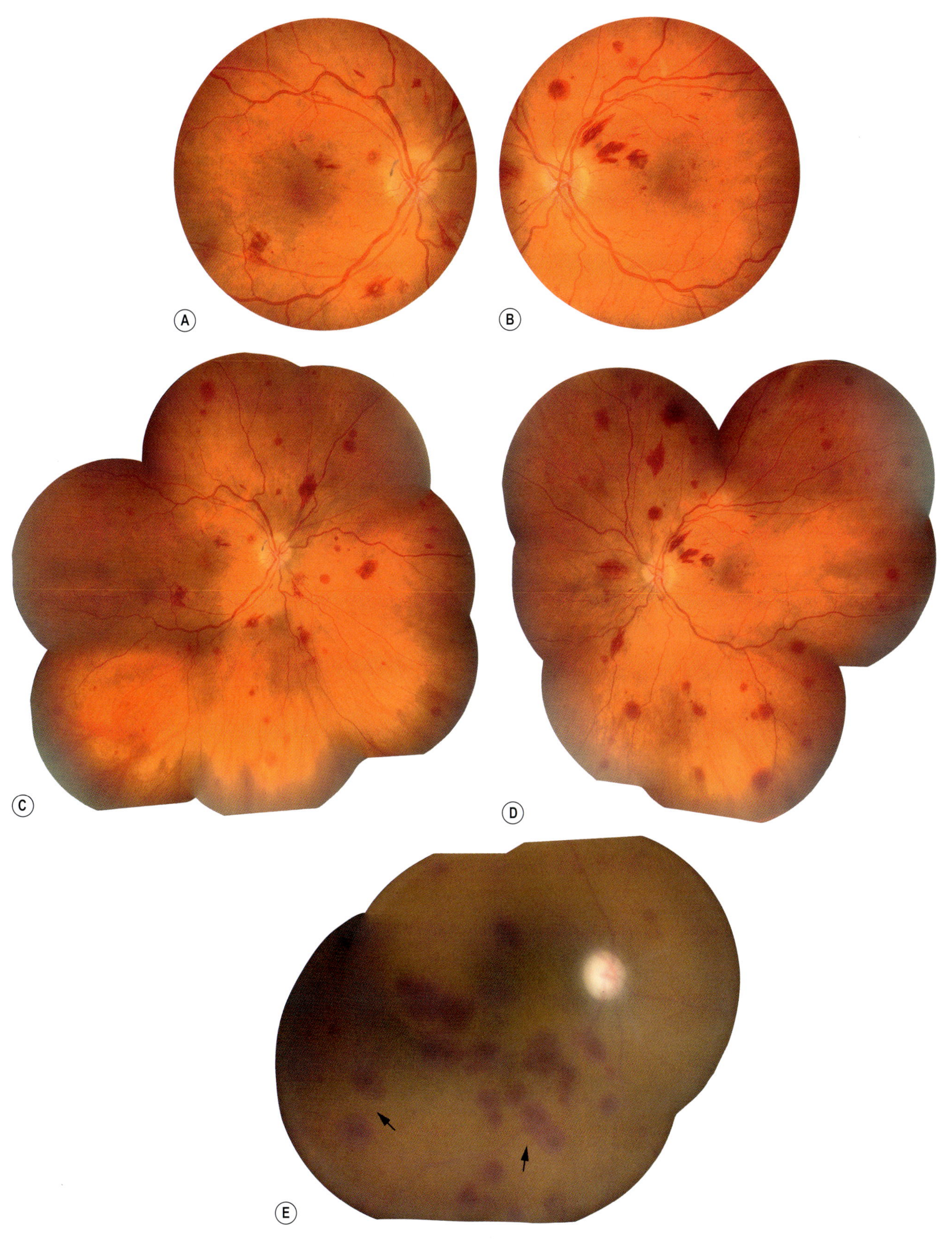
A
B
C
D
E

Retinopathy Associated with Hyperviscosity

The hyperviscosity syndrome consists of a bleeding diathesis, neurologic dysfunction, and retinopathy that may be associated with monoclonal gammopathies such as Waldenström's macroglobulinemia. Patients who have Waldenström's macroglobulinemia have a high intravascular concentration of an abnormal monoclonal IgM protein that causes increased blood viscosity and intravascular volume. This may produce the hyperviscosity syndrome associated with fatigue; headaches; epistaxis; visual impairment; sausagelike dilation of retinal veins; increased venous tortuosity; dot, blot, and flame-shaped retinal hemorrhages; retinal and optic disc edema; and retinal detachment (Figure 6.84J–L).[1345–1348] In addition to increased retinal circulation time, angiography may demonstrate areas of capillary nonperfusion and microaneurysms. Serous detachment of the retina in the macula may occur in some patients with Waldenström's macroglobulinemia and other dysproteinemias (see Figure 3.60). Plasmapheresis can lower serum viscosity and reverse the retinopathy.[1346,1348] Ocular signs of serum hyperviscosity may also occur in patients with multiple myeloma, polycythemia, or leukemia, and in patients with polyclonal gammopathies, most of whom have rheumatoid arthritis.[1349,1350] Severe occlusive and proliferative retinal vasculopathy may occasionally occur in association with systemic light-chain deposition, a plasma cell dyscrasia associated with a monoclonal paraprotein spike that may occur in the absence of the hyperviscosity syndrome.[1351]

6.84 Retinopathy associated with anemia and dysproteinemia.

A–F: Subconjunctival hemorrhage (A) and bilateral loss of central vision caused by macular hemorrhages in a patient with aplastic anemia. Note the fine white dots on the surface of the blood (arrows, B and C), which probably lies just beneath the internal limiting membrane. Several small, white-centered, superficial retinal hemorrhages were present (D). Angiography (E and F) showed no evidence of vascular permeability alterations.

G–I: Retinal vascular leakage associated with platelet abnormality in both eyes of this asymptomatic 6-year-old black boy who had elevated beta-thromboglobulins, hyperaggregable platelets, increased platelet factor IV, and microcytosis. Visual acuity was 20/20. The posterior fundi appeared normal (G). There were no cells in the vitreous. Angiography demonstrated marked retinal venous and capillary vascular permeability alterations in both eyes (H and I). Extensive medical and hematologic evaluations were otherwise negative.

J–L: Retinal hemorrhages and venous engorgement in a patient with Waldenström's macroglobulinemia. Note the link-sausage changes (arrows, L) and mottled fluorescence within the dilated retinal veins.

(G–I, courtesy of Dr. Saunders L. Hupp.)

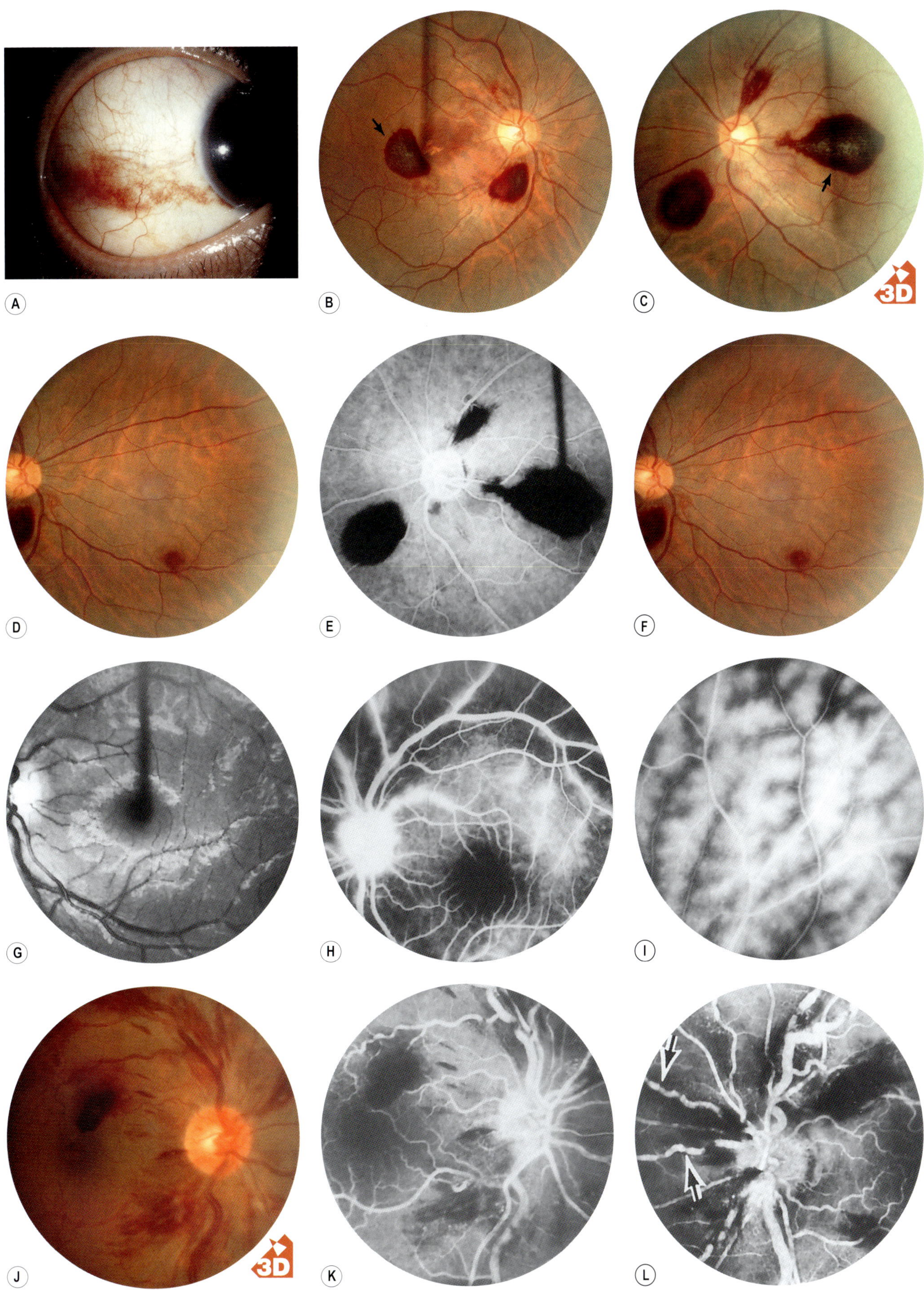
A
B
C
3D
D
E
F
G
H
I
J
3D
K
L

Hyperlipoproteinemia

Five types of hyperlipoproteinemia are described.[1352] Each has an abnormality of one or more of the plasma lipoproteins, chylomicrons, beta-lipoproteins, or pre-beta-lipoproteins. Each may occur as a heritable disorder or secondary to other diseases, particularly diabetes mellitus. Lipemia retinalis and lid xanthomas may occur as complications of types 4 and 5, both of which are characterized by increased very-low-density lipoproteins (pre-beta-lipoproteins) and increased serum triglyceride levels (Figure 6.85A–C). Cholesterol levels are increased in type 5 and may be normal in type 4. Lipemia retinalis is believed to be directly correlated with the level of serum triglycerides.[1353,1354] It usually develops when serum triglyceride levels reach 2500 mg/dl. The retinal arteries and veins develop an identical salmon-pink color that may progress to an ivory or cream color when the triglyceride level exceeds 5000 mg/dl (Figure 6.85A–C). Ordinarily, this is unassociated with a visual deficit, and the fundus rapidly returns to a normal appearance as serum lipid levels return toward normal. These patients usually do not develop retinal hemorrhages, cotton-wool patches, or exudation.[1355]

When hyperlipidemia is associated with other diseases affecting capillary permeability, unusual amounts of intraretinal hemorrhage and extravascular intraretinal accumulation of lipid may occur.[1356,1357] Some patients who have excessive accumulation of yellowish, lipid-rich exudate in or beneath the retina associated with frequently encountered disorders, such as choroidal neovascularization, diabetic retinopathy, and branch retinal vein occlusion, may have an underlying hyperlipoproteinemia (Figure 6.85G–L).[1330] Reduction of the amount of circulating blood lipid may reduce the severity of the exudation.[836] Hyperlipidemia in patients with proliferative retinopathy may occasionally result in lipid transudation into the vitreous, producing a picture simulating endophthalmitis.[1343] There is some evidence that patients with hyperlipidemia, particularly types 4 and 5, have an increased risk of developing retinal venous obstruction.[1358]

Parenteral hyperalimentation of lipid may occasionally result in focal intraretinal extravasation of lipid and blood (Figure 6.85G–I).[1359,1360]

6.85 Retinopathy associated with hyperlipidemia.

A–C: Lipemia retinalis in a patient before (A) and after (B and C) development of lipemia retinalis. Note the pallor of the major retinal vessels, which had a salmon-pink hue (B and C).

D–F: Cherry-red spot maculopathy and visual loss to 6/30 occurred bilaterally after 3 weeks of hyperalimentation in this 23-year-old man with weight loss and fever caused by Crohn's disease (D). Angiography was normal (E). The retinal whitening disappeared and the acuity returned to normal within 2 weeks after discontinuing parenteral nutrition (F). The retinal whitening was presumed to be caused by temporary accumulation of lipid by the ganglion cells during hyperalimentation.

G–I: This patient, who had diabetes, hypertension, and hyperlipidemia, developed focal mounds of intraretinal hemorrhage and lipid exudation (G) and angiographic evidence of dilated microvascular changes along the major vascular arcades in both eyes (H). Angiography demonstrated minimal evidence of diabetic and hypertensive retinopathy outside the focal areas of exudation and hemorrhage. The exudation and hemorrhage progressed to involve the central macular area of both eyes within 9 months (I).

J–L: Progressive loss of visual acuity occurred within 6 months in this 63-year-old woman with diabetes mellitus, hypertriglyceridemia, arthritis, gout, and an inferotemporal branch retina vein obstruction. Note the increase in the lipid exudation and the juxtapapillary hemorrhages when her visual acuity had declined to 20/400 (L).

(D–F, from Yassur et al.[1360]; J–L, courtesy of Dr. Frank J. Cullotta.)

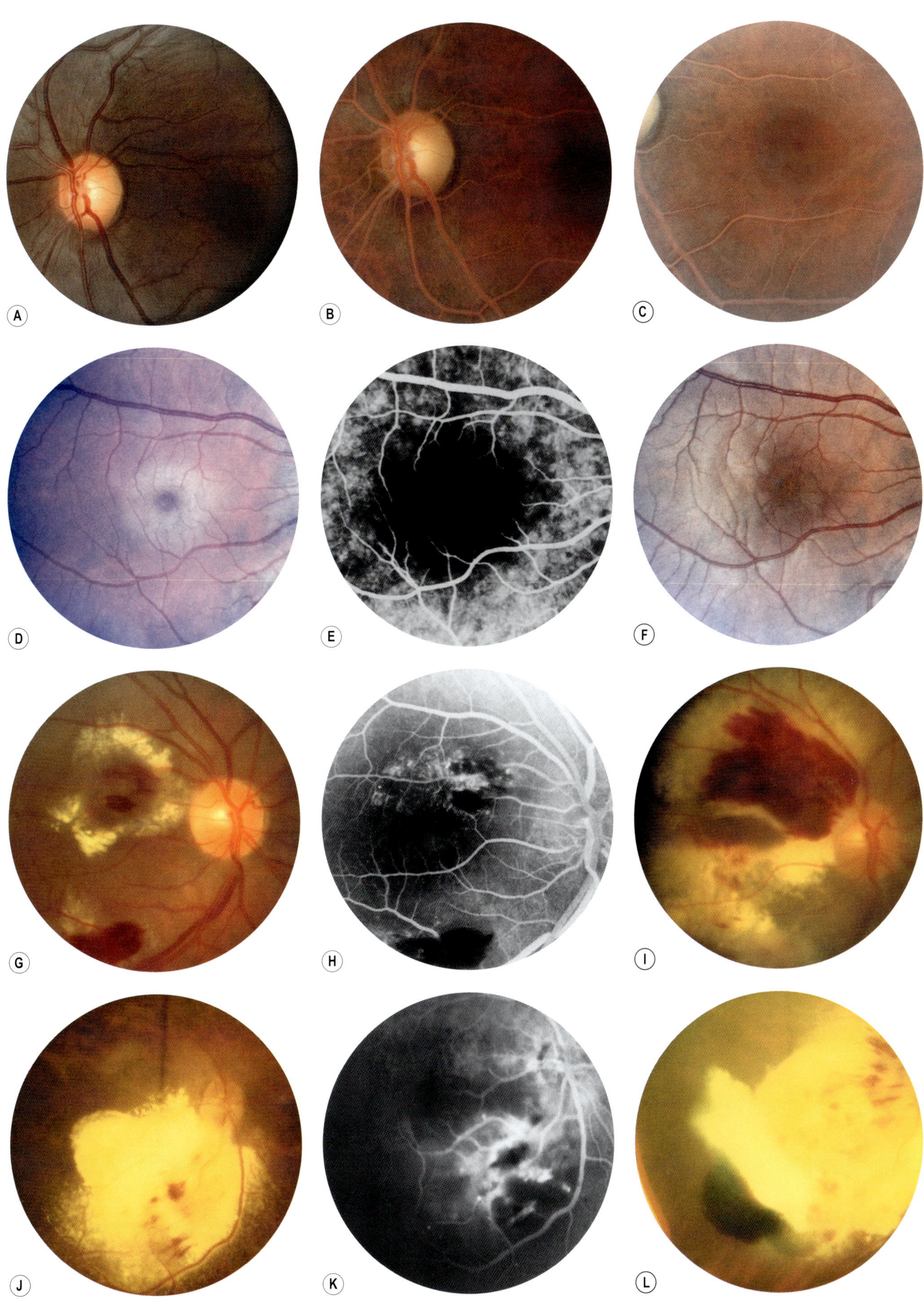
A
B
C
D
E
F
G
H
I
J
K
L

References

1. Beyer E-M. Familiäre Tortuositas der kleinen Netzhautarterien mit Makulablutung. Klin Monatsbl Augenheilkd 1958;132:532–40.
2. Werner H, Gafner F. Beitrag zur familiären Tortuositas der kleinen Netzhautarterien. Ophthalmologica 1961;141:350–6.
3. Cagianut B. Zum Krankheitsbild der familiären Tortuositas der kleinen Netzhautgefässe. Ophthalmologica 1968;156:322–4.
4. Cagianut B, Werner H. Zum Krankheitsbild der familiären Tortuositas der kleinen Netzhautarterien mit Maculablutung. Klin Monatsbl Augenheilkd 1968;153:533–42.
5. Goldberg MF, Pollack IP, et al. Familial retinal arteriolar tortuosity with retinal hemorrhage. Am J Ophthalmol 1972;73:183–91.
6. Wells CG, Kalina RE. Progressive inherited retinal arteriolar tortuosity with spontaneous retinal hemorrhages. Ophthalmology 1985;92:1015–24.
7. Kayazawa F, Machida T. Retinal arteriolar tortuosity with macular hemorrhage. Ann Ophthalmol 1983;15:42–3.
8. Wells CG, Kalina RE. Progressive inherited retinal arteriolar tortuosity with spontaneous retinal hemorrhages. Ophthalmology 1985;92:1015–24.
9. Faisal ZK, Abboud EB. New hemorrhages during scleral buckling in inherited retinal arteriolar tortuosity. Arch Ophthalmol 1995;113:853–4.
10. Gekeler F, Shinoda K, Junger M, et al. Familial retinal arterial tortuosity associated with tortuosity in nail bed capillaries. Arch Ophthalmol 2006;124:1492–4.
11. Plaisier E, Alamowitch S, Gribouval O, et al. Autosomal-dominant familial hematuria with retinal arteriolar tortuosity and contractures: a novel syndrome. Kidney Int 2005;67:2354–60.
12. Seo JH, Kim I, Yu HG. A case of carotid aneurysm in familial retinal arterial tortuosity. Korean J Ophthalmol 2009;23:57–8.
13. Johns KJ, Johns JA, Feman SS. Retinal vascular abnormalities in patients with coarctation of the aorta. Arch Ophthalmol 1991;109:1266–8.
14. Meredith TA. Inherited retinal venous beading. Arch Ophthalmol 1987;105:949–53.
15. Stewart MW, Gitter KA. Inherited retinal venous beading. Am J Ophthalmol 1988;106:675–81.
16. Beratis NG, Varvarigou A, Katsibris J, et al. Vascular retinal abnormalities in neonates of mothers who smoked during pregnancy. J Pediatr 2000;136:760–6.
17. Mansour AM, Bitar FF, Traboulsi EI, et al. Ocular pathology in congenital heart disease. Eye (Lond) 2005;19:29–34.
18. Bär C. Ein Fall von in den Glaskörper vordringender Arterienschlinge in einem durch Embolie der Centralarterie erblindeten Auge. Klin Monatsbl Augenheilkd 1901;39:307–15.
19. Brown GC, Magargal L, Augsburger JJ, et al. Preretinal arterial loops and retinal arterial occlusion. Am J Ophthalmol 1979;87:646–51.
20. Brucker AJ, Michels RG, Fine SL. Congenital retinal arterial loops and vitreous hemorrhage. Am J Ophthalmol 1977;84:220–3.
21. Degenhart W, Brown GC, Augsburger JJ, et al. Prepapillary vascular loops. Ophthalmology 1981;88:1126–31.
22. Grossniklaus H, Thall E, Annable W. Familial prepapillary vascular loops. Arch Ophthalmol 1986;104:1755–6.
23. Harcourt RB, Locket NA. Occlusion of a pre-retinal arterial loop. Br J Ophthalmol 1967;51: 562–5.
24. Lambert HM, Sipperley JO, Shacklett DE. Autosomal dominant preretinal vascular loops. Retina 1983;3:258–60.
25. Liebreich R. Demonstrations of diseases of the eye: persistent hyaloid artery and vein. Trans Pathol Soc Lond 1871;22:221.
26. Limaye SR, Tang RA, Pilkerton AR. Cilioretinal circulation and branch arterial occlusion associated with preretinal arterial loops. Am J Ophthalmol 1980;89:834–9.
27. Regenbogen L, Godel V, Spierer A, et al. Retinal arterial loop occlusion. Ann Ophthalmol 1981;13:729–32.
28. Shakin EP, Shields JA, Augsburger JJ, et al. Clinicopathologic correlation of a prepapillary vascular loop. Retina 1988;8:55–8.
29. Walker CH. Thrombosis of the inferior temporal branch of the arteria centralis retinae in an eye with a persistent hyaloid artery and vein; ? caused by exposure to direct sunlight. Trans Ophthalmol Soc UK 1903;23:279–81.
30. Brown GC, Donoso LA, Magargal LE. Congenital retinal macrovessels. Arch Ophthalmol 1982;100:1430–6.
31. Mauthner L. Lehrbuch der Ophthalmoscopie. Vienna: Tendler; 1868. p. 249
32. Han JR, Jeon GS, Park JH, et al. Congenital retinal macrovessel and foveal dysplasia of retinopathy of prematurity. Jpn J Ophthalmol 2009;53:277–9.
33. Mansour AM, Walsh JB, Henkind P. Arteriovenous anastomosis of the retina. Ophthalmology 1987;94:35–40.
34. Archer DB, Deutman A, Ernest JT, et al. Arteriovenous communications of the retina. Am J Ophthalmol 1973;75:224–41.
35. Augsburger JJ, Goldberg RE, Shields JA. Changing appearance of retinal arteriovenous malformation. Albrecht von Graefes Arch Klin Exp Ophthalmol 1980;215:65–70.
36. Baurmann H, Meyer F, Oberhoff P. Komplikationen bei der arteriovenösen anastomose der Netzhaut. Klin Monatsbl Augenheilkd 1968;153:562–71.
37. Bech K, Jensen OA. On the frequency of co-existing racemose haemangiomata of the retina and brain. Acta Psychiatr Neurol Scand 1961;36:47–56.
38. Bellhorn RW, Friedman AH, Henkind P. Racemose (cirsoid) hemangioma in rhesus monkey retina. Am J Ophthalmol 1972;74:517–22.
39. Cagianut B. Das arterio-venöse Aneurysma der Netzhaut. Klin Monatsbl Augenheilkd 1962;140:180–91.
40. Cameron ME, Greer CH. Congenital arterio-venous aneurysm of the retina; a post mortem report. Br J Ophthalmol 1968;52:768–72.
41. JDM Gass. Differential diagnosis of intraocular tumors; a stereoscopic presentation. St. Louis: CV Mosby; 1974. p. 307–9.
42. Gregersen E. Arteriovenous aneurysm of the retina; a case of spontaneous thrombosis and "healing". Acta Ophthalmol 1961;39:937–9.
43. Hayasaka S, Kanamori M, Morihiro K-I, et al. Anomalous macular vessels: case report and review of the recent Japanese literature. Ann Ophthalmol 1990;22:454–6.
44. Hopen G, Smith JL, Hoff JT, et al. The Wyburn-Mason syndrome; concomitant chiasmal and fundus vascular malformations. J Clin Neuro-Ophthalmol 1983;3:53–62.
45. Horiuchi T, Gass JDM, David NJ. Arteriovenous malformation in the retina of a monkey. Am J Ophthalmol 1976;82:896–904.
46. LaDow CS, Henefer EP, McFall TA. Central hemangioma of the maxilla, with von Hippel's disease: report of a case. J Oral Surg Anesth Hosp Dent Ser 1964;22:252–9.
47. Magnus H. Aneurysma arterioso-venosum retinale. Virchows Arch Pathol Anat 1874;60:38–45.
48. Mozetti M. Sulle anomolie dei vasi retinici ed in particolar modo sull'aneurisma cirsoide della retina. Boll Oculist 1939;18:455–68.
49. Pauleikhoff D, Wessing A. Arteriovenous communications of the retina during a 17-year follow-up. Retina 1991;11:433–6.
50. Schatz H, Chang LF, Ober RR. Central retinal vein occlusion associated with retinal arteriovenous malformation. Ophthalmology 1993;100:24–30.
51. Tilanus MD, Hoyng C, Deutman AF. Congenital arteriovenous communications and the development of two types of leaking retinal macroaneurysms. Am J Ophthalmol 1991;112:31–3.
52. Wyburn-Mason R. Arteriovenous aneurysm of mid-brain and retina, facial naevi and mental changes. Brain 1943;65:163–203.
53. Effron L, Zakov ZN, Tomsak RL. Neovascular glaucoma as a complication of the Wyburn-Mason syndrome. J Clin Neuro-Ophthalmol 1985;5:95–8.
54. Bonnet P, Dechaume J, Blanc E. L'anévrisme cirsoïde de la rétine (anévrisme racémeux); ses relations avec l'anévrisme cirsoïde de la face et l'anévrisme cirsoïde du cerveau. Bull Mem Soc Fr Ophtalmol 1938;51:521–4.
55. Brodsky MC, Hoyt WF, Higashida RT. Bonnet–Dechaume–Blanc syndrome with large facial angioma. Arch Ophthalmol 1987;105:854–5.
56. de Crecchio G, Pacente L, Alfieri MC, et al. Valsalva retinopathy associated with a congenital retinal macrovessel. Arch Ophthalmol 2000;118:146–7.
57. Koizumi H, Iida T, Mori T, et al. Retinal arteriolar macroaneurysm and congenital retinal macrovessel. Ophthalmic Surg Lasers Imag 2009;40:513–5.
58. Chen T-L, Yarng S-S. Vitreous hemorrhage from a persistent hyaloid artery. Retina 1993;13: 148–51.
59. Mansour AM, Wells CG, Jampol LM, et al. Ocular complications of arteriovenous communications of the retina. Arch Ophthalmol 1989;107:232–6.
60. Muñoz FJ, Rebolleda G, Cores FJ, et al. Congenital retinal arteriovenous communication associated with a full-thickness macular hole. Acta Ophthalmol 1991;69:117–20.
61. Dekking HM. Arteriovenous aneurysm of the retina with spontaneous regression. Ophthalmologica 1955;130:113–5.
62. Bolling JP, Buettner H. Acquired retinal arteriovenous communications in occlusive disease of the carotid artery. Ophthalmology 1990;97:1148–52.
63. Mintz-Hittner HA, Knight-Nanan DM, Satriano DR, et al. A small foveal avascular zone may be an historic mark of prematurity. Ophthalmology 1999;106:1409–13.
64. Provis JM, Hendrickson AE. The foveal avascular region of developing human retina. Arch Ophthalmol 2008;126:507–11.
65. Gariano RF. Special features of human retinal angiogenesis. Eye (Lond) 2010;24:401–7.
66. Hendrickson A, Troilo D, Possin D, et al. Development of the neural retina and its vasculature in the marmoset *Callithrix jacchus*. J Comp Neurol 2006;497:270–86.
67. Hendrickson A, Djajadi H, Erickson A, et al. Development of the human retina in the absence of ganglion cells. Exp Eye Res 2006;83:920–31.
68. Provis JM, Sandercoe T, Hendrickson AE. Astrocytes and blood vessels define the foveal rim during primate retinal development. Invest Ophthalmol Vis Sci 2000;41:2827–36.
69. van Genderen MM, Riemslag FC, Schuil J, et al. Chiasmal misrouting and foveal hypoplasia without albinism. Br J Ophthalmol 2006;90:1098–102.
70. Appen RE, Wray SH, Cogan DG. Central retinal artery occlusion. Am J Ophthalmol 1975;79: 374–81.
71. Ball CJ. Atheromatous embolism to the brain, retina, and choroid. Arch Ophthalmol 1966;76:690–5.
72. Brownstein S, Font RL, Alper MG. Atheromatous plaques of the retinal blood vessels; histologic confirmation of ophthalmoscopically visible lesions. Arch Ophthalmol 1973;90:49–52.
73. Carlson MR, Pilger IS, Rosenbaum AL. Central retinal artery occlusion after carotid angiography. Am J Ophthalmol 1976;81:103–4.
74. Gold D. Retinal arterial occlusion. Trans Am Acad Ophthalmol Otolaryngol 1977;83:OP392–OP408.
75. Hartel WC, Spoor TC, Hammer ME. Retinal embolism following percutaneous femoral cerebral angiography. J Clin Neuro-Ophthalmol 1982;2:49–54.
76. Ivan DJ, May DR, Evans RM. Active central retinal artery embolization. Ophthalmology 1981;88:673–5.
77. Karjalainen K. Occlusion of the central retinal artery and retinal branch arterioles; a clinical, tonographic and fluorescein angiographic study of 175 patients. Acta Ophthalmol Suppl 1971:109.
78. Kotsuka N. A case of retinal embolism with bright plaques in retinal artery. Jpn J Clin Ophthalmol 1966;20(947–948):89–92.
79. Schmidt D, Schumacher M, Wakhloo AK. Microcatheter urokinase infusion in central retinal artery occlusion. Am J Ophthalmol 1992;113:429–34.
80. Schwarcz TH, Eton D, Ellenby MI. Hollenhorst plaques: retinal manifestations and the role of carotid endarterectomy. J Vasc Surg 1990;11:635.
81. Tsutsumi A. Retinopathy in cyanotic congenital heart disease. Jpn J Clin Ophthalmol 1983;37:933–8.
82. Whiteman DW, Rosen DA. Pinkerton RMH. Retinal and choroidal microvascular embolism after intranasal corticosteroid injection. Am J Ophthalmol 1980;89:851–3.

83. Wiznia RA, Pearson WN. Use of transesophageal echocardiography for detection of a likely source of embolization to the central retinal artery. Am J Ophthalmol 1991;111:104–5.
84. Wolter JR, Ryan RW. Atheromatous embolism of the central retinal artery; secondary hemorrhagic glaucoma. Arch Ophthalmol 1972;87:301–4.
85. Brown GC, Magargal LE, Shields JA. Retinal arterial obstruction in children and young adults. Ophthalmology 1981;88:18–25.
86. Bucci Jr FA, Dimitsopulos TM, Krohel GB. Branch retinal artery occlusion secondary to percutaneous transluminal coronary angioplasty. Br J Ophthalmol 1989;73:309–10.
87. Pe'er J, Milgalter E, Matamoros N. Retinal emboli after open heart surgery. Arch Ophthalmol 1986;107:317.
88. Shimizu T, Kiyosawa M, Miura T. Acute obstruction of the retinal and choroidal circulation as a complication of interventional angiography. Graefes Arch Clin Exp Ophthalmol 1993;231:43–7.
89. Arruga J, Sanders MD. Ophthalmologic findings in 70 patients with evidence of retinal embolism. Ophthalmology 1982;89:1336–47.
90. Brown GC, Magargal LE. Sudden occlusion of the retinal and posterior choroidal circulations in a youth. Am J Ophthalmol 1979;88:690–3.
91. De Potter P, Zografos L. Survival prognosis of patients with retinal artery occlusion and associated carotid artery disease. Graefes Arch Clin Exp Ophthalmol 1993;231:212–6.
92. Kollarits CR, Lubow M, Hissong SL. Retinal strokes. I. Incidence of carotid atheromata. JAMA 1972;222:1273–5.
93. Bergen RL, Cangemi FE, Glassman R. Bilateral arterial occlusion secondary to Barlow's syndrome. Ann Ophthalmol 1982;14:673–5.
94. Caltrider ND, Irvine AR, Kline HJ, et al. Retinal emboli in patients with mitral valve prolapse. Am J Ophthalmol 1980;90:534–9.
95. Brown GC, Magargal LE, Simeone FA. Arterial obstruction and ocular neovascularization. Ophthalmology 1982;89:139–46.
96. Brown GC, Magargal LE. Central retinal artery obstruction and visual acuity. Ophthalmology 1982;89:14–19.
97. Brown GC, Shields JA. Cilioretinal arteries and retinal arterial occlusion. Arch Ophthalmol 1979;97:84–92.
98. Oji EO, McLeod D. Partial central retinal artery occlusion. Trans Ophthalmol Soc UK 1978;98:156–9.
99. Dahrling II BE. The histopathology of early central retinal artery occlusion. Arch Ophthalmol 1965;73:506–10.
100. Kroll AJ. Experimental central retinal artery occlusion. Arch Ophthalmol 1968;79:453–69.
101. JDM Gass. A fluorescein angiographic study of macular dysfunction secondary to retinal vascular disease. I. Embolic retinal artery obstruction. Arch Ophthalmol 1968;80:535–49.
102. McLeod D, Marshall J, Kohner EM, et al. The role of axoplasmic transport in the pathogenesis of retinal cotton-wool spots. Br J Ophthalmol 1977;61:177–91.
103. Burde RM, Smith ME, Black JT. Retinal artery occlusion in the absence of a cherry red spot. Surv Ophthalmol 1982;27:181–6.
104. Cherny M, O'Day J, Currie J. Intraretinal gray lesions as a sign of reversible visual loss following prolonged ophthalmic artery hypoperfusion. J Clin Neuro-Ophthalmol 1991;11:228–32.
105. Brown GC, Moffat K, Cruess A. Cilioretinal artery obstruction. Retina 1983;3:182–7.
106. Ros MA, Magargal LE, Uram M. Branch retinal-artery obstruction: a review of 201 eyes. Ann Ophthalmol 1989;21:103–7.
107. Zylbermann R, Rozenman Y, Ronen S. Functional occlusion of a cilioretinal artery. Ann Ophthalmol 1981;13:1269–72.
108. Hollenhorst RW. Significance of bright plaques in the retinal arterioles. Trans Am Ophthalmol Soc 1961;59:252–73.
109. Hollenhorst RW. Vascular status of patients who have cholesterol emboli in the retina. Am J Ophthalmol 1966;61:1159–65.
110. Younge BR. The significance of retinal emboli. J Clin Neuro-Ophthalmol 1989;9:190–4.
111. Sadun AA, Green RL, Nobe JR, et al. Papillopathies associated with unusual calcifications in the retrolaminar optic nerve. J Clin Neuro-Ophthalmol 1991;11:175–80.
112. Hayreh SS, Zimmerman MB. Central retinal artery occlusion: visual outcome. Am J Ophthalmol 2005;140:376–91.
113. David NJ, Gilbert DS, JDM Gass. Fluorescein angiography in retinal arterial branch obstructions. Am J Ophthalmol 1970;69:43–55.
114. David NJ, Norton EWD, Gass JDM, et al. Fluorescein angiography in cenral retinal artery occlusion. Arch Ophthalmol 1967;77:619–29.
115. Sano H, Kaneko H, Tani M. Clinical studies on occlusion of the retinal artery by fluorescein fundus photography. Jpn J Ophthalmol 1968;12:190–200.
116. Jacobs DS, Lessell S, Grove AS. Acquired arterial collateral vessels at the optic disc. Arch Ophthalmol 1992;110:20–1.
117. Klein R, Klein B, Henkind P, et al. Retinal collateral vessel formation. Invest Ophthalmol 1971;10:471–80.
118. Tsacopoulos M, Baker R. Characteristics of fluorescein leakage from retinal arterioles following microembolization. Exp Eye Res 1975;20:23–32.
119. Duker JS, Brown GC. Iris neovascularization associated with obstruction of the central retinal artery. Ophthalmology 1988;95:1244–50.
120. Duker JS, Brown GC. The efficacy of panretinal photocoagulation for neovascularization of the iris after central retinal artery obstruction. Ophthalmology 1989;96:92–5.
121. Duker JS, Brown GC. Neovascularization of the optic disc associated with obstruction of the central retinal artery. Ophthalmology 1989;96:87–91.
122. Duker JS, Sivalingam A, Brown GC, et al. A prospective study of acute central retinal artery obstruction; the incidence of secondary ocular neovascularization. Arch Ophthalmol 1991;109:339–42.
123. Hayreh SS, Podhajsky PA, Zimmerman MB. Retinal artery occlusion associated systemic and ophthalmic abnormalities. Ophthalmology 2009;116:1928–36.
124. Hayreh SS. Intra-arterial thrombolysis for central retinal artery occlusion. Br J Ophthalmol 2008;92:585–7.
125. Hayreh SS, Zimmerman MB. Fundus changes in central retinal artery occlusion. Retina 2007;27:276–89.
126. Hayreh SS. Neovascular glaucoma. Prog Retin Eye Res 2007;26:470–85.
127. Mizener JB, Podhajsky P, Hayreh SS. Ocular ischemic syndrome. Ophthalmology 1997;104:859–64.
128. Foster RE, Gutman FA, Meyers SM, et al. Acute multifocal inner retinitis. Am J Ophthalmol 1991;111:673–81.
129. Orzalesi N, Ricciardi L. Segmental retinal periarteritis. Am J Ophthalmol 1971;72:55–9.
130. Hayreh SS, Kolder HE, Weingeist TA. Central retinal artery occlusion and retinal tolerance time. Ophthalmology 1980;87:75–8.
131. Duker JS, Brown GC. Recovery following acute obstruction of the retinal and choroidal circulations; a case history. Retina 1988;8:257–60.
132. Younge BR, Rosenbaum TJ. Treatment of acute central retinal artery occlusion. Mayo Clin Proc 1978;53:408–10.
133. De La Paz MA, Patrinely JR, Marines HM, et al. Adjunctive hyperbaric oxygen in the treatment of bilateral cerebro-rhino-orbital mucormycosis. Am J Ophthalmol 1992;114:208–11.
134. Peyman GA, Gremillion Jr CM. Surgical removal of a branch retinal artery embolus: a case report. Int Ophthalmol 1990;14:295–8.
135. Watson PG. The treatment of acute retinal arterial occlusion. In: Cant JS, editor. The William Mackenzie centenary symposium on the ocular circulation in health and disease. St. Louis: CV Mosby; 1969. p. 234–45.
136. Blair NP, Baker DS, Rhode JP, et al. Vitreoperfusion; a new approach to ocular ischemia. Arch Ophthalmol 1989;107:417–23.
137. Jampol LM. Oxygen therapy and intraocular oxygenation. Trans Am Ophthalmol Soc 1987;85:407–37.
138. Vine AK, Maguire PT, Martonyi C, et al. Recombinant tissue plasminogen activator to lyse experimentally induced retinal arterial thrombi. Am J Ophthalmol 1988;105:266–70.
139. Rudkin AK, Lee AW, Chen CS. Central retinal artery occlusion: timing and mode of presentation. Eur J Neurol 2009;16:674–7.
140. Chen CS, Lee AW. Management of acute central retinal artery occlusion. Nat Clin Pract Neurol 2008;4:376–83.
141. Biousse V. Thrombolysis for acute central retinal artery occlusion: is it time? Am J Ophthalmol 2008;146:631–4.
142. Augsurger JJ, Magargal LE. Visual prognosis following treatment of acute central retinal artery obstruction. Br J Ophthalmol 1980;64:913–7.
143. Jorizzo PA, Klein ML, Shults WT, et al. Visual recovery in combined central retinal artery and central retinal vein occlusion. Am J Ophthalmol 1987;104:358–63.
144. Greven CM, Weaver RG, Harris WR. Transesophageal echocardiography for detecting mitral valve prolapse with retinal artery occlusions. Am J Ophthalmol 1991;111:103–4.
145. Wisotsky BJ, Engel HM. Transesophageal echocardiography in the diagnosis of branch retinal artery obstruction. Am J Ophthalmol 1993;115:653–6.
146. Campo RV, Aaberg TM. Digital subtraction angiography in the diagnosis of retinal vascular disease. Am J Ophthalmol 1983;96:632–40.
147. Shah HG, Brown GC, Goldberg RE. Digital subtraction carotid angiography and retinal arterial obstruction. Ophthalmology 1985;92:68–72.
148. Duker JS, Magargal LE, Stubbs GW. Quadrantic venous-stasis retinopathy secondary to an embolic branch retinal artery obstruction. Ophthalmology 1990;97:167–70.
149. Magargal LE, Sanborn GE, Zimmerman A. Venous stasis retinopathy associated with emboli obstruction of the central retinal artery. J Clin Neuro-Ophthalmol 1982;2:113–8.
150. Eckardt C, Götze O, Utermann D. Über die Lebenserwartung von Patienten mit Zirkulationsstörungen am hinteren Bulbusabschnitt. Ophthalmologica 1983;187:34–42.
151. Pfaffenbach DD, Hollenhorst RW. Morbidity and survivorship of patients with embolic cholesterol crystals in the ocular fundus. Am J Ophthalmol 1973;75:66–72.
152. Savino PJ, Glaser JS, Cassady J. Retinal stroke. Is the patient at risk? Arch Ophthalmol 1977;95:1185–9.
152A. Rudkin AK, Lee AW, Chen CS. Vascular risk factors for central retinal artery occlusion. Eye 2009;24:678–81.
153. Jahan R, Murayama Y, Gobin YP, et al. Embolization of arteriovenous malformations with Onyx: clinicopathological experience in 23 patients. Neurosurgery 2001;48:984–95. [discussion 995–7.]
154. Murayama Y, Vinuela F, Tateshima S, et al. Endovascular treatment of experimental aneurysms by use of a combination of liquid embolic agents and protective devices. AJNR Am J Neuroradiol 2000;21:1726–35.
155. Asouhidou I, Katsaridis V, Meng L, et al. Desaturation during Onyx embolization. Br J Anaesth 2010;105:385–6.
156. Jampol LM, Wong AS, Albert DM. Atrial myxoma and central retinal artery occlusion. Am J Ophthalmol 1973;75:242–9.
157. Kennedy RH, Flanagan JC, Eagle Jr RC, et al. The Carney complex with ocular signs suggestive of cardiac myxoma. Am J Ophthalmol 1991;111:699–702.
158. Lewis JM. Multiple retinal occlusions from a left atrial myxoma. Am J Ophthalmol 1994;117:674–5.
159. Matamoros N, BenEzra D. Bilateral retinopathy and encephalopathy. Graefes Arch Clin Exp Ophthalmol 1989;227:39–41.
160. Taylor RH, Deutsch J. Myxoma mix-up; a case report. J Clin Neuro-Ophthalmol 1992;12:207–9.
161. Tönz M, Laske A, Carrel T. Convulsions, hemiparesis, and central retinal artery occlusion due to left atrial myxoma in child. Eur J Pediatr 1992;151:652–4.
162. Yasuma F, Tsuzuki M, Yasuma T. Retinal embolism from left atrial myxoma. Jpn Heart J 1989;30:527–32.
163. Cogan DG, Wray SH. Vascular occlusions in the eye from cardiac myxomas. Am J Ophthalmol 1975;80:396–403.
164. Lee SY, Loo JL, Ang CL. Ischemic oculopathy as a complication of surgery for an atrial myxoma. Arch Ophthalmol 2004;122:130–1.

165. Rafuse PE, Nicolle DA, Hutnik CM, et al. Left atrial myxoma causing ophthalmic artery occlusion. Eye (Lond) 1997;11:25–9.
166. Tarkkanen A, Merenmies L, Mäkinen J. Embolism of the central retinal artery secondary to metastatic carcinoma. Acta Ophthalmol 1973;51:25–33.
167. Chuang EL, Miller III FS, Kalina RE. Retinal lesions following long bone fractures. Ophthalmology 1985;92:370–4.
168. DeVoe AG. Ocular fat embolism. A clinical and pathological report. Trans Am Ophthalmol Soc 1949;47:254–62.
169. Fritz MH, Hogan MJ. Fat embolization involving the human eye. Am J Ophthalmol 1948;31: 527–34.
170. Hogan MJ, Zimmerman LE. Ophthalmic pathology; an atlas and textbook, 2nd ed. Philadelphia: WB Saunders; 1962. p. 492.
171. Kearns TP. Fat embolism of the retina; demonstrated by a flat retinal preparation. Am J Ophthalmol 1956;41:1–2.
172. Chaine G, Davies J, Kohner EM. Ophthalmologic abnormalities in the hypereosinophilic syndrome. Ophthalmology 1982;89:1348–56.
173. Weinstein JM, Chui H, Lane S. Churg–Strauss syndrome (allergic granulomatous angiitis); neuro-ophthalmologic manifestations. Arch Ophthalmol 1983;101:1217–20.
174. Cho YP, Kwon TW, Ahn JH, et al. Protein C and/or S deficiency presenting as peripheral arterial insufficiency. Br J Radiol 2005;78:601–5.
175. Loh BK, Lee SY, Goh KY. Protein S deficiency manifesting simultaneously as central retinal artery occlusion, oculomotor nerve palsy, and systemic arterial occlusive diseases. Eye 2007;21:684–6.
176. Greiner K, Hafner G, Dick B, et al. Retinal vascular occlusion and deficiencies in the protein C pathway. Am J Ophthalmol 1999;128:69–74.
177. Ambati J, Hanuch OE, Bresnick GH. Protein C and protein S deficiency associated with retinal, optic nerve, and cerebral ischaemia. Br J Ophthalmol 1999;83:754–5.
178. Vignes S, Wechsler B, Elmaleh C, et al. Retinal arterial occlusion associated with resistance to activated protein C. Br J Ophthalmol 1996;80:1111.
179. Greven CM, Weaver RG, Owen J, et al. Protein S deficiency and bilateral branch retinal artery occlusion. Ophthalmology 1991;98:33–4.
180. Golub BM, Sibony PA, Coller BS. Protein S deficiency associated with central retinal artery occlusion. Arch Ophthalmol 1990;108:918.
181. Nelson ME, Talbot JF, Preston FE. Recurrent multiple-branch retinal arteriolar occlusions in a patient with protein C deficiency. Graefes Arch Clin Exp Ophthalmol 1989;227:443–7.
182. Glenn AM, Shaw PJ, Howe JW, et al. Complicated migraine resulting in blindness due to bilateral retinal infarction. Br J Ophthalmol 1992;76:189–90.
183. Inkeles DM, Walsh JB. Retinal fat emboli as a sequela to acute pancreatitis. Am J Ophthalmol 1975;80:935–8.
184. Jacob HS, Craddock PR, Hammerschmidt DE, et al. Complement-induced granulocyte aggregation; an unsuspected mechanism of disease. N Engl J Med 1980;302:789–94.
185. Kincaid MC, Green WR, Knox DL, et al. A clinicopathological case report of retinopathy of pancreatitis. Br J Ophthalmol 1982;66:219–26.
186. Purtscher O. Noch unbekannte Befunde nach Schädeltrauma. Ber Dtsch Ophthalmol Ges 1911;36:294–301.
187. Purtscher O. Angiopathia retinae traumatica. Lymphorrhagien des Augengrundes. Albrecht von Graefes Arch Ophthalmol 1912;82:347–71.
188. Shapiro I, Jacob HS. Leukoembolization in ocular vascular occlusion. Ann Ophthalmol 1982;14:60–2.
189. Snady-McCoy L, Morse PH. Retinopathy associated with acute pancreatitis. Am J Ophthalmol 1985;100:246–51.
190. Farmer SG, Kinyoun JL, Nelson JL, et al. Retinal vasculitis associated with autoantibodies to Sjögren's syndrome A antigen. Am J Ophthalmol 1985;100:814–21.
191. Levine SR, Crofts JW, Lesser GR. Visual symptoms associated with the presence of a lupus anticoagulant. Ophthalmology 1988;95:686–92.
192. Wong K, Ai E, Jones JV, et al. Visual loss as the initial symptom of systemic lupus erythematosus. Am J Ophthalmol 1981;92:238–44.
193. Arora N, Lambrou Jr FH, Stewart MW. Sudden blindness associated with central nervous system symptoms in a hemodialysis patient. Nephron 1991;59:490–2.
194. Sullivan KL, Brown GC, Forman AR. Retrobulbar anesthesia and retinal vascular obstruction. Ophthalmology 1983;90:373–7.
195. Siegler RL, Brewer ED, Swartz M. Ocular involvement in hemolytic-uremic syndrome. J Pediatr 1988;112:594–7.
196. Gum KB, Carter KD, Vine AK. Massive bilateral retinal vascular occlusion secondary to thrombotic thrombocytopenic purpura. Retina 1988;8:185–7.
197. Ong T, Nolan W, Jagger J. Purtscher-like retinopathy as an initial presentation of thrombotic thrombocytopenic purpura: a case report. Eye 2005;19:359–61.
198. Patel MR, Bains AK, O'Hara JP, et al. Purtscher retinopathy as the initial sign of thrombotic thrombocytopenic purpura/hemolytic uremic syndrome. Arch Ophthalmol 2001;119:1388–9.
199. Tajunisah I, Patel DK, Subrayan V. Purtscher retinopathy as an initial presentation of thrombotic thrombocytopenic purpura. J Thromb Thrombolysis 2009;30:112–3.
200. Okwuosa TM, Lee EW, Starosta M, et al. Purtscher-like retinopathy in a patient with adult-onset Still's disease and concurrent thrombotic thrombocytopenic purpura. Arthritis Rheum 2007;57:182–5.
201. Blodi BA, Johnson MW, JDM Gass. Purtscher's-like retinopathy after childbirth. Ophthalmology 1990;97:1654–9.
202. Chang M, Herbert WNP. Retinal arteriolar occlusions following amniotic fluid embolism. Ophthalmology 1984;91:1634–7.
203. Fischbein FI. Ischemic retinopathy following amniotic fluid embolism. Am J Ophthalmol 1969;67:351–7.
204. Stewart MW, Brazis PW, Guier CP, et al. Purtscher-like retinopathy in a patient with HELLP syndrome. Am J Ophthalmol 2007;143:886–7.
205. Roden D, Fitzpatrick G, O'Donoghue H, et al. Purtscher's retinopathy and fat embolism. Br J Ophthalmol 1989;73:677–9.
206. Nayak H, Harun S, Palimar P. Purtscher's retinopathy after fracture dislocation of shoulder joint. Emerg Med J 2005;22:831–2.
207. Kozlowski JMD, Peters AL. Purtscher's-like retinopathy associated with a cardiac aneurysm. Arch Ophthalmol 1992;110:880–1.
208. Parc C. Purtscher-like retinopathy as an initial presentation of a thrombotic microangiopathy associated with antineoplastic therapy. Am J Hematol 2007;82:486–8.
209. Banach MJ, Williams GA. Purtscher retinopathy and necrotizing vasculitis with gemcitabine therapy. Arch Ophthalmol 2000;118:726–7.
210. Lemagne J-M, Michiels X, Van Causenbroeck S, et al. Purtscher-like retinopathy after retrobulbar anesthesia. Ophthalmology 1990;97:859–61.
211. Lim BA, Ang CL. Purtscher-like retinopathy after retrobulbar injection. Ophthalmic Surg Lasers 2001;32:477–8.
212. Blodi BA, Williams CA. Purtscher-like retinopathy after uncomplicated administration of retrobulbar anesthesia. Am J Ophthalmol 1997;124:702–3.
213. Burton TC. Unilateral Purtscher's retinopathy. Ophthalmology 1980;87:1096–105.
214. Goldstein IM, Cala D, Radin A. Evidence of complement catabolism in acute pancreatitis. Am J Med Sci 1978;275:257–64.
215. Mellembakken JR, Aukrust P, Olafsen MK, et al. Activation of leukocytes during the uteroplacental passage in preeclampsia. Hypertension 2002;39:155–60.
216. Shaw Jr HE, Osher RH, Smith JL. Amaurosis fugax associated with SC hemoglobinopathy and lupus erythematosus. Am J Ophthalmol 1979;87:281–5.
217. Bruce GM. Retinitis in dermatomyositis. Trans Am Ophthalmol Soc 1938;36:282–97.
218. Cohen BH, Sedwick LA, Burde RM. Retinopathy of dermatomyositis. J Clin Neuro-Ophthalmol 1985;5:177–9.
219. Coppeto J, Lessell S. Retinopathy in systemic lupus erythematosus. Arch Ophthalmol 1977;95:794–7.
220. Dougal MA, Evans LS, McClellan KR, et al. Central retinal artery occlusion in systemic lupus erythematosus. Ann Ophthalmol 1983;15:38–40.
221. Gold D, Feiner L, Henkind P. Retinal arterial occlusive disease in systemic lupus erythematosus. Arch Ophthalmol 1977;95:1580–5.
222. Graham EM, Spalton DJ, Barnard RO. Cerebral and retinal vascular changes in systemic lupus erythematosus. Ophthalmology 1985;92:444–8.
223. Jabs DA, Fine SL, Hochberg MC. Severe retinal vaso-occlusive disease in systemic lupus erythematosus. Arch Ophthalmol 1986;104:558–63.
224. Liebman S, Cook C, Donaldson DD. Retinopathy with dermatomyositis. Arch Ophthalmol 1965;74:704–5.
225. Provost TT, Reichlin M. Antinuclear antibody-negative systemic lupus erythematosus. I. Anti-Ro (SSA) and anti-La (SSB) antibodies. J Am Acad Dermatol 1981;4:84–9.
226. Reichlin M, Wasicek CA. Clinical and biologic significance of antibodies to Ro/SSA. Hum Pathol 1983;14:401–5.
227. Snyers B, Lambert M, Hardy J-P. Retinal and choroidal vaso-occlusive disease in systemic lupus erythematosus associated with antiphospholipid antibodies. Retina 1990;10:255–60.
228. Solomon SM, Solomon JH. Bilateral central retinal artery occlusions in polyarteritis nodosa. Ann Ophthalmol 1978;10:567–9.
229. Stoumbos VD, Klein ML, Goodman S. Purtscher's-like retinopathy in chronic renal failure. Ophthalmology 1992;99:1833–9.
230. Cordes FC, Aiken SD. Ocular changes in acute disseminated lupus erythematosus; report of a case with microscopic findings. Am J Ophthalmol 1947;30:1541–55.
231. Diddie KR, Aronson AJ, Ernest JT. Chorioretinopathy in a case of systemic lupus erythematosus. Trans Am Ophthalmol Soc 1977;75:122–31.
232. Hammami H, Streiff EB. Altérations vasculaires rétiniennes dans un cas de lupus érythémateux disséminé; Evolution après traitement aux immunosuppresseurs. Ophthalmologica 1973;166:16–35.
233. Karpik AG, Schwartz MM, Dickey LE. Ocular immune reactants in patients dying with systemic lupus erythematosus. Clin Immunol Immunopathol 1985;35:295–312.
234. Koffle D, Bieserber G. Immunopathogenesis of tissue injury. In: Schur PH, editor. The clinical management of systemic lupus erythematosus. New York: Grune & Stratton; 1983. p. 29.
235. Nichols CJ, Mieler WF. Severe retinal vaso-occlusive disease secondary to procainamide-induced lupus. Ophthalmology 1989;96:1535–40.
236. Vine AK, Barr CC. Proliferative lupus retinopathy. Arch Ophthalmol 1984;102:852–4.
237. Bishko F. Retinopathy in systemic lupus erythematosus; a case report and review of the literature. Arthritis Rheum 1972;15:57–63.
238. Kincaid MC, Green WR, Knox DL, et al. A clinicopathological case report of retinopathy of pancreatitis. Br J Ophthalmol 1982;66:219–26.
239. Jampol LM, Rabb MF. Vasoocclusive diseases of the posterior pole. Int Ophthalmol Clin 1981;21:201–13.
240. Friberg TR, Gragoudas ES, Regan CDJ. Talc emboli and macular ischemia in intravenous drug abuse. Arch Ophthalmol 1979;97:1089–91.
241. Kaga N, Tso MOM, Jampol LM. Talc retinopathy in primates: a model of ischemic retinopathy. III. An electron microscopic study. Arch Ophthalmol 1982;100:1649–57.
242. Kresca LJ, Goldberg MF, Jampol LM. Talc emboli and retinal neovascularization in a drug abuser. Am J Ophthalmol 1979;87:334–9.
243. Murphy SB, Jackson WB, Pare JAP. Talc retinopathy. Can J Ophthalmol 1978;13:152–6.
244. Schatz H, Drake M. Self-injected retinal emboli. Ophthalmology 1979;86:468–83.
245. Tse DT, Ober RR. Talc retinopathy. Am J Ophthalmol 1980;90:624–40.
246. Brucker AJ. Disk and peripheral retinal neovascularization secondary to talc and cornstarch emboli. Am J Ophthalmol 1979;88:864–7.
247. Sharma MC, Ho AC. Macular fibrosis associated with talc retinopathy. Am J Ophthalmol 1999;128:517–9.
248. Jampol LM, Setogawa T, Rednam KRV, et al. Talc retinopathy in primates; a model of ischemic retinopathy. I. Clinical studies. Arch Ophthalmol 1981;99:1273–80.
249. Kaga N, Tso MOM, Jampol LM. Talc retinopathy in primates: a model of ischemic retinopathy. II. A histopathologic study. Arch Ophthalmol 1982;100:1644–8.

250. Tarantola R, Reichstein D, Morrison D, et al. Talc retinopathy presenting as multiple retinal arteriolar occlusions. Retinal Cases Brief Rep 2010;4:120–2.
251. Michelson JB, Whitcher JP, Wilson S, et al. Possible foreign body granuloma of the retina associated with intravenous cocaine addiction. Am J Ophthalmol 1979;87:278–80.
252. Siepser SB, Magargal LE, Augsburger JJ. Acute bilateral retinal microembolization in a heroin addict. Ann Ophthalmol 1981;13:699–702.
253. Wallace RT, Brown GC, Benson W, et al. Sudden retinal manifestations of intranasal cocaine and methamphetamine abuse. Am J Ophthalmol 1992;114:158–60.
254. Kumar RL, Kaiser PK, Lee MS. Crystalline retinopathy from nasal ingestion of methamphetamine. Retina 2006;26:823–4.
255. Rush JA, Kearns TP, Danielson GK. Cloth-particle retinal emboli from artificial cardiac valves. Am J Ophthalmol 1980;89:845–50.
256. Byers B. Blindness secondary to steroid injections into the nasal turbinates. Arch Ophthalmol 1979;97:79–80.
257. Ellis PP. Occlusion of the central retinal artery after retrobulbar corticosteroid injection. Am J Ophthalmol 1978;85:352–6.
258. Garland PE, Crandall AS, Creel DJ. Visual disturbance resulting from intranasal steroid injection. Arch Ophthalmol 1989;107:22–3.
259. Mieler WF, Bennett SR, Platt LW, et al. Localized retinal detachment with combined central retinal artery and vein occlusion after retrobulbar anesthesia. Retina 1990;10:278–83.
260. Ruttum MS, Abrams GW, Harris GJ, et al. Bilateral retinal embolization associated with intralesional corticosteroid injection for capillary hemangioma of infancy. J Pediatr Ophthalmol Strabismus 1993;30:4–7.
261. Shorr N, Seiff SR. Central retinal artery occlusion associated with periocular corticosteroid injection for juvenile hemangioma. Ophthalmic Surg 1986;17:229–31.
262. Thomas EL, Laborde RP. Retinal and choroidal vascular occlusion following intralesional corticosteroid injection of a chalazion. Ophthalmology 1986;93:405–7.
263. Wesley RE, Johnston DT, Gutow GS. Central retinal artery occlusion. Ophthalmic Surg 1987;18:123–5.
264. Wilkinson WS, Morgan CM, Baruh E, et al. Retinal and choroidal vascular occlusion secondary to corticosteroid embolisation. Br J Ophthalmol 1989;73:32–4.
265. Wilson RS, Havener WH, McGrew RN. Bilateral retinal artery and choriocapillaris occlusion following the injection of long-acting corticosteroid suspensions in combination with other drugs. I. Clinical studies. Ophthalmology 1978;85:967–73.
266. Evans DE, Zahorchak JA, Kennerdell JS. Visual loss as a result of primary optic nerve neuropathy after intranasal corticosteroid injection. Am J Ophthalmol 1980;90:641–4.
267. Martin PA, Church CA, Petti Jr GH, et al. Visual loss after intraturbinate steroid injection. Otolaryngol Head Neck Surg 2003;128:280–1.
268. Moshfeghi DM, Lowder CY, Roth DB, et al. Retinal and choroidal vascular occlusion after posterior sub-tenon triamcinolone injection. Am J Ophthalmol 2002;134:132–4.
269. Gupta V, Sharma SC, Gupta A, et al. Retinal and choroidal microvascular embolization with methylprednisolone. Retina 2002;22:382–6.
270. Wilson RS, McGrew RN, White HJ. Bilateral retinal artery and choriocapillaris occlusion following the injection of long-acting corticosteroid suspensions in combination with other drugs. II. Animal experimental studies. Ophthalmology 1978;85:975–85.
271. Dreizen NG, Framm L. Sudden unilateral visual loss after autologous fat injection into the glabellar area. Am J Ophthalmol 1989;107:85–7.
272. Mames RN, Snady-McCoy L, Guy J. Central retinal and posterior ciliary artery occlusion after particle embolization of the external carotid artery system. Ophthalmology 1991;98:527–31.
273. Greven CM, van Rens E, Slusher MM. Branch retinal artery occlusion after platelet transfusion. Am J Ophthalmol 1990;109:105–6.
274. Sachsenweger R. Luftembolie und Auge. Klin Monatsbl Augenheilkd 1957;130:813–23.
275. Brancato R, Pece A, Carassa R. Central retinal artery occlusion after local anesthesia for blepharoplasty. Graefes Arch Clin Exp Ophthalmol 1991;229:593–4.
276. Hogan MJ, Alvarado JA, Weddell JE. Histology of the human eye; an atlas and textbook. Philadelphia: WB Saunders; 1971. p. 508–19.
277. Strassman I, Silverstone BZ, Seelenfreund MH. Essential thrombocythemia: a rare cause of central retinal artery occlusion. Metab Pediatr Syst Ophthalmol 1991;14:18–20.
278. Percival SPB. The eye and Moschcowitz's disease (thrombotic thrombocytopenic purpura); a review of 182 cases. Trans Ophthalmol Soc UK 1970;90:375–82.
279. van den Berg W, Verbraak FD, Bos PJM. Homocystinuria presenting as central retinal artery occlusion and longstanding thromboembolic disease. Br J Ophthalmol 1990;74:696–7.
280. Wenzler EM, Rademakers AJJM, Boers GHJ. Hyperhomocysteinemia in retinal artery and retinal vein occlusion. Am J Ophthalmol 1993;115:162–7.
281. Asherson RA. Letter. Retina 1989;9:155–6.
282. Jonas J, Kölble K, Völcker HE, et al. Central retinal artery occlusion in Sneddon's disease associated with antiphospholipid antibodies. Am J Ophthalmol 1986;102:37–40.
283. Kleiner RC, Najarian LV, Schatten S. Vaso-occlusive retinopathy associated with antiphospholipid antibodies (lupus anticoagulant retinopathy). Ophthalmology 1989;96:896–904.
284. Pulido JS, Ward LM, Fishman GA. Antiphospholipid antibodies associated with retinal vascular disease. Retina 1987;7:215–8.
285. Lightman DA, Brod RD. Branch retinal artery occlusion associated with Lyme disease. Arch Ophthalmol 1991;109:1198–9.
286. Bernauer W, Gratwohl A. Bone marrow transplant retinopathy. Am J Ophthalmol 1992; 113:604–5.
287. Bray LC, Carey PJ, Proctor SJ. Ocular complications of bone marrow transplantation. Br J Ophthalmol 1991;75:611–4.
288. Lopez PF, Sternberg Jr P, Dabbs CK. Bone marrow transplant retinopathy. Am J Ophthalmol 1991;112:635–46.
289. Stuckenschneider BJ, Mieler WF. Ocular findings following bone marrow transplantation. (Scientific poster 250). Ophthalmology 1992;99(Suppl):152.
290. Coskuncan NM, Jabs DA, Dunn JP. The eye in bone marrow transplantation. VI. Retinal complications. Arch Ophthalmol 1994;112:372–9.
291. Parsons MR, Merritt DR, Ramsay RC. Retinal artery occlusion associated with tranexamic acid therapy. Am J Ophthalmol 1988;105:688–9.
292. Braunstein RA, Gass JDM. Branch artery obstruction caused by acute toxoplasmosis. Arch Ophthalmol 1980;98:512–3.
293. Dagi LR, Currie J. Branch retinal artery occlusion in the Churg–Strauss syndrome. J Clin Neuro-Ophthalmol 1985;5:229–37.
294. Font RL, Mehta RS, Streusand SB. Bilateral retinal ischemia in Kawasaki disease; postmortem findings and electron microscopic observations. Ophthalmology 1983;90:569–77.
295. Perry HD, Mallen FJ, Wright Jr GD, et al. Retinal arteriolar occlusion in multiple sclerosis. Ann Ophthalmol 1986;18:168–70.
296. Ashton N, Coomes EN, Garner A, et al. Retinopathy due to progressive systemic sclerosis. J Pathol Bacteriol 1968;96:259–68.
297. Capone Jr A, Meredith TA. Profound central visual loss and ocular neovascularization in idiopathic recurrent branch retinal arterial occlusion. Retina 1990;10:265–8.
298. Digre KB, Blodi CF, Bale JB. Cytomegalovirus infection in a healthy adult associated with recurrent branch retinal artery occlusion. Retina 1987;7:230–2.
299. Gass JDM, Tiedemann J, Thomas MA. Idiopathic recurrent branch retinal arterial occlusion. Ophthalmology 1986;93:1148–57.
300. Johnson MW, Flynn Jr HW, Gass JDM. Idiopathic recurrent branch retinal arterial occlusion. Arch Ophthalmol 1989;107:757.
301. Johnson MW, Thomley ML, Huang SS, et al. Idiopathic recurrent branch retinal artery occlusion; natural history and laboratory evaluation. Ophthalmology 1994;101:480–9.
302. Lusky M, Wysenbeek Y, Weinberger D, et al. Idiopathic bilateral branch-artery occlusion in a young woman. Ann Ophthalmol 1989;21:170–2.
303. Kayazawa F, Sonoda K. Segmental retinal periarteritis with branch arterial occlusion. Ann Ophthalmol 1983;15:584–6.
304. Egan RA, Hills WL, Susac JO. Gass plaques and fluorescein leakage in Susac Syndrome. J Neurol Sci 2010;299:97–100.
305. Susac JO, Egan RA, Rennebohm RM, et al. Susac's syndrome: 1975–2005 microangiopathy/autoimmune endotheliopathy. J Neurol Sci 2007;257:270–2.
306. Egan RA, Ha Nguyen T, Gass JD, et al. Retinal arterial wall plaques in Susac syndrome. Am J Ophthalmol 2003;135:483–6.
307. Hanscom TA. Indirect treatment of peripheral retinal neovascularization. Am J Ophthalmol 1982;93:88–91.
308. Jampol LM, Isenberg SJ, Goldberg MF. Occlusive retinal arteriolitis with neovascularization. Am J Ophthalmol 1976;81:583–9.
309. Pawate S, Agarwal A, Moses H, et al. The spectrum of Susac's syndrome. Neurol Sci 2009;30:59–64.
310. Allmendinger AM, Spektor V, Destian S. CT and MR imaging of Susac syndrome in a young male presenting with acute disorientation. Clin Imaging 2010;34:138–42.
311. Jarius S, Neumayer B, Wandinger KP, et al. Anti-endothelial serum antibodies in a patient with Susac's syndrome. J Neurol Sci 2009;285:259–61.
312. Susac JO. Susac's syndrome: the triad of microangiopathy of the brain and retina with hearing loss in young women. Neurology 1994;44:591–3.
313. Rennebohm RM, Lubow M, Rusin J, et al. Aggressive immunosuppressive treatment of Susac's syndrome in an adolescent: using treatment of dermatomyositis as a model. Pediatr Rheumatol Online J 2008;6:3.
314. Rennebohm RM, Egan RA, Susac JO. Treatment of Susac's Syndrome. Curr Treat Options Neurol 2008;10:67–74.
315. Conomy JP, Kellermeyer RW. Delayed cerebrovascular consequences of therapeutic radiation; a clinicopathologic study of a stroke associated with radiation-related carotid arteriopathy. Cancer 1975;36:1702–8.
316. Evans LS, Van de Graaff WB, Baker WH, et al. Central retinal artery occlusion after neck irradiation. Am J Ophthalmol 1992;114:224–5.
317. Irvine AR, Alvarado JA, Wara WM. Radiation retinopathy: an experimental model for the ischemic-proliferative retinopathies. Trans Am Ophthalmol Soc 1981;79:103–22.
318. Fisher M. Transient monocular blindness associated with hemiplegia. Arch Ophthalmol 1952;47:167–203.
319. Humphrey WT. Central retinal artery spasm. Ann Ophthalmol 1979;11:877–81.
320. Katz B. Migrainous central retinal artery occlusion. J Clin Neuro-Ophthalmol 1986;6:69–71.
321. Victor DI, Welch RB. Bilateral retinal hemorrhages and disk edema in migraine. J Ophthalmol 1977;84:555–8.
322. Wolter JR, Burchfield WJ. Ocular migraine in a young man resulting in unilateral transient blindness and retinal edema. J Pediatr Ophthalmol 1971;8:173–6.
323. Gray JA, Carroll JD. Retinal artery occlusion in migraine. Postgrad Med J 1985;61:517–8.
324. Grosberg BM, Solomon S, Friedman DI, et al. Retinal migraine reappraised. Cephalalgia 2006;26:1275–86.
325. Doyle E, Vote BJ, Casswell AG. Retinal migraine: caught in the act. Br J Ophthalmol 2004;88:301–2.
326. Hykin PG, Gartry D, Brazier DJ, et al. Bilateral cilio-retinal artery occlusion in classic migraine. Postgrad Med J 1991;67:282–4.
327. Daroff RB. Retinal migraine. J NeuroOphthalmol 2007;27:83.
328. Grosberg BM, Solomon S. Retinal migraine: two cases of prolonged but reversible monocular visual defects. Cephalalgia 2006;26:754–7.
329. Beversdorf D, Stommel E, Allen C, et al. Recurrent branch retinal infarcts in association with migraine. Headache 1997;37:396–9.
330. Brown GC, Tasman WS. Retinal arterial obstruction in association with presumed Toxocara canis neuroretinitis. Ann Ophthalmol 1981;13:1385–7.
331. Kelly PW, May DR. Central retinal artery occlusion following cosmetic blepharoplasty. Br J Ophthalmol 1980;64:918–22.
332. Gupta A, Jalali S, Bansal RK, et al. Anterior ischemic optic neuropathy and branch retinal artery occlusion in cavernous sinus thrombosis. J Clin Neuro-Ophthalmol 1990;10: 193–6.

499. Jampol LM. Pharmacologic therapy of aphakic and pseudophakic cystoid macular edema; 1985 update. Ophthalmology 1985;92:807–10.
500. Kraff MC, Sanders DR, Jampol LM. Prophylaxis of pseudophakic cystoid macular edema with topical indomethacin. Ophthalmology 1982;89:885–90.
501. McEntyre JM. A successful treatment for aphakic cystoid macular edema. Ann Ophthalmol 1978;10:1219–24.
502. Melberg NS, Olk RJ. Corticosteroid-induced ocular hypertension in the treatment of aphakic or pseudophakic cystoid macular edema. Ophthalmology 1993;100:164–7.
503. Fung WE.Vitrectomy-ACME Study Group Vitrectomy for chronic aphakic cystoid macular edema; results of a national, collaborative, prospective, randomized investigation. Ophthalmology 1985;92:1102–11.
504. Cox SN, Hay E, Bird AC. Treatment of chronic macular edema with acetazolamide. Arch Ophthalmol 1988;106:1190–5.
505. Marmor MF. Hypothesis concerning carbonic anhydrase treatment of cystoid macular edema: example with epiretinal membrane. Arch Ophthalmol 1990;108:1524–5.
506. Tripathi RC, Fekrat S, Tripathi BJ, et al. A direct correlation of the resolution of pseudophakic cystoid macular edema with acetazolamide therapy. Ann Ophthalmol 1991;23:127–9.
507. Coscas G. Maculopathies oedemateuses, Sociétés d'Ophtalmologie de France, 1972, rapport annuel. Bull Soc Ophtalmol Fr, numero special 1972.
508. Ffytche TJ, Blach RK. The aetiology of macular oedema. Trans Ophthalmol Soc UK. 1970;90:637–56.
509. François J, De Laey JJ, Verbraeken H. Das zystoide Ödem der Macula. Klin Monatsbl Augenheilkd 1973;162:125–38.
510. Irvine AR. Cystoid maculopathy. Surv Ophthalmol 1976;21:1–17.
511. Lakhanpal V, Schocket SS. Pseudophakic and aphakic retinal detachment mimicking cystoid macular edema. Ophthalmology 1987;94:785–91.
512. Bonnet M, Payan X. Pronostic à long terme de l'oedème cystoïde de la macula après microchirurgie du decollement rhegmatogène de la rètine. J Fr Ophthalmol 1993;16: 259–63.
513. Gass JDM. Fluorescein angiography: an aid to the retinal surgeon. In: Pruett RC, Regan CDJ, editors. Retina Congress; 25th anniversary meeting of the Retina Service Massachusetts Eye and Ear Infirmary (1972). New York: Appleton-Century-Crofts; 1974. p. 181–201.
514. Meredith TA, Reeser FH, Topping TM, et al. Cystoid macular edema after retinal detachment surgery. Ophthalmology 1980;87:1090–5.
515. Ryan Jr SJ. Cystoid maculopathy in phakic retinal detachment procedures. Am J Ophthalmol 1973;76:519–22.
516. Lobes Jr LA, Grand MG. Incidence of cystoid macular edema following scleral buckling procedure. Arch Ophthalmol 1980;98:1230–2.
517. Kimball RW, Morse PH, Benson WE. Cystoid macular edema after cryotherapy. Am J Ophthalmol 1978;86:572–3.
518. Kramer SG. Cystoid macular edema after aphakic penetrating keratoplasty. Ophthalmology 1981;88:782–7.
519. West CE, Fitzgerald CR, Sewell JH. Cystoid macular edema following aphakic keratoplasty. Am J Ophthalmol 1973;75:77–81.
520. Price Jr FW, Whitson WE. Natural history of cystoid macular edema in pseudophakic bullous keratopathy. J Cataract Refract Surg 1990;16:163–9.
521. Choplin NT, Bene CH. Cystoid macular edema following laser iridotomy. Ann Ophthalmol 1983;15:172–3.
522. Gass JDM. Lamellar macular hole: a complication of cystoid macular edema after cataract extraction: a clinicopathologic case report. Trans Am Ophthalmol Soc 1975;73:231–50.
523. Trese MT, Foos RY. Infantile cystoid maculopathy. Br J Ophthalmol 1980;64:206–10.
524. Brownstein S, Orton R, Jackson WB. Cystoid macular edema with equatorial choroidal melanoma. Arch Ophthalmol 1978;96:2105–7.
525. Kolker AE, Becker B. Epinephrine maculopathy. Arch Ophthalmol 1968;79:552–62.
526. Mackool RJ, Muldoon T, Fortier A, et al. Epinephrine-induced cystoid macular edema in aphakic eyes. Arch Ophthalmol 1977;95:791–3.
527. Thomas JV, Gragoudas ES, Blair NP, et al. Correlation of epinephrine use and macular edema in aphakic glaucomatous eyes. Arch Ophthalmol 1978;96:625–8.
528. Watanabe K, Hayasaka S, Hayasaka Y, et al. Cystoid macular edema associated with latanoprost use in a pseudophakic eye with a history of surgical complications. Jpn J Ophthalmol 2003;47:110–2.
529. Jager M, Jonas JB. Cystoid macular edema associated with latanoprost therapy in a pseudophakic vitrectomized patient after removal of silicone oil endotamponade. Eur J Ophthalmol 2003;13:221–2.
530. Gass JDM. Nicotinic acid maculopathy. Am J Ophthalmol 1973;76:500–10.
531. Harris JL. Toxic amblyopia associated with administration of nicotinic acid. Am J Ophthalmol 1963;55:133–4.
532. Millay RH, Klein ML, Illingworth DR. Niacin maculopathy. Ophthalmology 1988;95:930–6.
533. Parsons Jr WB, Flinn JH. Reduction in elevated blood cholesterol levels by large doses of nicotinic acid; preliminary report. JAMA 1957;165:234–8.
534. Tamási G, Borsy J, Gyenge R. Changes in serum triglyceride and cholesterol levels independently of free fatty acid after lipolysis inhibitors. Biochem Pharmacol 1970;19:1826–30.
535. Spirn MJ, Warren FA, Guyer DR, et al. Optical coherence tomography findings in nicotinic acid maculopathy. Am J Ophthalmol 2003;135:913–4.
536. Dajani HM, Lauer AK. Optical coherence tomography findings in niacin maculopathy. Can J Ophthalmol 2006;41:197–200.
537. Callanan D, Blodi BA, Martin DF. Macular edema associated with nicotinic acid (niacin). JAMA 1998;279:1702.
538. Jampol LM. Cystoid macular edema following cataract surgery. Arch Ophthalmol 1988;106:894–5.
539. Gass JD. Nicotinic acid maculopathy. Am J Ophthalmol 1973;76:500–10.
540. Deutman AF, AJLG Pinckers, Aan de Kerk AL. Dominantly inherited cystoid macular edema. Am J Ophthalmol 1976;82:540–8.
541. Fishman GA, Goldberg MF, Trautmann JC. Dominantly inherited cystoid macular edema. Ann Ophthalmol 1979;11:21–7.
542. Loeffler KU, Li Z-L, Fishman GA, et al. Dominantly inherited cystoid macular edema; a histopathologic study. Ophthalmology 1992;99:1385–92.
543. Pinckers A, Cruysberg JR, Kremer H, et al. Acetazolamide in dominant cystoid macular dystrophy. A pilot study. Ophthalmic Paediatr Genet 1993;14:95–9.
544. Hogewind BF, Pieters G, Hoyng CB. Octreotide acetate in dominant cystoid macular dystrophy. Eur J Ophthalmol 2008;18:99–103.
545. Reese AB. Telangiectasis of the retina and Coats' disease. Am J Ophthalmol 1956;42:1–8.
546. Campbell FP. Coats' disease and congenital vascular retinopathy. Trans Am Ophthalmol Soc 1976;74:365–424.
547. Casswell AG, Chaine G, Rush P, et al. Paramacular telangiectasis. Trans Ophthalmol Soc UK 1986;105:683–92.
548. Coats G. Forms of retinal disease with massive exudation. R Lond Ophthalmic Hosp Rep 1907–1908;17:440–525.
549. Gass JDM. A fluorescein angiographic study of macular dysfunction secondary to retinal vascular disease. V. Retinal telangiectasis. Arch Ophthalmol 1968;80:592–605.
550. Gass JDM. Differential diagnosis of intraocular tumors; a stereoscopic presentation. St. Louis: CV Mosby; 1974. p. 248.
551. Gass JDM, Blodi BA. Idiopathic juxtafoveolar retinal telangiectasis; update of classification and follow-up study. Ophthalmology 1993;100:1536–46.
552. Gomez Morales A. Coats' disease; natural history and results of treatment. Am J Ophthalmol 1965;60:855–65.
553. McGrand JC. Photocoagulation in Coats' disease. Trans Ophthalmol Soc UK 1970;90:47–56.
554. Ridley ME, Shields JA, Brown GC, et al. Coats' disease; evaluation of management. Ophthalmology 1982;89:1381–7.
555. Egerer I, Tasman W, Tomer TL. Coats disease. Arch Ophthalmol 1974;92:109–12.
556. Ehlers N, Jensen VA. Hereditary central retinal angiopathy. Acta Ophthalmol 1973;51:171–8.
557. Judisch GF, Apple DJ. Orbital cellulitis in an infant secondary to Coats' disease. Arch Ophthalmol 1980;98:2004–6.
558. Tripathi R, Ashton N. Electron microscopical study of Coats's disease. Br J Ophthalmol 1971;55:289–301.
559. McCormick WF, Hardman JM, Boulter TR. Vascular malformations ("angiomas") of the brain, with special reference to those occurring in the posterior fossa. J Neurosurg 1968;28:241–51.
560. Gass JDM, Oyakawa RT. Idiopathic juxtafoveolar retinal telangiectasis. Arch Ophthalmol 1982;100:769–80.
561. Chopdar A. Retinal telangiectasis in adults: fluorescein angiographic findings and treatment by argon laser. Br J Ophthalmol 1978;62:243–50.
562. Hutton WL, Snyder WB, Fuller D, et al. Focal parafoveal retinal telangiectasis. Arch Ophthalmol 1978;96:1362–7.
563. Diago T, Valls B, Pulido JS. Coats' disease associated with muscular dystrophy treated with ranibizumab. Eye (Lond) 2010, Jan 15
564. Lin CJ, Hwang JF, Chen YT, et al. The effect of intravitreal bevacizumab in the treatment of coats disease in children. Retina 2010;24:1295–6.
565. Peyman GA, Dellacroce JT, Ebrahim SA. Removal of submacular exudates in a patient with Coats disease: a case report. Retina 2006;26:836–9.
566. Farkas TG, Potts AM, Boone C. Some pathologic and biochemical aspects of Coats' disease. Am J Ophthalmol 1973;75:289–301.
567. Goel SD, Augsburger JJ. Hemorrhagic retinal macrocysts in advanced Coats' disease. Retina 1991;11:437–40.
568. Shields JA, Shields CL, Honavar SG, et al. Classification and management of Coats disease: the 2000 Proctor Lecture. Am J Ophthalmol 2001;131:572–83.
569. Black GC, Perveen R, Bonshek R, et al. Coats' disease of the retina (unilateral retinal telangiectasis) caused by somatic mutation in the NDP gene: a role for norrin in retinal angiogenesis. Hum Mol Genet 1999;8:2031–5.
570. Lin P, Shankar SP, Duncan J, et al. Retinal vascular abnormalities and dragged maculae in a carrier with a new NDP mutation (c.268delC) that caused severe Norrie disease in the proband. J AAPOS 2010;14:93–6.
571. Gass JDM, Harbin Jr TS, Del Piero EJ. Exudative stellate neuroretinopathy and Coats' syndrome in patients with progressive hemifacial atrophy. Eur J Ophthalmol 1991;1:2–10.
572. Muchnick RS, Aston SJ, Rees TD. Ocular manifestations and treatment of hemifacial atrophy. Am J Ophthalmol 1979;88:889–97.
573. Chijiiwa T, Nishimura M, Inomata H. Ocular manifestations of congenital muscular dystrophy (Fukuyama type). Ann Ophthalmol 1983;15:921–8.
574. Desai UR, Sabates FN. Long-term follow-up of facioscapulohumeral muscular dystrophy and Coats' disease. Am J Ophthalmol 1990;110:568–9.
575. Dickey JB, Daily MJ. Retinal telangiectasis in scapuloperoneal muscular dystrophy. Am J Ophthalmol 1991;112:348–9.
576. Fitzsimons RB, Gurwin EB, Bird AC. Retinal vascular abnormalities in facioscapulohumeral muscular dystrophy. Brain 1987;110:631–48.
577. Gurwin EB, Fitzsimons RB, Sehmi KS, et al. Retinal telangiectasis in facioscapulohumeral muscular dystrophy with deafness. Arch Ophthalmol 1985;103:1695–700.
578. Pauleikhoff D, Bornfeld N, Bird AC, et al. Severe visual loss associated with retinal telangiectasis and facioscapulohumeral muscular dystrophy. Graefes Arch Clin Exp Ophthalmol 1992;230:362–5.
579. Wulff JD, Lin JT, Kepes JJ. Inflammatory facioscapulohumeral muscular dystrophy and Coats' syndrome. Ann Neurol 1982;12:398–401.
580. Small RG. Coats' disease and muscular dystrophy. Trans Am Acad Ophthalmol Otolaryngol 1968;72:225–31.
581. Kondra L, Cangemi FE, Pitta CG. Alport's syndrome and retinal telangiectasia. Ann Ophthalmol 1983;15:550–1.
582. Burch JV, Leveille AS, Morse PH. Ichthyosis hystrix (epidermal nevus syndrome) and Coats' disease. Am J Ophthalmol 1980;89:25–30.

583. Jost BF, Olk RJ. Atypical retinitis proliferans, retinal telangiectasis, and vitreous hemorrhage in a patient with tuberous sclerosis. Retina 1986;6:53–6.
584. Haritoglou C, Gandorfer A, Kampik A. Indocyanine green can distinguish posterior vitreous cortex from internal-limiting membrane during vitrectomy with removal of epiretinal membrane. Retina 2003;23:262.
585. Morgan III WE, Crawford JB. Retinitis pigmentosa and Coats' disease. Arch Ophthalmol 1968;79:146–9.
586. Gass JDM. Stereoscopic atlas of macular diseases; diagnosis and treatment, 3rd ed. St. Louis: CV Mosby; 1987. p. 410–11.
587. Frenkel M, Russe HP. Retinal telangiectasia associated with hypogammaglobulinemia. Am J Ophthalmol 1967;63:215–20.
588. Shields CL, Zahler J, Falk N, et al. Neovascular glaucoma from advanced Coats disease as the initial manifestation of facioscapulohumeral dystrophy in a 2-year-old child. Arch Ophthalmol 2007;125:840–2.
589. Taylor DA, Carroll JE, Smith ME. Facioscapulohumeral muscular dystrophy associated with hearing loss and Coats' syndrome. Ann Neurol 1982;12:395–8.
590. Fishman GA, Trimble S, Rabb MF, et al. Pseudovitelliform macular degeneration. Arch Ophthalmol 1977;95:73–6.
591. Green WR, Quigley HA, De La Cruz Z, et al. Parafoveal retinal telangiectasis; light and electron microscopy studies. Trans Ophthalmol Soc UK 1980;100:162–70.
592. Lim JI, Bressler NM. Atypical parafoveal telangiectasis with subsequent anterior and posterior segment neovascularization. Retina 1992;12:351–4.
593. Gass JDM. A fluorescein angiographic study of macular dysfunction secondary to retinal vascular disease. VI. X-ray irradiation, carotid artery occlusion, collagen vascular disease, and vitritis. Arch Ophthalmol 1968;80:606–17.
594. Chew EY, Murphy RP, Newsome DA, et al. Parafoveal telangiectasis and diabetic retinopathy. Arch Ophthalmol 1986;104:71–5.
595. Moisseiev J, Lewis H, Bartov E. Superficial retinal refractile deposits in juxtafoveal telangiectasis. Am J Ophthalmol 1990;109:604–5.
596. Patel B, Duvall J, Tullo AB. Lamellar macular hole associated with idiopathic juxtafoveolar telangiectasia. Br J Ophthalmol 1988;72:550–1.
597. Gillies MC, Zhu M, Chew E, et al. Familial asymptomatic macular telangiectasia type 2. Ophthalmology 2009;116:2422–9.
598. Minnella AM, Yannuzzi LA, Slakter JS, et al. Bilateral perifoveal ischemia associated with chronic granulocytic leukemia. Arch Ophthalmol 1988;106:1170–1.
599. Grand MG, Kaine J, Fulling K. Cerebroretinal vasculopathy; a new hereditary syndrome. Ophthalmology 1988;95:649–59.
600. Gutmann DH, Fischbeck KH, Sergott RC. Hereditary retinal vasculopathy with cerebral white matter lesions. Am J Med Genet 1989;34:217–20.
601. Storimans CWJM, Oosterhuis JA, van Schooneveld MJ. Familial vascular retinopathy; a preliminary report. Doc Ophthalmol 1990;75:259–61.
602. Storimans CWJM, Van Schooneveld MJ, Oosterhuis JA, et al. A new autosomal dominant vascular retinopathy syndrome. Eur J Ophthalmol 1991;1:73–8.
603. van Effenterre G, Haut J, Brezin A. Retinal and choroidal ischemic syndrome, digestive tract and renal small vessel hyalinosis, intracerebral calcifications and phenotypic abnormalities: a new family syndrome. Graefes Arch Clin Exp Ophthalmol 1989;227:315–22.
604. Mateen FJ, Krecke K, Younge BR, et al. Evolution of a tumor-like lesion in cerebroretinal vasculopathy and TREX1 mutation. Neurology 2010;75:1211–3.
605. Qian Y, Kosmorsky G, Kaiser PK. Retinal manifestations of cerebroretinal vasculopathy. Semin Ophthalmol 2007;22:163–5.
606. Storimans CW, Fekkes D, van Dalen A, et al. Serotoninergic status in patients with hereditary vascular retinopathy syndrome. Br J Ophthalmol 1998;82:897–900.
607. Kernt M, Gschwendtner A, Neubauer AS, et al. Effects of intravitreal bevacizumab treatment on proliferative retinopathy in a patient with cerebroretinal vasculopathy. J Neurol 2010;257:1213–4.
608. Niedermayer I, Graf N, Schmidbauer J, et al. Cerebroretinal vasculopathy mimicking a brain tumor. Neurology 2000;54:1878–9.
609. Niedermayer I, Reiche W, Graf N, et al. Cerebroretinal vasculopathy and leukoencephalopathy mimicking a brain tumor. Report of two early-onset cases with Fanconi's anemia-like phenotypes suggesting an autosomal-recessive inheritance pattern. Clin Neuropathol 2000;19:285–95.
610. Weil S, Reifenberger G, Dudel C, et al. Cerebroretinal vasculopathy mimicking a brain tumor: a case of a rare hereditary syndrome. Neurology 1999;53:629–31.
611. Siveke JT, Schmid H. Evidence for systemic manifestations in cerebroretinal vasculopathy. Am J Med Genet A 2003;123A:309.
612. Ophoff RA, DeYoung J, Service SK, et al. Hereditary vascular retinopathy, cerebroretinal vasculopathy, and hereditary endotheliopathy with retinopathy, nephropathy, and stroke map to a single locus on chromosome 3p21.1-p21.3. Am J Hum Genet 2001;69:447–53.
613. Jen J, Cohen AH, Yue Q, et al. Hereditary endotheliopathy with retinopathy, nephropathy, and stroke (HERNS). Neurology 1997;49:1322–30.
614. Brant AM, Schachat AP, White RI. Ocular manifestations in hereditary hemorrhagic telangiectasia (Rendu-Osler-Weber disease). Am J Ophthalmol 1989;107:642–6.
615. Forker EL, Bean WB. Retinal arteriovenous aneurysm in hereditary hemorrhagic telangiectasia. Arch Intern Med 1963;111:778–83.
616. Meyer-Schwickerath G, von Barsewisch B. Gefässveränderungen an Haut und Retina. Ber Dtsch Ophthalmol Ges 1968;68:525–9.
617. Roubin IV. Telangiectasia of the disc in Osler's disease. Vestn Oftalmol 1957;70:29–30.
618. Vase I, Vase P. Ocular lesions in hereditary haemorrhagic telangiectasia. Acta Ophthalmol 1979;57:1084–90.
619. Geisthoff UW, Hille K, Ruprecht KW, et al. Prevalence of ocular manifestations in hereditary hemorrhagic telangiectasia. Graefes Arch Clin Exp Ophthalmol 2007;245:1141–4.
620. Mahmoud TH, Deramo VA, Kim T, et al. Intraoperative choroidal hemorrhage in the Osler-Rendu-Weber syndrome. Am J Ophthalmol 2002;133:282–4.
621. Tsai DC, Wang AG, Lee AF, et al. Choroidal telangiectasia in a patient with hereditary hemorrhagic telangiectasia. Eye (Lond) 2002;16:92–4.
622. Letteboer TG, Mager HJ, Snijder RJ, et al. Genotype-phenotype relationship for localization and age distribution of telangiectases in hereditary hemorrhagic telangiectasia. Am J Med Genet A 2008;146A:2733–9.
623. Lesca G, Olivieri C, Burnichon N, et al. Genotype-phenotype correlations in hereditary hemorrhagic telangiectasia: data from the French-Italian HHT network. Genet Med 2007;9:14–22.
624. Chang T.S.Aylward GW, Davis JL, editors. Idiopathic retinal vasculitis aneurysms and neuro-retinitis (IRVAN) syndrome, 102; 1995 p. 1089–97.
625. Karel I, Pelesska M, Divisová G. Fluorescence angiography in retinal vasculitis in children's uveitis. Ophthalmologica 1973;166:251–64.
626. Kincaid J, Schatz H. Bilateral retinal arteritis with multiple aneurysmal dilatations. Retina 1983;3:171–8.
627. Owens SL, Gregor ZJ. Vanishing retinal arterial aneurysms: a case report. Br J Ophthalmol 1992;76:636–8.
628. Samuel MA, Equi RA, Chang TS, et al. Idiopathic retinitis, vasculitis, aneurysms, and neuroretinitis (IRVAN): new observations and a proposed staging system. Ophthalmology 2007;114(1526–1529):e1.
629. Yeshurun I, Recillas-Gispert C, Navarro-Lopez P, et al. Extensive dynamics in location, shape, and size of aneurysms in a patient with idiopathic retinal vasculitis, aneurysms, and neuroretinitis (IRVAN) syndrome. Idiopathic retinal vasculitis, aneurysms, and neuroretinitis. Am J Ophthalmol 2003;135:118–20.
630. DiLoreto Jr DA, Sadda SR. Idiopathic retinal vasculitis, aneurysms, and neuroretinitis (IRVAN) with preserved perfusion. Retina 2003;23:554–7.
631. Riley WJ, Maclaren NK, Krischer J. A prospective study of the development of diabetes in relatives of patients with insulin-dependent diabetes. N Engl J Med 1990;323:1167–72.
632. Aiello LM, Rand LI, Briones JC. Diabetic retinopathy in Joslin Clinic patients with adult-onset diabetes. Ophthalmology 1981;88:619–23.
633. Frank RN. On the pathogenesis of diabetic retinopathy. Ophthalmology 1984;91:626–34.
634. Little HL. Alterations in blood elements in the pathogenesis of diabetic retinopathy. Ophthalmology 1981;88:647–54.
635. Little HL, Sacks A, Vassiliadis A, et al. Current concepts on pathogenesis of diabetic retinopathy: a dysproteinemia. Trans Am Ophthalmol Soc 1977;75:397–426.
636. Patz A. Clinical and experimental studies on retinal neovascularization. Am J Ophthalmol 1982;94:715–43.
637. Rubinstein K, Myska V. Pathogenesis and treatment of diabetic maculopathy. Br J Ophthalmol 1974;58:76–84.
638. Bresnick GH. Diabetic retinopathy viewed as a neurosensory disorder. Arch Ophthalmol 1986;104:989–90.
639. Frank RN. On the pathogenesis of diabetic retinopathy; a 1990 update. Ophthalmology 1991;98:586–93.
640. Catalano RA, Tanenbaum HL, Majerovics A. White centered retinal hemorrhages in diabetic retinopathy. Ophthalmology 1987;94:388–92.
641. Hardy KJ, Lipton J, Scase MO. Detection of colour vision abnormalities in uncomplicated type 1 diabetic patients with angiographically normal retinas. Br J Ophthalmol 1992;76:461–4.
642. Prager TC, Garcia CA, Mincher CA. The pattern electroretinogram in diabetes. Am J Ophthalmol 1990;109:279–84.
643. Ashton N. Studies of the retinal capillaries in relation to diabetic and other retinopathies. Br J Ophthalmol 1963;47:521–38.
644. Bresnick GH, Davis MD, Myers FL, et al. Clinicopathologic correlations in diabetic retinopathy. II. Clinical and histologic appearances of retinal capillary microaneurysms. Arch Ophthalmol 1977;95:1215–20.
645. Bresnick GH, Haight B, de Venecia G. Retinal wrinkling and macular heterotopia in diabetic retinopathy. Arch Ophthalmol 1979;97:1890–5.
646. Cogan DG, Kuwabara T. Capillary shunts in the pathogenesis of diabetic retinopathy. Diabetes 1963;12:293–300.
647. Cogan DG, Toussaint D, Kuwabara T. Retinal vascular patterns. IV. Diabetic retinopathy. Arch Ophthalmol 1961;66:366–78.
648. de Venecia G, Davis M, Engerman R. Clinicopathologic correlations in diabetic retinopathy. I. Histology and fluorescein angiography of microaneurysms. Arch Ophthalmol 1976;94:1766–73.
649. Kohner EM, Dollery CT. Fluorescein angiography of the fundus in diabetic retinopathy. Br Med Bull 1970;26:166–70.
650. Kohner EM, Dollery CT, Paterson JW, et al. Arterial fluorescein studies in diabetic retinopathy. Diabetes 1967;16:1–10.
651. Kohner EM, Henkind P. Correlation of fluorescein angiogram and retinal digest in diabetic retinopathy. Am J Ophthalmol 1970;69:403–14.
652. Norton EWD, Gutman F. Diabetic retinopathy studied by fluorescein angiography. Ophthalmologica 1965;150:5–17.
653. Scott DJ, Dollery CT, Hill DW. Fluorescein studies of the retinal circulation in diabetics. Br J Ophthalmol 1963;47:588–9.
654. Shimizu K, Kobayashi Y, Muraoka K. Midperipheral fundus involvement in diabetic retinopathy. Ophthalmology 1981;88:601–12.
655. Bertram B, Wolf S, Fiehöfer S. Retinal circulation times in diabetes mellitus type 1. Br J Ophthalmol 1991;75:462–5.
656. Rimmer T, Fallon TJ, Kohner EM. Long-term follow-up of retinal blood flow in diabetes using the blue light entoptic phenomenon. Br J Ophthalmol 1989;73:1–5.
657. Rimmer T, Fleming J, Kohner EM. Hypoxic viscosity and diabetic retinopathy. Br J Ophthalmol 1990;74:400–4.
658. Sinclair SH. Macular retinal capillary hemodynamics in diabetic patients. Ophthalmology 1991;98:1580–6.
659. Diabetic Retinopathy Study Research Group A modification of the Airlie House classification of diabetic retinopathy. Invest Ophthalmol Vis Sci 1981;21:210–26. [Report 7.]
660. Kohner EM, Dollery CT, Bulpitt CJ. Cotton-wool spots in diabetic retinopathy. Diabetes 1969;18:691–704.

661. Bodansky HJ, Cudworth AG, Whitelocke RAF, et al. Diabetic retinopathy and its relation to type of diabetes: review of a retinal clinic population. Br J Ophthalmol 1982;66:496–9.
662. Bresnick GH. Diabetic maculopathy; a critical review highlighting diffuse macular edema. Ophthalmology 1983;90:1301–17.
663. Bresnick GH. Diabetic macular edema; a review. Ophthalmology 1986;93:989–97.
664. Ferris III FL, Patz A. Macular edema. A complication of diabetic retinopathy. Surv Ophthalmol 1984;28:452–61.
665. Kearns M, Hamilton AM, Kohner EM. Excessive permeability in diabetic maculopathy. Br J Ophthalmol 1979;63:489–97.
666. Klein R, Klein BEK, Moss SE. The Wisconsin Epidemiologic Study of Diabetic Retinopathy. IV. Diabetic macular edema. Ophthalmology 1984;91:1464–74.
667. Klein R, Klein BEK, Moss SE. The Wisconsin Epidemiologic Study of Diabetic Retinopathy. VII. Diabetic nonproliferative retinal lesions. Ophthalmology 1987;94:1389–400.
668. Klein R, Meuer SM, Moss SE, et al. The Wisconsin Epidemiologic Study of Diabetic Retinopathy. XI. The incidence of macular edema. Ophthalmology 1989;96:1501–10.
669. Kohner EM. The evolution and natural history of diabetic retinopathy. Int Ophthalmol Clin 1978;18:1–16.
670. Patz A, Schatz H, Berkow JW. Macular edema – an overlooked complication of diabetic retinopathy. Trans Am Acad Ophthalmol Otolaryngol 1973;77:OP34–42.
671. Sigelman J. Diabetic macular edema in juvenile- and adult-onset diabetes. Am J Ophthalmol 1980;90:287–96.
672. Bec T, Lund-Andersen H. Cotton-wool spots and retinal light sensitivity in diabetic retinopathy. Br J Ophthalmol 1991;75:13–17.
673. Tani M. Cotton-wool patch in diabetic retinopathy. Folia Ophthalmol Jpn 1964;15:674–80.
674. Chihara E, Matsuoka T, Ogura Y, et al. Retinal nerve fiber layer defect as an early manifestation of diabetic retinopathy. Ophthalmology 1993;100:1147–51.
675. Brown GC, Ridley M, Haas D. Lipemic diabetic retinopathy. Ophthalmology 1984;91:1490–5.
676. Robertson DM, Misch DM. Pseudo-endophthalmitis caused by intravitreal lipid transudation in association with proliferative diabetic retinopathy and hyperlipidemia. Retina 1986;6:73–6.
677. Gass JDM. A fluorescein angiographic study of macular dysfunction secondary to retinal vascular disease. IV. Diabetic retinal angiopathy. Arch Ophthalmol 1968;80:583–91.
678. Schatz H, Patz A. Cystoid maculopathy in diabetics. Arch Ophthalmol 1976;94:761–8.
679. Mansour AM, Schachat A, Bodiford G, et al. Foveal avascular zone in diabetes mellitus. Retina 1993;13:125–8.
680. Morgado PB, Chen HC, Patel V. The acute effect of smoking on retinal blood flow in subjects with and without diabetes. Ophthalmology 1994;101:1220–6.
681. Diabetic Retinopathy Study Research Group. Photocoagulation treatment of proliferative diabetic retinopathy: the second report of diabetic retinopathy study findings. Ophthalmology 1978;85:82–106.
682. Davis MD. The natural course of diabetic retinopathy. Trans Am Acad Ophthalmol Otolaryngol 1968;72:237–40.
683. Foos RY, Kreiger AE, Forsythe AB, et al. Posterior vitreous detachment in diabetic subjects. Ophthalmology 1980;87:122–8.
684. Takahashi M, Trempe CL, Maguire K, et al. Vitreoretinal relationship in diabetic retinopathy; a biomicroscopic evaluation. Arch Ophthalmol 1981;99:241–5.
685. Bresnick GH, Smith V, Pokorny J. Visual function abnormalities in macular heterotopia caused by proliferative diabetic retinopathy. Am J Ophthalmol 1981;92:85–102.
686. Hersh PS, Green WR, Thomas JV. Tractional venous loops in diabetic retinopathy. Am J Ophthalmol 1981;92:661–71.
687. Jalkh A, Takahashi M, Topilow HW. Prognostic value of vitreous findings in diabetic retinopathy. Arch Ophthalmol 1982;100:432–4.
688. Lewis H, Abrams GW, Blumenkranz MS, et al. Vitrectomy for diabetic macular traction and edema associated with posterior hyaloidal traction. Ophthalmology 1992;99:753–9.
689. Nasrallah FP, Jalkh AE, Van Coppenolle F. The role of the vitreous in diabetic macular edema. Ophthalmology 1988;95:1335–9.
690. Nasrallah FP, Van de Velde F, Jalkh AE. Importance of the vitreous in young diabetics with macular edema. Ophthalmology 1989;96:1511–7.
691. Finkelstein D, Patz A, Fine SL. Abortive foveal retinal neovascularization in diabetic retinopathy. Retina 1981;1:62–6.
692. Hiscott P, Cooling RJ, Rosen P, et al. The pathology of abortive neovascular outgrowths from the retina. Graefes Arch Clin Exp Ophthalmol 1992;230:531–6.
693. Joondeph BC, Joondeph HC, Flood TP. Foveal neovascularization in diabetic retinopathy. Arch Ophthalmol 1987;105:1672–5.
694. Wong H-C, Sehmi KS, McLeod D. Abortive neovascular outgrowths discovered during vitrectomy for diabetic vitreous hemorrhage. Graefes Arch Clin Exp Ophthalmol 1989;227:237–40.
695. Palmberg P, Smith M, Waltman S. The natural history of retinopathy in insulin-dependent juvenile-onset diabetes. Ophthalmology 1981;88:613–8.
696. Yanko L, Goldbourt U, Michaelson IC. Prevalence and 15-year incidence of retinopathy and associated characteristics in middle-aged and elderly diabetic men. Br J Ophthalmol 1983;67:759–65.
697. Bertram B, Wolf S, Schulte K. Retinal blood flow in diabetic children and adolescents. Graefes Arch Clin Exp Ophthalmol 1991;229:336–40.
698. Klein R. The epidemiology of diabetic retinopathy: findings from the Wisconsin Epidemiologic Study of Diabetic Retinopathy. Int Ophthalmol Clin 1987;27:230–8.
699. Murphy RP, Nanda M, Plotnick L. The relationship of puberty to diabetic retinopathy. Arch Ophthalmol 1990;108:215–8.
700. Verougstraete C, Toussaint D, De Schepper J. First microangiographic abnormalities in childhood diabetes – types of lesions. Graefes Arch Clin Exp Ophthalmol 1991;229:24–32.
701. Klein R, Klein BEK, Moss SE. The Wisconsin Epidemiologic Study of Diabetic Retinopathy. IX. Four-year incidence and progression of diabetic retinopathy when age at diagnosis is less than 30 years. Arch Ophthalmol 1989;107:237–43.
702. Klein R, Klein BEK, Moss SE, et al. The Beaver Dam Eye Study. Retinopathy in adults with newly discovered and previously diagnosed diabetes mellitus. Ophthalmology 1992;99:58–62.
703. Klein R, Klein BEK, Moss SA. The Wisconsin Epidemiologic Study of Diabetic Retinopathy. X. Four-year incidence and progression of diabetic retinopathy when age at diagnosis is 30 years or more. Arch Ophthalmol 1989;107:244–9.
704. Chen M-S, Kao C-S, Chang C-J. Prevalence and risk factors of diabetic retinopathy among noninsulin-dependent diabetic subjects. Am J Ophthalmol 1992;114:723–30.
705. Wiznia RA. Photocoagulation of nonproliferative exudative diabetic retinopathy. Am J Ophthalmol 1979;88:22–7.
706. Klein R, Klein BEK, Moss SE, et al. The Wisconsin Epidemiologic Study of Diabetic Retinopathy. XIV. Ten-year incidence and progression of diabetic retinopathy. Arch Ophthalmol 1994;112:1217–28.
707. Cruickshanks KJ, Ritter LL, Klein R, et al. The association of microalbuminuria with diabetic retinopathy; the Wisconsin Epidemiologic Study of Diabetic Retinopathy. Ophthalmology 1993;100:862–7.
708. Chase HP, Garg SK, Jackson WE. Blood pressure and retinopathy in type I diabetes. Ophthalmology 1990;97:155–9.
709. Marshall G, Garg SK, Jackson WE. Factors influencing the onset and progression of diabetic retinopathy in subjects with insulin-dependent diabetes mellitus. Ophthalmology 1993;100:1133–9.
710. Kishi S, Shimizu K. Clinical manifestations of posterior precortical vitreous pocket in proliferative diabetic retinopathy. Ophthalmology 1993;100:225–9.
711. Shahidi M, Ogura Y, Blair NP. Retinal thickness analysis for quantitative assessment of diabetic macular edema. Arch Ophthalmol 1991;109:1115–9.
712. Moss SE, Klein R, Meuer MB, et al. The association of iris color with eye disease in diabetes. Ophthalmology 1987;94:1226–31.
713. Marshall J, Clover G, Rothery S. Some new findings on retinal irradiation by krypton and argon lasers. Doc Ophthalmol Proc Ser 1984;36:21–37.
714. Mühlhauser I, Sawicki P, Berger M. Cigarette-smoking as a risk factor for macroproteinuria and proliferative retinopathy in type I (insulin-dependent) diabetes. Diabetologia 1986;29:500–2.
715. Haffner SM, Klein R, Dunn JF. Increased testosterone in type I diabetic subjects with severe retinopathy. Ophthalmology 1990;97:1270–4.
716. Viebahn M, Barricks ME, Osterloh MD. Synergism between diabetic and irradiation retinopathy: case report and review. Br J Ophthalmol 1991;75:629–32.
717. Bresnick GH, Engerman R, Davis MD. Patterns of ischemia in diabetic retinopathy. Trans Am Acad Ophthalmol Otolaryngol 1976;81:OP694–OP709.
718. Haffner SM, Fong D, Stern MP. Diabetic retinopathy in Mexican Americans and non-Hispanic Whites. Diabetes 1988;37:878–84.
719. DAMAD Study Group Effect of aspirin alone and aspirin plus dipyridamole in early diabetic retinopathy; a multicenter randomized controlled clinical trial. Diabetes 1989;38:491–8.
720. Jaffe GJ, Burton TC. Progression of nonproliferative diabetic retinopathy following cataract extraction. Arch Ophthalmol 1988;106:745–9.
721. Jaffe GJ, Burton TC, Kuhn E. Progression of nonproliferative diabetic retinopathy and visual outcome after extracapsular cataract extraction and intraocular lens implantation. Am J Ophthalmol 1992;114:448–56.
722. Pollack A, Dotan S, Oliver M. Progression of diabetic retinopathy after cataract extraction. Br J Ophthalmol 1991;75:547–51.
723. Pollack A, Leiba H, Bukelman A. The course of diabetic retinopathy following cataract surgery in eyes previously treated by laser photocoagulation. Br J Ophthalmol 1992;76:228–31.
724. Ruiz RS, Saatci OA. Posterior chamber intraocular lens implantation in eyes with inactive and active proliferative diabetic retinopathy. Am J Ophthalmol 1991;111:158–62.
725. Schatz H, Atienza D, McDonald HR, et al. Severe diabetic retinopathy after cataract surgery. Am J Ophthalmol 1994;117:314–21.
726. Bierly JR, Dunn JP. Macular edema after carotid endarterectomy in ocular ischemic syndrome. Am J Ophthalmol 1992;113:105–7.
727. Duker JS, Brown GC, Bosley TM. Asymmetric proliferative diabetic retinopathy and carotid artery disease. Ophthalmology 1990;97:869–74.
728. Gay AJ, Rosenbaum AL. Retinal artery pressure in asymmetric diabetic retinopathy. Arch Ophthalmol 1966;75:758–62.
729. Bresnick GH, Condit R, Syrjala S. Abnormalities of the foveal avascular zone in diabetic retinopathy. Arch Ophthalmol 1984;102:1286–93.
730. Bresnick GH, de Venecia G, Myers FL. Retinal ischemia in diabetic retinopathy. Arch Ophthalmol 1975;93:1300–10.
731. Brinchmann-Hansen O, Dahl-Jorgensen K, Hanssen KF, et al. The response of diabetic retinopathy to 41 months of multiple insulin injections, insulin pumps, and conventional insulin therapy. Arch Ophthalmol 1988;106:1242–6.
732. Hill DW, Dollery CT, Mailer CM, et al. Arterial fluorescein studies in diabetic retinopathy. Proc R Soc Med 1965;58:535–7.
733. Merin S, Ber I, Ivry M. Retinal ischemia (capillary nonperfusion) and retinal neovascularization in patients with diabetic retinopathy. Ophthalmologica 1978;177:140–5.
734. Kincaid MC, Green WR, Fine SL. An ocular clinicopathologic correlative study of six patients from the Diabetic Retinopathy Study. Retina 1983;3:218–38.
735. Kuwabara T, Cogan DG. Retinal vascular patterns. VI. Mural cells of the retinal capillaries. Arch Ophthalmol 1963;69:492–502.
736. Ticho U, Patz A. The role of capillary perfusion in the management of diabetic macular edema. Am J Ophthalmol 1973;76:880–6.
737. Freyler H, Prskavec F, Stelzer N. Diabetische Chorioidopathie – eine retrospektive fluoreszenzangiographische Studie; Vorläufige Mitteilung. Klin Monatsbl Augenheilkd 1986;189:144–7.
738. Fryczkowski AW, Hodes BL, Walker J. Diabetic choroidal and iris vasculature scanning electron microscopy findings. Int Ophthalmol 1989;13:269–79.
739. Williams B. Angiotensin II, VEGF, and diabetic retinopathy. Lancet 1998;351:837–8.
740. Stoschitzky K. Angiotensin II, VEGF, and diabetic retinopathy. Lancet 1998;351:836–7.
741. Paques M, Massin P, Gaudric A. Growth factors and diabetic retinopathy. Diabetes Metab 1997;23:125–30.

742. Amalric P. Nouvelles considérations concernant l'évolution et le traitement de la rétinopathie diabétique. Ophthalmologica 1967;154:151–60.
743. Blankenship GW. Diabetic macular edema and argon laser photocoagulation: a prospective randomized study. Ophthalmology 1979;86:69–75.
744. Diabetic Retinopathy Study Research Group. Preliminary report on effects of photocoagulation therapy. Am J Ophthalmol 1976;81:383–96.
745. Diabetic Retinopathy Study Research Group. Four risk factors for severe visual loss in diabetic retinopathy; the third report from the Diabetic Retinopathy Study. Arch Ophthalmol 1979;97:654–5.
746. Hamilton AM. Management of diabetic retinopathy. Trans Ophthalmol Soc UK 1977;97:494–6.
747. Hercules BL, Gayed II, Lucas SB, et al. Peripheral retinal ablation in the treatment of proliferative diabetic retinopathy: a three-year interim report of a randomised, controlled study using the argon laser. Br J Ophthalmol 1977;61:555–63.
748. Marcus DF, Aaberg TM. Argon laser photocoagulation treatment of diabetic cystoid maculopathy. Ann Ophthalmol 1977;9:365–72.
749. McDonald HR, Schatz H. Grid photocoagulation for diffuse macular edema. Retina 1985;5: 65–72.
750. Merin S, Yanko L, Ivry M. Treatment of diabetic maculopathy by argon-laser. Br J Ophthalmol 1974;58:85–91.
751. Meyers SM. Macular edema after scatter laser photocoagulation for proliferative diabetic retinopathy. Am J Ophthalmol 1980;90:210–6.
752. Meyer-Schwickerath GRE, Schott K. Diabetic retinopathy and photocoagulation. Am J Ophthalmol 1968;66:597–603.
753. Okun E, Cibis PA. The role of photocoagulation in the therapy of proliferative diabetic retinopathy. Arch Ophthalmol 1966;75:337–52.
754. Patz A, Schatz H, Ryan SJ. Argon laser photocoagulation for treatment of advanced diabetic retinopathy. Trans Am Acad Ophthalmol Otolaryngol 1972;76:984–9.
755. Plumb AP, Swan AV, Chignell AH, et al. A comparative trial of xenon arc and argon laser photocoagulation in the treatment of proliferative diabetic retinopathy. Br J Ophthalmol 1982;66:213–8.
756. Reeser F, Fleischman J, Williams GA, et al. Efficacy of argon laser photocoagulation in the treatment of circinate diabetic retinopathy. Am J Ophthalmol 1981;92:762–7.
757. Spalter HF. Photocoagulation of circinate maculopathy in diabetic retinopathy. Am J Ophthalmol 1971;71:242–50.
758. Welch RB. The treatment of diabetic retinopathy. In: Goldberg MF, Fine SL, editors. Symposium on the treatment of diabetic retinopathy. Airlie House, Warrenton, Virginia: Public Health Service Publication No. 1890, Washington, DC, 1969, U.S. Department of Health, Education and Welfare; September 29 to October 1, 1968. p. 563–68.
759. Whitelocke RAF, Kearns M, Blach RK, et al. The diabetic maculopathies. Trans Ophthalmol Soc UK 1979;99:314–20.
760. British Multicentre Study Group. Photocoagulation for diabetic maculopathy; a randomized controlled clinical trial using the xenon arc. Diabetes 1983;32:1010–6.
761. Diabetic Retinopathy Study Research Group. Photocoagulation treatment of proliferative diabetic retinopathy; clinical application of Diabetic Retinopathy Study (DRS) findings, DRS report number 8. Ophthalmology 1981;88:583–600.
762. Diabetic Retinopathy Study Research Group. Two-year course of visual acuity in severe diabetic proliferative retinopathy with conventional management. Diabetic Retinopathy Vitrectomy Study (DRVS) Report number 1. Ophthalmology 1985;92:492–502.
763. Diabetic Retinopathy Study Research Group. Early vitrectomy for severe vitreous hemorrhage in diabetic retinopathy; two-year results of a randomized trial; Diabetic Retinopathy Vitrectomy Study report 2. Arch Ophthalmol 1985;103:1644–52.
764. Diabetic Retinopathy Study Research Group. Early vitrectomy for severe proliferative diabetic retinopathy in eyes with useful vision; results of a randomized trial – Diabetic Retinopathy Vitrectomy Study report 3. Ophthalmology 1988;95:1307–20.
765. Diabetic Retinopathy Vitrectomy Study Research Group. Early vitrectomy for severe proliferative diabetic retinopathy in eyes with useful vision; clinical application of results of a randomized trial – Diabetic Retinopathy report 4. Ophthalmology 1988;95:1321–34.
766. Diabetic Retinopathy Vitrectomy Study Research Group. Early vitrectomy for severe vitreous hemorrhage in diabetic retinopathy; four-year results of a randomized trial: diabetic Retinopathy Study report 5. Arch Ophthalmol 1990;108:958–64.
767. Early Treatment Diabetic Retinopathy Study Research Group. Photocoagulation for diabetic macular edema. Early Treatment Diabetic Retinopathy Study report number 1. Arch Ophthalmol 1985;103:1796–806.
768. Early Treatment Diabetic Retinopathy Study Research Group. Treatment techniques and clinical guidelines for photocoagulation of diabetic macular edema. Early Treatment Diabetic Retinopathy Study report number 2. Ophthalmology 1987;94:761–74.
769. Early Treatment Diabetic Retinopathy Study Research Group. Techniques for scatter and local photocoagulation treatment of diabetic retinopathy: early Treatment Diabetic Retinopathy Study report no 3. Int Ophthalmol Clin 1987;27:254–64.
770. Early Treatment Diabetic Retinopathy Study Research Group. Early treatment diabetic retinopathy study design and baseline patient characteristics. ETDRS report number 7. Ophthalmology 1991;98:741–56.
771. Early Treatment Diabetic Retinopathy Study Research Group. Effects of aspirin treatment on diabetic retinopathy. ETDRS report number 8. Ophthalmology 1991;98:757–65.
772. Early Treatment Diabetic Retinopathy Study Research Group. Early photocoagulation for diabetic retinopathy. ETDRS report number 9. Ophthalmology 1991;98:766–85.
773. Early Treatment Diabetic Retinopathy Study Research Group. Fluorescein angiographic risk factors for progression of diabetic retinopathy. ETDRS report number 13. Ophthalmology 1991;98:834–40.
774. Ferris III FL, Podgor MJ, Davis MD. Macular edema in diabetic retinopathy study patients. Diabetic Retinopathy Study report number 12. Ophthalmology 1987;94:754–60.
775. Lee CM, Olk RJ. Modified grid laser photocoagulation for diffuse diabetic macular edema; long-term visual results. Ophthalmology 1991;98:1594–602.
776. Olk RJ. Modified grid argon (blue-green) laser photocoagulation for diffuse diabetic macular edema. Ophthalmology 1986;93:938–50.
777. Striph GG, Hart Jr WM, Olk RJ. Modified grid laser photocoagulation for diabetic macular edema; the effect on the central visual field. Ophthalmology 1988;95:1673–9.
778. McDonald HR, Schatz H. Visual loss following panretinal photocoagulation for proliferative diabetic retinopathy. Ophthalmology 1985;92:388–93.
779. Blankenship GW. A clinical comparison of central and peripheral argon laser panretinal photocoagulation for proliferative diabetic retinopathy. Ophthalmology 1988;95:170–7.
780. Gardner TW, Eller AW, Friberg TR. Reduction of severe macular edema in eyes with poor vision after panretinal photocoagulation for proliferative diabetic retinopathy. Graefes Arch Clin Exp Ophthalmol 1991;229:323–8.
781. Aylward GW, Pearson RV, Jagger JD, et al. Extensive argon laser photocoagulation in the treatment of proliferative diabetic retinopathy. Br J Ophthalmol 1989;73:197–201.
782. Doft BH, Metz DJ, Kelsey SF. Augmentation laser for proliferative diabetic retinopathy that fails to respond to initial panretinal photocoagulation. Ophthalmology 1992;99:1728–35.
783. Blankenship GW, Gerke E, Batlle JF. Red krypton and blue-green argon laser diabetic panretinal photocoagulation. Graefes Arch Clin Exp Ophthalmol 1989;227:364–8.
784. Bressler SB. Does wavelength matter when photocoagulating eyes with macular degeneration or diabetic retinopathy? Arch Ophthalmol 1993;111:177–80.
785. Canning C, Polkinghorne P, Ariffin A, et al. Panretinal laser photocoagulation for proliferative diabetic retinopathy: the effect of laser wavelength on macular function. Br J Ophthalmol 1991;75:608–10.
786. Capoferri C, Bagini M, Chizzoli A. Electroretinographic findings in panretinal photocoagulation for diabetic retinopathy; a randomized study with blue-green argon and red krypton lasers. Graefes Arch Clin Exp Ophthalmol 1990;228:232–6.
787. Casswell AG, Canning CR, Gregor ZJ. Treatment of diffuse macular oedema: a comparison between argon and krypton lasers. Eye 1990;4:668–72.
788. Olk RJ. Argon green (514 nm) versus krypton red (647 nm) modified grid laser photocoagulation for diffuse diabetic macular edema. Ophthalmology 1990;97:1101–12.
789. Abu El Asrar AM, Morse PH. Laser photocoagulation control of diabetic macular oedema without fluorescein angiography. Br J Ophthalmol 1991;75:97–9.
790. Adamis AP, Miller JW, Bernal M-T. Increased vascular endothelial growth factor levels in the vitreous of eyes with proliferative diabetic retinopathy. Am J Ophthalmol 1994;118:445–50.
791. Stefansson E. Oxygen and diabetic eye disease. Graefes Arch Clin Exp Ophthalmol 1990;228:120–3.
792. Stefansson E, Machemer R, de Juan Jr E. Retinal oxygenation and laser treatment in patients with diabetic retinopathy. Am J Ophthalmol 1992;113:36–8.
793. Weiter JJ, Zuckerman R. The influence of the photoreceptor-RPE complex on the inner retina; an explanation for the beneficial effects of photocoagulation. Ophthalmology 1980;87:1133–9.
794. Wilson CA, Stefansson E, Klombers L. Optic disk neovascularization and retinal vessel diameter in diabetic retinopathy. Am J Ophthalmol 1988;106:131–4.
795. Blankenship GW, Machemer R. Long-term diabetic vitrectomy results; report of 10 year follow-up. Ophthalmology 1985;92:503–6.
796. Vander JF, Duker JS, Benson WE. Long-term stability and visual outcome after favorable initial response of proliferative diabetic retinopathy to panretinal photocoagulation. Ophthalmology 1991;98:1575–9.
797. Berger AR, Boniuk I. Bilateral subretinal neovascularization after focal argon laser photocoagulation for diabetic macular edema. Am J Ophthalmol 1989;108:88–90.
798. Lewis H, Schachat AP, Haimann MH. Choroidal neovascularization after laser photocoagulation for diabetic macular edema. Ophthalmology 1990;97:503–11.
799. Varley MP, Frank E, Purnell EW. Subretinal neovascularization after focal argon laser for diabetic macular edema. Ophthalmology 1988;95:567–73.
800. Guyer DR, D'Amico DJ, Smith CW. Subretinal fibrosis after laser photocoagulation for diabetic macular edema. Am J Ophthalmol 1992;113:652–6.
801. Han DP, Mieler WF, Burton TC. Submacular fibrosis after photocoagulation for diabetic macular edema. Am J Ophthalmol 1992;113:513–21.
802. Rutledge BK, Wallow IHL, Poulsen GL. Sub-pigment epithelial membranes after photocoagulation for diabetic macular edema. Arch Ophthalmol 1993;111:608–13.
803. Wallow IHL, Bindley CD. Focal photocoagulation of diabetic macular edema; a clinicopathologic case report. Retina 1988;8:261–9.
804. Elliott A, Flanagan D. Macular detachment following laser treatment for proliferative diabetic retinopathy. Graefes Arch Clin Exp Ophthalmol 1990;228:438–41.
805. Schatz H, Madeira D, McDonald HR, et al. Progressive enlargement of laser scars following grid laser photocoagulation for diffuse diabetic macular edema. Arch Ophthalmol 1991;109: 1549–51.
806. Benedett R, Olk RJ, Arribas NP. Transconjunctival anterior retinal cryotherapy for proliferative diabetic retinopathy. Ophthalmology 1987;94:612–9.
807. Ross WH, Gottner MJ. Peripheral retinal cryopexy for subtotal vitreous hemorrhage. Am J Ophthalmol 1988;105:377–82.
808. Vernon SA, Cheng H. Panretinal cryotherapy in neovascular disease. Br J Ophthalmol 1988;72:401–5.
809. Cordido M, Fernández-Vigo J, Fandiño J, et al. Natural evolution of massive vitreous hemorrhage in diabetic retinopathy. Retina 1988;8:96–101.
810. Flynn Jr HW, Chew EY, Simons BD. Pars plana vitrectomy in the early treatment diabetic retinopathy study; ETDRS report number 17. Ophthalmology 1992;99:1351–7.
811. Gollamudi SR, Smiddy WE, Schachat AP. Long-term survival rate after vitreous surgery for complications of diabetic retinopathy. Ophthalmology 1991;98:18–22.
812. Sato Y, Shimada H, Aso S, et al. Vitrectomy for diabetic macular heterotopia. Ophthalmology 1994;101:63–7.
813. Thompson JT, de Bustros S, Michels RG. Results of vitrectomy for proliferative diabetic retinopathy. Ophthalmology 1986;93:1571–4.
814. Thompson JT, de Bustros S, Michels RG, et al. Results and prognostic factors in vitrectomy for diabetic traction retinal detachment of the macula. Arch Ophthalmol 1987;105:497–502.

815. Thompson JT, de Bustros S, Michels RG, et al. Results and prognostic factors in vitrectomy for diabetic vitreous hemorrhage. Arch Ophthalmol 1987;105:191–5.
816. Miller SA, Butler JB, Myers FL, et al. Pars plana vitrectomy; treatment for tractional macula detachment secondary to proliferative diabetic retinopathy. Arch Ophthalmol 1980;98:659–64.
817. Rice TA, Michels RG, Rice EF. Vitrectomy for diabetic traction retinal detachment involving the macula. Am J Ophthalmol 1983;95:22–33.
818. Charles S, Flinn CE. The natural history of diabetic extramacular traction retinal detachment. Arch Ophthalmol 1981;99:66–8.
819. Blankenship GW, Flynn Jr HW, Kokame GT. Posterior chamber intraocular lens insertion during pars plana lensectomy and vitrectomy for complications of proliferative diabetic retinopathy. Am J Ophthalmol 1989;108:1–5.
820. Mirshahi A, Shenazandi H, Lashay A, et al. Intravitreal triamcinolone as an adjunct to standard laser therapy in coexisting high-risk proliferative diabetic retinopathy and clinically significant macular edema. Retina 2010;30:254–9.
821. Cho WB, Moon JW, Kim HC. Intravitreal triamcinolone and bevacizumab as adjunctive treatments to panretinal photocoagulation in diabetic retinopathy. Br J Ophthalmol 2010;94:858–63.
822. Machemer R, Sugita G, Tano Y. Treatment of intraocular proliferations with intravitreal steroids. Trans Am Ophthalmol Soc 1979;77:171–80.
823. Silva PS, Sun JK, Aiello LP. Role of steroids in the management of diabetic macular edema and proliferative diabetic retinopathy. Semin Ophthalmol 2009;24:93–9.
824. Zacks DN, Johnson MW. Combined intravitreal injection of triamcinolone acetonide and panretinal photocoagulation for concomitant diabetic macular edema and proliferative diabetic retinopathy. Retina 2005;25:135–40.
825. Erdol H, Turk A, Akyol N, et al. The results of intravitreal bevacizumab injections for persistent neovascularizations in proliferative diabetic retinopathy after photocoagulation therapy. Retina 2010;30:570–7.
826. Yeh PT, Yang CM, Lin YC, et al. Bevacizumab pretreatment in vitrectomy with silicone oil for severe diabetic retinopathy. Retina 2009;29:768–74.
827. Appen RE, Chandra SR, Klein R, et al. Diabetic papillopathy. Am J Ophthalmol 1980;90:203–9.
828. Barr CC, Glaser JS, Blankenship G. Acute disc swelling in juvenile diabetes; clinical profile and natural history of 12 cases. Arch Ophthalmol 1980;98:2185–92.
829. Pavan PR, Aiello LM, Wafai MZ. Optic disc edema in juvenile-onset diabetes. Arch Ophthalmol 1980;98:2193–5.
830. Stransky TJ. Diabetic papillopathy and proliferative retinopathy. Graefes Arch Clin Exp Ophthalmol 1986;224:46–50.
831. Doft BH, Kingley LA, Orchard TJ. The association between long-term diabetic control and early retinopathy. Ophthalmology 1984;91:763–9.
832. Goldstein DE, Blinder KJ, Ide CH. Glycemic control and development of retinopathy in youth-onset insulin-dependent diabetes mellitus; results of a 12-year longitudinal study. Ophthalmology 1993;100:1125–32.
833. Kroc Collaborative Study Group. Diabetic retinopathy after two years of intensive insulin treatment; follow-up of the Kroc Collaborative Study. JAMA 1988;260:37–41.
834. Reichard P, Sule J, Rosenqvist U. Capillary loss and leakage after five years of intensified insulin treatment in patients with insulin-dependent diabetes mellitus. Ophthalmology 1991;98:1587–93.
835. Diabetes Control and Complications Trial Research Group. The effect of intensive treatment of diabetes on the development and progression of long-term complications in insulin-dependent diabetes mellitus. N Engl J Med 1993;329:977–86.
836. Gordon B, Chang S, Kavanagh M. The effects of lipid lowering on diabetic retinopathy. Am J Ophthalmol 1991;112:385–91.
837. Klein BEK, Moss SE, Klein R, et al. The Wisconsin Epidemiologic Study of Diabetic Retinopathy. XIII. Relationship of serum cholesterol to retinopathy and hard exudate. Ophthalmology 1991;98:1261–5.
838. Sorbinil Retinopathy Trial Research Group. A randomized trial of sorbinil, an aldose reductase inhibitor, in diabetic retinopathy. Arch Ophthalmol 1990;108:1234–44.
839. TIMAD Study Group. Ticlopidine treatment reduces the progression of nonproliferative diabetic retinopathy. Arch Ophthalmol 1990;108:1577–83.
840. Perkovich BT, Meyers SM. Systemic factors affecting diabetic macular edema. J Ophthalmol 1988;105:211–2.
841. Ulbig M, Kampik A, Thurau S. Long-term follow-up of diabetic retinopathy for up to 71 months after combined renal and pancreatic transplantation. Graefes Arch Clin Exp Ophthalmol 1991;229:242–5.
842. Boone MI, Farber ME, Jovanovic-Peterson L, et al. Increased retinal vascular tortuosity in gestational diabetes mellitus. Ophthalmology 1989;96:251–4.
843. Johnston GP. Pregnancy and diabetic retinopathy. Am J Ophthalmol 1980;90:519–24.
844. Moloney JBM, Drury MI. The effect of pregnancy on the natural course of diabetic retinopathy. Am J Ophthalmol 1982;93:745–56.
845. Sinclair SH, Nesler C, Foxman B. Macular edema and pregnancy in insulin-dependent diabetes. Am J Ophthalmol 1984;97:154–67.
846. Gray RS, Starkey IR, Rainbow S. HLA antigens and other risk factors in the development of retinopathy in type 1 diabetes. Br J Ophthalmol 1982;66:280–5.
847. Johnston PB, Kidd M, Middleton D. Analysis of HLA antigen association with proliferative diabetic retinopathy. Br J Ophthalmol 1982;66:277–9.
848. Klein R, Klein BEK, Moss SE. Diabetes, hyperglycemia and age-related maculopathy; the Beaver Dam Study. Ophthalmology 1992;99:1527–34.
849. Zhang X, Saaddine JB, Chou CF, et al. Prevalence of diabetic retinopathy in the United States, 2005–2008. JAMA 2010;304:649–56.
850. Rigoli L, Lombardo F, Di Bella C. Wolfram syndrome and WFS1 gene. Clin Genet 2011;79(Feb):103–17.
851. Barrett TG, Bundey SE, Fielder AR, et al. Optic atrophy in Wolfram (DIDMOAD) syndrome. Eye (Lond) 1997;11:882–8.
852. Van den Bergh L, Zeyen T, Verhelst J, et al. Wolfram syndrome: a clinical study of two cases. Doc Ophthalmol 1993;84:119–26.
853. Mets RB, Emery SB, Lesperance MM, et al. Congenital cataracts in two siblings with Wolfram syndrome. Ophthalmic Genet 2010;31:227–9.
854. Dhalla MS, Desai UR, Zuckerbrod DS. Pigmentary maculopathy in a patient with Wolfram syndrome. Can J Ophthalmol 2006;41:38–40.
855. Kinsley BT, Swift M, Dumont RH, et al. Morbidity and mortality in the Wolfram syndrome. Diabetes Care 1995;18:1566–70.
856. Amoaku WMK, Archer DB. Cephalic radiation and retinal vasculopathy. Eye 1990;4:195–203.
857. Amoaku WMK, Archer DB. Fluorescein angiographic features, natural course and treatment of radiation retinopathy. Eye 1990;4:657–67.
858. Bagan SM, Hollenhorst RW. Radiation retinopathy after irradiation of intracranial lesions. Am J Ophthalmol 1979;88:694–7.
859. Bedford MA, Bedotto C, MacFaul PA, et al. Radiation retinopathy after the application of a cobalt plaque. Br J Ophthalmol 1970;54:505–9.
860. Brown GC, Shields JA, Sanborn G. Radiation optic neuropathy. Ophthalmology 1982;89:1489–93.
861. Brown GC, Shields JA, Sanborn G. Radiation retinopathy. Ophthalmology 1982;89:1494–501.
862. Chaudhuri PR, Austin DJ, Rosenthal AR. Treatment of radiation retinopathy. Br J Ophthalmol 1981;65:623–5.
863. Chee PHY. Radiation retinopathy. Am J Ophthalmol 1968;66:860–5.
864. Egbert PR, Fajardo LF, Donaldson SS, et al. Posterior ocular abnormalities after irradiation for retinoblastoma: a histopathological study. Br J Ophthalmol 1980;64:660–5.
865. Fitzgerald CR, Enoch JM, Temme LA. Radiation therapy in and about the retina, optic nerve, and anterior visual pathway; psychophysical assessment. Arch Ophthalmol 1981;99:611–23.
866. Gragoudas ES, Zakov NZ, Albert DM, et al. Long-term observations of proton-irradiated monkey eyes. Arch Ophthalmol 1979;97:2184–91.
867. Guyer DR, Mukai S, Egan KM. Radiation maculopathy after proton beam irradiation for choroidal melanoma. Ophthalmology 1992;99:1278–85.
868. Hayreh SS. Post-radiation retinopathy; a fluorescence fundus angiographic study. Br J Ophthalmol 1970;54:705–14.
869. Hudgins PA, Newman NJ, Dillon WP, et al. Radiation-induced optic neuropathy: characteristic appearances on gadolinium-enhanced MR. AJNR 1992;13:235–8.
870. Kinyoun JL, Chittum ME, Wells CG. Photocoagulation treatment of radiation retinopathy. Am J Ophthalmol 1988;105:470–8.
871. Midena E, Segato T, Piermarocci S. Retinopathy following radiation therapy of paranasal sinus and nasopharyngeal carcinoma. Retina 1987;7:142–7.
872. Miller ML, Goldberg SH, Bullock JD. Radiation retinopathy after standard radiotherapy for thyroid-related ophthalmopathy. Am J Ophthalmol 1991;112:600–1.
873. Noble KG, Kupersmith MJ. Retinal vascular remodelling in radiation retinopathy. Br J Ophthalmol 1984;68:475–8.
874. Roden DBT, Fowble B. Delayed radiation injury to the retrobulbar optic nerves and chiasm; clinical syndrome and treatment with hyperbaric oxygen and corticosteroids. Ophthalmology 1990;97:346–51.
875. Shukovsky LJ, Fletcher GH. Retinal and optic nerve complications in a high dose irradiation technique of ethmoid sinus and nasal cavity. Radiology 1972;104:629–34.
876. Tomsak RL, Smith JL. Radiation retinopathy in a patient with lung carcinoma metastatic to brain. Ann Ophthalmol 1980;12:619–22.
877. Boozalis GT, Schachat AP, Green WR. Subretinal neovascularization from the retina in radiation retinopathy. Retina 1987;7:156–61.
878. Archer DB, Amoaku WMK, Gardiner TA. Radiation retinopathy – clinical, histopathological, ultrastructural and experimental correlations. Eye 1991;5:239–51.
879. Atsumi O, Sakuraba T, Kimura S. A case of presumed radiation optic neuropathy. Acta Soc Ophthalmol Jpn 1991;95:504–10.
880. Borruat F-X, Schatz NJ, Glaser JS. Visual recovery from radiation-induced optic neuropathy. J Clin Neuro-Ophthalmol 1993;13:98–101.
881. Kline LB, Kim JY, Ceballos R. Radiation optic neuropathy. Ophthalmology 1985;92:1118–26.
882. Lovato AA, Char DH, Quivey JM, et al. Evaluation of acute radiation optic neuropathy by B-scan ultrasonography. Am J Ophthalmol 1990;110:233–6.
883. Young WC, Thornton AF, Gebarski SS, et al. Radiation-induced optic neuropathy: correlation of MR imaging and radiation dosimetry. Radiology 1992;185:904–7.
884. Zimmerman CF, Schatz NJ, Glaser JS. Magnetic resonance imaging of radiation optic neuropathy. Am J Ophthalmol 1990;110:389–94.
885. Elmassri A. Radiation chorioretinopathy. Br J Ophthalmol 1986;70:326–9.
886. Gall N, Leiba H, Handzel R, et al. Severe radiation retinopathy and optic neuropathy after brachytherapy for choroidal melanoma, treated by hyperbaric oxygen. Eye (Lond) 2007;21:1010–2.
887. Finger PT, Kurli M. Laser photocoagulation for radiation retinopathy after ophthalmic plaque radiation therapy. Br J Ophthalmol 2005;89:730–8.
888. Finger PT. Tumour location affects the incidence of cataract and retinopathy after ophthalmic plaque radiation therapy. Br J Ophthalmol 2000;84:1068–70.
889. Gunduz K, Shields CL, Shields JA, et al. Radiation retinopathy following plaque radiotherapy for posterior uveal melanoma. Arch Ophthalmol 1999;117:609–14.
890. Irvine AR, Wood IS. Radiation retinopathy as an experimental model for ischemic proliferative retinopathy and rubeosis iridis. Am J Ophthalmol 1987;103:790–7.
891. Guy J, Schatz NJ. Hyperbaric oxygen in the treatment of radiation-induced optic neuropathy. Ophthalmology 1986;93:1083–8.
892. Finger RP, Charbel Issa P, Ladewig M, et al. Intravitreal bevacizumab for choroidal neovascularisation associated with pseudoxanthoma elasticum. Br J Ophthalmol 2008;92: 483–7.
893. Arriola-Villalobos P, Donate-Lopez J, Calvo-Gonzalez C, et al. Intravitreal bevacizumab (Avastin) for radiation retinopathy neovascularization. Acta Ophthalmol 2008;86:115–6.
894. Finger PT, Chin K. Anti-vascular endothelial growth factor bevacizumab (avastin) for radiation retinopathy. Arch Ophthalmol 2007;125:751–6.
895. Duker JS, Brown GC, Ballas SK. Peripheral retinal neovascularization associated with hemoglobin C B° thalassemia. Am J Ophthalmol 1989;108:328–9.

896. Condon PI, Serjeant GR. Photocoagulation and diathermy in the treatment of proliferative sickle retinopathy. Br J Ophthalmol 1974;58:650–62.
897. Condon PI, Serjeant GR. Ocular findings in elderly cases of homozygous sickle-cell disease in Jamaica. Br J Ophthalmol 1976;60:361–4.
898. Condon PI, Serjeant GR. Behaviour of untreated proliferative sickle retinopathy. Br J Ophthalmol 1980;64:404–11.
899. Condon PI, Serjeant GR. Photocoagulation in proliferative sickle retinopathy: results of a 5-year study. Br J Ophthalmol 1980;64:832–40.
900. Cruess AF, Stephens RF, Magargal LE, et al. Peripheral circumferential retinal scatter photocoagulation for treatment of proliferative sickle retinopathy. Ophthalmology 1983; 90:272–8.
901. Eagle Jr RC, Yanoff M, Fine BS. Hemoglobin SC retinopathy and fat emboli to the eye; a light and electron microscopical study. Arch Ophthalmol 1974;92:28–32.
902. Fox PD, Dunn DT, Morris JS, et al. Risk factors for proliferative sickle retinopathy. Br J Ophthalmol 1990;74:172–6.
903. Gagliano DA, Goldberg MF. The evolution of salmon-patch hemorrhages in sickle cell retinopathy. Arch Ophthalmol 1989;107:1814.
904. Gass JDM. Stereoscopic atlas of macular diseases; diagnosis and treatment, 2nd ed. St. Louis: CV Mosby; 1977. p. 278.
905. Goldberg MF. Classification and pathogenesis of proliferative sickle retinopathy. Am J Ophthalmol 1971;71:649–65.
906. Goldberg MF. Natural history of untreated proliferative sickle retinopathy. Arch Ophthalmol 1971;85:428–37.
907. Goldberg MF. Retinal neovascularization in sickle cell retinopathy. Trans Am Acad Ophthalmol Otolaryngol 1977;83:OP409–OP431.
908. Goldberg MF, Galinos S, Lee C-B. Macular ischemia and infarction in sickling. Invest Ophthalmol 1973;12:633–5.
909. Kimmel AS, Magargal LE, Maizel R, et al. Proliferative sickle cell retinopathy under age 20: a review. Ophthalmic Surg 1987;18:126–8.
910. Knapp JW. Isolated macular infarction in sickle cell (SS) disease. Am J Ophthalmol 1972;73:857–9.
911. Nagpal KC, Goldberg MF, Rabb MF. Ocular manifestations of sickle haemoglobinopathies. Surv Ophthalmol 1977;21:391–411.
912. Raichand M, Goldberg MF, Nagpal KC. Evolution of neovascularization in sickle cell retinopathy; a prospective fluorescein angiographic study. Arch Ophthalmol 1977;95:1543–52.
913. Talbot JF, Bird AC, Maude GH. Sickle cell retinopathy in Jamaican children: further observations from a cohort study. Br J Ophthalmol 1988;72:727–32.
914. Talbot JF, Bird AC, Serjeant GR, et al. Sickle cell retinopathy in young children in Jamaica. Br J Ophthalmol 1982;66:149–54.
915. Sanders RJ, Brown GC, Rosenstein RB, et al. Foveal avascular zone diameter and sickle cell disease. Arch Ophthalmol 1991;109:812–5.
916. Clarkson JG. The ocular manifestations of sickle-cell disease: a prevalence and natural history study. Trans Am Ophthalmol Soc 1992;90:481–504.
917. Fox PD, Vessey SJR, Forshaw ML, et al. Influence of genotype on the natural history of untreated proliferative sickle retinopathy – an angiographic study. Br J Ophthalmol 1991;75:229–31.
918. Lee CM, Charles HC, Smith RT. Quantification of macular ischaemia in sickle cell retinopathy. Br J Ophthalmol 1987;71:540–5.
919. van Meurs JC. Relationship between peripheral vascular closure and proliferative retinopathy in sickle cell disease. Graefes Arch Clin Exp Ophthalmol 1991;229:543–8.
920. Khwarg SG, Feldman S, Ligh J, et al. Exchange transfusion in sickling maculopathy. Retina 1985;5:227–9.
921. Merritt JC, Risco JM, Pantell JP. Bilateral macular infarction in SS disease. J Pediatr Ophthalmol Strabismus 1982;19:275–8.
922. Asdourian GK, Goldberg MF, Rabb MF. Macular infarction in sickle cell B + thalassemia. Retina 1982;2:155–8.
923. Asdourian GK, Nagpal KC, Busse B. Macular and perimacular vascular remodelling in sickling haemoglobinopathies. Br J Ophthalmol 1976;60:431–53.
924. Stevens TS, Busse B, Lee C-B. Sickling hemoglobinopathies; macular and perimacular vascular abnormalities. Arch Ophthalmol 1974;92:455–63.
925. Acacio I, Goldberg MF. Peripapillary and macular vessel occlusions in sickle cell anemia. Am J Ophthalmol 1973;75:861–6.
926. Raichand M, Dizon RV, Nagpal KC. Macular holes associated with proliferative sickle cell retinopathy. Arch Ophthalmol 1978;96:1592–6.
927. Frank RN, Cronin MA. Posterior pole neovascularization in a patient with hemoglobin SC disease. Am J Ophthalmol 1979;88:680–2.
928. Jampol LM, Goldberg MF. Retinal breaks after photocoagulation of proliferative sickle cell retinopathy. Arch Ophthalmol 1980;98:676–9.
929. Bergren RL, Brown GC. Neovascular glaucoma secondary to sickle-cell retinopathy. Am J Ophthalmol 1992;113:718–9.
930. Perlman JI, Forman S, Gonzalez ER. Retrobulbar ischemic optic neuropathy associated with sickle cell disease. J Neuro Ophthalmol 1994;14:45–8.
931. Durant WJ, Jampol LM, Daily M. Exudative retinal detachment in hemoglobin SC disease. Retina 1982;2:152–4.
932. Carney MD, Jampol LM. Epiretinal membranes in sickle cell retinopathy. Arch Ophthalmol 1987;105:214–7.
933. Moriarty BJ, Acheson RW, Serjeant GR. Epiretinal membranes in sickle cell disease. Br J Ophthalmol 1987;71:466–9.
934. Moriarty BJ, Acheson RW, Condon PI, et al. Patterns of visual loss in untreated sickle cell retinopathy. Eye 1988;2:330–5.
935. Moriarty BJ, Webb DK, Serjeant GR. Treatment of subretinal neovascularization associated with angioid streaks in sickle cell retinopathy. Arch Ophthalmol 1987;105:1327–8.
936. Nagpal KC, Asdourian G, Goldbaum M. Angioid streaks and sickle haemoglobinopathies. Br J Ophthalmol 1976;60:31–4.
937. Ober RR, Michels RG. Optic disk neovascularization in hemoglobin SC disease. J Ophthalmol 1978;85:711–4.
938. McLeod DS, Goldberg MF, Lutty GA. Dual-perspective analysis of vascular formations in sickle cell retinopathy. Arch Ophthalmol 1993;111:1234–45.
939. Liang JC, Jampol LM. Spontaneous peripheral chorioretinal neovascularisation in association with sickle cell anaemia. Br J Ophthalmol 1983;67:107–10.
940. Dizon RV, Jampol LM, Goldberg MF, et al. Choroidal occlusive disease in sickle cell hemoglobinopathies. Surv Ophthalmol 1979;23:297–306.
941. Goldbaum MH, Galinos SO, Apple D. Acute choroidal ischemia as a complication of photocoagulation. Arch Ophthalmol 1976;94:1025–35.
942. Galinos SO, Smith TR, Brockhurst RJ. Angioma-like lesion in hemoglobin sickle cell disease. Ann Ophthalmol 1979;11:1549–52.
943. Goldberg MF. The diagnosis and treatment of secondary glaucoma after hyphema in sickle cell patients. Am J Ophthalmol 1979;87:43–9.
944. Radius RL, Finkelstein D. Central retinal artery occlusion (reversible) in sickle trait with glaucoma. Br J Ophthalmol 1976;60:428–30.
945. Wax MB, Ridley ME, Magargal LE. Reversal of retinal and optic disc ischemia in a patient with sickle cell trait and glaucoma secondary to traumatic hyphema. Ophthalmology 1982;89:845–51.
946. Slavin ML, Barondes MJ. Ischemic optic neuropathy in sickle cell disease. Am J Ophthalmol 1988;105:212–3.
947. Goldbaum MH, Jampol LM, Goldberg MF. The disc sign in sickling hemoglobinopathies. Arch Ophthalmol 1978;96:1597–600.
948. Goldbaum MH. Retinal depression sign indicating a small retinal infarct. Am J Ophthalmol 1978;86:45–55.
949. Condon PI, Serjeant GR. Ocular findings in sickle cell-haemoglobin O Arab disease. Br J Ophthalmol 1979;63:839–41.
950. Daneshmend TK. Ocular findings in a case of haemoglobin H disease. Br J Ophthalmol 1979;63:842–4.
951. Gartaganis S, Ismiridis K, Papageorgiou O. Ocular abnormalities in patients with β thalassemia. Am J Ophthalmol 1989;108:699–703.
952. Peachey NS, Charles HC, Lee CM. Electroretinographic findings in sickle cell retinopathy. Arch Ophthalmol 1987;105:934–8.
953. Peachy NS, Gagliano DA, Jacobson MS. Correlation of electroretinographic findings and peripheral retinal nonperfusion in patients with sickle cell retinopathy. Arch Ophthalmol 1990;108:1106–9.
954. Roy MS, Rodgers G, Gunkel R. Color vision defects in sickle cell anemia. Arch Ophthalmol 1987;105:1676–8.
955. van Meurs JC, Schwoerer J, Schwartz B. Retinal vessel autoregulation in sickle cell patients. Graefes Arch Clin Exp Ophthalmol 1992;230:442–5.
956. Nagpal KC, Patrianakos D, Asdourian GK. Spontaneous regression (autoinfarction) of proliferative sickle retinopathy. Am J Ophthalmol 1975;80:885–92.
957. Farber MD, Jampol LM, Fox P. A randomized clinical trial of scatter photocoagulation of proliferative sickle cell retinopathy. Arch Ophthalmol 1991;109:363–7.
958. Jacobson MS, Gagliano DA, Cohen SB. A randomized clinical trial of feeder vessel photocoagulation of sickle cell retinopathy. Ophthalmology 1991;98:581–5.
959. Jampol LM, Condon P, Farber M. A randomized clinical trial of feeder vessel photocoagulation of proliferative sickle cell retinopathy. I. Preliminary results. Ophthalmology 1983;90:540–5.
960. Jampol LM, Farber M, Rabb MF, et al. An update on techniques of photocoagulation treatment of proliferative sickle cell retinopathy. Eye 1991;5:260–3.
961. Kimmel AS, Magargal LE, Stephens RF, et al. Peripheral circumferential retinal scatter photocoagulation for the treatment of proliferative sickle retinopathy; an update. Ophthalmology 1986;93:1429–34.
962. Rednam KRV, Jampol LM, Goldberg MF. Scatter retinal photocoagulation for proliferative sickle cell retinopathy. Am J Ophthalmol 1982;93:594–9.
963. Dizon-Moore RV, Jampol LM, Goldberg MF. Chorioretinal and choriovitreal neovascularization; their presence after photocoagulation of proliferative sickle cell retinopathy. Arch Ophthalmol 1981;99:842–9.
964. Fox PD, Acheson RW, Serjeant GR. Outcome of iatrogenic choroidal neovascularisation in sickle cell disease. Br J Ophthalmol 1990;74:417–20.
965. Acheson RW, Fox PD, Chuang EL, et al. Treatment of iatrogenic choriovitreal neovascularization in sickle cell disease. Br J Ophthalmol 1991;75:729–30.
966. Carney MD, Paylor RR, Cunha-Vaz JG. Iatrogenic choroidal neovascularization in sickle cell retinopathy. Ophthalmology 1986;93:1163–8.
967. Condon PI, Jampol LM, Ford SM, et al. Choroidal neovascularisation induced by photocoagulation in sickle cell disease. Br J Ophthalmol 1981;65:192–7.
968. Hrisomalos NF, Jampol LM, Moriarty BJ. Neodymium-YAG laser vitreolysis in sickle cell retinopathy. Arch Ophthalmol 1987;105:1087–91.
969. Jampol LM, Green Jr JL, Goldberg MF, et al. An update on vitrectomy surgery and retinal detachment repair in sickle cell disease. Arch Ophthalmol 1982;100:591–3.
970. Pulido JS, Flynn Jr HW, Clarkson JG, et al. Pars plana vitrectomy in the management of complications of proliferative sickle retinopathy. Arch Ophthalmol 1988;106:1553–7.
971. Weissman H, Nadel AJ, Dunn M. Simultaneous bilateral retinal arterial occlusions treated by exchange transfusions. Arch Ophthalmol 1979;97:2151–3.
972. Goldbaum MH. Retinal depression sign indicating a small retinal infarct. Am J Ophthalmol 1978;86:45–55.
973. Lima CS, Rocha EM, Silva NM, et al. Risk factors for conjunctival and retinal vessel alterations in sickle cell disease. Acta Ophthalmol Scand 2006;84:234–41.
974. Bigar F, Witmer R. Progrediente aneurysmatische retinale Arteriopathie. Fortschr Ophthalmol 1983;79:488–91.
975. Boase DL, Gale RE, Huehns ER. Oxygen dissociation curve in Eales's disease. Br J Ophthalmol 1980;64:745–50.
976. Eales H. Primary retinal haemorrhage in young men. Ophthalmic Rev 1882;1:41–6.

1137. Johnson CA, Hatfield M, Pulido JS. Retinal vasculopathy in a family with autosomal dominant dyskeratosis congenita. Ophthalmic Genet 2009;30:181–4.
1138. Bessler M, Wilson DB, Mason PJ. Dyskeratosis congenita. FEBS Lett 2010 Sep 10;584: 3831–8.
1139. Mason PJ, Wilson DB, Bessler M. Dyskeratosis congenita – a disease of dysfunctional telomere maintenance. Curr Mol Med 2005;5:159–70.
1140. Blinder KJ, Khan JA, Giangiacomo J, et al. Optociliary veins and visual prognosis after central retinal vein occlusion. Ann Ophthalmol 1989;21:192–7.
1141. Fujino T, Curtin VT, Norton EWD. Experimental central retinal vein occlusion; a comparison of intraocular and extraocular occlusion. Arch Ophthalmol 1969;81:395–406.
1142. Hamilton AM, Kohner EM, Rosen D, et al. Experimental venous occlusion. Proc R Soc Med 1974;67:1045–8.
1143. Hamilton AM, Kohner EM, Rosen D, et al. Experimental retinal branch vein occlusion in rhesus monkeys. I. Clinical appearances. Br J Ophthalmol 1979;63:377–87.
1144. Hayreh SS. Discussion: an experimental study of the central retinal vein occlusion. Trans Ophthalmol Soc UK 1964;84:586–93.
1145. Hayreh SS, van Heuven WAJ, Hayreh MS. Experimental retinal vascular occlusion. I. Pathogenesis of central retinal vein occlusion. Arch Ophthalmol 1978;96:311–23.
1146. Hockley DJ, Tripathi RC, Ashton N. Experimental retinal branch vein occlusion in the monkey; histopathological and ultrastructural studies. Trans Ophthalmol Soc UK 1976;96:202–9.
1147. Hockley DJ, Tripathi RC, Ashton N. Experimental retinal branch vein occlusion in rhesus monkeys. III. Histopathological and electron microscopical studies. Br J Ophthalmol 1979;63:393–411.
1148. Kohner EM, Dollery CT, Shakib M, et al. Experimental retinal branch vein occlusion. Am J Ophthalmol 1970;69:778–825.
1149. Rubinstein K. Arterial insufficiency in retinal venous occlusion (a short symposium). Trans Ophthalmol Soc UK 1964;84:564–81.
1150. Keyser BJ, Flaharty PM, Sergott RC, et al. Color Doppler imaging of arterial blood flow in central retinal vein occlusion. Ophthalmology 1994;101:1357–61.
1151. Williamson TH, Baxter GM. Central retinal vein occlusion, an investigation by color Doppler imaging; blood velocity characteristics and prediction of iris neovascularization. Ophthalmology 1994;101:1362–72.
1152. Gass JDM. A fluorescein angiographic study of macular dysfunction secondary to retinal vascular disease. II. Retinal vein obstruction. Arch Ophthalmol 1968;80:550–68.
1153. Gass JDM. Stereoscopic atlas of macular diseases; diagnosis and treatment, 2nd ed. St. Louis: CV Mosby; 1977. p. 282.
1154. Gutman FA. Evaluation of a patient with central retinal vein occlusion. Ophthalmology 1983;90:481–3.
1155. Hayreh SS. So-called "central retinal vein occlusion." I. Pathogenesis, terminology, clinical features. Ophthalmologica 1976;172:1–13.
1156. Hayreh SS. Classification of central retinal vein occlusion. Ophthalmology 1983;90:458–74.
1157. Hayreh SS, Zimmerman MB, Podhajsky P. Incidence of various types of retinal vein occlusion and their recurrence and demographic characteristics. Am J Ophthalmol 1994;117:429–41.
1158. Hill DW, Griffiths JD. The prognosis in retinal vein thrombosis. Trans Ophthalmol Soc UK 1970;90:309–22.
1159. Joffe L, Goldberg RE, Magargal LE, et al. Macular branch vein occlusion. Ophthalmology 1980;87:91–8.
1160. Kohner EM, Laatikainen L, Oughton J. The management of central retinal vein occlusion. Ophthalmology 1983;90:484–7.
1161. Laatikainen L, Kohner EM. Fluorescein angiography and its prognostic significance in central retinal vein occlusion. Br J Ophthalmol 1976;60:411–8.
1162. McAllister IL, Constable IJ. Laser-induced chorioretinal venous anastomosis for treatment of nonischemic central retinal vein occlusion. Arch Ophthalmol 1995;113:456–62.
1163. McLeod D, Kohner EM. Hemorrhages after central retinal vein occlusion. Arch Ophthalmol 1978;96:1921.
1164. Priluck IA, Robertson DM, Hollenhorst RW. Long-term follow-up of occlusion of the central retinal vein in young adults. Am J Ophthalmol 1980;90:190–202.
1165. Smith VH. Arterial insufficiency in retinal venous occlusion (a short symposium). Trans Ophthalmol Soc UK 1964;84:581–6.
1166. Zegarra H, Gutman FA, Zakov N, et al. Partial occlusion of the central retinal vein. Am J Ophthalmol 1983;96:330–7.
1167. Kearns TP. Differential diagnosis of central retinal vein obstruction. Ophthalmology 1983;90:475–80.
1168. Reyes ME, Barr CC, Gamel JW. Blood levels in macular cystoid spaces and their relationship to retinal vein obstruction. Retina 1994;14:14–18.
1169. Foss AJE, Headon MP, Hamilton AM, et al. Transient vessel wall sheathing in acute retinal vein occlusions. Eye 1992;6:313–6.
1170. Hayreh SS, March W, Phelps CD. Ocular hypotony following retinal vein occlusion. Arch Ophthalmol 1978;96:827–33.
1171. Sabates R, Hirose T, McMeel JW. Electroretinography in the prognosis and classification of central retinal vein occlusion. Arch Ophthalmol 1983;101:232–5.
1172. Minturn J, Brown GC. Progression of nonischemic central retinal vein obstruction to the ischemic variant. Ophthalmology 1986;93:1158–62.
1173. Welch JC, Augsburger JJ. Assessment of angiographic retinal capillary nonperfusion in central retinal vein occlusion. Am J Ophthalmol 1987;103:761–6.
1174. Hayreh SS, Klugman MR, Beri M, et al. Differentiation of ischemic from non-ischemic central retinal vein occlusion during the early acute phase. Graefes Arch Clin Exp Ophthalmol 1990;228:201–17.
1175. Servais GE, Thompson HS, Hayreh SS. Relative afferent pupillary defect in central retinal vein occlusion. Ophthalmology 1986;93:301–3.
1176. Grey RHB, Bloom PA. Retinal ischaemia and relative afferent pupil defects in central retinal vein occlusion. Eur J Ophthalmol 1991;1:85–8.
1177. Hayreh SS, Klugman MR, Podhajsky P, et al. Electroretinography in central retinal vein occlusion; correlation of electroretinographic changes with pupillary abnormalities. Graefes Arch Clin Exp Ophthalmol 1989;227:549–61.
1178. Johnson MA, McPhee TJ. Electroretinographic findings in iris neovascularization due to acute central retinal vein occlusion. Arch Ophthalmol 1993;111:806–14.
1179. Grant WM. Shallowing of the anterior chamber following occlusion of the central retinal vein. Am J Ophthalmol 1973;75:384–9.
1180. Hyams SW, Neumann E. Transient angle-closure glaucoma after retinal vein occlusion. Br J Ophthalmol 1972;56:353–5.
1181. Weber PA, Cohen JS, Baker ND. Central retinal vein occlusion and malignant glaucoma. Arch Ophthalmol 1987;105:635–6.
1182. Ravalico G, Parodi MB. Exudative retinal detachment subsequent to retinal vein occlusion. Ophthalmologica 1992;205:77–82.
1183. Weinberg D, Jampol LM, Schatz H, et al. Exudative retinal detachment following central and hemicentral retinal vein occlusions. Arch Ophthalmol 1990;108:271–5.
1184. Quinlan PM, Elman MJ, Bhatt AK, et al. The natural course of central retinal vein occlusion. Am J Ophthalmol 1990;110:118–23.
1185. Walters RF, Spalton DJ. Central retinal vein occlusion in people aged 40 years or less: a review of 17 patients. Br J Ophthalmol 1990;74:30–5.
1186. Zegarra H, Gutman FA, Conforto J. The natural course of central retinal vein occlusion. Ophthalmology 1979;86:1931–9.
1187. Chan C-C, Little HL. Infrequency of retinal neovascularization following central retinal vein occlusion. Ophthalmology 1979;86:256–62.
1188. Hayreh SS, Rojas P, Podhajsky P, et al. Ocular neovascularization with retinal vascular occlusion. III. Incidence of ocular neovascularization with retinal vein occlusion. Ophthalmology 1983;90:488–506.
1189. Magargal LE, Brown GC, Augsburger JJ, et al. Neovascular glaucoma following central retinal vein obstruction. Ophthalmology 1981;88:1095–101.
1190. Sinclair SH, Gragoudas ES. Prognosis for rubeosis iridis following central retinal vein occlusion. Br J Ophthalmol 1979;63:735–43.
1191. Akiba J, Kado M, Kakehashi A, et al. Role of the vitreous in posterior segment neovascularization in central retinal vein occlusion. Ophthalmic Surg 1991;22:498–502.
1192. Pollack A, Dottan S, Oliver M. The fellow eye in retinal vein occlusive disease. Ophthalmology 1989;96:842–5.
1193. D'Amato RJ, Miller NR, Fine SL, et al. The effect of age and initial visual acuity on the systemic and visual prognosis of central retinal vein occlusion. Aust NZ J Ophthalmol 1991;19:119–22.
1194. Rubinstein K, Jones EB. Retinal vein occlusion: long-term prospects; ten years' follow-up of 143 patients. Br J Ophthalmol 1976;60:148–50.
1195. Humayun M, Kattah J, Cupps TR, et al. Papillophlebitis and arteriolar occlusion in a pregnant woman. J Clin Neuro-Ophthalmol 1992;12:226–9.
1196. Lyle TK, Wybar K. Retinal vasculitis. Br J Ophthalmol 1961;45:778–88.
1197. Winterkorn JMS, Odel JG, Behrens MM, et al. Large optic nerve with central retinal artery and vein occlusions from optic neuritis/perineuritis rather than tumor. J Clin Neuro-Ophthalmol 1994;14:157–9.
1198. Duker JS, Sergott RC, Savino PJ, et al. Optic neuritis with secondary retinal venous stasis. Ophthalmology 1989;96:475–80.
1199. Keyser BJ, Hass AN. Retinal vascular disease in ulcerative colitis. Am J Ophthalmol 1994;118:395–6.
1200. Fong ACO, Schatz H, McDonald HR, et al. Central retinal vein occlusion in young adults (papillophlebitis). Retina 1991;11:3–11.
1201. Green WR, Chan CC, Hutchins GM, et al. Central retinal vein occlusion: a prospective histopathologic study of 29 eyes in 28 cases. Retina 1981;1:27–55.
1202. Appiah AP, Greenidge KC. Factors associated with retinal-vein occlusion in Hispanics. Ann Ophthalmol 1987;19:307–12.
1203. Appiah AP, Trempe CL. Risk factors associated with branch vs. central retinal vein occlusion. Ann Ophthalmol 1989;21:153–7.
1204. Brunette I, Boghen D. Central retinal vein occlusion complicating spontaneous carotid-cavernous fistula. Arch Ophthalmol 1987;105:464–5.
1205. Elman MJ, Bhatt AK, Quinlan PM, et al. The risk for systemic vascular diseases and mortality in patients with central retinal vein occlusion. Ophthalmology 1990;97:1543–8.
1206. Gilmer G, Swartz M, Teske M, et al. Over-the-counter phenylpropanolamine: a possible cause of central retinal vein occlusion. Arch Ophthalmol 1986;104:642.
1207. Glacet-Bernard A, Chabanel A, Coscas G, et al. Elévation de l'agrégation érythrocytaire au cours des occlusions veineuses rétiniennes. J Fr Ophtalmol 1990;13:500–5.
1208. Hitchings RA, Spaeth GL. Chronic retinal vein occlusion in glaucoma. Br J Ophthalmol 1976;60:694–9.
1209. Jørgensen JS, Guthoff R. Ophthalmoscopic findings in spontaneous carotid cavernous fistula: an analysis of 20 patients. Graefes Arch Clin Exp Ophthalmol 1988;226:34–6.
1210. Kohner EM, Cappin JM. Do medical conditions have an influence on central retinal vein occlusion? Proc R Soc Med 1974;67:1052–4.
1211. Krüger K, Anger V, Haas D. Der Thrombin-Anti-thrombin-III-Komplex; Ursache bei venösen Gefässverschlüssen der Netzhaut. Ophthalmologe 1992;89:67–70.
1212. Mansour AM, Walsh JB, Goldberger S, et al. Role of diabetes mellitus on the natural history of central retinal vein occlusion. Ophthalmologica 1992;204:57–62.
1213. McGrath MA, Wechsler F, Hunyor ABL, et al. Systemic factors contributory to retinal vein occlusion. Arch Intern Med 1978;138:216–20.
1214. Rath EZ, Frank RN, Shin DH, et al. Risk factors for retinal vein occlusions; a case-control study. Ophthalmology 1992;99:509–14.
1215. Ross Russell RW, Ikeda H. Clinical and electrophysiological observations in patients with low pressure retinopathy. Br J Ophthalmol 1986;70:651–6.
1216. Schmidt D, Schumacher M. Zentralvenenverschluss als Folge von spontanen arteriovenösen Fisteln der Arteria carotis zum Sinus cavernosus. Fortsch Ophthalmol 1991;88:683–6.

1217. Slamovits TL, Klingele TG, Burde RM, et al. Moyamoya disease with central retinal vein occlusion; case report. J Clin Neuro-Ophthalmol 1981;1:123–7.
1218. Smith P, Green WR, Miller NR, et al. Central retinal vein occlusion in Reye's syndrome. Arch Ophthalmol 1980;98:1256–60.
1219. Snir M, Axer-Siegel R, Buckman G, et al. Central venous stasis retinopathy following the use of tranexamic acid. Retina 1990;10:181–4.
1220. Stowe III GC, Zakov ZN, Albert DM. Central retinal vascular occlusion associated with oral contraceptives. Am J Ophthalmol 1978;86:798–801.
1221. Mansour AM, Walsh JB, Henkind P. Mortality and morbidity in patients with central retinal vein occlusion. Ophthalmologica 1992;204:199–203.
1222. Chern S, Magargal LE, Annesley WH. Central retinal vein occlusion associated with drusen of the optic disc. Ann Ophthalmol 1991;23:66–9.
1223. Chern S, Magargal LE, Brav SS. Bilateral central retinal vein occlusion as an initial manifestation of pseudotumor cerebri. Ann Ophthalmol 1991;23:54–7.
1224. Kline LB, Kirkham TH, Belanger G, et al. Traumatic central retinal vein occlusion. Ann Ophthalmol 1978;10:587–91.
1225. Noble MJ, Alvarez EV. Combined occlusion of the central retinal artery and central retinal vein following blunt ocular trauma: a case report. Br J Ophthalmol 1987;71:834–6.
1226. Ring CP, Pearson TC, Sanders MD, et al. Viscosity and retinal vein thrombosis. Br J Ophthalmol 1976;60:397–410.
1227. Trope GE, Lowe GDO, McArdle BM, et al. Abnormal blood viscosity and haemostasis in long-standing retinal vein occlusion. Br J Ophthalmol 1983;67:137–42.
1228. Wolf S, Arend O, Bertram B, et al. Hemodilution therapy in central retinal vein occlusion; one-year results of a prospective randomized study. Graefes Arch Clin Exp Ophthalmol 1994;232:33–9.
1229. Glacet-Bernard A, Chabanel A, Lelong F, et al. Elevated erythrocyte aggregation in patients with central retinal vein occlusion and without conventional risk factors. Ophthalmology 1994;101:1483–7.
1230. Brown GC. Central retinal vein obstruction with lipid exudate. Arch Ophthalmol 1989;107:1001–5.
1231. Dodson PM, Galton DJ, Hamilton AM, et al. Retinal vein occlusion and the prevalence of lipoprotein abnormalities. Br J Ophthalmol 1982;66:161–4.
1232. Dodson PM, Westwick J, Marks G, et al. β-Thromboglobulin and platelet factor 4 levels in retinal vein occlusion. Br J Ophthalmol 1983;67:143–6.
1233. Cole MD, Dodson PM, Hendeles S. Medical conditions underlying retinal vein occlusion in patients with glaucoma or ocular hypertension. Br J Ophthalmol 1989;73:693–8.
1234. Gusek GC, Jonas JB, Naumann GO. Retinale Gefässverschlüsse sind unabhängig von der Papillengrösse; Eine morphometrische Untersuchung von 140 Patienten. Klin Monatsbl Augenheilkd 1990;197:14–17.
1235. Mansour AM, Walsh JB, Henkind P. Optic disc size in central retinal vein occlusion. Ophthalmology 1990;97:165–6.
1236. Strahlman ER, Quinlan PM, Enger C, et al. The cup-to-disc ratio and central retinal vein occlusion. Arch Ophthalmol 1989;107:524–5.
1237. Giuffrè G. Tilted discs and central retinal vein occlusion. Graefes Arch Clin Exp Ophthalmol 1993;231:41–2.
1238. Hayreh SS, Zimmerman MB, Podhajsky P. Seasonal variations in the onset of retinal vein occlusion. Br J Ophthalmol 1992;76:706–10.
1239. Lavin MJ, Dhillon BJ. Cyclic variation in onset of central retinal vein occlusion. Br J Ophthalmol 1987;71:18–20.
1240. Glacet-Bernard A, Coscos G, Chabanel A, et al. A randomized, double-masked study on the treatment of retinal vein occlusion with troxerutin. Am J Ophthalmol 1994;118:421–9.
1241. Hansen LL, Wiek J, Wiederhold MA. Randomised prospective study of treatment of non-ischaemic central retinal vein occlusion by isovolaemic haemodilution. Br J Ophthalmol 1989;73:895–9.
1242. Kohner EM, Pettit JE, Hamilton AM, et al. Streptokinase in central retinal vein occlusion: a controlled clinical trial. Br Med J 1976;1:550–3.
1243. Central Vein Occlusion Study Group. A randomized clinical trial of early panretinal photocoagulation for ischemic central vein occlusion. The Central Vein Occlusion Study Group N Report. Ophthalmology 1995;102:1434–44.
1244. Central Vein Occlusion Study Group. Baseline and early natural history report. The Central Vein Occlusion Study. Arch Ophthalmol 1993;111:1087–95.
1245. Central Vein Occlusion Study Group. Evaluation of grid pattern photocoagulation for macular edema in central vein occlusion. The Central Vein Occlusion Study Group M Report. Ophthalmology 1995;102:1425–33.
1246. Clarkson JG. Photocoagulation for ischemic central retinal vein occlusion; Central Vein Occlusion Study. Arch Ophthalmol 1991;109:1218–9.
1247. Klein ML, Finkelstein D. Macular grid photocoagulation for macular edema in central retinal vein occlusion. Arch Ophthalmol 1989;107:1297–302.
1248. Ip MS, Scott IU, VanVeldhuisen PC, et al. A randomized trial comparing the efficacy and safety of intravitreal triamcinolone with observation to treat vision loss associated with macular edema secondary to central retinal vein occlusion: the Standard Care vs Corticosteroid for Retinal Vein Occlusion (SCORE) study report 5. Arch Ophthalmol 2009;127:1101–14.
1249. Wolf-Schnurrbusch UE, Ghanem R, Rothenbuehler SP, et al. Predictors for short term visual outcome after anti-VEGF therapy of macular edema due to central retinal vein occlusion. Invest Ophthalmol Vis Sci 2010 Nov;18.
1250. Kinge B, Stordahl PB, Forsaa V, et al. Efficacy of ranibizumab in patients with macular edema secondary to central retinal vein occlusion: results from the sham-controlled ROCC study. Am J Ophthalmol 2010;150:310–4.
1251. Cinal A, Ziemssen F, Bartz-Schmidt KU, et al. Intravitreal bevacizumab for treatment of serous macular detachment in central retinal vein occlusion. Graefes Arch Clin Exp Ophthalmol 2010 Nov;4.
1252. Vasco-Posada J. Modification of the circulation in the posterior pole of the eye. Ann Ophthalmol 1972;4:48–59.
1253. McAllister IL, Yu D-Y, Vijayasekaran S, et al. Induced chorioretinal venous anastomosis in experimental retinal branch vein occlusion. Br J Ophthalmol 1992;76:615–20.
1254. McAllister IL, Gillies ME, Smithies LA, et al. The Central Retinal Vein Bypass Study: a trial of laser-induced chorioretinal venous anastomosis for central retinal vein occlusion. Ophthalmology 2010;117:954–65.
1255. Branch Vein Occlusion Study Group. Argon laser photocoagulation for macular edema in branch vein occlusion. Am J Ophthalmol 1984;98:271–82.
1256. Branch Vein Occlusion Study Group. Argon laser scatter photocoagulation for prevention of neovascularization and vitreous hemorrhage in branch vein occlusion; a randomized clinical trial. Arch Ophthalmol 1986;104:34–41.
1257. Archer DB. Natural course of branch retinal vein obstruction. Trans Ophthalmol Soc UK 1974;94:623–35.
1258. Archer DB, Ernest JT, Newell FW. Classification of branch retinal vein obstruction. Trans Am Acad Ophthalmol Otolaryngol 1974;78:OP148–OP165.
1259. Birchall CH, Harris GS, Drance SM, et al. Visual field changes in branch retinal 'vein' occlusion. Arch Ophthalmol 1976;94:747–54.
1260. Blankenship GW, Okun E. Retinal tributary vein occlusion; history and management by photocoagulation. Arch Ophthalmol 1973;89:363–8.
1261. Clemett RS. Retinal branch vein occlusion; changes at the site of obstruction. Br J Ophthalmol 1974;58:548–54.
1262. Clemett RS, Kohner EM, Hamilton AM. The visual prognosis in retinal branch vein occlusion. Trans Ophthalmol Soc UK 1973;93:523–35.
1263. Gass JDM. Stereoscopic atlas of macular diseases; diagnosis and treatment, 3rd ed. St. Louis: CV Mosby; 1987. p. 428–34.
1264. Gutman FA. Macular edema in branch retinal vein occlusion: prognosis and management. Trans Am Acad Ophthalmol Otolaryngol 1977;83:OP488–OP493.
1265. Gutman FA, Zegarra H. The natural course of temporal retinal branch vein occlusion. Trans Am Acad Ophthalmol Otolaryngol 1974;78:OP178–OP192.
1266. Henkind P, Wise GN. Retinal neovascularization, collaterals, and vascular shunts. Br J Ophthalmol 1974;58:413–22.
1267. Joondeph HC, Goldberg MF. Rhegmatogenous retinal detachment after tributary retinal vein occlusion. Am J Ophthalmol 1975;80:253–7.
1268. Lang GE, Freissler K. Klinische und fluoreszenzangiographische Befunde bei Patienten mit retinalen Venenastverschlüssen; Eine unizentrische Studie über 211 Patienten. Klin Monatsbl Augenheilkd 1992;201:234–9.
1269. Rosen J, Tanenbaum HL. Venous shunting and macular edema. Can J Ophthalmol 1973;8:349–52.
1270. Shilling JS, Kohner EM. New vessel formation in retinal branch vein occlusion. Br J Ophthalmol 1976;60:810–5.
1271. Takeda M, Tanabe H, Kimura S, et al. Fluorescein angiographic analysis of late changes after retinal branch vein occlusion. Jpn J Clin Ophthalmol 1980;34:309–20.
1272. Frangieh GT, Green WR, Barraquer-Somers E, et al. Histopathologic study of nine branch retinal vein occlusions. Arch Ophthalmol 1982;100:1132–40.
1273. Duker JS, Brown GC. Anterior location of the crossing artery in branch retinal vein obstruction. Arch Ophthalmol 1989;107:998–1000.
1274. Feist RM, Ticho BH, Shapiro MJ, et al. Branch retinal vein occlusion and quadratic variation in arteriovenous crossings. Am J Ophthalmol 1992;113:664–8.
1275. Michels RG, Gass JDM. The natural course of retinal branch vein obstruction. Trans Am Acad Ophthalmol Otolaryngol 1974;78:OP166–OP177.
1276. Sekimoto M, Hayasaka S, Setogawa T. Type of arteriovenous crossing at site of branch retinal vein occlusion. Jpn J Ophthalmol 1992;36:192–6.
1277. Weinberg D, Dodwell DG, Fern SA. Anatomy of arteriovenous crossings in branch retinal vein occlusion. Am J Ophthalmol 1990;109:298–302.
1278. Weinberg DV, Egan KM, Seddon JM. Asymmetric distribution of arteriovenous crossings in the normal retina. Ophthalmology 1993;100:31–6.
1279. Zhao J, Sastry SM, Sperduto RD, et al. Arteriovenous crossing patterns in branch retinal vein occlusion. Ophthalmology 1993;100:423–8.
1280. Gutman FA, Zegarra H. Retinal detachment secondary to retinal branch vein occlusions. Trans Am Acad Ophthalmol Otolaryngol 1976;81:OP491–OP496.
1281. Serop S, De Laey JJ. Décollement séreux de la rétine, secondaire à l'occlusion veineuse rétinienne. Bull Soc Belge Ophtalmol 1991;241:113–9.
1282. Schatz H, Yannuzzi L, Stransky TJ. Retinal detachment secondary to branch vein occlusion: parts I and II. Ann Ophthalmol 1976;8:1437–52. 61–71
1283. Cousins SW, Flynn Jr HW, Clarkson JG. Macroaneurysms associated with retinal branch vein occlusion. Am J Ophthalmol 1990;109:567–70.
1284. Magargal LE, Augsburger JJ, Hyman D, et al. Venous macroaneurysm following branch retinal vein obstruction. Ann Ophthalmol 1980;12:685–8.
1285. Sanborn GE, Magargal LE. Venous macroaneurysm associated with branch retinal vein obstruction. Ann Ophthalmol 1984;16:464–8.
1286. Schulman J, Jampol LM, Goldberg MF. Large capillary aneurysms secondary to retinal venous obstruction. Br J Ophthalmol 1981;65:36–41.
1287. Takeda M, Kimura S. Large capillary aneurysms secondary to retina branch vein occlusion. Jpn J Clin Ophthalmol 1982;36:315–22.
1288. Finkelstein D. Ischemic macular edema; recognition and favorable natural history in branch vein occlusion. Arch Ophthalmol 1992;110:1427–34.
1289. Finkelstein D, Clarkson J, Diddie K, et al. Branch vein occlusion; retinal neovascularization outside the involved segment. Ophthalmology 1982;89:1357–61.
1290. Pournaras CJ, Tsacopoulos M, Strommer K, et al. Scatter photocoagulation restores tissue hypoxia in experimental vasoproliferative microangiopathy in miniature pigs. Ophthalmology 1990;97:1329–33.

1291. Kado M, Hirokawa H, Yoshida A. Role of the vitreous in retinal neovascularization evaluated by a comparison of central retinal vein occlusion and branch retinal vein occlusion. Acta Soc Ophthalmol Jpn 1989;93:812–6.
1292. Kado M, Trempe CL. Role of the vitreous in branch retinal vein occlusion. Am J Ophthalmol 1988;105:20–4.
1293. Trempe CL, Takahashi M, Topilow HW. Vitreous changes in retinal branch vein occlusion. Ophthalmology 1981;88:681–7.
1294. Joondeph HC, Joondepth BC. Posterior tractional retinal breaks complicating branch retinal vein occlusion. Retina 1988;8:136–40.
1295. Murakami K, Ho PC, Trempe CL, et al. Tractional detachment of the macula following branch retinal vein occlusion. Ann Ophthalmol 1983;15:760–5.
1296. Regenbogen L, Godel V, Feiler-Ofry V, et al. Retinal breaks secondary to vascular accidents. Am J Ophthalmol 1977;84:187–96.
1297. Ernest JT, Stern WH. Internal limiting membrane detachment in branch retinal vein obstruction. Am J Ophthalmol 1974;78:324–6.
1298. Cohen G. Rhegmatogenous retinal detachment secondary to branch retinal vein occlusion; a case report. Retina 1981;1:186–9.
1299. Richmond PP, Orth DH. Branch retinal vein occlusion associated with optic nerve drusen; a case report. Ophthalmic Surg 1989;20:38–41.
1300. Denis P, Nordmann J-P, Laroche L, et al. Branch retinal vein occlusion associated with a sarcoid choroidal granuloma. Am J Ophthalmol 1992;113:333–4.
1301. Miller SA, Bresnick GH. Retinal branch vessel occlusion in acute intermittent porphyria. Ann Ophthalmol 1979;11:1379–83.
1302. Bowers DK, Finkelstein D, Wolff SM, et al. Branch retinal vein occlusion; a clinicopathologic case report. Retina 1987;7:252–9.
1303. Danis RP, Wallow IHL. Microvascular changes in experimental branch retinal vein occlusion. Ophthalmology 1987;94:1213–21.
1304. de Juan Jr E, Stefánsson E, Dickson JS. Capillary endothelial-cell mitogenic activity in experimental branch vein occlusion. Graefes Arch Clin Exp Ophthalmol 1990;228:191–4.
1305. Rosen DA, Marshall J, Kohner EM, et al. Experimental retinal branch vein occlusion in rhesus monkeys. II. Retinal blood flow studies. Br J Ophthalmol 1979;63:388–92.
1306. Wallow IHL, Danis RP, Bindley C, et al. Cystoid macular degeneration in experimental branch retinal vein occlusion. Ophthalmology 1988;95:1371–9.
1307. Cairns JD. Photocoagulation in the treatment of retinal branch vein occlusion. Aust J Ophthalmol 1974;2:5–9.
1308. Cox MS, Whitmore PV, Gutow RF. Treatment of intravitreal and prepapillary neovascularization following branch retinal vein occlusion. Trans Am Acad Ophthalmol Otolaryngol 1975;79:0P387–0P393.
1309. Finkelstein D. Argon laser photocoagulation for macular edema in branch vein occlusion. Ophthalmology 1986;93:975–7.
1310. Flindall RJ. Photocoagulation in chronic cystoid macular oedema secondary to branch vein occlusion. Can J Ophthalmol 1972;7:395–404.
1311. Gitter KA, Cohen G, Baber BW. Photocoagulation in venous occlusive disease. Am J Ophthalmol 1975;79:578–81.
1312. Kelley JS, Patz A, Schatz H. Management of retinal branch vein occlusion: the role of argon laser photocoagulation. Ann Ophthalmol 1974;6:1123–34.
1313. Krill AE, Archer D, Newell FW. Photocoagulation in complications secondary to branch vein occlusion. Arch Ophthalmol 1971;85:48–60.
1314. Laatikainen L. Photocoagulation in retinal venous occlusion. Acta Ophthalmol 1977;55: 478–88.
1315. Wetzig PC. The treatment of acute branch vein occlusion by photocoagulation. Am J Ophthalmol 1979;87:65–73.
1316. Oncel M, Peyman GA, Khoobehi B. Tissue plasminogen activator in the treatment of experimental retinal vein occlusion. Retina 1989;9:1–7.
1317. Osterloh MD, Charles S. Surgical decompression of branch retinal vein occlusions. Arch Ophthalmol 1988;106:1469–71.
1318. Pollock S, Miller NR. Central retinal vein occlusion complicating spontaneous carotid-cavernous fistula. Arch Ophthalmol 1986;104:331.
1319. Fechtner RD, Minckler D, Weinreb RN, et al. Complications of glaucoma surgery; ocular decompression retinopathy. Arch Ophthalmol 1992;110:965–8.
1320. Vijayasekaran S, McAllister IL, Morgan WH, et al. Intravitreal triamcinolone acetonide induced changes in the anterior segment in a pig model of branch retinal vein occlusion. Graefes Arch Clin Exp Ophthalmol 2010;249:215–22.
1321. Rouvas A, Petrou P, Ntouraki A, et al. Intravitreal ranibizumab (Lucentis) for branch retinal vein occlusion-induced macular edema: nine-month results of a prospective study. Retina 2010;30:893–902.
1322. Parveen S, Narayanan R, Sambhav K, et al. Bevacizumab compared with macular laser grid photocoagulation for cystoid macular edema in branch retinal vein occlusion. Retina 2010;30:1324–5.
1323. Campochiaro PA, Hafiz G, Shah SM, et al. Sustained ocular delivery of fluocinolone acetonide by an intravitreal insert. Ophthalmology 2010;117(1393–1399):e3.
1324. Scott IU, Ip MS, VanVeldhuisen PC, et al. A randomized trial comparing the efficacy and safety of intravitreal triamcinolone with standard care to treat vision loss associated with macular Edema secondary to branch retinal vein occlusion: the Standard Care vs Corticosteroid for Retinal Vein Occlusion (SCORE) study report 6. Arch Ophthalmol 2009;127:1115–28.
1325. Russo V, Barone A, Conte E, et al. Bevacizumab compared with macular laser grid photocoagulation for cystoid macular edema in branch retinal vein occlusion. Retina 2009;29:511–5.
1326. Hayreh SS, Hayreh MS. Hemi-central retinal vein occlusion; pathogenesis, clinical features, and natural history. Arch Ophthalmol 1980;98:1600–9.
1327. Appiah AP, Trempe CL. Differences in contributory factors among hemicentral, central, and branch retinal occlusions. Ophthalmology 1989;96:364–6.
1328. Chopdar A. Hemi-central retinal vein occlusion; pathogenesis, clinical features, natural history and incidence of dual trunk central retinal vein. Trans Ophthalmol Soc UK 1982;102:241–8.
1329. Chopdar A. Dual trunk central retinal vein incidence in clinical practice. Arch Ophthalmol 1984;102:85–7.
1330. Brod RD, Shields JA, Shields CL, et al. Unusual retinal and renal vascular lesions in the Klippel-Trenaunay-Weber syndrome. Retina 1992;12:355–8.
1331. Aisen ML, Bacon BR, Goodman AM, et al. Retinal abnormalities associated with anemia. Arch Ophthalmol 1983;101:1049–52.
1332. Holt JM, Gordon-Smith EC. Retinal abnormalities in diseases of the blood. Br J Ophthalmol 1969;53:145–60.
1333. Golnik KC, Newman SA. Anterior ischemic optic neuropathy associated with macrocytic anemia. J Clin Neuro-Ophthalmol 1990;10:244–7.
1334. Klewin KM, Appen RE, Kaufman PL. Amaurosis and blood loss. Am J Ophthalmol 1978;86:669–72.
1335. Yap E-Y, Gleaton MS, Buettner H. Visual loss associated with pseudoxanthoma elasticum. Retina 1992;12:315–9.
1336. Vargiami E, Zafeiriou DI, Gombakis NP, et al. Hemolytic anemia presenting with idiopathic intracranial hypertension. Pediatr Neurol 2008;38:53–4.
1337. Biousse V, Rucker JC, Vignal C, et al. Anemia and papilledema. Am J Ophthalmol 2003;135:437–46.
1338. Taylor HR, Tikellis G, Robman LD, et al. Vitamin E supplementation and macular degeneration: randomised controlled trial. BMJ 2002;325:11.
1339. Singh R, Gupta V, Gupta A, et al. Spontaneous closure of microaneurysms in diabetic retinopathy with treatment of co-existing anaemia. Br J Ophthalmol 2005;89:248–9.
1340. Foster RM. The incidence of retinal haemorrhages in severe anaemia. Trans R Soc Trop Med Hyg 1970;64:99–101.
1341. Mansour AM. Aplastic anemia simulating central retinal vein occlusion. Am J Ophthalmol 1985;100:478–9.
1342. Merin S, Freund M. Retinopathy in severe anemia. Am J Ophthalmol 1968;66:1102–6.
1343. Rubenstein RA, Yanoff M, Albert DM. Thrombocytopenia, anemia, and retinal hemorrhage. Am J Ophthalmol 1968;65:435–9.
1344. Vaiser A, Hutton WL, Marengo-Rowe AJ, et al. Retinal hemorrhage associated with thrombasthenia. Am J Ophthalmol 1975;80:258–62.
1345. Ashton N, Kok D'A, Foulds WS. Ocular pathology in macroglobulinaemia. J Pathol Bacteriol 1963;86:453–61.
1346. Carr RE, Henkind P. Retinal findings associated with serum hyperviscosity. Am J Ophthalmol 1963;56:23–31.
1347. Friedman AH, Marchevsky A, Odel JG, et al. Immunofluorescent studies of the eye in Waldenström's macroglobulinemia. Arch Ophthalmol 1980;98:743–6.
1348. Thomas EL, Olk RJ, Markman M, et al. Irreversible visual loss in Waldenström's macroglobulinaemia. Br J Ophthalmol 1983;67:102–6.
1349. Sanders TE, Podos SM, Rosenbaum LJ. Intraocular manifestations of multiple myeloma. Arch Ophthalmol 1967;77:789–94.
1350. Sarnat RL, Jampol LM. Hyperviscosity retinopathy secondary to polyclonal gammopathy in a patient with rheumatoid arthritis. Ophthalmology 1986;93:124–7.
1351. Enzenauer RJ, Stock JG, Enzenauer RW, et al. Retinal vasculopathy associated with systemic light chain deposition disease. Retina 1990;10:115–8.
1352. Fredrickson DS, Levy RI. Familial hyperlipoproteinemia. In: Stanbury JB, Wyngaarden JB, Fredrickson DS, editors. The metabolic basis of inherited disease. New York: McGraw-Hill; 1972. p. 92, 3rd ed. 545.
1353. Dunphy EB. Ocular conditions associated with idiopathic hyperlipemia. Am J Ophthalmol 1950;33:1579–86.
1354. Martinez KR, Cibis GW, Tauber JT. Lipemia retinalis. Arch Ophthalmol 1992;110:1171.
1355. Orlin C, Lee K, Jampol LM, et al. Retinal arteriolar changes in patients with hyperlipidemias. Retina 1988;8:6–9.
1356. Blodi FC. Retinal involvement in idiopathic hyperlipemia. Trans Am Acad Ophthalmol Otolaryngol 1960;64:720–5.
1357. Kurz GH, Shakib M, Sohmer KK, et al. The retina in type 5 hyperlipoproteinemia. Am J Ophthalmol 1976;82:32–43.
1358. Dodson PM, Galton DJ, Winder AF. Retinal vascular abnormalities in the hyperlipidaemias. Trans Ophthalmol Soc UK 1981;101:17–21.
1359. Stock JG, Pope Jr J, Enzenauer RW. Retinal findings in the fat overload syndrome. Arch Ophthalmol 1990;108:329.
1360. Yassur Y, Smir M, Ben-Sira I. Cherry red spot maculopathy after hyperalimentation for Crohn's disease. In: Fine SL, Owens SL, editors. Management of retinal vascular and macular disorders. Baltimore: Williams & Wilkins; 1983. p. 156–8.
1361. Jager RD, Timothy NH, Coney JM, et al. Congenital retinal macrovessel. Retina 2005;25: 538–40.
1362. Schwartz SG, Hickey M, Puliafito CA. Bilateral CRAO and CRVO from thrombotic thrombocytopenic purpura: OCT findings and treatment with triamcinolone acetonide and bevacizumab. Ophthalmic Surg Lasers Imaging 2006;37:420–2.
1363. Hall S, Buettner H, Luthra HS. Occlusive retinal vascular disease in systemic lupus erythematosus. J Rheumatol 1984;11:846–50.

CHAPTER 7

Macular Dysfunction Caused by Vitreous and Vitreoretinal Interface Abnormalities

Diseases affecting primarily the vitreous and vitreoretinal interface are associated with a variety of macular lesions causing loss of central vision. These lesions may be detected ophthalmoscopically and biomicroscopically and should be differentiated from the other causes of macular dysfunction. In no other area of macular disease is the use of a fundus contact lens more important to detect and define the anatomic changes. Recently introduced techniques that improve our ability in this regard are optical coherence tomography (OCT) and kinetic ultrasonography.[1–9]

ANATOMIC CONSIDERATIONS

The vitreous is a semisolid gel containing a hyaluronic acid network interspersed in a framework of randomly spaced collagen fibrils. The framework is most apparent histologically in the region of the pars plana, where it is strongly anchored to the ciliary epithelium in an area referred to as the vitreous base. Posterior to the pars plana the concentration of collagen and hyaluronic acid is greatest in the ill-defined outer part of the vitreous gel, referred to as the vitreous cortex, that lies along the inner retinal surface. The collagen fibrils, which are condensed to form an outer layer of the vitreous cortex, are adherent to the internal limiting membrane (ILM: basement membrane, or basal lamina of the Müller cells) of the retina (Figures 7.01 and 7.02). The basal lamina thickness increases from the vitreous base posteriorly, to where it reaches maximal thickness at the crest of the foveal clivus. From there it rapidly becomes thinner, reaching a thickness of 200 Å or less in the foveal center.[10] At the margin of the optic disc, the basal lamina abruptly thins to approximately 450 Å, where it covers the disc surface. Here the basal lamina is associated with multiple gaps associated with glial epipapillary membranes that are probably of developmental origin.[11] Attachment plaques or hemidesmosomes are evident electron microscopically along the vitreoretinal junction in the peripheral and equatorial zones but are absent posteriorly except in the foveal area.[10] These findings indicate greater adherence of the basal lamina to the Müller cells in these zones with attachment plaques but do not necessarily reflect greater adherence of the vitreous to the basal lamina in these areas.[12] There is other evidence, however, to indicate greater adherence of cortical vitreous to the basal lamina in these areas, including the central macular region.[13–15] Progressive liquefaction of the posterior vitreous occurs with aging, giving rise to a large optically empty cavity of liquified vitreous in the premacular area, referred to as the premacular bursa, or prefoveolar pocket (Figure 7.03).[15–21] The thin layer of the posterior cortical vitreous gel lying on the inner surface of the macula is not visible biomicroscopically, and the anterior interface of the bursa may be visible and misinterpreted biomicroscopically as the posterior hyaloid of the separated vitreous.

7.01 Vitreoretinal attachment in the macular region.

The collagen fibrillae making up the vitreous cortex (vc) are adherent to the internal limiting membrane (basement membrane of Müller cells). This membrane is thick in the perifoveal area but extremely thin in the foveal region. Arrow indicates vitreocyte lying on the internal limiting membrane at the vitreoretinal interface.

7.02 Vitreoretinal interface at the electron microscopic level.

The collagen fibrillae making up the vitreous cortex (vc) are adherent to the basement membrane (bm, basal lamina, internal limiting membrane) of the Müller cells (M). On separation of the vitreous, the collagen fibrillae realign to form the posterior hyaloid membrane (phm). Some of the vitreous cortex may remain adherent to the basement membrane (arrow).

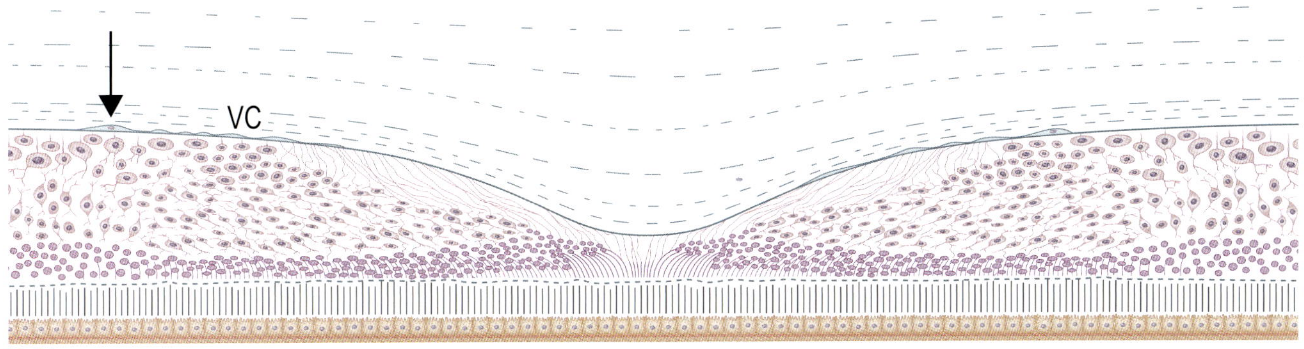

7.01

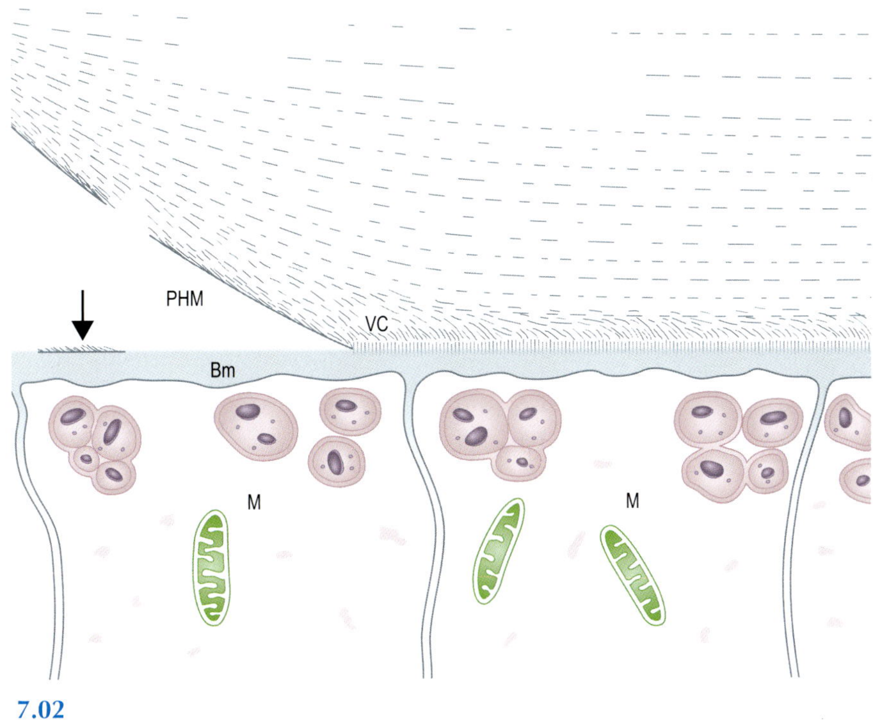

7.02

The degree of vitreoretinal adherence varies with age as well as location in the eye. OCT illustrates the change in the contour of the vitreous attachment to the posterior pole with age. Children and young adults show no separation of the posterior hyaloid from the retinal surface (Figure 7.04D). From the fifth decade onwards the posterior hyaloid shows a gentle curve away from the retina, still being attached to the fovea and the optic disc (Figure 7.04E, arrows). There are no visible effects of traction on any structure at this stage. As the posterior hyaloid tries to separate from the retina, various configurations occur in different eyes that include incomplete separation with residual vitreofoveal or vitreopapillary traction, and anomalous separation with vitreoschisis resulting in epiretinal membrane and full-thickness or lamellar macular hole (Figure 7.05A–E, G, I, and J). A normal vitreous separation shows the posterior hyaloid membrane separated from the retina with a normal foveal contour (Figure 7.04F). Generally the adherence decreases with age. The attachment of the vitreous to the retina is greatest at those sites where the ILM of the retina is the thinnest (Figure 7.01). These sites include the vitreous base, the major retinal vessels, the optic nerve head, the 1500-μm-diameter rim surrounding the fovea, and the 500-μm-diameter foveola. The latter two sites of attachment are probably important in the development of idiopathic age-related macular hole. Forces generated by movement of the vitreous and the premacular bursa as the eye moves may also play a role in the pathogenesis of posterior vitreous detachment (PVD), epiretinal membranes, and macular holes (Figure 7.03).

7.03 Diagrams of vitreous structure in older adults.

A–C: Optically empty premacular bursa, sites of maximum vitreoretinal attachment (larger arrows indicate greater attachment) and dynamics of vitreous movement with gaze left and right (B and C).

Kishi and coworkers found anatomic evidence that the prefoveolar vitreous cortex (PVC) may be focally condensed and tightly adherent to the inner surface of the foveolar retina.[13] They examined 59 eyes with spontaneous PVD with scanning electron microscopy. In 44% of the eyes they found three patterns of vitreous remnants on the surface of the foveolar area. The most common pattern, type 1, found in one-half of these eyes, was a 500-μm-diameter disc of condensed cortical vitreous adherent to the foveolar retina (Figure 7.06A). In 30% of cases (type 2) a 500-μm-diameter ring of remnants was found adherent to the margin of the foveolar retina (Figure 7.06B and C). In some eyes the authors also noted a 1500-μm-diameter ring of vitreous remnants at the foveal margin (Figure 7.06A). Twenty percent of the eyes (type 3) showed a pseudocyst formation consisting of a focal 200–300-μm-diameter disc of contracted vitreous cortex bridging the foveolar area. These findings suggest that the structures of the PVC and the vitreoretinal interface in the foveolar area are probably different from that elsewhere in the macular area.

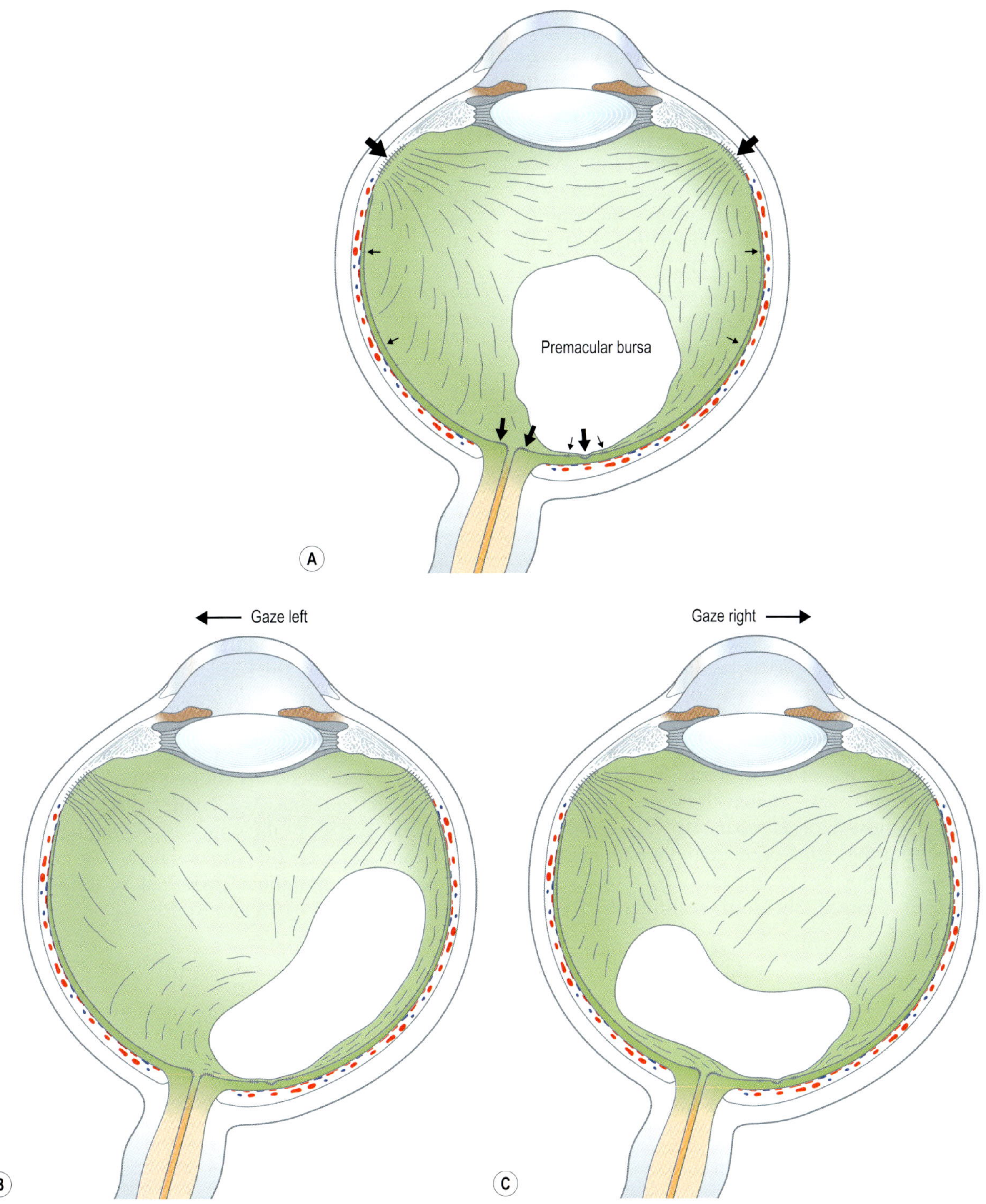
Premacular bursa
A
Gaze left
Gaze right
B
C

The cells that are part of the normal vitreous are widely scattered within the vitreous cortex along the surface of the retina and ciliary body. Their concentration is maximal within the vitreous base and near the posterior pole. These cells, termed "hyalocytes," show phagocytic properties, have a high metabolic activity, and may be responsible for both the formation and the maintenance of several vitreous components. They are probably mesenchymal cells with macrophage-like properties. When properly stimulated, they are capable of cell migration, proliferation, collagen formation, and membrane contraction. The membrane contraction (collagen) may be mediated via transforming growth factor (TGF)-β_2 since using anti-TGF-β_2 neutralizing antibodies experimentally can block the contraction.[22] This capability of fibrous metaplasia may supplement the process of collapse, condensation, and shrinkage of the normal collagen framework in the production of pathologic vitreous membranes. Much of the posterior vitreous becomes liquefied by the seventh decade (synchysis senilis). This process of syneresis may be accompanied by spontaneous separation of the vitreous cortex from the retina, a process referred to as PVD.[10,23–29] Following vitreous separation, there is condensation and realignment of the collagen molecules comprising the outer surface of the cortical vitreous to form a distinct membrane, the so-called posterior hyaloid membrane, which may be visible biomicroscopically and histologically (Figure 7.02). PVD is present in over 25% of persons by the seventh decade and approximately 65% by the eighth decade. It is more common in women. PVD most frequently begins in the macular region following spontaneous dehiscence of the posterior hyaloid near the center of the macula.[23,24,30] It may, however, begin more peripherally. In most patients separation of the posterior hyaloid face from the retina occurs rapidly and smoothly and may or may not be accompanied by symptoms of photopsia and floaters. Slit-lamp examination reveals anterior displacement of the posterior hyaloid membrane. A gray-white ring of vitreous condensation (Weiss ring) that marks the site of previous vitreous attachment to the margins of the optic disc is usually visible and is the single most important biomicroscopic sign of posterior vitreous separation from the optic disc and macular area (Figure 7.04). In cases where the posterior hyaloid face tears near the site of attachment to the crest of the fovea, a similar condensation ring may lie in front of the macula (Figure 7.06). These condensation rings are often distorted and twisted. PVD usually occurs without producing any visible alterations in the retina. As the vitreous separates, traction on the inner surface of the optic disc, along the major vascular arcades, or near the vitreous base may occasionally produce a focal intraretinal, preretinal, or diffuse vitreous hemorrhage (Figure 7.07A and B).[31,32]

7.04 Diagram showing stages of posterior vitreous separation.

A: Top, Vitreofoveal detachment. Arrow indicates contracted and condensed prefoveolar vitreous cortex (pseudo-operculum) suspended on the posterior surface (arrowheads) of the vitreous cortical gel.
B: Middle, Vitreomacular detachment. The posterior hyaloid (arrowheads) is separated from the macula but not the optic disc.
C: Bottom, Posterior vitreous detachment with hyaloid (arrowheads) separated from the retina and optic disc. Arrows indicate prepapillary condensation ring.
D and E: Optical coherence tomography of a 40-year-old woman with intact vitreous completely filling the vitreous cavity with its posterior wall abutting the retinal surface, (D). A 50-year-old woman with early signs of prefoveal vitreous changes that makes the posterior hyaloid somewhat taut, and it begins to show as a convex bulge towards the retina, (E).
F: An older patient with complete posterior hyaloid separation that is seen freely floating in front of the retina (arrow).

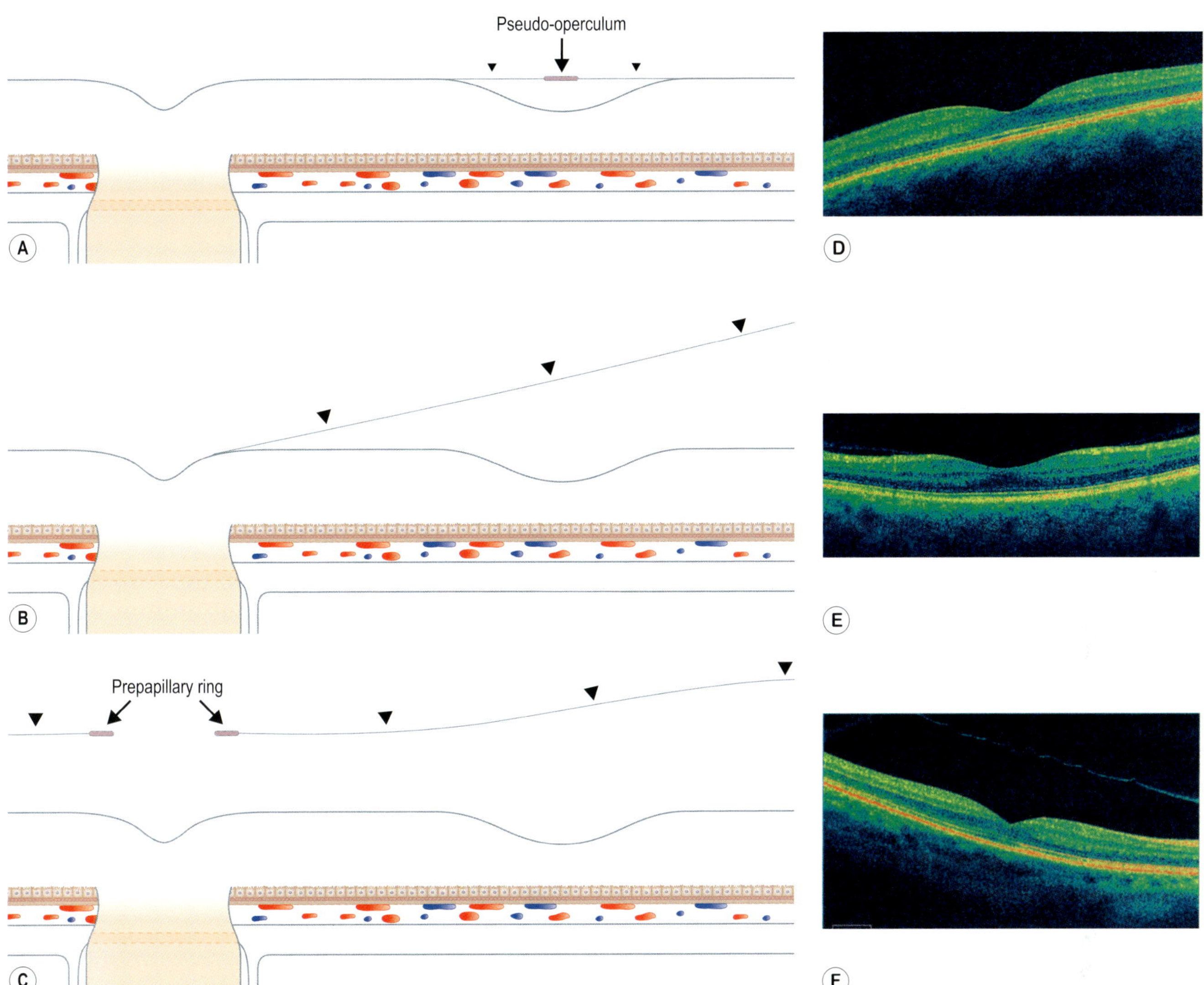
Pseudo-operculum
A
D
B
E
Prepapillary ring
C
F

PVD is the primary cause of peripheral retinal tears and rhegmatogenous retinal detachment. Pathologic alterations in the vitreous gel unrelated to aging may be responsible for vitreous shrinkage and premature PVD. Patients with high myopia are more likely to develop PVD early.[33] Anomalous PVD may result in either vitreoschisis leading to macular hole, macular pucker or diabetic traction detachment (see next section) or partial (incomplete) PVD with residual traction in the periphery causing peripheral retinal tears,[10,12] in the macula causing vitreomacular traction, or the optic disc resulting in vitreopapillary traction.[22]

7.05 Anatomic changes in the macula caused by traction exerted by incomplete posterior detachment of the vitreous.

A: Transient macular distortion. Arrow indicates the area where vitreous remains adherent and is exerting traction on the retina.
B: Posterior vitreous detachment is complete. Note rarefaction of the posterior hyaloid anterior to the foveal area.
C: Macular traction, edema, degeneration, and detachment.
D: Paramacular traction, retinal vessel avulsion, and retinal detachment.
E: Macular hole.
F: Juxtapapillary traction and retinal detachment.

Vitreoschisis

Posterior vitreous cortex is composed of lamellae running tangential to the ILM. These lamellae are the site of potential cleavage when the vitreous detaches. Anomalous PVD results in vitreoschisis whereby a split occurs within the posterior hyaloid leaving a membrane adherent to, or in close proximity to, the retinal ILM. Contraction of this membrane may result in anteroposterior or tangential traction at various points of adherence to the inner retinal surface (Figure 7.08A–C). The pathogenesis of macular hole and macular pucker may be explained at least in part via this phenomenon. Hyalocytes are located approximately 50 μm from the retinal surface within the cortical vitreous. It has been postulated that the split occurs at different levels in patients with macular hole and pucker. A split posterior to the hyalocytes is likely to play a role in macular hole formation where a thin acellular membrane is left adherent to the ILM. Taut contraction of this membrane over the fovea likely pops up the foveal depression which may cause a dehiscence in the continuity of the foveal tissue, initiating the process of a macular hole. A split in the cortical vitreous anterior to the hyalocytes leaves behind a thicker cellular membrane on the retinal surface. Hyalocytes stimulate migration of monocytes from the circulation and glial cells from the retina. Cytokines, platelet-derived growth factor, and other chemokines stimulate proliferation of these cells, resulting in hypercellular epiretinal membranes. Hyalocytes are also known to cause collagen contraction, resulting in a pucker. Recurrence of epiretinal membranes may also be explained by vitreoschisis wherein the anterior wall may be removed at surgery and the cells in the residual posterior wall proliferate and contract. OCT is able to detect these membranes and their interplay with the retina, except when the membranes are extremely thin.[22,34–36]

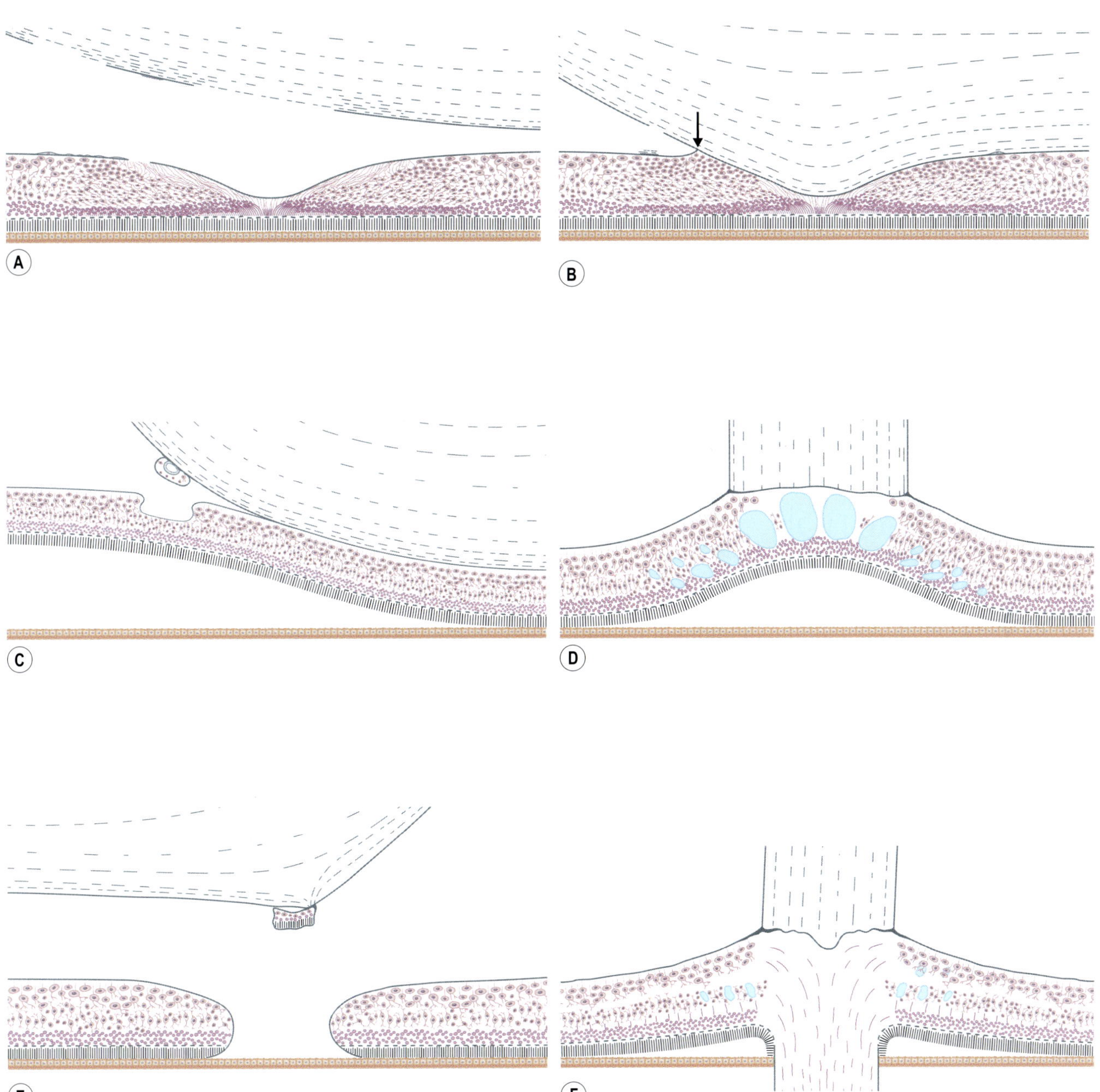
A
B
C
D
E
F

Two distinct clinicopathological features of membranes removed from eyes with vitreomacular traction syndrome without obvious PVD suggest different forms of epiretinal fibrocellular proliferation: (1) multilayered cellular membranes separated from the ILM by a layer of intervening native vitreous collagen in eyes with visible epiretinal membrane; and (2) single cells or a cellular monolayer directly on the ILM with no visible epiretinal membrane. The predominant cell type is myofibroblast that contributes to the contractility, in both types. The higher number in the multilayered membranes may explain the cystoid macular edema and progressive vitreomacular traction characteristic of this disorder.[37] Overall, it appears that the location of the split in the posterior vitreous cortex and variable cellular proliferation determine the nature and severity of vitreofoveal traction and epiretinal membrane formation.

VITREOUS TRACTION MACULOPATHIES

Changes in the vitreous gel may cause traction on the retinal surface and macular distortion through several different mechanisms, including: (1) incomplete PVD in which the vitreous remains attached focally to the macular surface, resulting in macular cysts or macular detachment; (2) anomalous posterior vitreous separation resulting in vitreoschisis with continued broad foveal traction causing macular cysts; (3) vitreoschisis with proliferation of the posterior layer into epiretinal membrane causing macular distortion; (4) vitreous gel condensation and shrinkage caused by inflammatory, vascular, and metabolic diseases in the absence of hyaloid separation; (5) complete PVD with subsequent epiretinal membrane formation; and (6) a peculiar form of traction maculopathy that is related to focal tangential contraction of the PVC, anterior displacement of the foveal retina, resulting in idiopathic macular hole.

7.05 Continued

G and **H**: This 78-year-old diabetic woman complained of central visual change and difficulty reading for 4 weeks. Her vision dropped from 20/20 to 20/40. Optical coherence tomography revealed focal vitreofoveal traction causing foveal cysts that did not spontaneously resolve on observation for 3 months (G). A pars plana vitrectomy resolved the macular edema and vision returned to 20/20 (H).
I–L: This 70-year-old woman's vision decreased to 20/40 and 20/50 respectively. Small cysts in both foveas were seen secondary to focal vitreofoveal traction (I and J). Absence of spontaneous improvement with continued observation for 3 months in the right eye and 9 months in the left eye prompted a vitrectomy in both eyes, which resulted in restoration of foveal contour and visual improvement to 20/20 in each eye (K and L).

7.06 Vitreous remnants on inner retinal surface in the fovea following spontaneous vitreoretinal separation.

A: Scanning electron micrograph showing 500-µm-diameter disc of condensed vitreous cortex (white arrow) adherent to foveolar retina. Open arrow indicates 1500-µm-diameter ring of vitreous remnants at the margin of the foveal retina.
B: Scanning electron micrograph showing 500-µm-diameter ring of vitreous cortical remnants (white arrow) at the margin of the foveola.
C: Higher magnification of open arrow shown in B. Note aligned collagen fibers of vitreous origin in contrast to smooth appearance of underlying internal limiting membrane.

(From Kishi et al.[13])

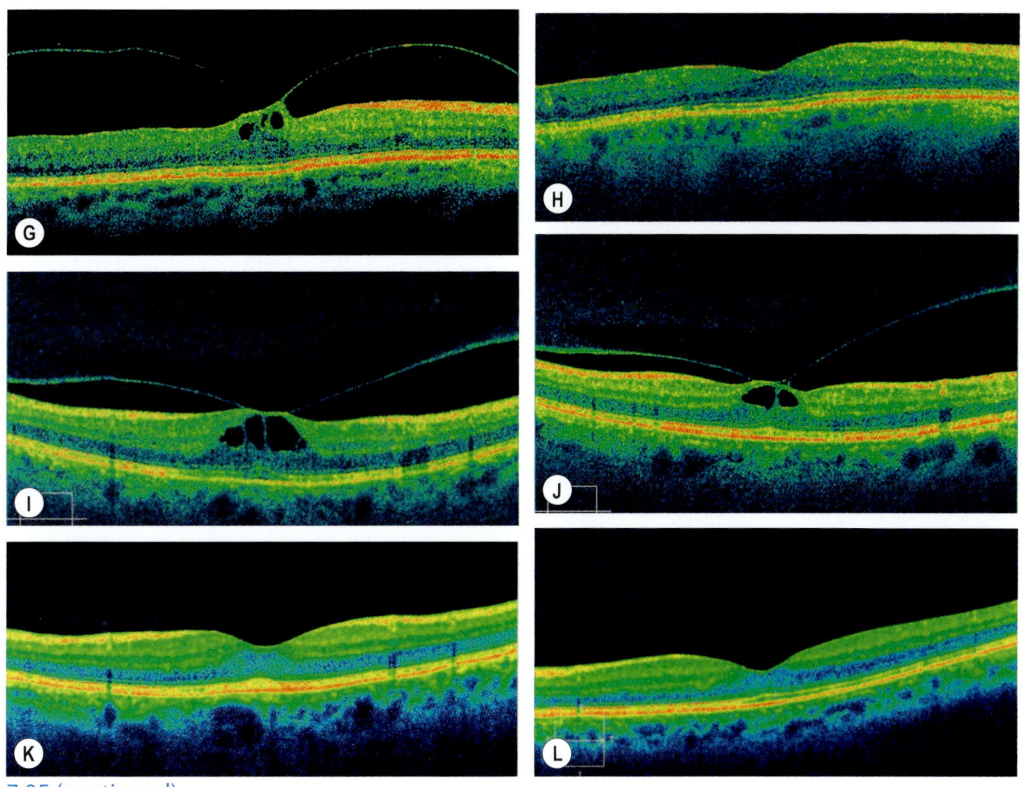

7.05 (continued)

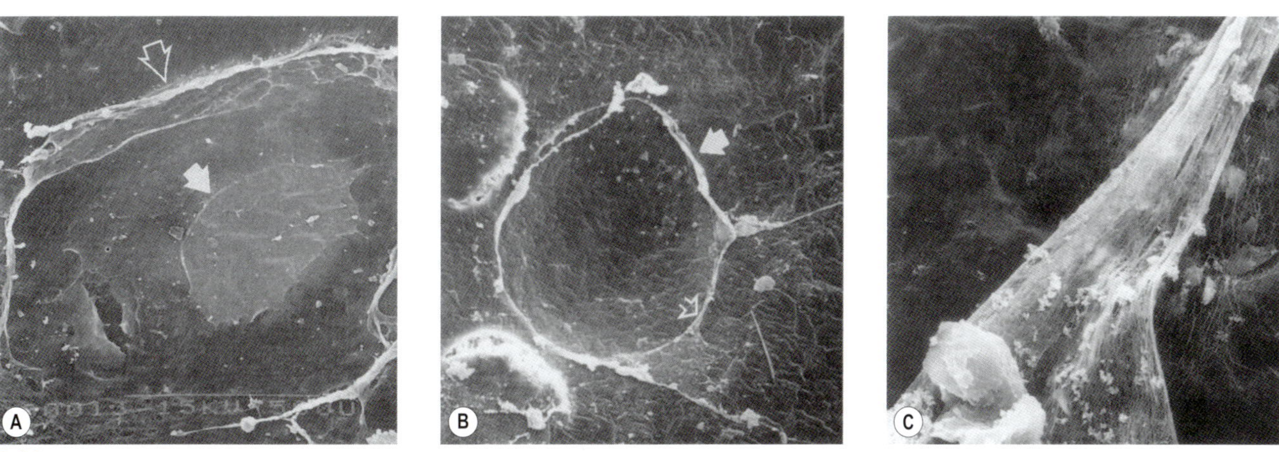

7.06

Traction Maculopathy Caused by Incomplete Posterior Vitreous Detachment

Approximately 30% of patients (average age 60 years) who develop a symptomatic PVD will have evidence of vitreous hemorrhage or a peripheral retinal tear or both. This affects twice as many women as men. In all, 10–15% of these patients will develop a PVD in the second eye, usually within 2 years. Vitreous hemorrhage that is usually caused by a demonstrable peripheral full- or partial-thickness retinal tear is the most frequent cause of transient loss of vision in patients after an acute PVD (Figures 7.05D and 7.07A). In most cases the macula is unaffected by the PVD. Small hemorrhages around the optic disc, along the major vascular arcades, and less frequently in the macula may be the only sign of microtrauma to the retina caused by the PVD (Figure 7.07A and B).[31,32] When the PVD is impeded by abnormal vitreoretinal adhesions in the macular area, traction and distortion of the macula may cause blurring of vision, metamorphopsia, and occasionally a scotoma (Figures 7.05A, G, I, and J, and 7.07C–F and J–L). Ophthalmoscopic and biomicroscopic examination reveals a partial PVD and tenting of the retina at the site of the vitreoretinal adhesion.[25,30,38–40] This site may be localized in the parafoveal region rather than directly in the foveal area. If the onset of symptoms is recent, the vitreoretinal adhesion may separate in a matter of days or weeks and visual function may be restored to normal (Figure 7.07E, F, and L). These patients, however, may subsequently develop evidence of epiretinal membrane (Figure 7.07G). In a few cases an epiretinal membrane may develop before PVD (a visible Weiss ring) occurs (Figure 7.08A–C).

7.07 Vitreous traction maculopathy.

A and B: This woman experienced sudden blurring of vision associated with a preretinal hemorrhage caused by posterior vitreous detachment and avulsion of a small capillary in the vicinity of the superotemporal retinal vein (arrows).

C–G: A 41-year-old man noted sudden onset of blurred vision and metamorphopsia in the right eye as a result of incomplete separation of the vitreous, which remained attached to the superior nasal portion of the macula (arrow, C and D; see Figure 7.05A). Fine retinal striae radiated outward from the macula. Visual acuity was 20/70. Angiography revealed no definite abnormality. Eight days later spontaneous separation of the vitreous was associated with a circular tear in the posterior hyaloid in the foveal area (E and F). The condensation of the edges of the hole in the posterior hyaloid indicated in the fundus painting (F) is not visible in E (see Figure 7.05B). Visual acuity returned to 20/25. The retinal wrinkles noted in C were no longer visible. Eighteen months later he developed metamorphopsia caused by contraction of an epiretinal membrane in the nasal half of the macula. Note the fine retinal folds radiating from the temporal edge of the membrane (G).

H: Paramacular vitreous traction causing retinal vessel avulsion (arrow) and serous detachment of the macula (see Figure 7.05D).

I: Vitreous traction on the optic disc and juxtapapillary retina was responsible for the misdiagnosis of papilledema in this patient (see Figure 7.05F).

J–L: Blurred vision in a 62-year-old woman with macular edema and detachment resulting from prolonged vitreous traction (see Figure 7.05C). Visual acuity was 20/200. Arrows indicate margin of the detachment. Angiography revealed evidence of cystoid macular edema (K). Twenty-nine months later the vitreous separated and visual acuity returned to 20/40 (L).

(H, from Benson and Tasman.[49];

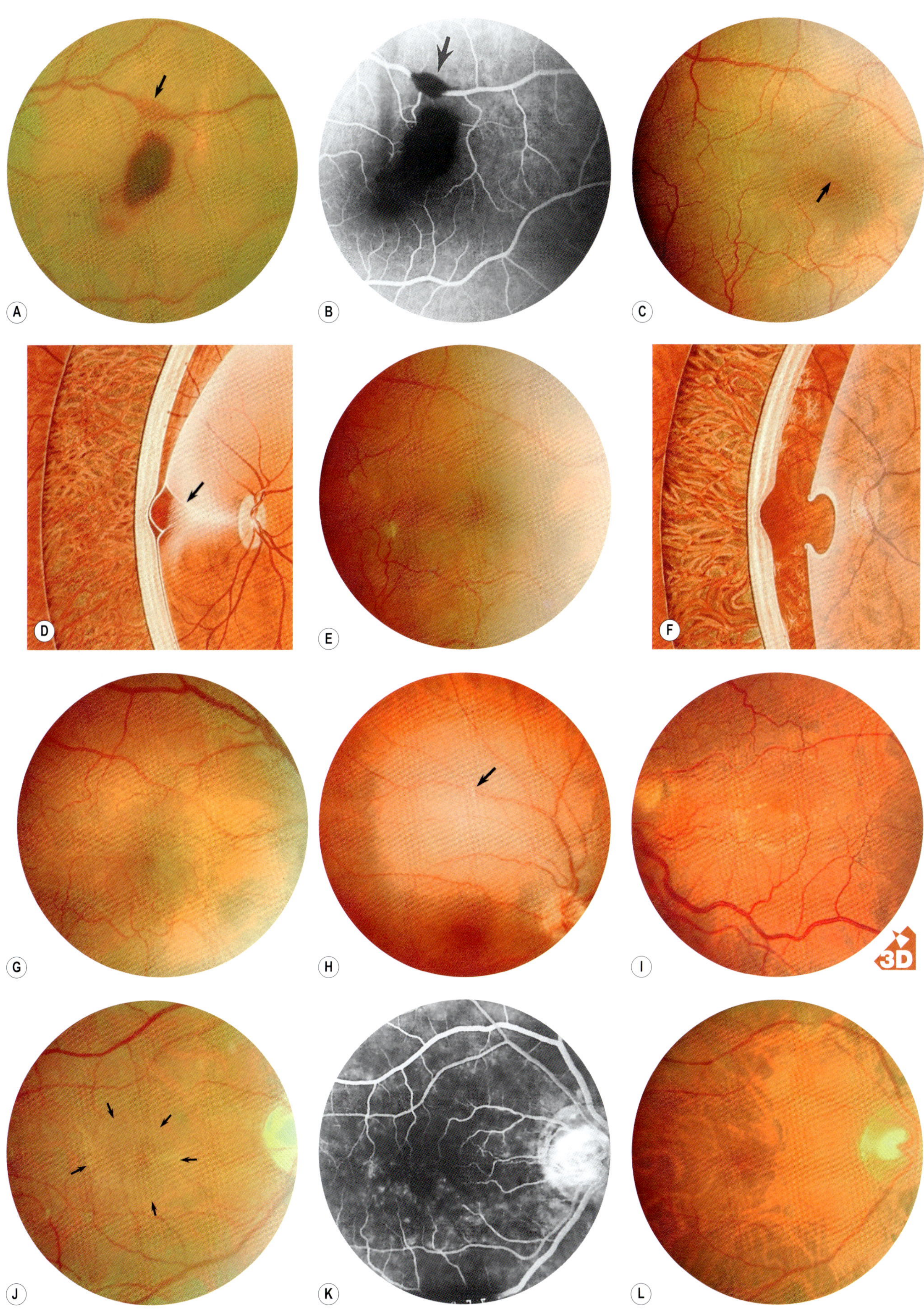
A
B
C
D
E
F
G
H
I
3D
J
K
L

In some patients vitreoretinal adhesion in the macular area is sufficiently dense that prolonged traction causes distortion, cystic edema, degeneration, and detachment of the macula. This may be caused by a linear area of attachment of the posterior hyaloid to the retinal surface (Figure 7.07C), a single condensed strand of vitreous attached to the paracentral retina, a cone-shaped mass of condensed vitreous with attachment to the entire foveal inner surface (Figures 7.05C and 7.07J and L), and paracentral traction at the major vascular arcades (Figure 7.07A and H). Vitreoschisis with splitting of the posterior hyaloid into two layers and persistent broad attachment of the posterior layer to the retina may be responsible for this (Figure 7.08I). When the partly detached vitreous remains attached to the center of the macula, the retina is tented anteriorly, causing a localized tractional serous retinal detachment that is surrounded by radiating retinal folds (Figures 7.05C, and 7.07J and L, 7.08C, E–H). Cystic changes are often evident centrally (Figure 7.08B).[41] Prolonged vitreous traction may be associated with angiographic evidence of retinal capillary permeability alterations, and development of an epiretinal membrane in the area of vitreoretinal adhesion. Spontaneous separation of the adhesion may eventually occur (Figure 7.07J–L). Surgical separation of the vitreoretinal attachment may be required to reattach the macula (Figure 7.09J–L).[26,42–47] Lysis of vitreoretinal adhesions may be accomplished in some cases with Q-switched neodymium laser.[48]

Vitreous traction at the site of a major retinal vessel may cause not only a tractional retinal detachment that extends into the macula but also avulsion of the blood vessel (Figures 7.05D and 7.07H), vitreous hemorrhage, proliferative retinopathy (Figure 7.09), and infrequently a full-thickness retinal hole.[49–53]

Vitreous traction on the optic nerve head and juxtapapillary retina may cause a fundus picture that simulates papilledema, optic disc capillary angioma, astrocytoma, or combined retinal pigment epithelium (RPE) and retinal hamartoma (Figures 7.05E and 7.07I, 7.09D–G, and see Figure 7.26).[54]

7.08 Vitreofoveal traction causing macular edema and macular detachment.

A–D: A 76-year-old male with glaucoma and a visual decline to 20/80 in his right eye showing a partial ring in the prefoveal vitreous (arrow) (A). Angiography revealed cystoid macular edema (B). Optical coherence tomography (OCT) revealed tractional foveal detachment and cysts (C). A vitrectomy caused prompt resolution of the cysts and the detachment, with vision recovering to 20/30.

E–H: This 35-year-old type 1 diabetic with prior panretinal photocoagulation for severe proliferative diabetic retinopathy complained of floaters and rapid loss of vision in his left eye over 2 weeks. He had a foveal detachment with a preretinal hemorrhage overhanging his fovea within a vitreous traction band (E). The traction band was connected to an area of gliosis above the superotemporal arcade (F). OCT shows discontinuity of the elevated retina due to shadowing from the prefoveal blood and membrane (G). A OCT section through the edge of the vitreous band shows the foveal detachment and the attachment of the band to the retina (H).

Vitreoschisis causing macular edema.

I–K: This 56-year-old male shows evidence of splitting of the posterior hyaloid (arrow) (I) with macular traction caused by the adherence of the posterior layer to the retina resulting in diffuse macular edema (J). Postvitrectomy the macular edema resolved with restoration of vision to 20/25 (K).

L: Ultrastructure of the foveolar area lying between the small arrows shows a significant population of Müller cells (pale-staining cells indicated by the large arrow) in the umbo region.

(L, from Hogan et al.[74])

In some cases with unusual adherence of the center of the fovea to the vitreous, a PVD that begins in the extramacular area may cause either a partial (lamellar) or full-thickness macular hole as it extends through the macular area (Figures 7.05E and 7.09H, J–L). This, however, is an infrequent mechanism for causing a macular hole (see discussion of idiopathic macular hole in a subsequent section).

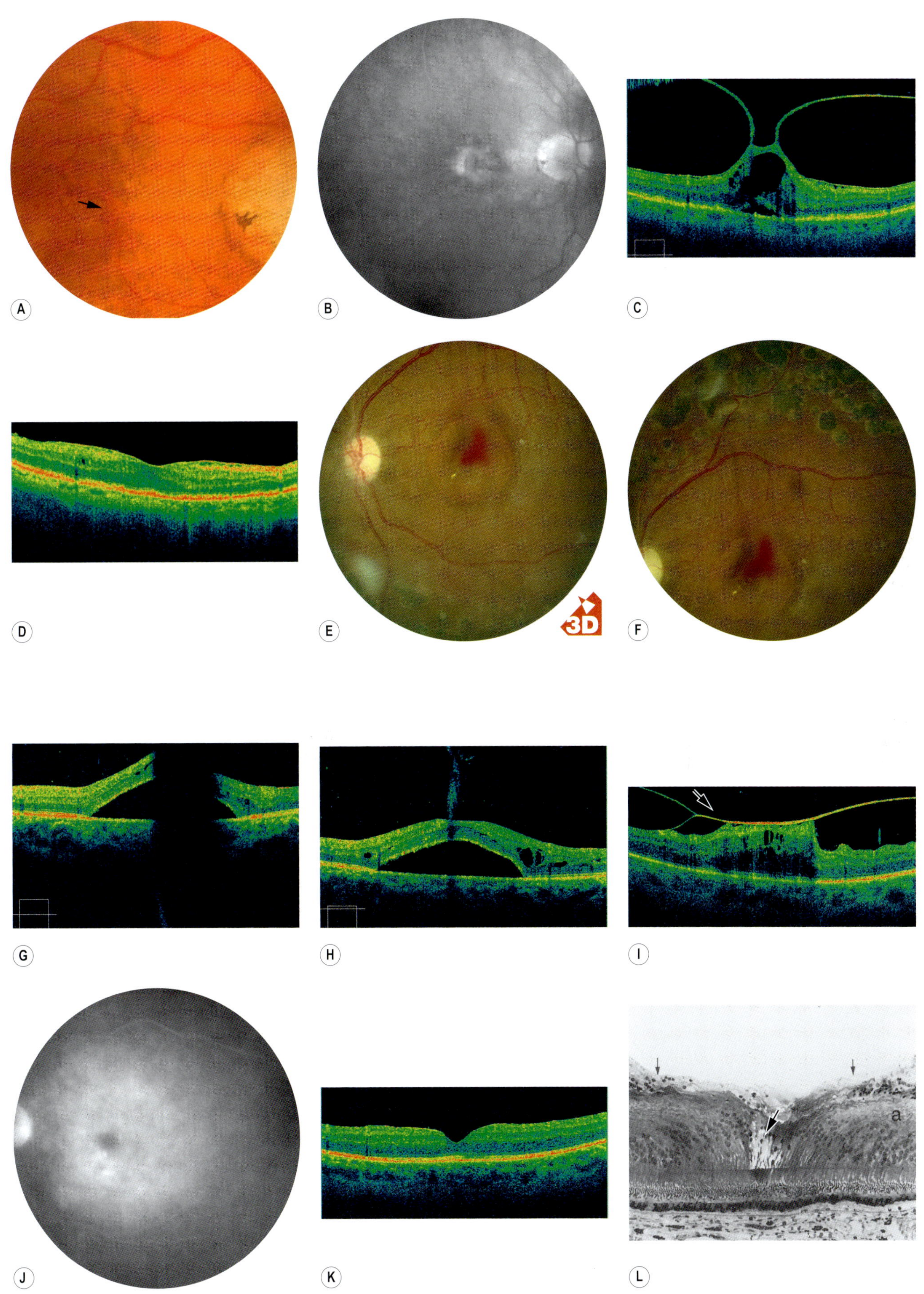
A
B
C
D
E
3D
F
G
H
I
J
K
a
L

Idiopathic Traction Maculopathy Unassociated with Posterior Vitreous Detachment

There is some evidence to suggest that subtle changes may occasionally occur in the vitreous body, causing it to contract and to exert anterior traction on the retinal surface posteriorly, without any biomicroscopic evidence of posterior separation, or discrete vitreous bands attached to the inner retinal surface (Figure 7.10E–I). This traction may be associated with cystoid macular edema and angiographic evidence of retinal capillary leakage in the macular area or serous detachment of the sensory retina. (See discussion of diabetic traction maculopathy, p. 544, and congenital pit of the optic nerve head, p. 1260.) Vascular leakage or inflammation with or without secondary vascular permeability alteration can result in vitreous contraction without posterior separation in conditions such as pars planitis (Figure 7.10A–D), retinal capillary hemangioma (see Chapter 13), Coats' disease, and others.

7.09 Vitreous traction maculopathy associated with epiretinal membrane formation.

A–C: A 26-year-old patient initially was seen because of blurred vision caused by vitritis associated with an active focus of toxoplasmosis in the peripheral fundus. Three months later the vitreous cleared and visual acuity returned to 20/20. One month later he developed crinkling of the inner retinal surface caused by an epiretinal membrane (arrows, A). Seven weeks later he was seen because of metamorphopsia. The vitreous along with the epiretinal membrane had detached superiorly and was adherent to the center of the macula (arrows, B). Visual acuity was 20/30. One week later the vision had improved to 20/20. The vitreous detachment had extended further inferiorly. Six years later the condensed ball of epiretinal membrane (arrow, C) and the posterior hyaloid were still attached to the retina inferonasally.
D–G: This 65-year-old patient developed blurred vision associated with a macular pucker that appeared to have pulled free from its attachment to a branch retinal artery inferior to the macula inferiorly (arrow, D). Note the suggestion of a small vascular tuft (arrow, D). Seven months later the patient returned with a semiopaque angiomatous preretinal lesion resembling an astrocytoma (E). Angiography revealed a neovascular frond within this lesion (F). Over the next 6 months the tumor enlarged (G). Following photocoagulation the patient developed subretinal neovascularization.
H: Macular hole caused by vitreous traction. Note irregular inferior edge of hole where the flap has torn free. The operculum (arrow) was attached to the posterior hyaloid face.
I: In 1989, this 40-year-old man with high myopia noted a paracentral scotoma in the right eye. One year later his visual acuity was 20/25 bilaterally. There was an incomplete posterior vitreous detachment and adherence of the vitreous to a focal area of epiretinal membrane condensation and tractional retinal detachment. Angiography demonstrated evidence of mild underlying depigmentation of the pigment epithelium. Over the subsequent 4 years he developed a focal area of geographic atrophy beneath the focal area of tractional retinal detachment (I). The visual acuity was 20/30.
J and K: Macular detachment and hole caused by vitreous traction. Note in the stereoscopic views (J) the focal adherence of the vitreous strand to the edge of the hole. Because of persistence of the detachment a vitrectomy was done and the retina was reattached (K).
L: Optical coherence tomography of a patient with a full-thickness macular hole with a complete posterior vitreous detachment.

(B, from Jaffe[38]; D–G, courtesy of Dr. Robert Machemer.)

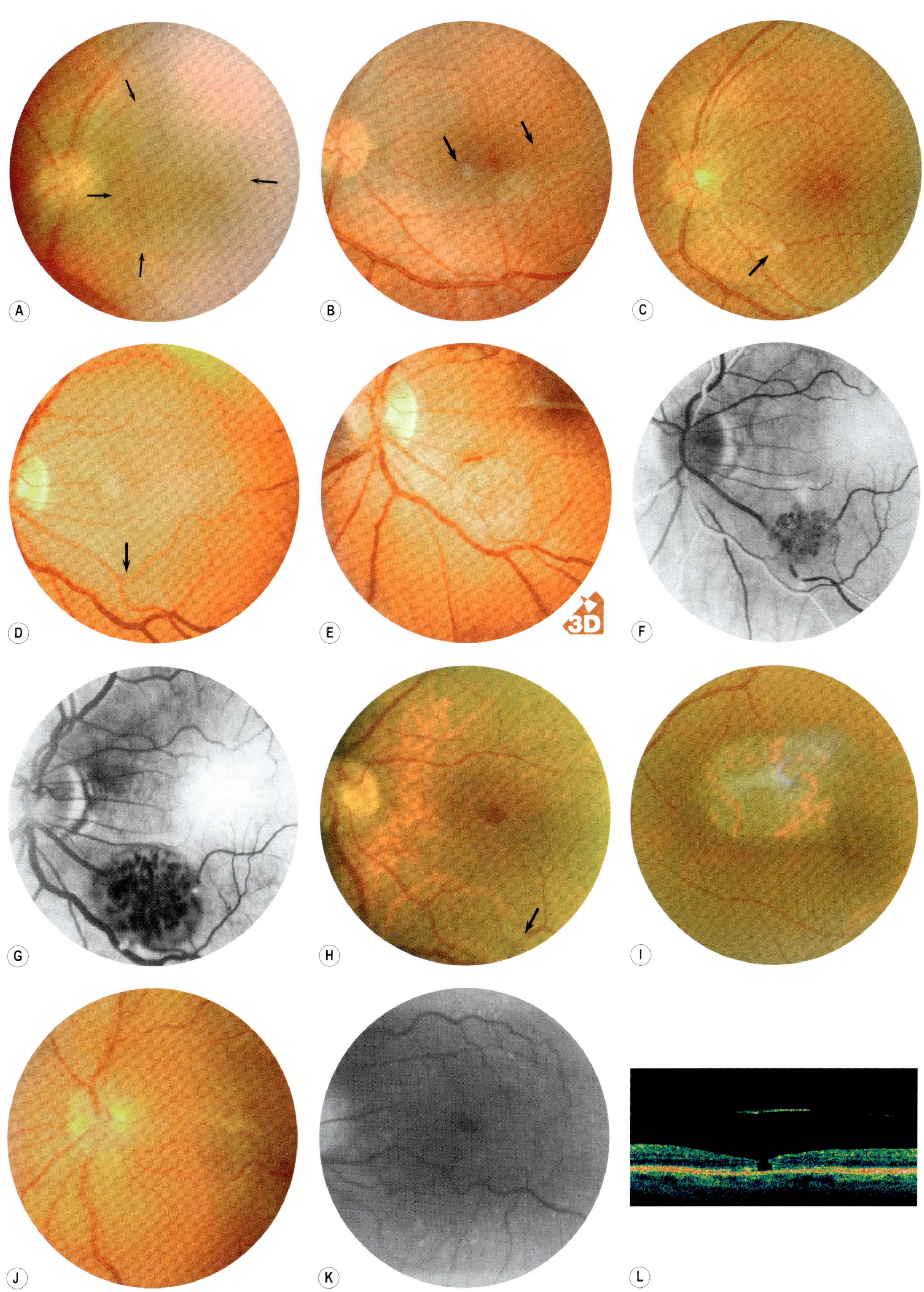
A
B
C
D
E
3D
F
G
H
I
J
K
L

Traction Maculopathy Caused by Spontaneous Contraction of the Prefoveolar Vitreous Cortex Unassociated with a Posterior Vitreous Detachment

Idiopathic Age-Related Macular Hole

Idiopathic age-related macular hole, referred to henceforth in this section as macular hole, affects predominantly older patients, more often women at a ratio of 2 or 3:1.[55] They often discover blurred vision and metamorphopsia when they cover the fellow normal eye.[56–66] Most patients report that both eyes were normal during their last eye examination 1 or 2 years previously. From the pathogenetic and therapeutic standpoint, it is important to differentiate idiopathic age-related macular hole from the less common causes of macular hole, such as trauma or macular traction resulting from incomplete posterior vitreous separation, transvitreal bands of vitreous condensation, or neighboring epiretinal membranes. An understanding of the structure of the vitreous and aging changes in its structure discussed previously in this chapter, and the ultrastructure of the foveolar retina (Figure 7.08L) are important in considering the pathogenesis of age-related macular hole, which typically begins in eyes with an optically empty liquefied premacular vitreous and no evidence of posterior vitreous separation.

It is likely no other condition in ophthalmology has elicited as much debate and controversy about its pathogenesis as macular hole, since the original description by Gass. It is important to bear in mind that Gass described the mechanism much before OCT was available. With the advent of OCT we began to view the interplay between the fovea and the vitreous, a concept that Don Gass had visualized by his keen observation with a fundus contact lens and interpretation. The earliest observations with the first-generation OCT were made by Alain Gaudric, where he introduced the terms "foveal cyst" and "anteroposterior traction forces" at the vitreofoveal junction associated with localized perifoveal vitreous detachment.[67] Subsequent reports have continued to use this as the basis of macular hole formation.[68,69] Gass, who constantly reappraised the understanding of various diseases, in 1999 wrote about the forgotten "Müller cell cone" (Figure 7.11B) and postulated dissolution of the Müller cells in eyes destined to develop a macular hole.[70] An inverted cone of Müller cells occupying the inner half of the fovea centralis was first shown by Yamada et al. histopathologically in a 45-year-old woman (Figure 7.08L).[71] Gass postulated breakdown of the compact arrangement of the Müller cells and perhaps their movement into the prefoveal vitreous cortex initiating centripetal contraction that pops the foveal depression up (Figure 7.10J–L). It is likely that the dissolution of the Müller cell cone weakens the fovea which splits by the contracting forces of the overlying vitreous. The concentric contraction of the prefoveal vitreous cortex can explain the localized perifoveal vitreous detachment seen on OCT (Figure 7.11C) by foreshortening the vitreous cortex. Subsequent reports have alluded to this concept.[72] The role of the Müller cell cone changes in eyes destined to form a macular hole is further strengthened by the observation of various other anatomic appearances such as foveal cysts, foveal detachment, and diffuse foveal/macular thickening (Figures 7.07 and 7.08), in eyes with vitreomacular traction alone, none of which leads to a macular hole. Figure 7.11F also illustrates that tangential, rather than anteroposterior, forces play a role in macular hole formation; the operculum is lying close to the foveola rather than being drawn more anteriorly which should have occurred if anteroposterior traction forces were predominant.

Table 7.1 and the diagrams in Figures 7.10 (J–L) and 7.11 summarize the characteristic biomicroscopic features and the presumed anatomic changes accompanying each of the stages of development of a macular hole.[73]

Stage 1-A: Impending Macular Hole

Although the earliest precipitating event responsible for the progression of changes leading to a macular hole has not been identified, the author believes that proliferation of Müller cells located in the center of the normal foveola (Figures 7.8 and 7.10J–L)[74] and their extension through the ILM at the umbo into the outer part of the layer of formed PVC is most likely responsible for causing contraction, condensation, and partial loss of transparency of the outer part of vitreous cortex in the foveolar and perifoveolar region. Retinal astrocytes and vitreocytes would seem to be less likely candidates as cells responsible for inducing contracture of the PVC.[75,76] Tangential contraction of the outer part of the prefoveolar cortical vitreous causes anterior displacement and serous detachment of the foveolar retina (Figures 7.10K and 7.11B). Biomicroscopically

7.10 Traction maculopathy unassociated with posterior vitreous detachment

A–D: This 21-year-old suffered a gradual decline in his right-eye vision to 20/200 over a year secondary to pars planitis that responded to anterior sub-Tenon triamcinalone injection. The densely adherent vitreous in the posterior pole contracted, resulting in retinal puckering and telangiectasia of the small retinal vessels (A and B). Optical coherence tomography revealed traction over the disc and posterior pole (C). A tedious and long vitrectomy resulted in removal of the densely adherent vitreous and improvement in vision to 20/30. Note the residual papillomacular fold from retinal redundancy secondary to stretching by the adherent vitreous (D).

E–I: This 35-year-old woman underwent a vitrectomy with membrane peel after being symptomatic for more than 9 years from idiopathic (spontaneous) macular pucker. Her visual acuity was count fingers that improved to 20/100. There was no posterior hyaloid separation; the vitreous was continuous with the membrane that was multilayered and densely adherent to the retinal surface (G and H). Residual striations were seen at the retinal pigment epithelium level following vitrectomy (I).

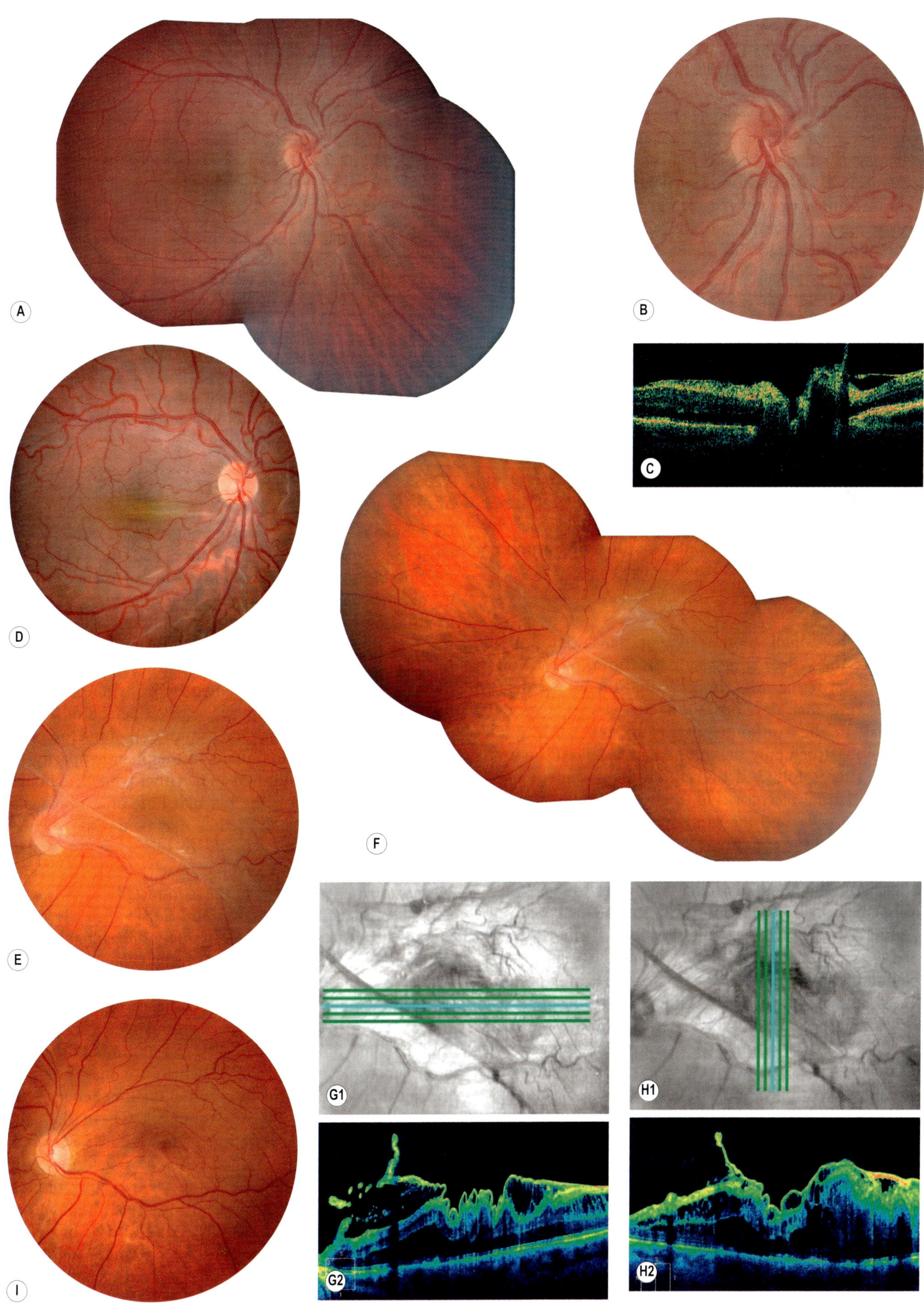
A
B
C
D
E
F
G1
H1
G2
H2
I

displacement of the relatively normal complement of retinal receptors; (2) this dehiscence occurs soon after the change from a yellow spot (stage 1-A impending hole) to a yellow ring lesion (stage 1-B impending hole), but in most cases it is not detectable with a thin slit beam as a defect in the center of the ring because of the presence of the semitranslucent condensed cortical vitreous bridging the hole (stage 1-B occult hole); (3) most of the prehole opacities overlying stage 2 and stage 3 holes are condensed prefoveal vitreous cortex (pseudo-opercula), not opercula; and (4) following successful vitreous surgery, which includes tamponade of the hole with an intravitreal gas bubble, if done within 1 year of commencement of hole formation, the anatomy of the central retina and its visual function may be restored to nearly normal levels in some patients as a result of retinal reattachment and centripetal repositioning of the retinal receptors. If these concepts of the anatomic changes occurring in macular hole development are correct, histopathologic examination of the prehole opacities should determine that most of them contain no retinal receptor cells but are composed of vitreous collagen, reactive Müller cell and astrocytic proliferation, and in some cases ILM of the retina. Although retinal opercula have been described histopathologically in two eyes, one with posttraumatic and the other with an idiopathic macular hole, it is uncertain whether the "opercula" contained retinal receptor cells.[85] Opercula have not been observed in most idiopathic macular holes studied histopathologically.

Spontaneous Abortion of Macular Hole Formation

In approximately 50% of cases, patients with stage 1-A and early stage 1-B lesions may experience rapid improvement in visual symptoms because of spontaneous separation of the vitreous from the fovea without developing a full-thickness macular hole (Figure 7.14).[58,86–88] In such cases, the patient usually notices improvement in the symptoms and biomicroscopy may show several different pictures, all of which are accompanied by return of the foveal depression and a good visual prognosis.

Vitreofoveal Separation and Pseudo-operculum Formation

The foveal area returns to a normal appearance except for the presence of a semitranslucent, operculum-like structure or pseudo-operculum (condensed, contracted prefoveal vitreous cortex) immediately in front of the fovea (Figure 7.14A–C). When viewed obliquely with a thin slit beam, the pseudo-operculum in a few patients will cast a yellow shadow on the pigment epithelium.[89] Some patients with a pseudo-operculum will notice a small scotoma when reading and a few will describe it as having a yellow color.

Vitreofoveal Separation without Pseudo-operculum Formation

After spontaneous vitreofoveal separation the fundus returns to a normal appearance and no pseudo-operculum is evident.

7.11 Continued

C: The asymptomatic fellow eye of a patient with a full-thickness macular hole showing early perifoveal vitreous detachment; this eye subsequently developed a macular hole.
D and E: Stage 2, A 68-year-old woman dropped her vision to 20/80– in her left eye. Optical coherence tomography shows the edge of an operculum as depicted in A.
F: Stage 3 hole with an operculum lying just anterior to the hole.
G: Stage 4 hole with the operculum pulled away from the hole due to subsequent posterior vitreous detachment.

(A, from Gass[73]; B, adapted from Gass.[70];)

Vitreofoveal Separation and Lamellar Hole Formation

Separation of the vitreous from the fovea in these patients is associated with a break in the continuity of the ILM and the biomicroscopic appearance of one or more sharply defined reddish defects in the inner retinal surface in the foveolar area (Figures 7.14D–F and I and J, and 7.15H). An operculum is usually evident overlying the defect. The defect may be minute and simulate that seen after sun gazing or in patients with no recognizable cause (Figure 7.14J).[90] Larger lamellar holes often have a scalloped border (Figure 7.14D). Unlike full-thickness holes there is no rim of retinal detachment. The visual acuity is usually 20/30 or better. Fluorescein angiography shows minimal or no fluorescence in the area of the lamellar hole (Figure 7.14E). The demonstration of a focus of bright fluorescence within the area of the lamellar hole suggests the possible presence of a full-thickness hole without a rim of detachment (Figure 7.13D–F). This type of full-thickness hole appears identical biomicroscopically to a lamellar hole, may be associated with visual acuity of 20/30 or better, and is likely to develop a rim of retinal detachment and be associated with visual loss at a later date. The visual prognosis for patients with a lamellar hole is excellent.

Incomplete Separation of the Contracted Prefoveolar Vitreous Cortex

A portion or all of the contracted PVC may remain as a small stellate opacity on the surface of the center of the foveolar retina and be associated with fine stellate retinal folds simulating X-linked foveomacular schisis (Figure 7.14K and L).[84]

It is important to use a fundus contact lens to look for signs of vitreofoveal separation not only in the symptomatic eye but also in the fellow eye of any patient with evidence of a macular hole in one eye. Spectral domain OCT is very useful in detecting the relation of the posterior hyaloid to the fovea. Fellow eyes with evidence of vitreofoveal separation probably have less than a 5% chance of developing a macular hole.[57,58,91,92] Some patients who have reportedly developed a hole after demonstration of a PVD

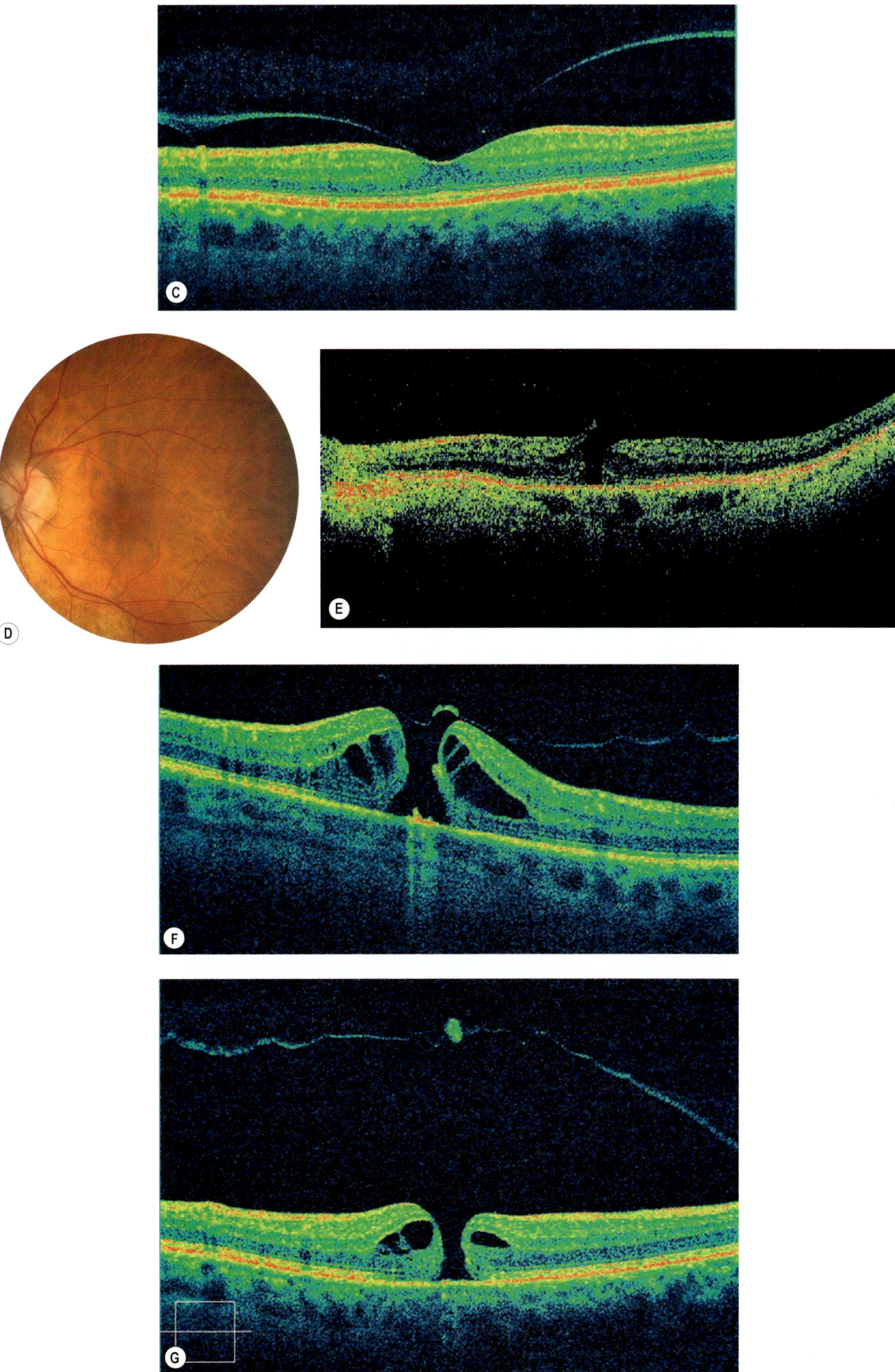
C
D
E
F
G

probably had small occult holes that developed at the time of PVD.[93] Others probably had residual vitreous cortex on the inner retinal surface centrally after separation of the vitreous from the optic disc and paracentral macular area.

Natural Course

The time course from the development of symptoms and stage 1 impending macular hole to a fully developed stage 3 or 4 hole varies but in most patients is within 6 months. In some patients the course may be complete within a matter of weeks, and in others hole formation may not have progressed beyond stage 2 till several years later. The visual acuity usually stabilizes after the first 6–12 months at a mean level of 20/200.[94,95] A few patients with stage 3 and 4 holes may maintain excellent visual function of 20/40 to 20/50 for years.

Spontaneous reattachment of the retina surrounding the hole may occur (Figures 7.15G and 7.16) and the biomicroscopic appearance may be identical with that of a lamellar macular hole. In some cases the hole may disappear and recovery of vision may be excellent.[96–98] Closure of a macular hole occurs occasionally as the result of development of an epiretinal membrane (Figure 7.16).[99]

Approximately 25% of patients with a macular hole have evidence of posterior vitreous separation from the optic disc and macula in the fellow eye. The macula of the asymptomatic eye is usually normal but it may show evidence of previous spontaneous separation of the vitreous that is limited to the foveal area.[95] In addition, other minor changes may occur at the vitreoretinal interface, including epiretinal membrane formation, small irregular folds of the inner retinal surface, and absence of the foveal reflex. Fluorescein angiography in the "asymptomatic eye" is typically normal. The value of focal electroretinography in detecting predilection for hole development in the fellow eye is uncertain.[100] The only finding of definite prognostic significance in the fellow eye is the presence or absence of a PVD.[58,101–103] The reported risk for development of a hole in the normal fellow eye has varied from 1% to 22%.[55,58,63,65,66,87,98,103–108] The probable risk is between 10% and 15%. The presence of a PVD or vitreofoveal separation probably reduces the risk of developing a hole to 1% or less. Possible explanations for the occasional patient with a PVD who develops a hole include: a tear in the posterior hyaloid at the time of PVD, leaving vitreous cortex attached to the central macular area, and a subclinical full-thickness microhole caused by traction during the PVD.[109] In most patients the second eye becomes involved within 2 years.[56] Those with bilateral involvement usually retain moderately useful central vision, and most can read successfully with high-power spectacles.

7.12 Stages of development of idiopathic macular hole.

A and **B**: Progression of stage 1-A impending macular hole with yellow spot (arrow, A) to stage 3 hole with prehole opacity (arrow, B).
C: Stage 4 macular hole with posterior vitreous detachment.
D–F: Progression stage 1-B yellow ring lesion (D), to early stage 2 hole (note small eccentric round hole and underlying yellow fleck at the 10 o'clock edge of the yellow ring, E), to stage 3 hole (F). Prehole opacity barely visible overlying the inferotemporal border of hole.
G–J: Progressive enlargement of can opener-type stage 2 hole (arrows) that began at the 2:30 to 3:30 o'clock margin of the yellow ring (G). (See Figure 7.11G.) When last examined the hole extended from 1:30 to 8 o'clock (J). Note the serrated inner edge of the yellow ring in H and I.
K and **L**: This eccentric can-opener tear extended 11 clock hours from 9:30 to 8:30.

(D–F and G–K, from Gass.[58];)

Table 7.1 Biomicroscopic classification of age-related macular hole

Stage	Biomicroscopic findings	Anatomic interpretation
1-A (impending hole)	Central yellow spot, loss of foveolar depression, no vitreofoveolar separation	Early serous detachment of foveolar retina
1-B (impending or occult hole)	Yellow ring with bridging interface, loss of foveolar depression, no vitreofoveolar separation	Small ring – serous foveolar detachment with lateral displacement of xanthophyll. Large ring – central occult foveolar hole with centrifugal displacement of foveolar retina and xanthophyll, with bridging contracted prefoveolar vitreous cortex. Cannot detect transition from impending to occult hole
2	Eccentric oval, crescent, or horseshoe retinal defect inside edge of yellow ring	Hole (tear) in periphery of contracted prefoveolar vitreous cortex bridging round retinal hole, no loss of foveolar retina. Central round retinal defect with rim of elevated retina
	With prefoveolar opacity	Hole with pseudo-operculum,* rim of retinal detachment, no posterior vitreous detachment from optic disc and macula
	Without prefoveolar opacity	Hole without pseudo-operculum or posterior vitreous detachment
3		Central round $\geq$ 400-μm-diameter retinal defect, no Weiss's ring, rim of elevated retina
	With prefoveolar opacity	Hole with pseudo-operculum, no posterior vitreous detachment from optic disc and periphery of macula
	Without prefoveolar opacity	Hole without pseudo-operculum, no posterior vitreous detachment from optic disc and macula
4	Central round retinal defect, rim of elevated retina, Weiss's ring	
	With small vitreous opacity near temporal edge of ring	Hole with pseudo-operculum, posterior vitreous detachment from optic disc and macula with mobile Weiss ring and pseudo-operculum†
	Without small opacity	Hole and posterior vitreous detachment from optic disc and macula without pseudo-operculum

*Pseudo-operculum contains no retinal receptors.
†Usually found near temporal border of Weiss's ring.

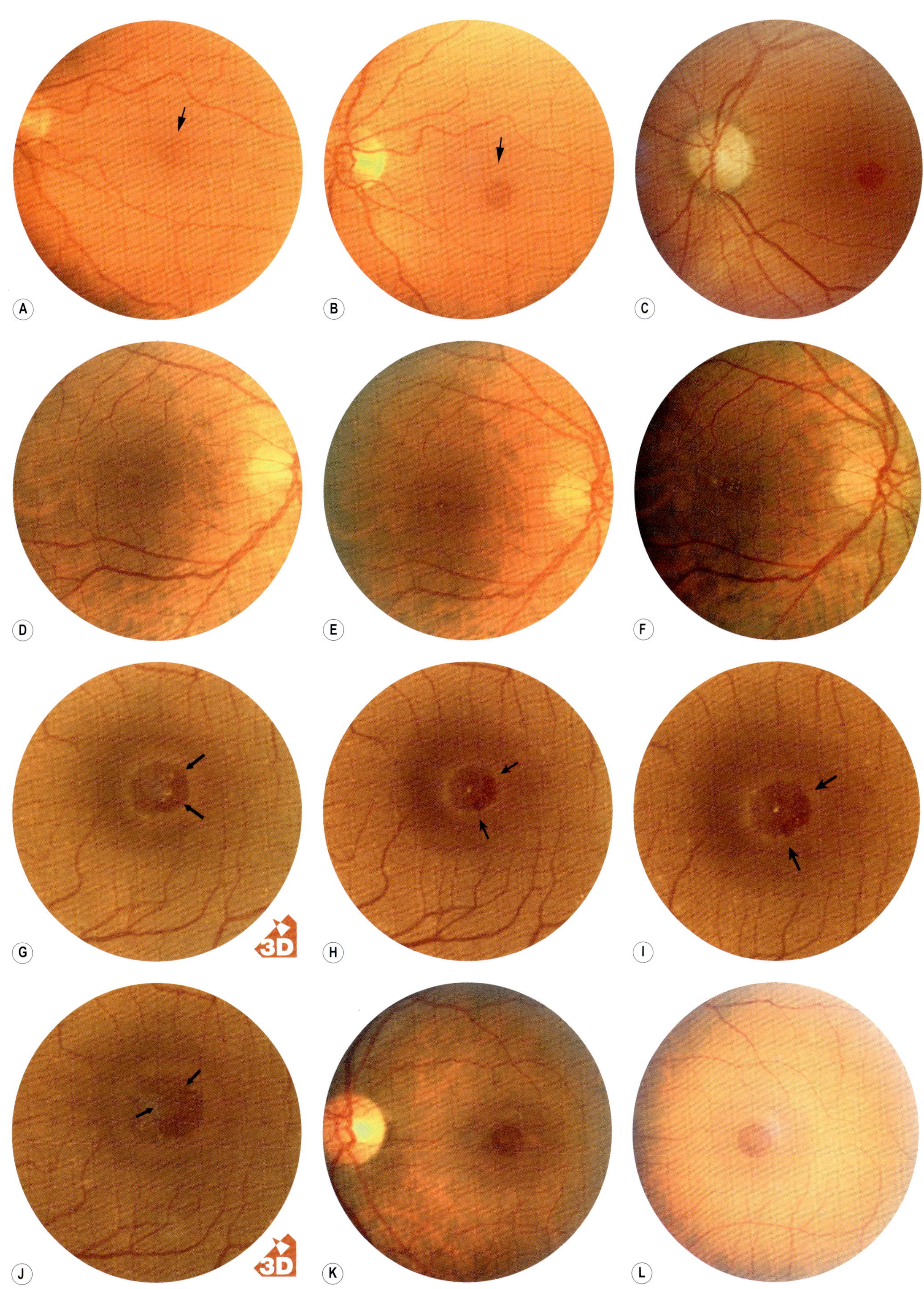
A
B
C
D
E
F
G
3D
H
I
J
3D
K
L

Pathology and Pathogenesis

Immunocytochemical labeling and electron microscopic examination of vitreous removed at the time of surgery for impending macular holes has demonstrated cortical vitreous containing RPE and glial cells.[75,110,111] Histopathologic examination of a macular hole has failed to demonstrate any evidence of either retinal or choroidal vascular disease as a cause for the development of a macular hole (Figure 7.15).[83,85,107,112] The edges of the hole are typically rounded, some cystic spaces in the outer plexiform and inner nuclear layers are often present, and there is frequently cellular proliferation from the edges of the hole on to the neighboring inner retinal surface (Figure 7.15E).[107] A cellular prehole opacity may occasionally be observed (Figure 7.15A and B). It is not known whether or not retinal receptor cells are included.

Nodular proliferations of the RPE overlying an eosinophilic material probably account for the yellowish deposits noted biomicroscopically in the depth of the macular hole (Figure 7.15C and D). These appear to be identical in structure to the reactive, proliferative type of drusen noted histopathologically in eyes with long-standing retinal detachment. Proliferation of the RPE is probably caused by loss of the RPE's contact with the outer segments of the retinal photoreceptors as well as its exposure to the vitreous.[85] There are two reports in which histopathologic examination of the second eye in patients with unilateral macular hole found cystic spaces in the outer plexiform layer in the paracentral macular area.[85,113] The fact that fluorescein angiography in asymptomatic second eyes, as well as in the affected eyes, shows no permeability alterations suggests that these cysts probably are not caused by abnormal retinal vascular permeability. In spite of these findings, which suggest that a slow process of cystic degeneration of the center of the fovea may predate the development of a macular hole, Gass's observations suggest that macular hole development is not preceded by a gradual change in either the appearance of the macula or visual function. On the contrary, its formation begins abruptly, although its full development usually occurs over a period of 2–3 months. There is no evidence to incriminate either the underlying RPE or the choroid in the pathogenesis of macular hole formation.[60,112,113] As discussed previously the primary tissues involved in macular hole formation involve the vitreoretinal interface region in the foveolar area. Electron microscopic study of a series of prefoveolar operculum-like structures collected at the time of macular hole surgery are needed to confirm the anatomic interpretation of the biomicroscopic stages of hole development suggested here by the author.[73]

The predilection for hole development to occur in women has suggested that ingestion of estrogenic compounds may be of importance in the pathogenesis of macular hole.[59,62,114]

7.13 Angiographic findings in stages of macular hole development.

A–C: A stage 1-A impending macular hole developed in a 62-year-old woman with a 4-day history of metamorphopsia in the left eye. She had previously developed a macular hole in the right eye (see I and J). Visual acuity in the left eye was 20/40. Note central yellow lesion (A). There were no cystic changes or evidence of a dehiscence in the retina. Angiography revealed slight fluorescence centrally (B). Twenty-six months later (C) a macular hole with an operculum was present and the patient's visual acuity was 20/70.
D–F: What appeared to be an inner lamellar macular hole (D) showed focal hyperfluorescence (E), suggesting the presence of an occult small stage 2 hole. Eight months later she showed evidence of the small stage 2 hole with a rim of retinal detachment.
G and H: Stage 3 macular hole in a 64-year-old woman with a visual acuity of 20/100. Note sharp margins of the hole, surrounding halo caused by retinal elevation and cystic degeneration of the retina, small yellow deposits that appear to lie on the surface of the retinal pigment epithelium, and small prehole opacity lying just anterior to the retina and partly obscuring the underlying yellow deposits from view. The retinal vessels are within normal limits. Fluorescein angiography (H) revealed a circumscribed area of hyperfluorescence corresponding to the size of the retinal hole. This fluorescence faded within 1 hour. The parafoveal capillary bed was within normal limits.
I and J: Stage 3 macular hole with prehole opacity in a 62-year-old woman with a 3-year history of loss of vision in the right eye and a 4-day history of distortion of vision in the left eye (see A–C). Vision in the right eye was 20/200. Angiography (J) revealed hyperfluorescence corresponding to the area of the hole and obstruction of this fluorescence by the prehole opacity.
K and L: A long-standing macular hole and localized retinal detachment surrounded by an epiretinal membrane. Angiography showed that the white opacities within the hole were nonfluorescent (L). Note rim of hyperfluorescence around the hole showing evidence of loss of pigment from the retinal pigment epithelium in the area of long-standing retinal detachment surrounding the hole.

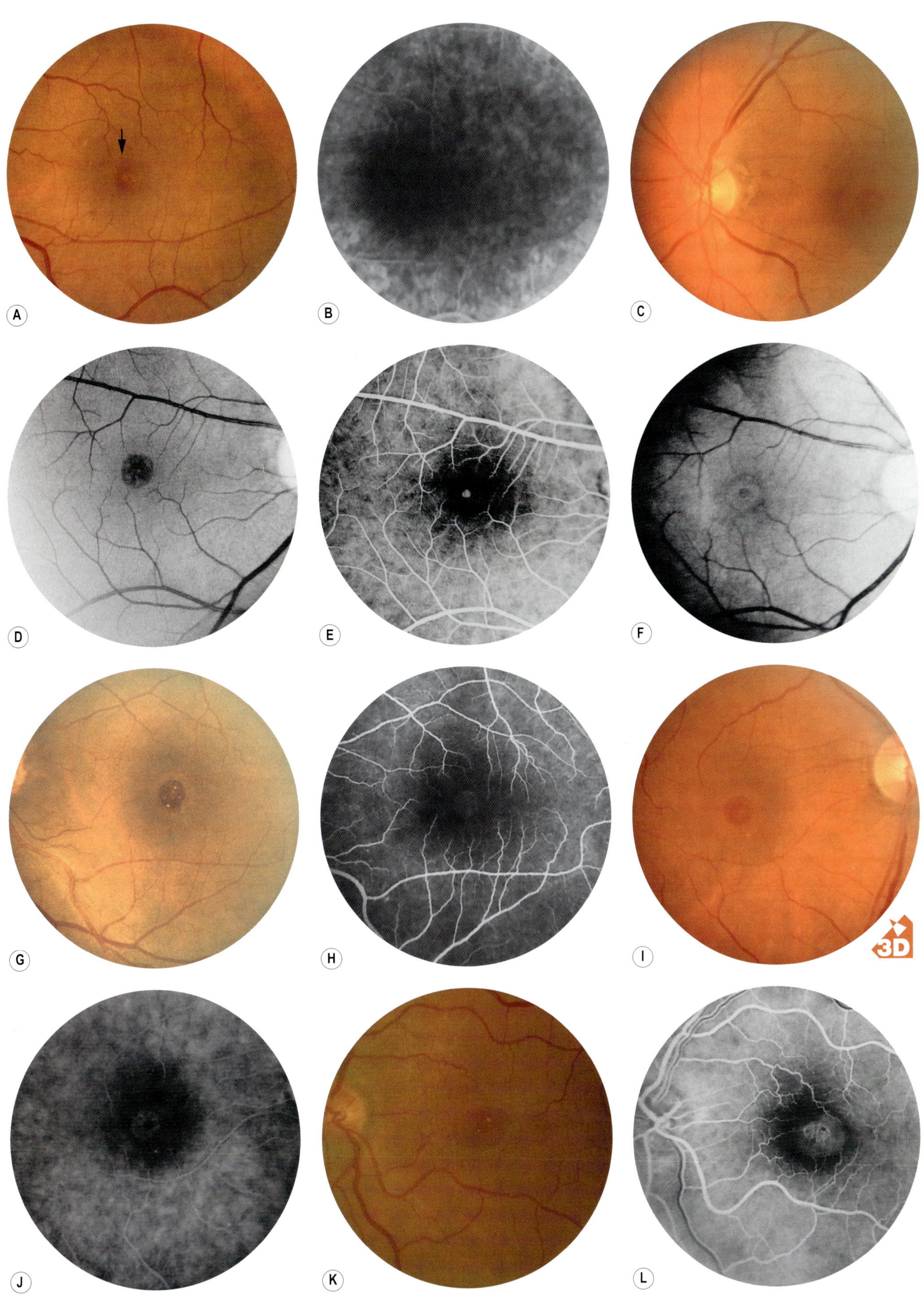
A
B
C
D
E
F
G
H
I
3D
J
K
L

Treatment

In 1988 surgical separation of the PVC was suggested as a possible treatment to prevent hole formation in patients with stage 1 impending macula holes.[58] Uncontrolled pilot studies of vitreous surgery for treatment of impending macular holes suggested that the surgery might be of benefit.[47,111,121–125] The criteria used for an impending hole by these authors, however, were not confined to those of a stage 1 impending hole as defined by this author.[58] Furthermore, there are many lesions that may simulate a stage 1 hole and misdiagnosis of an impending hole is frequent.[84] A randomized, multicenter clinical trial to evaluate the effectiveness of surgical peeling of the vitreous for treatment of an impending macular hole in one eye in patients with a stage 3 or 4 hole in the fellow eye was organized in 1988.[126] The results of this study of 62 patients showed that approximately 40% of eyes in both groups developed a full-thickness hole. The study was discontinued before definite conclusions could be reached because of a dramatic drop in patient recruitment coinciding with enthusiastic reports concerning treatment of full-thickness holes. With the following available information: (1) that 40–60% of stage 1 holes spontaneously abort; (2) that there is a high incidence of misdiagnosis of stage 1 holes; and (3) the apparently favorable results of surgery for full-thickness holes, it is probably prudent to observe patients with a stage 1 impending hole, particularly when the fellow eye is normal.

7.14 Aborted stages of development of a macular hole.

A–C: This woman with a macular hole in the fellow eye developed blurred vision and a stage 1-B lesion in the right eye (A and top part of C). Several weeks later her symptoms disappeared and her visual acuity and fundus returned to normal (B and bottom part of C1). Arrow in C1 indicates pseudo-operculum that was faintly visible biomicroscopically. This 70-year-old man noted metamorphopsia while reading, of 3 weeks' duration. His visual acuity had decreased to 20/40 and careful biomicroscopic examination revealed vitreous traction over the foveola. Optical coherence tomography confirmed foveolar elevation secondary to posterior hyaloid traction (arrow C2 above). He was observed and returned 6 weeks later with a Weiss ring and restoration of visual acuity to 20/20 (C2, below).

D–F: This man with a macular hole in his fellow eye developed metamorphopsia and blurred vision in the left eye caused by a stage 1-A impending macular hole. His symptoms improved spontaneously and examination revealed a large inner lamellar macular hole and prehole opacity (D). Note the sharply defined scalloped edges and absence of a rim of detachment. Angiography showed only faint fluorescence (E). F indicates the probable anatomy of this lesion. His visual acuity in this eye has remained 20/25+ for 5 years.

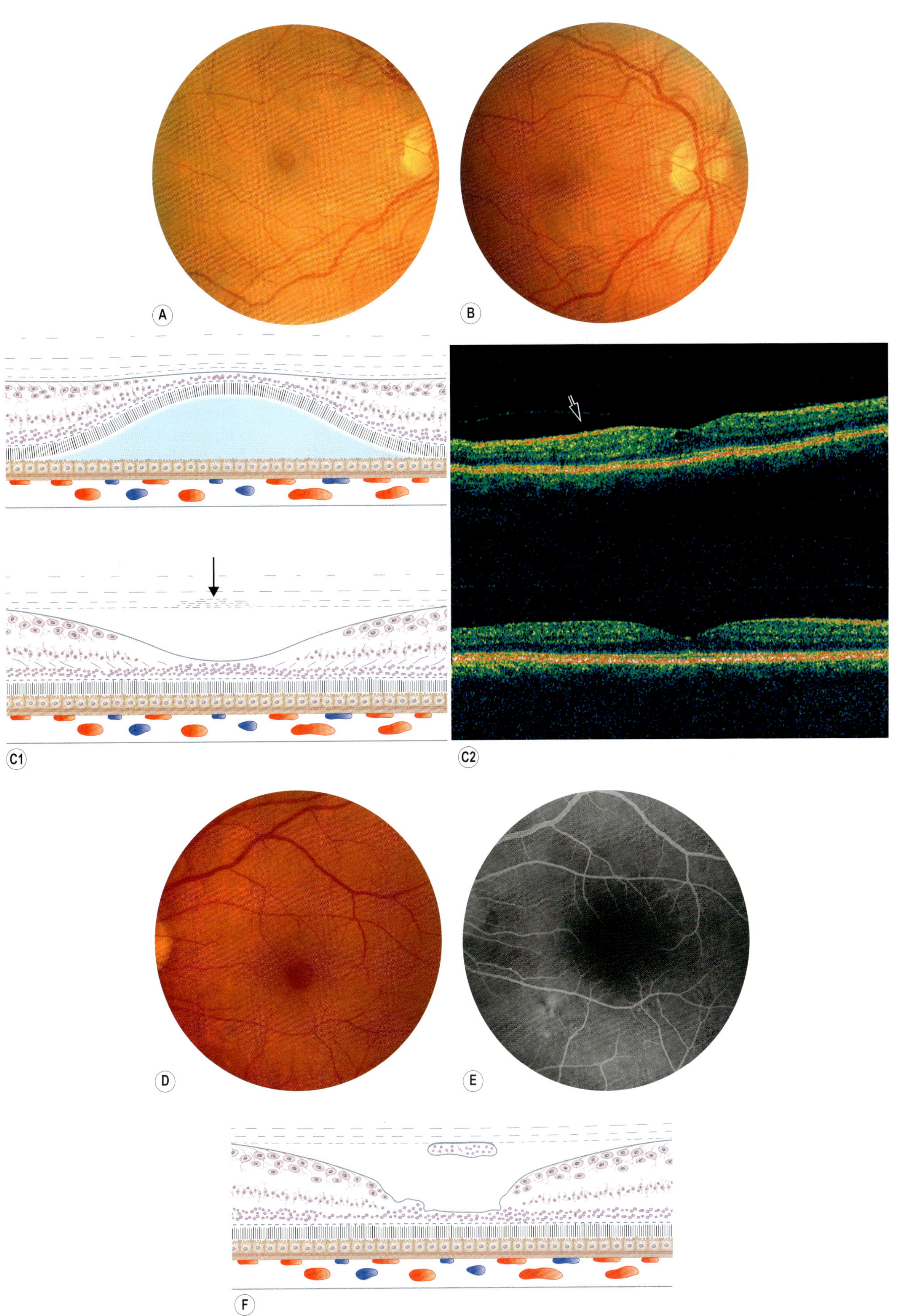
A
B
C1
C2
D
E
F

7.14 Continued

G–I: This woman noted blurred vision and metamorphopsia in the right eye associated with a stage 1-B lesion (G). She improved spontaneously and her visual acuity improved to 20/30. Note the pair of paracentral inner lamellar holes (arrow, I).

J: Note the small inner lamellar hole (arrow) associated with 20/20 visual acuity in this man with a stage 3 hole and 20/200 visual acuity in his fellow eye.

K and L: Radiating retina folds associated with stellate contracted prefoveolar vitreous cortex associated with 20/30 visual acuity in a woman who probably spontaneously aborted an impending macular hole.

Kelly and Wendel in 1991,[127] Glaser and colleagues in 1992,[128] Poliner and Tornambe in 1992,[129] and others,[45,130–134] in uncontrolled pilot studies, reported successful closure of macular holes and visual improvement using pars plana vitrectomy, intraocular gas, and 1–2 weeks of face-down positioning (Figure 7.18). Glaser's group used a tissue growth factor, TGF-β, to stimulate proliferation of glial cells to seal the hole. Some surgeons have used the patient's serum in lieu of TGF-β.[135] The visual results obtained by all of these investigators were similar in those eyes with successful reattachment of the retina. Approximately 70% obtained improvement of two lines of visual acuity or better, and 20–40% regained 20/40 or better. These same authors, who originally obtained only approximately a 50% reattachment rate, have reported at recent meetings successful reattachment in 90–95% of cases and return of acuity to 20/40 or better in approximately 50% of cases (Figure 7.19A–F). Reoperation of eyes with failed macular hole surgery may result in visual improvement.[136,137]

Since first conceptualized in 1999, removal of the ILM at the time of the vitrectomy has vastly improved the rate of hole closure and decreased the need for repeat surgery. Various methods to stain or delineate the transparent ILM have been employed using indocyanine green (ICG), trypan blue, and triamcinolone. Toxicity with use of ICG appears to be variable and related to the longer duration of the surgery and the higher intensity of the illuminating light. Surgical complications have included retinal tears with and without retinal detachment; retinal vascular occlusion; light toxicity pigment epitheliopathy; cataract; acute permanent loss of temporal visual field, probably caused by damage to the nasal part of the optic disc during fluid–gas exchange; and reopening of the macular hole.[127–129,136,138–141] A controlled clinical trial randomizing patients with full-thickness holes to surgery or to observation is under way, and over 150 patients have been randomized.[142]

Following successful reattachment of the retina after surgery for a macular hole, the macula may return to a nearly normal appearance, the hyperfluorescence corresponding with the hole preoperatively often disappears, and a central scotoma may no longer be demonstrable.[76,80] A few patients may regain 20/20 visual acuity.[96] These surgical results were difficult to explain on the basis of the initial anatomic interpretation of the biomicroscopic stages of hole development.[58] The prehole opacity seen in 75–80% of patients was originally thought to represent an operculum containing the foveolar retina; this operculum was thought to be derived from a circumferential tear occurring in the periphery of a stage 1-B lesion, and significant improvement of vision even with reattachment of the retina around the hole was thought unlikely. Evidence now strongly suggests that nearly all macular holes begin as an occult central foveolar dehiscence at the umbo and that hole development is the result of centrifugal sliding and retraction of the receptors away from the center of the hole analogous to the opening of a lens diaphragm. It is understandable that surgical reattachment of the retina around the hole, when accompanied by reactive glial cell proliferation and contraction, may result in "closure of the lens diaphragm" and return of the foveal retina to its near-normal anatomic position and function in some patients (Figures 7.18 and 7.19). The disappearance of the focal hyperfluorescence corresponding with the hole, and of the absolute central scotomas that occur in some patients after successful macular hole surgery, is further evidence in support of the concept of centripetal movement of the paracentral retinal receptors and the xanthophyll.[76]

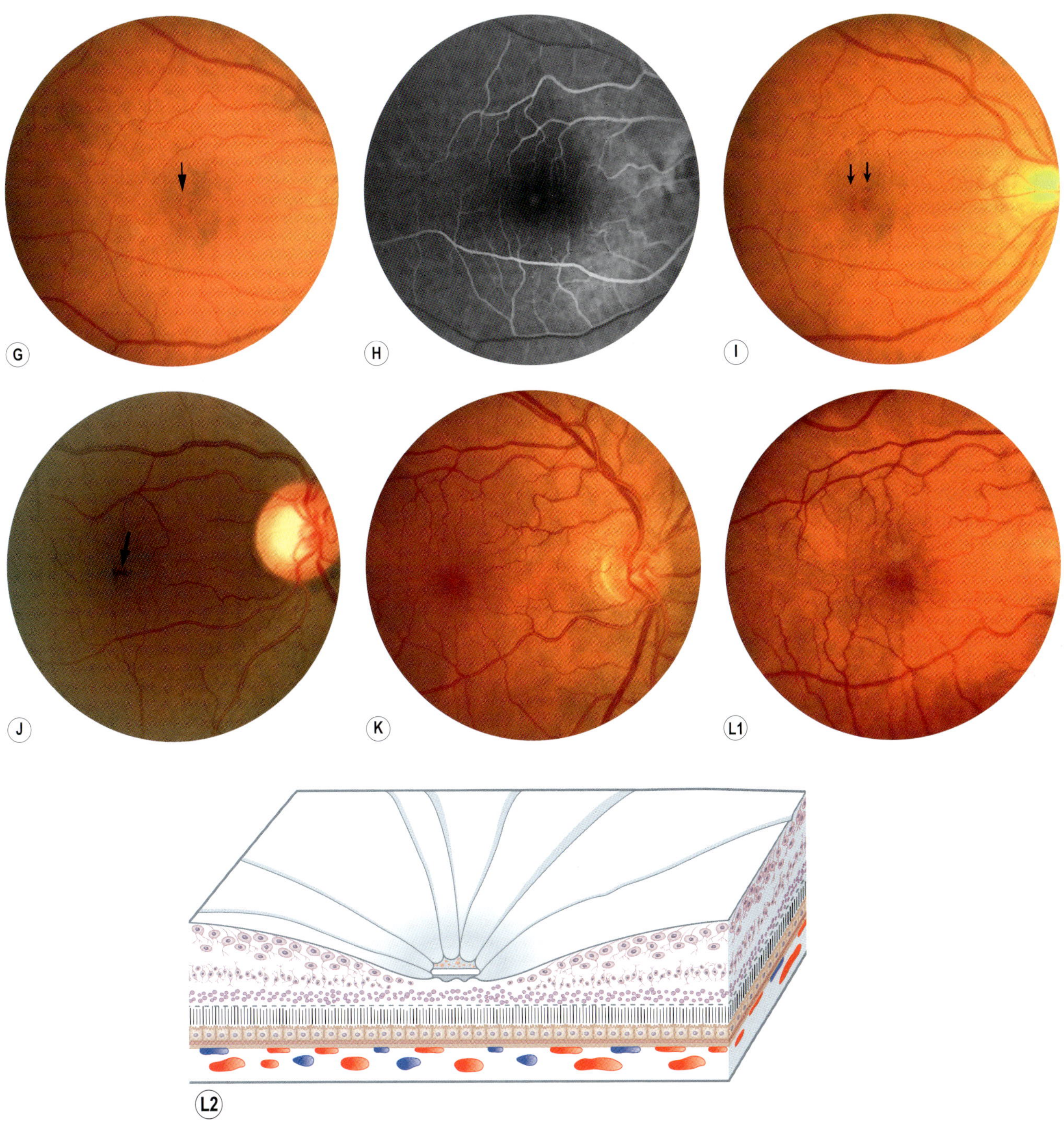
G
H
I
J
K
L1
L2

The criteria for recommending surgery for a macular hole have evolved over the past 20 years. At the start most patients undergoing surgery had symptoms for a year or less, visual acuity of 20/70 or worse, and a large stage 2 or stage 3 or 4 macular hole. The results of a randomized study and other reports broadened to include early stage 2 holes and holes of longer duration. Although the likelihood for progression to a stage 2 hole is probably directly related to the diameter of the stage 1-B yellow ring and the level of visual acuity loss, there is no reliable information or method at this time to determine which stage 1-B lesions will progress to hole formation.[58]

The patient considering surgery for a macular hole in one eye and having normal function in the fellow eye should be aware of the following: (1) chances of developing a hole in the fellow eye are 10–15% and probably less than 5% in the presence of vitreofoveal separation; and (2) treatment usually involves two operations, including cataract surgery.[145,146]

Laser treatment to the edge of macular holes has had minimal success in improving visual function.[147,148] The treatment has no rationale as far as preventing further retinal detachment in patients with senile macular holes is concerned since the detachment involves only the central macular area and is unlikely to cause extensive detachment in these patients with relatively emmetropic eyes.[95] There is less chance for visual improvement following surgical treatment of macular holes associated with other diseases, such as diabetic retinopathy, Behçet's disease, or for holes caused by trauma.[149]

7.15 Histopathology of an idiopathic senile macular hole.

A: Gross photograph showing retinal "operculum" (arrow) suspended in front of the hole.
B: Photomicrograph of retinal "operculum" shown in A demonstrates glial cells but no definite evidence of retinal photoreceptor cells. This may be the balled-up nodule of contracted prefoveolar fibroglial membrane and not an operculum.
C: Histopathology of full-thickness macular hole with nodular proliferations of the retinal pigment epithelium (RPE) in the base of the hole (arrows).
D: High-power view of change in the RPE shown in A (arrows). Note that the underlying choroid is within normal limits.
E: High-power view of the edge of the hole shown in C. Note the extension of retinal glial cells (arrow) on to the anterior surface of the retina.
F: Long-standing macular hole with demarcation ring (arrows) composed of proliferated RPE cells. GR2 IJRT, grade 2 idiopathic juxtafoveolar retinal telangiectasia.
G: Macular hole with reattachment of its edges.
H: Inner lamellar macular hole.

(A and B, from Frangieh et al.[85]; G and H, from Guyer et al.[107])

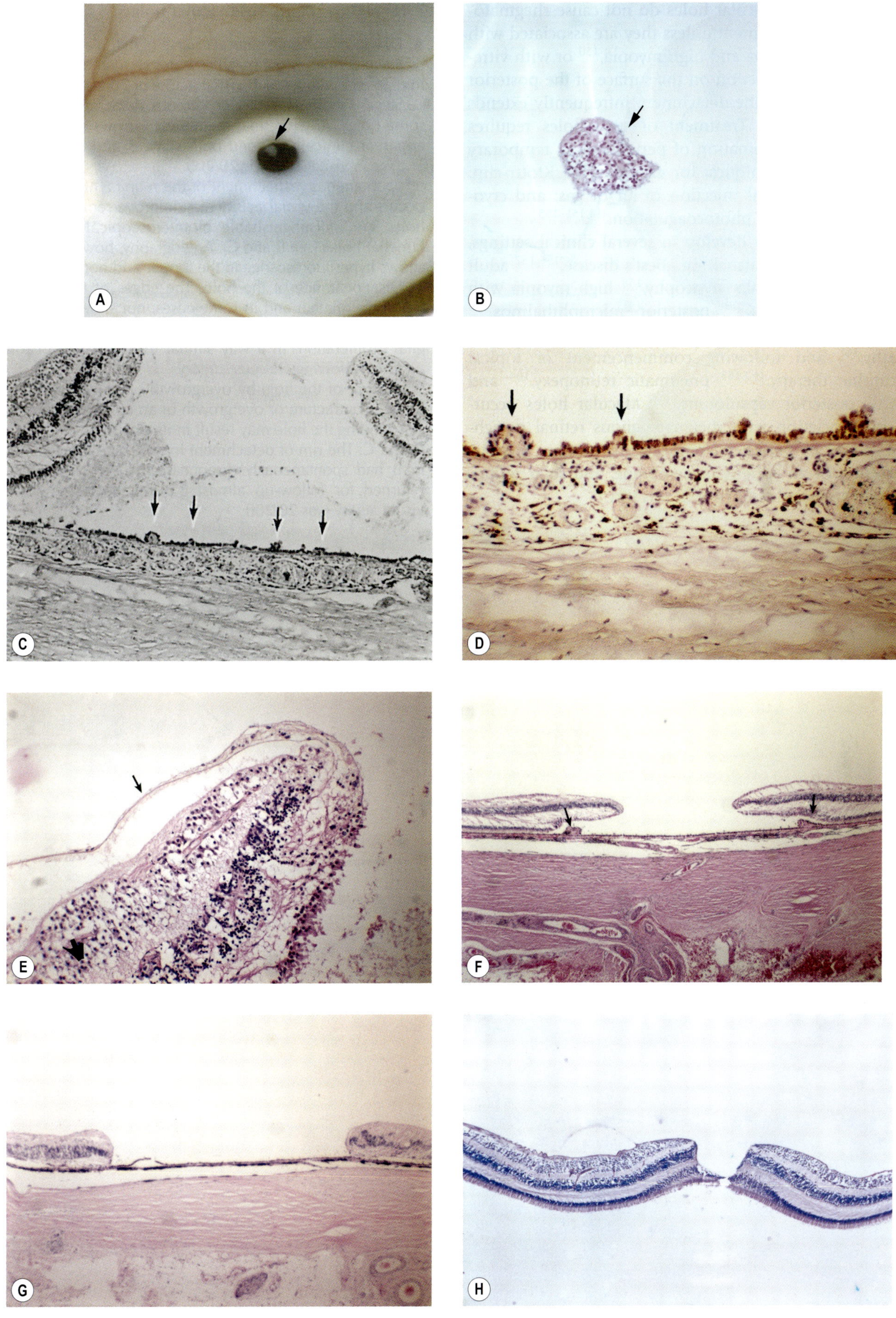
A
B
C
D
E
F
G
H

Differential Diagnosis

Most patients referred to the author with a diagnosis of a stage 1-A impending hole have had a foveolar yellow lesion caused by one of the following: solitary drusen, small RPE detachment, idiopathic central serous chorioretinopathy, foveolar detachment with epiretinal membrane, bilateral idiopathic juxtafoveolar retinal telangiectasis, pattern dystrophy, cystoid macular edema, and solar maculopathy (Figure 7.17).[84]

Lesions that may simulate a full-thickness macula hole include an inner lamellar macular hole (Figure 7.14D), a hole in an epiretinal membrane (Figures 7.17J–L and see Figure 7.21A), geographic atrophy of the RPE (Figure 7.17G–I), choroidal neovascularization, a small focal area of central serous chorioretinopathy, cystoid macular edema with a large central cyst (Figure 7.17A–C), focal retinal atrophy associated with bilateral juxtafoveal retinal telangiectasis (Figure 7.17D and E) congenital optic pit, and a solitary macular cyst, a lesion that rarely occurs.[105,115–117] Features of a full-thickness macular hole that differentiate it from most simulating lesions are the presence of a halo of retinal detachment surrounding the hole, yellow deposits within the depth of the hole, and a zone of hyperfluorescence corresponding to the size of the hole during the early stages of angiography. Use of the slit-beam test (Watzke sign), 50-μm-size aiming beam laser perimetry, OCT, and fluorescein angiography are helpful adjuncts to contact lens examination in arriving at the correct diagnosis. Echography is capable of detecting PVD and the presence of pseudo-opercula but appears to be no better than contact lens examination in this regard.[118–120]

7.17 Lesions simulating a macular hole.

A–C: Idiopathic cystoid macular edema (CME) was associated with a large central cyst (A and C) that was mistaken for a macular hole in this man. Angiography revealed the correct diagnosis (B).
D–F: Bilateral idiopathic juxtafoveolar telangiectasis was the cause of the focal atrophy of the retina (D and F) that was incorrectly diagnosed as a macular hole, before the angiogram (E) was obtained.
G–I: Geographic atrophy of the outer retina and retinal pigment epithelium caused by age-related macular degeneration (G and I) and focal hyperfluorescence (H) was responsible for the incorrect diagnosis of a macular hole in this elderly patient.

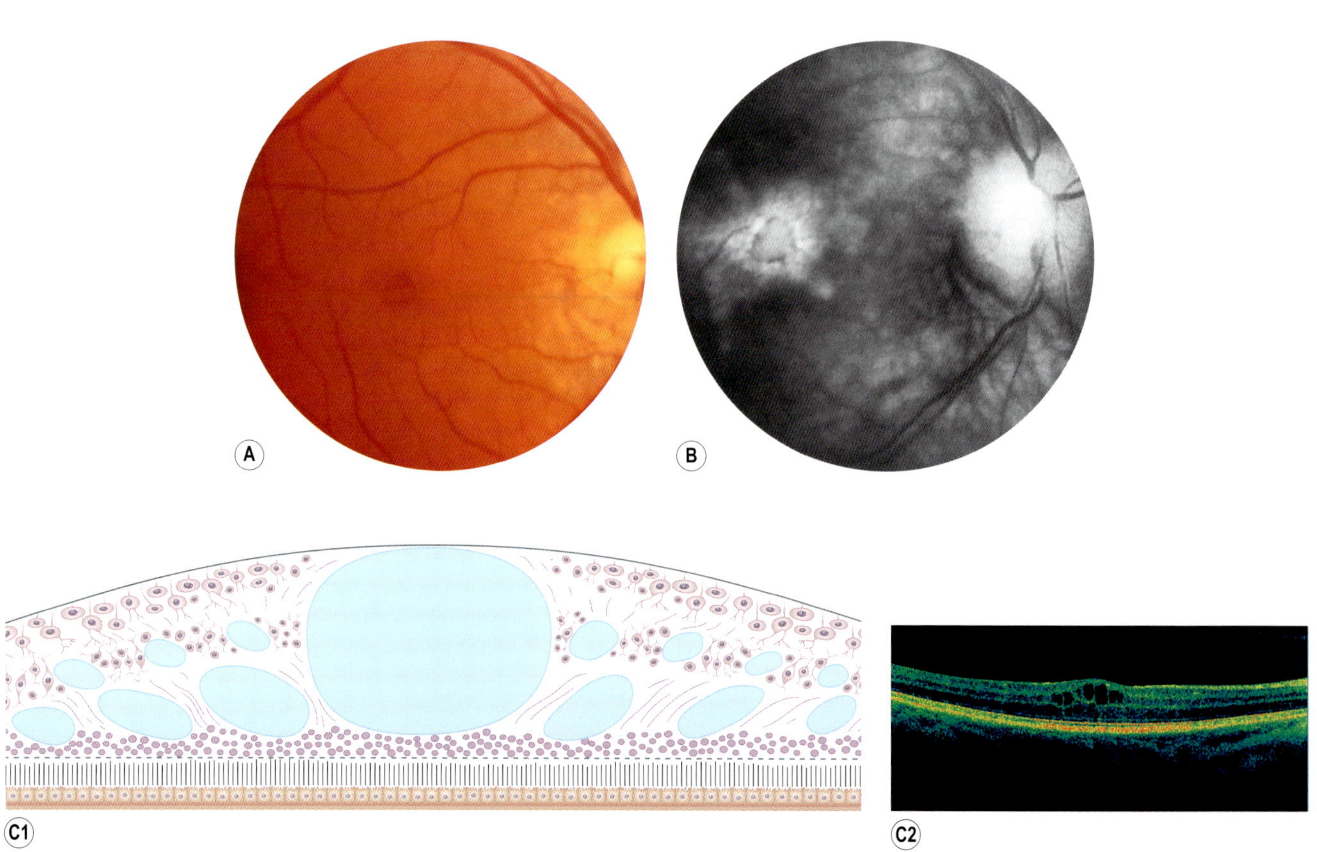

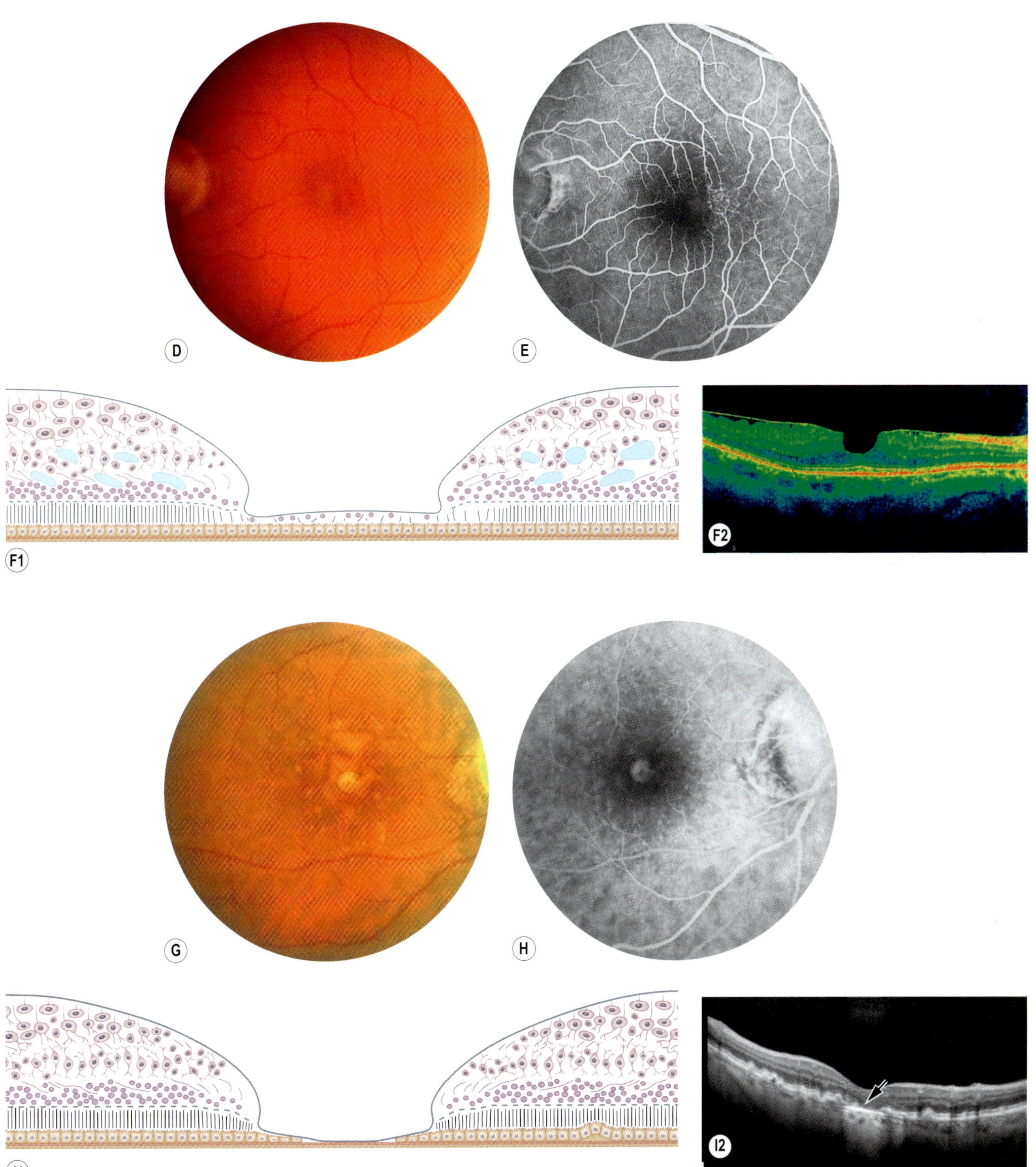
D
E
F1
F2
G
H
I1
I2

7.17 Continued

J–L: This patient, who had a macular hole in the right eye, had no complaints in the left eye. Visual acuity was 20/20. A circular rim of condensed vitreous lying on the inner retinal surface centrally (J) and minimal evidence of crinkling of the inner retinal surface suggested the presence of an occult perifoveolar epiretinal membrane (L). There was no evidence of posterior vitreous detachment. She soon developed a posterior vitreous separation, mild visual blurring, and definite evidence of a pericentral epiretinal membrane (K).

7.18 Diagram of surgical repair of macular hole.

A: Preoperative appearance of stage 3 hole. Arrow indicates contracted vitreous cortex (pseudo-operculum) attached to the layer of vitreous gel lying between the liquefied vitreous (premacular bursa) and the retinal hole.
B: Postoperative appearance after vitrectomy, surgical peeling of cortical vitreous, and intravitreal gas injection. With the patient in the face-down position, the bubble compresses the edges of the hole against the retinal pigment epithelium.
C–E: Enlarged views to show that proliferation and contraction of retinal glial cells cause centripetal movement of the retina and closure of the hole.
F–I: This 68-year-old woman had a visual decline to 20/80– over 3 months. She had a stage 2 hole with an eccentric operculum still attached to the foveal edge (F and G). Her vision improved to 20/30 following a vitrectomy with internal limiting membrane peel leading to hole closure (H).
J and K: This 60-year-old woman showed closure of hole and gain of full foveal thickness over 6 months following a vitrectomy and internal limiting membrane peel.

(J and K, courtesy of Dr. Franco Recchia.)

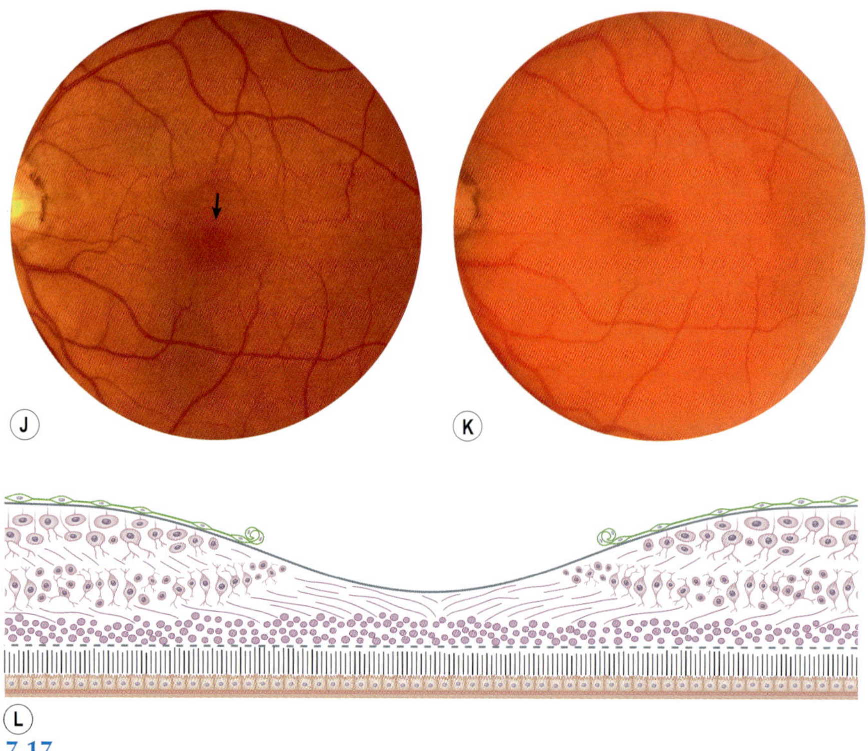

7.17

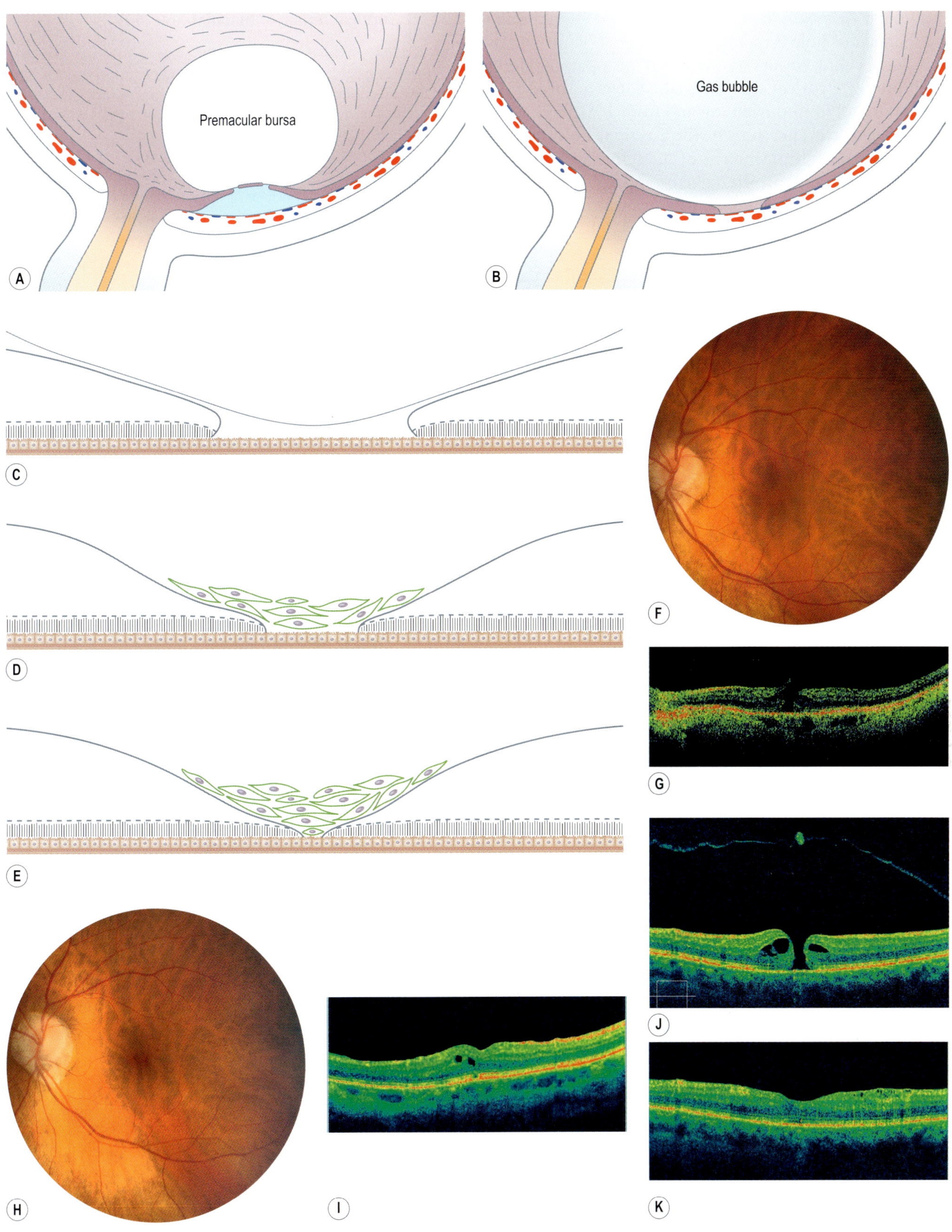
Premacular bursa
Gas bubble
A
B
C
D
E
F
G
H
I
J
K

Limited histopathologic information also supports this mechanism of hole formation and closure (Figure 7.19D–G). Funata and coworkers examined histopathologically both eyes of a patient whose visual acuity improved from 20/400 to 20/30 in the left eye and from 20/400 to 20/40 in the right eye after surgery for a retinal hole.[143] They found successful reattachment of the retina in both eyes. Closure of the hole in the right eye was associated with glial proliferation and probable centripetal inward drawing of the retinal receptors (Figure 7.19D–F). In the left eye retinal reattachment was unassociated with gliosis. Madreperla et al. reported their findings in another patient whose preoperative visual acuity was 20/80 and postoperative acuity was 20/40.[144] One month postoperatively the patient died and histopathologic examination showed closure of the hole and close approximation of the retinal receptors centrally by proliferating Müller cells (Figure 7.19G).

7.19 Surgical repair of macular hole.

A–C: Preoperative appearance of stage 3 macular hole (A). Visual acuity, 20/80. Angiogram showed fluorescence centrally. Postoperative appearance (B). Visual acuity, 20/20. The hole was no longer evident. Angiogram (C) showed a ring of persistent fluorescence.
D–F: Preoperative appearance of a stage 3 hole (D). Visual acuity was 20/200. Postoperative appearance (E). Visual acuity was 20/40. Histopathologic examination of the eye obtained at autopsy shows closure of hole by proliferating glial cells (arrow, F).
G: Histopathology of a macular hole following surgical repair shows reapproximation of the hole edges (arrows) by Müller cell proliferation.

(A–D, courtesy of Dr. William E. Smiddy; E–G from Funata et al.[143])

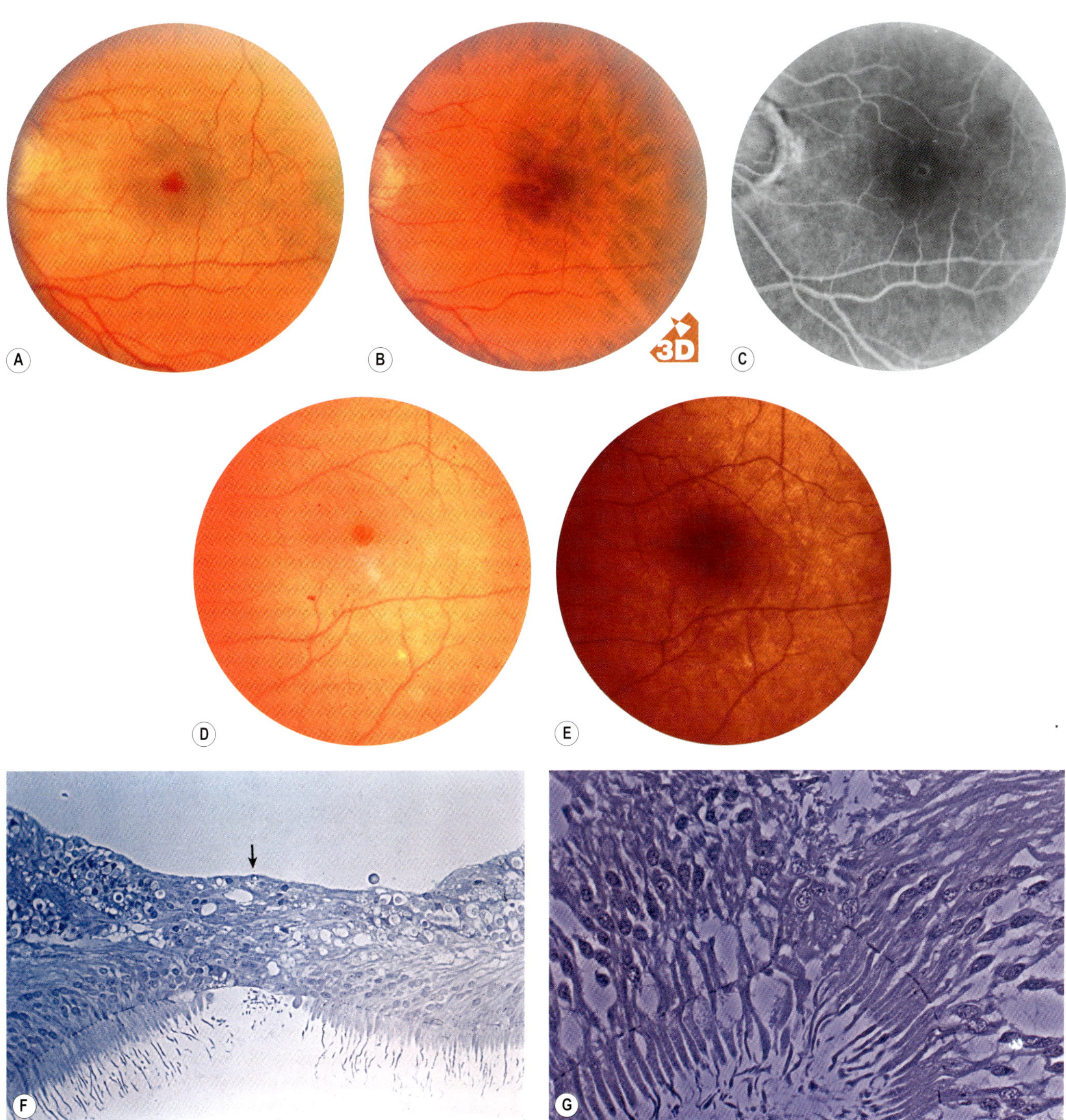
A
B
3D
C
D
E
F
G

MACULAR DYSFUNCTION CAUSED BY EPIRETINAL MEMBRANE CONTRACTION

After partial or complete PVD, a translucent or semitranslucent fibrocellular membrane may become apparent ophthalmoscopically and biomicroscopically on the inner retinal surface in the macular area (Figure 7.07C–G). In approximately 25% of cases similar membranes may develop before development of a PVD (Figure 7.09A–C). Anomalous PVD due to splitting of the cortical vitreous lamellae may leave a residual cellular membrane over the retinal surface that proliferates and contracts, resulting in an epiretinal membrane.[22,35,166]

The contraction or shrinkage of this epiretinal membrane produces varying degrees of distortion, intraretinal edema, and degeneration of the underlying retina (Figures 7.20 and 7.21).[83,167–170]

Epiretinal membranes may be classified according to the severity of retinal distortion, associated biomicroscopic changes, and associated ocular disorders.

Classification of Epiretinal Membranes According to Severity of Retinal Distortion

Grade 0: "Cellophane Maculopathy"

In cellophane maculopathy the membrane may be completely translucent and may be unassociated with any distortion of the inner retinal surface. The only ophthalmoscopic or biomicroscopic clue to its presence is a "cellophane" light reflex coming from the inner retinal surface.

7.20 Epiretinal membrane.

A: Diagram showing crinkled cellophane maculopathy associated with fine irregular wrinkles of the inner retinal layers.
B: Diagram showing macular pucker. Coarse retinal folds often associated with retinal edema, cystic degeneration, and localized detachment.
C–E: This patient developed metamorphopsia caused by a small juxtafoveolar epiretinal membrane (arrows). Note retinal folds radiating outward from the region of the membrane. Some of these pass through the macula. Fundus painting (D) of the same patient illustrating the relationship of the epiretinal membrane (arrow) to the underlying retina. Angiography revealed mild tortuosity of the retinal vessels in the region of the membrane (E).
F: Semitranslucent epiretinal membrane causing distortion of the macula of this 55-year-old patient, who had no other evidence of intraocular disease. Contraction of the membrane has pulled the paramacular vessels toward the horizontal raphe.
G: Epiretinal membrane lying in the central area of the macula in this 14-year-old girl, who had no other evidence of ocular disease. Note retinal folds radiating outward from the macula.
H: Prominent epiretinal membrane in a 40-year-old man whose visual acuity was 20/20.
I–K: Epiretinal membrane causing macular pucker in a 72-year-old man who had no other evidence of intraocular disease. Visual acuity was 20/400. Several small holes with an appearance similar to Swiss cheese were present in the retina superior to the macula (arrow, I). Beneath these holes was a small amount of subretinal fluid. This patient has been observed for approximately 8 years with no change. Angiography revealed marked central displacement of the paramacular retinal vessels (J), early leakage of dye from the retinal capillaries, and an irregular pattern of fluorescein staining in the retina (K and L). The typical cystoid pattern is not apparent because of the marked distortion of the retinal architecture.

Grade 1: "Crinkled Cellophane Maculopathy"

Following contraction or shrinkage of the epiretinal membrane, the underlying inner retinal surface may be gathered into a series of small irregular folds. These alterations produce an irregular, iridescent light reflex, which may be likened to that stemming from the surface of cellophane that has been rolled into a ball and reopened into a sheet containing many fine irregular crinkles on its surface (Figures 7.7G, 7.9A, and 7.20A, C, and F). Biomicroscopically, details of the underlying small retinal vessels may be indistinct. Fine, superficial radiating retinal folds extend outward from the margins of the contracted membrane and are often the most prominent sign indicating the presence of an epiretinal membrane (Figure 7.20C and D). OCT demonstrates fine superficial wrinkles in the inner retina (Figure 7.20L). The membrane is often centered in the perifoveal area but may occasionally extend across the full width of the macula. The wrinkling may be sufficient to produce tortuosity of the fine macular capillaries. If the area of membrane contraction is sufficiently large, it produces tortuosity of the underlying paramacular vessels and displaces the surrounding retinal vessels toward the fovea (Figure 7.20F). Some patients show multiple focal areas of preretinal membrane contraction in the posterior pole. Cystoid macular

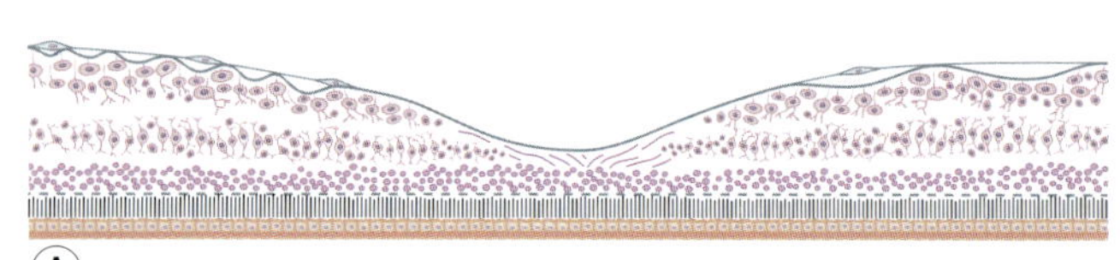

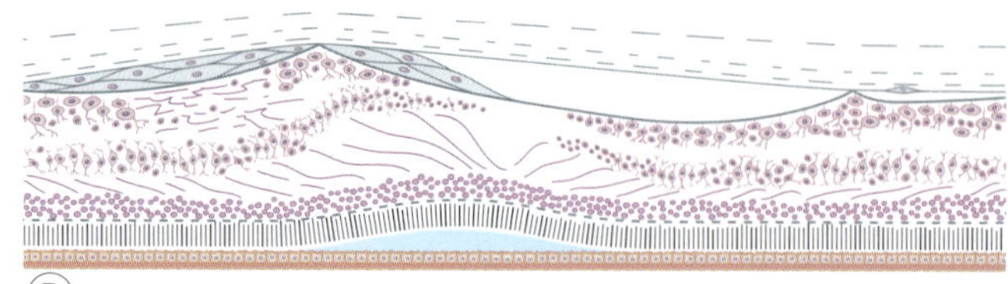

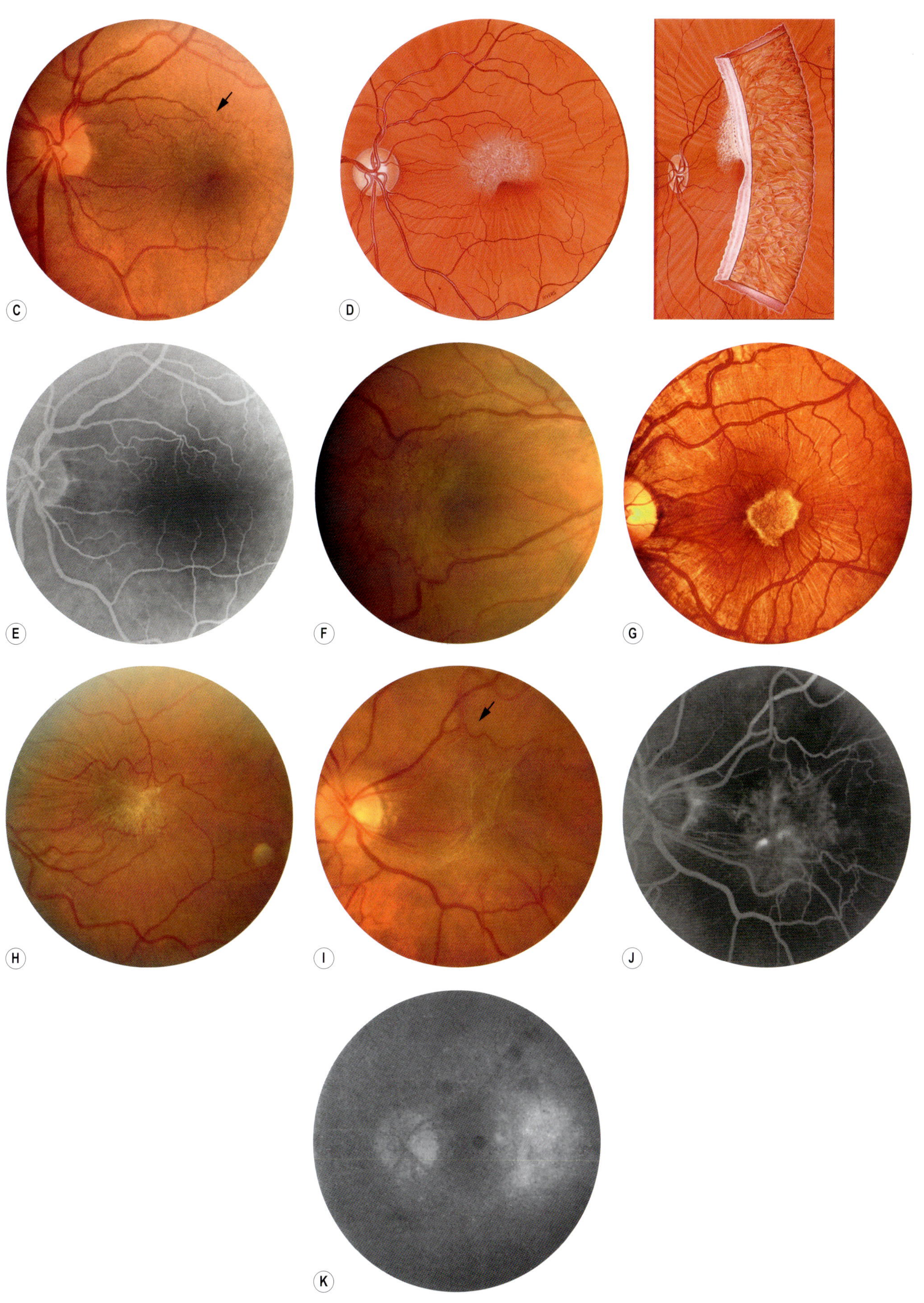
C
D
E
F
G
H
I
J
K

edema, retinal hemorrhages, retinal exudates, and disturbances of the RPE are typically absent except in those cases in which the vitreoretinal interface changes are either secondary to or incidental to other choroidal and retinal diseases. Vitreous degenerative changes and a PVD are often present. Inflammatory cells are usually not present. When seen they suggest that an underlying inflammatory disease is present and that the inflammation is more likely the cause of, rather than the result of, the epiretinal membrane. Many patients with grade 1 membranes have normal acuity and are asymptomatic. OCT may show mild flattening of the foveal depression, without retinal thickening or cysts (Figure 7.20L). Some patients are seen because of a mild visual disturbance in one eye. The patient is often unable to date the onset of the visual complaint. Acuity is typically reduced to a level no worse than 20/40. Metamorphopsia is demonstrable in patients with reduced acuity. The reduction in acuity caused by an epiretinal membrane is primarily related to the distortion produced in the outer retinal layers (photoreceptors) and not to the size or degree of translucency of the membrane. Visual acuity may be unaffected in some patients with prominent centrally located membranes (Figure 7.20H). This latter type of membrane probably is caused by centripetal sliding of the contracting membrane along the ILM.

Grade 2: "Macular Pucker"

The epiretinal membrane may be sufficiently dense to be visible as a distinct grayish membrane on the inner retinal surface (Figures 7.20B, G–I, and 7.22A). It may partly obscure the underlying retinal vessels. In such cases the degree of retinal distortion and crinkling is usually marked, and gross puckering of the macula may be present (Figures 7.20I, 7.22A and C–E, and 7.23C). Retinal edema, small retinal hemorrhages, cotton-wool exudates, and localized serous detachment of the retina may accompany prominent preretinal vitreous membrane formation and contraction. A Weiss ring is present in over 90% of cases.

Soon after the development of severe macular distortion, angiography usually shows leakage of dye from the underlying retinal vessels and evidence of retinal edema (Figure 7.20J and K). Because of retinal distortion, the pattern of dye staining is irregular and not typical of cystoid macular edema. In a matter of weeks or months there is usually a reduction in the amount of retinal edema and dye leakage. Visual acuity is usually significantly affected. It may be less than 20/200 if the macula is severely puckered. In many instances patients are unable to date the onset of their symptoms. In others, they may suddenly experience central photopsia and loss of central vision (Figure 7.23C). Metamorphopsia is usually demonstrable in these cases in which the entire thickness of the retina is affected by wrinkling.

Epiretinal membranes responsible for puckering of the retina may be eccentrically located in the paracentral region, including the area of the optic disc, in which case loss of macular function is primarily caused by tractional displacement as well as distortion of the foveal area (Figure 7.22C–E). Contraction of a juxtapapillary epiretinal membrane may occasionally be mistaken for papilledema or juxtapapillary combined RPE and retinal hamartoma.

7.21 Spontaneous contraction of a perifoveolar epiretinal membrane causing a picture simulating a macular hole.

A–C: Hole in epiretinal membrane simulating a macular hole in an asymptomatic 64-year-old woman who had 20/15 visual acuity and normal Amsler grid, static, and kinetic perimetric findings in this eye. Note the fine crinkling of the inner retinal surface surrounding the hole in an epiretinal membrane and the fine retinal folds radiating outward from the macular area (A). Angiography showed no abnormality (B). OCT and diagram (C) shows fibrocellular epiretinal membrane (arrow, above) before contraction, and after contraction (below) and formation of a pseudomacular hole. The membrane surrounds but does not cover the foveal area. B, Following spontaneous contraction of the epiretinal membrane. Shortening of the cells making up the epiretinal membrane produces an anterior and central displacement of the inner retinal layers to produce the clinical picture of a pseudomacular hole. Note that there is minimal or no distortion of the outer retinal layers or the retinal pigment epithelium.

D–F: Spontaneous partial closure of a hole in an epiretinal membrane occurred in this 69-year-old woman with a 2-month history of floaters in the right eye. Visual acuity in the right eye was 20/25 and in the left eye was 20/20. A posterior vitreous detachment and a few cells in the anterior and posterior vitreous in the right eye were present. Note the oval hole surrounded by an epiretinal membrane (D). Fluorescein angiography was normal. Fifteen months later visual acuity in the right eye was 20/50. Further contraction of the epiretinal membrane has narrowed the oval hole in the membrane to a horizontal slit that is now displaced temporal to the center of the macula (E). Diagram (F) illustrates the contraction of the epiretinal membrane and partial closure of the pseudomacular hole.

Classification of Epiretinal Membranes According to Associated Biomicroscopic Findings

Foveolar Hole in Epiretinal Membrane Simulating a Macular Hole (Pseudomacular Hole)

Spontaneous contraction of an epiretinal membrane that surrounds but does not cover the foveolar area may produce a biomicroscopic appearance simulating a full-thickness macular hole (Figures 7.17J–L, 7.21, and 7.24).[115,171–173] Most of these membranes probably develop before PVD and fail to cover the foveolar area because of the unusual degree of vitreoretinal adherence there. The patient usually has no complaints, and visual acuity is normal or nearly normal. Biomicroscopy reveals crinkling of the inner retinal surface surrounding the hole in the epiretinal membrane and a punched-out appearance in the area of the hole. As the slit beam is moved across the hole, there is usually a light reflex that is evidence of retinal tissue in the base of the hole. The foveal

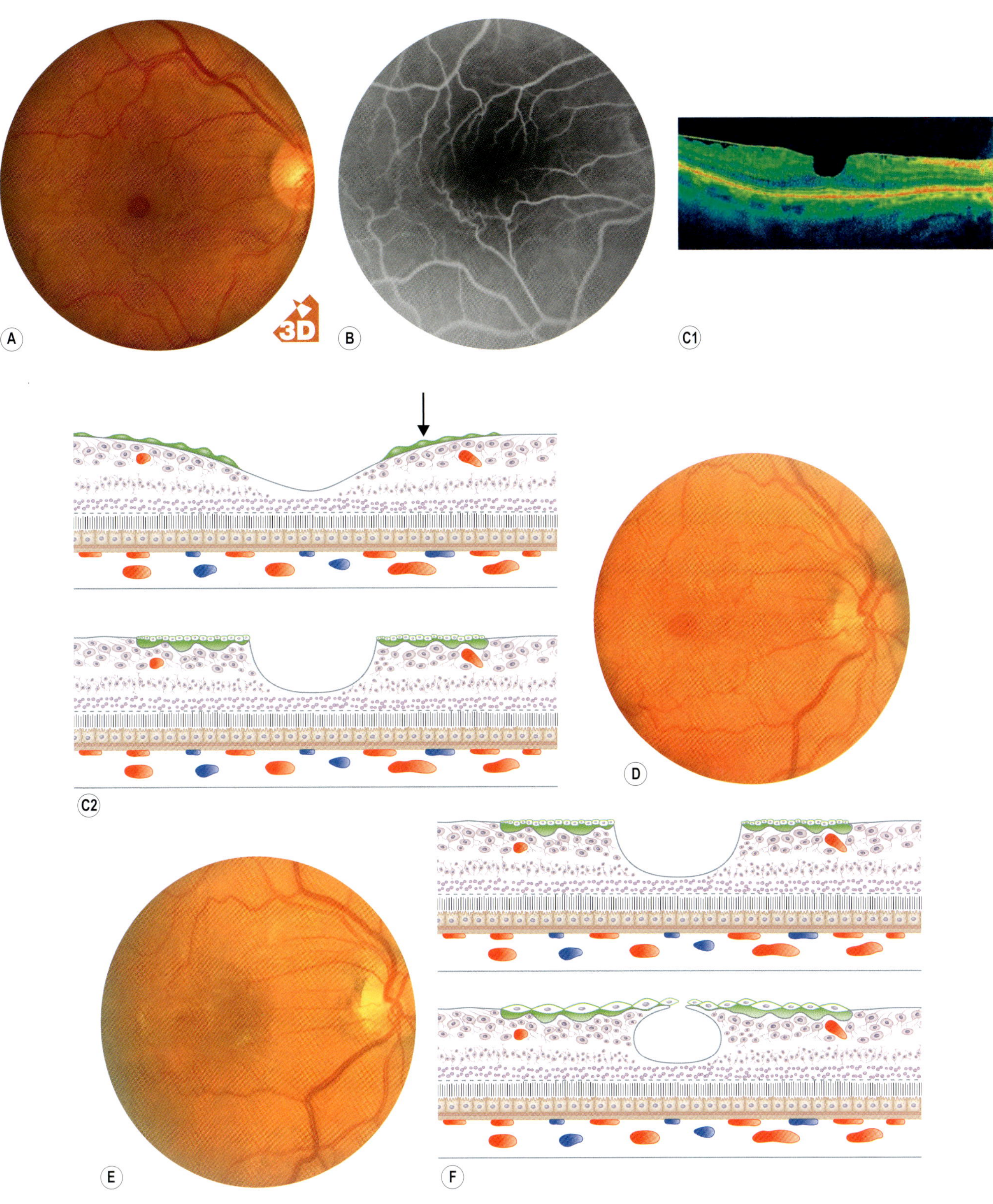
A
3D
B
C1
D
C2
E
F

reflex is usually absent. Fluorescein angiography is generally normal (Figure 7.21B) but may show a very faint zone of hyperfluorescence corresponding with the pseudohole. This zone of hyperfluorescence is typically much less prominent than the finely granular area of hyperfluorescence seen with a full-thickness hole (Figure 7.13I–L). The presence of the semitransparent perifoveolar epiretinal membrane probably causes the foveolar area to appear faintly hyperfluorescent by contrast to the perifoveolar area. Features of a full-thickness macular hole, including the halo of marginal detachment, yellow deposits within the hole, and a translucent operculum in front of some holes, are not seen in a pseudomacular hole. OCT will reveal retention of photoreceptors (Figure 7.22C), unlike a full-thickness macular hole (Figure 7.11F and G). The visual prognosis in these patients is good. In a few patients additional contraction of an eccentrically located perifoveal epiretinal membrane may distort the foveal area (Figure 7.21D and E). In others the epiretinal membrane may peel free from the inner retinal surface (Figures 7.21J–L). Teardrop-shaped or slitlike pseudomacular holes frequently accompany a severe macular pucker. Contraction of a pericentral epiretinal membrane that remains firmly adherent to the inner retinal surface may cause an anterior herniation of the foveolar retina through the hole in the membrane (Figure 7.21G–I).[117,174] This lesion may also be mistaken for a full-thickness macular hole. Bonnet and Fleury noted the development of this foveolar prolapse in three eyes that developed recurrent epiretinal membrane following surgical peeling of an epiretinal membrane.[175]

Epiretinal Membrane Formation Associated with Full-Thickness Macular Hole

Occasionally vitreous contraction on the retinal surface around the foveal area may be sufficient to mechanically cause a full-thickness hole in the macula (Figure 7.24G–I) or in the paracentral region (Figure 7.20J). Macular holes produced by this mechanism are typically oval or irregular in shape. They simulate closely a hole that involves the epiretinal membrane alone (pseudomacular hole). Angiography in the former case, however, shows striking hyperfluorescence corresponding with the full-thickness hole (Figure 7.24J). It is usually impossible to determine whether the macular hole occurred before the development of an epiretinal membrane or developed as a complication of the membrane. Mild degrees of crinkled cellophane retinopathy often accompany a full-thickness macular hole (Figure 7.13K).

Pigmentation of Epiretinal Membranes

Hyperpigmentation of an idiopathic epiretinal membrane may occur spontaneously in the absence of a retinal hole (Figure 7.22C and D).[176] Pigmented epiretinal membranes caused by a proliferation of RPE cells may occur, usually in the extramacular region, in as many as 3% of patients following repair of rhegmatogenous retinal detachment.[177] Similar pigmented membranes may occur in the macula of patients with peripheral retinal holes.[167,177–180] They also have been observed overlying photocoagulation scars.[180] Proliferation of pigmented as well as nonpigmented RPE cells has been demonstrated histopathologically in epiretinal membranes.[167,181] In some cases, pigmentation of epiretinal membranes may be caused by the incorporation of macrophages containing either melanin or hemosiderin.

7.21 Continued

G–I: Anterior herniation of the foveolar retina following spontaneous contraction of a perifoveolar epiretinal membrane (G and I) was misinterpreted as a macular hole. Following surgical excision of the membrane the visual acuity improved from 20/400 to 20/60 (H). Diagram (I) illustrates the progression of an epiretinal membrane (above) to retinal herniation (below) after contraction of the epiretinal membrane.

J–L: This 57-year-old woman complained of mild blurring of the right eye. Visual acuity in the right eye was 20/25 and J-1. Vision in the left eye was 20/20 and J-1. Note the pseudomacular hole (J) surrounded by an epiretinal membrane. Fifteen months later the patient was asymptomatic. Visual acuity was 20/15. The epiretinal membrane had spontaneously peeled from the retinal surface (K). Diagram (L) shows epiretinal membrane before (above) and after (arrow, below) peeling.

(A and B, from Gass[115] and G–I, from Smiddy and Gass.[117]),

Choroidal Neovascularization Underlying Epiretinal Membranes

Gass observed the development of choroidal neovascularization in two patients several years after they developed an idiopathic macular pucker. An unsuspected choroidal neovascular membrane (CNVM) was discovered by fluorescein angiography beneath the pucker of another patient referred for surgical peeling of the epiretinal membrane (Figure 7.22E and F). In these three patients there was no evidence of any abnormality in the macula of the opposite eye or of any other cause for the choroidal neovascularization in the affected eye. Stereoscopic fluorescein angiograms and OCT should be obtained in all patients scheduled for surgical peeling of opacified epiretinal membranes to exclude the presence of occult choroidal neovascularization.

Spontaneous Separation of an Epiretinal Membrane

Occasionally the peripheral portions of the contracting membrane detach from or slide along the retinal surface and curl up into a roll or ridge at one edge of the membrane (Figures 7.21J–L, 7.22A, and 7.23C and D).[169–171,176,182–185] This process of spontaneous peeling of a preretinal membrane often stops along the course of a major retinal vessel, where the vitreoretinal adhesion may be maximum. In some instances the membrane may spontaneously detach from the entire macular surface and remain as an adherent localized mass in the extramacular

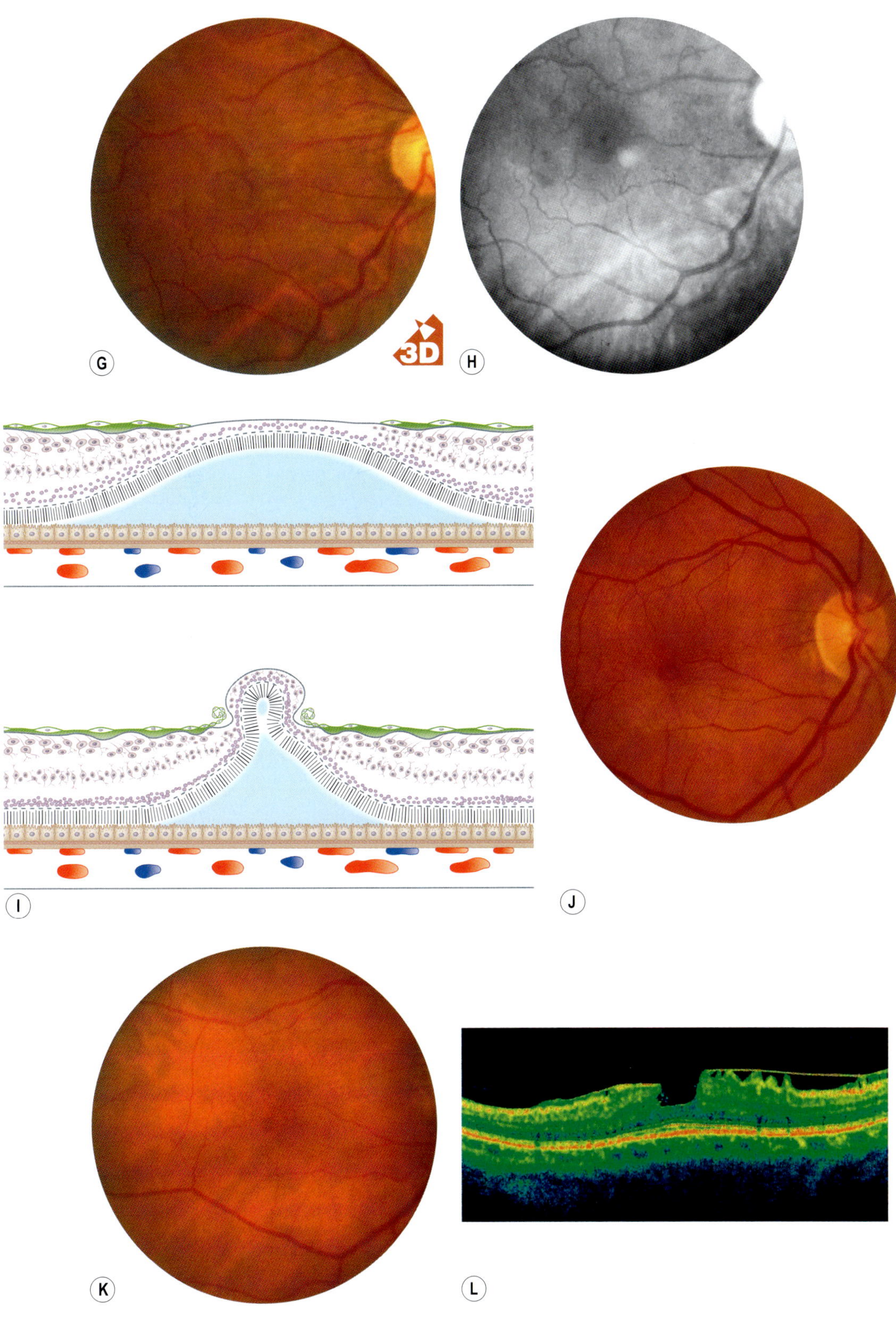
G
3D
H
I
J
K
L

region (Figures 7.09A–C and 7.23D). Distortion of the macula may disappear and visual function improves in such instances. Spontaneous detachment of more peripherally located epiretinal membranes that are the cause of tractional retinal detachment may also occur.[186]

Classification of Epiretinal Membranes According to Associated Disorders

Idiopathic Epiretinal Membranes

Crinkled cellophane maculopathy and macular pucker may occur in healthy patients without evidence of other intraocular disease.[169,170,176,183,187–190] These membranes usually occur in one eye of patients 50 years of age or older. Both sexes are affected equally. Bilateral loss of central vision from severe pucker occurs infrequently. The peripheral fundus should be examined to rule out peripheral tears or retinal vascular lesions. In 90% of the patients a PVD is present.[189]

Macular dysfunction caused by an epiretinal membrane is occasionally seen in asymptomatic children and young adults in the absence of any history to explain their presence (Figure 7.20G and 7.23I–L).[183,190–195] These membranes in younger patients are generally nonprogressive, are frequently centered over major retinal vessels, and are unassociated with a PVD. Occasionally they can be extensive, multilayered, and strongly adherent to the underlying retina (Figure 7.10E–H).

Retinal Vascular Diseases

Epiretinal membrane formation occurs frequently in association with retinal vascular diseases causing intraretinal exudation, such as diabetes, hypertension (see Figure 6.26H and L), venous obstruction, telangiectasis, angiomatosis (see Figure 13.19), and aphakic cystoid edema.[196] Macular distortion caused by the development of an epiretinal membrane may occasionally occur early following photocoagulation of retinal vascular diseases, particularly when the treatment is done in the paramacular area.

Retinal Tears and Rhegmatogenous Retinal Detachment

Crinkled cellophane maculopathy and macular pucker are frequently encountered in patients either before or after treatment for a peripheral retinal hole or a rhegmatogenous retinal detachment.[197–201] Macular pucker is a major cause of poor central vision after successful repair of a retinal detachment.[198,201–204] It typically occurs 8–16 weeks following surgery. Its development is probably determined primarily by the events occurring at the time of vitreous contraction and retinal hole formation rather than by the type of treatment used. Nevertheless, various authors have incriminated a variety of factors in its pathogenesis, including preoperative findings of macular detachment, vitreous hemorrhage, low visual acuity, rolled edges of retinal holes, star folds, equatorial folds, cryotherapy, age greater than 30 years,[203] and multiple operations,[201–205] as well as intraoperative complications such as loss of vitreous and multiple attempts at subretinal fluid drainage.[204] Focal areas of epiretinal membrane formation in the periphery of the fundus identical to that occurring in the macula are responsible for the star-shaped retinal folds that may accompany detachment. Macular pucker and star-shaped folds represent mild forms of the more severe disorder of proliferative vitreoretinopathy (massive vitreous proliferation), which is caused by cellular proliferation, predominantly that of RPE cells and astrocytes, on both the anterior and posterior surfaces of the retina.[206,207]

Approximately 20% of patients who develop a macular pucker after a scleral buckling procedure will experience improvement in visual acuity.[202] Part of this improvement is caused by relaxation or partial peeling of the epiretinal membrane, and part is caused by partial resolution of the intraretinal edema, which is more likely to be severe early after its development, particularly in aphakic patients.

Vitreous Inflammatory Diseases

Any disease producing an inflammatory cellular infiltrate in the vitreous, such as toxoplasmosis retinitis (Figure 7.09A–C), uveitis, trauma, intraocular tumor, or tapetoretinal dystrophies, may be associated with development of epiretinal membranes in the macula.

7.22 Pseudomacular hole.

A: A 68-year-old asymptomatic woman had 20/20 vision and a Weiss ring. The foveal center appears red against the gray contrast of the epiretinal membrane that spares the foveola, giving it the appearance of a pseudomacular hole.
B and **C**: Similar appearance of a pseudomacular hole in this 65-year-old woman who also had optic disc drusen (B). Optical coherence tomography shows preservation of the foveal cones and early partial separation of the epiretinal membrane from the retinal surface (C).

Macular pucker.
D and **E**: Macular pucker with partial separation and rolled edge of epiretinal membrane (arrow, D). Note marked distortion and displacement of the retinal vessels toward the horizontal raphe (E).
F and **G**: Delayed pigmentation occurring in an idiopathic epiretinal membrane in a healthy woman who was 57 years old when seen initially in 1965 because of recent loss of vision in the right eye. Her visual acuity was 20/400. She had a nonpigmented macular pucker (F). She was observed at yearly intervals until 1975, during which time her visual acuity improved to 20/70 and the epiretinal membrane became progressively pigmented (G). There were no holes in the retina.
H–J: This patient was referred to the Bascom Palmer Eye Institute for surgical removal of an idiopathic epiretinal membrane in the right eye (H and I). There was no biomicroscopic evidence of choroidal neovascularization. Angiography, however, unexpectedly revealed its presence (J).
K and **L**: Idiopathic juxtapapillary pucker and retinal neovascularization in a 35-year-old man who noted metamorphopsia of 2 years' duration. His visual acuity was 20/25. Note capillary dilation and leakage (K and L) within the area of the epiretinal membrane, whose peripheral edges have contracted toward the papillomacular bundle.

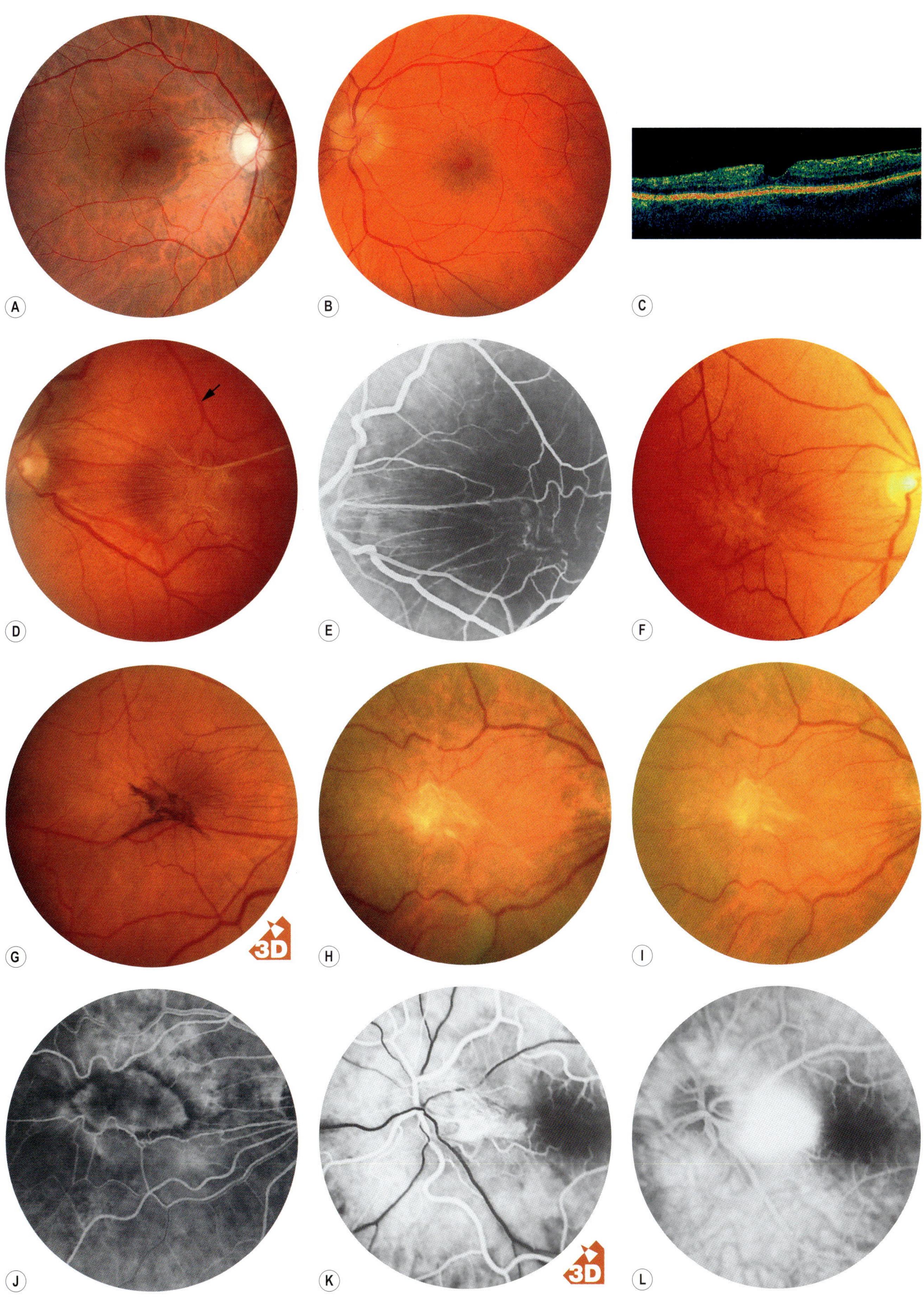
A
B
C
D
E
F
G
3D
H
I
J
K
3D
L

Pathology and Pathogenesis

Histopathologically, epiretinal membranes are composed of a fibrocellular sheet that varies in thickness from a single layer of collagen and interspersed cells (Figure 7.25A) to a thicker, multilayer of fibrocellular proliferation that often bridges coarse folds on the retinal surface (Figure 7.25B). The latter is often associated with intraretinal edema.[115,167,178,179,196,199,208–210] The precise morphologic identification of the cells of origin of epiretinal membranes by either electron or light microscopy is difficult because of the ability of astrocytes, hyalocytes, fibrocytes, macrophages,[178,211] and RPE cells to change into cells with a similar appearance and function.[168,177,178,181,211–228] Most epiretinal membranes are composed of a variety of cell types, including one or more of the following: myofibroblasts, RPE cells, fibrous astrocytes, fibrocytes, and macrophages. Few fragments of the footplates of Müller cells are seen on the retinal side of the membrane.[229] Several, and perhaps all, cell types have the capability of developing myofibroblastic properties that are probably responsible for the contractile properties of epiretinal and vitreous membranes.[211,216,228,230–232] Epiretinal membranes can be produced experimentally by a variety of techniques, including intravitreal injection of blood, carbon particles, fibroblasts, and RPE cells.[225,233–237]

The stimuli for epiretinal membrane formation are poorly understood. A PVD appears to be one important stimulus.[34,36,166,169,200,238–241]

Approximately 75% of epiretinal membranes are found in eyes with a PVD.[187,238,242] These membranes are particularly prone to develop in eyes following transient vitreomacular traction soon after separation of the vitreous from the retina and within weeks or several months after vitreous detachment and rhegmatogenous retinal detachment.[200] Two different mechanisms for epiretinal membrane formation and contraction after vitreous detachment have been proposed. One mechanism (more recently, believed to be the less common) is the proliferation and contraction of fibrous astrocytes that extend from the retina and optic nerve through either pre-existing dehiscences in the ILM of the retina and optic nerve head, or dehiscences caused by vitreous separation. These dehiscences are most likely to occur on the optic nerve head or along the major retinal vessels where the ILM is attenuated. These fibrocellular membranes are composed of a syncytium of cells with small, spindle-shaped nuclei and scanty cytoplasm arranged in either a single or a multilayered fashion along the inner retinal surface (Figure 7.25A). Contraction and interaction of the cells rather than contraction of the extracellular component of the membrane are probably most important in causing retinal wrinkling.[243] Electron microscopic studies of idiopathic epiretinal membranes have demonstrated that RPE cells and fibrous astrocytes are the predominant cell type composing these membranes.[244] Membranes in younger patients, ones in patients with a history of recent development of symptoms, and recurrent membranes are more likely to contain RPE cells with myoblastic differentiation as well as myofibroblasts.[193,194,234] Other cell types that occasionally predominate are fibrocytes and myofibroblasts.

7.23 Spontaneous separation and movement of epiretinal membranes.

A and B: Note partial peeling and superotemporal displacement of an epiretinal membrane (arrows) that occurred over 5 years in this 44-year-old man.
C and D: Spontaneous detachment of the epiretinal membrane occurred in this 66-year-old man who developed acute loss of vision, photopsia, and metamorphopsia caused by macular pucker (C) 28 months after cataract extraction. Eleven months after his initial examination, his visual acuity had returned to 20/30 and the condensed remnant of the membrane remained attached to the retina in the papillomacular bundle area (D).
E–H: This woman with a history of a scleral buckle in the left eye developed loss of central vision caused by an epiretinal membrane in the macula (E). On the buckle inferiorly she had an angiomatous proliferation of capillaries in the retina. Angiography revealed mild tortuosity of the retinal vessels in the area of the pucker (F) and staining of the peripheral neovascular lesion. Several months following laser treatment of the neovascular lesion (G), she noted spontaneous improvement in the vision and the epiretinal membrane in the left macula had peeled off the central macular area (H).
I–L: This 11-year-old boy developed loss of central vision in the right eye caused by a pucker (I). Angiography revealed tortuosity and central displacement of the macular retinal vessels (stereo, J and K). Following surgical excision of the membrane (L) the visual acuity improved from 20/200 to 20/25.

(I–L, courtesy of Dr. Patrick E. Rubsamen.)

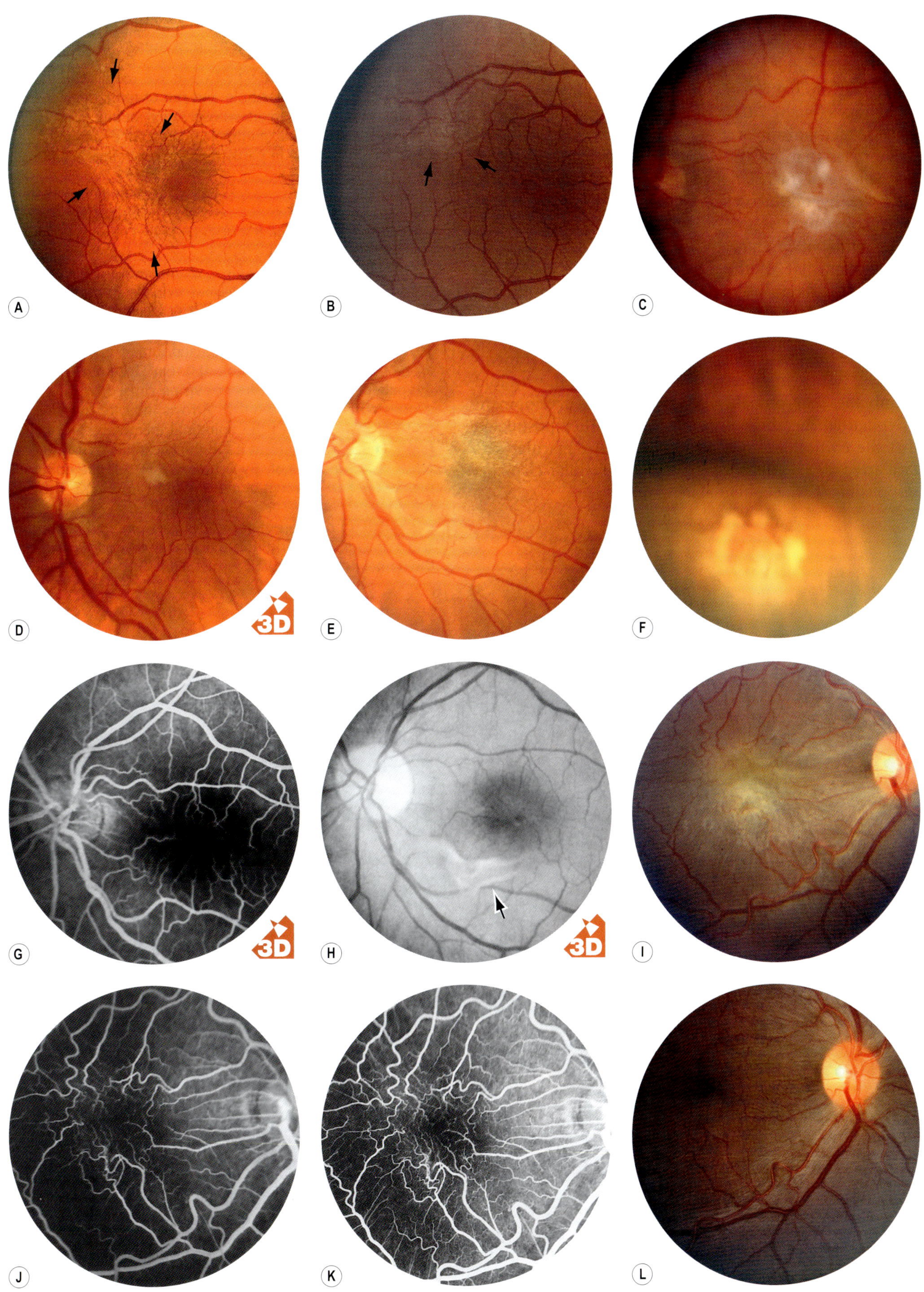
A
B
C
D
3D
E
F
G
3D
H
3D
I
J
K
L

Prognosis

Patients with macular distortion caused by contraction of an epiretinal membrane usually show little or no progression of distortion after their initial examination.[176,183,189] A few patients, however, experience a progressive loss of visual function over a period of months or years.[211,246] The infrequency with which the distortion worsens suggests that membrane contraction usually occurs rapidly and is self-limiting. Angiographic evidence of retinal capillary permeability is more likely to be present soon after contraction of the epiretinal membrane has occurred, and in eyes with membranes that are more likely to progress.[247] Approximately 50% of patients maintain good visual acuity, and in over 80% the visual function is either stable or improves. Fewer than 10% show a decline in visual acuity. Spontaneous peeling of the membrane occasionally results in dramatic visual improvement (Figures 7.08A–C, 7.21J–L, and 7.23C and D).[193,244,248–250] Spontaneous separation of a preretinal membrane in the macula is particularly likely to occur following laser or cryotherapy of a peripheral retinal angioma (Figure 13.19A–F).[248,250] Angiographic evidence of leakage may be the result of epiretinal membrane formation, or may be the precursor of epiretinal membrane as in branch retinal vein occlusion or retinal hemangioma.

Treatment

In the absence of any evidence of intravitreal inflammation, there is no reason to believe that corticosteroid treatment is beneficial in treating patients with intraretinal edema that may accompany a severe pucker. Surgical peeling of epiretinal membranes from the macular surface has been successfully accomplished (Figure 7.23I–L).[244,251–268] The best surgical candidates are those patients with moderate to severe visual loss, and a short duration of macular puckering. Approximately 75% of patients experience two lines of visual acuity improvement after surgery. Membrane peel with and without dye (ICG and trypan blue) assistance seems to have similar results.[269–272] Surgical complications include cataract (approximately 50–75% within 2 years), peripheral retinal tears, retinal detachment, posterior retinal tears, photic maculopathy particularly with ICG dye assistance, anterior ischemic optic neuropathy, and endophthalmitis.[254,256–259,261,273,274] Regrowth of epiretinal tissue occurs in a small percentage of cases. Failure to remove all layers of the epiretinal membrane in multilayered vitreoschisis cases may contribute to the recurrence.[34]

7.25 Histopathology of macular distortion caused by epiretinal membranes.

A: Photomicrograph of crinkled cellophane maculopathy showing fine wrinkling of the inner retinal surface resulting from contraction of an epiretinal membrane. A fine fibrocellular membrane (arrow) lies on the surface of the folded internal limiting membrane.

B: Photomicrograph showing macular pucker, cystoid macular edema, and degeneration secondary to contraction of an epiretinal membrane. The membrane is artifactitiously detached near the large retinal folds (arrow).

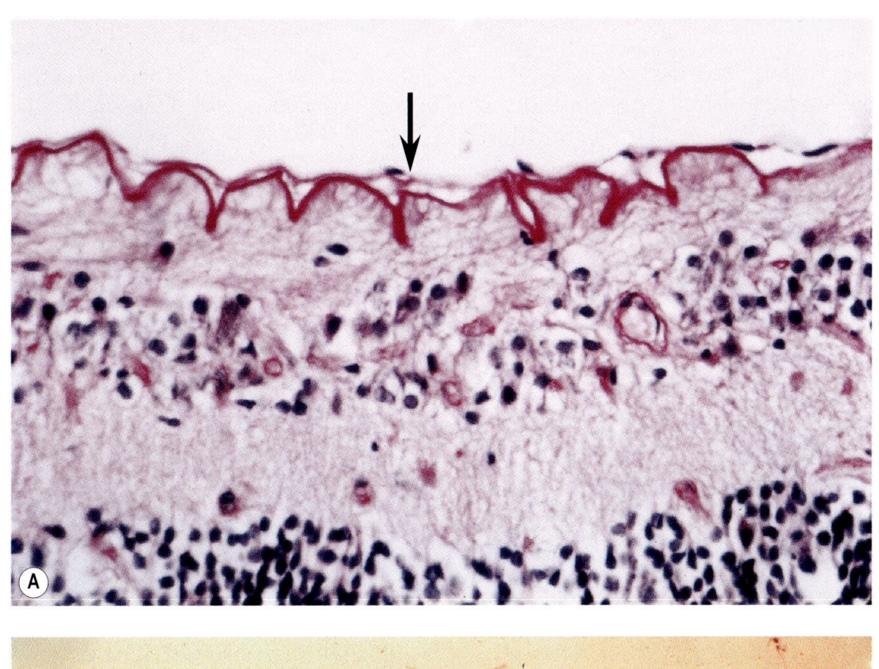
A

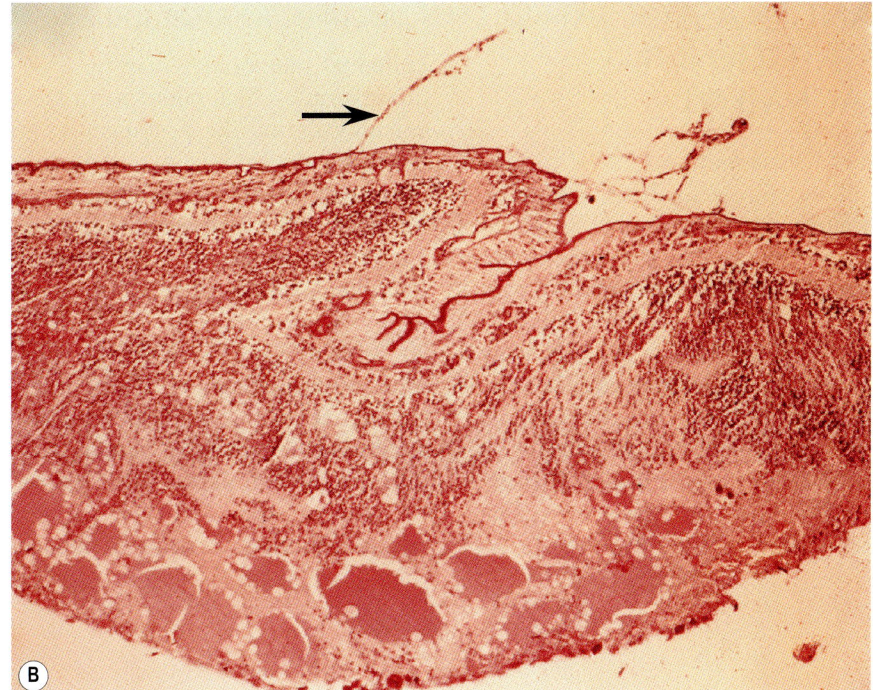
B

Vitreopapillary Traction

Subretinal hemorrhage (Figure 7.26), decreased visual acuity, swollen optic nerve head, peripapillary traction detachment, and intrapapillary and epipapillary hemorrhages are all signs that may be associated with vitreopapillary traction.[6,275–278] Careful biomicroscopy with a 78-D or a fundus contact lens often reveals an oval vitreous condensation located eccentrically anterior to the optic disc with the absence of a CNVM as the cause of the subretinal hemorrhage. OCT is an invaluable tool in confirming the traction exerted by the vitreous attached to the disc, but detached elsewhere (Figure 7.26C and F). Vitreopapillary traction in proliferative diabetic retinopathy may contribute to the visual loss in addition to other causes such as poor macular perfusion, macular edema, and vitreous hemorrhage.[6,279] Surgical removal with pars plana vitrectomy is indicated for decreased visual acuity and/or a field defect.

7.26 Vitreopapillary traction.

A–F: An 80-year-old woman was followed for mild cystoid macular edema and vitreopapillary traction for 6 years with a visual acuity of 20/30 in both eyes that remained stable (A). She developed an asymptomatic juxtapapillary subretinal hemorrhage in the right eye with no change in her vision (B). Optical coherence tomography demonstrated attachment of the vitreous to the disc surface bilaterally (C). Fluorescein angiography was unremarkable (D and E). She received one injection of bevacizumab for an erroneous diagnosis of juxtapapillary choroidal neovascularization with no change in the hemorrhage. She had moderate cataracts and the vision and vitreopapillary traction (F) remained unchanged over 6 years.

RETINAL CHANGES ASSOCIATED WITH RHEGMATOGENOUS RETINAL DETACHMENT

Rhegmatogenous retinal detachment is one of the most important disorders of the vitreoretinal interface, and it may cause or be associated with a variety of abnormalities in the macular area. Approximately 30–40% of patients in whom retinal detachment includes the macula will regain good visual acuity after successful reattachment.[280–289] Most patients who fail to regain good visual acuity will show biomicroscopic and fluorescein angiographic lesions that account for the loss.[172,198,290] In some, however, usually those with macular detachment of 2 months' or longer duration, the macular area will show minimal changes, and visual loss is probably caused by failure of regeneration and realignment of photoreceptors.[291]

Epiretinal Membrane

Epiretinal membranes may be present before the development of a retinal detachment but often become apparent only during the postoperative course. Preoperatively, patients with detachment and epiretinal membranes in the macular area will usually show a stellate arrangement of multiple, white, retinal folds (Figure 7.27A and B). These are often accompanied by peripheral star folds, meridional folds, and rolled edges of retinal tears. Postoperatively, epiretinal membranes are the most frequently recognized abnormality in the macula.[172,198] Approximately 5% of patients undergoing scleral buckling procedures will develop severe macular pucker that may or may not be associated with massive periretinal proliferation and failure of standard scleral buckling procedures. Vitrectomy and surgical removal of these membranes are successful in salvaging the sight in some of these patients.

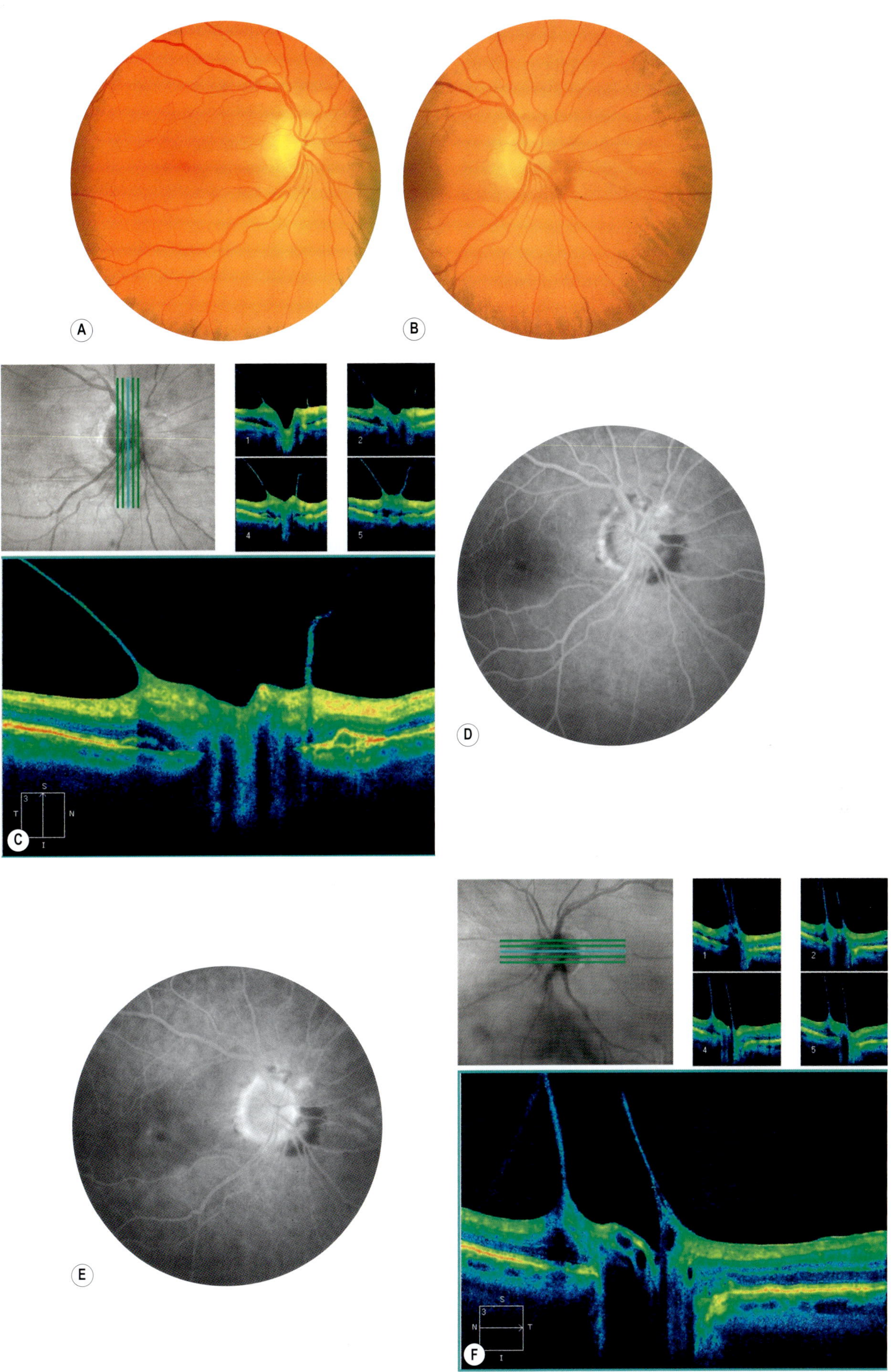
A
B
C
D
E
F
S
T
N
I
3
1
2
4
5

Cystoid Macular Edema

Cystoid macular edema may be present either when the patient is seen initially with a retinal detachment (Figure 7.27C) or postoperatively. It occurs most frequently, but not exclusively, in aphakic eyes. Cystoid macular edema and epiretinal membranes are the most frequent macular findings in patients with poor acuity after buckling procedures.

In most patients with rhegmatogenous retinal detachment, fluorescein angiography shows no evidence of retinal vascular permeability alterations. In long-standing retinal detachment, however, angiography may demonstrate evidence of capillary dilation, increased permeability, and areas of capillary nonperfusion. In myopic children with recent onset of detachment, angiography may demonstrate large areas of diffuse leakage of dye (Figure 7.27D–F).[172]

Macular and Paramacular Holes

Rhegmatogenous detachments caused by holes in the macula or paramacular region usually occur in highly myopic patients with posterior staphylomata or in patients with direct vitreous traction on the posterior retina.[150,292,293] In most cases these detachments are confined to the posterior half of the eye, and they infrequently extend out to the ora serrata. When the detachment is confined to the macula in patients with a posterior staphyloma and myopia, the detachment may be caused by traction rather than a hole, and spontaneous reattachment may occur.[294] See discussion in Chapter 3.

Approximately 0.5–1% of patients with rhegmatogenous retinal detachment and a peripheral retinal hole will also have a macular hole.[292,295] During the course of surgery or immediately following surgery a macular hole may develop in another 1–2% of patients.[295] Fluorescein angiography may be helpful in differentiating macular holes from macular cysts, pseudomacular hole caused by an epiretinal membrane (Figure 7.21A and B), or partial-thickness macular holes (see Figure 6.36).

Macular holes in nonmyopic eyes without evidence of vitreous traction do not require treatment at the time of surgery for retinal detachment caused by peripheral retinal tears.[296] A variety of techniques has been employed in the repair of retinal detachments caused by macular and paramacular holes in patients with myopic staphylomata or posterior vitreous traction (Figure 7.09J–L).[2,93,151,152,154,155,297–299]

7.27 Macular changes in rhegmatogenous retinal detachment.

A: Early stellate pattern of retinal folds indicative of the presence of epiretinal membrane.
B: Advanced stellate retinal folds in a patient who developed massive periretinal proliferation.
C: Cystoid macular edema (arrows).
D–F: A 17-year-old myopic female with recent onset of rhegmatogenous retinal detachment and multiple peripheral retinal tears. Note cloudiness of subretinal fluid and angiographic evidence of leaking retinal blood vessels.
G–I: Long-standing superior rhegmatogenous retinal detachment and outer retinal cyst (arrow, H) in a 56-year-old man who was asymptomatic until several days before admission, when he noted loss of central vision caused by extension of the detachment into the macula. Angiography showed early hyperfluorescence caused by attenuation of the retinal pigment epithelium and late staining caused by retinal capillary leakage in the area of long-standing detachment (I).
J: Subretinal fibrous proliferative bands and fenestrated membranes in a patient with long-standing retinal detachment.
K and L: Subretinal fibrous strands (arrows) associated with a long-standing inferior rhegmatogenous retinal detachment that spontaneously reattached. Similar findings were present in the opposite eye.

(G–I, from Gass.[172])

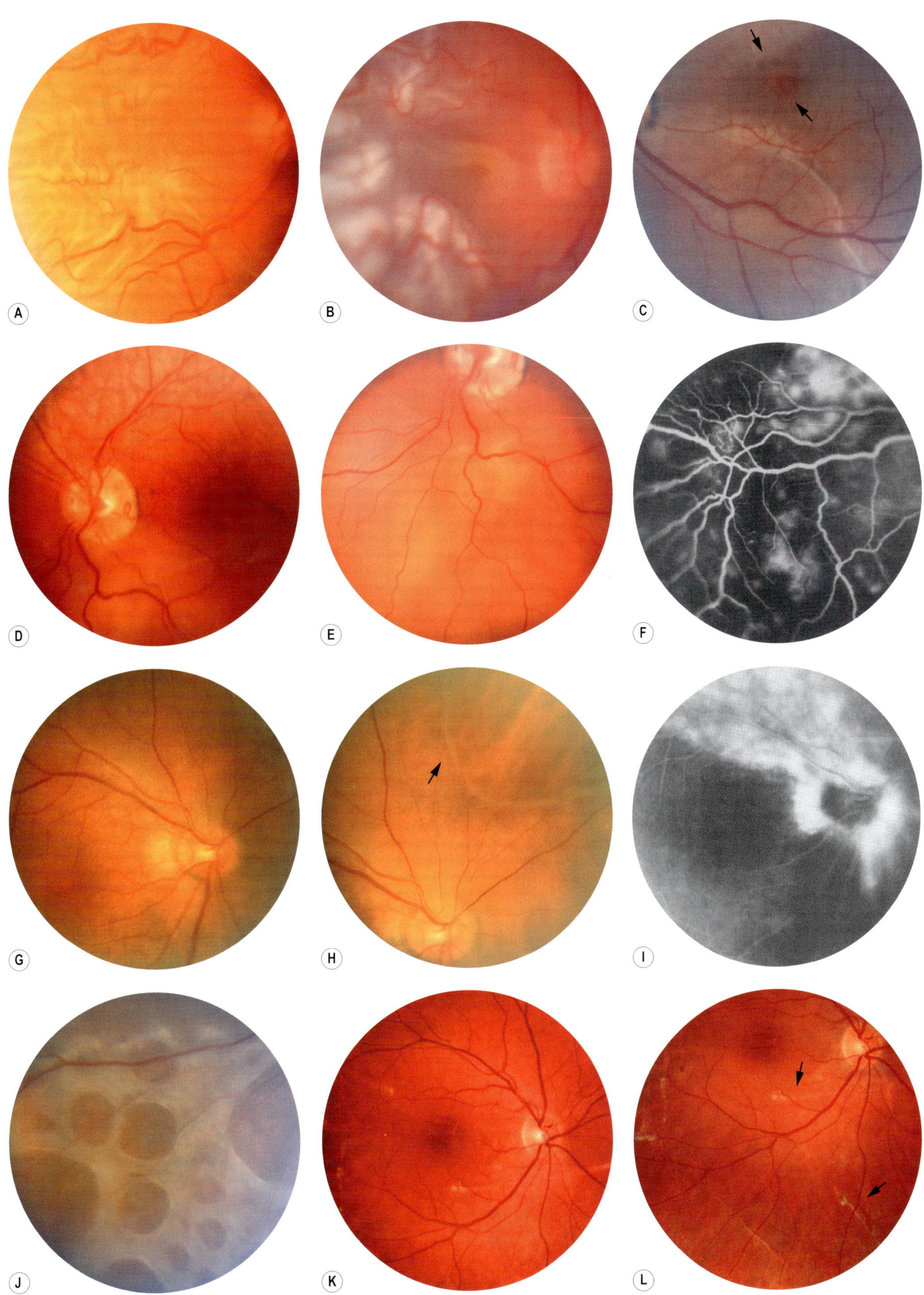
A
B
C
D
E
F
G
H
I
J
K
L

Pigment Epithelial Atrophy, Demarcation Lines, and Subretinal Neovascularization

With prolonged retinal detachment (usually beyond a period of 6 months), the RPE becomes partly depigmented within the area of detachment (Figures 7.27G–I and 7.28K), and it may proliferate along the junction of detached and attached retina to form a demarcation line (Figures 7.28A, F, and K, and 7.28A–D). A series of these lines may occur as the detachment spreads over a period of months or years. They may eventually extend into the macular area (Figure 7.28L). Similar demarcation lines may occur along the posterior border of a chronic choroidal detachment (Figure 7.29F). These RPE changes are more easily detected with fluorescein angiography (Figures 7.27I and 7.28K).[172,300] Angiography is helpful in differentiating a long-standing retinal detachment from retinoschisis. The latter condition is not associated with RPE changes unless it is associated with retinal detachment from holes developing in the outer and usually the inner layer of retinoschisis (Figure 7.30).[172]

I have seen three patients with loss of central vision caused by choroidal neovascularization at the edge of a demarcation line lying adjacent to the foveal area (Figure 7.29A–D).[301–303]

Subretinal Fibrosis

A light gray fenestrated sheet or multiple opaque strands may be present on the posterior surface of the detached retina in approximately 3% of patients with a rhegmatogenous detachment (Figure 7.27J).[304–307] Subretinal strands are frequently arranged in a reticular or other geometric pattern. In some cases they may be separated from the posterior retinal surface. They are most often seen in long-standing detachment and are often associated with demarcation lines. They result from fenestrations developing in large, thin fibrocellular sheets growing on the back surface of the retina. In contrast to epiretinal membranes, these usually do not affect the incidence of surgical success.[306] Occasionally, however, one or more of these strands may remain taut after scleral buckling and prevent complete reattachment of the macula.

7.28 Complications of long-standing rhegmatogenous retinal detachment.

A–E: This young myopic woman presented with bilateral inferior retinal detachments and prominent pigmented demarcation lines that extended only to the peripheral macular region in both eyes. A scleral buckling procedure was done in the left eye. The patient elected to have reinforcement of the demarcation lines with laser photocoagulation rather than surgery in the right eye (A). She had no further trouble for 10 years, when she developed evidence of intraretinal neovascularization and angiomatous formation within the area of retinal detachment in the area indicated by the arrow in A. No further treatment was done until 2 years later when the retinal tumor enlarged (B) and caused symptomatic vitreous cells and mild cystoid macular edema (C, D). Following argon laser treatment of the angiomatous lesion (B), the lipid exudate disappeared (E) and the vitreous cells and cystoid macular edema improved.

F–J: Retinal angiomatous proliferation (arrows, I–K) and yellow intraretinal and subretinal exudation developed in a 24-year-old woman with long-standing bilateral inferior rhegmatogenous retinal detachments and demarcation lines (G and H). The retina reattached after cryotherapy of the angiomatous proliferation and retinal holes. Note the hyperfluorescence on the detachment side of the demarcation line (arrow) in the left eye (K). The demarcation line in the left eye was reinforced using argon laser.

K: Large retinal fold running through the macula in this patient following a vitrectomy and scleral buckle repair of a macula off retinal detachment. Note the subretinal perfluorcarbon bubbles within the fold (arrow).

(K, courtesy of Dr. Baker Hubbard.)

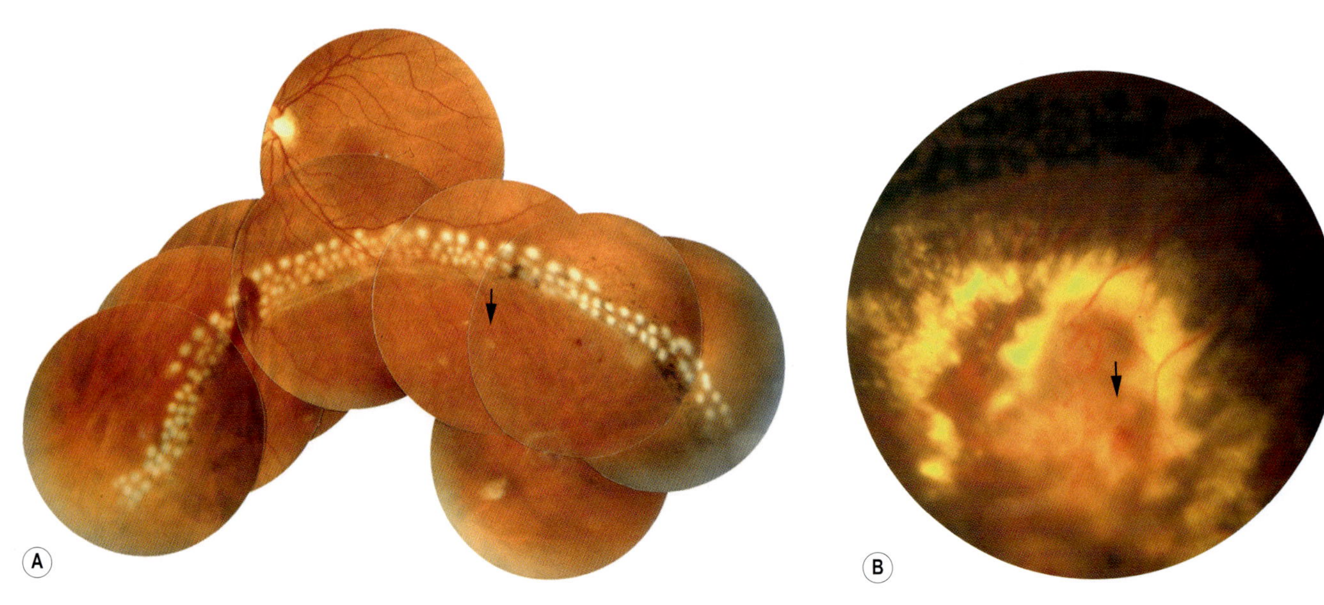

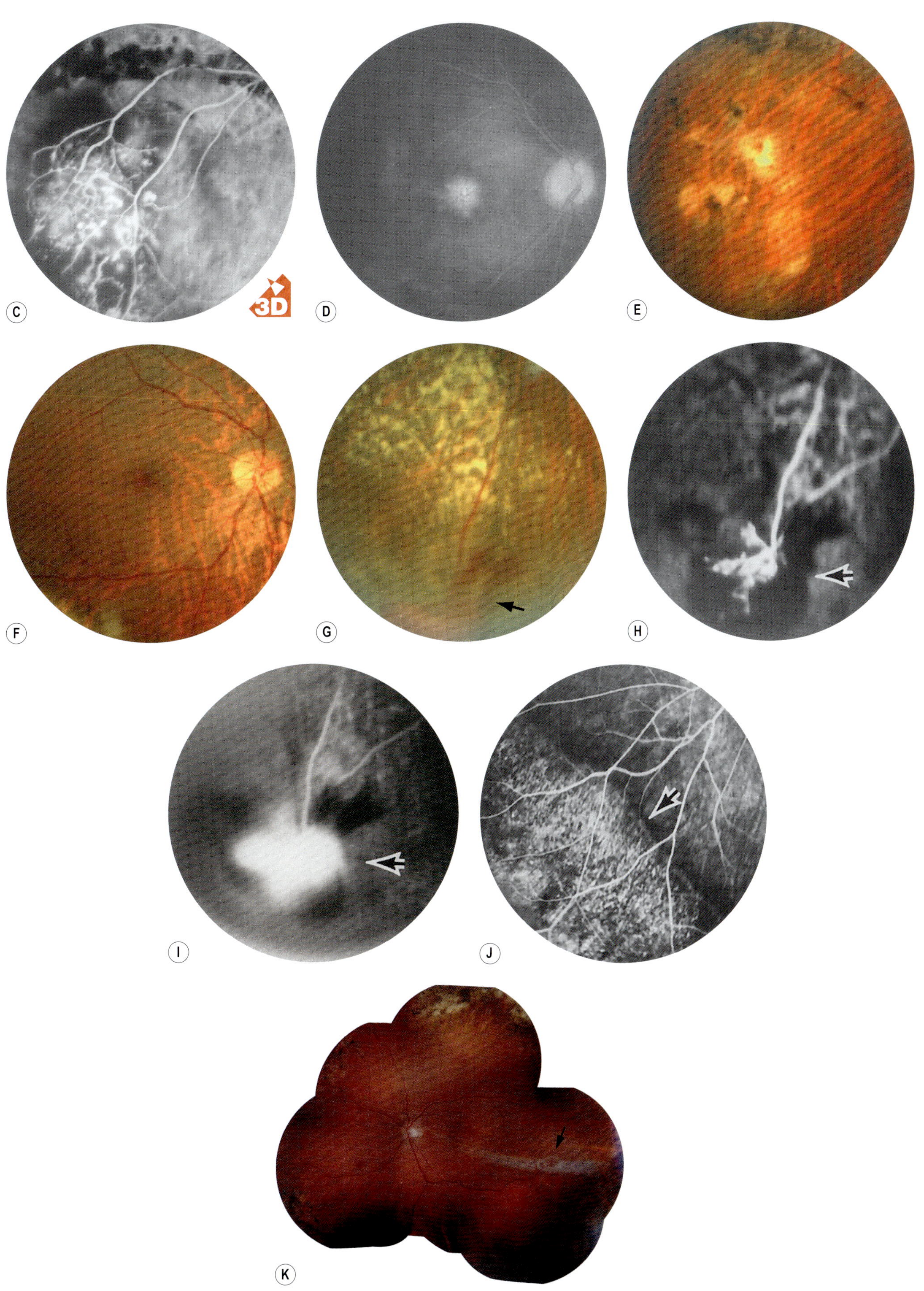
C
3D
D
E
F
G
H
I
J
K

Gravitation of Subretinal Pigment Following Cryotherapy

RPE pigment liberated at the time of vigorous cryotherapy, usually to superotemporal holes in patients with retinal detachments involving the macula, may gravitate within the subretinal fluid to the macular area. This pigment deposit may remain static or may become diminished to some degree. It is probably not associated with any significant morbidity in regard to visual recovery.[198,308–312] This granular, polymorphic deposition of pigment should be distinguished from the pigmentation caused by proliferation and fibrous metaplasia of the RPE on the inner retinal surface (Figure 7.29K and L).

Lesions Simulating Serous Detachments of the Retinal Pigment Epithelium

Early in the postoperative course following successful repair of a retinal detachment, the physician may notice one or more lesions with the biomicroscopic features of serous detachments of the RPE in the macular region or elsewhere in the fundus (Figure 7.29G–I).[313,314] Angiographically, however, these lesions do not show staining with fluorescein, and they probably represent focal areas of cloudy serous detachment of the sensory retina. They vary in size from one-fourth to four disc diameters. Several months or a year may be required before resolution occurs. When these lesions are large and solitary, they are most likely to be misdiagnosed as serous detachments of the RPE. When they are multiple they may be mistaken for multifocal areas of choroiditis.[315] Similar lesions have been observed in experimental retinal detachment.[316]

Retinal Neovascularization and Angiomatous Proliferation Caused by Chronic Retinal Detachment

Long-standing rhegmatogenous retinal detachment may cause retinal vascular occlusion and focal proliferation of preretinal as well as intraretinal capillaries that may simulate a capillary hemangioma (Figure 7.28A–F).[317,318] These lesions may cause intraretinal and subretinal exudation and occasionally vitreous hemorrhage. Similar proliferative vascular lesions as well as choroidal neovascularization may occur at drainage sites made during scleral buckling procedures.[319,320]

7.29 Macular complications associated with long-standing retinal detachment.

A–C: Subretinal neovascularization (arrow, B) developed within a pigmented demarcation line in a patient who had previous successful surgery for a long-standing retinal detachment.
D and **E**: This patient was followed for 8 years with recurrent subfoveal bleeding caused by subretinal neovascularization occurring within a demarcation line (D). Eight years after the photograph in D she returned with evidence of intraretinal vascular proliferation and exudation temporal to the macula (E) occurring within the area of intraretinal migration of retinal pigment epithelium caused by long-standing retinal detachment.
F: Angiographic evidence of demarcation lines (arrows) caused by long-standing choroidal and retinal detachment.
G: Sharply circumscribed puddle of subretinal fluid simulating serous retinal pigment epithelium (RPE) detachment after successful scleral buckling operation.
H–J: Similar large puddle of cloudy subretinal fluid (arrows, H and I) remained for 3–4 weeks after a successful buckling operation. Note the multiloculated appearance superiorly (I). Angiography showed no evidence of RPE detachment (J).
K and **L**: Pigmented epiretinal membranes causing macular pucker in two patients following scleral buckling procedures.

Submacular Hemorrhage During Surgery

Choroidal hemorrhage occurring at the time of drainage of the subretinal fluid is the most common cause of subretinal blood extending into the macular area. It may occur occasionally, however, because of spontaneous rupture of an occult CNVM in the macular or juxtapapillary area. Many patients who have spread of subretinal blood into the macula from adjacent sources (e.g., CNVMs or choroidal ruptures) regain good acuity after clearing of the blood. This is less likely to occur, however, in patients with rhegmatogenous retinal detachment.

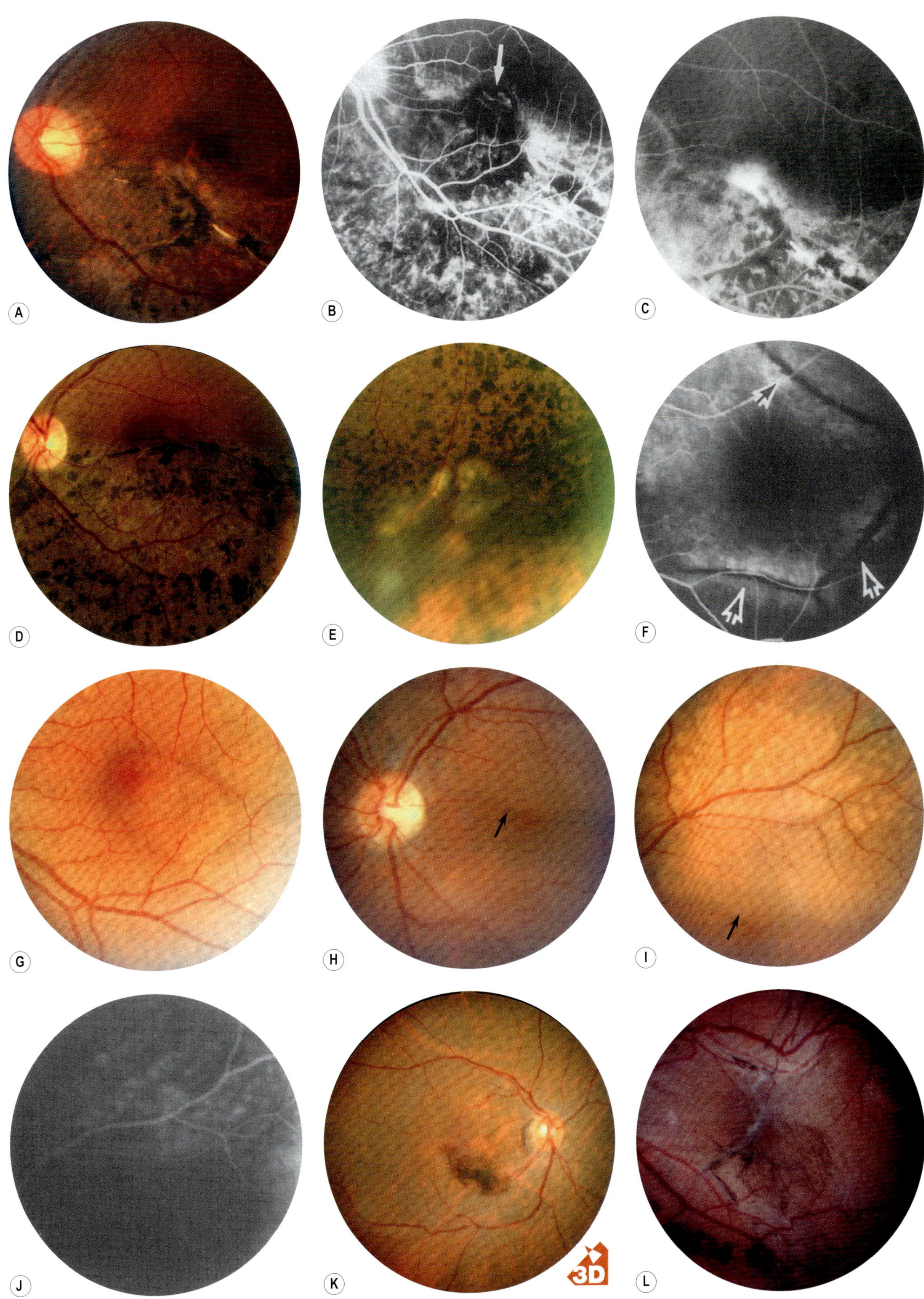
A
B
C
D
E
F
G
H
I
J
K
L
3D

Postscleral Buckle Macular Folds

Retinal folds extending into the macular area may be the cause of a poor visual result after a scleral buckling procedure. These may be either radial or curvilinear folds at the posterior edge of a radial buckle that was placed too far posteriorly; radial folds extending from a drainage site associated with retinal incarceration; or folds caused by posterior slippage of the retina following the use of intraocular gas in the repair of a large retinal tear (see Figures 7.28K and 4.06C).

Retinal Crystals

Eyes with longstanding retinal detachment very occasionally develop shiny fine crystals in the macula (Figure 7.31A and B). The constituents of these crystals are not clearly known; the possibility of them being calcium oxalate crystals is most believed. Whether they represent hemosiderin-laden macrophages, eythrocyte breakdown products, or photoreceptor outer segments is still debated. They do not affect vision, and often prompt exploration for a localized peripheral retinal detachment.[321–323]

DEGENERATIVE RETINOSCHISIS

Degenerative retinoschisis is present in approximately 1–4% of healthy adult patients.[172,324–328] It most frequently involves the inferotemporal peripheral fundus and is often bilateral. Anatomically, the splitting of the retina usually occurs at the outer plexiform layer but it may occur more superficially (Figure 7.31C). It typically is seen clinically as a sharply circumscribed, smooth, nonmobile elevation of the inner retina extending posteriorly from the ora serrata (Figure 7.31D and E). It is not associated with changes in the RPE, which is in contact with the retinal receptor layer in the area of the split retina. The outer layer is difficult to see without scleral depression. Retinoschisis in most patients is asymptomatic and nonprogressive.[329] Posterior extension of retinoschisis into the macular area occurs rarely and is most likely to develop in patients with the reticular form of degenerative retinoschisis, which has an extremely thin inner retinal layer (Figure 7.31D and E).[325,327] It has been estimated that the chance of retinal detachment developing in a patient with retinoschisis is 0.04%.[325]

7.30 Senile schisis detachment.

A and B: This woman had peripheral retinoschisis with large outer retinal holes (arrows). There was no evidence of extension of the shallow retinal detachment surrounding the holes posterior to the zone of schisis.
C–J: Extension of fluid from within the schisis cavity through holes in the outer retinal layer (arrow, C) into the subretinal space in the macula occurred in a 66-year-old man who noted loss of vision in the right eye. His visual acuity was 20/60. He had a large bullous area of peripheral retinoschisis temporally, associated with several large holes (small arrows, D and E) in the outer retinal layer posteriorly. A shallow serous retinal detachment extended from the edge of the outer retinal holes into the center of the macula (large arrow, D and F). Angiography revealed a large area of early hyperfluorescence indicative of retinal pigment epithelium depigmentation within the areas of the outer retinal holes (arrows, G) and in a zone of long-standing shallow retinal detachment that extended from the posterior edge of the holes into the temporal macula (H). Argon green laser was used to treat the edge of the outer retinal holes and along the posterior edge of the schisis (I) in an effort to close the neck of the detachment. Because of incomplete closure the same area was retreated several months later, and was successful in reattaching the retina in the macular area (J). His acuity returned to 20/30.

(A and B, courtesy of Dr. Gerald A. Brooksby; C–J, from Ambler et al.[330])

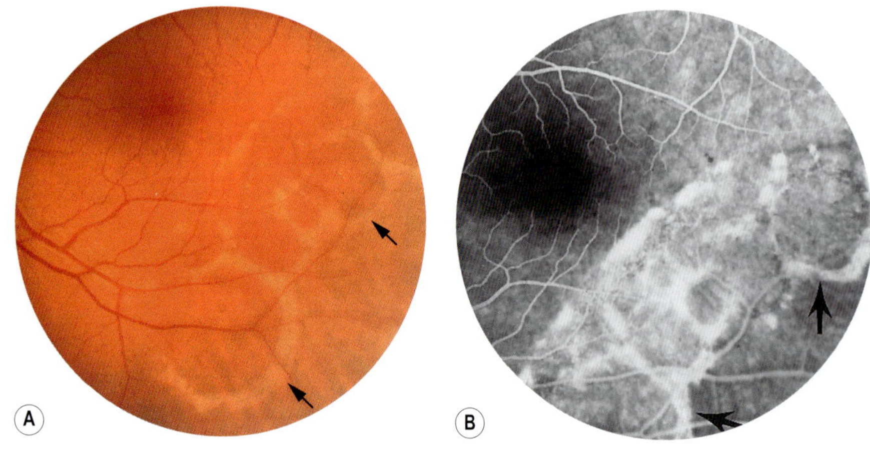

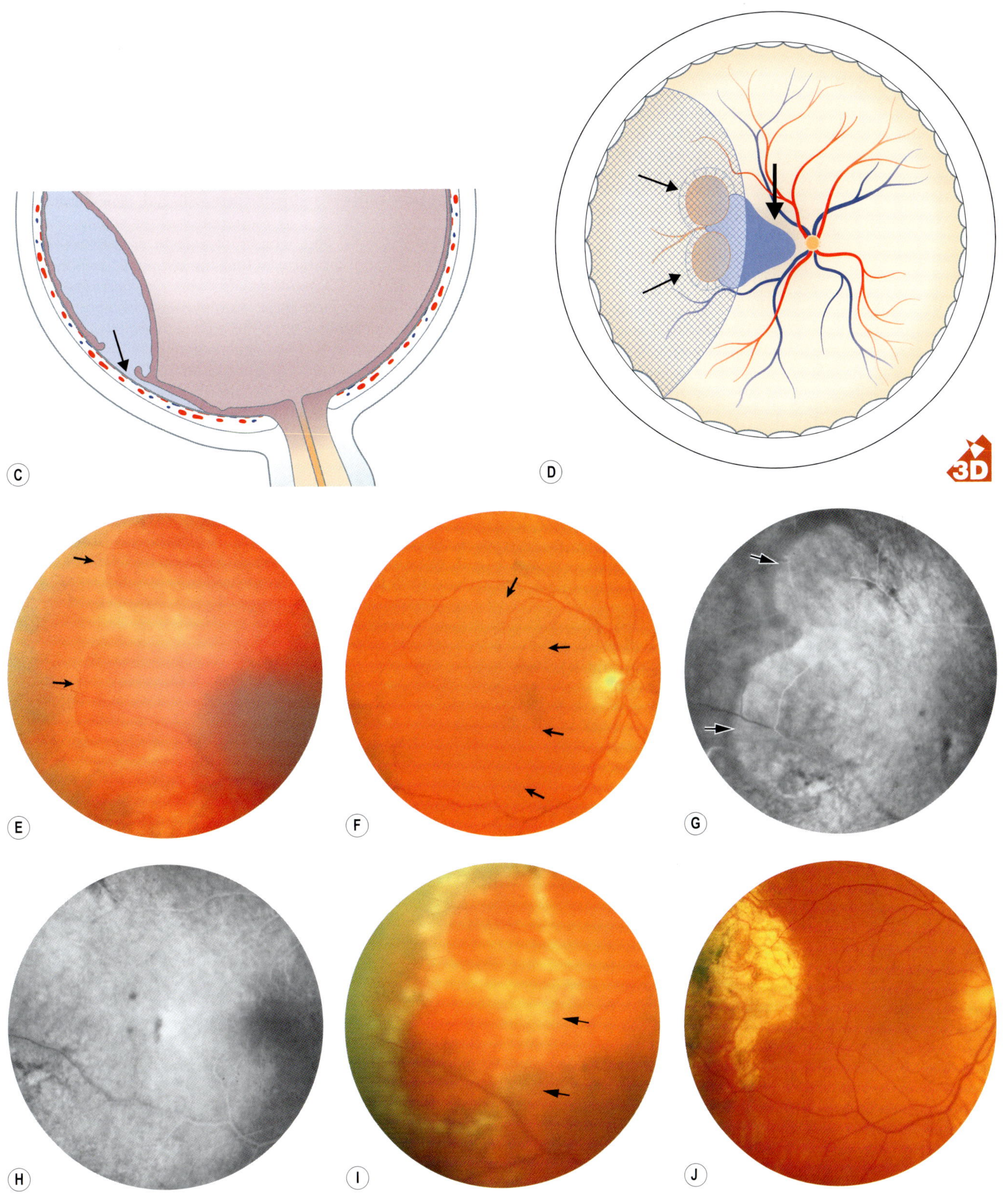
C
D
3D
E
F
G
H
I
J

Schisis Detachment

There is some predilection for large areas of posterior extension of schisis to develop large outer-wall holes and a shallow retinal detachment that may slowly extend into the macula (Figures 7.30 and 7.32A–C, and F).[328,330,331] Before posterior extension of the retinal detachment beyond the edge of the schisis, the detachment may be difficult to detect. The presence of hypopigmentation of the RPE around the outer retinal holes or one or more pigmented demarcation lines indicates retinal detachment (Figure 7.30B and G). The retinal detachment extending into the macula may be shallow and it may be possible to close the communication between the macular detachment and the outer-wall holes with one or more sessions of moderately intense laser photocoagulation across the neck of the detachment along the posterior edge of the schisis as well as along the edge of the outer-wall holes (Figures 7.30C–J and 7.32G and H).[330] In other cases, it may be necessary to employ vitrectomy and intravitreal gas injection to achieve resolution of the detachment.[328,330–332] Schisis detachment, when confined to the peripheral fundus, rarely progresses and requires no treatment.[329] The author believes, however, that posterior extension of schisis to near the macula, particularly when associated with large outer-wall holes, constitutes a threat to central vision and should be delimited with several rows of laser photocoagulation (Figure 7.32J and K) without waiting to demonstrate progression.

7.31 Retinal crystals associated with retinal detachment.

A and B: Perifoveal distribution of shiny white crystals in this patient with a long-standing inferior retinal detachment. His visual acuity was 20/20.

Degenerative retinoschisis.

C: Photomicrograph showing split at the level of the nerve fiber layer (arrow) and extensive cystoid degeneration of the peripheral retina.

D: Stereoscopic photographs of a large area of retinoschisis that extends posteriorly into the temporal portion of the macula in this 52-year-old man, who also had retinoschisis in the other eye. Note there is no evidence of retinal pigment epithelium degeneration in the area of the retinoschisis.

E–H: In November 1975, bilateral retinoschisis was noted in this asymptomatic 68-year-old woman. In the left eye it extended almost to the macula (E). One year later she lost central vision in the left eye because of macular detachment caused by a large posterior outer-wall tear at the posterior edge of the retinoschisis. A scleral buckle supplemented with postoperative photocoagulation (F and G) was used in closing the tear (arrows). Ten years later her visual acuity was 20/30 (H).

I and J: Spontaneous collapse of degenerative retinoschisis in this middle-aged woman. The retinoschisis was present in June 1979 (I) and had disappeared in September 1979 (J).

(A and B, courtesy of Dr. David Weinberg; C, courtesy of Dr. Robert Y. Foos.)

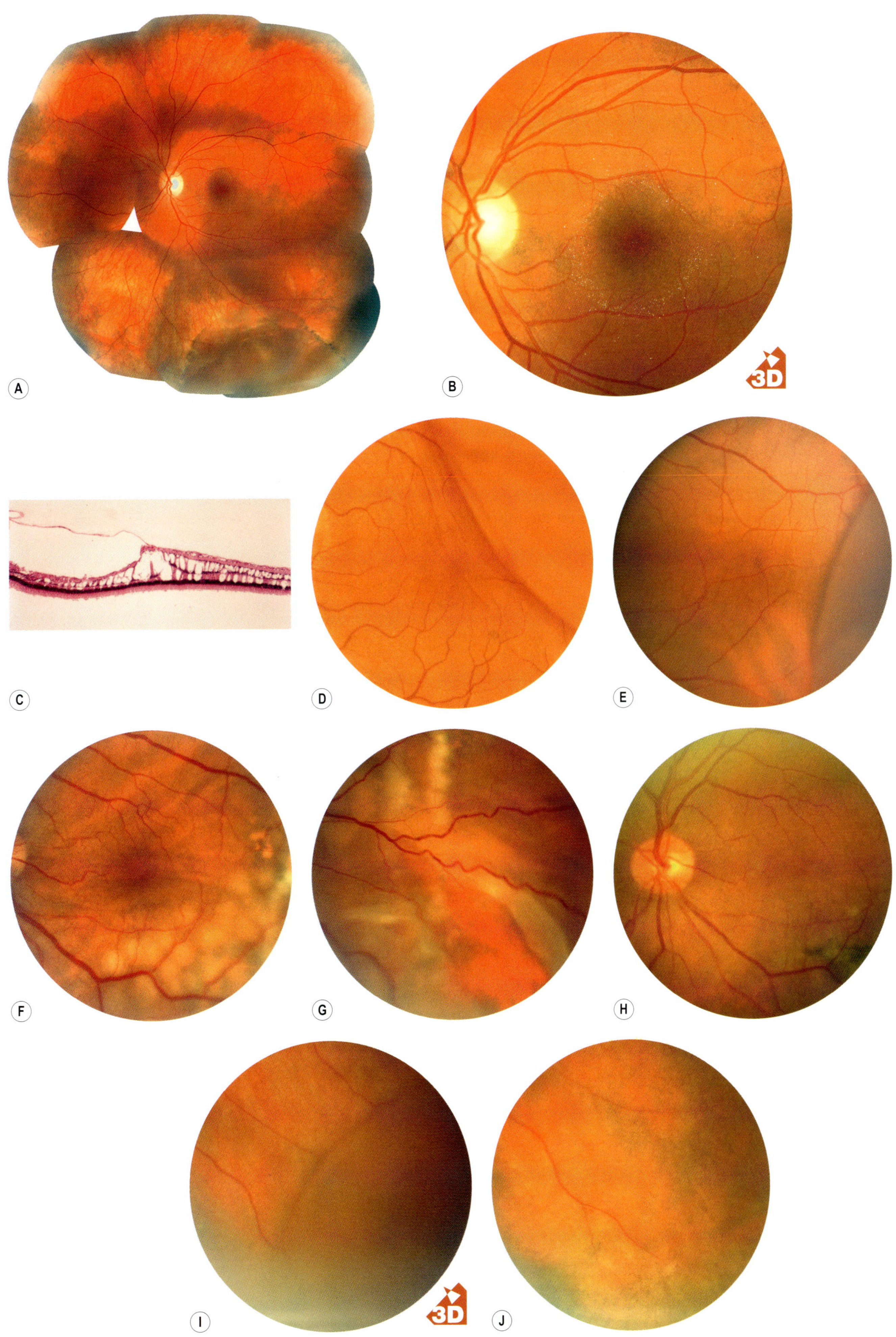
A
B
3D
C
D
E
F
G
H
I
3D
J

Unlike patients with X-linked juvenile retinoschisis, there is no evidence of any specific macular abnormality in patients with degenerative retinoschisis. Detailed macular function tests in these patients are comparable to those in unaffected patients.[326]

Fluorescein angiography shows no abnormality in the background choroidal fluorescence in the area of retinoschisis (Figure 7.29B and C) as long as there is no hole or detachment in the outer retinal layer. In some cases there may be evidence of retinal capillary dilation, leakage, and dropout in the inner retinal layers.

The pathogenesis of degenerative retinoschisis is unknown, but chronic vitreous traction on the peripheral retina that is predisposed to microcystoid degeneration, particularly on the temporal side, is probably important. The schisis begins with coalescence of the cysts of Blessig–Iwanoff microcystoid degeneration resulting in a system of tunnel-like spaces in the outer plexiform layer. Subsequently a second independent system of spaces develops at the level of the inner nuclear layer. At first the inner and outer systems are separated by the junction of the neurons with the horizontal cells that lie between the inner and outer plexiform layers (Figure 7.32A–F). Gradually the supporting columns between the cysts disintegrate, splitting the remaining retinal elements into two layers with sparse cellular connections in between them, mostly made up of Müller cells. At this stage, the surface of the retinoschisis shows pitting corresponding to the footplates of the Müller cells (Figure 7.32B). Eventually when the tissue pillars undergo complete necrosis, the layers separate completely.[333] The material that fills the cavity is composed of mucopolysaccharide and is believed to result from the breakdown of the tissue elements.[334]

7.32 Retinoschisis.

A–F: A 38-year-old male with recent decrease in vision in the left eye to 20/100. The right eye saw 20/20. A large retinoschisis was seen in the inferotemporal region of the left eye extending to the foveal center, in addition to flecks of fundus flavimaculatus in the posterior pole in both eyes (A–C). An outer retinal break with adjacent subretinal fluid was found at the superior edge of the schisis (C, arrow). Optical coherence tomography through the foveal center and elsewhere revealed vertically oriented schisis cavities (D and E). A section through the area of the outer break demonstrated subretinal fluid beneath the schisis cavity (F). He was treated with oral and topical acetazolamide and refracted to 20/40 with a hyperopic correction.

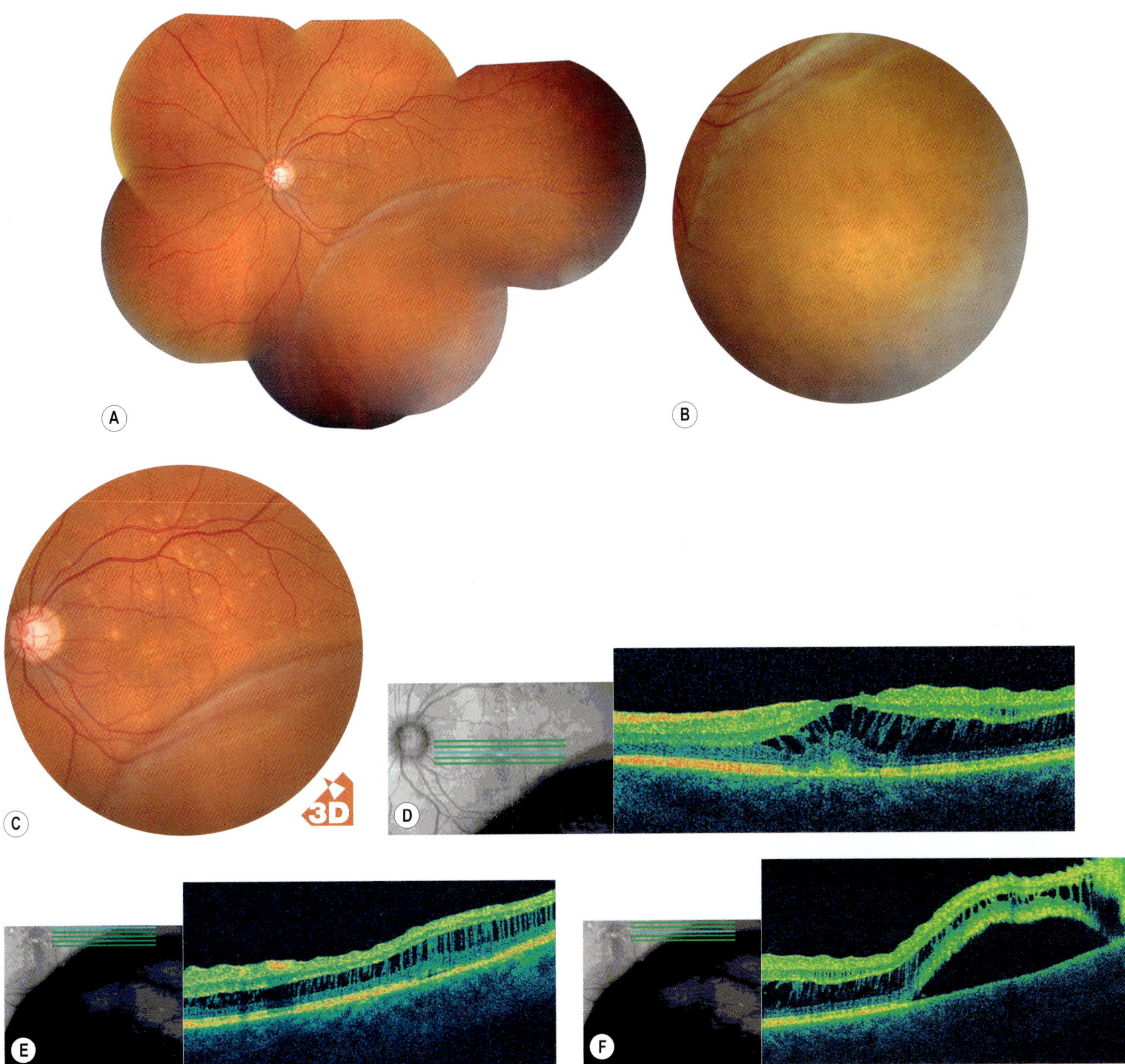
A
B
C
3D
D
E
F

Spontaneous reattachment of the inner layer occasionally occurs (Figure 7.29H and I). No treatment is indicated unless a retinal detachment associated with inner and outer retinal holes develops, or unless there is demonstrated progression of schisis (Figures 7.32 I to K) or a schisis detachment with outer-wall holes into the macular area.

Most degenerative retinoschisis occur independently; however association with nanophthalmos, high myopia, and tilted discs has been reported.[335–338] Acquired retinoschisis and retinal folds occur as a sequel to the retinopathy in children suffering nonaccidental trauma.[339]

Retinoschisis is most likely to be mistaken for a localized rhegmatogenous retinal detachment or occasionally the reverse. The typical configuration of the elevated inner retinal surface, absence of evidence of visible and angiographic changes in the underlying RPE, and presence of an absolute scotoma are features suggesting retinoschisis. The presence of a demarcation line is strong evidence of a rhegmatogenous detachment, which in the presence of schisis may be difficult to identify. Angiographic evidence of depigmentation of the RPE peripheral to the demarcation line indicates present or past retinal detachment in that area.

7.32 Continued

G and **H**: Laser applied to an outer retinal break in an eye with extreme thinning of the schisis layers.
I–K: This 40-year-old high myope was found to have a large schisis in the inferotemporal quadrant on routine examination (I and J). Two years later the cavity had enlarged in height and extended posteriorly (K). She underwent laser demarcation of the retina posterior to the schisis in an attempt to prevent further progression.

(G and H, courtesy of Dr. Franco Recchia.)

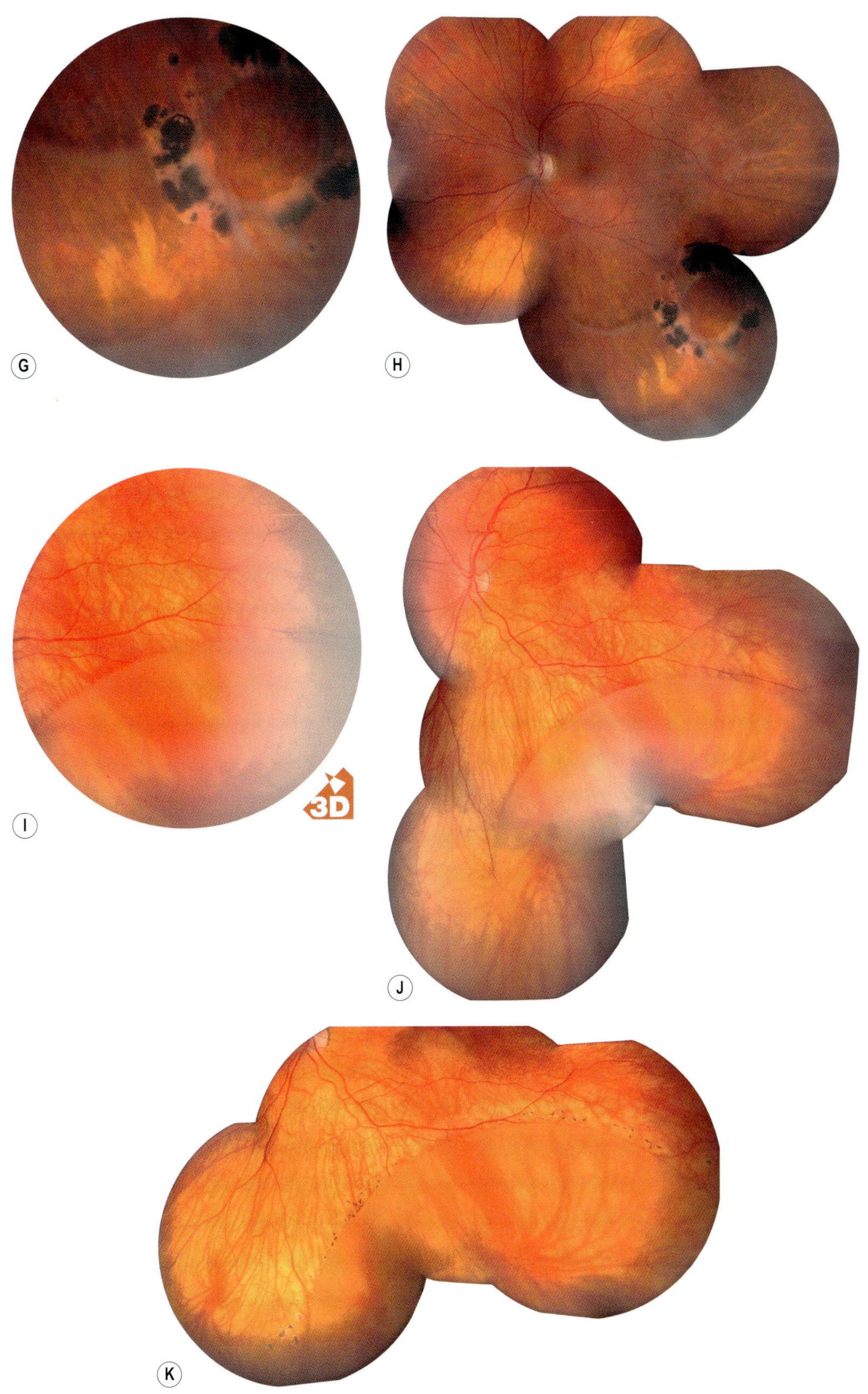
G
H
3D
I
J
K

AMYLOIDOSIS

Loss of vision caused by accumulation of amyloid in the vitreous may occur in primary familial amyloidosis with or without systemic involvement and occasionally in patients with neither systemic nor familial involvement.[340–354]

The amyloid is probably produced in the retinal vessels and secreted into the vitreous. Early, it may produce prominent perivascular sheathing and localized vitreous veils.[353] Later, as the vitreous becomes more opacified, it has been described biomicroscopically as having a cotton-wool, glass-wool, or cobweb appearance (Figures 7.33A and 7.34A, B, and E). It may be misdiagnosed as inflammatory exudate or resolving retinal and vitreous blood. Cotton-wool spots unassociated with hypertension occurred in one patient.[346]

Histopathologically, amyloid may be demonstrated within and surrounding retinal vessels as well as within large choroidal vessels and the choriocapillaris (Figure 7.33E).[347,355]

Vitreous deposits in amyloidosis occur primarily in patients with dominantly inherited amyloidosis associated with peripheral neuropathy, amyloid nephropathy, and cardiomyopathy (familial amyloidotic polyneuropathy) (Figures 7.33B and C and 7.34A, B, and E).[341,350] Most of these patients have a mutant form of the protein transthyretin associated with a mutation in the transthyretin gene.[351,354,356,357] This mutation may be present in patients with vitreous opacification and no family history of the disorder.[358] Retinal neovascularization and vitreous hemorrhages occur in some patients associated with elevated vascular endothelial growth factor levels.[340,354,359,360] Patients with vitreous opacities should be checked for the transthyretin mutation even when they have no definite family history of amyloidosis. Additional means of diagnosis include biopsy of affected organs, including the eye, kidney, or rectum. Liver transplantation is promising by eliminating production of the abnormal transthyretin in the liver. Ocular involvement has increased or occurred after liver transplantation in some patients secondary to continued retinal production of transthyretin.[361,362]

Familial oculoleptomeningeal amyloidosis (heredo-oto-ophthalmo-encephalopathy) is characterized by hemiplegic migraine, periodic obtundation, psychosis, seizures, carpal tunnel syndrome, intracerebral hemorrhage, myelopathy, deafness, cerebellar ataxia, peripheral neuropathy, visual loss associated with retinal and vitreous infiltration with amyloid and cataract, and systemic organ involvement (Figure 7.33G–L).[345,352,363] The retinal lesions resemble cotton-wool patches but histologically are amyloid infiltration of the retina (Figure 7.33G and I).

Crawford reported cotton-wool exudates in a patient with nonfamilial systemic amyloidosis and no evidence of systemic hypertension.[344] Histologically, these retinal lesions were swollen, degenerated, necrotic axons in the nerve fiber layer unassociated with amyloid deposits in either the retina or the vitreous. Amyloid is known to deposit in and around the retinal and choroidal vessels, sometimes causing a severe chorioretinopathy.[364]

7.33 Primary amyloidosis.

A–F: Slit-lamp photograph of this 62-year-old man who experienced painless progressive loss of vision for several years because of amyloid deposition (arrow) in the vitreous of both eyes (A). His past medical history was positive for severe peripheral neuropathy and the carpal tunnel syndrome. Note the atrophy of the skin and muscles of the hands and feet (B and C). His family history was negative. An open-sky lensectomy and vitrectomy were done. His visual acuity improved from counting fingers at 1 foot (30 cm) to 20/30. Note the remnants of amyloid on the optic disc (arrow, D) and on the retinal surface temporal to the macula (arrow, E). He subsequently died of a coronary thrombosis. Photomicrograph (F) showing amyloid deposits occluding much of the choriocapillaris and within the wall of the large choroidal vessels (arrows).

G and **H**: This 51-year-old woman with dominantly inherited oculoleptomeningeal amyloidosis had a 20-year history of progressive peripheral neuropathy, carpal tunnel syndrome, hyperreflexia, dysarthria, nystagmus, and memory loss. Visual acuity was 20/25 bilaterally. In the perimacular area she had numerous superficial gray-white lesions that stained angiographically (G and H). One year later she developed visual loss, vitreous opacification, and thickening of the tongue. Visual acuity improved from 20/400 to 20/40 in both eyes following vitrectomy. The vitreous exhibited dichroism and stained positively for amyloid.

I–L: The 28-year-old son of the patient in G and H had a history of hemiplegic migraine and seizures beginning in his teenage years. He died at age 29 years from complications of intracerebral hemorrhage. Pathologic examination of the eyes revealed birefringent amyloid deposits in the blood vessel walls and perivascular spaces of the retina (arrows, I (Congo red stain) and J (polarized light)), extensive amyloid deposition in the leptomeninges and the blood vessel walls within the leptomeninges (arrows, K and L (Congo red stain)). Other organ involvement included the heart, alimentary tract, skeletal muscle, and nerves.

(D and E, from Kasner et al.[347]; J–L, from Uitti et al.[352];

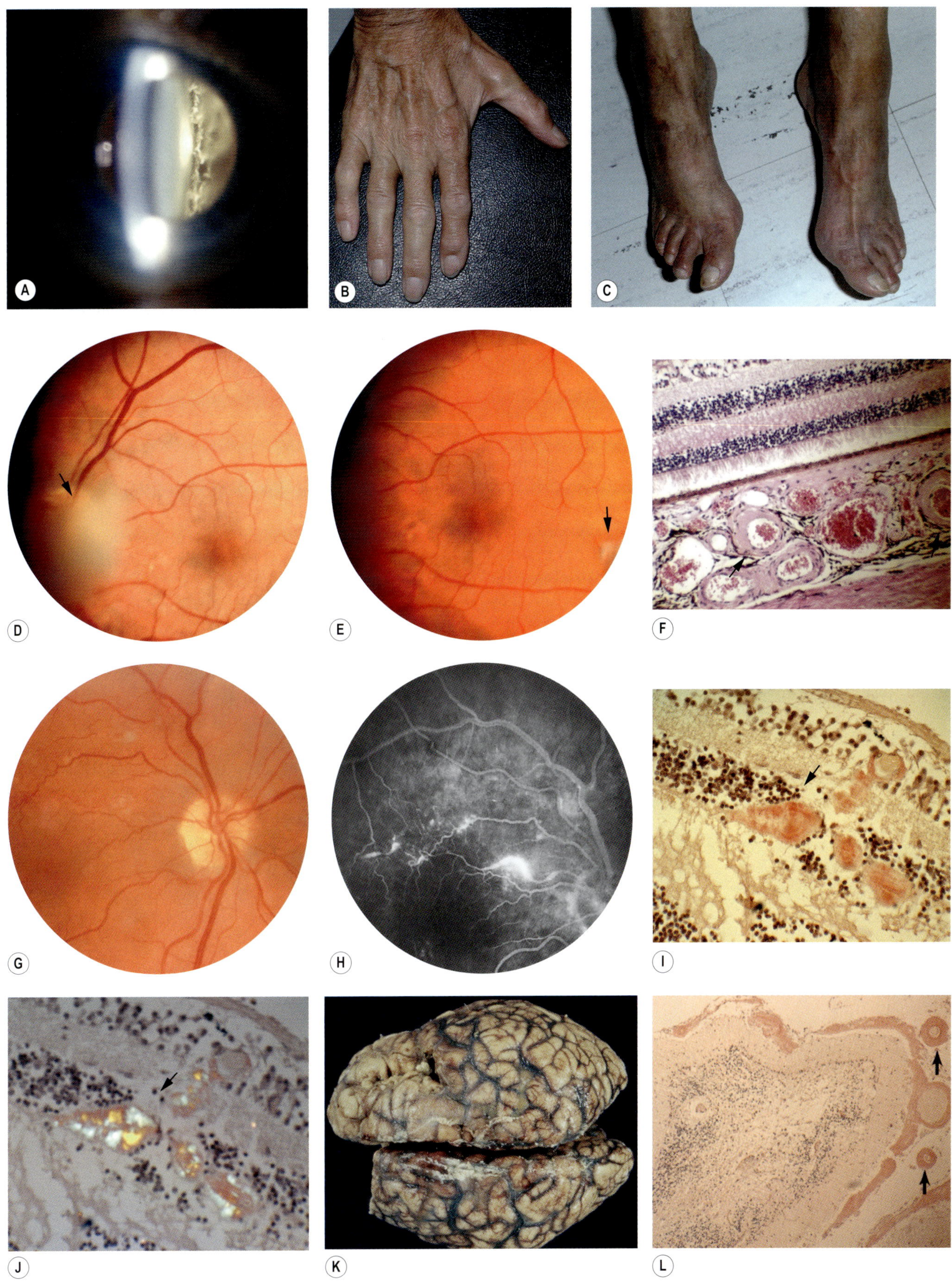
A
B
C
D
E
F
G
H
I
J
K
L

Vitrectomy is the only effective means of restoring vision in patients with amyloidosis (Figures 7.33D and E and 7.34C and D).[347,357,365] Removal of as much of the vitreous framework as possible is indicated since recurrence of the amyloid deposits may occur.[343,366] The material will stain with Congo red and show typical yellow-green bi-refringence with polarized light (Figure 7.34F). Panretinal photocoagulation is required for eyes with retinal neovascularization and vitreous hemorrhages.

ASTEROID HYALOSIS

Asteroid hyalosis is a degenerative disease of the vitreous of unknown cause.[377–384] It is characterized by the development of white or yellow-white spherical or disc-shaped bodies (asteroid bodies) composed of calcium soap within the collagen framework of the vitreous (Figure 7.35I and K). They develop initially in the vicinity of the retinal blood vessels and may eventually be present in such large numbers throughout the vitreous that visualization of the ocular fundus is not possible. In spite of this, however, the patient's visual function is only minimally affected. Fluorescein angiography may provide an excellent view of the fundus when it is obscured ophthalmoscopically (Figure 7.35I and F).[379] Histopathologically, the asteroid bodies have a crystalline appearance and they stain positively with fat and acid mucopolysaccharides that are unaffected by pretreatment with hyaluronidase.[382] Though asteroid bodies have been extensively investigated, their origin, mode of formation, and composition are incompletely elucidated. Ultrastructurally they are composed primarily of multilaminar membranes typical of complex acidic lipids, particularly phospholipids, and are associated with calcium phosphate complexes lying in a homogeneous background matrix.[383,384] In addition to calcium and phosphorus, the most detectable elements, sulfur and potassium, may be found. Chondroitin 6 sulfate and carbohydrates specific for hyaluronic acid have been found.[385] Experimentally asteroid hyalosis has been produced in galactose-fed beagles which develop a retinopathy similar to diabetic retinopathy.[386]

Asteroid hyalosis typically develops in later life and most often affects only one eye. Its association with diabetes mellitus is a subject of debate given the significant numbers with unilateral involvement.[377,380] Abnormal vitreoretinal adhesions with vitreoschisis and anomalous PVD have been documented by OCT.[387] Vitrectomy is rarely needed to restore vision but may be necessary in the occasional patient who has unexplained visual loss.[379,382] In spite of a visible Weiss ring, these eyes may have adherent residual vitreous cortex which should be sought for during surgery.

7.34 Amyloidosis

A–F: A 32-year-old Korean male noted floaters and progressive diminution of vision over 2 years. His visual acuity was count fingers in the right and 20/50 in the left eye. Dense vitreous opacities, neovascularization of the retina, and retinal hemorrhages were noted in both eyes (A, B, and E). White deposits around blood vessels were also seen (C). He underwent a pars plana vitrectomy and focal laser with improvement in vision to 20/30 in 1 week and 20/20 in 1 month in his right eye. Subsequently the left eye suffered a vitreous hemorrhage prompting a vitrectomy with improvement of vision to 20/30. The vitreous deposits showed apple-green birefringence on polarized microscopy with Congo red (F). His vitreous vascular endothelial growth factor levels were highly elevated. His 30-year-old brother was examined and found to have similar findings, requiring a vitrectomy in his left eye. Both brothers were positive for Glu54Gly transthyretin mutation (DNA change: 221 A > G), confirming familial amyloidotic polyneuropathy.

(Courtesy Dr. Jennifer Lim. Reproduced from O'Hearn et al.[354])

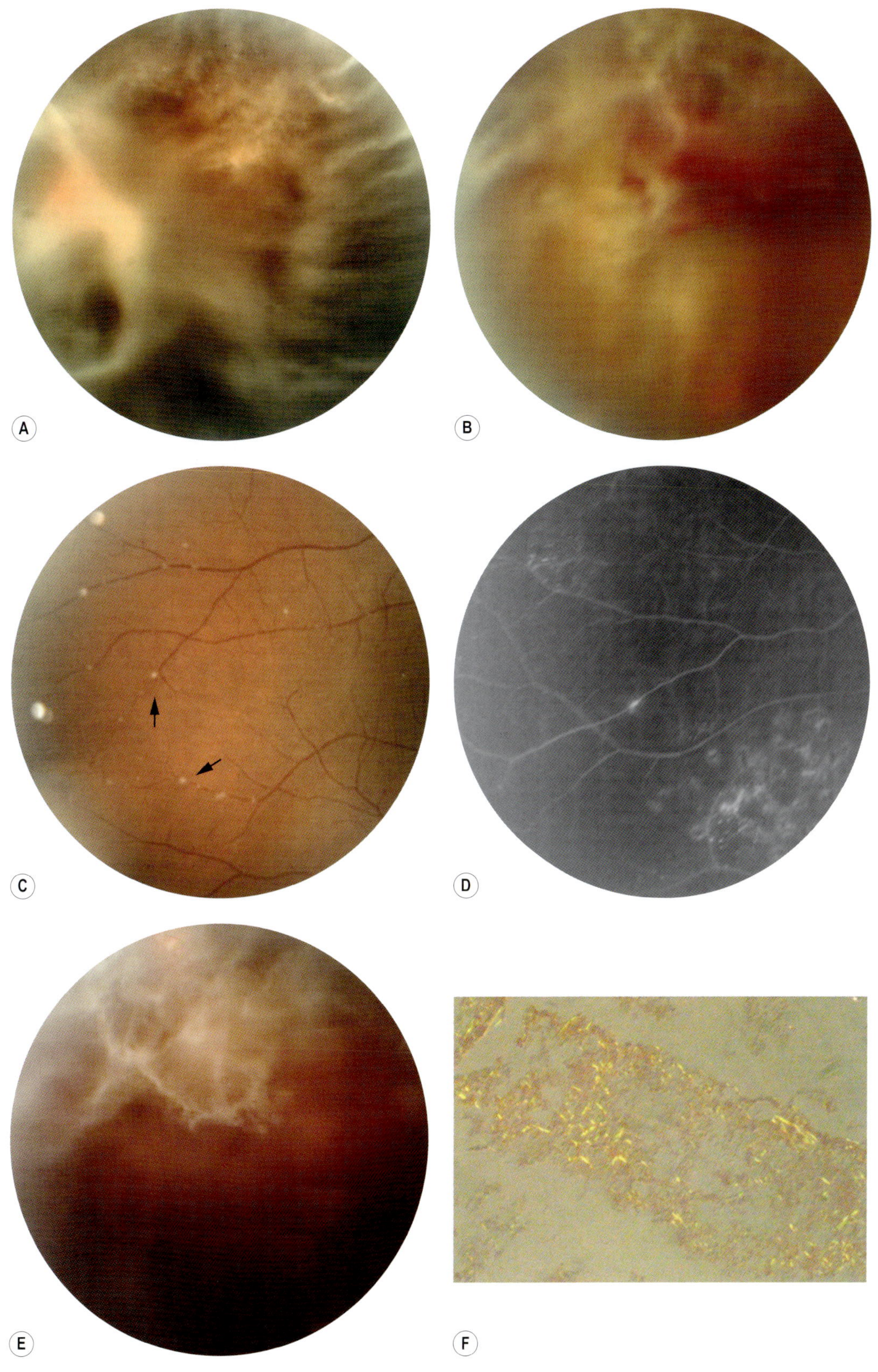
A
B
C
D
E
F

VITREOUS CYSTS

Vitreous cysts may arise in otherwise normal eyes, in diseased eyes, or in association with remnants of the hyaloid system.[367–375] Those occurring in normal or diseased eyes are typically round or lobulated, partly pigmented or nonpigmented, translucent structures lying free in the vitreous cavity (Figure 7.35A–D). Cysts associated with the hyaloid system are usually sessile, nonpigmented gray cysts attached to the surface of the optic disc (Fig. 7.35C). Most free-floating cysts probably remain unchanged for many years, cause no symptoms, and require no treatment.[372] Pigmented cysts located close to the retinal surface can be mistaken for a pigmented tumor. They occasionally interfere with visual function, and in such cases aspiration of the cyst or disruption with laser (D1 and D2) may provide symptomatic relief.[367,371]

The cyst wall in most cases is probably composed of retinal pigment epithelial cells (Fig. 7.35E and F).[370,376] Nork and Millecchia found a single layer of pigment laden epithelial cells on a basement membrane that resembled Bruch's membrane with a lamina rara, lamina densa and a thick collagenous layer (Fig. 7-35 E and F). The cells were positive for carbonic anhydrase (Fig. 7.35G), and on electron microscopy showed microvilli, zonula adherens and occludens, all features of retinal pigment epithelial cells (Fig. 7.35H). There were premelanosomes (Fig. 7.35H, inset, open arrow), which are of fetal origin, and not produced postnatally in RPE cells, suggesting the cyst to be a choristoma of the primary hyaloidal system with sequestered RPE cells.[376]

METASTATIC CARCINOMA AND MELANOMA TO THE VITREOUS

See Chapter 13.

7.35 Vitreous cysts.

A: Irregular, translucent, pigmented, free-floating vitreous cyst.

B: Free-floating pigmented cyst located just inferior to the macula.

C: Nonpigmented cyst attached to the optic nerve head.

D to H: This 35 year old otherwise healthy Caucasian woman had noted a floater in her left eye since childhood. The floater was now constant and vision declined to 20/40. A partly pigmented vitreous cyst was seen tethered to Cloquet's canal and was associated with a Mittendorf's dot (D1). Argon laser done to perforate the cyst wall collapsed the cyst (D2) but the cyst then hung in front of her macula requiring a pars plana vitrectomy and cyst removal. The cyst wall is made up of a basement membrane with pigment laden cells consistent with RPE (Toluidine blue) (E and F). Staining for carbonic anhydrase is positive confirming RPE origin of the cyst cells (G). Electron microscopy revealed zonula occludens (H, arrow) and pre-melanosomes (H, inset) that is considered to be fetal in origin suggesting arrested development of the RPE cells.

Asteroid Hyalosis.

I and J: Asteroid bodies were sufficiently concentrated that a view of the fundus details was difficult in this patient, who was complaining of visual loss in the left eye (I). Angiography (J), however, provided a clear view of evidence of age-related macular degeneration and subfoveal neovascularization.

K: Gross eye specimen showing asteroid bodies suspended in the vitreous framework.

L: Histopathology of asteroid hyalosis showing spherical and ovoid PAS-positive amorphous bodies suspended in the vitreous framework.

Courtesy: D to H, Dr. Michael Nork. Reprinted with permission from Ophthalmology (Nork, T. M. and L. L. Millecchia. Treatment and histopathology of a congenital vitreous cyst. Ophthalmology 1998: 105(5); 825-830.)

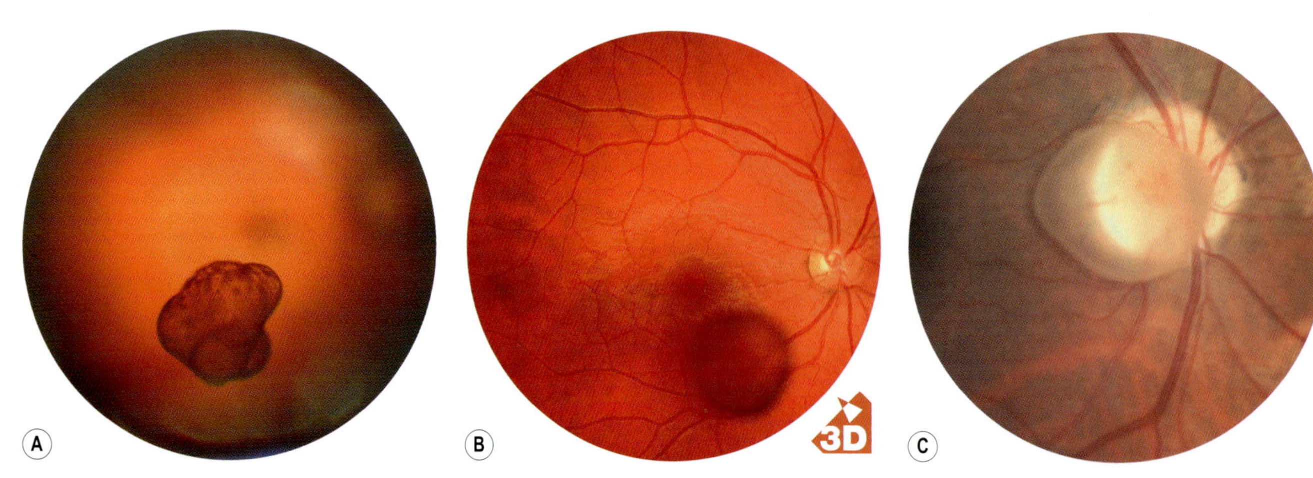

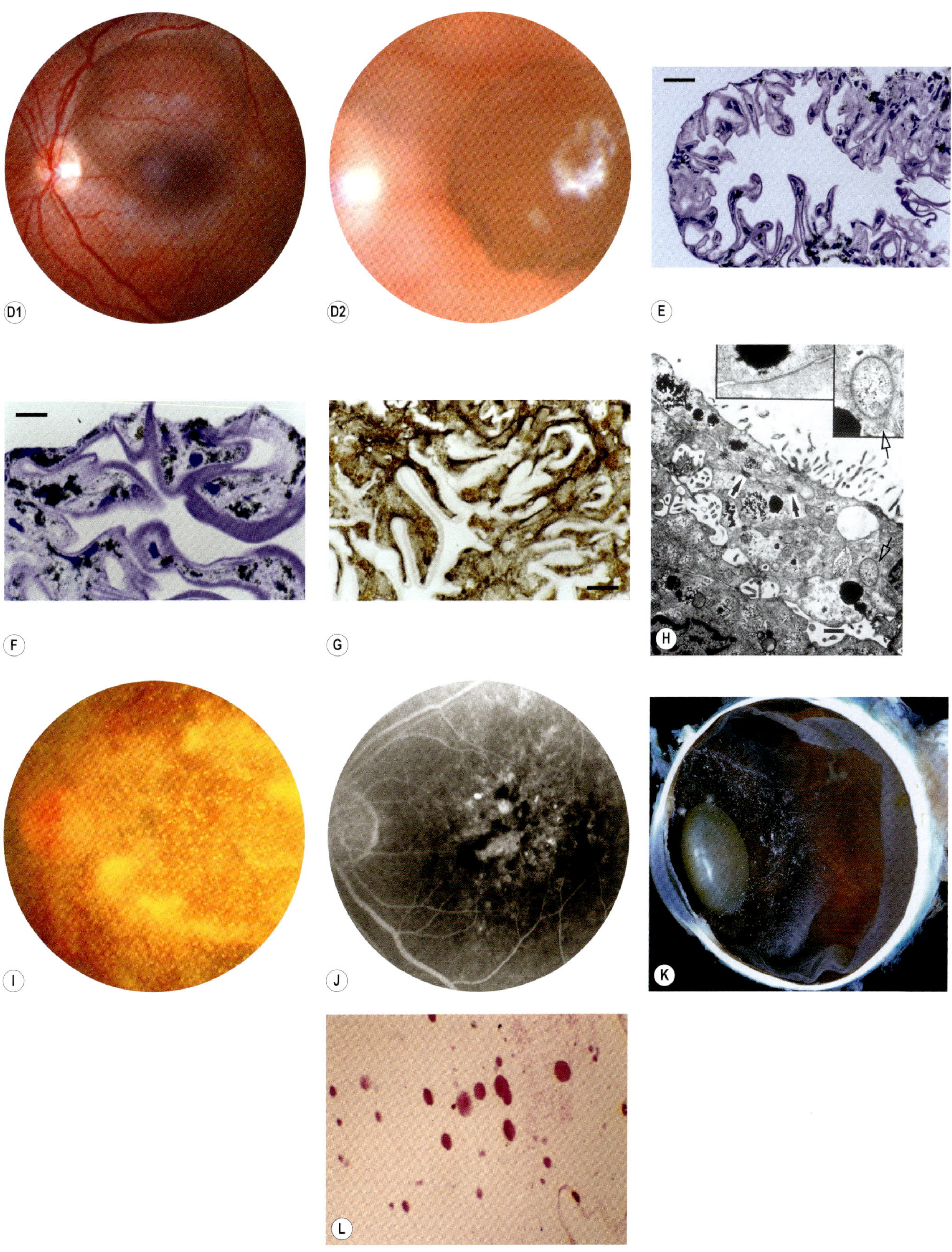
D1
D2
E
F
G
H
I
J
K
L

References

1. Bartsch D-U, Intaglietta M, Bille JF, et al. Confocal laser tomographic analysis of the retina in eyes with macular hole formation and other focal macular diseases. Am J Ophthalmol 1989;108:277–87.
2. Hee MR, Puliafito CA, Wong C, et al. Optical coherence tomography of macular holes. Ophthalmology 1995;102:748–56.
3. Kiryu J, Shahidi M, Ogura Y, et al. Illustration of the stages of idiopathic macular holes by laser biomicroscopy. Arch Ophthalmol 1995;113:1156–60.
4. Ogura Y, Shahidi M, Mori MT, et al. Improved visualization of macular hole lesions with laser biomicroscopy. Arch Ophthalmol 1991;109:957–61.
5. Mirza RG, Johnson MW, Jampol LM. Optical coherence tomography use in evaluation of the vitreoretinal interface: a review. Surv Ophthalmol 2007;52:397–421.
6. Karatas M, Ramirez JA, Ophir A. Diabetic vitreopapillary traction and macular oedema. Eye (Lond) 2005;19:676–82.
7. Drexler W, Morgner U, Ghanta RK, et al. Ultrahigh-resolution ophthalmic optical coherence tomography. Nat Med 2001;7:502–7.
8. Huang D, Swanson EA, Lin CP, et al. Optical coherence tomography. Science 1991;254: 1178–81.
9. Coleman DJ, Daly SW, Atencio A, et al. Ultrasonic evaluation of the vitreous and retina. Semin Ophthalmol 1998;13:210–8.
10. Foos RY. Vitreoretinal juncture; topographical variations. Invest Ophthalmol 1972;11:801–8.
11. Roth AM, Foos RY. Surface structure of the optic nerve head. 1. Epipapillary membranes. Am J Ophthalmol 1972;74:977–85.
12. Foos RY. Subhyaloid hemorrhage illustrating a mechanism of macular hole formation. Arch Ophthalmol 1992;110:598.
13. Kishi S, Demaria C, Shimizu K. Vitreous cortex remnants at the fovea after spontaneous vitreous detachment. Int Ophthalmol 1986;9:253–60.
14. Nork TM, Gioia VM, Hobson RR, et al. Subhyaloid hemorrhage illustrating a mechanism of macular hole formation. Arch Ophthalmol 1991;109:884–5.
15. Sebag J. Age-related changes in human vitreous structure. Graefes Arch Clin Exp Ophthalmol 1987;225:89–93.
16. Kishi S, Shimizu K. Posterior precortical vitreous pocket. Arch Ophthalmol 1990;108:979–82.
17. Kishi S, Shimizu K. Reply to letter by JGF Worst. Arch Ophthalmol 1991;109:1060.
18. Kishi S, Yokozuka K, Tobe K. Bursa premacularis. Acta Soc Ophthalmol Jpn 1988;92:1881–8.
19. Worst J. Extracapsular surgery in lens implantation (Binkhorst lecture). Part IV: Some anatomical and pathophysiological implications. Am Intra-Ocular Implant Soc J 1978;4:7–14.
20. Worst JGF. Cisternal systems of the fully developed vitreous body in the young adult. Trans Ophthalmol Soc UK 1977;97:550–4.
21. Worst JGF. Posterior precortical vitreous pocket. Arch Ophthalmol 1991;109:1058–9.
22. Sebag J. Vitreous: the resplendent enigma. Br J Ophthalmol 2009;93:989–91.
23. Eisner G. Biomicroscopy of the peripheral fundus: an atlas and textbook. Berlin: Springer; 1973. p. 45.
24. Foos RY, Wheeler NC. Vitreoretinal juncture: synchysis senilis and posterior vitreous detachment. Ophthalmology 1982;89:1502–12.
25. Jaffe NS. Complications of acute posterior vitreous detachment. Arch Ophthalmol 1968;79: 568–71.
26. Reese AB, Jones IS, Cooper WC. Macular changes secondary to vitreous traction. Am J Ophthalmol 1967;64:544–9.
27. Sebag J. Age-related differences in the human vitreoretinal interface. Arch Ophthalmol 1991;109:966–71.
28. Tabotabo MM, Karp LA, Benson WE. Posterior vitreous detachment. Ann Ophthalmol 1980;12:59–61.
29. Tasman WS. Posterior vitreous detachment and peripheral retinal breaks. Trans Am Acad Ophthalmol Otolaryngol 1968;72:217–24.
30. Linder B. Acute posterior vitreous detachment and its retinal complications; a clinical biomicroscopic study. Acta Ophthalmol Suppl 1966:87.
31. Cibis GW, Watzke RC, Chua J. Retinal hemorrhages in posterior vitreous detachment. Am J Ophthalmol 1975;80:1043–6.
32. Schachat AP, Sommer A. Macular hemorrhages associated with posterior vitreous detachment. Am J Ophthalmol 1986;102:647–9.
33. Yonemoto J, Ideta H, Sasaki K, et al. The age of onset of posterior vitreous detachment. Graefes Arch Clin Exp Ophthalmol 1994;232:67–70.
34. Sebag J. To see the invisible: the quest of imaging vitreous. Dev Ophthalmol 2008;42:5–28.
35. Johnson MW. Perifoveal vitreous detachment and its macular complications. Trans Am Ophthalmol Soc 2005;103:537–67.
36. Sebag J. Classifying posterior vitreous detachment: a new way to look at the invisible. Br J Ophthalmol 1997;81:521.
37. Gandorfer A, Rohleder M, Kampik A. Epiretinal pathology of vitreomacular traction syndrome. Br J Ophthalmol 2002;86:902–9.
38. Jaffe NS. Vitreous traction at the posterior pole of the fundus due to alterations in the vitreous posterior. Trans Am Acad Ophthalmol Otolaryngol 1967;71:642–51.
39. Kanski JJ. Complications of acute posterior vitreous detachment. Am J Ophthalmol 1975;80:44–6.
40. Novak MA, Welch RB. Complications of acute symptomatic posterior vitreous detachment. Am J Ophthalmol 1984;97:308–14.
41. Boniuk M. Cystic macular edema secondary to vitreoretinal traction. Surv Ophthalmol 1968;13:118–21.
42. Machemer R, Williams Sr JM. Pathogenesis and therapy of traction detachment in various retinal vascular diseases. Am J Ophthalmol 1988;105:170–81.
43. McDonald HR, Johnson RN, Schatz H. Surgical results in the vitreomacular traction syndrome. Ophthalmology 1994;101:1397–403.
44. Reese AB, Jones IS, Cooper WC. Vitreomacular traction syndrome confirmed histologically. Am J Ophthalmol 1970;69:975–7.
45. Smiddy WE, Green WR, Michels RG, et al. Ultrastructural studies of vitreomacular traction syndrome. Am J Ophthalmol 1989;107:177–85.
46. Smiddy WE, Michels RG, Glaser BM, et al. Vitrectomy for macular traction caused by incomplete vitreous separation. Arch Ophthalmol 1988;106:624–8.
47. Smiddy WE, Michels RG, Green WR. Morphology, pathology, and surgery of idiopathic vitreoretinal macular disorders; a review. Retina 1990;10:288–96.
48. Jagger JD, Hamilton AMP, Polkinghorne P. Q-switched neodymium YAG laser vitreolysis in the therapy of posterior segment disease. Graefes Arch Clin Exp Ophthalmol 1990;228:222–5.
49. Benson WE, Tasman W. Rhegmatogenous retinal detachments caused by paravascular vitreoretinal traction. Arch Ophthalmol 1984;102:669–70.
50. de Bustros S, Welch RB. The avulsed retinal vessel syndrome and its variants. Ophthalmology 1984;91:86–8.
51. Folk JC, Ma C, Blodi CF, et al. Occlusion of bridging or avulsed retinal vessels by repeated photocoagulation. Ophthalmology 1987;94:1610–3.
52. Robertson DM, Curtin VT. Norton EWD. Avulsed retinal vessels with retinal breaks; a cause of recurrent vitreous hemorrhage. Arch Ophthalmol 1971;85:669–72.
53. Vine AK. Avulsed retinal veins without retinal breaks. Am J Ophthalmol 1984;98:723–7.
54. Bonnet M. Hyperfluorescence papillaire par tardif du vitré. J Fr Ophtalmol 1991;14:529–36.
55. Aaberg TM. Macular holes; a review. Surv Ophthalmol 1970;15:139–62.
56. Aaberg TM, Blair CJ. Gass JDM. Macular holes. Am J Ophthalmol 1970;69:555–62.
57. Avila MP, Jalkh AE, Murakami K, et al. Biomicroscopic study of the vitreous in macular breaks. Ophthalmology 1983;90:1277–83.
58. Gass JDM. Idiopathic senile macular hole; its early stages and pathogenesis. Arch Ophthalmol 1988;106:629–39.
59. James M, Feman SS. Macular holes. Albrecht von Graefes Arch Klin Exp Ophthalmol 1980;215:59–63.
60. Kruis JA, Bastiaensen LAK, Hoefnagels KLJ. Senile idiopathic macular holes. Doc Ophthalmol 1983;55:81–9.
61. Margherio RR, Schepens CL. Macular breaks. I. Diagnosis, etiology, and observations. Am J Ophthalmol 1972;74:219–32.
62. McDonnell PJ, Fine SL, Hillis AI. Clinical features of idiopathic macular cysts and holes. Am J Ophthalmol 1982;93:777–86.
63. Morgan CM, Schatz H. Idiopathic macular holes. Am J Ophthalmol 1985;99:437–44.
64. Murakami K. Biomicroscopic observation of macular breaks. Hokkaido Igaku Zasshi 1985;60:335–41.
65. Yaoeda H. Clinical observation on macular hole. Acta Soc Ophthalmol Jpn 1967;71:1723–36.
66. Yoshioka H. Clinical studies on macular hole. III. On the pathogenesis of the senile macular hole. Acta Soc Ophthalmol Jpn 1968;72:575–84.
67. Gaudric A, Haouchine B, Massin P, et al. Macular hole formation: new data provided by optical coherence tomography. Arch Ophthalmol 1999;117:744–51.
68. Spaide RF, Wong D, Fisher Y, et al. Correlation of vitreous attachment and foveal deformation in early macular hole states. Am J Ophthalmol 2002;133:226–9.
69. Ezra E. Idiopathic full thickness macular hole: natural history and pathogenesis. Br J Ophthalmol 2001;85:102–8.
70. Gass JD. Müller cell cone, an overlooked part of the anatomy of the fovea centralis: hypotheses concerning its role in the pathogenesis of macular hole and foveomacualr retinoschisis. Arch Ophthalmol 1999;117:821–3.
71. Yamada Y, Miljkovic D, Wehrli P, et al. A new type of corrin synthesis. Angew Chem Int Ed Engl 1969;8:343–8.
72. Spaide RF. Closure of an outer lamellar macular hole by vitrectomy: hypothesis for one mechanism of macular hole formation. Retina 2000;20:587–90.
73. Gass JDM. Reappraisal of biomicroscopic classification of stages of development of a macular hole. Am J Ophthalmol 1995;119:752–9.
74. Hogan MJ, Alvarado JA, Weddell JE. Histology of the human eye; an atlas and textbook. Philadelphia: WB Saunders; 1971. p. 491–92.
75. Campochiaro PA, Van Niel E, Vinores SA. Immunocytochemical labeling of cells in cortical vitreous from patients with premacular hole lesions. Arch Ophthalmol 1992;110:371–7.
76. Thompson JT, Hiner CJ, Glaser BM, et al. Fluorescein angiographic characteristics of macular holes before and after vitrectomy with transforming growth factor beta-2. Am J Ophthalmol 1994;117:291–301.
77. Hikichi T, Trempe CL. Risk of decreased visual acuity in full-thickness idiopathic macular holes. Am J Ophthalmol 1993;116:708–12.
78. Smith RG, Hardman Lea SJ, Galloway NR. Visual performance in idiopathic macular holes. Eye 1990;4:190–4.
79. Sjaarda RN, Frank DA, Glaser BM, et al. Assessment of vision in idiopathic macular holes with macular microperimetry using the scanning laser ophthalmoscope. Ophthalmology 1993;100:1513–8.
80. Sjaarda RN, Frank DA, Glaser BM, et al. Resolution of an absolute scotoma and improvement of relative scotoma after successful macular hole surgery. Am J Ophthalmol 1993;116: 129–39.
81. Acosta F, Lashkari K, Reynaud X, et al. Characterization of functional changes in macular holes and cysts. Ophthalmology 1991;98:1820–3.
82. Callanan DG, Blodi BA, Lubinski WP, et al. S (blue) cone perimetry in macular holes before and after vitrectomy. ARVO Abstract 1415. Invest Ophthalmol Vis Sci 1993;34:990.
83. Gass JDM. Stereoscopic atlas of macular diseases; diagnosis and treatment, 2nd ed. St. Louis: CV Mosby; 1977. p. 334.
84. Gass JDM, Joondeph BC. Observations concerning patients with suspected impending macular holes. Am J Ophthalmol 1990;109:638–46.
85. Frangieh GT, Green WR, Engel HM. A histopathologic study of macular cysts and holes. Retina 1981;1:311–36.

86. de Bustros S. The Vitrectomy for Prevention of Macular Hole Study Group. Vitrectomy for prevention of macular holes; results of a randomized multicenter clinical trial. Ophthalmology 1994;101:1055–9.
87. Guyer DR, de Bustros S, Diener-West M, et al. Observations on patients with idiopathic macular holes and cysts. Arch Ophthalmol 1992;110:1264–8.
88. Wiznia RA. Reversibility of the early stages of idiopathic macular holes. Am J Ophthalmol 1989;107:241–5.
89. Gass JDM, Van Newkirk M. Xanthic scotoma and yellow foveolar shadow caused by a pseudo-operculum after vitreofoveal separation. Retina 1992;12:242–4.
90. Cairns JD, MacCombe MF. Microholes of the fovea centralis. Aust NZ J Ophthalmol 1988;16:75–9.
91. Akiba J, Quiroz MA, Trempe CL. Role of posterior vitreous detachment in idiopathic macular holes. Ophthalmology 1990;97:1610–3.
92. Akiba J, Yoshida A, Trempe CL. Risk of developing a macular hole. Arch Ophthalmol 1990;108:1088–90.
93. Gordon LW, Glaser BM, Darmakusuma I, et al. Full-thickness macular hole formation in eyes with a pre-existing complete posterior vitreous detachment. Ophthalmology 1995;102:1702–5.
94. Hikichi T, Trempe CL. Relationship between floaters, light flashes, or both, and complications of posterior vitreous detachment. Am J Ophthalmol 1994;117:593–8.
95. Johnson RN. Gass JDM. Idiopathic macular holes; observations, stages of formation, and implications for surgical intervention. Ophthalmology 1988;95:917–24.
96. Bidwell AE, Jampol LM. Macular holes and excellent visual acuity. Arch Ophthalmol 1988;106:1350–1.
97. Hikichi T, Trempe CL. Resolution of an absolute scotoma after spontaneous disappearance of idiopathic full-thickness macular hole. Am J Ophthalmol 1994;118:121–2.
98. Yuzawa M, Watanabe A, Takahashi Y, et al. Observation of idiopathic full-thickness macular holes; follow-up observation. Arch Ophthalmol 1994;112:1051–6.
99. Lewis H, Cowan GM, Straatsma BR. Apparent disappearance of a macular hole associated with development of an epiretinal membrane. Am J Ophthalmol 1986;102:172–5.
100. Birch DG, Jost BF, Fish GE. The focal electroretinogram in fellow eyes of patients with idiopathic macular holes. Arch Ophthalmol 1988;106:1558–63.
101. Gass JDM. Risk of developing macular hole. Arch Ophthalmol 1991;109:610–1.
102. Kishi S, Yokozuka K, Kamei Y. The state of the vitreous in idiopathic macular holes. Acta Soc Ophthalmol Jpn 1991;95:678–85.
103. Trempe CL, Weiter JJ, Furukawa H. Fellow eyes in cases of macular hole; biomicroscopic study of the vitreous. Arch Ophthalmol 1986;104:93–5.
104. Bronstein MA, Trempe CL, Freeman HM. Fellow eyes of eyes with macular holes. Am J Ophthalmol 1981;92:757–61.
105. Fish RH, Anand R, Izbrand DJ. Macular pseudoholes; clinical features and accuracy of diagnosis. Ophthalmology 1992;99:1665–70.
106. Fisher YL, Slakter JS, Yannuzzi LA, et al. A prospective natural history study and kinetic ultrasound evaluation of idiopathic macular holes. Ophthalmology 1994;101:5–11.
107. Guyer DR, Green WR, de Bustros S, et al. Histopathologic features of idiopathic macular holes and cysts. Ophthalmology 1990;97:1045–51.
108. Lewis ML, Cohen S, Smiddy WE, et al. Bilaterality of idiopathic macular holes. Graefes Arch Clin Exp Ophthalmol 1996;234:241–5.
109. Smiddy WE. Atypical presentations of macular holes. Arch Ophthalmol 1993;111:626–31.
110. Sebag J. Tissue analysis from two patients with premacular hole lesions. Arch Ophthalmol 1993;111:22.
111. Smiddy WE, Michels RG, de Bustros S, et al. Histopathology of tissue removed during vitrectomy for impending idiopathic macular holes. Am J Ophthalmol 1989;108:360–4.
112. Morgan CM, Schatz H. Involutional macular thinning; a pre-macular hole condition. Ophthalmology 1986;93:153–61.
113. Kornzweig AL, Feldstein M. Studies of the eye in old age. II. Hole in the macula: a clinico-pathologic study. Am J Ophthalmol 1950;33:243–7.
114. Larsson L, Österlin S. Posterior vitreous detachment; a combined clinical and physicochemical study. Graefes Arch Clin Exp Ophthalmol 1985;223:92–5.
115. Gass JDM. Lamellar macular hole: a complication of cystoid macular edema after cataract extraction: clinicopathologic case report. Trans Am Ophthalmol Soc 1975;73:231–50. [Also Arch Ophthalmol 1976;94:793–800.]
116. Martinez J, Smiddy WE, Kim J, et al. Differentiating macular holes from macular pseudoholes. Am J Ophthalmol 1994;117:762–7.
117. Smiddy WE, Gass JDM. Masquerades of macular holes. Ophthalmic Surg 1995;26:16–24.
118. Dugel PU, Smiddy WE, Byrne SF, et al. Macular hole syndromes; echographic findings with clinical correlation. Ophthalmology 1994;101:815–21.
119. Fisher YL, Slakter JS, Friedman RA, et al. Kinetic ultrasound evaluation of the posterior vitreoretinal interface. Ophthalmology 1991;98:1135–8.
120. Van Newkirk MR, Gass JDM, Callanan D, et al. Follow-up and ultrasonographic examination of patients with macular pseudo-operculum. Am J Ophthalmol 1994;117:13–18.
121. Chambers RB, Davidorf FH, Gresak P, et al. Modified vitrectomy for impending macular holes. Ophthalmic Surg 1991;22:730–4.
122. Gass JDM, Discussion of Glaser BM, Michels RG, Kuppermann BD, et al. Transforming growth factor-β_2 for the treatment of full-thickness macular holes; a prospective randomized study. Ophthalmology 1992;99:1173.
123. Jost BF, Hutton WL, Fuller DG, et al. Vitrectomy in eyes at risk for macular hole formation. Ophthalmology 1990;97:843–7.
124. Margherio RR, Trese MT, Margherio AR, et al. Surgical management of vitreomacular traction syndromes. Ophthalmology 1989;96:1437–45.
125. Smiddy WE, Michels RG, Glaser BM, et al. Vitrectomy for impending idiopathic macular holes. Am J Ophthalmol 1988;105:371–6.
126. de Bustros S. Editorial: early stages of macular holes; to treat or not to treat. Arch Ophthalmol 1990;108:1085.
127. Kelly NE, Wendel RT. Vitreous surgery for idiopathic macular holes; results of a pilot study. Arch Ophthalmol 1991;109:654–9.
128. Glaser BM, Michels RG, Kuppermann BD, et al. Transforming growth factor-β_2 for the treatment of full-thickness macular holes; a prospective randomized study. Ophthalmology 1992;99:1162–72.
129. Poliner LS, Tornambe PE. Retinal pigment epitheliopathy after macular hole surgery. Ophthalmology 1992;99:1671–7.
130. Mein CE, Flynn Jr HW. Recognition and removal of the posterior cortical vitreous during vitreoretinal surgery for impending macular hole. Am J Ophthalmol 1991;111:611–3.
131. Ruby AJ, Williams DF, Grand MG, et al. Pars plana vitrectomy for treatment of stage 2 macular holes. Arch Ophthalmol 1994;112:359–64.
132. Smiddy WE, Glaser BM, Green WR, et al. Transforming growth factor beta; a biologic chorioretinal glue. Arch Ophthalmol 1989;107:577–80.
133. Smiddy WE, Glaser BM, Thompson JT, et al. Transforming growth factor-β_2 significantly enhances the ability to flatten the rim of subretinal fluid surrounding macular holes; preliminary anatomic results of a multicenter prospective randomized study. Retina 1993;13:296–301.
134. Wendel RT, Patel AC, Kelly NE, et al. Vitreous surgery for macular holes. Ophthalmology 1993;100:1671–6.
135. Liggett PE, Alfaro DV, Horio B, et al. Autologous serum as a tissue adhesive in the treatment of idiopathic macular holes. Ophthalmology 1993;100(Suppl.):73.
136. Duker JS, Wendel R, Patel AC, et al. Late re-opening of macular holes after initially successful treatment with vitreous surgery. Ophthalmology 1994;101:1373–8.
137. Ie D, Glaser BM, Thompson JT, et al. Retreatment of full-thickness macular holes persisting after prior vitrectomy; a pilot study. Ophthalmology 1993;100:1787–93.
138. Charles S. Retinal pigment epithelial abnormalities after macular hole surgery. Retina 1993;13:176.
139. Duker JS. Retinal pigment epitheliopathy after macular hole surgery. Ophthalmology 1993;100:1604–5.
140. Lansing MB, Glaser BM, Liss H, et al. The effect of pars plana vitrectomy and transforming growth factor-beta 2 without epiretinal membrane peeling on full-thickness macular holes. Ophthalmology 1993;100:868–72.
141. Melberg NS, Thomas MA. Visual field loss after pars plana vitrectomy with air/fluid exchange. Am J Ophthalmol 1995;120:386–8.
142. Freeman WR. Editorial: Vitrectomy surgery for full-thickness macular holes. Am J Ophthalmol 1993;116:233–5.
143. Funata M, Wendel RT, de la Cruz Z, et al. Clinicopathologic study of bilateral macular holes treated with pars plana vitrectomy and gas tamponade. Retina 1992;12:289–98.
144. Madreperla SA, Geiger GL, Funata M, et al. Clinicopathologic correlation of a macular hole treated by cortical vitreous peeling and gas tamponade. Ophthalmology 1994;101: 682–6.
145. Fine SL. Editorial: Vitreous surgery for macular hole in perspective. Is there an indication?. Arch Ophthalmol 1991;109:635–6.
146. de Bustros S, Thompson JT, Michels RG, et al. Nuclear sclerosis after vitrectomy for idiopathic epiretinal membranes. Am J Ophthalmol 1988;105:160–4.
147. Schocket SS, Lakhanpal V, Xiaoping M, et al. Laser treatment of macular holes. Ophthalmology 1988;95:574–82.
148. Makabe R. Kryptonlaserkoagulation bei idiopathischem Makulaloch. Klin Monatsbl Augenheilkd 1990;196:202–4.
149. Flynn Jr HW. Macular hole surgery in patients with proliferative diabetic retinopathy. Arch Ophthalmol 1994;112:877–8.
150. Siam A-L. Macular hole with central retinal detachment in high myopia with posterior staphyloma. Br J Ophthalmol 1969;53:62–3.
151. Blodi CF, Folk JC. Treatment of macular hole retinal detachments with intravitreal gas. Am J Ophthalmol 1984;98:811.
152. Gonvers M, Machemer R. A new approach to treating retinal detachment with macular hole. Am J Ophthalmol 1982;94:468–72.
153. Klöti R. Erfahrungen mit der Silberklemme bei Makulaloch-bedingten Netzhautablösungen. Ophthalmologica 1970;161:210–6.
154. Miyake Y. A simplified method of treating retinal detachment with macular hole. Am J Ophthalmol 1984;97:243–5.
155. Schulenburg WE, Cooling RJ, McLeod D. Management of retinal detachments associated with macular breaks. Trans Ophthalmol Soc UK 1983;103:360–4.
156. Mehta M, Katsumi O, Tetsuka S, et al. Best's macular dystrophy with a macular hole. Acta Ophthalmol 1991;69:131–4.
157. Schachat AP, de la Cruz Z, Green WR, et al. Macular hole and retinal detachment in Best's disease. Retina 1985;5:22–5.
158. Noble KG, Chang S. Adult vitelliform macular degeneration progressing to full-thickness macular hole. Arch Ophthalmol 1991;109:325.
159. Lee S, Ai E, Lowe M, Wang T. Bilateral macular holes in sporadic posterior microphthalmos. Retina 1990;10:185–8.
160. Muñoz FJ, Rebolleda G, Cores FJ, et al. Congenital retinal arteriovenous communication associated with a full-thickness macular hole. Acta Ophthalmol 1991;69:117–20.
161. Cohen SM, Gass JDM. Macular hole following severe hypertensive retinopathy. Arch Ophthalmol 1994;112:878–9.
162. Benedict WL, Shami M. Impending macular hole associated with topical pilocarpine. Am J Ophthalmol 1992;114:765–6.
163. Garlikov RS, Chenoweth RG. Macular hole following topical pilocarpine. Ann Ophthalmol 1975;7:1313–6.
164. Avins LR, Krummenacher TR. Macular holes after pneumatic retinopexy. Arch Ophthalmol 1988;106:724–5.
165. Blacharski PA, Newsome DA. Bilateral macular holes after Nd:YAG laser posterior capsulotomy. Am J Ophthalmol 1988;105:417–8.

166. Gupta P, Yee KM, Garcia P, et al. Vitreoschisis in macular diseases. Br J Ophthalmol 2011;95:376–80.
167. Clarkson JG, Green WR, Massof D. A histopathologic review of 168 cases of preretinal membrane. Am J Ophthalmol 1977;84:1–17.
168. Gloor BP. Cellular proliferation on the vitreous surface after photocoagulation. Albrecht von Graefes Arch Klin Exp Ophthalmol 1969;178:99–113.
169. Jaffe NS. Macular retinopathy after separation of vitreoretinal adherence. Arch Ophthalmol 1967;78:585–91.
170. Wise GN. Clinical features of idiopathic preretinal macular fibrosis. Am J Ophthalmol 1975;79:349–57.
171. Allen Jr AW, Gass JDM. Contraction of a perifoveal epiretinal membrane simulating a macular hole. Am J Ophthalmol 1976;82:684–91.
172. Gass JDM. Fluorescein angiography: an aid to the retinal surgeon. In: Pruett RC, Regan CDJ, editors. Retina Congress; 25th Anniversary Meeting of the Retina Service, Massachusetts Eye and Ear Infirmary. New York: Appleton-Century-Crofts; 1972. p. 181–201.
173. Mandelcorn MS, Lipton N. Epi-macular holes: a cause of decreased vision in the elderly. Can J Ophthalmol 1977;12:182–7.
174. Zarbin MA, Michels RG, Green WR. Epiretinal membrane contracture associated with macular prolapse. Am J Ophthalmol 1990;110:610–8.
175. Bonnet M, Fleury J. Pseudo-trou maculaire tardif après pelage chirurgical d'une membrane prémaculaire. J Fr Ophtalmol 1992;15:123–30.
176. Gass JDM. Stereoscopic atlas of macular diseases; diagnosis and treatment, 2nd ed. St. Louis: CV Mosby; 1977. p. 344.
177. Robertson DM, Buettner H. Pigmented preretinal membranes. Am J Ophthalmol 1977;83: 824–9.
178. Kampik A, Green WR, Michels RG, et al. Ultrastructural features of progressive idiopathic epiretinal membrane removed by vitreous surgery. Am J Ophthalmol 1980;90:797–809.
179. Laqua H. Pigmented macular pucker. Am J Ophthalmol 1978;86:56–8.
180. Wallow IHL, Miller SA. Preretinal membrane by retinal pigment epithelium. Arch Ophthalmol 1978;96:1643–6.
181. Machemer R, van Horn D, Aaberg TM. Pigment epithelial proliferation in human retinal detachment with massive periretinal proliferation. Am J Ophthalmol 1978;85:181–91.
182. Curtin VT. Pathologic changes following retinal detachment surgery. Symposium on retina and retinal surgery: transactions of the New Orleans Academy of Ophthalmology. St. Louis: CV Mosby; 1969. p. 147–70.
183. Gass JDM. Stereoscopic atlas of macular diseases a funduscopic and angiographic presentation. St. Louis: CV Mosby; 1970. p. 215.
184. Messner KH. Spontaneous separation of preretinal macular fibrosis. Am J Ophthalmol 1977;83:9–11.
185. Sumers KD, Jampol LM, Goldberg MF, et al. Spontaneous separation of epiretinal membranes. Arch Ophthalmol 1980;98:318–20.
186. Byer NE. Spontaneous disappearance of early postoperative preretinal retraction; a sequel of retinal detachment surgery. Arch Ophthalmol 1973;90:133–5.
187. Roth AM, Foos RY. Surface wrinkling retinopathy in eyes enucleated at autopsy. Trans Am Acad Ophthalmol Otolaryngol 1971;75:1047–58.
188. Scudder MJ, Eifrig DE. Spontaneous surface wrinkling retinopathy. Ann Ophthalmol 1975;7:333–41.
189. Sidd RJ, Fine SL, Owens SL, et al. Idiopathic preretinal gliosis. Am J Ophthalmol 1982;94:44–8.
190. Wise GN. Congenital preretinal macular fibrosis. Am J Ophthalmol 1975;79:363–5.
191. Barr CC, Michels RG. Idiopathic nonvascularized epiretinal membranes in young patients: report of six cases. Ann Ophthalmol 1982;14:335–41.
192. Kimmel AS, Weingeist TA, Blodi CF, et al. Idiopathic premacular gliosis in children and adolescents. Am J Ophthalmol 1989;108:578–81.
193. Mulligan TG, Daily MJ. Spontaneous peeling of an idiopathic epiretinal membrane in a young patient. Arch Ophthalmol 1992;110:1367–8.
194. Smiddy WE, Michels RG, Gilbert HD, et al. Clinicopathologic study of idiopathic macular pucker in children and young adults. Retina 1992;12:232–6.
195. Tetsumoto K, Nakahashi K, Tsukahara Y, et al. Two cases of idiopathic preretinal macular fibrosis in children. Acta Soc Ophthalmol Jpn 1990;94:875–81.
196. Gass JDM. A fluorescein angiographic study of macular dysfunction secondary to retinal vascular disease. III. Hypertensive retinopathy. Arch Ophthalmol 1968;80:569–82.
197. Appiah AP, Hirose T. Secondary causes of premacular fibrosis. Ophthalmology 1989;96:389–92.
198. Cleary PE, Leaver PK. Macular abnormalities in the reattached retina. Br J Ophthalmol 1978;62:595–603.
199. Gloor BP. On the question of the origin of macrophages in the retina and the vitreous following photocoagulation (autoradiographic investigations by means of ^{3}H-thymidine). Albrecht von Graefes Arch Klin Exp Ophthalmol 1974;190:183.
200. Sabates NR, Sabates FN, Sabates R, et al. Macular changes after retinal detachment surgery. Am J Ophthalmol 1989;108:22–9.
201. Uemura A, Ideta H, Nagasaki H, et al. Macular pucker after retinal detachment surgery. Ophthalmic Surg 1992;23:116–9.
202. Hagler WS, Aturaliya U. Macular puckers after retinal detachment surgery. Br J Ophthalmol 1971;55:451–7.
203. Lobes Jr LA, Burton TC. The incidence of macular pucker after retinal detachment surgery. Am J Ophthalmol 1978;85:72–7.
204. Tanenbaum HL, Schepens CL, Elzeneiny I, et al. Macular pucker following retinal detachment surgery. Arch Ophthalmol 1970;83:286–93.
205. Bishara SA, Buzney SM. Dispersion of retinal pigment epithelial cells from experimental retinal holes. Graefes Arch Clin Exp Ophthalmol 1991;229:195–9.
206. Machemer R, Aaberg TM, Freeman HM, et al. An updated classification of retinal detachment with proliferative vitreoretinopathy. Am J Ophthalmol 1991;112:159–65.
207. Machemer R, Laqua H. Pigment epithelium proliferation in retinal detachment (massive periretinal proliferation). Am J Ophthalmol 1975;80:1–23.
208. Green WR, Kenyon KR, Michels RG, et al. Ultrastructure of epiretinal membranes causing macular pucker after retinal re-attachment surgery. Trans Ophthalmol Soc UK 1979;99: 63–77.
209. Hamilton CW, Chandler D, Klintworth GK, et al. A transmission and scanning electron microscopic study of surgically excised preretinal membrane proliferations in diabetes mellitus. Am J Ophthalmol 1982;94:473–88.
210. Laqua H, Machemer R. Clinical-pathological correlation in massive periretinal proliferation. Am J Ophthalmol 1975;80:913–29.
211. Kampik A, Kenyon KR, Michels RG, et al. Epiretinal and vitreous membranes; comparative study of 56 cases. Arch Ophthalmol 1981;99:1445–54.
212. Bellhorn MB, Friedman AH, Wise GN, et al. Ultrastructure and clinicopathologic correlation of idiopathic preretinal macular fibrosis. Am J Ophthalmol 1975;79:366–73.
213. Cherfan GM, Smiddy WE, Michels RG, et al. Clinicopathologic correlation of pigmented epiretinal membranes. Am J Ophthalmol 1988;106:536–45.
214. Hiscott PS, Grierson I, McLeod D. Retinal pigment epithelial cells in epiretinal membranes; an immunohistochemical study. Br J Ophthalmol 1984;68:708–15.
215. Hiscott PS, Grierson I, Trombetta CJ, et al. Retinal and epiretinal glia – an immunohistochemical study. Br J Ophthalmol 1984;68:698–707.
216. Jiang DY, Hiscott PS, Grierson I, et al. Growth and contractility of cells from fibrocellular epiretinal membranes in primary tissue culture. Br J Ophthalmol 1988;72:116–26.
217. Kenyon KR, Michels RG. Ultrastructure of epiretinal membrane removed by pars plana vitreoretinal surgery. Am J Ophthalmol 1977;83:815–23.
218. Laqua H, Machemer R. Glial cell proliferation in retinal detachment (massive periretinal proliferation). Am J Ophthalmol 1975;80:602–18.
219. Machemer R. Pathogenesis and classification of massive periretinal proliferation. Br J Ophthalmol 1978;62:737–47.
220. Maguire AM, Smiddy WE, Nanda SK, et al. Clinicopathologic correlation of recurrent epiretinal membranes after previous surgical removal. Retina 1990;10:213–22.
221. Maumenee AE. Further advances in the study of the macula. Arch Ophthalmol 1967;78: 151–65.
222. Mittleman D, Green WR, Michels RG, et al. Clinicopathologic correlation of an eye after surgical removal of an epiretinal membrane. Retina 1989;9:143–7.
223. Morino I, Hiscott P, McKechnie N, et al. Variation in epiretinal membrane components with clinical duration of the proliferative tissue. Br J Ophthalmol 1990;74:393–9.
224. Newsome DA, Rodrigues MM, Machemer R. Human massive periretinal proliferation; in vitro characteristics of cellular components. Arch Ophthalmol 1981;99:873–80.
225. Rentsch FJ. Preretinal proliferation of glial cells after mechanical injury of the rabbit retina. Albrecht von Graefes Arch Klin Exp Ophthalmol 1973;188:79–90.
226. Rentsch FJ. The ultrastructure of preretinal macular fibrosis. Albrecht von Graefes Arch Clin Exp Ophthalmol 1977;203:321–37.
227. Singh AK, Glaser BM, Lemor M, et al. Gravity-dependent distribution of retinal pigment epithelial cells dispersed into the vitreous cavity. Retina 1986;6:77–80.
228. Smiddy WE, Maguire AM, Green WR, et al. Idiopathic epiretinal membranes; ultrastructural characteristics and clinicopathologic correlation. Ophthalmology 1989;96:811–21.
229. Snead MP, Snead DR, James S, et al. Clinicopathological changes at the vitreoretinal junction: posterior vitreous detachment. Eye (Lond) 2008;22:1257–62.
230. Hui Y-N, Goodnight R, Zhang X-J, et al. Glial epiretinal membranes and contraction; immunohistochemical and morphological studies. Arch Ophthalmol 1988;106:1280–5.
231. Wallow IHL, Greaser ML, Stevens TS. Actin filaments in diabetic fibrovascular preretinal membrane. Arch Ophthalmol 1981;99:2175–81.
232. Wallow IHL, Stevens TS, Greaser ML, et al. Actin filaments in contracting preretinal membranes. Arch Ophthalmol 1984;102:1370–5.
233. Algvere P, Kock E. Experimental epiretinal membranes induced by intravitreal carbon particles. Am J Ophthalmol 1983;96:345–53.
234. Lean JS. Origin of simple glial epiretinal membranes in an animal model. Graefes Arch Clin Exp Ophthalmol 1987;225:421–5.
235. Miller B, Miller H, Ryan SJ. Experimental epiretinal proliferation induced by intravitreal red blood cells. Am J Ophthalmol 1986;102:188–95.
236. Radke ND, Tano Y, Chandler D, et al. Simulation of massive periretinal proliferation by autotransplantation of retinal pigment epithelial cells in rabbits. Am J Ophthalmol 1981;91: 76–87.
237. Stern WH, Fisher SK, Anderson DH, et al. Epiretinal membrane formation after vitrectomy. Am J Ophthalmol 1982;93:757–72.
238. Hirokawa H, Jalkh AE, Takahashi M, et al. Role of the vitreous in idiopathic preretinal macular fibrosis. Am J Ophthalmol 1986;101:166–9.
239. Sebag J. Imaging vitreous. Eye (Lond) 2002;16:429–39.
240. Sebag J. Anomalous posterior vitreous detachment: a unifying concept in vitreo-retinal disease. Graefes Arch Clin Exp Ophthalmol 2004;242:690–8.
241. Sebag J. Vitreoschisis. Graefes Arch Clin Exp Ophthalmol 2008;246:329–32.
242. Wiznia RA. Posterior vitreous detachment and idiopathic preretinal macular gliosis. Am J Ophthalmol 1986;102:196–8.
243. Glaser BM, Cardin A, Biscoe B. Proliferative vitreoretinopathy; the mechanism of development of vitreoretinal traction. Ophthalmology 1987;94:327–32.
244. Sivalingam A, Eagle Jr RC, Duker JS, et al. Visual prognosis correlated with the presence of internal-limiting membrane in histopathologic specimens obtained from epiretinal membrane surgery. Ophthalmology 1990;97:1549–52.
245. Kishi S, Shimizu K. Oval defect in detached posterior hyaloid membrane in idiopathic preretinal macular fibrosis. Am J Ophthalmol 1994;118:451–6.
246. Thomas EL, Michels RG, Rice TA, et al. Idiopathic progressive unilateral vitreous fibrosis and secondary traction retinal detachment. Retina 1982;2:134–44.

247. Akiba J, Yoshida A, Trempe CL. Prognostic factors in idiopathic preretinal macular fibrosis. Graefes Arch Clin Exp Ophthalmol 1991;229:101–4.
248. Gass JDM. Photocoagulation of macular lesions. Trans Am Acad Ophthalmol Otolaryngol 1971;75:580–2.
249. Greven CM, Slusher MM, Weaver RG. Epiretinal membrane release and posterior vitreous detachment. Ophthalmology 1988;95:902–5.
250. Schwartz PL, Trubowitsch G, Fastenberg DM, et al. Macular pucker and retinal angioma. Ophthalmic Surg 1987;18:677–9.
251. de Bustros S, Rice TA, Michels RG, et al. Vitrectomy for macular pucker; use after treatment of retinal tears or retinal detachment. Arch Ophthalmol 1988;106:758–60.
252. de Bustros S, Thompson JT, Michels RG, et al. Vitrectomy for idiopathic epiretinal membranes causing macular pucker. Br J Ophthalmol 1988;72:692–5.
253. Margherio RR, Cox Jr MS, Trese MT, et al. Removal of epimacular membranes. Ophthalmology 1985;92:1075–83.
254. McDonald HR, Verre WP, Aaberg TM. Surgical management of idiopathic epiretinal membranes. Ophthalmology 1986;93:978–83.
255. Michels RG. Vitreous surgery for macular pucker. Am J Ophthalmol 1981;92:628–39.
256. Michels RG. Vitrectomy for macular pucker. Ophthalmology 1984;91:1384–8.
257. Michels RG, Gilbert HD. Surgical management of macular pucker after retinal reattachment surgery. Am J Ophthalmol 1979;88:925–9.
258. Pesin SR, Olk RJ, Grand MG, et al. Vitrectomy for premacular fibroplasia; prognostic factors, long-term follow-up, and time course of visual improvement. Ophthalmology 1991;98: 1109–14.
259. Poliner LS, Olk RJ, Grand MG, et al. Surgical management of premacular fibroplasia. Arch Ophthalmol 1988;106:761–4.
260. Rice TA, de Bustros S, Michels RG, et al. Prognostic factors in vitrectomy for epiretinal membranes of the macula. Ophthalmology 1986;93:602–10.
261. Shea M. The surgical management of macular pucker in rhegmatogenous retinal detachment. Ophthalmology 1980;87:70–4.
262. Stallman JB, Meyers SM. Spontaneous disappearance of white retinal changes after dissection of epiretinal macular membranes. Retina 1988;8:165–8.
263. Thompson JT. Epiretinal membrane removal in eyes with good visual acuities. Retina 2005;25:875–82.
264. Meyer CH, Rodrigues EB, Kroll P. Trypan blue has a high affinity to cellular structures such as epiretinal membrane. Am J Ophthalmol 2004;137:207–8.
265. Perrier M, Sebag M. Epiretinal membrane surgery assisted by trypan blue. Am J Ophthalmol 2003;135:909–11.
266. Benhamou N, Massin P, Spolaore R, et al. Surgical management of epiretinal membrane in young patients. Am J Ophthalmol 2002;133:358–64.
267. Potter MJ, Lee AS, Moshaver A. Improvement in macular function after epiretinal membrane removal in a patient with Stargardt disease. Retina 2000;20:560–1.
268. Meredith TA. Epiretinal membrane delamination with a diamond knife. Arch Ophthalmol 1997;115:1598–9.
269. Yuson RM, Nigam N, Mojana F, et al. The use of intraoperative indocyanine green dye to assist in epiretinal membrane removal: a novel application of indocyanine green surgical use. Retina 2009;29:1367–70.
270. Konstantinidis L, Berguiga M, Beknazar E, et al. Anatomic and functional outcome after 23-gauge vitrectomy, peeling, and intravitreal triamcinolone for idiopathic macular epiretinal membrane. Retina 2009;29:1119–27.
271. Fang X, Zheng X, Weng Y, et al. Anatomical and visual outcome after vitrectomy with triamcinolone acedonide-assisted epiretinal membrane removal in highly myopic eyes with retinal detachment due to macular hole. Eye (Lond) 2009;23:248–54.
272. Habib MS, Steel DH, Ling R, et al. Vitrectomy with membrane peeling for vasocentric idiopathic epiretinal membranes. Retina 2008;28:981–6.
273. Cherfan GM, Michels RG, de Bustros S, et al. Nuclear sclerotic cataract after vitrectomy for idiopathic epiretinal membranes causing macular pucker. Am J Ophthalmol 1991;111:434–8.
274. Kozak I, Freeman WR. Nonprogressive extrafoveal retinal hole after foveal epiretinal membrane removal. Am J Ophthalmol 2006;141:769–71.
275. Sibony P, Fourman S, Honkanen R, et al. Asymptomatic peripapillary subretinal hemorrhage: a study of 10 cases. J Neuroophthalmol 2008;28:114–9.
276. Aras C, Arici C, Akova N. Peripapillary serous retinal detachment preceding complete posterior vitreous detachment. Graefes Arch Clin Exp Ophthalmol 2008;246:927–9.
277. Kokame GT, Yamamoto I, Kishi S, et al. Intrapapillary hemorrhage with adjacent peripapillary subretinal hemorrhage. Ophthalmology 2004;111:926–30.
278. Wisotsky BJ, Magat-Gordon CB, Puklin JE. Vitreopapillary traction as a cause of elevated optic nerve head. Am J Ophthalmol 1998;126:137–9.
279. Kroll P, Wiegand W, Schmidt J. Vitreopapillary traction in proliferative diabetic vitreoretinopathy [see comments]. Br J Ophthalmol 1999;83:261–4.
280. Chisholm IA, McClure E, Foulds WS. Functional recovery of the retina after retinal detachment. Trans Ophthalmol Soc UK 1975;95:167–72.
281. Davidorf FH, Havener WH, Lang JR. Macular vision following retinal detachment surgery. Ophthalmic Surg 1975;6:74–81.
282. Davies EWG, Gundry MF. Failure of visual recovery following retinal surgery. Mod Probl Ophthalmol 1974;12:58–63.
283. Friberg TR, Eller AW. Prediction of visual recovery after scleral buckling of macula-off retinal detachments. Am J Ophthalmol 1992;114:715–22.
284. Grupposo SS. Visual acuity following surgery for retinal detachment. Arch Ophthalmol 1975;93:327–30.
285. Gundry MF. Davies EWG. Recovery of visual acuity after retinal detachment surgery. Am J Ophthalmol 1974;77:310–4.
286. Isernhagen RD, Wilkinson CP. Visual acuity after the repair of pseudophakic retinal detachments involving the macula. Retina 1989;9:15–21.
287. McPherson AR, O'Malley RE, Butner RW, et al. Visual acuity after surgery for retinal detachment with macular involvement. Ann Ophthalmol 1982;14:639–45.
288. Tani P, Robertson DM, Langworthy A. Prognosis for central vision and anatomic reattachment in rhegmatogenous retinal detachment with macula detached. Am J Ophthalmol 1981;92: 611–20.
289. Wilkinson CP. Visual results following scleral buckling for retinal detachments sparing the macula. Retina 1981;1:113–6.
290. Jarrett WH, Brockhurst RJ. Unexplained blindness and optic atrophy following retinal detachment surgery. Arch Ophthalmol 1965;73:782–91.
291. Enoch JM, Van Loo Jr JA, Okun E. Realignment of photoreceptors disturbed in orientation secondary to retinal detachment. Invest Ophthalmol 1973;12:849–53.
292. Morita H, Ideta H, Ito K. Causative factors of retinal detachment in macular holes. Retina 1991;11:281–4.
293. Stirpe M, Michels RG. Retinal detachment in highly myopic eyes due to macular holes and epiretinal traction. Retina 1990;10:113–4.
294. Bonnet M, Semiglia R. Evolution spontanée du décollement de la rétine du pôle postérieur du myope fort. J Fr Ophtalmol 1991;14:618–23.
295. Brown GC. Macular hole following rhegmatogenous retinal detachment repair. Arch Ophthalmol 1988;106:765–6.
296. Riordan-Eva P, Chignell AH. Full thickness macular breaks in rhegmatogenous retinal detachment with peripheral retinal breaks. Br J Ophthalmol 1992;76:346–8.
297. Greco GM, Bonavolonta G. Treatment of retinal detachments due to macular holes. Retina 1987;7:177–9.
298. Laqua H. Die Behandlung der Ablatio mit Maculaforamen nach der Methode von Gonvers und Machemer. Klin Monatsbl Augenheilkd 1985;186:13–17.
299. Rashed O, Sheta S. Evaluation of the functional results after different techniques for treatment of retinal detachments due to macular holes. Graefes Arch Clin Exp Ophthalmol 1989;227:508–12.
300. Aaberg TM, Machemer R. Correlation of naturally occurring detachments with long-term retinal detachment in the owl monkey. Am J Ophthalmol 1970;69:640–50.
301. Gass JDM. Stereoscopic atlas of macular diseases; diagnosis and treatment, 3rd ed. St. Louis: CV Mosby; 1987. p. 716–17.
302. Lopez PF, Aaberg TM, Lambert HM, et al. Choroidal neovascularization occurring within a demarcation line. Am J Ophthalmol 1992;114:101–2.
303. Matsumura M, Yamakawa R, Yoshimura N, et al. Subretinal strands; tissue culture and histological study. Graefes Arch Clin Exp Ophthalmol 1987;225:341–5.
304. Machemer R. Surgical approaches to subretinal strands. Am J Ophthalmol 1980;90:81–5.
305. Sternberg Jr P, Machemer R. Subretinal proliferation. Am J Ophthalmol 1984;98:456–62.
306. Wallyn RH, Hilton GF. Subretinal fibrosis in retinal detachment. Arch Ophthalmol 1979;97:2128–9.
307. Wilkes SR, Mansour AM, Green WR. Proliferative vitreoretinopathy; histopathology of retroretinal membranes. Retina 1987;7:94–101.
308. Abraham RK, Shea M. Significance of pigment dispersion following cryoretinopexy: scotomata and atrophy. Mod Probl Ophthalmol 1969;8:455–61.
309. Hilton GF. Subretinal pigment migration; effects of cryosurgical retinal reattachment. Arch Ophthalmol 1974;91:445–50.
310. Shea M. Complications of cryotherapy in retinal detachment surgery. Can J Ophthalmol 1968;3:109–15.
311. Sudarsky RD, Yannuzzi LA. Cryomarcation line and pigment migration after retinal cryosurgery. Arch Ophthalmol 1970;83:395–401.
312. Theodossiadis GP, Kokolakis SN. Macular pigment deposits in rhegmatogenous retinal detachment. Br J Ophthalmol 1979;63:498–506.
313. Avins LR, Hilton GF. Lesions simulating serous detachment of the pigment epithelium; occurrence after retinal detachment surgery. Arch Ophthalmol 1980;98:1427–9.
314. Lobes Jr LA, Grand MG. Subretinal lesions following scleral buckling procedure. Arch Ophthalmol 1980;98:680–3.
315. Woldoff HS, Dooley Jr WJ. Multifocal choroiditis after retinal detachment surgery. Ann Ophthalmol 1979;11:1182–4.
316. Machemer R. Experimental retinal detachment in the owl monkey. II. Histology of retina and pigment epithelium. Am J Ophthalmol 1968;66:396–410.
317. Bonnet M. Peripheral neovascularization complicating rhegmatogenous retinal detachments of long duration. Graefes Arch Clin Exp Ophthalmol 1987;225:59–62.
318. Felder KS, Brockhurst RJ. Retinal neovascularization complicating rhegmatogenous retinal detachment of long duration. Am J Ophthalmol 1982;93:773–6.
319. Goldbaum MH, Weidenthal DT, Krug S, et al. Subretinal neovascularization as a complication of drainage of subretinal fluid. Retina 1983;3:114–7.
320. Gottlieb F, Fammartino JJ, Stratford TP, et al. Retinal angiomatosis mass; a complication of retinal detachment surgery. Retina 1984;4:152–7.
321. Habib MS, Byrne S, McCarthy JH, et al. Refractile superficial retinal crystals and chronic retinal detachment: case report. BMC Ophthalmol 2006;6:3.
322. Ahmed I, McDonald HR, Schatz H, et al. Crystalline retinopathy associated with chronic retinal detachment. Arch Ophthalmol 1998;116:1449–53.
323. Cogan DG, Kuwabara T, Silbert J, et al. Calcium oxalate and calcium phosphate crystals in detached retinas. AMA Arch Ophthalmol 1958;60:366–71.
324. Byer NE. Clinical study of senile retinoschisis. Arch Ophthalmol 1968;79:36–44.
325. Byer NE. The natural history of senile retinoschisis. Mod Probl Ophthalmol 1977;18:304–11.
326. Hauch TL, Straatsma BR, Andersen E, et al. Macular function in typical and reticular retinoschisis. Retina 1981;1:293–5.
327. Straatsma BR, Foos RY. Typical and reticular degenerative retinoschisis. Am J Ophthalmol 1973;75:551–75.
328. Sulonen JM, Wells CG, Barricks ME, et al. Degenerative retinoschisis with giant outer layer breaks and retinal detachment. Am J Ophthalmol 1985;99:114–21.

329. Byer NE. Long-term natural history study of senile retinoschisis with implications for management. Ophthalmology 1986;93:1127–36.
330. Ambler JS, Gass JDM, Gutman FA. Symptomatic retinoschisis-detachment involving the macula. Am J Ophthalmol 1991;112:8–14.
331. Sneed SR, Blodi CF, Folk JC, et al. Pars plana vitrectomy in the management of retinal detachments associated with degenerative retinoschisis. Ophthalmology 1990;97:470–4.
332. Ambler JS, Meyers SM, Zegarra H, et al. The management of retinal detachment complicating degenerative retinoschisis. Am J Ophthalmol 1989;107:171–6.
333. Zimmerman LE, Spencer WH. The pathologic anatomy of retinoschisis with a report of two cases diagnosed clinically as malignant melanoma. Arch Ophthalmol 1960;63:10–19.
334. Yanoff M, Kertesz Rahn E, Zimmerman LE. Histopathology of juvenile retinoschisis. Arch Ophthalmol 1968;79:49–53.
335. Pandita A, Guest SJ. Sectorial retinoschisis associated with field defect in a patient with tilted discs. Clin Experiment Ophthalmol 2010;38:317–20.
336. Dhrami-Gavazi E, Schiff WM, Barile GR. Nanophthalmos and acquired retinoschisis. Am J Ophthalmol 2009;147:108–10, e1.
337. Hotta K, Hirakata A, Hida T. Retinoschisis associated with disc coloboma. Br J Ophthalmol 1999;83:124.
338. Humayun MS, Fujii GY, Au Eong KG, et al. Bilateral retinoschisis, retinal neovascularization, and severe myopia in a young female. Ophthalmic Surg Lasers 2000;31:442–3.
339. Watts P, Obi E. Retinal folds and retinoschisis in accidental and non-accidental head injury. Eye 2008;22:1514–6.
340. Ando E, Ando Y, Maruoka S, et al. Ocular microangiopathy in familial amyloidotic polyneuropathy, type I. Graefes Arch Clin Exp Ophthalmol 1992;230:1–5.
341. Andrade C. A peculiar form of peripheral neuropathy; familial atypical generalized amyloidosis with special involvement of the peripheral nerves. Brain 1952;75:408–27.
342. Bene C, Kranias G. Ocular amyloidosis: Clinical points learned from one case. Ann Ophthalmol 1990;22:101–2.
343. Biswas J, Badrinath SS, Rao NA. Primary nonfamilial amyloidosis of the vitreous; a light microscopic and ultrastructural study. Retina 1992;12:251–3.
344. Crawford JB. Cotton wool exudates in systemic amyloidosis. Arch Ophthalmol 1967;78:214–6.
345. Goren H, Steinberg MC, Farboody GH. Familial oculoleptomeningeal amyloidosis. Brain 1980;103:473–95.
346. Hamburg A. Unusual cause of vitreous opacities; primary familial amyloidosis. Ophthalmologica 1971;162:173–7.
347. Kasner D, Miller GR, Taylor WH, et al. Surgical treatment of amyloidosis of the vitreous. Trans Am Acad Ophthalmol Otolaryngol 1968;72:410–8.
348. Monteiro JG, Martins AFF, Figueira A, et al. Ocular changes in familial amyloidotic polyneuropathy with dense vitreous opacities. Eye 1991;5:99–105.
349. Okayama M, Goto I, Ogata J, et al. Primary amyloidosis with familial vitreous opacities; an unusual case and family. Arch Intern Med 1978;138:105–11.
350. Rukavina JG, Block WD, Jackson CE, et al. Primary systemic amyloidosis: a review and an experimental, genetic, and clinical study of 29 cases with particular emphasis on the familial form. Medicine 1956;35:239–334.
351. Sandgren O, Holmgren G, Lundgren E. Vitreous amyloidosis associated with homozygosity for the transthyretin methionine-30 gene. Arch Ophthalmol 1990;108:1584–6.
352. Uitti RJ, Donat JR, Rozdilsky B, et al. Familial oculoleptomeningeal amyloidosis; report of a new family with unusual features. Arch Neurol 1988;45:1118–22.
353. Wong VG, McFarlin DE. Primary familial amyloidosis. Arch Ophthalmol 1967;78:208–13.
354. O'Hearn TM, Fawzi A, He S, et al. Early onset vitreous amyloidosis in familial amyloidotic polyneuropathy with a transthyretin Glu54Gly mutation is associated with elevated vitreous VEGF. Br J Ophthalmol 2007;91:1607–9.
355. Ts'o MOM, Bettman Jr JW. Occlusion of choriocapillaris in primary nonfamilial amyloidosis. Arch Ophthalmol 1971;86:281–6.
356. Sandgren O, Holmgren G, Lundgren E, et al. Restriction fragment length polymorphism analysis of mutated transthyretin in vitreous amyloidosis. Arch Ophthalmol 1988;106:790–2.
357. Schwartz MF, Green WR, Michels RG, et al. An unusual case of ocular involvement in primary systemic nonfamilial amyloidosis. Ophthalmology 1982;89:394–401.
358. Skinner M, Harding J, Skare I, et al. A new transthyretin mutation associated with amyloidotic vitreous opacities; asparagine for isoleucine at position 84. Ophthalmology 1992;99:503–8.
359. Baum MD, Weiss HS, Sanders RJ. Panretinal photocoagulation in the treatment of vitreoretinal amyloidosis. Arch Ophthalmol 1998;116:1534.
360. Savage DJ, Mango CA, Streeten BW. Amyloidosis of the vitreous. Fluorescein angiographic findings and association with neovascularization. Arch Ophthalmol 1982;100:1776–9.
361. Ando E, Ando Y, Haraoka K. Ocular amyloid involvement after liver transplantation for polyneuropathy. Ann Intern Med 2001;135:931–2.
362. Munar-Ques M, Salva-Ladaria L, Mulet-Perera P, et al. Vitreous amyloidosis after liver transplantation in patients with familial amyloid polyneuropathy: ocular synthesis of mutant transthyretin. Amyloid 2000;7:266–9.
363. Bek T. Ocular changes in heredo-oto-ophthalmo-encephalopathy. Br J Ophthalmol 2000;84:1298–302.
364. Pece A, Yannuzzi L, Sannace C, et al. Chorioretinal involvement in primary systemic nonfamilial amyloidosis. Am J Ophthalmol 2000;130:250–3.
365. Ferry AP, Lieberman TW. Bilateral amyloidosis of the vitreous body; report of a case without systemic or familial involvement. Arch Ophthalmol 1976;94:982–91.
366. Irvine AR, Char DH. Recurrent amyloid involvement in the vitreous body after vitrectomy. Am J Ophthalmol 1976;82:705–8.
367. Awan KJ. Biomicroscopy and argon laser photocystotomy of free-floating vitreous cysts. Ophthalmology 1985;92:1710–1.
368. Flynn WJ, Carlson DW. Pigmented vitreous cyst. Arch Ophthalmol 1994;112:1113.
369. Lusky M, Weinberger D, Kremer I. Vitreous cyst combined with bilateral juvenile retinoschisis. J Pediatr Ophthalmol Strabismus 1988;25:75–6.
370. Orellana J, O'Malley RE, McPherson AR, et al. Pigmented free-floating vitreous cysts in two young adults; electron microscopic observations. Ophthalmology 1985;92:297–302.
371. Ruby AJ, Jampol LM, Nd YAG. treatment of a posterior vitreous cyst. Am J Ophthalmol 1990;110:428–9.
372. Steinmetz RL, Straatsma BR, Rubin ML. Posterior vitreous cyst. Am J Ophthalmol 1990;109:295–7.
373. Taranath DA, Flaherty MP. Free-floating unilateral pigmented vitreous cyst in a child. J Pediatr Ophthalmol Strabismus 2007;44:243–4.
374. Narendran N, Doyle E, Laidlaw A. Anterior and posterior vitreous cysts. Clin Experiment Ophthalmol 2004;32:229–30.
375. Jones WL. Free-floating vitreous cyst. Optom Vis Sci 1998;75:171–3.
376. Nork TM, Millecchia LL. Treatment and histopathology of a congenital vitreous cyst. Ophthalmology 1998;105:825–30.
377. Bergren RL, Brown GC, Duker JS. Prevalence and association of asteroid hyalosis with systemic disease. Am J Ophthalmol 1991;111:289–93.
378. Feist RM, Morris RE, Witherspoon CD, et al. Vitrectomy in asteroid hyalosis. Retina 1990;10:173–7.
379. Hampton GR, Nelsen PT, Hay PB. Viewing through the asteroids. Ophthalmology 1981;88: 669–72.
380. Luxenberg M, Sime D. Relationship of asteroid hyalosis to diabetes mellitus and plasma lipid levels. Am J Ophthalmol 1969;67:406–13.
381. Renaldo DP. Pars plana vitrectomy for asteroid hyalosis. Retina 1981;1:252–4.
382. Rodman HI, Johnson FB, Zimmerman LE. New histopathological and histochemical observations concerning asteroid hyalitis. Arch Ophthalmol 1961;66:552–63.
383. Streeten BW. Vitreous asteroid bodies; ultrastructural characteristics and composition. Arch Ophthalmol 1982;100:969–75.
384. Topilow HW, Kenyon KR, Takahashi M, et al. Asteroid hyalosis; biomicroscopy, ultrastructure, and composition. Arch Ophthalmol 1982;100:964–8.
385. Winkler J, Lunsdorf H. Ultrastructure and composition of asteroid bodies. Invest Ophthalmol Vis Sci 2001;42:902–7.
386. Kador PF, Wyman M. Asteroid hyalosis: pathogenesis and prospects for prevention. Eye (Lond) 2008;22:1278–85.
387. Mochizuki Y, Hata Y, Kita T, et al. Anatomical findings of vitreoretinal interface in eyes with asteroid hyalosis. Graefes Arch Clin Exp Ophthalmol 2009;247:1173–7.

CHAPTER 8

Traumatic Retinopathy

BERLIN'S EDEMA (COMMOTIO RETINAE)

After a blunt contusion to the front of the eye, a patient may experience acute visual loss caused by Berlin's edema (commotio retinae). In this condition the retina develops a gray-white color that affects primarily the outer retina[1–5] that may be confined to the macular area (Figure 8.01A and E) or may involve extensive areas of the peripheral retina (Figure 8.01B). In some cases the whitening may be accompanied by retinal or preretinal hemorrhages (Figure 8.02A and B) or subretinal blood and choroidal rupture. The retinal whitening in the macular area may clear completely, and central vision may be restored (Figure 8.01F). In other instances, loss of central vision may be permanent and may be associated with no visible fundus change, mottling of the retinal pigment epithelium (RPE), migration of pigment into the overlying retina, or partial or full-thickness macular hole formation (Figures 8.02D, E and F, and 8.05). The whitening in the peripheral retina may be followed initially by pigment mottling and later by atrophy of the RPE and migration of pigment into the overlying retina, producing a peripheral change that clinically and histopathologically simulates retinitis pigmentosa (Figure 8.02E and F).[6,7]

Fluorescein angiography typically shows no evidence of retinal vascular or choroidal permeability alterations in the area of Berlin's edema (Figure 8.01C and D).[3,6,8,9] Angiography occasionally shows a transient leakage of dye from the retinal arterioles in the posterior pole or staining at the level of the RPE (Figure 8.02C).[10] Following resolution of the outer retinal whitening, angiography may or may not show evidence of window defects in the RPE. Vitreous fluorophotometry usually shows no evidence of breakdown of the blood–retinal barrier.[11] Optical coherence tomography (OCT) shows increased density of the photoreceptor layers initially (Figure 8.01J–L), followed by lucent areas if the receptors show cell death followed by thinning of the receptor layer.[12–15] If the injury is mild the receptors recover and the OCT findings resolve. Multifocal electroretinogram (ERG) shows depression of the amplitudes in the affected area which recover if the outer segments regenerate or remain permanently affected if the receptors do not recover.[14] Light and electron microscopic studies of Berlin's edema in humans as well as that produced experimentally in animals have shown that the outer retinal whitening is caused by fragmentation of the photoreceptor outer segments and acute damage to the receptor cells (Figure 8.01G and H).[4,8,16] OCT, if done during this stage, will show increased reflectivity of the photoreceptor layer and sometimes small clear spaces suggesting disruption of the photoreceptors.[13] This loss of transparency is associated with no or minimal extracellular or intracellular edema in the retinal cells and with minimal damage to the choriocapillaris.[2,4,16,17] Other changes may include breakdown of the outer blood–retinal barrier at the level of the RPE that is usually re-established between 7 and 14 days.[17] If only the outer segments of the receptor cells are involved, these will regenerate rapidly and the retina may regain its normal appearance and function. The OCT findings also normalize. A more severe contusion may cause contusion necrosis and atrophy of the outer retina (Figure 8.02G and H) and a macular hole. The contusion damage to the retinal receptor cells is probably caused by mechanical distortion of the retina by deformation of the vitreous as well as hydraulic forces.[16]

8.01 Berlin's edema (commotio retinae).

A–D: This 10-year-old boy was struck in the left eye by a rock. Visual acuity was 20/70. Note the zone of whitening involving the outer retinal layer in the macula (arrows, A). There was a large area of retinal whitening in the far periphery of the same eye (B). Angiography was normal and showed no evidence of retinal vascular abnormalities (C and D).

E and **F**: Berlin's edema of the left macula in a 20-year-old woman (E). Three days later the edema had disappeared and the macular function had returned to normal (F).

G–I: Photomicrographs of normal monkey retina (G), retina 4 hours (H), and retina 48 hours (I) after blunt trauma. Note disruption of photoreceptor cells outer segments (arrow, H), pyknotic nuclei in the outer nuclear layer (H and I), and vacuolization of inner-segment layer of photoreceptors (arrow, I, paraphenylenediamine dye).

J and **K**: A 28-year-old male was hit in the left eye by a cricket ball. The fovea was gray-white from commotio but maintained an acuity of 20/20. An OCT through the commotio shows edema and increased reflectivity (arrow, K) of the affected photoreceptors compared to the adjacent unaffected receptors (arrow heads).

L: A dart penetrated this 11-year-old's sclera and choroid causing a choroidal and subretinal hemorrhage and a gray-white patch of commotio (arrow) at its foveal edge. Spectralis OCT through the commotio demonstrates the thickening of the IS/OS junction (arrow) signifying trauma to the photoreceptors.

(G and H from Sipperley et al.[4],

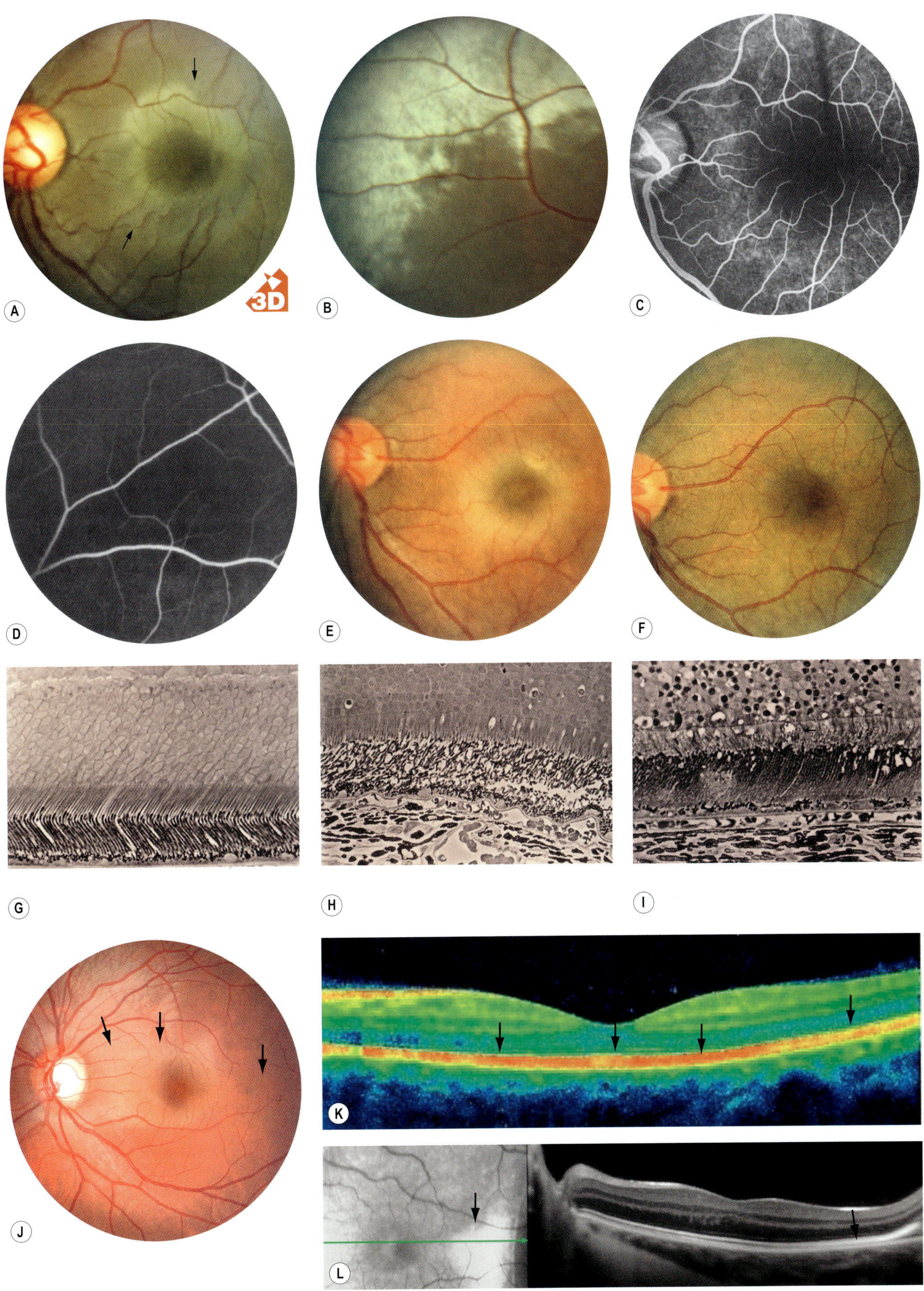
A
3D
B
C
D
E
F
G
H
I
J
K
L

Subretinal hemorrhage caused by choroidal rupture may occasionally accompany Berlin's edema (see Chapter 3). Trauma similar to that which causes Berlin's edema may also cause acute damage to the RPE and serous detachment of the macula (Figure 8.02C, and see Figure 8.03A–C), as well as acute tears in the RPE.[18]

POSTERIOR CHOROIDAL RUPTURE (TRAUMATIC CHOROIDOPATHY)

Acute contusion necrosis of the RPE or, more frequently, a rupture in the inner choroid and RPE at the posterior pole may cause a serous and/or hemorrhagic detachment of the retina often in the macula or juxtapapillary region (Figure 8.03).[19–28] In the case of contusion necrosis a localized serous detachment of the retina occurs and angiography shows multiple focal areas of diffusion of fluorescein from the choroid across the damaged RPE into the subretinal fluid (Figure 8.03A–C).[21] Following resolution of the detachment, varying degrees of RPE atrophy may develop. Tears in the RPE may be evident after a contusion injury.[29] When there is a choroidal rupture, the localized subretinal hematoma typically overlies and obscures the rupture (Figure 8.03D). In some cases, outer retinal whitening (Berlin's edema) accompanies the choroidal rupture (Figure 8.02B).[30] (See discussion of contusion maculopathy, Chapter 8.) As the subretinal blood disappears, the rupture involving the choroid and RPE becomes visible as a curvilinear yellowish line with tapered ends concentric with, but often remotely located from, the optic disc (Figure 8.03E, G, I, and J). The rupture typically involves only the inner layers of the choroid but may be full thickness in some cases. In many patients the choroidal rupture is outside the foveolar area and visual acuity often returns to near normal. Occasionally a macular hole or evulsion of the optic nerve head may accompany an underlying choroidal rupture.[25,31] Choroidal ruptures may occur after minor trauma in patients with angioid streaks (see Figure 3.38I).[22,32]

Intravenous fluorescein is helpful in detecting choroidal ruptures partly obscured by subretinal blood or in detecting small ruptures that may be difficult to visualize ophthalmoscopically (Figure 8.03F). If the rupture involves only the inner layers, angiography will show large choroidal vessels traversing the defect in the pigment epithelium, Bruch's membrane, and choriocapillaris (Figure 8.03K). Angiography may demonstrate evidence of chorioretinal vascular anastomosis at the site of the rupture (Figure 8.03L).

Histologically, the choroidal rupture involves at least the choriocapillaris, Bruch's membrane, and the RPE. (Figure 8.03H).[22,33] The inner layers of the retina overlying the rupture may or may not be damaged.[34]

8.02 Contusion necrosis of the retinal pigement epithelium (RPE) and retina.

A–C: This man sustained blunt trauma and visual loss in the right eye. Note outer retinal whitening and retinal and preretinal blood (A and B). Angiography (C) showed extensive staining caused by necrosis of the RPE, as well as evidence of curvilinear choroidal rupture underlying the blood.
D: Postcontusion macular hole (arrow) and retinal and RPE atrophy in a 19-year-old man previously struck in the eye with a baseball.
E: Macular hole (arrow) adjacent to two choroidal ruptures. The hole did not close following vitrectomy with internal limiting membrane peel due to contraction of the underlying Bruch's membrane by the choroidal rupture.
F: Peripheral retinal and RPE degeneration caused by blunt trauma. Note narrowing of the retinal vessels and migration of pigment into the retina (arrow) similar to that seen in retinitis pigmentosa.
G: Photomicrograph of the foveal area showing focal loss of receptor cells, cystic degeneration, and chorioretinal adhesions (arrows) following trauma. The separation of retina from the RPE is probably artifactitious.
H: Photomicrograph of the foveal area showing more severe postcontusion atrophy of the retina and RPE.
I and **J**: Appearance in a 15-year-old 1 year after blunt injury from a bottle rocket which left him with severe contusion necrosis of the macular retina and choroid (I). Visual acuity was count fingers at 0.6 meters (2 feet). Optical coherence tomography of the macula shows atrophic retina (J).
K: Picture 2 months after an assault in a 22-year-old male showing several choroidal ruptures, resolving subretinal hemorrhages and organization into fibrous scars.

(I and J, courtesy of Dr. Franco Recchia; K, courtesy of Dr. Paul Sternberg Jr.)

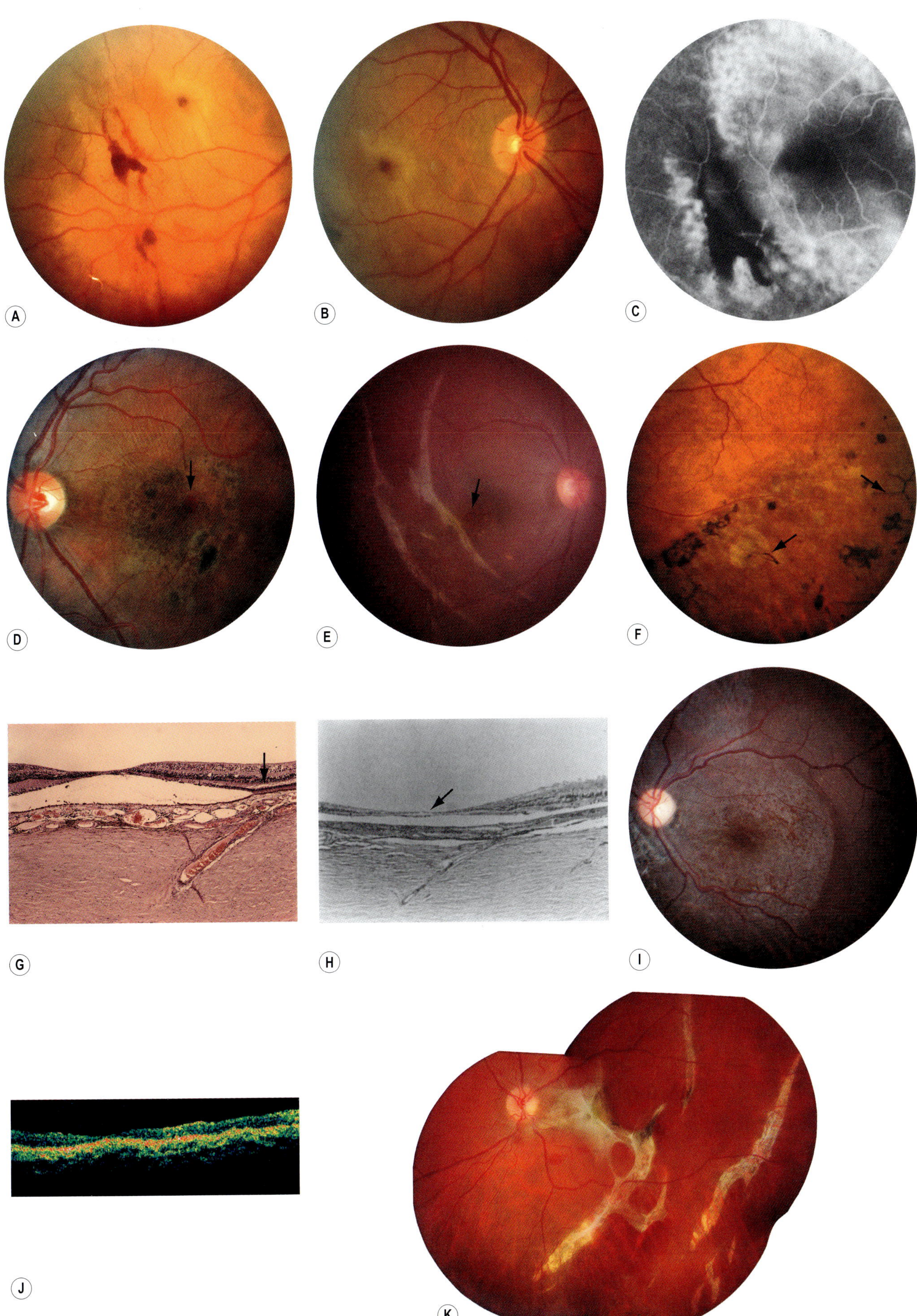
A
B
C
D
E
F
G
H
I
J
K

Some patients may develop visual loss within several months or years after trauma because of spontaneous bleeding or serous exudation from choroidal neovascularization arising at the site of an old choroidal rupture (Figure 8.03I and J).[23,31,35–40] This neovascularization is usually type II and often produces a pigment halo at the site of ingrowth of the vessels into the subsensory retinal space. Similar delayed neovascularization may occur at the site of a choroidal rupture caused by the impact of an intraocular foreign body, or at a surgically produced choroidal perforation made during the course of scleral buckling for retinal detachment.[41] Extensive organization of subretinal blood may produce a variety of disciform scars, some of which may simulate a melanoma.

Gass has seen several patients who, following contusion injury to the head, have developed a typical ophthalmoscopic and angiographic picture of idiopathic central serous chorioretinopathy within several days of the accident. Probably these are patients predisposed to this disease who, as a result of the emotional stress rather than direct trauma to the eye, develop a detachment. The prognosis for spontaneous recovery is excellent.[42,43]

8.03 Postcontusion maculopathy (choroidal rupture).

A–C: Serous retinal detachment in the macula noted immediately after severe blunt contusion to the right eye in a 7-year-old girl. Angiograms show evidence of multiple focal areas of leaking of fluorescein from choroidal vessels into the subretinal fluid.

D–F: Submacular hemorrhage secondary to choroidal rupture following a contusion to the right eye in a young adult (D). Several weeks later the subretinal blood has cleared (E). Note the small choroidal rupture (arrow). Angiography revealed fluorescence in the region of the choroidal rupture (F).

G: Large choroidal rupture in the papillomacular bundle region of a 21-year-old man who experienced loss of vision several months previously in an automobile accident. The visual acuity at the time of this photograph was 20/30.

H: Histopathology of a broad choroidal rupture in the papillomacular bundle of another patient. Note the hyperplasia of the retinal pigment epithelium at the site of the break in Bruch's membrane (arrow).

I: A hemorrhagic detachment of the macula secondary to choroidal neovascularization (arrow) developing at the site of an old choroidal rupture in a 54-year-old man who had sustained blunt trauma to the eye 2 years previously. At that time, he had evidence of a subretinal hemorrhage that had subsequently cleared. Approximately 6 weeks before this photograph the patient experienced sudden loss of central vision in his left eye.

J–L: Serous detachment of the retina caused by type II subretinal choroidal neovascular membrane (arrows) arising in old choroidal rupture.

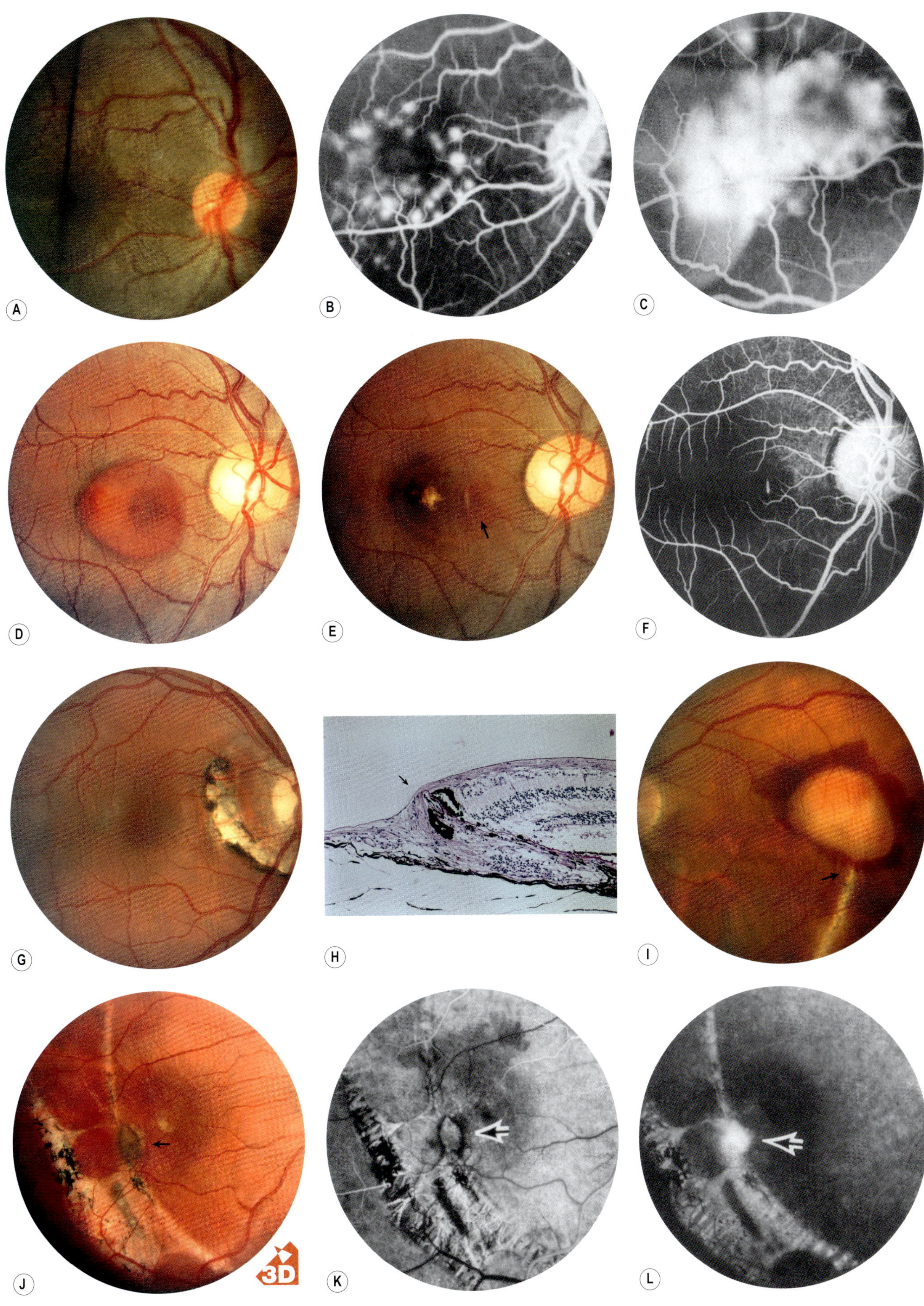
A
B
C
D
E
F
G
H
I
J
3D
K
L

MACULAR COMPLICATIONS OF PERIPHERAL CHORIORETINAL CONTUSION AND RUPTURE (SCLOPETARIA)

Contusion and rupture of the peripheral choroid and retina caused by a high-velocity missile striking or passing close to but not penetrating the globe (sclopetaria) is an infrequent manifestation of nonpenetrating ocular trauma.[44–46] A large, often ragged retinal and choroidal break associated with surrounding retinal whitening and varying amounts of blood are the cardinal fundoscopic features (Figure 8.04A–F). The white sclera may be visible within the break. In spite of the break in the retina, rhegmatogenous detachment occurs infrequently. Loss of macular function may occur acutely because of extension of the damage posteriorly (Figure 8.04A), associated macular hole,[47] or it may develop many months after the injury as a result of vascular proliferative and exudative changes occurring within the peripheral scar (Figure 8.04G–L). Late fundus appearance is characterized by plaque-like fibrous proliferation with variable amount of pigment with scalloped margins. The pathogenesis of the loss of tissue seems to be partially from dissolution and partly from retraction of the retinal and choroidal tissue.[48] Retinal detachment is uncommon due to scarring and fibrous proliferation that follow the injury.[48–50]

8.04 Contusion injury to the peripheral retina and choroid.

A–F: Sclopetaria with rupture of the peripheral choroid and retina caused by a bullet passing adjacent to the eye wall. Note the stellate choroidal ruptures, scarring, and subretinal blood extending into the macula (A) from the peripheral site of chorioretinal rupture (B). Six months later: note the extensive scarring posteriorly (C and D) and peripherally in the area of retinal (E) and chorioretinal dehiscence (F).
G–K: Delayed loss of vision occurred in this young woman who developed an exudative retinal detachment (G) caused by a peripheral fibrovascular subretinal mass (H) several years following a contusion injury to the retina inferotemporally. The subretinal exudate resolved following transscleral cryopexy (I and J). Six months later she noted mild metamorphopsia caused by traction of an epiretinal membrane that over a period of several months partly peeled from the retinal surface (J and K).
L: A large zone of retinal and retinal pigment epithelium atrophy with bone corpuscular pigmentation (arrows) developed over a period of several years following an inferotemporal contusion injury to the right eye.

(L, courtesy of Dr. Maurice F. Rabb.)

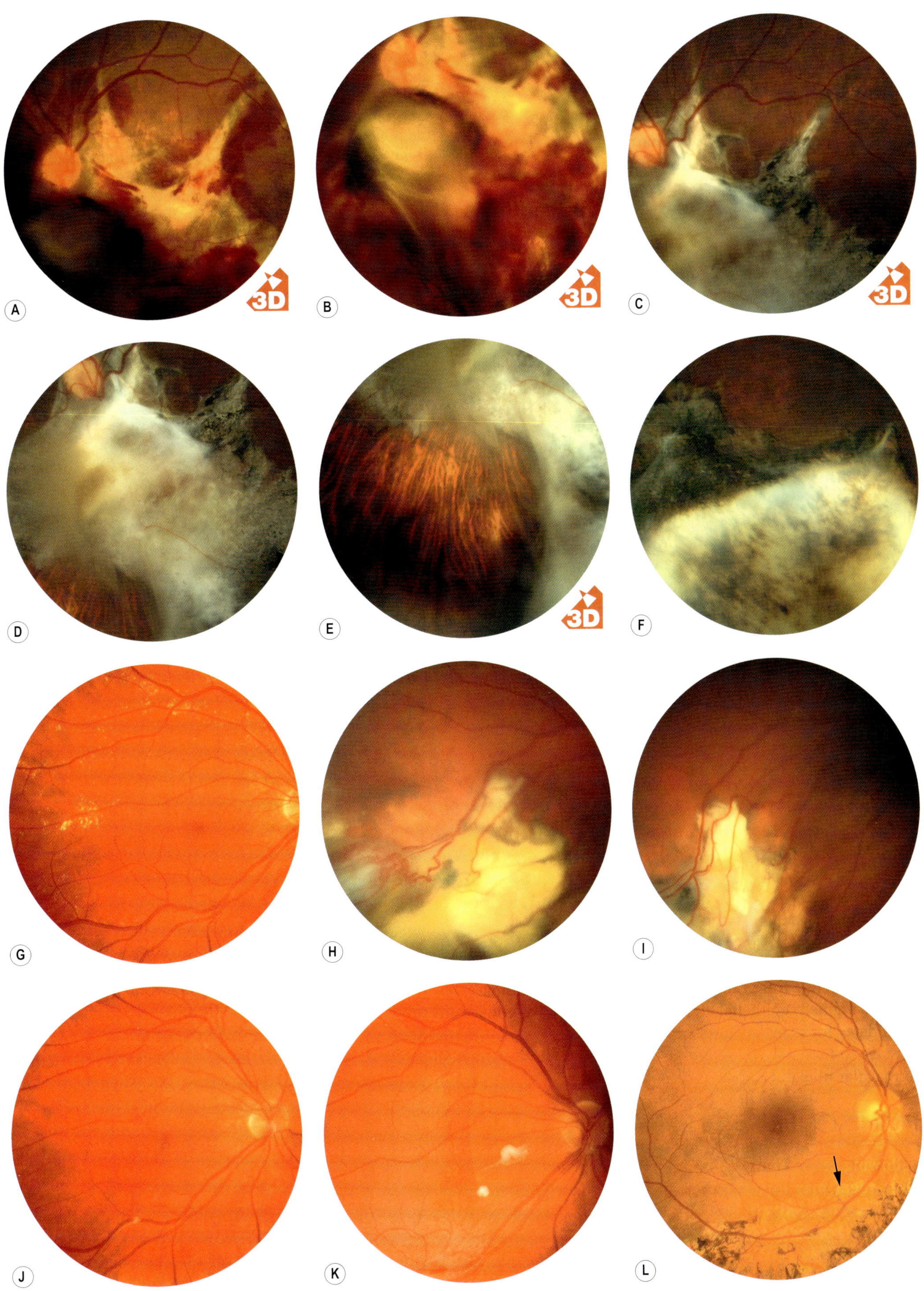
A
3D
B
3D
C
3D
D
E
3D
F
G
H
I
J
K
L

these two layers, and a fourth layer of capillaries exists within the most superficial aspect of the nerve fiber layer around the disc. This fourth layer of peripapillary capillaries extends for two disc diameters nasal to the disc and for four disc diameters temporal to the disc, although for only one disc diameter along the horizontal meridian.[74]Unlike the other capillaries in the retina, the peripapillary capillaries have fewer feeding arterioles and fewer anastamoses.[75] As a result they may be more susceptible to embolic occlusion. Histopathologic examination of an eye 34 months after development of Purtscher's retinopathy has demonstrated inner retinal atrophy compatible with retinal arterial occlusion.[71]

A fundoscopic picture virtually identical to that of Purtscher's retinopathy may occur in patients with central retinal artery obstruction, acute pancreatitis, lupus erythematosus, dermatomyositis, scleroderma, and amniotic fluid embolism (see discussion in Chapter 6).

RETINAL AND VITREOUS HEMORRHAGE ASSOCIATED WITH SUBARACHNOID AND SUBDURAL HEMORRHAGE (TERSON'S SYNDROME)

Terson described vitreous hemorrhage occurring in patients with subarachnoid hemorrhage and attributed it to a sudden increase in venous pressure that ruptures epipapillary and peripapillary capillaries.[76–78] Others have attributed the intraocular hemorrhages to a rapid increase in intracranial pressure causing compression of the central retinal vein and its choroidal anastomotic channels.[76] Approximately 20% of patients suffering either spontaneous or posttraumatic subarachnoid or subdural hemorrhages develop intraocular hemorrhages that in most cases are confined to the juxtapapillary and macular areas (Figure 8.07A–D).[79,80] Intraretinal and subretinal bleeding occurs primarily from the optic disc and retinal blood vessels. The intraretinal hemorrhages can be superficial or deep, blot or flame-shaped. Often some of the deep intraretinal hemorrhages appear petalloid with feathery margins due to dissection of blood into the outer plexiform layer (Figure 8.07G–I). Intraretinal and subretinal bleeding occurs primarily from the optic disc and retinal blood vessels. Elevated mounds of blood either beneath the internal limiting membrane of the retina or in the subhyaloid space may occur (Figure 8.06K).[81,82] In most cases these hemorrhages clear spontaneously and visual function is unaffected. Occasionally the vitreous hemorrhage fails to clear and vitrectomy may be necessary to restore vision.[83–85] The surgeon may find some evidence of retinal blood vessel and RPE damage (Figure 8.07E and F).

8.06 Purtscher's retinopathy.

A–F: This 45-year-old man noted blurred vision after falling out of a racing boat going at high speed. Visual acuity was 20/30. Note patchy swelling of the retina surrounding the optic nerve head (A). The white material appeared to lie mostly anterior to the retinal vessels. It was associated with superficial hemorrhage. Note relative sparing of the macula (B). There were no lesions in the peripheral fundus. Arteriovenous-phase angiograms showed lack of filling and obscuration of the capillary bed in the region of the white lesions (C) and later showed evidence of fluorescein leakage into the retina (D). Ten days later there had been considerable clearing of the retinopathy (E). Five months later there was mild temporal pallor (F). Visual acuity was 20/30.

G–I: This 28-year-old man was thrown from his car and sustained a basilar and ethmoidal fracture. Note the large area of ischemic whitening and hematomas that probably lie beneath the internal limiting membrane (G and H). The left eye was normal. Note the superficial retinal scar (arrow, I) and traction lines extending through the macula approximately 5 weeks later.

J–L: This patient received cardiopulmonary resuscitation following a motor vehicle accident. Bilateral subconjunctival hemorrhages with preretinal hemorrhage and nerve fiber infarcts in the right eye and peripapillary retinal whitening and retinal hemorrhages in the left eye seen 2 weeks postevent. Visual acuity was 20/20 in the right eye and 4/200 in the left eye. He had a left traumatic optic neuropathy in addition and the vision remained at 6/200.

(J–L, courtesy of Dr. Paul Sternberg, Jr.)

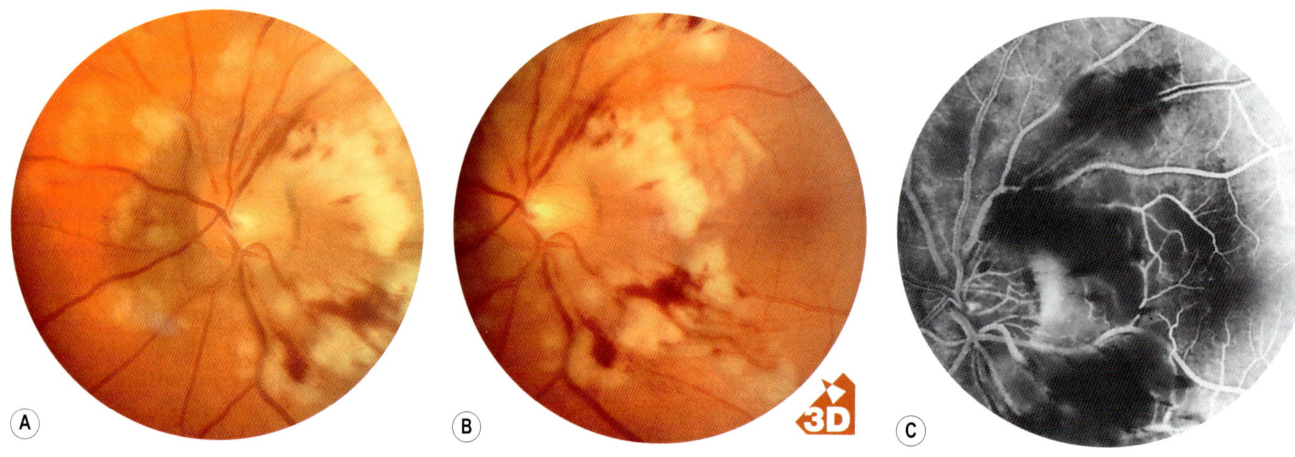

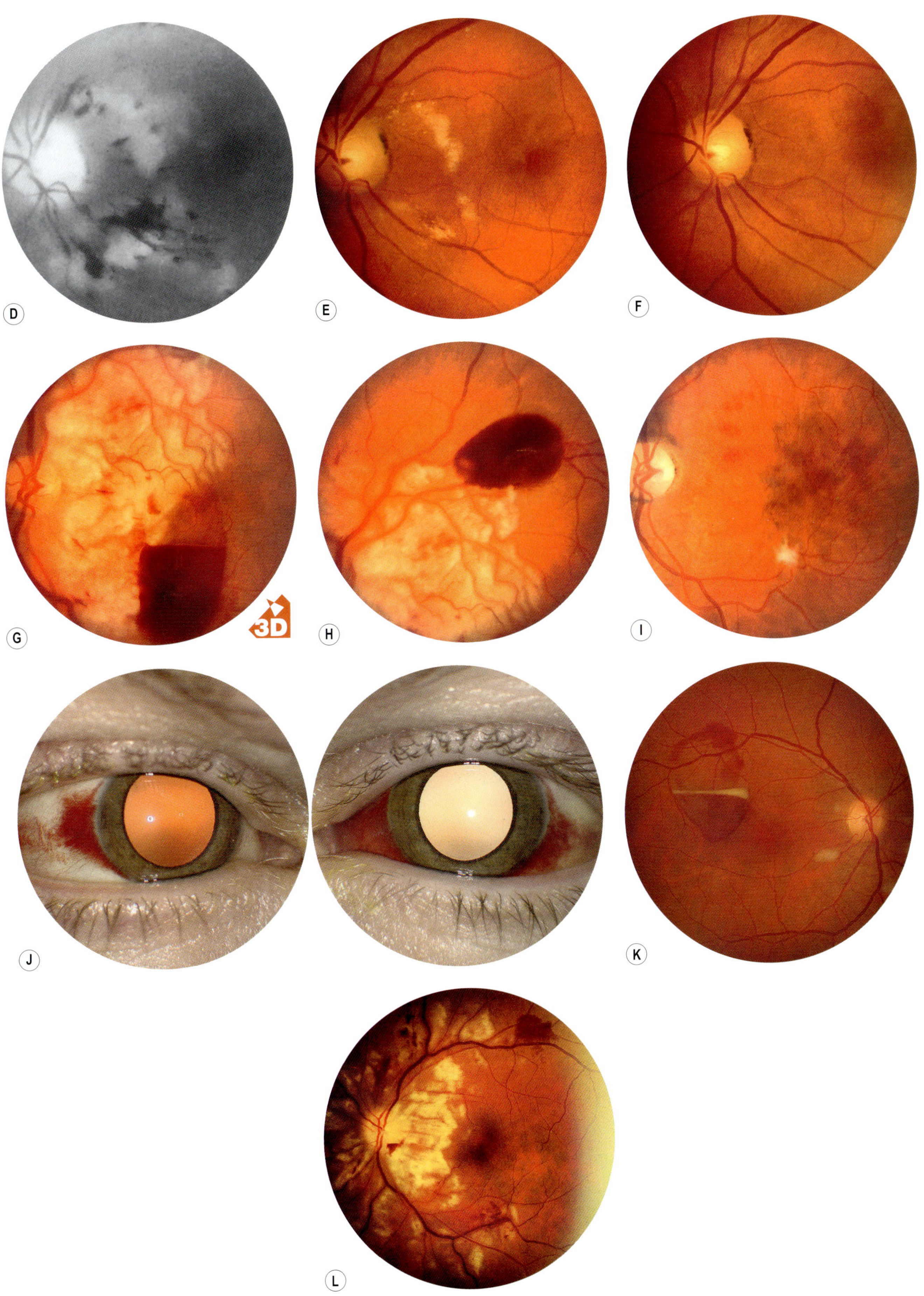
D
E
F
G
3D
H
I
J
K
L

The amount of blood in the eye is not necessarily related to the severity of the subarachnoid hemorrhage.[86] A perimacular retinal fold may develop after resolution of the subinternal limiting membrane hematoma in some patients.[87] Epiretinal membrane in the macula is the most common sequela of Terson's syndrome but is not associated with visual morbidity.[88] Because severe proliferative vitreoretinopathy occasionally develops, patients should be monitored periodically with ultrasonography while awaiting clearance of the blood, and prompt vitrectomy carried out if needed.[89]

Terson's syndrome is seen with ruptured aneurysms (Figure 8.07G–J), arteriovenous malformations, head trauma, including gunshot injuries, post epidural injections, and post endoscopic ventricular colloid cyst removal and dissecting aneurysms of the vertebrobasilar system.[90–94] Children with subarachnoid hemorrhage are less likely to develop vitreous and retinal hemorrhages compared to adults.[95] This may be due to better resilience of the vessels in children compared to adults.

HEMORRHAGIC MACULOPATHY CAUSED BY SUBARACHNOID AND EPIDURAL INJECTIONS

Patients may develop multiple scotomas caused by retinal hemorrhages in one or both eyes immediately after the injection of oxygen into the subarachnoid space during the course of myelography,[96] or following epidural injection of corticosteroids for relief of back pain.[97,98] These hemorrhages often occur as the result of bleeding from the deep retinal capillary plexus and cause a petalloid pattern of blood with tapered edges centrally surrounding the center of the macula. Sudden elevation of the cerebrospinal fluid pressure and elevation of retinal venous pressure are the most likely explanations for the hemorrhages, some of which may occur from the superficial as well as the deep retinal capillaries in a pattern similar to that seen in Terson's syndrome. The prognosis for the spontaneous return of normal visual function is good.

POSTCONTUSION NEURORETINOPATHY

Blunt trauma to the eye or periorbital region may cause acute visual loss associated with a swollen optic disc, and optic disc and retinal hemorrhages that are usually confined to the posterior fundus (Figure 8.08A–C). Some of the blood is derived from the deep plexus of retinal blood vessels and may extend into the outer plexiform layer of Henle to form a radiating pattern centrally. The fundus picture may simulate that seen in patients with papillophlebitis, with Terson's syndrome (see Figure 8.07H–J), and following epidural injections. A sudden elevation in the central retinal venous pressure caused by the trauma is presumed to be important in the pathogenesis of the optic disc and retinal hemorrhages. A similar pattern of inner and outer retinal hemorrhages occasionally occurs unilaterally in healthy patients, with no explanation for them (see Figure 8.07K and L).

8.07 Terson's syndrome.

A–D: This 45-year-old woman noted visual blurring in both eyes soon after admission to the hospital because of a subarachnoid hemorrhage. Note the multiple darker superficial subinternal limiting membrane retinal hemorrhages (arrow), lighter subretinal hemorrhages, and optic disc edema in both eyes (A–C). Fluorescein angiography revealed evidence of optic disc edema (D).

E and **F**: This 50-year-old man experienced an acute hypertensive crisis, headache, neck pain, and coma. Fresh superficial globular juxtapapillary hemorrhages were noted in both eyes. Six days later he had bilateral dense vitreous hemorrhages. Over the subsequent 6 years his vision was hand motions only because of the persistence of the vitreous blood. When seen at the Bascom Palmer Eye Institute neither fundus could be visualized because of old vitreous blood. He had a vitrectomy in both eyes. Postoperatively, his visual acuity in the right eye was 20/25 and in the left eye was 20/40. The right fundus was normal except for hypertensive retinal arterial narrowing and two white choroidal vessels in the macular area (E). In the left fundus, similar choroidal vessels were associated with a zone of retinal pigment epithelial atrophy in the macula (F).

G–J: This 48-year-old man developed sudden severe headache and lost consciousness transiently while driving his truck. He was difficult to rouse when examined in the emergency room. A computed tomography scan of the head showed subarachnoid hemorrhage and magnetic resonance angiography confirmed an anterior communicating artery aneurysm. His visual acuity was 20/70 in the right eye and 20/20 in the left eye at the bedside, when examined after a coil was placed in the aneurysm. Multiple preretinal and deep retinal hemorrhages, some of which were petalloid in the outer plexiform layer, were seen in the right eye (G and H). The left eye had a few deep retinal hemorrhages. Note similarity of the distribution of the hemorrhages to that shown in Figures 8.07K and L and 8.08A and B. Ten weeks later his vision was still 20/70 in the right eye, and the hemorrhages were clearing, with a residual small preretinal hemorrhage over his fovea (J). Optical coherence tomography confirms the preretinal location of the hemorrhage and rules out a macular hole (J)

Idiopathic unilateral deep retinal hemorrhages.

K and **L**: Unilateral visual loss and multiple deep retinal hemorrhages occurred in the left eye of this otherwise healthy young adult who gave no history of trauma or illness. Note the petalloid arrangement of the hemorrhages that probably are located in the outer plexiform layer.

(K and L, courtesy of Dr. Maurice Rabb.)

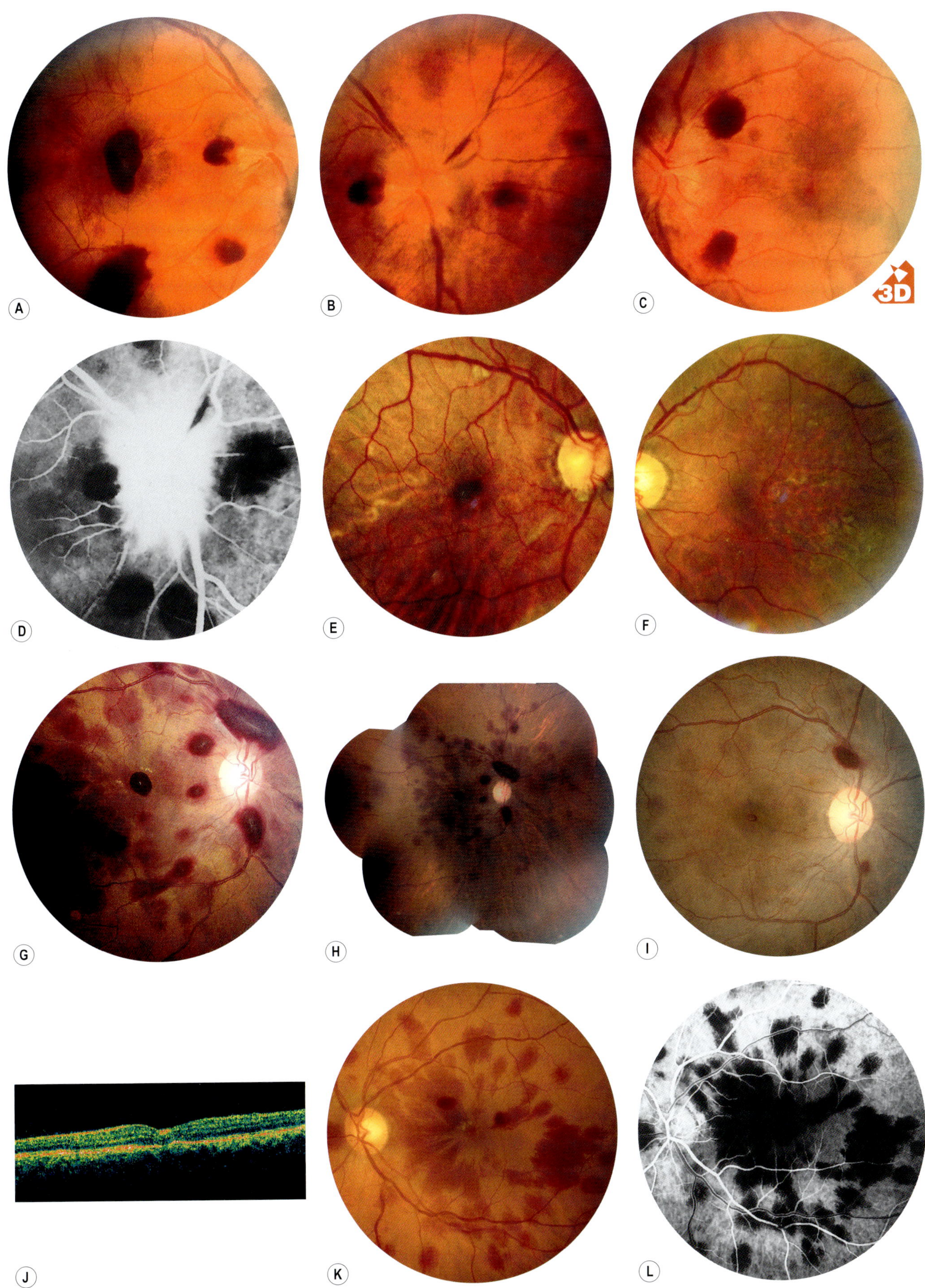
A
B
C
3D
D
E
F
G
H
I
J
K
L

SHAKEN-BABY SYNDROME

Shaken-baby syndrome results from severe shaking of infants, often as a form of punishment. The signs and symptoms are nonspecific and may mimic infection, intoxication, or metabolic abnormalities. These include (1) bradycardia, apnea, and hypothermia; (2) lethargy, irritability, seizures, hypotonia, full or bulging fontanelle, and increased head size; (3) scattered superficial retinal hemorrhages, dome-shaped subinternal limiting membrane or subhyaloid hematomas, and cotton-wool patches; and (4) skin bruises.[99–113] A history of a recent minor accident or shaking in an effort to resuscitate may be obtained in some cases. The retinopathy may simulate that seen in Terson's syndrome, Purtscher's retinopathy, or central retinal vein occlusion (Figure 8.08D–L). Late fundoscopic changes include a circular retinal fold that may create a crater-like depression in the macula and traumatic retinoschisis.[101,104,105,114,115] The circular retinal fold may be a product of abrupt vitreoretinal traction associated with shaking,[114] vitreous traction after partial separation of the vitreous in the central macular region,[115] or contraction of the internal limiting membrane or the posterior hyaloid membrane after resolution of a subinternal limiting membrane or subhyaloid hematoma. Laboratory findings include bloody cerebrospinal fluid and subdural tap and, in almost all cases, computed tomographic evidence of at least one of the following: subdural hemorrhage, subarachnoid hemorrhage, or cerebral contusion.[116] The prognosis is poor, and many children are left with severe neurologic and developmental defects, including visual deficits and in some cases blindness.

The histopathologic findings in the eyes of these patients reveal evidence of intraretinal blood, subhyaloid and subinternal limiting membrane hematomas, as well as blood in the subdural and subarachnoid spaces around the optic nerve (Figure 8.08F–J).[99,101,108,115,117,118] The subdural and subarachnoid hemorrhage in the optic nerve may be subtle and the only manifestation of the shaken-baby syndrome. Special stains for iron may be helpful in detecting evidence of previous blood in these areas occurring many months before the eyes are obtained at autopsy.

The finding of retinal hemorrhages in a child with suspected injury is more likely to be caused by shaking than by blunt trauma,[99,100,112,118] and it is an important predictor of neurologic injury.[119]

8.08 Postcontusion hemorrhagic neuroretinopathy.

A–C: This young woman experienced loss of vision after being shoved against a wall. Note the swollen optic disc, and superficial and deep retinal hemorrhages, which gradually cleared. Mild optic atrophy was associated with 20/50 acuity.

Shaken-baby syndrome (nonaccidental trauma)

D and **E**: Shaken-baby syndrome with multiple superficial retinal hemorrhages (arrow, D) in a 6-month-old infant.

F: Photomicrograph of subinternal limiting membrane hemorrhage in an infant who died of complications of shaken-baby syndrome.

G and **H**: Gross findings in a 42-week-old infant with extensive intraretinal hemorrhages and papilledema (G) and blood in the perineural sheath of the optic nerve (arrow, H). Similar changes were present in both eyes.

I and **J**: Photomicrographs of another physically abused infant with gross findings similar to G and H in both eyes. Note peripapillary subretinal blood (upper arrow, I) and hemorrhagic infarction of the retina (J). There was blood in the subarachnoid and subdural space (lower arrow, I) in both eyes.

K and **L**: Retinal hemorrhages are widespread and extend up to the ora serrata. Widespread extent of retinal and preretinal hemorrhages documented on Retcam images (L).

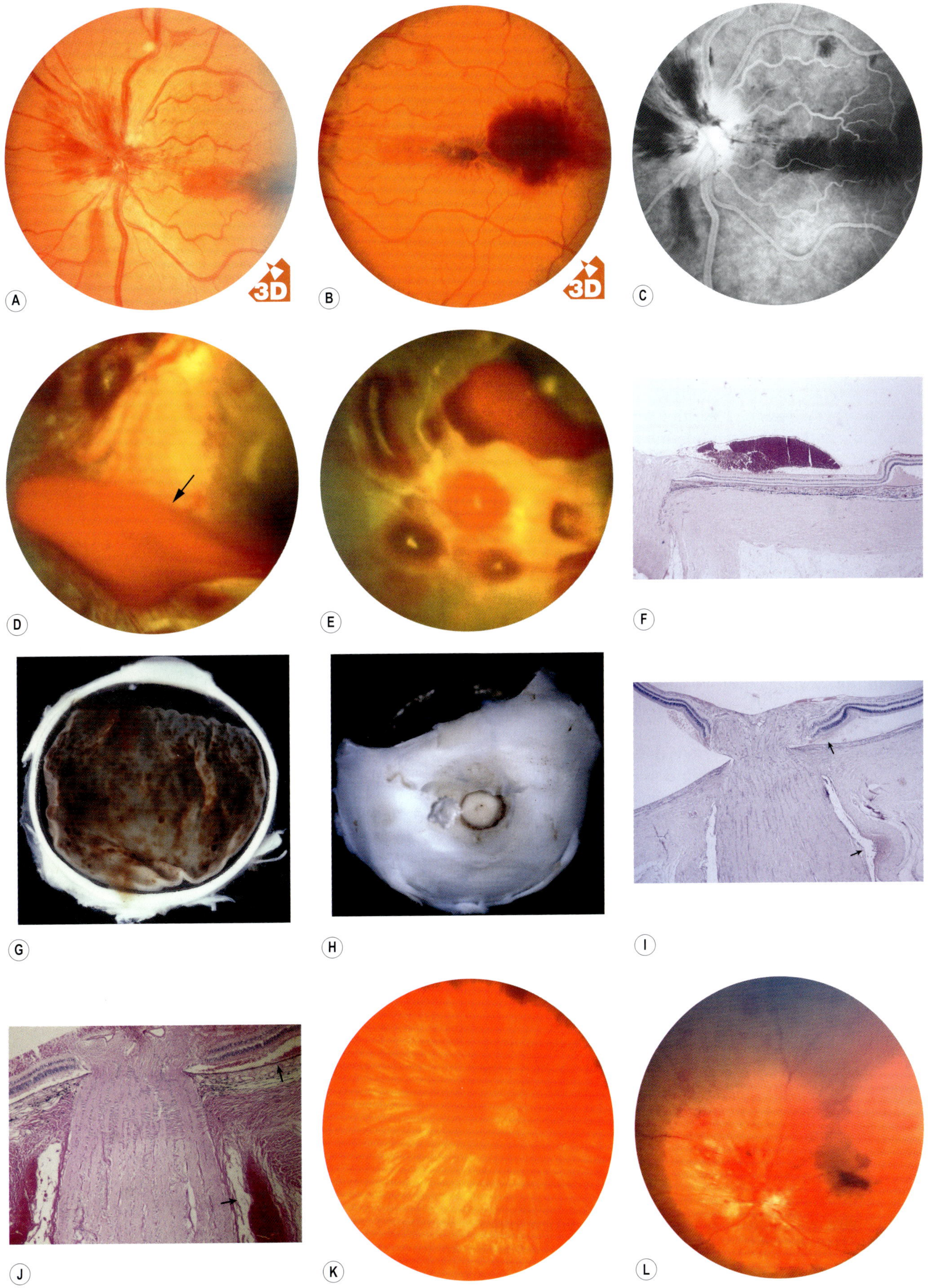
3D
3D
A
B
C
D
E
F
G
H
I
J
K
L

RETINAL VESSEL RUPTURE ASSOCIATED WITH PHYSICAL EXERTION (VALSALVA RETINOPATHY)

A sudden rise in intrathoracic or intra-abdominal pressure, particularly against a closed glottis (Valsalva's maneuver) during lifting, bowel movement, coughing, or vomiting, may cause a rapid rise of intravenous pressure within the eye and spontaneous rupture of superficial retinal capillaries in otherwise normal eyes or in eyes associated with acquired retinal vascular abnormalities (diabetic or hypertensive retinal angiopathy) or congenital retinal vascular disease (retinal telangiectasis and congenital retinal artery tortuosity) (Figure 8.09).[120–126] Sudden loss of vision may result from hemorrhagic detachment of the internal limiting membrane, vitreous hemorrhage, or, if bleeding occurs near the foveal region, dissection of blood beneath the retina. The author has seen one moderate myope develop extensive choroidal hemorrhage following violent incessant vomiting (Figure 8.09A and B). These patients typically have a circumscribed, round or dumbbell-shaped, bright red mound of blood beneath the internal limiting membrane in or near the central macular area (Figure 8.09D, F, H, and J). A glistening light reflex is present on the surface. A few fine striae indicative of wrinkling of the internal limiting membrane may be present on the surface of the hematoma. Part of the blood turns yellow after several days. The shape and color of these lesions may suggest an intraocular parasite (Figure 8.09D and E). A fluid level caused by settling of the formed blood elements may develop soon after the hemorrhage (Figure 8.09H and J). As the blood resolves, the serous detachment of the internal limiting membrane may persist for several days or weeks (Figure 8.09I).[127] Spontaneous reattachment occurs, and the appearance of the macula and visual acuity usually return to normal.

Occasionally, a small (less than one disc diameter), round, preretinal hemorrhage centered in the foveal area occurs.[120,123] The surface may show multiple yellow-white dots simulating that of a strawberry (see Figure 8.09D). Its surface usually does not show a reflex suggestive of the presence of an internal limiting membrane. It may represent a small amount of blood lying between the internal limiting membrane and the posterior hyaloid interface. In addition, patients with these small central lesions often have a thin layer of blood lying beneath the retina in the paramacular area. Complete recovery of vision usually occurs spontaneously. In unusual circumstances where a subinternal limiting membrane hematoma is responsible for visual loss in the patient's only normally functioning eye, neodymium-YAG laser disruption of the internal limiting membrane allowing the blood to gravitate into the inferior vitreous cavity may restore central vision more promptly (Figure 8.09K and L).[128–130] Subinternal limiting membrane hemorrhage and preretinal hemorrhage identical to that just described occasionally occur in the normal individual in the absence of a clear-cut history of unusual exertion or Valsalva's maneuver.[131,132] Some patients may have evidence of retinal vascular disease, for example, diabetes or hypertension (Figure 6.26G). Other apparently healthy patients may give a history of multiple previous episodes of loss of central or paracentral vision secondary to spontaneous retinal hemorrhages. Their family members may give a similar history.[133] Tortuosity of the second- and third-order retinal arterioles may or may not be present in these patients with a familial history (Figure 6.01A–C). No specific hematologic disorder has been described in this condition, which is probably inherited as an autosomal-dominant trait. Recovery of vision is the rule.

8.09 Valsalva retinopathy.

A–C: This healthy 59-year-old myopic woman developed sudden onset of blurring of vision of the right eye after several bouts of vomiting following food poisoning. She had a retinal detachment in this repaired by a scleral buckle previously. Her visual acuity was 20/40 with extensive choroidal hemorrhage (A and B). Four weeks later the hemorrhage had cleared completely and the visual acuity returned to 20/20 (C).

D and E: This young man, who was on a respirator because of acute respiratory distress syndrome of unknown cause, experienced loss of central vision in the left eye. He was referred to the eye clinic because of a suspected intraocular parasite. Note the superficial retinal blood that probably lies beneath the internal limiting membrane (D). Angiography revealed no retinal or choroidal vascular abnormality (E). The blood cleared, and the visual acuity returned to normal.

F and G: This 56-year-old man was lifting a heavy box when he suddenly lost central vision in his right eye 3 months before examination at Bascom Palmer Eye Institute. His local physician suspected an intraocular cysticercus larva. Visual acuity was 20/200. Note the parasite-like shape of the subinternal limiting membrane blood (F). Angiography revealed no evidence of retinal vascular change (G).

H and I: Serous and hemorrhagic detachment of the internal limiting membrane of the retina in a 33-year-old man who experienced sudden loss of vision during a bout of vomiting (H). Visual acuity was 20/80. There was no other evidence of retinal vascular disease. Three months later a shallow serous detachment of the internal limiting membrane remained (I). Visual acuity was 20/15.

J: This 30-year-old woman had a cardiac arrest during surgery on her hand. Cardiac resuscitation was successful and, when she regained consciousness 2 days later, she noted blurred vision in the right eye. Three weeks later her visual acuity in the right eye was 20/40. She had a subinternal limiting membrane hematoma in the macula and blood in the vitreous inferiorly in the right eye (J). The left eye was normal. Within 4 months the blood cleared and her acuity returned to 20/20.

K and L: Pre and post Yag laser disruption of subhyaloid hemorrhage to speed up resolution.

K and L, courtesy of Dr. Susan Malinowski

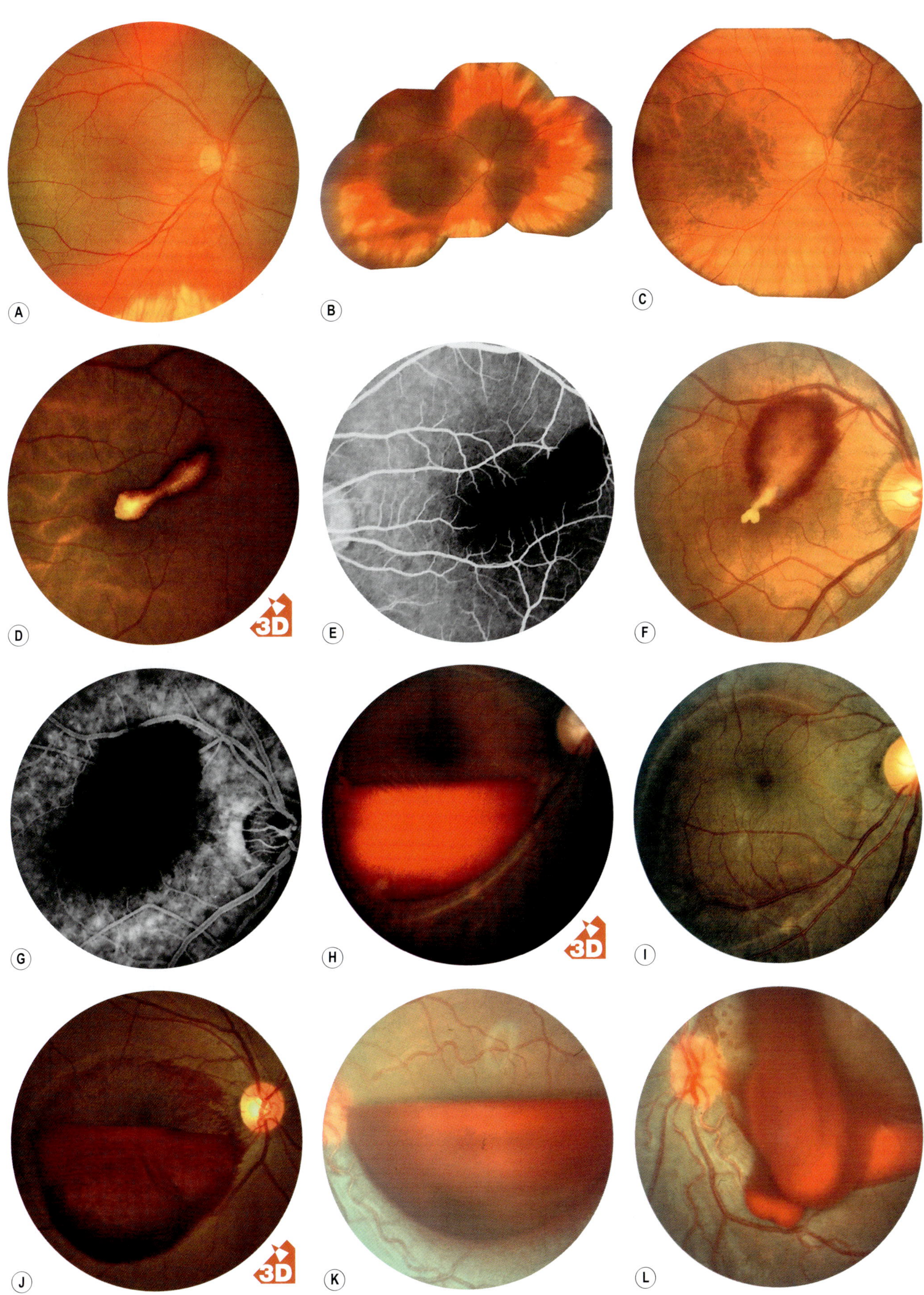
A
B
C
D
3D
E
F
G
H
3D
I
J
3D
K
L

EVULSION OF THE OPTIC DISC

A forceful backward dislocation of the optic nerve from the scleral canal can occur under several circumstances, including: (1) extreme rotation and forward displacement of the globe; (2) penetrating orbital injury causing a backward pull on the optic nerve; or (3) sudden increase in intraocular pressure causing a rupture of the lamina cribrosa.[134–137] This latter mechanism might be more appropriately termed "expulsion" rather than "evulsion." In all cases a tear in the lamina cribrosa and nerve fibers at the disc margin occurs. This tear may be partial or complete and may be associated with massive intraocular hemorrhage (Figure 8.10G and H) or only minimal bleeding (Figure 8.10A–C, E, and F).[138] In the latter case the dark, pit-like deformity caused by a partial evulsion may simulate an optic pit (Figure 8.10A).[135,136] Visual loss from these injuries is usually great. Over a period of weeks or months, fibroglial proliferation obliterates the cavity caused by the evulsion (Figure 8.10D).

A penetrating injury of the optic nerve head may simulate a partial evulsion (Figure 8.10I).

OCULAR DECOMPRESSION RETINOPATHY

Some patients following glaucoma surgery will develop superficial and deep retinal hemorrhages as a result of the pressure lowering[139] (Figure 8.10J and L). Most often, even though there is an increase in the retinal and choroidal blood flow due to the sudden low intraocular pressure; retinal bleeding is not seen. However, if the increased blood flow is excessive, autoregulation of retinal vessels cannot tolerate the volume, which overwhelms the capacitance of the capillary bed and retinal veins, resulting in retinal bleeding. A sudden decrease in intraocular pressure also induces forward shifting of the lamina cribrosa and acute blockage of axonal transport. This indirectly compresses the central retinal vein and precipitates hemorrhagic retinopathy resembling a retinal vein occlusion (Figure 8.10J and L).[140–146]

8.10 Evulsion of the optic nerve head.

A–D: Partial evulsion of the optic nerve head in a man who sustained sudden loss of vision in the left eye during a brawl. His visual acuity was 8/200. There was a large, gray, optic pit-like depression (arrows, A) involving the temporal half of the optic disc. There was juxtapapillary retinal and subretinal blood. Angiography showed an intact cilioretinal artery in the area of the partly evulsed optic disc (B and C, stereo). Eleven years later extensive fibroglial proliferation obscured the optic nerve head from view (D).

E and **F**: Contusion necrosis and partial evulsion of the inferior half of the optic nerve head in an 8-year-old boy immediately after the injury (E) and 4 months later (F).

G and **H**: Severe evulsion of the optic nerve head and contusion necrosis of the surrounding retina.

I: Perforating wound of the eye simulating a partial evulsion of the optic nerve head in a 6-year-old boy who was hit in the eye with a homemade safety-pin dart that entered the eye adjacent to the inferior limbus, missed the lens, and perforated the juxtapapillary eye wall (arrow). The child withdrew the dart himself. His visual acuity was 20/200. Two months later he developed cells, flare, and keratitic precipitates in the opposite eye.

Decompression retinopathy

J and **K**: A 50-year-old on first postoperative day with retinal and preretinal hemorrhages following trabeculectomy with mitomycin C for elevated intraocular pressure secondary to herpetic trabeculitis (J). All hemorrhages resolved in 2 months and vision improved to 20/40 with pinhole (K).

L and **M**: A 69-year-old high myope Caucasian woman developed retinal and preretinal hemorrhages noted first postoperative day following trabeculectomy with mitomycin C for primary open-angle glaucoma (L). Her preoperative intraocular pressure was 46 mm and dropped to 6 mm on day 1 postoperatively. She also had peripheral choroidal detachments. Optical coherence tomography shows increased reflectivity from the superficial foveal hemorrhage and shadowing posterior to it (M). All retinal hemorrhages resolved in 2 months.

(J and K, courtesy of Dr. Franco Recchia; L and M, courtesy of Dr. Jeffrey Kammer.)

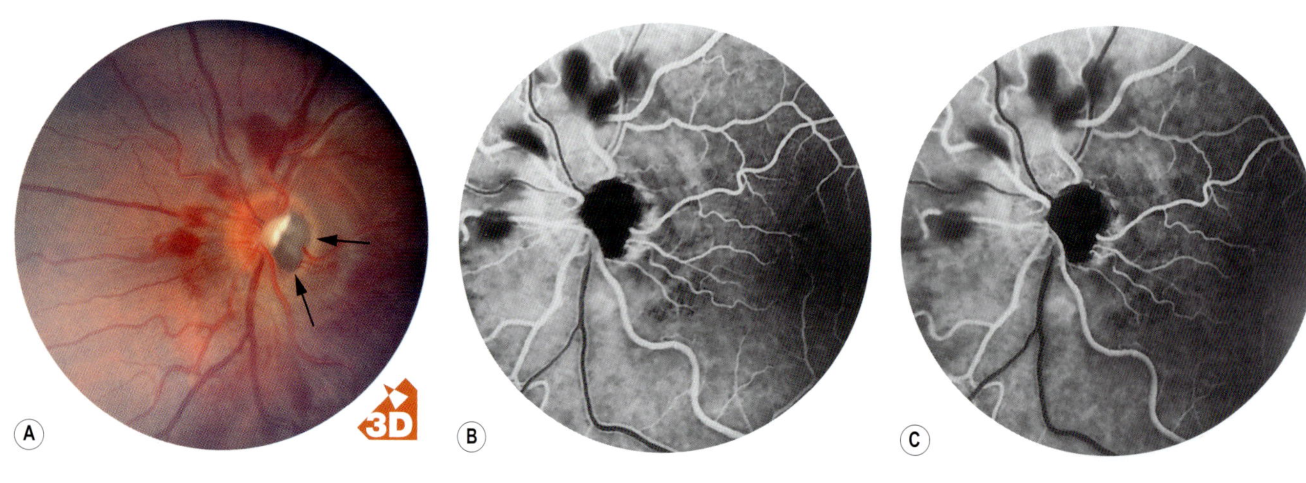

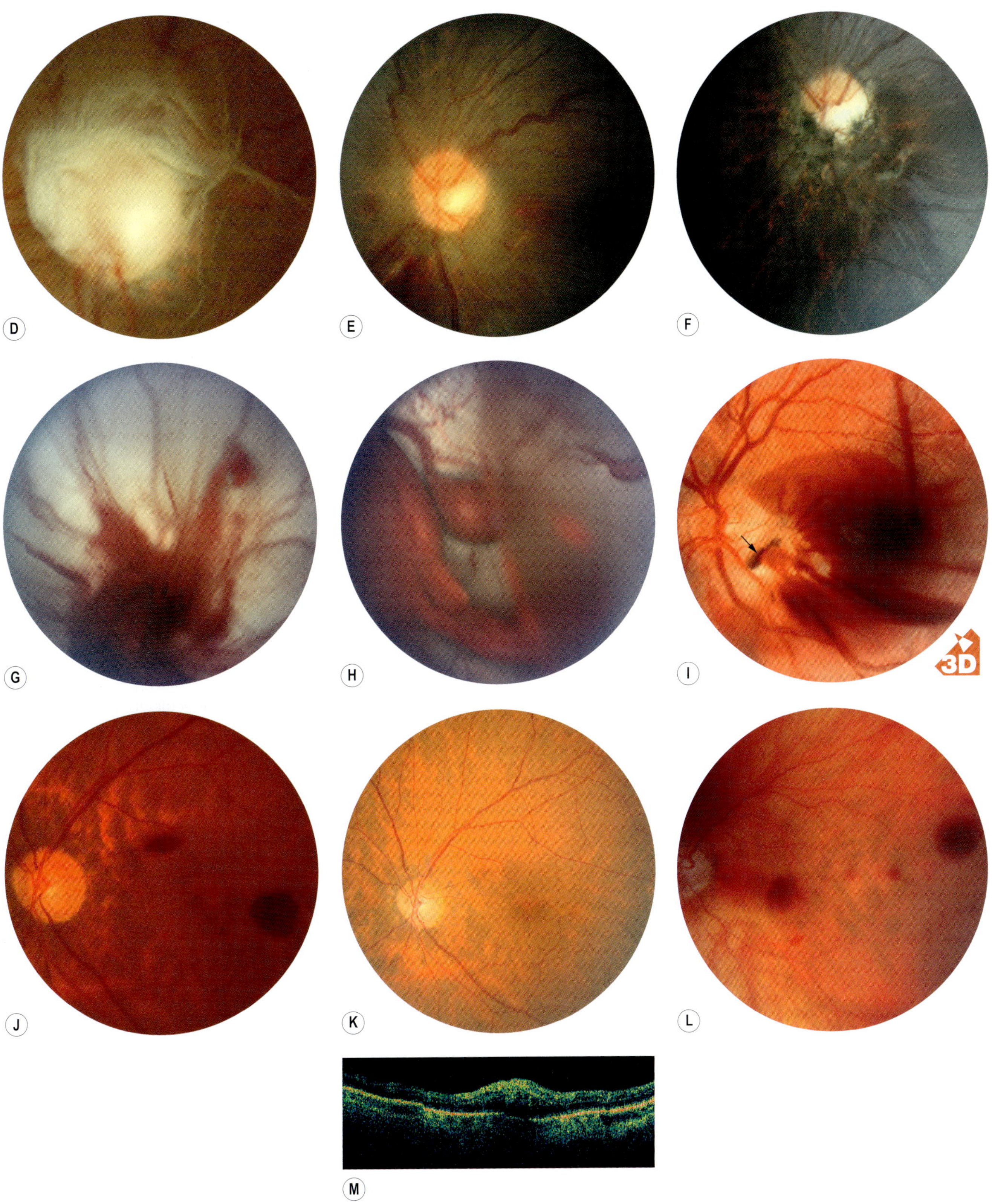
D
E
F
G
H
I
3D
J
K
L
M

Some of the hemorrhages may be white-centered. The visual acuity is typically unaffected by these changes, unless a significant central retinal vein occlusion occurs.[147]

INTRAOCULAR FOREIGN BODIES

A great variety of foreign bodies may penetrate the ocular wall and become lodged within the choroid and retina. In most instances their identity is known and measures for removal are often undertaken promptly. In some cases, however, the invasion of the foreign body may not be recognized until months or years later, when the patient experiences signs or symptoms related to breakdown of the foreign body (e.g., siderosis or chalcosis; Figure 8.11B, C, I, and J) or when a mass lesion in the fundus is discovered on routine eye examination (Figure 8.11B–E). Occasionally it may simulate a melanoma and result in removal of the eye (Figure 8.11B–E).[135,148,150] The use of ultrasonography, radiography, and electroretinography in mass lesions of uncertain etiology can reduce the chances of this mistake (Figure 8.11B). The late development of subretinal neovascularization occurring at a foreign-body impact site may occur[151] (see Chapter 9).

8.11 Intraocular foreign bodies.

A: Metallic foreign body lying on the inner retinal surface.
B: Juxtapapillary pigmented tumor that was suspected to be a melanoma. An orbital roentgenogram, however, revealed a metallic foreign body within the pigmented mass.
C–E: A juxtapapillary pigmented mass that was diagnosed as a choroidal melanoma and the eye was enucleated. Gross photographs show the mass (arrows, C). Photomicrographs show the juxtapapillary mass that lies within the sclera and choroid beneath the atrophic retina (D). It stained positively for iron and calcium, and polarization (E) revealed evidence of hemosiderin. These changes probably resulted from the impact and subsequent disintegration of an unsuspected iron foreign body.
F–H: Intraocular iron foreign body sustained while hammering on metal. Stereoscopic angiogram shows elevation at the site of the embedded foreign body that was still present following an attempt to remove it after pars plana vitrectomy and lensectomy.
I and J: Chalcosis in a 40-year-old schizophrenic man who had visual acuity of 20/25, a mild sunflower cataract (I), mild vitritis, and a yellow mass in the superotemporal quadrant of the left eye (J). There was no history of a foreign-body injury, and no site of entry was found. Orbital roentgenogram revealed a foreign body that proved to be brass after removal via the pars plana.

(C–E, Rones and Zimmerman.[150])

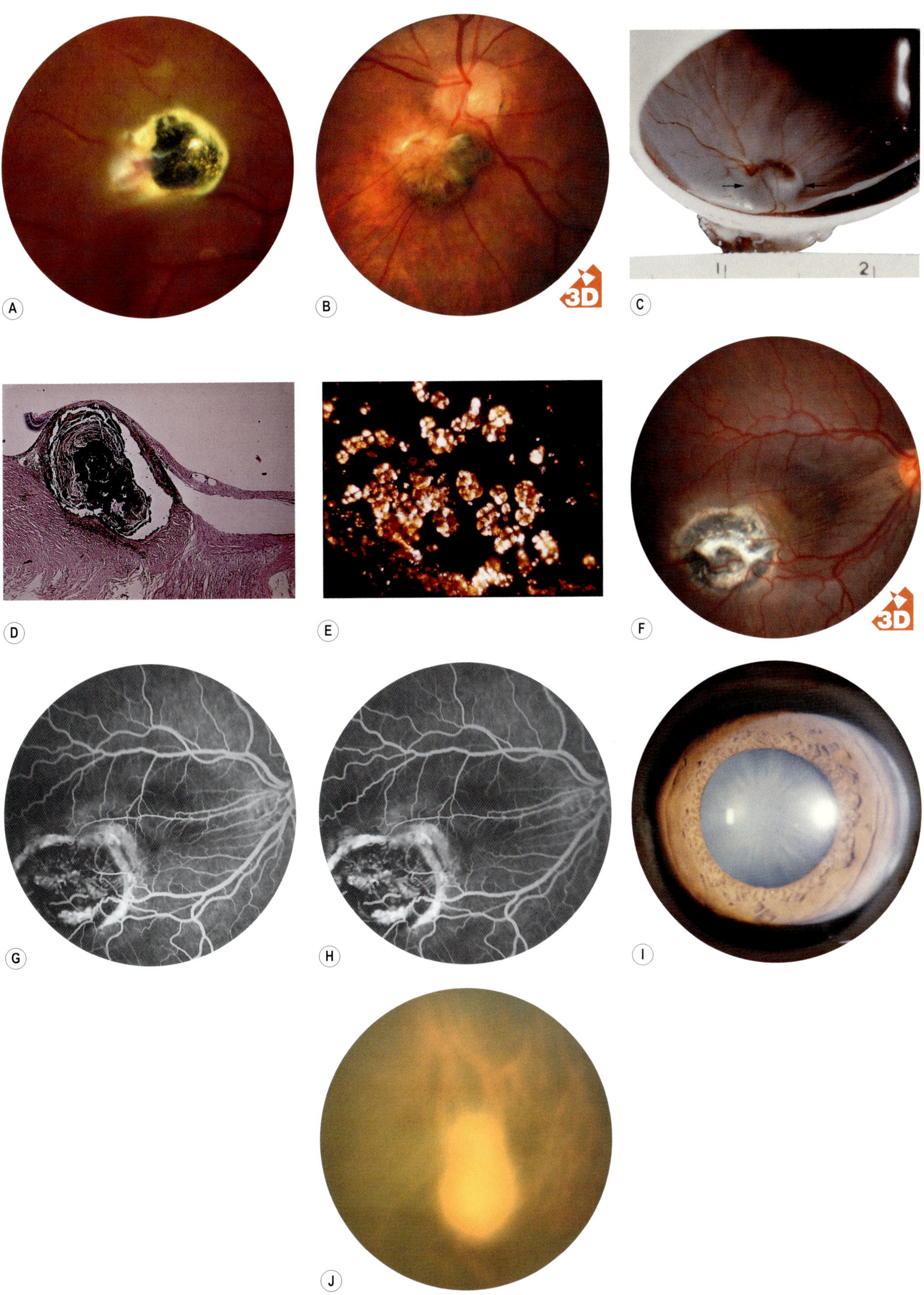
1
2
3D
3D
A
B
C
D
E
F
G
H
I
J

CHORIORETINOPATHY AND OPTIC NEUROPATHY ASSOCIATED WITH RETROBULBAR INJECTIONS

Acute visual loss may be associated with retrobulbar local anesthetic injections. There are a variety of mechanisms causing visual loss. These include penetration of the eye wall,[152–159] penetration of the optic nerve,[155,157,158] compression of the optic nerve, intra-arterial injection of anesthesia,[158] and spasm of the central retinal artery (Figure 8.12).[160] In cases of perforation of the eye the site of exit is often visible in the posterior pole and is associated with variable amounts of intraretinal, subretinal, and vitreous blood (Figure 8.12A and B). Retinal detachment, vitreous traction, and subretinal neovascularization may occur as late complications (Figure 8.12A–D). Penetration of the optic nerve sheaths may be associated with intrasheath injection, brainstem anesthesia, respiratory arrest,[161–166] and anterior extension of the anesthetic into the subretinal space.[157,158] Intrasheath injection as well as injection into the optic nerve may cause occlusion of the central retinal artery and vein,[157,158,167] or severe ischemic optic neuropathy (Figure 8.12E–L). Risk factors include: sharp needles, needles longer than 1.25 inches (3.17 cm), axial myopia, multiple injections, injections by nonophthalmologists, enophthalmos, previous scleral buckling procedure, traditional superonasal gaze position during the injection, and poor patient cooperation.[153,159,168] Use of blunted retrobulbar needles 1.25 inches (3.17 cm) or less in length and injection with the eye in the straight-ahead position may be helpful in preventing visual loss.[157,168]

Penetration of the anterior ocular coats during peribulbar anesthetic injections, particularly with sharp, small-gauge needles, may occur and often is unassociated with permanent visual loss.[152] The author has seen one patient who sustained immediate loss of vision associated with subretinal injection of Xylocaine and epinephrine local anesthetic (see Figure 9.14I–L).

8.12 Complications of retrobulbar anesthesia.

A–D: Ocular perforation with a needle occurred during local anesthesia in this elderly woman scheduled for cataract extraction. She noted a dark violaceous spot at the time of the retrobulbar injection and poor central vision postoperatively. Three weeks later her visual acuity in the left eye was 20/300. There was an entrance site inferiorly and an exit site just superior to the center of the macula (arrows, A and B). Ten months later her visual acuity in the right eye was 5/200. There was evidence of subretinal neovascularization surrounding the exit site (C and D).

E and **F**: Combined central retinal artery and central retinal vein occlusion was present on the first day after cataract surgery under local anesthesia.

G and **H**: This patient noted marked visual loss on the first postoperative day after cataract extraction done several months before these photographs were taken. Note pallor of the optic disc and narrowing and cuffing of the inferior branch retinal arteries. Angiography revealed a large inferior zone of capillary nonperfusion (H).

I: Subretinal and intravitreal depo-prednisolone following a scleral buckling procedure.

J – L: This hypertensive woman noted loss of vision in this eye during the course of cataract extraction. On the first postoperative day her visual acuity was light perception only and the fundus showed a picture simulating Purtscher's retinopathy. The visual function gradually improved and several months later her visual acuity was 20/30. There was mild optic atrophy (J and K). Healed laser scars around the site of perforation (L).

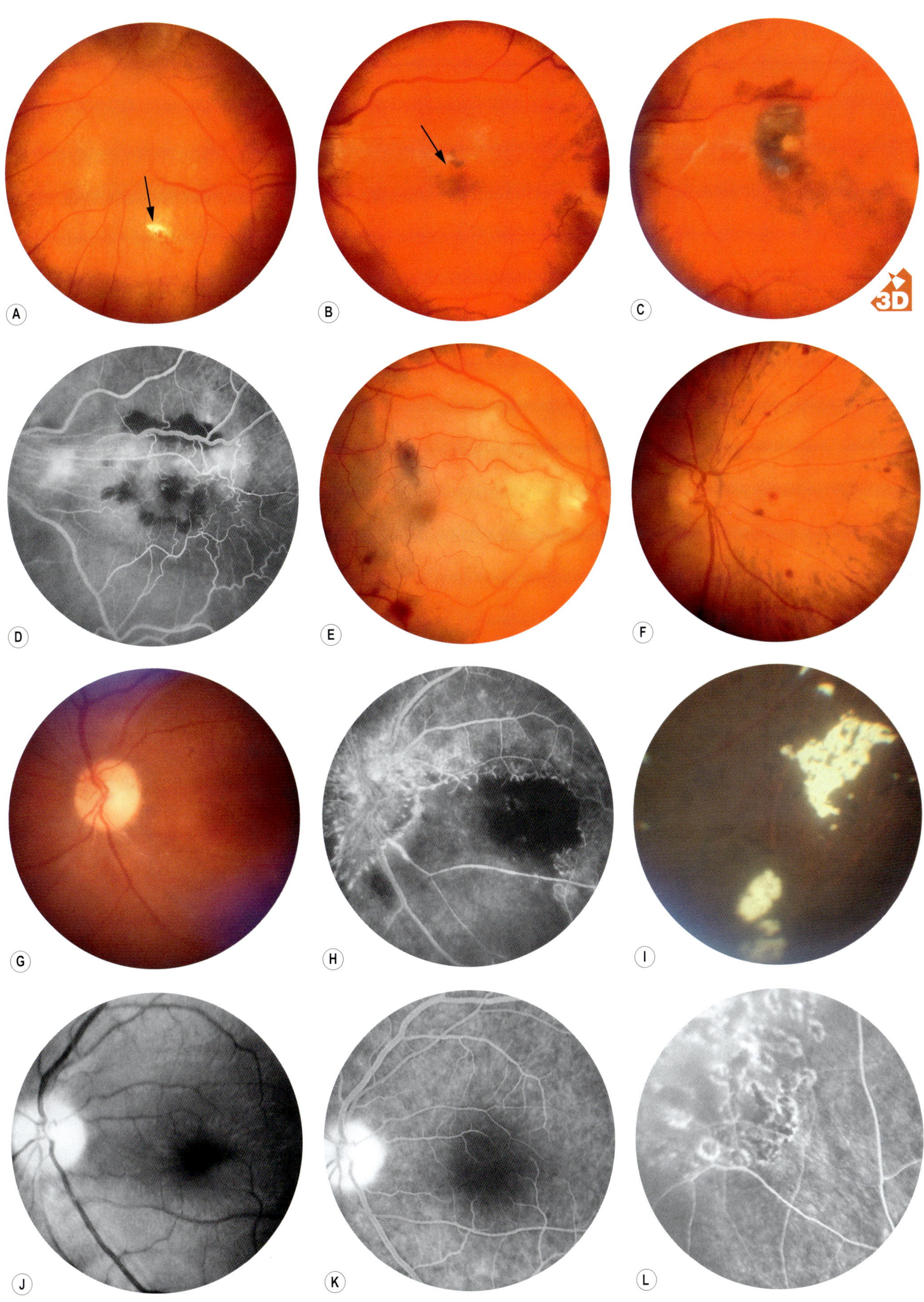
A
B
C
3D
D
E
F
G
H
I
J
K
L

PHOTIC MACULOPATHY

Light may cause damage to retinal tissues by means of three basic mechanisms: photochemical, photocoagulative, and mechanical.[169,170] Photochemical damage occurs when light of the visible spectrum, particularly the blue end, causes photochemical changes and retinal injury without significantly raising the tissue temperature. Photocoagulation occurs when light generates a temperature of more than 10°F above body temperature and causes coagulation of retinal proteins. Mechanical injury is caused by acoustic waves or gaseous formation after rapid tissue absorption of light. Many factors, including pigmentation, clarity and nature of the media, wavelength of light, dose rate, and body temperature, are important in determining the nature of the injury.

Solar Retinopathy

The terms "solar retinopathy," "eclipse burns," and "foveomacular retinitis," which most authors believe are synonymous, refer to a specific foveolar lesion that occurs: (1) in certain patients following viewing of an eclipse[171,172]; (2) after direct sun gazing by lookouts,[173] sunbathers,[174] malingerers,[175,176] or schizophrenics[177]; (3) as part of a religious ritual[178,179]; (4) in young people under the influence of hallucinogenic agents, particularly LSD (Figures 8.13 and 8.14)[180–182]; and (5) in patients, typically children or young adults, who deny a history of unusual exposure to sun.[183,184] Those who admit to sun gazing often develop, soon after exposure, a central scotoma, chromatopsia, metamorphopsia, and headache. The visual acuity is reduced to 20/40 to 20/70. In most cases visual acuity returns to between 20/20 and 20/40 within a period of 3–6 months.[172]

During the first few days after exposure a small yellow-white spot with a surrounding faint gray zone develops in the center of the foveolar area (Figure 8.13A). This spot fades after several days and is replaced by a reddish spot with a pigment halo. After approximately 10–14 days this often fades from view and is usually replaced by a small (25–50 μm), reddish, sharply circumscribed, often irregularly shaped, faceted lamellar hole or depression in the foveolar area (Figure 8.13B–F). This defect may lie immediately beneath or just adjacent to the foveal reflex that is typically present. It is not associated with an overlying operculum or evidence of posterior vitreous separation. Occasionally the diameter of this pit may be 100–200 μm (Figure 8.13E and F). This pit is probably caused by focal loss of the retinal receptors.[184,185] OCT is invaluable in demonstrating the focal loss of photoreceptors with sharply circumscribed edges (Figure 8.13I and J, 8.14G and H). It is permanent and is highly suggestive of previous sun gazing. Similar lesions, however, may occur after spontaneous vitreous separation, usually in patients 50 years or older (see discussion of macular holes, Chapter 7), and in some patients after whiplash-like injuries (see Figure 8.05 H, p. 722).[52,53]

In some patients sustaining prolonged or repeated exposures, particularly those under the influence of hallucinogenic agents, a larger lesion with mottling of the RPE may occur (Figure 8.13A).[181,182,184] Possible factors predisposing to macular damage from the sun include younger age (lens clearer), pupil dilation, relative emmetropia, high body temperature, and geophysical conditions allowing increase in the atmospheric transmission of ultraviolet B radiation to the Earth's surface.[186]

Fluorescein angiography in most patients shows no abnormality during either the early or the late phases of the disease. In a few patients seen within the first 48 hours, a small focal area of staining may be present. Days to weeks later there may be a small spot of hyperfluorescence caused by a window defect in the RPE. The presence of xanthophyll pigment in the foveal area may be responsible for the difficulty in demonstrating angiographic evidence of minor RPE damage in these cases.

8.13 Solar maculopathy.

A–D: This 16-year-old boy noted blurred vision in both eyes soon after having gazed at the sun. When seen initially, his visual acuity was 20/30 in the right eye and 20/100 in the left eye. He had a small yellow spot in the foveal center of both eyes (A). Fluorescein angiography was normal. Thirteen weeks later, visual acuity was 20/20 in the right eye and 20/100 in the left eye. In the center of both foveas there was a sharply circumscribed inner lamellar hole (B and C). Two months later the pits had enlarged slightly (D) and they remained unchanged 7 years later when his visual acuity was 20/15 in the right eye and 20/20 in the left eye.

E and **F**: Large foveolar pits many years after sun gazing. The patient's visual acuity was 20/30.

G–J: A 20-year-old man with bipolar disorder on antipsychotics. Visual acuity was 20/30 in each eye. Both macula show central yellow change (G and H) with corresponding photoreceptor disruption on optical coherence tomography (I and J).

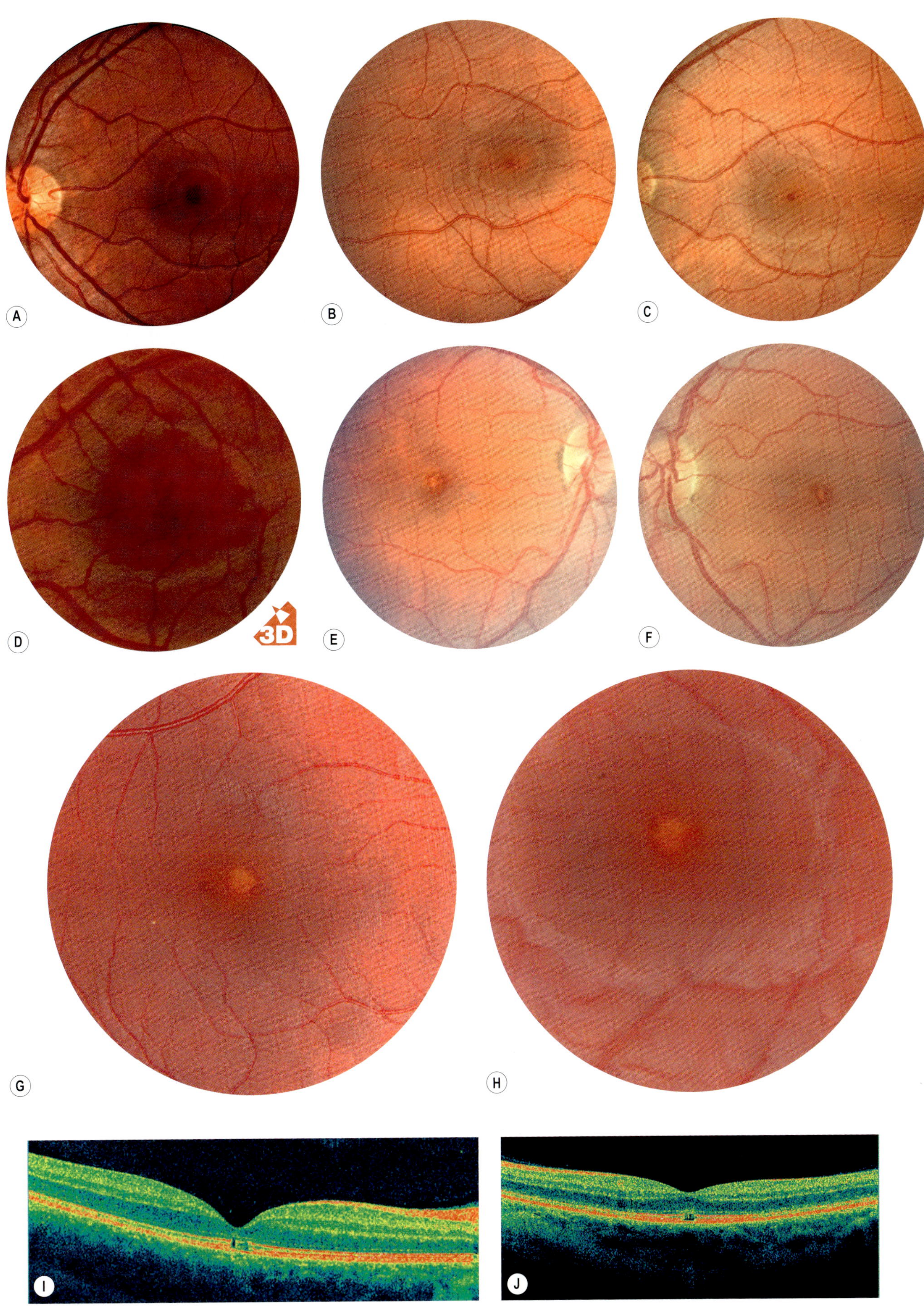
A
B
C
D
3D
E
F
G
H
I
J

There is experimental evidence to suggest that the blue wavelengths of light are chiefly responsible for producing a photochemical injury that during the first 48 hours manifests itself primarily as damage to the apical melanosomes of the RPE followed by macrophage phagocytosis of the melanosomes in the subretinal space. Between 48 hours and 5 days after exposure, disruption of the receptor elements becomes more apparent. Much of this damage is reversible and thus explains why many patients regain good acuity.[187–194] In severe cases, depigmentation of the RPE and permanent loss of the receptor elements may occur (Figure 8.14K and L).[184] There is also evidence to suggest that there is great individual variation in susceptibility for developing solar retinopathy. Some patients with minimal exposure to the sun (e.g., during sunbathing) may develop a macular lesion,[174,183] whereas others, even after purposely staring at the sun for as long as an hour, may develop only a minimal lesion.[194] Most patients recover normal or nearly normal acuity, and no treatment has been proved to be of value.

It is probable that acute visual loss in naval personnel attributed to foveomacular retinitis was caused primarily by sun gazing.[195] It is also probable that some reported cases of idiopathic foveolar lesions, identical to solar maculopathy, occurred in patients who for a variety of reasons may have denied sun gazing.[183] The possibility still exists, however, that there are other as yet unidentified causes for this clinical picture.

8.14 Probable solar burn.

A–H: This 42-year-old FBI detective complained of gradual onset of paracentral small scotomas of 1–2 years' duration in both eyes. Visual acuity was 20/25 in each eye. Foveal thinning (outer lamellar hole) is noted in each eye of approximately 100-μm size (A and B). The foveal defects are more discernible on the redfree photographs (C and D). Fluorescein angiography revealed no corresponding defects. Optical coherence tomography done 1 year later shows focal loss of foveal photoreceptors corresponding to the red lesions in each eye (G and H). Visual acuity and fundus appearance have remained unchanged over 3 years. He denied sun gazing.

Clinicopathologic correlation of a probable solar macular burn.

J–L: A 20-year-old Air Force-enlisted man with a 2-week history of blurred vision in the right eye and a 1-week history of blurred vision in the left eye. He admitted being under the influence of LSD but denied sun gazing. Visual acuity in the right eye was 20/200 and in the left eye was 20/60. In the right eye he had a large oval area of retinal pigment epithelium (RPE) derangement centered in the macula (I). In the left macula he had a small yellow lesion similar to the one in the right eye. Fluorescein angiography showed evidence of a window defect in the RPE in the right macula (J). It showed no abnormality in the left eye. Seven days later the visual acuity in the left eye had improved to 20/30. Approximately 6 months later he was killed in an automobile accident, and his eyes were obtained at autopsy. Histopathologic examination of the eye depicted in A showed focal loss of the rod and cone nuclei and receptor elements in the central macular area (arrows, K). There was focal thinning and depigmentation of the otherwise viable RPE cells in the foveal region (L). Arrow indicates the junction between the normal and depigmented RPE. Note that Bruch's membrane, the choriocapillaris, and the remaining choroidal vessels are normal. Serial sections of the left eye failed to reveal a definite abnormality in the foveal area.

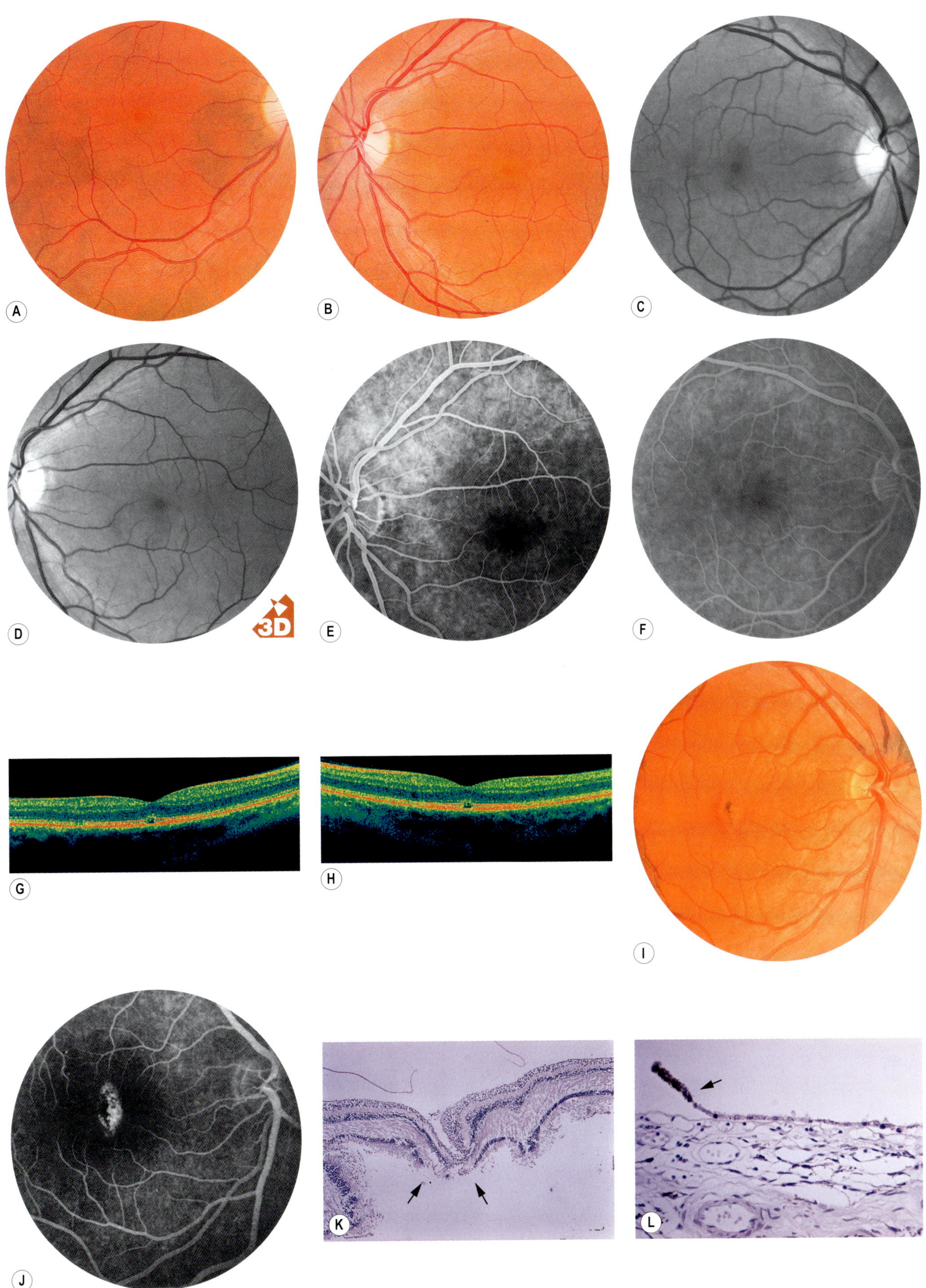
A
B
C
D
3D
E
F
G
H
I
J
K
L

Welding-Arc Maculopathy

Exposure to a welding arc commonly causes keratoconjunctivitis, but only rarely does it cause visual loss. In certain instances, however, there is some evidence that prolonged exposure over a period of minutes or more may cause facial burn, decreased pupillary response to light, decreased acuity with a central scotoma, a concentric peripheral field loss, and biomicroscopic changes in the macula that appear almost identical to those seen following exposure to the sun (Figure 8.15A–D).[184,196–199] Depending on the severity of the disease, visual acuity usually returns to normal in a matter of days or weeks. The course of visual recovery and fundus changes closely parallels solar maculopathy. As in the case of solar maculopathy, there is evidence to suggest that the retinal damage secondary to a welding arc is probably explained on a photochemical rather than a thermal basis and is primarily caused by the wavelengths at the blue end of the visible spectrum.[200] Similar photochemical macular burns may occur after brief exposure to the flash associated with short-circuiting a high-tension electric current (Figure 8.15E–H).[201] Dolphin and Lincoff reported homonymous, oval, white retinal lesions in a patient exposed to a 700-V electric discharge that occurred when two electric rails generated an arc of light.[202]

In case of metal-arc inert gas (MIG) welding, the arc is ensheathed in a stream of inert gas to prevent oxidation of molten metal. The gas changes the emitted radiation into the visible and near-infrared range and can be absorbed by the retina, resulting in thermal and photochemical damage (Figure 8.15I–M). This is in contrast to electrical welding arc where the radiation is predominantly in the ultraviolet range.[203,204]

Unusual fundus lesions reported in two patients exposed to electric arc welding appear to be unrelated RPE detachments in one patient and nonspecific chorioretinal scars in the other.[205,206] There is one report of a macular hole occurring after exposure to electric welding arc.[207]

8.15 Photic maculopathy.

A–D: Photic maculopathy caused by welding in this 19-year-old man who developed marked pain in the eyes and progressive visual loss soon after spending 2 hours "tacking" with a helium welder 2 weeks before his initial examination at the Bascom Palmer Eye Institute. He had symmetric, small, yellow, foveolar lesions at the level of the retinal pigment epithelium (RPE) (A and B). His visual acuity in the right eye was 20/100 and in the left eye was 20/200. Angiography in both eyes showed a small focal window defect in the RPE centrally (C). Ten months later the patient's visual acuity had returned in the right eye to 20/30+ and in the left eye to 20/50+. Note the slight enlargement of the area of depigmentation in the center of the macular area (D).

E–H: Photic maculopathy and facial burns caused by electric arc flash occurred in this workman (E) when he drove a spike into a high-voltage line. Forty-eight hours after the injury, his visual acuity in the left eye was 20/50. He had a yellow spot in the center of the fovea (F). Two weeks after injury his acuity was 20/40 and the spot was less prominent (G). Eight months after injury his visual acuity was 20/20. There was a circular zone of depigmentation of the RPE (H) that was readily apparent as a ring of hyperfluorescence angiographically.

Welding arc maculopathy in metal-arc inert gas (MIG) welders.

I–M: A 36-year-old Caucasian welder complained of photopsias and central scotoma for 5 days in his right eye following an arc welding flash while using a MIG. His vision was 20/30 in the right and 20/20 in the left eye. Fundus showed foveal detachments in both eyes (I and J) confirmed on optical coherence tomography (L and M). Fluorescein angiogram showed no leakage into the subretinal space (K). Observation was recommended; his vision improved to 20/25 at 6 weeks and 20/20 at 6 months with resolution of the serous retinal detachment.

(E–H, From Gardner et al.,[201] I–M, courtesy of Dr. Amy Noffke.)

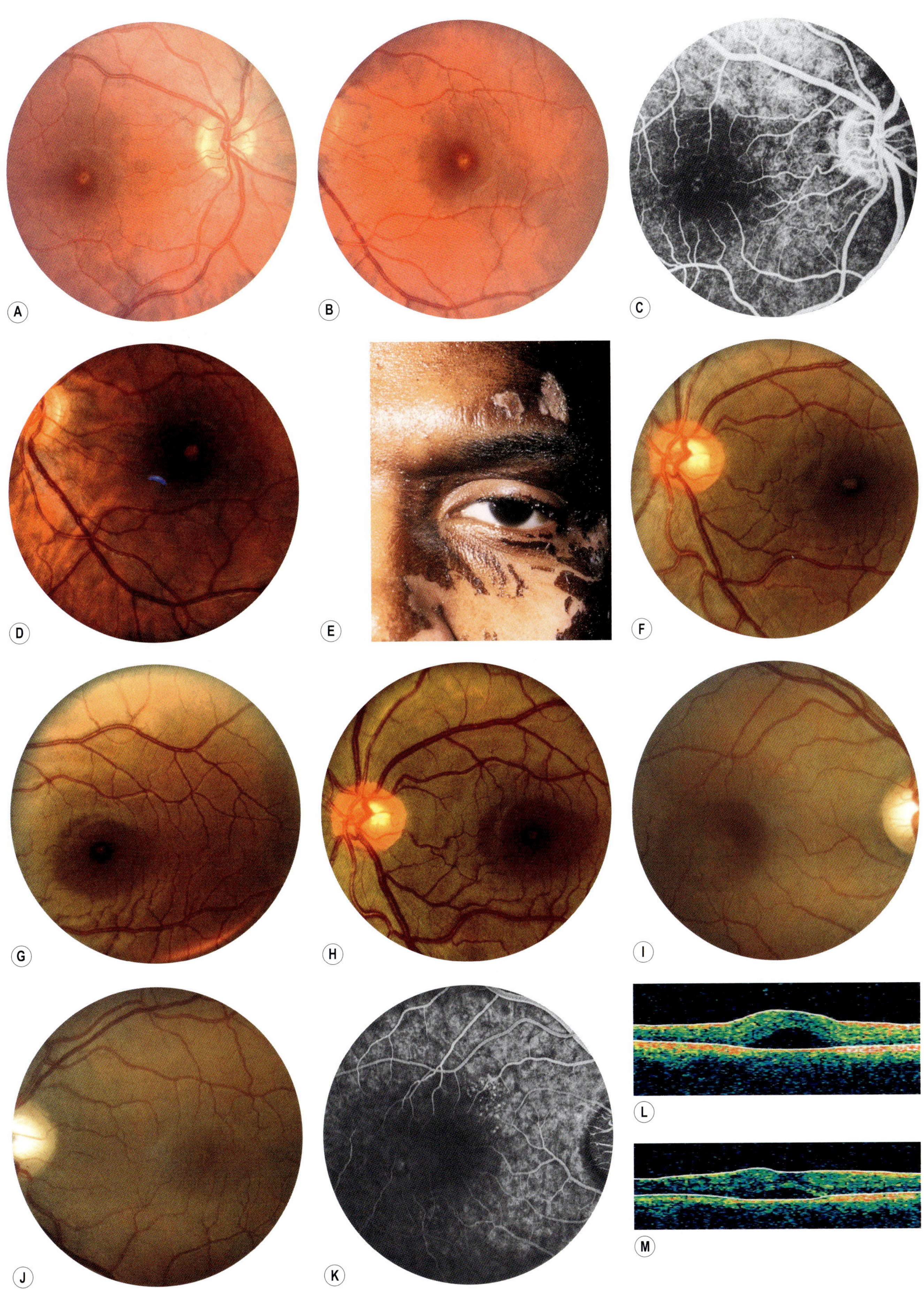
A
B
C
D
E
F
G
H
I
J
K
L
M

Lightning and Electrocution Retinopathy

Lightning, with a force of up to 1 million V and 30 000 A, causes significant mortality and morbidity to those in its path. Lightning reaches its victim by four routes: (1) direct strike; (2) side flash – lightning strikes a nearby object and arcs through the path of least resistance; (3) ground current – lightning strikes the ground and travels along its surface; and (4) rarely, by current traveling through wires or pipes reaching people in bath tubs or on the phone. Ophthalmic injury from lightning has three proposed mechanisms.[208,209] The electrical current passes through ocular tissues, causing disruption of cell membranes, converts to heat causing damage, and vasoconstricts causing tissue ischemia. Industrial accidents or occupational injuries from high-voltage electricity cause similar effects.[210–215] The cardiovascular and nervous systems offer paths of lesser resistance and thus are more susceptible, though any organ system can be affected.

Lightning-induced ocular injuries include thermal keratopathy, uveitis, hyphema, anterior and posterior subcapsular cataract, and dislocated lens in the anterior segment. Posterior-segment injuries include vitreous hemorrhage, retinal edema, maculopathy, macular cyst (Figure 8.16), macular hole, central retinal vein occlusion, central retinal artery occlusion, thermal papillitis, and optic neuropathy. The foveal changes seem to result from dissolution of retinal photoreceptors and adjacent neuritis (Figure 8.16G, H, J, and L). Multiple cranial nerve palsies and nystagmus can also occur.[209]

Coming in contact with, or in close proximity to, a high-voltage electric current results in acute visual loss associated with macular changes.[208,209,216–223] Macular edema simulating Berlin's edema seen early may be replaced by lesions described as a "cyst" (Figure 8.16), "macular hole," or solar maculopathy over time. Eventually the macula is noted to be thin on OCT; a macular hole may spontaneously close or persist. Diffuse retinal thinning and necrosis can result in atrophic retinal tears and retinal detachment (Figure 8.17). Optic nerve pallor and diffusely constricted vessels are noted in severely affected eyes (Figure 8.17 C, D, G, and H).

8.16 Lightning maculopathy.

A–L: This 44-year-old female lost consciousness after being struck by lightning while jogging. She awoke 4 days later and complained of decreased vision and hearing and suffered burns to her left side and leg. Her vision with pinhole was 20/70– and 20/50+ in the two eyes. She had bilateral central scotoma on the Amsler grid. The right foveola showed a yellowish change and the left eye a vitreous opacity and reddish appearance to the foveola (A–D). There were dark nonfluorescent dots in the fovea of both eyes on the angiogram (E and F). Optical coherence tomography (OCT) of right eye showed increased density of the yellow lesion and the photoreceptors underneath it and small cystic spaces outside the foveola (G). The left eye OCT showed a cystic space (H). The vision in the right eye dropped to 20/100 and the yellow lesion turned more diffuse and granular (I). The OCT now showed dissolution of the foveolar cells and receptors and the residual internal limiting membrane bridging the space (J). The left eye maintained 20/50 visual acuity and the fovea showed a contracted yellow change to its surface with underlying empty cavities left over from loss of cells K and L).

(A–L, courtesy of Dr. David Fintak.)

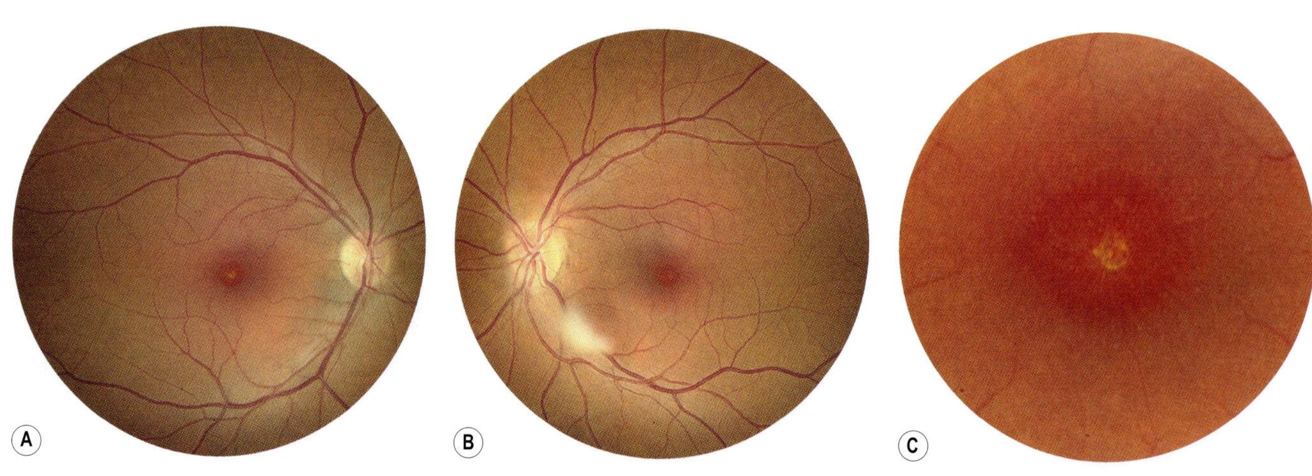

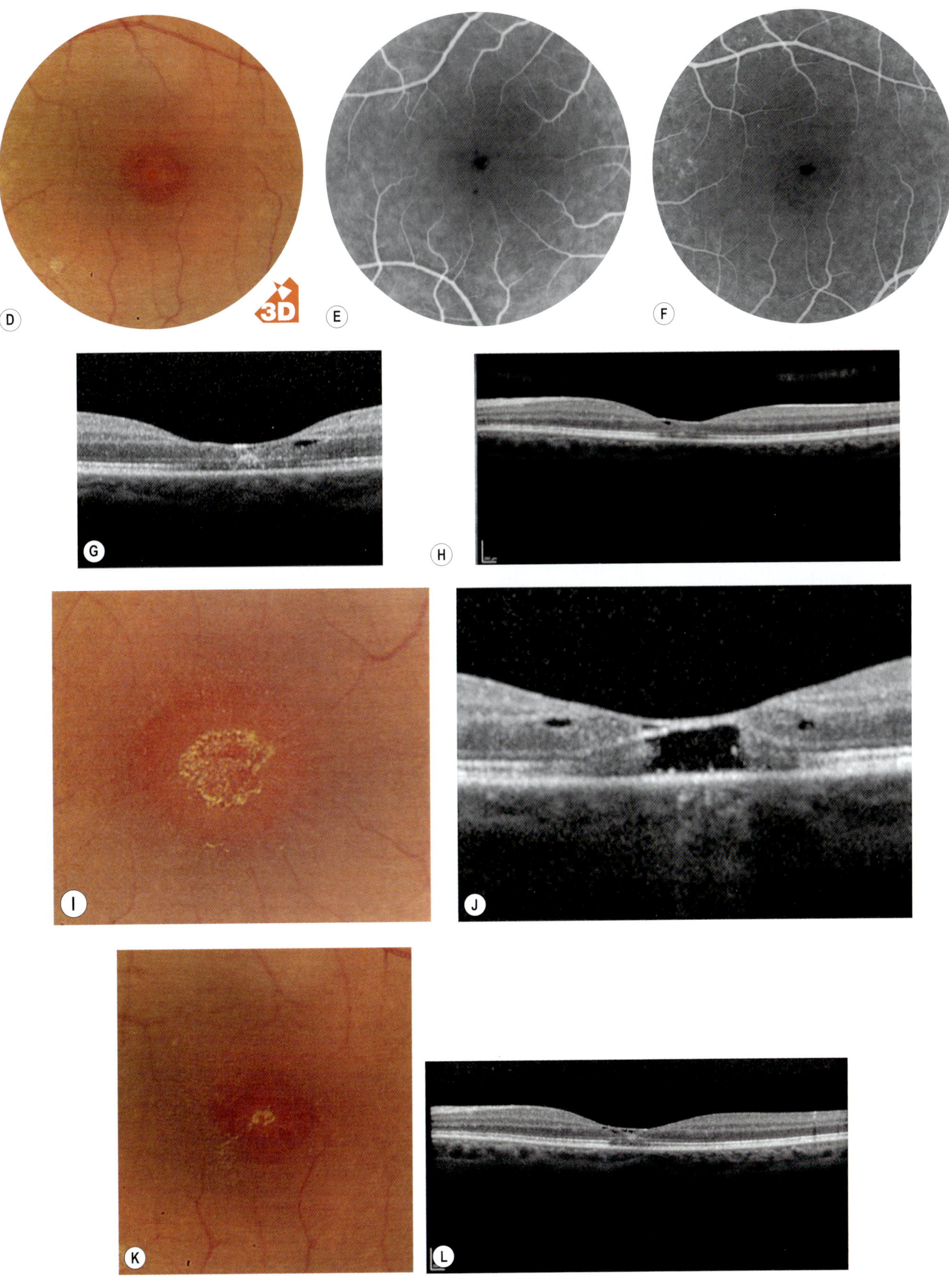
D
3D
E
F
G
H
I
J
K
L

Acute Retinal Damage Caused by Ophthalmic Instruments

The toxic effects of light on the retina in experimental animals have been documented in the case of the indirect ophthalmoscope,[224–227] intraocular fiberoptic light,[170,228] and the operating microscope.[229–236] The visible and infrared wavelengths of light are probably most important in causing instrument-induced retinal damage.[200] Lesions similar to those produced experimentally in animals using the operating microscope and corneal contact lens have been observed in humans following extracapsular cataract extraction with and without intraocular lens implantation.[237–247] On the first and second postoperative days these patients may have a paracentral scotoma associated with an irregularly oval, yellow-white, deep retinal lesion that is most frequently located just above, below, or temporal to the center of the fovea (Figure 8.18A). Because of the frequent use of a bridle stay suture superiorly the lesion has been reported most often just below the center of the macula. The lesion stains intensely with fluorescein (Figure 8.18B). This is replaced over several days and weeks by a zone of fine mottling of the RPE (Figure 8.18C) that is most easily visualized as a focal area of hyperfluorescence angiographically. One case, reported as an example of "pseudophakic serous maculopathy," was probably also caused by phototoxicity.[242] Although in most patients central visual acuity is unaffected, the scotoma may be permanent.[237,248] The retinal xanthophyll may play a role in ameliorating the effects of light damage to the center of the macula.[233,237] The reported incidence of photic maculopathy following extracapsular cataract extraction varies from 7 to 28%.[239,249] The most significant risk factor is the perioperative exposure time to the operating microscope light.[249] A variety of measures may prove effective in reducing chances of photic maculopathy in humans, including reduction of operating time, frequent covering of the cornea, oblique illumination, ultraviolet filters, utilization of an air bubble in the anterior chamber, and insertion of the intraocular lens with the plano surface forward.[230] Retinal burns, however, have occurred in spite of all of these precautions, except the last mentioned.[250]

Retinal lesions identical to those produced experimentally with endoilluminators have occurred during the course of pars plana vitrectomy in humans.[228,251–256] Typically the burns are sharply defined, less than two disc diameters in size, and assume the shape of the light source used: oval if by filament and round if by fiberoptic. Larger more pleomorphic burns, however, may occur. The greatest risk appears to occur during surgical removal of epiretinal membranes and cortical vitreous.[255,256] Reduction of time of exposure, use of low-power source, and avoidance of blue light and high temperature of infusion media are recommended to reduce the risk of a retinal burn.[255] Light damage to the retina may occur in the detached as well as the attached retina.[170]

8.17 Electrocution retinopathy.

A–J: This 41-year-old window installer lost consciousness and fell following electrocution with a live wire. His visual acuity was 20/200 in the right eye and 5/200 in the left eye. He complained of decreased color vision and mild anisocoria. Both lenses showed symmetrical stellate cataracts. Two weeks after onset, the fundus showed pallor of the optic disc and cotton-wool spots inferior to the disc bilaterally (C and D). Angiogram showed foveal thinning on the right and occlusion of small vessels corresponding to the nerve fiber infarcts (E and F). Three months after onset, the cotton-wool spots had resolved (G and H). The optic disc continued to be pale. He developed a retinal detachment in the left eye requiring a vitrectomy and a buckle. His Goldmann visual field showed residual inferior fields in the left eye and a nasal field only in the right eye. Humphrey visual field showed bilateral nasal field defect. Optical coherence tomography at 1 year showed symmetrical severe retinal thinning with progressive cataract in both eyes (I and J). His right eye improved to 20/70. The left eye remained at 20/200. Further history revealed he was cherry picking and moved into a high-tension line, receiving 15 000V electrocution to the shoulder.

(A–J, courtesy of Dr. Michael Goldbaum.)

Histopathologic findings in animals and humans exposed to the operating microscope have shown evidence of photoreceptor and RPE damage in the area of the visible retinal burn.[236,241,257] Animal models have demonstrated that high oxygen tension in the blood is associated with worsening of light damage to the retina[238]; high levels of serum vitamin C, corticosteroids, and dimethylthiourea exert a protective effect.[258–260] Mitochondria are particularly susceptible to light damage, perhaps because they contain cytochromes that absorb the light.[261]

Although the operating microscope light has been suggested as a possible cause for clinically significant cystoid macular edema, there is little evidence to support this idea.[193,225,240,262–264]

Retinal Injury from Laser Exposure

Accidental photocoagulation burns with ruby, argon, neodymium-YAG, and rhodamine dye lasers, femtosecond laser, have been reported.[250,265–274] Fortunately, in most cases good visual function has been retained. Figure 8.18D–F illustrates how a moderately intense solitary laser burn to the center of the fovea is compatible with return of good acuity in spite of destruction of the central photoreceptors.

Ophthalmologists who use operating microscopes or who do laser photocoagulation may have decreased color discrimination for colors in a tritan color confusion axis.[248,275,276] There is a correlation between the years of laser use and the chronic reduction in color contrast sensitivity.

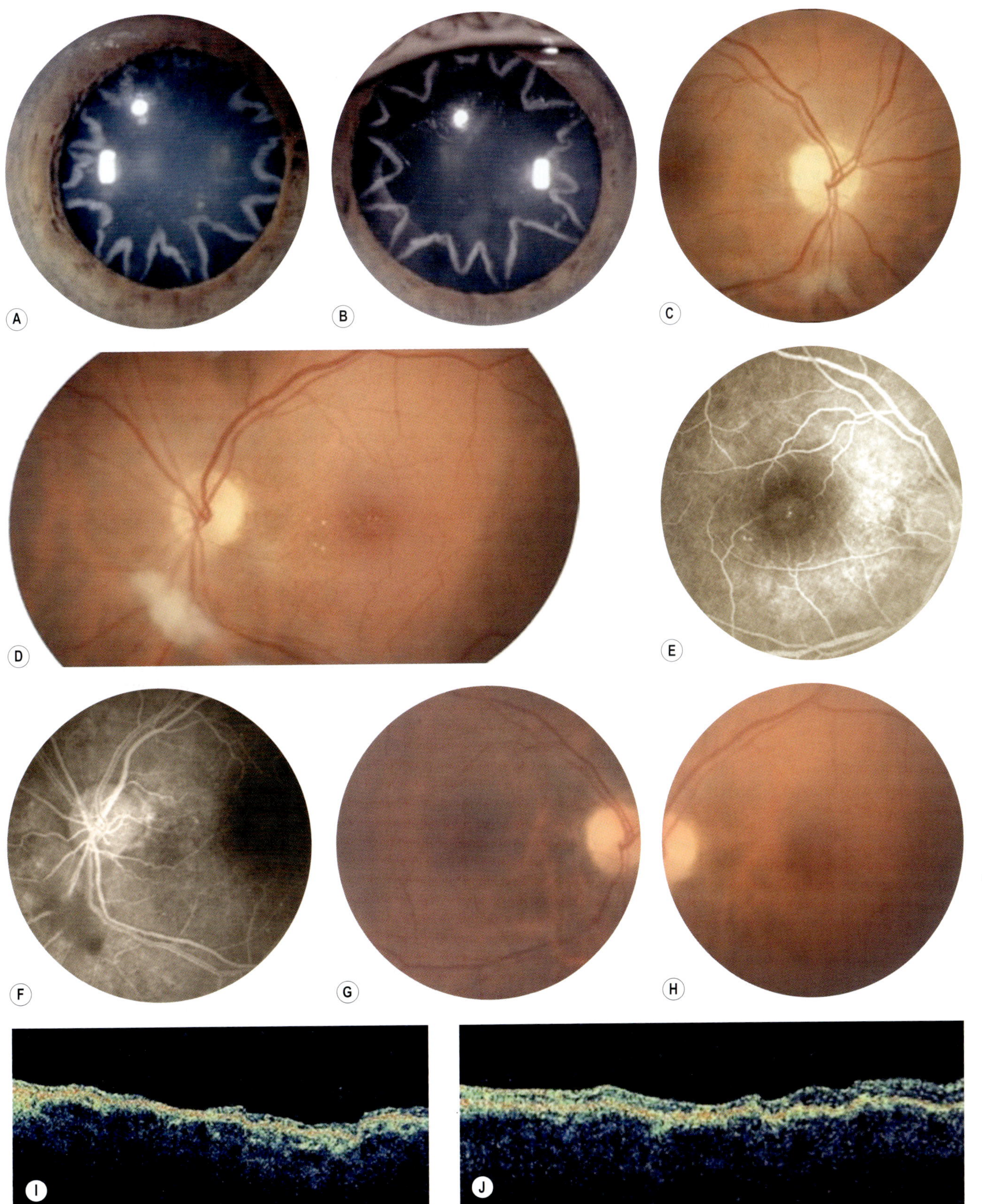
A
B
C
D
E
F
G
H
I
J

Wiebers et al. reported four patients with bilateral high-grade carotid artery stenosis who experienced episodic visual impairment related exclusively to light exposure.[277] They postulated that this may be related to delay in regeneration of visual pigments caused by ischemia.

Accidental macular injury from YAG laser disruption of subhyaloid hemorrhage can occur due to the photodisruptive effect of the YAG laser. A macular hole or cyst is seen due to loss and dissolution of tissue (Figure 8.18G–L). The macular holes can spontaneously close or remain open. Secondary choroidal neovascularization can occur due to breaks in the Bruch's membrane. Visual prognosis after closure of the macular hole is variable and depends on collateral damage to adjacent cells and tissue.[274]

Laser Pointers

Red laser pointers are safer than green laser pointers. Robertson et al. evaluated clinically and histopathologically effects on three eyes with red laser pointers and one with green laser pointer.[278,279] Patients with melanoma scheduled to undergo enucleation were exposed to the laser pointers for 1 minute with foveola fixation, 5 minutes below fixation, and 15 minutes above fixation. The eyes exposed to red laser pointers showed no clinically or angiographically discernible changes. The eye exposed to green laser showed a yellow change at the level of the RPE at 1-minute exposure in the foveal center, and 15 minutes superior to the fovea. OCT showed thickening at the level of the RPE at 24 hours at both locations. Histological examination 20 days after laser exposure showed focal clumping of pigment granules and apical movement of nuclei in some RPE cells. There was some displacement of RPE cells into the subretinal space with minimal changes in the overlying photoreceptors and none in the choriocapillaris. In spite of these histological changes the patient was asymptomatic. The eye that received red laser exposure showed no such change. Overall, transient exposure to laser pointers, either green or red with the normal blink response, evokes minimal risk.[278,279] However children should be warned against playing with laser pointers where they may stare at the laser light for a prolonged period.

Retinal Damage Caused by Chronic Exposure to Sunlight

The effect of long-term exposure to ambient light on the retina is the subject of considerable controversy. There is some evidence to suggest that age-related macular degeneration may be aggravated by the amount of exposure to the visible wavelengths of sunlight but not to ultraviolet light.[280–283]

8.18 Photic maculopathy from microscope light.

A–C: One day after exposure of the right macula of a phakic eye to the operating microscope for a period of 1 hour. The eye was blind because of a craniopharyngioma. Note the gray-white lesion located at the level of the retinal pigment epithelium (RPE) (A) and the intense fluorescein staining of the outer retina (B). Eight days after the exposure there was mottling of the RPE in the area of the lesion (C).

D–F: Acute ruby laser burn in the center of the fovea of a man with a ciliary body melanoma. Visual acuity before the burn was 20/20 and the fundus was normal (D). Five minutes after a moderately intense one-degree burn that generated a small steam bubble, there was a central gray foveal opacity (E). The visual acuity was 20/70. Two weeks later the acuity had returned to 20/25 at the time of enucleation. (F) Partial destruction of the central foveal area.

Laser induced foveal burn.

G–L: A 42-year-old man was seen with complaints of decreased vision in his right eye of 1 month's duration. He had suffered a vitreous hemorrhage following head injury 2 months previously. On recovering consciousness, the treating ophthalmologist performed laser photocoagulation of the posterior hyaloid for premacular hemorrhage. On examination, his best-corrected visual acuity was 20/200. Fundoscopy of the right eye (G) showed a central macular hole (arrowhead) with demarcation lines extending temporally (arrows). The hole was better appreciated on optical coherence tomography imaging (H). Fluorescein angiography (I and J) showed transmission hyperfluorescence in the center (arrowhead) with prominent demarcation lines (arrows). Raster line scan (K) passing through the foveal center showed elevated internal limiting membrane (ILM) (arrows) corresponding to the demarcation lines seen temporally, indicating that the patient might have had Terson's syndrome following head injury. The foveal center shows an outer macular hole (arrowhead) that most likely resulted from the laser disruption attempted by the treating physician to drain sub-ILM blood. Overlay RPE-fit scan (L) shows the hole.

(A–C, From Robertson and Feldman[245] published with permission from the American Journal of Ophthalmology; copyright Ophthalmic Publishing Co.; G–L, courtesy of Dr. Vishali Gupta and Dr. Amod Gupta.)

Specific Circumstances Resulting in Chorioretinal Trauma

- Recreational: firework, paint ball, fishing hook and louvre, golf club and golf ball (more often club than ball), baseball, soft ball, hockey puck, basketball, BB gun pellet
- Occupational: intraocular foreign body, explosives, improvised explosive devices, war injuries, blast injury, electrical/welding arc
- Domestic: bungee cord, air bag, pencil, scissors, dog bites
- Homicidal: gunshot, knife, bottle, fist.

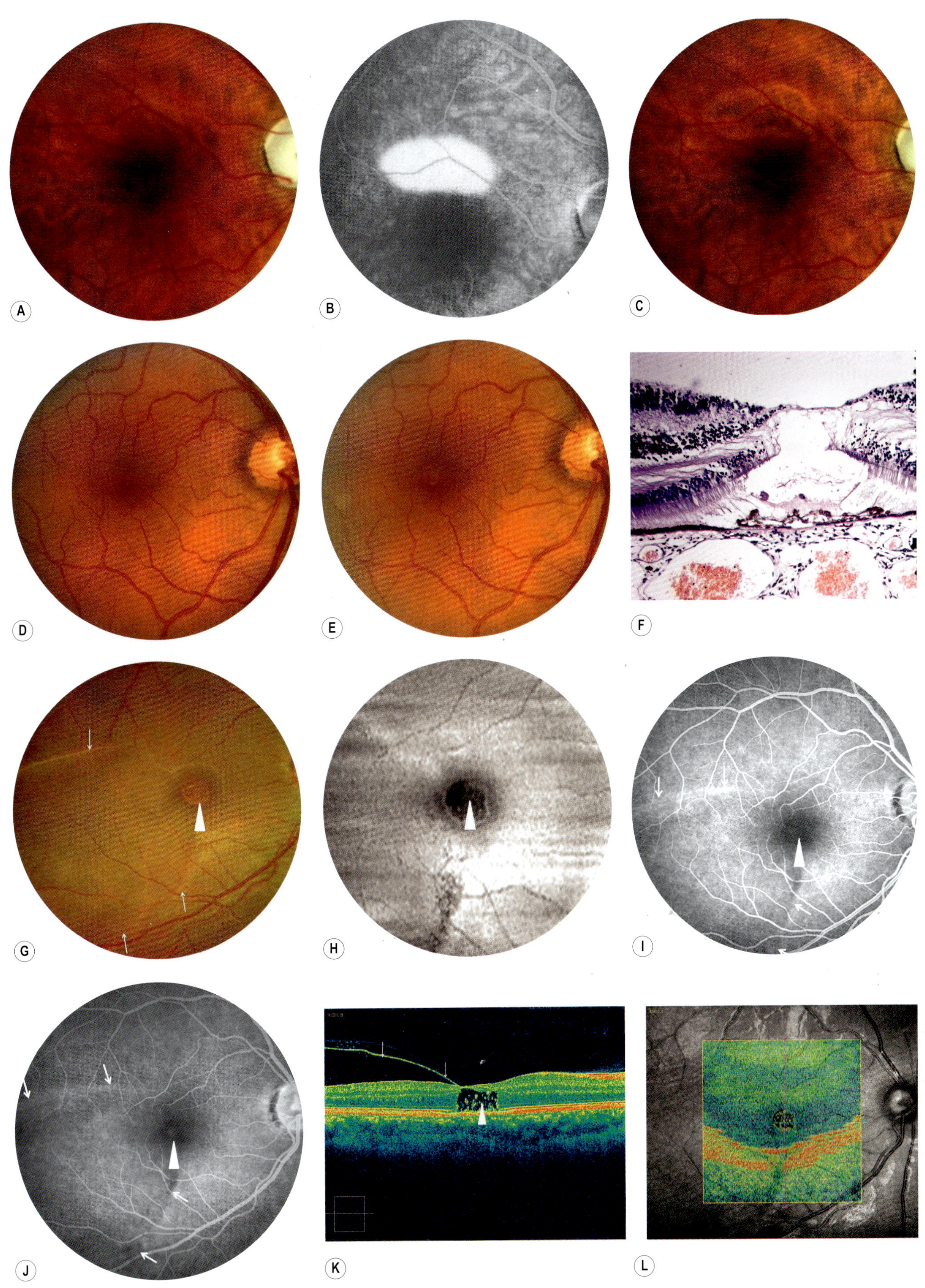
A
B
C
D
E
F
G
H
I
J
K
L

References

1. Berlin R. Zur sogenannten Commotio retinae. Klin Monatsbl Augenheilkd 1873;11:42–78.
2. Blight R, Hart JCD. Structural changes in the outer retinal layers following blunt mechanical non-perforating trauma to the globe: an experimental study. Br J Ophthalmol 1977;61:573–87.
3. Gass JDM. Stereoscopic atlas of macular diseases; diagnosis and treatment, 2nd ed. St. Louis: CV Mosby; 1977. p. 314.
4. Sipperley JO, Quigley HA, Gass JDM. Traumatic retinopathy in primates; the explanation of commotio retinae. Arch Ophthalmol 1978;96:2267–73.
5. Williams DF, Mieler WF, Williams GA. Posterior segment manifestations of ocular trauma. Retina 1990;10:S35–44.
6. Bastek JV, Foos RY, Heckenlively J. Traumatic pigmentary retinopathy. Am J Ophthalmol 1981;92:621–4.
7. Cogan DG. Pseudoretinitis pigmentosa; report of two traumatic cases of recent origin. Arch Ophthalmol 1969;81:45–53.
8. Kohno T, Ishibashi T, Inomata H, et al. Experimental macular edema of commotio retinae: preliminary report. Jpn J Ophthalmol 1983;27:149–56.
9. Hart JCD, Frank HJ. Retinal opacification after blunt non-perforating concussional injuries to the globe; a clinical and retinal fluorescein angiographic study. Trans Ophthalmol Soc UK 1975;95:94–100.
10. Beckingsale AB, Rosenthal AR. Early fundus fluorescein angiographic findings and sequelae in traumatic retinopathy: case report. Br J Ophthalmol 1983;67:119–23.
11. Pulido JS, Blair NP. The blood–retinal barrier in Berlin's edema. Retina 1987;7:233–6.
12. Seider M, Lujan BJ, Gregori G, et al. Ultra-high resolution spectral domain optical coherence tomography of traumatic maculopathy. Ophthalmic Surg Lasers Imaging 2009;40:516–21.
13. Sony P, Venkatesh P, Gadaginamath S, et al. Optical coherence tomography findings in commotio retina. Clin Experiment Ophthalmol 2006;34:621–3.
14. Lai TY, Yip WW, Wong VW, et al. Multifocal electroretinogram and optical coherence tomography of commotio retinae and traumatic macular hole. Eye 2005;19:219–21.
15. Carpineto P, Ciancaglini M, Aharrh-Gnama A, et al. Optical coherence tomography and fundus microperimetry imaging of spontaneous closure of traumatic macular hole: a case report. Eur J Ophthalmol 2005;15:165–9.
16. Mansour AM, Green WR, Hogge C. Histopathology of commotio retinae. Retina 1992;12:24–8.
17. Bunt-Milam AH, Black RA, Bensinger RE. Breakdown of the outer blood–retinal barrier in experimental commotio retinae. Exp Eye Res 1986;43:397–412.
18. Levin LA, Seddon JM, Topping T. Retinal pigment epithelial tears associated with trauma. Am J Ophthalmol 1991;112:396–400.
19. Beyrer CR. Traumatic serous detachments of the retinal pigment epithelium. Ann Ophthalmol 1978;10:51–4.
20. Collier M. La chorio-retinopathie post-traumatique de Hutchinson-Siegrist. Ann Oculist 1973;206:193–220.
21. Friberg TR. Traumatic retinal pigment epithelial edema. Am J Ophthalmol 1979;88:18–21.
22. Gass JDM. Stereoscopic atlas of macular diseases; a fundoscopic and angiographic presentation. St. Louis: CV Mosby; 1970. p. 94.
23. Gitter KA, Slusher M, Justice Jr J. Traumatic hemorrhagic detachment of retinal pigment epithelium. Arch Ophthalmol 1968;79:729–32.
24. Gross JG, Freeman WR. Post-traumatic yellow maculopathy. Retina 1990;10:37–41.
25. Hart JCD, Natsikos VE, Raistrick ER, et al. Indirect choroidal tears at the posterior pole: a fluorescein angiographic and perimetric study. Br J Ophthalmol 1980;64:59–67.
26. Lewis RA, Donaldson DD. Traumatic retinal hemorrhage. Arch Ophthalmol 1973;90:502–3.
27. Rimmer S, Shuler JD. Severe ocular trauma from a driver's-side air bag. Arch Ophthalmol 1991;109:774.
28. von Graefe A. Zwei Fälle von Ruptur der Chorioidea. Albrecht von Graefes Arch Ophthalmol 1854;1:402–3.
29. Levin LA, Seddon JM, Topping T. Retinal pigment epithelial tears associated with trauma. Am J Ophthalmol 1991;112:396–400.
30. Sipperley JO, Quigley HA, Gass JDM. Traumatic retinopathy in primates; the explanation of commotio retinae. Arch Ophthalmol 1978;96:2267–73.
31. Hart CD, Raistrick R. Indirect choroidal tears and late onset serosanguinous maculopathies. Graefes Arch Clin Exp Ophthalmol 1982;218:206–10.
32. Levin DB, Bell DK. Traumatic retinal hemorrhages with angioid streaks. Arch Ophthalmol 1977;95:1072–3.
33. Aguilar JP, Green WR. Choroidal rupture; a histopathologic study of 47 cases. Retina 1984;4:269–75.
34. Maberley AL, Carvounis EP. The visual field in indirect traumatic rupture of the choroid. Can J Ophthalmol 1977;12:147–52.
35. Fuller B, Gitter KA. Traumatic choroidal rupture with late serous detachment of macula; report of successful argon laser treatment. Arch Ophthalmol 1973;89:354–5.
36. Gass JDM. Pathogenesis of disciform detachment of the neuroepithelium. VI. Disciform detachment secondary to heredodegenerative, neoplastic and traumatic lesions of the choroid. Am J Ophthalmol 1967;63:689–711.
37. Hilton GF. Late serosanguineous detachment of the macula after traumatic choroidal rupture. Am J Ophthalmol 1975;79:997–1000.
38. Pearlstone AD. Delayed loss of central vision following multiple posterior segment trauma. Ann Ophthalmol 1980;12:409–11.
39. Wood CM, Richardson J. Indirect choroidal ruptures: aetiological factors, patterns of ocular damage, and final visual outcome. Br J Ophthalmol 1990;74:208–11.
40. Zografos L, Chamero J. Evolution au long cours des ruptures indirectes traumatiques de la choroïde. J Fr Ophtalmol 1990;13:269–75.
41. Weidenthal DT. Choroidal neovascularization (CNV) arising from drainage site after scleral buckling surgery. In: Fine SL, Owens SL, editors. Management of retinal vascular and macular disorders. Baltimore: Williams & Wilkins; 1983. p. 199–207.
42. Anshu A, Chee SP. Diffuse unilateral subacute neuroretinitis. Int Ophthalmol 2008;28:127–9.
43. Aiello LP, Arrigg PG, Shah ST, et al. Solar retinopathy associated with hypoglycemic insulin reaction. Arch Ophthalmol 1994;112:982–3.
44. Goldzieher W. Beiträg zur Pathologie der orbitalen Schussverletzungen. Z Augenheilkd 1901;6:277–85.
45. Martin DF, Awh CC, McCuen II BW, et al. Treatment and pathogenesis of traumatic chorioretinal rupture (sclopetaria). Am J Ophthalmol 1994;117:190–200.
46. Perry HD, Rahn EK. Chorioretinitis sclopetaria; choroidal and retinal concussion injury from a bullet. Arch Ophthalmol 1977;95:328–9.
47. Grosso A, Panico C. Surgical management of sclopetaria associated with macular hole in a young patient: long term results. Eye 2009;23:1875–6.
48. Dubovy SR, Guyton DL, Green WR. Clinicopathologic correlation of chorioretinitis sclopetaria. Retina 1997;17:510–20.
49. Ahmadabadi MN, Karkhaneh R, Roohipoor R, et al. Clinical presentation and outcome of chorioretinitis sclopetaria: a case series study. Injury 2010;41:82–5.
50. Martin DF, Awh CC, McCuen II BW, et al. Treatment and pathogenesis of traumatic chorioretinal rupture (sclopetaria). Am J Ophthalmol 1994;117:190–200.
51. Daily L. Macular and vitreal disturbances produced by traumatic vitreous rebound. South Med J 1970;63:1197–8.
52. Grey RHB. Foveo-macular retinitis, solar retinopathy, and trauma. Br J Ophthalmol 1978;62:543–6.
53. Kelly JS, Hoover RE, George T. Whiplash maculopathy. Arch Ophthalmol 1978;96:834–5.
54. Burke JP, Orton HP, West J, et al. Whiplash and its effect on the visual system. Graefes Arch Clin Exp Ophthalmol 1992;230:335–9.
55. Daily L. Further observations on foveolar splinter and macular wisps. Arch Ophthalmol 1973;90:102–3.
56. Mitamura Y, Saito W, Ishida M, et al. Spontaneous closure of traumatic macular hole. Retina 2001;21:385–9.
57. Arevalo JF. Posterior segment complications after laser-assisted in situ keratomileusis. Curr Opin Ophthalmol 2008;19:177–84.
58. Yamada H, Sakai A, Yamada E, et al. Spontaneous closure of traumatic macular hole. Am J Ophthalmol 2002;134:340–7.
59. Yeshurun I, Guerrero-Naranjo JL, Quiroz-Mercado H. Spontaneous closure of a large traumatic macular hole in a young patient. Am J Ophthalmol 2002;134:602–3.
60. Lange AP, Vandekerckhove K, Becht C, et al. Spontaneous closure of a traumatic macular hole. Klin Monatsbl Augenheilkd 2009;226:359–60.
61. Valmaggia C, Pfenninger L, Haueter I. Spontaneous closure of a traumatic macular hole. Klin Monatsbl Augenheilkd 2009;226:361–2.
62. Amari F, Ogino N, Matsumura M, et al. Vitreous surgery for traumatic macular holes. Retina 1999;19:410–3.
63. Hwang YS, Lai CC, Yang KJ, et al. A rapid and successful treatment for airbag-related traumatic macular hole. Chang Gung Med J 2001;24:530–5.
64. Chen YP, Chen TL, Chao AN, et al. Surgical management of traumatic macular hole-related retinal detachment. Am J Ophthalmol 2005;140:331–3.
65. Burton TC. Unilateral Purtscher's retinopathy. Ophthalmology 1980;87:1096–105.
66. Gass JDM. Stereoscopic atlas of macular diseases; diagnosis and treatment, 2nd ed. St. Louis: CV Mosby; 1977. p. 185.
67. Jacob HS, Craddock PR, Hammerschmidt DE, et al. Complement-induced granulocyte aggregation; an unsuspected mechanism of disease. N Engl J Med 1980;302:789–94.
68. Kelley JS. Purtscher's retinopathy related to chest compression by safety belts; fluorescein angiographic findings. Am J Ophthalmol 1972;74:278–83.
69. Madsen PH. Traumatic retinal angiopathy (Purtscher). Ophthalmologica 1972;165:453–8.
70. Marr WG, Marr EG. Some observations on Purtscher's disease: traumatic retinal angiopathy. Am J Ophthalmol 1962;54:693–705.
71. Pratt MV, de Venecia G. Purtscher's retinopathy: a clinicohistopathological correlation. Surv Ophthalmol 1970;14:417–23.
72. Purtscher O. Angiopathia retinae traumatica. Lymphorrhagien des Augengrundes. Albrecht von Graefes Arch Ophthalmol 1912;82:347–71.
73. Urbanek J. Fettembolie des Auges. Albrecht von Graefes Arch Ophthalmol 1934;131:147–73.
74. Henkind P. Radial peripapillary capillaries of the retina. I. Anatomy: human and comparative. Br J Ophthalmol 1967;51:115–23.
75. Agrawal A, McKibbin MA. Purtscher's and Purtscher-like retinopathies: a review. Surv Ophthalmol 2006;51:129–36.
76. Khan SG, Frenkel M. Intravitreal hemorrhage associated with rapid increase in intracranial pressure (Terson's syndrome). Am J Ophthalmol 1975;80:37–43.
77. Terson A. De l'hémorrhagie dans le corps vitré au cours de l'hémorrhagie cérébrale. Clin Ophtalmol 1900;6:309.
78. Terson A. Le syndrome de l'hématome du corps vitré et de l'hémorrhagie intracranienne spontanés. Ann Oculist 1926;163:666–73.
79. Shaw Jr HE, Landers III MB, Sydnor CF. The significance of intraocular hemorrhages due to subarachnoid hemorrhage. Ann Ophthalmol 1977;9:1403–5.
80. Walsh FB, Hoyt WF. Clinical neuro-ophthalmology, 3rd ed. Baltimore: Williams & Wilkins; 1969. p. 1786.
81. Morris DA, Henkind P. Relationship of intracranial optic-nerve sheath and retinal hemorrhage. Am J Ophthalmol 1967;64:853–9.
82. Weingeist TA, Goldman EJ, Folk JC, et al. Terson's syndrome; clinicopathologic correlations. Ophthalmology 1986;93:1435–42.
83. Castrén JA. Pathogeneses and treatment of Terson-syndrome. Acta Ophthalmol 1963;41:430–4.
84. Clarkson JG, Flynn Jr HW, Daily MJ. Vitrectomy in Terson's syndrome. Am J Ophthalmol 1980;90:549–52.
85. Shaw Jr HE, Landers III MB. Vitreous hemorrhage after intracranial hemorrhage. Am J Ophthalmol 1975;80:207–13.

86. Garfinkle AM, Danys IR, Nicolle DA, et al. Terson's syndrome; a reversible cause of blindness following subarachnoid hemorrhage. J Neurosurg 1992;76:766–71.
87. Keithahn MAZ, Bennett SR, Cameron D, et al. Retinal folds in Terson syndrome. Ophthalmology 1993;100:1187–90.
88. Schultz PN, Sobol WM, Weingeist TA. Long-term visual outcome in Terson syndrome. Ophthalmology 1991;98:1814–9.
89. Velikay M, Datlinger P, Stolba U, et al. Retinal detachment with severe proliferative vitreoretinopathy in Terson syndrome. Ophthalmology 1994;101:35–7.
90. Boogaarts H, Grotenhuis A. Terson's syndrome after endoscopic colloid cyst removal: case report and a review of reported complications. Minim Invasive Neurosurg 2008;51:303–5.
91. Inoue T, Tsutsumi K, Shigeeda T. Terson's syndrome as the initial symptom of subarachnoid hemorrhage caused by ruptured vertebral artery aneurysm. Case report. Neurol Med Chir (Tokyo) 2006;46:344–7.
92. Choudhari KA, Pherwani AA, Gray WJ. Terson's syndrome as the sole presentation of aneurysmal rupture. Br J Neurosurg 2003;17:355–7.
93. Gibran S, Mirza K, Kinsella F. Unilateral vitreous haemorrhage secondary to caudal epidural injection: a variant of Terson's syndrome. Br J Ophthalmol 2002;86:353–4.
94. Naseri A, Blumenkranz MS, Horton JC. Terson's syndrome following epidural saline injection. Neurology 2001;57:364.
95. Schloff S, Mullaney PB, Armstrong DC, et al. Retinal findings in children with intracranial hemorrhage. Ophthalmology 2002;109:1472–6.
96. Oberman J, Cohn H, Grand MG. Retinal complications of gas myelography. Arch Ophthalmol 1979;97:1905–6.
97. Kushner FH, Olson JC. Retinal hemorrhage as a consequence of epidural steroid injection. Arch Ophthalmol 1995;113:309–13.
98. Ling C, Atkinson PL, Munton CGF. Bilateral retinal haemorrhages following epidural injection. Br J Ophthalmol 1993;77:316–7.
99. Budenz DL, Farber MG, Mirchandani HG, et al. Ocular and optic nerve hemorrhages in abused infants with intracranial injuries. Ophthalmology 1994;101:559–65.
100. Buys YM, Levin AV, Enzenauer RW, et al. Retinal findings after head trauma in infants and young children. Ophthalmology 1992;99:1718–23.
101. Elner SG, Elner VM, Arnall M, et al. Ocular and associated systemic findings in suspected child abuse; a necropsy study. Arch Ophthalmol 1990;108:1094–101.
102. Friendly DS. Ocular manifestations of physical child abuse. Trans Am Acad Ophthalmol Otolaryngol 1971;75:318–32.
103. Gilkes MJ, Mann TP. Fundi of battered babies. Lancet 1967;2:468–9.
104. Greenwald MJ, Weiss A, Oesterle CS, et al. Traumatic retinoschisis in battered babies. Ophthalmology 1986;93:618–25.
105. Han DP, Wilkinson WS. Late ophthalmic manifestations of the shaken baby syndrome. J Pediatr Ophthalmol Strabismus 1990;27:299–303.
106. Harley RD. Ocular manifestations of child abuse. J Pediatr Ophthalmol Strabismus 1980;17:5–13.
107. Jensen AD, Smith RE, Olson MI. Ocular clues to child abuse. J Pediatr Ophthalmol 1971;8:270–2.
108. Ober RR. Hemorrhagic retinopathy in infancy: a clinicopathologic report. J Pediatr Ophthalmol Strabismus 1980;17:17–20.
109. San Martin R, Steinkuller PG, Nisbet RM. Retinopathy in the sexually abused battered child. Ann Ophthalmol 1981;13:89–91.
110. Spaide RF. Shaken baby syndrome; ocular and computed tomographic findings. J Clin Neuro-Ophthalmol 1987;7:108–11.
111. Tongue AC. Editorial: The ophthalmologist's role in diagnosing child abuse. Ophthalmology 1991;98:1009–10.
112. Garcia CA, Gomes AH, Vianna RN, et al. Late-stage diffuse unilateral subacute neuroretinitis: photocoagulation of the worm does not improve the visual acuity of affected patients. Int Ophthalmol 2005;26:39–42.
113. Vedantham V, Vats MM, Kakade SJ, et al. Diffuse unilateral subacute neuroretinitis with unusual findings. Am J Ophthalmol 2006;142:880–3.
114. Gaynon MW, Koh K, Marmor MF, et al. Retinal folds in the shaken baby syndrome. Am J Ophthalmol 1988;106:423–5.
115. Massicotte SJ, Folberg R, Torczynski E, et al. Vitreoretinal traction and perimacular retinal folds in the eyes of deliberately traumatized children. Ophthalmology 1991;98:1124–7.
116. Ludwig S, Warman M. Shaken baby syndrome: a review of 20 cases. Ann Emerg Med 1984;13:104–7.
117. Lambert SR, Johnson TE, Hoyt CS. Optic nerve sheath and retinal hemorrhages associated with the shaken baby syndrome. Arch Ophthalmol 1986;104:1509–12.
118. Riffenburgh RS, Sathyavagiswaran L. Ocular findings at autopsy of child abuse victims. Ophthalmology 1991;98:1519–24.
119. Wilkinson WS, Han DP, Rappley MD, et al. Retinal hemorrhage predicts neurologic injury in the shaken baby syndrome. Arch Ophthalmol 1989;107:1472–4.
120. Duane TD. Valsalva hemorrhagic retinopathy. Am J Ophthalmol 1973;75:637–42.
121. Gass JDM. Options in the treatment of macular diseases. Trans Ophthalmol Soc UK 1972;92:449–68.
122. Gass JDM. Stereoscopic atlas of macular diseases; diagnosis and treatment, 2nd ed. St. Louis: CV Mosby; 1977. p. 320.
123. Kassoff A, Catalano RA, Mehu M. Vitreous hemorrhage and the Valsalva maneuver in proliferative diabetic retinopathy. Retina 1988;8:174–6.
124. Linde R, Record R, Ferguson J. Resolution of preretinal hemorrhage. Arch Ophthalmol 1977;95:1466–7.
125. de Crecchio G, Pacente L, Alfieri MC, et al. Valsalva retinopathy associated with a congenital retinal macrovessel. Arch Ophthalmol 2000;118:146–7.
126. Cortez R, Denny JP, Muci-Mendoza R, et al. Diffuse unilateral subacute neuroretinitis in Venezuela. Ophthalmology 2005;112:2110–4.
127. Perez-Rico C, Montes-Mollon A, Castro-Rebollo M, et al. Optical coherence tomography features of sub-internal limiting membrane hemorrhage and temporary premacular cavity following Nd-YAG laser membranotomy in Valsalva retinopathy. Jpn J Ophthalmol 2008;52:513–5.
128. Gabel V-P, Birngruber R, Gunther-Koszka H, et al. Nd:YAG laser photodisruption of hemorrhagic detachment of the internal limiting membrane. Am J Ophthalmol 1989;107:33–7.
129. Sahu DK, Namperumalsamy P, Kim R, et al. Argon laser treatment for premacular hemorrhage. Retina 1998;18:79–82.
130. Chen HP, Kuo HK, Tsai SH, et al. Acute retinal necrosis syndrome: clinical manifestations and visual outcomes. Chang Gung Med J 2004;27:193–200.
131. Pitta CG, Steinert RF, Gragoudas ES, et al. Small unilateral foveal hemorrhages in young adults. Am J Ophthalmol 1980;89:96–102.
132. Pruett RC, Carvalho ACA, Trempe CL. Microhemorrhagic maculopathy. Arch Ophthalmol 1981;99:425–32.
133. Kalina RE, Kaiser M. Familial retinal hemorrhages. Am J Ophthalmol 1972;74:252–5.
134. Archer DB, Canavan YM. Contusional injuries of the distal optic nerve. Trans Ophthalmol Soc NZ 1983;35:14–23.
135. Chang M, Eifrig DE. Optic nerve avulsion. Arch Ophthalmol 1987;105:322–3.
136. Park JH, Frenkel M, Dobbie JG, et al. Evulsion of the optic nerve. Am J Ophthalmol 1971;72:969–71.
137. Salzmann M. Die Ausreissung des Sehnerven (Evulsio nervi optici). Z Augenheilkd 1903;9: 489–505.
138. Williams DF, Williams GA, Abrams GW, et al. Evulsion of the retina associated with optic nerve evulsion. Am J Ophthalmol 1987;104:5–9.
139. Fechtner RD, Minckler D, Weinreb RN, et al. Complications of glaucoma surgery; ocular decompression retinopathy. Arch Ophthalmol 1992;110:965–8.
140. Nonoyama S, Tanito M, Katsube T, et al. Decompression retinopathy and serous retinal detachment after trabeculotomy in a patient with systemic amyloidosis. Jpn J Ophthalmol 2009;53:73–5.
141. Bansal A, Ramanathan US. Ocular decompression retinopathy after trabeculectomy with mitomycin-C for angle recession glaucoma. Indian J Ophthalmol 2009;57:153–4.
142. Arevalo JF, Mendoza AJ, Millan FA, et al. Simultaneous bilateral ocular decompression retinopathy after trabeculectomy with mitomycin C for uveitic glaucoma. Graefes Arch Clin Exp Ophthalmol 2008;246:471–3.
143. Wakita M, Kawaji T, Ando E, et al. Ocular decompression retinopathy following trabeculectomy with mitomycin C associated with familial amyloidotic polyneuropathy. Br J Ophthalmol 2006;90:515–6.
144. Bui CM, Recchia FM, Recchia CC, et al. Optical coherence tomography findings in ocular decompression retinopathy. Ophthalmic Surg Lasers Imaging 2006;37:333–5.
145. Nah G, Aung T, Yip CC. Ocular decompression retinopathy after resolution of acute primary angle closure glaucoma. Clin Experiment Ophthalmol 2000;28:319–20.
146. Danias J, Rosenbaum J, Podos SM. Diffuse retinal hemorrhages (ocular decompression syndrome) after trabeculectomy with mitomycin C for neovascular glaucoma. Acta Ophthalmol Scand 2000;78:468–9.
147. Suzuki R, Nakayama M, Satoh N. Three types of retinal bleeding as a complication of hypotony after trabeculectomy. Ophthalmologica 1999;213:135–8.
148. Ferry AP. Lesions mistaken for malignant melanoma of the posterior uvea; a clinicopathologic analysis of 100 cases with ophthalmoscopically visible lesions. Arch Ophthalmol 1964;72: 463–9.
149. Lipper S, Eifrig DE, Peiffer RL, et al. Chorioretinal foreign body simulating malignant melanoma. Am J Ophthalmol 1981;92:202–5.
150. Rones B, Zimmerman LE. An unusual choroidal hemorrhage simulating malignant melanoma. Arch Ophthalmol 1963;70:30–2.
151. Bego B, Turut P, Malthieu D, et al. Neo-vaisseaux sous-retiniens après plaie chorio-retinienne par corps étranger intra-oculaire (1 cas). Bull Soc Ophtalmol Fr 1989;89:263–5.
152. Duker JS, Belmont JB, Benson WE, et al. Inadvertent globe perforation during retrobulbar and peribulbar anesthesia; patient characteristics, surgical management, and visual outcome. Ophthalmology 1991;98:519–26.
153. Grizzard WS, Kirk NM, Pavan PR, et al. Perforating ocular injuries caused by anesthesia personnel. Ophthalmology 1991;98:1011–6.
154. Hay A, Flynn Jr HW, Hoffman JI, et al. Needle penetration of the globe during retrobulbar and peribulbar injections. Ophthalmology 1991;98:1017–24.
155. Hersch M, Baer G, Dieckert JP, et al. Optic nerve enlargement and central retinal-artery occlusion secondary to retrobulbar anesthesia. Ann Ophthalmol 1989;21:195–7.
156. Martin DF, Meredith TA, Topping TM, et al. Perforating (through-and-through) injuries of the globe; surgical results with vitrectomy. Arch Ophthalmol 1991;109:951–6.
157. Mieler WF, Bennett SR, Platt LW, et al. Localized retinal detachment with combined central retinal artery and vein occlusion after retrobulbar anesthesia. Retina 1990;10:278–83.
158. Morgan CM, Schatz H, Vine AK, et al. Ocular complications associated with retrobulbar injections. Ophthalmology 1988;95:660–5.
159. Schneider ME, Milstein DE, Oyakawa RT, et al. Ocular perforation from a retrobulbar injection. Am J Ophthalmol 1988;106:35–40.
160. Klein ML, Jampol LM, Condon PI, et al. Central retinal artery occlusion without retrobulbar hemorrhage after retrobulbar anesthesia. Am J Ophthalmol 1982;93:573–7.
161. Ahn JC, Stanley JA. Subarachnoid injection as a complication of retrobulbar anesthesia. Am J Ophthalmol 1987;103:225–30.
162. Brookshire GL, Gleitsmann KY, Schenk EC. Life-threatening complication of retrobulbar block; a hypothesis. Ophthalmology 1986;93:1476–8.
163. Cohen SM, Sousa FJ, Kelly NE, et al. Respiratory arrest and new retinal hemorrhages after retrobulbar anesthesia. Am J Ophthalmol 1992;113:209–11.
164. Friedberg HL, Kline Jr OR. Contralateral amaurosis after retrobulbar injection. Am J Ophthalmol 1986;101:688–90.

165. Javitt JC, Addiego R, Friedberg HL, et al. Brain stem anesthesia after retrobulbar block. Ophthalmology 1987;94:718–24.
166. Lee DS, Kwon NJ. Shivering following retrobulbar block. Can J Anaesth 1988;35:294–6.
167. Pautler SE, Grizzard WS, Thompson LN, et al. From retrobulbar injection into the optic nerve. Ophthalmic Surg 1986;17:334–7.
168. Katsev DA, Drews RC, Rose BT. An anatomic study of retrobulbar needle length. Ophthalmology 1989;96:1221–4.
169. Agarwal LP, Malik SRK. Solar retinitis. Br J Ophthalmol 1959;43:366–70.
170. Zilis JD, Machemer R. Light damage in detached retina. Am J Ophthalmol 1991;111:47–50.
171. Cordes FC. Eclipse retinitis. Am J Ophthalmol 1948;31:101–3.
172. Penner R, McNair JN. Eclipse blindness; report of an epidemic in the military population of Hawaii. Am J Ophthalmol 1966;61:1452–7.
173. Marlor RL, Blais BR, Preston FR, et al. Foveomacular retinitis, an important problem in military medicine: Epidemiology. Invest Ophthalmol 1973;12:5–16.
174. Gladstone GJ, Tasman W. Solar retinitis after minimal exposure. Arch Ophthalmol 1978;96:1368–9.
175. Ewald RA, Ritchey CL. Sun gazing as the cause of foveomacular retinitis. Am J Ophthalmol 1970;70:491–7.
176. Freedman J, Gombos GM. Fluorescein fundus angiography in self-induced solar retinopathy; a case report. Can J Ophthalmol 1971;6:124–7.
177. Anaclerio AM, Wicker HS. Self-induced solar retinopathy by patients in a psychiatric hospital. Am J Ophthalmol 1970;69:731–6.
178. Cangelosi GC, Newsome DA. Solar retinopathy in persons on religious pilgrimage. Am J Ophthalmol 1988;105:95–7.
179. Hope-Ross MTS, Mooney D. Solar retinopathy following religious rituals. Br J Ophthalmol 1988;72:931–4.
180. Ewald RA. Sun gazing associated with the use of LSD. Ann Ophthalmol 1971;3:15–17.
181. Fuller DG. Solar maculopathy associated with the use of lysergic acid diethylamide (LSD). Am J Ophthalmol 1976;81:413–6.
182. Schatz H, Mendelblatt F. Solar retinopathy from sun-gazing under the influence of LSD. Br J Ophthalmol 1973;57:270–3.
183. Cialdini AP, Jalkh AE, Tolentino FI. Acute foveal outer retinopathy. Arch Ophthalmol 1987;105:1490.
184. Gass JDM. Stereoscopic atlas of macular diseases; diagnosis and treatment, 2nd ed. St. Louis: CV Mosby; 1977. p. 322.
185. Hope-Ross MW, Mahon GJ, Gardiner TA, et al. Ultrastructural findings in solar retinopathy. Eye 1993;7:29–33.
186. Yannuzzi LA, Fisher YL, Slakter JS, et al. Solar retinopathy; a photobiologic and geophysical analysis. Retina 1989;9:28–43.
187. Ham Jr WT, Mueller HA, Ruffolo Jr JJ, et al. Action spectrum for retinal injury from near-ultraviolet radiation in the aphakic monkey. Am J Ophthalmol 1982;93:299–306.
188. Ham Jr WT, Mueller HA, Ruffolo Jr JJ, et al. Solar retinopathy as a function of wavelength: its significance for protective eyewear. In: Williams TP, Baker BN, editors. The effects of constant light on visual processes. New York: Plenum Press; 1980. p. 319–46.
189. Ham Jr WT, Mueller HA, Sliney DH. Retinal sensitivity to damage from short wavelength light. Nature 1976;260:153–4.
190. Ham Jr WT, Mueller HA, Williams RC, et al. Ocular hazard from viewing the sun unprotected and through various windows and filters. Appl Optics 1973;12:2122–9.
191. Ham Jr WT, Ruffolo Jr JJ, Mueller HA, et al. Histologic analysis of photochemical lesions produced in rhesus retina by short-wavelength light. Invest Ophthalmol Vis Sci 1978;17: 1029–35.
192. Lawwill T. Three major pathologic processes caused by light in the primate retina: a search for mechanisms. Trans Am Ophthalmol Soc 1982;80:517–79.
193. Li Z-L, Tso MOM, Jampol LM, et al. Retinal injury induced by near-ultraviolet radiation in aphakic and pseudophakic monkey eyes; a preliminary report. Retina 1990;10:301–14.
194. Tso MOM, LaPiana FG. The human fovea after sungazing. Trans Am Acad Ophthalmol Otolaryngol 1975;79:OP788–OP795.
195. Kerr LM, Little HL. Foveomacular retinitis. Arch Ophthalmol 1966;76:498–504.
196. Naidoff MA, Sliney DH. Retinal injury from a welding arc. Am J Ophthalmol 1974;77:663–8.
197. Power WJ, Travers SP, Mooney DJ. Welding arc maculopathy and fluphenazine. Br J Ophthalmol 1991;75:433–5.
198. Terrien F. Du pronostic des troubles visuels d'origine électrique. Arch Ophthalmol (Paris) 1902;22:692–738.
199. Uniat L, Olk RJ, Hanish SJ. Arc-welding maculopathy. Am J Ophthalmol 1986;102:394–5.
200. Michaels M, Dawson WW, Feldman RB, et al. Infrared; an unseen and unnecessary hazard in ophthalmic devices. Ophthalmology 1987;94:143–8.
201. Gardner TW, Ai E, Chrobak M, et al. Photic maculopathy secondary to short-circuiting of a high-tension electric current. Ophthalmology 1982;89:865–8.
202. Dolphin K, Lincoff H. Bilateral radiant damage to the cornea and retina after exposure to a 700-V electric discharge. Am J Ophthalmol 1992;114:775–6.
203. Magnavita N. Photoretinitis: an underestimated occupational injury? Occup Med (Lond) 2002;52:223–5.
204. Brittain GP. Retinal burns caused by exposure to MIG-welding arcs: report of two cases. Br J Ophthalmol 1988;72:570–5.
205. Beaumont P. Retinal burns from MIG-welding arcs. Br J Ophthalmol 1989;73:852.
206. Brittain GPH. Retinal burns caused by exposure to MIG-welding arcs: report of two cases. Br J Ophthalmol 1988;72:570–5.
207. Würdemann HV. The formation of a hole in the macula; light burn from exposure to electric welding. Am J Ophthalmol 1936;19:457–60.
208. Moon SJ, Kim JE, Han DP. Lightning-induced maculopathy. Retina 2005;25:380–2.
209. Norman ME, Albertson D, Younge BR. Ophthalmic manifestations of lightning strike. Surv Ophthalmol 2001;46:19–24.
210. Biro Z, Pamer Z. Electrical cataract and optic neuropathy. Int Ophthalmol 1994;18:43–7.
211. Boozalis GT, Purdue GF, Hunt JL, et al. Ocular changes from electrical burn injuries. A literature review and report of cases. J Burn Care Rehabil 1991;12:458–62.
212. Miller BK, Goldstein MH, Monshizadeh R, et al. Ocular manifestations of electrical injury: a case report and review of the literature. CLAO J 2002;28:224–7.
213. Moore MC. Ocular injury from electric current and lightning flash. Trans Ophthalmol Soc Aust 1956;16:87–92.
214. Mutlu FM, Duman H, Cil Y. Early-onset unilateral electric cataract: a rare clinical entity. J Burn Care Rehabil 2004;25:363–5.
215. Reddy SC. Electric cataract: a case report and review of the literature. Eur J Ophthalmol 1999;9:134–8.
216. Campo RV, Lewis RS. Lightning-induced macular hole. Am J Ophthalmol 1984;97:792–4.
217. Duke-Elder S, MacFaul PA. System of ophthalmology, vol. 14, part 2: Non-mechanical injuries. St Louis: CV Mosby; 1971. pp. 813–35.
218. Handa JT, Jaffe GJ. Lightning maculopathy; a case report. Retina 1994;14:169–72.
219. Noel L-P, Clarke WN, Addison D. Ocular complications of lightning. J Pediatr Ophthalmol Strabismus 1980;17:245–6.
220. Espaillat A, Janigian Jr R, To K. Cataracts, bilateral macular holes, and rhegmatogenous retinal detachment induced by lightning. Am J Ophthalmol 1999;127:216–7.
221. Yi C, Liang Y, Jiexiong O, et al. Lightning-induced cataract and neuroretinopathy. Retina 2001;21:526–8.
222. Lee MS, Gunton KB, Fischer DH, et al. Ocular manifestations of remote lightning strike. Retina 2002;22:808–10.
223. Rivas-Aguino PJ, Garcia RA, Arevalo JF. Bilateral macular cyst after lightning visualized with optical coherence tomography. Clin Experiment Ophthalmol 2006;34:893–4.
224. Friedman E, Kuwabara T. The retinal pigment epithelium. IV. The damaging effects of radiant energy. Arch Ophthalmol 1968;80:265–79.
225. Tso MOM. Photic maculopathy in rhesus monkey; a light and electron microscopic study. Invest Ophthalmol 1973;12:17–34.
226. Tso MOM. Wallow IHL, Powell JO, et al. Recovery of the rod and cone cells after photic injury. Trans Am Acad Ophthalmol Otolaryngol 1972;76:1247–61.
227. Tso MOM, Woodford BJ. Effect of photic injury on the retinal tissues. Ophthalmology 1983;90:952–63.
228. Fuller D, Machemer R, Knighton RW. Retinal damage produced by intraocular fiber optic light. Am J Ophthalmol 1978;85:519–37.
229. Brod RD, Olsen KR, Ball SF, et al. The site of operating microscope light-induced injury on the human retina. Am J Ophthalmol 1989;107:390–7.
230. Fechner PU, Barth R. Effect on the retina of an air cushion in the anterior chamber and coaxial illumination. Am J Ophthalmol 1983;96:600–4.
231. Hochheimer BF, D'Anna SA, Calkins JL. Retinal damage from light. Am J Ophthalmol 1979;88:1039–44.
232. Irvine AR, Wood I, Morris BW. Retinal damage from the illumination of the operating microscope; an experimental study in pseudophakic monkeys. Arch Ophthalmol 1984;102:1358–65.
233. Jaffe GJ, Wood IS. Retinal phototoxicity from the operating microscope: a protective effect by the fovea. Arch Ophthalmol 1988;106:445–6.
234. Johnson RN, Schatz H, McDonald HR. Photic maculopathy: early angiographic and ophthalmoscopic findings and late development of choroidal folds. Arch Ophthalmol 1987;105:1633–4.
235. Khwarg SG, Linstone FA, Daniels SA, et al. Incidence, risk factors, and morphology in operating microscope light retinopathy. Am J Ophthalmol 1987;103:255–63.
236. Parver LM, Auker CR, Fine BS. Observations on monkey eyes exposed to light from an operating microscope. Ophthalmology 1983;90:964–72.
237. Hupp SL. Delayed, incomplete recovery of macular function after photic retinal damage associated with extracapsular cataract extraction and posterior lens insertion. Arch Ophthalmol 1987;105:1022–3.
238. Jaffe GJ, Irvine AR, Wood IS, et al. Retinal phototoxicity from the operating microscope; the role of inspired oxygen. Ophthalmology 1988;95:1130–41.
239. Khwarg SG, Geoghegan M, Hanscom TA. Light-induced maculopathy from the operating microscope. Am J Ophthalmol 1984;98:628–30.
240. Kraff MC, Sanders DR, Jampol LM, et al. Effect of an ultraviolet-filtering intraocular lens on cystoid macular edema. Ophthalmology 1985;92:366–9.
241. Kramer T, Brown R, Lynch M, et al. Molteno implants and operating microscope-induced retinal phototoxicity; a clinicopathologic report. Arch Ophthalmol 1991;109:379–83.
242. Macy JI, Baerveldt G. Pseudophakic serous maculopathy. Arch Ophthalmol 1983;101: 228–31.
243. McDonald HR, Irvine AR. Light-induced maculopathy from the operating microscope in extracapsular cataract extraction and intraocular lens implantation. Ophthalmology 1983;90:945–51.
244. Michels M, Sternberg Jr P. Operating microscope-induced retinal phototoxicity: pathophysiology, clinical manifestations and prevention. Surv Ophthalmol 1990;34:237–52.
245. Robertson DM, Feldman RB. Photic retinopathy from the operating room microscope. Am J Ophthalmol 1986;101:561–9.
246. Ross WH. Light-induced maculopathy. Am J Ophthalmol 1984;98:488–93.
247. Stamler JF, Blodi CF, Verdier D, et al. Microscope light-induced maculopathy in combined penetrating keratoplasty, extracapsular cataract extraction, and intraocular lens implantation. Ophthalmology 1988;95:1142–6.
248. Arden GB, Berninger T, Hogg CR, et al. A survey of color discrimination in German ophthalmologists; changes associated with the use of lasers and operating microscopes. Ophthalmology 1991;98:567–75.
249. Byrnes GA, Antoszyk AN, Mazur DO, et al. Photic maculopathy after extracapsular surgery; a prospective study. Ophthalmology 1992;99:731–8.

250. Boldrey EE, Ho BT, Griffith RD. Retinal burns occurring at cataract extraction. Ophthalmology 1984;91:1297–302.
251. Kuhn F, Morris R, Massey M. Photic retinal injury from endoillumination during vitrectomy. Am J Ophthalmol 1991;111:42–6.
252. McDonald HR, Harris MJ. Operating microscope-induced retinal phototoxicity during pars plana vitrectomy. Arch Ophthalmol 1988;106:521–3.
253. McDonald HR, Verre WP, Aaberg TM. Surgical management of idiopathic epiretinal membranes. Ophthalmology 1986;93:978–83.
254. Meyers SM, Bonner RF. Retinal irradiance from vitrectomy endoilluminators. Am J Ophthalmol 1982;94:26–9.
255. Michels M, Lewis H, Abrams GW, et al. Macular phototoxicity caused by fiberoptic endoillumination during pars plana vitrectomy. Am J Ophthalmol 1992;114:287–96.
256. Poliner LS, Tornambe PE. Retinal pigment epitheliopathy after macular hole surgery. Ophthalmology 1992;99:1671–7.
257. Green WR, Robertson DM. Pathologic findings of photic retinopathy in the human eye. Am J Ophthalmol 1991;112:520–7.
258. Lam STM, Gurne DH. Amelioration of retinal photic injury in albino rats by dimethylthiourea. Arch Ophthalmol 1990;108:1751–7.
259. Rosner M, Lam TT, Fu J, et al. Methylprednisolone ameliorates retinal photic injury in rats. Arch Ophthalmol 1992;110:857–61.
260. Tso MOM. Retinal photic injury in normal and scorbutic monkeys. Trans Am Ophthalmol Soc 1987;85:498–556.
261. Lawwill T. Effects of prolonged exposure of rabbit retina to low-intensity light. Invest Ophthalmol 1973;12:45–51.
262. Henry MM, Henry LM, Henry LM. A possible cause of chronic cystic maculopathy. Ann Ophthalmol 1977;9:455–7.
263. Hochheimer BF. A possible cause of chronic cystic maculopathy; the operating microscope. Ann Ophthalmol 1981;13:153–5.
264. Mannis MJ, Becker B. Retinal light exposure and cystoid macular edema. Arch Ophthalmol 1980;98:1133.
265. Alhalel A, Glovinsky Y, Treister G, et al. Long-term follow up of accidental parafoveal laser burns. Retina 1993;13:152–4.
266. Anderson DR, Knighton RW, Feuer WJ. Evaluation of phototoxic retinal damage after argon laser iridotomy. Am J Ophthalmol 1989;107:398–402.
267. Boldrey EE, Little HL, Flocks M, et al. Retinal injury due to industrial laser burns. Ophthalmology 1981;88:101–7.
268. Fowler BJ. Accidental industrial laser burn of macula. Ann Ophthalmol 1983;15:481–3.
269. Hirsch DR, Booth DG, Schocket S, et al. Recovery from pulsed-dye laser retinal injury. Arch Ophthalmol 1992;110:1688–9.
270. Liu HF, Gao GH, Wu DC, et al. Ocular injuries from accidental laser exposure. Health Phys 1989;56:711–6.
271. Zuclich JA, Stolarski DJ. Retinal damage induced by red diode laser. Health Phys 2001; 81:8–14.
272. Hagemann LF, Costa RA, Ferreira HM, et al. Optical coherence tomography of a traumatic neodymium:YAG laser-induced macular hole. Ophthalmic Surg Lasers Imaging 2003;34:57–9.
273. Cooper BA, Blinder KJ, Shah GK, et al. Femtosecond laser-induced premacular hemorrhage. Retina 2004;24:812–4.
274. Ying HS, Symons RC, Lin KL, et al. Accidental Nd:YAG laser-induced choroidal neovascularization. Lasers Surg Med 2008;40:240–2.
275. Berninger TA, Canning CR, Gündüz K, et al. Using argon laser blue light reduces ophthalmologists' color contrast sensitivity; argon blue and surgeons' vision. Arch Ophthalmol 1989;107:1453–8.
276. Gündüz K, Arden GB. Changes in colour contrast sensitivity associated with operating argon lasers. Br J Ophthalmol 1989;73:241–6.
277. Wiebers DO, Swanson JW, Cascino TL, et al. Bilateral loss of vision in bright light. Stroke 1989;20:554–8.
278. Robertson DM, Lim TH, Salomao DR, et al. Laser pointers and the human eye: a clinicopathologic study. Arch Ophthalmol 2000;118:1686–91.
279. Robertson DM, McLaren JW, Salomao DR, et al. Retinopathy from a green laser pointer: a clinicopathologic study. Arch Ophthalmol 2005;123:629–33.
280. Cruickshanks KJ, Klein R. Klein BEK. Sunlight and age-related macular degeneration; the Beaver Dam Eye Study. Arch Ophthalmol 1993;111:514–8.
281. Taylor HR, Muñoz B, West S, et al. Visible light and risk of age-related macular degeneration. Trans Am Ophthalmol Soc 1990;88:163–73.
282. Taylor HR, West S, Muñoz B, et al. The long-term effects of visible light on the eye. Arch Ophthalmol 1992;110:99–104.
283. West SK, Rosenthal FS, Bressler NM, et al. Exposure to sunlight and other risk factors for age-related macular degeneration. Arch Ophthalmol 1989;107:875–9.

Index

A

B

C

E

F

G

H

I

J

K

L

M

N

O

P

S

T

U

V

W

X

Z

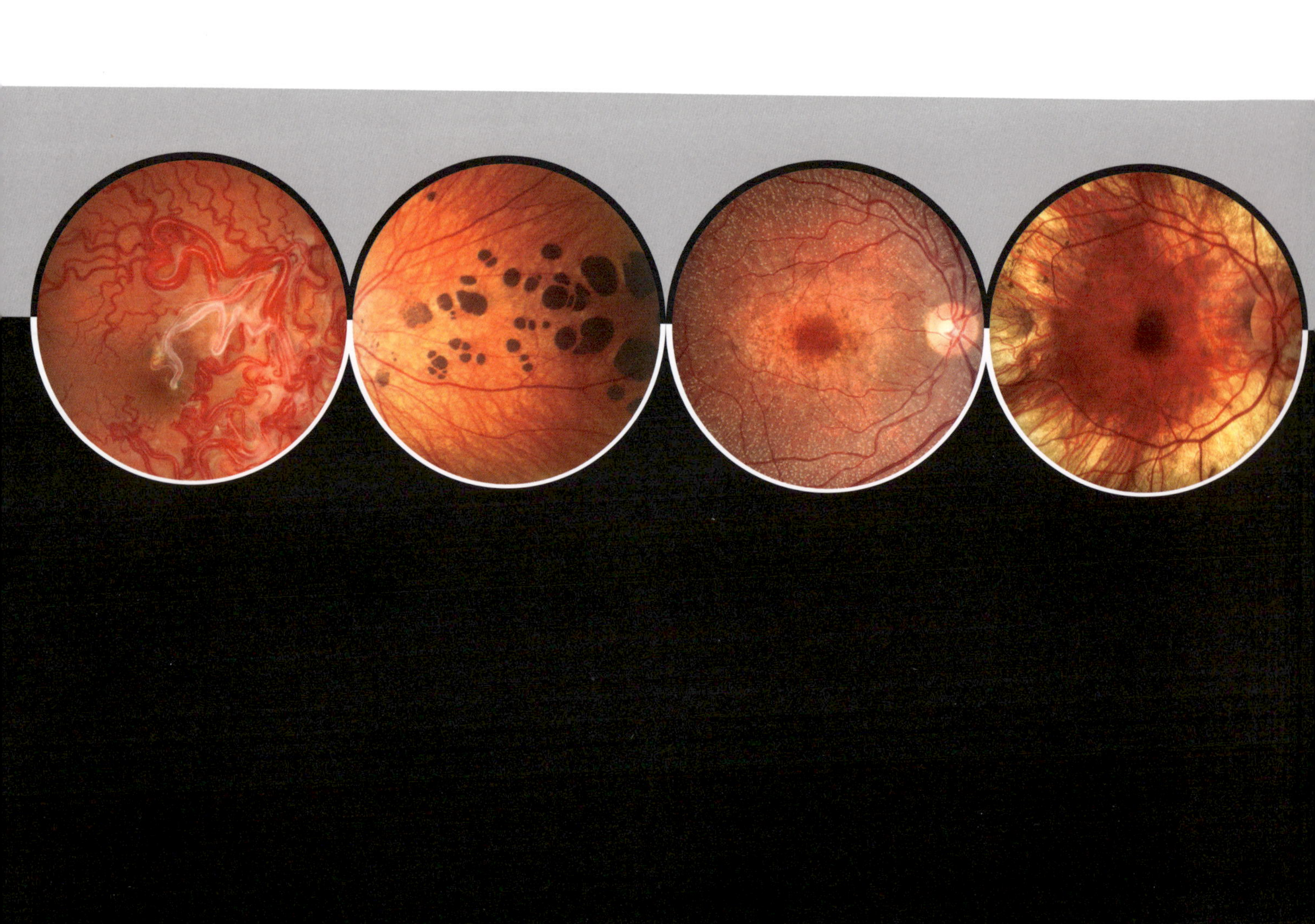

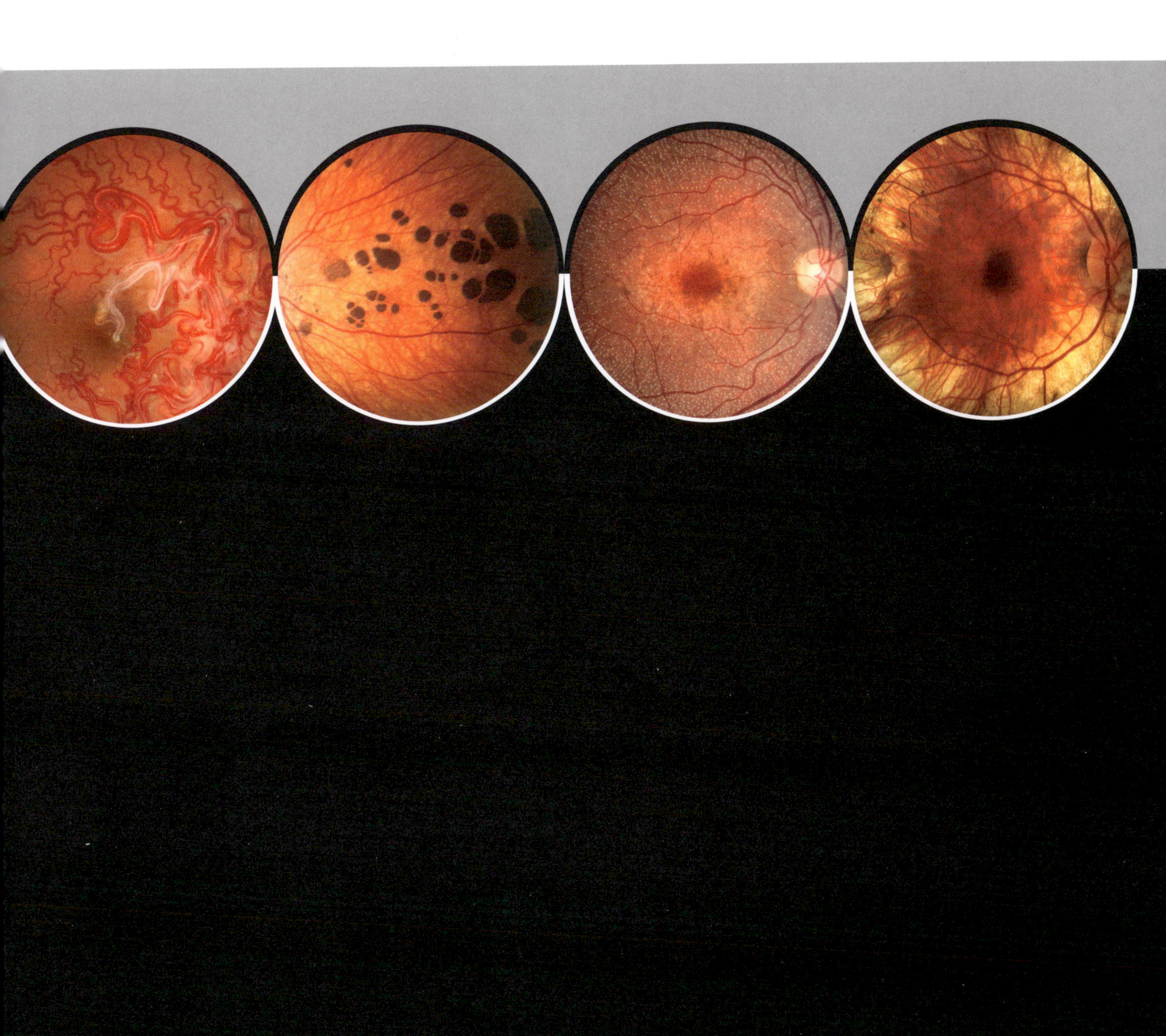

Gass' Atlas of
MACULAR
DISEASES

Dedication

To my parents, grandmother and siblings

Vimala Chandraiah
Daksha Chandraiah
M.C. Chandraiah
B. S. Puttamma
Dinesh, Suchita, Vinuta and Mamata
for their unending love and faith in me

To my teachers

J. Donald M. Gass
Amod Gupta
for their inspiration and teaching

and to their spouses and children
Margy Ann Gass and Gunita Gill Gupta
John, Carlton, Media, Dean and Sumedha
for supporting their careers and allowing me to borrow their time

To my colleagues and friends
for selflessly sharing their cases and knowledge

To our patients
for giving us the privilege of learning through them

Commissioning Editor: Russell Gabbedy
Development Editor: Sharon Nash
Editorial Assistant: Kirsten Lowson
Project Manager(s): Jess Thompson/Andrew Riley
Design: Stewart Larking
Illustration Manager: Gillian Richards
Illustrator: Martin Woodward
Multimedia Producer: Nathan Wiles
Marketing Manager(s) (UK/USA): Gaynor Jones/Helena Mutak

VOLUME TWO

FIFTH EDITION

Gass' Atlas of MACULAR DISEASES

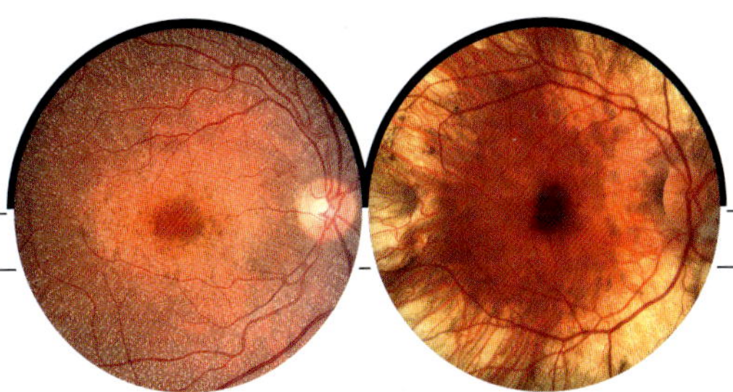

ANITA AGARWAL, MD

Associate Professor of Ophthalmology

Vanderbilt Eye Institute

Vanderbilt University School of Medicine

Nashville, TN

USA

ELSEVIER
SAUNDERS

ELSEVIER
SAUNDERS

SAUNDERS is an imprint of Elsevier Inc.

First edition 1970
Second edition 1977
Third edition 1987
Fourth edition 1997
Fifth edition 2012

Notices
Knowledge and best practice in this field are constantly changing. As new research and experience broaden our understanding, changes in research methods, professional practices, or medical treatment may become necessary. Practitioners and researchers must always rely on their own experience and knowledge in evaluating and using any information, methods, compounds, or experiments described herein. In using such information or methods they should be mindful of their own safety and the safety of others, including parties for whom they have a professional responsibility.

With respect to any drug or pharmaceutical products identified, readers are advised to check the most current information provided (i) on procedures featured or (ii) by the manufacturer of each product to be administered, to verify the recommended dose or formula, the method and duration of administration, and contraindications. It is the responsibility of practitioners, relying on their own experience and knowledge of their patients, to make diagnoses, to determine dosages and the best treatment for each individual patient, and to take all appropriate safety precautions.

To the fullest extent of the law, neither the Publisher nor the authors, contributors, or editors, assume any liability for any injury and/or damage to persons or property as a matter of products liability, negligence or otherwise, or from any use or operation of any methods, products, instructions, or ideas contained in the material herein.

Saunders

British Library Cataloguing in Publication Data
Agarwal, Anita.
Gass' atlas of macular diseases. – 5th ed.
1. Macula lutea Diseases Atlases.
I. Title II. Gass, J. Donald M. (John Donald M.), 1928-2005
Stereoscopic atlas of macular diseases.
617.7'3-dc22

Library of Congress Cataloging in Publication Data
A catalog record for this book is available from the Library of Congress

ISBN: 978-1-4377-1580-4

Printed in China
Last digit is the print number: 9 8 7 6 5 4 3 2 1

CONTENTS

VOLUME ONE

Figures with 3D indicate bonus stereoscopic images available online at www.expertconsult.com

Figures with 3D indicate bonus stereoscopic images available online at www.expertconsult.com

CONTENTS

VOLUME TWO

9 Toxic Diseases Affecting the Pigment Epithelium and Retina 755

Anita Agarwal

Figures with 3D indicate bonus stereoscopic images available online at www.expertconsult.com

10 Infectious Diseases of the Retina and Choroid 805

Anita Agarwal

Forewords

This fifth edition of the Gass Atlas of Macular Diseases by Dr. Anita Agarwal brilliantly combines the best of the previous editions with new technical advances, new entities and international perspective. The Atlas is a guide to help the clinician to arrive at a diagnosis of both common and uncommon diseases and to understand the pathogenesis. The online version continues the tradition for viewing stereo photographs. A hallmark of Dr. Gass' teaching style is a simple yet detailed description of clinical observations. This technique is preserved in the current edition and enhanced through electronic illustrations and Optical Coherence Tomography (OCT) which frequently depicts precisely what Dr. Gass envisaged.

The table of contents is reorganized to reflect the explosion of information, particularly in areas such as inflammatory and infectious diseases and tumors addressed in separate chapters. Updates on manifestations of tuberculosis and syphilis are included along with new viral diseases such as Epstein–Barr and West Nile virus. Chapter 11 contains a description of some new diagnostic entities including acute idiopathic maculopathy and persistent and relentless placoid pigment epitheliopathy. Tumors are presented in three chapters – Retinal Pigment Epithelium (12), Retina (13) and Choroid (14).

Dr. Agarwal and her co-author, Dr. Arun D Singh, have updated and extended the extraordinary work of Dr. J. Donald M. Gass, an individual recognized as one of the outstanding ophthalmologists of the 20th century, and helped to catapult his work into the future. In a time of increasing paperless communication this wonderful text will serve all physicians interested in macular disease as a continuing reference to improve their diagnostic acumen and provide better care for their patients.

John G. Clarkson, MD
Professor, Chair and Dean Emeritus
Bascom Palmer Eye Institute, Miami, FL

What a task it would be to rewrite the Bible! What about the Bible of retinal disease – Donald Gass' stereoscopic atlas? For the last three decades this book has informed us, helped us in the diagnosis and treatment of difficult cases, and served as the foundation for the evolution of the entire field of medical retina. The brilliant pattern recognition, memory, and synthesizing skills of Donald Gass allowed him to document an unimaginable amount of important information in his book. He described for the first time scores of new diseases and physical findings. His photographic collection – built over years of seeing patients, providing mail consultations, and attending innumerable meetings, is unparalleled. His knowledge of ocular pathology added to the value of these archives. Even today, time and time again, when we suspect we have a new observation, perusal of the atlas shows us to be way behind Don.

As expected, the Atlas aged and illness prevented Don from completing a new edition. In most circumstances an editor or many editors, (but not a single author) would try to live up to the original and usually not succeed. Fortunately one of Don's most talented disciples has stepped into the breach.

Anita Agarwal was a fellow with Don and worked side by side with him at Vanderbilt University. Since his death, at conferences and in her publications, she has shown immense grasp of Don's knowledge base and has taken his place in educating us about the diseases that Don had mastered. She has an excellent knowledge of systemic diseases, genetics and many aspects of internal medicine very rare in ophthalmology. Now we are grateful that she has devoted years of her life to updating this precious text. Using Don's original files and her encyclopedic knowledge of the retina, a new version of the Bible appears. (Dr. Arun D. Singh has assisted her on the chapters on tumors.) The figures, including colour photographs, OCTs, angiographies, X-rays, and histopathologic specimens are still unparalleled; multiple images are often available of the same entity, demonstrating the variability of these diseases. Anita has also added an international flavour to the book with discussions of diseases rarely or not seen in the USA. The book covers common diseases (e.g. age-related macular degeneration) in detail, but also discusses very rare entities (e.g. diffuse unilateral subacute neuroretinitis).

There are other great books and atlases of medical retina but this book remains the Bible. Thank you Anita

Lee M. Jampol, MD
Louis Feinberg Professor and Chair Emeritus
Northwestern University, Chicago, IL

Of all my ophthalmology books, the Gass Atlas of Macular Diseases has been the most treasured, and most dog-eared, possession. Since I first acquired my copy of the second edition as a resident, I avidly awaited the publication of the more recent version, then immediately purchased it to replace my worn copy of the previous edition. When Dr. Gass became too ill to write a fifth edition, I made a personal commitment to ensure that the legacy of this impactful book would not pass away as well. Thus, it is with great pride that I write this foreword, celebrating the continuance of the Gass Atlas, acknowledging the importance of careful clinical examination in the diagnosis of retinal disease, and recognizing the "passing of the baton" to the next generation.

Most of the ophthalmic community links J. Donald M. Gass to the Bascom Palmer Eye Institute. Dr. Gass was one of the founding physicians there, and forever changed our understanding of the macula. He opened our eyes to the complexity of macular diseases, by creating logical, well-defined classifications, based on carefully made clinical observations and a remarkable recollection of patients with similar histories and examinations. He passed on this knowledge to a world of residents, fellows, and colleagues across the globe. In fact, virtually every retina specialist considers himself or herself to be a student of Dr. Gass, even if they never had the opportunity to meet him. Fortunate were those who trained at BPEI and had the privilege of seeing patients with him and attending the weekly fluorescein conferences. It is no coincidence that Bascom Palmer became the breeding ground for many of the future leaders of the retina community.

However, the rest of us still learned from him. For some, it was attending lectures at conferences like the Annual Meeting of the American Academy of Ophthalmology. For others, they had the good fortune to work beside him as part of multicenter collaborative trials. I vividly remember my first meeting as an investigator in the Macular Photocoagulation Study in the 1980s. As the day concluded, they held a session where the Reading Center shared cases that were more difficult or confusing. The various experts would put forward their thoughts; however, the case was not settled until Dr. Gass weighed in. Even in a room filled with the "giants" in our field, Dr. Gass had the final word.

Here at Vanderbilt, we feel privileged to share some of the credit for the legacy of Dr. Gass' impact on ophthalmology. While J. Donald M. Gass was born in Canada, he was raised in Nashville, Tennessee when his father accepted a job in the state department of public health. He attended Vanderbilt as an undergraduate and as a medical student, winning the Founder's Medal as the top student in his graduating class. He married his high school sweetheart, Margy Ann, and it was anticipated that they would return to Nashville when he completed his training.

However, his return to Nashville was delayed for over 30 years until 1995 when he retired from his long-time faculty position as Professor of Ophthalmology at the University of Miami. Fortunately, his retirement was short-lived. Dr. Denis O'Day, the chair at Vanderbilt at that time, was able to convince Dr. Gass to join the faculty here. He returned to clinical practice, writing, and teaching. Dr. O'Day writes, "The image that will forever endure for me is the one I saw every week. It is of a man sitting, surrounded by colleagues, residents, students, and fellows. All are peering at photographs of the retina and the conversation is animated: all are engaged. As I walk by, I recognize our singular good fortune in having such a true academician in our midst."

One of those individuals surrounding Dr. Gass is Dr. Anita Agarwal. Drawn to Vanderbilt for a medical retina fellowship to learn under Dr. Gass, Anita developed an almost photographic memory of the Gass Atlas, and an encyclopedic knowledge of the retina literature. She came to evaluate a case in a brilliant Gass-like manner. Over time, her interest in the diversity of retinal diseases and her ability to make challenging diagnoses led her to earn a position of respect among the small community of similar experts.

It is highly appropriate that Dr. Anita Agarwal should be authoring this fifth edition. As well as any retina specialist in the world, she knows the previous editions from cover to cover. She has had the good fortune to have daily access to the Gass Archives: Dr. Gass' slides, patient charts, and personal notes that were bequested to the Vanderbilt Eye Institute upon his death. In fact, much of her writing has been conducted in a faculty office devoted to the Gass material: a room in which Dr. Gass' white coat hangs on the door and where the space is dominated by the large wooden cabinet with sliding trays that Dr. Gass would use to prepare his lectures and his manuscripts.

Dr. Agarwal has spent the better part of two years preparing this magnificent fifth edition. While she has restructured the chapters, updated the material to include newer conditions and new testing modalities like OCT, and engaged her talented friend and colleague, Dr. Arun D. Singh to write the chapters on intraocular tumors, this new edition retains the format of the previous editions. Most importantly, she has retained "the voice" of Dr. Gass. The words may be new or the condition may have been described subsequent to Dr. Gass's death, but Dr. Gass still speaks to us in this new edition.

I am hopeful that the Gass Atlas will live on through many future generations. The editors and publishers at Elsevier have done the ophthalmic community a wonderful service by investing in the creation of this fifth edition. I am grateful for their confidence in Dr. Agarwal, and certain that the readers will agree that this is a worthy successor to the previous editions.

Paul Sternberg, Jr., M.D.
G. W. Hale Professor and Chair,
Vanderbilt Eye Institute, Nashville, TN

World Map

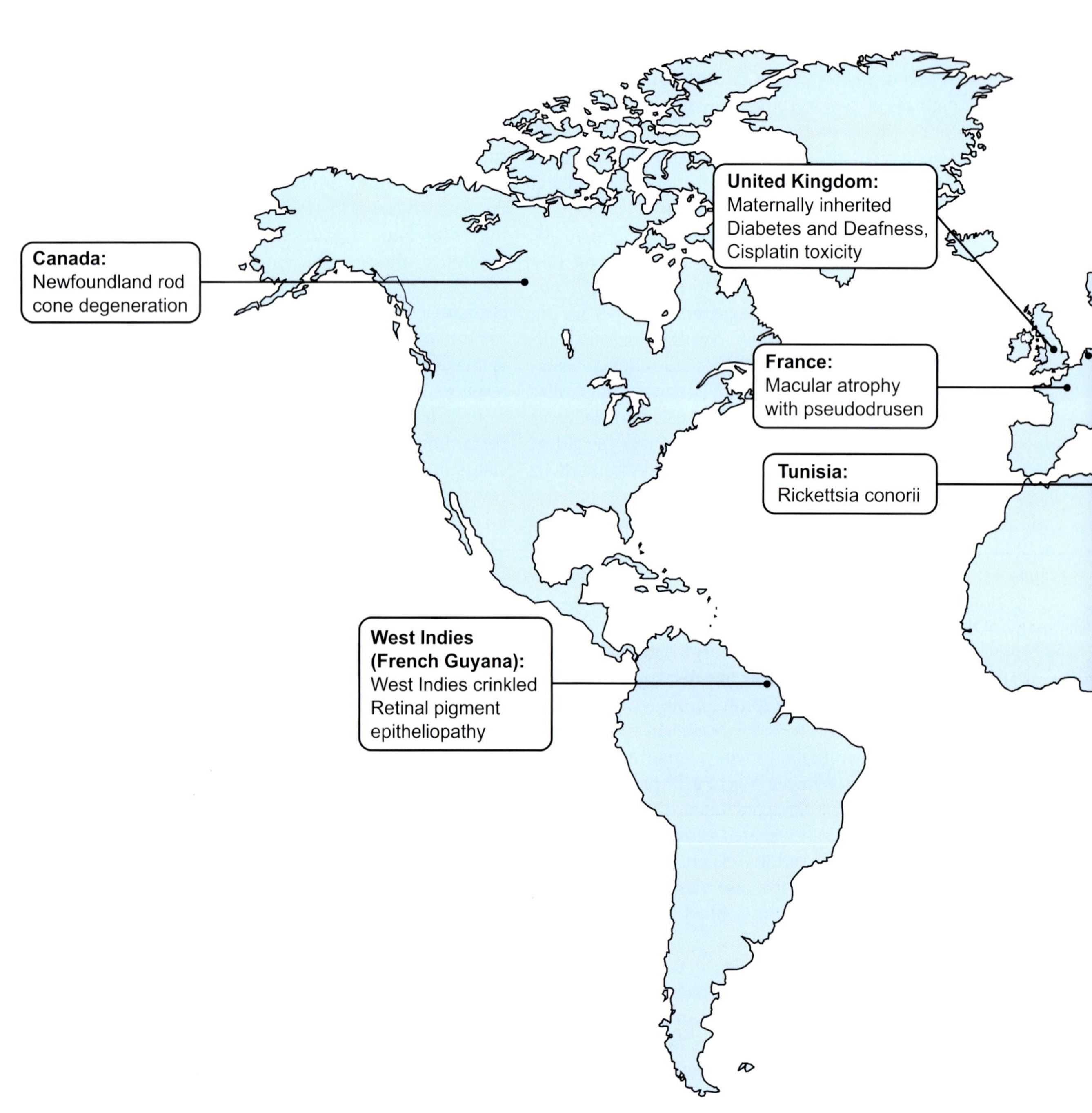
International Cases Presented in the Fifth Edition
Canada:
Newfoundland rod cone degeneration
United Kingdom:
Maternally inherited Diabetes and Deafness, Cisplatin toxicity
France:
Macular atrophy with pseudodrusen
Tunisia:
Rickettsia conorii
West Indies (French Guyana):
West Indies crinkled Retinal pigment epitheliopathy

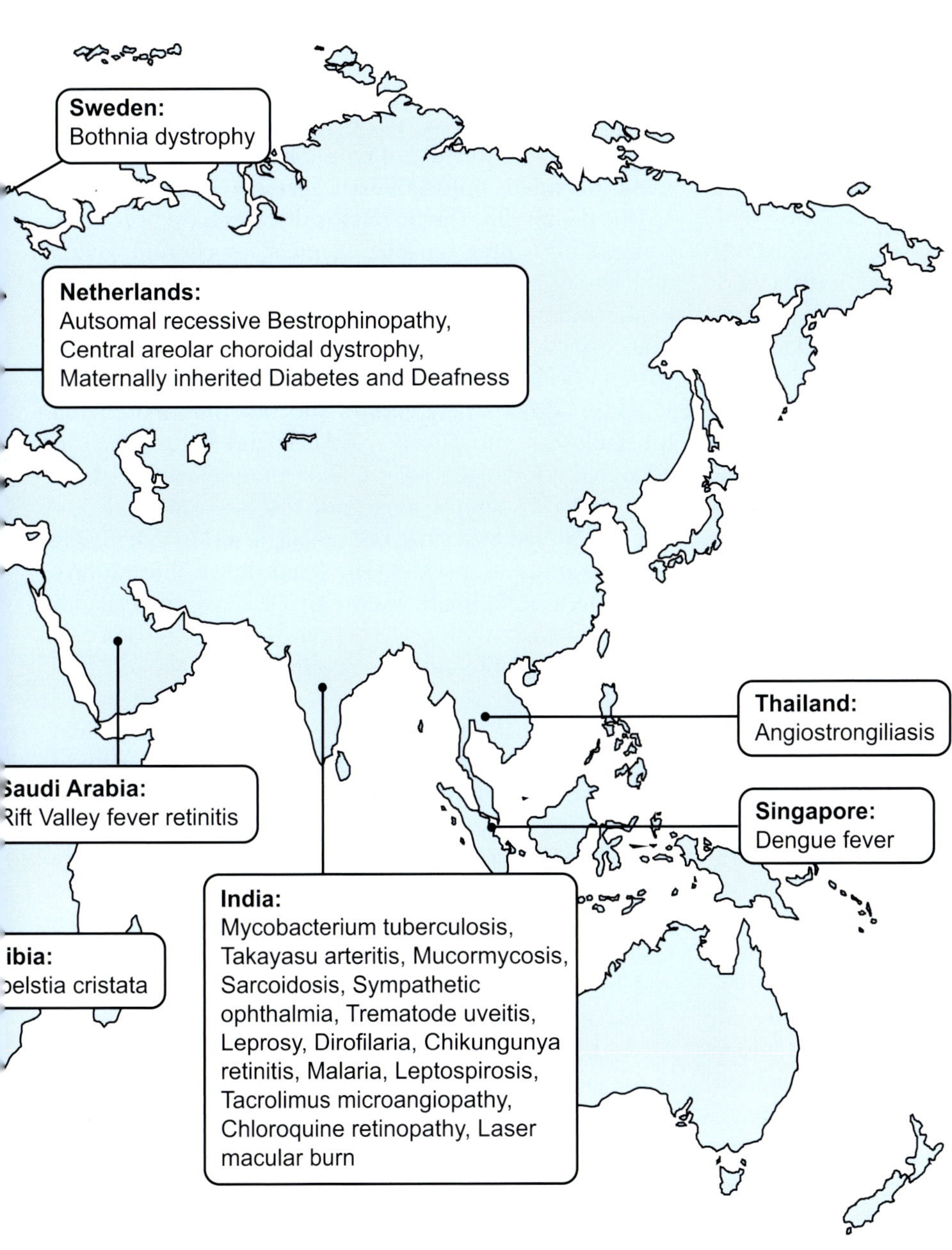

Sweden:
Bothnia dystrophy
Netherlands:
Autsomal recessive Bestrophinopathy,
Central areolar choroidal dystrophy,
Maternally inherited Diabetes and Deafness
Thailand:
Angiostrongiliasis
Saudi Arabia:
Rift Valley fever retinitis
Singapore:
Dengue fever
India:
Mycobacterium tuberculosis,
Takayasu arteritis, Mucormycosis,
Sarcoidosis, Sympathetic
ophthalmia, Trematode uveitis,
Leprosy, Dirofilaria, Chikungunya
retinitis, Malaria, Leptospirosis,
Tacrolimus microangiopathy,
Chloroquine retinopathy, Laser
macular burn
ibia:
elstia cristata

Preface to the Fifth Edition

One of the most fortunate turns in life landed me square in front of J. Donald M. Gass, my idol from a distance, whose work I had read, studied and admired since the beginning of my ophthalmology training in India. In 1997, I entered my medical retina fellowship, initiating an unending, rewarding lesson from this giant. As known to the entire world of retinal physicians, Don Gass has had a truly profound impact on our understanding of retinal and macular diseases. His keen observation skills, photographic memory of ocular features, and ability to integrate clinical findings with pathological changes led him to describe several diseases for the first time and help us understand the pathogenic mechanisms of many other previously described conditions. Two of his singularly important qualities – meticulous attention to clinical details and analysis of stereoscopic images of the retina – became the hallmark of his defining publication, his 'Stereoscopic Atlas of Macular Diseases'. The evolution of the Atlas over its multiple editions has captured and illustrated the tremendous growth our field has experienced over the decades between the first and fourth version.

It is the greatest privilege of my professional life to be selected to edit this new 5th edition of Gass' Atlas of Macular Diseases . In this publication, I have tried to retain the "voice" of Dr. Gass, and continue his work, presenting new disease entities, consolidating known diseases, and discussing new concepts in the pathogenesis of existing conditions.

This edition incorporates a number of structural modifications.

First, each chapter includes an expanded table of contents to facilitate locating the individual conditions. The contents of the Atlas in Chapters 3, 5, 7, 10 and 11 of the 4th edition have been reorganized. Previously, Chapter 3 was quite exhaustive and lengthy, containing all disorders that caused a serous or hemorrhagic retinal detachment, be it inflammatory (such as VKH and sympathetic ophthalmia), infectious (such as Toxocara or certain fungal diseases), neoplastic (such as choroidal tumors), degenerative (such as age-related macular degeneration) or inherited (such as Malattia levantinese and Sorsby's dystrophy). The various infectious, inflammatory, neoplastic and inherited disorders have been moved to individual chapters, with the current Chapter 3 discussing only idiopathic, degenerative and miscellaneous causes of serous and hemorrhagic retinal detachment. The contents of Chapter 7, that included both infectious and inflammatory retinal diseases, have been split into two separate chapters, one on infectious diseases (Chapter 10) and a second on inflammatory diseases (Chapter 11). Chapter 5 addresses heredo-dystrophic conditions of the retina, choroid and pigment epithelium; it includes several new disorders including Bothnia dystrophy, Newfoundland rod cone degeneration, and pattern dystrophy associated with newly identified systemic diseases such as maternally inherited mitochondrial diseases and hereditary spastic paraplegia. The neoplastic diseases have been reorganized into three separate chapters for choroid, retina and retinal pigment epithelium and include the various benign tumors and hamartomas. The chapter on infectious diseases (Chapter 10) includes previously discussed bacterial followed by fungal, parasitic and viral diseases. However, various new entities and new information on tuberculosis, leptospirosis, parasites, and viruses such as chikungunya, dengue, west nile and rift valley fever have been added. Attempts to include diseases prevalent outside the United States has been made to aid in diagnosing rare and unusual diseases. The hand drawn illustrations, which were a hallmark feature of Dr. Gass' understanding of disease pathology, have been skillfully converted to electronic artwork, and fundus photographs are now presented in color.

The Atlas has maintained the case descriptive format of Gass' teaching method, encompassing history, clinical exam and follow up when available. The online version features stereoscopic images that are notated by a 3D sign. A stereo viewer accompanies the book.

Overall, the Atlas emphasizes clinical features, pathogenesis, information about genetics and its role in disease pathogenesis where known, differential diagnosis, and limited information on treatment. Extensive elaboration on results of clinical trials, controversies on medical management and surgery are not discussed; the Atlas is designed to be an exhaustive guide in arriving at the proper diagnosis of common and uncommon diseases and understanding their pathogenesis.

Anita Agarwal

Preface to the First Edition

The accessibility of the tissues of the inner eye to close scrutiny by the physician is unequaled by any other organ of the body. Having acquired a knowledge of ocular pathology and the skills of ophthalmoscopy and biomicroscopy, the physician is able to record his in vivo observations of the ocular fundus in gross pathologic terms with reasonable accuracy. This becomes of particular importance in evaluating the patient with loss of central vision resulting from alterations in the structure of the macula. The physician should attempt to determine as far as possible the anatomic changes present, such as choroidal atrophy, choroidal thickening, choroidal wrinkling, change in color of the pigment epithelium, serous detachment of the pigment epithelium, serous detachment of the retina, hemorrhagic detachment of the pigment epithelium and retina, cystoid retinal edema, intraretinal hemorrhage, loss of retinal transparency, retinal wrinkling, and preretinal membrane. He should also attempt to determine the locus of the primary disease process–choroid, retinal pigment epithelium, retinal, or vitreous. Only after making these determinations can the physician evaluate the significance of the patient's ocular, medical, and family history in arriving at a diagnosis, prognosis, and course of therapy.

A variety of ancillary studies may be helpful in certain instances. The use of intravenous fluorescein is of particular value in detecting and defining certain physiologic as well as anatomic changes in the ocular fundus.

The purpose of this atlas is to utilize black and white fundus photographs, stereo color fundus photographs, fluorescein angiographs, and photomicrographs to illustrate some of the anatomic and physiologic alterations produced by a variety of intraocular disease processes affecting the macular region.

After a discussion of the normal macular region (Chapter 1), the diseases affecting this region will be considered in the following order according to the primary tissue involved: diseases of the choroid (Chapters 2 to 4), pigment epithelium (Chapter 5), retina (Chapters 6 to 10), vitreous (Chapter 11), and congenital pit of the optic nerve head (Chapter 12). This subdivision is somewhat arbitrary in that it is not possible in some instances to know which of the ocular tissues is primarily involved by a particular disease process. Stereophotographs of some of the fundus photographs are included in fifteen reels, each containing seven views, attached to the back cover of the book. The appropriate reel number (Roman numeral) and view number (Arabic numeral) are indicated in the lower right-hand corner of the black and white photographs.

All fundus photographs were made with the Zeiss fundus camera. Fluorescein angiography was done utilizing modifications[1,2] of the technique described by Novotny and Alvis.[3] Kodak Kodachrome II and Kodak Tri-X film was used.

With a single exception, the fundus photographs used in this atlas were obtained from the photographic files of the Bascom Palmer Eye Institute of the University of Miami. Most of the patients were examined by me.

I wish to thank Dr. Edward W.D. Norton, Chairman of the Department of Ophthalmology, the members of the full-time and resident staff, and the many other physicians whose patients are illustrated in this book. I am particularly indebted to Mr. Johnny Justice, Jr. and his assistants, Mr. Kenneth Peterson, Mrs. Dixie Sparks Gilbert, and Mr. Earl Choromokos for their skill in fundus photography, and to Mr. Joseph Goren and Miss Barbara French for preparation of the illustrations. Finally, I wish to thank Mrs. Margaret Bertolami, Dr. Alexander R. Irvine, Mrs. Reva Hurtes, and Miss Beth Railinshafer for their help in preparing and editing the manuscript.

J. Donald M. Gass

In Remembrance of Dr Gass

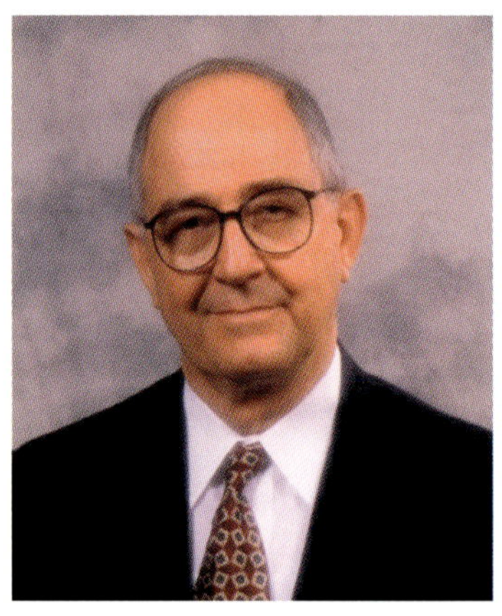

As a teenager growing up on Key Biscayne, I would awake on school days and leave the house in time to catch a 6:15 a.m. school bus into town. On the way out, I would find my father, up since before dawn, hard at work in the downstairs den of our home. The images of him pecking away on his electric typewriter with his four finger technique, peering up at slides, rummaging through piles of index cards, and painstakingly drawing illustrations of the macula remain imprinted in my memory. This scene repeated itself for many years beginning in the late sixties. "The book", as we called it around the house (we didn't know it as the "Atlas" back then), was taking shape. In those days, we were always aware of the presence of the book in the background of daily life around the Gass household. My father was usually careful not to let it intrude on other family priorities, but from time to time an increased sense of urgency to meet some deadline would become evident. My mother would often wonder out loud, sometimes with a tinge of irritation, if the book would ever be finished. As it turned out, the answer was not for at least forty years and I am now honored to contribute this foreword for the fifth edition of **Gass' Atlas of Macular Diseases** by Anita Agarwal MD.

I'm not sure when I became fully aware of the profound impact on the world of ophthalmology that my father's work at Bascom Palmer was having. The family received hints of this from time to time, hearing stories about my father from his colleagues and friends who would appear at our house. A modest and unassuming person, we would never hear a thing about any of this directly from him. Not being a doctor myself, it took me some years to piece together the full picture, but over time I became cognizant of the fact that the man I called "Dad" had become a giant in his field.

My job has taken me all over the world and I have lived on five continents. Over the years and until now, I have been amazed by the number of encounters I have had around the world with former colleagues, residents, fellows, students or patients who knew my father personally or were somehow influenced by his work, in many cases via the Gass Atlas. There are always the comments about the impact of his research, his skill as a teacher, or the brilliance of his scientific insights. But I also find, without exception, that the comments from those who knew him personally are accompanied by a story about some kindness my father had shown them or an anecdote about how he had somehow touched their lives. They always want to tell me something that I already know... that in addition to being a renowned physician, Don Gass was a very special human being.

Indeed, my father was an extraordinary person apart from all of his contributions to ophthalmology. He was first and foremost a loving husband, father, and grandfather who cherished his family. To my brothers and sister and me, he was "Dad". To everyone else in the family, including his five grandchildren, he was "Don". Growing up, there was nothing I wanted more than to be doing something with him. I can remember him teaching me how to fly a kite, ride a bike, throw a spiral, shoot a free throw underhanded, and how to fish. He took me to baseball games, taught me how to read a box score, and turned me into a lifelong Orioles fan. More importantly, I learned from him what it means to live one's life well, by observing over the years the most powerful example of this I have ever seen. Whether one knew my father as a physician, colleague, mentor, friend, neighbor or family, he was respected and loved for his kindness, his gentleness, his patience, his sense of humor, his integrity, his steadfast faith in the Lord, and a genuine humility rarely seen in others.

When I was younger, I often thought about what motivated my father to get up every day before dawn to write a book. I knew it was not a desire for fame or recognition or money. I could always see the constancy of purpose and his passion for what he was doing that remained unabated until the day he died. I could also sense the personal responsibility he felt for the continued stewardship of his work, including the Gass Atlas, because he understood it was important. But as I observed my father over the years, I came to understand there was also something else that made him tick. It was the simple yet deep satisfaction and joy that he got from creating something, solving a problem, and completing a task well. In his later years, I watched him become an accomplished wood craftsman by applying the same creativity, curiosity, dexterity, attention to detail, and patience that made him a great doctor. He spent much of his spare time in his wood shop crafting toys for the grandchildren, furniture for the house, or incredibly detailed model sailing ships. Some of these projects took hours; others took several years to complete. I loved seeing the smile on his face and the twinkle in his eyes which gave away the pure joy and sense of accomplishment he felt after completing even the simplest of these projects. I am certain that is the same feeling he had in completing each successive edition of the Gass Atlas.

I am delighted and grateful that Dr. Anita Agarwal who worked with my father in his final years at

Vanderbilt agreed to take on the challenge of authoring the fifth edition of the Gass Atlas more than four decades after the first edition was published. I know that my father would be very proud of her. The Gass Atlas represents a significant piece of my father's life's work and an important part of his legacy. However, the most enduring legacy of Dr. J. Donald M. Gass is the one that lives on in the lives, the careers, and the memories of the people touched by this remarkable man over the course of a lifetime.

John D. Gass on behalf of my mother Margy Ann, my brothers Carlton and Dean, and my sister Media

J. Donald M. Gass

Gentleman, Scholar and Genius

John Donald McIntyre Gass was born on Prince Edward Island, Canada on August 2nd 1928. At 2 weeks of age, he rode on a train with his mother from Canada to Nashville to join his father, a chest physician who had been named to direct the tuberculosis hospitals in Tennessee. He attended the two-room Grassland primary school, which housed 3 grades in each room. Being exposed to the same lessons for 3 years, Don Gass mastered 3rd grade while still in first grade, leaving himself plenty of time to learn more. He always fondly recalled his 1st grade teacher, who loaded her station wagon every month with books from the library for her students to read. Thus, was born his interest in reading. Several years later, he met his first and only love, Margy Ann Loser, on their high school bus; they were married in 1950. He attended Vanderbilt University for his undergraduate education and was deployed to Korea soon after being married. On his return, he began medical school at Vanderbilt, graduating with the highest honor: the Founder's medal.

Much to his father's puzzlement, Don Gass chose ophthalmology, a field then in its infancy. He spent his internship at the University of Iowa, and went on to be a resident at the Wilmer Eye Institute at the Johns Hopkins Hospital. There, he idolized Dr. Frank Walsh; whom he recognized the instant Dr. Walsh walked in for morning rounds on day one. While a resident, he wrote several papers on topics ranging from the optic chiasm to corneal iron lines. Between his senior residency and year as Chief Resident, he completed a fellowship in ophthalmic pathology at the Armed Forces institute of Pathology. This experience gave him an insight into disease pathology that he used skillfully through his entire career. He became quite facile in describing and postulating the pathogenesis of many diseases, most often accurately. Many of these insights were confirmed subsequently, using sophisticated tests such as OCT and autofluorescence imaging.

His numerous clinical contributions resulted from a unique combination of keen observation skills including the evaluation of stereoscopic images, attention to details, ability to comprehend and explain symptoms, and an uncanny memory for clinical findings among patients that he may have seen decades apart. He could not rest until he figured out all aspects of a new disease. Dr. Gary Abrams once told me that when Don Gass came upon a new disease, he talked about it incessantly till he figured it out completely in his mind. His excitement on seeing a new or rare disease was palpable and spread to his trainees. I recall the twinkle in his eyes and the excitement in his voice when he found the 250 micron DUSN worm coiled up in the midst of several retinal scars. His approach to understanding findings was simple and straightforward, and he used common objects to describe the analogy: a bagel for ring shaped sub RPE neovascularization and the petalloid appearance of fluorescein staining in cystoid macular edema. Fluorescein angiography was just introduced as Don Gass began his career in Miami, his study and interpretation of this investigative modality in retinal and choroidal diseases has helped us understand a majority of them. To this end, the talented photographer Johnny Justice at Bascom Palmer Eye Institute aided him.

Don Gass had a *simple but diligent* method to make notes about the various patients' findings. He carried 4×6″ note cards in his pocket and wrote down salient information about a hitherto undescribed condition that he saw. He cataloged them alphabetically. When he saw a few more patients with similar findings, he gathered all his cards and began deciphering the findings. In this manner, he described more than 30 original diseases and new features of several others. The descriptive names he gave to these diseases such as acute posterior multifocal placoid pigment epitheliopathy, acute exudative polymorphous vitelliform maculopathy, and acute zonal occult outer retinopathy would provide the clinician insight towards their pathogenesis or pattern of involvement. His understanding of disease pathology was cemented by his drawings. Many of his drawings are exact replica of what we now see on OCT imaging; a feat that Don Gass achieved several decades before the availability of OCT imaging. Renderings of the pathogenesis of a macular hole, vitreofoveal traction, type 1 and type 2 choroidal neovascularization, and the appearance of RPE detachments are just a few examples.

This giant in our field was kind, humble and generous. The transcriptionist at Vanderbilt told me of the largest fruit basket that she had ever seen in her life arrive at her doorstep when she was ill, sent by Dr. Gass. He enjoyed simple pleasures, such as fishing and woodworking. His knowledge and interest in sports was evident during animated discussions on Monday at lunch about the weekend's various sporting events and results. Most of all, he was a healer and teacher, who made each one of us a better doctor, a better teacher and a better human being. We were so privileged to have known him.

Written on behalf of all his students, past, present and future.

Anita Agarwal

Medications or other substances that find their way into the eye may cause visual dysfunction by virtue of a toxic effect on the sensory retina, the retinal pigment epithelium (RPE), and the optic nerve. In some instances (e.g., digitalis toxicity) visual symptoms may be unassociated with ophthalmoscopic changes in the fundus. In other instances the ophthalmoscopic changes may involve any one or a combination of the RPE, retina, and optic nerve head. Fluorescein angiography is particularly valuable in detecting mild toxic alterations of the RPE before they are apparent ophthalmoscopically. Optical coherence tomography (OCT), autofluorescence imaging, full-field, and multifocal electroretinography help localize the defect in many instances.

CHLOROQUINE (ARALEN) AND HYDROXYCHLOROQUINE (PLAQUENIL) RETINOPATHY

Chloroquine initially was used as an antimalarial agent in World War II, but since 1959 it has been used in the treatment of amebiasis, rheumatoid arthritis, scleroderma, and systemic lupus erythematosus. Hydroxychloroquine has largely replaced chloroquine due to lower incidence of toxicity. Degeneration of the RPE and sensory retina caused by prolonged use of chloroquine or hydroxychloroquine is one of the most important of the retinotoxic diseases.[1-22] Most patients who have developed retinopathy have received daily doses of chloroquine in excess of 250 mg or hydroxychloroquine in excess of 750 mg for at least a total dose of between 100 and 300 g.[21] There is evidence that the incidence of retinotoxic effects is lower following hydroxychloroquine than following chloroquine therapy.[18,21,23-25] Four unequivocal cases of hydroxychloroquine retinopathy were reported prior to 1991.[23,25,26] All had normal or reduced visual acuity, paracentral scotomata, and bull's-eye maculopathy. Some have evidence of peripheral retinopathy.[25] Although it has been suggested that patients receiving daily dosages of hydroxychloroquine up to 400 mg or 6.5 mg/kg of body weight per day may tolerate massive cumulative doses (for example 3923 g) without developing retinopathy,[23] such did occur in one patient who received 400 mg/day and a total dose of less than 2920 g.[25] Gass has seen another woman who, after taking a total of 146 g (200 mg/day × 730 days) of hydroxychloroquine, experienced rapid development of paracentral visual field loss and early bull's-eye maculopathy. The retinopathy caused by both drugs is probably a general toxic effect but some eyes have developed toxicity after minimal exposure while others with long usage show no ill effects. This implies that some eyes may be predisposed to toxicity sooner than others by unknown factors. A study of eight patients with chloroquine and hydroxychloroquine retinopathy for *ABCA4* mutations revealed two patients with heterozygous *ABCR* missense mutations, but none in 80 controls, suggesting some patients with *ABCR* mutations may be predisposed to retinal toxicity.[27] Vitreous fluorophotometry has demonstrated a breakdown in the blood–retinal barrier in patients receiving chloroquine but not hydroxychloroquine.[24] The earliest sign of toxicity, which may occur before development of any other ophthalmoscopic or electrophysiologic abnormality, is a paracentral visual field loss. The patient's use of the Amsler grid may be helpful in detecting these early field defects.[5]

The earliest ophthalmoscopic and angiographic alterations in the RPE occur in the parafoveal area (Figure 9.01A–C and E–K). At this stage a paracentral scotoma and minimal or no loss of visual acuity are characteristic. An enlarging ring of atrophy of the RPE surrounding the fovea produces a bull's-eye-like lesion that is indistinguishable ophthalmoscopically from other causes of this lesion (see Chapter 5). As the RPE alterations extend into the foveolar area, the patient loses central vision. Weiter et al. have suggested that the retinal xanthophyll in the foveolar area may exert a photoprotective effect in the various causes of bull's-eye maculopathy.[28] In addition to changes in the

9.01 Chloroquine and hydroxychloroquine retinopathy.

A and **B**: After receiving chloroquine, 250 mg daily for 27 years for discoid disseminated lupus erythematosus, this 50-year-old woman noted blurring of vision in both eyes. Visual acuity was 20/30. She had a symmetric bull's-eye pattern of atrophy of the retinal pigment epithelium (RPE) in both eyes (A). Early arteriovenous-phase angiography revealed evidence of preservation of the choriocapillaris within the area of RPE atrophy centrally (B). Electroretinographic findings were normal.

C and **D**: This 53-year-old woman received a total dose of 454 g hydroxychloroquine and chloroquine over a 36-month period. She showed progressive RPE and retinal degeneration for 16 years after stopping the medication.

E–H: This 50-year-old woman, who received chloroquine 500 mg/day for 13 years for rheumatoid arthritis, began to notice a "halo" scotoma and nyctalopia in both eyes in February 1977. Her visual acuity at that time was 20/30. She had a bull's-eye pattern of RPE atrophy bilaterally (E). Her electroretinographic findings were normal. The chloroquine was discontinued. Seven years later the bull's-eye pattern of atrophy had enlarged slightly and her visual acuity had decreased to 20/50 (F and G). Two years later she had experienced further loss of vision. The central island of RPE showed further evidence of atrophy angiographically (H). Visual acuity at that time was 20/200.

I: Histopathology of chloroquine maculopathy showing focal loss of the outer nuclear layer and the receptor elements, irregular depigmentation of the RPE, and preservation of the choriocapillaris.

J–L: A 45-year-old woman with lupus since age 4 shows widespread photoreceptor and pigment epithelial loss in addition to the bull's-eye change, which progressed despite cessation of chloroquine after more than 20 years of use. Her visual acuity was 20/40 and 20/50. An electroretinogram showed moderate reduction of rod and cone function.

(C and D, courtesy of Dr. Ray T. Oyakawa, were made 6 years after photographs in a previous report by Brinkley et al.[2] I, from Wetterholm and Winter[22])

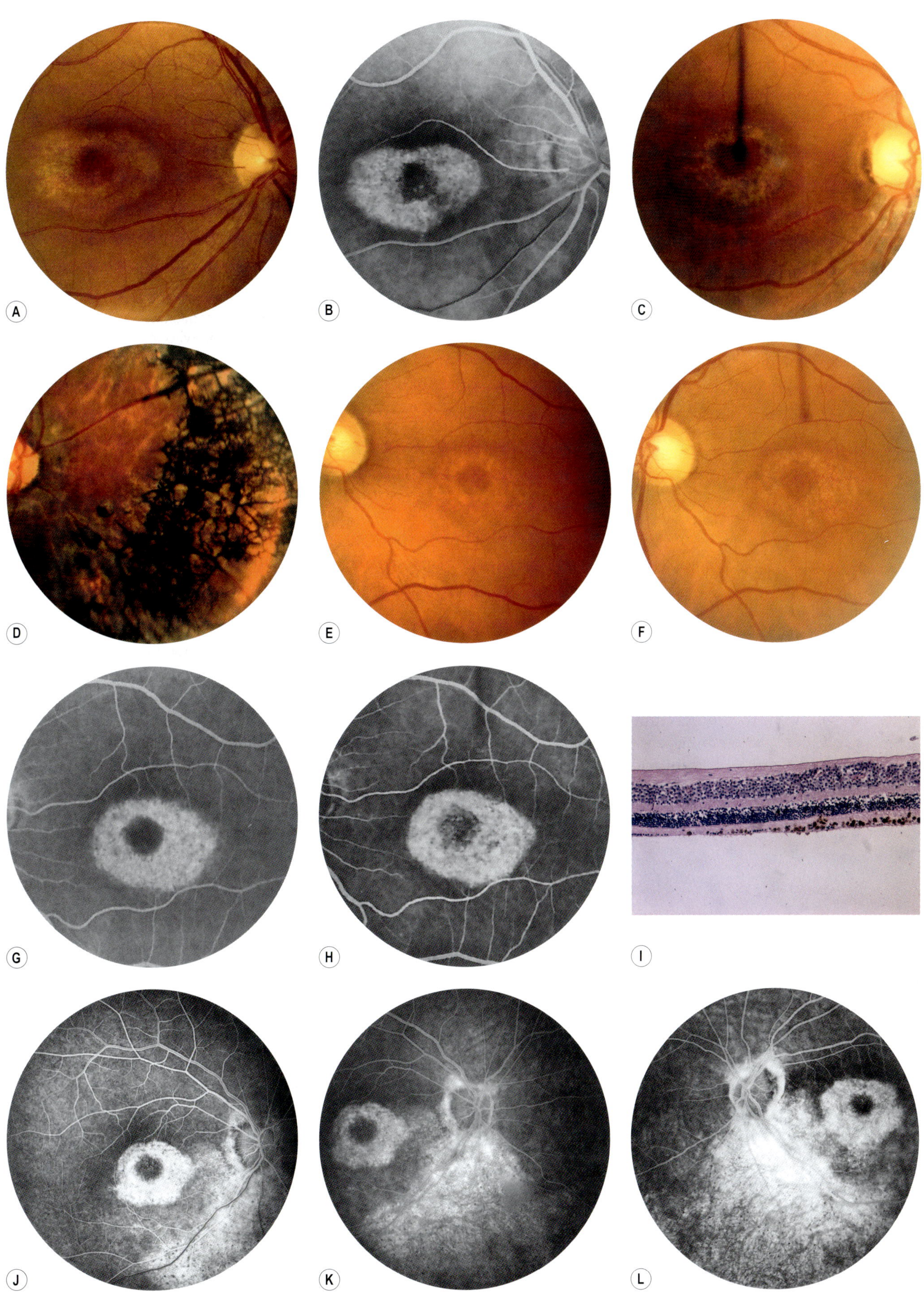
A
B
C
D
E
F
G
H
I
J
K
L

posterior pole, continued use of the drug may cause extensive alterations in the RPE and retina peripherally (Figure 9.01D, J–L). These changes, together with narrowing of the retinal vessels and optic disc pallor, may resemble primary tapetoretinal dystrophies. Severe visual loss and blindness may eventually occur. Other ocular changes caused by chloroquine include whitening of the lashes, a whorl-like pattern of subepithelial corneal deposits, decreased corneal sensitivity, and extraocular muscle palsies.[7,12]

Fluorescein angiography and fundus autofluorescence imaging (Figure 9.02C–E, K, and L) are helpful in demonstrating the faint bull's-eye pattern of hyperfluorescence before its detection biomicroscopically, particularly in patients with blond fundi. In patients with darkly pigmented fundi, biomicroscopic evidence of RPE changes may precede angiographic changes.[29] The area of RPE depigmentation (Figure 9.01B, F, H, and I) in general corresponds to the area of field loss. There is minimal angiographic evidence of damage to the choriocapillaris in the areas of RPE depigmentation (Figure 9.01B, G, J, and K) (see discussion in Chapter 2). The detection of small paracentral scotomata to red light is one of the earliest findings in chloroquine toxicity. Use of static perimetry through the vertical meridian may be the most sensitive means of detecting the early visual field damage.[8] Multifocal electroretinogram (ERG) may be able to detect early drop in receptor amplitudes in the parafoveolar region.[30–36] OCT is often able to detect loss of photoreceptors before angiographic changes (Figure 9.02G and H). The electro-oculogram (EOG) may initially be supernormal (200–350%).[9]

Ideally patients requiring more than 200 mg chloroquine or 350 mg hydroxychloroquine daily should have a baseline complete eye examination, including visual acuity, visual fields, and fundus photography. If there is any biomicroscopic evidence of abnormality of the RPE or other signs of retinal degeneration or a family history of retinal degeneration, fluorescein angiography, multifocal ERG, full-field ERG and EOG should be considered as part of the baseline workup.

In the first 5 years of chloroquine or hydroxychloroquine therapy the American Academy of Ophthalmology recommendations suggest exams at periods appropriate for the patient's age. After 5 years of therapy annual exam including central 10° visual field optical coherence tomography (OCT), color vision, and dilated fundus exam is recommended. However any suggestion of early field defects, changes in color perception, and other degenerative changes at the RPE/outer retina should warrant a prompt evaluation with autofluorescence, central visual field testing, fluorescein angiography, and discontinuation of the drug. At the present time, multifocal ERG may be the most useful means to detect early changes, even before visual field and angiographic changes appear.[30,31,33,34] OCT can show loss of perifoveolar receptors much earlier than discernible changes on fundus examination or fluorescein angiography. Most of all, attention should be paid to the patient's symptoms – variously described as changes in color perception, areas of their face missing when looking into the mirror, or parts of the TV image missing, and difficulty with dark adaptation.

9.02 Chloroquine retinopathy.

A–H: This 34-year-old African American woman was treated with chloroquine for 10 years at a dose of 250 mg once daily. She had difficulty focusing for the past year but could read 20/25 with a correction of −3.00 D. She could only see the test plate on the Ishihara chart in each eye. Fundus photographs show a ring-shaped retinal pigment epithelium (RPE) atrophy sparing the foveal center (A and B), corresponding decreased autofluorescence (C and D) and window defects on the angiogram (E and F). Optical coherence tomography of both eyes shows disruption of photoreceptors and loss of inner segment/outer segment (IS/OS) junction in the fovea (arrows) with patchy preservation of receptors in the foveal center.

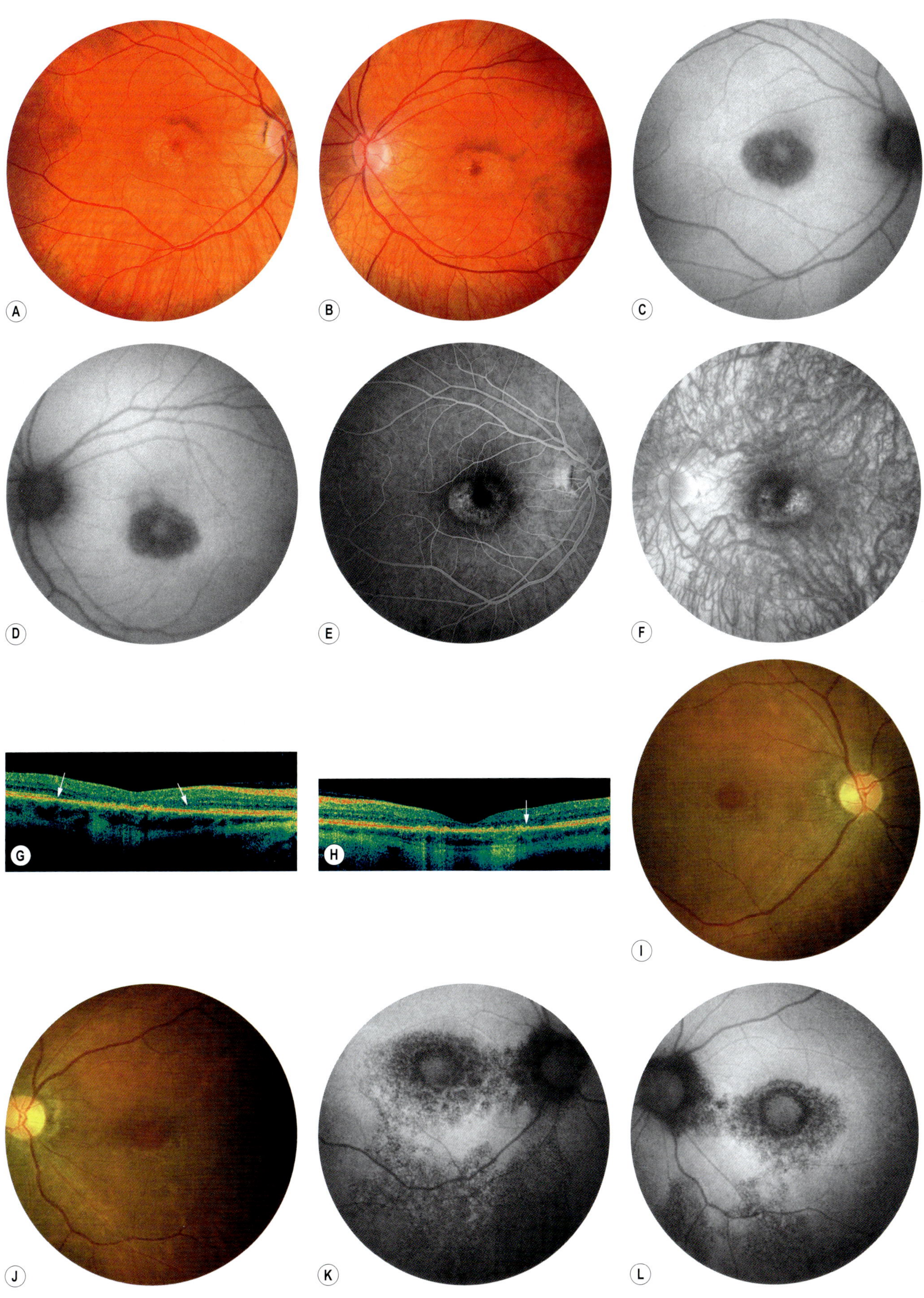
A
B
C
D
E
F
G
H
I
J
K
L

Histopathologically, depigmentation of the RPE, loss of the rod and cone receptor elements, and subretinal clumping of pigment occur in the macular area (Figure 9.01L).[22,37] Electron microscopic studies have revealed widespread changes in the retina, with the most severe occurring in the ganglion cells in spite of their relatively normal appearance by light microscopy.[16] There is experimental evidence that chloroquine is concentrated in the RPE and remains there long after cessation of treatment.[1,17] In experimental mice given intraperitoneal chloroquine, there was marked abnormality of the outer retinal layers with complete loss of the outer plexiform layer, photoreceptors, and photoreceptor nuclei. The RPE demonstrated focal atrophy, loss of nuclei, and pigment irregularity. The inner retina showed loss of Müller cells and the presence of membranous cytoplasmic bodies. In contrast, those experimental animals given the drug orally have shown much less damage with most changes limited to the RPE and photoreceptors. This suggests that the appearance of toxicity at variable durations of treatment and at variable cumulative doses in some patients may be related to the difference in absorption and bioavailability of the drug.[38] Although there is some evidence that the early electrophysiologic changes may be reversible, in most cases, once visual loss has occurred, it is irreversible and may progress long after cessation of treatment (Figure 9.01E–L).[11,14,20,39] There may be an interval of 7 years or longer after cessation of chloroquine and the development of the first signs of retinopathy.[39] Some patients with disease attributed to late onset and progression of chloroquine retinopathy may in fact have had a genetically determined disease that can cause fundus changes identical to chloroquine retinopathy (e.g., cone dystrophy, rod–cone dystrophy, ceroid lipofuscinosis, and Stargardt's disease).

9.02 Continued

I–N: A 34-year-old Indian woman received chloroquine for 2 years. Both macula have an incomplete bull's-eye appearance (I and J) that are more visible and widespread on auto fluorescence imaging (K and L). Multifocal electroretinogram shows patchy photoreceptor dysfunction with reduced amplitudes in the fovea in both eyes (M and N).

(I–N, courtesy of Dr. Vishali Gupta and Dr. Amod Gupta.)

Amplitudes P1(b)

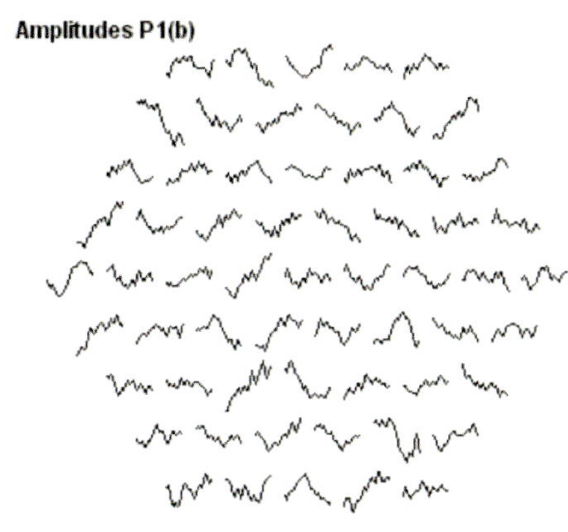

3D Amplitudes P1(b)

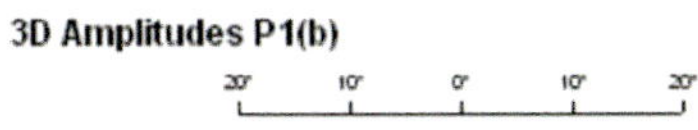

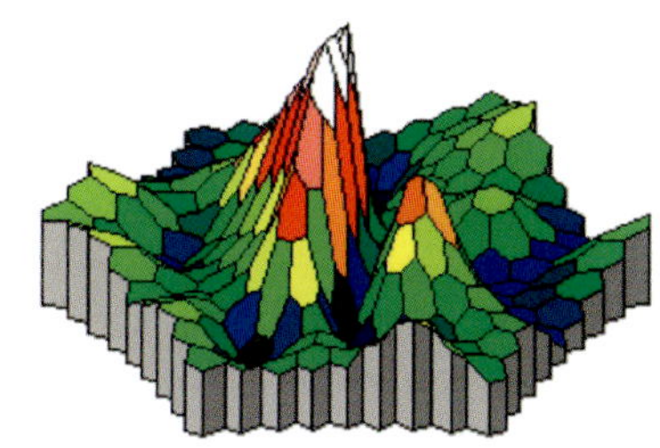

(M) OD

Amplitudes P1(b)

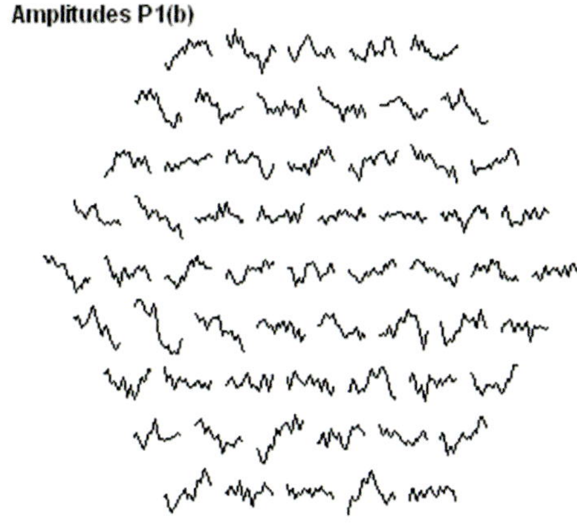

3D Amplitudes P1(b)

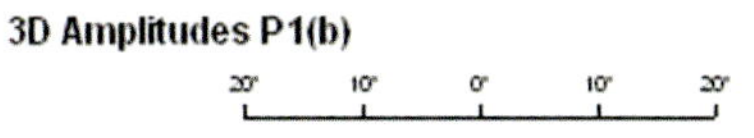

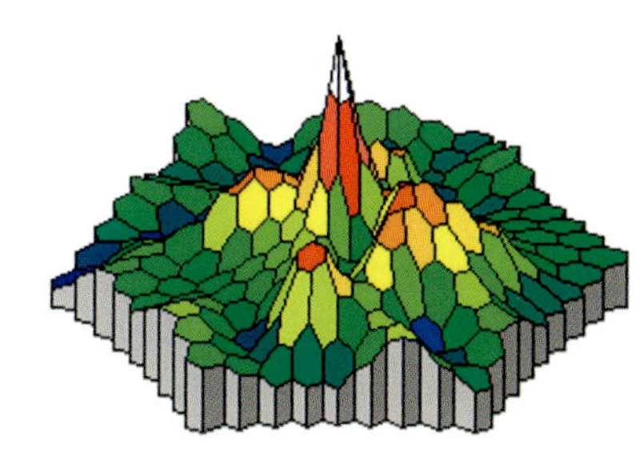

(N) OS

THIORIDAZINE (MELLARIL) RETINOPATHY

Patients with acute thioridazine retinopathy typically experience blurred vision, dyschromatopsia (brownish coloration), or nyctalopia 3–8 weeks after receiving the drug in excess of 800 mg/day[40–53] and less frequently in lower doses.[40,46] Maximum daily dose seems more critical than cumulative dose. The fundus may be normal initially. Later a mild, fine, then coarse granular salt-and-pepper pigmentary retinopathy with a relatively uniform distribution involving the macula and sometimes the midperiphery as well, may occur (Figure 9.03A). In some patients this may progress to include patchy or nummular areas of loss of the RPE and choriocapillaris (Figure 9.03D–L)[2,48–50] and may eventually progress to a severe diffuse tapetoretinal degeneration. Progression of the pigmentary changes but not necessarily functional changes may occur after the medication is discontinued.[42,49,54] Visual function may occasionally improve after cessation of toxic levels of the drug.[54] Other patients, however, may experience a late, slow progression of functional as well as anatomic changes. The progressive enlargement and confluence of patches of extrafoveal geographic atrophy of the RPE and choriocapillaris are similar to those seen in gyrate atrophy, Bietti's crystalline dystrophy, and choroideremia. Fluorescein angiography may be helpful in detecting mild RPE alterations (Figure 9.03B and C). The ERG responses may be normal early but become attenuated later in more severe cases.

Histopathologically, thioridazine retinopathy is associated with atrophy and disorganization of the photoreceptor outer segments followed by loss of the RPE and choriocapillaris.[50]

Retinotoxicity has been attributed to concentration of the drug within melanin granules in the uveal melanocytes and RPE.[50,51] The drug inhibits oxidative phosphorylation, resulting in abnormal rhodopsin synthesis, which causes disintegration of rod outer segments.[55] The RPE is overtaxed with accumulation of lipofuscin as abnormal pigment granules. In addition it is believed that thioridazine and other phenothiazines block the D4 dopamine receptors with subsequent increase in retinal melatonin synthesis and activity. This occurs in the photoreceptors and RPE where the D4 subtype of the D2-receptor family is predominant.[56] Thioridazine has a structure similar to NP-207, an experimental drug that was never marketed because of severe retinotoxicity.[57] There is no specific treatment other than stopping the medication.

9.03 Thioridazine (Mellaril) retinopathy.

A–C: Mild visual loss occurred in a 21-year-old woman with schizophrenia who received thioridazine, 800 mg/day, for 3 years. The mild pigment epithelial alterations (A) were more apparent angiographically (B and C).

D–G: This 60-year-old woman received thioridazine daily for 11 years beginning at age 25 years. She was asymptomatic visually and had 20/20 visual acuity bilaterally until age 55, when she developed nyctalopia and paracentral scotomas. Her visual acuity was 20/25, right eye, and 20/50, left eye. She had widely scattered areas of geographic atrophy of the retinal pigment epithelium (RPE) that included the macular area (D–F).

G–L: This 48-year-old woman complained of progressive constriction of her visual fields for years, more prominent in the past 6 months. Her vision was 20/40 OD and 20/80 OS. She had received thioridazine for 2 years, which was discontinued 15 years prior following development of retinal and visual field changes. She had nummular areas of RPE loss in both eyes (G, H, and L) progressing to choroidal and retinal vascular attenuation and optic atrophy (I–K).

(G–L, courtesy of Dr. Michael Altaweel.)

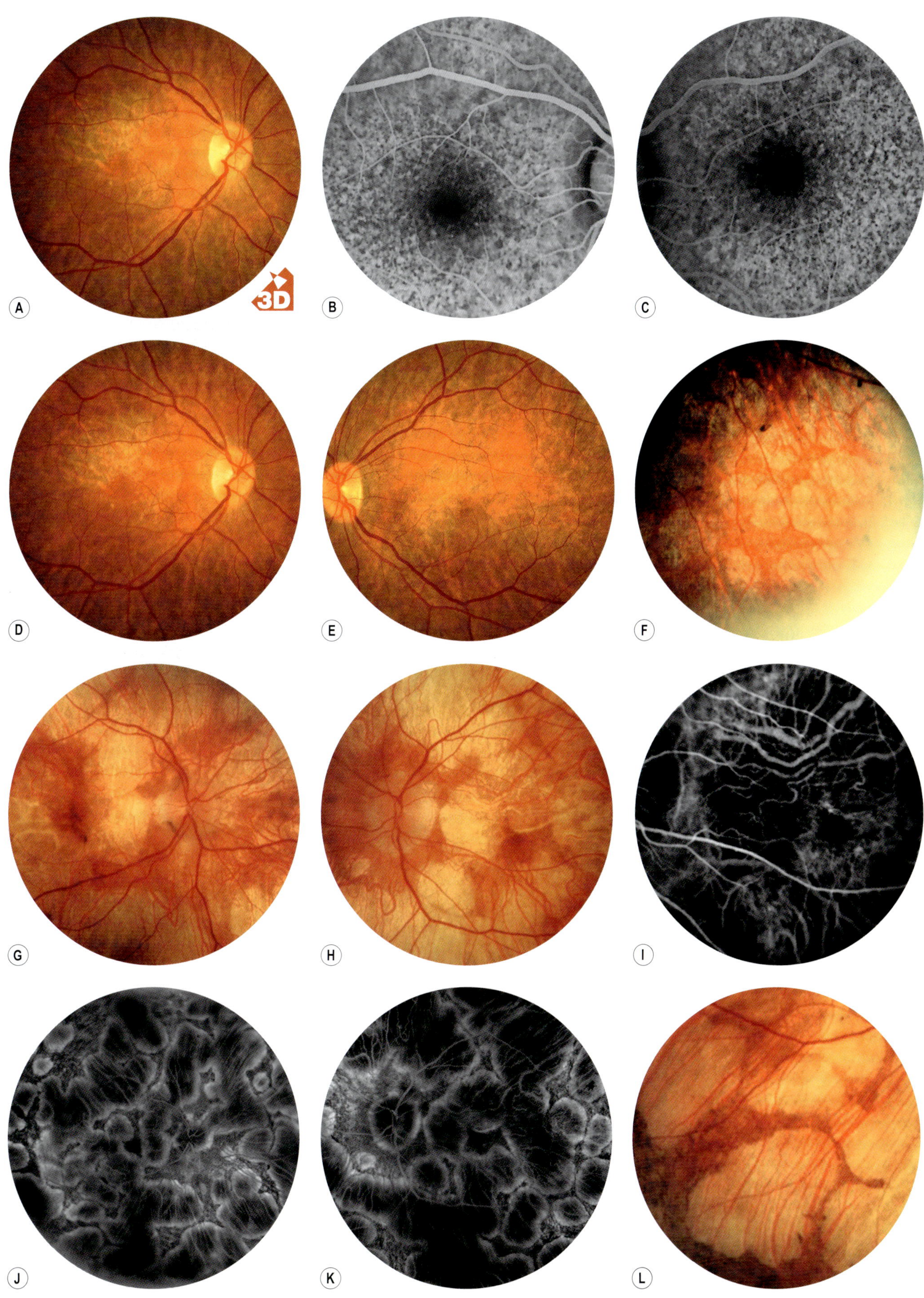
3D
A
B
C
D
E
F
G
H
I
J
K
L

CHLORPROMAZINE (THORAZINE) RETINOPATHY

Chlorpromazine rarely causes retinal toxicity. When taken in large doses in the range of 2400 mg/day over 12 months it may cause mild pigmentary changes in the retina (Figure 9.04A and B).[58–60] These rarely are associated with visual or functional deficits. Because patients receiving chlorpromazine have often received other medications that may have included potentially retinotoxic drugs, assignment of the exact cause of the retinopathy may be difficult. White and yellow-white granular deposits may occur in the axial part of the anterior subcapsular region of the lens, and in the posterior layers of the cornea in patients receiving 300 mg/day of chlorpromazine for 3 years or more.[59] The usual dosage of chlorpromazine is 40–75 mg/day, although dosages up to 800 mg/day are not uncommon.

CLOFAZIMINE RETINOPATHY

Clofazimine is a red iminophenazine dye used concurrently with dapsone and rifampin as the treatment of choice for lepromatous leprosy, for treatment of dapsone-resistant leprosy, and for *Mycobacterium avium* complex infections in patients with acquired immunodeficiency syndrome (AIDS). After several months of treatment, clofazimine crystals may accumulate in the ocular tissues. Reversible side-effects include a superficial whorl pattern of anterior corneal pigmented lines, brownish discoloration of the conjunctiva and tears, and crystals in the iris and sclera. A large bull's-eye pattern of pigment epithelial atrophy (Figure 9.04C and D) has occurred in two patients following 200 mg/day (total dose of approximately 48 g) and after 300 mg/day (total dose of approximately 40 g).[61,62] This was associated with reduced ERG b-waves and full-field photopic and scotopic as well as flicker amplitudes.

9.04 Chlorpromazine and trifluoperazine retinopathy.

A–B: This 41-year-old schizophrenic woman received chlorpromazine (Thorazine) and trifluoperazine (Stelazine) for many years. There was no definite history of treatment with thioridazine. Her visual acuity in both eyes was 20/30. She had diminished photopic and scotopic responses electroretinographically. The patchy and nummular areas of atrophy of the retinal pigment epithelium (RPE) (arrows A and B) were similar to those caused by thioridazine toxicity.

Clofazimine retinopathy.

C and **D**: After 8 months of treatment with 48 g clofazimine for *Mycobacterium avium* complex associated with acquired immunodeficiency syndrome (AIDS), this patient developed a bull's-eye pattern of RPE mottled depigmentation in the macula bilaterally. His visual acuity was 20/25. There was some generalized reduction of all components of his electroretinogram (ERG) responses. His color vision (AOHRR pseudoisochromatic plates) was normal.

Deferoxamine toxicity.

E–L: This 72-year-old woman complained of gradual onset of blurred vision in both eyes and yellowish discoloration of vision for 2 months. Her visual acuity was 20/20 2 months prior to presentation. Her vision had dropped now to 20/25 in the right eye and 20/40 in the left eye. The fundus in both eyes showed peripapillary areas of RPE mottling that were more visible on the red-free photographs (E and F). A fluorescein angiogram showed leopard spot-like pigmentary changes corresponding to the pigment mottling (G and H). She had a history of sideroblastic anemia and had received intravenous desferrioxamine for 5 months for iron overload secondary to blood transfusions. She continued to develop pigmentary changes in the macula (I to L). Her ERG showed subnormal rod and cone function with decreased amplitudes and increased latency. Humphrey visual field showed enlarged blind spot with central visual field suppression.

(C and D, From Cunningham et al.[62]) (E–L, courtesy of Dr. Seenu Hariprasad.)

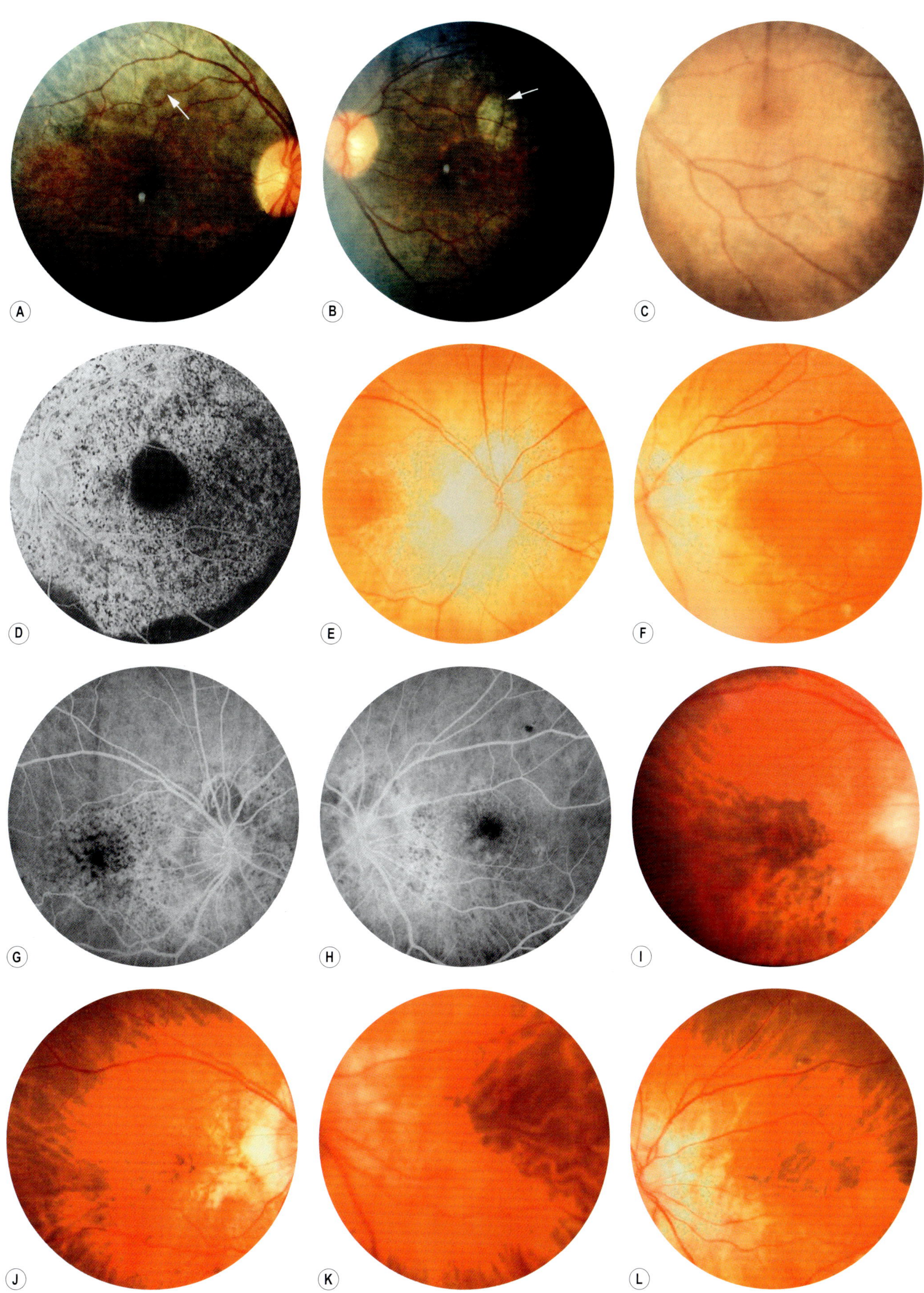
A
B
C
D
E
F
G
H
I
J
K
L

DEFEROXAMINE MACULOPATHY

Intravenous administration of deferoxamine mesylate (DFO), 3–12 g/24 hours, for the treatment of transfusional hemosiderosis has produced rapid onset of visual loss; color vision abnormalities; nyctalopia; a ring scotoma; reduced electroretinographic, electro-oculographic, dark adaptation, and visual evoked responses; and mid- to high-frequency hearing loss of cochlear type.[63–70] The fundi may be normal initially or there may be a slight graying of the macula (Figure 9.05A). Both eyes are affected. Visual symptoms usually begin 7–10 days after the last treatment. Development of maculopathy may occur after chronic subcutaneous injection of deferoxamine.[71] Fluorescein angiography soon after the onset of visual symptoms in the presence of a normal-appearing fundus may show progressive staining at the level of the RPE in the macular areas, and in some cases leakage of dye from the optic disc vessels (Figure 9.05B and C). Pigmentary changes usually appear within several weeks (Figure 9.05D). After cessation of treatment, return of visual function occurs over 3–4 months and approximately 70% of patients recover normal acuity. Two 70-year-old patients developed pseudovitelliform lesions in the macula of both eyes while on low-dose deferoxamine.[72] Reversible EOG changes have been noted,[68] and a drop in the Arden ratio to less than 1.5 was seen in another patient on DFO for 2 years. On cessation of DFO following splenectomy her EOG and visual acuity returned to normal, hence EOG at regular intervals may be used as a monitor for toxicity.[73] Some patients show increase in both rod and cone implicit times and reduction of a- and b-wave amplitudes.[74] The mechanism of retinal toxicity is unknown. Although chelation of iron is unlikely to be the explanation, removal of other metals, particularly copper, from the RPE may be important.[65,68] Copper fluxes may cause oxidative cell membrane resulting in lipid peroxidation products that are toxic to the RPE. Copper movement into extracellular fluids may interrupt monoaminergic neurotransmission in the retina.[75] Light microscopic and ultrastructural changes in the RPE in an eye of a patient studied after recovery of visual function included patchy depigmentation and thinning, loss of microvilli from the apical surface, vacuolization of the cytoplasm, swelling and calcification of mitochondria, disorganization of the plasma membrane, and thickening of Bruch's membrane.[69]

More recently an oral agent Exjade is being used as a chelating agent in patients receiving repeated blood transfusions. Figure 9.05E–L shows a patient who continued to develop macular and extramacular pigmentary changes even after being switched to Exjade. High-frequency sensorineural loss and bone dysplasia are other features of deferoxamine toxicity.

9.05 Deferoxamine retinopathy.

A–D: This 64-year-old woman with chronic renal failure and renal dialysis developed severe osteoporosis that was thought to be related to excessive absorption of aluminum from the dialysate used to treat her renal insufficiency.[67] Following intravenous deferoxamine the patient noted dyschromatopsia, blurring of vision, and difficulty in reading. At the time of examination 15 days after her intravenous therapy her visual acuity was 20/30. She had 10° central relative scotomata. Fundoscopic examination showed slight graying of the retina paracentrally (A). Fluorescein angiography showed a mottled pattern of hyperfluorescence throughout the macula and a central area of staining at the level of the RPE (B and C). She noted rapid improvement of her vision soon after her examination. When seen 8 months later, her only complaint was mild dyschromatopsia and her visual acuity was 20/20 in the right eye and 20/25 in the left eye. There was mottling of the RPE in the macular areas of both eyes (D).

E–L: This 80-year-old male suffered from myelofibrosis for the previous 3 years and received deferoxamine (Desferal) a year later. Six to eight weeks following initiation of Desferal he noticed rapid development of circumscribed circular scotomas in both eyes with progressive worsening. He underwent cataract extraction in both eyes 3 months later with improvement of vision to 20/60 OU. Visual deterioration continued, he was switched to deferasirox (Exjade) 9 months later when his vision was 20/200 in both eyes. Coarse pigment clumping in the fovea and diffuse pigment mottling throughout the postequatorial fundus were noted. Fluorescein angiogram revealed pigment alteration and disrupted RPE in the fovea. Goldmann visual fields were full peripherally with central scotomas of 10–15° OU. Electroretinogram showed marked decrease in rod function and mild to moderate decrease in cone function. His copper and zinc levels were normal, he had no hearing problem, and Exjade could not be discontinued due to iron overload. He was started on AREDS (age-related eye disease study) vitamins.

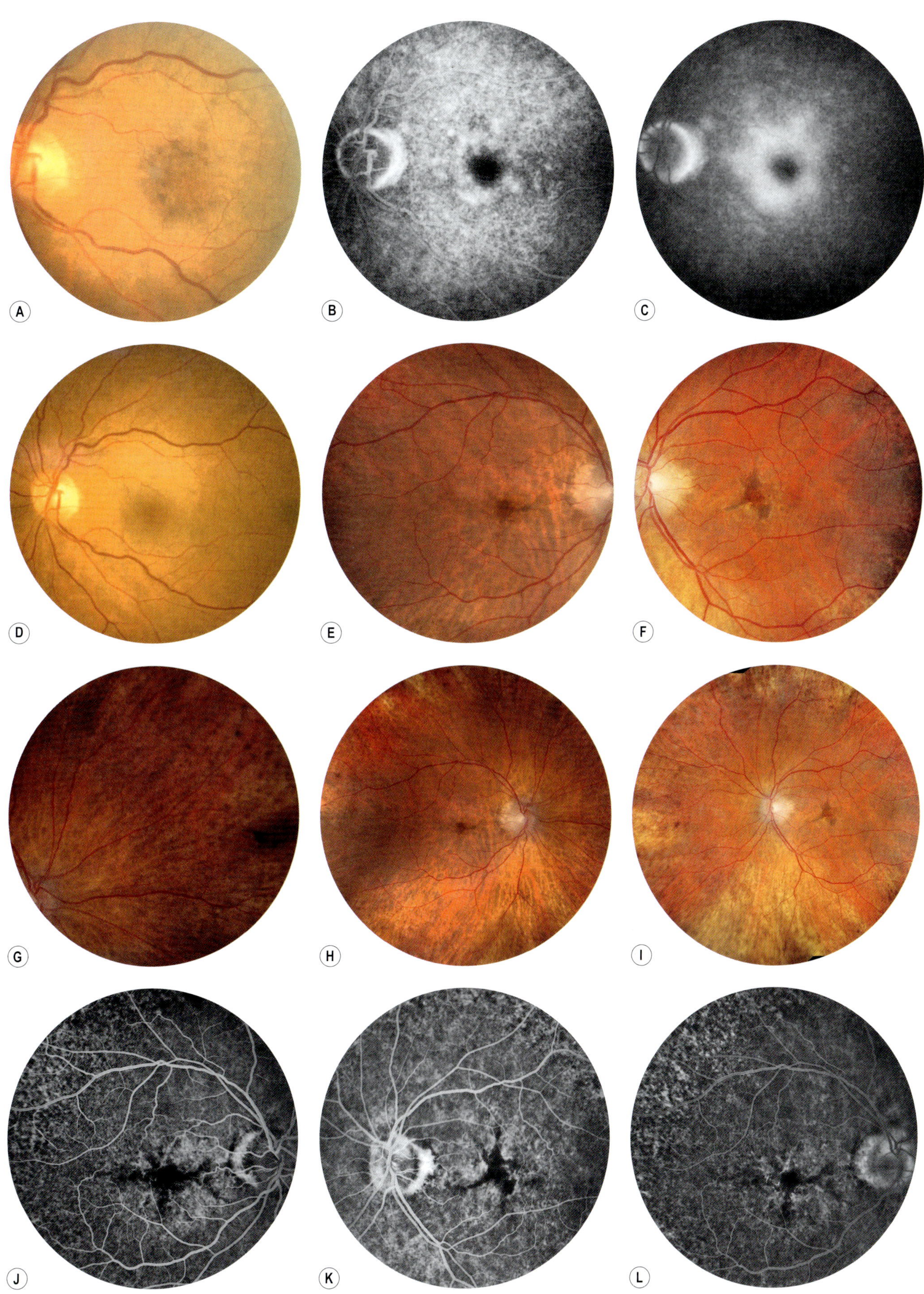
A
B
C
D
E
F
G
H
I
J
K
L

SIDEROTIC RETINOPATHY

If iron-containing foreign bodies enter the eye, the iron may become oxidized and be bound to the ocular tissues, producing either localized siderosis or, particularly when the foreign body lodges in the vitreoretinal region, diffuse ocular siderosis (Figure 9.06A–E).[76–78] Evidence of ocular siderosis includes pupillary mydriasis, darkening of the iris (Figure 9.06D), and orange deposits in the anterior subcapsular region of the lens. Posteriorly, hazy ocular media may preclude visualization of the fundus. Early optic disc hyperemia and fluorescein angiographic evidence of leakage may be present. Later a picture simulating pigmentary degeneration of the retina and progressive loss of peripheral visual fields may occur (Figure 9.06A and B). These changes may be associated with optic disc hyperemia. Retinal vascular narrowing, and occasionally microangiopathy with vascular occlusion and leakage are seen.[79,80] Abnormalities in the ERG eventually occur (Figure 9.06E) and may be reversible following early removal of the intraocular iron foreign body.[81–84] Histopathologically, the iron is initially deposited primarily in the inner retina and RPE. Eventually, however, degeneration may affect all layers of the retina.

The natural course of a retained intraocular iron foreign body is variable. In some cases the foreign body may be absorbed or become encapsulated and the siderosis may stabilize or regress.[85,86] In some cases the hyperpigmentation of the encapsulated mass may simulate a choroidal melanoma (Figure 8.11B–E).[87] In general, intraocular iron foreign bodies should be removed, particularly from an eye showing evidence of siderosis.[88] Removal of foreign bodies deeply embedded in the ocular wall or of largely oxidized foreign bodies may be difficult or impossible.

An acute pigment epitheliopathy, serous retinal detachment, and transient visual loss occurred in a patient with systemic hypertension and chronic glomerulonephritis after intravenous administration of iron dextran.[89]

Experimental injection of iron powder or iron-containing solutions into the vitreous may produce acute geographic areas of retinal whitening (Figure 9.06F–K), fluorescein angiographic evidence of severe disruption of the RPE (Figure 9.06G), and a diminished or nonrecordable ERG within the first 24 hours of the injection.[90] A zone of focal atrophy of the RPE surrounded by a zone of pigment epithelial clumping develops within a few weeks (Figure 9.06H and I). Histologically, the primary damage is to the receptor cells and RPE (Figure 9.06J and K). Retinal damage is much more severe with ferrous than with ferric compounds.

9.06 Siderosis bulbi.

A–C: This man was blind in the left eye because of siderosis following two unsuccessful attempts at removal of a retained intraocular foreign body 8 years previously. Note the severe atrophy of the retina and retinal pigment epithelium (RPE) and the delayed perfusion of the retina and choroidal blood vessels angiographically (A and B). Ultrasonography (C) confirmed the presence of the foreign body. The electroretinogram (ERG) was extinguished in the left eye.
D and **E**: This 44-year-old construction worker who hammers metal on metal noted "his eyes were changing." The left iris is siderotic (D). His visual acuity was 20/20 in the right eye and 20/70 in the left. Visual field was full on the right and constricted on the left side. An ERG shows significant decrease in scotopic and photopic function with delayed rod implicit time and decreased rod and cone amplitudes (E).

Acute siderotic maculopathy in a primate.

F–K: This squirrel monkey developed a circular white area in the macula 1 day after the intravitreal injection of 0.01 mg iron as ferrous chloride (F). Fluorescein angiography revealed transmission of the choroidal fluorescence and later intense staining in the area of this whitening (G). Twenty-eight days later there was a circumscribed area of RPE depigmentation surrounded by a halo of hyperpigmentation in the macular area (H). A window defect in the RPE was evident angiographically (I). A phase-contrast micrograph made 1 day after intravitreal injection of iron powder showed pyknosis of the outer retinal cell nuclei and edema of the inner retina (J). A phase-contrast micrograph 28 days following intravitreal injection showed a sharp demarcation between the normal and atrophic outer retinal layers in the macular region (K).

(A–C, courtesy of Dr. Scot R. Sneed; D and E, courtesy of Dr. Timothy Olsen; J and K from Masciulli et al.[90] Published with permission from The American Journal of Ophthalmology; copyright Ophthalmic Publishing Co.)

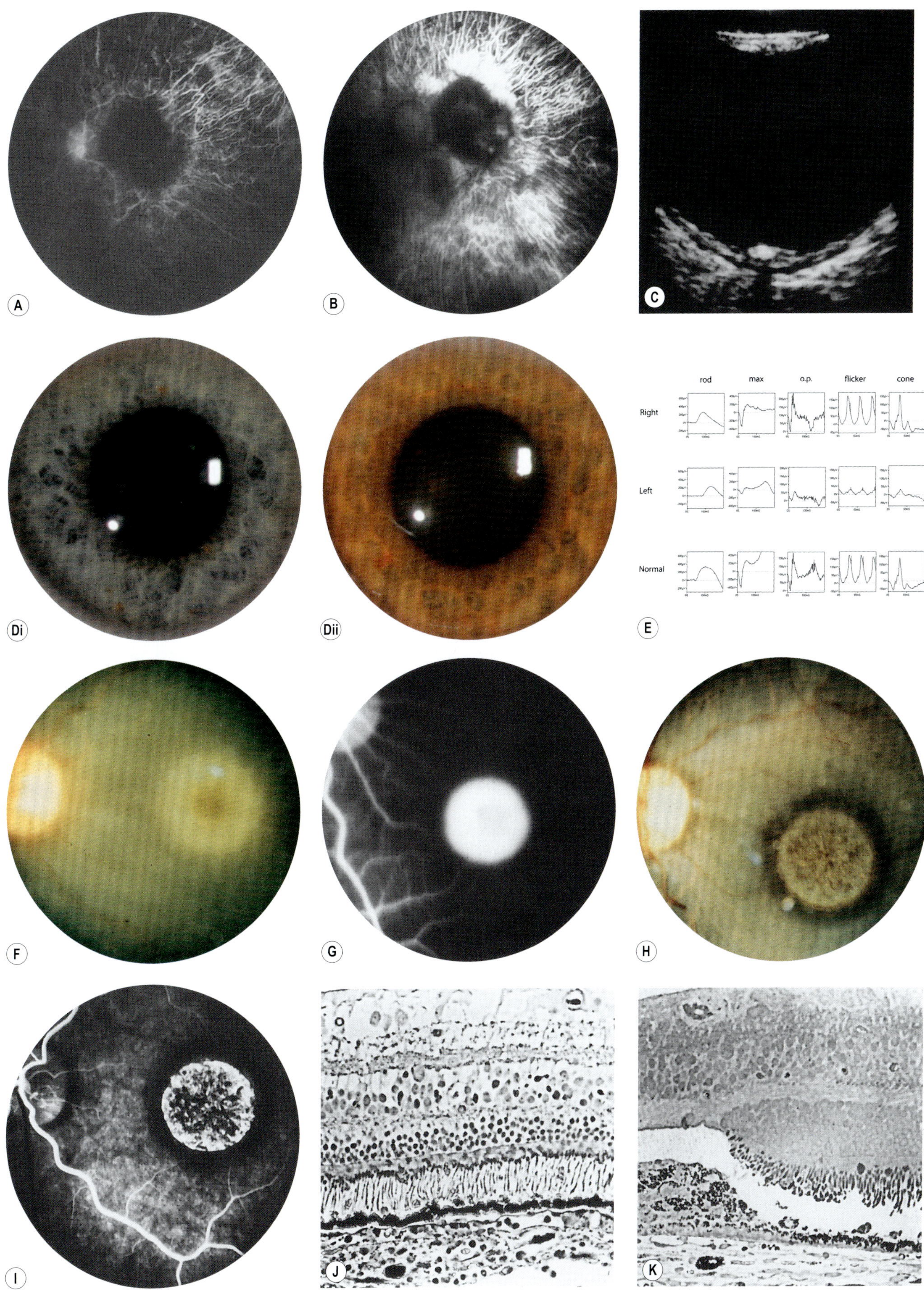
A
B
C
Di
Dii
E
rod
max
o.p.
flicker
cone
Right
Left
Normal
F
G
H
I
J
K

CHALCOSIS MACULOPATHY

Patients with an intraocular copper foreign body may show a wide spectrum of reactions to its presence. In the case of a copper alloy, the inflammatory reaction may be minimal and a slow diffusion of copper occurs and impregnates limiting membranes of the eye to produce the picture of chalcosis that may include peripheral corneal ring, sunflower cataract (see Figure 8.11I), and heterochromia of the iris.[91–93] In addition, irregular yellowish-golden flakes may be deposited in the macular area away from the site of the foreign body (Figure 9.07A and B).[91,92] It is presumed that these apparently inert deposits are either copper carbonates or oxides. They appear to have little effect on visual acuity. Their location is uncertain, but they appear to be deep to the retinal vessels. These flakes disappear after removal of the foreign body (Figure 9.07C).[91,92] The ERG is subnormal in approximately 50% of patients with chalcosis.

Experimentally, copper has been found in the macrophages within the retina, in Müller cells, and in granular clumps scattered throughout the retina.[93,94] Clinicopathologic study in eyes with retained copper foreign bodies show copper deposits in Descemet's membrane, vitreous, internal limiting membrane of the retina, and fibrous capsule around the foreign bodies. Eyes with foreign bodies containing more than 85% copper show more disseminated copper deposits and eyes with alloy containing less than 85% copper show more localized deposits. Retinal structures are usually well preserved, even in eyes with an intraocular copper foreign body retained for 22 years.[95]

ARGYROSIS

Argyrosis may be associated with discoloration of the skin, mucous membranes, and many of the body organs occurring with application of colloidal silver-containing eye drops, eyelash tint, in photographers, photochemists, miners, silversmiths and industrial workers using silver-containing compounds. When this discoloration is confined to the eye following topical application of silver compounds to the eye, the blue-gray discoloration of the conjunctiva and cornea (Figure 9.07D) is referred to as argyria. The discoloration is caused by deposition of silver in the basement membrane of the conjunctiva and cornea, as well as in Descemet's membrane. Occupational exposure in a silversmith from Italy was found to deposit the metal in the endothelial basement membranes of the conjunctiva and deep corneal stroma just anterior to the endothelium.[96] Peripheral and central or diffuse corneal deposition has been noted, with the central involvement occurring with longer exposure. Patients with argyrosis caused by chronic ingestion of silver-containing compounds may develop discoloration of the skin and body organs, as well as loss of the normal choroidal markings in the ocular fundus, a "dark" choroid fluorescein angiographically, and a leopard-spot mottling of the ocular fundus when viewed with red-free light (Figure 9.07E–G).[97] These fundus changes are probably caused by loss of transparency of Bruch's membrane as a result of deposition of silver in the membrane (Figure 9.07H).[97,98] The discoloration is permanent and chelation therapy is ineffective.

9.07 Chalcosis.

A–C: Copper deposits in the macula of an 18-year-old patient with a posterior dislocated lens. He sustained an intraocular copper foreign-body injury 5 years previously. These deposits disappeared 14 months after removal of the foreign body (C). His visual acuity was 20/20.

Argyrosis.

D: Bluish discoloration of the conjunctiva (argyrosis).

E–G: Dark choroid (G) associated with argyrosis of Bruch's membrane in a patient with systemic argyrosis caused by using a mouth wash containing silver (Collargent Acetarsol, Sarbach, Suresnes, France) 3 times a day for 3 years. Red light photograph shows no details of choroidal circulation and leopard spot pattern of the fundus temporally (E) that is accentuated in the infrared light photograph (F).

H: Photomicrographs showing argyrosis of the retinal pigment epithelium and Bruch's membrane (arrows).

(A–C, From Delaney,[91] E and G, from Cohen et al.,[97] H, from Spencer et al.[98])

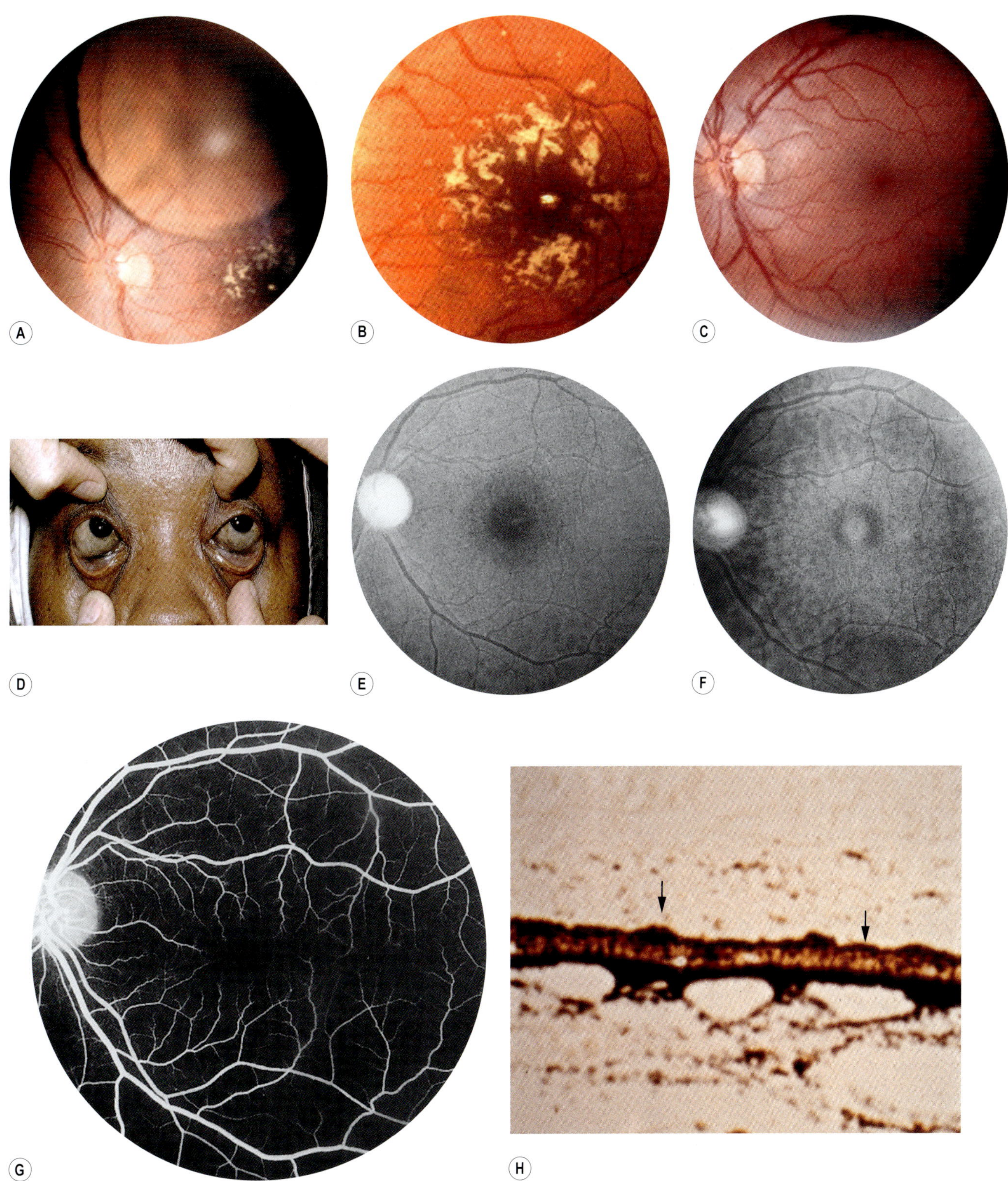
A
B
C
D
E
F
G
H

CISPLATINUM AND BCNU (CARMUSTINE) RETINOPATHY

Intracarotid arterial chemotherapy with BCNU (1,3-*bis*-(9,2-chlorethyl)-1-nitrosourea), 300–400 mg, and cisplatinum (*cis*-diammine dichloroplatinum(II)), 200 mg, is used for treatment of recurrent malignant gliomas of the brain. This may cause precipitous ipsilateral visual loss and fundus changes of two different types. Patients receiving BCNU either alone or in combination with cisplatinum may develop visual loss associated with ophthalmoscopic signs of retinal infarction, retinal periarteritis and phlebitis, and papillitis.[99–106] A retinopathy similar to interferon retinopathy with severe bilateral retinal ischemia leading to retinal neovascularization has been described (Figure 9.08G–J).[107] The mechanism of the vasculopathy is believed to be from increased platelet reactivity to nonaggregating concentration of the agonists involved in the arachidonic acid metabolism (increased thromboxane synthesis and early onset of platelet aggregation wave). The retinopathy was found to be reversible or stable; however the field defect and vision loss from optic neuropathy progressed even after discontinuation of the drug.[108] Other findings may include cavernous sinus syndrome, partial sixth- and third-nerve palsies, severe conjunctival injection and chemosis, pain, and secondary glaucoma. Approximately 65% of patients treated develop these findings accompanied by visual loss about 6 weeks after the start of treatment. Once visual loss begins it is usually progressive and severe.

Intracarotid injection above the level of the ophthalmic artery does not protect from development of ocular complications.[103] Those treated with cisplatinum alone or in combination with BCNU may develop visual loss associated with a pigmentary retinopathy, with a central scotoma, and later diffuse constriction of the visual field.[99,102,109] The ERG may be nonrecordable in some patients.[104,109] The visual symptoms and pigmentary changes are usually mild following administration of cisplatinum alone and appear to be potentiated with the addition of BCNU.[109] Figure 9.08A–F shows pigmentary retinopathy in two patients treated with cisplatinum and bleomycin. A similar pigmentary maculopathy has been reported after a combination of intracarotid injection of mannitol and methotrexate together with intravenous administration of cyclophosphamide.[110] Mannitol disruption of the blood–ocular barrier was thought to be instrumental in the macular changes, which typically do not occur with use of the two drugs alone (see Chapter 13).

9.08 Cisplatinum and bleomycin chorioretinal toxicity.

A–E: This 46-year-old man had a right-sided intracarotid injection of cisplatinum and bleomycin for treatment of a glioblastoma of the brain. He noted the immediate sensation of heat behind the ipsilateral eye, and transient paralysis of the right arm. One day later he noted visual loss in the right eye. Eight days later visual acuity in the right eye was light perception only. The left eye was normal. Examination of the right fundus revealed swelling of the optic disc, narrowing of the retinal vessels, and subtle retinal pigment epithelium (RPE) mottling that was more apparent angiographically (A and B). Eight days later visual acuity was hand movements and there was prominent mottling of the RPE (C–E).

F: This 36-year-old man experienced rapid visual loss 2 weeks previously several days following a left-sided intracarotid injection of cisplatinum and bleomycin. His visual acuity was 20/20 right eye and 20/400 left eye. Note the mottling of the RPE in the left macula.

G–J: This patient received polychemotherapy (bleomycin, etoposide, and cisplatin) for a recurrence of germ cell testicular tumor. Ten weeks after treatment, he lost vision in his left eye. He had bilateral widespread retinal ischemia with cotton-wool spots, superficial retinal hemorrhages, microaneurysm formation, and neovascularization in the left eye (G, H). Fluorescein angiography revealed patchy bilateral retinal ischemia, leaking capillaries and microaneurysms and enlarged foveal avascular zone with areas of NVE on the left (I and J). Systemic causes were thoroughly investigated and excluded.

(G–J, From Kwan et al.[107])

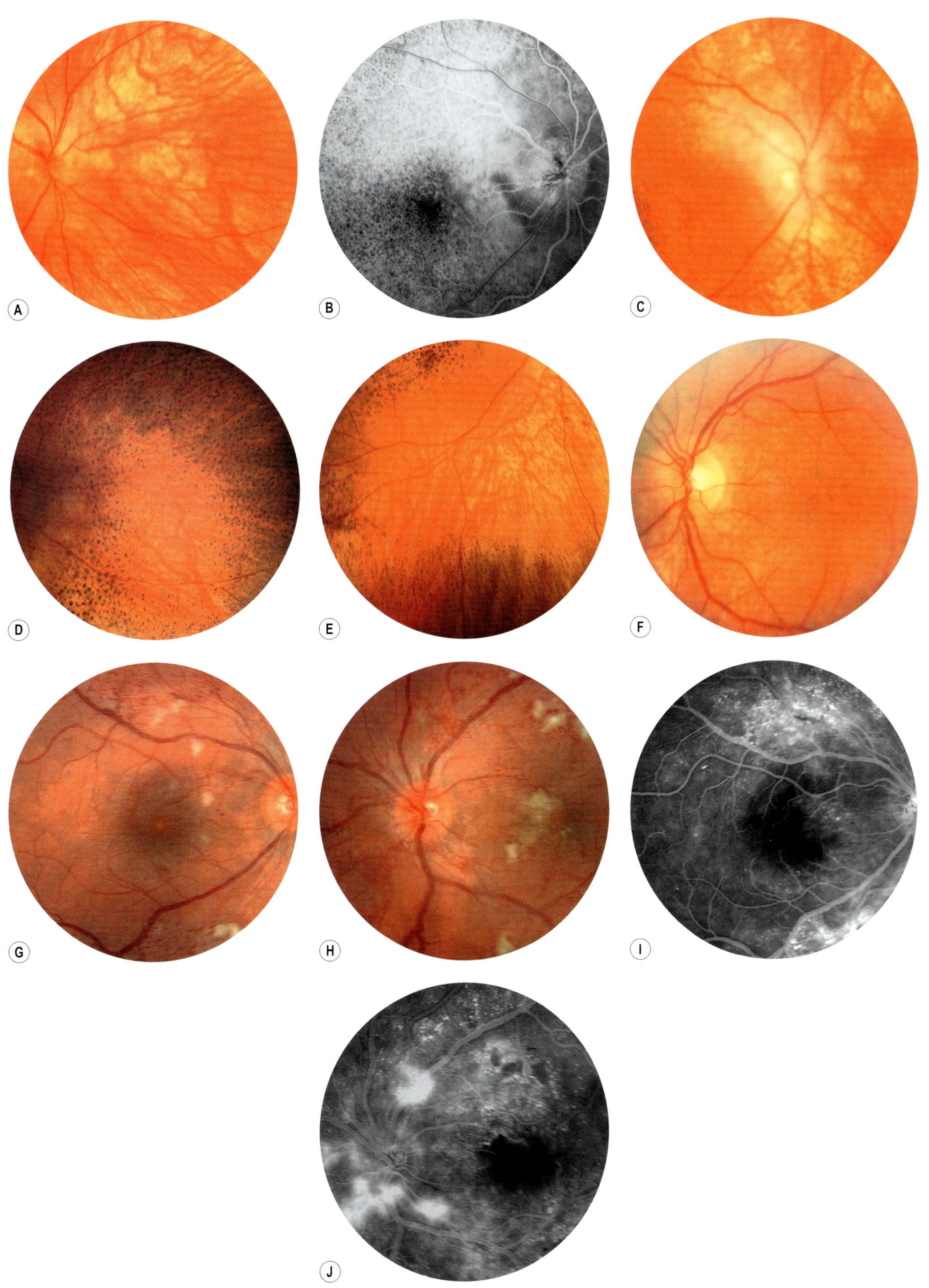
A
B
C
D
E
F
G
H
I
J

TAMOXIFEN RETINOPATHY

Tamoxifen citrate, a nonsteroidal antiestrogen, is used to treat patients with breast carcinoma and more recently as high-dose therapy for brain tumors.[111] Patients who receive high doses of tamoxifen (total amount of drug in excess of 90g) may develop loss of central vision, macular edema, and superficial white refractile deposits that are located primarily in the inner layers of the retina (Figure 9.09A, B, D, and E).[112–115] There may be punctate gray lesions at the level of the outer retina and RPE that appear nonfluorescent (hypofluorescent) angiographically (Figure 9.09F). Refractile lesions are more numerous and larger in the paramacular area, are more heavily concentrated temporal to the macula, and show some tendency to clump. Peripheral crystals can occur in some cases. OCT confirms the inner retinal loation.[116,117] The number and size of the lesions do not change after cessation of tamoxifen. Light microscopy and electron microscopy show that the retractile lesions are located in the nerve fiber and inner plexiform layers.[112] They are intracellular and stain positively for glycosaminoglycans. The lesions appear to represent products of axonal degeneration. Histopathologically they are similar to corpora amylacea but are larger and more numerous in the paramacular area than the peripapillary area.

There is evidence that long-term low-dosage tamoxifen may cause retinopathy.[118–122] In a prospective study of 63 patients receiving a median dose of 20mg/day tamoxifen for a median duration of 25 months, four patients developed retinopathy and/or keratopathy 10, 27, 31, and 35 months after commencement of treatment.[122] The mean total dose in these four patients was 14.4g. Decreased acuity, bilateral macular edema, and yellow-white dots in the paramacular and foveal areas occurred in all four patients and corneal opacities occurred in one patient. After withdrawal of drug, almost all ocular complications were reversible.[118,122]

Heier and coworkers found mild deposition of intraretinal crystals in only two of 135 visually asymptomatic tamoxifen-treated patients (mean cumulative dose 17.2g).[121] The two patients with crystals had a cumulative dose of 10.9 and 21.9g, respectively. In severe cases OCT shows intraretinal pseudocyst formation similar to those seen in idiopathic type 2 juxtafoveolar telangiectasia, likely from axonal degeneration of Müller cells and photoreceptors.[116,117,123] The pseudocyst gradually enlarges with rupture of the inner layer to result in a macular hole.[124] Transient bilateral optic disc edema, retinal hemorrhages, and macular edema may occasionally occur after starting low-dose tamoxifen daily.[111,118,120] Multifocal ERG done prospectively to monitor for macular toxicity is not useful even in patients who develop crystals.[125]

OXALOSIS

Oxalosis is the deposition of calcium oxalate in various tissues of the body. The eye may be solely involved or may be involved as part of systemic oxalosis. Systemic oxalosis may be the result of: (1) a primary hyperoxaluria secondary to an inborn error of metabolism types 1 and 2 (see Chapter 5); (2) a toxic reaction to ethylene glycol or methoxyflurane general anesthesia;[126–128] or (3) chronic renal failure and hemodialysis.[129] Ocular involvement in secondary systemic oxalosis has been observed after use of methoxyflurane, which is a nonflammable anesthetic. When administered to patients with renal dysfunction and particularly if administered over a prolonged period of time, it may cause irreversible renal failure secondary to the metabolic breakdown of the anesthetic to oxalic acid and fluoride ions (Figure 9.09K). These patients, as well as those with primary hyperoxaluria, may develop numerous yellow-white, punctate, crystalline lesions diffusely scattered throughout the posterior pole and midperiphery of the eyes (see Figures 5.67 and 9.09G and H). In some, the crystals appear to be most prominent in the pigment epithelium with surrounding areas of hypertrophic and hyperplastic RPE (Figure 9.09I),[126,127] and in others, along the retinal arteries (Figure 9.09G).[128,129] Less commonly the crystals are intraretinal, and optic atrophy is seen occasionally. In patients with methoxyflurane toxicity the retinal and pigment epithelial crystals may occur in the absence of changes in the optic disc, the macula, and the caliber of the retinal vessels seen in primary hyperoxaluria (see Figure 5.67). Histopathologically, the flecks seen ophthalmoscopically are calcium oxalate crystals in the RPE, neurosensory retina, and ciliary epithelium (Figure 9.09J and K).[127]

9.09 Tamoxifen retinopathy.

A–C: Following a mastectomy for breast carcinoma this woman received a total dose of 67.5g tamoxifen over a period of 9 years. Her visual acuity was 20/200 in both eyes. Note the intraretinal crystals are more prominent in the left eye.
D–F: This 63-year-old woman, who received a total dose of between 90 and 158g tamoxifen over a period of 29 months for treatment of metastatic breast carcinoma, noted loss of central vision. Visual acuity was 20/50. There were superficial white refractile deposits that appeared to be in the inner layers of the retinas of both eyes (D and E). Note also the white spots in the periphery of the macula that angiographically appeared nonfluorescent (F). Later phase angiograms showed cystoid macular edema. Five months previously her visual acuity had been 20/30 in the right eye and 20/25 in the left eye and the fundi were normal.

Secondary oxalosis.

G and H: Retinal oxalosis in a 34-year-old woman after 2 years of inhalation abuse of methoxyflurane. There were multiple bright yellow-white crystals throughout the retina and pigment epithelium with a retinal arterial and periarterial predilection. She subsequently developed renal failure. Kidney biopsy revealed birefringent crystals in the renal tubule lumens.
I–L: Retinal oxalosis in a 63-year-old man who developed renal failure following methoxyflurane anesthesia (I). He subsequently died, and his eyes were obtained at autopsy. Note the birefringent oxalate crystals present in the retina (J), in the macular region, in the retinal pigment epithelium (K), and in the kidney (L).

(D–F, From McKeown et al.[114] G and H, from Novak et al.[128] I–L,From Bullock and Albert[127])

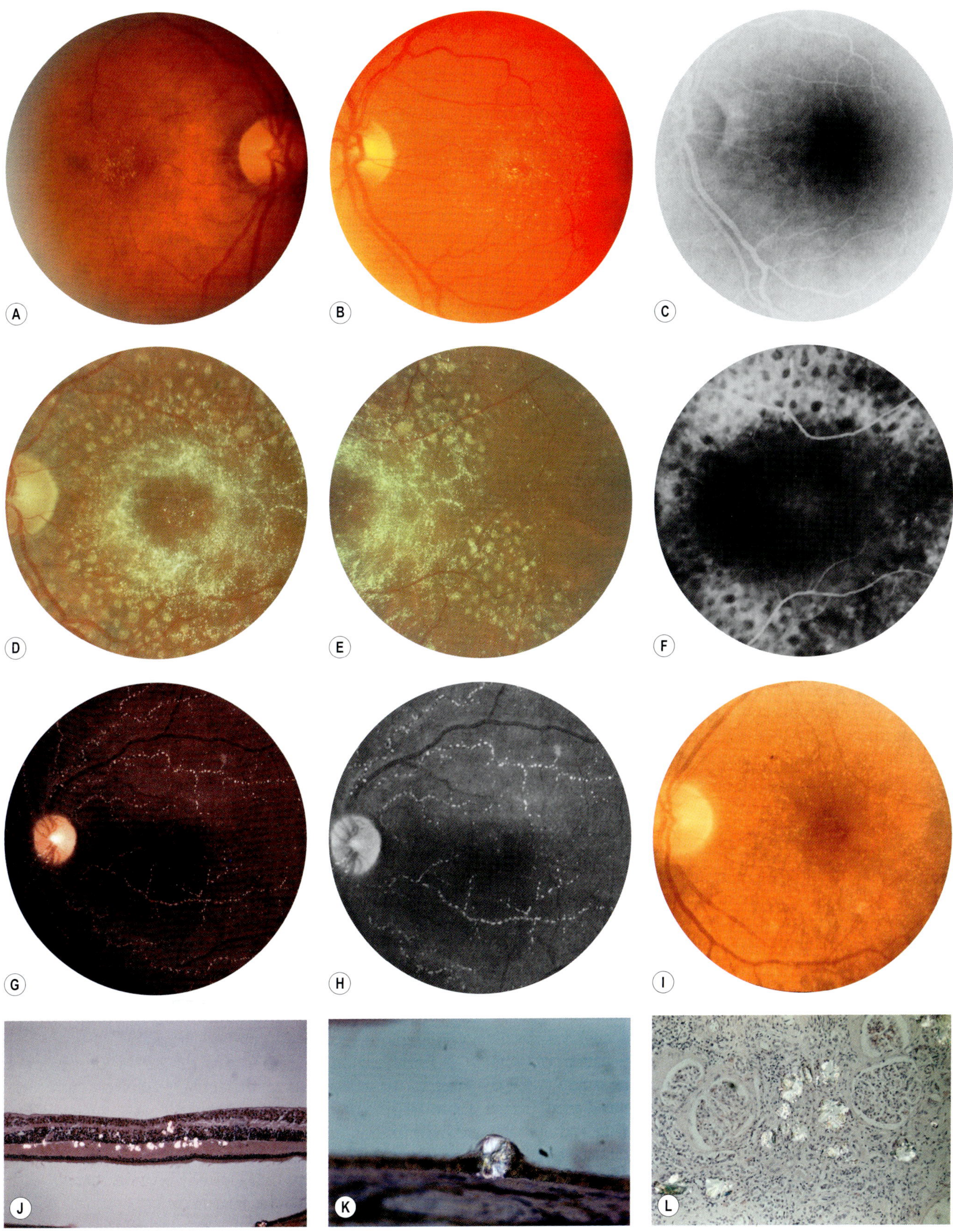
A
B
C
D
E
F
G
H
I
J
K
L

The differential diagnosis includes the other forms of so-called flecked retina, including Bietti's crystalline dystrophy, nephropathic cystinosis, canthaxanthine retinopathy, West African crystalline maculopathy, Sjögren–Larsson's syndrome, talc retinopathy, fundus albi punctatus, retinitis punctata albescens, Stargardt's disease, Alport's syndrome, bilateral acquired juxtafoveolar telangiectasis, and vitamin A deficiency.

Calcium oxalate crystals may be found within the retina as an incidental finding in patients with long-standing retinal detachment (see Chapter 7, Figure 7.31A and B) and with morgagnian cataracts unassociated with evidence of systemic oxalosis.

CANTHAXANTHINE MACULOPATHY

Canthaxanthine is a carotenoid dye used in food and drug coloration. Some patients who use it orally (usually a total dose of 19 g or more within 24 months) as a tanning agent may develop a symmetric distribution of golden particles in a doughnut pattern in the superficial retina in the macular areas (Figure 9.10).[130–137] The retinal crystals may be exaggerated in eyes with other diseases of the fundus (Figure 9.10D–I).[138] A few patients may develop similar crystals in the cornea at the level of Descemet's membrane.[139] Retrospective studies of pure canthaxanthine (Orobronze) consumers revealed an incidence of retinal deposits varying from 12% to 14%.[130,132] The occurrence of the deposits correlates with the total dose ingested. In two studies 37 g canthaxanthine induced retinal deposits in 50% of the patients[130] and 60 g induced deposits in 100% of patients.[140] Predisposing factors that lead to onset of retinopathy at much lower dosage include focal disease of the RPE,[131,132] ocular hypertension,[131] and concurrent use of beta carotene (Figure 9.10D–I).[131] Hennekes reported the development of canthaxanthine retinopathy in a patient with retinitis pigmentosa after ingestion of 12–14 g over a period of 4 months.[141] The maculopathy is usually associated with normal visual acuity but reduced retinal sensitivity.[142] Some patients may demonstrate subnormal dark adaptation and electroretinographic responses.[135,137,143,144] The ERG changes in most patients are reversible after the ingestion of canthaxanthine is stopped.[145] EOG responses are normal.[134,140,141,144,146,147] Fluorescein angiography is typically normal but may show a bull's-eye pattern of faint hyperfluorescence (Figure 9.10C). Morphologically these red, birefringent, and lipid-soluble carotenoid crystals are located in the inner layers of the entire retina and the ciliary body.[148] They are particularly large and numerous perifoveally, where they are clinically visible. They are located in a spongy degeneration of the inner neuropil and are associated with atrophy of the inner parts of Müller cells. They presumably represent a canthaxanthine–lipoprotein complex.[148]

The retinal crystals may gradually disappear a year or more after ingestion of canthaxanthine is discontinued, and some may remain for at least 7 years.[134,140,149] The delay in reversibility is in keeping with the observation that the plasma concentration of canthaxanthine takes at least 9 months to recover to normal levels in patients having received daily oral dosage of 100 mg for 3 months.[147] The return to normal values of static perimetry threshold in some patients suggests that the abnormality is not the result of an irreversible anatomic alteration, as suggested in experimental studies in rabbits.[150,151]

Retinopathy identical to that of canthaxanthine retinopathy may occur in some patients without a history of extradietary intake of canthaxanthine (Figure 9.08J and K).[152] Similar retinopathy has developed in one patient receiving long-term nitrofurantoin therapy.[153]

Administration of amounts of canthaxanthine comparable to those ingested by patients developing canthaxanthine retinopathy produced morphologic changes in the retina of rabbits and cats, but no retinal crystals.[150,151,154] The cats developed a progressive orange sheen to the ocular fundus that morphologically was associated with increased RPE cell height and vacuolization caused by enlargement and disruption of phagosomes.[154] Dose-dependent ingestion of canthaxanthine in cynomolgus monkeys has shown accumulation of the crystals in nests and rods within ganglion cells near the ora serrata and in the macula.[155] An ultrahigh-frequency OCT showed the crystals to be in superficial retina.[156]

9.10 Canthaxanthine retinopathy.

A–C: Note the glistening yellow crystals arranged in a doughnut shape in the superficial and deep retina in the macula of this patient who was a long-term user of skin-tanning agents. Note the perifoveolar ring of hyperfluorescence, which probably is caused by obstruction of the background fluorescence by the crystals rather than depigmentation of the retinal pigment epithelium (RPE).

D–F: Unilateral deposition of canthaxanthine in the right eye of a patient with recurrent idiopathic central serous chorioretinopathy in the ipsilateral eye (D and F). Left eye is unaffected (E).

G: Asymmetric canthaxanthine retinopathy occurred in an asymptomatic 58-year-old woman with an old inferior temporal branch retinal vein obstruction in the left macula. She was complaining of blurred vision and "lemon-yellow pinwheel" photopsia in the left eye. Visual acuity was 20/20, right eye, and 20/40, left eye. There were more crystals in the left macula and there were intracorneal crystals in both eyes. She had taken oral canthaxanthine for many years.

H and **I**: Canthaxanthine retinopathy associated with chronic recurrent bilateral idiopathic central serous chorioretinopathy. He took canthaxanthine, one tablet per day for 4 months, 15 years before these photographs. Visual acuity was 20/300, right eye, and 20/25, left eye.

J and **K**: Crystalline retinopathy identical to that caused by canthaxanthine in a 48-year-old man with no history of supplemental canthaxanthine.

L: Mild unilateral crystalline retinopathy (arrow) of unknown cause in a middle-aged man.

(A and B, From Cortin et al.[131])

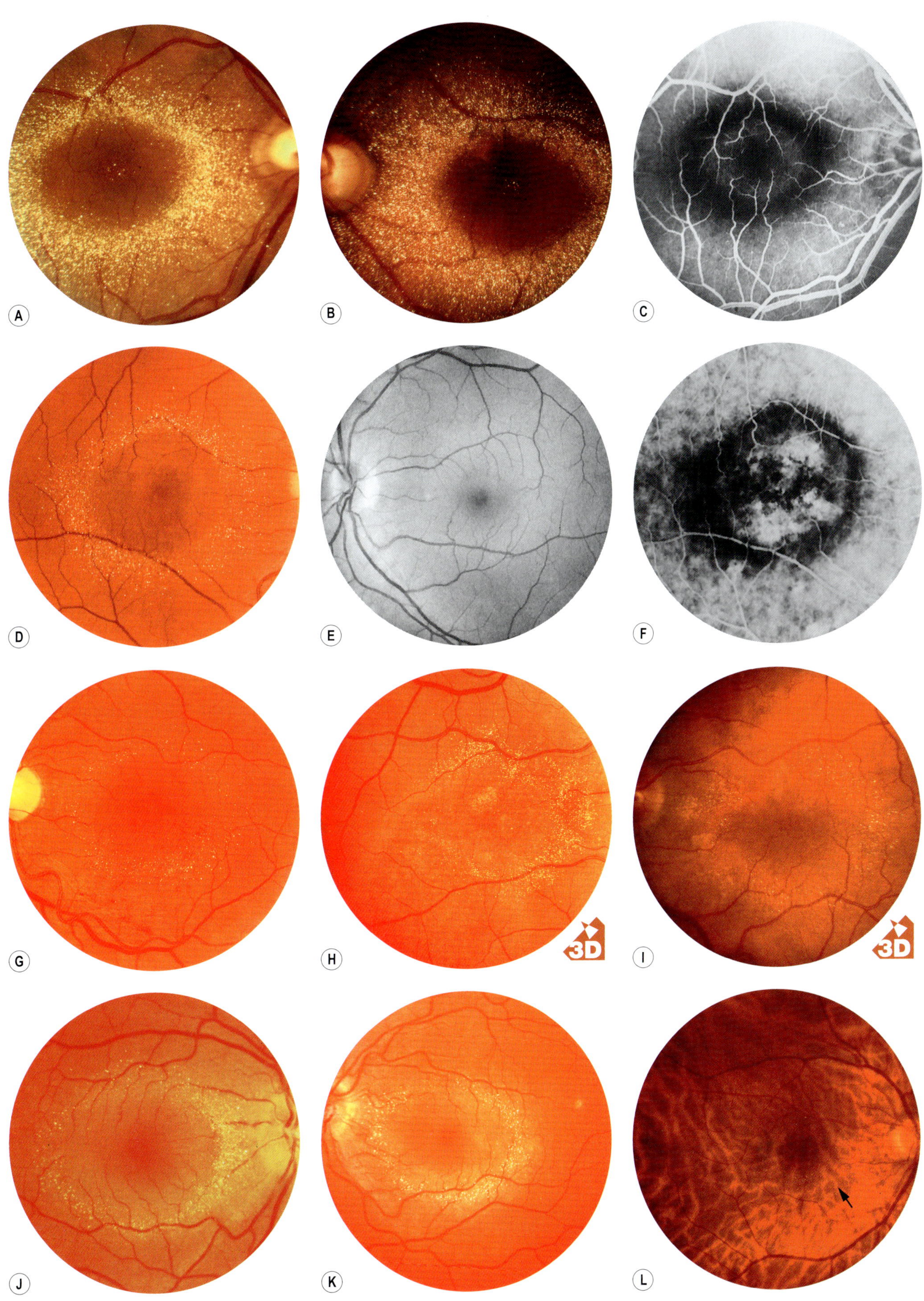
A
B
C
D
E
F
G
H
3D
I
3D
J
K
L

WEST AFRICAN CRYSTALLINE MACULOPATHY

Elderly patients from the Igbo tribe in Southeastern Nigeria in West Africa have been found to deposit green or yellow, refractile, foveal crystals that are bilateral and asymmetric in distribution.[157] Subsequent reports have found the crystals in several West African tribes, including those in Liberia, Ghana, and Sierra Leone.[157–159] These crystals are found in the inner retina, mostly in the foveal inner plexiform layer, and do not affect vision or electrophysiology of the eyes (Figure 9.11A–E).[157–159] OCT can demonstrate the location of the crystals, seen in the superficial retina in Figure 9.11L. Most patients are older than 50 years of age. The original description of the condition attributed the crystals to ingestion of kola nuts. However,[157,159] only one of three patients had a history of ingestion of kola nuts more than 20 years previously. Fifteen of the 20 patients reported so far and two others (Figure 9.11A–I) had diabetic retinopathy, one sickle-cell retinopathy, one branch retinal vein occlusion (BRVO), one familial exudative vitreoretinopathy (FEVR), and one other patient of Dr. Edwin Ryan had a branch retinal vein occlusion; it is conceivable that the hyperpermeability of their retinal vessels may have facilitated the deposition of the crystals. All reported cases thus far have found crystals in the macula; however Figure 9.11F–H illustrates extramacular deposition of crystals in the vicinity of the flat new vessels in this patient with proliferative diabetic retinopathy. Her brother with nonproliferative diabetic retinopathy has macular crystals only.

NITROFURANTOIN CRYSTALLINE RETINOPATHY

Nitrofurantoin macrocrystal used for a prolonged period (19 years) in a patient resulted in deposition of the shiny crystals in and around the disc and macula in both eyes. The antimicrobial is used to treat urinary tract infections. Its chemical structure delays dissolution and hence remains in a crystalline form and may become deposited on prolonged use.[160]

9.11 West African crystalline maculopathy.

A–C: An asymptomatic 46-year-old man from Lagos, Nigeria, with a 4-year history of noninsulin-dependent diabetes mellitus and hypertension was seen in May 2003. He had been living in the USA for 5 years. He denied renal disease, intravenous drug use, history of exposure to general anesthesia, nitrofurantoin use, or ingestion of canthaxanthine or tamoxifen. A history of kola nut ingestion was remote and infrequent. Visual acuities were 20/20 OU. Fundus showed moderate nonproliferative diabetic retinopathy bilaterally. In addition to macular exudates most prominent temporally, refractile yellow green crystals were noted in the fovea of both eyes (A and B). No crystals were noted outside the macular region. He subsequently developed clinically significant macular edema bilaterally requiring focal laser treatment in 2004 with resolution of the macular exudates and edema. Four years later, despite resolution of macular edema and absence of leakage on fluorescein angiography, the foveal crystals have persisted with some shift in their distribution (C). D–L: His 59-year-old sister was evaluated in March 2008. She had a 12-year history of diabetes mellitus with insulin use over the previous 2 years. She was also from Lagos, Nigeria, and had been living in the USA for 3 years. No definitive history of kola nut ingestion could be elicited. Visual acuities are 20/50 OD and 20/40 OS. She had 2+ nuclear sclerotic cataracts bilaterally. Fundus exam showed nonproliferative diabetic retinopathy bilaterally with similar refractile yellow green crystals in the fovea of both eyes (D and E). There were no macular exudates or edema in either eye. Very little extramacular crystalline deposits were present. She underwent uncomplicated cataract extraction with posterior-chamber lens implantation in both eyes in July 2008. In September 2009 visual acuities were 20/40 OD and 20/30 OS. She developed early proliferative diabetic retinopathy with areas of flat NVE in the nasal and temporal midperiphery of both eyes. The crystals were now noted both in the macula as well as the midperiphery with clustering of the deposits adjacent to areas of flat NVE (F–I). Angiogram confirmed the NVE (J and K). Optical coherence tomography examination demonstrated that the crystalline deposits were located in the superficial inner retina (L). Another 55-year-old sister (one of six other siblings) who was visiting from Nigeria was examined in February 2009. She had no ocular complaints and no history of diabetes, hypertension, or other vascular disease. Her retinal examination was entirely normal with no evidence of crystalline deposits.

(A–L, courtesy of Dr. Everton Arrindell.)

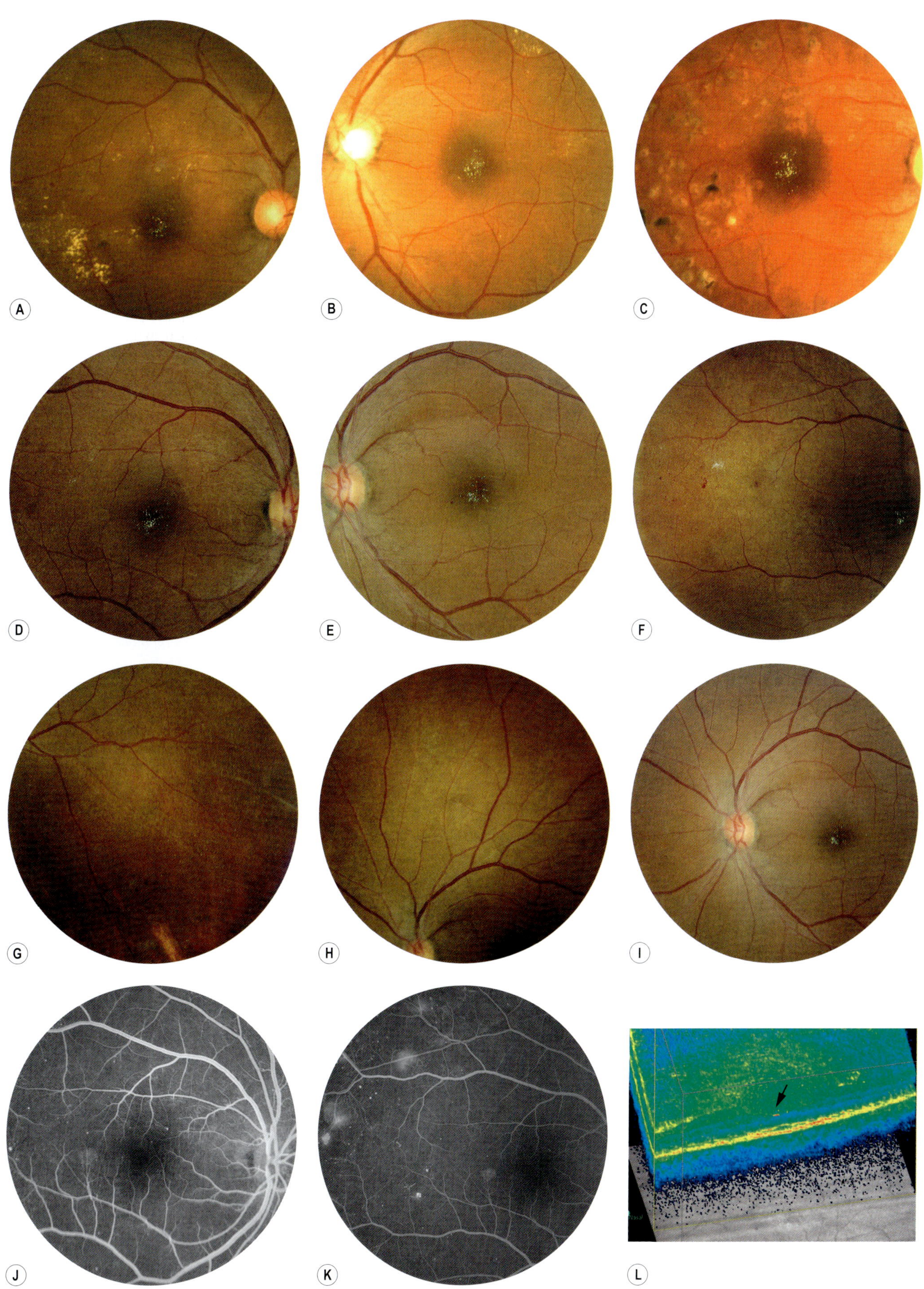
A
B
C
D
E
F
G
H
I
J
K
L

FLECKED RETINA ASSOCIATED WITH VITAMIN A DEFICIENCY

Patients with vitamin A deficiency secondary to inadequate dietary intake, malabsorption states resulting from celiac sprue, regional enteritis, jejunal bypass surgery, chronic liver disease, hepatic transplantation and more recently with bariatric surgery may develop night blindness, corneal xerosis, and a peculiar peripheral retinal change characterized by the presence of multiple, yellow-white, somewhat granular spots in the outer retina Figure 9.12A, C, D, F, and K) (fundus xerophthalmicus; Uyemura's syndrome).[161–172] These flecks are of various sizes and shapes and simulate drusen. The retinal changes have been associated with marked constriction of the visual fields (Figure 9.12H and I), abnormal dark adaptation, and electroretinographic changes, including disappearance of the a-wave followed by loss of the b-wave and greater reduction of the scotopic than the photopic responses. Following administration of vitamin A, there may be either complete or partial (Figure 9.12A and J–L) reversal of the fundus and electrophysiologic changes, depending on the chronicity of the deficiency.[169,171,172] The fundus changes are more likely to occur in those patients with vitamin A deficiency who develop evidence of corneal xerosis.

Fluorescein angiography shows only a mild variable fluorescence of the flecks (Figure 9.12G), suggesting the location of the flecks to be primarily at the photoreceptor layer; only some of these may cause secondary RPE change, accounting for the patchy hyperfluorescence.

Animals with vitamin A deficiency histopathologically develop disorganization of the rod outer segments and eventual loss of the visual cells.[163] It is probable that the transient yellow-white spots occurring in humans are related to the macrophagic response to loss of rod outer segments and RPE cell disruption similar to that which has been demonstrated histopathologically to account for the peculiar yellow-white spots that may be seen in patients with Leber's congenital amaurosis soon after birth. Malabsorption syndromes, including gluten enteropathy or celiac disease (Figure 9.12J and K), nutritional and other causes of malabsorption, liver dysfunction such as cirrhosis (Figure 9.12K and L), and most recently gastric bypass surgery are common clinical settings for vitamin A deficiency. Concomitant zinc deficiency has also been implicated in the pathogenesis of xerophthalmia.

9.12 Xerophthalmia.

A–L: A 65-year-old male with a known history of pernicious anemia for 10 years presented with progressive night blindness for 18 months. He was receiving biweekly shots of vitamin B_{12}. His visual acuity was 20/30 OU; color vision was subnormal. Fine gray white dots were seen in both fundi, distinct on red-free images (A–F (arrows)). Angiogram showed variable fluorescence of the flecks suggesting these changes were at the photoreceptor level rather than at the pigment epithelium (G). Rod and cone functions were decreased on electroretinogram (ERG) testing. Serum vitamin A level measured 0.06 mg/l (normal 0.30–1.20 mg/l) and retinyl palminate 0.00 mg/l (normal <0.11). An upper and lower gastrointestinal study was done. There was almost total villous atrophy, and the lamina propria was infiltrated with mixed inflammatory cells consisting of lymphocytes, plasma cells, and granulocytes (H and I). The gastric and esophageal mucosa was normal, thus the previous diagnosis of pernicious anemia was erroneous. A diagnosis of celiac disease was made. He received daily intramuscular injections of Aquasol A 100 000 units for 3 days followed by every 2 weeks. He was advised to follow a gluten-free diet. Three months following the diagnosis and treatment his nyctalopia had resolved, the ERG and visual field defects had improved, and the white flecks had mostly resolved (J).

K and **L**: A 64-year-old woman with IgA nephropathy requiring dialysis, and cirrhosis secondary to medications noted difficulty in the dark and in dim lighting over 1 year. Her uncorrected visual acuity was 20/40 and 20/50; color vision was 3/11 in each eye. Upper nasal retina shows white punctate flecks of xerophthalmia (arrow, K). Her vitamin level was 0.06 mg/l (normal 0.3–1.2 mg/l). She received oral vitamin A supplement at 80 000 units ×2 and her symptoms improved in 3 days. Upper nasal retina of right eye shows resolution of most of the flecks at 9 weeks (L).

(A, G and J; Yannuzzi, Lawrence J., The Retinal Atlas, Saunders 2010, 978-0-7020-3320-9, p.861. K and L, courtesy or Dr. Wayne Wu and Dr. Franco Recchia.)

One 50-year-old man with acquired night blindness associated with steatorrhea was noted to have the typical changes of fundus albipunctatus.[167] His abnormal dark adaptation curves improved after vitamin A administration, but the fundus remained unchanged. Although it was postulated that the albipunctate spots may have resulted from photoreceptor damage after chronic vitamin A deficiency, this seems unlikely since other investigators who have studied this disease have not noted persistence of the white spots following therapy.

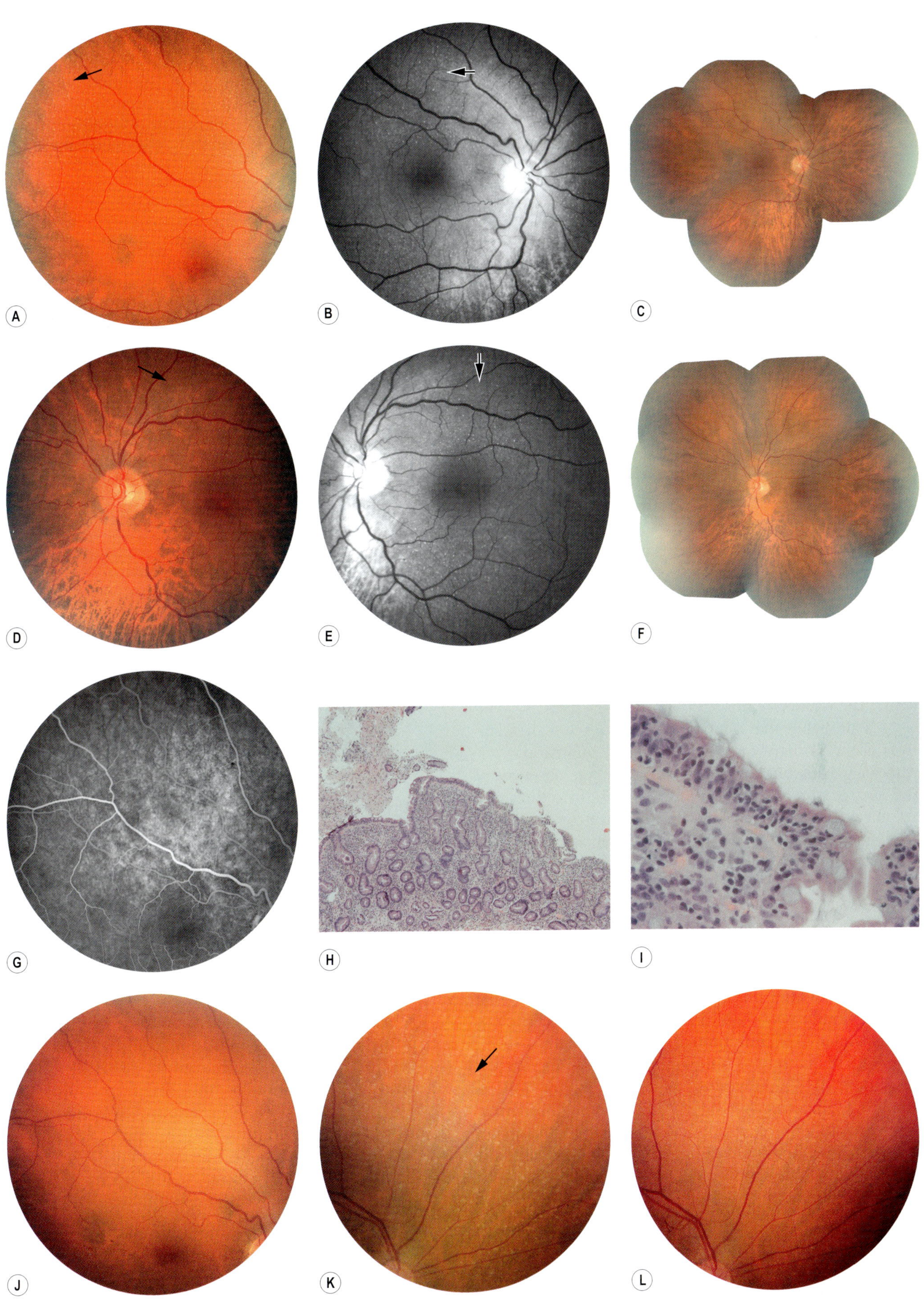
A
B
C
D
E
F
G
H
I
J
K
L

AMINOGLYCOSIDE MACULOPATHY

The inadvertent injection of large doses of gentamicin into either the anterior chamber after cataract extraction or the vitreous during a sub-Tenon's injection may produce a rapid and severe visual loss associated with a peculiar retinopathy that is most marked in the macular area (Figure 9.13).[173–182] The patient is usually aware of profound loss of vision on the first postoperative day. Initially the fundus picture may simulate that seen in central retinal artery occlusion. There is marked whitening and swelling of the retina in the macular area associated with a cherry-red spot (Figure 9.13D, F, and I). Other surrounding areas of patchy retinal whitening may be evident. Retinal hemorrhages develop and become more numerous (Figure 9.13A, F, and I). Although intravitreal injection of levels of gentamicin up to 200 µg were previously considered safe for the treatment of endophthalmitis, macular infarction may occur in some patients after intravitreal injection of 0.1 or 0.2 mg gentamicin sulfate.[183–185] Repetitive injections of nontoxic doses may produce retinal damage.[186] Fluorescein angiography typically shows a sharply defined zone of retinal vascular nonperfusion in the macular area associated with dye leakage from the neighboring retinal vessels (Figure 9.13B, C, E, G, H, K, and L).[177,178] The retinal whitening and hemorrhages may persist for many weeks or several months (Figure 9.13J). Optic atrophy and retinal pigmentary changes develop later and may be accompanied by rubeosis irides and hemorrhagic glaucoma. The visual prognosis is poor.

It is probable that gentamicin and not the preservatives is the primary cause of the retinal infarction.[174,177] Although experimentally the presence or absence of the lens or vitreous does not change the toxic threshold to injected aminoglycosides, there is concern clinically that nontoxic doses of aminoglycosides may be toxic if injected intravitreally into vitrectomized eyes.[187,188] Although tobramycin and amikacin are less toxic than gentamicin, both have produced fundus findings similar to those caused by gentamicin.[183,189] The retinopathy has been observed most frequently following intravitreal injections of 0.4 mg gentamicin after vitrectomy, but also in some cases after injection of 0.1 or 0.2 mg, doses that had previously been considered safe.[183] Prophylactic use of subconjunctival injection of gentamicin after routine surgery was the second most frequent cause of macular infarction. The retinopathy has been observed following the inadvertent intraocular injection of tobramycin after cataract extraction.[173,174,176] In one case this apparently resulted from diffusion of the subconjunctivally injected drug through the cataract wound.[176] The same maculopathy has occurred after intravitreal injections of amikacin.[174] With the advent of sutureless vitrectomy, surgery using subconjunctival gentamicin is fraught with the same risk.[190] Because of the frequency and severity of the complication, Campochiaro and Lim[174] recommended: (1) abandonment of prophylactic use of subconjunctival aminoglycosides after routine surgery, and (2) avoidance of intravitreal aminoglycosides in the prophylaxis of penetrating ocular trauma. Ceftazidime has replaced intravitreal amikacin for treatment of endophthalmitis.

9.13 Gentamicin retinal toxicity.

A–E: This 67-year-old man had accidental irrigation of the anterior chamber with 0.5 ml gentamicin instead of acetylcholine after cataract extraction and placement of an intraocular lens. A posterior capsulotomy was done. Twenty minutes later the mistake was discovered, and the anterior chamber was irrigated. The next day the vision in the eye was light perception only. Two days postoperatively there was corneal edema and a semiopaque retina with peripheral retinal hemorrhages (A). Fluorescein angiography revealed extensive areas of nonperfusion of the retina in the posterior pole (B and C) and selective periarterial leakage (arrows, C). One month postoperatively the cornea was clear. There was a cherry-red spot surrounded by a milky white retina, dilated tortuous veins, many retinal hemorrhages, and pigmentary sheathing of the arteries (D). Angiography revealed persistence of the retinal vascular hypoperfusion (E). Visual acuity was hand movements. Six weeks later the patient developed evidence of neovascular glaucoma.

F–I: This 29-year-old man sustained an intraocular metallic foreign-body injury. After removal of the foreign body transsclerally with a magnet, clindamycin 250 µg and gentamicin 400 µg were injected intravitreally. Ten hours postoperatively visual acuity was 20/200. Thirty-two hours postoperatively, the patient noted a dark central scotoma. Six days postoperatively there was whitening of the retina in the macular area associated with several blot hemorrhages (F). Angiography revealed nonperfusion of the retina in the macular area and leakage of dye from the surrounding vessels (G and H). Ten days postoperatively visual acuity was 5/200 and there was an increase in the area of retinal whitening and hemorrhages (I). Six months later the visual acuity was 10/200. There were atrophic retinal and retinal pigment epithelium changes in the macula.

J–L: This woman had an extracapsular cataract extraction that was complicated by vitreous loss. Four days later she developed a hypopyon. A vitreous biopsy and intravitreal injection of gentamicin, vancomycin, and dexamethasone were done. Postoperatively she noted only bare light perception with the right eye. Four months postoperatively her visual acuity was 6/200. Fundoscopic examination revealed pigment cells in the vitreous, scattered retinal hemorrhages, whitening of the retina centrally (J), and several cotton-wool patches around the nasal aspect of the optic disc. Angiographically there was marked loss of the retinal blood vessels (K and L).

(A–I, From McDonald et al.[177]; F–I, courtesy of Dr. Matthew D. Davis.)

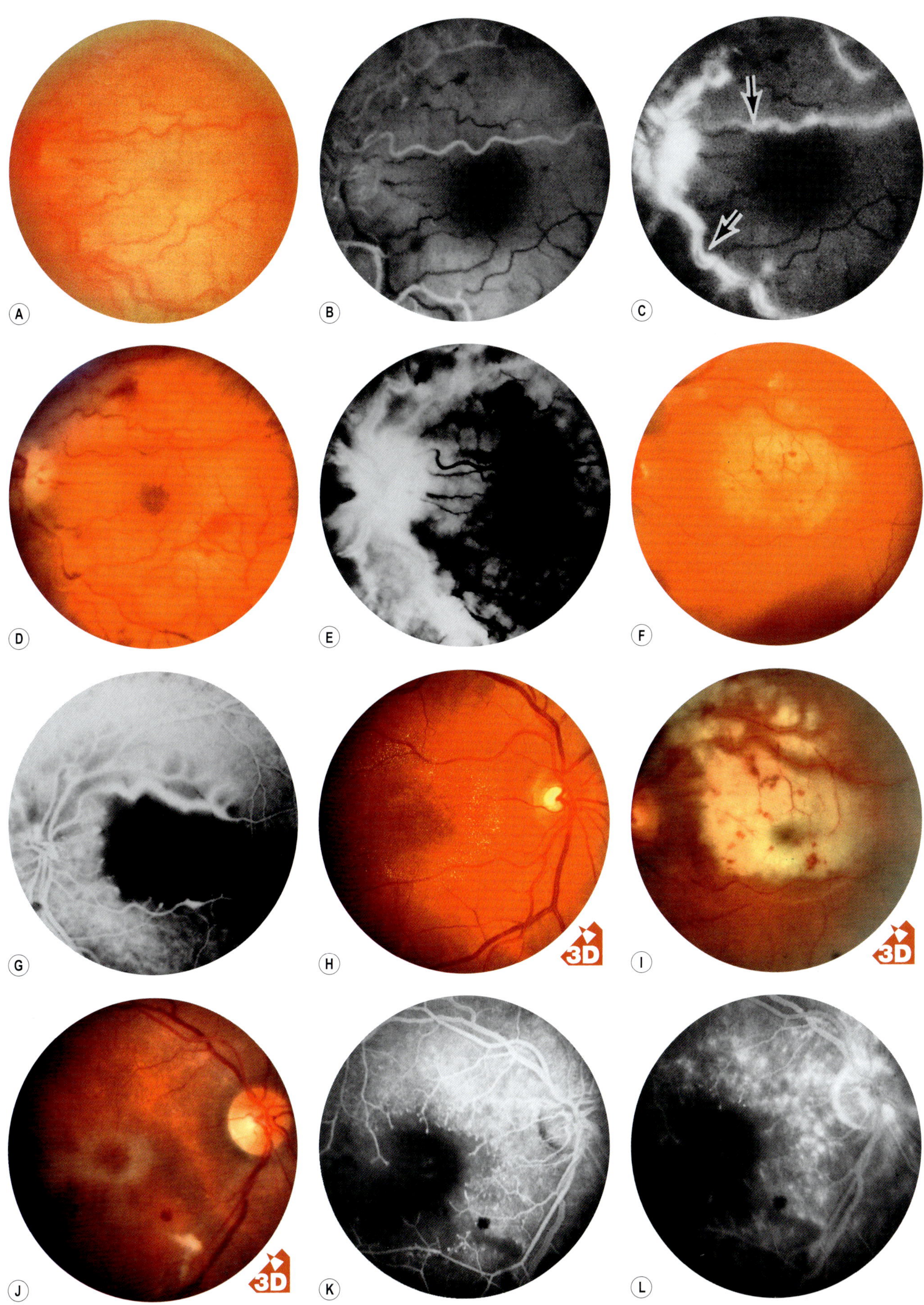
A
B
C
D
E
F
G
H
3D
I
3D
J
3D
K
L

Experimentally, retinal toxicity to gentamicin may occur at levels as low as 100 μg injected into the vitreous.[191] In the rabbit model D'Amico et al.[191] found lamellar storage material in the liposomes of RPE and macrophages after injection of 100 μg into the vitreous; disruption of pigment epithelial cell organelles and loss of photoreceptors after 400 μg; and full-thickness retinal necrosis after 800 μg. These findings implicate the RPE as the primary site of toxicity.[191] Aminoglycoside maculopathy similar to that seen in humans has been produced in subhuman primates following intravitreal injection of 1000–10 000 μg gentamicin.[192,193] Evidence suggests that the retinal whitening and the isoelectric electroretinographic findings that occur within minutes or hours of the injection are caused by direct damage to the inner retina by the drug before development of occlusion of the retinal vasculature. Rabbit and rat retinas both in vitro and in vivo, exposed to escalating small doses of gentamicin, showed reversible loss of b-waves but preserved a-waves. The reduced b-wave may be from metabolic effect on the bipolar cells or secondarily via effect on glutamate transport by the Müller cells. It is possible that aminoglyocosides induce metabolic change in the inner neurons that secondarily affect vascular perfusion. Alternately or in addition the toxic metabolic effects may occur at the vascular endothelial cells. Histology of the retina showed diffuse vacuolization of the nerve fiber, ganglion cell, and inner plexiform layers.[194] The latter is accompanied by retinal hemorrhages, damage to retinal pericytes and endothelial cells, and thrombosis. A possible mechanism to explain the retinal vascular occlusion was granulocytic plugging of the retinal capillary bed.[193]

In some patients aminoglycoside macular toxicity may be difficult to differentiate from that produced as a complication of intraneural injection during retrobulbar anesthesia or that resulting from spontaneous occlusion of the central retinal artery and vein. The vitreous inflammatory cell reaction, shallow retinal detachment, and delayed onset of retinal hemorrhages, as well as the characteristic angiographic pattern and prolonged retinal whitening associated with aminoglycoside toxicity are helpful in this regard.[175,176,195]

9.14 Interferon retinopathy.

A–C: Bilateral nerve fiber infarcts in this 30-year-old male who was healthy till he was diagnosed with nonmetastatic cutaneous melanoma 5 months previously (A and B). He had noticed mild visual distortion in his left eye for several weeks while receiving high-dose intravenous, followed by subcutaneous, interferon alfa 2-b. His visual acuity was 20/20 in both eyes. Fluorescein angiogram of both eyes showed occluded precapillary arterioles and capillary nonperfusion (C). He also developed a left caudate nucleus infarct resulting in a right-sided stroke and was found to have an ejection fraction of 30% secondary to cardiomyopathy. Interferon was discontinued, the nerve fiber infarcts resolved, he recovered completely from the stroke, and the cardiac function improved dramatically.

Methamphetamine and cocaine retinopathy.

D and **E**: This 39-year-old man with a history of essential hypertension noted acute loss of vision in the left eye. He admitted snorting cocaine before his visual loss. Visual acuity was 20/20 right eye, and light perception only in the left eye. Note evidence of central retinal artery occlusion in the left eye and multiple cotton-wool patches in both eyes.

F–H: This man noted blurred vision in the left eye after snorting cocaine and an argument with his wife. He denied trauma. The right eye was normal. Note the multiple superficial retinal hemorrhages, one of which has a white center (arrow, G), boat-shaped preretinal hematomas, and intravitreal blood.

Lidocaine–epinephrine toxicity.

I–L: This 27-year-old man noted immediate pain and loss of vision during an anterior peribulbar injection of lidocaine and epinephrine in the upper nasal quadrant in preparation for pterygium removal. Fundus examination revealed a retinal detachment (presumably the anesthetic) that extended from the injection site into the posterior fundus. Laser photocoagulation was placed in the area of the subretinal blood and within 48 hours the subretinal fluid had resolved. Two weeks later the optic disc was pale and its margin was blurred (I). There were fine radiating lines in the macula. Angiography was unremarkable except for irregular hyperfluorescence in the area of laser treatment (J) and staining of the optic disc (K). Five weeks later his visual acuity was 20/80 and the optic disc was pale (L).

(A–C, courtesy of Dr. Arun D. Singh.)

INTERFERON-ASSOCIATED RETINOPATHY

Patients receiving interferon alfa 2-a subcutaneously or interferon alfa 2-b intravenously (Figure 9.14A–C) may develop multiple cotton-wool ischemic patches in the retina associated with retinal hemorrhages.[196] The pattern of the retinopathy may simulate Purtscher's retinopathy and be associated with decreased visual acuity. The fundus changes are reversible after discontinuing the interferon therapy. Mild diabetes and systemic hypertension were present in 50% of patients developing the retinopathy.[196] Similar fundus changes with retinal hemorrhages and cotton-wool spots with visual field changes have been seen, though less frequently, in patients receiving interferon beta-1b for multiple sclerosis. The fundus changes and field defects reverse once the drug is discontinued.[197–199] These observations suggest that patients with moderately severe diabetic, hypertensive, or other retinopathy associated with retinal capillary nonperfusion may be at greater risk of progression of the retinopathy and permanent visual loss following the administration of large amounts of interferon such as might be used in the treatment of patients with malignancies.[200] Circulating C5a levels have been found to be elevated in some patients developing retinopathy on interferon alpha; whether this is the cause or the result of the vasculopathy is undetermined.[201]

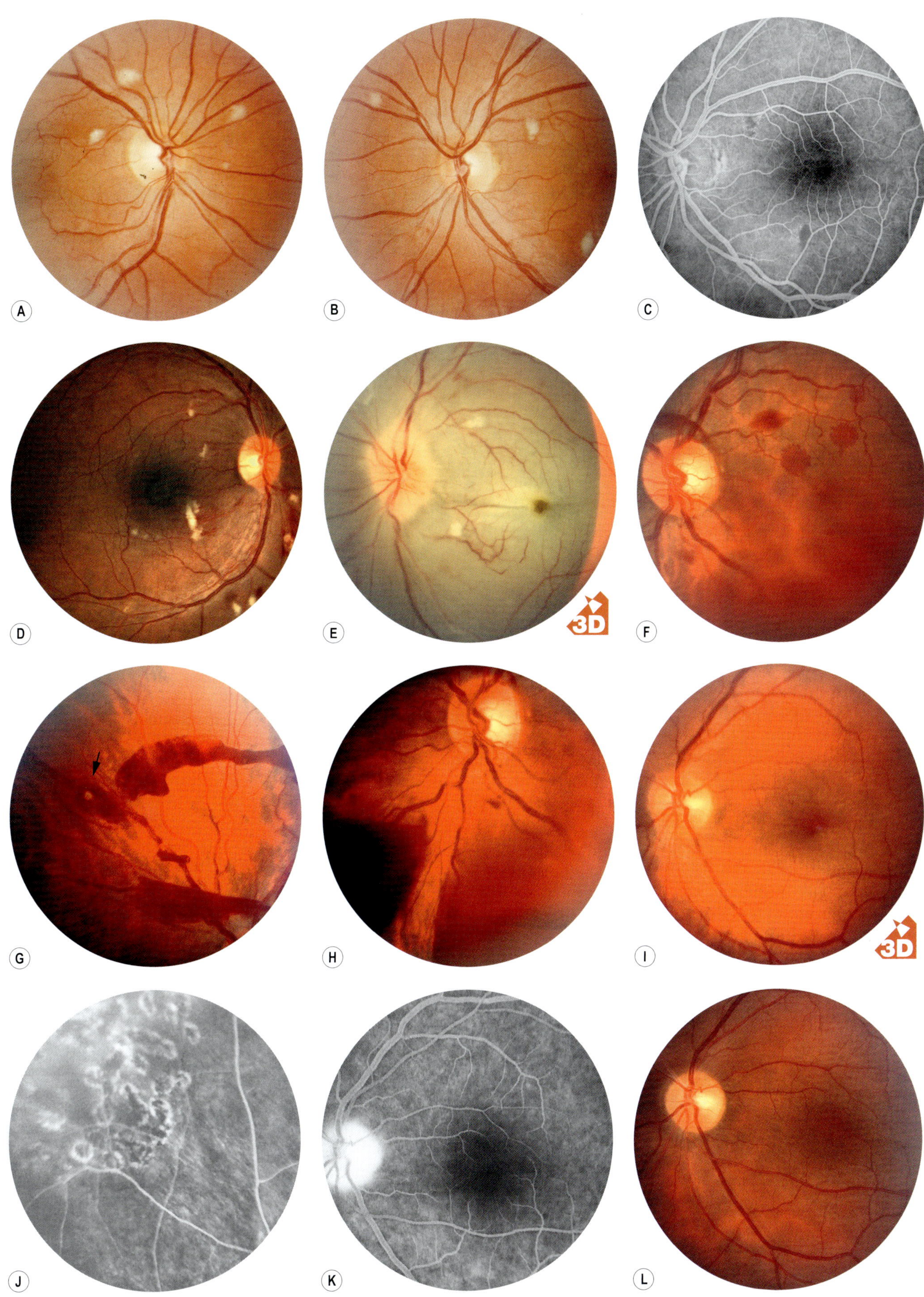
A
B
C
D
E
3D
F
G
H
I
3D
J
K
L

METHAMPHETAMINE AND COCAINE RETINOPATHY

Inhalation of methamphetamine and cocaine may be followed by acute visual loss in one or both eyes. The route of acquisition of the drugs determines to an extent the clinical manifestations. Subconjunctival placement of methamphetamine results in conjunctivitis, episcleritis, and scleritis. Intravenous and intranasal snorting is associated with amaurosis fugax, retinal vasculitis with perivenous exudation and vitritis,[202] retinal and optic disc hemorrhages,[203] multiple cotton-wool patches, Purtscher-like retinopathy,[204] and central retinal artery occlusion (Figure 9.14D–H).[203,205] A case of severe retinal and choroidal ischemia has been seen with large wedge-shaped choroidal infarcts corresponding to the Amalric triangles in a chronic cocaine user (Figure 9.15C and F). The adrenomimetic response and sudden increase in blood pressure after use of these drugs probably contribute to these retinal manifestations.[204,206–210] Retinopathy similar to talc retinopathy has been seen in one patient with intranasal snorting of methamphetamine.[211] Chronic cocaine users develop vascular remodeling with increase in retinal arteriolar branching angle and venous caliber.[212]

PRESUMED DEXTROAMPHETAMINE MACULOPATHY

A patient who was on dextroamphetamine (Dexedrine) for 18 years at a dose of 15 mg/day for 10 years, followed by10 mg/day, developed gradual difficulty with dark adaptation and translucent holes in her vision.

Her posterior pole showed symmetric mottling at the RPE level in the two eyes (Figure 9.15G and H). Fluorescein angiogram showed window defects (Figure 9.15I and J). Her rod ERG was mildly reduced but cone ERG was within the range for her age. EOGs measured 2.9 and 3.6 in the right and left eye respectively. Discontinuation of the medication showed improvement in symptoms subjectively by 2 months. She was subsequently switched to an alternate drug to treat her narcolepsy. Amphetamines release dopamine, and to a lesser extent serotonin and epinephrine at low doses in the retina. Long-term use of dextroamphetamine in this patient may have had deleterious effects on the RPE.

LIDOCAINE–EPINEPHRINE TOXICITY

The inadvertent injection of lidocaine into the inner eye typically causes immediate corneal clouding, pupillary dilation, pupillary paralysis, and profound visual loss, all of which usually revert to normal within 24 hours.[213] In one patient there was persistence of a large central scotoma that was attributed to possible intraocular bleeding. Experimentally, intraocular lidocaine was not associated with evidence of permanent retinal damage. Figure 9.14I–L illustrates the findings in a young man who apparently had an injection of 0.5 ml lidocaine–epinephrine into the subretinal space in preparation for pterygium excision. Immediately after the injection his visual acuity was 1/200. When examined by a retinal specialist 2 hours later, the intraocular pressure was 16 mmHg and the visual acuity was no light perception. There was mild whitening of the retina at the site of the injection and in the macular area. The retina was detached, presumably by the injected lidocaine, nasally from the site of sclerochoroidal perforation near the equator to the posterior pole. The subretinal fluid was no longer evident when examined 2 days later. He experienced partial recovery of vision but was left with a large temporal and central scotoma corresponding with the area of retinal detachment and mild optic atrophy. The nature of the visual field defect suggests that the subretinal lidocaine–epinephrine rather than the transient rise in intraocular pressure was responsible for the permanent retinal visual loss.

9.15 Cocaine-induced retinal and choroidal ischemia.

A–F: A 50-year-old male lost vision in his left eye acutely associated with abdominal pain and right-sided weakness. He could see 20/25 with his right eye and could not perceive light with his left eye. There was a cotton-wool spot in his right eye (A); the left eye had several patches of full-thickness retinal whitening associated with broken-up blood columns in both veins and arterioles diffusely throughout the fundus (B and D). In the temporal periphery there were triangles of retinal whitening (C) corresponding to Pierre Amalric's triangles. An angiogram showed poor blood flow through the retinal arteries and veins and wedge-shaped areas of increased choroidal fluorescence in the areas intervening the white triangles (arrows), which are watershed zones of the posterior ciliary arteries (E–F). This patient showed multiple occlusions of both the short and long posterior ciliary arteries and branches of the central retinal artery due to a combination of vasospasm and emboli from cocaine use.

Probable dextroamphetamine retinopathy

G–M: This 38-year-old Caucasian woman with a scar in her right eye since childhood began noticing "translucent defects" with her left eye and progressive difficulty at night over 4 years. She saw 20/100 eccentrically in her right eye and 20/40 in her left eye. She missed half the Ishihara color plates with each eye. Goldmann visual field revealed a central scotoma in the right eye and full fields peripherally in both eyes. Both retinas showed mottling of the pigment epithelium in the macula and nasal to the disc (G and H), more visible on the angiogram with late staining (I and J). Diffuse reduction in autofluorescence was seen corresponding to the retinal pigment epithelium change (K and L). An optical coherence tomography through the left macula showed disruption of the photoreceptors and possible thin layer of subretinal fluid (M). This patient had been on dextroamphetamine (Dexedrine) for 18 years at a dose of 15 mg/day for 10 years, followed by 10 mg/day for narcolepsy. An electroretinogram showed mild reduction in rod amplitudes and cone amplitudes at the lower end of normal. Arden ratio was 3.5 on the right and 2.1 on the left. Dexedrine was discontinued and the patient reported improvement in her symptoms at 2 months.

(A–F, courtesy of Dr. David Sarraf and Dr. Shantan Reddy[214] (Reprinted from Retina Cases and Brief Reports 5(1):91-93, Winter 2011.)

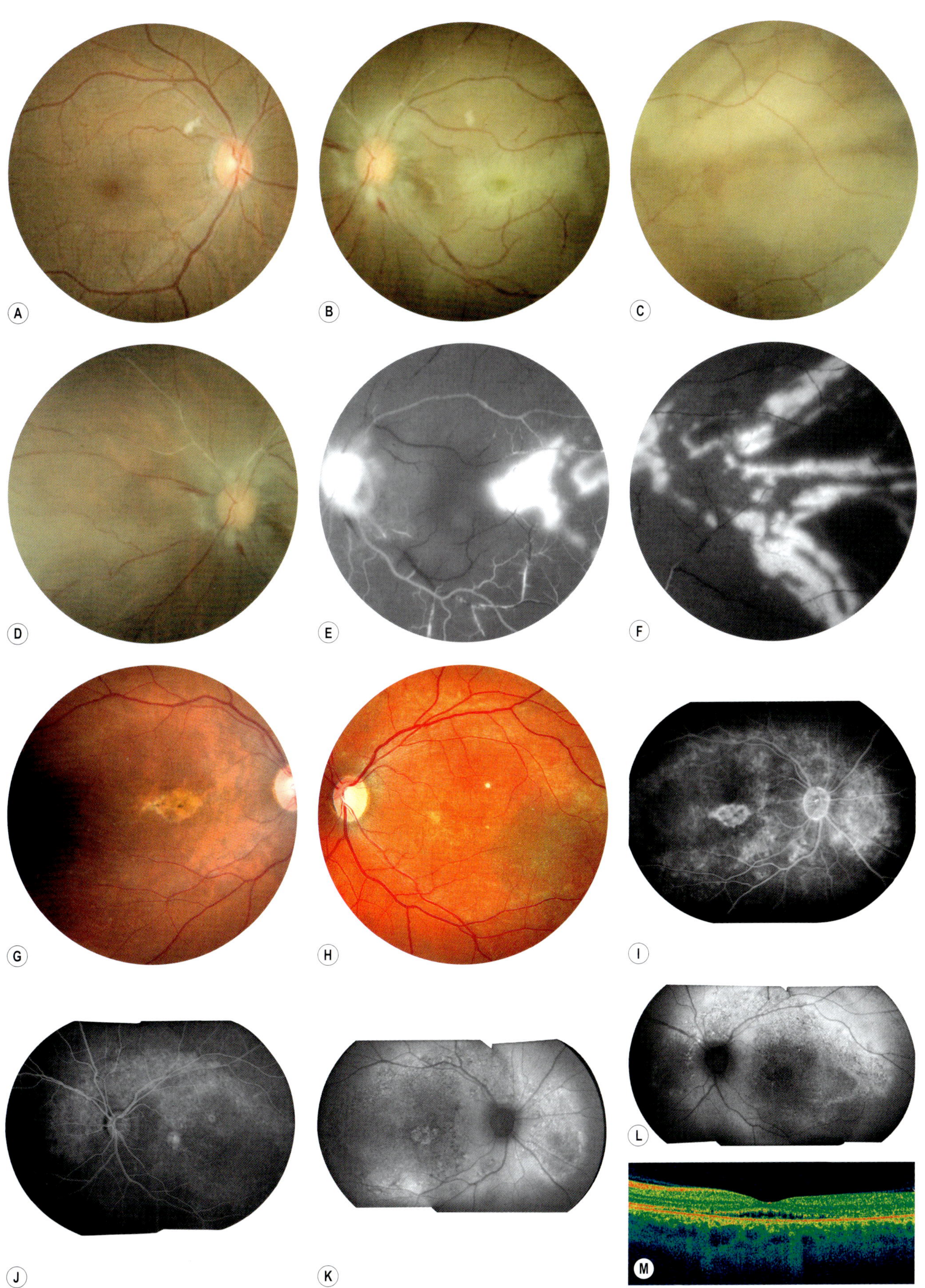
A
B
C
D
E
F
G
H
I
J
K
L
M

QUININE TOXICITY

Following an overdose of quinine, whether by accidental ingestion or from attempts at abortion or suicide, patients develop nausea, vomiting, headache, tremor, tinnitus, and hypotension and may become obtunded or even comatose. When they awake within the first 24 hours, they may be totally blind. Examination of the fundus at that time reveals a slight loss of retinal transparency, mild dilation of the retinal veins, and normal-caliber retinal arteries (Figure 9.16A).[215–217] Fluorescein angiography shows no abnormality other than slight obstruction of the background choroidal fluorescence (Figure 9.16B). Electroretinography may be normal or show slight changes such as slowing of the a-wave, transient increase in the depth of the a-wave, decrease in the b-wave, and loss of oscillatory potentials.[216] The EOG usually shows no light rise.[218] Within several days the patient often recovers normal visual acuity but retains only a small island of central vision. The EOG becomes progressively normal. The ERG shows progressive loss of the b-wave. Recovery of retinal transparency, progressive narrowing of the retinal arteries, and pallor of the optic disc begin within several days of recovery of central vision (Figure 9.16C–F). Visual evoked potentials are abnormal. Dark adaptation usually shows delayed cone adaptation and little or no rod function. It is probable that the increase in background choroidal fluorescence that occurs soon after the acute visual loss is caused primarily by the return of normal retinal transparency, rather than loss of pigment from the RPE. A patient with a failed suicide attempt 49 years prior using quinine tablets presented with pallor of the optic nerve, narrowed retinal arteries and veins, and constricted visual fields resembling fields secondary to open-angle glaucoma. The ERG showed reduced amplitudes and increased latency for both scotopic and photopic function.[219]

ERG done on children with cerebral malaria from *Plasmodium falciparum* receiving therapeutic doses of quinine shows a reversible decrease in the a-wave amplitude of maximal photoreceptor response and cone response from the time of quinine infusion.[220]

In animals with experimentally induced quinine retinal toxicity histopathologic examination of the early changes shows evidence of photoreceptor cell as well as ganglion cell alterations.[221,222] In later stages of the disease in humans, histopathologic examination shows loss of ganglion cells, nerve fiber layer, and photoreceptors.

Pupillary abnormalities that may be permanent in these patients include poor reaction to light, tonic pupillary reaction, vermiform pupillary motion, and denervation supersensitivity.[217,218,223]

The normal caliber of the retinal arteries and the normal retinal and choroidal circulation time seen during the acute stages of the disease suggest that vascular changes play little role in causing the retinal damage. The progressive narrowing of the retinal arterial tree that usually does not begin until after the patient has recovered central vision is probably caused by atrophy of the inner retinal layers as well as increased oxygen tension related to greater diffusion of oxygen from the choroid due to loss of photoreceptors. Thus, there is no rationale for retinal vascular dilators in the treatment of quinine toxicity. Lowering of the plasma level of quinine with repeated oral administration of activated charcoal theoretically may be beneficial.[224] There is, however, no treatment of proven value.

Quinine toxicity typically occurs with oral doses greater than 4 g, but there have been many case reports of toxicity with smaller doses. The recommended daily therapeutic dose is no more than 2 g, and the fatal oral dose for adults is approximately 8 g.

9.16 Quinine retinal toxicity.

This 25-year-old woman swallowed 12–15 tablets (3.7–4.7 g) of quinine as a suicidal gesture. This was followed by vomiting, buzzing in the ears, and blindness approximately 9 hours later. Examination $14^1/_2$ hours after ingestion revealed no light perception in both eyes, mild loss of retinal transparency, and slight venous distension (A). Fluorescein angiography showed venous distension and slight loss of details of the choroidal fluorescence (B). Thirty-five hours after ingestion, she noted return of a small island of central vision. Her acuity was 20/20. The fundi were unchanged. Five days after ingestion there were optic disc pallor, narrowing of the retinal vessels, and partial clearing of the retinal haziness (C). Nine days after ingestion there was further clearing of the retina and pallor of the optic disc (D and E). Angiography was normal except for retinal vascular narrowing (F). After 6 months, visual acuity was 20/15 and 20° of visual field remained in both eyes.

Methyl alcohol ocular toxicity.

G–J: This 53-year-old man experienced rapid loss of vision following the ingestion of methyl alcohol. Note the swelling and opacification of the optic nerve head and juxtapapillary retina (G). Angiography showed minimal staining of the optic nerve head (H). Eight weeks later the optic disc was pale and the visual loss persisted (I). Angiography showed hypofluorescence of the optic nerve head and evidence of juxtapapillary atrophy of the retinal pigment epithelium (J) that was probably present at the time of the initial photographs (compare with H).

Bisphosphonates

K and L: Scleritis in the left eye within 1 week of receiving intravenous bisphonate (Reclast) for steroid-induced osteopenia in a 74-year-old physician.

(A–F from Brinton et al.[216] published with permission from American Journal of Ophthalmology; copyright The Ophthalmic Publishing Co.)

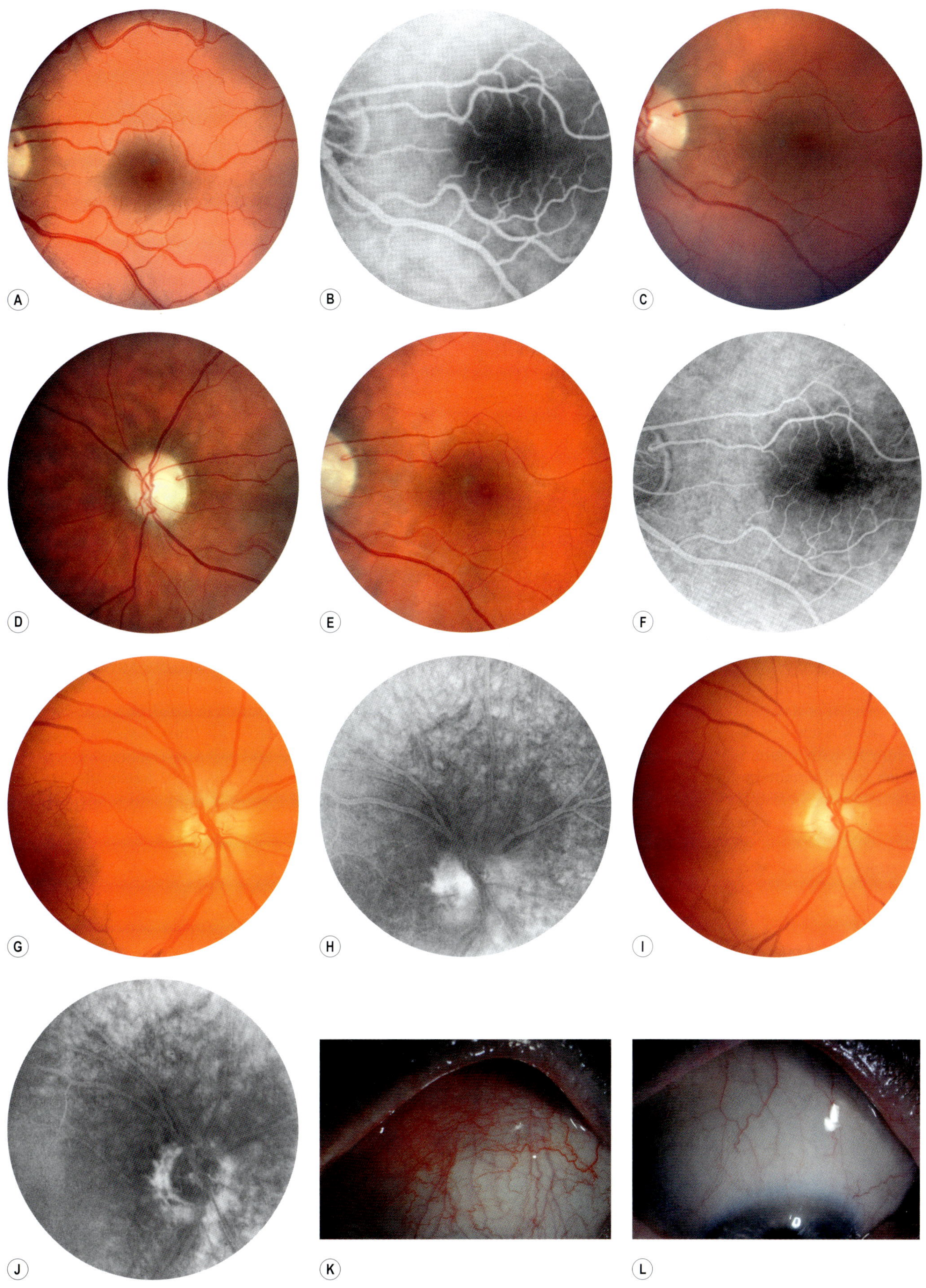
A
B
C
D
E
F
G
H
I
J
K
L

METHYL ALCOHOL TOXICITY

Within 18–48 hours of the ingestion of methyl alcohol, which is metabolized to formaldehyde and formic acid, patients may experience symptoms ranging from spots before the eyes to complete blindness.[225] Diminution of pupillary reaction to light may occur in patients with impaired visual acuity as well as in some patients with normal acuity. The degree of pupillary light reflex impairment is of considerable prognostic significance. Patients with dilated, fixed pupils usually die or suffer severe visual damage. Fundoscopic examination shows hyperemia of the optic disc, whitish striated edema of the disc margins and along the course of the major retinal vessels, and engorgement of the retinal veins (Figure 9.16G). Patients who survive and sustain severe visual damage develop optic atrophy in approximately 1–2 months (Figure 9.16I). A dense cecocentral scotoma, often sparing central fixation, is the most frequent field defect. Nerve fiber bundle defects and peripheral field constriction develop frequently and blindness may occur. ERG abnormalities involving the a- and b-waves occur.[226,227]

Experimental findings in rhesus monkeys suggest that the primary lesion in methyl alcohol poisoning is disruption of axoplasmic flow just at or behind the lamina cribrosa.[228–230] It is postulated that toxic metabolic breakdown products of methanol exert adverse effects on cytochrome oxidase and other oxidative enzymes, which causes swelling of the oligodendroglial cells in the retrolaminar optic nerve. This results in axonal compression, axoplasmic flow stasis, and optic disc edema.[228]

Recent reports of experimental methanol toxicity in rats and electrophysiologic and histopathologic studies in a human with methanol toxicity have demonstrated evidence that the retinal receptors and RPE are affected.[231,232] The absorption, distribution, and metabolism of methanol and ethanol are similar. Since ethanol has a 100-fold greater affinity for alcohol dehydrogenase than methanol, treatment consists of early administration of ethanol and correction of metabolic acidosis.

BISPHOSPHONATES

Bisphosphonates used to treat osteoporosis inhibit bone resorption by binding to hydroxyapatite crystals and inhibit their dissolution. Intravenous preparations pamidronate disodium and zoledronic acid cause conjunctivitis, anterior uveitis, episcleritis, anterior and posterior scleritis and acute retinal pigment epitheliitis.[311–318] The onset of ocular symptoms occurs within 24–48 hours of infusion. All cases of iridocyclitis respond to topical steroids and the scleritis to oral steroids. The one case of retinal pigment epitheliitis resolved spontaneously.

Oral preparations alendronate, risedronate, and etidronate have been associated with blurred vision, eye pain, conjunctivitis, uveitis, and scleritis (Figure 9.16K). The onset of symptoms occurs 2 days to 2 weeks after starting therapy. They are self-limited if mild, and moderate cases respond to topical steroids.

9.17 Drug-induced cystoid macular edema.

Glucophage

A–F: This 48-year-old type 2 diabetic with proliferative diabetic retinopathy had no macular edema and a visual acuity of 20/25 + in his left eye (A). He returned complaining of fluctuating vision 4 months later when his vision had decreased to 20/40 due to cystoid macular edema (B–E). He was also noted to have evidence of fluid retention with pedal edema. He was on glucophage in addition to insulin. Glucophage was discontinued and he returned 5 weeks later with return of vision to 20/25 and complete resolution of the cystoid edema on optical coherence tomography (OCT) (F) and significant improvement in his pedal edema.

Paclitaxel.

G–L: A 60-year-old woman with bilateral gradual decrease in vision over 6 months to 20/30 in the right eye and 20/70 in the left eye. Both macula showed cystoid swelling more visible on the OCT images (G–J). An angiogram showed no dye leakage in either fovea (K and L). The patient was receiving Abraxane (albumin-bound paclitaxel nanoparticles) for metastatic breast cancer, the cause of cystic maculopathy.

(G–L, courtesy of Dr. David Weinberg.)

PACLITAXEL TOXICITY

Paclitaxel and docetaxel are antimicrotubule agents that inhibit mitosis and are used as chemotherapeutic agents for breast and lung carcinoma. Nonleaking cystoid macular edema that is reversible on discontinuation of the drug is seen with the protein-bound form of paclitaxel (Figure 9.17 G to L).[238–240] One patient experienced photopsias and visual field defects.[241]

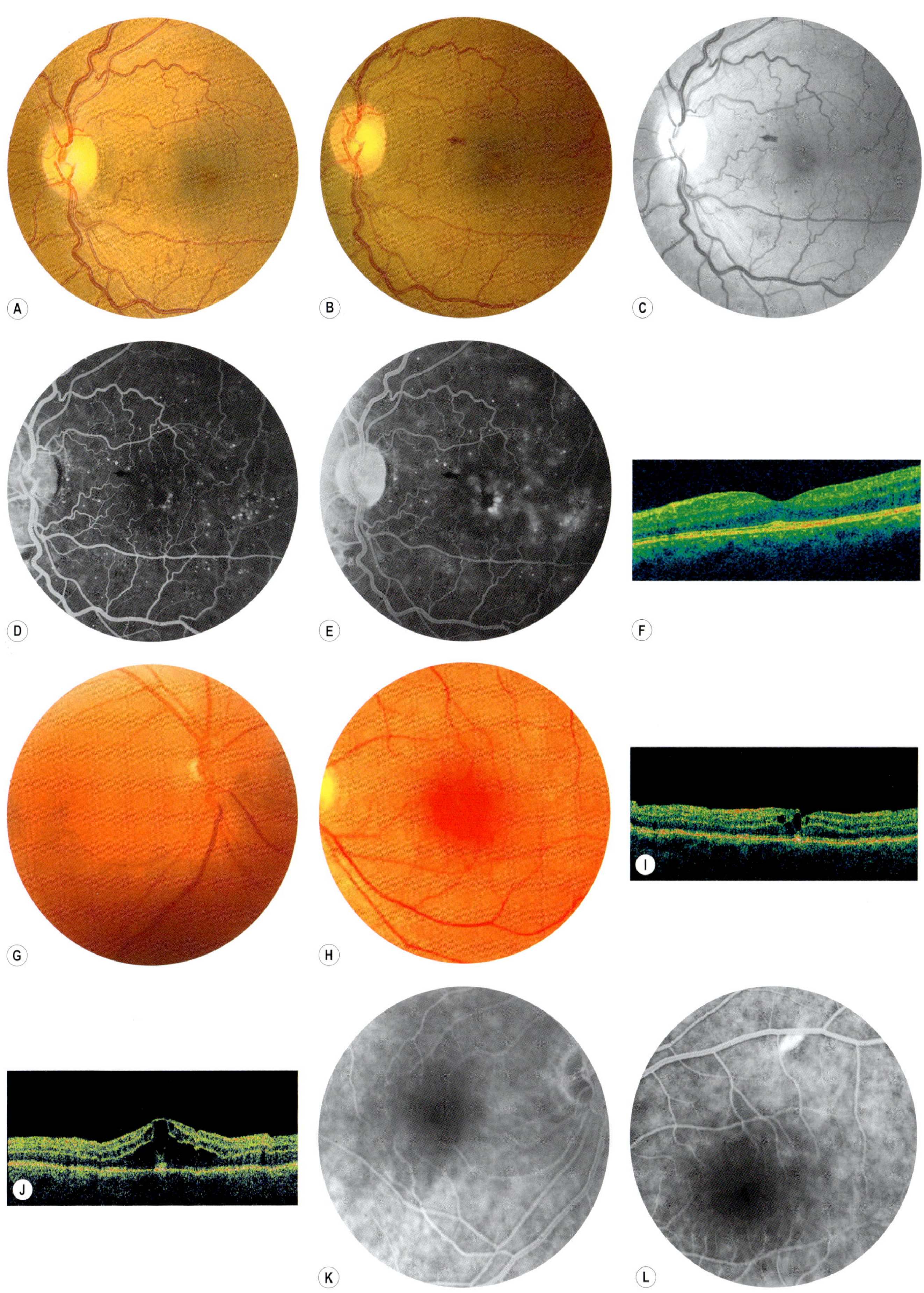
A
B
C
D
E
F
G
H
I
J
K
L

IMATINIB MESYLATE (GLEEVEC) TOXICITY

Imatinib mesylate used in the treatment of leukemia causes fluid retention and conjunctival and periorbital edema in almost 30% of patients. Cystoid macular edema with or without subretinal fluid that is reversible if the drug is discontinued early has been reported in three cases.[242–244] The mechanism is still speculative. If stereo fluorescein angiography demonstrates intraretinal fluid accumulation from RPE dysfunction, oral acetazolamide may be useful in treating the cystoid edema.

GLITAZONE TOXICITY

Glitazones (rosiglitazone and pioglitazone) used to reduce insulin resistance in type 2 diabetics cause fluid retention and pedal edema in 4–7% of patients when used alone and up to 15% when used with insulin.[245] These patients show pedal edema and rapid weight gain, which improves after discontinuing the drug. Cystoid macular edema secondary to diffuse leakage occurs in some of these patients and is refractory to laser treatment and diuretics.[246–248] Discontinuation of the medication helps if done early. Similar occurrence of cystoid macular edema in a type 2 diabetic patient on metformin which resolved within 6 weeks following discontinuation of metformin is illustrated in Figure 9.17A–F.

NICOTINIC ACID MACULOPATHY

See Chapter 6.

EPINEPHRINE AND PROSTAGLANDIN ANALOG-INDUCED CYSTOID MACULAR EDEMA

Topical epinephrine drops and prostaglandin analogs such as latanoprost, travaprost, and bimetoprost can cause angiographically evident cystoid macular edema, often reversible on discontinuation of the medication.

VENLAFAXINE

Venlafaxine (Effexor), an antipsychotic drug, is reported to cause blepharedema. The author has seen a patient who developed bilateral cystoid macular edema (Figure 9.18A, B, E, and F) associated with other systemic signs of intolerance to venlafaxine. The edema persisted in spite of discontinuation of the drug, and recurred 2 months following bilateral intravitreal triamcinalone injections. Fluorescein angiography demonstrated leakage of dye at the RPE (Figure 9.18C and D) prompting treatment with oral acetazolamide for 3 months, which resulted in resolution of cystoid macular edema (Figure 9.18G and H).

9.18 Venlafaxine (Effexor)-induced cystoid macular edema (CME).

A–H: This 48-year-old woman showed worsening of her situational depression and developed bilateral blurred vision over 2 months following a switch of her antidepressant from Lexapro to venlafaxine (Effexor XR). After 3 months of being on the medication venlafaxine was changed to Wellbutrin, which helped her depression. Her vision remained affected and she was found to have bilateral cystoid macular edema, that on angiography showed accumulation of dye via the retinal pigment epithelium and visible on optical coherence tomography (A–F). The CME responded to bilateral intravitreal triamcinalone (4 mg) but recurred in 2 months when she also developed bilateral posterior subcapsular cataracts and persistent elevated intraocular pressures that required bilateral trabeculectomies. Topical Pred Forte did not help the CME. Since the dye accumulated from incompetence of the pigment epithelium, she was started on oral acetazolamide at 250 mg three times a day. The CME responded and resolved over 2 months (G and H). She was slowly tapered off the acetazolamide over 4 months and CME did not recur.

Dehydration/marathon retinopathy.

I–K: This 30-year-old Asian-Indian orthopedic resident awoke with decreased vision in the right eye. He had run 20 miles a day and half before. He was a −9D myope and was otherwise healthy. Visual acuity was counting fingers at 1.2 meter (4 feet) in the right eye and 20/25 in the left eye. He had a central scotoma on the Goldmann visual field; there were several cotton-wool spots, dot-blot hemorrhages, and cilio-retinal artery occlusion on the right (I and J). Fluorescein angiogram showed slowing of flow through the cilio-retinal artery on this side (L). Probable risk factors included homozygosity for MTHFR A1298C mutation and recent dehydration, all of which caused him to develop the central retinal vein/ciliary retinal artery occlusion. A week later, his visual acuity improved to 20/20. He had a small inferotemporal relative paracentral scotoma and ended up running the Chicago marathon 3 weeks later.

High-altitude retinopathy

L–N: A 26-year-old male noted blurring of his right eye vision 3 nights into his climb of Mount Muztagata (at 20 000 feet (6096 meters)). The highest point is at 24 757 feet (7546 meters). The picture was taken 10 days later when his vision was recorded at 20/80 in the right and 20/20 in the left eye. He had two macular preretinal hemorrhages on the right and few intraretinal hemorrhages in the left eye (L and M). Fluorescein angiogram only showed blocked fluorescence from the hemorrhage (N). His hemorrhages cleared and vision returned to 20/20 in both eyes.

(I–K, courtesy of Dr. Mathew MacCumber and Dr. Kirk Packo, L–N, courtesy of Dr. Ron Adelman.)

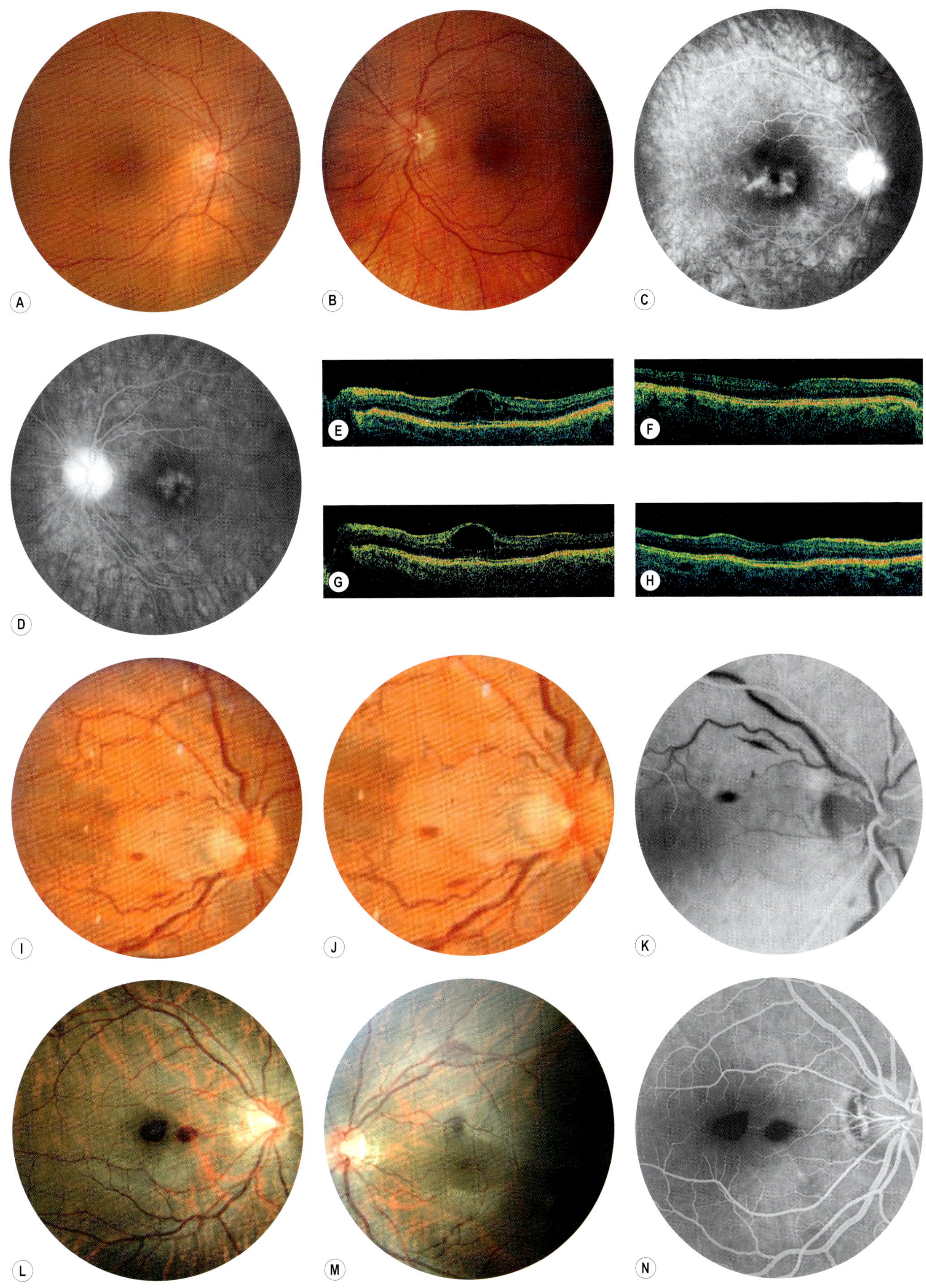
A
B
C
D
E
F
G
H
I
J
K
L
M
N

INDOCYANINE GREEN TOXICITY

The use of indocyanine green dye during chromovitrectomy to stain the internal limiting membrane has improved the success rate of macular hole closure. However various instances of retinal toxicity have been noted. The postulated mechanisms include direct biochemical toxicity to the neural retinal cells and RPE, osmolarity effect on the vitreoretinal interface, mechanical cleavage effect to the inner limiting membrane/inner retinal surface and light-induced injury.[233,234] The direct damage to, and induction of apoptosis of, neuroretinal and RPE cells appear to be dose-dependent. Indocyanine green absorption of light is in the near-infrared range (780–830 nm) and induces photooxidation type I (increased local temperature of tissue) and photo-oxidation type II (photodynamic effects).[235,236]

Biochemical changes in the inner limiting membrane with increased stiffening has also been noted.[237] To minimize toxicity, a low concentration, short duration, and low illumination are recommended.[234,236]

TACROLIMUS TOXICITY

Thrombotic microangiopathy of various organs is a side-effect of tacrolimus (FK506) and presents as a retinal infarct with cotton-wool spots and retinal hemorrhages in the eye (Figures 9.19A and B and 9.20A and B).[259] The underlying mechanism is thrombotic thrombocytopenia and hemolysis, which require discontinuation of the drug, plasmapheresis, and fresh frozen plasma as rescue. Endothelial swelling and intraluminal fibrin are seen in the glomeruli on kidney biopsy. Fluorescein angiogram reveals occluded macular vessels (Figures 9.19C–F and 9.20C–E). Schisis-like changes are sometimes seen due to loss of retinal tissue from infarction (Figure 9.20H and I). The microangiopathy usually occurs within a few days posttransplant and is seen post solid organ and bone marrow transplant. Similar microangiopathy is seen with cyclosporine, sirolimus, and systemic antivascular endothelial growth factor therapy (VEGF) with bevacizumab.

AMIODARONE OPTIC NEUROPATHY

Patients receiving amiodarone, an antiarrhythmic drug, may develop verticillate keratopathy, tremor, ataxia, pulmonary fibrosis, and occasionally visual loss associated with optic disc swelling and hemorrhages. These changes may be followed by optic atrophy and narrowing of the retinal arteries in some patients.[260–262] It is uncertain whether or not this optic neuropathy is a peculiar complication of the drug or is a routine nonarteritic anterior ischemic optic neuropathy occurring in the group of patients who are predisposed to this complication.[263] The corneal deposits may result in blue-green rings or colored halos around lights. A maculopathy attributed to accumulation of the drug in the RPE has been described; however the cases were not well documented and may not be related to amiadarone.[264]

9.20 Tacrolimus microangiopathy

A–K: This 43-year-old Indian male presented with sudden progressive decrease in vision in both eyes for 4 weeks. He had received a live related renal allograft 6 weeks previously. He was on tacrolimus 5 mg twice a day, mycophenolate mofetil 1 g twice a day and prednisolone 15 mg once daily. He was also on blood pressure medication and his blood pressure read 130/80 mmHg. His visual acuity was count fingers at 0.5 meter. Both macula showed whitening with retinal hemorrhages. An angiogram showed macular infarction with occlusion of the perifoveal arterioles. He showed no evidence of thrombocytopenia, renal failure, or hemolysis. Four months later the retinal whitening had mostly resolved and by 11 months his vision had stabilized at 20/200 in both eyes. Optical coherence tomography of both macula showed schisis-like cavities without significant overall thickening, signifying loss of retinal substance.

(A–K, courtesy of Dr. Vishali Gupta and Dr. Amod Gupta.)

SILDENAFIL (VIAGRA)

The commonest side-effect of Viagra is a transient bluish discoloration of vision and impaired blue/green discrimination. Serous retinal detachments simulating idiopathic central serous chorioretinopathy have been seen in patients taking sildenafil for erectile dysfunction.[265–267] It is a cyclic guanosine monophosphate-specific phosphodiesterase type 5 inhibitor, which is a potent vasodilator that increases choroidal thickness by 30% by increasing choroidal blood flow by 20–30%.[268] Choroidal engorgement as an idiosyncratic effect may be the underlying mechanism of exudative retinal detachment.[266] In most patients the serous detachment resolved on discontinuation of the drug (dechallenge) and recurred in a few on rechallenge.[265,266] Ischemic optic neuropathy, branch retinal artery occlusion, and an acute third-nerve palsy have also been seen; however these may be related to vascular compromise in patients already predisposed to vascular accidents.[269–271]

CORTICOSTEROID-ASSOCIATED CENTRAL SEROUS CHORIORETINOPATHY

See Chapter 3.

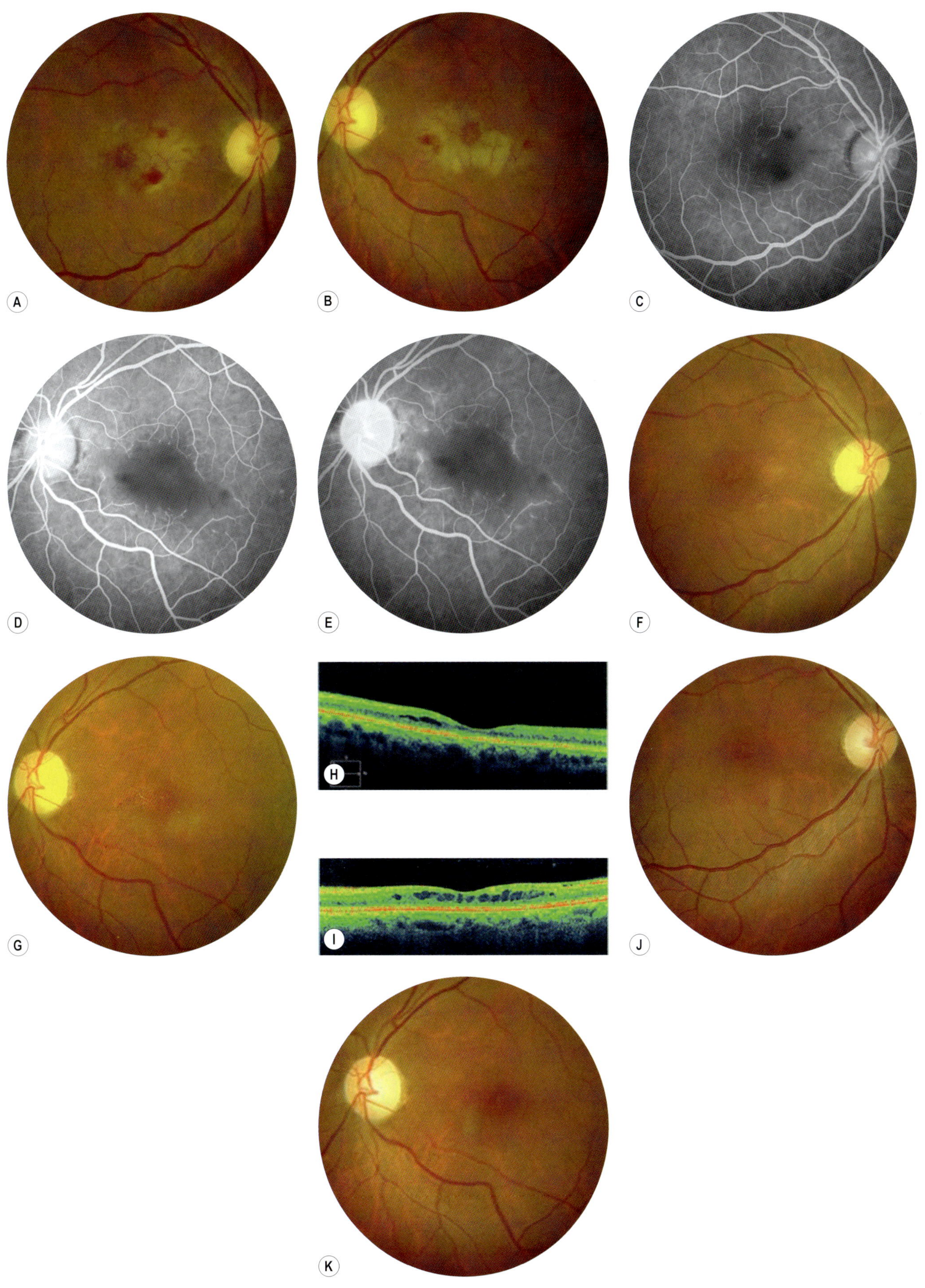
A
B
C
D
E
F
G
H
I
J
K

RETINOIDS

A few patients on isotretinoin therapy for acne complain of poor night vision and difficulty with dark adaptation. Two patients had abnormal ERGs and dark adaptation, which recovered slowly over 25 months in one patient and 6–12 months in the other.

CIDOFOVIR

Cidofovir is an anti-cytomegalovirus (CMV) anucleotide analog and shows broad-spectrum activity against CMV, varicella-zoster virus, herpes simplex virus types 1 and 2, and Epstein–Barr virus. After uptake into cells it is converted into an active, long-acting metabolite, an analog to cytosine. It blocks viral DNA polymerase relatively selectively. Uveitis and hypotony are common (25–50%) after both intravenous and intravitreal cidofovir. Direct cytotoxicity to ciliary epithelium is considered to be the cause of decreased aqueous production. A break in the blood–retinal and blood–ocular barrier, especially in eyes with chronic smoldering CMV retinitis, is likely responsible for the iritis and anterior uveitis. Reducing the dose of cidofovir in these eyes with higher bioavailability can decrease the intensity of the inflammation. The uveitis responds to cycloplegics and topical steroids. Cystoid macular edema is seen during immune recovery.[272]

RIFABUTIN

Rifabutin is used in the treatment or prophylaxis of systemic *Mycobacterium avium* complex infections in patients with AIDS, and sometimes in immunocompetent people.[273] Hypopyon uveitis can begin within a few days to a few weeks of beginning treatment in both immunosuppressed and immunocompetent individuals.[274–278] Panuveitis with retinal vasculitis is seen rarely in patients with pulmonary tuberculosis.[279] Bilateral corneal endothelial deposits, in the absence of inflammation, have also been reported with rifabutin use in human immunodeficiency virus (HIV)-positive adults and children.[280,281] The stellate, refractile endothelial deposits are first observed in the periphery, and may eventually extend to involve the central cornea. These deposits are associated with flare and can occur in eyes without associated infections such as CMV retinitis. Over time, the deposits may take on a golden hue and progress despite cessation of rifabutin. Anterior lens deposition, vitreous opacities,[276] cystoid macular edema,[282] and a reversible retinal dysfunction have been documented in experimental studies.[283]

The mechanism for uveitis is not clearly understood: possibilities include deposition of immunoglobulins or antirifabutin antibodies, although rifabutin in vivo does not alter cell-mediated immunity. The inflammatory response can be exacerbated by concomitant use of macrolides[278,284] or azole drugs such as fluconazole. The uveitis responds to discontinuation of rifabutin and institution of topical steroids and cycloplegics.

VIGABATRIN

Vigabatrin is a gamma-aminobutyric acid transaminase inhibitor used to treat children with infantile spasms and adults with partial seizures. The drug is not approved by the US Food and Drug Administration but is used extensively in Europe and Canada for treating infantile spasms and partial epilepsy. It is the drug of choice in treating infantile spasms in tuberous sclerosis. The ocular toxicity in the form of peripheral visual field changes[285] resulting from retinal nerve fiber toxicity with consecutive optic atrophy was first noted in 1997.[285–291] About 40–50% of adults and children on the medication show evidence of toxicity. The drug crosses the blood–retinal barrier and is found to be 18.5 times more concentrated in the retina. The 30-Hz photopic flicker is the earliest affected ERG parameter. The drug is specifically taken up by amacrine, horizontal, bipolar, and Müller cells of the retina where it exerts its toxicity. Monitoring with serial visual fields and optical coherence measurement of retinal nerve fiber thickness are recommended.[292]

INDOMETHACIN RETINOPATHY

There are a few reports of retinal changes attributed to indomethacin (Indocin); however, none presents convincing evidence of a causal relationship between indomethacin therapy and the fundus changes.[298–300]

DIGITALIS AND DIGOXIN RETINAL TOXICITY

Digitalis and digoxin may cause defective color vision, xanthopsia, and other aberrations of color vision, as well as abnormal dark adaptation and reduced photopic flicker ERG amplitudes.[301–303] The fundus appearance is unaffected. The patient may or may not complain of dyschromatopsia. Color vision testing is a useful measure in the diagnosis of toxicity of these drugs and may reveal both red–green and blue–yellow deficiencies. Long-term use of digitalis even at therapeutic doses causes red–green and tritan deficiency in 20–30% of patients.[304]

GLYCINE RETINAL TOXICITY ASSOCIATED WITH TRANSURETHRAL RESECTION

Glycine is the most commonly used irrigating substance during transurethral resection and endometrial ablations. Exposure of the prostate venous sinuses may allow excessive absorption of glycine, which, when reaches levels of approximately 4000 μmol/l (>30 mg/dl), may cause transient visual disturbances such as "darkening" of vision, or severe visual loss for up to several hours.[305] Glycine absorption results in excess fluid absorption and dilutional hyponatremia, resulting in pulmonary edema and encephalopathy.[306–310] Fundoscopic examination is normal. Visual loss is associated with ERG changes consisting of loss of oscillatory potentials and attenuation of 30-Hz "flicker following." This retinal dysfunction may be the result of glycine's role as an inhibitory neurotransmitter.

FLUDARABINE TOXICITY

Fludarabine is a purine analog antineoplastic agent which has been tried in patients with a variety of lymphoproliferative malignancies and as an immune suppressor before stem cell transplant. Ocular toxicity is not common at the low-dose regimen. However a phase I study showed loss of vision in all but two of the 13 patients who received high-dose fludarabine. The visual loss is irreversible and progressive, except in rare instances where vision improves. Loss of bipolar cell function on ERG is first noted. Histology shows dramatic loss of ganglion and bipolar cells, loss of myelin, and severe necrosis of the optic nerve.[319] In addition, reactivation of acute retinal necrosis and other opportunistic viral and fungal infections are seen.[320]

GEMCITABINE PURTSCHER-LIKE RETINOPATHY

Gemcitabine is a nucleoside analog used to treat osteosarcoma, nonsmall cell lung cancer, breast, ovarian, transitional, and pancreatic cancers. A 59-year-old male treated for nonsmall cell lung cancer developed Purtscher-like retinopathy and peripheral vascular occlusions involving the digits and dorsal penis along with positive antinuclear antibodies and an elevated sedimentation rate. Discontinuation of the drug and systemic steroids quietened the lesions, though they persisted for 8–10 months with loss of the fourth digit.[321]

ACUTE MACULAR NEURORETINOPATHY AFTER INJECTION OF SYMPATHOMIMETICS

See Chapter 11.

DRUG-INDUCED ACUTE MYOPIA

Chlorthalidone, hydrochlorothiazide, triamterine, and topiramate are known to induce acute myopia with retinal folds. A variable degree of ciliary body swelling, ciliary muscle spasm, peripheral choroidal effusions, and forward movement of the iris lens diaphragm contribute towards the myopic change. Most of these are transient and correctable on discontinuation of the drug.[322–324] Patients on topiramate often develop bilateral or unilateral acute angle closure glaucoma requiring medications, and sometimes peripheral iridectomy or iridoplasty.[325–330]

References

1. Bernstein H, Zvaifler N, Rubin M, et al. The ocular deposition of chloroquine. Invest Ophthalmol 1963;2:384–92.
2. Brinkley Jr JR, Dubois EL, Ryan SJ. Long-term course of chloroquine retinopathy after cessation of medication. Am J Ophthalmol 1979;88:1–11.
3. Carr RE, Gouras P, Gunkel RD. Chloroquine retinopathy; early detection by retinal threshold test. Arch Ophthalmol 1966;75:171–8.
4. Carr RE, Henkind P, Rothfield N, et al. Ocular toxicity of antimalarial drugs; long-term follow-up. Am J Ophthalmol 1968;66:738–44.
5. Easterbrook M. The use of Amsler grids in early chloroquine retinopathy. Ophthalmology 1984;91:1368–72.
6. François J, de Rouck A, Cambie E, et al. Rétinopathie chloroquinique. Ophthalmologica 1972;165:81–99.
7. Grant WM. Toxicology of the eye, 4th ed. Springfield, IL: CC Thomas; 1993. p. 371–82.
8. Hart Jr WM, Burde RM, Johnston GP, et al. Static perimetry in chloroquine retinopathy; perifoveal patterns of visual field depression. Arch Ophthalmol 1984;102:377–80.
9. Heckenlively JR, Martin D, Levy J. Chloroquine retinopathy. Am J Ophthalmol 1980;89:150.
10. Henkind P, Carr RE, Siegel IM. Early chloroquine retinopathy: clinical and functional findings. Arch Ophthalmol 1964;71:157–65.
11. Henkind P, Gold DH. Ocular manifestations of rheumatic disorders; natural and iatrogenic. Rheumatology 1973;4:13–59.
12. Henkind P, Rothfield NF. Ocular abnormalities in patients treated with synthetic antimalarial drugs. N Engl J Med 1963;269:433–9.
13. Kearns TP, Hollenhorst RW. Chloroquine retinopathy; evaluation by fluorescein fundus angiography. Arch Ophthalmol 1966;76:378–84.
14. Martin LJ, Bergen RL, Dobrow HR. Delayed onset chloroquine retinopathy: case report. Ann Ophthalmol 1978;10:723–6.
15. Percival SPB, Behrman J. Ophthalmological safety of chloroquine. Br J Ophthalmol 1969;53:101–9.
16. Ramsey MS, Fine BS. Chloroquine toxicity in the human eye; histopathologic observations by electron microscopy. Am J Ophthalmol 1972;73:229–35.
17. Rubin M, Bernstein HN, Zvaifler NJ. Studies on the pharmacology of chloroquine; recommendations for the treatment of chloroquine retinopathy. Arch Ophthalmol 1963;70:474–81.
18. Rynes RI, Krohel G, Falbo A, et al. Ophthalmologic safety of long-term hydroxychloroquine treatment. Arthritis Rheum 1979;22:832–6.
19. Sachs DD, Hogan MJ, Engleman EP. Chorioretinopathy induced by chronic administration of chloroquine phosphate (abstract). Arthritis Rheum 1962;5:318–9.
20. Sassani JW, Brucker AJ, Cobbs W, et al. Progressive chloroquine retinopathy. Ann Ophthalmol 1983;15:19–22.
21. Tobin DR, Krohel GB, Rynes RI. Hydroxychloroquine seven-year experience. Arch Ophthalmol 1982;100:81–3.
22. Wetterholm DH, Winter FC. Histopathology of chloroquine retinal toxicity. Arch Ophthalmol 1964;71:82–7.
23. Johnson MW, Vine AK. Hydroxychloroquine therapy in massive doses without retinal toxicity. Am J Ophthalmol 1987;104:139–44.
24. Raines MF, Bhargava SK, Rosen ES. The blood–retinal barrier in chloroquine retinopathy. Invest Ophthalmol Vis Sci 1989;30:1726–31.
25. Weiner A, Sandberg MA, Gaudio AR, et al. Hydroxychloroquine retinopathy. Am J Ophthalmol 1991;112:528–34.
26. Shearer RV, Dubois EL. Ocular changes induced by long-term hydroxychloroquine (Plaquenil) therapy. Am J Ophthalmol 1967;64:245–52.
27. Shroyer NF, Lewis RA, Lupski JR. Analysis of the ABCR (ABCA4) gene in 4-aminoquinoline retinopathy: is retinal toxicity by chloroquine and hydroxychloroquine related to Stargardt disease? Am J Ophthalmol 2001;131:761–6.
28. Weiter JJ, Delori F, Dorey CK. Central sparing in annular macular degeneration. Am J Ophthalmol 1988;106:286–92.
29. Cruess AF, Schachat AP, Nicholl J, et al. Chloroquine retinopathy; is fluorescein angiography necessary? Ophthalmology 1985;92:1127–9.
30. Chang WH, Katz BJ, Warner JE, et al. A novel method for screening the multifocal electroretonogram in patients using hydroxychloroquine. Retina 2008;28:1478–86.
31. Gilbert ME, Savino PJ. Missing the bull's eye. Surv Ophthalmol 2007;52:440–2.
32. Teoh SC, Lim J, Koh A, et al. Abnormalities on the multifocal electroretinogram may precede clinical signs of hydroxychloroquine retino-toxicity. Eye 2006;20:129–32.
33. Lai TY, Chan WM, Li H, et al. Multifocal electroretinographic changes in patients receiving hydroxychloroquine therapy. Am J Ophthalmol 2005;140:794–807.
34. Neubauer AS, Stiefelmeyer S, Berninger T, et al. The multifocal pattern electroretinogram in chloroquine retinopathy. Ophthalmic Res 2004;36:106–13.
35. Maturi RK, Yu M, Weleber RG. Multifocal electroretinographic evaluation of long-term hydroxychloroquine users. Arch Ophthalmol 2004;122:973–81.
36. Penrose PJ, Tzekov RT, Sutter EE, et al. Multifocal electroretinography evaluation for early detection of retinal dysfunction in patients taking hydroxychloroquine. Retina 2003;23:503–12.
37. Bernstein HN, Ginsberg J. The pathology of chloroquine retinopathy. Arch Ophthalmol 1964;71:238–45.
38. Gaynes BI, Torczynski E, Varro Z, et al. Retinal toxicity of chloroquine hydrochloride administered by intraperitoneal injection. J Appl Toxicol 2008;28:895–900.
39. Ehrenfeld M, Nesher R, Merin SL. Delayed-onset chloroquine retinopathy. Br J Ophthalmol 1986;70:281–3.
40. Applebaum A. An ophthalmoscopic study of patients under treatment with thioridazine. Arch Ophthalmol 1963;69:578–80.
41. Connell MM, Poley BJ, McFarlane JR. Chorioretinopathy associated with thioridazine therapy. Arch Ophthalmol 1964;71:816–21.
42. Davidorf FH. Thioridazine pigmentary retinopathy. Arch Ophthalmol 1973;90:251–5.
43. de Margerie J. Ocular changes produced by a phenothiazine drug: thioridazine. Trans Can Ophthalmol Soc 1962;25:160–75.
44. Fishman GA. Thioridazine hydrochloride (Mellaril) toxic pigmentary chorioretinopathy. In: Smith JL, editor. Neuro-ophthalmology focus 1982. New York: Masson; 1981. p. 109–18.
45. Gregory MH, Rutty DA, Wood RD. Differences in the retinotoxic action of chloroquine and phenothiazine derivatives. J Pathol 1970;102:139–50.
46. Heshe J, Engelstoft FH, Kirk L. Retinal injury developing under thioridazine therapy. Nord Psykiatr T 1961;15:442–7.
47. Kimbrough BO, Campbell RJ. Thioridazine levels in the human eye. Arch Ophthalmol 1981;99:2188–9.
48. Kozy D, Doft BH, Lipkowitz J. Nummular thioridazine retinopathy. Retina 1984;4:253–6.
49. Meredith TA, Aaberg TM, Willerson WD. Progressive chorioretinopathy after receiving thioridazine. Arch Ophthalmol 1978;96:1172–6.
50. Miller III FS, Bunt-Milam AH, Kalina RE. Clinical-ultrastructural study of thioridazine retinopathy. Ophthalmology 1982;89:1478–88.
51. Potts AM. Uveal pigment and phenothiazine compounds. Trans Am Ophthalmol Soc 1962;60:517–52.
52. Potts AM. The reaction of uveal pigment in vitro with polycyclic compounds. Invest Ophthalmol 1964;3:405–16.
53. Scott AW. Retinal pigmentation in a patient receiving thioridazine. Arch Ophthalmol 1963;70:775–8.
54. Marmor MF. Is thioridazine retinopathy progressive? Relationship of pigmentary changes to visual function. Br J Ophthalmol 1990;74:739–42.
55. Kimbrough BO, Campbell RJ. Thioridazine levels in the human eye. Arch Ophthalmol 1981;99:2188–9.
56. Fornaro P, Calabria G, Corallo G, et al. Pathogenesis of degenerative retinopathies induced by thioridazine and other antipsychotics: a dopamine hypothesis. Doc Ophthalmol 2002;105: 41–9.
57. Burian HM, Fletcher MC. Visual functions in patients with retinal pigmentary degeneration following the use of NP 207. Arch Ophthalmol 1958;60:612–29.
58. DeLong SL, Poley BJ, McFarlane JR. Ocular changes associated with long-term chlorpromazine therapy. Arch Ophthalmol 1965;73:611–7.
59. Mathalone MBR. Eye and skin changes in psychiatric patients treated with chlorpromazine. Br J Ophthalmol 1967;51:86–93.
60. Weekley RD, Potts AM, Reboton J, et al. Pigmentary retinopathy in patients receiving high doses of a new phenothiazine. Arch Ophthalmol 1960;64:65–76.
61. Craythorn JM, Swartz M, Creel DJ. Clofazimine-induced bull's-eye retinopathy. Retina 1986;6:50–2.
62. Cunningham CA, Friedberg DM, Carr RE. Clofazimine-induced generalized retinal degeneration. Retina 1990;10:131–4.
63. Blake DR, Winyard P, Lunec J, et al. Cerebral and ocular toxicity induced by desferrioxamine. Q J Med 1985;56:345–55.
64. Cases A, Kelly J, Sabater F, et al. Ocular and auditory toxicity in hemodialyzed patients receiving desferrioxamine. Nephron 1990;56:19–23.
65. Davies SC, Marcus RE, Hungerford JL, et al. Ocular toxicity of high-dose intravenous desferrioxamine. Lancet 1983;2:181–4.
66. Lakhanpal V, Schocket SS, Jiji R. Deferoxamine (Desferal(Rx))-induced toxic retinal pigmentary degeneration and presumed optic neuropathy. Ophthalmology 1984;91:443–51.
67. O'Hare JA, Murnaghan DJ. Evidence of increased parathyroid activity on discontinuation of high-aluminum dialysate in patients undergoing hemodialysis. Am J Med 1984;77:229–32.
68. Pall H, Blake DR, Winyard P, et al. Ocular toxicity of desferrioxamine – an example of copper promoted auto-oxidative damage? Br J Ophthalmol 1989;73:42–7.
69. Rahi AHS, Hungerford JL, Ahmed AI. Ocular toxicity of desferrioxamine: light microscopic histochemical and ultrastructural findings. Br J Ophthalmol 1986;70:373–81.
70. Ravelli M, Scaroni P, Mombelloni S, et al. Acute visual disorders in patients on regular dialysis given desferrioxamine as a test. Nephrol Dial Transplant 1990;5:945–9.
71. Mehta AM, Engstrom Jr RE, Kreiger AE. Deferoxamine-associated retinopathy after subcutaneous injection. Am J Ophthalmol 1994;118:260–2.
72. Gonzales CR, Lin AP, Engstrom RE, et al. Bilateral vitelliform maculopathy and deferoxamine toxicity. Retina 2004;24:464–7.
73. Hidajat RR, McLay JL, Goode DH, et al. EOG as a monitor of desferrioxamine retinal toxicity. Doc Ophthalmol 2004;109:273–8.
74. Haimovici R, D'Amico DJ, Gragoudas ES, et al. The expanded clinical spectrum of deferoxamine retinopathy. Ophthalmology 2002;109:164–71.
75. Pall H, Blake DR, Winyard P, et al. Ocular toxicity of desferrioxamine – an example of copper promoted auto-oxidative damage? Br J Ophthalmol 1989;73:42–7.
76. Cibis PA, Brown EB, Hong SM. Ocular effects of systemic siderosis. Am J Ophthalmol 1957;44:158–72.
77. Cibis PA, Yamashita T, Rodrigues F. Clinical aspects of ocular siderosis and hemosiderosis. Arch Ophthalmol 1959;62:180–7.
78. Schocket SS, Lakhanpal V, Varma SD. Siderosis from a retained intraocular stone. Retina 1981;1:201–7.
79. Cleary G, Sheth HG, Laidlaw AH. Delayed transient macular ischaemia due to ocular siderosis. Eye 2007;21:1132–3.
80. Shaikh S, Blumenkranz MS. Fluorescein angiographic findings in ocular siderosis. Am J Ophthalmol 2001;131:136–8.
81. Knave B. Electroretinography in eyes with retained intraocular metallic foreign bodies; a clinical study. Acta Ophthalmol Suppl 1969:100.
82. Kuhn F, Witherspoon CD, Skalka H, et al. Improvement of siderotic ERG. Eur J Ophthalmol 1992;2:44–5.
83. Imaizumi M, Matsumoto CS, Yamada K, et al. Electroretinographic assessment of early changes in ocular siderosis. Ophthalmologica 2000;214:354–9.

84. O'Duffy D, Salmon JF. Siderosis bulbi resulting from an intralenticular foreign body. Am J Ophthalmol 1999;127:218–9.
85. Broendstrup P. Two cases of temporary siderosis bulbi with spontaneous resorption and without impairment of function. Acta Ophthalmol 1944;22:311–6.
86. Konstantinidis L, Borruat FX, Wolfensberger TJ. Long-term stability of retinal function despite retained intraocular metallic foreign body. Klin Monatsbl Augenheilkd 2008;225:482–5.
87. Sneed SR. Ocular siderosis. Arch Ophthalmol 1988;106:997.
88. Sneed SR, Weingeist TA. Management of siderosis bulbi due to a retained iron-containing intraocular foreign body. Ophthalmology 1990;97:375–9.
89. Hodgkins PR, Morrell AJ, Luff AJ, et al. Pigment epitheliopathy with serous detachment of the retina following intravenous iron dextran. Eye 1992;6:414–5.
90. Masciulli L, Anderson DR, Charles S. Experimental ocular siderosis in the squirrel monkey. Am J Ophthalmol 1972;74:638–61.
91. Delaney Jr WV. Presumed ocular chalcosis: a reversible maculopathy. Ann Ophthalmol 1975;7:378–80.
92. Felder KS, Gottlieb F. Reversible chalcosis. Ann Ophthalmol 1984;16:638–41.
93. Rao NA, Tso MOM, Rosenthal AR. Chalcosis in the human eye; a clinicopathologic study. Arch Ophthalmol 1976;94:1379–84.
94. Rosenthal AR, Appleton B. Histochemical localization of intraocular copper foreign bodies. Am J Ophthalmol 1975;79:613–25.
95. Rao NA, Tso MO, Rosenthal AR. Chalcosis in the human eye. A clinicopathologic study. Arch Ophthalmol 1976;94:1379–84.
96. Pala G, Fronterre A, Scafa F, et al. Ocular argyrosis in a silver craftsman. J Occup Health 2008;50:521–4.
97. Cohen SY, Quentel G, Egasse D, et al. The dark choroid in systemic argyrosis. Retina 1993;13:312–6.
98. Spencer WH, Garron LK, Contreras F, et al. Endogenous and exogenous ocular and systemic silver deposition. Trans Ophthalmol Soc UK 1980;100:171–8.
99. Caruso R, Wilding G, Ballintine E, et al. Cisplatin retinopathy. ARVO Abstracts. Invest Ophthalmol Vis Sci 1985;26(Suppl.):34.
100. Greenberg HS, Ensminger WD, Chandler WF, et al. Intra-arterial BCNU chemotherapy for treatment of malignant gliomas of the central nervous system. J Neurosurg 1984;61:423–9.
101. Grimson BS, Mahaley Jr MS, Dubey HD, et al. Ophthalmic and central nervous system complications following intracarotid BCNU (Carmustine). J Clin Neuro-Ophthalmol 1981;1:261–4.
102. Kupersmith MJ, Frohman LP, Choi IS, et al. Visual system toxicity following intra-arterial chemotherapy. Neurology 1988;38:284–9.
103. Margo CE, Murtagh FR. Ocular and orbital toxicity after intracarotid cisplatin therapy. Am J Ophthalmol 1993;116:508–9.
104. Miller DF, Bay JW, Lederman RG, et al. Ocular and orbital toxicity of BCNU (Carmustine) and cisplatinum for malignant gliomas. Ophthalmology 1985;92:402–6.
105. Ostrow S, Hahn P, Wiernik PH, et al. Ophthalmologic toxicity after cis-dichlorodiammine platinum(II) therapy. Cancer Treat Rep 1978;62:1591–4.
106. Shingleton BJ, Bienfang DC, Albert DM, et al. Ocular toxicity associated with high-dose carmustine. Arch Ophthalmol 1982;100:1766–72.
107. Kwan AS, Sahu A, Palexes G. Retinal ischemia with neovascularization in cisplatin related retinal toxicity. Am J Ophthalmol 2006;141:196–7.
108. Khawly JA, Rubin P, Petros W, et al. Retinopathy and optic neuropathy in bone marrow transplantation for breast cancer. Ophthalmology 1996;103:87–95.
109. Kupersmith MJ, Seiple WH, Holopigian K, et al. Maculopathy caused by intra-arterially administered cisplatin and intravenously administered carmustine. Am J Ophthalmol 1992;113:435–8.
110. Millay RH, Klein ML, Shults WT, et al. Maculopathy associated with combination chemotherapy and osmotic opening of the blood-brain barrier. Am J Ophthalmol 1986;102:626–32.
111. Bourla DH, Sarraf D, Schwartz SD. Peripheral retinopathy and maculopathy in high-dose tamoxifen therapy. Am J Ophthalmol 2007;144:126–8.
112. Kaiser-Kupfer MI, Kupfer C, Rodrigues MM. Tamoxifen retinopathy; a clinicopathologic report. Ophthalmology 1981;88:89–93.
113. Kaiser-Kupfer MI, Lippman ME. Tamoxifen retinopathy. Cancer Treat Rep 1978;62:315–20.
114. McKeown CA, Swartz M, Blom J, et al. Tamoxifen retinopathy. Br J Ophthalmol 1981;65:177–9.
115. Vinding T, Nielsen NV. Retinopathy caused by treatment with tamoxifen in low dosage. Acta Ophthalmol 1983;61:45–50.
116. Mauget-Faysse M, Gambrelle J, Quaranta-El Maftouhi M. Optical coherence tomography in tamoxifen retinopathy. Breast Cancer Res Treat 2006;99:117–8.
117. Gualino V, Cohen SY, Delyfer MN, et al. Optical coherence tomography findings in tamoxifen retinopathy. Am J Ophthalmol 2005;140:757–8.
118. Ashford AR, Donev I, Tiwari RP, et al. Reversible ocular toxicity related to tamoxifen therapy. Cancer 1988;61:33–5.
119. Chang T, Gonder JR, Ventresca MR. Low-dose tamoxifen retinopathy. Can J Ophthalmol 1992;27:148–9.
120. Griffiths MFP. Tamoxifen retinopathy at low dosage. Am J Ophthalmol 1987;104:185–6.
121. Heier JS, Dragoo RA, Enzenauer RW, et al. Screening for ocular toxicity in asymptomatic patients treated with tamoxifen. Am J Ophthalmol 1994;117:772–5.
122. Pavlidis NA, Petris C, Briassoulis E, et al. Clear evidence that long-term low-dose tamoxifen treatment can induce ocular toxicity. A prospective study of 63 patients. Cancer 1992;69:2961–4.
123. Cronin BG, Lekich CK, Bourke RD. Tamoxifen therapy conveys increased risk of developing a macular hole. Int Ophthalmol 2005;26:101–5.
124. Bernstein PS, DellaCroce JT. Diagnostic & therapeutic challenges. Tamoxifen toxicity. Retina 2007;27:982–8.
125. Salomao SR, Watanabe SE, Berezovsky A, et al. Multifocal electroretinography, color discrimination and ocular toxicity in tamoxifen use. Curr Eye Res 2007;32:345–52.
126. Albert DM, Bullock JD, Lahav M, et al. Flecked retina secondary to oxalate crystals from methoxyflurane anesthesia: clinical and experimental studies. Trans Am Acad Ophthalmol Otolaryngol 1975;79:OP817–OP826.
127. Bullock JD, Albert DM. Flecked retina; appearance secondary to oxalate crystals from methoxyflurane anesthesia. Arch Ophthalmol 1975;93:26–30.
128. Novak MA, Roth AS, Levine MR. Calcium oxalate retinopathy associated with methoxyflurane anesthesia. Retina 1988;8:230–6.
129. Wells CG, Johnson RJ, Qingli L, et al. Retinal oxylosis; a clinicopathologic report. Arch Ophthalmol 1989;107:1638–43.
130. Boudreault G, Cortin P, Corriveau L-A, et al. La rétinopathie à la canthaxanthine: 1. Étude clinique de 51 consommateurs. Can J Ophthalmol 1983;18:325–8.
131. Cortin P, Boudreault G, Rousseau AP, et al. La rétinopathie à la canthaxanthine: 2. Facteurs prédisposants. Can J Ophthalmol 1984;19:215–9.
132. Cortin P, Corriveau LA, Rousseau A, et al. Canthaxanthine retinopathy. J Ophthalmic Photogr 1983;6:68.
133. Cortin P, Corriveau LA, Rousseau AP, et al. Maculopathie en paillettes d'or. Can J Ophthalmol 1982;17:103–6.
134. Harnois C, Samson J, Malenfant M, et al. Canthaxanthin retinopathy; anatomic and functional reversibility. Arch Ophthalmol 1989;107:538–40.
135. Lonn LI. Canthaxanthin retinopathy. Arch Ophthalmol 1987;105:1590–1.
136. Metge P, Mandirac-Bonnefoy C, Bellaube P. Thésaurismose rétinienne à la canthaxanthine. Bull Mem Soc Fr Ophtalmol 1984;95:547–9.
137. Ros AM, Leyon H, Wennersten G. Crystalline retinopathy in patients taking an oral drug containing canthaxanthine. Photodermatol 1985;2:183–5.
138. Chang TS, Aylward GW, Clarkson JG, et al. Asymmetric canthaxanthin retinopathy. Am J Ophthalmol 1995;119:801–2.
139. Philip W. Carotinoid-Einlagerungen in der Netzhaut. Klin Monatsbl Augenheilkd 1985;187:439–40.
140. Hennekes R, Weber U, Küchle HJ. Über canthaxanthinschäden der Netzhaut. Z Prackt Augenheilkd 1985;6:7.
141. Hennekes R. Periphere Netzhautdystrophie nach Canthaxanthin-Einnahme?. Fortschr Ophthalmol 1986;83:600–1.
142. Harnois C, Cortin P, Samson J, et al. Static perimetry in canthaxanthin maculopathy. Arch Ophthalmol 1988;106:58–60.
143. Barker FM, Arden GB, Bird AC, et al. The ERG in canthaxanthin therapy. ARVO Abstracts. Invest Ophthalmol Vis Sci 1987;28(Suppl.):304.
144. McGuinness R, Beaumont P. Gold dust retinopathy after the ingestion of canthaxanthine to produce skin-bronzing. Med J Aust 1985;143:622–3.
145. Arden GB, Oluwole JO, Polkinghorne P, et al. Monitoring of patients taking canthaxanthin and carotene: an electroretinographic and ophthalmological survey. Hum Toxicol 1989;8:439–50.
146. Saraux H, Laroche L. Maculopathie à paillettes d'or après absorption de canthaxanthine. Bull Soc Ophtalmol Fr 1983;83:1273–5.
147. Weber U, Goerz G. Augenschaden durch Carotinoid-Einnahme. Dtsch Arzteblatt 1985;25:181.
148. Daicker B, Schiedt K, Adnet JJ, et al. Canthaxanthin retinopathy; an investigation by light and electron microscopy and physicochemical analysis. Graefes Arch Clin Exp Ophthalmol 1987;225:189–97.
149. Leyon H, Ros AM, Nyberg S, et al. Reversibility of canthaxanthin deposits within the retina. Acta Ophthalmol 1990;68:607–11.
150. Weber U, Kern W, Novotny GEK, et al. Experimental carotenoid retinopathy. I. Functional and morphological alterations of the rabbit retina after 11 months dietary carotenoid application. Graefes Arch Clin Exp Ophthalmol 1987;225:198–205.
151. Weber U, Michaelis L, Kern W, et al. Experimental carotenoid retinopathy. II. Functional and morphological alterations of the rabbit retina after acute canthaxanthin application with small unilamellar phospholipid liposomes. Graefes Arch Clin Exp Ophthalmol 1987;225:346–50.
152. Oosterhuis JA, Remky H, Nijman NM, et al. Canthaxanthin-retinopathie ohne Canthaxanthin-Einnahme. Klin Monatsbl Augenheilkd 1989;194:110–6.
153. Ibanez HE, Williams DF, Bonuik I. Crystalline retinopathy associated with long-term nitrofurantoin therapy. Arch Ophthalmol 1994;112:304–5.
154. Scallon LJ, Burke JM, Mieler WF, et al. Canthaxanthine-induced retinal pigment epithelial changes in the cat. Curr Eye Res 1988;7:687–93.
155. Goralczyk R, Barker FM, Buser S, et al. Dose dependency of canthaxanthin crystals in monkey retina and spatial distribution of its metabolites. Invest Ophthalmol Vis Sci 2000;41:1513–22.
156. Chan A, Ko TH, Duker JS. Ultrahigh-resolution optical coherence tomography of canthaxanthine retinal crystals. Ophthalmic Surg Lasers Imaging 2006;37:138–9.
157. Sarraf D, Ceron O, Rasheed K, et al. West African crystalline maculopathy. Arch Ophthalmol 2003;121:338–42.
158. Rajak SN, Mohamed MD, Pelosini L. Further insight into West African crystalline maculopathy. Arch Ophthalmol 2009;127:863–8.
159. Browning DJ. West African crystalline maculopathy. Ophthalmology 2004;111:921–5.
160. Ibanez HE, Williams DF, Boniuk I. Crystalline retinopathy associated with long-term nitrofurantoin therapy. Arch Ophthalmol 1994;112:304–5.
161. Bors F, Fells P. Reversal of the complications of self-induced vitamin A deficiency. Br J Ophthalmol 1971;55:210–4.
162. Brown GC, Felton SM, Benson WE. Reversible night blindness associated with intestinal bypass surgery. Am J Ophthalmol 1980;89:776–9.
163. Dowling JE. Night blindness, dark adaptation, and the electroretinogram. Am J Ophthalmol 1960;50:875–89.
164. Fells P, Bors F. Ocular complications of self-induced vitamin A deficiency. Trans Ophthalmol Soc UK 1969;89:221–8.
165. Fuchs A. White spots of the fundus combined with night blindness and xerosis (Uyemura's syndrome). Am J Ophthalmol 1959;48:101–3.
166. Grey RHB. Visual field changes following hepatic transplantation in a patient with primary biliary cirrhosis. Br J Ophthalmol 1991;75:377–80.
167. Levy NS, Toskes PP. Fundus albipunctatus and vitamin A deficiency. Am J Ophthalmol 1974;78:926–9.
168. O'Donnell M, Talbot JF. Vitamin A deficiency in treated cystic fibrosis: case report. Br J Ophthalmol 1987;71:787–90.

169. Sommer A, Tjakrasudjatma S, Djunaedi E, et al. Vitamin A-responsive panocular xerophthalmia in a healthy adult. Arch Ophthalmol 1978;96:1630–4.
170. Teng-Khoen-Hing. Fundus changes in hypovitaminosis A. Ophthalmologica 1959;137:81–5.
171. Teng-Khoen-Hing. Further contributions to the fundus xerophthalmicus. Ophthalmologica 1965;150:219–38.
172. Uyemura M. Ueber eine merkwürdige Augenhintergrundveränderung bei zwei Fällen von idiopathischer Hemeralopie. Klin Monatsbl Augenheilkd 1928;81:471–3.
173. Balian JV. Accidental intraocular tobramycin injection: a case report. Ophthalmic Surg 1983;14:353–4.
174. Campochiaro PA, Lim JI. The Aminoglycoside Toxicity Study Group: aminoglycoside toxicity in the treatment of endophthalmitis. Arch Ophthalmol 1994;112:48–53.
175. Grizzard WS. Aminoglycoside macular toxicity after subconjunctival injection. Arch Ophthalmol 1990;108:1206.
176. Judson PH. Aminoglycoside macular toxicity after subconjunctival injection. Arch Ophthalmol 1989;107:1282–3.
177. McDonald HR, Schatz H, Allen AW, et al. Retinal toxicity secondary to intraocular gentamicin injection. Ophthalmology 1986;93:871–7.
178. Snider III JD, Cohen HB, Chenoweth RG. Acute ischemic retinopathy secondary to intraocular injection of gentamicin. In: Ryan SJ, Dawson AK, Little HL, editors. Retinal diseases. Orlando, FL: Grune & Stratton; 1985. p. 227–32.
179. Loewenstein A, Zemel E, Vered Y, et al. Retinal toxicity of gentamicin after subconjunctival injection performed adjacent to thinned sclera. Ophthalmology 2001;108:759–64.
180. Rosenbaum JD, Krumholz DM, Metz DM. Gentamicin retinal toxicity after cataract surgery in an eye that underwent vitrectomy. Ophthalmic Surg Lasers 1997;28:236–8.
181. Seawright AA, Bourke RD, Cooling RJ. Macula toxicity after intravitreal amikacin. Aust N Z J Ophthalmol 1996;24:143–6.
182. Green K, Chapman J, Cheeks L. Ocular toxicity of subconjunctival gentamicin. Lens Eye Toxic Res 1992;9:439–46.
183. Campochiaro PA, Conway BP. Aminoglycoside toxicity – a survey of retinal specialists. Arch Ophthalmol 1991;109:946–50.
184. Pflugfelder SC, Hernández E, Fliesler SJ, et al. Intravitreal vancomycin; retinal toxicity, clearance, and interaction with gentamicin. Arch Ophthalmol 1987;105:831–7.
185. Zachary IG, Forster RK. Experimental intravitreal gentamicin. Am J Ophthalmol 1976;82: 604–11.
186. Oum BS, D'Amico DJ, Kwak HW, et al. Intravitreal antibiotic therapy with vancomycin and aminoglycoside: Examination of the retinal toxicity of repetitive injections after vitreous and lens surgery. Graefes Arch Clin Exp Ophthalmol 1992;230:56–61.
187. Peyman GA. Aminoglycoside toxicity. Arch Ophthalmol 1992;110:446.
188. Talamo JH, D'Amico DJ, Hanninen LA, et al. The influence of aphakia and vitrectomy on experimental retinal toxicity of aminoglycoside antibiotics. Am J Ophthalmol 1985;100:840–7.
189. D'Amico DJ, Caspers-Velu L, Libert J, et al. Comparative toxicity of intravitreal aminoglycoside antibiotics. Am J Ophthalmol 1985;100:264–75.
190. Cardascia N, Boscia F, Furino C, et al. Gentamicin-induced macular infarction in transconjunctival sutureless 25-gauge vitrectomy. Int Ophthalmol 2008;28:383–5.
191. D'Amico DJ, Libert J, Kenyon KR, et al. Retinal toxicity of intravitreal gentamicin; an electron microscopic study. Invest Ophthalmol Vis Sci 1984;25:564–72.
192. Brown GC, Eagle RC, Shakin EP, et al. Retinal toxicity of intravitreal gentamicin. Arch Ophthalmol 1990;108:1740–4.
193. Conway BP, Tabatabay CA, Campochiaro PA, et al. Gentamicin toxicity in the primate retina. Arch Ophthalmol 1989;107:107–12.
194. Hancock HA, Guidry C, Read RW, et al. Acute aminoglycoside retinal toxicity in vivo and in vitro. Invest Ophthalmol Vis Sci 2005;46:4804–8.
195. Waltz K, Margo CE. Intraocular gentamicin toxicity. Arch Ophthalmol 1991;109:911.
196. Guyer DR, Tiedeman J, Yannuzzi LA, et al. Interferon-associated retinopathy. Arch Ophthalmol 1993;111:350–6.
197. Ohira M, Ito D, Shimizu T, et al. Retinopathy: an overlooked adverse effect of interferon-beta treatment of multiple sclerosis. Keio J Med 2009;58:54–6.
198. Folden DV, Lee MS, Ryan Jr EH. Interferon beta-associated retinopathy in patients treated for multiple sclerosis. Neurology 2008;70:1153–5.
199. Saito H, Suzuki M, Asakawa T, et al. Retinopathy in a multiple sclerosis patient undergoing interferon-therapy. Mult Scler 2007;13:939–40.
200. Okuse C, Yotsuyanagi H, Nagase Y, et al. Risk factors for retinopathy associated with interferon alpha-2b and ribavirin combination therapy in patients with chronic hepatitis C. World J Gastroenterol 2006;12:3756–9.
201. Sugano S, Suzuki T, Watanabe M, et al. Retinal complications and plasma C5a levels during interferon alpha therapy for chronic hepatitis C. Am J Gastroenterol 1998;93:2441–4.
202. Shaw HEJR, Lawson JG, Stulting RD. Amaurosis fugax and retinal vasculitis associated with methamphetamine inhalation. J Clin Neuro-Ophthalmol 1985;5:169–76.
203. Wallace RT, Brown GC, Benson W, et al. Sudden retinal manifestations of intranasal cocaine and methamphetamine abuse. Am J Ophthalmol 1992;114:158–60.
204. Rahman W, Thomas S, Wiselka M, et al. Cocaine-induced chorioretinal infarction. Br J Ophthalmol 2008;92:150–1.
205. Zeiter JH, Corder DM, Madion MP, et al. Sudden retinal manifestations of intranasal cocaine and methamphetamine abuse. Am J Ophthalmol 1992;114:780–1.
206. Pinilla I, Abecia E, Borque E, et al. Cocaine-induced preretinal haemorrhage in a young adult. Acta Ophthalmol Scand 2007;85:343–4.
207. Michaelides M, Larkin G. Cocaine-associated central retinal artery occlusion in a young man. Eye 2002;16:790–2.
208. Sleiman I, Mangili R, Semeraro F, et al. Cocaine-associated retinal vascular occlusion: report of two cases. Am J Med 1994;97:198–9.
209. Wallace RT, Brown GC, Benson W, et al. Sudden retinal manifestations of intranasal cocaine and methamphetamine abuse. Am J Ophthalmol 1992;114:158–60.
210. Devenyi P, Schneiderman JF, Devenyi RG, et al. Cocaine-induced central retinal artery occlusion. CMAJ 1988;138:129–30.
211. Kumar RL, Kaiser PK, Lee MS. Crystalline retinopathy from nasal ingestion of methamphetamine. Retina 2006;26:823–4.
212. Leung IY, Lai S, Ren S, Kempen J, et al. Early retinal vascular abnormalities in African-American cocaine users. Am J Ophthalmol 2008;146:612–9.
213. Lincoff H, Zweifach P, Brodie S, et al. Intraocular injection of lidocaine. Ophthalmology 1985;92:1587–91.
214. Reddy S, Goldman DR, Hubschman J-P, et al. Cocaine and choroidal infarction. Revisiting the triangular sign of Amalric. [Report] Retinal Cases and Brief Reports Winter 2011;5(1):91–3.
215. Bacon P, Spalton DJ, Smith SE. Blindness from quinine toxicity. Br J Ophthalmol 1988;72: 219–24.
216. Brinton GS, Norton EWD, Zahn JR, et al. Ocular quinine toxicity. Am J Ophthalmol 1980;90:403–10.
217. Canning CR, Hague S. Ocular quinine toxicity. Br J Ophthalmol 1988;72:23–6.
218. Gangitano JL, Keltner JL. Abnormalities of the pupil and visual-evoked potential in quinine amblyopia. Am J Ophthalmol 1980;89:425–30.
219. Danias J, Brodie S. Delayed quinine toxicity mimicking open angle glaucoma. Br J Ophthalmol 2001;85:245–6.
220. Lochhead J, Movaffaghy A, Falsini B, et al. The effect of quinine on the electroretinograms of children with pediatric cerebral malaria. J Infect Dis 2003;187:1342–5.
221. Caffi M, Rapizzi A. Sull'intossicazione sperimentale da chinino; ricerche sperimentali istologiche ed istochimiche sulla retina e sul nervo ottico di coniglio. Minerva Oftalmol 1966;8:65–8.
222. Casini F. Il metabolismo respiratorio della retina nell' intossicazione sperimentale da chinino. Arch Ottalmol 1939;46:263–79.
223. Knox DL, Palmer CAL, English F. Iris atrophy after quinine amblyopia. Arch Ophthalmol 1966;76:359–62.
224. Guly U, Driscoll P. The management of quinine-induced blindness. Arch Emerg Med 1992;9:317–22.
225. Benton Jr CD, Calhoun Jr FP. The ocular effects of methyl alcohol poisoning: report of a catastrophe involving 320 persons. Am J Ophthalmol 1953;36:1677–85.
226. Potts AM, Praglin J, Farkas I, et al. Studies on the visual toxicity of methanol. VIII. Additional observations on methanol poisoning in the primary test object. Am J Ophthalmol 1955;40: 76–83.
227. Ruedemann Jr AD. The electroretinogram in chronic methyl alcohol poisoning in human beings. Am J Ophthalmol 1962;54:34–53.
228. Baumbach GL, Cancilla PA, Martin-Amat G, et al. Methyl alcohol poisoning. IV. Alterations of the morphological findings of the retina and optic nerve. Arch Ophthalmol 1977;95:1859–65.
229. Hayreh MS, Hayreh SS, Baumbach GL, et al. Methyl alcohol poisoning. III. Ocular toxicity. Arch Ophthalmol 1977;95:1851–8.
230. Martin-Amat G, Tephly TR, McMartin KE, et al. Methyl alcohol poisoning. II. Development of a model for ocular toxicity in methyl alcohol poisoning using the rhesus monkey. Arch Ophthalmol 1977;95:1847–50.
231. Fells JT, Murray TG, Lewandowski MF, et al. Methanol poisoning: clinical evidence of direct retinal dysfunction. ARVO Abstracts. Invest Ophthalmol Vis Sci 1991;32:689.
232. Murray TG, Burton TC, Rajani C, et al. Methanol poisoning; a rodent model with structural and functional evidence for retinal involvement. Arch Ophthalmol 1991;109:1012–6.
233. Querques G, Prascina F, Iaculli C, et al. Intravitreal pegaptanib sodium (Macugen) for radiation retinopathy following episcleral plaque radiotherapy. Acta Ophthalmol 2008;86:700–1.
234. Tokuda K, Zorumski CF, Izumi Y. Involvement of illumination in indocyanine green toxicity after its washout in the ex vivo rat retina. Retina 2009;29:371–9.
235. Narayanan R, Kenney MC, Kamjoo S, et al. Toxicity of indocyanine green (ICG) in combination with light on retinal pigment epithelial cells and neurosensory retinal cells. Curr Eye Res 2005;30:471–8.
236. Rodrigues EB, Meyer CH, Mennel S, et al. Mechanisms of intravitreal toxicity of indocyanine green dye: implications for chromovitrectomy. Retina 2007;27:958–70.
237. Haritoglou C, Kreutzer T, Tadayoni R, et al. Staining and peeling of the internal limiting membrane using a fluorescent dye (Rhodamine 6 G). Br J Ophthalmol 2008;92:1265–8.
238. Smith SV, Benz MS, Brown DM. Cystoid macular edema secondary to albumin-bound paclitaxel therapy. Arch Ophthalmol 2008;126:1605–6.
239. Joshi MM, Garretson BR. Paclitaxel maculopathy. Arch Ophthalmol 2007;125:709–10.
240. Teitelbaum BA, Tresley DJ. Cystic maculopathy with normal capillary permeability secondary to docetaxel. Optom Vis Sci 2003;80:277–9.
241. Hofstra LS, de Vries EG, Willemse PH. Ophthalmic toxicity following paclitaxel infusion. Ann Oncol 1997;8:1053.
242. Georgalas I, Pavesio C, Ezra E. Bilateral cystoid macular edema in a patient with chronic myeloid leukaemia under treatment with imanitib mesylate: report of an unusual side effect. Graefes Arch Clin Exp Ophthalmol 2007;245:1585–6.
243. Masood I, Negi A, Dua HS. Imatinib as a cause of cystoid macular edema following uneventful phacoemulsification surgery. J Cataract Refract Surg 2005;31:2427–8.
244. Fraunfelder FW, Solomon J, Druker BJ, et al. Ocular side-effects associated with imatinib mesylate (Gleevec). J Ocul Pharmacol Ther 2003;19:371–5.
245. Mudaliar S, Chang AR, Henry RR. Thiazolidinediones peripheral edema, and type 2 diabetes: incidence, pathophysiology, and clinical implications. Endocr Pract 2003;9:406–16.
246. Fong DS, Contreras R. Glitazone use associated with diabetic macular edema. Am J Ophthalmol 2009;147:583–6.
247. Liazos E, Broadbent DM, Beare N, et al. Spontaneous resolution of diabetic macular oedema after discontinuation of thiazolidenediones. Diabet Med 2008;25:860–2.
248. Ryan Jr EH, Han DP, Ramsay RC, et al. Diabetic macular edema associated with glitazone use. Retina 2006;26:562–70.
249. Labriola LT, Friberg TR, Hein A. Marathon runner's retinopathy. Semin Ophthalmol 2009;24:247–50.

250. Gaudard A, Varlet-Marie E, Monnier JF, et al. Exercise-induced central retinal vein thrombosis: possible involvement of hemorheological disturbances. A case report. Clin Hemorheol Microcirc 2002;27:115–22.
251. Rennie D, Morrissey J. Retinal changes in Himalayan climbers. Arch Ophthalmol 1975;93: 395–400.
252. Shults WT, Swan KC. High altitude retinopathy in mountain climbers. Arch Ophthalmol 1975;93:404–8.
253. Wiedman M. High altitude retinal hemorrhage. Arch Ophthalmol 1975;93:401–3.
254. Lubin JR, Rennie D, Hackett P, et al. High altitude retinal hemorrhage: a clinical and pathological case report. Ann Ophthalmol 1982;14:1071–6.
255. Wiedman M. High altitude retinal hemorrhage. Arch Ophthalmol 1975;93:401–3.
256. Chang B, Nolan H, Mooney D. High-altitude flight retinopathy. Eye 2004;18:653–6.
257. Wiedman M, Tabin GC. High-altitude retinopathy and altitude illness. Ophthalmology 1999;106:1924–6. [discussion 1927.]
258. Bandyopadhyay S, Singh R, Gupta V, et al. Anterior ischaemic optic neuropathy at high altitude. Indian J Ophthalmol 2002;50:324–5.
259. Mohsin N, Nooyi C, Jha A, et al. Retinal injury as an early manifestation of posttransplant thrombotic microangiopathy: recovery with plasma exchanges and conversion to sirolimus – case report and review of the literature. Transplant Proc 2007;39:1272–5.
260. Garrett SN, Kearney JJ, Schiffman JS. Amiodarone optic neuropathy. J Clin Neuro-Ophthalmol 1988;8:105–10.
261. Gittinger Jr JW, Asdourian GK. Papillopathy caused by amiodarone. Arch Ophthalmol 1987;105:349–51.
262. Nazarian SM, Jay WM. Bilateral optic neuropathy associated with amiodarone therapy. J Clin Neuro-Ophthalmol 1988;8:25–8.
263. Younge BR. Amiodarone optic neuropathy. J Clin Neuro-Ophthalmol 1988;8:29.
264. Thystrup JD, Fledelius HC. Retinal maculopathy possibly associated with amiodarone medication. Acta Ophthalmol (Copenh) 1994;72:639–41.
265. Fraunfelder FW, Fraunfelder FT. Central serous chorioretinopathy associated with sildenafil. Retina 2008;28:606–9.
266. Quiram P, Dumars S, Parwar B, et al. Viagra-associated serous macular detachment. Graefes Arch Clin Exp Ophthalmol 2005;243:339–44.
267. Allibhai ZA, Gale JS, Sheidow TS. Central serous chorioretinopathy in a patient taking sildenafil citrate. Ophthalmic Surg Lasers Imaging 2004;35:165–7.
268. Grunwald JE, Siu KK, Jacob SS, et al. Effect of sildenafil citrate (Viagra) on the ocular circulation. Am J Ophthalmol 2001;131:751–5.
269. Oguz H. Sildenafil-associated vascular CASUALTIES. Eye (Lond) 2007;21:676–7. [author reply 677–8.]
270. Tripathi A, O'Donnell NP. Branch retinal artery occlusion; another complication of sildenafil. Br J Ophthalmol 2000;84:934–5.
271. Marmor MF, Kessler R. Sildenafil (Viagra) and ophthalmology. Surv Ophthalmol 1999;44:153–62.
272. Kersten AJ, Althaus C, Best J, et al. Cystoid macular edema following immune recovery and treatment with cidofovir for cytomegalovirus retinitis. Graefes Arch Clin Exp Ophthalmol 1999;237:893–6.
273. Awotesu O, Missotten T, Pitcher MC, et al. Uveitis in a patient receiving rifabutin for Crohn's disease. J R Soc Med 2004;97:440–1.
274. Schimkat M, Althaus C, Becker K, et al. Rifabutin-associated anterior uveitis in patients infected with human immunodeficiency virus. Ger J Ophthalmol 1996;5:195–201.
275. Lowe SH, Kroon FP, Bollemeyer JG, et al. Uveitis during treatment of disseminated Mycobacterium avium-intracellulare complex infection with the combination of rifabutin, clarithromycin and ethambutol. Neth J Med 1996;48:211–5.
276. Chaknis MJ, Brooks SE, Mitchell KT, et al. Inflammatory opacities of the vitreous in rifabutin-associated uveitis. Am J Ophthalmol 1996;122:580–2.
277. Rifai A, Peyman GA, Daun M, et al. Rifabutin-associated uveitis during prophylaxis for Mycobacterium avium complex infection. Arch Ophthalmol 1995;113:707.
278. Shafran SD, Singer J, Zarowny DP, et al. Determinants of rifabutin-associated uveitis in patients treated with rifabutin, clarithromycin, and ethambutol for Mycobacterium avium complex bacteremia: a multivariate analysis. Canadian HIV Trials Network Protocol 010 Study Group. J Infect Dis 1998;177:252–5.
279. Skolik S, Willermain F, Caspers LE. Rifabutin-associated panuveitis with retinal vasculitis in pulmonary tuberculosis. Ocul Immunol Inflamm 2005;13:483–5.
280. Haider D, Dhawahir-Scala FE, Strouthidis NG, et al. Acute panuveitis with hypopyon in Crohn's disease secondary to medical therapy: a case report. J Med Case Reports 2007;1:42.
281. Smith JA, Mueller BU, Nussenblatt RB, et al. Corneal endothelial deposits in children positive for human immunodeficiency virus receiving rifabutin prophylaxis for Mycobacterium avium complex bacteremia. Am J Ophthalmol 1999;127:164–9.
282. Vaudaux JD, Guex-Crosier Y. Rifabutin-induced cystoid macular oedema. J Antimicrob Chemother 2002;49:421–2.
283. Myers AC, Kjellstrom S, Bruun A, et al. Rifabutin accumulates in the lens and reduces retinal function in the rabbit eye. Retina 2009;29:106–11.
284. Kelleher P, Helbert M, Sweeney J, et al. Uveitis associated with rifabutin and macrolide therapy for Mycobacterium avium intracellulare infection in AIDS patients. Genitourin Med 1996;72:419–21.
285. Malmgren K, Ben-Menachem E, Frisen L. Vigabatrin visual toxicity: evolution and dose dependence. Epilepsia 2001;42:609–15.
286. Durbin S, Mirabella G, Buncic JR, et al. Reduced grating acuity associated with retinal toxicity in children with infantile spasms on vigabatrin therapy. Invest Ophthalmol Vis Sci 2009;50:4011–6.
287. Kinirons P, Cavalleri GL, O'Rourke D, et al. Vigabatrin retinopathy in an Irish cohort: lack of correlation with dose. Epilepsia 2006;47:311–7.
288. Rebolleda G, Garcia Perez JL, Munoz Negrete FJ, et al. Vigabatrin toxicity in children. Ophthalmology 2005;112:1322–3.
289. Best JL, Acheson JF. The natural history of Vigabatrin associated visual field defects in patients electing to continue their medication. Eye 2005;19:41–4.
290. Buncic JR, Westall CA, Panton CM, et al. Characteristic retinal atrophy with secondary "inverse" optic atrophy identifies vigabatrin toxicity in children. Ophthalmology 2004;111:1935–42.
291. Frisen L, Malmgren K. Characterization of vigabatrin-associated optic atrophy. Acta Ophthalmol Scand 2003;81:466–73.
292. Lawthom C, Smith PE, Wild JM. Nasal retinal nerve fiber layer attenuation: a biomarker for vigabatrin toxicity. Ophthalmology 2009;116:565–71.
293. Dempsey LC, O'Donnell JJ, Hoff JT. Carbon monoxide retinopathy. Am J Ophthalmol 1976;82:692–3.
294. Ferguson LS, Burke MJ, Choromokos EA. Carbon monoxide retinopathy. Arch Ophthalmol 1985;103:66–7.
295. Kelley JS, Sophocleus GJ. Retinal hemorrhages in subacute carbon monoxide poisoning; exposures in homes with blocked furnace flues. JAMA 1978;239:1515–7.
296. Murray WR. Amblyopia caused by inhalation of carbon monoxide gas. Minn Med 1926;9:561–4.
297. von Restorff W, Hebisch S. Dark adaptation of the eye during carbon monoxide exposure in smokers and nonsmokers. Aviat Space Environ Med 1988;59:928–31.
298. Burns CA. Indomethacin, reduced retinal sensitivity, and corneal deposits. Am J Ophthalmol 1968;66:825–35.
299. Graham CM, Blach RK. Indomethacin retinopathy: case report and review. Br J Ophthalmol 1988;72:434–8.
300. Henkes HE, van Lith GHM, Canta LR. Indomethacin retinopathy. Am J Ophthalmol 1972;73:846–56.
301. Chuman MA, LeSage J. Color vision deficiencies in two cases of digoxin toxicity. Am J Ophthalmol 1985;100:682–5.
302. Robertson DM, Hollenhorst RW, Callahan JA. Receptor function in digitalis therapy. Arch Ophthalmol 1966;76:852–7.
304. Weleber RG, Shults WT. Digoxin retinal toxicity; clinical and electrophysiologic evaluation of a cone dysfunction syndrome. Arch Ophthalmol 1981;99:1568–72.
304. Lawrenson JG, Kelly C, Lawrenson AL, et al. Acquired colour vision deficiency in patients receiving digoxin maintenance therapy. Br J Ophthalmol 2002;86:1259–61.
305. Creel DJ, Wang JM, Wong KC. Transient blindness associated with transurethral resection of the prostate. Arch Ophthalmol 1987;105:1537–9.
306. Propst AM, Liberman RF, Harlow BL, et al. Complications of hysteroscopic surgery: predicting patients at risk. Obstet Gynecol 2000;96:517–20.
307. Taskin O, Buhur A, Birincioglu M, et al. Endometrial Na^+, K^+-ATPase pump function and vasopressin levels during hysteroscopic surgery in patients pretreated with GnRH agonist. J Am Assoc Gynecol Laparosc 1998;5:119–24.
308. Taskin O, Yalcinoglu A, Kucuk S, et al. The degree of fluid absorption during hysteroscopic surgery in patients pretreated with goserelin. J Am Assoc Gynecol Laparosc 1996;3:555–9.
309. Fraser IS, Angsuwathana S, Mahmoud F, et al. Short and medium term outcomes after rollerball endometrial ablation for menorrhagia. Med J Aust 1993;158:454–7.
310. Osborne GA, Rudkin GE, Moran P. Fluid uptake in laser endometrial ablation. Anaesth Intensive Care 1991;19:217–9.
311. Colucci A, Modorati G, Miserocchi E, et al. Anterior uveitis complicating zoledronic acid infusion. Ocul Immunol Inflamm 2009;17:267–8.
312. Sharma NS, Ooi JL, Masselos K, et al. Zoledronic acid infusion and orbital inflammatory disease. N Engl J Med 2008;359:1410–1.
313. Kilickap S, Ozdamar Y, Altundag MK, et al. A case report: zoledronic acid-induced anterior uveitis. Med Oncol 2008;25:238–40.
314. Santaella RM, Fraunfelder FW. Ocular adverse effects associated with systemic medications: recognition and management. Drugs 2007;67:75–93.
315. Gilhotra JS, Gilhotra AK, Holdaway IM, et al. Acute retinal pigment epitheliitis associated with intravenous bisphosphonate. Br J Ophthalmol 2006;90:798–9.
316. Benderson D, Karakunnel J, Kathuria S, et al. Scleritis complicating zoledronic acid infusion. Clin Lymphoma Myeloma 2006;7:145–7.
317. El Saghir NS, Otrock ZK, Bleik JH. Unilateral anterior uveitis complicating zoledronic acid therapy in breast cancer. BMC Cancer 2005;5:156.
318. Durnian JM, Olujohungbe A, Kyle G. Bilateral acute uveitis and conjunctivitis after zoledronic acid therapy. Eye 2005;19:221–2.
319. Ding X, Herzlich AA, Bishop R, et al. Ocular toxicity of fludarabine: a purine analog. Expert Rev Ophthalmol 2008;3:97–109.
320. Bowyer JD, Johnson EM, Horn EH, et al. Oochroconis gallopava endophthalmitis in fludarabine treated chronic lymphocytic leukaemia. Br J Ophthalmol 2000;84:117.
321. Banach MJ, Williams GA. Purtscher retinopathy and necrotizing vasculitis with gemcitabine therapy. Arch Ophthalmol 2000;118:726–7.
322. Mahesh G, Giridhar A, Saikumar SJ, et al. Drug-induced acute myopia following chlorthalidone treatment. Indian J Ophthalmol 2007;55:386–8.
323. D'Alena P, Robinson M. Hygroton-induced myopia. Calif Med 1969;110:134–5.
324. Ericson LA. Hygroton-induced myopia and retinal edema. Acta Ophthalmol (Copenh) 1963;41:538–43.
325. Zalta AH, Smith RT. Peripheral iridoplasty efficacy in refractory topiramate-associated bilateral acute angle-closure glaucoma. Arch Ophthalmol 2008;126:1603–5.
326. Parikh R, Parikh S, Das S, et al. Choroidal drainage in the management of acute angle closure after topiramate toxicity. J Glaucoma 2007;16:691–3.
327. Sachi D, Vijaya L. Topiramate induced secondary angle closure glaucoma. J Postgrad Med 2006;52:72–3.
328. Sankar PS, Pasquale LR, Grosskreutz CL. Uveal effusion and secondary angle-closure glaucoma associated with topiramate use. Arch Ophthalmol 2001;119:1210–1.
329. Rhee DJ, Goldberg MJ, Parrish RK. Bilateral angle-closure glaucoma and ciliary body swelling from topiramate. Arch Ophthalmol 2001;119:1721–3.
330. Banta JT, Hoffman K, Budenz DL, et al. Presumed topiramate-induced bilateral acute angle-closure glaucoma. Am J Ophthalmol 2001;132:112–4.

CHAPTER 10

Infectious Diseases of the Retina and Choroid

Infectious agents may be carried from elsewhere in the body and cause one or more foci of infection in the retina and less often in the choroid in one or both eyes. If treated early with specific antibiotics, the ocular damage may be minimized (Figure 10.01). Infectious diseases can be caused by bacteria, fungi, viruses, and parasites. They can involve both the retina and the choroid. Certain agents can contiguously spread to the vitreous cavity causing endophthalmitis, while certain others are limited to the retina and choroid. In some instances when bacteria and fungi gain entrance into the vitreous, either endogenously or exogenously, vitritis with or without periphlebitis may be the earliest sign of an endophthalmitis.[1]

PYOGENIC CHORIORETINITIS

Septic emboli containing bacteria derived from focal areas of infection such as diseased heart valves, or focal abscesses involving the teeth, skin, or other organs, may lodge in the retina and produce focal white areas of retinitis and overlying vitritis (Figures 10.01 and 10.02). These may be accompanied by white-centered hemorrhages (Figures 10.01, B; 10.02, E). Less frequently the septic emboli lodge in the choroid and may produce a subretinal abscess (see Figure 10.03, A–C). Most patients with bacterial retinitis will have signs and symptoms of systemic illness, including fever, chills, elevated white blood cell counts, petechiae, splinter hemorrhages of the nail bed, and physical findings pointing to the primary site of the infection. Roth described white retinal lesions and separate hemorrhages in patients with sepsis.[1–9] Litten described white-centered hemorrhages in patients with endocarditis and called them 'Roth's spots'.[5] The white center may contain organisms, although most are sterile and are composed of white blood cells. In many instances the white center is composed of fibrin occurring at the site of extravasation of blood from the retinal blood vessels.[8,10] Roth's spots occur most frequently in patients with severe anemia from any cause, including leukemia and subacute bacterial endocarditis. If bacterial sepsis is suspected, prompt medical evaluation, including blood cultures, a search for the primary site of the infection, and institution of antibiotic therapy, may succeed in preservation of useful vision in some patients (Figure 10.01). Overt endophthalmitis may require pars plana vitrectomy in addition to intravenous therapy if progression occurs. The majority of patients with metastatic bacterial retinitis are already hospitalized for their systemic illness, but a high index of suspicion is necessary to detect those who are ambulatory with evidence of disseminated sepsis in their eyes.[11]

10.01 Bacterial septic embolization of the retina and optic nerve head.

A to **F**: This 12-year-old girl noted blurred vision during an acute febrile illness. Visual acuity was 15/400. There was massive intraretinal and subretinal exudation in the macular and juxtapapillary regions (A). There were peripheral patches of retinitis surrounded by multiple Roth's spots (B and C). Angiography revealed leakage of dye from the lesion at the temporal margin of the optic disc (D). Coagulase-positive staphylococci were cultured from the blood and a dental root abscess. She received intravenous antibiotic therapy. One year later (E and F), visual acuity had improved to 20/25. *Arrow* indicates a vitreous veil on the optic nerve head secondary to posterior separation of the vitreous. Focal chorioretinal scars remained at the site of some of the areas of retinitis (compare C and F).

G to **L**: Metastatic bacterial retinitis, macular star, and papillitis (G and H) occurring in a 32-year-old man who was receiving zidovudine (AZT) and aciclovir (Zovirax) because of HIV positivity for 10 years. He complained of decreasing vision in his right eye of 2 months' duration. Medical workup, including blood cultures, was negative. Visual acuity was 20/400 in the right eye. There were minimal vitreous cells. Six weeks after treatment with doxycycline the lesions showed evidence of early resolution. Note the angiomatous appearance of the optic disc lesion (I and K). Three months later the lesions had resolved (L). His visual acuity, however, had improved only slightly to 20/80.

FOCAL INDOLENT METASTATIC BACTERIAL RETINITIS IN ACQUIRED IMMUNE DEFICIENCY SYNDROME (AIDS)

Patients with AIDS may develop multifocal, discrete, yellow–white patches of bacterial retinitis that enlarge slowly over weeks, and accumulate large amounts of subretinal fluid and fibrinous exudate with minimal inflammatory cell reaction in the overlying vitreous (Figure 10.01, G–L).[12] This form of indolent bacterial retinitis is caused by relatively nonpathogenic bacteria, such as *Rhinococcus equi* and *Bartonella* (see discussion of cat-scratch disease in the next section), that usually respond to oral doxycycline. In immunosuppressed patients the retinal lesions may be mistaken for the more frequently encountered retinal infections caused by Herpes viruses, *Candida*, *Cryptococcus*, and *Toxoplasma* organisms.

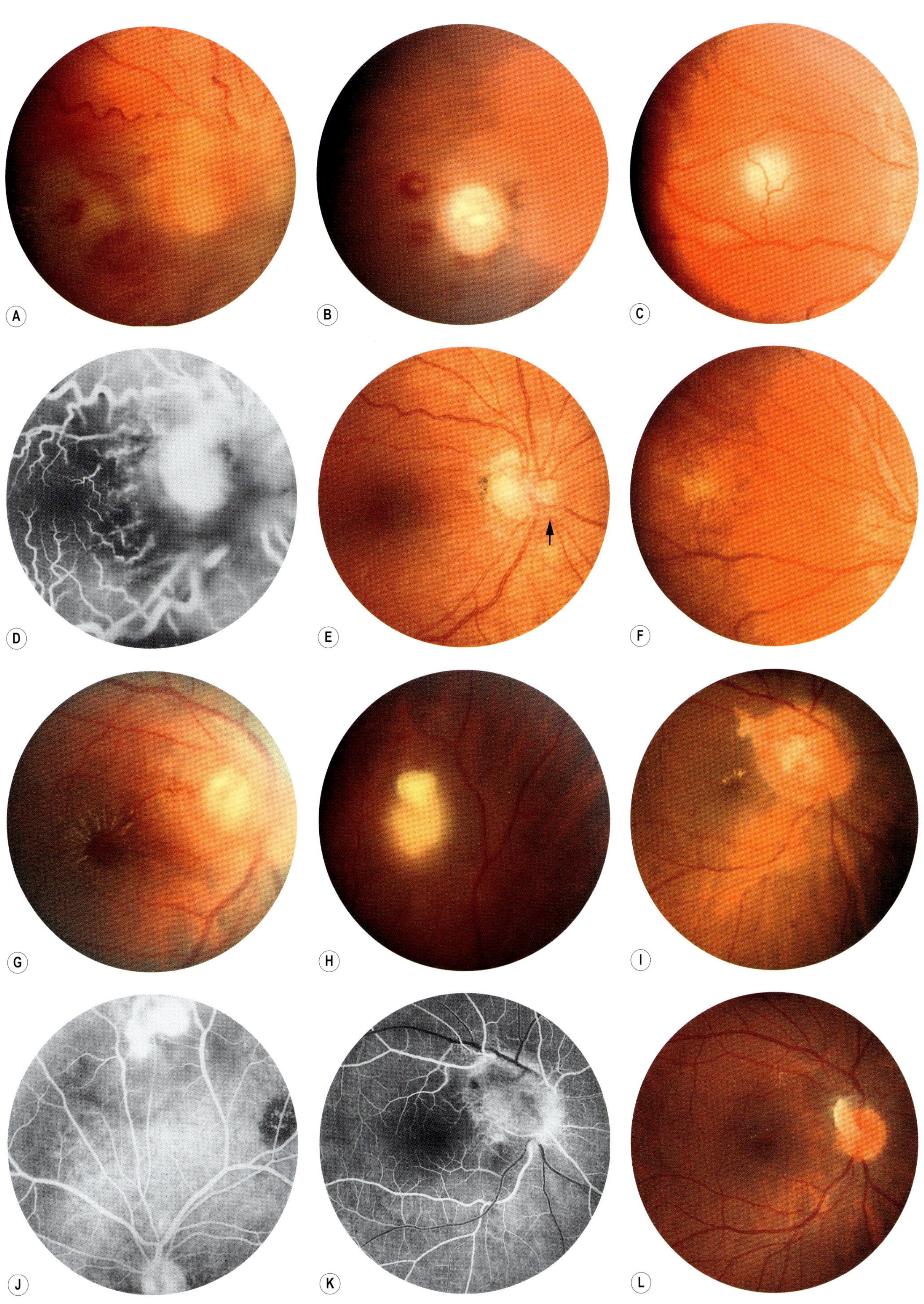
A
B
C
D
E
F
G
H
I
J
K
L

BACTERIAL CHOROIDAL ABSCESS

Patients with focal bacterial infections may develop septic emboli that may lodge in either the retinal or the choroidal circulation. In the latter case a choroidal and subretinal abscess may develop (Figures 10.02, A–C; Figure 10.03, A–C).[13,14]

10.02 Metastatic bacterial retinitis.

A to **D**: This 32-year-old woman presented with 3-week history of visual blur in the left eye. There was a focal area of outer retinitis surrounded by exudates (A). The fluorescein angiogram showed hyperfluorescence and late staining and leakage of the lesion (B and C). She had a small area of swelling of the tip of her middle finger on the left hand, diagnosed initially as cellulitis and treated with oral antibiotics. The infection did not respond and spread quickly and she was subsequently found to have meticillin-resistant *Staphylococcus aureus* (MRSA). She was started on IV vancomycin. There was no history of immunocompromise or visits to hospital or nursing homes. She responded to vancomycin and the lesion resolved, leaving a flat pigmented scar (D).
E to **H**: This 42-year-old man presented with fever, night sweats, spots on his legs (F and G), and blurred vision for 2 weeks. Six weeks after his initial visit to the emergency room a punch biopsy of the spot on his leg showed endothelial swelling of the small vessels, fibrin deposits and infiltrate of red cells, neutrophils and nuclear dust diagnosed as leukocytoclastic vasculitis (Henoch–Schönlein purpura, HSP). He was given a methylprednisolone (Medrol) dose pack that he took off and on for 4 months. He continued to have fever and night sweats, and had a 40 lb (18 kg) weight loss. His visual acuity was 20/25 in the right eye and 20/400 in the left eye with an afferent papillary defect. The left fundus showed several nerve fiber infarcts and retinal hemorrhages (E). He returned to the emergency room when he was found to have a heart murmur and a history of rheumatic fever. Echocardiogram revealed vegetations, he was anemic with a hemoglobin of 6.1 g/dL, and had urinary red blood cells and granular casts. Blood culture grew *Actinobacillus actinomycetemcomitans*, an organism found in the oral cavity. He underwent replacement of his mitral and aortic valve; the hemorrhages and nerve fiber infarcts cleared. The mechanism of the Purtscher-like retinopathy is likely from the vasculitis associated with HSP and the immunological changes from subacute bacterial endocarditis. Representative gross picture of a vegetation on the aortic valve (I).
J to **L**: This 46-year-old white man presented with a painless decrease in vision in both eyes for 2 months. He had a history of diabetes, cocaine use, and chronic deep vein thrombosis, and was hospitalized 2 weeks prior to loss of vision with fevers, elevated white cell count, and diabetic ketoacidosis. His blood cultures grew *Staph. aureus*, which was resistant to penicillin. He had had a 3.1 cm prostatic abscess which required surgical drainage. He was treated with nafcillin and rifampin (rifampicin). The patient stopped his antibiotics and the fevers and bacteremia recurred which was felt to be from an infected thrombus in the leg. The thrombus was excised and he was restarted on antibiotics. His visual acuity was counting fingers at 6 feet in the right eye and counting fingers at 4 feet in the left eye. There were 2+ anterior vitreous cells, vitreous hemorrhage in the right eye, preretinal gliosis, and an area of chorioretinovitreal neovascularization (J). In the left macula, he had an area of chorioretinovitreal new vessels (K). The fluorescein angiogram of the left eye shows a lacy pattern to the vessels that were present on the surface of the retina (L). This patient developed a chorioretinovitreal neovascularization in areas of atrophic scars caused by *Staph. aureus* retinitis. The neovascularization continued to grow and showed evidence of bleeding. Optical coherence tomography (OCT) showed the presence of vessels on the surface of the retina with contraction of the posterior hyaloid and shadowing effect from the blood. He underwent panretinal photocoagulation with partial involution of the chorioretinovitreal neovascularization.

(Courtesy: A–D, Dr Robert Mittra; E–H, Dr Mark Daily; I, Dr. J to K, Dr Culver Boldt and Dr James Folk.)

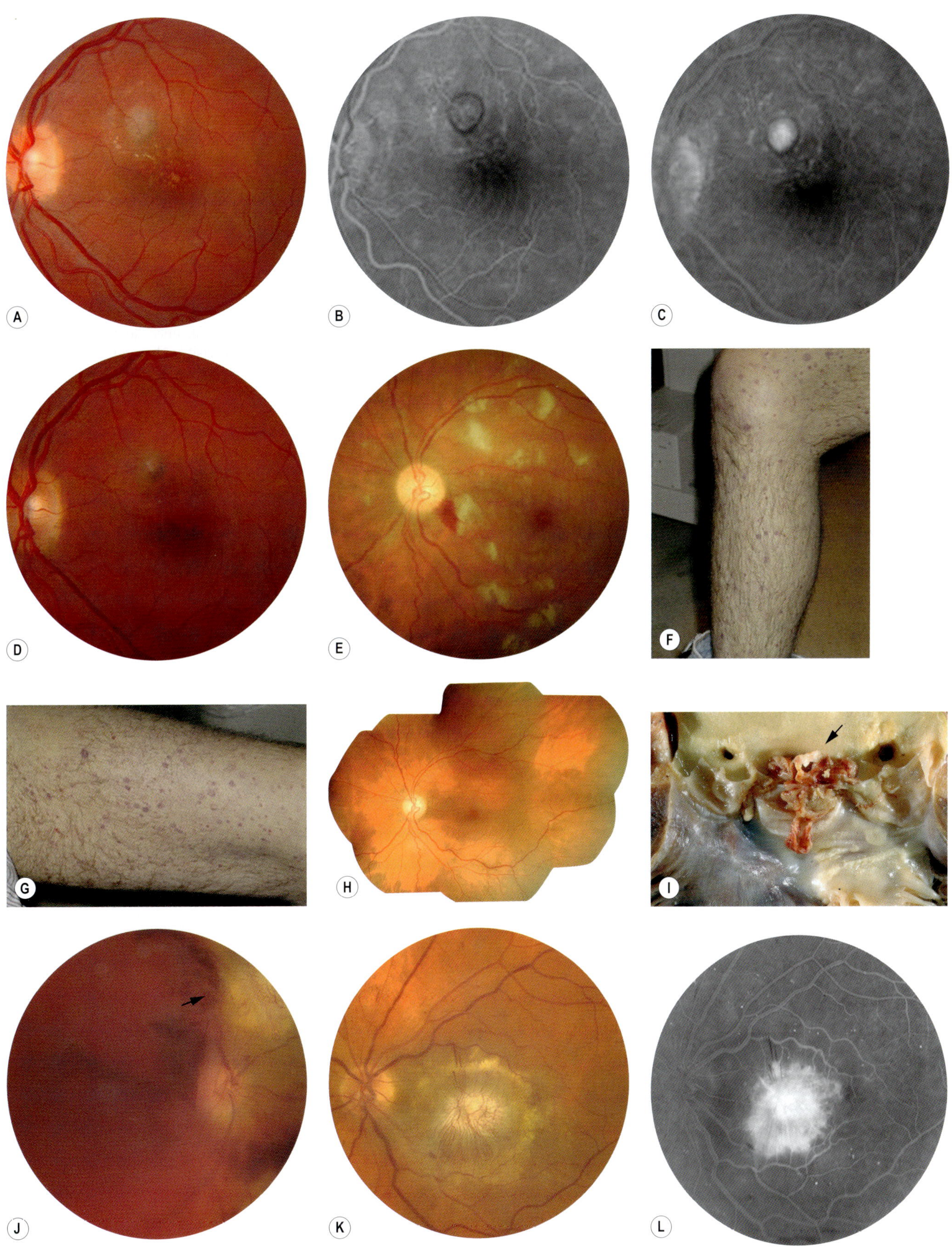
A
B
C
D
E
F
G
H
I
J
K
L

NOCARDIA

Nocardia asteroides is a gram-positive filamentous bacterium found in soil and decaying vegetable matter that shares some features with fungi. It is an opportunistic pathogen known to affect the retina and choroid in a small number of solid organ transplant recipients.[15–18] *N. asteroides* accounts for 80–90% of human infections, followed by *N. brasiliensis*, *N. farcinica*, and *N. nova*. The infection is generally disseminated with abscesses involving the lung, brain, skin, eye, and other sites. It begins as a solitary subretinal or choroidal yellow lesion that grows in size with new satellite lesions appearing over days (Figure 10.03 D and I). Overlying retinal hemorrhages are seen (Figure 10.03, D–H).[19–26] Diagnosis is based on demonstrating the organism by a transvitreal fine needle retinal biopsy, blood cultures, or biopsy of any other affected site.[16] Ring lesions are quite characteristic of Nocarida on MRI (Figure 10.03 J). The organism is a gram-positive branching hypha. Treatment consists of reduction or discontinuation of immunosuppressives and institution of appropriate antibiotics/a such as trimethoprim–sulfamethoxazole, amoxicillin–clavulanate, imipenem–cilastatin, cefotaxime, clarithromycin, and ciprofloxacin.[27,28]

10.03 Bacterial submacular abscesses.

A to **C**: Submacular bacterial abscess (A) in a 32-year-old woman hospitalized with disseminated lupus erythematosus, gram-positive bacterial endocarditis, septicemia, petechiae, and a 1-day history of loss of central vision in the left eye. Fluorescein angiography revealed evidence of a nonvascularized, nonfluorescent submacular exudate and late leakage of dye from the overlying retinal vessels (B and C). Several days later she developed massive purulent endophthalmitis.

Nocardia Retinitis.

D to **H**: *Nocardia* sub-retinal pigment epithelium (RPE) abscess (D) in a 70-year-old man with Hodgkin's disease. Angiography showed a nonvascularized subretinal mass with late leakage of dye from retinal vessels into the vitreous (E and F). There was a sub-RPE abscess lying between the necrotic retina and the choroid (G). Filamentous branching organisms (*arrows*) were present in the choriocapillaris and along Bruch's membrane (*arrows*, H).

I to **K**: This 35 year old east Indian male with a 2 year history of nephrotic syndrome secondary to MPGN was on 10 mg of prednisone daily. He presented with bilateral simultaneous acute visual loss to light perception in each eye associated with periocular pain, redness and chemosis. Both fundi showed multiple subretinal yellow infiltrates with exudative retinal detachment and scattered retinal hemorrhages (I). He developed hypotonia and seizures within 2 days. He was treated variously for tuberculosis, toxoplasmosis and fungal infections with no improvement. His neurological and ocular conditions worsened. Vitrectomy, orbital biopsy and serial CSF examinations did not yield a causative organism. MRI showed ring lesions (J) initially and a right parieto occipital mass (K) later. Eventually, biopsy of the parietal mass revealed nocardia. The patient was then treated with imipenem; his infection cleared up but he was blind in both eyes.

(D and H from Lissner GS et al.,[23]; published with permission from the American Journal of Ophthalmology; copyright by the Ophthalmic Publishing Co.; I to K, Dr. Hemant Trehan.)

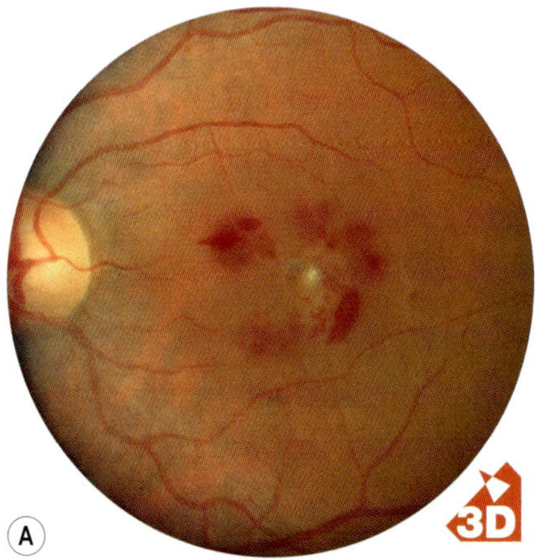

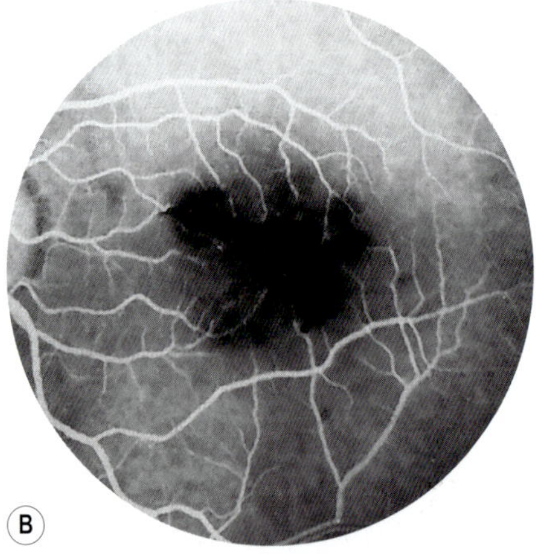

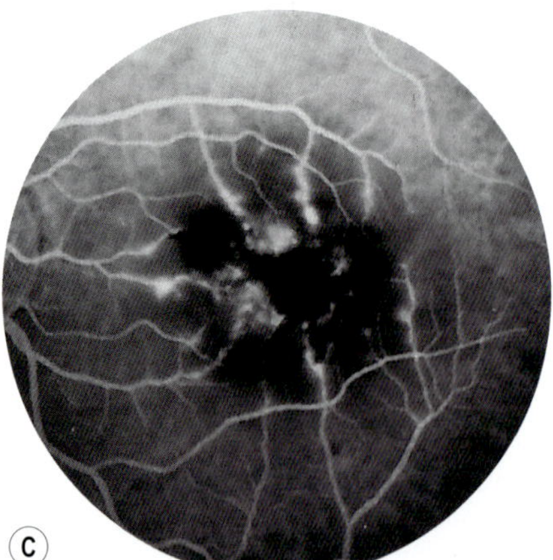

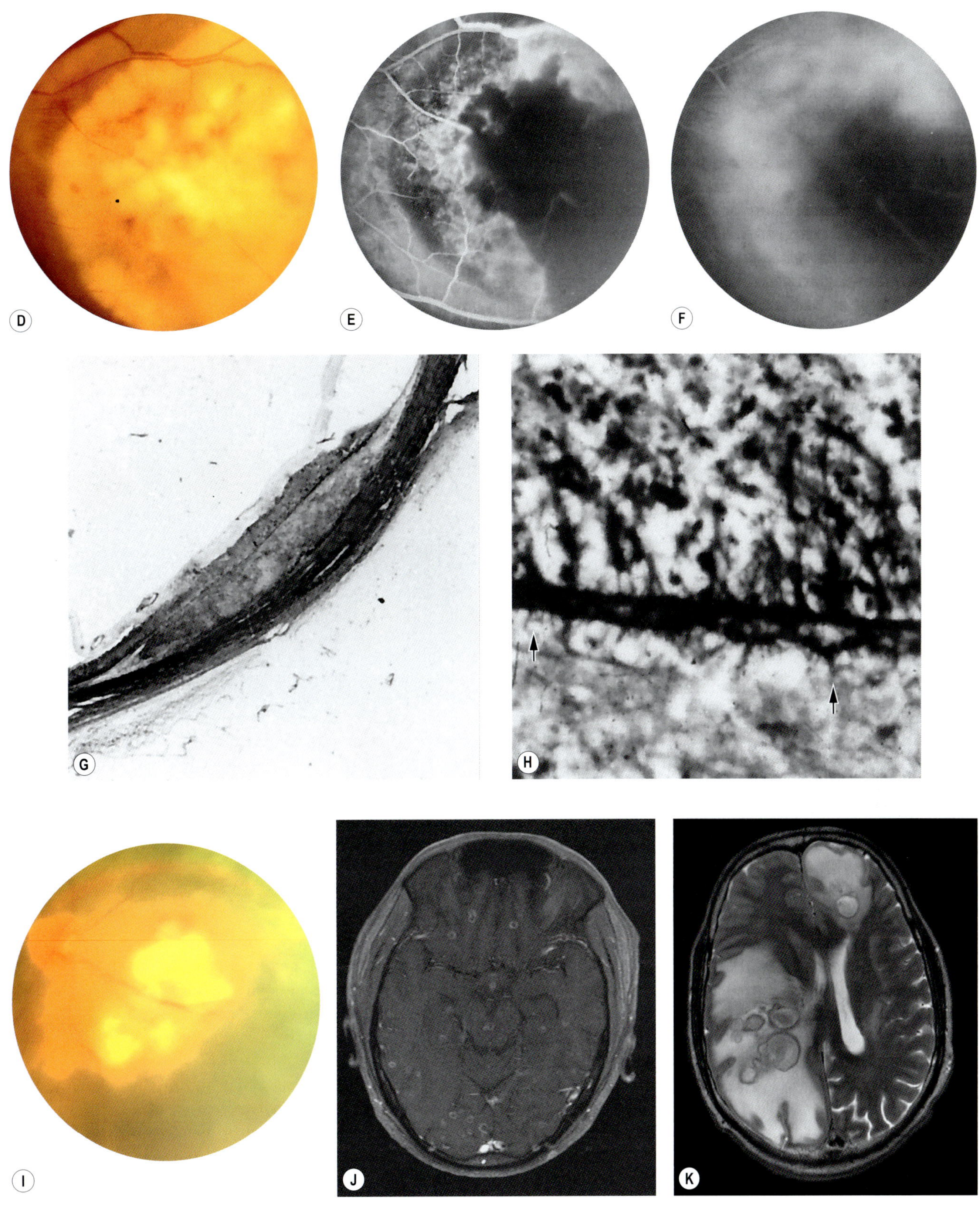
D
E
F
G
H
I
J
K

CAT-SCRATCH DISEASE

Cat-scratch disease (CSD) classically is described as tender regional lymphadenopathy developing in association with a primary skin lesion received as a result of contact with cats, termed Parinaud's oculoglandular fever. This may be accompanied by generalized ache, malaise, anorexia, and occasionally fever. Whereas a scratch is the common mode of transmission of CSD, it may be transmitted by cat bites, licking, or handling of objects associated with cats, particularly kittens. CSD is caused by a pleomorphic gram-negative bacillus, referred to previously as the English–Wear bacillus, the *Rochalimaea* bacillus, and recently *Bartonella*.[29,30] It is a worldwide zoonotic disease; the cat flea *Ctenocephalides felis* is the transmission vector between cats. Twenty-one species of *Bartonella* have been identified either by culture or polymerase chain reaction (PCR), eight of which are known to cause human disease including CSD, trench fever, endocarditis, myocarditis, Oroya fever (Carrion's disease), and retinitis. *Bartonella henselae, B. quintana, B. elizabethae,* and *B. grahamii* cause ocular lesions.[29] The focal white retinal lesions may occur anywhere in the fundus but have some predilection to occur adjacent to and obstruct major retinal arteries and, less often, veins (Figure 10.04, A–H).

These retinal lesions, as well as similar lesions involving the optic nerve head, may be associated with an angiomatous proliferation of capillaries (Figure 10.04, I–L).[31,32] The white lesions typically involve the inner half of the retina and may or may not be associated with overlying vitreous cells. They may simulate cotton-wool ischemic spots, but their distribution in the fundus is not necessarily associated with the distribution of a first-order arteriole as is the case with cotton-wool spots.

The focal white retinal and optic disc lesions, swelling of the optic disc, and macular star figure typically clear spontaneously within several weeks or months and the visual acuity usually returns to normal or near normal. Most of the retinal lesions resolve without causing retinal pigment epithelium (RPE) damage.[32a–32d] In 1977 and 1987 the author noted the association of CSD in patients with Leber's stellate neuroretinitis and multifocal retinitis, and this relationship has been documented by several subsequent reports (Figure 10.05, A–I).[33–41] CSD is probably an important, but not the only, cause of the clinical syndrome of self-limited acute idiopathic multifocal retinitis and neuroretinitis (Figure 10.05, A–F) (see Leber's idiopathic stellate neuroretinitis, Chapter 15, p. 1278). Occasionally severe occlusive vasculitis with involvement of both arteries and veins can be seen.[42] A case of unilateral elevated intraocular pressure associated with anterior synechiae secondary to possible involvement of the angle structures from CSD has been documented.[43] Isolated optic disc neovascularization without evidence of retinal ischemia in one patient hypothesizes the predilection of the bacillus to multiply in vascular endothelium and result in inflammatory neovascularization.[44]

10.04 Benign multifocal retinitis and papillitis caused by cat-scratch bacillus and other bacteria or viruses of low pathogenicity.

A to **D**: This 32-year-old woman noted floaters and a paracentral scotoma in the right eye soon after two episodes of chills and fever. Her visual acuity was 20/20 in the right eye and 20/25 in the left eye. In both eyes she had multiple focal areas of inner retinal whitening. One of these (*arrows*, A) was associated with obstruction of an inferior temporal branch retinal artery. A focal lesion was present nasally on the left optic disc (*arrow*, B). All of the lesions stained (*arrows*, C and D). Medical evaluation was unremarkable except for some elevation of cardiolipin antibody. One year later she was well and had 20/20 visual acuity bilaterally.

E: This 21-year-old woman in the second trimester of pregnancy noted floaters and visual loss in the left eye 2 weeks following an episode of fever of unknown origin. She owned seven cats but could recall no history of being scratched. Visual acuity in the left eye was counting fingers only. One to 2+ vitreous cells were present in the left eye. Multifocal white lesions interpreted as inner retinitis were present in both eyes (*arrows*). One of these was associated with obstruction of the superotemporal branch retinal artery in the left eye. Medical evaluation, including blood cultures, was negative.

F to **H**: This 28-year-old man with AIDS noted blurred vision in the left eye associated with multiple foci of retinitis and papillitis (*arrows*, F–H). One lesion (*lower arrow*, F) caused obstruction of the inferior branch retinal artery.

I to **L**: This healthy 22-year-old man had a 3-week history of blurred vision in the right eye. He owned many household cats, was frequently scratched, but denied recent illness. Visual acuity was 20/200 in the right eye and 20/20 in the left eye. Note the hemimacular star, exudative retinal detachment, and focal retinitis (*arrow*, I) enveloping but not obstructing the inferior branch retinal artery. A similar but smaller focal area of retinitis was present in the left eye (*arrow*, J). Note the pseudoangiomatous appearance of the active lesion angiographically (*arrow*, K). Both lesions stained (L). Within several weeks he recovered normal vision without treatment.

The CSD bacillus may also cause acute encephalopathy and other neurologic and systemic manifestations in otherwise healthy patients and in patients with AIDS.[32–34] Ocular and central nervous system (CNS) involvement typically occurs in children or young adults. Patients with CNS involvement may manifest convulsions and fever in approximately 50% of cases and neuroretinitis in 10–15% of cases.[34] Spontaneous recovery of vision and neurologic deficits occurs in nearly all cases, usually within 3 months. Biopsy of enlarged lymph nodes may reveal evidence of the infection. The bacillus may be demonstrated by the Warthin–Starry stain or culture from skin or lymph node specimens. Detection of antibodies to the cat-scratch bacillus is helpful in the diagnosis.[33,34] The indirect fluorescent antibody assay for *Bartonella henselae* and *B. quintana*, available through the Centers for Disease Control and Prevention (CDC) in Atlanta, is sensitive for the diagnosis of CSD.[29] The favorable prognosis without treatment

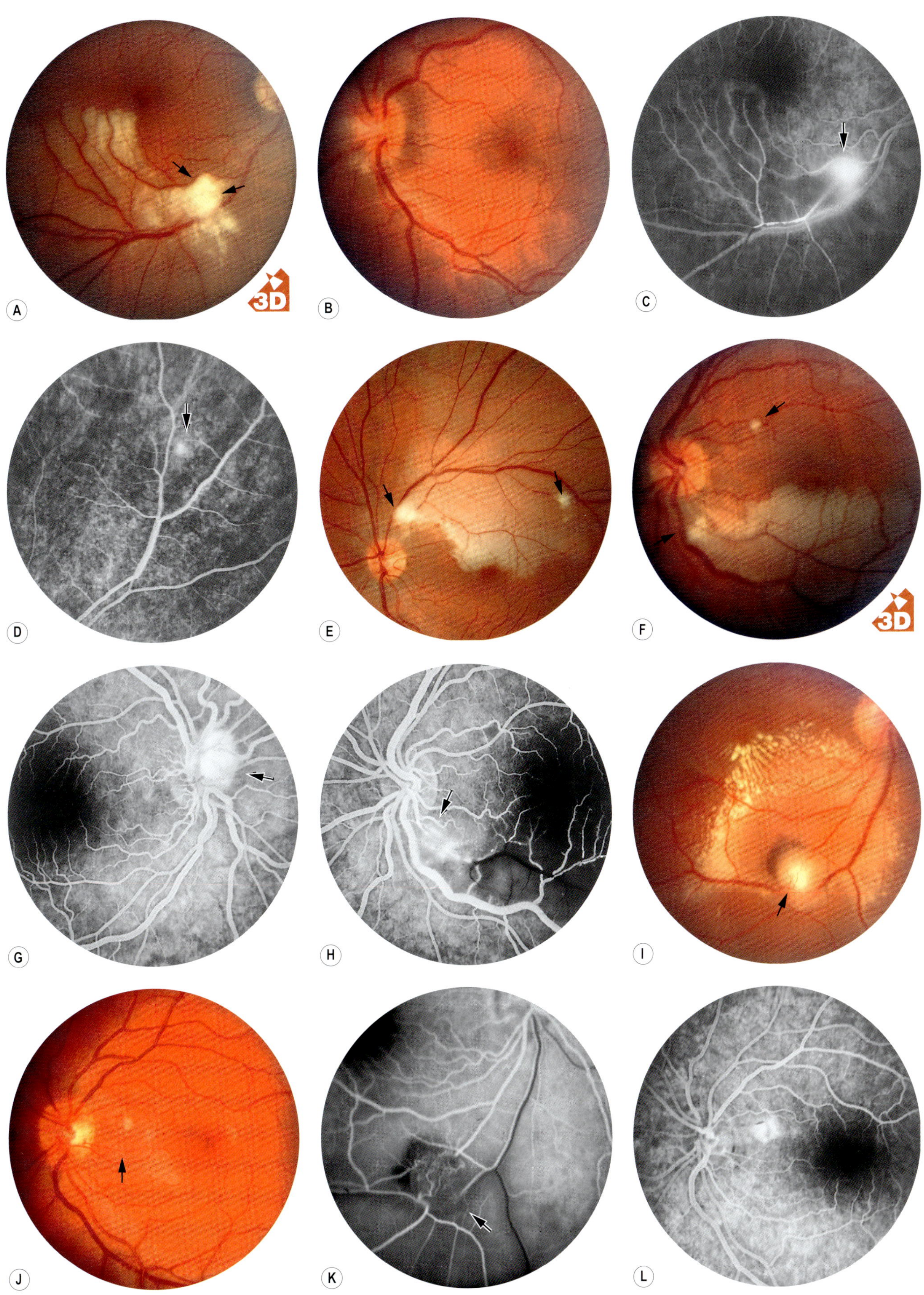
3D
A
B
C
D
E
F
3D
G
H
I
J
K
L

makes evaluation of treatment with doxycycline, ciprofloxacin, and prednisone difficult.

The tendency for some of the retinal and optic nerve inflammatory lesions to appear very vascular biomicroscopically and angiographically may be an important feature of cat-scratch infection (Figure 10.04, J–L). Angioma like masses referred to as epithelioid angiomatosis and caused by the cat-scratch bacillus have occurred on the skin and mucous membranes of patients with AIDS.[32,41,45–47] In these patients the lesions may appear clinically similar to Kaposi's sarcoma. In the eye the lesions may simulate capillary angiomas or astrocytic hamartomas of the retina (Figure 10.04, I–L). Treatment is indicated only for those with significant loss of vision or when associated with the immunocompromised state as in patients with AIDS. The organism is susceptible to several antibiotics including trimethoprim and sulfamethoxazole, rifampin (rifampicin), azithromycin, doxycycline, ciprofloxacin and others.

10.05 *Bartonella* neuroretinitis.

A to **H**: This 25-year-old woman presented with a 2-week loss of vision in the right eye, 1 week following a fever. She owned two cats, but denied a lick or scratch. Her visual acuity was 20/200 in the right eye and 20/20 in the left eye. The right eye showed disc edema, dilated vessels on the disc surface, and a perfect lipid star in the macula; the left eye had a small line of lipid temporal to the disc. OCT of the right macula showed retinal edema and intraretinal lipid in the outer plexiform layer (*arrow*) and subretinal fluid with precipitates. She was treated with azithromycin dose pack given the significant loss of vision. Her *Bartonella* titer was positive 1:256. Her vision in the right eye improved to 20/25 by 4 months and 20/20 by 9 months with complete resolution of lipid (H).

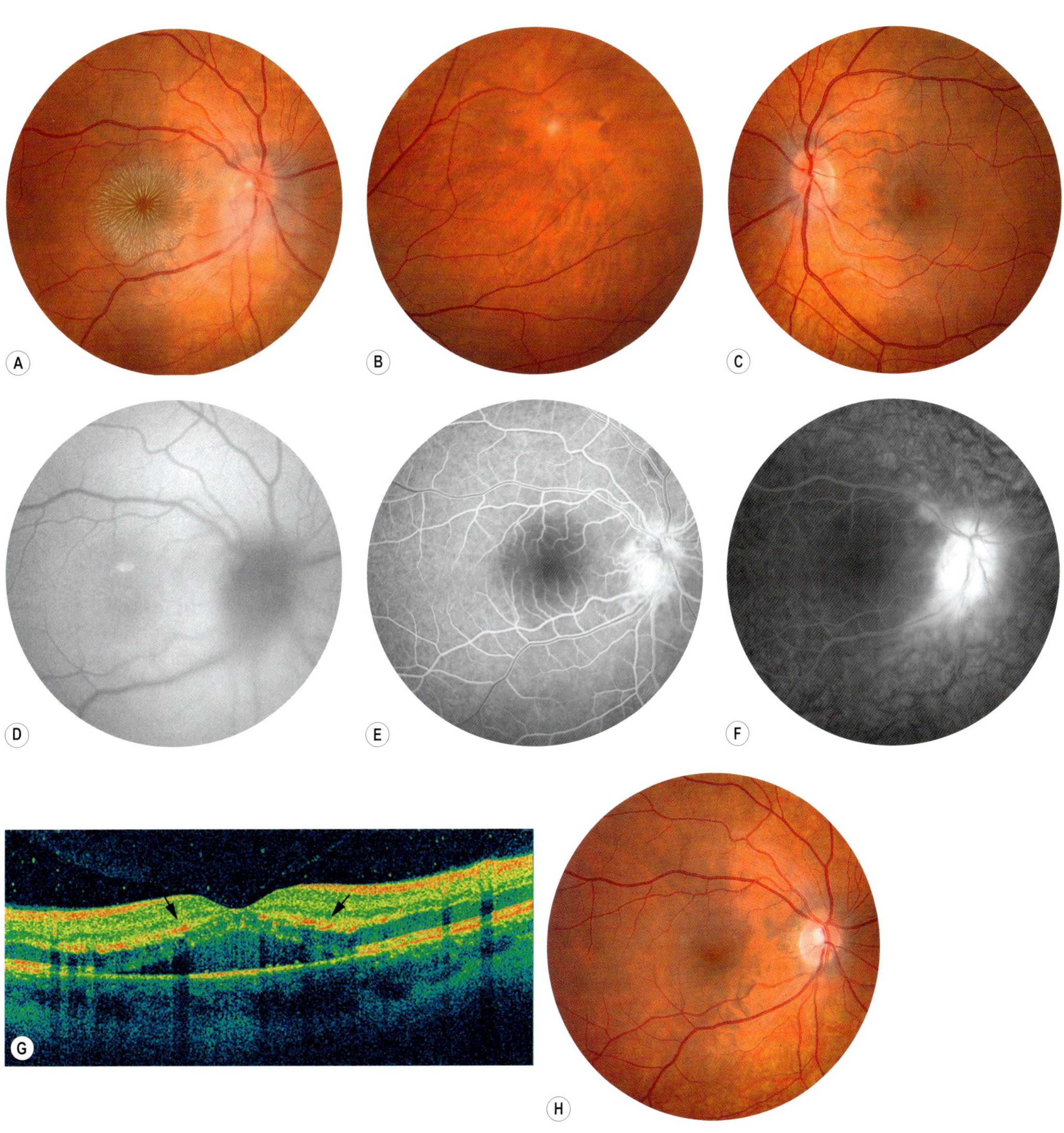
A
B
C
D
E
F
G
H

LUETIC CHORIORETINITIS

Many different fundus lesions have been described in congenital and acquired syphilis (Figures 10.07–10.11). Salt-and-pepper changes affecting primarily the peripheral retina are the most frequent alterations described with congenital syphilis. Severe involvement of the ocular fundus, however, may occur and produce a picture simulating retinitis pigmentosa (Figure 10.11, E and F). In acquired syphilis, particularly in patients with secondary syphilis, several acute fundoscopic pictures should suggest the possibility of syphilis. Secondary syphilis occurs 6 weeks to 6 months after the primary inoculation, which particularly in homosexuals may be overlooked. During the secondary stage of syphilis there is widespread dissemination of the spirochetes, and the patient often experiences malaise, fever, hair loss, papular macular rash, condyloma lata, mucous patches, and generalized lymphadenopathy (Figures 10.07, J–L; 10.11, J and K). Approximately 5% of patients with secondary syphilis will show evidence of panuveitis.[71,72] Probably the most common fundus change is that of vitreous cellular infiltration and either single or multiple, nonelevated (placoid), geographic, yellow–white, ill-defined, chorioretinal lesions that often are confluent in the posterior pole and mid periphery of the fundus (Figures 10.07, B and G; 10.10, H; 10.11, I and L).[73–85] Both eyes are affected in half of all cases. In some patients the chorioretinal lesions may be largely confined to the area around the optic disc. They may be associated with superficial, flame-shaped hemorrhages. The fundus picture may simulate the early stages of the acute retinal necrosis syndrome.[86–89] Secondary retinal detachment and choroidal detachment develop in some patients.[90] The active yellow–gray placoid outer retinal and choroidal lesions fade centrally, and often there is clumping of the RPE in a leopard-spot configuration (Figures 10.07, D, H, and I; 10.10).[80] These pigment clumps may become less apparent over a period of months. The clinical course is variable. In some cases the chorioretinitis resolves spontaneously, and the appearance of the fundus and retinal function may return to near normal. In others widespread areas of chorioretinal atrophy and loss of retinal function occur (Figure 10.11, A–C). Migration of RPE into the overlying retina in a bone-spicule pattern may occur many months later. Choroidal neovascularization developing at the edge of a chorioretinal scar may be a late complication (Figure 10.11, D).[91]

10.07 Luetic chorioretinitis.

A to **F**: Acute posterior placoid chorioretinitis in both eyes of this 42-year-old homosexual man with a 2-week history of blurred vision and floaters in both eyes. Approximately 6 weeks previously he had noted a skin eruption on the sole of his left foot and perirectal pruritus. Visual acuity was 20/20 in the right eye and 20/30 in the left eye. There was evidence of bilateral anterior and posterior uveitis, with many vitreous cells and opacities in the left eye (A). Because of the presence of irregular retinal whitening in the periphery of the left eye, a diagnosis of possible acute retinal necrosis was made. Four weeks later he noted marked visual loss in the right eye. Visual acuity was 8/200. There were several large zones of gray–white change at the level of the RPE and outer retina in the macula (B) and periphery (C) of the right eye. Angiography (D and E) revealed these lesions to be hypofluorescent early and to stain later. A leopard-spot pattern of background hypofluorescence was apparent in the macular area (D). The blood and cerebrospinal fluid serology were positive for syphilis. Following IV penicillin, the fundus changes and uveitis cleared promptly, leaving a coarsely mottled pattern of pigmentation in the macular area. He experienced a rapid recovery of vision. Four months later his visual acuity was 20/15 in the right eye and 20/20 in the left eye. There was mild pigment mottling in both macular areas.
G to **I**: Acute posterior placoid chorioretinitis, vitritis, and maculopapular dermatitis caused by secondary syphilis in a 48-year-old man whose visual acuity was 6/200. Fluorescein angiography revealed a leopard-spot pattern of nonfluorescence in the area of partial fading of the gray–white lesion that was nonfluorescent early and stained late (H and I). His left eye became involved several days later. The lesions resolved promptly after treatment with penicillin and his acuity returned to 20/30 in the right eye and 20/20 in the left eye within 4 weeks.
J to **L**: Alopecia (J), and maculopapular dermatitis (K and L) in patients with acute visual loss associated with acute posterior placoid chorioretinitis caused by secondary syphilis.

(G–K from Gass et al.[80]; L from Passo and Rosenbaum.[94])

Fluorescein angiography in the region of the active yellow–white chorioretinal lesions initially shows evidence of hypofluorescence, followed by late staining at the level of the RPE (Figure 10.07, D, E, H, and I). Fluorescein staining of the optic disc and major retinal veins is frequent. During the early stages of resolution of the active chorioretinal lesions, the leopard-spot change in the RPE may be more apparent angiographically than ophthalmoscopically.

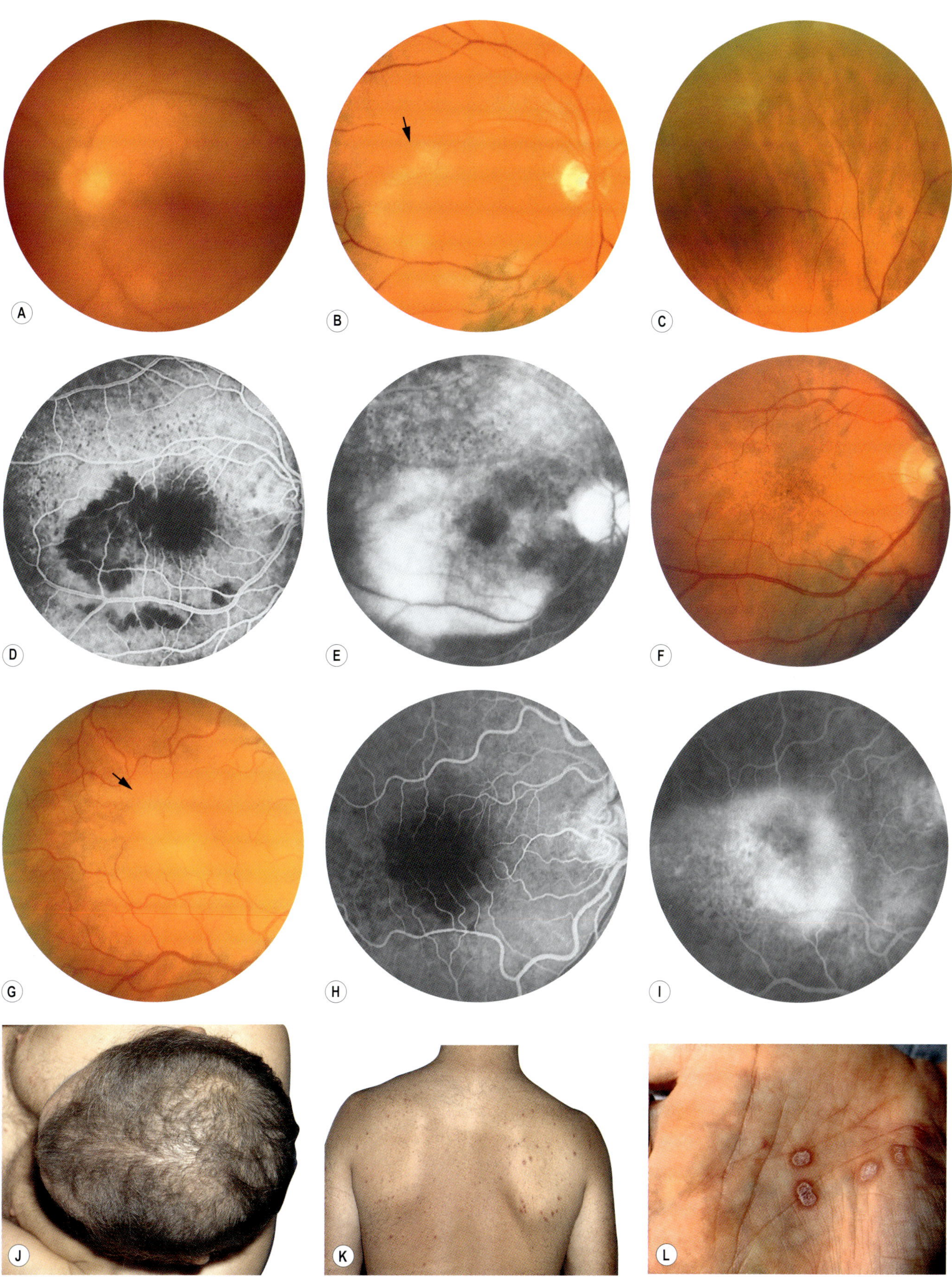
A
B
C
D
E
F
G
H
I
J
K
L

The acute placoid chorioretinal lesions of secondary syphilis may be mistaken for those of acute placoid multifocal pigment epitheliopathy and serpiginous choroiditis.[80] Eliciting a history and/or the detection of any of the nonocular manifestations of secondary syphilis, and institution of prompt treatment with penicillin, is important in making the correct diagnosis and in preventing permanent visual loss. Return of visual function may be dramatic. The patient should be evaluated for evidence of AIDS, which often accompanies secondary lues.[80,92–95] Syphilis may be accelerated and neurosyphilis encountered earlier in patients with AIDS.[92]

In the past 5 years there have been several cases of ocular syphilis with a specific clinical presentation that resembles acute retinal necrosis, most often seen in homosexual and heterosexual men who have sex with men (MSM). The findings include a characteristic ground glass appearance of multifocal whitish lesions present in the inner retina and at the preretinal level, associated with occlusive vasculitis of the vessels in their vicinity[87,96–98] (Figures 10.08, B, D, and I; 10.09, H–J). The inner retinal and preretinal collection, along with the perivascular infiltration, resolve with treatment (Figures 10.08, E–G and K; 10.09, M and N). This presentation is now seen in nearly 35% of cases of ocular syphilis, with the placoid lesion making up another third, and the remaining third accounted for by nonspecific anterior uveitis, disc edema, vasculitis, and other lesions (Figures 10.09, O–X; 10.10, A–G). Whether different serotypes of *Treponema pallidum* cause different clinical manifestations is the explanation of the diverse manifestations is not known.

10.08 Syphilitic inner retinitis and vasculitis.

A to **G**: A 28-year-old Hispanic man noted blurring of vision in his left eye 1 day after a dental procedure. He was on amoxicillin and miconazole. He presented a week later with a vision of 20/20 on the right and 0/30 on the left. There were numerous keratic precipitates, anterior chamber cell and flare, Koeppe iris nodules, and anterior vitreous cells. There were collections of white cells on the posterior hyaloid temporal to the macula and in the inferior vitreous base (A and D). The inferotemporal retinal vessels showed whitening of their walls (B and C). He was HIV-positive and blood and cerebrospinal fluid rapid plasma reagin (CSF RPR) were grossly elevated. He received IV penicillin for 14 days, following which signs and symptoms resolved with return of vision to 20/25 and gradual melting off of the white cells of the retina and the vessel walls.

H to **L**: This 44-year-old Caucasian man presented with cystoid macular edema and a vision of 20/25. Fluorescein was unremarkable except for dye accumulation in the cysts (H). He was treated with one intravitreal injection of triamcinolone, and vision improved and the macular edema resolved. Two months later he noted recurrence of the visual blur in the right eye, and returned after a further 2 months with count fingers vision, several areas of preretinal collection of white cells, and vascular narrowing (I). Angiogram showed leopard-spot pigment change (J and K). His VDRL was positive and HIV was negative. He received IV penicillin for 21 days, but vision remained poor due to optic atrophy and arterial occlusion (L).

(Courtesy: A–G, Dr Pauline Merrill; H–L, Dr Ivan Batlle. J, Also, Yannuzzi, Lawrence J., The Retinal Atlas, Saunders 2010, 978-0-7020-3320-9, p.348.)

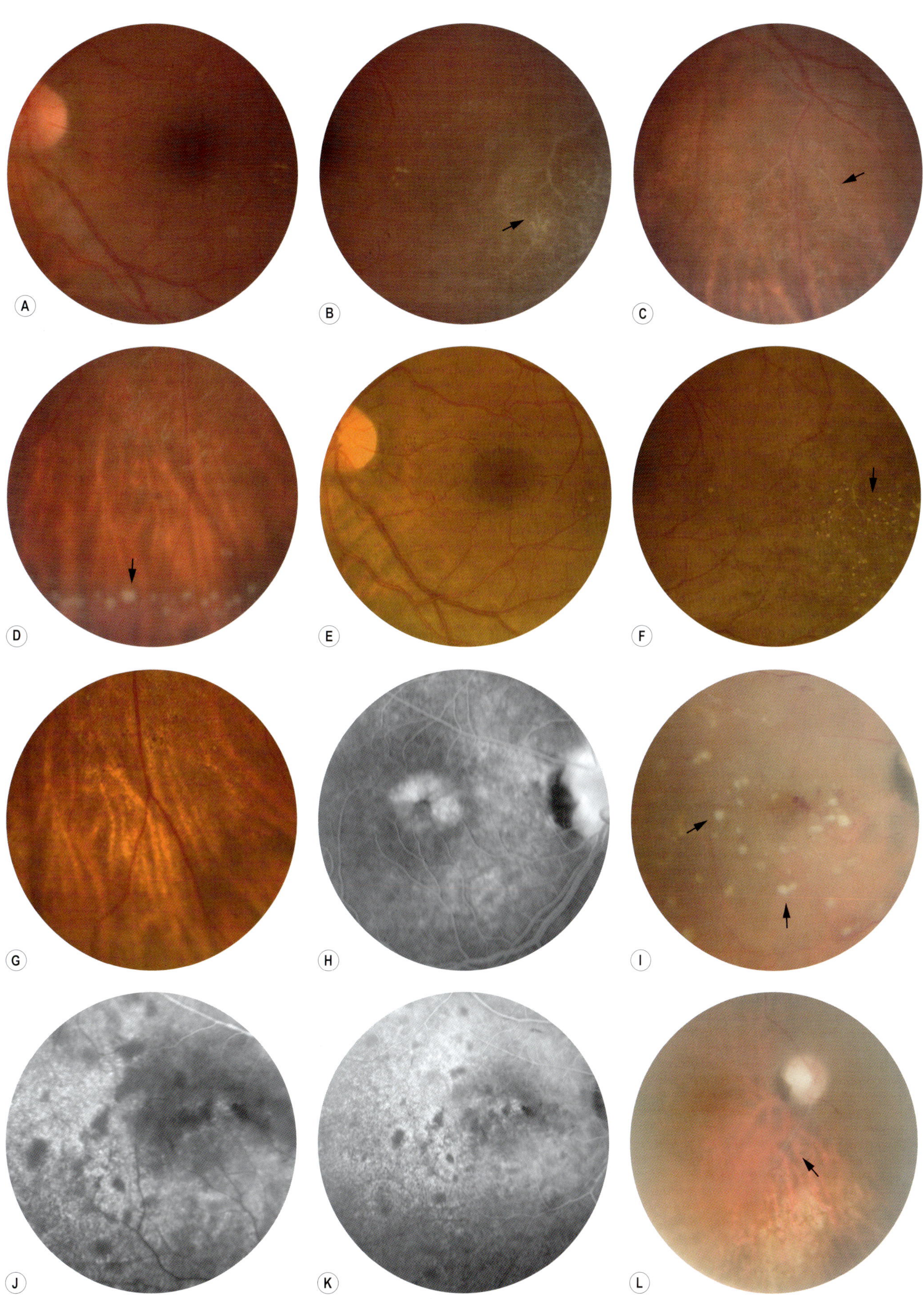
A
B
C
D
E
F
G
H
I
J
K
L

In some patients with acquired syphilis the fundus picture is primarily that of retinal vasculitis with retinal hemorrhages,[71,81,86,99–103] occlusive arterial disease, and retinitis proliferans (see Figure 10.11, G and H).[81,99] Many different fundoscopic changes have been attributed to syphilis, including neuroretinitis,[104] disciform scar,[105] acute retinal necrosis,[89] pseudo-retinitis pigmentosa, Kyrieleis' plaques,[106] and optic atrophy.[107] Syphilis has been called the 'great imitator'.[84] Anterior segment involvement with a syphilitic gumma (Figure 10.10, G) presents with an iris mass. It is often difficult to determine the stage of syphilis based on the ocular findings, though most inflammatory presentations of syphilis occur in the secondary stage. Similar findings have been seen in patients with neurosyphilis, tertiary syphilis, and latent syphilis.[108] The incidence of syphilis has been on the rise since 2000 with a 33.5% increase noted between 2000 and 2004. Several outbreaks have been reported from New York City, Miami-Dade County, Washington, Houston, San Francisco, and Southern California. A CDC analysis estimates that 64% of the early stage syphilis cases in 2004 were in MSM compared to 5% in 1999.[109]

Since it is a common infection, however, care must be used in assigning it as the cause of an ocular disease solely on the basis of positive serologic tests for syphilis. These include the nonspecific reagin tests, such as VDRL, or more specific tests, including fluorescent treponemal antibody-absorption (FTA-Abs) and microhemagglutination assay-*Treponema pallidum* (MHA-TP). There is some controversy concerning the criteria for diagnosis of neurosyphilis and for the dosage and route of administration of penicillin in these patients.[110] Because of the high incidence of positive reaction of the cerebrospinal fluid (CSF) to the serologic tests for syphilis during the secondary stages of the disease, CSF examination is usually not recommended for patients presenting with the ocular manifestations of secondary syphilis. Recommended treatment for patients with active chorioretinal disease caused by syphilis is aqueous crystalline penicillin G (18–24 million U IV daily) or procaine penicillin (2.4 million U IM daily) with oral probenecid (500 mg four times daily) for 10–14 days. If CSF pleocytosis has been noted, these patients should be monitored at 6-monthly intervals with CSF studies until the cell count normalizes. In patients allergic to penicillin, IV or IM ceftriaxone (2 g per day for 10–14 days) can be used.[111] All patients with syphilis should be tested for HIV status and the treatment in HIV-positive patients lasts for 3 weeks. Those who are HIV-positive should be monitored for treatment failure at 6, 12, 18, and 24 months.

10.09 Syphilitic placoid chorioretinitis and retinitis.

A to N: A 65-year-old diabetic and hypertensive man reported a 1-day sudden visual loss to 20/80 in his left eye. There was an afferent papillary defect but no anterior chamber or vitreous cells. Placoid lesions at the level of the choroid or pigment epithelium with a few blot retinal hemorrhages were noted in the left eye (B). Angiogram showed mild late irregular hyperfluorescence of the placoid lesion (C). A diagnosis of 'choroidal ischemia' was made; carotid and cardiac echo were normal. His vision declined to 20/150 at week 1 when oral prednisone was begun at 40 mg per day. At week 2 the vision worsened in his right eye and did not improve in his left. The right eye now had placoid lesions while the lesions in the left eye had faded (D and E). An angiogram showed late hyperfluorescence of the placoid lesion in both eyes (F and G). Oral prednisone was increased to 100 mg per day and laboratory tests were ordered. He skipped his appointment and returned after a week with a drop in vision to hand motions in his right eye and 20/100 in the left. He now had several focal areas of superficial retinal whitening and vascular narrowing in both eyes in addition to the placoid lesion that had extended under the fovea in the right eye (H–J). An angiogram showed early blocked fluorescence of the placoid lesion with late staining and leopard-spot change (K and L). RPR and FTA-Abs returned positive.

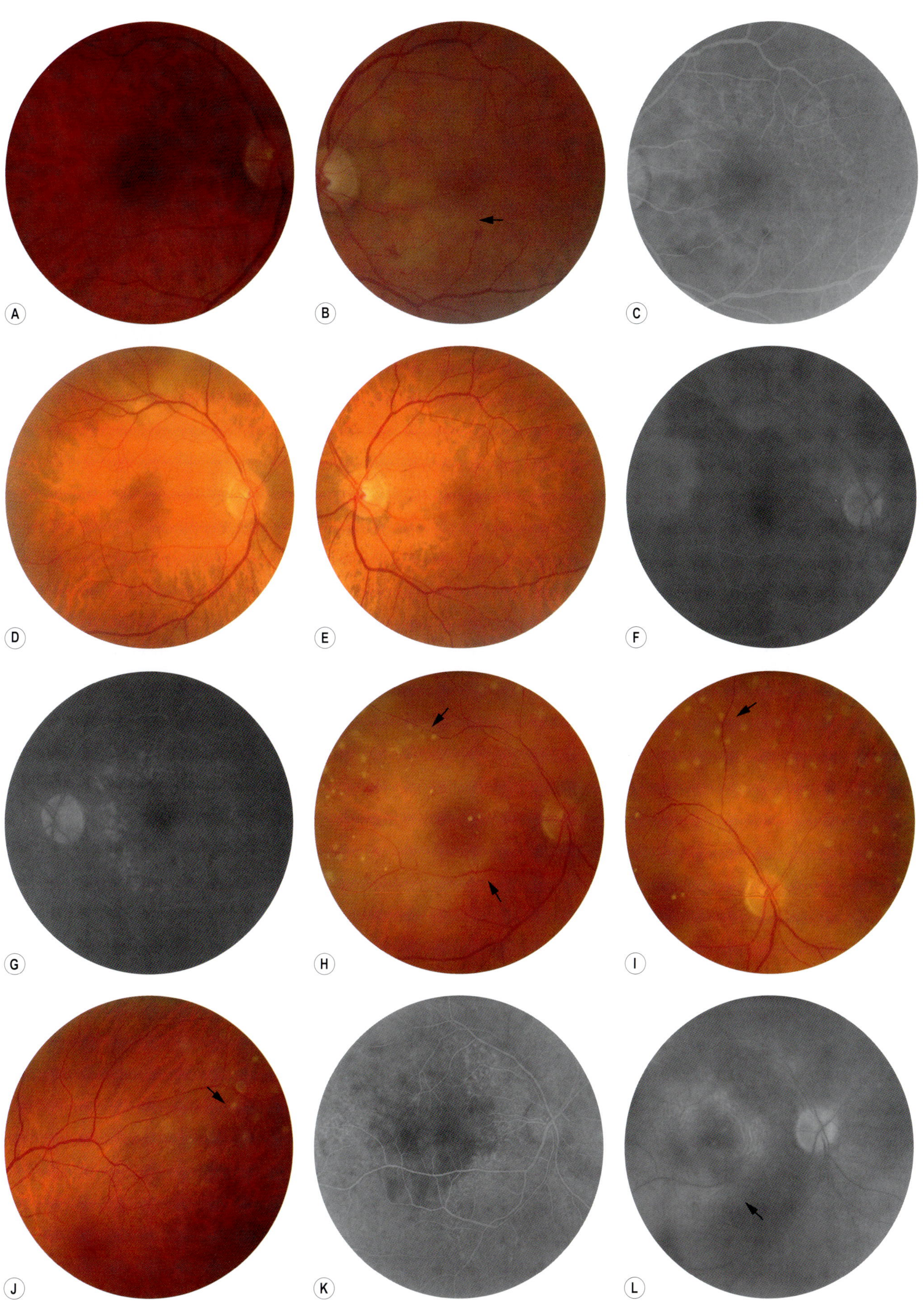
A
B
C
D
E
F
G
H
I
J
K
L

10.09 Continued

He reported several internet sexual partners over 2 years following the death of his wife from cancer. He was hospitalized and received 2 million units every 4 h of IV crystalline penicillin followed by benzathine penicillin G 2.4 million units IM for 3 weeks. All white and placoid lesions resolved with residual vascular narrowing (M and N).

O to **X**: A 44-year-old Hispanic woman had several months of declining vision in both eyes associated with some pain around the eyes. Her daughter reported that the mother's personality had recently changed; she had become short tempered and forgetful. Her best corrected visual acuity was 20/60 on the right and 20/25 on the left. There were 2–3 + vitreous cells in both eyes. She had had a whole body rash 15 years prior and had two lifetime sexual partners. Both optic discs were swollen with dilated telangiectatic vessels on their surface (O and P). There were old inactive perivascular chorioretinal scars in both eyes in the mid periphery (Q and R). The red-free images showed the abnormal disc vessels better (S and T). Angiogram delineated the dilated vessels over the disc and surrounding retina early, which leaked profusely in the mid and late phases (U–W). The peripheral chorioretinal scars showed staining of the edges with no new activity (X). Further history revealed her first partner had a sore on his penis 15 years ago, after which she had developed the whole body rash that resolved with no sequelae. She had felt normal until recently with the onset of visual blur and personality change. Her RPR was negative but her *Treponema pallidum* particle agglutination (TPPA) test was positive, confirming a diagnosis of tertiary syphilis. She received 24 million units of IV penicillin for 14 days. At 3 weeks her vision had improved to 20/50 on the right and remained at 20/25 on the left. Her personality returned to normal.

(Courtesy: A–N, Dr Sundeep Dev; O–X, Dr Jeffrey Whitehead. O, P, R, V, Also, Yannuzzi, Lawrence J., The Retinal Atlas, Saunders 2010, 978-0-7020-3320-9, p.352.)

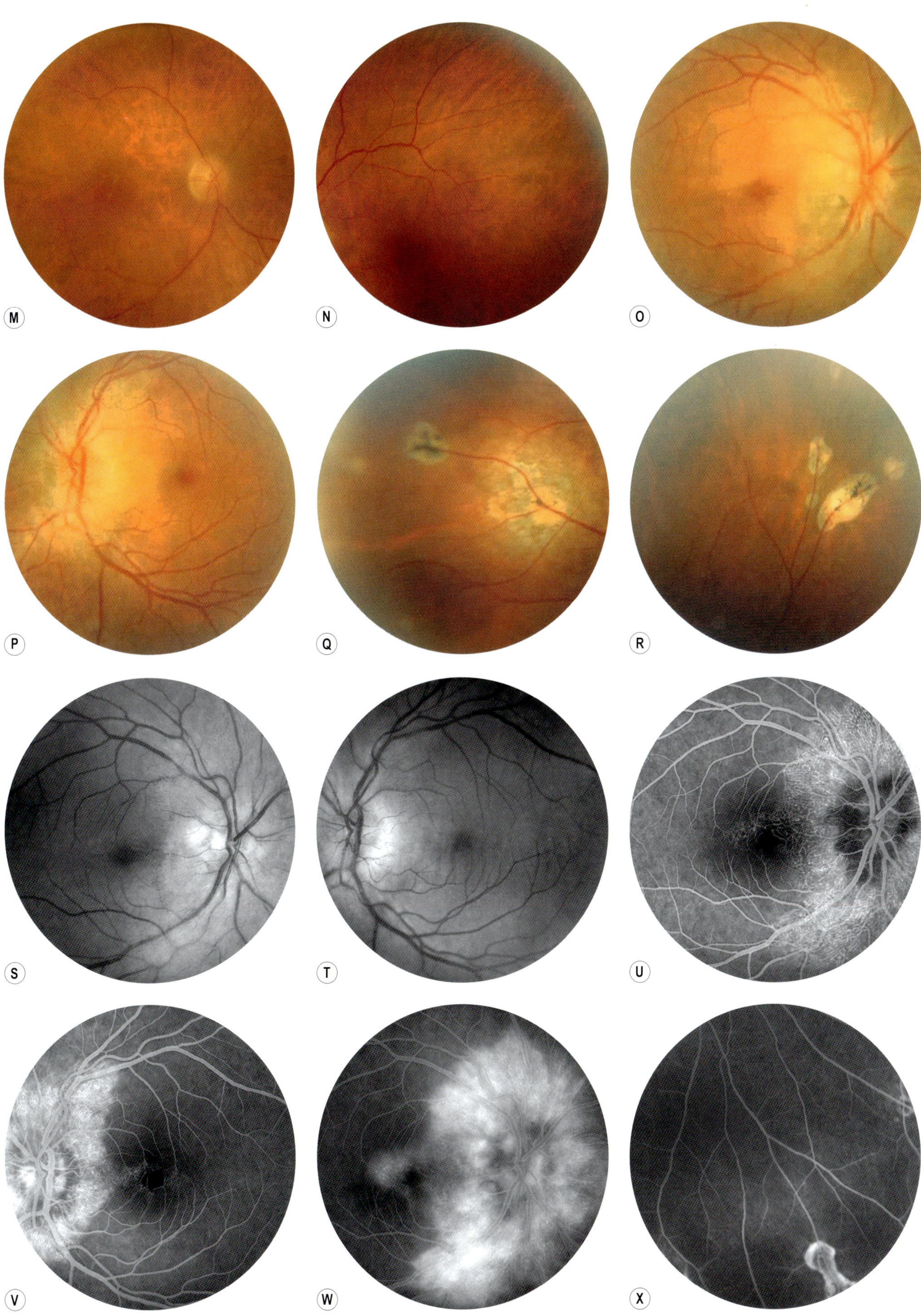
M
N
O
P
Q
R
S
T
U
V
W
X

10.10 Syphilitic optic neuritis.

A to F: This 58-year-old elementary school teacher woke up with a circular yellow light in her central vision. Visual acuity was 20/20 in both eyes. Anterior segment was normal. A Humphrey visual field showed an enlarged blind spot in the right eye. The right fundus showed a swollen optic disc (A and B) and the left was normal (C). An MRI of the brain and orbits revealed no abnormalities. Observation was recommended, and a test for syphilis returned positive, as did her husband's subsequently. Visual acuity dropped to 20/40 in the right eye, the disc edema persisted (D), and an angiogram showed dilated vessels on its surface (E). She was desensitized to penicillin and treated with 2 weeks of IV penicillin and doxycycline. The disc edema improved (F) and the visual acuity returned to 20/25 in the right eye and remained at 20/20 in the left eye.

Syphilitic gumma.

G to L: This 53-year-old man presented with a history of scratching his left eye while changing his contact lenses. He was diagnosed with a corneal ulcer and started on gatifloxacin (Zymar) drops. Two weeks later his visual acuity had dropped to hand motions in the left eye and he was noted to have an anterior chamber granuloma with blood and dilated iris vessels with posterior synechia and uveitis (G). Fundus examination of the right eye revealed a placoid lesion in the inferonasal fundus (H). A fluorescein angiogram of this eye showed late hyperfluorescence (I). A VDRL was done which confirmed syphilitic gumma. He was known to be HIV-positive and was on nevirapine (Viramune) with a CD4 count of 283 and an undetectable viral load. His CSF VDRL was positive at 1:4 and RPR was positive at 1:512. He was started on IV penicillin G every 4 h. A week later his gumma had decreased in size by half and the placoid lesion in the fundus had almost resolved, leaving mild pigment mottling (J). A fluorescein angiogram done 4 weeks later revealed leopard-spot pigment change at the site of the placoid lesion (L) and complete resolution of the syphilitic gumma (K).

(Courtesy: A–F, Dr Mark Daily; G–L, Dr Charlie Barr.)

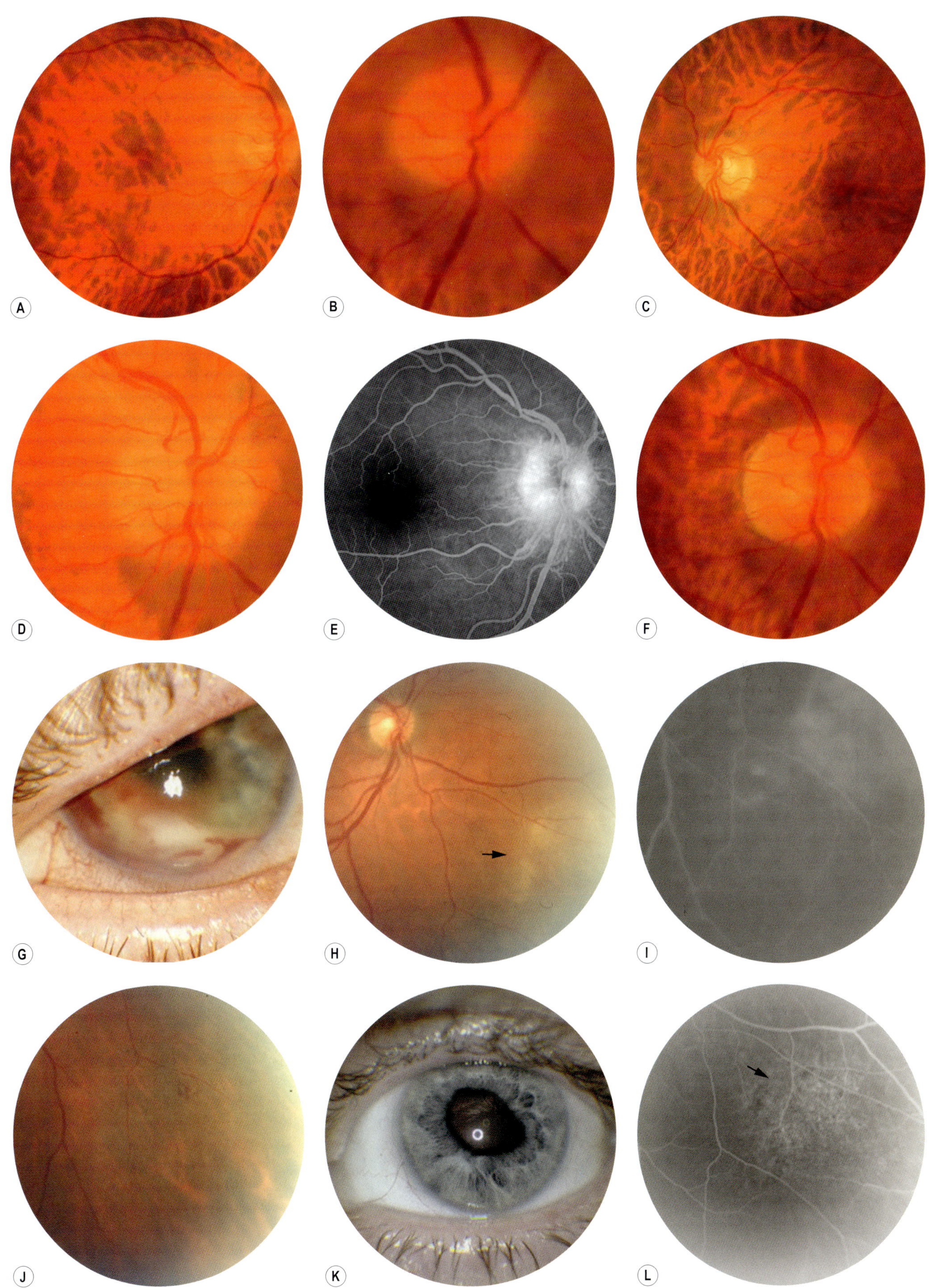
A
B
C
D
E
F
G
H
I
J
K
L

10.11 Luetic chorioretinitis.

A to **C**: Bilateral chorioretinal scars caused by secondary luetic chorioretinitis.
D: Subretinal neovascularization (*arrow*) in the macula of a patient with chorioretinal scars following chorioretinitis caused by secondary syphilis.
E and **F**: Congenital luetic chorioretinopathy in a 41-year-old woman with poor vision all of her life, interstitial keratitis, positive fluorescent treponemal antibody (FTA), and 20/80 visual acuity. Note the narrowing of the retinal vessels, optic disc pallor, and pseudo-retinitis pigmentosa change peripherally.
G and **H**: Presumed luetic retinal vasculitis in this 30-year-old homosexual man with a 10-day history of blurred vision in his right eye. The left eye was amblyopic since birth. Five years previously he had primary syphilis. Sixteen months previously he developed a skin rash on the feet and hands. This was diagnosed as syphilis 3 months before the onset of visual symptoms and he received IM penicillin. His visual acuity was 20/50 in his right eye and hand motions only in the left eye. He had widely scattered retinal hemorrhages, perivascular exudation (G), and angiographic evidence of multiple sites of retinal vascular obstruction, predominantly affecting the veins (H). There was perivascular staining in the late photographs.
I to **L**: Placoid chorioretinitis in this HIV-positive 45-year-old man with generalized rash over his trunk, abdomen, and palms. He complained of decreased vision in his right eye for 2 weeks; visual acuity was 4/200 in the right and 20/25 in the left eye. He had a faint placoid lesion in the left superior macula. His CD4 count was in the 200s and viral load was undetectable. He was admitted and received IV penicillin for 3 weeks. The placoid lesion appeared much less distinct within a week (L) and his vision improved to 20/70. He did not return for further follow up.

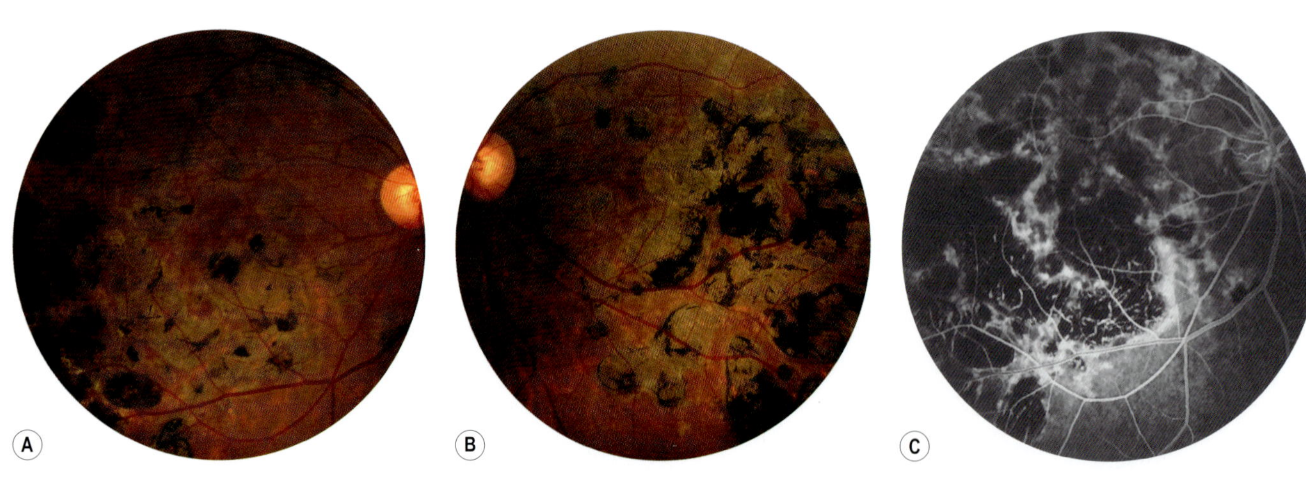

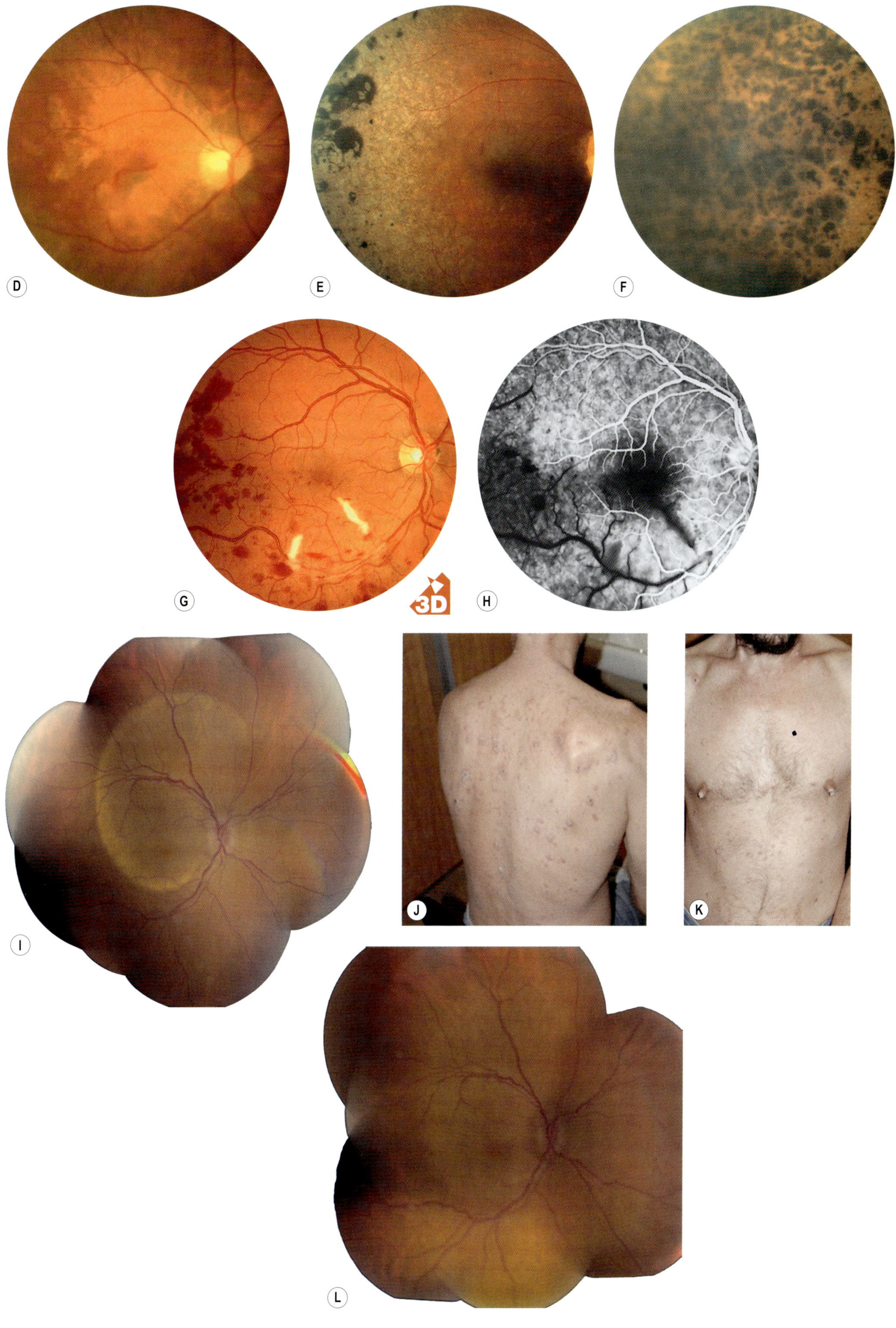
D
E
F
G
3D
H
I
J
K
L

TUBERCULOSIS

Even though pulmonary and extrapulmonary tuberculosis (TB) has been prevalent worldwide for hundreds of years, reports of ocular TB apart from Eales' disease have been meager until the past 10 years. This is likely due to the inability to confirm the diagnosis accurately, lack of knowledge among the ophthalmic personnel in countries with a high prevalence of the disorder, and less access to specialized care in these countries. Several new manifestations of intraocular TB have been reported.[63,112–124] With an increase in the number of HIV patients, ocular TB is on the rise. Extrapulmonary involvement is seen in 50% of patients with both TB and AIDS.

Tuberculosis is a systemic disease caused by *Mycobacterium tuberculosis* and is characterized by caseating granuloma formation in the affected tissues. Although pulmonary TB is the commonest manifestation, extrapulmonary involvement can include the gastrointestinal, genitourinary, cardiovascular, skin and central nervous system including the eyes. Pathogenesis of tuberculous infection evolves through five stages following implantation of inhaled mycobacteria in a respiratory bronchiole or alveolus.

- Stage 1: The alveolar macrophage phagocytoses the bacteria and either destroys them or the bacteria grow and destroy the macrophage.
- Stage 2: Circulating monocytes are recruited to this nidus and phagocytose the bacteria. The bacteria prevent the fusion of the lysosome to the phagosome, thus preventing their destruction.
- Stage 3: A delayed type hypersensitivity reaction develops destroying the bacteria, resulting in caseous necrosis. This lesion contains central caseation surrounded by activated and nonactivated macrophages, T lymphocytes, and other immune cells. If the cell-mediated immunity is good, the highly activated macrophages destroy the bacteria, thus halting the progression of the lesion at this subclinical stage.
- Stage 4: If the cell-mediated immunity is poor, the bacteria escape from the edge of the caseation and multiply within macrophages, causing more caseation and growth of the tubercle. A few bacteria-laden macrophages may enter the lymphatics or blood vessels and reach other parts of the lung and other organs including the eye.
- Stage 5: The central caseous material liquefies and relentless multiplication of the bacteria ensues in spite of good cell-mediated immunity. The bacteria erode the bronchial wall and spread to other organs.[113]

Ocular Tuberculosis

Anterior Uveitis

Acute and chronic granulomatous uveitis with mutton fat keratic precipitates, iris and angle nodules, and anterior chamber granulomas are features of tuberculous anterior uveitis (see Figure 10.15, D). Sometimes a hypopyon may be seen and the iris nodules may become vascularized. Essential iris atrophy has also been reported. Tubercular anterior uveitis may also present as a mild or moderate recurrent iridocyclitis; granulomas are absent in these eyes but small translucent nodules may be seen at the pupillary margin (Koeppe nodules).[113,125,126]

10.12 Tubercular multifocal chorioretinitis.

A to **F**: A 30-year-old woman in India complained of insidious onset, gradually progressive loss of vision in the left eye over 18 months. This was associated with pain and redness. She was treated for acute anterior uveitis elsewhere with topical and oral steroids up to 60 mg per day. She was otherwise healthy. Her vision in the left eye was 20/100, with anterior chamber cell and flare. She had several deep choroidal lesions in the posterior pole with overlying exudative retinal detachment (A). An angiogram showed early hypofluorescence of the choroidal lesions and late hyperfluorescence beginning at the edge of the lesions and pooling of dye into the subretinal space (B–D). She had no contact with a person with active tuberculosis. Mantoux test was positive at 20 × 23 mm, sedimentation rate was 5 mm, chest X-ray was normal, and QuantiFERON-TB Gold was positive. She received four-drug anti-TB therapy, along with 60 mg of prednisone and 10 mg of pyridoxine. Three weeks later her vision had improved to 20/25 and the lesions appear healed (E and F).

G to **L**: A 17-year-old Indian girl with decrease in right eye vision for 3 months to counting finger at 3 meters and a relative afferent defect. She had a subretinal lesion with intense full-thickness retinitis in the center and adjacent small retinal hemorrhages. Fluorescein angiogram showed gradual hyperfluorescence and leakage of dye from the choroidal lesion (H and I). The lesion remained nonfluorescent on ICG angiography (J and K). Resolution of inflammation and flat atrophic scar seen following treatment with anti TB medications.

(Courtesy: Dr Vishali Gupta and Dr Amod Gupta.)

Intermediate Uveitis

Patients present with low-grade smoldering chronic uveitis, vitritis, snowball opacities, snow banking, peripheral vascular sheathing, and peripheral retinochoroidal granulomas. Fluorescein gonioangiography shows early hyperfluorescence of small, discrete, whitish lesions in the ciliary body band near the iris root. Cystoid macular edema is often present.[113]

Retinochoroiditis Caused by *Mycobacterium Tuberculosis* in Immunosuppressed Patients

The eye in the immunocompetent individual with pulmonary tuberculosis is infrequently affected. Patients with miliary tuberculosis may develop multifocal choroidal granulomas and, less often, endophthalmitis. Patients with AIDS and tuberculosis, however, may develop severe multifocal retinochoroiditis, caused by *M. tuberculosis* as well as by the ordinarily less pathogenic *M. avium*.[2]

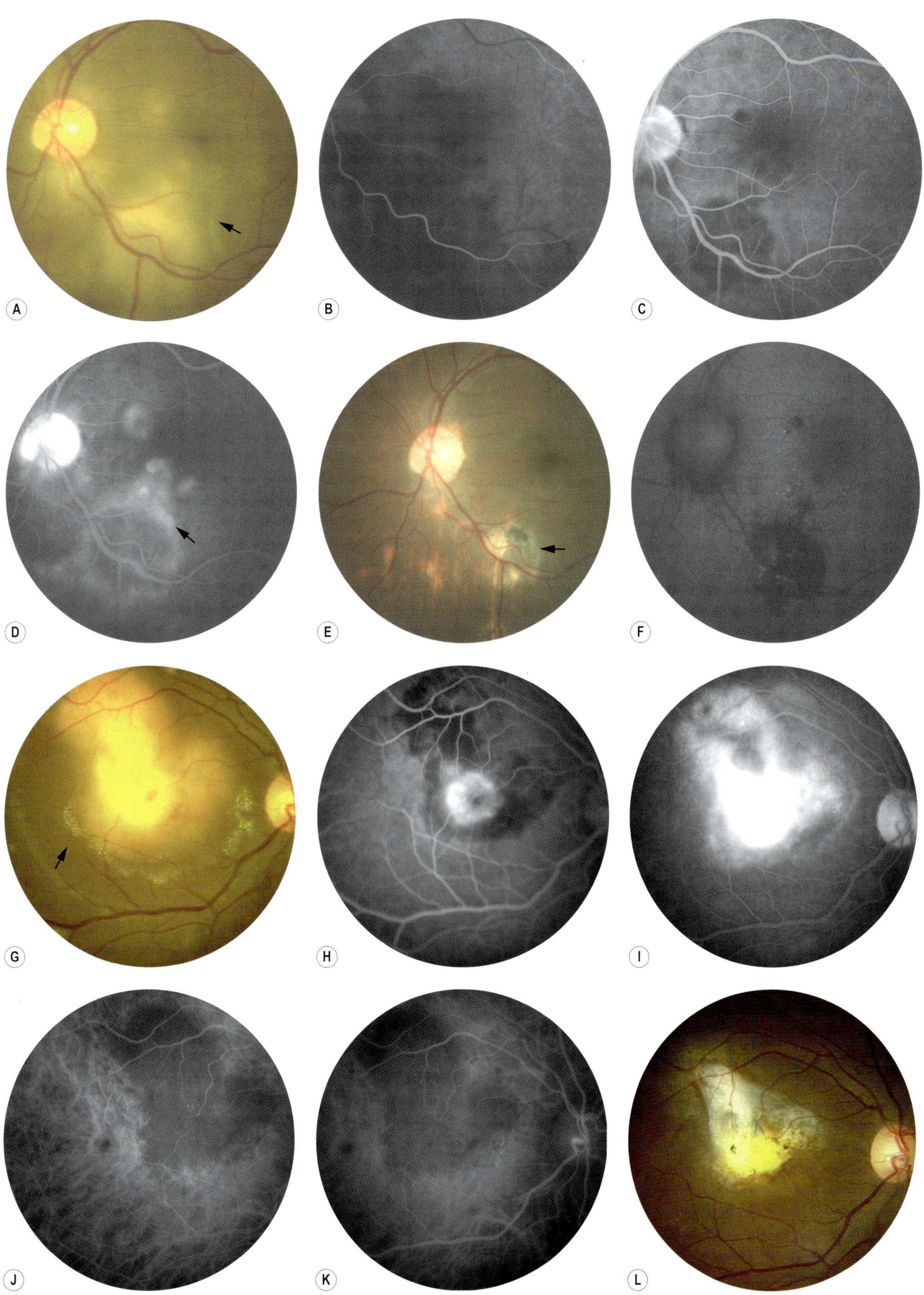
A
B
C
D
E
F
G
H
I
J
K
L

Posterior Uveitis and Panuveitis

Choroidal Tubercles

Multifocal small choroidal tubercles is the commonest manifestation, being either unilateral or bilateral and sarcoid-like, suggesting hematogenous spread of the organism.[127–137] They vary from one-fourth to one disc area in size, have a grayish-yellow color, and very occasionally may have adjacent retinal hemorrhages (Figure 10.12, A–D). This presentation is also a feature of miliary TB. Once treatment is instituted, the yellow–gray lesions turn whiter with sharp borders and eventually get pigmented (Figure 10.12, E).[113,115,118,119,126,138–141]

Subretinal Abscess

The caseous material can liquefy secondary to rapid multiplication of the bacilli, resulting in necrosis and abscess formation. These may be seen in disseminated TB or in isolation without evidence of TB in other parts of the body. A high index of suspicion and prevalence in endemic countries should alert the physician to the diagnosis. Chorioretinal anastomosis or subretinal neovascularization can occur over healing lesions (Figure 10.12, G–K).

Choroidal Tuberculoma

This is a solitary mass that is yellow–white, elevated, sometimes with overlying retinal folds and retinal hemorrhage.[128,129,133,136,142–145] The mass can be located anywhere in the fundus and continues to grow both in height and diffuse spread.

Serpiginous-Like Choroiditis

The hallmark of this presentation is the relentless progression of the active edge, with the initial lesion being: (1) multifocal choroiditis that progresses to become confluent and has several advancing active edges (Figure 10.13, A–F); (2) an initial plaque-like lesion with ameboidal spread (Figure 10.13, G and H); and (3) inactive healed scars that show new activity at their edges and progress (Figure 10.13, I–K). When any of these serpiginous choroiditis-like presentations continue to progress despite oral steroids and other immunosuppressives, one should suspect tubercular choroiditis. Workup should include Mantoux skin test, chest X-ray and CT scan, and QuantiFERON-TB Gold (QFT-G) to establish the diagnosis of TB. In the event that all of these are negative, PCR of aqueous or vitreous fluid should be performed to establish the diagnosis.[113,121]

10.13 Serpiginous-like tuberculosis.

A to **K**: Decline in left eye vision to 20/40 over 6 weeks in this 25-year-old Indian man. There were multifocal and confluent creamy lesions with evidence of central healing in some of them (A–C). Angiogram showed hypofluorescence of the creamy edges and patchy transmission hyperfluorescence of the center (D–F). A montage of the lesions showed both serpiginous and multifocal lesions (G and H). His Mantoux test was positive with 24 × 20 mm of induration, chest X- ray showed hilar adenopathy. *Treponema pallidum* haemagglutination (TPHA) test was negative. He received four-drug anti-TB therapy for 4 months, followed by two-drug therapy for 1 year, along with oral steroids at 1.5 mg/kg per day that was tapered over 6 months. Vision improved to 20/30 at 3 months with a decrease in lesion activity (I and J) and to 20/20 at 24 months with complete clearing (K).

(Courtesy: Dr Vishali Gupta and Dr Amod Gupta.)

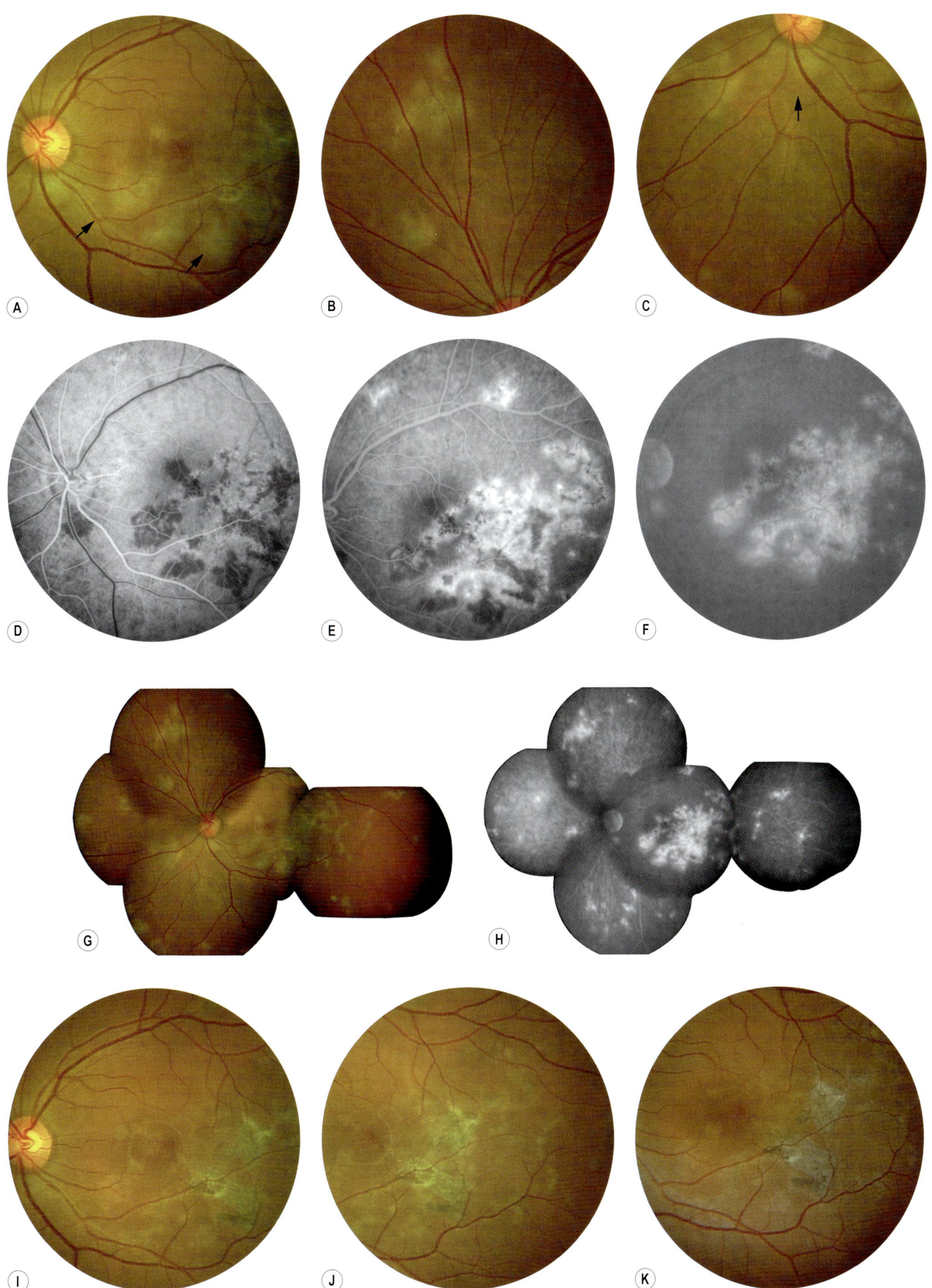
A
B
C
D
E
F
G
H
I
J
K

Tubercular Retinal Vasculitis

Active exudation around the veins and sometimes arteries, associated with retinal hemorrhages, lipid leakage, and occasionally with focal chorioretinitis, should alert one to the diagnosis of tubercular vasculitis (Figure 10.14).[113] This should be differentiated from sarcoid vasculitis and Behçet's disease, which are more arterial than venular. With time, retinal nonperfusion and neovascularization of the retina may occur. Whether the vasculitis is infective per se or represents a hypersensitivity response to *M. tuberculosis* antigens remains speculative. These patients should also undergo various diagnostic tests to confirm TB and rule out sarcoid and Behçet's disease. They require anti-TB therapy and monitoring for future neovascularization that warrants laser ablation of the ischemic retina. Hypersensitivity reaction to TB antigens is likely in a subgroup of patients with Eales' disease (see Chapter 6).

All patients suspected of ocular TB should undergo Mantoux testing, chest X-ray, chest CT if needed, and QuantiFERON-TB Gold test initially.[113,146,147] PCR of tissue fluid can help establish the diagnosis when the other tests are inconclusive. Patients begun on corticosteroids alone when all these tests are negative should be monitored closely for persistence or progression of the lesions, in which case invasive testing with a fine needle biopsy should be performed to demonstrate presence of the organism. All patients with ocular TB should be started on four drugs for the first 2 months and continued on two drugs for a total of 18 months.[112,113] Both 9- and 12-month treatments are inadequate and the lesions are likely to recur after completion of treatment. The bacilli divide very slowly in solid organs, unlike in the lung, hence the need for the longer duration of treatment. Oral steroids at a dose of 0.5–1 mg/kg are also started along with the anti-TB regimen, and tapered slowly over 9–12 months depending on the response.

10.14 Tubercular vasculitis.

A to **W**: Vision declined rapidly to count fingers at 3 meters in this 26-year-old man who had widely distributed nerve fiber infarcts, retinal hemorrhages, perivenous exudation, and mild vitritis (A–E). Fluorescein angiogram showed blockage from the retinal hemorrhages, and staining and leakage from the venous endothelium (F–I). His Mantoux test was

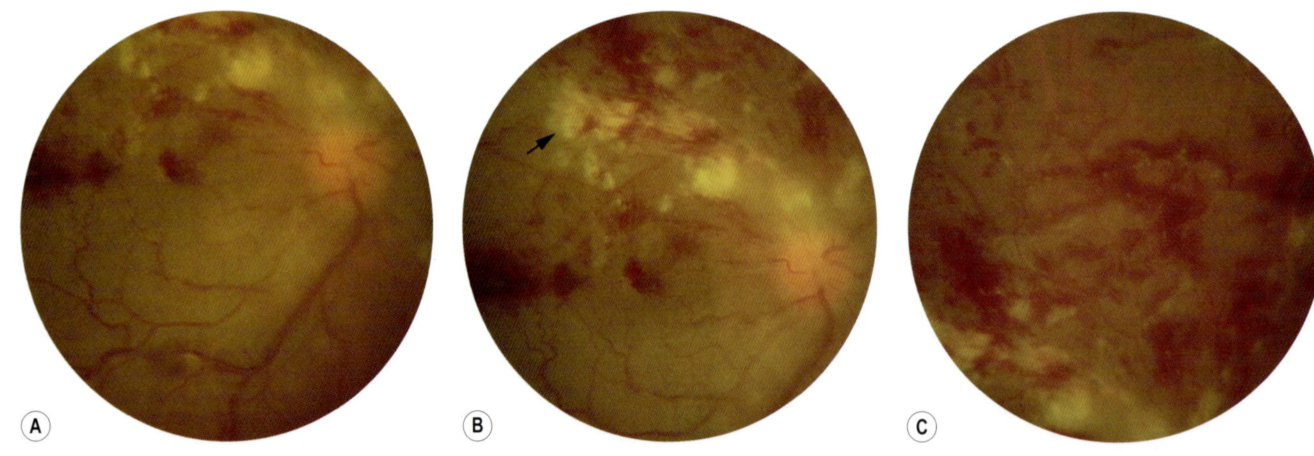

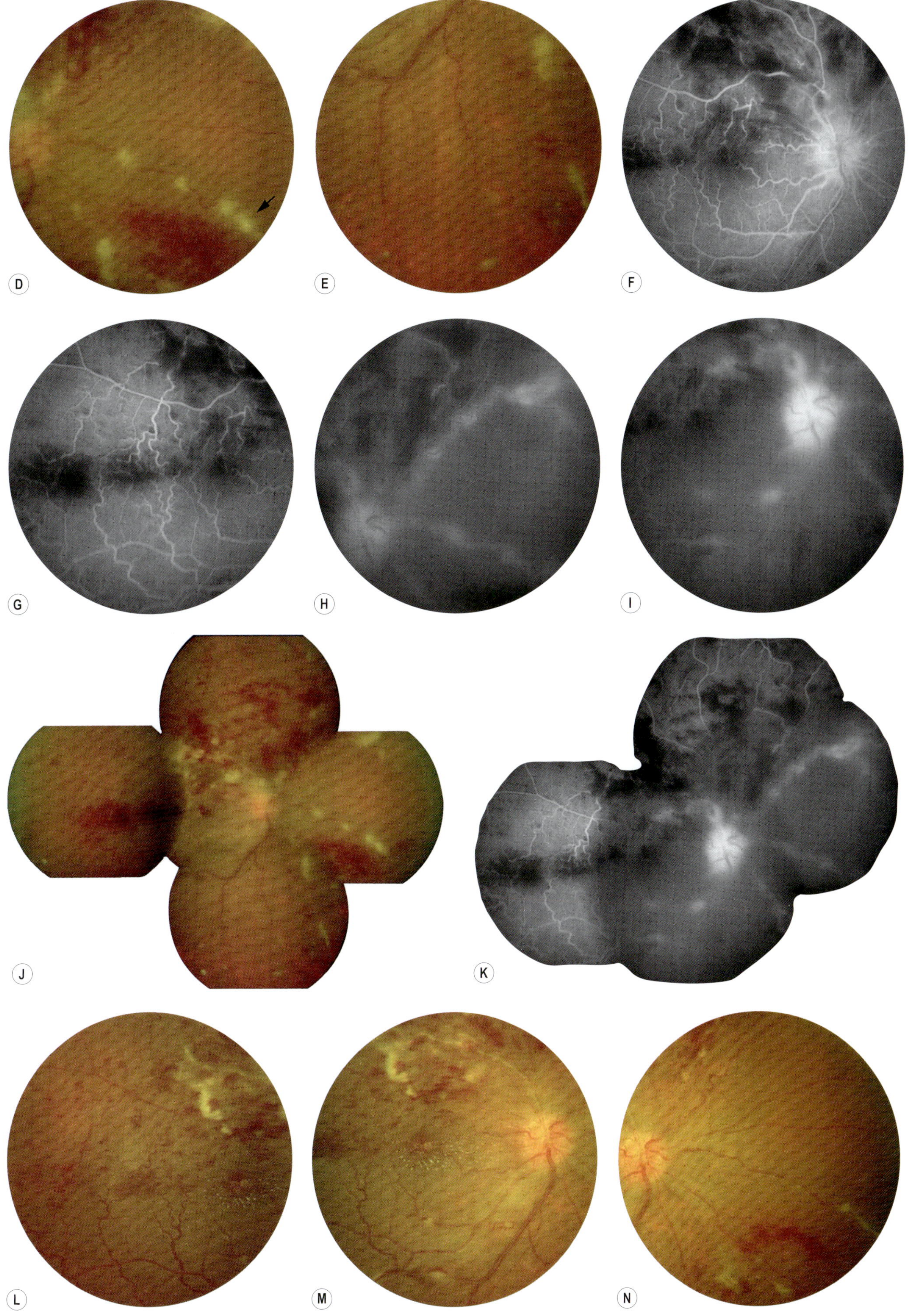
D
E
F
G
H
I
J
K
L
M
N

A paradoxical reaction similar in mechanism to Jarisch–Herxheimer may be seen after initiation of anti-TB therapy that requires an increase in the dose of steroids for a few weeks until the lesions begin to involute.

Nearly 2 billion people are infected with *M. tuberculosis* worldwide, though only 10% develop active disease in their lifetime. Twenty-two countries have been identified that harbor 80% of the world's TB population: India, China, Indonesia, Bangladesh, Pakistan, Nigeria, the Philippines, South Africa, the Russian Federation, Ethiopia, Vietnam, the Democratic Republic of the Congo, Brazil, Tanzania, Kenya, Thailand, Myanmar, Afghanistan, Uganda, Peru, Zimbabwe, and Cambodia.[148,149]

When it occurs focally in the choroid, it produces a nonspecific choroidal inflammatory mass similar to that seen in cryptococcosis, nocardiosis, or other inflammatory diseases of the choroid including sarcoidosis (Figure 10.15, A–C). A large choroidal tuberculoma mass may simulate a melanoma and may fail to respond to anti-TB therapy.[20,144] Barondes et al. described a healthy patient with a negative tuberculin skin test and a focal choroidal lesion which on trans pars plana biopsy contained acid-fast bacilli.[129,150] In some apparently healthy patients the disease may progress rapidly to produce a picture of panophthalmitis. *Mycobacterium avium-intracellulare*, in addition to *M. tuberculosis*, may cause multifocal choroiditis as well as retinitis in patients with AIDS.[127,129]

Eales' Disease

A small subgroup of Eales' disease patients who present with recurrent vitreous hemorrhages, peripheral venous sheathing, and retinal neovascularization may have a hypersensitivity response to tuberculous antigen (see Chapter 6).

Phlyctenular conjunctivitis is an allergic response to various microbial proteins including tuberculous protein (Figure 10.15, E).

10.14 Continued

positive and measured 20 × 20 mm, chest X-ray showed pleural effusion, VDRL was nonreactive, and TPHA test was negative. He was treated with four-drug anti-TB therapy and the lesions began to resolve, with a decrease in retinal hemorrhages and edema, and sheathing of the veins at 3 months (L–P) and 6 months (Q and R). Angiogram showed patchy nonfluorescence and vascular remodeling (S–U). He developed neovascularization of the retina requiring scatter laser photocoagulation in the upper temporal quadrant initially (S) and inferonasal quadrant subsequently (T, V, and W).

(Courtesy: Dr Vishali Gupta and Dr Amod Gupta.)

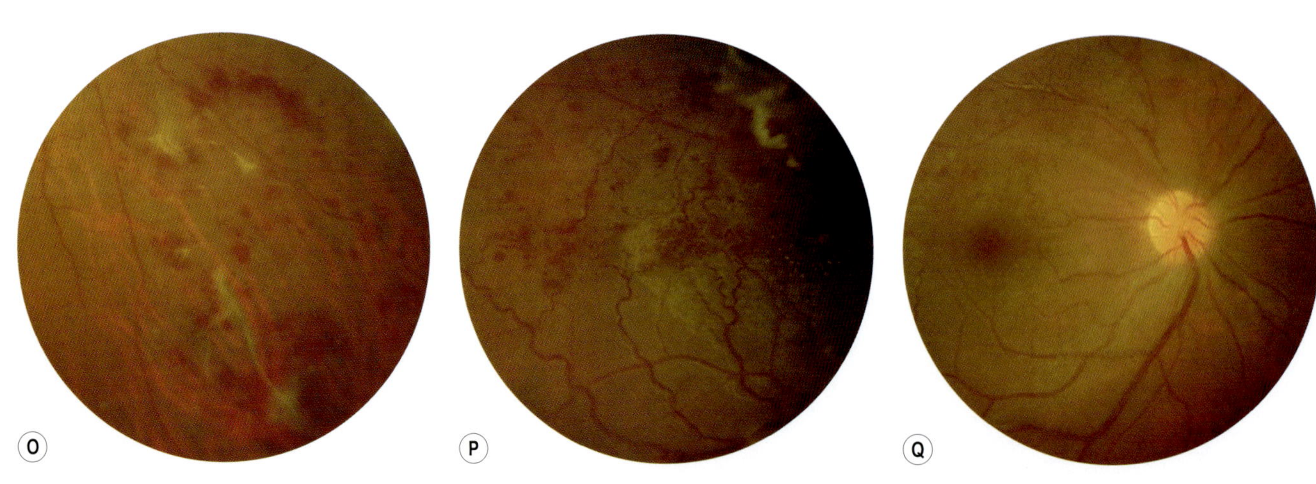

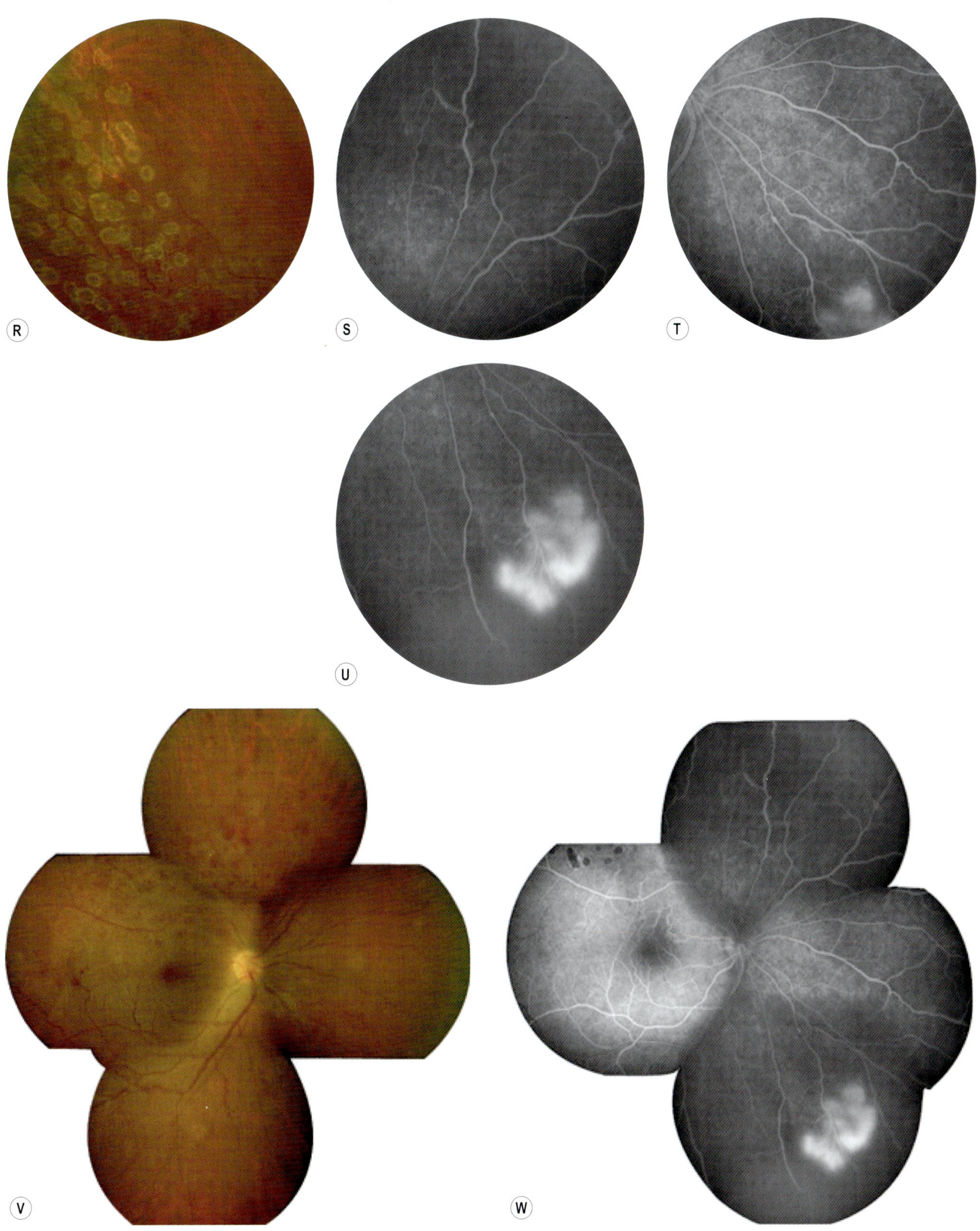
R
S
T
U
V
W

LEPROSY

Leprosy is a chronic granulomatous disease caused by *Mycobacterium leprae*. Depending on the immunologic status of the patient the disease presents in three forms: lepromatous with poor cell-mediated immunity, tuberculoid with good cellular immunity, and borderline (tuberculoid or lepromatous). Polar lepromatous leprosy is the anergic form of the disease with marked lack of cell-mediated immunity. These patients have a high bacterial index; the bacilli grow and multiply within foamy macrophages and are transported to all parts of the body. The bacteria are known not to tolerate warm temperatures and are found in the cooler parts of the body – skin, peripheral nerves, cornea and iris in the eye. Hence there are no firmly documented cases of leprosy affecting the retina and choroid.[151] A case with fundus involvement in the form of heaped-up, highly reflective, white material reported in the literature by Choyce and another fundus lesion by Chatterjee in 1964[152,153] have never been further substantiated, though a couple of enucleated eyes have shown the presence of *M. leprae* within macrophages in the retina and choroid. This is very unusual and extremely rare.[154]

Ocular involvement is mostly limited to madarosis, lack of corneal sensation, beaded corneal nerves, keratitis, granulomatous anterior uveitis with iris atrophy, keratic precipitates, lepra pearls in the iris, and involvement of the skin, lacrimal sac, and lid muscles resulting in lagophthalmos (Figure 10.15, F). Glaucoma occurs secondary to iris changes and uveitis. Low intraocular pressure has also been found due to infiltration of the ciliary body and decreased aqueous production.[155–157]

Histology of enucleated blind eyes has found bacteria and foamy macrophages laden with *M. leprae* in the cornea, iris, anterior uveal tissue, and anterior choroid due to its affinity to cooler areas. The retina was found to be free of the bacilli.[155,156]

This acid-fast bacillus cannot be grown in vitro and has only been cultured in the foot pads of the nine-banded armadillo. Recent use of reverse transcriptase-polymerase chain reaction (RT-PCR) has enabled confirmation of the diagnosis in several cases.[158] The disease is endemic in India, Nepal, Brazil, and the tropics of Asia and Africa, with 70% of affected individuals residing here.

10.15 Tubercular choroidal granuloma.

A to **C**: This 26-year-old HIV-negative Indian man complained of a progressive decrease in vision over 3 months. He had a recent loss of weight and respiratory illness. His visual acuity was count fingers on the right and 20/20 on the left side. A large tuberculoma occupied the entire macula (A) with smaller tubercles in the mid periphery. A fine needle aspiration biopsy was positive for *Mycobacterium tuberculosis* by PCR. He received four-drug anti-TB therapy; 2 weeks later signs of resolution began (B). The lesions looked much less active at 2 months (C).

D: Large mutton fat keratic precipitates suggesting granulomatous uveitis in this 17-year-old Indian man recently migrated to the United States from India. In addition, he had severe vitritis. His chest X-ray was negative but Mantoux was positive with a necrotic reaction at 24 × 20 mm. He received four-drug anti-TB medication and topical steroids for 18 months, with resolution of all signs and visual recovery to 20/20.

E: Phlyctenular conjunctivitis, an immune response seen in patients with tuberculosis.

Leprosy.

F: Madarosis, peripheral corneal scarring, signs of uveitis, and loss of nasal cartilage in this Indian patient with lepromatous leprosy.

(Courtesy: A–C, Dr J. Biswas; E and F, Dr S.R. Rathinam.)

FUNGAL RETINOCHOROIDITIS

Certain fungi either involve primarily the retina or extend rapidly from the choroid into the retina where they produce white intraretinal fungal abscesses (*Aspergillus fumigatus, Candida albicans, Trichosporon beigelii, Scedosporium apiospermum,* and *Sporothrix schenckii*). Others produce primarily yellow–white multifocal choroidal infiltrates that may cause serous and hemorrhagic retinal detachment (*Histoplasma capsulatum, Blastomyces dermatitidis, Coccidioides immitis,* and *Cryptococcus neoformans*). These latter diseases may be associated with disciform retinal detachment. Mucormycosis invades blood vessels and presents with vascular obstruction such as central or branch retinal artery or ophthalmic artery obstruction, due to the rather large size of the hyphae.[159–162]

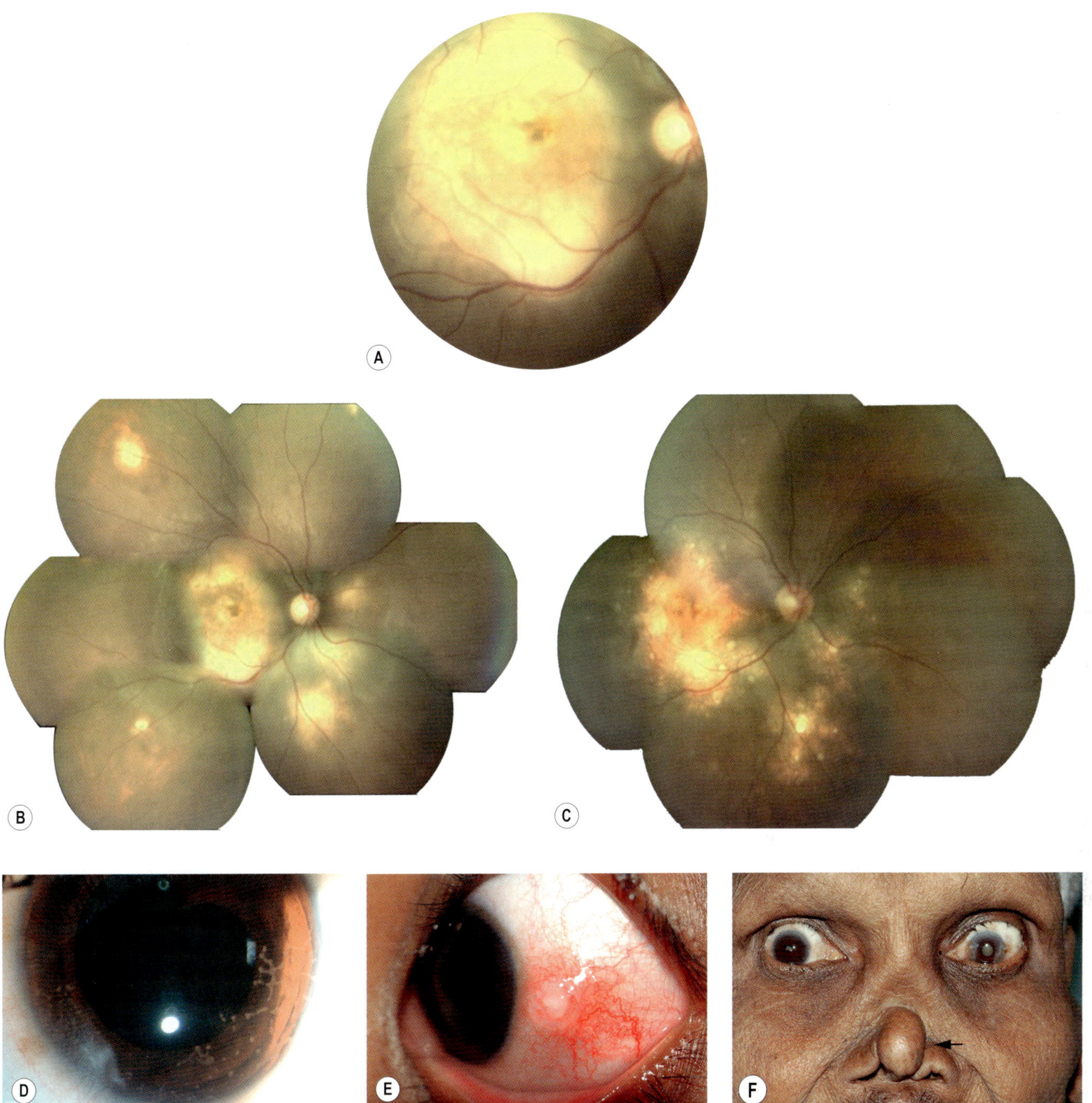
A
B
C
D
E
F

CANDIDA RETINOCHOROIDITIS

Hospitalized patients, particularly those with postoperative complications of abdominal surgery receiving prolonged intensive antibiotic treatment by an intravenous catheter, are prone to develop candidemia and focal white retinal abscesses (Figure 10.16, A–F).[163–178] The focal white retinal lesions are typically superficially located in the retina and are frequently associated with small cottony balls in the vitreous overlying the primary lesion (Figure 10.16, D). Other predisposing factors for development of retinal candidiasis include IV drug abuse, chemotherapy, corticosteroid administration, malignancy, bone marrow transplantation, diabetes, severe burns, endocrine hypofunction, other debilitating diseases, contaminated intravenously administered medications, and maternal birth canal infection.[163–165,167,168,179–183] The author has seen two diabetic patients developing *Candida* retinitis following ureteral stent placement whose urine culture grew *Candida albicans*.

The appearance of the fundus lesion is strongly suggestive of the diagnosis. The diagnosis may be confirmed by cultures of the site of IV administration, blood cultures, or vitreous aspiration. Multiple white-centered superficial retinal hemorrhages may also occur.[164] The white centers may be caused by microabscesses containing the fungi,[178] or by sterile fibrin–platelet aggregates (see previous discussion of pyogenic bacterial infection). The disease may respond to systemically administered amphotericin B or 5-fluorocytosine, or both.[175–177,179,184] Intravitreal injection of amphotericin B has been used successfully as a primary form of treatment[177,184–186] and as an adjunct to systemic treatment (Figure 10.16, C–F).[175] More recently, fluconazole, voriconazole, and caspofungin have been successful in treating *Candida* retinitis in addition to, or with no response to, amphotericin.[187–189] Spontaneous resolution of *Candida* retinal abscesses may occur.[165] For this reason patients with mild retinal involvement and no evidence of other organ involvement may be followed for evidence of progression.[166] The development of retinal striae around a focal retinal monilial abscess is a sign suggesting early resolution of the lesion.[190] If the retinal lesion(s) progresses, or if evidence of more advanced disease is present, the administration of fluconazole, itraconazole, voriconazole, posaconazole, or caspofungin may be effective. To avoid renal toxicity associated with treatment with systemic amphotericin B, some patients with ocular involvement in the absence of evidence of other organ involvement with monilial infection may be managed successfully with pars plana vitrectomy and intravitreal injection of amphotericin B.[175,177,179,186,191]

Candida retinitis is more common in patients post gastrointestinal surgery, hyperalimentation, toxic megacolon, and in diabetics, whereas *Aspergillus* infections are more commonly seen post organ transplant or cardiac surgery. In an outpatient setting, *Candida* is seen in IV drug abusers and often can be mistaken for *Toxoplasma* retinitis. Presence of a 'string of pearls' and absence of Kyrieleis' arteriolitis and old scars adjacent to active retinitis should raise the suspicion of *Candida*; efforts should be made to confirm a history of IV drug abuse since the treatment for the two conditions is vastly different.

The development of epiretinal membranes may be the cause of visual loss in some patients otherwise successfully treated for chorioretinal monilial infection. Surgical removal of these membranes may result in partial restoration of visual function.[192]

10.16 Candida septic chorioretinitis.

A: Focal *Candida* retinal abscess with 'cotton ball' vitreous opacities in this 28-year-old woman with a history of IV drug use. She was diagnosed initially with toxoplasmosis until the history of drug use was unearthed while she was trying to buy drugs on the hospital campus from a 'visitor'. She underwent a vitrectomy, and fungal stains and cultures were positive for *Candida albicans*.
B and C: Histopathology of focal *Candida* chorioretinitis. Note the predominantly granulomatous inflammation of the retina and vitreoretinal juncture. The overlying vitreous contains predominantly histiocytes. Special stains revealed evidence of *Monilia* (*arrow*, B). Both yeast and hyphae are seen in the overlying vitreous of a patient with *Candida* retinitis (C).
D to G: *Candida* endophthalmitis in a 50-year-old man with chronic alcoholism who noted pain and redness in his right eye. Visual acuity was 20/50. Note the string of white vitreous opacities (D and E). *Candida albicans* was cultured from the vitreous and from an ulcer on the bottom of his foot (F). At the time of vitrectomy, intravitreal amphotericin B was given and systemic administration of ketoconazole was begun. Six weeks later visual acuity was 20/25 and the fundus was normal (G).

Aspergillus chorioretinitis.

H to I: This 33-year-old man, with a history of 'bruised ribs and chills', IV drug abuse, and a 1-day history of eye pain and visual loss in the right eye, had a visual acuity of 2/200 in the right eye and 20/20 in the left eye, mild iritis, vitritis, and a subhyaloid (*top arrow*, H) and subretinal hypopyon (*bottom arrow*, H) associated with a subretinal hemorrhagic inflammatory mass in the right macula. Cultures of the aqueous humor and blood, echocardiography, and HIV serology were negative. An intravitreal injection of amphotericin B, 5 μg, was done. Vitreous culture was positive for *Aspergillus flavus*. He received IV amphotericin B for 3 weeks. Eleven months later his visual acuity was 20/400 and there was a flat scar in the right macula (I).

Histoplasmosis retinochoroiditis.

J to L: This 29-year-old-man with AIDS died because of complications associated with cytomegalovirus pneumonitis and systemic histoplasmosis. He complained of a hazy spot in his left eye. He had multiple white foci of retinitis in both eyes (J). Microscopic examination of his eyes revealed multifocal areas of necrotizing perivascular retinitis (K) and choroiditis associated with *H. capsulatum* organisms (*arrow*, L).

(B, courtesy Dr Narsing Rao; C, courtesy Dr Ralph Eagle; J–L from Specht et al.[224])

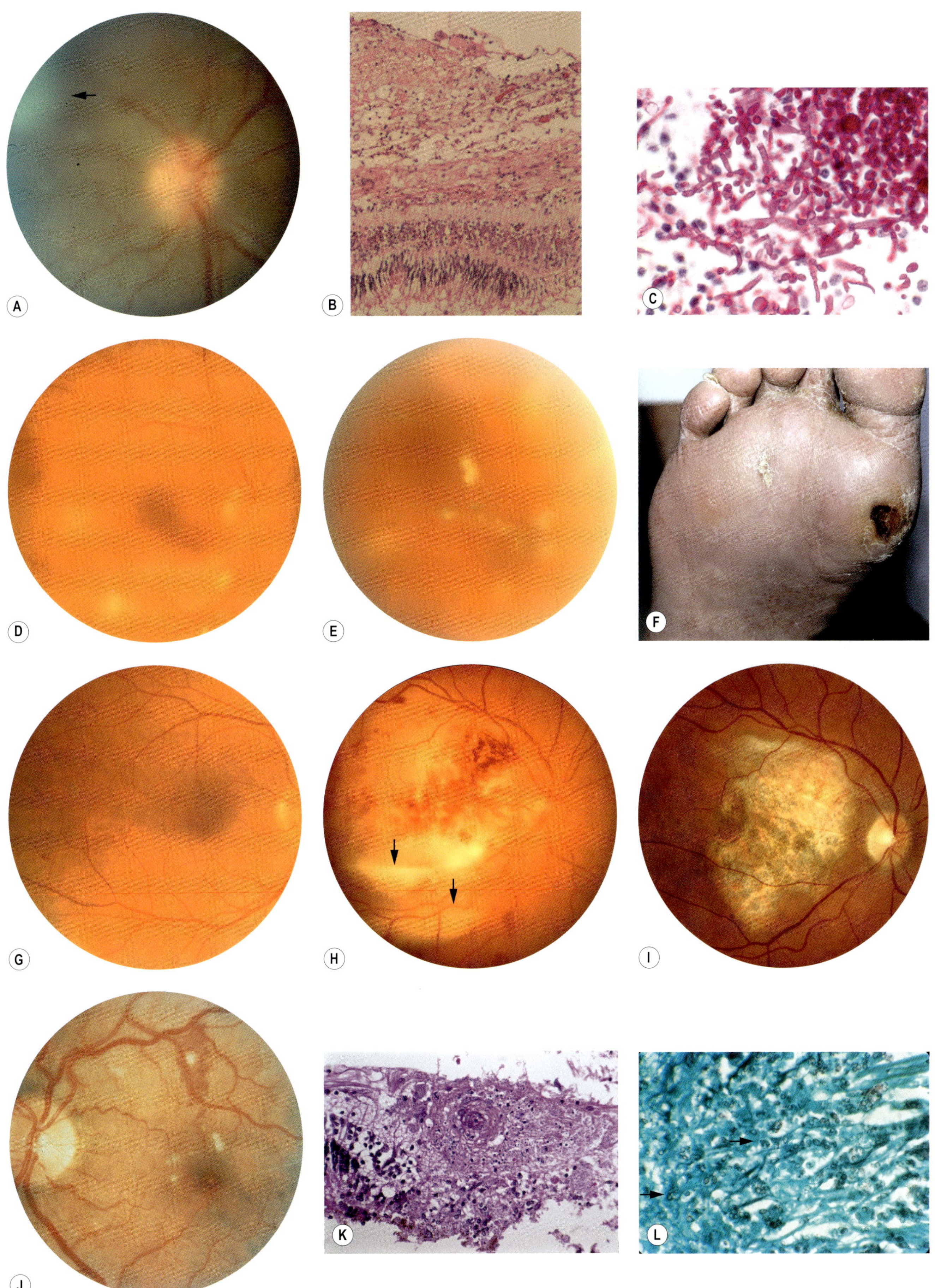
A
B
C
D
E
F
G
H
I
J
K
L

ASPERGILLUS RETINITIS

Intravenous drug abuse is the primary cause of intraocular infection with *Aspergillus.* In these patients it ranks only behind *Candida* as the cause of endogenous fungus endophthalmitis. It is also acquired in an organ transplant immunosuppressed state, whereas *Candida* is seen in patients after gastrointestinal surgery and hyperalimentation.[193,194] Ocular involvement is typically the first manifestation of the infection except when it occurs in immune incompetent individuals.[182,195–199] The patients present with subacute visual loss, mild pain, and redness of the eye that may be associated with a varying degree of anterior chamber reaction. Chorioretinitis and endophthalmitis caused by *Aspergillus* have characteristic clinical features. Deep retinal or chorioretinitis with progressive horizontal enlargement of the lesion is characteristic of *Aspergillus* as compared to *Candida* that has a small retinal focus and grows progressively into the vitreous.[193,194] Preretinal or subretinal exudation may be accompanied by a hypopyon as a result of layering of inflammatory cells (Figure 10.16, G and H).[200] A hemorrhagic retinal vasculitis may be present.[197,198] Isolated retinal hemorrhages and preretinal fluffy vitreous opacities may obscure fundus details. In some cases only a mild vitritis may be present initially. A variety of species of *Aspergillus* may be responsible for human infection. Pars plana vitrectomy and systemic azoles such as fluconazole, voriconazole, and posaconazole are the first choice in treatment of *Aspergillus* infection of the inner eye. Intravitreal injection of voriconazole can be used as an adjunct to systemic therapy.

Rao and Hidayat found *Aspergillus* to grow preferentially in the sub-RPE and subretinal space and to invade choroidal and retinal blood vessels, whereas *Candida* grew preferentially into the vitreous cavity in eyes enucleated for fungal endophthalmitis.[193,194]

Retinochoroiditis Caused by Other Fungi

Other fungal diseases, such as trichosporonosis[201] and sporotrichosis,[196,202–211] *Scedosporium apiospermum,*[212–216] and *Fusarium,*[217–221] may cause chorioretinal lesions and endophthalmitis similar to that produced by *Candida.*

COCCIDIOIDOMYCOSIS

Primary infection with the fungus *Coccidioides immitis,* like that with *Histoplasma capsulatum,* is a common cause of an acute, benign, self-limiting pulmonary disease. It is most prevalent in the interior valleys of California. It is unknown whether it is a common cause of subclinical chorioretinal scars and late visual complications similar to those found in areas where histoplasmosis is endemic (Figure 10.18, A–C).[225,226] As part of the primary infection, this fungus does occasionally cause loss of vision secondary to focal infectious granulomatous choroiditis, retinitis, and endophthalmitis (Figures 10.17, A–C and J; 10.18, D and E).[225,227–236] Patients inhale the anthrospores causing pneumonia, which secondarily may spread via the bloodstream, most often to the CNS and bones. Flu-like symptoms, cough, erythema nodosum, and arthralgias are often the presenting symptoms. Hydrocephalus and meningitis have been reported (Figure 10.17, A–F).

10.17 Coccidioidomycosis.

A to **F**: This 42-year-old woman noted a paracentral blur in her right eye while hospitalized for communicating hydrocephalus. She was previously diagnosed and treated with fluconazole for coccidioidomycosis pneumonia and meningitis in California. Her visual acuity was 20/15 in both eyes. She had an old choroidal scar temporal to the macula and a newer lesion inferior to fixation in her right eye (A). The fellow eye had a faint lesion in the posterior pole and several in the mid periphery (B and C). Angiogram showed staining of the lesions (D and E). She underwent a ventriculoperitoneal shunt and received systemic antifungals; the paracentral scotoma improved over 6 weeks.

G to **N**: A flu-like illness developed 1 month after a trip to Arizona in this 48-year-old man which resolved in 2 weeks. Three months later he experienced progressively worsening low back pain, which on MRI showed a ring-enhancing abscess in the disc between L2 and L3 (G). A biopsy of the abscess revealed chronic granulomatous inflammation with thick-walled spherules containing endospores (GMS stain) (H and I). Four months later he noted metamorphopsia in the left eye and a decline in vision to 20/80. There were no signs of inflammation. Left fundus showed two creamy choroidal lesions (J), one of which showed intense leakage consistent with a choroidal neovascular membrane (K and L). An OCT showed heaped-up cells anterior to the pigment epithelium (M). His visual acuity improved to 20/50 after intravitreal injections of bevacizumab and the lesion improved on OCT (N).

(Courtesy: A–F, Dr Hua Gao; G–N, Dr Mathew MacCumber and Dr Sachin Mudvari. A, C, E, J, M, N, Also, Yannuzzi, Lawrence J., The Retinal Atlas, Saunders 2010, 978-0-7020-3320-9, p.361.)

CRYPTOCOCCOSIS

Cryptococcosis is a chronic or subacute pulmonary systemic or meningitic infection caused by *Cryptococcus neoformans.*[234,237–239] Patients with the meningitic form of the disease may develop papilledema, papillitis, optic atrophy, and extraocular muscle palsies (Figure 10.18, G–I). Spread to the juxtapapillary choroid and retina may occur directly or via the bloodstream. Multifocal irregular yellow–white choroidal lesions, focal subretinal masses, and vitreoretinal abscesses have been described, usually in debilitated or immunosuppressed patients (Figure 10.18, F).[14,127,238,240–246] Simultaneous chorioretinal infection with *Cryptococcus* and cytomegalovirus has occurred.[228,241] Cryptococcal chorioretinitis may occasionally occur in apparently healthy patients prior to their developing evidence of meningitis.[225,246] When confined to the choroid and outer retina, the lesion may simulate a variety of diseases, including a melanoma, focal granuloma, or a disciform exudative process (Figure 10.18, F).[234,238,240,247–249] It is important to consider the possibility of cryptococcosis before placing

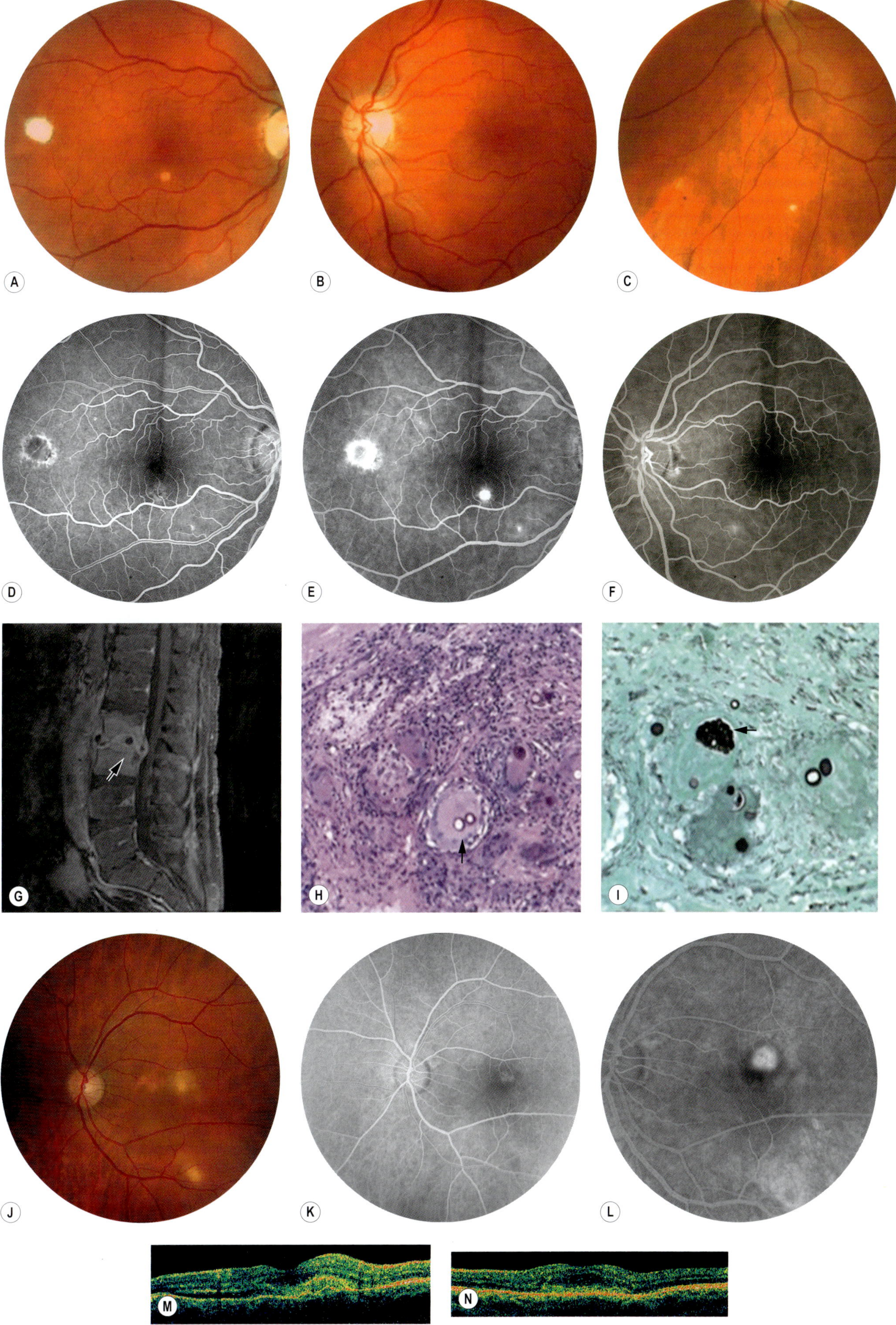

A
B
C
D
E
F
G
H
I
J
K
L
M
N

a patient on corticosteroid treatment, which may cause a fulminant and fatal spread of the infection.[233,245] The diagnosis may be confirmed by examination of the CSF and vitreous. Treatment with the newer azole antifungal agents will cause resolution of the infection.[229,231,242,243] Spontaneous resolution of intraocular lesions occasionally occurs.[230,250]

PHYCOMYCOSIS (MUCORMYCOSIS)

Though rare, mucormycosis is a severe, often fatal fungal infection unless diagnosed early, caused by fungi of the Zygomycetes class. Its classic presentation is in an immunocompromised host, often with severe diabetes and ketoacidosis, cancers, cirrhosis, or renal failure, and in patients on immunosuppressives and steroids. The route of entry is mostly through inhalation of fungal spores, though percutaneous entry can occur. Ocular involvement is usually due to contiguous spread from rhinocerebral mucormycosis, and patients present with ophthalmoplegia, rapid decrease in vision due to central retinal artery or ophthalmic artery occlusion, multiple large nerve fiber infarcts, and hypotony.[160,161,251,252] Intravenous entry can result in endogenous endophthalmitis (Figure 10.19, A–I).[253] 253 Early diagnosis is by clinical examination of the oral and nasal cavity and confi rmation by obtaining scrapings or biopsy from the dark eschar in these areas. The hyphae, which are large, nonseptate, and highly invasive, spread rapidly into soft tissue and blood vessels (Figure 10.19, B and C). They exert their effect by occluding ocular and orbital vessels and the vasa nervorum, resulting in proptosis, phthalmoplegia, and choroidal and retinal infarcts. Treatment consists of early extensive debridement, local and IV amphotericin, and newer antifungals such as posaconazole.[254–256]

10.18 Coccidioidomycosis, cryptococcosis, and blastomycosis.

A to **C**: Presumed ocular coccidioidomycosis in a 46-year-old man who lived most of his life in southern California and Arizona. He had a diagnosis of pulmonary coccidioidomycosis as a young man. He was visually asymptomatic until recently, when he noted distorted vision in the left eye. He had bilateral multifocal chorioretinal and juxtapapillary scars identical to that seen in presumed ocular histoplasmosis syndrome (POHS). A type II subretinal neovascular membrane and subfoveal blood were present in the left eye.
D and **E**: Focal granuloma observed clinically in the fundus of a 28-year-old man who died of disseminated coccidioidomycosis. High-power view shows multiple spherule-containing endospores (*arrow*, E).
F: Focal chorioretinitis caused by *Cryptococcus neoformans* in a nonimmunosuppressed 41-year-old man with obstructive hydrocephalus. There were no vitreous cells. The eye became blind from endophthalmitis. Diagnostic enucleation established the diagnosis.
G and **H**: Severe bilateral papilledema caused by *Cryptococcus* meningitis with optic nerve involvement in a 36-year-old nonimmunosuppressed woman with severe headaches and fever of unknown etiology. She died and histopathologic examination revealed encapsulated *Cryptococcus* organisms (*arrow*) in the optic nerve (H) and brain.
I: Electron micrograph of encapsulated *Cryptococcus* organisms in the choroid.
J to **K**: Multifocal blastomycosis choroiditis in a 43-year-old man who developed fever, chills, cough, and blurred vision soon after a hunting trip. He had multifocal lesions in the lung, skin, and choroid bilaterally (J and K). He failed to respond to anti-TB medication. Biopsy of skin revealed blastomycosis. The ocular and systemic disease responded promptly to amphotericin B therapy.

(D and E from Boyden and Yee[229]; F from Shields[238]; I from Avendaño[237]; F and I published with permission from the American Journal of Ophthalmology; copyright by the Ophthalmic Publishing Co.; J and K, courtesy Dr Froncie A. Gutman.)

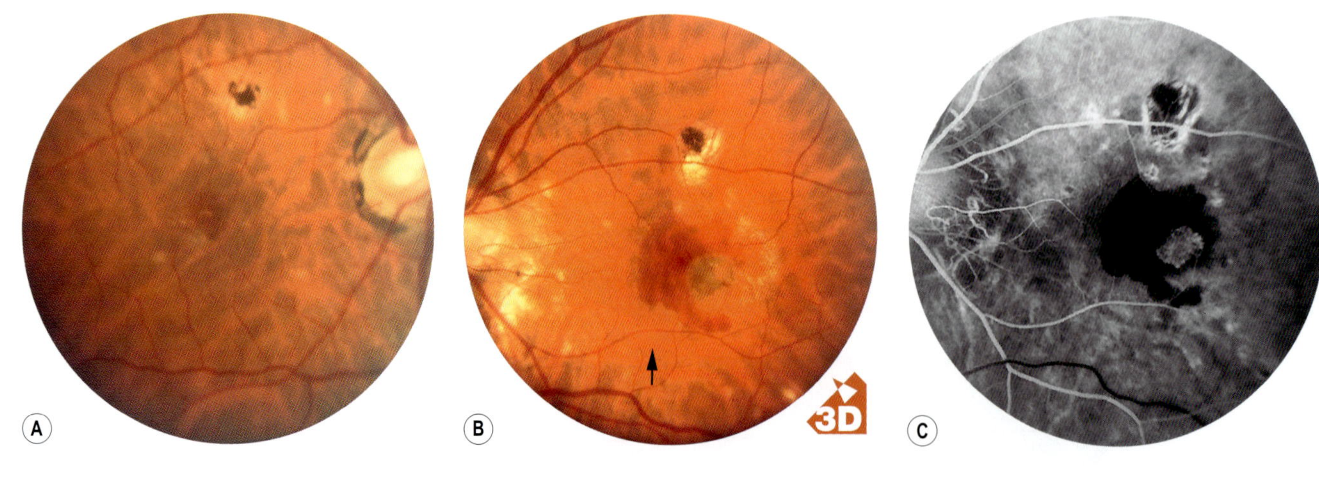

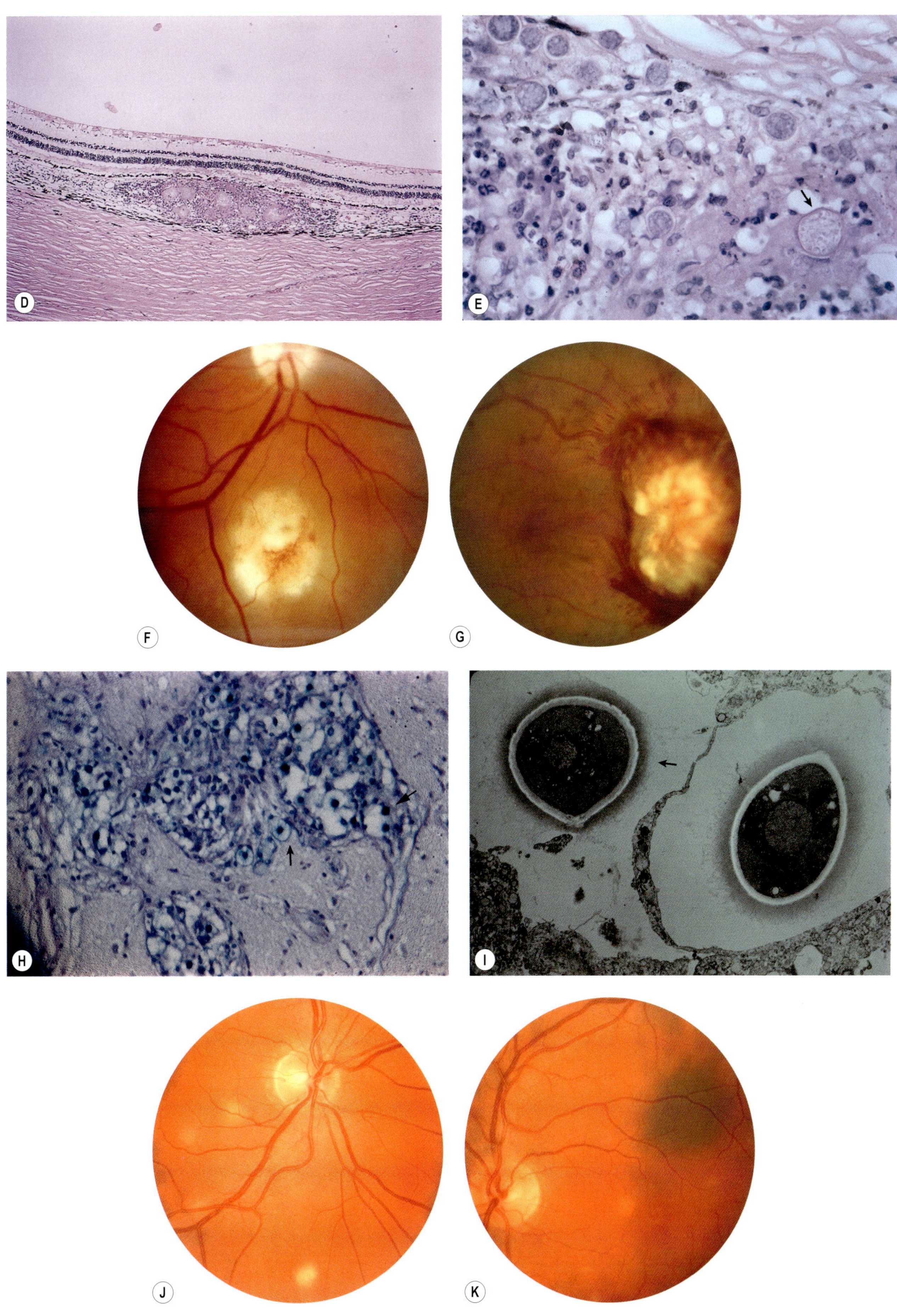
D
E
F
G
H
I
J
K

BLASTOMYCOSIS

Endogenous infection with *Blastomyces dermatitidis* following inhalation of conidia into the lungs may cause multifocal choroiditis (Figure 10.18, J and K), endophthalmitis, and panophthalmitis.[235–237] Whereas pulmonary and cutaneous granulomas are the most frequent manifestations of systemic blastomycosis, ocular involvement occasionally occurs and may affect otherwise apparently healthy patients.[225,235] Biopsy of skin lesions, if present, is helpful in establishing the diagnosis. The ocular as well as the systemic infection may respond favorably to ketoconazole, amphotericin, and newer azole therapy.

HISTOPLASMOSIS RETINITIS AND CHOROIDITIS IN IMMUNE INCOMPETENT PATIENTS

Histoplasma capsulatum may cause multifocal, active, white, retinal, subretinal, and choroidal lesions in one or both eyes of patients with AIDS (Figure 10.16, J–L) or other immune incompetent states (see Figure 3.43, A–C).[127,224,257,258] In immune incompetent individuals histoplasmosis may cause focal choroiditis that typically results in multiple focal atrophic chorioretinal scars without producing ocular symptoms. These scars later in life may be the site of development of subretinal neovascularization and visual loss (see presumed ocular histoplasmosis syndrome in Chapter 3).

Though rare, mucormycosis is a severe, often fatal fungal infection unless diagnosed early, caused by fungi of the *Zygomycetes* class. Its classic presentation is in an immunocompromised host, often with severe diabetes and ketoacidosis, cancers, cirrhosis, or renal failure, and in patients on immunosuppressives and steroids. The route of entry is mostly through inhalation of fungal spores, though percutaneous entry can occur. Ocular involvement is usually due to contiguous spread from rhinocerebral mucormycosis, and patients present with ophthalmoplegia, rapid decrease in vision due to central retinal artery or ophthalmic artery occlusion, multiple large nerve fiber infarcts, and hypotony.[160,161,251,252] Intravenous entry can result in endogenous endophthalmitis (Figure 10.19, A–I).[253]

Early diagnosis is by clinical examination of the oral and nasal cavity and confirmation by obtaining scrapings or biopsy from the dark eschar in these areas. The hyphae, which are large, nonseptate, and highly invasive, spread rapidly into soft tissue and blood vessels (Figure 10.19, B, C). They exert their effect by occluding ocular and orbital vessels and the vasa nervorum, resulting in proptosis, ophthalmoplegia, and choroidal and retinal infarcts.

Treatment consists of early extensive debridement, local and IV amphotericin, and newer antifungals such as posaconazole.[254–256]

10.19 Mucormycosis.

A to **I**: A 28-year-old man in India with 10-day history of sudden onset decrease in vision, 5 days after receiving IV fluids during a hydrocele repair. His vision was 20/20 in the right eye and count fingers in the left eye. The right eye was normal. The left vitreous was extremely hazy and no fundus details were seen (A). He underwent a pars plana vitrectomy for a diagnosis of endogenous endophthalmitis and received intravitreal vancomycin, amphotericin, ceftazidime, and dexamethasone. Cytology revealed mucor with broad hyphae branching at right angles (B and C, arrow). An ear, nose, and throat evaluation for sinus disease was negative. He was treated with oral itraconazole, topical steroids, and antibiotics. Postoperatively multiple foci of retinitis and periarterial plaques (D, E, and H) were noted that scarred over 3 months (I).

(Copyright *International Ophthalmology*, Springer Science + Business Media B.V. 2008; Dr Amod Gupta. Gupta P, Sachdev N, Kaur J, et al. Endogenous mycotic endophthalmitis in an immunocompetent patient. Int Ophthalmol. 2009;29(4):315-8. Epub 2008 Jun 5.)

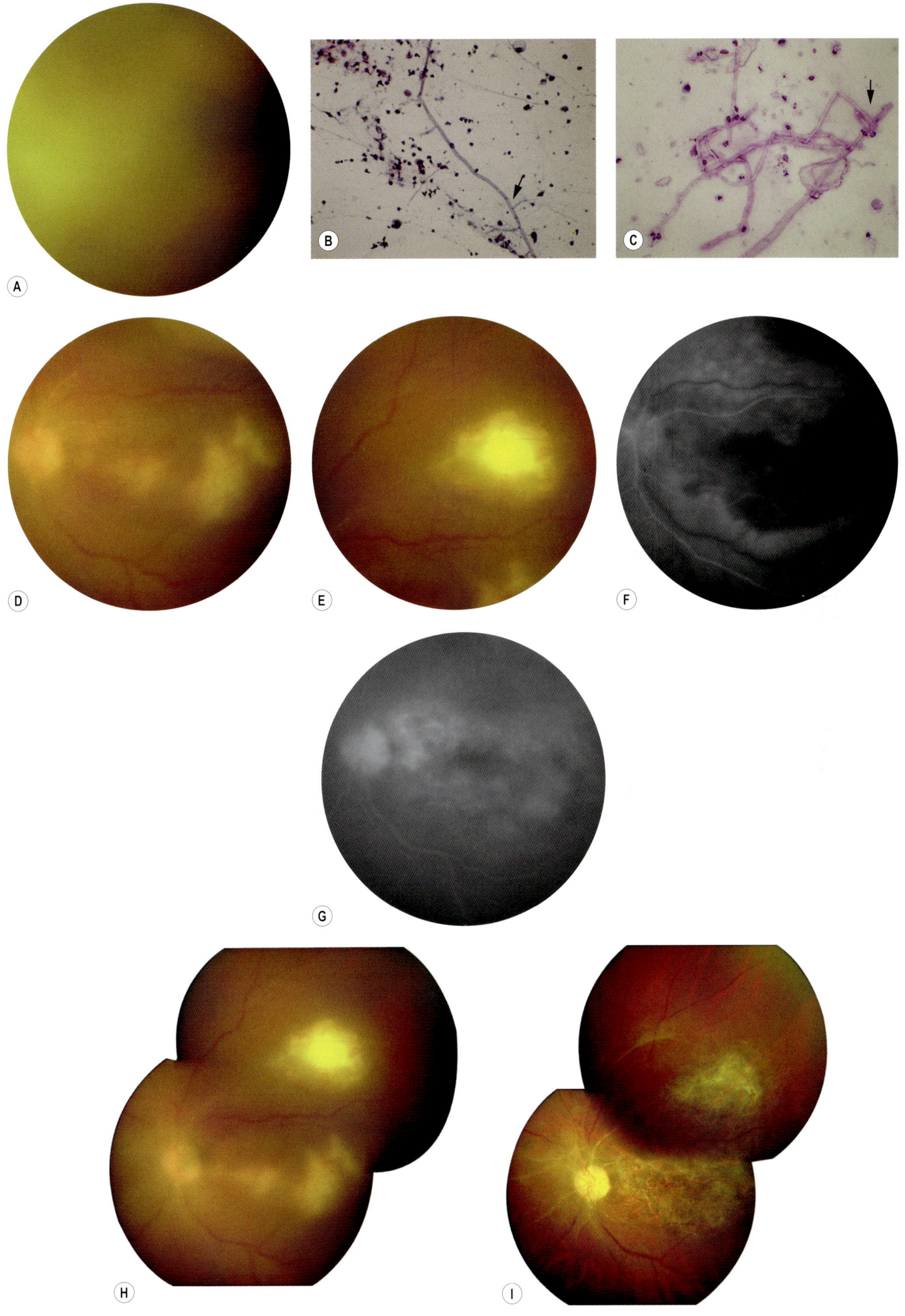
A
B
C
D
E
F
G
H
I

TOXOPLASMOSIS RETINITIS

Toxoplasmosis is the most frequent cause of focal necrotizing retinitis in otherwise healthy human individuals (Figures 10.21–10.23).[259–292] The protozoan *Toxoplasma gondii* is either transmitted to the fetus in utero when the mother acquires the infection during pregnancy or, less commonly, it infects the retina following ingestion of the organism. There is a predilection for infection of the CNS and the retina. In congenital toxoplasmosis the retinal lesion may occur as part of a generalized severe infection (encephalomyelitis, convulsions, fever, jaundice, cerebral calcification, hydrocephalus, and paralyses of various types) or more frequently as part of a mild subclinical infection. Large, atrophic, often excavated, chorioretinal scars centered in or near the macular area or elsewhere in the fundus in children and adults are probably caused in many cases by congenital toxoplasmosis (Figure 10.20, B, C, H, J, and K). When they are symmetric, however, these macular lesions must be differentiated from similar-appearing inherited dystrophic lesions.

10.20 Congenital toxoplasmosis retinitis.

A to D: Heterotopia of the macula and dragging of the retinal vessels of the right eye (A and B) caused by congenital toxoplasmosis retinitis in a 29-year-old woman with intracranial calcification and focal chorioretinal scars (B and C). Note angiographic evidence of retinochoroidal anastomosis at the site of the scar in the left eye (*arrow*, D).

E and F: Macular scars in an HIV-positive infant presumed to be caused by congenital toxoplasmosis. Visual acuity was 20/20, right eye, and 20/40, left eye.

G to I: Presumed congenital toxoplasmosis in a 32-year-old woman with poor vision since birth. Note the deep excavation of the scar in the right macula.

J and K: Multiple chorioretinal scars of uncertain cause in both eyes of this 9-year-old child who had good vision until recently when she developed evidence of subretinal neovascularization in the left macula. She was the product of an 8-month pregnancy that was terminated because of retarded intrauterine growth.

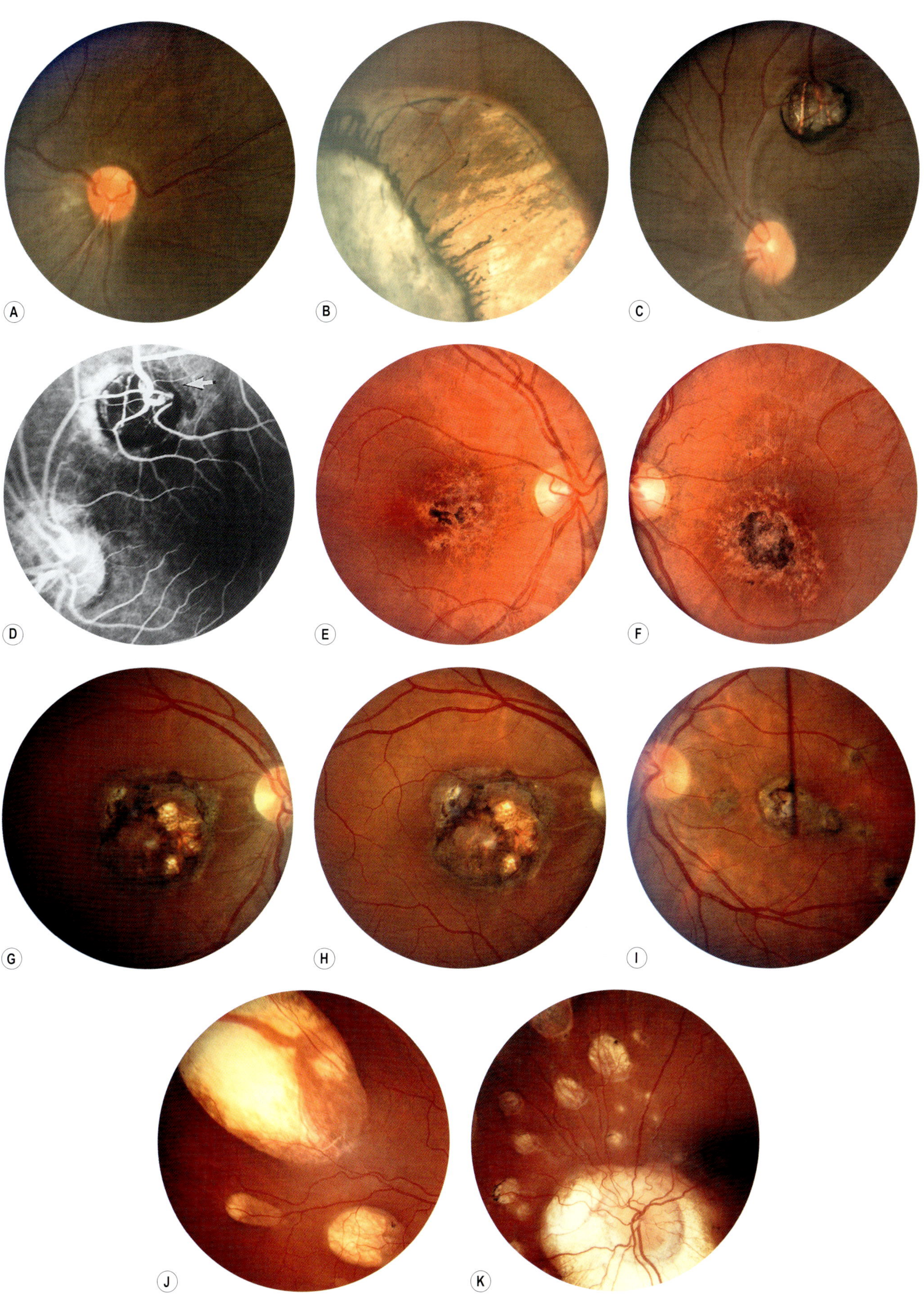
A
B
C
D
E
F
G
H
I
J
K

Whether acquired in utero or postnatally, the *Toxoplasma* organisms may lie dormant in the encysted form in the apparently normal retina, either adjacent to or remote from chorioretinal scars. When the organisms become unencysted, one or more acute, white, necrotizing lesions may occur in a previously normal-looking retina or at the margin of an old chorioretinal scar (Figure 10.21). The lesions usually involve the full thickness of the retina but in some cases may be confined to either the inner or, less frequently, the outer half of the retina. In the former they are associated with overlying vitreous inflammatory cell infiltration. When the retinitis involves primarily the outer retina, serous detachment of the underlying retina is frequently present (Figure 10.21, A–I). When the acute lesion includes a major retinal vessel, it may cause either a branch retinal arterial occlusion (Figure 10.22, A–C)[262,267,270] or a venous occlusion (Figure 10.22, D and E).[270]

Most patients with acute retinitis are seen initially because of a history of floaters and less often because of loss of central vision caused by foveal involvement by focal retinitis (Figure 10.21), cystoid macular edema, or detachment associated with paracentral focal retinitis. Focal periarterial exudates and arterial atheromatous plaques (Kyrieleis' arteriolitis) simulating arterial emboli may occur either in the immediate vicinity of the acute retinitis or remote from it (Figure 10.22, F–I).[267–269,275,282,293] Fluorescein angiography shows no permeability alterations or evidence of artery obstruction in the area of the arterial plaques but demonstrates marked fluorescein staining in the area of the retinitis (Figures 10.21, B, C, E, H, and I; 10.22, C). The periarterial plaques may fade or may persist following resolution of the retinitis. Occasionally acute multifocal arterial wall opacification is widespread throughout the fundus and may be accompanied by similar multifocal gelatinous-appearing opacities scattered along the major retinal veins. Ophthalmoscopic and angiographic evidence of diffuse perivenous exudation may occasionally occur in areas remote from the acute retinitis. The presence in those patients with retinal vasculitis of reduced levels of antibody affinity to retinal S-antigen with normal levels of circulating immune complexes suggests a defective regulation of antiretinal autoimmunity.[294] Swelling of the optic disc and angiographic evidence of staining of the disc may accompany focal areas of retinitis or, in some cases, may be the presenting manifestation of toxoplasmosis (Figure 10.22, J–L). Multiple, small, gray deposits (presumably inflammatory cells) may develop along the inner retinal surface in the vicinity of the acute retinitis, and it may be difficult to distinguish these from small foci of active retinitis. If the vitreous separates from the retina near the acute lesion, these gray deposits usually remain attached to the posterior surface of the vitreous.

10.21 Serous macular detachment caused by active outer retinal toxoplasmosis and by subretinal neovascularization arising at a toxoplasmosis chorioretinal scar.

A to **E**: This 18-year-old woman developed floaters associated with a focal area of acute retinitis (*arrow*, A) and widespread periphlebitis in the right eye. Angiography showed intense staining in the area of the retinitis and leakage of dye from the major retinal veins and optic disc (B and C). Several years later, she developed visual loss caused by serous retinal detachment in the macula associated with multiple foci of outer retinitis near the edge of the old scar and in the papillomacular bundle area (*arrows*, D). Angiography (E) revealed early staining of the foci of retinitis and late diffuse staining of the subretinal fluid.
F to **I**: Serous macular detachment caused by recurrence of retinitis (*arrows*, F and G) near a scar. Note late staining of the subretinal fluid.
J and **K**: Serous macular detachment caused by recurrence of retinitis (*arrow*, J) in a patient with bilateral macular scars.
L: Serosanguinous retinal detachment caused by subretinal neovascularization arising at the inferior edge of a toxoplasmosis scar.

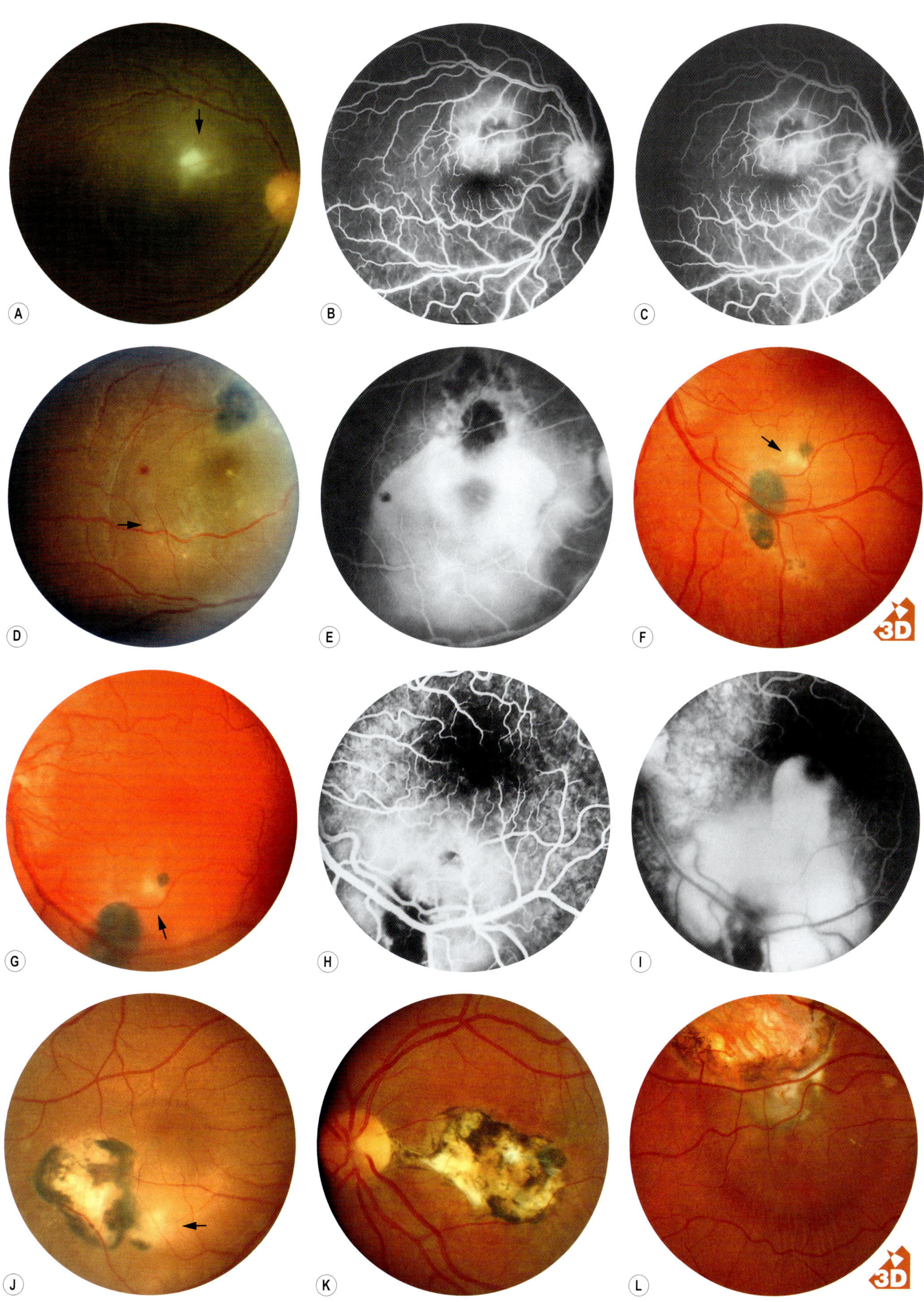
A
B
C
D
E
F
3D
G
H
I
J
K
L
3D

The active focus of retinitis usually enlarges for a period of 1–2 weeks before gradually fading over a period of several months, usually leaving in its wake a pigmented atrophic chorioretinal scar. Segmental optic disc pallor may develop in the zone of nerve fiber atrophy caused by the retinitis.

In some patients the onset of the disease is characterized by the development of multifocal small foci of retinitis, largely confined to the outer retinal layers (Figure 10.23, A).[264,295] After resolution, some of these small lesions may leave no chorioretinal scarring. There may be a series of remissions and exacerbations before development of the larger, more typical, full-thickness focus of acute retinitis (Figure 10.23, A–D). Another atypical presentation is that of an acute papillitis before the development of a focal area of retinitis (Figure 10.22, J–L).[266,278,292,296] Findings that suggest that disc swelling may be caused by toxoplasmosis are severe vitreous inflammation, fluffy white peripapillary lesions, nerve fiber bundle defect, and often good visual acuity.[266,296]

The clinical diagnosis of ocular toxoplasmosis is always a presumptive one. Most patients will demonstrate skin test and serologic evidence of previous contact with the organism with positive IgG titers.[297] The diagnosis of acute toxoplasmosis is very likely in otherwise healthy patients with a focus of acute retinitis in an eye with one or more chorioretinal scars. Even in the absence of another scar, a solitary focus of acute retinitis in a healthy patient occurs most often in patients with serologic evidence of the infection with positive IgM antibodies; a few do not, and the titers may be low in many patients. In addition to the enzyme-linked immunosorbent assay (ELISA) test, the immunofluorescent antibody test, and the Sabin–Feldman dye test (rarely done anymore), detection of evidence of toxoplasmosis in the aqueous humor may be accomplished using PCR.[298–300] Cytologic diagnosis of toxoplasmosis may occasionally be made from vitreous biopsy.[301]

Most chorioretinal scars caused by toxoplasmosis are atrophic, partly pigmented, and associated with postinflammatory changes in the overlying vitreous and a nerve fiber bundle visual field defect. Hypertrophic disciform scars, however, develop in some patients (Figure 10.23, E and F). In rare cases reactive proliferation of the RPE in these scars may be mistaken for a melanoma.[302] Remodeling of the retinal circulation caused by previous occlusion of vessels passing through the area of retinitis is often present (Figure 10.22, D and E). Evidence of retinochoroidal anastomosis may develop due to full-thickness retinal involvement and subsequent atrophy, thus bringing the retinal vessels in close proximity to the choroidal vessels (Figure 10.22, D).[274,282,303] Development of subretinal neovascularization, usually type 2, at the edge of an inactive scar may cause loss of central vision (Figure 10.21, L).[268,304] The large macular chorioretinal scars seen in children and attributed to congenital toxoplasmosis usually do not show evidence of postinflammatory changes in the vitreous. Unusual and unexplained associations with toxoplasmosis retinitis are the development of Fuchs' heterochromic cyclitis and either unilateral or bilateral zones of retinitis pigmentosa-like fundus changes.[276,305–307] Gary Holland has categorized the location of *Toxoplasma* retinitis into three zones: zone 1 (3000 microns from the fovea center or 1500 microns from the optic disc margin), zone 2 (from zone 1 to the anterior borders of the vortex veins), and zone 3 (from the anterior border of zone 2 to the ora serrata).

Familial involvement with ocular toxoplasmosis is rare. In southern Brazil (Alto Uruguai region), however, familial ocular toxoplasmosis is endemic.[308,309] The prevalence of ocular toxoplasmosis there is 30 times higher than elsewhere,[308] with 85% of the population being infected and 18% of them have evidence of *Toxoplasma* retinochoroiditis. The frequent ingestion of raw or undercooked pork has been suggested as a possible explanation for this. In the United States, the prevalence of *T. gondii* infection is 22.5%, although the prevalence of ocular involvement in these is only 2%.

This difference in the prevalence rates in different parts of the world is likely related to the prevalence of the different genotypes. Three genotypes have been isolated in humans and animals: types I, II, and III. Type II is the mildest genotype and is seen in the United States and Europe. South America, especially southern Brazil, has the more virulent type I and atypical genotypes. Sexual recombinants (atypical genotypes) also have increased virulence.[310]

10.22 Toxoplasmosis retinitis.

A to C: Branch retinal arterial occlusion caused by acute retinitis, presumed to be toxoplasmosis (A). Angiography showed evidence of branch artery obstruction (*arrow*, B) and late staining in the area of retinitis (C).

D and E: Retinochoroidal anastomosis (*arrows*) in two patients following venous obstruction caused by toxoplasmosis retinitis.

F to I: Chorioretinal scars (H) and marked periarterial plaque deposition persisting for years following multiple areas of acute retinitis presumed to be caused by toxoplasmosis in a 30-year-old man whose visual acuity was 20/20 in both eyes. Angiography showed evidence of the periarterial plaques and minimal evidence of obstruction to blood flow (I).

J to L: Presumed toxoplasmosis papillitis in a 7-year-old boy with acute loss of vision in the right eye (J). Angiography revealed staining of the optic disc (K). Within several months the disc swelling resolved and optic atrophy was evident. Twenty-one months later he had further loss of vision in the right eye caused by acute retinitis in the macula (L).

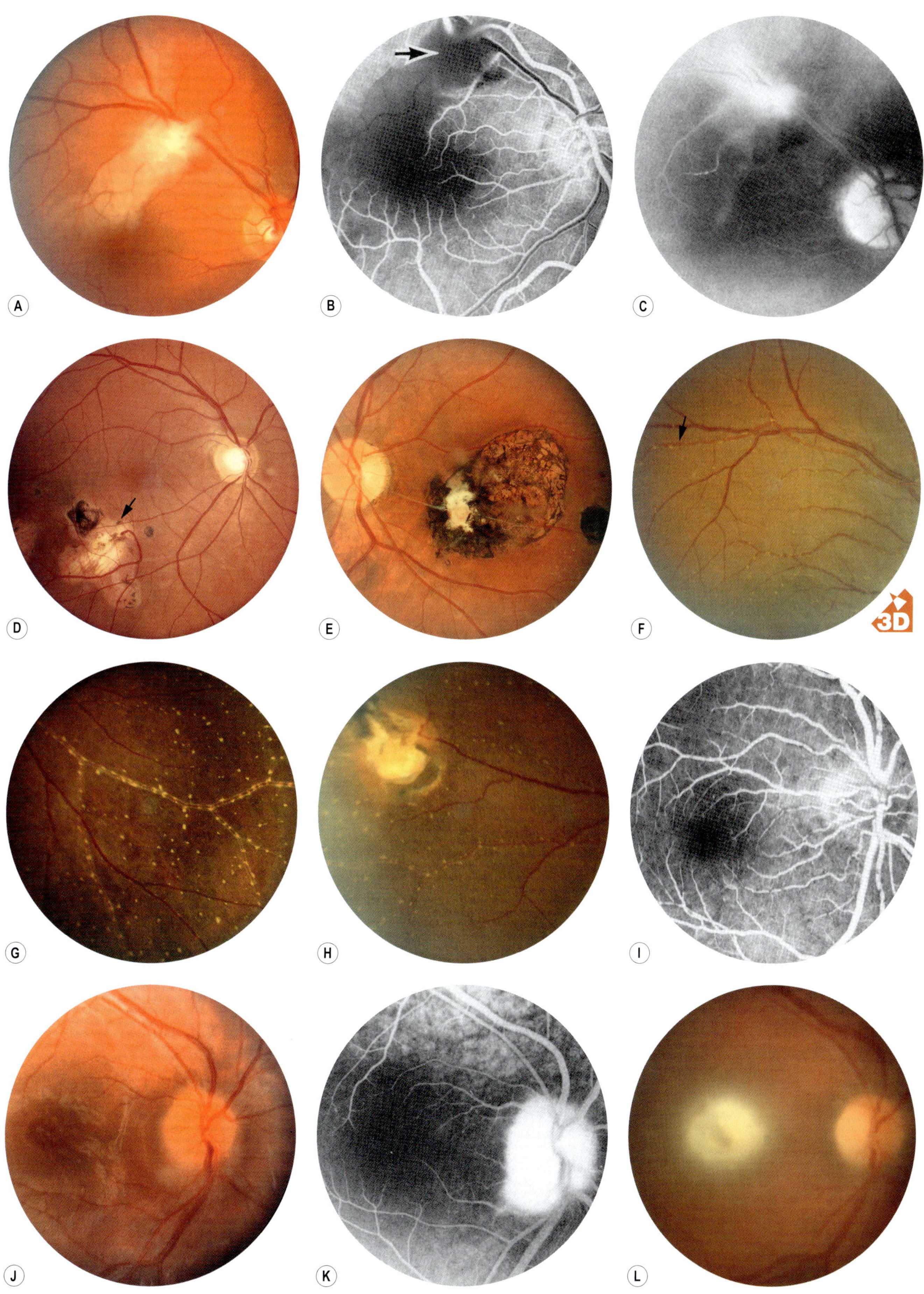
A
B
C
D
E
F
3D
G
H
I
J
K
L

Even though toxoplasmosis is considered an endemic disease, there have been a few outbreaks around the world[311–316] and a recent epidemic in Coimbatore, a city in southern India.[310,317,318] These outbreaks and clustering of cases have been linked to a source – either contaminated municipal water or infected kittens and a feral cat harboring the more virulent genotype. The largest epidemic has been reported from one center in southern India where 248 patients (254 eyes) with retinochoroiditis were seen between August 2004 and July 2005. Of the 230 eyes (90.5%) with unifocal retinitis, 67% were located in zone 1, 25% in zone 2, and the remainder in zone 3.

Although recurrence is a hallmark of *Toxoplasma* retinochoroiditis, no definite factor(s) has been found to trigger recurrences. The risk of recurrence decreases as the disease-free interval increases; however, once a reactivation occurs, the risk of further recurrences increases (clusters). This is likely from some of the oocysts degenerating over time and hence the smaller load of dormant cysts, but with a recurrence the number of organisms increases, thus increasing the chance of another recurrence. Patients greater than 40 years of age had a higher chance of recurrence, likely from altered immunologic state. The longer the duration of infection, the greater the chance of recurrence, again implying organism load.[319]

Histopathologic examination of an acute toxoplasmosis lesion in eyes of immunocompetent patients reveals a focal necrotizing retinitis associated with an underlying acute and chronic granulomatous choroiditis and scleritis (Figures 10.23, G and H; 10.24, A and B).[320] The inflammatory reaction surrounding the necrotizing retinitis is markedly reduced in immunosuppressed patients (Figure 10.23, I). In spite of the presence of scleritis that may be evident ultrasonographically beneath the focal retinitis in immunocompetent patients, only occasionally do they complain of pain.[321] The encysted and free forms of *Toxoplasma* organisms are found in the relatively normal retina surrounding the necrotic retina (Figure 10.23, J and K).[280,322] They are occasionally found in the choroid in immunosuppressed patients.

The value of pyrimethamine (Daraprim), sulfadiazine, clindamycin, minocycline, trimethoprim–sulfamethoxazole, and corticosteroids in the treatment of active lesions in immunocompetent humans is uncertain.[259,323–328] Treatment probably has no value in preventing recurrences.[328] These drugs have been demonstrated to be effective in experimental infections with *Toxoplasma* in animals. There is only minimal evidence, however, that they are of value in the treatment of toxoplasmosis in immunocompetent humans.[263] Most authors agree that treatment is unnecessary and inadvisable in lesions outside the macular area. In cases where the center of the macula is threatened, use of one or more of the antibiotics in combination with systemic corticosteroids is advisable. Intravitreal clindamycin at a dose of 1 mg is a rapid means of treating *Toxoplasma* retinitis, and can be used in fovea-threatening cases, in severely immunosuppressed patients for a quick onset, and in pregnant women.[329,330] Topical corticosteroids and mydriatics are indicated in the presence of accompanying iridocyclitis. Those children born to mothers who acquired *Toxoplasma* during pregnancy should be on anti-*Toxoplasma* treatment up to their first birthday.

10.23 Toxoplasmosis retinitis.

A to **D**: Multifocal subacute recrudescent retinitis presumed to be caused by toxoplasmosis in a 17-year-old girl who was seen initially with a 1-month history of blurred vision in the right eye (A). Visual acuity was 20/100 in the right eye and 20/20 in the left eye. There were no vitreous cells. Note the multiple, small, gray lesions in the foveolar area (*arrows*). Angiography at that time showed no evidence of fluorescein staining. Photographs taken at 2- to 3-month intervals over the subsequent several years showed a frequent change in the position of the gray lesions and no evidence initially of residual RPE changes (B). The visual acuity remained unchanged. Seven years after her initial examination, she returned with acute loss of vision in the right eye. There was a large area of acute retinitis in the right macula (C). Over the subsequent 9 years, she had other acute attacks. When the patient was last seen, visual acuity was 20/200 and a large atrophic macular scar was present (D).
E and **F**: Active toxoplasmosis retinitis (E) resolved and produced an elevated hypertrophic scar with retinochoroidal anastomosis (F).
G: Acute toxoplasmosis retinochoroiditis in an immunocompetent patient. Note the necrotic retina separated by Bruch's membrane (*arrow*) from a focal area of thickening of the choroid by granulomatous inflammation.
H: Focal area of granulomatous choroiditis and scleritis underlying toxoplasmosis retinitis in an immunocompetent adult.
I to **K**: Photomicrographs of acute focal necrotizing *Toxoplasma* retinochoroiditis in an immunosuppressed patient. Note the loss of nuclei in all layers with patchy preservation of a few photoreceptor nuclei and nongranulomatous inflammatory reaction in the underlying choroid (I). A high-power view of the lesion shows encysted organisms (J) and free tachyzoites (K, *arrow*).

(G, courtesy Dr Andrew P. Ferry, presented at Verhoeff Society, 1987; H from Hogan and Zimmerman[320]; I–K, courtesy Dr Ralph Eagle.)

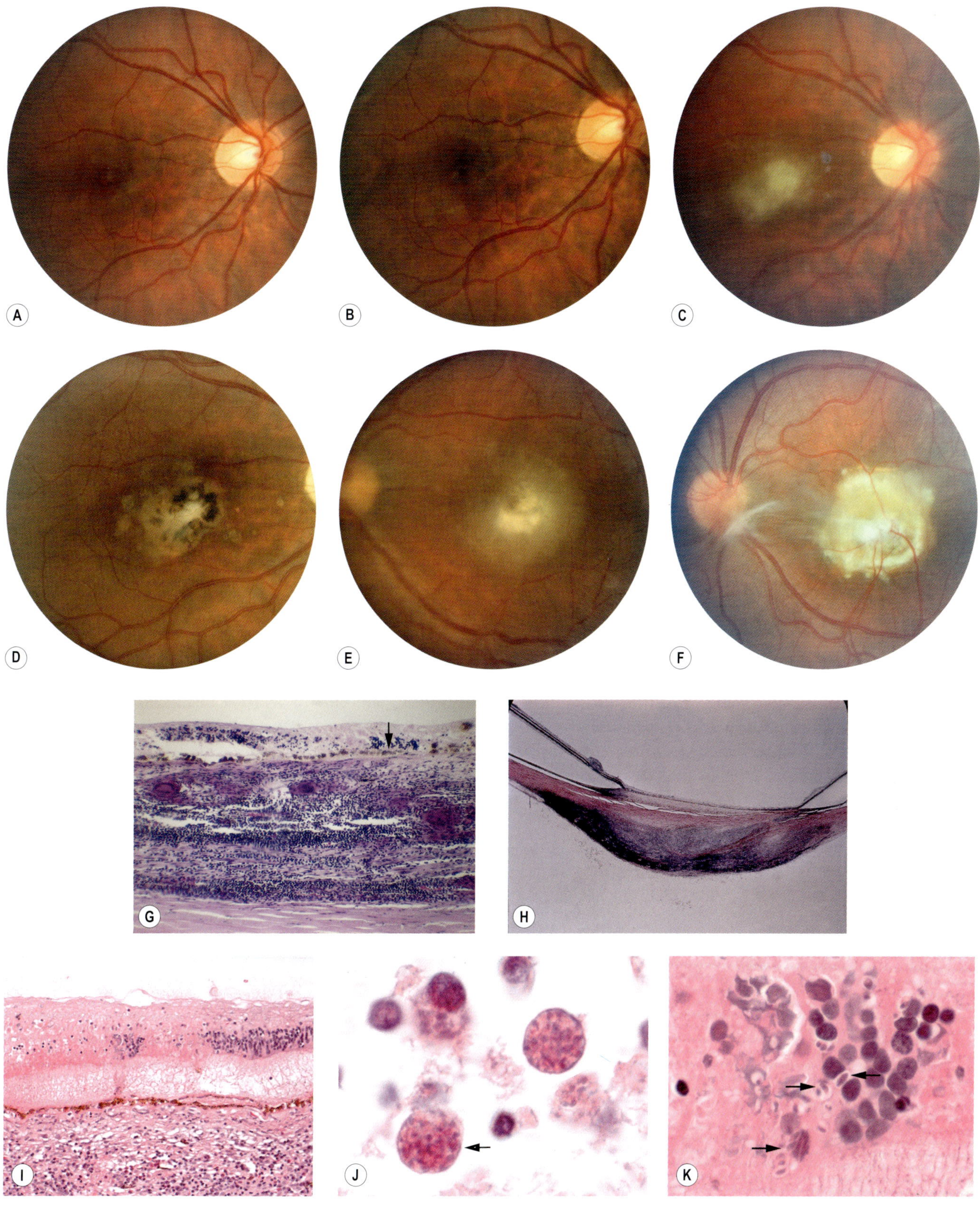
A
B
C
D
E
F
G
H
I
J
K

In patients with AIDS or who are immunocompromised for other reasons, toxoplasmosis may cause a fulminant and widespread necrotizing retinitis as well as encephalitis.[183,281,331–342] Features of toxoplasmosis retinitis in patients with AIDS that differ from those in immunocompetent patients are multiple active lesions, infrequency of acute lesions arising adjacent to inactive scars, frequent involvement of both eyes, and frequent evidence of CNS involvement. Some of these patients present with multifocal, small, widely scattered lesions that may rapidly become confluent and produce a clinical picture identical to acute retinal necrosis.[338] Vitritis is usually present but may be less than that seen in immunocompetent patients with similar size retinal lesions. Clinically, the retinal lesions may simulate those caused by cytomegalic inclusion disease,[335] although typically retinal hemorrhages are less prominent and vitritis more evident in lesions caused by toxoplasmosis. Toxoplasmosis encephalitis is a leading cause of death in patients with AIDS. Approximately 10–20% of patients with intracranial toxoplasmosis develop retinal lesions.[336] Involvement of the brain often occurs in the absence of ocular involvement. Toxoplasmosis may cause either a diffuse necrotizing encephalitis or discrete space-occupying intracranial lesions. In the former, computed tomography may be normal; in the latter, it may show focal lesions with ring-shaped enhancement after contrast infusion.[336] Coinfections of the retina and choroid may occur.[335,336] The retinal and the brain lesions caused by *Toxoplasma* respond favorably to pyrimethamine and sulfadiazine, but recurrence of the infection is common after cessation of treatment.[335,336] Corticosteroid treatment may be necessary to reduce cerebral edema but probably is unnecessary in the treatment of retinitis since the intensity of the inflammation is less than in normal patients.[336] The results of serologic tests in patients with AIDS are unreliable. The presence of elevated IgM in as many as 12% of these patients suggests a high incidence of acquired infection.[279]

Solitary active toxoplasmosis retinitis may be simulated by other infections (*Candida*, pyogenic bacteria, bacteria of low pathogenicity in patients with AIDS, cat-scratch disease bacillus), ischemic retinopathy, and neoplasia (large-cell lymphoma, metastatic carcinoma to the retina). Retinal artery occlusion caused by a focal area of toxoplasmosis may appear similar to that occurring in patients with acute multifocal retinitis associated with cat-scratch disease or of unknown cause (see Figure 10.04), and patients with bilateral idiopathic recurrent branch retinal artery occlusion (see Figures 6.10 and 6.11). Multifocal outer toxoplasmosis may simulate punctate inner choroiditis (pseudo-presumed ocular histoplasmosis) (see Figure 11.21-11.23), and diffuse unilateral subacute neuroretinitis (see Figures 10.28 and 10.29).

10.24 *Toxoplasma gondii* retinochoroiditis.

A to **C**: Necrotic retina displays cysts of *Toxoplasma gondii*. The choroid reveals chronic granulomatous inflammation (A, hematoxylin and eosin). Multiple toxoplasmic cysts are present in the retina and the cysts show presence of bradyzoites (B, *arrow*, periodic acid–Schiff). Ultrastructural features of a retinal *Toxoplasma gondii* cyst containing bradyzoites (C).

Malaria retinopathy.

D to **J**: A 20-year-old Indian man with high intermittent fevers diagnosed clinically as malaria complained of visual loss in his left eye 10 days after fever onset. A patch of retinitis with decreased axoplasmic flow was seen adjacent to the disc (D). The angiogram showed nonfluorescence of the area with late staining of the edges (E and F). Four weeks later the retinal opacification had improved with lipid exudates in a star pattern. A branch coming off the inferotemporal artery showed sheathing (G). The follow-up angiogram shows narrowed flow through the affected arteriole with no late staining of the affected retina (H–J).

(Courtesy: A–C, Dr Narsing Rao; D–J, Dr Vishali Gupta.)

MALARIA

Plasmodium vivax, *P. falciparum*, *P. ovale*, *P. malariae*, and *P. knowlesi* are the parasites causing malaria characterized by intermittent fevers – chills that recur on a regular basis every 24–48 h depending on the parasite subtype. Each year up to 3 million deaths and 5 billion episodes of clinical illness are reported, with 90% of them occurring in Africa.

Cerebral involvement with *Plasmodium falciparum* malaria major is an important cause of mortality, particularly in children in tropical regions.[343] Those manifesting papilledema and outer retinal edema outside the major retinal vascular arcades are more likely to die or survive with neurologic sequelae. Other fundus findings include retinal hemorrhages (orange color hemorrhages due to the associated anemia), cotton-wool spots, intraretinal edema, narrowed and obstructed arteries and small capillaries in the macula, and venous distension and tortuosity. The erythrocytes that have engulfed the parasites are less pliable and block small vessels causing the small retinal infarcts and hemorrhages (Figure 10.24, A–C). The retinal whitening resolves over time, as do the lipid exudates (Figure 10.24, D–F).[344–350]

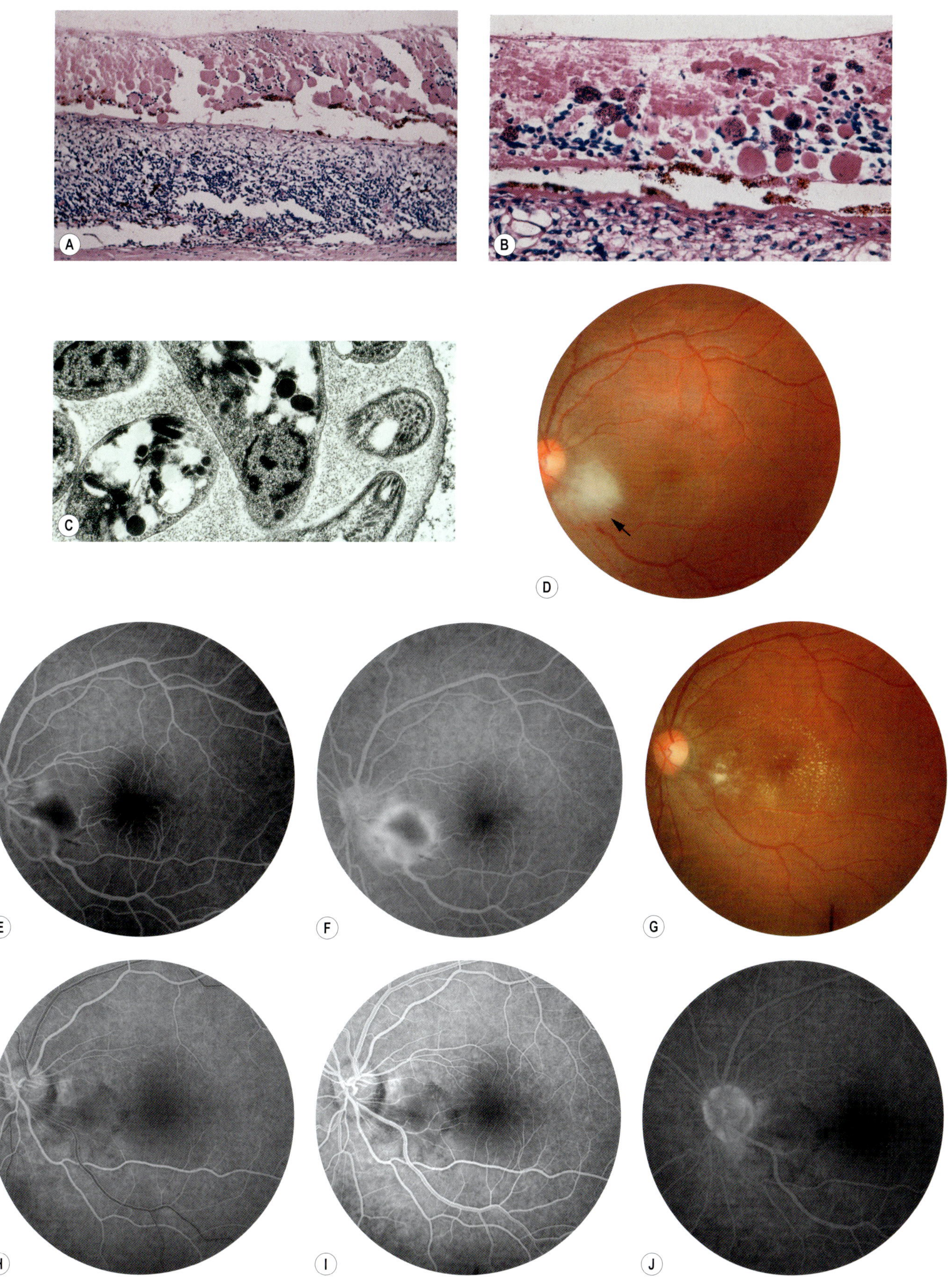
A
B
C
D
E
F
G
H
I
J

PNEUMOCYSTIS JIROVECI CHOROIDITIS

Pneumocystis jiroveci (pronounced "yee-row-vetsee", previously known as *P. carinii*) is an opportunistic pathogen in patients with various humoral and cell-mediated immunologic abnormalities and is the most common infection in patients with AIDS (over 80%).[351] It was previously classified as a protozoan, but reclassified in 1998 as a yeast-like fungus based on nucleic acid and biochemical analysis. Its name was changed in 2001 to *Pneumocystis jiroveci*, a species specific to humans. It is a normal commensal of the pulmonary system and becomes pathogenic in immunocompromised states. *Pneumocystis jiroveci* infection is the initial manifestation of AIDS in over 50% of patients. Those with T- and B-cell abnormalities appear more susceptible than patients with B-cell deficiency alone. Infection with *Pneumocystis* may be life threatening. In humans infection is primarily limited to lungs, lymph nodes, spleen, and less often liver, bone marrow, small and large intestine, pericardium, myocardium, hard palate, periureteral soft tissue, and choroid. *Pneumocystis jiroveci* choroiditis often occurs in patients receiving long-term aerosolized pentamidine therapy.[352–361] Clinically the multifocal choroidal lesions are placoid or slightly elevated, yellow–white, round or oval, multilobulated, and variably sized, with finely granular RPE that may simulate lesions seen in large cell lymphoma, metastatic carcinoma, atypical mycobacterial infection, sarcoidosis, or Dalen–Fuchs nodules (Figure 10.25, A–F). The choroidal lesions progress slowly and are associated with minimal vitreous reaction and visual loss. Although both eyes are usually affected, unifocal unilateral lesions may occur.[130,353] Angiographically these focal lesions are hypofluorescent early, and stain late (Figure 10.25, B and C).[352–354,357]

Pneumocystis is a unicellular organism with many morphologic features but it is considered to be a fungus (Figure 10.25, H and I).[134,362] It exists exclusively in extracellular spaces. It is not readily cultured. There is no reliable serologic test for identification; most recently PCR for its DNA is being used. Diagnosis depends upon demonstration of organisms with special stains – methenamine silver, toluidine blue, or Giemsa. Silver stains primarily the mature cysts (Figure 10.25, I). Choroidal infiltrates are acellular, eosinophilic, vacuolated, and frothy, and involve the full-thickness choroid including choriocapillaris (Figure 10.25, G and H).[131,132,134,354,355,362] Foci of hemorrhage and calcification may be present. Silver stains show *Histoplasma*-like organisms (Figure 10.25, I). Electron microscopy (EM) provides a definitive diagnosis and shows trophozoites and thick-walled cystic organisms (Figure 10.25, J). The overlying RPE is usually minimally affected.

Treatment consists of IV or oral therapy with trimethoprim–sulfamethoxazole, dapsone, pentamidine, or co-trimoxazole.[129,354,355,362] Potential side effects include neutropenia, thrombocytopenia, skin rash, fever, nephrotoxicity, hepatotoxicity, and others. Early ophthalmoscopic detection of choroiditis may save sight as well as prevent a fatal outcome. Failure of the choroidal lesions to respond to treatment should suggest the possibility of a coexisting infection of the choroid, e.g., *Mycobacterium avium-intracellulare, Cryptococcus neoformans, Mycobacterium tuberculosis,* and *Histoplasma capsulatum*.[353,357,361]

Ocular as well as other sites of infection with *Pneumocystis* probably occur at the time of spread from pneumonitis. These lesions become inactivated but not sterilized and may reactivate at a later time. Patients receiving prophylactic aerosolized pentamidine therapy are not protected against extrapulmonary disease, hence immuno-compromised patients are on prophylaxis with trimethoprim–sulfamethoxazole or co-trimoxazole. Presumed *P. jiroveci* choroiditis served as a marker for disseminated infection[353] before oral prophylaxis. The number of HIV cases developing *P. jirovecii* choroiditis has since dropped dramatically. Only two case reports have been seen in the past decade, one an HIV patient on a low dose of co-trimoxazole and another a post transplant leukemic patient.[363,364]

10.25 ***Pneumocystis jiroveci*** **choroiditis in patients with AIDS.**

A to **E**: This 24-year-old HIV-positive man presented with a 3-month history of *Pneumocystis* pneumonitis and a 1-month history of severe headaches related to central nervous system cryptococcosis. He had no visual complaints. Visual acuity was 20/20 bilaterally. The fundi of both eyes showed widely scattered, multifocal, partly confluent, slightly elevated, cream-colored lesions (A). Angiography revealed early blockage of choroidal fluorescence and late staining of the choroidal lesions (B and C). The patient was treated with trimethoprim, sulfamethoxazole, amphotericin B, and fluconazole IV. Over the following 2 weeks he noted progressive loss of vision in both eyes. The choroidal lesions were unchanged but he developed early papillitis (D). His vision declined to counting fingers only in both eyes. Six weeks later there was evidence of partial resolution of the choroiditis but the papillitis had increased (E).

F to **J**: This 34-year-old man with AIDS and pulmonary pneumocystosis had received multiple medications including pentamidine inhalation treatment. He had no visual complaints when he was discovered to have multiple cream-colored choroidal lesions in both eyes (F). His visual acuity in the right eye was 20/30. He died 3 weeks later. Gross examination of an eye removed from a 35-year-old patient with AIDS and *Pneumocystis* pneumonia revealed multiple yellowish placoid lesions involving the choroid (*arrows*, G). Histopathologically the choroidal lesions consisted of eosinophilic, acellular, vacuolated lesions (H) that when stained with methenamine silver stain demonstrated cystic organisms (*arrow*, I). Electron microscopy revealed cysts, some of which contained intracystic bodies (*arrows*, J).

(F–J from Rao et al.[362])

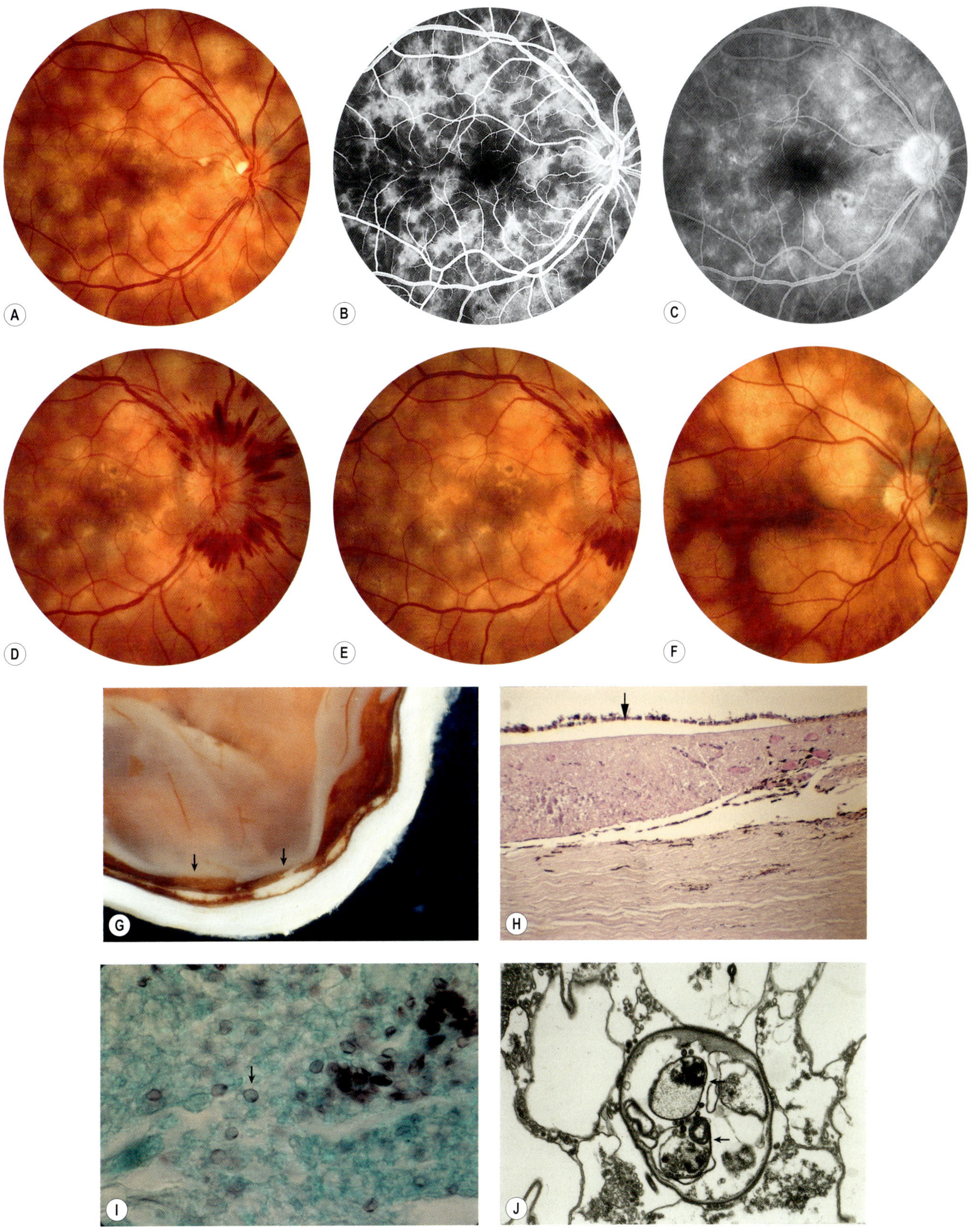
A
B
C
D
E
F
G
H
I
J

TOXOCARIASIS

Patients, typically healthy children or young adults, may experience unilateral loss of vision secondary to invasion of the eye by a single second-stage larval form of the *Toxocara canis* ascarid (Figure 10.26).[365–376] The eggs of the dog ascarid are deposited in the soil, where they undergo a change required before they become infectious to humans, who contract the disease primarily by ingestion of contaminated soil and not by direct contact with dogs. Following hatching of the eggs in the gastrointestinal tract, the second-stage larvae invade the blood vessels of the gastrointestinal tract and enter the eye, probably via the uveal tract. Bilateral ocular invasion probably occurs rarely. The patients manifest a variety of clinical pictures, including: (1) localized disciform macular detachment (Figure 10.26, A–C);[365] (2) multifocal granulomas with interconnecting tracks, so-called meandering toxocariasis (Figure 10.26, F–I);[377,378] (3) peripheral disciform retinal detachment; (4) papillitis;[359,366,379–382] (5) optic nerve head tumor (Figure 10.26, D and E);[354,366,381,383] (6) peripheral retinal or pars plana mass with vitritis (unilateral pars planitis; Figure 10.26, I–K);[362,368,370,375] (7) retinal detachment; (8) endophthalmitis;[367,368,375,384] and (9) cataract. These patients typically have externally quiet eyes in spite of having endophthalmitis. The organism, which measures approximately 300–400 μm in length, is at the subbiomicroscopic level in size.[357,360,371,385] It presumably enters the subretinal space by way of the choriocapillaris, where it may incite an eosinophilic granulomatous reaction and cause a serous and hemorrhagic disciform detachment of the retina (Figure 10.26, A).[365,386] The reaction may destroy the overlying retina and extend into the vitreous (Figure 10.26, C).[366,370,375] On healing, a gray or white umbilicated disciform scar, often with retinochoroidal vascular anastomosis, may result (Figure 10.26, B and C).[365,386]

The diagnosis of a subretinal granuloma caused by *Toxocara canis* is presumptive. Eosinophilia can be demonstrated in some patients. The ocular disease rarely occurs in children with other clinical evidence of visceral larva migrans (coughing, wheezing, pulmonary infiltration, hepatomegaly, leukocytosis, persistent eosinophilia, elevation of isohemagglutinins, and elevated serum immunoglobulin levels). Visceral larva migrans occurs presumably with ingestion of a large number of eggs.[387] *Toxocara catis* is rarely if ever the cause of ocular toxocariasis. The ELISA test may detect serum IgG antibodies in as high as 90% of patients with clinically suspected ocular disease.[361,366,388,389] The ELISA test titer of aqueous humor and vitreous is usually higher than that demonstrated in the serum and in some cases may be positive when the serum shows no evidence of antibodies.[390–394] This is likely due to intraocular antibody production. Monoclonal antibodies to larval excretory–secretory antigens that bind with species specificity to the cuticular surface of infective larvae may prove to be of value in the laboratory diagnosis of toxocariasis.[378,395]

10.26 Intraocular toxocariasis.

A: Subretinal granuloma with surrounding subretinal hemorrhage in a 14-year-old girl with presumed *Toxocara canis*.
B: Organized subretinal granuloma with retinochoroidal anastomosis in a 10-year-old girl with presumed *Toxocara canis*.
C: Organized subretinal granuloma with extension of the mass into the vitreous in an 8-year-old boy with presumed *Toxocara canis*.
D and E: Peripapillary *Toxocara* granuloma and exudative macular detachment in a 4-year-old girl. The eye was enucleated because of the possibility of retinoblastoma. Histopathologic examination revealed a peripapillary subretinal eosinophilic granuloma surrounding a *Toxocara* organism (*arrow*, E).
F to H: Probable meandering toxocariasis in a 25-year-old woman who first noted loss of central vision in the right eye at age 16 years. This was associated with serosanguinous retinal detachment in the right macula and multiple choroidal lesions superotemporal to the macula, including the elevated white lesion seen in F. Her *Toxocara* ELISA test was positive. Her visual acuity improved and she was asymptomatic until 9 years later, when she had recurrence of symptoms in the right eye. Note the hypertrophic scar surrounded by a shallow serous retinal detachment (*large arrows*, G and H) and the track-like pattern of scars indicating probable movement (*small arrows*, G) of worm 9 years previously (G). The larva was probably encapsulated within the large scar in the superotemporal macular area (*large arrows*, G and H). This scar appeared to contain calcium ultrasonographically.
I: Peripheral inflammatory mass causing a macular hole and macular displacement in a boy with presumed *Toxocara* granuloma. Note demarcation lines caused by previous retinal detachment.
J and K: *Toxocara* granuloma posterior to the iris and ciliary body of a child who presented with a white pupil. Note the eosinophilic granulomas (*arrows*, J), one of which contained the *Toxocara* larva (*white arrow*), shown in higher power in K.

(D and E from Bird et al.[366]; published with permission from the American Journal of Ophthalmology; copyright by the Ophthalmic Publishing Co.)

The clinical finding of a localized subretinal exudative lesion in the macula or a localized disciform scar, usually associated with retinochoroidal anastomosis of one eye of a child with no other evidence of ocular disease, should suggest the diagnosis of *Toxocara canis*. It must be remembered, however, that occasionally focal areas of retinitis associated with toxoplasmosis may also produce a proliferative subretinal scar that resembles in every way that produced by *Toxoplasma* (see Figure 10.23, F). Bilateral disciform detachments occurring in children are unlikely to be caused by *Toxocara canis*. In such a case, other family members should be studied for evidence of a macular dystrophy. Serous and hemorrhagic disciform detachments in children may occur occasionally as a complication of Best's vitelliform disease (see Chapter 5), other hereditary dystrophies (see Chapter 5), rubella retinitis (see p. 918), and diffuse unilateral subacute neuroretinitis (see pp. 864–872), and in patients with idiopathic panuveitis, vitritis, and multifocal chorioretinitis (see Chapter 11).

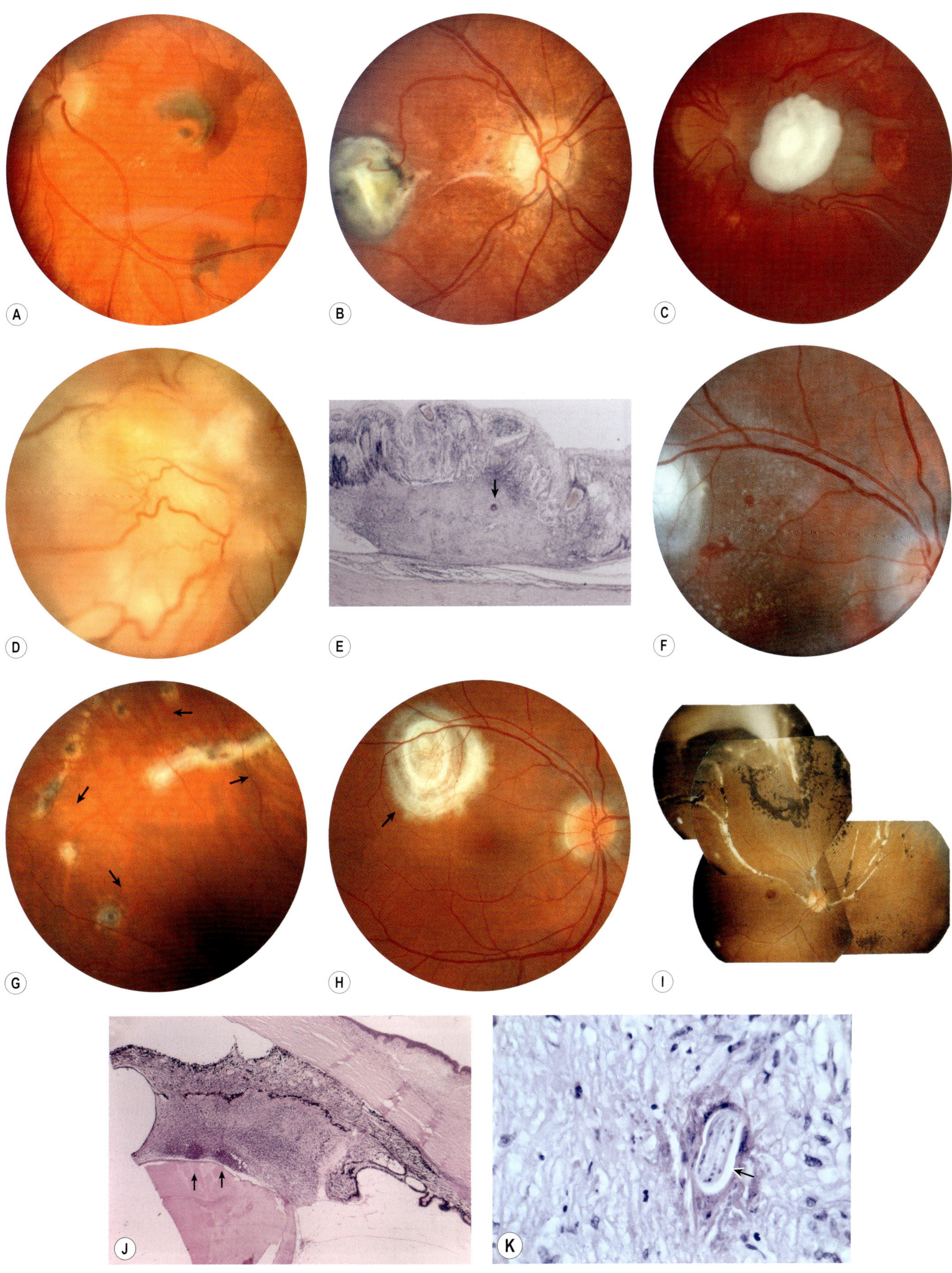
A
B
C
D
E
F
G
H
I
J
K

Histopathologically, material left in the wake of the migrating larvae may cause a strongly eosinophilic granulomatous reaction along its path. The organism is usually identified in the center of an eosinophilic abscess (Figure 10.26, E and J).[366,370,375,396,397] Ocular toxocariasis has been produced experimentally.[355,357,385,398]

There is no satisfactory medical treatment for ocular *Toxocara canis.* Photocoagulation may be of some value in the treatment of subretinal granulomas in the paracentral region causing macular detachment. Vitrectomy procedures have been used successfully in the treatment of retinal detachment associated with vitreous traction caused by intravitreal or more peripherally located subretinal granulomas.[379,399–400]

CYSTICERCOSIS

Cysticercosis is caused by human ingestion of the eggs of *Taenia solium* (pork tapeworm). The eggs disintegrate in the gastrointestinal tract, the embryos invade the intestinal wall and are carried throughout the body, where they undergo metamorphosis to become *Cysticercus cellulosae* (Figure 10.27, A). Most patients have several larvae in the body though only one may be seen in the eye. Often larvae are seen in the brain and subcutaneous tissue.[401] Some of the integumental and brain cysts can calcify and can be detected by plain X-ray of the abdomen, forearms, and skull. Seizures and headache may be the presenting signs of CNS cysticercus. These larvae may enter the eye (more frequently the left) by way of either the central retinal artery or the ciliary arteries.[373,391,402,403] They may gain entrance to the subretinal space (Figure 10.27, B and C), the vitreous cavity (Figure 10.27, G), or the anterior chamber (Figure 10.27, H). Over a period of many months they grow into a large cystic structure. When they are located beneath the retina, they may be mistakenly diagnosed as a serous detachment of the RPE or retina, as a choroidal tumor (Figure 10.27, B, C, and I),[383,385,397,404–406] or a retinoblastoma.[407]

Recognition of the white head or scolex that is often invaginated and moving within the cystic body permits accurate clinical diagnosis (Figure 10.27, A–C). The scolex reacts and moves to light shone into the eye. Echography may be helpful in localization and differential diagnosis in some cases associated with retinal detachment and vitreous opacification.[372,408] Multiple organisms may occasionally be found in one or both eyes.[392,409] During its early growth the organism may incite minimal reaction. Eventually, however, secondary inflammation, usually caused by the death of the organism, may destroy the eye, or leakage of cyst fluid through the wall may cause inflammatory debris. Extraocular locations often seen are in the subconjunctiva, along the rectus muscles, eyelids, and in the orbit.[410] In endemic areas ocular involvement is encountered most frequently during the early decades of life,[398,411] though other studies have found them predominantly in the third and fourth decades.[412] There is a male predilection of 2:1, suggesting that working men are more exposed to unhygienic food and water.[412] Almost 30% of affected individuals are vegetarians; hence contaminated water and uncooked vegetables may carry the eggs in addition to poorly cooked pork. Approximately one half of patients will show evidence of antibodies to cysticercus. The infestation is common in Mexico, India, Pakistan, and other developing countries.[401,407,410–414]

Because of the predilection for inflammation after death of the organism, surgical excision of the living organism is the ideal treatment.[415–419] When located in the far periphery of the eye, the larvae may be removed transsclerally (Figure 10.27, B–E). Transscleral removal of larvae located in the posterior pole is difficult. Photocoagulation of small larvae that do not exceed two disc diameters in size has been reported by Barsante.[383,404] Even when small, however, photocoagulation treatment results in considerable inflammation and scar tissue reaction. When in the vitreous the organism may be removed by vitrectomy.[415,416,418] Even though it is best to remove the organism intact, meticulous washout following accidental rupture during vitrectomy has resulted in preservation of the eye and visual recovery. All patients should be evaluated for additional extraocular cysticerci.[401] Praziquantel is an anthelmintic used in treating intracranial cysticerci along with systemic steroids to quell the inflammatory response to the death of the organisms.

10.27 Ocular cysticercosis.

A: Drawing of *Cysticercus cellulosae* larvae with the scolex extended (*left*) and invaginated (*right*).

B to F: Subretinal *Cysticercus* larva in a 78-year-old woman from south Florida. She complained of progressively worsening floaters in the left eye of 5 months' duration. Note the invaginated scolex (*arrows*) and change in shape of the cysticercus in the subretinal space inferior to the left macula (B and C). Laser photocoagulation applications were placed around the organism several days before its surgical removal by the author via a posterior sclerotomy and choroidotomy. Note the ring of photocoagulation scars and the sclerotomy scar (D and *arrow*, E) several weeks after its removal. Photomicrograph of the cysticercus (F) shows invaginated scolex with hooklets (*upper arrow*) and sucker (*lower arrow*). Her visual acuity was 20/20 18 months after surgery.

G: Subretinal *Cysticercus* with scolex extended anteriorly through the foveal center into the vitreous. *Black arrow* indicates sucker; *white arrow* indicates ring of hooklets.

H and I: *Cysticercus* in the anterior chamber.

J: Subretinal *Cysticercus* with invaginated scolex (*arrows*) in a 6-year-old patient whose eye was removed with the mistaken diagnosis of retinoblastoma.

(G from Barsante[404]; H, courtesy Dr J. Arce; I, courtesy Dr Myron Yanoff.)

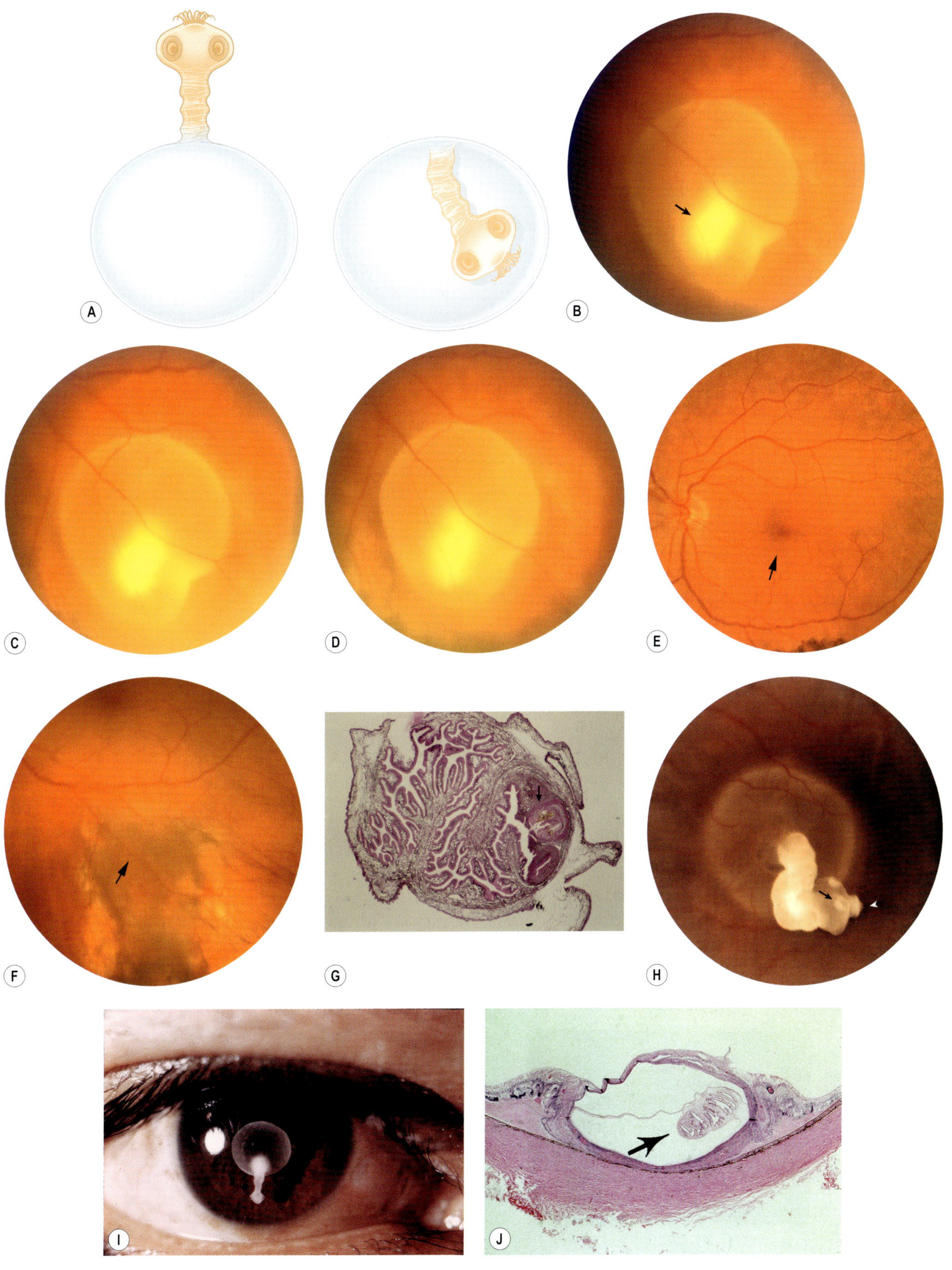
A
B
C
D
E
F
G
H
I
J

DIFFUSE UNILATERAL SUBACUTE NEURORETINITIS

Diffuse unilateral subacute neuroretinitis (DUSN) is a clinical syndrome characterized early by visual loss, vitritis, papillitis, retinal vasculitis, and recurrent crops of evanescent gray–white outer retinal lesions and later by progressive visual loss, optic atrophy, retinal vessel narrowing, and diffuse RPE degeneration occurring in one eye of otherwise healthy patients (Figures 10.28–10.31).[420–422] DUSN is caused by at least two as yet unidentified species of nematodes: a smaller one believed to be the third-stage larva of the dog hookworm and a larger worm, the larva of a raccoon roundworm, that may wander in the subretinal space for 4 years or longer and cause progressive ocular damage.[420,421,423–426]

Patients may be seen initially during the early or subacute stage of the disease because of persistent vitritis and/or acute visual loss in one eye. Vitreous cells are invariably present but in some patients may be few in number. There may be mild to moderate swelling of the optic disc in the affected eye. There may or may not be any other visible changes in the fundus at that time. Visual acuity may be mildly or severely affected. A Marcus Gunn pupil reaction is usually present. A few patients may demonstrate a mild ciliary flush, anterior chamber cells, flare, and keratic precipitates. An occasional patient may have a hypopyon. Usually within several days or weeks, careful observation of these patients will disclose focal, gray–white or yellow–white lesions (with the smaller worm) and more gray–brown (with the larger worm) with fuzzy borders that involve the external layers of the retina and RPE (Figures 10.28, A and D; 10.29, A, B, D, F, G, and J; 10.30, A–C).

The lesions are typically confined to a single zone, frequently in the macular or juxtamacular areas. They typically fade from view, usually within several days, leaving minimal or mild ophthalmoscopic evidence of change in the underlying RPE. Successive crops of these lesions may occur from week to week in the same or adjacent areas of the fundus (Figure 10.29) and in some cases these may completely resolve only to recur again. Focal retinal hemorrhages, perivenous exudation similar to that seen in sarcoidosis (Figure 10.28, J), and occasionally localized serous detachment of the retina may occur. In some patients during the early course of the disease the visual acuity may be normal or minimally affected. Over a period of weeks (larger worm) or months (smaller worm), diffuse as well as focal depigmentation of the RPE occurs (Figure 10.28, G–I). These changes are usually least prominent in the central macular area. The multifocal areas of depigmentation, which are most numerous in the mid peripheral fundus, may simulate those seen in the presumed ocular histoplasmosis syndrome.

Accompanying these progressive changes in the RPE is a gradual narrowing of the retinal arterioles and increasing pallor of the optic disc (Figure 10.28, D–I). Pigment migration into the overlying retina is uncommon. In many cases, particularly in young children, the disease is not detected until the defective vision is found on a school vision examination. Choroidal neovascularization and disciform lesions may occur in some patients. One young boy in Florida was found to have large macular subretinal fibrosis. In general, the degree of optic disc pallor and retinal vessel narrowing parallels that of central visual loss, but striking exceptions occur.

10.28 Diffuse unilateral subacute neuroretinitis (DUSN).

A to **C**: Note the subretinal motile nematode (*arrows*) and the subretinal gray–white inflammatory lesions in the inferior portion of the macula of a 14-year-old boy with acute visual loss in his right eye. Visual acuity was 20/200.

D to **G**: This young girl experienced rapid loss of vision in the right eye and was misdiagnosed as having acute posterior multifocal placoid pigment epitheliopathy. Note the coiled subretinal nematode (*arrow*, D). Angiography showed the subretinal lesions to be nonfluorescent early (E) and to stain later (F). Note also evidence of retinal perivasculitis. The presence of the worm was unrecognized at the time of initial examination. Twenty-eight months later the patient's visual acuity was counting fingers only. Note the optic atrophy, narrowing of the retinal vessels, and diffuse degenerative changes in the RPE (G).

H and **I**: Late stages of DUSN in a 15-year-old black boy whose visual acuity was 20/400. Note the optic atrophy, severe narrowing, and sheathing of the retinal arteries (H), and widespread mottled depigmentation of the RPE with relative sparing of the macula angiographically (I).

J to **L**: Perivasculitis in a 27-year-old man with mild loss of vision in the right eye. The left eye was normal. The candle wax-dripping exudates suggested sarcoidosis (J). Medical evaluation was negative. Angiography revealed extensive staining (K). Four months later the exudates had cleared (L). There was a vitreous tag (*arrow*), pallor of the optic disc, and multiple focal as well as diffuse changes in the peripheral RPE. A 700 μm motile subretinal nematode was found at the equator and was killed with argon laser. Six weeks later the visual acuity was 20/25 and there was no evidence of active retinitis.

(D–G from Gass et al.[421])

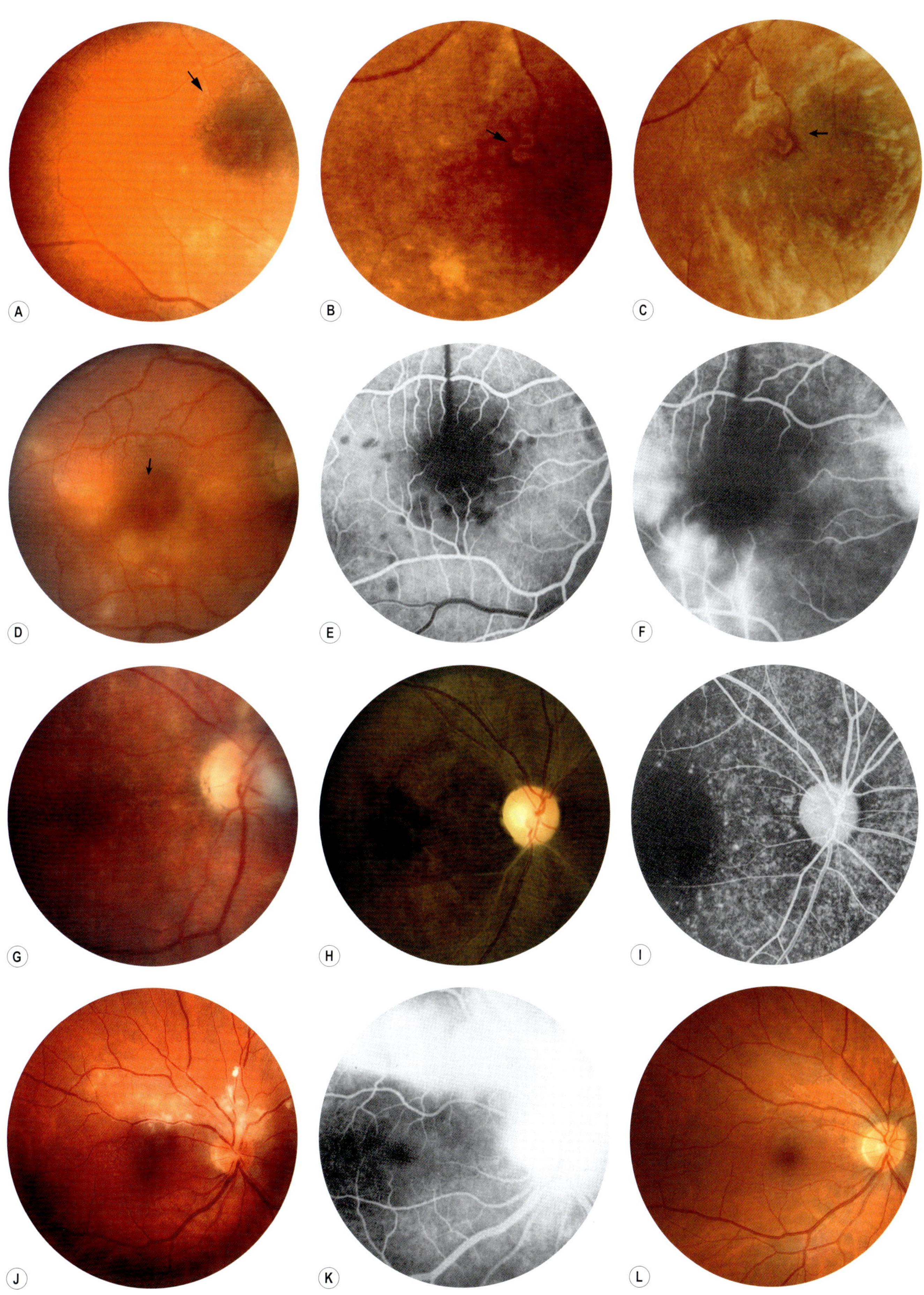
A
B
C
D
E
F
G
H
I
J
K
L

The disease is caused by a motile, white, often glistening nematode that is gently tapered at both ends and varies in length from 400 to 2000 μm, with its largest diameter being approximately one-twentieth of its length (Figures 10.28, A–D; 10.29, B, C, F, and G; 10.30, A–D, and G–L; 10.31).[420,421,423–427] It propels itself by a series of slow coiling and uncoiling movements and less often by slithering, snake-like movements in the subretinal space. It may be found during any stage of the disease and should be looked for even in patients with advanced optic atrophy, narrowing of the retinal vessels, and degenerative changes in the RPE.[421] The second eye is rarely affected; only one such incidence has been reported.[428] There are at least two endemic areas in the United States for this disease. In the southeastern United States, the Caribbean islands, and Latin America the nematode varies in length from approximately 400 to 700 μm.[420,429] In the other endemic area, the north midwestern United States, and in other parts of the United States, it measures approximately 1500–2000 μm in length (Figures 10.30, A–F; 10.31). Individual cases have been reported from Germany, Venezuela, India, Bangladesh, Europe, and Ghana.[340,430–438] A careful search with a fundus contact lens, a 70 or 90 diopter lens, is required to locate the smaller worm. The larger worm is relatively easy to detect using indirect ophthalmoscopy and a fundus contact lens. The worm is most likely to be found somewhere in the vicinity of active deep retinal white lesions that probably are caused by a toxic inflammatory reaction to material left in the wake of the wandering nematode. These lesions and the worm are more frequently located in the extramacular areas. The magnification and wide field of view provided by a fundus contact lens and the fundus camera are ideal for locating these worms.

Fluorescein angiography in the early stages of the disease usually demonstrates leakage of dye from the capillaries on the optic nerve head. The gray–white areas of active retinitis are nonfluorescent early but stain during the later phases of angiography (Figures 10.28, E and F; 10.29, E). Prominent perivenous leakage of dye may occur in some patients in the earliest stage of the disease (Figure 10.28, K), and there may be minimal or no angiographic evidence of damage to the RPE. As the disease progresses, greater evidence of loss of pigment from the RPE is manifested angiographically as an irregular increase in the background choroidal fluorescence (Figure 10.28, I).

The electroretinogram in the affected eye is usually reduced in all stages of the disease and often is moderately or severely reduced, with the b-wave being affected more than the a-wave in the later stages of the disease.[421,422,439] Rarely the electroretinogram may be extinguished.

The identification of the worm is unknown. Serologic tests for *Toxocara canis* are typically negative.[420] The stools are free of ova and parasites. Eosinophilia is infrequently detected. These patients do not manifest evidence of systemic disease. A small nematode was excised by means of eye-wall biopsy in one patient (Figure 10.30, G–I). Although there were some features that suggested the possibility of *Ancylostoma caninum*, its precise identification could not be made.[440] Cunha de Souza et al. extracted a subretinal nematode through a retinotomy after pars plana vitrectomy (Figure 10.30, L).[429] Unfortunately, because of poor fixation, definite identification of the worm was not possible. Grossly it showed similar features to the worm removed in Miami,[440] and to a 380 μm long subretinal worm successfully aspirated from the eye of a patient by Professor Kuhnt in 1886 (Figure 10.30, K).[441] Dr Dwight D. Bowman recently reviewed the pictures of the worm removed by Cunha de Souza (Figure 10.30, L) and concluded that it is most likely *Ancylostoma caninum*.[442] It is of interest that three of the last 10 patients with a subretinal worm identified at the Bascom Palmer Eye Institute had cutaneous larval migrans months or several years before the onset of ocular symptoms. *Ancylostoma caninum*, a hookworm of dogs, is a common cause of cutaneous larval migrans in the southeastern United States. The infective third-stage larva of *A. caninum* is approximately 650 μm in length and is capable of surviving in host tissue, including that of humans, many months and probably years without changing size or shape.[443] The second-stage larvae of *Baylisascaris procyonis* (larger worm), a nematode found in the intestinal tract of raccoons, has been suggested as a possible cause for DUSN.[430,444–450] Although

10.29 Diffuse unilateral subacute neuroretinitis.

A to **C**: This 14-year-old boy was hospitalized because of suspected ocular histoplasmosis or toxoplasmosis. He had noted rapid loss of vision in the left eye. Over a 5-week period, crops of evanescent gray–white subretinal lesions appeared and disappeared (A) before a motile subretinal nematode (*arrows*, B and C) was noted. The nematode disappeared, and 3 years later the patient's visual acuity was counting fingers only. He had optic atrophy, some narrowing of the retinal vessels, and diffuse changes in the RPE.

D to **I**: This young man developed acute visual loss in the right eye associated with a few vitreous cells and multiple outer retinal lesions confined to the macula of the right eye. These lesions obstructed choroidal fluorescence early and stained late (E). The diagnosis was acute posterior placoid multifocal pigment epitheliopathy. Over the next 11 days the crops of white lesions moved inferotemporally. The subretinal worm (*arrow*, D, and *inset*, F and G) was found in retrospective review of photographs, and photocoagulation (H) resulted in a focal scar (I) and resolution of the disorder.

J to **L**: This 16-year-old girl presented with a 3-month history of visual loss in the right eye. Visual acuity was 20/40 and there was a 2+ afferent pupillary defect. Vitreous inflammation and multifocal outer retinal lesions were present in the right macula. A subretinal worm was suspected (*arrow*, J) but did not show movement. One week after 2 g thiabendazole per day for 2 days, all of the subretinal lesions had disappeared except for the area of intense retinitis and vitreous reaction (K), presumably caused by death of the worm. Five months later her acuity was 20/25. Note the scar at the site of the focal retinitis (*arrow*, L).

(A–C from Gass et al.[421]; J–L from Gass et al.[454],).

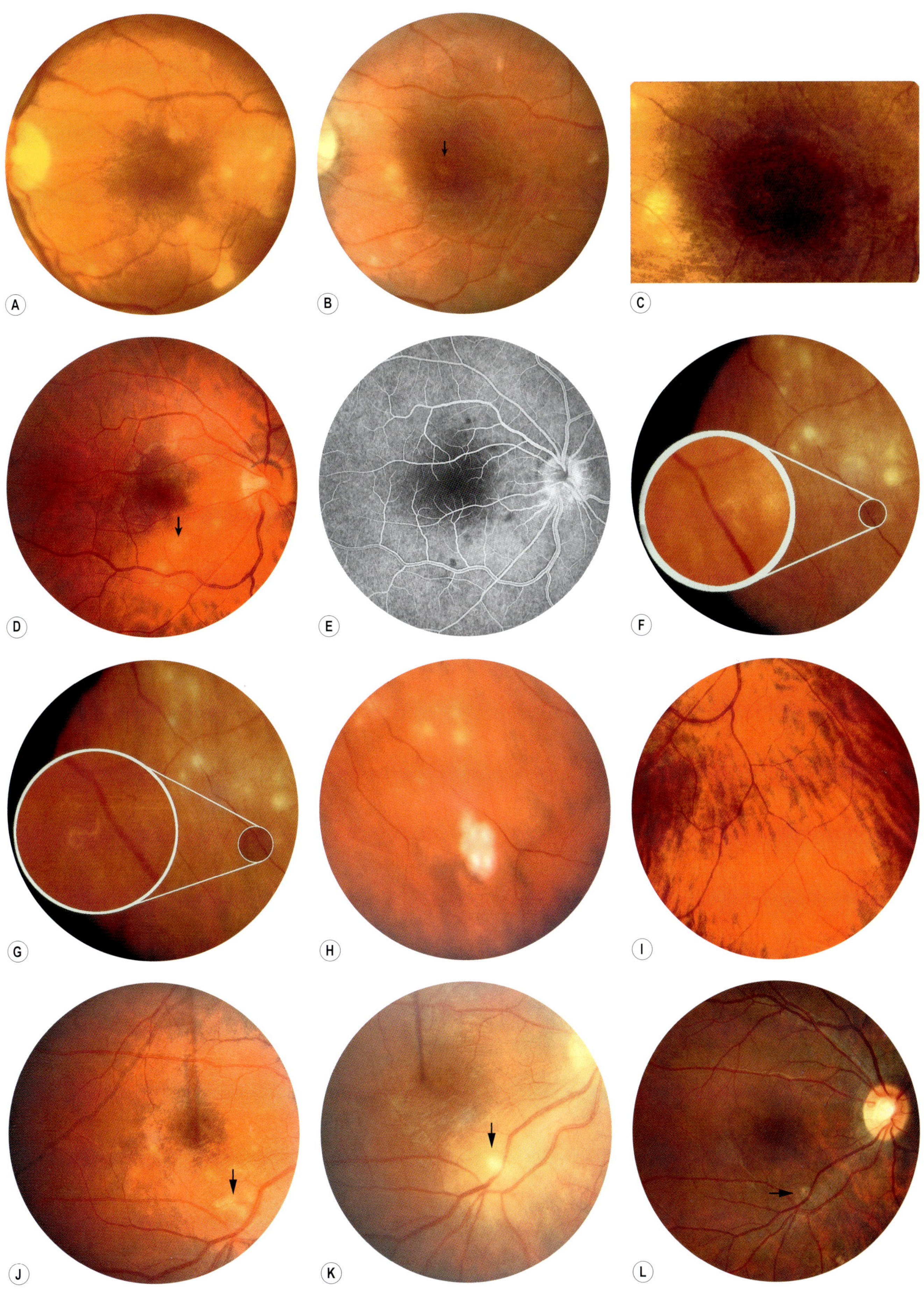
A
B
C
D
E
F
G
H
I
J
K
L

this nematode, whose larval stage measures 1000–1500 μm in length, is a common cause for meningoencephalitis in other animals, it has been rarely incriminated in similar disease in humans except a few cases in children.[430,444] The infrequent history of exposure to raccoons and the absence of CNS involvement in over 100 patients with DUSN seen at the Bascom Palmer Eye Institute make *Baylisascaris* highly unlikely as a cause for DUSN in the southeastern United States, the Caribbean, and Latin America.[451] In DUSN the size of the nematodes, the geographic distribution of reported cases, the clinical picture, and the infrequency of serologic evidence of infection with *Toxocara canis* make it unlikely that *T. canis* is the cause of DUSN.

The pathogenesis of DUSN appears to involve a local toxic tissue effect on the outer retina caused by worm byproducts left in its wake, as well as a more diffuse toxic reaction affecting both the inner and outer retinal tissues.[420–422,452] This latter reaction is manifest initially by rapid loss of visual function and alteration of the electroretinogram, and later by evidence of loss of the ganglion cells (optic atrophy) and narrowing of the retinal vessels. Optical coherence tomography has shown disruption of the photoreceptor layer within weeks of onset of visual loss both at the site of the lesions and in the fovea (Figure 10.31, E, N, and O). Subsequently the inner retinal layers thin out (Figure 10.31, N). The variability of the inflammatory signs and tissue damage seen in these patients suggests great differences in host immune response to the organism.

There are differences in the color of the lesions, the motility speed, and the rate of progression of the disease between the smaller *Ancylostoma caninum* hookworm larva and the larger *Baylisascaris procyonis* ascarid larva. The lesions caused by *Ancylostoma* are gray–white (Figures 10.28 A, D, and J; 10.29, A, B, G, H, and K) and hence more visible than the lesions secondary to *Baylisascaris* where the lesions are gray–brown and more difficult to discern (Figure 10.31, C, I, and J). The larger worm travels much faster than the smaller worm. In the author's experience, those patients who harbor the *Baylisascaris* worm show a more rapid rate of progression of the disease (the vision dropped to the 20/80–20/100 level within a month and to count fingers by 2 months) while in the patients with the smaller worm, the visual loss was slower and took approximately 4 or more months to drop to the 20/80–20/100 level. A possible explanation for this phenomenon is likely from the more rapid movement of the larger worm resulting in widespread release of toxic products.

Childhood infection with *Baylisascaris procyonis* can be associated with neural larva migrans featured by severe neurologic degeneration. Four cases have been described with ocular and neural larva migrans. The neural degeneration is progressive and widespread, with developmental delay and cerebellar and cerebral degeneration resulting in being confined to a wheelchair, incontinent, and fed by gastrostomy tubes.[453]

10.30 Diffuse unilateral subacute neuroretinitis (DUSN).

A to **F**: These figures illustrate large subretinal nematodes associated with DUSN in patients, all of whom were from the midwestern United States. A shows the nematode (*arrow*) in a 65-year-old woman who experienced rapid loss of vision in her right eye. B and C illustrate movement of a similar-sized subretinal worm (*arrows*) in a 13-year-old boy with rapid loss of vision in the right eye. Note the blurred optic disc margin and coarse mottling of the RPE. D to F illustrate argon laser photocoagulation of a large worm (*upper arrow*, D) in a 23-year-old man. Note that the S-shaped RPE imprint of the worm (*lower arrow*, D, and *arrow*, E) in the central macular area, where it apparently had lain for some time before moving superiorly, has disappeared in F.
G to **J**: Small subretinal nematode (*arrow*) that initially was located in the macula of an 18-year-old Puerto Rican boy (G). Several months later the patient's visual acuity was counting fingers and the nematode had migrated to the mid periphery of the fundus. Reversed C-shaped applications of argon laser photocoagulation (H) were used to chase the worm anterior to the equator. An eye-wall resection was done. Note the worm lying in the subretinal space (*arrows*, I and J).
K: In January 1886 Professor H. Kuhnt in Jena aspirated a nematode from the posterior vitreous eye of a 31-year-old man (his drawing, K). He interpreted the worm, which was 0.38 mm in length, as either a filarial worm or adolescent form of *Strongylus*. In 1986 Dr P.C. Beaver's interpretation of Kuhnt's drawing was probable *Toxocara canis* (personal communication).
L: This worm (600 μm long and 30 μm wide) was extracted from the subretinal space via pars plana vitrectomy in a patient with the typical findings of DUSN. On gross examination it was initially interpreted as a probable third stage of *Toxocara canis* but more recently has been interpreted as *Ancylostoma caninum*. Unfortunately, the worm decomposed before microscopic examination could be done. The patient had no serologic evidence of having toxocariasis.

(A–C and G from Gass and Braunstein[420], © 1983, American Medical Association. All rights reserved. D–F from Raymond et al.[425]; K from Kuhnt[441]; L from Cunha de Souza et al.[943], Bowman.[442])

Only one eye believed to be affected by DUSN has been studied histopathologically.[422] The eye was enucleated 15 months after the onset of the disease, which was clinically suggestive of the early acute and subacute phases of DUSN. This occurred at a time before recognition of the cause of this syndrome, and it is probable that the subretinal worm was lost during sectioning of the eye during gross examination. Histopathologically the eye showed evidence of a nongranulomatous vitritis, retinitis, and retinal and optic nerve perivasculitis with extensive degeneration of the peripheral retina, mild degeneration of the posterior retina, mild optic atrophy, mild degenerative changes in the RPE, and a low-grade, patchy, nongranulomatous choroiditis. No evidence of eosinophilia or a worm was present. Failure to find sufficient structural retinal and optic nerve damage to account for the patient's light perception-only vision at the time of enucleation suggested that the loss of visual function was partly explained on a pathophysiologic rather than an anatomic basis.

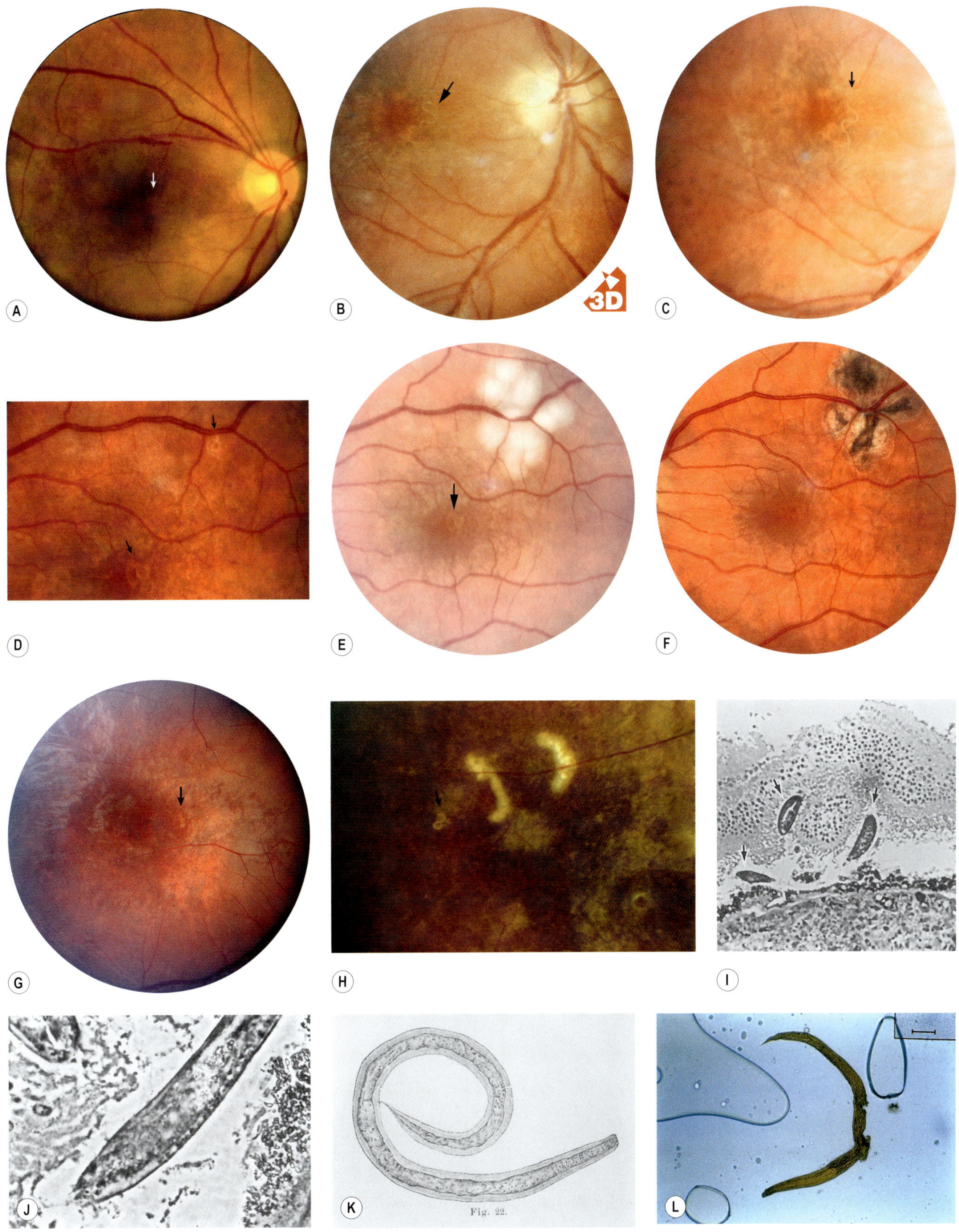
A
B
3D
C
D
E
F
G
H
I
J
K
Fig. 22.
L

Photocoagulation, the treatment of choice, is effective in destroying the worm without causing significant intraocular inflammation (Figures 10.29, H; 10.30, E; 10.31, J and K). Locating the worm, which is always found in the vicinity of the white outer retinal lesions when they are present, may require prolonged and repeated examinations. The destruction of the *Ancylostoma* worm is very quick and complete with laser due to its smaller size and slower mobility. However, the larger *Baylisascaris* worm is far more motile and will run when laser touches it, hence it is wise to wait until it moves to an area some distance from the fovea and use fairly intense white burns to stun it and then complete the laser photocoagulation. Obtaining photographs of the laser site post treatment is important in ensuring the worm is completely dead; it often survives and can move to a new area (Figure 10.31, J and K). When migrating in the subretinal space, the worm is relatively isolated from the effect of orally administered thiabendazole or diethylcarbamazine, except in those patients with moderate to severe vitreous inflammation.[420] In these latter patients, thiabendazole has been successful in causing death of the worm (Figure 10.29, J–L).[454] The presence of a focal area of intense retinitis and fading of the other white lesions 7–10 days after oral administration of thiabendazole is evidence of success of the treatment, and is followed by rapid and permanent resolution of the disease. Another strategy for treatment that has proved successful in one patient, after numerous unsuccessful attempts to locate the worm in an eye with minimal inflammation, was the application of scatter laser applications surrounding and within the zone of outer retinal white lesions to disrupt the blood–retinal barrier before administration of thiabendazole (Figure 10.32, A and B).

Diffuse unilateral subacute neuroretinitis is a great imitator. In the acute and subacute stages, it may simulate diseases associated with unilateral papillitis, papilledema, retrobulbar neuritis, and vitritis. When associated with perivasculitis, it may simulate retinal sarcoidosis (Figure 10.28, J–L). When associated with active outer retinal white lesions, it may mimic acute multifocal posterior placoid pigment epitheliopathy (Figure 10.28, D),

10.31 Diffuse unilateral subacute neuroretinitis (DUSN) (*Baylisascaris procyonis*).

A to **O**: A 58-year-old physician noted a rapid onset of visual loss associated with psychedelic photopsias and deep discomfort around the left eye of 2–3 days' duration. Her visual acuity was 20/200, and she had small multifocal brown lesions with indistinct borders around both arcades. A fluorescein angiogram showed these lesions better and the ones straddling the inferior arcade showed activity (A and B). A diagnosis of MEWDS was made and she was kept under observation. A fundus photograph done at that time was noted only for the indistinct lesions and the coiled worm that was present was not noticed (C). The lesions were hypoautofluorescent in the center surrounded by a hyper autofluorescent border (D). An OCT through the inferior fovea showed patchy loss and diffuse disruption of the photoreceptors (E). Her visual loss, photopsias and eye pain continued and an angiogram 2 weeks later shows new lesions nasal to the disc not present previously (F, *arrows*). She was considered to have atypical multiple evanescent white dot syndrome (MEWDS) and was offered consultation by an expert on MEWDS. A week later the patient noted further worsening of her vision and visual field. A repeat angiogram showed fresh lesions now straddling the ST arcade (G and H). She was suspected to have Lyme disease, and serology, lumbar puncture, and an infectious disease workup was performed. Lyme titer and CSF studies returned negative. Four and half weeks from her first presentation and about 12 days after she saw him, the expert realized this could be DUSN. Her previous fundus photographs were reviewed by the expert and her first retina doctor, both of whom could find the large DUSN worm, *Baylisascaris procyonis* in the pictures (I). The patient was asked to return to her first retina specialist who lasered the worm (J). This worm moves rapidly compared to the smaller *Ancylostoma caninum* larva and is difficult to immobilize. A photograph done immediately after the laser showed the worm was still alive and moving, though slowly (J). Further laser was applied immediately and the worm was killed (K). The patient's vision and visual field improved over 6 weeks and then remained stationary. Her eye pain and photopsias resolved without recurrence. Autofluorescence and OCT findings of photoreceptor outer and inner segments loss and retinal thinning did not change significantly (M–O). The patient showed partial improvement in her vision and visual field by 6 weeks, but no further.

(Courtesy: Dr Robert Wendel.)

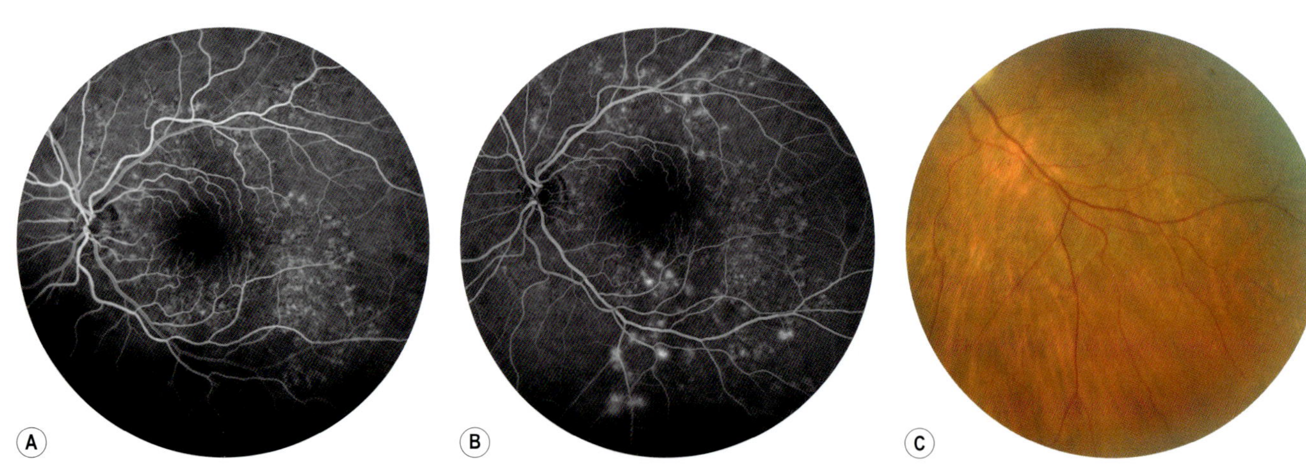

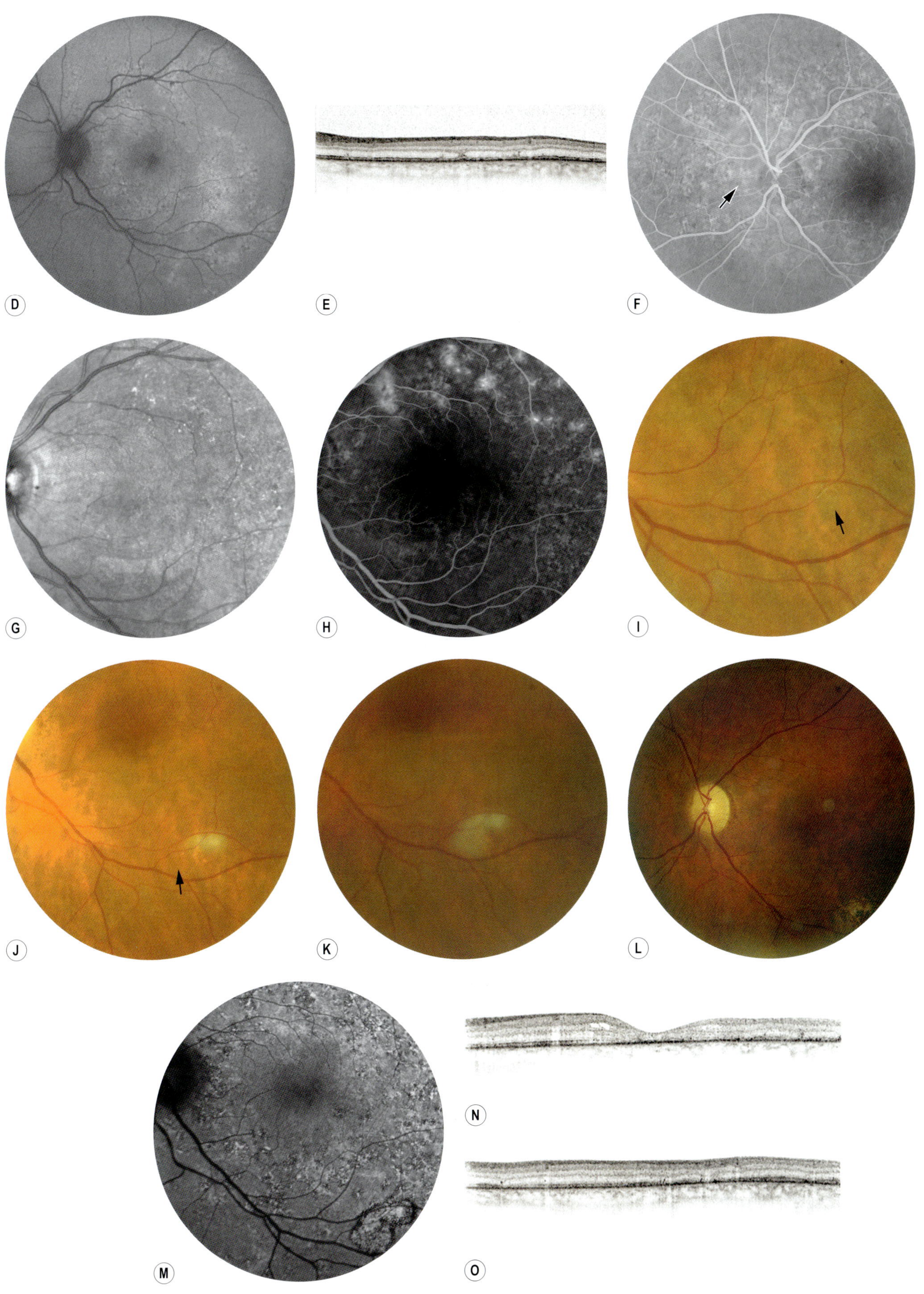

D
E
F
G
H
I
J
K
L
M
N
O

serpiginous choroiditis, evanescent white dot syndrome, Behçet's disease, multifocal outer toxoplasmosis, and the pseudo-presumed ocular histoplasmosis syndrome (Figure 10.29, A and B). In the later stages it may be misdiagnosed as unilateral optic atrophy caused by retrobulbar or intracranial lesions, the presumed ocular histoplasmosis syndrome, unilateral retinitis pigmentosa, posttraumatic chorioretinopathy, and chorioretinal atrophy after ophthalmic artery occlusion (Figure 10.28, H and I). It is important to consider the diagnosis in patients with the early findings of the disease because photocoagulation of the worm will prevent further loss of visual function and occasionally will be followed by visual improvement.

It is imperative to suspect the diagnosis in those eyes that do not seem to fit the profile of multiple evanescent white dot syndrome (MEWDS), which is most often the misdiagnosis, since both diseases are unilateral and 'photopsia' is a common symptom in both. The fluorescein angiogram shows mild hyperfluorescence early and gets more intense in the late phase. One has to think of DUSN in any patient diagnosed as MEWDS who does not improve within 3 weeks, and if fluorescein changes persist or new lesions appear after 3 weeks (Figure 10.31, A, B, and H). Questions about outdoor activity, cutaneous larva migrans, travel to South and Central America, Florida, etc. should be explored. Unless one has a high index of suspicion, the diagnosis is missed until irreversible visual loss has occurred.

FILARIASIS AND GUINEA WORM

These belong to the same order and resemble each other closely. *Dirofilaria* inhabits animals while humans are the natural hosts for *Onchocerca*, *Loa loa*, *Wuchereria bancrofti*, and *Brugia malayi*.

ONCHOCERCIASIS

Also known as river blindness, onchocerciasis is caused by a nematode filarial worm called *Onchocerca volvulus*. It causes blindness and debilitating skin lesions infecting more than 18 million people, 99% of whom live in Africa, especially in Central and East Africa.[455–462] More than 300 000 are blind and double that number are visually impaired. The remaining patients are in Latin America: Mexico, Guatemala, Brazil, Colombia, Venezuela, and Ecuador. The parasite is transmitted by small blackflies of the genus *Simulium*, which breed in fast-flowing streams and rivers. The microfilaria is deposited by the fly during a bloody meal and it grows into an adult worm in about a year. They live in the subcutaneous tissues over bony prominences. The adult female has a lifespan of 12–15 years and produces millions of microfilariae when fertilized by an adult male. The microfilariae swarm into the dermal layers throughout the body, have a lifespan of about 2 years themselves, and are taken by blackflies during a bloody meal.

10.32 Diffuse unilateral subacute neuroretinitis (DUSN).

A and **B**: Scatter laser applied to the quadrant with recent lesions from DUSN when the worm could not be found on repeated examination. She was given oral albendazole for 3 days. A photograph 3 days later showed three active lesions (*arrows*), suggesting sites where the staggering worm moved to, before dying.

Chorioretinal degenerative changes seen in patients with onchocerciasis.

C to **G**: Chorioretinal degeneration presumed to be caused by onchocerciasis in an African. Note in the composite (C) and macular area (D) of the left fundus, the narrowing of the retinal vessels, pallor of the optic disc, and the large geographic areas of atrophy and hyperplasia of the RPE. Similar changes were present in the right eye (E). Angiography reveals some loss of the choriocapillaris in the areas of geographic RPE atrophy (F and G).

H to **J**: Similar but less severe changes with relative sparing of the central macular area in another patient with onchocerciasis.

(A and B, reprinted with permission from Gupta A, Gupta V, Herbort CP, Khairallah M (eds). *Uveitis: Text and Imaging*. Delhi: Jaypee; 2009. Courtesy: H–J, Dr Hugh R. Taylor.)

Symptomatically and ophthalmoscopically this syndrome closely simulates some of the tapetoretinal dystrophies and begins 1–3 years after infection. The patient's primary complaints are loss of peripheral vision and night blindness. The primary fundoscopic findings consist of varying degrees of atrophy of the RPE, choroid, and retina, with the most prominent involvement being initially in the posterior fundus, particularly in the juxtapapillary area and often in rather discretely outlined zones temporal to the macular area (Figure 10.32). The chorioretinal changes are secondary to the inflammation produced by the thousands of microfilariae in the choroid, and it is only rarely that a worm is seen in the retina or vitreous. It is uncertain whether autoimmune mechanisms play a role in the pathogenesis of onchocercal chorioretinitis.[441,455,463,464] These changes are usually associated with progressive pallor of the optic disc and occasional optic disc swelling and focal areas of slight swelling of the choroid. Longitudinal studies of lesions of the posterior segment in patients with untreated onchocerciasis have demonstrated progressive changes that include live microfilariae, intraretinal hemorrhages, cotton-wool patches, intraretinal pigment, white and shiny intraretinal deposits, RPE window defects, and progressive depigmentation at the edge of chorioretinal scarring at rates up to 200 μm/year.[465] Ivermectin and mebendazole therapy did not appear to alter the progression of depigmentation of the scars.

These observations suggest that onchocercal chorioretinitis is associated with early changes in the retina and RPE, and that the retinal disease may progress rapidly. Angiographically, both the optic disc and the area of choroidal swelling show evidence of fluorescein staining. Varying degrees of RPE hyperplasia and subretinal fibrosis occur.

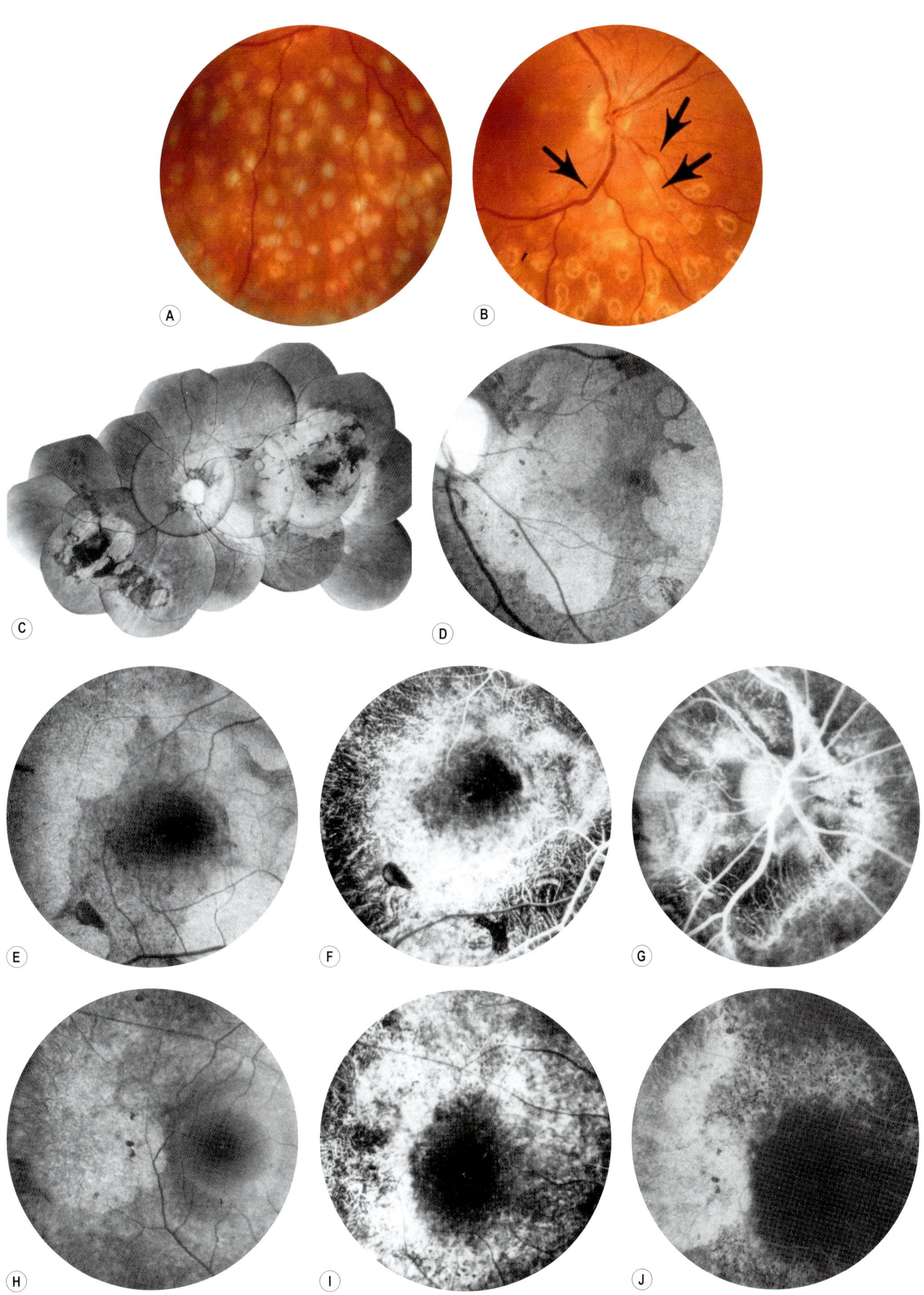
A
B
C
D
E
F
G
H
I
J

Disciform detachment of the macula is not part of the picture. Peripheral visual field loss is often out of proportion to the atrophy of the choroid and retina, and much of the visual loss is believed to be caused by optic nerve damage. Microfilariae 100–200 μm in length have been observed biomicroscopically within or beneath the retina in patients with normal fundi and visual function.[458] The fact that organisms occur in the choroid of these patients who have filariae throughout the body does not necessarily prove that they are the cause of the fundus changes. The observations of acute transient multifocal areas of staining at the level of the RPE and progressive changes in the optic nerve in these patients following treatment with diethylcarbamazine citrate, however, lend some support to the concept that *Onchocerca volvulus* is responsible for the fundus changes occurring chronically in these patients.[457,462] There is some evidence to suggest that these fundus changes may be more prominent in patients who have received treatment over a prolonged period of time, compared to those who have not. Thus, it appears that onchocerciasis, either alone or in concert with some other organisms or genetic factors, is responsible for a night-blinding disease and, in at least some endemic areas, is responsible for severe disabling posterior ocular disease. The pathogenesis of this disease may prove to share some features with that of the pseudo-retinitis pigmentosa sine pigmenti that occurs in patients with diffuse unilateral subacute neuroretinitis (see pp. 864–872).

Unlike diethylcarbamazine, which quickly eliminates microfilaria from the eye and is associated with reactive and occasionally functional ocular changes, ivermectin eliminates microfilariae slowly from the anterior chamber of the eye over a period of 6 months and causes minimal ocular inflammatory reaction or functional deficit. This slow action of ivermectin may be attributed in part to its inability to cross the blood–aqueous barrier[466] and/or the mode of action of ivermectin, which may inactivate (paralyze) rather than kill the microfilaria.[467,468] A single dose of ivermectin, 150 μg/kg, repeated once a year leads to a marked reduction in skin microfilaria counts and ocular involvement. It has no long-term effect on adult worms. There is no significant exacerbation of either anterior or posterior segment eye disease. Treatment leads to a marked and prolonged improvement in ocular status. Safety and effectiveness permit its use on a massive scale and it promises to revolutionize treatment of this disease.[469,470]

10.33 Filariasis.

A to **F**: A 28-year-old man living in India complained of a constant floater with snake-like movements for 3 months. There was no associated visual deficit, photopsia, redness, watering, prior ocular surgery, trauma, or previous such episodes. He had increased appetite and stomach ache. He had eaten raw meat a few days prior, and there was no history of recent travel or contact with pets. The vision in both eyes was 6/6 with no inflammatory reaction. A 6 DD long (9 mm) cylindrical worm with an unsegmented smooth body was seen in the vitreous cavity (A and B). The worm showed slow movements. There were chorioretinal atrophic patches in the retina (B–D). Angiogram showed transmission defects (E and F). Systemic investigations, including stool examination, for three consecutive days were unremarkable. The live worm was removed via pars plana vitrectomy and was identified as a dirofilaria.

G: Subconjunctival microfilaria in a patient from South India endemic for *Wuchereria bancrofti*.

Probable blowfly larva (Calliphoridae).

H to **M**: A 33-year-old woman from Western Pennsylvania presented with blurred vision in the right eye. An oval yellow lesion was seen inferotemporal to the optic disc (H). A fluorescein angiogram was interpreted as a choroidal neovascular membrane (I and J) and she received an intravitreal injection of bevacizumab. Three weeks later her vision improved to 20/25. The lesion now looked like a linear track with a worm that had a central black line at its anterior end (K and L). Over the next 4 weeks the worm moved further (M). She was otherwise healthy. She drank unpasteurized goat's milk and lived with goats, cat, dog, guinea fowl, fish, and turtle, and in the proximity of wild deer and turkeys. This worm may be a first stage larva of Calliphoridae, a blowfly.

N: Internet public domain image of Calliphoridae larvae showing a black line in their middle similar to the worm in the patient's eye.

(Courtesy: A–F, Dr Subina Narang; G, Dr S.R. Rathinam; H–M, Dr Roy Tuller; N, public domain on the web. A, Also, Yannuzzi, Lawrence J., The Retinal Atlas, Saunders 2010, 978-0-7020-3320-9, p.375.)

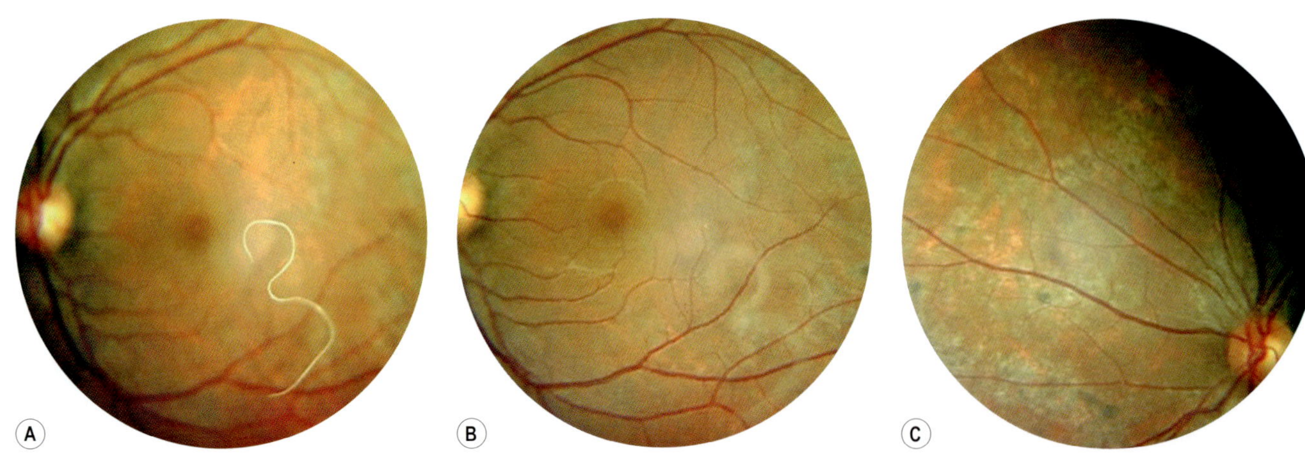

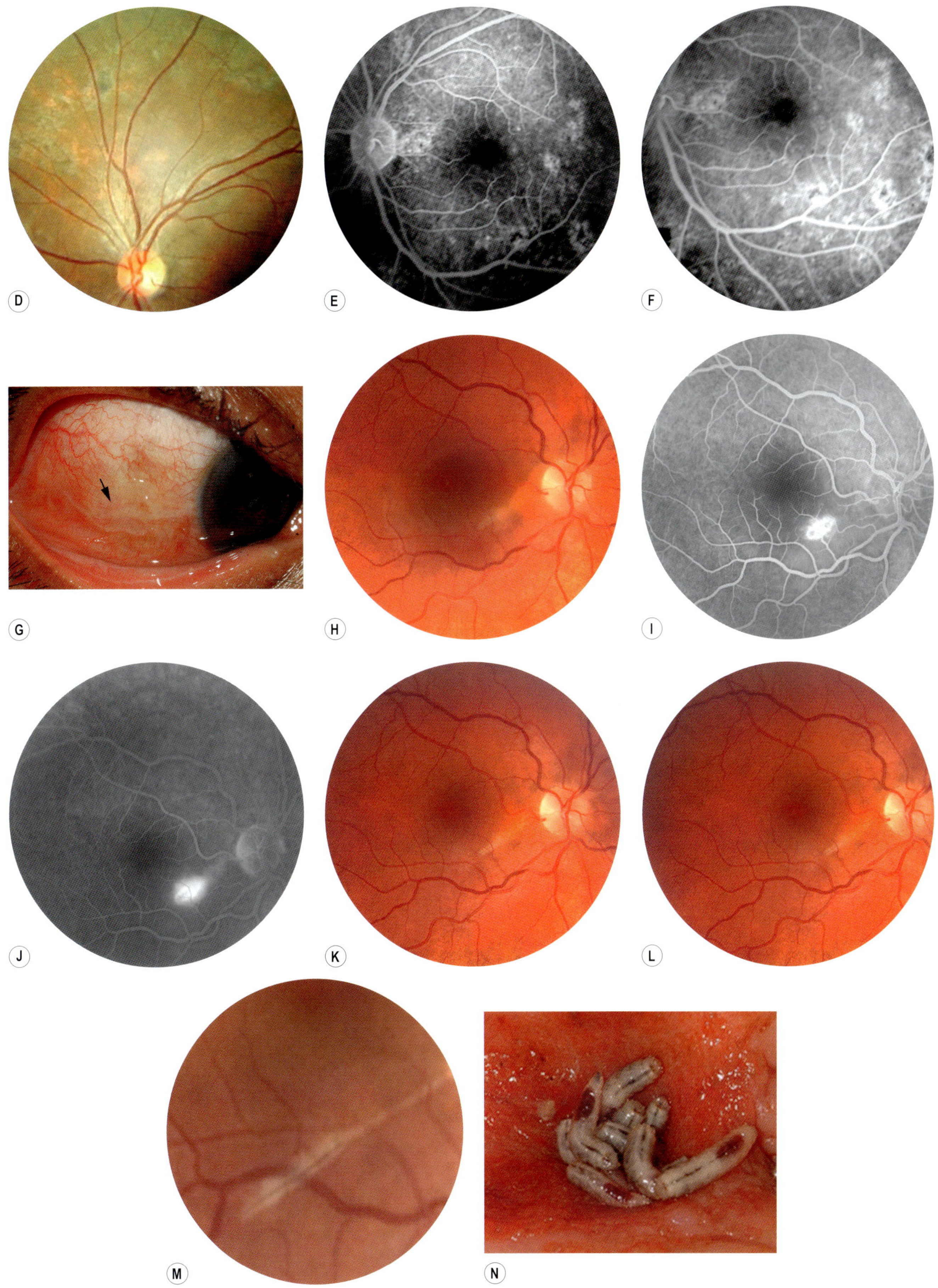
D
E
F
G
H
I
J
K
L
M
N

The bacterium *Wolbachia* has been known to infest the parasite in a symbiotic relationship. Recent findings of depleting the bacterium *Wolbachia* by use of doxycycline has made the adult worm sterile and affected worm development.

LOAIASIS

Loa loa is a human filaria endemic in central and western Africa. The adult worm resides in the subcutaneous tissue rather than in the lymphatics. It sheds microfilariae into the bloodstream and is transmitted by the bite of a blood-sucking fly *Chrysops*. The microfilariae mature in the fly and move into its brain and proboscis, and are deposited in a human by the bite of the fly. They are commonly found under the skin causing 'Calabar swelling', that is, painful nodules. The adult worm may be seen under the conjunctiva and over the sclera. It is not known to migrate intraocularly. Those patients that are coinfected with *Onchocerca* and *Loa loa* react with significant inflammation when treated with ivermectin, resulting in severe neurologic symptoms including coma, encephalitis, retinal hemorrhages, and membranous glomerulonephritis. This is believed to be from the rapid death of a large number of microfilariae.[471,472] Systemic steroids and supportive care are required in this situation.[472]

DIROFILARIASIS

There are over 40 species of *Dirofilaria* in wild (foxes) and domestic animals such as dogs and cats worldwide. All four species found in the subcutaneous tissues of humans are accidental zoonotic infections: *D. immitis* (dog heart worm), *D. repens*, *D. tenuis* (raccoons), and *D. ursi* (bears). Cases have been reported mostly in the Mediterranean region, Southern Europe, the Russian Federation, Sri Lanka, India, and the Middle East. Though subconjunctival and orbital locations are the common sites,[473–477] *D. repens* and *D. immitis* have been removed from the vitreous of the human eye.[478–484]

In its natural host the adult female lives in the subcutaneous tissues or the heart, and sheds microfilariae into the bloodstream. The infective third-stage larva (microfilaria) is transmitted into human subcutaneous tissue by the bite of an adult *Culex* or *Aedes* mosquito. Subcutaneous, subconjunctival, and orbital granulomatous reaction is the most common human manifestation.[473,474,476,477,485–487] Sometimes, the larva grows into a small adult and has been recovered from the vitreous (Figure 10.33, A and B), subconjunctival space (Figure 10.33, G) and anterior chamber of the eye.[483,488,489] The worm can be in the subretinal space and the vitreous cavity. Chorioretinal scars are seen diffusely all over the fundus; these do not typically look like tracks that are seen with the maggots of the botfly (Figure 10.33, C–F). It is possible that the dirofilarial larva moves around haphazardly in the vitreous cavity and subretinal space causing the diffuse chorioretinal changes. The visual loss appears to be moderate compared to DUSN worms, which are very toxic to the retina, and the ophthalmomyiasis from botfly larvae where patients are often asymptomatic even though the maggot has traversed the length and breadth of the subretinal space (Figures 10.35, G and H; 10.36, A–I). The adult *D. immitis* varies in length from a few centimeters to 35 cm. Surgical removal of the subconjunctival or intravitreal worm is the treatment of choice. It is possible that the large intraocular nematode illustrated in Figure 10.34 (J–L) may have been a dirofilarial worm.

10.34 Gnathostomiasis.

A to **C**: Faintly visible macular star (A) and intravitreal *Gnathostoma* (B and C) in a young Vietnamese girl complaining of blurred vision in the right eye. Her visual acuity was 20/60. *Arrows* indicate the mouth of this nematode, whose body is filled with red blood. Note the stomal end of the worm is attached to a vitreous strand. The worm was initially mistaken for a partly occluded retinal vascular anomaly. The worm was successfully removed via the pars plana.
D and **E**: Intravitreal *Gnathostoma* with arrows indicating the stoma.

Subretinal Porrocaceum or Hexametra.

F to **I**: This large subretinal nematode was surgically removed via the pars plana in this 27-year-old man who presented with a 3-week history of blurred vision and floaters and a 3-day history of only light perception in his left eye. A 9000 μm long nematode (*arrows*, G) was found in the subretinal space at the time of surgery. After a retinotomy the nematode was grasped with forceps (H) and was extracted from the eye. Ten months later the vitreous was clear (I) and his visual acuity was 20/80.

Large subretinal nematode of uncertain type.

J to **L**: A long, coiled, motile subretinal nematode, estimated to be approximately 25 mm long (*arrows*, J), was found in the eye of this Latin American air force pilot who noted recent loss of vision in his left eye. Note the unusual pattern of fluorescein staining of the subretinal exudate enveloping the nematode. Several weeks later, examination in Miami revealed a pigment figure in the left macula, and a nonmotile, partly decomposed worm in the subretinal space (*arrows*, K and L) at the temporal edge of the left macula. Note the swollen end segment of the worm (*small arrows*) and the small diameter, tightly coiled loops of the worm (*large arrow*, L). The type of nematode could not be identified.

(A–C, courtesy Dr Stephen R. Fransen; D and E from Bathrick et al.[507]; F–I from Goodhart et al.[519])

BRUGIA MALAYI AND *WUCHERERIA BANCROFTI*

These are human filarial worms endemic in Asia, Latin America, and Africa. The adult worm lives in the lymphatics of humans and can block lymph flow causing elephantiasis. The adult periodically sheds microfilariae into the bloodstream. Very rarely the microfilariae can gain entrance intraocularly, likely via the choroidal circulation, and has been found in the vitreous cavity and anterior chamber,[490–500] or the subcutaneous tissue of

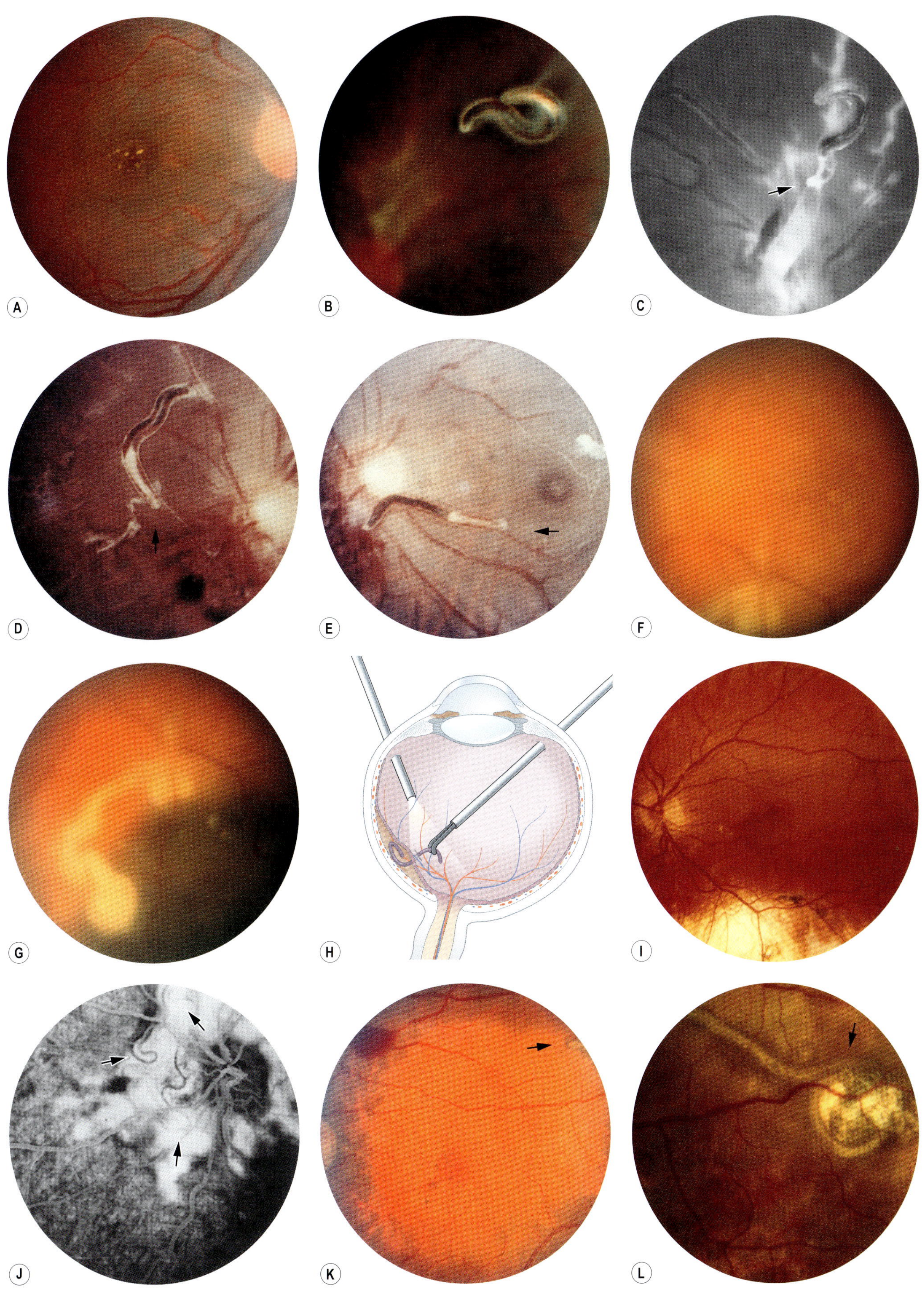
A
B
C
D
E
F
G
H
I
J
K
L

the eye and orbit.[501,502] A case of placoid pigment epitheliopathy and retinal vasculitis causing neovascularization of the retina was seen by the author in a patient with *W. bancrofti* microfilariae in his peripheral blood. The chorioretinopathy did not respond to systemic steroids alone, but did respond to oral diethylcarbamazine citrate and the subsequent retinal neovascularization to panretinal photocoagulation.[503]

GNATHOSTOMIASIS

Gnathostoma spinigerum is the most common species known to cause human gnathostomiasis. Others causing human infestation are *G. hispidum*, *G. nipponicum*, *G. doloresi*, and recently *G. binucleatum* and *G. malaysiae*.[504,505] The worm is primarily found in Asia and Central and South America. The definitive hosts are cats and dogs. It has been reported in mammals in North America. Its life cycle involves three larval stages that develop in fresh water. In the first stage, as a free-living form, it is ingested by copepods and matures to the second larval stage. The copepods are ingested by fish, snakes, and other animals that drink contaminated water. The worm completes its third larval stage in them. At this stage humans may become facultative hosts by eating the raw infected intermediate host. Second-stage larvae can also be ingested from eating or handling raw fish. Outbreaks of visceral and cutaneous migrans have been reported due to consumption of raw fish in certain areas.[505,506] It is at the third stage that the larvae may migrate for many years in humans, causing inflammation in multiple organ systems, including the skin, lungs, CNS, and eye (Figure 10.34, A–E).[507–510]

Nineteen cases of intraocular gnathostomiasis have been reported and the worm has involved the posterior ocular segment in six instances.[460,469,504,511–517] The commonest symptom is the sudden onset of a moving vertical or curved floater in the eye following an episode of significant eye ache. The ache in the eye subsides with the onset of the floater. Visual acuity is usually normal or only mildly affected, suggesting that the worm does not liberate any toxins early on. The parasite likely enters the eye through the retinal artery at the optic nerve head or elsewhere. The head is the broader end with a mouthpart consisting of two broad lips with two papillae on each. There are four rows of 40–48 hooklets soon after the lips. The rest of the body has transverse rows of cuticles with minute spines. The worm attaches its mouth to the retina and feeds off the blood vessels; one can see a blood column through its translucent body. The larva is alive most of the time and has been successfully removed by vitrectomy (Figure 10.34, A–E),[460,504,516] with recovery of vision in most instances. At vitrectomy, efforts to suck the parasite into a soft tip cannula may be met with resistance by its tenacious attachment to the retina. Bleeding from the site(s) of its attachment is also common. A report of several retinal holes resulting in a retinal detachment by Bathrick et al. alludes to this feature.[518] Once the worm is removed, no specific anthelmintic is necessary.

10.35 Angiostrongyliasis.

A: A 27-year-old man in Thailand developed progressive visual loss in his left eye for 3 weeks following eosinophilic meningitis 2 months prior. He had a history of eating raw *Pila* sp. snails. Vision in this eye was 1/200, with an afferent pupillary defect, cells and flare in the anterior chamber, subretinal tracks, pale disc, and generalized retinal pigment epithelial alteration. An immature male *Angiostrongylus cantonensis* was removed from the vitreous cavity by pars plana vitrectomy. His vision improved to 20/200.
B: A 36-year-old Thai man lost vision in his right eye over a week to the 2/200 level. A subretinal live parasite was treated with diode laser. His vision improved to 20/200.

Ophthalmomyiasis interna.

C to E: This asymptomatic 16-year-old girl had a visual acuity of 20/10 bilaterally. Her left eye was normal. Note the crisscrossing tracks throughout the right eye. These tracks were demonstrated best with fluorescein angiography (D and E). The maggot had exited the eye.
F: Submacular hemorrhage caused by a maggot that has migrated into the vitreous cavity.
G: Maggot lying on the anterior surface of the retina. Note the surrounding subretinal tracks and the round retinal hemorrhages (*arrows*).
H to J: Subretinal tracks in a black woman with a history of loss of central vision for many months in the right eye. Visual acuity in the right eye was 20/200 and in the left eye was 20/20. Note the crosshatched subretinal tracks and optic atrophy in the right eye (H and I); left fundus was normal (J). No maggot was identified in the right eye.
K: Scanning electron micrograph of first instar larva of the rodent botfly, *Cuterebra*.
L: *Cuterebra jellisoni* botfly.

(A and B, courtesy Dr S. Sinawat; F, courtesy Dr T.F. Schlaegel Jr; G, courtesy Dr W.S. Grizzard; H–J, courtesy Dr Ralph F. Hamilton Jr; J from Custis et al.[531]; L from Baird.[535])

OTHER NEMATODE INFECTIONS OF THE EYE

Goodart and associates[519] have reported the successful removal of a 9 mm nematode, either *Porrocaceum* or *Hexametra*, from the subretinal space of a young man with uveitis and total retinal detachment (Figure 10.34, F–I). The adult stages of these large ascarid larvae are found in the stomach and intestine of carnivorous reptiles, birds, or mammals. The larvae ordinarily develop within the tissues of small mammals before becoming infective for the final host. This patient probably ingested the eggs from soil or water contaminated with the feces of an owl, hawk, snake, or other carnivorous final host.

Angiostrongyliasis

Angiostrongylus cantonensis is very rarely seen in the eye, and can be found in the anterior chamber, vitreous cavity or subretinally.[520–523] The patients may be asymptomatic, mildly symptomatic, or present with significant decline in vision, pain, and redness. These patients can have uveitis, subretinal tracks, necrotizing retinitis, disc

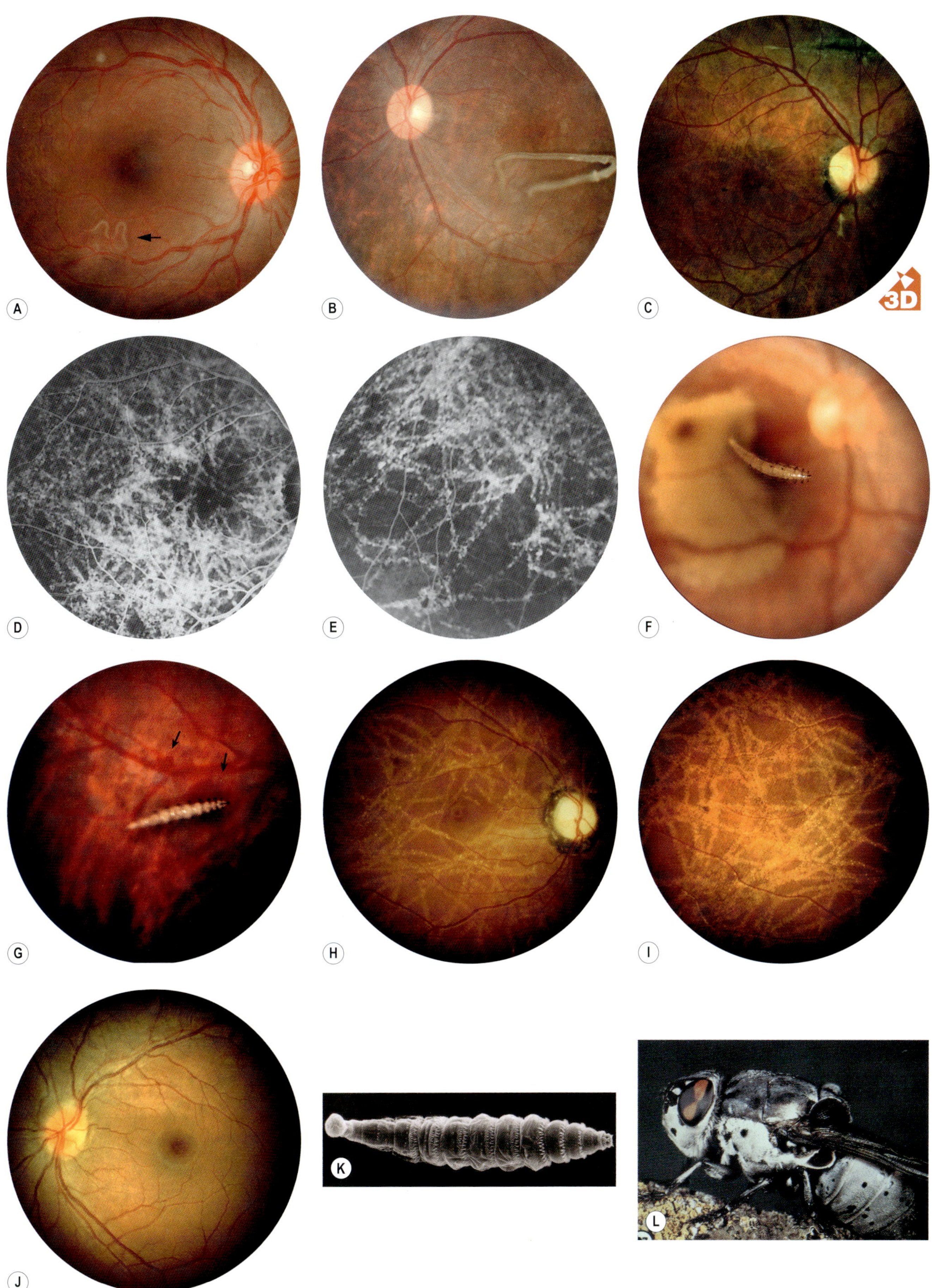
A
B
C
3D
D
E
F
G
H
I
J
K
L

swelling, papillitis, macular and retinal edema, retinal pigment alteration, and retinal detachment.[521,523] The severe pigmentary alteration is probably from inflammation of the choroid and retina due to subretinal migration of the worm prior to access into the vitreous cavity. The intermediate host is *Pila* sp. snail and other aquatic animals, and infection is acquired by eating raw snails, shrimp, and monitor lizards. The incubation period is between 2 weeks and 2 months.[520–522,524]

Eosinophilic meningitis and encephalitis are other disorders caused by this nematode; the latter is fatal. It is prevalent in tropical countries, mainly Thailand, Vietnam, Japan, Taiwan, and Papua New Guinea, although ocular infestation has been seen occasionally in India and Sri Lanka.[521,523–526] Headache, associated CSF eosinophilia, and serologic evidence of antibodies, along with a history of ingesting raw snails, help in making the diagnosis. Most reports are from Thailand. Persistent headache for more than 7 days and elderly age differentiate meningitis from encephalitis. The *A. cantonensis* larvae are in the meninges and subarachnoid space and cause inflammatory damage. Treatment involves albendazole and systemic steroids.[520,525,527,528] The worms in the eye have all been removed surgically given the size of the worm.[521,523,526]

OPHTHALMOMYIASIS

Calliphoridae

In the summer of 2009, three cases of a new larva that measured approximately 2000 microns in length with a characteristic central black line through its middle (Figure 10.33, H, K–M) were seen in Western Pennsylvania (two in Pittsburgh and one in Williamsburg). All patients were asymptomatic or had mild symptoms. The larva leaves a track that is partly pigmented (Figure 10.33, K–M) and seems to move slower than the botfly larva that leaves several crisscross tracks (see Figures 10.35, A–C, G, and H; 10.36, A–I). There was mild inflammation at the site of entry into the subretinal space with a decrease in vision to the 20/50 level (Figure 10.33, I and J). Vision recovered following one injection of intravitreal bevacizumab and has remained at 20/20. The two other patients also had a similar larva and were mostly asymptomatic since the track was away from the fovea in both cases.

In order to establish the identity of the worm, exclusive search of the literature (both human and veterinary) and the Internet resulted in the larva being identified as possibly Calliphoridae, a blowfly larva (Figure 10.33, N).

Ophthalmomyiasis Interna

The term 'myiasis' describes the invasion of the living vertebrate organism by the larval form (maggot) of certain flies in the order Diptera. The larvae responsible for intraocular invasion (ophthalmomyiasis interna) belong mostly to those genera that are obligatory tissue parasites, that is, those that exclusively require living host tissue for the completion of their larval development. These include the cattle, sheep, horse, deer, reindeer, rodent, squirrel, chipmunk, rabbit, and human botflies.[529] Flies identified as causes of ophthalmomyiasis interna include *Hypoderma bovis*, *Hypoderma tarandi*, *Cuterebra* sp., *Gasterophilus intestinalis*, *H. lineatum*, *Oedemagena tarandi*, *Oestrus ovis*, *Cochliomyia hominivorax*, *Rhinoestrus purpureus*, and *Gedoelstia cristata*.[529–534] The rodent botfly maggot *Cuterebra* (Figure 10.35, J and K) and *Hypoderma* are probably responsible for most cases of ophthalmomyiasis interna in the United States.[531–533,535,536] The eggs or larvae may be transported to the human corneal or conjunctival surface by the adult fly, by a secondary vector such as a tick or mosquito, or by the patient's hands. Most patients give no history of being struck in the eye by a fly. The maggots may either remain in the periocular tissues (ophthalmomyiasis externa),[537–540] or bore their way through the ocular coats and come to lie in the anterior chamber, posterior chamber, or subretinal space (Figures 10.35 and 10.36).[531,532,534,541–555]

The reaction of the eye to the larval invasion varies. Signs of inflammation usually develop only after the death of the maggot. In some cases the maggot gains entrance into the subretinal space and over a period of months makes many excursions back and forth across the breadth of the fundus, creating an unusual pattern of

10.36 *Ophthalmomyiasis interna.*

A to **G**: This 40-year-old asymptomatic man was seen for a routine eye examination for glasses. The left fundus has several crisscross tracks made by a botfly larva that is visible along the inferotemporal vessels (A–E). Note the movement of the larva with change in its head position. By the time the patient returned after photographs, the larva had moved to the superotemporal quadrant where it was photocoagulated using argon green laser (F). A composite picture showing extensive excursions of the larva throughout the fundus without causing many symptoms (G). There are two dot hemorrhages on the disc.
H: Time-lapse composite photographs showing movement of a maggot (*arrow*) in the subretinal space. This worm was destroyed with photocoagulation without causing significant intraocular inflammation.
I: A composite photograph of an asymptomatic patient who was seen for glasses. His visual acuity was 20/20. Note the extensive pattern of subretinal tracks and the clumps of pigmentation temporal to the macula and surrounding the optic disc (*arrows*). No maggot was visible in the eye. The patient was seen again several years later, and the visual function and fundi were unchanged.

Subretinal tracks in Lytico-Bodig.

J and **K**: Subretinal tracks (J and K) presumed to have been caused by a fly maggot in two Chomoro Indians from Guam. Note the 'dead-end' track (*arrow*, J).
L: Histopathology of a track observed clinically in a Chomoro Indian shows hypopigmentation of the pigment epithelium (between the arrows), a few subretinal pigment-laden macrophages, and some thickening of Bruch's membrane.

(Courtesy: A–G, Dr Juan Astruc; H, Dr Constance R. Fitzgerald; I from Gass and Lewis[552], J and K, courtesy Dr S.D. Thomas Hanlon.)

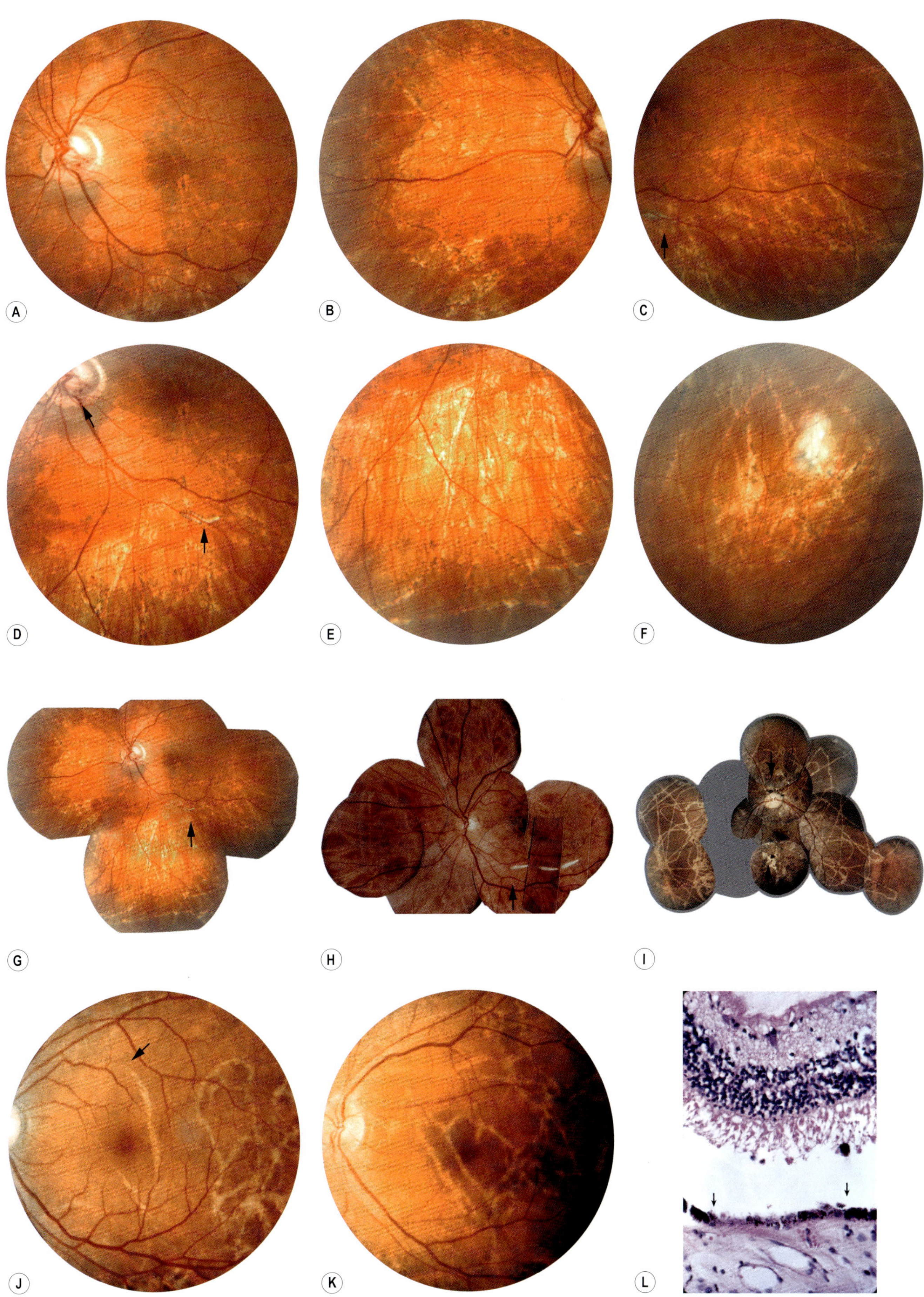
A
B
C
D
E
F
G
H
I
J
K
L

crosshatching or 'railroad' tracks in the RPE (Figures 10.35 and 10.36).[532,550,552,555a] During its entrance through the sclera and choroid and its course beneath the retina it may cause one or more small subretinal hemorrhages (see Figure 7.16, D–F). In some cases it exits from the eye without causing any symptoms, despite widespread damage to the RPE in the macular area (Figures 10.35, A–C; 10.36, A and B).[552,556] In one case a *Cuterebra* maggot was found in the conjunctiva of a boy who presented with a subconjunctival and a subretinal hemorrhage and tracks.[556] In some cases the maggot may die in the subretinal space and cause a localized toxic reaction and a scar. In other cases it may enter the vitreous cavity, where usually it dies soon afterward, probably from lack of nutrition. The inflammatory reaction that follows varies from a minimal vitritis to an intense endophthalmitis. The caliber of the retinal vessels and the color of the optic nerve head are usually unaffected; however, optic atrophy and visual loss may occur in a few cases (Figure 10.35, G).[548] Invasion of the cornea has occurred.[557] Only rarely are both eyes affected, and this occurred in a patient from Guam[542] (see discussion of Lytico-Bodig after this section).

Linear and arcuate tracks in the ocular fundus should always suggest the possibility of ophthalmomyiasis. The tracks are less numerous and more easily recognized in the peripheral fundus. In the posterior pole the tracks may be so numerous that their confluence may be mistaken for a variety of diffuse inflammatory, traumatic, or degenerative diseases affecting the RPE (Figures 10.35, A; 10.36, A and B). In such cases fluorescein angiography is especially valuable in silhouetting the tracks (Figure 10.35, B and C). Although other organisms such as *Toxocara canis* (the nematodes responsible for diffuse unilateral subacute neuro-retinitis) and trematodes may migrate into the subretinal space, they do not produce the widespread pattern of broad RPE tracks that are believed to be pathognomonic for myiasis. The transverse rings that are present on its body leave a characteristic track with crosshatchings The curvilinear depigmented bands or bead-like arrangement of atrophic chorioretinal scars that may occur, usually at the equator in the presumed ocular histoplasmosis syndrome (POHS) and pseudo-POHS, may be mistaken for the tracks in myiasis.[555] The author has seen two patients with an extensive network of subretinal fibrous strands and demarcation lines following spontaneous reattachment of a chronic rhegmatogenous retinal detachment incorrectly diagnosed as myiasis. A positive clinical diagnosis of ophthalmo-myiasis can be made only with visualization of the white or semitranslucent segmented maggot, tapered slightly at both ends (Figures 10.35, D–F; 10.36, A and D–I).

In the presence of significant intraocular inflammation, the initial treatment of intraocular myiasis should be directed toward the reduction of inflammation with the use of corticosteroids. If inflammation cannot be controlled, surgical removal of the maggot is indicated. If the maggot is alive and the eye is free of inflammation, the clinician may elect to observe the patient carefully for spontaneous exit of the maggot from the eye. If treatment of a subretinal maggot is elected, photocoagulation is probably preferable to removal of the organism by sclerotomy (Figure 10.36, F). The maggot should be watched until it moves beyond the macular and juxtapapillary area before photocoagulation treatment is begun. In three patients treated with photocoagulation, no unusual inflammatory reaction occurred.[550,551]

10.37 Lytico-Bodig.

A to **C**: This 43-year-old Guamian gentleman with Chomoro ancestry migrated to the United States at age 28. On an examination for possible welder's flash burn he was found to have tracks in his left eye. His vision was 20/20 OU. The right fundus was normal. The left eye showed subretinal tracks, some of which were dead-end tracks, throughout the posterior pole. No larva was visible. He had grown up near a beach in Guam and had reared cows, goats, and chickens. He did not recall an episode of visual loss or being bitten by an insect. He had no evidence of neurological disease or dementia.

***Ophthalmomyiasis interna* (Gedoelstia cristata).**

D to **G**: A 21-year-old gardener presented in Namibia, Africa, with severe pain and redness in his right eye that began as soon as a fly hovering in front of him darted into his right eye. He had proptosis, conjunctival hemorrhage, and chemosis, and limitation of eye movements in all directions (D). His visual acuity was hand motions. The right fundus had a large serous retinal detachment and areas of retinal whitening (E). He was treated with systemic steroids. The orbital cellulitis and serous detachment slowly improved over a few weeks with visible subretinal yellow curvilinear lines (F). Further resolution of the subretinal fluid clearly shows the subretinal tracks of the larvae (G). No larva(e) was visible and the patient's vision improved to 20/20.

H to **J**: This 29-year-old man was seen in Namibia 24 h after a gray fly hovered in front of his eye and flew into it. This was followed immediately by significant pain. He had conjunctival hemorrhage, chemosis, injection, and limitation of elevation (H). The following day he developed severe orbital pain with vomiting, 5 mm proptosis, and an intraocular pressure elevation to 40 mmHg. He was afebrile. He developed progressive exudative retinal detachment over the next few days (I). There were subretinal white dots and progressive linear marks suggestive of tracks (*arrows, J*) and one site of subretinal and epiretinal hemorrhage (not seen in the picture). He was treated with systemic steroids, ivermectin, and pressure-lowering medications. An MRI of the brain and orbit was normal except for proptosis. His clinical picture and serous retinal detachment resolved over the next couple of weeks and vision returned to 20/20. Curvilinear tracks and white dots remained (*arrows J*); no larva was seen.

(Courtesy: D to J Dr L.S. Petrick; and Dr Jannes Brandt.)

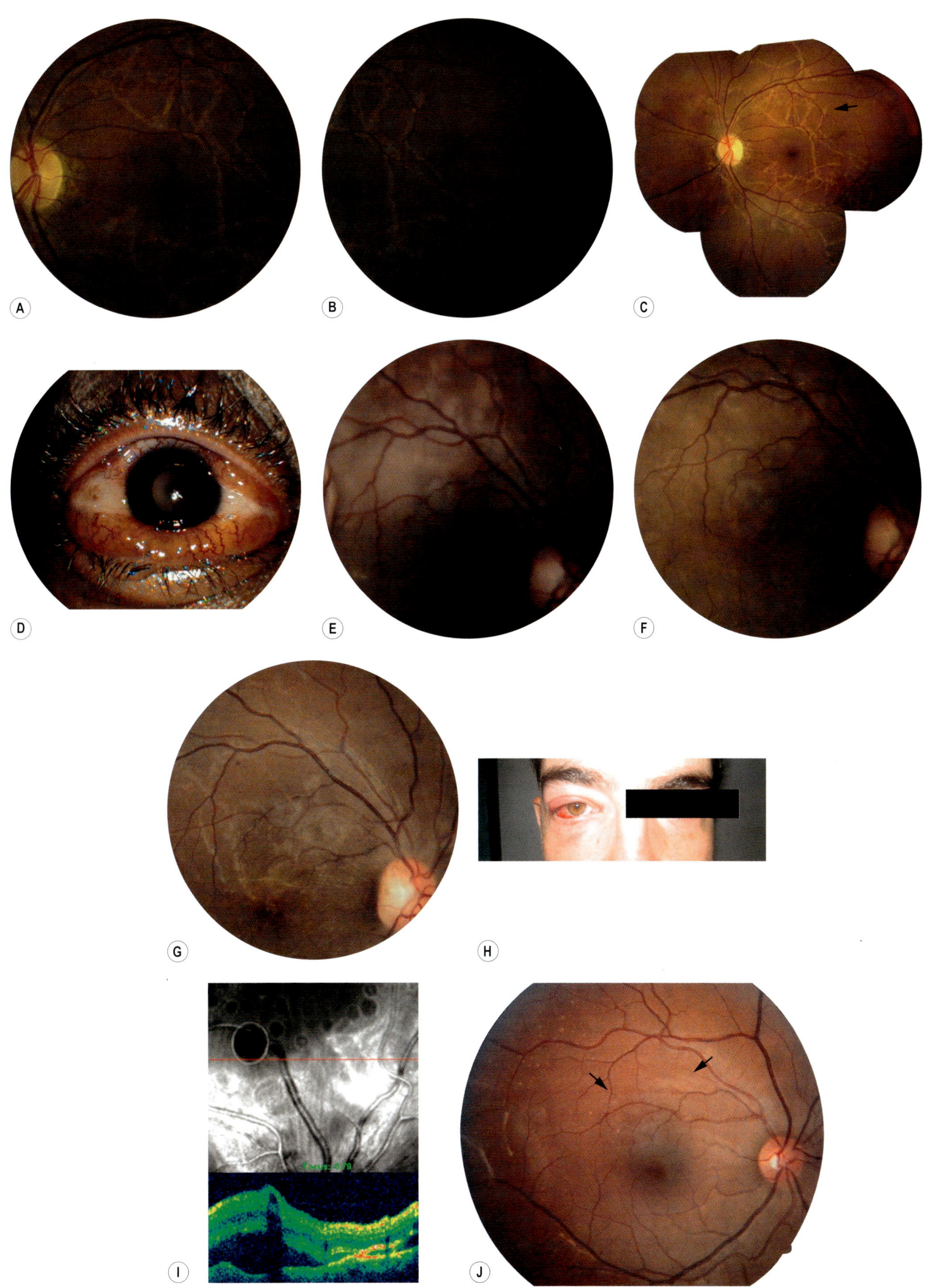
A
B
C
D
E
F
G
H
I
J

Schistosomiasis

Trematodes that inhabit the blood vessels of humans are referred to as schistosomes. Dickinson and coworkers reported a unique case of eccentric multifocal choroiditis that resembled acute posterior multifocal placoid pigment epitheliopathy and serpiginous choroiditis in a 17-year-old man with visual loss and an itchy rash on his forehead of 2 weeks' duration. He had recently returned from Tanzania.[564] Histologic examination of the skin lesions revealed ova of *Schistosoma mansoni.* Other cases of *Schistosoma* causing subretinal granuloma,[568–570] subconjunctival nodules, and intraocular granuloma have been reported.[568,569]

Fasciola Hepatica (Liver Fluke)

Fasciola hepatica is a zoonotic helminth seen in sheep-raising countries. Reports of human infestation vary from 2.4 million to 17 million. At least three cases of intraocular *F. hepatica* associated with significant intraocular inflammation have been seen.[563] The patient presented with pain, redness, and loss of vision of 10 days' duration in the Caspian sea region. The anterior chamber showed bloody hypopyon and the anterior vitreous was full of debris. A flatworm was seen moving in the anterior chamber. Washout of the anterior chamber followed by lensectomy and vitrectomy revealed an immature *F. hepatica*. There was patchy retinal whitening, vitritis, and vitreous hemorrhage. Once the worm was removed and the debris cleared, the eye quietened with improvement in vision to 20/200.

10.38 Continued

F to **I**: Vitritis and periphlebitis caused by a subretinal trematode in a healthy 38-year-old Asian man complaining of visual loss in the left eye. His visual acuity was 4/200. Following treatment with sub-Tenon's capsular corticosteroids his vision improved and irregular pigmentary tracks became evident (F). Twenty-one months after recurrent episodes of vitreous inflammation, a motile trematode (*arrow*, H) that was encysted was found in the vitreous (H) and was removed via pars plana vitrectomy. The trematode was identified as *Alaria mesocercaria* (I). Note the oral sucker (*left arrow*), ventral sucker (*right arrow*), and penetration glands (*P*). The patient's visual acuity returned to 20/50.
J and **K**: A 10-year-old boy from a village in South India presented with redness and a white lesion in his right eye for 3 months. A white granuloma that was partly gliotic and partly vascular was seen in the anterior chamber of the right eye, consistent with a clinical diagnosis of trematode granuloma.

(A–I from McDonald et al.[566]. J and K, courtesy of Dr. S.R. Rathinam.)

The eggs or metacercariae are ingested with uncooked watercress or other aquatic plants. The metacercariae excyst in the duodenum and migrate through the intestinal wall, enter the liver and make their way into the biliary ducts to grow into maturity. Occasionally the metacercariae enter the blood vessels and travel to other organs, and can enter the eye.

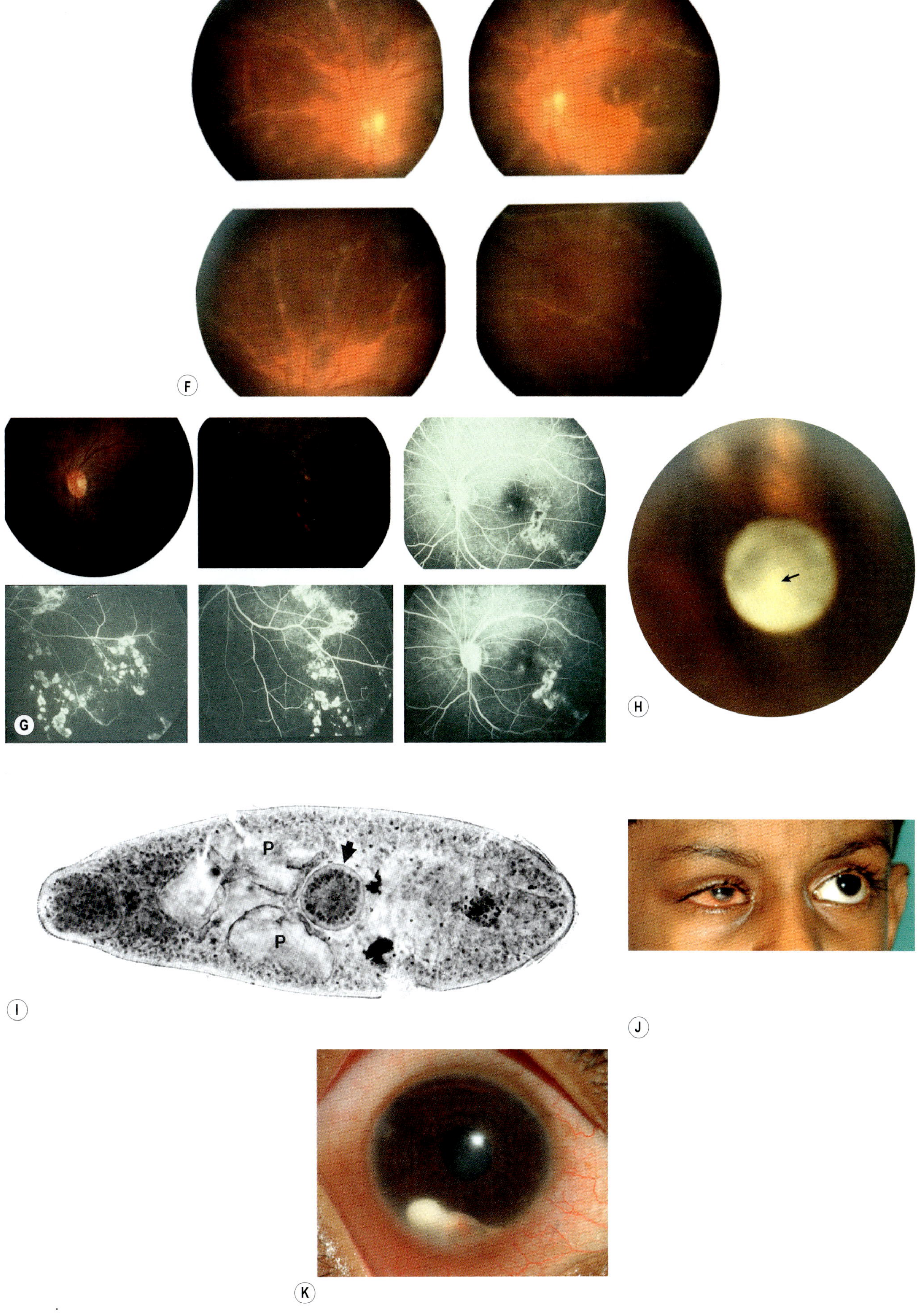
F
G
H
P
P
I
J
K

Trematodes in South India

Rathinam and coworkers reported a series (41 patients) of mostly young males aged 16 or younger (38 boys and 3 girls) with conjunctival allergic granulomas, occasionally with anterior chamber inflammatory granuloma (Figure 10.38, J and K). Thirty-four of the patients were from a single village. Surgical excision of 13 granulomas revealed a zonal granulomatous inflammation admixed with eosinophilic leukocytes in nine; four of the nine displayed fragments of the tegument and internal structures of a trematode and Splendore–Hoeppli phenomenon (central deposit of granular, acellular eosinophilic material surrounded by eosinophilic leukocytes, epithelioid cells, histiocytes, and lymphocytes in response to foreign material such as caterpillar hairs, tarantula hairs, synthetic fibers, etc.). The remaining five revealed nongranulomatous inflammation made up of lymphocytes, histiocytes, and eosinophils. These children bathed or swam in the local village pond and acquired the infection. The trematode is likely *Philophthalmus* which has three intermediate hosts: mollusks, snails, and frogs. The infected birds lay eggs in the water, the eggs hatch in the water to miracidia that enter the mollusks and snails where they grow into cercariae.[571–573] Children swimming in the ponds infested with these mollusks acquire the infection. Treatment is surgical excision of the granuloma if in the subconjunctival space; intraocular granuloma may require topical steroids and surgical excision. Prevention by avoiding swimming in trematode-infested ponds is likely the most effective method of controlling this infection.

RETINOPATHY ASSOCIATED WITH RICKETTSIAL DISEASES

Rickettsial agents are classified into three major categories: the spotted fever group, the typhus group, and the other diseases group.

Rocky Mountain spotted fever (RMSF) is an acute febrile eczematous disease caused by *Rickettsia rickettsii*, a gram-negative bacterium transmitted by the wood and dog tick. It is not confined to the Rocky Mountain area, with nearly half of the cases occurring in the south Atlantic states.[574] Patients present with fever, headache, and a maculopapular or petechial rash on the extremities that spreads centripetally to involve the torso. The overall mortality rate is between 3% and 8%, indicating the need for prompt diagnosis and treatment with tetracycline or chloramphenicol. Ocular findings that may accompany the acute illness include petechial lesions on the bulbar conjunctiva, conjunctivitis, anterior uveitis, papilledema, retinal venous engorgement, cytoid bodies, retinal hemorrhages, and retinal vascular occlusion (Figure 10.39, A–C and E–H).[575–580] Fluorescein angiography shows evidence of capillary nonperfusion in the region of the cotton-wool patches, leakage of dye from the retinal vessels in the vicinity of the patches, and evidence of venous obstruction (Figure 10.39, B, C, and G). In exanthematous cutaneous lesions, the organisms invade the nuclei of the capillary endothelial cells, proliferate, and destroy the capillary endothelial cells. Necrosis of the intima and media causes thrombosis and microinfarcts. It is probable that the pathogenesis of the retinal vascular changes is similar. The fundus findings usually, but not always, resolve without causing visual loss following treatment of the disease with antibiotics such as chloramphenicol and tetracycline. The illustrated patient progressed to no light perception since the diagnosis was not suspected until very late and no specific treatment was given.

Similar fundus findings have been reported in other rickettsial diseases, including endemic typhus.[581–584]

The clinical suspicion can be confirmed by serologic testing for RMSF. Other organ system involvement can include hepatomegaly, renal failure, disseminated intravascular coagulation, shock, seizures, fluctuating neurologic status, coma, and death. A majority of cases occur in children due to exposure to outdoor recreational activities and affinity to dogs, and in hunters. In fact, most internists order Lyme and Rickettsial titers in cases of suspected tick bite.

10.39 Rocky Mountain spotted fever (*Rickettsia rickettsii*).

A to **I**: This 55-year-old man had a rapid decline in vision to 20/200 in his left eye. He had no light perception in his right eye for 5 years following a retinal detachment. He had a chorioretinitis with serous retinal detachment involving the left macula (A). An early phase angiogram showed good retinal perfusion and pooling of dye in the late phase (B and C). The OCT confirmed the serous elevation (D). He had a normal complete blood count, HIV test was negative, and PCR for *Herpes zoster*, *Herpes simplex*, and *Cytomegalovirus* was negative. An infectious disease consultation did not yield any clues. His vision loss continued and the lesion progressed to involve the entire fundus with diffuse retinal vascular obstruction and choroidal effusion (E–I). The vision dropped to no light perception. His family doctor ordered a *Rickettsia* titer when he discovered that the patient had been hunting prior to the onset of visual symptoms, which returned positive.

(Courtesy: Dr Gaurav Shah. G and H, Also, Yannuzzi, Lawrence J., The Retinal Atlas, Saunders 2010, 978-0-7020-3320-9, p.362.)

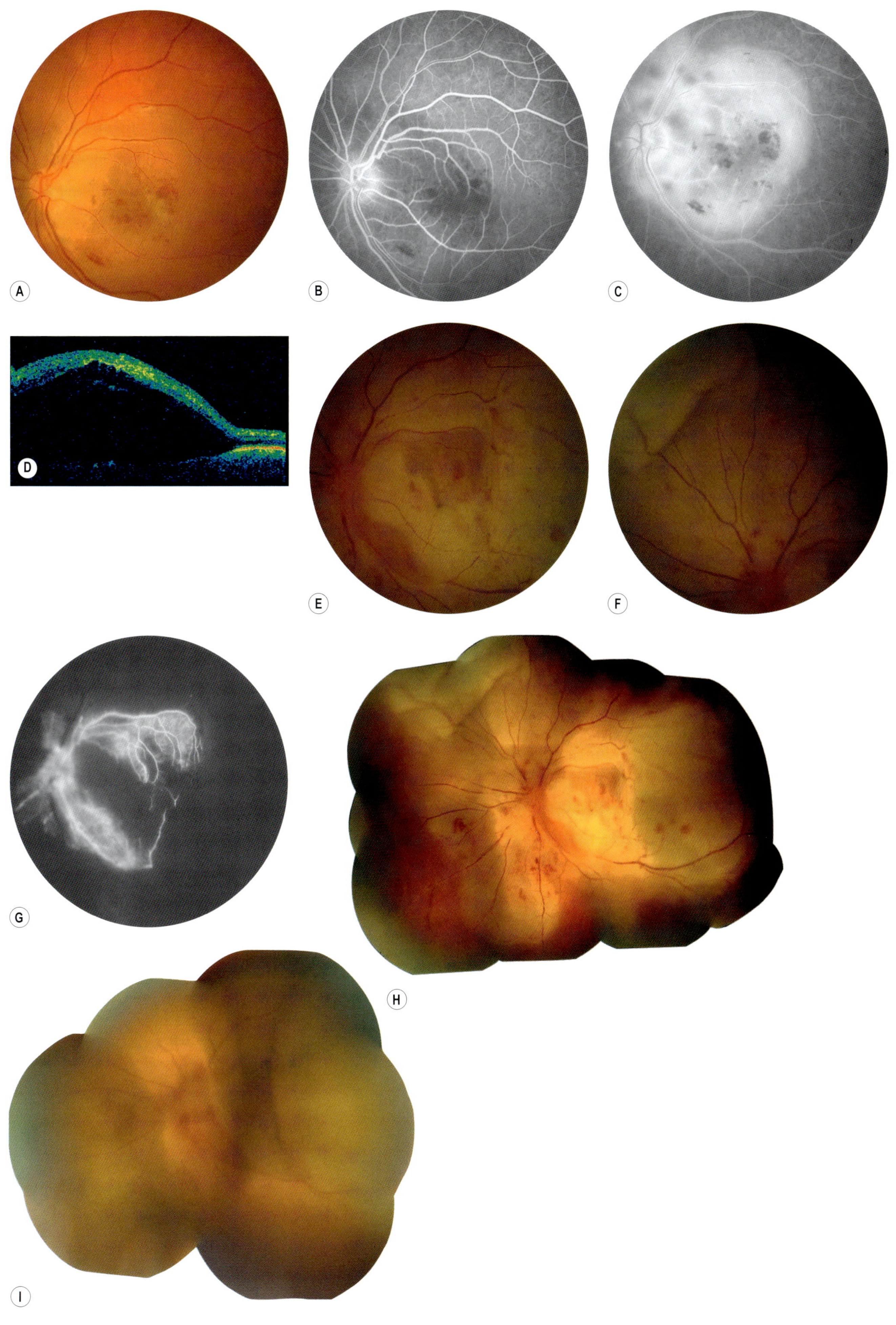

Rickettsia Conorii (Mediterranean Spotted Fever, MSF)

Rickettsia conorii is endemic in Mediterranean countries. It is transmitted by a dog tick *Rhipicephalus sanguineus*. Systemic signs are similar to RMSF with fever, headache, and a maculopapular rash that can involve the palms and soles. In one series of 30 patients (60 eyes) with serologically proven MSF, 80% showed chorioretinal involvement associated with mild vitritis. One-third of patients showed changes only on a fluorescein angiogram. Common findings were retinal hemorrhages and retinal vasculitis involving the vessels on the disc, posterior pole or periphery (Figure 10.40, A and E). Other findings were branch retinal artery occlusion, cystoid macular edema, arteriolar plaques similar to Kyrieleis arteritis seen in *Toxoplasma*, and serous retinal detachment in one eye each. The pathogenic hallmark is the invasion of the vascular endothelial cells by the organism, causing endothelial injury and necrosis (Figure 10.40, B).

Treatment involves early institution of oral tetracyclines in the form of doxycycline; fluoroquinolones and clarithromycin can be used if tetracyclines are contraindicated.

VIRAL DISEASES

Cytomegalovirus Retinochoroiditis and Optic Neuritis

Although as many as 81% of adults have complement fixation antibodies indicating previous exposure to cytomegalovirus (CMV), manifest disease is rare in otherwise healthy individuals and occurs primarily in the unborn infant and the immunosuppressed patient.[585–588]

Congenital CMV Infection

Cytomegalovirus is the commonest of all congenital and perinatal viral infections and occurs in 0.2–2.4% of all live births. The fetus may acquire the infection as a consequence of primary (40%) or recurrent (1%) maternal infection. The incidence is higher in lower socioeconomic groups. Fortunately, only 10% of the children are symptomatic. Prematurity, microcephaly, intracranial calcification (periventricular), increased CSF protein, chorioretinitis, optic atrophy, petechiae, jaundice, hearing impairment, hepatosplenomegaly, anemia, and thrombocytopenia constitute the clinical features.[589–591] The virus is shed in nasopharyngeal secretions, urine, saliva, cervical secretions, and breast milk for 2–5 years and is the means to demonstrate active infection. Most often the chorioretinitis is inactive since the children are immunocompetent. However, active retinitis should be treated with systemic ganciclovir until the lesions become inactive.[591]

10.40 Mediterranean spotted fever (*Rickettsia conorii* retinitis).

A to **D**: A 20-year-old man in Tunisia with a 3-week history of fever and skin rash complained of decreased vision in the left eye of 5 days' duration. Visual acuity was 20/20 (right eye) and 20/200 (left eye). The anterior segment in both eyes, and fundus of the right eye were unremarkable. There were 2 + vitreous cells in the left eye. The fundus of the left eye showed a superomacular focus of retinitis associated with retinal hemorrhages, optic disc edema, and hard exudates in a macular star configuration (A). Late-phase fluorescein angiogram of the left eye shows hyperfluorescence of the focus of retinitis, diffuse retinal vascular leakage, blockage of choroidal fluorescence by retinal hemorrhages, and optic disc staining (B). Optical coherence tomography shows hyperreflectivity of the focus of retinitis and a serous retinal detachment extending to the fovea (C). A diagnosis of Mediterranean spotted fever was confirmed by positive serologic testing (antibodies to *Rickettsia conorii* by indirect immunofluorescence). The patient was treated with doxycycline 200 mg per day and prednisone 1 mg/kg per day with gradual taper over a period of 4 weeks. Visual acuity improved gradually. Four months after presentation, visual acuity was 20/25 in the left eye. Fundus shows healing of the retinitis without scar formation, and resolution of associated findings (D).
E to **I**: A 57-year-old woman in Tunisia with a 1-week history of fever, headache, malaise, and lymphocytic meningitis complained of floaters in both eyes. Visual acuity was 20/20 in both eyes. The right fundus shows two small white retinal lesions juxtavascular in location (*arrows*), with associated retinal hemorrhages (E). Late-phase fluorescein angiography shows faint leakage of dye from the superotemporal vein and optic disc staining. Note the presence of an area of old RPE alteration inferonasal to the macula (F). Late-phase indocyanine green (ICG) angiography shows multiple small hypofluorescent dots (*arrows*) (G). Note the hypofluorescence of the area of old RPE alteration. The ocular findings were suggestive of a diagnosis of a rickettsial disease. Serologic testing confirmed the diagnosis of acute murine typhus, a rickettsial infection caused by *Rickettsia typhi*. The patient was treated with oral tetracyclines for 2 weeks. Two months later, fundus (H) and fluorescein and ICG (I) angiographic findings related to murine typhus had resolved.

(Courtesy: Dr Moncef Khairallah.)

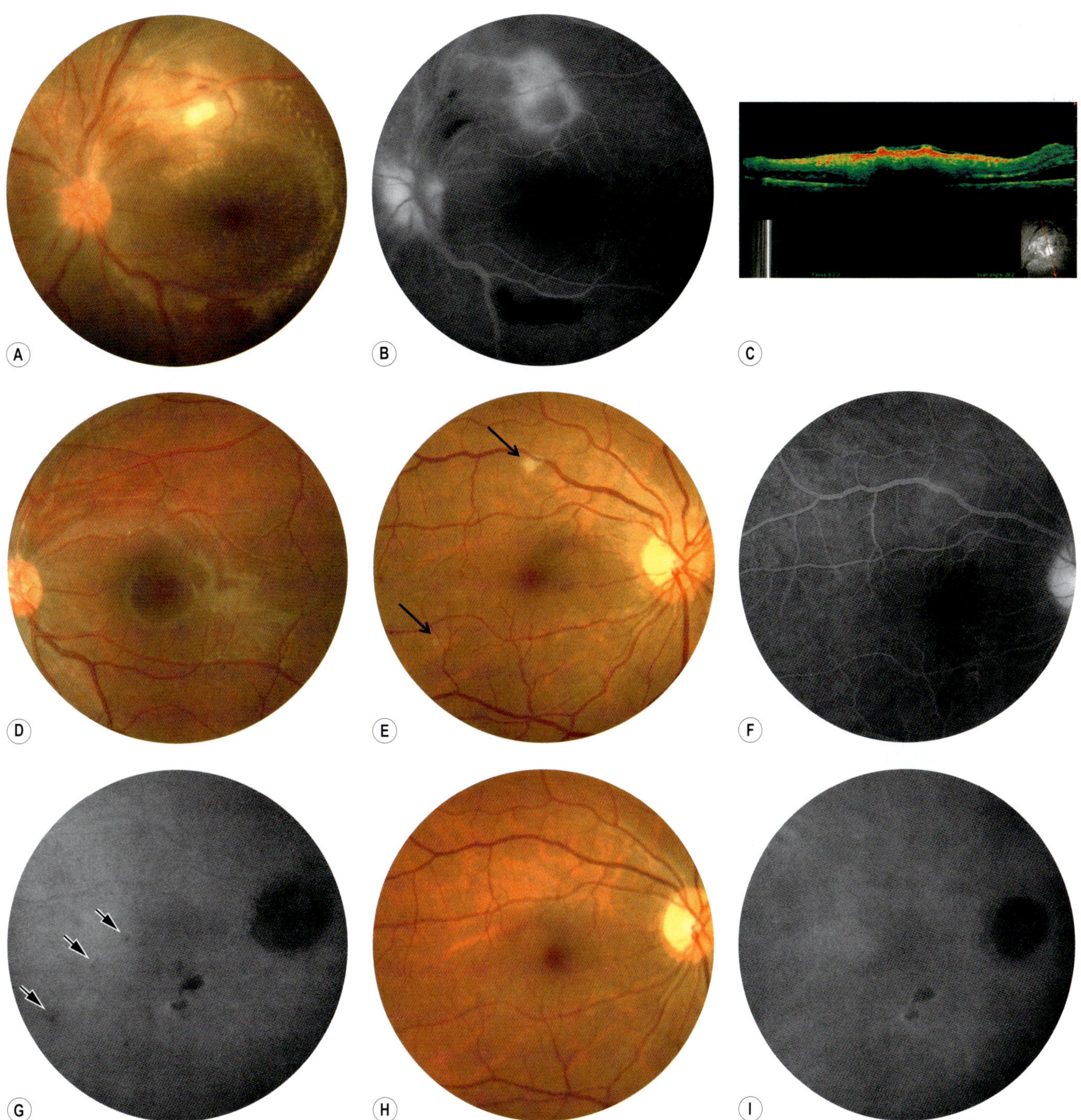
A
B
C
D
E
F
G
H
I

Postnatally acquired infections occur most commonly in immunosuppressed individuals with the acquired immune deficiency syndrome (AIDS; see p. 806), renal allografts, or systemic malignancies or while receiving high-dose corticosteroids. Approximately 30% of patients with AIDS will develop CMV retinitis.[589,592] Cytomegalovirus retinitis is the first manifestation of AIDS in approximately 2% of patients and results in the initial diagnosis of AIDS in approximately 15% of patients.[593,594] Survival after the diagnosis of AIDS may be significantly shorter if CMV retinopathy is the initial manifestation of syndrome.[595,596] The ophthalmoscopic features of the acute stage of necrotizing retinitis include multiple, granular, yellow–white areas that become confluent and are associated with retinal hemorrhages, vascular sheathing, and sharp margins separating the active area of necrotizing retinitis from the surrounding retina (Figure 10.41, A and D–G). The fundoscopic appearance has been likened to that of pizza. The segmental distribution of the hemorrhagic lesions along major retinal vessels may be mistaken for branch vein occlusion.[597] Cytomegalovirus retinitis infrequently begins in the central macular area.[588,598–600] The retinitis spreads much like a brush fire, leaving an atrophic retina and a mottled RPE along its trailing edges (Figure 10.41, P–R). Vitreous cells may or may not accompany the retinitis. Cytomegalovirus retinitis infrequently poses an immediate threat to loss of vision on presentation.[588,599,600] It is a slowly progressive, necrotizing retinitis that appears in either a fulminant hemorrhagic or granular pattern. As the infection progresses, the leading edge of the infection is followed by a healing process that results in a thin fibroglial scar. Small refractile deposits and larger yellow–white plaque-like deposits occur within areas of healed CMV retinitis. These large plaques do not appear calcified or refractile, yet histologically these fibroglial scars may be highly calcified (Figure 10.41, P–R).[601–604] Early spontaneous resolution of CMV retinitis may account for chorioretinal scars found on initial examination of patients with AIDS.[604]

Infection of the optic disc and juxtapapillary retina is often associated with severe visual loss (Figure 10.41, D and E).[605,606] In some cases involvement of the optic disc and juxtapapillary retina causes visual loss as the result of intraretinal exudation and macular star formation and with exudative macular detachment (Figure 10.41, E).[607,608] Patients with low CD4 + counts, usually less than 100, are at increased risk for developing CMV retinitis and HIV-related noninfectious retinal vasculopathy.[600,601] Fluorescein angiography demonstrates evidence of retinal vascular occlusion and permeability alterations in the areas of hemorrhagic and necrotizing retinitis (Figure 10.41, B and C).

Severe sheathing of the retinal vessels appearing like frosted branches of a tree, simulating that occurring in idiopathic frosted retinal periphlebitis, may accompany CMV retinitis (Figure 10.41, G–I).[595,609–612] This may be associated with signs of vitreous and anterior chamber inflammation. Fluorescein angiography shows no occlusion or stasis but does demonstrate late leakage from the sheathed vessels. This perivasculitis usually clears within several weeks after antiviral treatment.[610,613] Corticosteroids may not be necessary.[607,613] The CMV retinitis, however, often continues to show evidence of graying along its margin (Figure 10.41, P–R and T). This smoldering retinitis may extend slowly and is a sign of persistent activity. Cystoid macular edema occurs infrequently in patients with AIDS (Figure 10.41, X), particularly in those with less severe states of immunosuppression.

Disc neovascularization may develop in patients with CMV retinitis, and it may regress spontaneously.[614] Exudative and rhegmatogenous retinal detachment (Figure 10.41, L) may complicate CMV retinitis.[594,607,615–619] Approximately 15–30% of patients with CMV retinitis develop a rhegmatogenous retinal detachment. The differential diagnosis may be difficult because small or ragged holes may be difficult to visualize.[599,620] Patients with chronic vitritis may lose central vision because of cystoid macular edema.

Histopathologically, the areas of active retinitis are sharply circumscribed from the normal-appearing retina.[594,621,622] The retina is thickened, and its laminar architecture is markedly disrupted by the presence of many enlarged cells containing prominent Cowdry type A intranuclear eosinophilic inclusions with surrounding clear zones (Figure 10.41, J), giving the cells an owl's-eye

10.41 Cytomegalovirus (CMV) retinitis in patients receiving corticosteroid and antimetabolite therapy following renal transplantation.

A to **C**: This 35-year-old woman noted paracentral scotomata in both eyes. In the right eye she had an active wedge-shaped area of retinitis associated with hemorrhages and perivascular cuffing (A). In the left eye she had large geographic areas of chorioretinal scarring at sites of previous retinitis. Angiography of the area illustrated in A revealed widespread collapse of the retinal vascular bed in the area of acute retinitis, and multiple focal areas of staining within the lesion (B and C). Eleven years later, visual acuity in the right eye was 20/200. She had extensive peripheral chorioretinal scarring, vitritis, and cystoid macular edema. The left eye had a dense cataract, and visual acuity was only light perception.

Cytomegalovirus (CMV) retinitis in patients with AIDS.

D to **F**: Progressive CMV retinitis and optic neuritis occurring over a 2-month period. Note the extensive exudation into the macular area (D) 1 month after the photograph in E, and evidence of early resolution of the retinitis after ganciclovir treatment in F.

G to **I**: Frosted branch angiopathy accompanying CMV retinitis. The perivenous exudation is continuous along the venous wall and is different from the periarteriolar plaques seen in acute retinal necrosis, where the plaques are discontinuous and are on the arterioles (see Figure 10.44, B and E).

J and **K**: Thickened retina in which the normal retinal elements are replaced by extensive infiltration of large mononuclear cells containing prominent intranuclear and intracytoplasmic inclusions. Intranuclear inclusions (owl eyes) are seen in the retinal cells (K1) and within the RPE (K2).

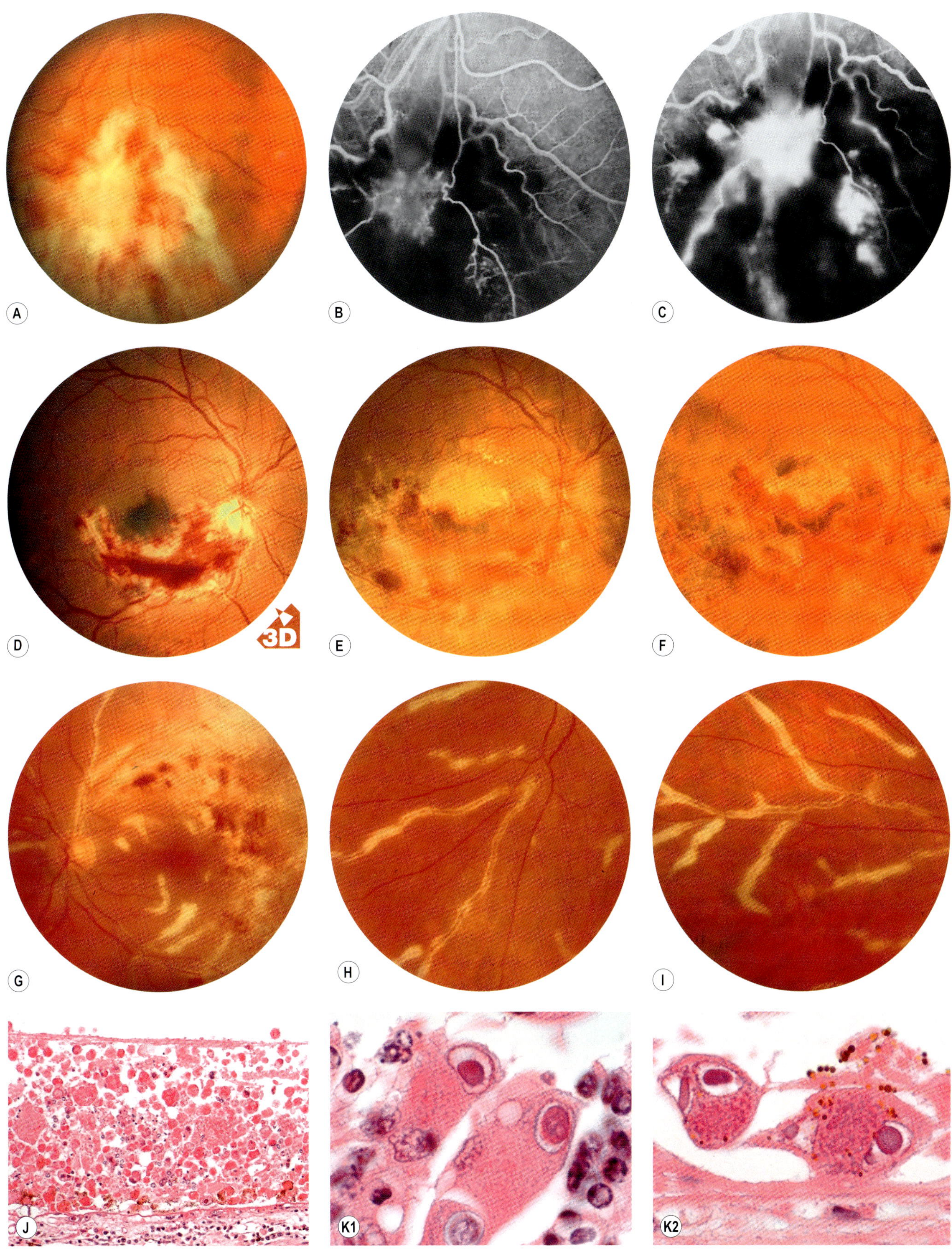
A
B
C
D
3D
E
F
G
H
I
J
K1
K2

appearance (Figure 10.41, K1 and K2). The underlying RPE is typically disrupted and varying degrees of chronic inflammatory cells are present in the underlying choroid. Intranuclear inclusions may be identified in RPE, optic nerve, and vascular endothelial cells of the choroid. Electron microscopy demonstrates viral particles typical of the DNA viruses as well as prominent electron-dense cytoplasmic bodies.[623,624]

The clinical diagnosis is made by demonstrating virus in the patient's urine and by a rise in complement fixation and neutralization titers. The virus can be cultured from the anterior chamber in eyes with hypopyon,[606,625–627] saliva, buffy coat of the blood, tears,[628,629] vitreous, and the retina.[608,614,623,630] Polymerase chain reaction for CMV in aqueous and vitreous fluid can be used to aid diagnosis in atypical cases.

Dual infection of the retina with human immunodeficiency virus type 1 (HIV-1) and CMV occurs but its role in producing fundus changes or in the enhancement of other infections is uncertain.[631–634] Autopsy studies of patients with AIDS have shown evidence suggesting that bilateral CMV retinitis may be a marker for HIV encephalitis.[631,633] These studies have failed to demonstrate evidence that HIV is a cause for cotton-wool patches.

Ganciclovir is the treatment of choice in patients with CMV retinitis,[588,589,592,595,614,620,634–637] 80–90% of whom will demonstrate evidence of prompt resolution of the retinitis following induction dosages of IV ganciclovir. Those with visual loss associated with exudative detachment often experience improvement in visual acuity.[607,608] Prior to the availability of highly active antiretroviral therapy (HAART), 30–50% of patients reactivated while on maintenance treatment.[585,625,634,636] Ganciclovir is a viral static drug that does not eliminate the virus or suppress expression of all virus genes.[616,638] It appears to function by limiting viral DNA synthesis and subsequent packaging of viral DNA into infectious units.[616,638] There is also evidence that decreasing the amount of corticosteroid therapy has a favorable effect on CMV retinitis in cases other than AIDS. Approximately 33% of patients with AIDS receiving ganciclovir for CMV retinitis in the past demonstrated evidence of persistent smoldering retinitis, that is, graying along margins of the zones of retinitis. The smoldering retinitis may slowly extend without evidence of other activity seen in the retina (Figure 10.41, P–R). In some cases, however, this persistent gray border may not progress and biopsy of such lesions has shown no evidence of viral particles.[639,640] Since the widespread use of antiretroviral therapy, this is mostly seen in developing countries where HAART is not universally available. Fundus photographs and visual fields are helpful in detecting evidence of progression.[588,595,596,599,641,642]

10.41 Continued

L: Rhegmatogenous retinal detachment occurring from small breaks in the area of inactive retinitis.

M to **R**: A 44-year-old poorly compliant man with cotton-wool spots from HIV retinopathy in both eyes (M and N) developed bilateral CMV retinitis 8 months later. Further spread and partial resolution of CMV retinitis in both eyes occurred over the next 8 months.

S to **U**: This 52-year-old woman with leukemia developed a patch of retinitis (S). She received systemic ganciclovir followed by placement of a ganciclovir implant (U). The retinitis healed with residual pigmented and gliotic scar.

V to **X**: An 18-year-old girl with acute lymphocytic leukemia developed CMV antigenemia. She was treated with oral valganciclovir for a few months and switched to aciclovir. Four months later she presented with floaters in both eyes. Smoldering CMV retinitis with some healed areas were noted in both eyes. She was in remission and was off chemotherapy for the leukemia. Visual acuity was 20/20 in each eye. She received IV ganciclovir followed by oral valganciclovir. The lesions became less active (V) and eventually resolved with residual pigmentary changes. Autofluorescence imaging shows pigment epithelial loss nasally in the left eye (W). Subsequently bilateral ganciclovir implants were placed. 6 months later she developed vitreous cells and cystoid macular edema (CME) in her left eye with decrease in vision to the 20/80 level. A fluorescein angiogram showed petalloid pooling of dye in the fovea (X). Topical prednisone acetate four times a day over 3 months resulted in resolution of vitreous cells and CME due to immune recovery uveitis with restoration of vision to 20/40. She had a central posterior subcapsular cataract accounting for the 20/40 visual acuity.

(J and K, courtesy Dr Ralph Eagle.)

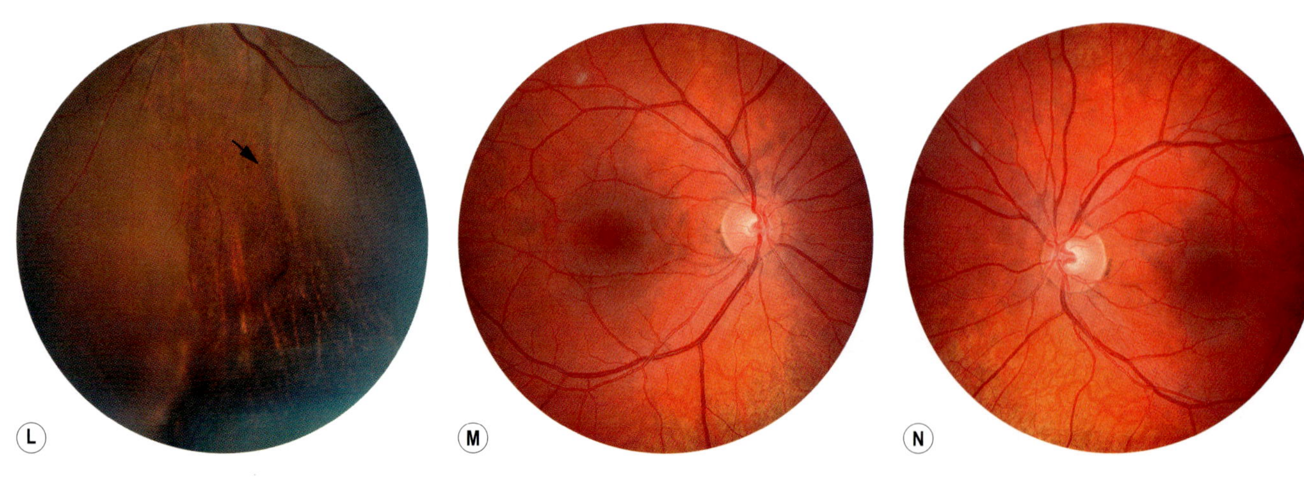

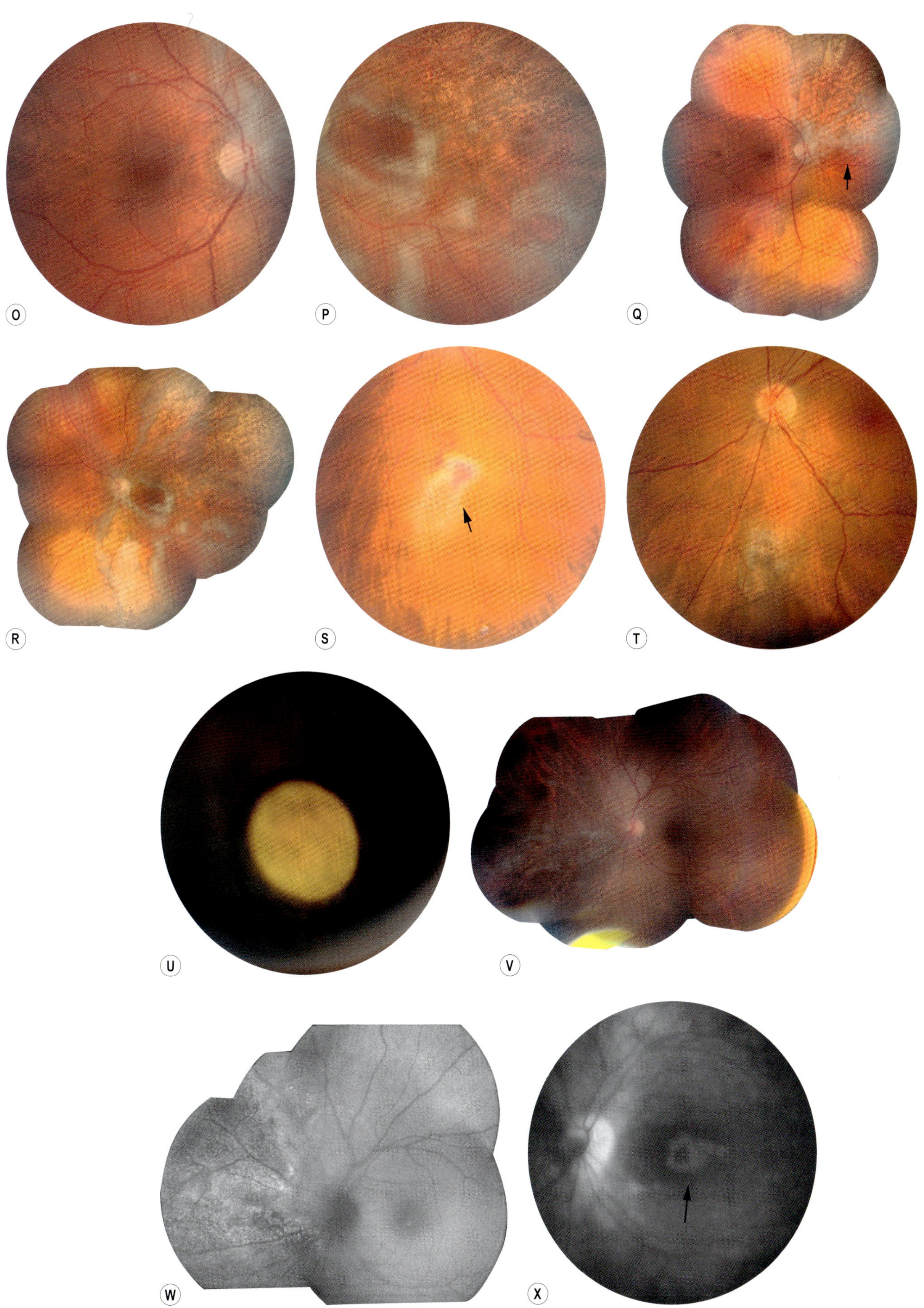
O
P
Q
R
S
T
U
V
W
X

Intravitreal administration of ganciclovir appears to be a safe and effective alternative in the management of CMV retinitis in patients with AIDS.[592,635,643,644] It is particularly useful in patients with severe neutropenia or as an adjuvant for systemic therapy.[592,596,645,646] Sustained-release intravitreal ganciclovir in the treatment of CMV retinitis has been demonstrated clinically, experimentally, and pathologically to be successful since its first use in 1996.[647–649] Combination treatment with foscarnet and ganciclovir may be helpful in the 10–20% of patients whose CMV retinitis is resistant to ganciclovir alone.[650–652] Side effects of ganciclovir therapy include frequent bone marrow toxicity, indefinite IV treatment, and frequent relapses on maintenance treatment unless used concurrently with HAART. The drug cannot be used with zidovudine (AZT) because of bone marrow toxicity.[610,651,653,654] Foscarnet may be used with AZT, which may also have a favorable effect on CMV retinitis.[604,647] Ganciclovir and foscarnet appear to be equivalent in controlling CMV retinitis and preserving vision; however, patient survival is somewhat longer with foscarnet.[654]

The mean survival of patients with AIDS after development of CMV retinitis has increased since 1981.[595] The location of retinal lesions appears to have no prognostic significance for survival. The interval from diagnosis of AIDS to diagnosis of CMV retinitis (median 9 months) has not increased.

Surgeons often use vitrectomy and silicone oil in the management of retinal detachment in patients with AIDS because this technique is effective in these complicated detachments and the operating time is reduced.[594,615,617–620,655] Disadvantages of this technique include hyperopic shift, reduction in accommodative amplitudes, and cataract. The visual results after surgery are generally poor and they continue to worsen after surgery. Indications for repair will change with advances in medical treatment of AIDS.[594,656] Ocular toxoplasmosis and herpes zoster virus (HZV) are other causes of detachment in AIDS. Retinal detachment occurs more frequently after HZV than after CMV retinitis. Use of laser treatment to prevent the progression of CMV retinitis appears to be ineffective.[639,657]

Herpes Virus Retinochoroiditis

The herpes family of viruses (DNA virus) under a variety of circumstances causes a fundoscopic picture of necrotizing retinochoroiditis that is sufficiently characteristic to suggest strongly the diagnosis. This family includes the herpesvirus simiae, which only rarely infects humans. These viruses also produce a similar histopathologic picture of necrotizing retinitis and underlying choroiditis. In areas adjacent to, as well as remote from, the areas of retinal necrosis, intranuclear inclusion bodies may be found by light microscopy, and viral particles by electron microscopy in the retina, RPE, and optic nerve cells. Specific identification of the particular herpesvirus depends on viral cultures, immunofluorescent histologic studies, and PCR for the detection of the virus genome.[658] Vitreous or chorioretinal biopsy and culture may be indicated in patients with suspected herpes infection or other infection, macular-threatening lesions, suspicion of malignancy, and when the results are expected to influence therapy or patient care. Ideally the specimen should be divided into three parts for light and electron microscopy study, immunohistochemistry, and microbiology and tissue culture. Biopsy should only be undertaken if there is support of an experienced immunopathologist and the availability of necessary laboratory capabilities, including immunohistochemistry, electron microscopy, and tissue culture.[659] The quality of the cytologic material obtained from vitreous biopsy is probably similar in specimens obtained by needle aspiration and vitreous suction cutter aspiration done without infusion solution.[660,661]

10.42 Herpes simplex retinochoroiditis and encephalitis.

A to F: This 18-month-old boy had a 4-day history of lethargy and low-grade fever accompanied by seizures on the second day of his illness. He was comatose on admission to the hospital. A lumbar puncture revealed 219 white blood cells with 63% monocytes in the cerebrospinal fluid; protein was 189 mg/dL. CT scan revealed a left temporal lobe lesion. Fundoscopic examination revealed multifocal areas of retinitis, perivasculitis, and hemorrhage (A and B). The patient died on the fourteenth day of his illness. Gross examination of the eyes revealed hemorrhagic retinitis (C). A photomicrograph showed retinal necrosis, retinitis (D), perivasculitis, choroiditis, and viral intranuclear inclusions (*arrow*, E) that were most common in the inner nuclear layer. Electron microscopy revealed intranuclear viral particles typical of herpesvirus (*arrow*, F). Similar findings were present in the brain.

G to I: A 66-year-old man had a history of right-sided herpes zoster ophthalmicus 4 months before developing visual loss in the ipsilateral eye. His visual acuity was 20/50 OD and 20/20 OS. Examination revealed iritis, vitritis, and multiple, slightly elevated white choroidal lesions in the right eye.

(A–F from Cibis et al.[662]

Herpes Simplex Retinochoroiditis

Herpes simplex retinochoroiditis occurs most often in neonates with herpes simplex encephalitis.[621,662–664] It is usually caused by herpes simplex type 2 and is acquired from the mother's genital tract at birth. The risk of a newborn acquiring infection from a mother with herpes infection is approximately 50%.[626] Ocular involvement occurs in approximately 20% of neonatal infants with herpes simplex virus (HSV). It varies widely in severity from conjunctivitis to necrotizing retinochoroiditis.[665] The retinitis begins as multicentric areas of retinal opacification that frequently become confluent (Figure 10.42, A–F). It is associated with variable amounts of retinal hemorrhage. The disease in infants is usually fatal. In some patients chorioretinal scars may be evident at birth.[664]

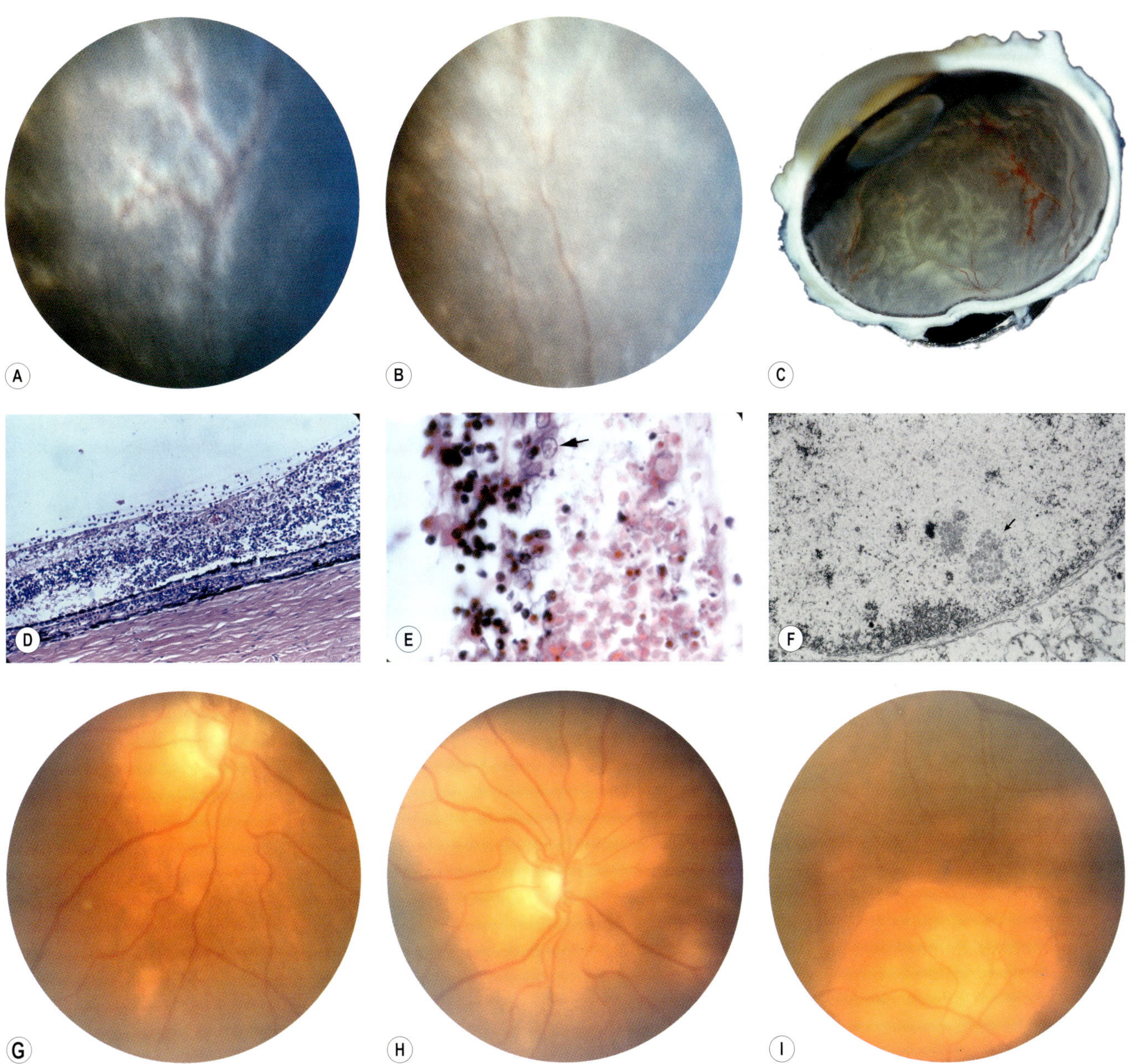
A
B
C
D
E
F
G
H
I

Hypopigmented skin lesions, brain lesions, and quiet retinal scars suggest that intrauterine infection probably occurred during the second trimester.[664] First trimester infection probably produces teratogenic defects. Third trimester infection produces active neonatal HSV infection. Late ophthalmologic manifestations of neonatal HSV infection include optic atrophy, chorioretinal scars, corneal scars, and cataract.[627,664,666] Coarse hyperpigmented areas may occur pre-equatorially in clinically silent cases. There is a high incidence of ocular changes in those patients with neurologic disease resulting from neonatal herpes simplex. Visual impairment in patients who are severely neurologically handicapped as a result of HSV infection is caused mainly by cortical blindness.[666,667]

Herpes simplex retinochoroiditis may occur alone or in association with encephalitis in both healthy adu lts[623,640,642,645,668–670] and immunosuppressed patients.[646,670] Herpes simplex virus has been isolated from eyes with the acute retinal necrosis syndrome in otherwise healthy adult patients with primary HSV-1 or recurrent HSV-1.[587,645] Magnetic resonance imaging studies may show evidence of spread of the virus posteriorly to both optic tracts and lateral geniculate ganglia.[623] Thus, the clinical disease shares many features with the 'von Szily' experimental model for HSV retinitis in the mouse.[629]

Herpesvirus B

Herpesvirus simiae (herpes B virus) is an alpha herpesvirus endemic in monkeys of the *Macaca* species, in which it causes stomatitis and conjunctivitis.[603,633,671,672] The virus is extremely virulent in humans, 75% of whom die of an ascending myelitis. It may cause multifocal necrotizing retinitis, optic neuritis, and panuveitis in one or both eyes of humans.[603,624,672]

HERPES ZOSTER CHOROIDOPATHY

Patients with primary (chicken pox) or secondary herpes zoster ophthalmicus develop one or more focal creamy white choroidal lesions that may be associated with serous retinal detachment, retinal vasculitis, vitritis, cystoid macular edema, and scleritis (Figure 10.41, G–I).[351,381,382,384,395] These may be associated with early blockage of fluorescence and late fluorescein staining. Focal chorioretinal scars may develop after their resolution. They may be accompanied by focal atrophic scars in the iris in patients after herpes zoster ophthalmicus.[351] In some cases it is difficult to determine whether the choroidal lesions are primarily infiltrative or atrophic or both. Ischemia related to ciliary nerve infection by the virus has been implicated in their causation in patients with herpes zoster ophthalmicus.[25,351] An immune-induced granulomatous choroidal vasculitis similar to that occurring in the brain and optic nerve is another possible explanation.

10.43 Herpes zoster-varicella virus chorioretinitis.

A and B: This 37-year-old woman with chicken pox developed episcleritis, visual loss, exudative macular detachment, and focal choroiditis in the left eye. She showed rapid improvement of all signs and symptoms following treatment with aciclovir.
C: This patient sustained marked visual loss following a severe episode of chicken pox when she was 4 years of age. Her visual acuity was 20/200 bilaterally.

Ischemic optic neuropathy in association with herpes zoster ophthalmicus.

D to G: Acute loss of vision in the right eye occurred 2 days after development of herpes zoster ophthalmicus in this 40-year-old HIV-positive man with evidence of ischemic optic neuropathy and mild central vein obstruction. His visual acuity was light perception and progressed to no light perception within several days. Doppler studies revealed evidence of stenosis of the ophthalmic artery. MRI scan of the brain was normal. Two months later he had some anterior chamber reaction in the right eye, which was still blind.
H and I: This 7-year-old boy with a 6-day history of herpes zoster ophthalmicus had acute loss of vision caused by anterior ischemic optic neuropathy (H). His visual acuity was 20/100. He had a dense superior altitudinal scotoma and marked contraction of the inferior visual field. He was treated with oral prednisone 50 mg per day. Four years later (I), note the optic atrophy. His acuity was 20/60.
J to L: Photomicrographs showing postischemic cavernous atrophy of the optic nerve (J) caused by granulomatous arteritis (K and L) in a blind, painful eye removed from a patient who had herpes zoster ophthalmicus.

Herpes Zoster Virus (HZV), Retinochoroiditis, and Optic Neuritis

Most patients with herpes zoster ophthalmicus and chicken pox demonstrate no involvement of the choroid, retina, or optic nerve. Nevertheless, there are several clinical syndromes in which chorioretinal and optic nerve involvement by the HZV may cause severe visual loss.[673–679]

Focal Choroiditis

During the convalescent stage of chicken pox or herpes zoster ophthalmicus an occasional patient may develop one or more yellow–white placoid choroidal lesions throughout the posterior fundus (Figure 10.43, A–C).[680]

Congenital Varicella Syndrome

Infants of mothers who had varicella infection during the second trimester may demonstrate, at birth or soon afterward, systemic findings including bulbar palsy, mild hemiparesis, cicatricial skin lesions, developmental delay, and learning difficulties, as well as ocular manifestations including chorioretinal atrophy, chorioretinal scars simulating toxoplasmosis, hypoplastic optic discs, attenuated electroretinographic and evoked occipital potential amplitudes, congenital cataract, and Horner's syndrome (Figure 10.43, C).[681] The HZV titer to IgM is typically negative.

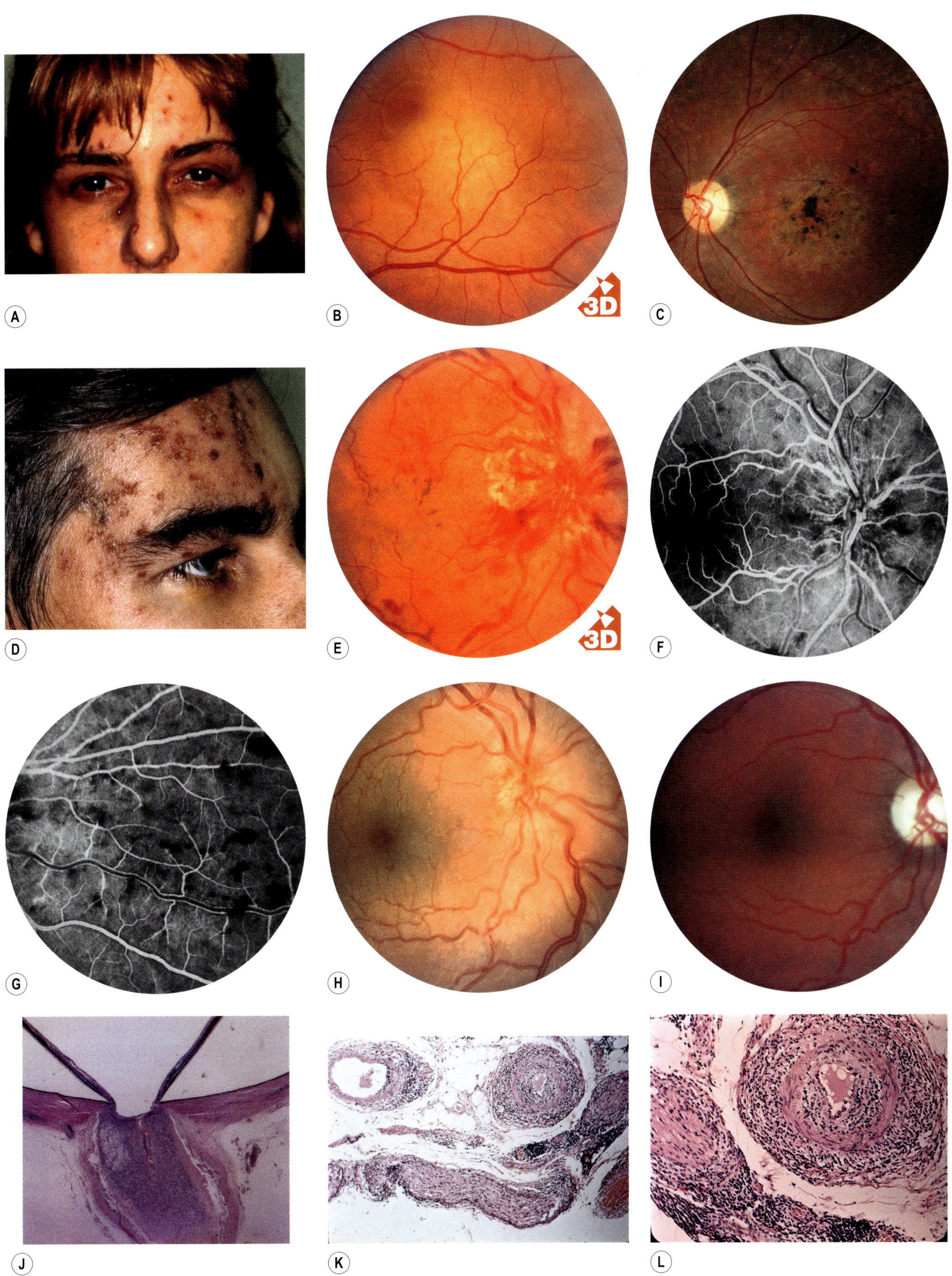
3D
3D
A
B
C
D
E
F
G
H
I
J
K
L

Focal Retinitis, Neuroretinopathy, Ischemic Optic Neuropathy, and Retinal Vascular Occlusion

In children and adults the external manifestation of herpes zoster ophthalmicus or chicken pox may be associated occasionally with optic disc swelling, macular star, branch or central retinal artery or vein occlusion, and multifocal retinitis (Figure 10.43, D–I).[682–686] In children and adults HZV can cause a granulomatous arteritis and an ocular syndrome similar to that produced by cranial arteritis, including ophthalmoplegia, ischemic optic neuropathy, hypotony, phthisis bulbi, and contralateral hemiplegia (Figure 10.43, J–K).[678,687–689]

Acute Retinal Necrosis (Herpetic Thrombotic Retinochoroidal Angiitis and Necrotizing Neuroretinitis)

Herpes zoster virus (varicella-zoster virus, VZV) is the primary cause of acute retinal necrosis, a clinical syndrome that develops in one or both eyes of typical healthy individuals of all ages. Herpes simplex virus 1 and 2 (HSV-1 and HSV-2) account for a smaller number of cases,[690–695] with the average age at presentation being 52.4 years for VZV, 44.3 years for HSV-1, and 24.3 years for HSV-2.[696] HSV-1 viral acute retinal necrosis generally follows recent or remote herpetic encephalitis.[692,697] There has been a rise in HSV-2 cases, especially in the late teenage years.[691,693,695,698] It is characterized by the development of mild anterior uveitis, followed within a few days by vitreous inflammation, pain, occasionally glaucoma, and usually a rapid decline in visual function caused by a rapidly progressing occlusive retinal arteritis, necrotizing retinitis, and optic neuritis associated with progressive inflammatory infiltration of the vitreous (Figures 10.44–10.46).[673,679,699–722]

10.44 Acute retinal necrosis syndrome.

A to **F**: A 50-year-old diabetic African American man presented with rapid decline in vision over 3 days, elevated intraocular pressure, several areas of focal and confluent retinitis, and retinal arterial narrowing with perivenous hemorrhages (A). His visual acuity was 20/80 in the affected eye. A clinical diagnosis of herpetic retinitis and panuveitis was made, and he received oral valaciclovir (Valtrex), followed 2–3 days later by oral prednisone. Aqueous PCR was positive for Herpes simplex virus. Two weeks later there continues to be vitritis; retinal arteries show periarterial plaques and sheathing (B). The multifocal lesions are now confluent in the periphery and mid periphery (C and D). He was continued on oral valaciclovir and the prednisone was slowly tapered over the next 6 months. At 5 months the optic disc is pale, the retinal arterioles continue to have periarteriolar plaques and sheathing, and the peripheral lesions show pigmentary changes and fibrosis (E and F). His vision improved to 20/50 and at last follow-up there were no retinal tears or detachment.

G to **J**: Extensive peripheral necrotizing retinitis in a healthy 79-year-old woman. Note the confluent areas of retinitis in the periphery associated with perivascular hemorrhage (G and H) and the patchy involvement posteriorly with sparing of the center of the macula (I). There was marked narrowing of the retinal vasculature and pallor of the optic disc. The right fundus was normal. The retinitis resolved spontaneously. Seven weeks later, visual acuity was 20/50. There was complete closure of all of the nasal retinal vessels (J) and extensive closure of the peripheral vasculature temporally. She maintained this vision over the subsequent 3 years, when she was lost to follow-up.

K: This man was blinded in both eyes by the acute retinal necrosis syndrome several years previously. Note the optic atrophy and thread-like remnants of the retinal vessels

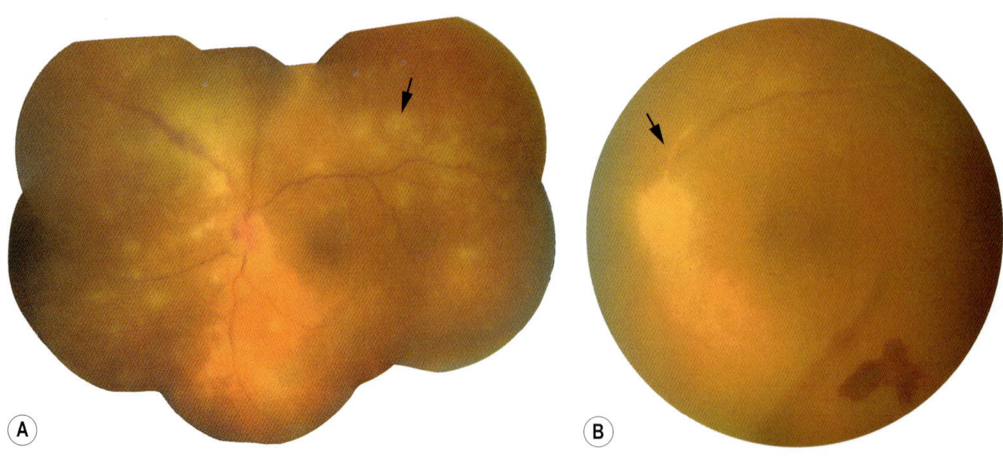

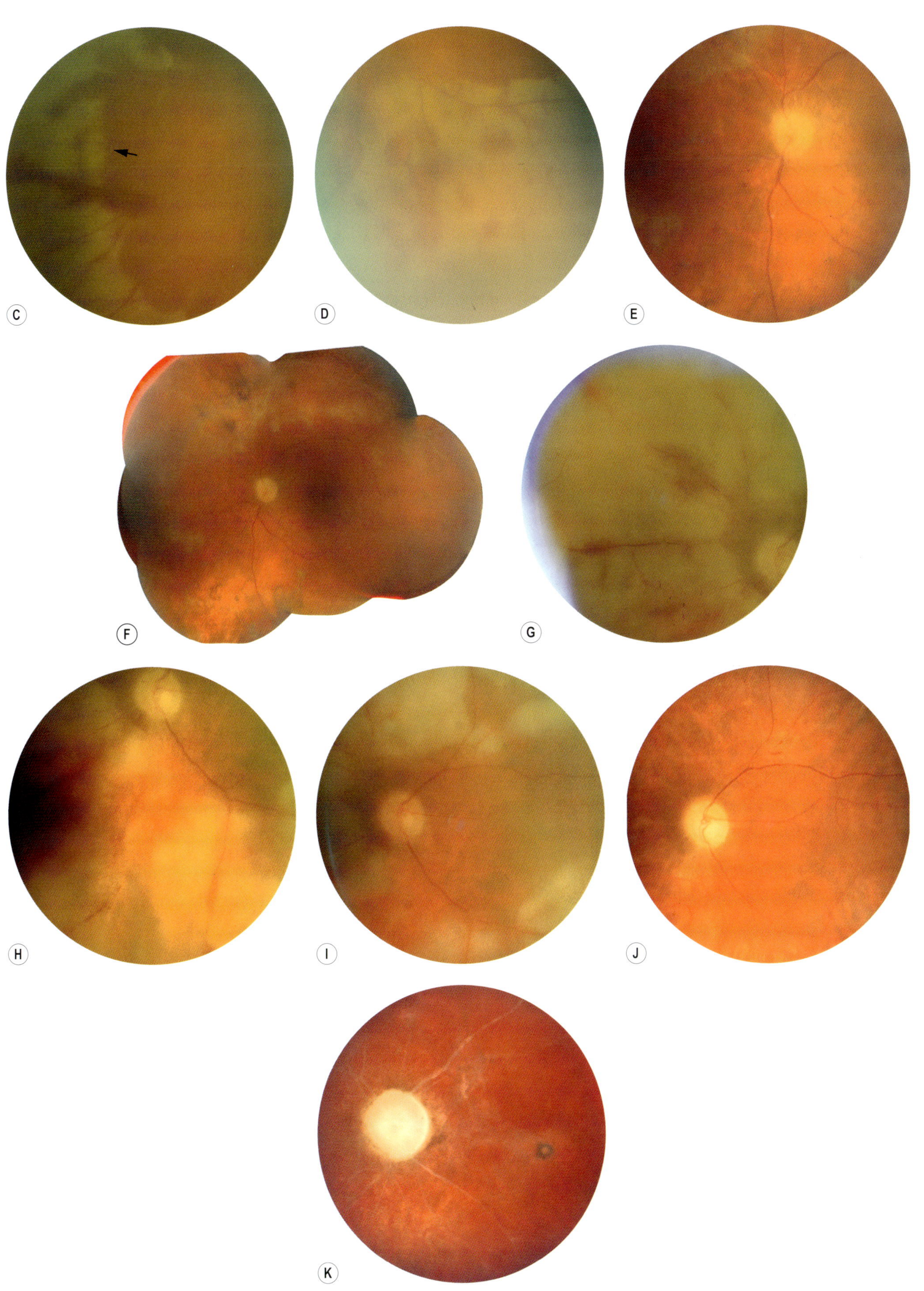
C
D
E
F
G
H
I
J
K

The retinal whitening often begins in multifocal areas that become confluent in the peripheral fundus (Figure 10.44, A–I). It is typically associated with perivascular infiltration, vascular occlusion, and hemorrhage (Figures 10.44, B–D; 10.45, A–H, O, and P). The occlusive vasculitis may affect the major retinal and optic nerve head arteries posterior to the zones of full-thickness necrotizing retinitis (Figures 10.44, B–D; 10.45, A and D–F). Retinal opacification rapidly spreads posteriorly, frequently sparing the macula (Figure 10.44, F and I). Multiple posterior white lesions occasionally occur early in the course of the disease. These may involve either or both the inner and outer retina. Marked yellow atheromatous cuffing, narrowing, and occlusion of the major branch retinal arteries may develop (Figure 10.44, B, I, and O). Widespread necrotizing retinitis is the predominant fundus finding in most patients; however, some show evidence of extensive retinal arteritis preceding development of large areas of retinal necrosis (Figure 10.45, J and Q). In some patients visual loss is caused primarily by branch or central retinal artery occlusion, and the presence of either an arcuate pattern or diffuse retinal whitening and cherry-red spot along with the atheromatous changes may be misinterpreted as embolic occlusion of the retinal arteries secondary to carotid artery disease.[705,723–725] Some patients may demonstrate a milder progression and severity of the disease.[726,727] An associated scleritis with underlying choroidal effusion is sometimes seen (Figure 10.45, M and N).

Fluorescein angiography demonstrates reduced perfusion in the areas of retinal necrosis and retinal capillary permeability alteration, as well as evidence of focal choroidal inflammatory cell infiltration and RPE damage in areas uninvolved by retinal necrosis (Figure 10.45, D–H). After a few days the necrotic retina crumbles and sheds into the vitreous and a sharply outlined pattern of usually mild pigment mottling is left in the area of previous retinal necrosis (Figure 10.45, P). Even as the areas of retinitis are clearing, the patient may experience further sudden and profound loss of vision caused by thrombotic arterial occlusion within or near the optic nerve head. In approximately two-thirds of eyes, large irregular retinal holes develop in the necrotic retina and are followed by vitreous organization, traction, and extensive retinal detachment (Figure 10.45, K, Q, and R). The detachment typically occurs 6–12 weeks after the onset of the disease. The overall prognosis for visual acuity is generally poor, with only 30% of affected eyes achieving an acuity of better than 20/200.

Risk factors for severity of the disorder early in the course of the disease are retinal arteritis, reduced electroretinographic amplitudes, and elevated circulating immune complexes.[728] Central vision, however, may be retained in those patients who do not develop retinal detachment because of the tendency for the retinitis and choroiditis to spare the posterior pole (Figure 10.44, A–F).

Approximately two-thirds of patients with the acute retinal necrosis syndrome are men. The second eye becomes involved in approximately one-third of patients, usually within 6 weeks of onset in the first eye. Involvement of the second eye may be delayed for as long as 19 years.[717,729] In patients receiving early treatment with aciclovir, the likelihood of involvement of the fellow eye is reduced.[730] Most patients have no antecedent systemic disease. Herpes zoster ophthalmicus, the Ramsay Hunt syndrome, and chicken pox may occur in some patients shortly before the onset of acute retinal necrosis.[679,701,703,710,721,731–736] Herpes simplex virus, aphthous ulcers, and IV cocaine have been implicated in the development of acute retinal necrosis in several patients.[702,721,737,738]

10.45 Acute retinal necrosis caused by herpes simplex virus type 2 (HSV-2).

A to **L**: An 18-year-old girl presented with photophobia, pain and redness, and a decrease in vision to 20/40 in the left eye. She was diagnosed with anterior uveitis and started on topical steroids and cycloplegics. Symptoms worsened over the next 4 days and the vision dropped to 20/80. A diagnosis of panuveitis with optic neuritis was made, and oral steroids at 80 mg per day were begun. She was referred the next day when her vision had decreased to count fingers. Cells were seen in the anterior chamber and vitreous cavity, along with a swollen optic disc, several areas of retinal whitening, macular whitening and scattered blot retinal hemorrhages (A–C, G). A diagnosis of acute retinal necrosis was made. Angiogram showed occlusion of several arterioles in the mid peripheral fundus inferiorly and inferonasally (D–F, H). Aqueous PCR was sent for varicella-zoster virus (VZV), HSV-1 and -2, and CMV, and oral steroids were discontinued and IV aciclovir was begun. By 2 days the media haze worsened and the lesions became more confluent (I). Aqueous PCR returned positive for HSV-2 and negative for VZV and HSV-1. Oral steroid was added at 40 mg, and a week later the vitreous cells had decreased, but the retinitis was still confluent with retinal infarcts (J). Ten days later the retina detached, with several large holes in the ischemic inferior retina confirmed on an ultrasound due to poor visibility from the vitreous haze (K). She underwent a vitrectomy, scleral buckle, and silicone oil placement, and her retina has remained flat under the oil. She was continued on systemic aciclovir for 9+ months, and oral and topical steroids tapered over 7–8 months. The optic nerve remained pale with narrowed retinal vasculature. Her vision stabilized at 20/200.

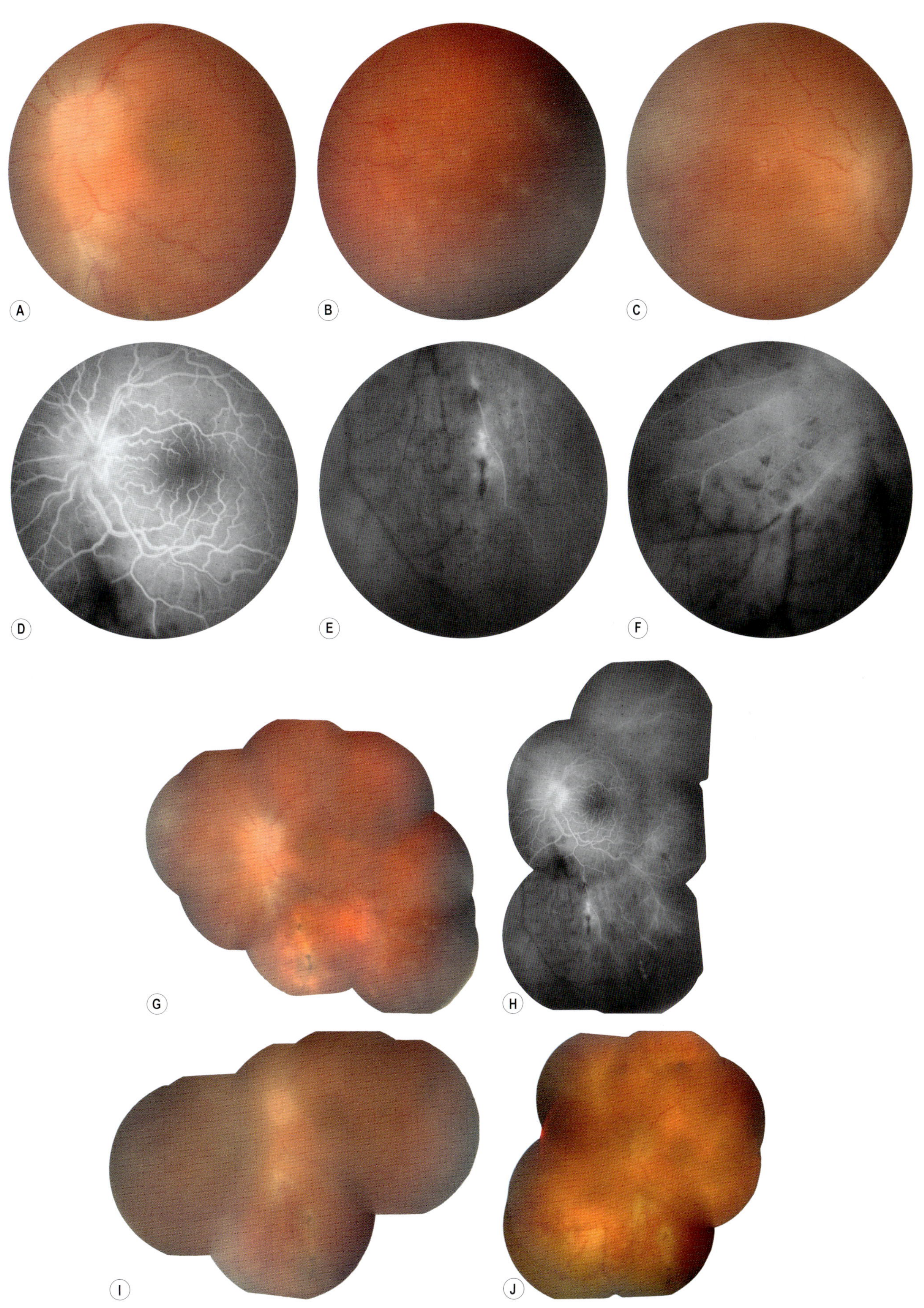
A
B
C
D
E
F
G
H
I
J

Histopathologic examination of the eyes of immunocompetent patients with the early stage of acute retinal necrosis caused by the HZV reveals two major components: (1) sharply defined zones of full-thickness necrotizing retinitis associated with replicating herpes virus (Figure 10.46); and (2) occlusive vasculitis affecting the choroidal and retinal vessels unassociated with evidence of replicating virus within the blood vessels (Figure 10.46, B).[705,723,731] The thickened necrotic retina involving all layers seen histopathologically corresponds with the zones of dense retinal whitening seen clinically (Figure 10.44, C, D, and G). In the areas adjacent to the necrotic retina where the retina is partly preserved, numerous intranuclear inclusion bodies typical of the herpesviruses are evident by light and electron microscopy in the retina and RPE (Figure 10.46, G and H). Immunocytopathologic staining techniques, immunofluorescence, and PCR techniques have been used to identify the virus as herpes zoster.[678,716,731,739,740] In areas where the white necrotizing retinitis has faded from view clinically, only skeletal remains of partly thrombosed major retinal vessels may be found (Figure 10.46, C). The major retinal arteries may be occluded as a result of infiltration of the arterial walls by acute and chronic inflammatory cells as well as lipid-laden macrophages (Figure 10.46, B). The choroid may be focally and diffusely thickened by acute and chronic inflammatory cells and occlusive vasculitis that involves both the choroidal arteries and the choriocapillaris (Figure 10.46, C, D, and F). This vasculitis may be associated with necrosis of the overlying pigment epithelium and outer retina (Figure 10.46, F). A necrotizing optic neuritis may be found (Figure 10.46, E). No virus has been identified in the uveal tract or in the walls of the retinal vessels. It is probable that the HZV does not invade the retinal and choroidal blood vessels but instead induces an acute reactive inflammatory granulomatous response within the retinal arterial wall, as well as in the choroidal vasculature, that plays an important role in the ischemic damage to the inner and outer retina apart from the necrosis inflicted by direct intraretinal spread of the replicating virus. This reactive immune-induced vasculitis is probably largely responsible for the panuveitis and necrotizing optic neuropathy accompanying this disorder (Figure 10.46, E).

The same explanation may be invoked for the giant cell arteritis associated with ischemic optic neuropathy (Figure 10.43, E–L) and contralateral hemiplegia that occurs in some patients with herpes zoster ophthalmicus.[688,708,741] Clinically the marked choroidal involvement (Figure 10.46, A, C, D, and F) in patients with acute retinal necrosis is largely occult because of the loss of transparency of the overlying ischemic retina. On histopathologic examination of two eyes enucleated many months after partial resolution of acute retinal necrosis caused by HZV, the author found a smoldering retinochoroiditis and a giant-cell reaction in the vicinity of Bruch's membrane and the internal limiting membrane of the retina.[716,742] This granulomatous response to these collagenous membranes is similar to that which may occur around Descemet's membrane in patients after HZV keratitis.[743,744]

Although most cases of acute retinal necrosis are probably caused by the herpes zoster virus, the herpes simplex virus, cytomegalovirus, Epstein–Barr virus, and *Toxoplasma* have been incriminated in a few cases.[737,738,745] Establishing the cause of acute retinal necrosis has been aided by recent success with PCR. Previously, serial determination of serum and intraocular fluid HZV antibody levels, viral culture, and immunocytopathologic techniques were used to identify HZV infection in tissue sections.[658,731,739,740] Biopsy of the retina at the junction of the necrotic and unaffected retina during pars plana vitrectomy is occasionally used for diagnosis.[746–748] Our failure to recognize the acute retinal necrosis (ARN) syndrome some 20 years ago suggests that a mutation in the HZV may have occurred. The genotypes HLA-DQw7A and HLA-BW62,DR4 occur in 55% and 16%, respectively (controls 19% and 3%), of patients with ARN.[749]

10.45 Continued

Varicella-zoster scleritis and acute retinal necrosis (ARN).

M to **R**: This 68-year-old man was seen elsewhere and treated with oral and topical steroids for 2 weeks with a diagnosis of panuveitis. He was found to have scleritis with severe pain and redness in the temporal quadrant of his right eye. A choroidal detachment was seen under the scleritis along with significant vitritis and arteriolar plaques (M–O). A diagnosis of ARN with scleritis secondary to varicella-zoster virus was made. He received oral valaciclovir (Valtrex), 1 g three times a day, and 48 h later oral steroids were added. Two weeks later there was some healing of the retinitis (P), but he subsequently developed a rhegmatogenous retinal detachment in the inferior and nasal quadrants (Q and R). He underwent a vitrectomy and repair of the retinal detachment with placement of silicone oil. His retina has remained attached though the arterioles showed occlusion with several periarteriolar plaques.

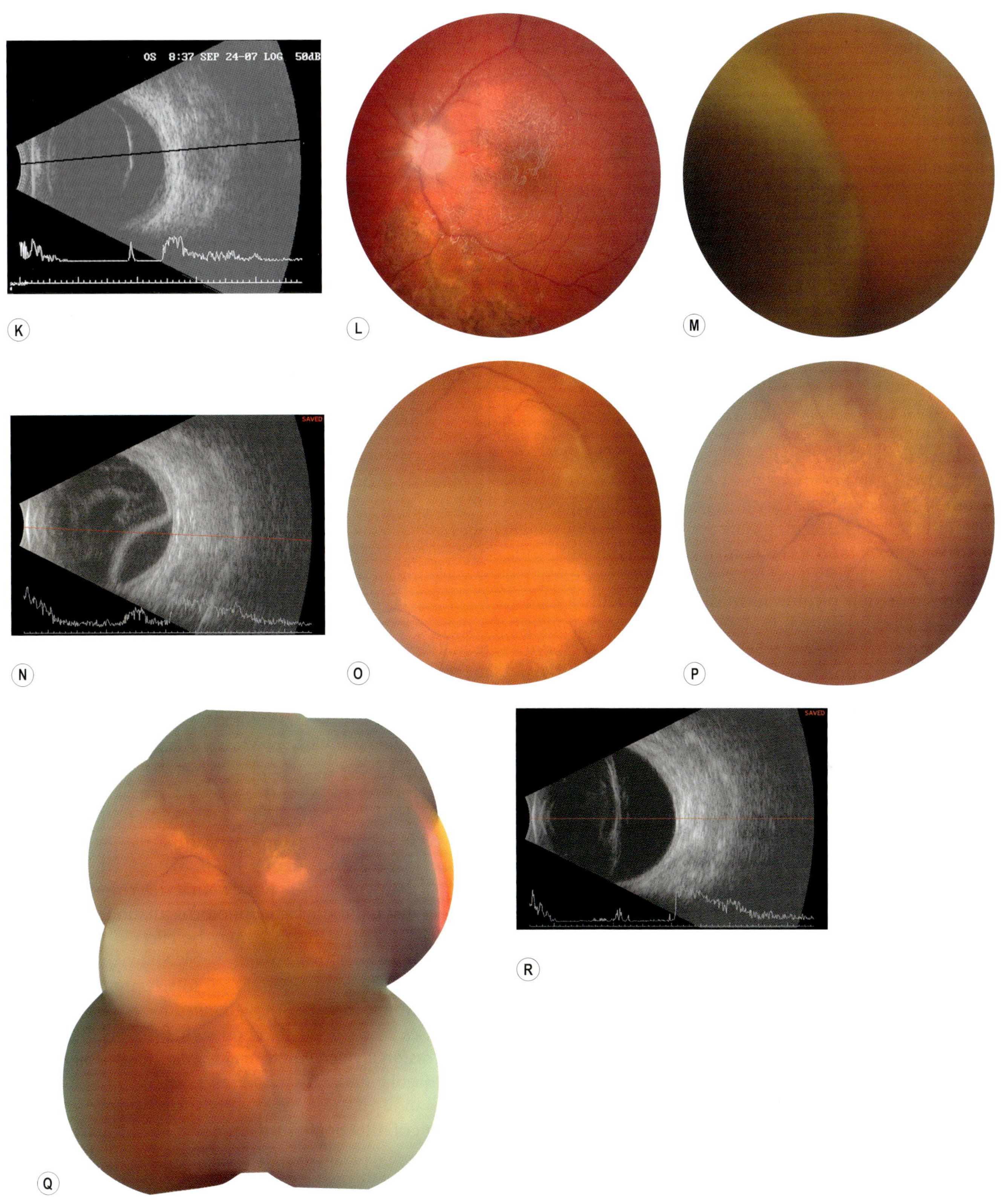
OS 8:37 SEP 24-07 LOG 50dB
SAVED
SAVED
K
L
M
N
O
P
Q
R

Acute Retinal Necrosis in Immune Incompetent Patients (Posterior Outer Retinal Necrosis)

Immune incompetent patients, particularly those with AIDS, often develop a distinct clinical picture of acute retinal necrosis characterized by fewer inflammatory signs, deep retinal opacification, frequent involvement of the macula, less involvement of the retinal and choroidal blood vessels, poor response to antiviral agents, and rapid progression to severe bilateral visual loss (Figure 10.47).[769–778] Though the fundus appearance appears to be outer retinal involvement (posterior outer retinal necrosis or PORN syndrome), there is clinical and histopathologic evidence that the necrotizing viral retinitis also involves the inner retina early in these patients (Figure 10.47, A–E and J–P).[773] Because these patients are immuno-suppressed, the acute reactive granulomatous retinal and choroidal arteritis typically seen in immune incompetent patients with HZV ARN is less severe, but the replicating virus causes severe, rapidly progressing retinal necrosis involving all retinal layers. Progression to loss of light perception occurs in two-thirds of patients. Early aggressive treatment of the retinitis and the immunocompromised state with HAART is recommended to salvage some vision.[776,779]

10.47 Progressive outer retinal necrosis (PORN) syndrome.

A to **G**: Acute visual loss occurred in this 49-year-old man who was HIV-positive. Note the multifocal lesions surrounding paracentral zones of retinal whitening that involved the inner as well as the outer retina (A and B). Angiography showed evidence of perifoveolar retinal vascular occlusion and incomplete staining of the white paracentral lesions (C to E). Two weeks later he had severe visual loss and progression of the retinitis (F), and 5 weeks after the onset of symptoms he was virtually blind. Note the severe retinal vascular narrowing, optic disc pallor, and relative sparing of the choroid (F). The left eye was enucleated and herpes zoster virus (HSV) was cultured and identified with immunofluorescent staining with a monoclonal antibody to varicella-zoster virus. **H** to **K**: Visual loss occurred in this 39-year-old man with AIDS and a history of two episodes of herpes zoster dermatitis. Note the multifocal white retinal lesions (H and I). There was minimal vitreous inflammation. One week later his visual acuity was 20/300 in the right eye and hand movements only in the left eye. Vision progressed rapidly to no light perception in the right eye, which was enucleated for diagnostic purposes. Histopathologic examination (J and K) revealed extensive necrosis of the retina that in many areas was more marked in the inner than outer retina. Note the absence of the retinal and choroidal vascular inflammatory response and compare it with the severe inflammatory response that occurs in the immunocompetent patient with ARN caused by HZV (see Figure 10.46).

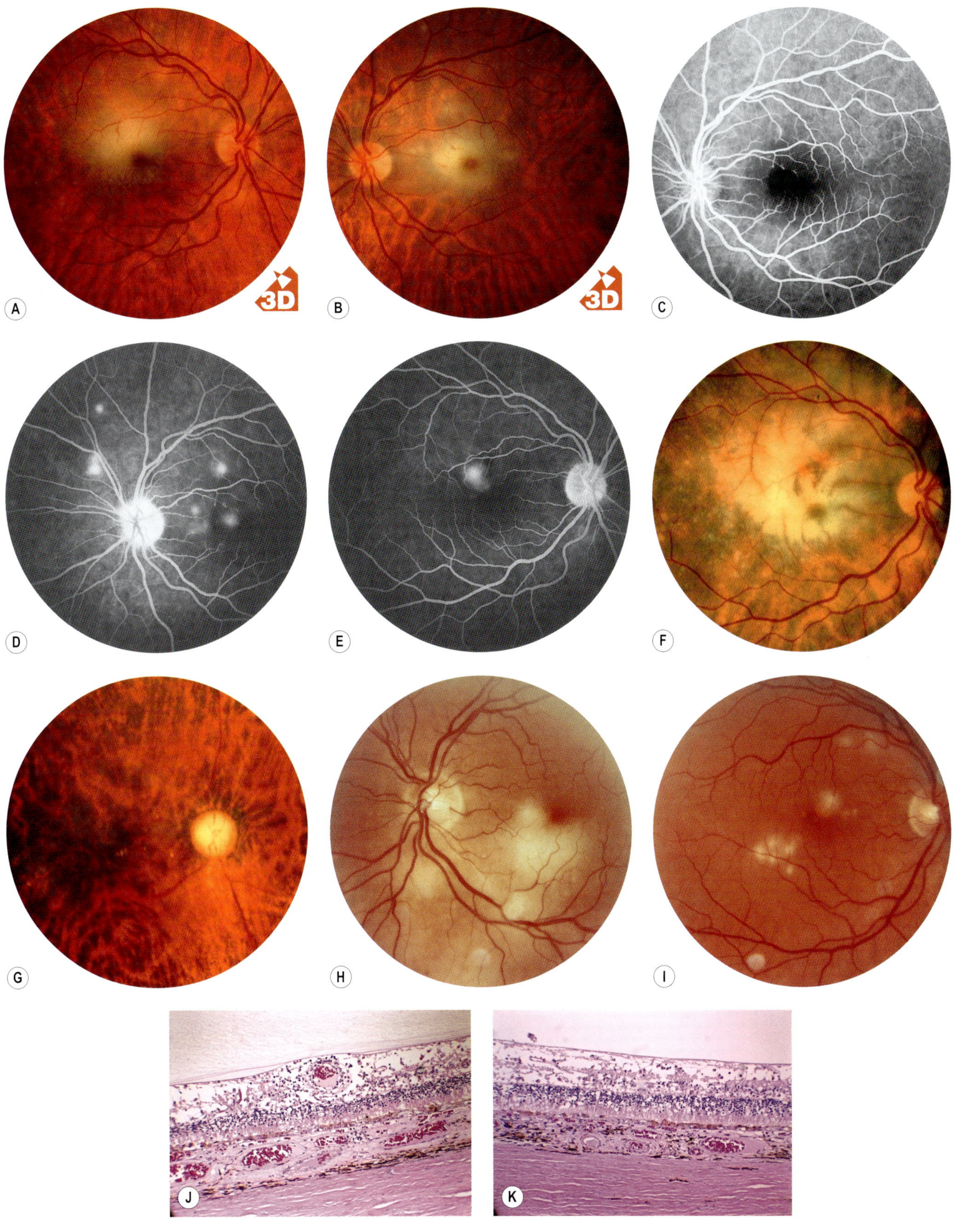
A
B
C
D
E
F
G
H
I
J
K
3D
3D

10.47 Continued

L to **P**: A 49-year-old African American woman complained of decreased vision in both eyes. She was diagnosed with HIV/AIDS 3 months prior with a CD4 count less than 20. She had a history of CMV viremia, esophageal ulcers, chronic gastritis, hypertension, and oral candidiasis. Her vision was 3/200 in the right eye and 20/80 in the left eye. Both eyes had widespread deep outer retinal whitening in the macula and periphery with retinal hemorrhages (L, M and O). There were areas of retinal atrophy anterior to the peripheral active lesions (O). Angiogram showed late staining of the active lesions and transmission defects of the atrophic zones (N and P). A vitreous biopsy was positive for varicella-zoster virus by PCR and negative for CMV and HSV. She received 2400 mg of intravitreal foscarnet in both eyes and oral valganciclovir 900 mg twice a day. The whitening disappeared and the lesions became pigmented.

(A and E from Margolis et al.[944]; G–J from Margo[773]; L–P, courtesy Dr Gaurav Shah.)

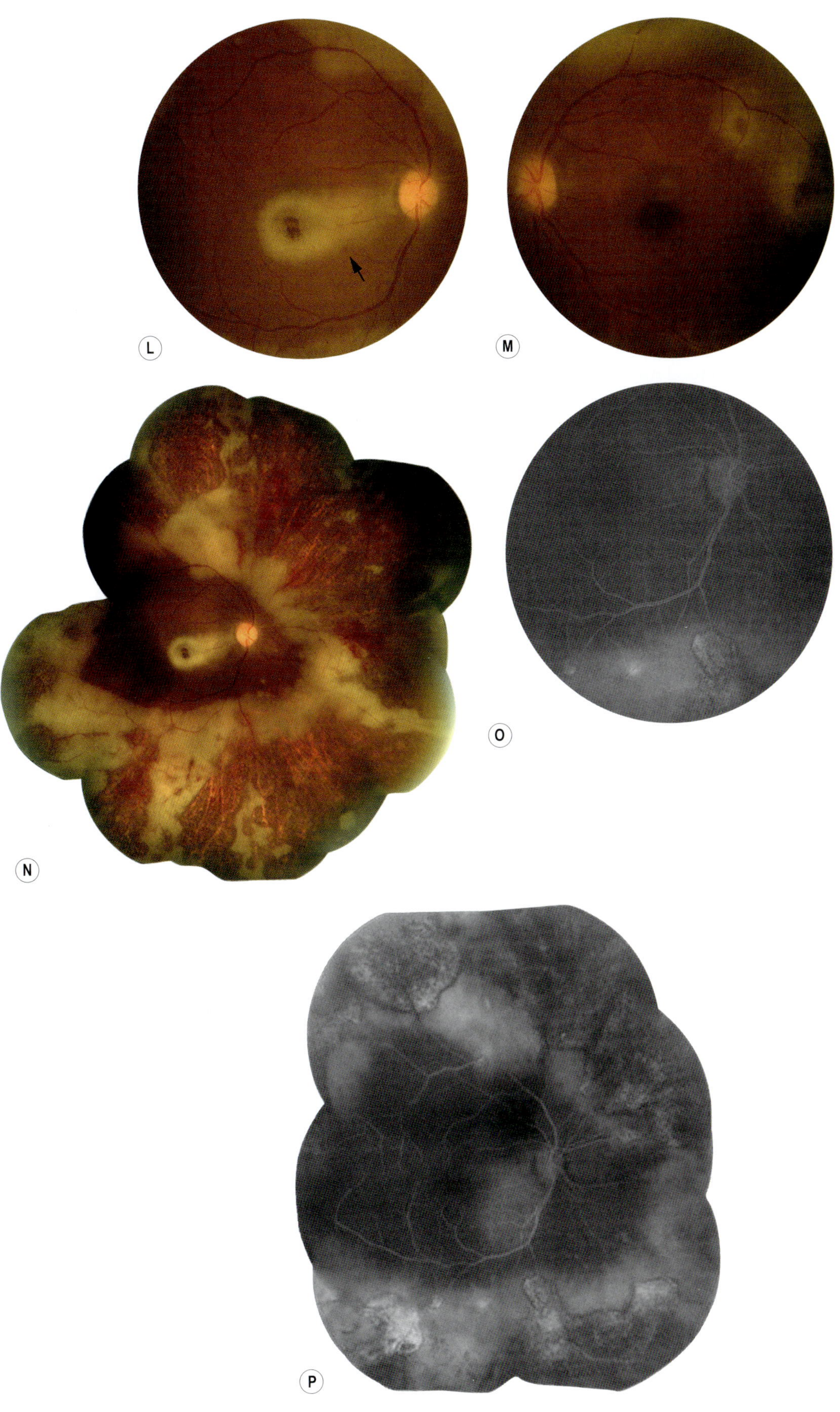
L
M
N
O
P

HUMAN IMMUNODEFICIENCY VIRUS (HIV) AND ACQUIRED IMMUNE DEFICIENCY SYNDROME

Acquired immune deficiency syndrome (AIDS) first became apparent in 1975 but has rapidly become a global pandemic. In the United States, the Centers for Disease Control and Prevention (CDC) made the first announcement of AIDS cases in five homosexual men in Los Angeles who were hospitalized with *P. carinii* pneumonia, CMV infection and candidiasis.[780] The disease is transmitted primarily by sexual contact that can be homosexual, bisexual, or heterosexual; by parenteral transmission, by transfusion of infected blood products, or by injection using blood-contaminated needles or syringes; and perinatally before, during, or after delivery.[12,183,258,781–813] The definition of AIDS that was formerly based primarily on the acquisition of one or more 'indicator diseases' associated with HIV infections, such as infection by opportunistic organisms, lymphomas, and encephalopathy, now includes asymptomatic patients with CD4+ T-lymphocyte counts of less than 200 cells/μL.[810]

AIDS is caused by infection with the retrovirus human immunodeficiency virus (HIV), which causes a profound immunodeficiency resulting primarily from a progressive quantitative and qualitative deficiency of the CD4+ subset of T lymphocytes referred to as the helper or inducer T cells. There is an associated elevation of circulating immune complexes and elevated serum IgA and IgG levels. The median time from HIV exposure to the development of AIDS is approximately 11 years.[790] Patients often are seen initially because of fever, generalized lymphadenopathy, a wide variety of severe opportunistic infections, and, in approximately 30% of patients, the development of a progressive form of Kaposi's sarcoma. Ocular findings occur in 50–70% of patients. The most common ocular finding is one or more cotton-wool patches (approximately 50–70% of cases) (Figure 10.48, A), retinal hemorrhages and Roth's spots (approximately 40%), microaneurysms (approximately 20%), and cytomegalic retinitis (approximately 25%) (Figures 10.41; 10.48, D–F).[786,793,797] The cotton-wool patches are similar to those occurring in other retinal vascular diseases except that they are generally smaller in size.[789] They regress in 4–6 weeks. They may appear early in the course of the disease, and their appearance is unrelated to specific infections or the general status of the patient. When these patches are viewed by fluorescein angiography, they are identical with cotton-wool patches seen from other causes.[788] Histopathologically, they are cytoid bodies associated with arteriolar obstruction, basal laminar thickening, endothelial cell swelling, and degeneration of the pericytes.[788] We have observed calcification histopathologically within cytoid bodies in two patients with AIDS (Figure 10.48, B and C).[814] Although structures resembling *Pneumocystis jirovecii* were identified in a cotton-wool patch in one case,[791] there is minimal evidence to support an infectious cause for the arteriolar obstruction. Vascular damage from a circulating immune complex deposition has been suggested as the cause.[788] HIV-1 has been demonstrated in the retina, conjunctiva, tears, iris, and cornea of patients with AIDS.[705,785,808] The role of this virus in causing cotton-wool patches, microaneurysms and hemorrhages,[786,815–819] nonstaining cystoid macular edema, macular star, optic neuropathy, or otherwise unexplained visual loss in some patients with AIDS,[771,806,818,820–822] and in potentiating the effects of opportunistic infections is uncertain.[817]

Most opportunistic infections occur in patients with a CD4+ T-lymphocyte count of less than 200 cells/μL. For opportunistic infections associated with AIDS, see the following: bacteria, p. 806; cytomegalovirus, p. 892; herpes zoster virus and acute retinal necrosis, pp. 900–910; mycobacterium, pp. 830–836; cat-scratch disease, pp. 812–814; cryptococcosis, p. 842; histoplasmosis, p. 846; *Pneumocystis*, p. 858.

10.48 Acquired immune deficiency syndrome.

A: Cotton-wool spots.
B and C: Photomicrographs of cotton-wool patch. Note cytoid body, which is partly calcified (*arrows*, B; hematoxylin and eosin). Some of the calcified tissue (pale area) was dislodged during sectioning. The whole cytoid body stained positively for calcium (C, von Kossa stain).
D and E: Cytomegalic inclusion disease retinitis.
F: Photomicrograph of the retina with many cytomegalic cells with intracytoplasmic (*arrow*) and intranuclear inclusions – 'owl's eye' (*arrowhead*) in a patient with CMV retinitis.
G: Cytomegalic inclusion papillitis.
H and I: Clinical photograph (H) and photomicrograph (I) of Kaposi's sarcoma of the inferior conjunctival cul-de-sac.
J: Kaposi's sarcoma of the lower eyelid.
K and L: Kaposi's sarcoma of the conjunctiva in a patient with AIDS before (K) and several weeks after (L) subconjunctival injection of 0.5 mL of 3 million units interferon alfa-2a.

(B and C from Tanenbaum et al.[814]; F, courtesy Dr Narsing Rao; K and L from Hummer et al.[796])

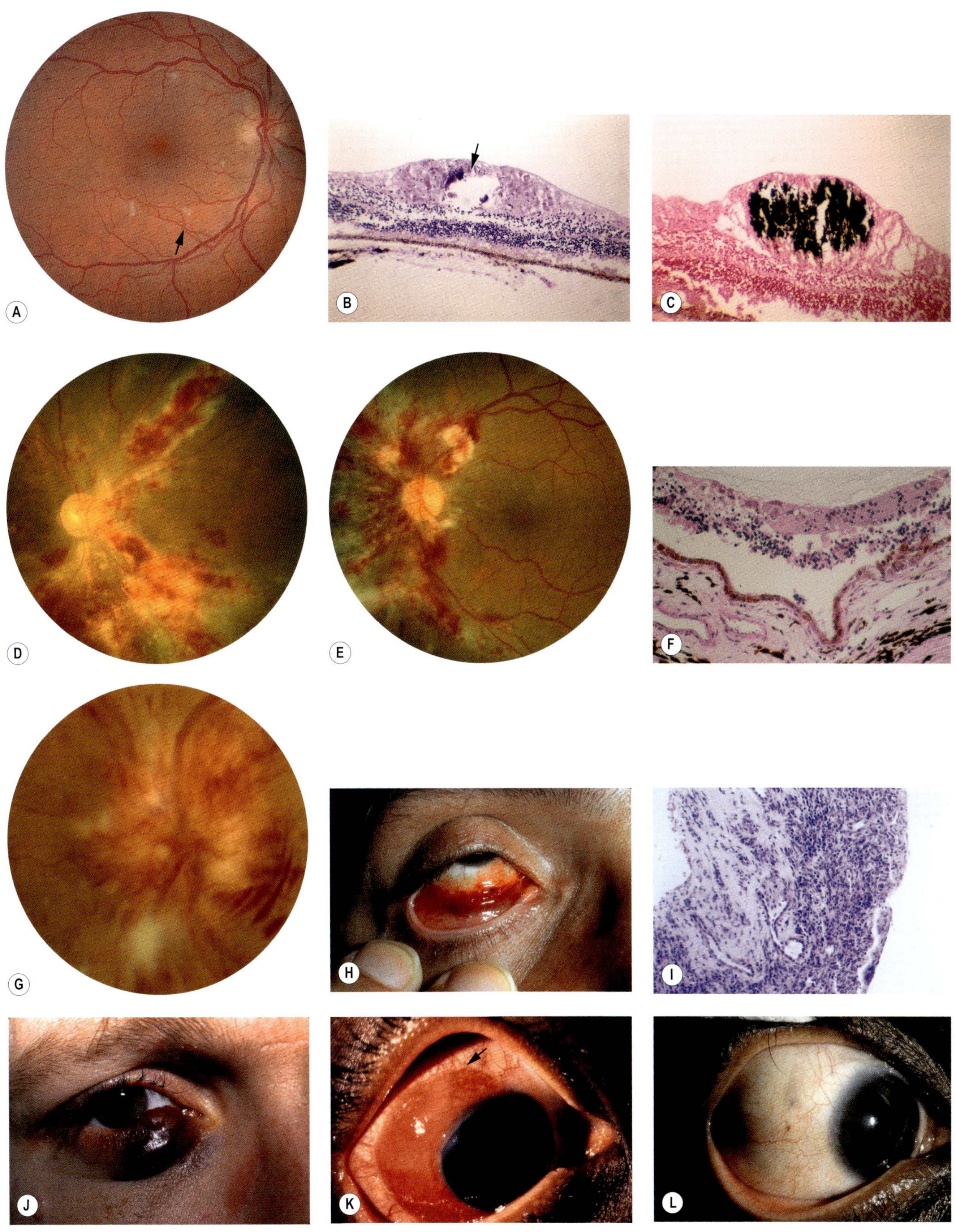
A
B
C
D
E
F
G
H
I
J
K
L

10.49 Epstein–Barr virus (EBV).

A to **I**: A 26-year-old woman developed sudden fever, diffuse myalgia, sore throat, and difficulty swallowing. Seven weeks later she noted ocular discomfort, fatigue, headache, tinnitus, mild hearing loss, and pericentral scotoma. Mild lympadenopathy and resolving pharyngitis was found on examination. Retinal veins in both eyes had patchy phlebitis (A–C) that on angiography showed leakage from the venous wall (D–G). All laboratory tests were negative except for positive IgM and IgG antibodies to EBV and a quantitative EBV PCR was positive in 500 copies/mL. The lesions responded to oral prednisone at 60 mg twice a day that was tapered at 20 mg per week with complete resolution of the phlebitis in both eyes (H and I).

J to **N**: A 65-year-old woman with pathologic myopia and a central scar in the left macula noted a rapid decrease in vision in her good right eye. She developed headache, neck stiffness, malaise, and cervical adenopathy. When examined a week later, the right eye showed faint yellow lesions in the macula, and the left was unchanged with a pre-existing atrophic scar (J). Nineteen days later her vision in the right eye

Cytomegalic retinitis and optic neuritis are the most serious ocular complications of AIDS from the visual as well as the overall prognostic standpoint (Figure 10.41, A–L and P–T). Cytomegalic retinitis develops late in the course of the disease, is progressive, and, before the use of antiviral agents, was usually followed several weeks after its discovery by death caused by systemic infection with CMV or one or more of the following: *Pneumocystis carinii* (*jiroveci*) pneumonia, *Cryptococcus neoformans* meningitis, *Toxoplasma gondii* encephalitis, and disseminated *Mycobacterium avium*, *Mycobacterium avium-intracellulare*, and *Candida albicans*.[258,782,786,797,823,824] With the introduction of HAART in the late 1990s, CMV retinitis can be cured or controlled in some patients, though they may have to be on chronic ganciclovir treatment or receive intravitreal ganciclovir implants. Immune recovery uveitis with vitreous inflammation and cystoid macular edema has emerged in the post HAART era, where immune reconstitution elicits an inflammatory response in patients recovering from CMV retinitis. This uveitis can be treated successfully with topical or local steroids.

Kaposi's sarcoma appears as one or more erythematous violaceous masses that may involve the conjunctiva, skin of the lids, and occasionally the orbits (Figure 10.48, H–L).[796,801,809] Progressive involvement of the skin, mucous membranes, internal organs, and lymph nodes may be the major cause of death in approximately 9% of patients. Burkitt's lymphoma of the orbit and a variety of neuro-ophthalmologic complications, usually caused by intracranial infections, may occur.[807] Intraocular lymphoma, squamous cell carcinoma of the conjunctiva, ocular surface disease such as microsporidia keratitis, molluscum contagiosum, and drug-induced uveitis (cidofovir and rifabutin) are other ocular manifestations seen in AIDS.

Therapy in patients with AIDS is directed toward inhibition of replication of HIV by antiretroviral medications and control of opportunistic infections. Chemotherapy, cryotherapy, local excision, and tumor injection with alpha-interferon are used to control Kaposi's sarcoma (Figure 10.48, K and L).[796]

Although HIV and AIDS initially were diseases of the developed countries and Africa, the incidence has risen dramatically in other parts of the world, with the largest rise occurring in South East Asia and India. HIV transmission in these countries is mostly heterosexual. By 2007, an estimated 33.2 million people worldwide and 1 million in the United States were HIV infected. Women and minorities have shown a rise in incidence, along with men who have sex with men (MSM) who continue to be a high-risk group.[780]

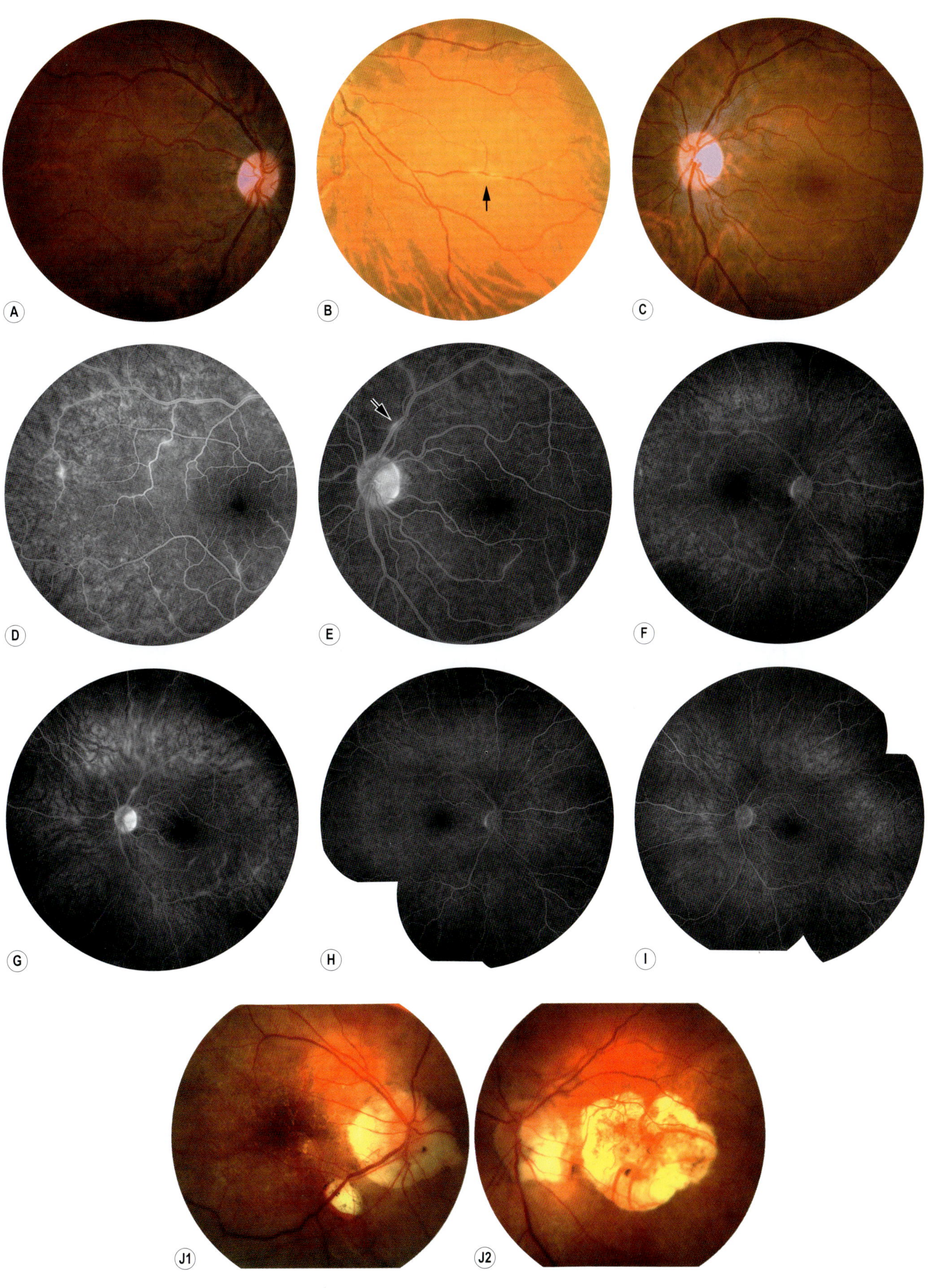
A
B
C
D
E
F
G
H
I
J1
J2

EPSTEIN–BARR VIRUS

Epstein–Barr virus (EBV) infects virtually everyone by adulthood, and a lifelong latency is maintained. It infects children silently, whereas the majority of adolescents develop infectious mononucleosis (IM). Thus the clinical outcome of EBV infection is age dependent. Children with primary immune insufficiency can have fatal or chronic IM, malignant B-cell lymphoma, virus-associated hemophagocytic syndrome, aplastic anemia, or acquired hypogammaglobulinemia. Part of the predilection for AIDS and other immunosuppressed patients to develop B-cell lymphomas may result from EBV infection. Aciclovir and immunoglobulin therapy can be of value in some patients with active EBV infection.[714,825] Ocular involvement seldom occurs in patients with other clinical manifestations of EBV. A variety of ocular disorders associated with EBV infection have been reported, including acute necrotizing retinitis,[658,826] outer punctate retinitis simulating toxoplasmosis,[714,825] multifocal choroiditis and panuveitis (Figure 10.49, J–L, and N),[730,827] anterior uveitis, severe panuveitis with optic disc swelling, macular edema,[828] and possibly retinal phlebitis (Figure 10.49, A–I). There is conflicting information concerning the incidence of serologic evidence of recent EBV infection in patients with multifocal choroiditis and panuveitis (see multifocal choroiditis and panuveitis, p. 988).

HUMAN T-LYMPHOTROPIC VIRUS TYPE 1

Human T-lymphotropic virus type 1 (HLTV-1) is a human retrovirus that causes adult T-cell leukemia and lymphoma and HTLV-1-associated myelopathy (HAM).

The virus is endemic in the Caribbean, Italy, Middle East, sub-Saharan Africa, and southwest Japan including Kyushu and Okinawa islands.[797,829–833] A small number of these patients develop adult T-cell leukemia/lymphoma and myelopathy. The remaining carriers may remain asymptomatic and otherwise healthy or develop uveitis or retinal vasculitis.[834–837] The uveitis can be granulomatous (75%) or nongranulomatous (25%). It is usually a panuveitis with white retinal lesions, vitreous cells, fluorescein leakage from the retinal vessels, and variable anterior segment involvement. It can have a waxing and waning course, usually responds to steroids, and can recur.[832,833,838–841] A small subset of patients with HTLV-1 antibodies develop a recalcitrant retinal vasculitis and progressive chorioretinal degeneration. This disease does not respond to steroids and appears to be at the severe end of the spectrum.[842] Some of these patients may eventually develop myelopathy. The clinical appearance resembles CMV retinitis, acute retinal necrosis, and frosted branch angiitis, but does not respond to ganciclovir. Vitreous and retinal biopsy with PCR identification of HTLV may be the only way to establish a diagnosis in nonendemic areas.

Adult T-cell leukemia (ATL) patients can develop a picture of retinal vasculitis and infiltrates confirmed by biopsy showing infiltration of leukemic/lymphoma cells in the retina.[830,842,843] These patients are not necessarily from the endemic areas (see Chapter 13, Fig. 13. 33). Intraocular lymphoma with yellow–white sub-RPE deposits has also been very rarely caused by HTLV-1.[844,845]

10.49 Continued

was 20/200 and the left was count fingers. There were a few vitreous cells bilaterally and coaelescing yellow lesions were noted in both macula with relative sparing of the peripheral retina and blood vessels (K and L). Laboratory testing showed lymphocytosis but negative for syphilis, Lyme disease, and *Toxoplasma*. She underwent a vitrectomy for a concern for lymphoma which showed atypical lymphocytes characteristic of EBV infection. She was started on valaciclovir 1 g PO three times a day and oral prednisone 50 mg per day. Over the next 2 weeks her inflammation subsided, the lesions turned atrophic (N) and the vision stabilized at 20/80 on the right and count fingers on the left.

(Courtesy: A–I, Dr Michael Altaweel; J–N, Dr Stephen Kim and Dr Daniel Martin. Reprinted with permission from Retina Cases and Brief Reports.)

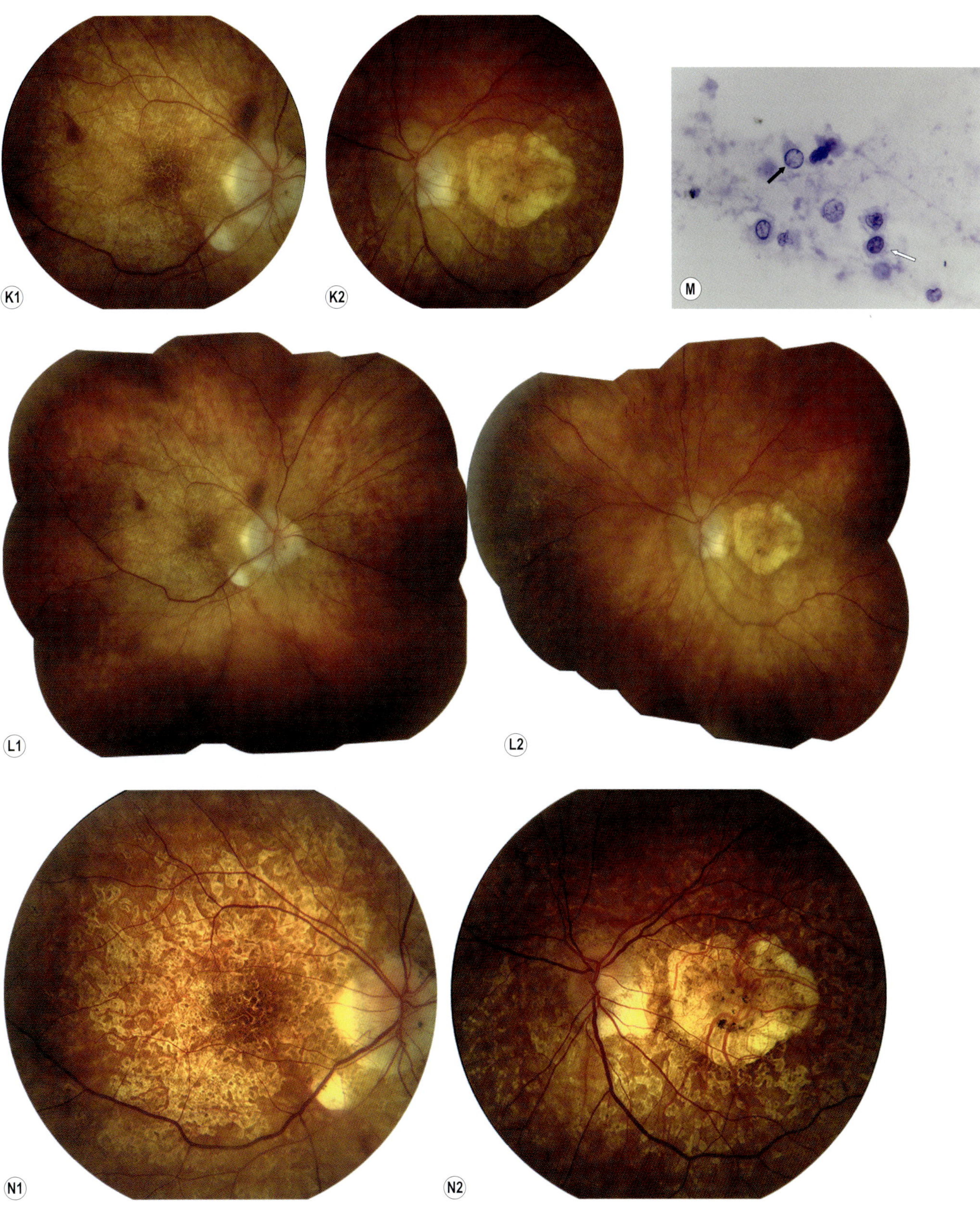
K1
K2
M
L1
L2
N1
N2

RUBELLA RETINITIS

Children born of mothers who contracted rubella during the first trimester of pregnancy may show a variety of anomalies of development of the eyes and other organs (Figure 10.50).[846–860] In these children there is a high incidence of what has been described as salt-and-pepper mottling of the RPE (Figure 10.50, D–K).[849,855] This is often most prominent in the posterior fundus. Both eyes are affected in 80% of cases.[855] Early progression of the pigment mottling in childhood may be caused by persistence of the rubella virus within the RPE. Pigment mottling, however, becomes less prominent in adulthood. This pigmentary change of the fundus may be accompanied by evidence of pigment loss from the pigment epithelium of the irides, which in some cases will transilluminate in an irregular fashion (Figure 10.50, C). These alterations of the RPE may occur alone or may be associated with other ocular abnormalities, such as cataracts and microphthalmos, and systemic abnormalities, including deafness and congenital heart disease (Figure 10.50, A and B). In patients with evidence of RPE involvement only, the visual acuity is usually normal. Choroidal neovascularization and disciform macular detachment may be a late complication of rubella retinopathy (Figure 10.50, F–I).[848,849,852,859,860a,860b] The electroretinographic and electro-oculographic findings, color vision, and visual fields in most patients are normal. Fluorescein angiography shows mottled hyperfluorescence caused by extensive and irregular loss of pigment from the RPE (Figure 10.50, H and I) and may be helpful in detecting early choroidal neovascularization (Figure 10.50, H). Autofluorescence imaging shows finely mottled decreased autofluorescence corresponding to the areas of RPE loss.[861] Pathologically, the salt-and-pepper changes in the fundus are caused by altered pigmentation and some atrophy of the RPE.[847] The retina and choroid are unaffected. Rubella retinopathy may be mimicked by inherited dystrophies of the RPE (see Figure 4.05), the carrier state of X-linked ocular albinism (see Figure 5.37, J), X-linked choroideremia (see Figure 5.28, E and F), and toxic diseases of the RPE (see Figure 9.03, A–E).[850]

10.50 Congenital rubella.

A: This child had microphthalmos and cataract in the left eye, rubella retinopathy in the right eye, hearing loss, dental hypoplasia, and congenital heart disease.
B to **E**: Dental hypoplasia (B), iris stromal and RPE atrophy (C), and rubella retinopathy (D) in a 4-year-old boy whose mother had rubella in the first trimester of pregnancy. Note the extensive derangement of the RPE (D). His visual acuity was normal. At age 11 years, the RPE changes were less apparent (E).
F to **I**: Rubella retinopathy (F and G) in a 9-year-old boy who developed loss of vision in the right eye secondary to subfoveal choroidal neovascularization (*arrow*, F). His mother received gammaglobulin injections during the first trimester of pregnancy because of exposure to an epidemic of rubella. His visual acuity in the left eye was 20/15. His electro-oculographic and electroretinographic findings were normal. Angiography in the right eye showed evidence of choroidal neovascularization (H) and widespread alterations of the RPE in both eyes (H and I).
J and **K**: Compare the prominent RPE mottling associated with rubella in an 11-year-old (J) with that of the more subtle mottling in a 37-year-old man (K). Angiography in the man shows evidence of marked hypopigmentation of the RPE. Visual acuity was normal in both patients.

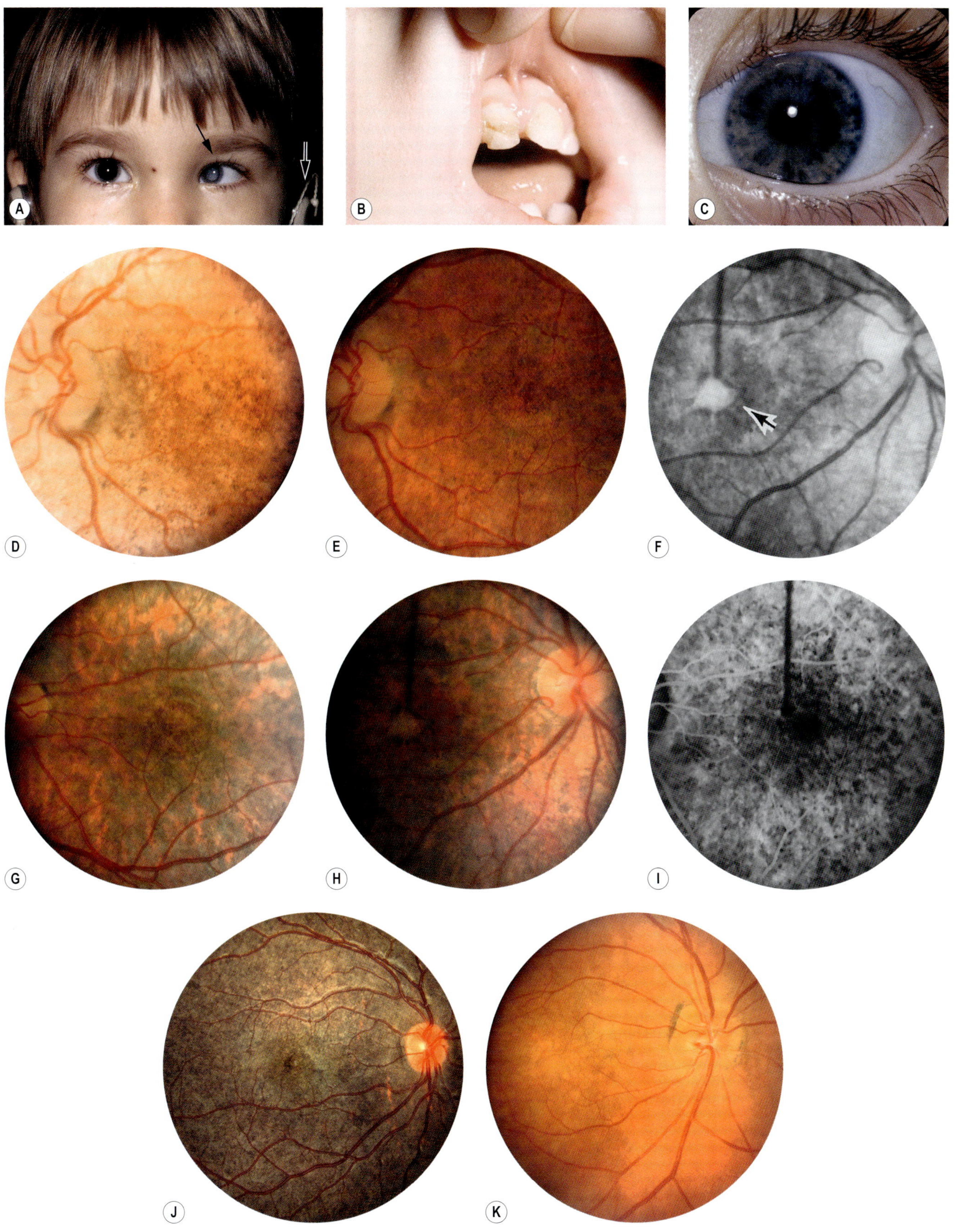
A
B
C
D
E
F
G
H
I
J
K

SUBACUTE SCLEROSING PANENCEPHALITIS

Subacute sclerosing panencephalitis (Dawson's encephalitis) is a progressive neurologic disease representing a slow viral disease caused by a defective measles virus. It typically follows a preceding measles infection in children and young adults by a mean interval of 7 years. Males are affected three times as often as females. Personality and behavioral changes are usually followed by dementia, seizures, myoclonus, and death. It occasionally occurs in young adults, who may recover with only minimal neurologic deficit (Figure 10.51, C–I). The disease can occasionally be seen in adults above age 25 and has been reported in a 49-year-old man.[862] Fifty percent of patients will have involvement of the visual system. Visual complaints often antedate the onset of neurologic symptoms by several weeks.[782,814,863] Neurologic symptoms may be delayed as long as 22 months.[781,782,864,865] Most patients have a history of preceding measles (rubeola infection), usually before 2 years of age.

The patients may be seen initially because of loss of central vision caused by one or more small, flat, focal, white retinal lesions or larger, more ragged, gray–white areas (Figure 10.51, A–D).[866–868] Either one or both eyes may be affected. When the retinitis involves the center of the macula, a cherry-red spot may be present.[834,835,869,870] The white retinal lesions resolve rapidly and are replaced by irregular areas of RPE atrophy, gliotic scarring of the retina, radiating retinal folds, and occasionally retinal hole formation (Figure 10.51, B and G–J). The pigmentary changes may be misinterpreted as heredomacular dystrophy. The pigmentary changes are not always confined to the macula.[836,871] There is minimal evidence of choroidal involvement. The vitreous is relatively free of inflammation. The optic disc may be swollen or atrophic.[866,872] Angiography is helpful in detecting subtle changes in the RPE.[873,874] Other causes of visual decline can present as homonymous hemianopia or cortical blindness.[875]

Histopathologically, the acute stage of subacute sclerosing panencephalitis is characterized by patchy focal areas of retinal necrosis, pigment-laden macrophages, minimal evidence of inflammation in the retina, loss of pigment from the RPE, and minimal inflammation in the choroid.[819,834,869,876] Later the retina may show focal areas of atrophy of the inner, outer, or both layers, with disruption and hyperplasia of the RPE and the presence of Cowdry type A and Cowdry type B intranuclear inclusions as well as some intracytoplasmic inclusions (Figure 10.51, K).[867,869,876] Viral particles typical for measles virus have been identified in both the retina and the brain of these patients.[822,834,867,869] It affects both the white and gray matter of the brain. Evidence of measles virus has been demonstrated in the retina utilizing immunofluorescent techniques.[869,876] The demonstration of high levels of measles antibody in the serum and CSF is helpful in establishing the diagnosis. The electroencephalogram shows bursts of high-amplitude, sharply contoured, slow-wave complexes. T2-weighted MRI shows diffuse or focal periventricular and subcortical white matter changes.[862] There is much evidence that subacute sclerosing panencephalitis is caused by an altered form of the measles virus. There is no effective treatment. High doses of intrathecal alpha- and beta-interferon or via an Omega reservoir with oral isoprinosine administered over 6 weeks has, however, subjectively improved symptoms, but has failed to prevent death.[862]

10.51 Retinitis caused by subacute sclerosing panencephalitis.

A and **B**: This 12-year-old boy had several patches of acute retinitis in the right macula (A). He had similar lesions in his left eye. His visual acuity was 20/400 in the right eye and finger counting at 4 feet in the left eye. Note the cherry-red spot. Ten days later there was partial clearing of the central lesion and evidence of a larger lesion temporally (B). At that time he had no neurologic symptoms and the neurologic evaluation was normal. During the next month, however, he became lethargic, mute, and blind. He died 2 months later of cardiopulmonary arrest. He had been exposed to measles at age 5 and had received attenuated measles virus vaccine 5 months before the onset of visual symptoms.

C to **I**: A healthy 21-year-old man had a 1-week history of blurred vision in his left eye. At that time there was evidence of retinal whitening associated with some hemorrhage (C). The right fundus was within normal limits except for the presence of a small hemorrhage in the macula. A medical evaluation that included spinal fluid examination revealed a rubeola IgG titer in the cerebrospinal fluid of 1:64, which was thought to be diagnostic of subacute sclerosing panencephalitis. The patient's past medical history was negative for measles or immunization against rubeola. Three years previously he had been hospitalized for brain fever of uncertain etiology. Two weeks after visual loss in the left eye he noted loss of vision in the right eye. Examination revealed an irregular area of necrotizing retinitis (D). A fluorescein angiogram revealed evidence of perivascular leakage of dye and some staining of the lesions (E and F). The retinal lesions in his left eye had partly faded (G). An electroencephalogram revealed findings compatible with subacute sclerosing panencephalitis. Six months later there was irregular scarring and thinning of the retina in the macular area of both eyes (H and I). Visual acuity was counting fingers at 3 feet.

J and **K**: Irregular pigmentary disturbances of the macula and mild papilledema caused by subacute sclerosing panencephalitis (J) in an 8-year-old boy who 4 weeks previously became lethargic, incontinent, and finally comatose. He died 3 weeks later, and histopathologic examination of the macular region revealed an atrophic thinned retina containing large masses of multinucleated syncytial giant cells containing numerous intranuclear eosinophilic inclusions (K).

(A and B from Landers and Klintworth[869], © 1971, American Medical Association. All rights reserved. C–I, courtesy Dr W. Sanderson Grizzard and Dr Andrew K. Vine; J and K from Font et al.[876], © 1973, American Medical Association. All rights reserved.)

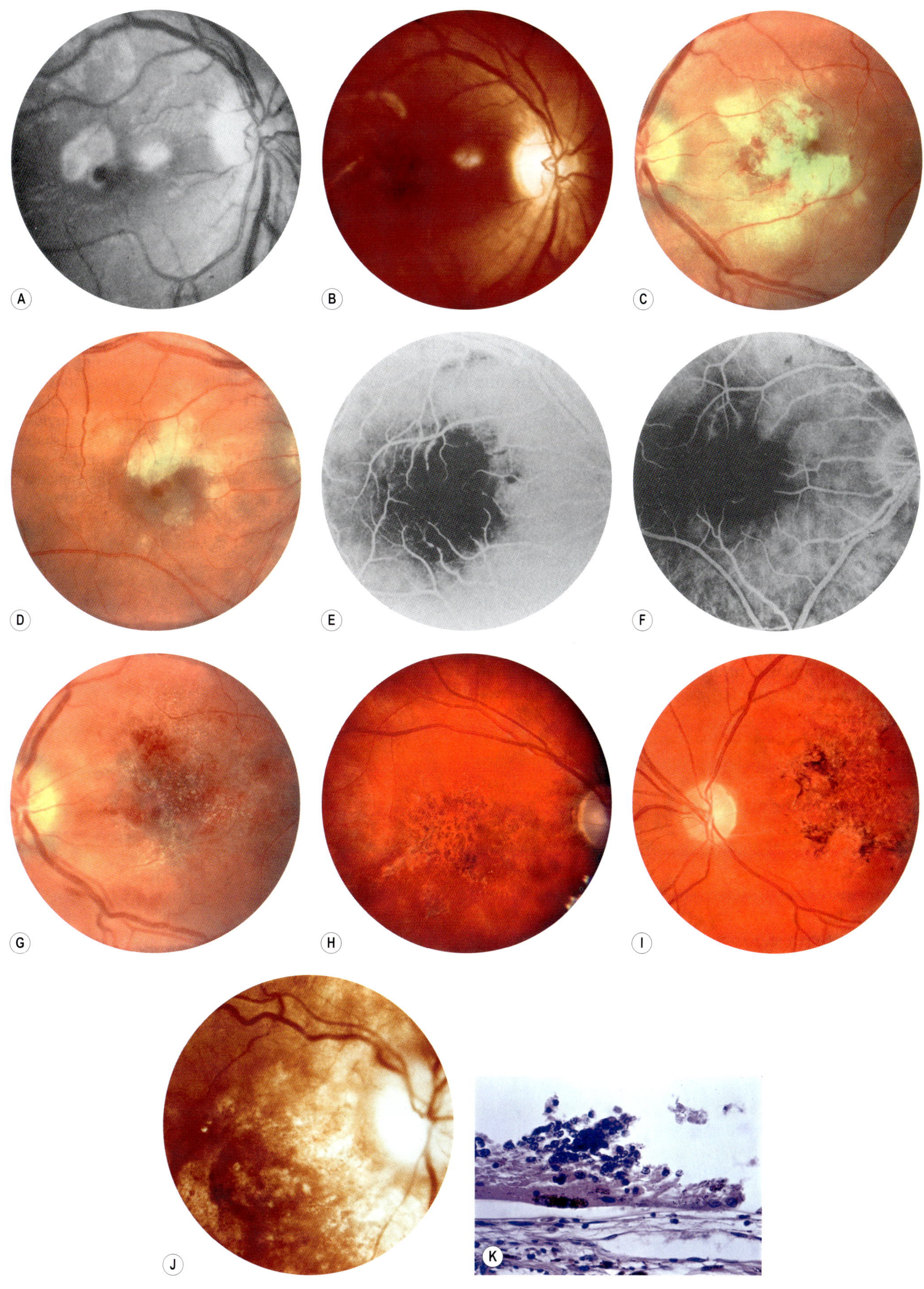
A
B
C
D
E
F
G
H
I
J
K

DENGUE FEVER

Dengue fever is a viral illness endemic in tropical and subtropical regions, including the Caribbean, South and Central America, Asia, Africa, and the Pacific. The female *Aedes aegyptii/albopictus* mosquito transmits the disease. Five clinical syndromes can occur: nonspecific febrile illness, classic dengue, dengue hemorrhagic fever, dengue shock syndrome, and unusual syndromes such as encephalopathy and hepatitis. Classic dengue presents with an abrupt onset of fever, severe headache, myalgias, arthralgias, nausea, vomiting, and a maculopapular rash. The rash eventually becomes confluent, sparing small islands of skin. Dengue hemorrhagic fever affects children less than 15 years of age in hyperendemic regions with increased capillary permeability and hemostatic disturbances as its hallmark. The most severe form (grade 4) is associated with profound shock and circulatory problems and is termed dengue shock syndrome. Thrombocytopenia causes petechial bleeding, epistaxis, and bleeding gums, and can manifest in the eye as retinal hemorrhages and loss of vision.[890] Macular hemorrhage, retinal edema, optic neuritis, ischemic optic neuropathy, decreased axoplasmic flow, macular exudates, and retinal pigment epithelial lesions are seen. Factors contributing to the circulatory disturbances can also cause choroidal effusions and secondary serous retinal detachments.[891]

10.53 Dengue retinopathy.

A to **F**: Bilateral disc edema, perivascular infiltrates, and retinal hemorrhages associated with mild anterior uveitis in a 33-year-old Chinese woman in Singapore, 6 days after the onset of dengue fever (A and B). Her best corrected visual acuity was 20/400 in each eye. Early knobby hyperfluorescence of the venular wall in the posterior pole and elsewhere (*arrows*) in both eyes, with late leakage was seen (C–F).
G to **L**: Bilateral retinal white dots in the macula in a 16-year-old girl with visual symptoms 7 days after fever onset. Her visual acuity was 20/40 in the right eye and 20/50 in the left eye. The white dots are hyperfluorescent on the fluorescein angiogram and hypofluorescent on indocyanine angiography (ICG) and remain so in the late phase. ICG shows more dots than seen on the angiogram.

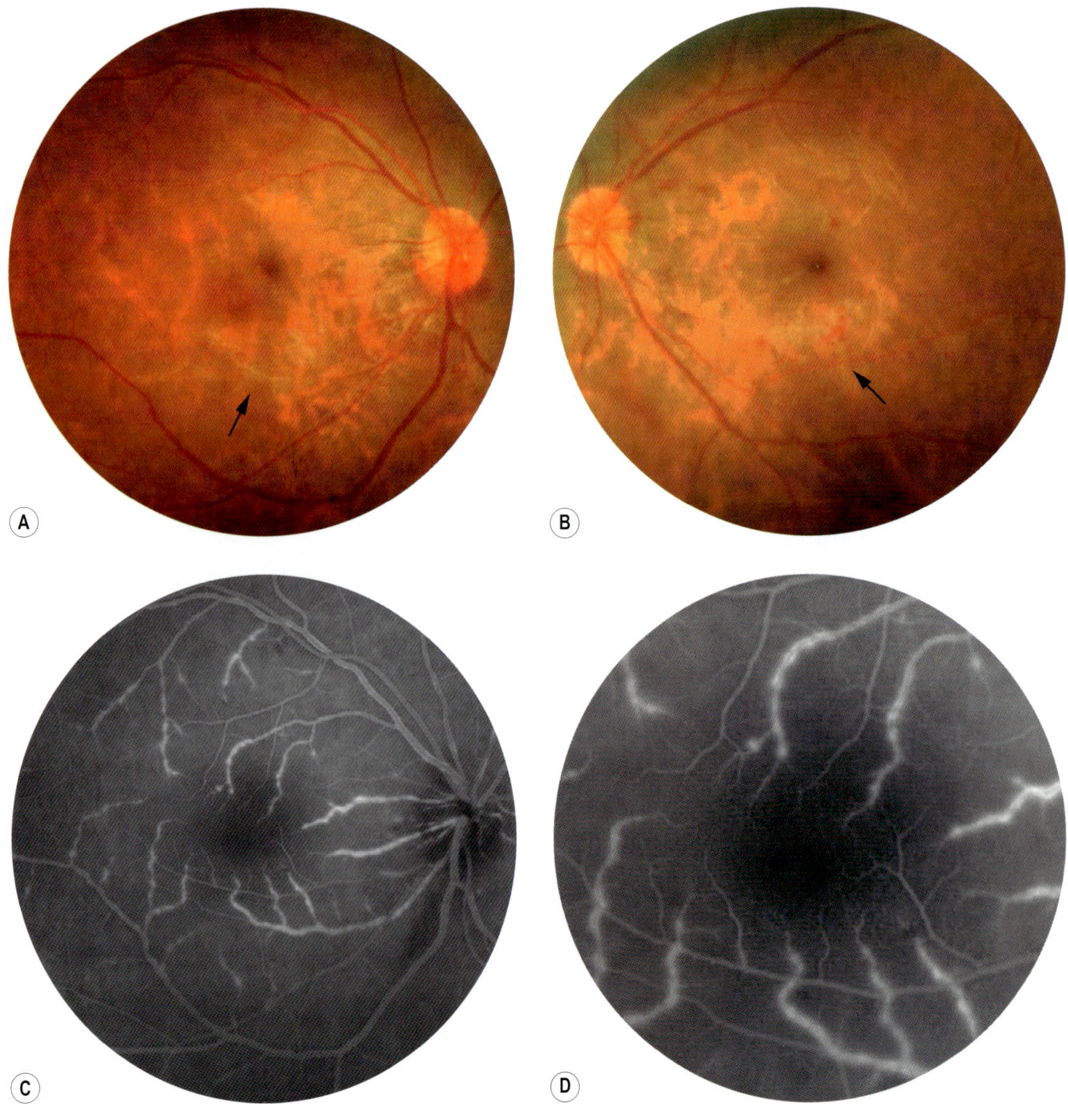

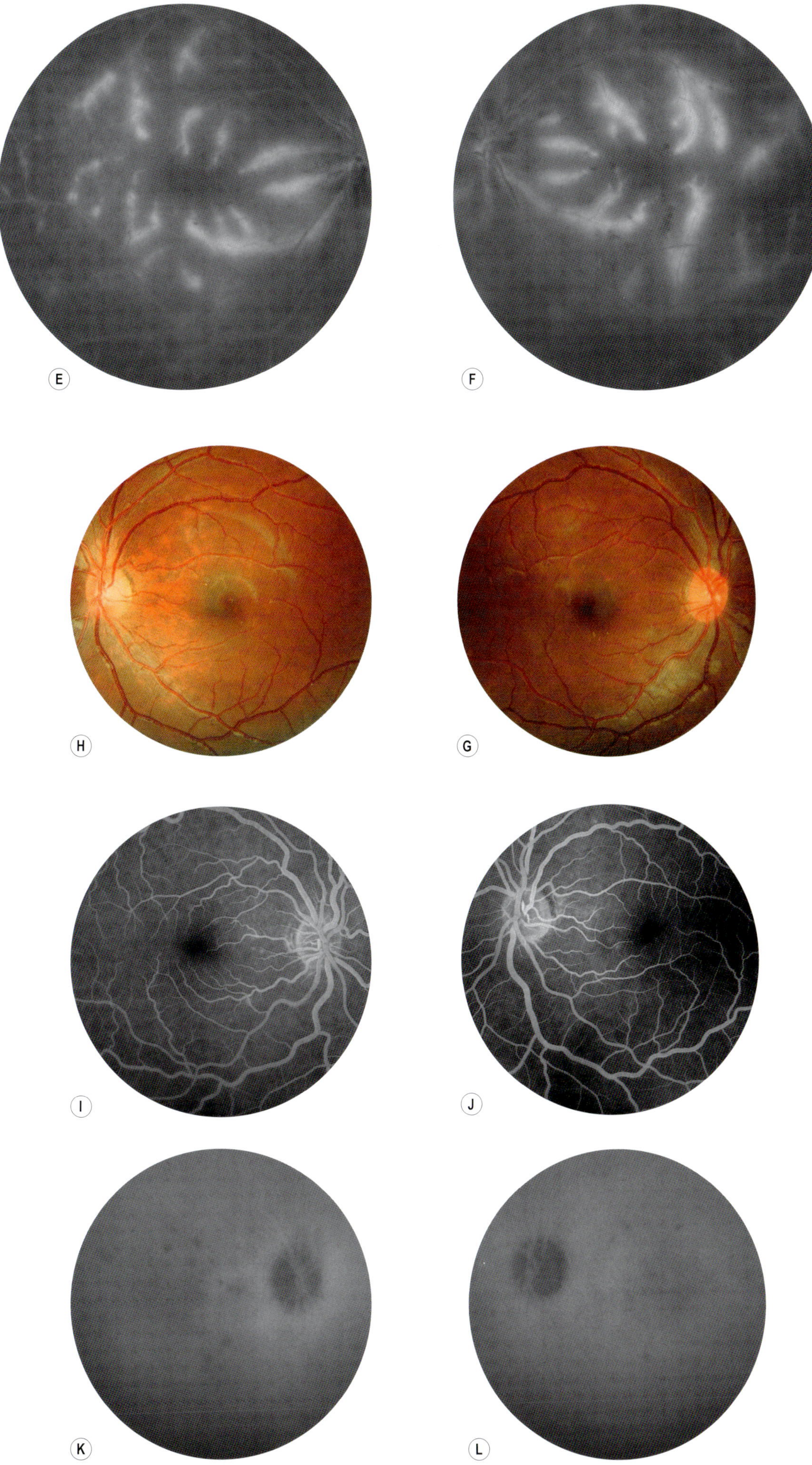
E
F
H
G
I
J
K
L

Ocular involvement occurs in a small subset of patients and manifests 1 week after fever onset. They present with retinitis, arteritis, and retinal hemorrhages, with or without associated anterior uveitis and vitritis. Cotton-wool spots, retinal hemorrhages, and branch retinal artery occlusions are common findings (Figure 10.53. A, B, M, N, and P).[890,892–902] Fluorescein angiography reveals leakage of dye from arteries and veins and evidence of arteriolar or venous obstruction (Figure 10.53, C–F, O, Q, and R). Indocyanine green angiography reveals additional dark spots not visible on the angiogram (Figure 10.53, K and L). Thrombocytopenia that accompanies the infection is responsible for the retinal hemorrhages in those eyes without florid vasculitis. Anterior uveitis is nongranulomatous. Although the fundus appearance can mimic Behçet's disease, the temporal relation of the ocular involvement to the systemic manifestations of dengue fever differentiates the two conditions. Stellate neuroretinitis, foveolitis, optic neuritis, macular edema, exudative retinal detachment, and macular infarction have all been noted.[890–893,895–901,903]

10.53 Continued

M to **O**: Serous macular detachment, nerve fiber infarcts and few white dots in the right eye of this 27-year-old (M). Angiogram shows involvement of the vessel wall and nonperfusion of the retinal capillaries corresponding to the nerve fiber infarct (O).

P to **S**: A 21-year-old Indian female complained of vision loss in her left eye 7 days after the onset of fever, clinically suspected to be secondary to dengue. Her visual acuity was 20/400. She had two patches of retinitis with retinal opacification, hemorrhages, and lipid exudates (P). The angiogram revealed associated microangiitis with late leakage of dye (Q and R). One month later her vision had improved to 20/100 with resolution of the retinitis and residual lipid exudates and retinal hemorrhage (S).

Courtesy: A–O, Dr Soon-Phaik Chee, reprinted from Bacsal et al.[899], P–S, Dr Vishali Gupta.)

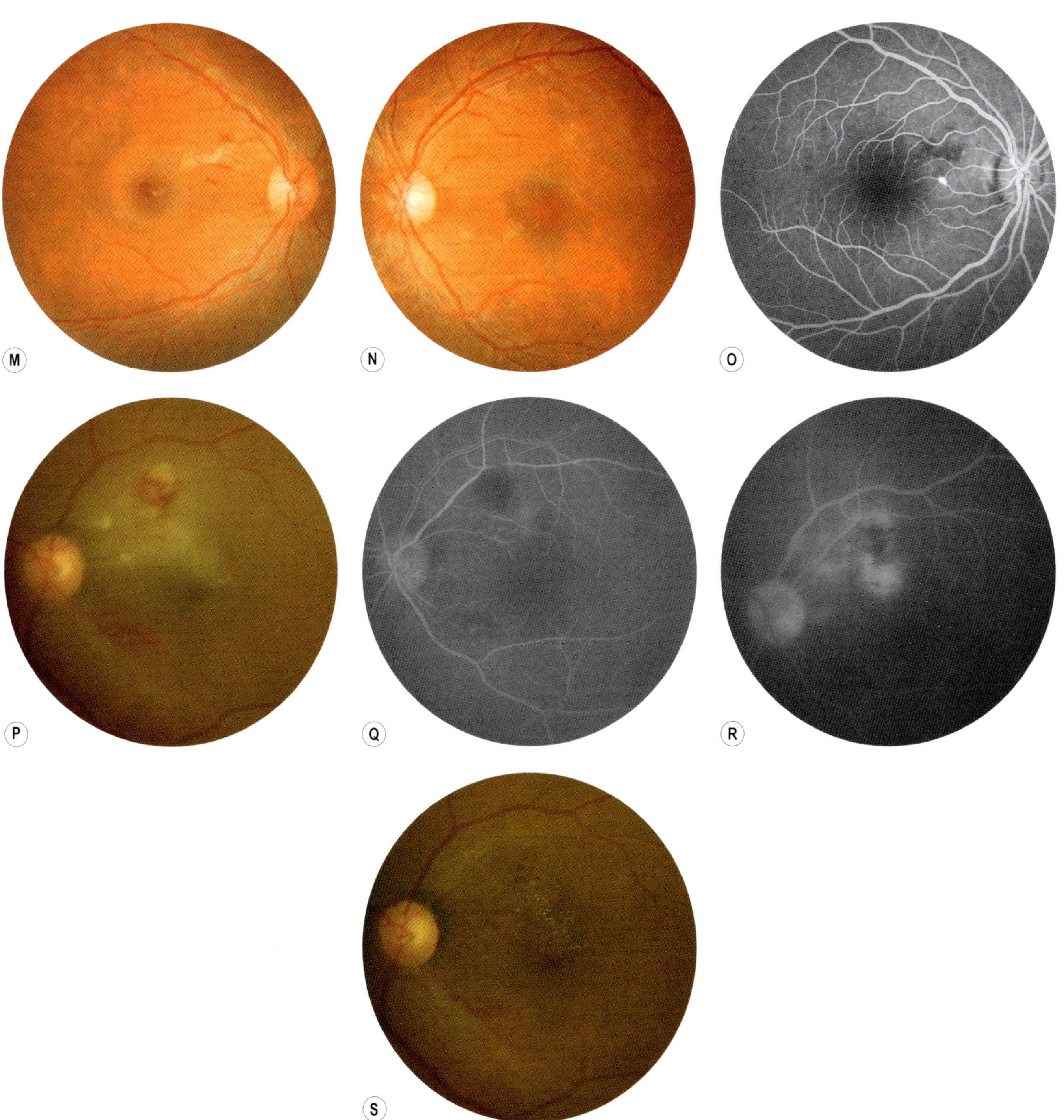
M
N
O
P
Q
R
S

CHIKUNGUNYA VIRUS

An outbreak of chikungunya occurred after 20 years since the previous episode in India and some islands of the Indian Ocean in 2006.[904,905] Chikungunya fever was first described in 1955 after an outbreak on the Makonde Plateau along the border between Mozambique and Tanzania. There have been subsequent outbreaks in India, Vietnam, Indonesia, Bangkok, and Myanmar. The virus is a single-stranded RNA virus of the genus *Alphavirus*, causing fever, headache, fatigue, nausea, vomiting, myalgia, rash, and joint pain.

Several reports from the Indian outbreak of 2006 have described the ocular manifestations which include conjunctivitis, unilateral or bilateral iridocyclitis, secondary glaucoma, retinitis, vitritis, retinal hemorrhages, neuroretinitis, and optic neuritis.[905–909] Focal areas of retinal whitening with adjacent retinal hemorrhages characterized the retinitis (Figure 10.54, A–F). An angiogram revealed vascular occlusion and leakage with late staining of the involved retina (Figure 10.54, G, H, and I) and serous retinal detachment (Figure 10.54, J and K). The ocular signs appeared approximately 3–4 weeks after the onset of the viral illness; hence it may be an immune-mediated rather than a direct viral infection. However, these mechanisms are not well understood given the rarity of the disease. Treatment is mostly supportive. Some patients received oral/IV aciclovir and systemic steroids, but whether this modified the clinical course is debatable. The visual recovery was moderate, with complete resolution of the conjunctivitis and uveitis. Those patients with optic neuritis had a less than favorable visual outcome.[904,905,907,908]

MUMPS NEURORETINITIS

Papillitis and neuroretinitis, usually associated with clinical evidence of meningoencephalitis, occasionally develop in patients with mumps.[910,911] One or more foci of retinitis may also be present. Most patients recover normal visual function.

10.54 Chikungunya retinitis.

A to **D**: A 48-year-old Indian man presented with gradual diminution in vision in both eyes for 15 days, 3 months after a bout of prolonged fever. His visual acuity was 8/200 in the right eye and count fingers at 3 feet in the left eye. Anterior segment was unremarkable. Both fundi had retinal infarction and hemorrhages in the macula and around the disc (A and B). Aqueous PCR for HSV, VZV, and CMV were negative. RT-PCR for Chikungunya virus detected nine copies of viral RNA/mL. He received oral valaciclovir and prednisone. Two months later his vision had improved to 20/60 and 20/80 in the right and left eyes, respectively. The retinal whitening and hemorrhages had improved (C and D)

E to **M**: A 42-year-old Indian man complained of blurred vision in both eyes for 2 weeks which began 2 weeks after a fever. His vision was 4/400 in each eye. There were fine pigment specks on the corneal endothelium and flare in both eyes. Both eyes had retinal whitening and hemorrhages and intraretinal edema, and the left had shallow serous detachment in addition (E and F). The optic discs were hyperemic bilaterally. Angiogram showed hypoperfusion in the early phase and late hyperfluorescence and leakage in both eyes (G–I). OCT of the right eye showed intraretinal edema and the left intraretinal and subretinal fluid (J and K). His Chikungunya IgM antibody was positive; dengue rapid test, treponemal hemagglutination, HSV-1 and -2, and *Toxoplasma* antibodies were negative. He received IV aciclovir for 1 week followed by oral aciclovir for 8 weeks, and 40 mg of oral prednisone tapered over 6 weeks. Ten weeks after onset his vision returned to 20/20 and the retina appeared almost normal in both eyes (L and M).

(A–D, courtesy Dr J. Biswas and Dr Sudharshan; E–K, courtesy Dr P. Mahendradas, reprinted from Mahendradas et al.[905])

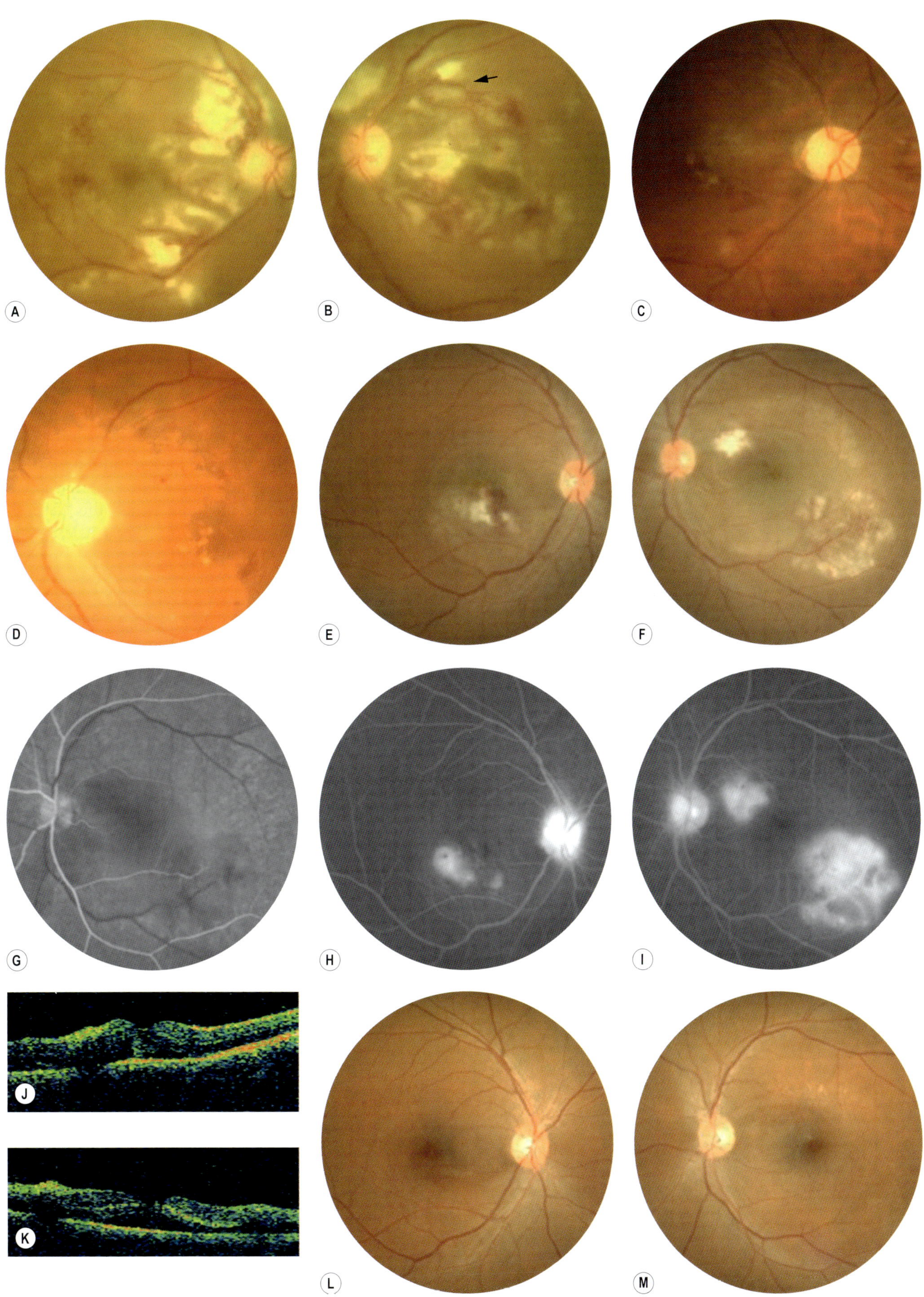
A
B
C
D
E
F
G
H
I
J
K
L
M

RIFT VALLEY FEVER RETINITIS

Rift Valley fever is an acute disease primarily affecting cattle and sheep caused by a specific arthropod-borne virus that is endemic in the western one-third of Africa. Epidemics involving humans have occurred, the most severe of which caused the death of over 600 people in Egypt during 1977 and 1978. In autumn of 2000 an outbreak occurred for the first time in Saudi Arabia (Figure 10.55).[912] In humans this is typically an acute febrile illness with biphasic temperature elevations mimicking dengue fever. It is associated with muscle and joint pains, headaches, and occasionally nausea and vomiting. Conjunctivitis and photophobia are common during the early phases of the disease. Visual loss occurs often days or weeks after subsidence of the fever and is associated with multiple areas of what appear to be acute necrotizing and hemorrhagic retinitis in the macular and paramacular areas (Figure 10.55, A and E), similar to that seen in subacute sclerosing panencephalitis and the herpes viruses.[913–917] Vitritis and occlusion of the major retinal arteries are common. This latter change is presumed to be related to proliferation of the retinal vascular endothelium. Vitreous hemorrhage and retinal detachment may occur in some patients. The natural course of the disease is variable: patients may recover normal acuity or may have severe permanent visual loss, depending on the location and severity of the retinal involvement. The most severe systemic complications are encephalitis and hemorrhagic hepatitis.

The virus is an RNA type and is believed to be transmitted by an insect, possibly the mosquito. Human infection can also occur by handling diseased or dead animals or contaminated specimens. The diagnosis is based on a demonstrated rise in the hemagglutination antibodies of the Rift Valley fever virus and the complement fixation test.

10.55 Rift Valley fever retinitis.

A to D: This 40-year-old Saudi woman had a sudden loss of vision 10 days after developing fever related to Rift valley fever (RVF). Serum IgM for RVF virus was positive. Her visual acuity was count fingers at 1 meter on the right and 20/20 on the left. She had 1+ anterior chamber and vitreous cells. A creamy macular lesion with two adjacent retinal hemorrhages was seen (A). The lesion scarred down over time with folds in the surrounding inner retina at 2 years (B). The visual acuity remained at count fingers. An angiogram showed staining of the foveal scar and a linear window defect extending to the disc edge (C and D).

E: Another patient with creamy full-thickness retinitis involving the macula, associated with positive titers for RVF virus.

F and G: Two other patients 1–2 years after presentation with atrophic and partly pigmented scar in the macula.

(Courtesy: Dr Ali Al-Hazami, reprinted from Al-Hazami et al.[912])

VITRITIS AND RETINITIS IN WHIPPLE'S DISEASE

Whipple's disease is a chronic multisystemic disease characterized by fever, diarrhea, weight loss, steatorrhea, polyserositis, arthralgia, and impaired intestinal absorption. Other features include mesenteric and peripheral adenopathy; cutaneous pigmentation; heart murmur; neurologic signs and symptoms including personality changes, dementia, and memory defect; myoclonus; ataxia; supranuclear ophthalmoplegia; and seizure disorders.[918–939] Ocular findings include vitreous opacities (Figure 10.56, A),[930,932,933,940] exudative material overlying the pars plana (Figure 10.56, B),[919,930] retinal hemorrhages, cotton-wool patches, scattered white exudates, chorioretinitis (Figure 10.56) C,[918,929] retinal vasculitis, and uveitis (Figure 10.56, B, D, and E),[919,927,930,938] papilledema,[926,937] and glaucoma. One patient studied with fluorescein angiography showed multifocal areas of retinal capillary closure, diffuse retinal vasculitis, and choroidal folds.[918]

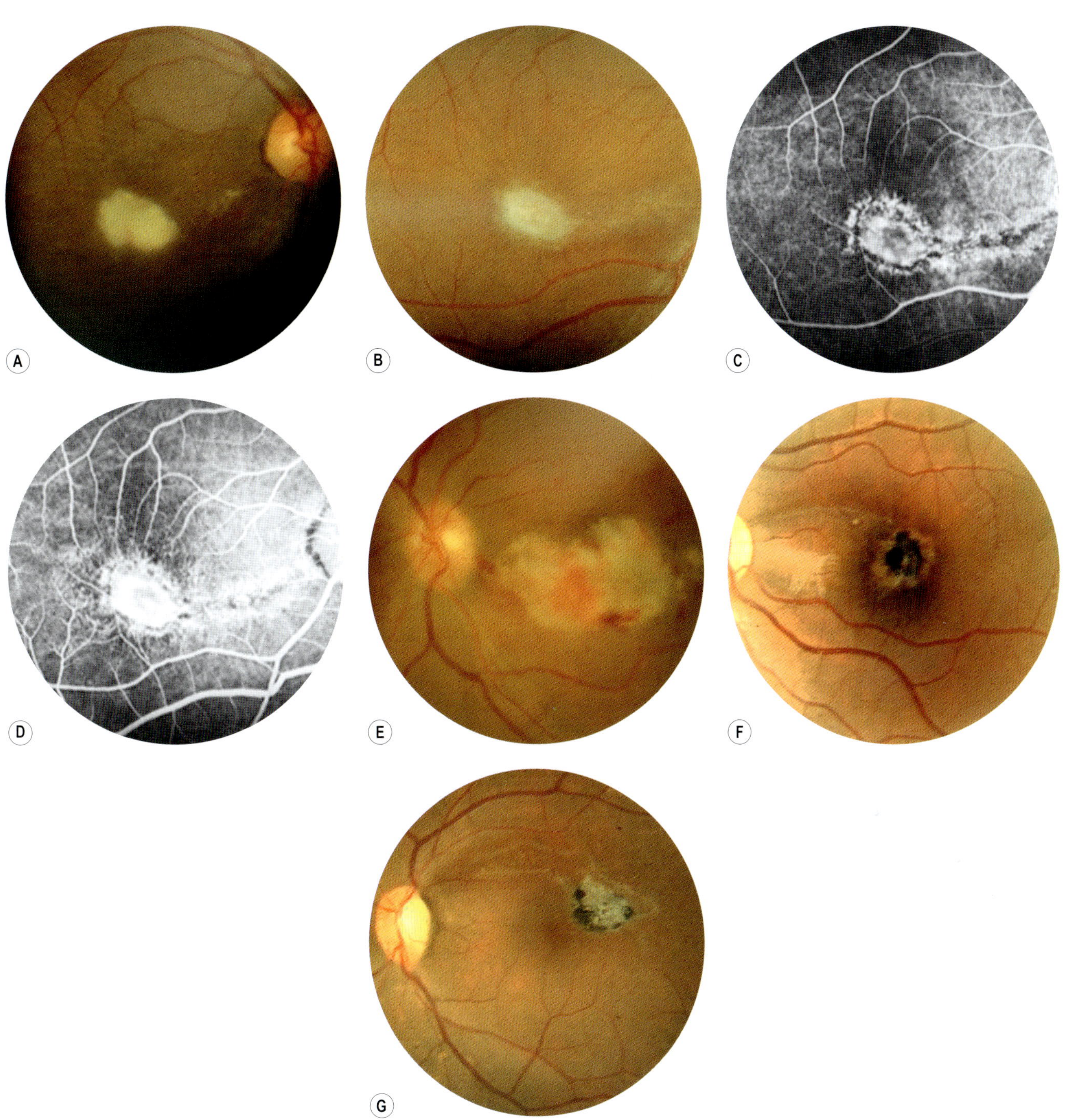
A
B
C
D
E
F
G

Histopathologically, foamy macrophages with many periodic acid–Schiff (PAS)-positive intercellular granules are found in many organs of the body including the brain and eye (Figure 10.56, L and M).[931,932,940] These are degradation products of *Tropheryma whippelii* that accumulate in the cells with little or no cell damage (Figure 10.56, J and K). Duodenal or jejunal biopsy is the usual method of diagnosis. The villi show widening with infiltration of the lamina propria with histiocytes and mononuclear inflammatory cells and dilation of lymphatic channels. Altered cell-mediated immunity and macrophage dysfunction is a feature of the condition. Vitrectomy has been employed in some cases.[919,930] Electron microscopy reveals degenerated rod-shaped bacteria within and adjacent to macrophages.

This gram-negative actinomycete with distinct morphologic characteristics is named *Tropheryma whippelii*. The organism is difficult to culture, but can be identified by polymerase PCR assay, as was done in the vitreous aspirate from a woman with uveitis and only minimal symptoms of Whipple's disease.[926,937] Margo and coworkers found macrophages filled with PAS-positive particles similar to those in Whipple's disease in the vitreous aspirate removed from the eye of a patient with coryneform bacterial endophthalmitis and no evidence of Whipple's disease.[925,936] Electron microscopy to demonstrate the thin bacillus within the cell wall surrounded by a membrane that confers a trilamellar aspect with a central nucleolus is pathognomonic of the agent that causes Whipple's disease.[941] The disease is more common in Caucasian males and has a higher incidence in HLA B27-positive patients.

Treatment of patients with Whipple's disease with antibiotics results in remission of symptoms and reduction in the PAS-positive macrophages. Antibiotic therapy including tetracycline, trimethoprim–sulfamethoxazole, sulfadiazine, penicillin and streptomycin, or ceftriaxone is the mainstay of therapy. An acute inflammatory reaction similar to the Jarisch–Herxheimer reaction in syphilis is sometimes seen following institution of therapy. This may be heralded by fever, chills, splenomegaly, erythema nodosum, leukocytosis with neutrophilia, arthritis, and arthralgia.[941,942] In severe cases, discontinuation of antibiotics results in resolution of findings. Whipple's disease should be considered in the differential diagnosis of patients with evidence of vitritis and retinitis and signs and symptoms of neurologic disease or inflammatory bowel disease such as Crohn's and ulcerative colitis. The differential diagnosis includes reticulum cell sarcoma, Behçet's disease, sarcoidosis, and other causes of vitritis.

10.56 Whipple's disease.

A to **K**: This 51-year-old Caucasian female presented with a 5-month history of floaters and hazy vision in the right eye. Over the previous month, she had noticed floaters in the left eye and further increase in the floaters in the right eye. She had undergone bilateral nephrectomy and renal transplant for polycystic kidney disease. She was on azathioprine (Imuran) 75 mg and prednisone 10 mg per day. She had pneumonia 3 years prior and had a coronary artery bypass graft (CABG) 2 months prior. She has had intermittent recent fungal skin lesions. She denied fevers and night sweats. She had mild arthritis in the knees. Two years prior, she was hospitalized and received IV antibiotics for a painful bout of migratory arthritis. No urinary, neurological, or cardiac symptoms were present. She has had problems with irritable bowel in the past but denied active gastrointestinal complaints at this time. Her visual acuity was 20/50 in the right eye and 20/25 in the left eye. The vitreous showed whitish, thick, snowball-like deposits, mostly on the retinal surface and some in the inferior vitreous, more in the right eye (A) than the left eye. The left eye showed perivascular white fluffy balls (B). Her urine culture, blood culture, PCR from aqueous and vitreous for fungus, HSV, HZV, and vitreous biopsy were negative for fungus or lymphoma. The vitreous biopsy was reported as rare macrophages with very rare lymphocytes. The fungal cultures and bacterial cultures were negative. She developed a retinal infarction temporal to the fovea (C), noted 1 day post vitrectomy, which included injection of amphotericin and fluconazole at the end of the surgery. She was started on oral fluconazole 400 mg per day, doxycycline 100 mg twice a day, and trimethoprim–sulfamethoxazole (Bactrim) twice a day. Silver stain for fungus was negative. There was no evidence of malignancy or viral inclusion particles. The acid-fast bacillus stain and PCR for CMV, HSV-1, HSV-2, EBV, and *Toxoplasma* were negative. Two weeks later, her visual acuity improved to 20/30 in the right eye. Vitreous was clearer. The area of retinal infarction had resolved. Fluorescein angiogram showed mild cystoid macular edema (D and E). Six weeks later, the inflammation worsened and the vision dropped to 20/50 in the right eye and 20/40 in the left eye (F and G). Fluorescein angiogram showed window defects corresponding to small mid peripheral chorioretinal scars (H and I). QuantiFERON-TB Gold test was negative. IgG was negative for *Toxoplasma*, CMV, EBV, and *Bartonella*. A repeat vitrectomy in the left eye showed cells containing large nuclei (J and K). The vitreous and blood PCR was positive for *Tropheryma whippelii*. Six months later, her vision had improved to 20/30 OU with nuclear sclerosis following a single vancomycin injection of 1 mg and IV ceftriaxone once a day for 1 month, followed by oral trimethoprim–sulfamethoxazole twice a day.

L: Photomicrograph showing clusters of macrophages within the inner retinal layers and in the vitreous (*arrow*).

M: Higher-power photomicrograph showing clusters of macrophages within the retina (*arrows*).

(A–K, from Razonable et al.[940]; L and M from Font et al.[920], © 1978, American Medical Association. All rights reserved.)

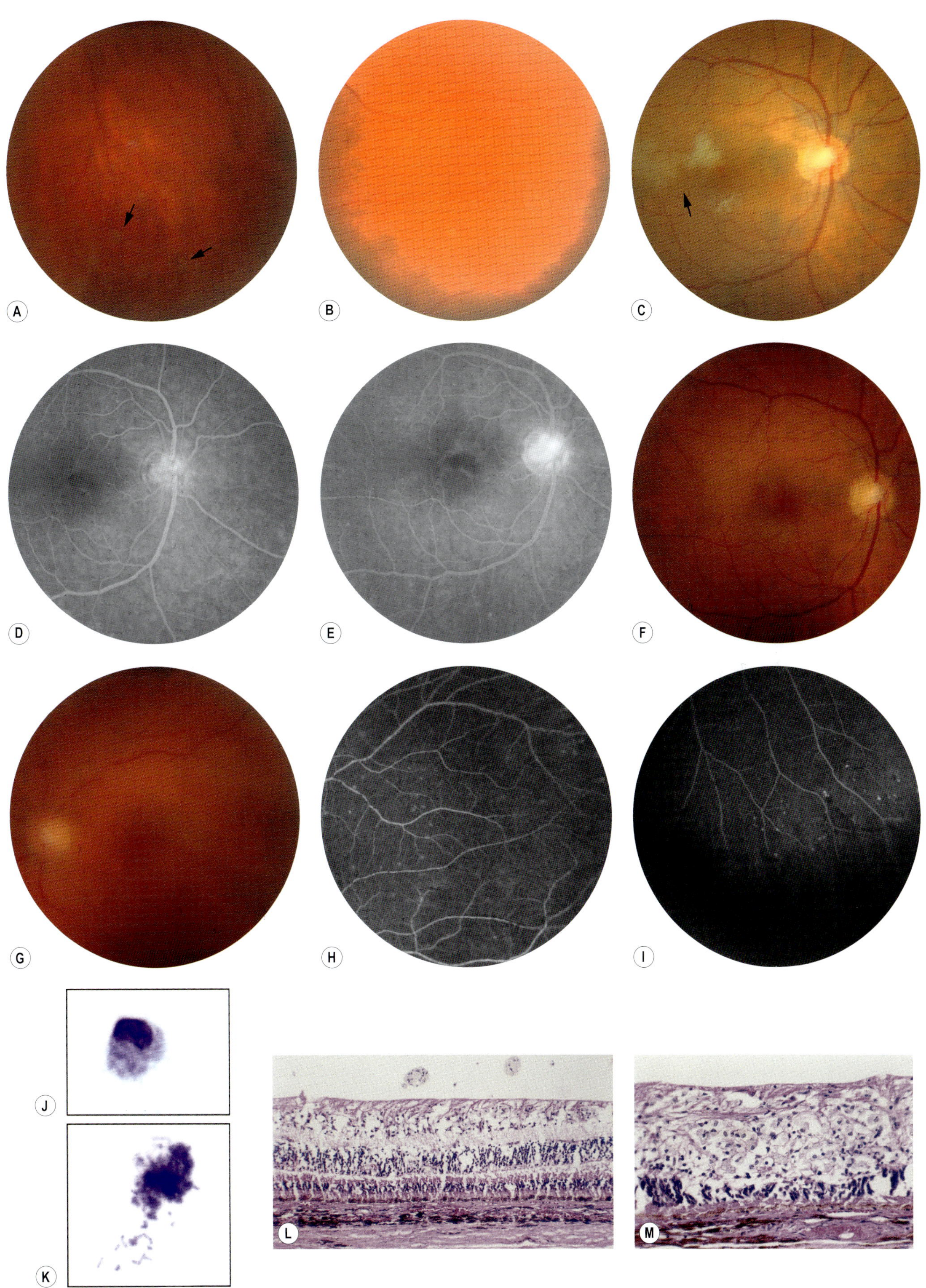
A
B
C
D
E
F
G
H
I
J
K
L
M

References

1. Packer AJ, Weingeist TA, Abrams GW. Retinal periphlebitis as an early sign of bacterial endophthalmitis. Am J Ophthalmol 1983;96:66–71.
2. Blodi BA, Johnson MW, McLeish WM, Gass JD. Presumed choroidal tuberculosis in a human immunodeficiency virus infected host. Am J Ophthalmol 1989;108:605–7.
3. Herschorn BJ, Brucker AJ. Embolic retinopathy due to Corynebacterium minutissimum endocardititis. Br J Ophthalmol 1985;69:29–31.
4. Kennedy JE, Wise GN. Clinicopathological correlation of retinal lesions; subacute bacterial endocarditis. Arch Ophthalmol 1965;74:658–62.
5. Litten M. Ueber die bei der acuten malignen Endocarditis und anderen septischen Erkrankungen vorkommenden Retinalveränderungen. Ber Ophthalmol Ges 1877;10:140–3.
6. Munier F, Othenin-Girard P. Subretinal neovascularization secondary to choroidal septic metastasis from acute bacterial endocarditis. Retina 1992;12:108–12.
7. Neudorfer M, Barnea Y, Geyer O, Siegman-Igra Y. Retinal lesions in septicemia. Am J Ophthalmol 1993;116:728–34.
8. Roth M. Beiträge zur Kenntniss der varicösen Hypertrophie der Nervenfasern. Arch Pathol Anat Physiol 1872;55:197–217.
9. Roth M. Ueber Netzhautaffection bei Wundfiebern. Dtsch Z Chir 1872;1:471.
10. Duane TD, Osher RH, Green WR. White centered hemorrhages: their significance. Ophthalmology 1980;87:66–9.
11. Hussain B, Lynn W, Lightman SL. Metastatic endophthalmitis. Br J Hosp Med (Lond) 2007;68:424–8.
12. Davis JL, Nussenblatt RB, Bachman DM, et al. Endogenous bacterial retinitis in AIDS. Am J Ophthalmol 1989;107:613–23.
13. Coll GE, Lewis H. Metastatic choroidal abscess and choroidal neovascular membrane associated with Staphylococcus aureus endocarditis in a heroin user. Retina 1994;14:256–9.
14. Carney MD, Combs JL, Waschler W. Cryptococcal choroiditis. Retina 1990;10:27–32.
15. Kim JE, Landon RE, Connor Jr TB, Kivlin JD. Endogenous ocular nocardiosis. J AAPOS 2004;8:194–5.
16. Bozbeyoglu S, Yilmaz G, Akova YA, et al. Choroidal abscess due to nocardial infection in a renal allograft recipient. Retina 2004;24:164–6.
17. Lakosha H, Pavlin CJ, Lipton J. Subretinal abscess due to Nocardia farcinica infection. Retina 2000;20:269–74.
18. Davitt B, Gehrs K, Bowers T. Endogenous Nocardia endophthalmitis. Retina 1998;18:71–3.
19. Ferry AP, Font RL, Weinberg RS, et al. Nocardial endophthalmitis: report of two cases studied histopathologically. Br J Ophthalmol 1988;72:55–61.
20. Gregor RJ, Chong CA, Augsburger JJ, et al. Endogenous Nocardia asteroides subretinal abscess diagnosed by transvitreal fine-needle aspiration biopsy. Retina 1989;9:118–21.
21. Ishibashi Y, Watanabe R, Hommura S, et al. Endogenous Nocardia asteroides endophthalmitis in a patient with systemic lupus erythematosus. Br J Ophthalmol 1990;74:433–6.
22. Jampol LM, Strauch BS, Albert DM. Intraocular nocardiosis. Am J Ophthalmol 1973; 76:568–73.
23. Lissner GS, O'Grady R, Choromokos E. Endogenous intraocular Nocardia asteroides in Hodgkin's disease. Am J Ophthalmol 1978;86:388–94.
24. Meyer SL, Font RL, Shaver RP. Intraocular nocardiosis; report of three cases. Arch Ophthalmol 1970;83:536–41.
25. Phillips WB, Shields CL, Shields JA, et al. Nocardia choroidal abscess. Br J Ophthalmol 1992;76:694–6.
26. Sher NA, Hill CW, Eifrig DE. Bilateral intraocular Nocardia asteroides infection. Arch Ophthalmol 1977;95:1415–8.
27. Naik S, Mateo-Bibeau R, Shinnar M, et al. Successful treatment of Nocardia nova bacteremia and multilobar pneumonia with clarithromycin in a heart transplant patient. Transplant Proc 2007;39:1720–2.
28. Bonifaz A, Flores P, Saul A, Carrasco-Gerard E, Ponce RM. Treatment of actinomycetoma due to Nocardia spp. with amoxicillin–clavulanate. Br J Dermatol 2007;156:308–11.
29. Dalton MJ, Robinson LE, Cooper J, et al. Use of Bartonella antigens for serologic diagnosis of cat-scratch disease at a national referral center. Arch Intern Med 1995;155:1670–6.
30. Wear DJ, Margileth AM, Hadfield TL, et al. Cat scratch disease: a bacterial infection. Science 1983;221:1403–5.
31. Fish RH, Hogan RN, Nightingale SD, Anand R. Peripapillary angiomatosis associated with cat-scratch neuroretinitis. Arch Ophthalmol 1992;110:323.
32. Schlossberg D, Morad Y, Krouse TB, et al. Culture-proved disseminated cat-scratch disease in acquired immunodeficiency syndrome. Arch Intern Med 1989;149:1437–9.
32a. Ormerod, Skolnick, et al. 1998.
32b. Solley, Martin, et al. 1999.
32c. Eggenberger. 2000.
32. Chang, Lee, et al. 2001.
33. Bar S, Segal M, Shapira R, Savir S. Neuroretinitis associated with cat scratch disease. Am J Ophthalmol 1990;110:703–5.
34. Carithers HA, Margileth AM. Cat-scratch disease; acute encephalopathy and other neurologic manifestations. Am J Dis Child 1991;145:98–101.
35. Chrousos GA, Drack AV, Young M, et al. Neuroretinitis in cat scratch disease. J Clin Neuro-Ophthalmol 1990;10:92–4.
36. Gass JDM. Stereoscopic atlas of macular diseases: diagnosis and treatment, 2nd ed. St Louis: CV Mosby; 1977. p. 376.
37. Gass JDM. Stereoscopic atlas of macular diseases: diagnosis and treatment, 3rd ed. St Louis: CV Mosby; 1987. p. 746–51.
38. Golnik KC, Marotto ME, Fanous MM, et al. Ophthalmic manifestations of Rochalimaea species. Am J Ophthalmol 1994;118:145–51.
39. Ulrich GG, Waecker Jr NJ, Meister SJ, et al. Cat scratch disease associated with neuroretinitis in a 6-year-old girl. Ophthalmology 1992;99:246–9.
40. Weiss AH, Beck RW. Neuroretinitis in childhood. J Pediatr Ophthalmol Strabismus 1989;26:198–203.
41. Angritt P, Tuur SM, Macher AM, et al. Epithelioid angiomatosis in HIV infection: neoplasm or cat-scratch disease? Lancet 1988;1:996.
42. Berguiga M, Abouzeid H, Bart PA, Guex-Crosier Y. Severe occlusive vasculitis as a complication of cat scratch disease. Klin Monatsbl Augenheilkd 2008;225:486–7.
43. Ziemssen F, Bartz-Schmidt KU, Gelisken F. Secondary unilateral glaucoma and neuroretinitis: atypical manifestation of cat-scratch disease. Jpn J Ophthalmol 2006;50:177–9.
44. Mason III JO. Retinal and optic nerve neovascularization associated with cat scratch neuroretinitis. Retina 2004;24:176–8.
45. Grossniklaus HE. The cat scratch disease–bacillary angiomatosis puzzle. Am J Ophthalmol 1994;118:246–8.
46. LeBoit PE, Berger TG, Egbert BM, et al. Epithelioid haemangioma-like vascular proliferation in AIDS: manifestation of cat scratch disease or bacillus infection? Lancet 1988;1:960–3.
47. Stoler MH, Bonfiglio TA, Steigbigel RT, Pereira M. An atypical subcutaneous infection associated with acquired immune deficiency syndrome. Am J Clin Pathol 1983;80:714–8.
48. Sauer A, Hansmann Y, Jaulhac B, et al. Five cases of paralytic strabismus as a rare feature of Lyme disease. Clin Infect Dis 2009;48:756–9.
48a. Mikkila, Seppala, et al. 2000.
48b. Rothermel, Hedges, et al. 2001.
48c. Krist, Wenkel, 2002.
49. Aaberg TM. The expanding ophthalmologic spectrum of Lyme disease. Am J Ophthalmol 1989;107:77–80.
50. Berglöff J, Gasser R, Feigl B. Ophthalmic manifestations of Lyme borreliosis: a review. J Neuro-Ophthalmol 1994;14:15–20.
51. Bialasiewicz AA, Ruprecht KW, Naumann GOH, Blenk H. Bilateral diffuse choroiditis and exudative retinal detachments with evidence of Lyme disease. Am J Ophthalmol 1988; 105:419–20.
52. Breeveld J, Rothova A, Kuiper H. Intermediate uveitis and Lyme borreliosis. Br J Ophthalmol 1992;76:181–2.
53. Jacobson DM, Frens DB. Pseudotumor cerebri syndrome associated with Lyme disease. Am J Ophthalmol 1989;107:81–2.
54. Lesser RL, Kornmehl EW, Pachner AR, et al. Neuro-ophthalmologic manifestations of Lyme disease. Ophthalmology 1990;97:699–706.
55. Schönherr U, Lang GE, Meythaler FH. Bilaterale Lebersche Neuroretinitis stellata bei Borrelia burgdorferi-Serokonversion. Klin Monatsbl Augenheilkd 1991;198:44–7.
56. Smith JL, Crumpton BC, Hummer J. The Bascom Palmer Eye Institute Lyme/syphilis survey. J Clin Neuro-Ophthalmol 1990;10:255–60.
57. Smith JL, Parsons TM, Paris-Hamlin AJ, Porschen RK. The prevalence of Lyme disease in a nonendemic area: a comparative serologic study in a south Florida eye clinic population. J Clin Neuro-Ophthalmol 1989;9:148–55.
58. Smith JL, Winward KE, Nicholson DF, Albert DW. Retinal vasculitis in Lyme borreliosis. J Clin Neuro-Ophthalmol 1991;11:7–15.
59. Suttorp-Schulten MSA, Luyendijk L, van Dam AP, et al. Birdshot chorioretinopathy and Lyme borreliosis. Am J Ophthalmol 1993;115:149–53.
60. Winward KE, Smith JL, Culbertson WW, Paris-Hamelin A. Ocular Lyme borreliosis. Am J Ophthalmol 1989;108:651–7.
61. Rathinam SR. Ocular manifestations of leptospirosis. J Postgrad Med 2005;51:189–94.
62. Rathinam SR. Ocular leptospirosis. Curr Opin Ophthalmol 2002;13:381–6.
63. Rathinam SR, Cunningham Jr ET. Infectious causes of uveitis in the developing world. Int Ophthalmol Clin 2000;40:137–52.
64. Martins MG, Matos KT, da Silva MV, de Abreu MT. Ocular manifestations in the acute phase of leptospirosis. Ocul Immunol Inflamm 1998;6:75–9.
65. Rathinam SR, Rathnam S, Selvaraj S, et al. Uveitis associated with an epidemic outbreak of leptospirosis. Am J Ophthalmol 1997;124:71–9.
66. Bal AM. Unusual clinical manifestations of leptospirosis. J Postgrad Med 2005;51:179–83.
67. Chu KM, Rathinam R, Namperumalsamy P, Dean D. Identification of Leptospira species in the pathogenesis of uveitis and determination of clinical ocular characteristics in south India. J Infect Dis 1998;177:1314–21.
68. Mancel E, Merien F, Pesenti L, et al. Clinical aspects of ocular leptospirosis in New Caledonia (South Pacific). Aust N Z J Ophthalmol 1999;27:380–6.
69. Priya CG, Bhavani K, Rathinam SR, Muthukkaruppan VR. Identification and evaluation of LPS antigen for serodiagnosis of uveitis associated with leptospirosis. J Med Microbiol 2003;52(Pt 8):667–73.
70. Rathinam SR, Namperumalsamy P. Leptospirosis. Ocul Immunol Inflamm 1999;7:109–18.
71. Kranias G, Schneider D, Raymond LA. A case of syphilitic uveitis. Am J Ophthalmol 1981;91:261–3.
72. Moore JE. Syphilitic iritis; a study of 249 patients. Am J Ophthalmol 1931;14:110–22.
73. Song JH, Hong YT, Kwon OW. Acute syphilitic posterior placoid chorioretinitis following intravitreal triamcinolone acetonide injection. Graefes Arch Clin Exp Ophthalmol 2008;246:1775–8.
74. Dodds EM, Lowder CY, Boskovich SA, Longworth DL, Foster RE. Simultaneous syphilitic necrotizing retinitis and placoid chorioretinitis in acquired immune deficiency syndrome. Retina 1995;15:354–6.
75. Gass JD, Braunstein RA, Chenoweth RG. Acute syphilitic posterior placoid chorioretinitis. Ophthalmology 1990;97:1288–97.
76. Arruga J, Valentines J, Mauri F, et al. Neuroretinitis in acquired syphilis. Ophthalmology 1985;92:262–70.
77. de Souza EC, Jalkh AE, Trempe CL, et al. Unusual central chorioretinitis as the first manifestation of early secondary syphilis. Am J Ophthalmol 1988;105:271–6.
78. Duke-Elder S, Dobree JH. Diseases of the retina. System of ophthalmology. St Louis: CV Mosby; 1967. p. 52, 72, 100, 221, 530.
79. Friberg TR. Photo essay. Syphilitic chorioretinitis. Arch Ophthalmol 1989;107:1676–7.

80. Gass JDM, Braunstein RA, Chenoweth RG. Acute syphilitic posterior placoid chorioretinitis. Ophthalmology 1990;97:1288–97.
81. Morgan CM, Webb RM, O'Connor GR. Atypical syphilitic chorioretinitis and vasculitis. Retina 1984;4:225–31.
82. Schlaegel Jr TF, Kao SF. A review (1970–1980) of 28 presumptive cases of syphilitic uveitis. Am J Ophthalmol 1982;93:412–4.
83. Shimuzu R, Numaga T, Kimura Y, Horiuchi T. Acute syphilitic retinochoroiditis. Jpn J Clin Ophthalmol 1989;43:13–19.
84. Walsh FB, Hoyt WF. Clinical neuro-ophthalmology, 3rd ed. Baltimore: Williams and Wilkins; 1969. p. 1551.
85. Yagasaki T, Akiyama K, Nomura H, Awaya S. Two cases of acquired syphilis with acute central chorioretinitis as initial manifestation. Jpn J Ophthalmol 1992;36:301–9.
86. Lobes Jr LA, Folk JC. Syphilitic phlebitis simulating branch vein occlusion. Ann Ophthalmol 1981;13:825–7.
87. Reddy S, Cunningham Jr ET, Spaide RF. Syphilitic retinitis with focal inflammatory accumulations. Ophthalmic Surg Lasers Imaging 2006;37:429–31.
88. Cunningham Jr ET, Schatz H, McDonald HR, Johnson RN. Acute multifocal retinitis. Am J Ophthalmol 1997;123:347–57.
89. Mendelsohn AD, Jampol LM. Syphilitic retinitis; a cause of necrotizing retinitis. Retina 1984;4:221–4.
90. DeLuise VP, Clark III SW, Smith JL, Collart P. Syphilitic retinal detachment and uveal effusion. Am J Ophthalmol 1982;94:757–61.
91. Halperin LS, Lewis H, Blumenkranz MS, et al. Choroidal neovascular membrane and other chorioretinal complications of acquired syphilis. Am J Ophthalmol 1989;108:554–62.
92. Levy JH, Liss RA, Maguire AM. Neurosyphilis and ocular syphilis in patients with concurrent human immunodeficiency virus infection. Retina 1989;9:175–80.
93. McLeish WM, Pulido JS, Holland S, et al. The ocular manifestations of syphilis in the human immunodeficiency virus type 1-infected host. Ophthalmology 1990;97:196–203.
94. Passo MS, Rosenbaum JT. Ocular syphilis in patients with human immunodeficiency virus infection. Am J Ophthalmol 1988;106:1–6.
95. Stoumbos VD, Klein ML. Syphilitic retinitis in a patient with acquired immunodeficiency syndrome-related complex. Am J Ophthalmol 1987;103:103–4.
96. Wickremasinghe S, Ling C, Stawell R, et al. Syphilitic punctate inner retinitis in immunocompetent gay men. Ophthalmology 2009;116:1195–200.
97. Huang C, Park S, Castellarin AA, et al. Diagnostic and therapeutic challenges. Retina 2007;27:385–90.
98. Doris JP, Saha K, Jones NP, Sukthankar A. Ocular syphilis: the new epidemic. Eye 2006;20:703–5.
99. Belin MW, Baltch AL, Hay PB. Secondary syphilitic uveitis. Am J Ophthalmol 1981;92:210–4.
100. Crouch Jr ER, Goldberg MF. Retinal periarteritis secondary to syphilis. Arch Ophthalmol 1975;93:384–7.
101. Duke-Elder S, Perkins ES. Diseases of the uveal tract System of ophthalmology. St Louis: CV Mosby; 1966. p. 292.
102. Halperin LS, Berger AS, Grand MG. Photoessay. Syphilitic disc edema and periphlebitis. Retina 1990;10:223–5.
103. Savir H, Kurz O. Fluorescein angiography in syphilitic retinal vasculitis. Ann Ophthalmol 1976;8:713–6.
104. Folk JC, Weingeist TA, Corbett JJ, et al. Syphilitic neuroretinitis. Am J Ophthalmol 1983;95:480–6.
105. Saari M. Disciform detachment of the macula. III. Secondary to inflammatory diseases. Acta Ophthalmol 1978;56:510–7.
106. Krishnamurthy R, Cunningham Jr ET. Atypical presentation of syphilitic uveitis associated with Kyrieleis plaques. Br J Ophthalmol 2008;92:1152–3.
107. Sacks JG, Osher RH, Elconin H. Progressive visual loss in syphilitic optic atrophy. J Clin Neuro-Ophthalmol 1983;3:5–8.
108. Tsimpida M, Low LC, Posner E, et al. Acute syphilitic posterior placoid chorioretinitis in late latent syphilis. Int J STD AIDS 2009;20:207–8.
109. Chao JR, Khurana RN, Fawzi AA, et al. Syphilis: reemergence of an old adversary. Ophthalmology 2006;113:2074–9.
110. Berger JR. Diagnosing neurosyphilis; the value of the cerebrospinal fluid VDRL or lack thereof. J Clin Neuro-Ophthalmol 1989;9:234–5.
111. Centers for Disease Control and Prevention. Sexually transmitted diseases treatment guidelines 2002. MMWR Recomm Rep 2002;51(RR-6):1–78.
112. Bansal R, Gupta A, Gupta V, et al. Role of anti-tubercular therapy in uveitis with latent/manifest tuberculosis. Am J Ophthalmol 2008;146:772–9.
113. Gupta V, Gupta A, Rao NA. Intraocular tuberculosis – an update. Surv Ophthalmol 2007;52:561–87.
114. Varma D, Anand S, Reddy AR, et al. Tuberculosis: an under-diagnosed aetiological agent in uveitis with an effective treatment. Eye (Lond) 2006;20:1068–73.
115. Rao NA, Saraswathy S, Smith RE. Tuberculous uveitis: distribution of Mycobacterium tuberculosis in the retinal pigment epithelium. Arch Ophthalmol 2006;124:1777–9.
116. Babu RB, Sudharshan S, Kumarasamy N, et al. Ocular tuberculosis in acquired immunodeficiency syndrome. Am J Ophthalmol 2006;142:413–8.
117. Mehta S, Gilada IS. Ocular tuberculosis in acquired immune deficiency syndrome (AIDS). Ocul Immunol Inflamm 2005;13:87–9.
118. Gupta V, Gupta A, Arora S, et al. Simultaneous choroidal tuberculoma and epididymo-orchitis caused by Mycobacterium tuberculosis. Am J Ophthalmol 2005;140:310–2.
119. Gupta A, Gupta V. Tubercular posterior uveitis. Int Ophthalmol Clin 2005;45:71–88.
120. Rathinam SR, Rao NA. Tuberculous intraocular infection presenting with pigmented hypopyon: a clinicopathological case report. Br J Ophthalmol 2004;88:721–2.
121. Gupta V, Gupta A, Arora S, et al. Presumed tubercular serpiginouslike choroiditis: clinical presentations and management. Ophthalmology 2003;110:1744–9.
122. Biswas J, Shome D. Choroidal tubercles in disseminated tuberculosis diagnosed by the polymerase chain reaction of aqueous humor. A case report and review of the literature. Ocul Immunol Inflamm 2002;10:293–8.
123. Bodaghi B, LeHoang P. Ocular tuberculosis. Curr Opin Ophthalmol 2000;11:443–8.
124. Bowyer JD, Gormley PD, Seth R, et al. Choroidal tuberculosis diagnosed by polymerase chain reaction. A clinicopathologic case report. Ophthalmology 1999;106:290–4.
125. Ang M, Htoon HM, Chee SP. Diagnosis of tuberculous uveitis: clinical application of an interferon-gamma release assay. Ophthalmology 2009;116:1391–6.
126. Tabbara KF. Tuberculosis. Curr Opin Ophthalmol 2007;18:493–501.
127. Morinelli EN, Dugel PU, Riffenburgh R, Rao NA. Infectious multifocal choroiditis in patients with acquired immune deficiency syndrome. Ophthalmology 1993;100:1014–21.
128. Abrams J, Schlaegel Jr TF. The role of the isoniazid therapeutic test in tuberculous uveitis. Am J Ophthalmol 1982;94:511–5.
129. Barondes MJ, Sponsel WE, Stevens TS, Plotnik RD. Tuberculous choroiditis diagnosed by chorioretinal endobiopsy. Am J Ophthalmol 1991;112:460–1.
130. Blodi BA, Johnson MW, McLeish WM, Gass JDM. Presumed choroidal tuberculosis in a human immunodeficiency virus infected host. Am J Ophthalmol 1989;108:605–7.
131. Cangemi FE, Friedman AH, Josephberg R. Tuberculoma of the choroid. Ophthalmology 1980;87:252–8.
132. Fountain JA, Werner RB. Tuberculous retinal vasculitis. Retina 1984;4:48–50.
133. Goldberg MF. Presumed tuberculous maculopathy. Retina 1982;2:47–50.
134. Inoue S, Ubuka M. A case of choroidal miliary tuberculosis as studied by fluorescence fundus photography. Folia Ophthalmol Jpn 1972;23:256–9.
135. Massaro D, Katz S, Sachs M. Choroidal tubercles; a clue to hematogenous tuberculosis. Ann Intern Med 1964;60:231–41.
136. Nakama T, Matsui K, Sugi K, Oshima K. Solitary tuberculosis of the choroid: report of a suspected case. Folia Ophthalmol Jpn 1969;20:873–8.
137. Shiono T, Abe S, Horiuchi T. A case of miliary tuberculosis with disseminated choroidal haemorrhages. Br J Ophthalmol 1990;74:317–9.
138. Reddy S, Roe R, Cunningham Jr ET, et al. Diagnostic and therapeutic challenges. Retina 2006;26:954–9.
139. Mehta S, Chauhan V, Hastak S, Jiandani P, Dalal P. Choroidal tubercles in neurotuberculosis: prevalence and significance. Ocul Immunol Inflamm 2006;14:341–5.
140. Mehta S. Ocular lesions in acute disseminated tuberculosis. Ocul Immunol Inflamm 2004;12:311–5.
141. Sharma PM, Singh RP, Kumar A, et al. Choroidal tuberculoma in miliary tuberculosis. Retina 2003;23:101–4.
142. Ayanru JO, Alli AF, Faal HB, et al. Tuberculoma of the eye; a case report. Trop Geogr Med 1986;38:301–4.
143. Kim JY, Carrol CP, Opremcak EM. Antibiotic-resistant tuberculous choroiditis. Am J Ophthalmol 1993;115:259–61.
144. Lyon CE, Grimson BS, Peiffer Jr RL, Merritt JC. Clinicopathological correlation of a solitary choroidal tuberculoma. Ophthalmology 1985;92:845–50.
145. Mansour AM, Haymond R. Choroidal tuberculomas without evidence of extraocular tuberculosis. Graefes Arch Clin Exp Ophthalmol 1990;228:382–5.
146. Itty S, Bakri SJ, Pulido JS, et al. Initial results of QuantiFERON-TB Gold testing in patients with uveitis. Eye (Lond) 2009;23:904–9.
147. Babu K, Satish V, Satish S, et al. Utility of QuantiFERON TB gold test in a south Indian patient population of ocular inflammation. Indian J Ophthalmol 2009;57:427–30.
148. Corbett EL, Watt CJ, Walker N, et al. The growing burden of tuberculosis: global trends and interactions with the HIV epidemic. Arch Intern Med 2003;163:1009–21.
149. Dye C, Scheele S, Dolin P, et al. Consensus statement. Global burden of tuberculosis: estimated incidence, prevalence, and mortality by country. WHO Global Surveillance and Monitoring Project. JAMA 1999;282:677–86.
150. Font RL, Spaulding AG, Green WR. Endogenous mycotic panophthalmitis caused by Blastomyces dermatitidis: report of a case and review of the literature. Arch Ophthalmol 1967;77:217–22.
151. Weerekoon L. Ocular leprosy in West Malaysia. Search for a posterior segment lesion. Br J Ophthalmol 1972;56:106–13.
152. Chatterjee S, Chaudhury DS. Pattern of eye diseases in leprosy patients of Northern Ghana. Int J Lepr 1964;32:53–63.
153. Chatterjee S, Chaudhury DS. Hypopigmented patches in fundus in leprosy. Lepr Rev 1964;35:88–90.
154. Robertson I, Weiner JM, Finkelstein E. Untreated Hansen's disease of the eye: a clinicopathological report. Aust J Ophthalmol 1984;12:335–9.
155. Rathinam SR, Khazaei HM, Job CK. Histopathological study of ocular erythema nodosum leprosum and post-therapeutic scleral perforation: a case report. Indian J Ophthalmol 2008;56:417–9.
156. Shamsi FA, Chaudhry IA, Moraes MO, et al. Detection of Mycobacterium leprae in ocular tissues by histopathology and real-time polymerase chain reaction. Ophthalmic Res 2007;39:63–8.
157. Daniel E, Sundar Rao PS, Ffytche TJ, et al. Iris atrophy in patients with newly diagnosed multibacillary leprosy: at diagnosis, during and after completion of multidrug treatment. Br J Ophthalmol 2007;91:1019–22.
158. Chaudhry IA, Shamsi FA, Elzaridi E, et al. Initial diagnosis of leprosy in patients treated by an ophthalmologist and confirmation by conventional analysis and polymerase chain reaction. Ophthalmology 2007;114:1904–11.
159. Thajeb P, Thajeb T, Dai D. Fatal strokes in patients with rhino-orbito-cerebral mucormycosis and associated vasculopathy. Scand J Infect Dis 2004;36:643–8.
160. Yang SW, Kim SY, Chung J, Kim KB. Two cases of orbital infarction syndrome. Korean J Ophthalmol 2000;14:107–11.
161. Balch K, Phillips PH, Newman NJ. Painless orbital apex syndrome from mucormycosis. J Neuroophthalmol 1997;17:178–82.

162. Lee BL, Holland GN, Glasgow BJ. Chiasmal infarction and sudden blindness caused by mucormycosis in AIDS and diabetes mellitus. Am J Ophthalmol 1996;122:895–6.
163. Aguilar GL, Blumenkranz MS, Egbert PR, McCulley JP. Candida endophthalmitis after intravenous drug abuse. Arch Ophthalmol 1979;97:96–100.
164. Brownstein S, Mahoney-Kinsner J, Harris R. Ocular Candida with pale-centered hemorrhages. Arch Ophthalmol 1983;101:1745–8.
165. Dellon AL, Stark WJ, Chretien PB. Spontaneous resolution of endogenous Candida endophthalmitis complicating intravenous hyperalimentation. Am J Ophthalmol 1975;79:648–54.
166. Donahue SP, Greven CM, Zuravleff JJ, et al. Intraocular candidiasis in patients with candidemia: clinical implications derived from a prospective multicenter trial. Ophthalmology 1994;101:1302–9.
167. Edwards Jr JE, Foos RY, Montgomerie JZ, Guze LB. Ocular manifestations of Candida septicemia: review of seventy-six cases of hematogenous Candida endophthalmitis. Medicine 1974;53:47–75.
168. Elliott JH, O'Day DM, Gutow GS, et al. Mycotic endophthalmitis in drug abusers. Am J Ophthalmol 1979;88:66–72.
169. Fishman LS, Griffin JR, Sapico FL, Hecht R. Hematogenous Candida endophthalmitis – a complication of candidemia. N Engl J Med 1972;286:675–81.
170. Fleming KO. Candida albicans abscess of retina. Can J Ophthalmol 1972;7:132–5.
171. Griffin JR, Pettit TH, Fishman LS, Foos RY. Blood-borne Candida endophthalmitis: a clinical and pathologic study of 21 cases. Arch Ophthalmol 1973;89:450–6.
172. Henderson DK, Edwards Jr JE, Montgomerie JZ. Hematogenous Candida endophthalmitis in patients receiving parenteral hyperalimentation fluids. J Infect Dis 1981;143:655–61.
173. Palmer EA. Endogenous Candida endophthalmitis in infants. Am J Ophthalmol 1980;89:388–95.
174. Parke II DW, Jones DB, Gentry LO. Endogenous endophthalmitis among patients with candidemia. Ophthalmology 1982;89:789–96.
175. Perraut Jr LE, Perraut LE, Bleiman B, Lyons J. Successful treatment of Candida albicans endophthalmitis with intravitreal amphotericin B. Arch Ophthalmol 1981;99:1565–7.
176. Snip RC, Michels RG. Pars plana vitrectomy in the management of endogenous Candida endophthalmitis. Am J Ophthalmol 1976;82:699–704.
177. Stern GA, Fetkenhour CL, O'Grady RB. Intravitreal amphotericin B treatment of Candida endophthalmitis. Arch Ophthalmol 1977;95:89–93.
178. Van Buren JM. Septic retinitis due to Candida albicans. AMA Arch Pathol 1958;65:137–46.
179. Axelrod AJ, Peyman GA, Apple DJ. Toxicity of intravitreal injection of amphotericin B. Am J Ophthalmol 1973;76:578–83.
180. Chess J, Kaplan S, Rubinstein A, et al. Candida retinitis in bare lymphocyte syndrome. Ophthalmology 1986;93:696–8.
181. Daily MJ, Dickey JB, Packo KH. Endogenous Candida endophthalmitis after intravenous anesthesia with propofol. Arch Ophthalmol 1991;109:1081–4.
182. McDonnell PJ, McDonnell JM, Brown RH, Green WR. Ocular involvement in patients with fungal infections. Ophthalmology 1985;92:706–9.
183. Morinelli EN, Dugel PU, Lee M, et al. Opportunistic intraocular infections in AIDS. Trans Am Ophthalmol Soc 1992;90:97–109.
184. Fisher JF, Taylor AT, Clark J, et al. Penetration of amphotericin B into the human eye. J Infect Dis 1983;147:164.
185. Barrie T. The place of elective vitrectomy in the management of patients with Candida endophthalmitis. Graefes Arch Clin Exp Ophthalmol 1987;225:107–13.
186. Brod RD, Flynn Jr HW, Clarkson JG, et al. Endogenous Candida endophthalmitis: management without intravenous amphotericin B. Ophthalmology 1990;97:666–74.
187. Shah CP, McKey J, Spirn MJ, Maguire J. Ocular candidiasis: a review. Br J Ophthalmol 2008;92:466–8.
188. Arriola-Villalobos P, Diaz-Valle D, Alejandre-Alba N, et al. Bilateral Candida chorioretinitis following etanercept treatment for hidradenitis suppurativa. Eye 2008;22:599–600.
189. Varma D, Thaker HR, Moss PJ, et al. Use of voriconazole in candida retinitis. Eye 2005;19:485–7.
190. Dunn ET, Mansour AM. Retinal striae as a sign of resolving candidal chorioretinitis. Graefes Arch Clin Exp Ophthalmol 1988;226:591–2.
191. Jones DB. Chemotherapy of experimental endogenous Candida albicans endophthalmitis. Trans Am Ophthalmol Soc 1980;78:846–95.
192. McDonald HR, De Bustros S, Sipperley JO. Vitrectomy for epiretinal membrane with Candida chorioretinitis. Ophthalmology 1990;97:466–9.
193. Rao NA, Hidayat AA. Endogenous mycotic endophthalmitis: variations in clinical and histopathologic changes in candidiasis compared with aspergillosis. Am J Ophthalmol 2001;132:244–51.
194. Rao NA, Hidayat A. A comparative clinicopathologic study of endogenous mycotic endophthalmitis: variations in clinical and histopathologic changes in candidiasis compared to aspergillosis. Trans Am Ophthalmol Soc 2000;98:183–93. [discussion 93–4.]
195. Bodoia RD, Kinyoun JL, Qingli L, Bunt-Milam AH. Aspergillus necrotizing retinitis: a clinico-pathologic study and review. Retina 1989;9:226–31.
196. Doft BH, Clarkson JG, Rebell G, Forster RK. Endogenous Aspergillus endophthalmitis in drug abusers. Arch Ophthalmol 1980;98:859–62.
197. Gross JG. Endogenous aspergillus-induced endophthalmitis: successful treatment without systemic antifungal medication. Retina 1992;12:341–5.
198. Halperin LS, Roseman RL. Successful treatment of a subretinal abscess in an intravenous drug abuser. Arch Ophthalmol 1988;106:1651–2.
199. Lance SE, Friberg TR, Kowalski RP. Aspergillus flavus endophthalmitis and retinitis in an intravenous drug abuser: a therapeutic success. Ophthalmology 1988;95:947–9.
200. Weishaar PD, Flynn Jr HW, Murray TG, et al. Endogenous Aspergillus endophthalmitis: clinical features and treatment outcomes. ARVO Abstracts. Invest Ophthalmol Vis Sci 1995;36:789.
201. Walsh TJ, Orth DH, Shapiro CM, et al. Metastatic fungal chorioretinitis developing during trichosporon sepsis. Ophthalmology 1982;89:152–6.
202. Curi AL, Felix S, Azevedo KM, et al. Retinal granuloma caused by Sporothrix schenckii. Am J Ophthalmol 2003;136:205–7.
203. Vieira-Dias D, Sena CM, Orefice F, et al. Ocular and concomitant cutaneous sporotrichosis. Mycoses 1997;40:197–201.
204. Cartwright MJ, Promersberger M, Stevens GA. Sporothrix schenckii endophthalmitis presenting as granulomatous uveitis. Br J Ophthalmol 1993;77:61–2.
205. Brunette I, Stulting RD. Sporothrix schenckii scleritis. Am J Ophthalmol 1992;114:370–1.
206. Witherspoon CD, Kuhn F, Owens SD, et al. Endophthalmitis due to Sporothrix schenckii after penetrating ocular injury. Ann Ophthalmol 1990;22:385–8.
207. Kurosawa A, Pollock SC, Collins MP, et al. Sporothrix schenckii endophthalmitis in a patient with human immunodeficiency virus infection. Arch Ophthalmol 1988;106:376–80.
208. Castro RM, de Sabogal MF, Cuce LC, Salebian A. Disseminate sporotrichosis – report of a clinical case with mucocutaneous, osteo-articular, and ocular lesions. Mykosen 1981;24:92–6.
209. Font RL, Jakobiec FA. Granulomatous necrotizing retinochoroiditis caused by Sporotrichum schenkii. Report of a case including immunofluorescence and electron microscopical studies. Arch Ophthalmol 1976;94:1513–9.
210. Levy JH. Intraocular sporotrichosis. Report of a case. Arch Ophthalmol 1971;85:574–9.
211. Cassady JR, Foerster HC. Sporotrichum schenckii endophthalmitis. Arch Ophthalmol 1971;85:71–4.
212. Taylor A, Wiffen SJ, Kennedy CJ. Post-traumatic Scedosporium inflatum endophthalmitis. Clin Experiment Ophthalmol 2002;30:47–8.
213. McKelvie PA, Wong EY, Chow LP, Hall AJ. Scedosporium endophthalmitis: two fatal disseminated cases of Scedosporium infection presenting with endophthalmitis. Clin Experiment Ophthalmol 2001;29:330–4.
214. Carney MD, Tabassian A, Guerry RK. Pseudo-Allescheria boydii endophthalmitis. Retina 1996;16:263–4.
215. Larocco Jr A, Barron JB. Endogenous Scedosporium apiospermum endophthalmitis. Retina 2005;25:1090–3.
216. Figueroa MS, Fortun J, Clement A, De Arevalo BF. Endogenous endophthalmitis caused by Scedosporium apiospermum treated with voriconazole. Retina 2004;24:319–20.
217. Spriet I, Delaere L, Lagrou K, et al. Intraocular penetration of voriconazole and caspofungin in a patient with fungal endophthalmitis. J Antimicrob Chemother 2009;64:877–8.
218. Wykoff CC, Flynn Jr HW, Miller D, et al. Exogenous fungal endophthalmitis: microbiology and clinical outcomes. Ophthalmology 2008;115:1501–7. [7 e1–2]
219. Tu EY, McCartney DL, Beatty RF, et al. Successful treatment of resistant ocular fusariosis with posaconazole (SCH–56592). Am J Ophthalmol 2007;143:222–7.
220. Rezai KA, Eliott D, Plous O, et al. Disseminated Fusarium infection presenting as bilateral endogenous endophthalmitis in a patient with acute myeloid leukemia. Arch Ophthalmol 2005;123:702–3.
221. Glasgow BJ, Engstrom Jr RE, Holland GN, et al. Bilateral endogenous Fusarium endophthalmitis associated with acquired immunodeficiency syndrome. Arch Ophthalmol 1996;114:873–7.
222. Klintworth GK, Hollingsworth AS, Lusman PA, Bradford WD. Granulomatous choroiditis in a case of disseminated histoplasmosis; histologic demonstration of Histoplasma capsulatum in choroidal lesions. Arch Ophthalmol 1973;90:45–8. [Correspondence 1974;91:237.]
223. Macher A, Rodrigues MM, Kaplan W, et al. Disseminated bilateral chorioretinitis due to Histoplasma capsulatum in a patient with the acquired immunodeficiency syndrome. Ophthalmology 1985;92:1159–64.
224. Specht CS, Mitchell KT, Bauman AE, Gupta M. Ocular histoplasmosis with retinitis in a patient with acquired immune deficiency syndrome. Ophthalmology 1991;98:1356–9.
225. Rodenbiker HT, Ganley JP, Galgiani JN, Axline SG. Prevalence of chorioretinal scars associated with coccidioidomycosis. Arch Ophthalmol 1981;99:71–5.
226. Wong VG. Focal choroidopathy in experimental ocular histoplasmosis. Trans Am Ophthalmol Soc 1972;70:615–30.
227. Alexander PB, Coodley EL. Disseminated coccidioidomycosis with intraocular involvement. Am J Ophthalmol 1967;64:283–9.
228. Blumenkranz MS, Stevens DA. Endogenous coccidioidal endophthalmitis. Ophthalmology 1980;87:974–84.
229. Boyden BS, Yee DS. Bilateral coccidioidal choroiditis: a clinicopathologic case report. Trans Am Acad Ophthalmol Otolaryngol 1971;75:1006–10.
230. Cutler JE, Binder PS, Paul TO, Beamis JF. Metastatic coccidioidal endophthalmitis. Arch Ophthalmol 1978;96:689–91.
231. Glasgow BJ, Brown HH, Foos RY. Miliary retinitis in coccidioidomycosis. Am J Ophthalmol 1987;104:24–7.
232. Levitt JM. Ocular manifestations of coccidioidomycosis. Am J Ophthalmol 1948;31:1626–8.
233. Pettit TH, Learn RN, Foos RY. Intraocular coccidioidomycosis. Arch Ophthalmol 1967;77:655–61.
234. Rodenbiker HT, Ganley JP. Ocular coccidioidomycosis. Surv Ophthalmol 1980;24:263–90.
235. Trowbridge DH. Ocular manifestations of coccidioidomycosis. Trans Pacif Cst Oto-Ophthalmol Soc 1952;33:229–46.
236. Zakka KA, Foos RY, Brown WJ. Intraocular coccidioidomycosis. Surv Ophthalmol 1978;22:313–21.
236a. Dublin AB, Philips HE. Computer tomography of disseminated coccidiodomycosis. Radiology 1980 May;135(2):361-8.
237. Avendaño J, Tanishima T, Kuwabara T. Ocular cryptococcosis. Am J Ophthalmol 1978;86:110–3.
238. Shields JA, Wright DM, Augsburger JJ, Wolkowicz MI. Cryptococcal chorioretinitis. Am J Ophthalmol 1980;89:210–8.
239. Coccidioidomycosis.
240. Agarwal A, Gupta A, Sakhuja V, et al. Retinitis following disseminated cryptococcosis in a renal allograft recipient. Efficacy of oral fluconazole. Acta Ophthalmol (Copenh) 1991;69:402–5.
241. Doft BH, Curtin VT. Combined ocular infection with cytomegalovirus and cryptococcosis. Arch Ophthalmol 1982;100:1800–3.

242. Hester DE, Kylstra JA, Eifrig DE. Isolated ocular cryptococcosis in an immunocompetent patient. Ophthalmic Surg 1992;23:129–31.
243. Hiss PW, Shields JA, Augsburger JJ. Solitary retinovitreal abscess as the initial manifestation of cryptococcosis. Ophthalmology 1988;95:162–5.
244. Khodadoust AA, Payne JW. Cryptococcal (torular) retinitis: a clinicopathologic case report. Am J Ophthalmol 1969;67:745–50.
245. Schulman JA, Leveque C, Coats M, et al. Fatal disseminated cryptococcosis following intraocular involvement. Br J Ophthalmol 1988;72:171–5.
246. Stone SP, Bending J, Hakim J, et al. Cryptococcal meningitis presenting as uveitis. Br J Ophthalmol 1988;72:167–70.
247. Arevalo JF, Fuenmayor-Rivera D, Giral AE, Murcia E. Indocyanine green videoangiography of multifocal Cryptococcus neoformans choroiditis in a patient with acquired immunodeficiency syndrome. Retina 2001;21:537–41.
248. Sheu SJ, Chen YC, Kuo NW, et al. Endogenous cryptococcal endophthalmitis. Ophthalmology 1998;105:377–81.
249. Biswas J, Gopal L, Sharma T, et al. Recurrent cryptococcal choroiditis in a renal transplant patient: clinicopathologic study. Retina 1998;18:273–6.
250. Hiles DA, Font RL. Bilateral intraocular cryptococcosis with unilateral spontaneous regression: report of a case and review of the literature. Am J Ophthalmol 1968;65:98–108.
251. Szalai G, Fellegi V, Szabo Z, Vitez LC. Mucormycosis mimicks sinusitis in a diabetic adult. Ann N Y Acad Sci 2006;1084:520–30.
252. Harrison AR, Wirtschafter JD. Ocular neuromyotonia in a patient with cavernous sinus thrombosis secondary to mucormycosis. Am J Ophthalmol 1997;124:122–3.
253. Gupta A, Gupta V, Dogra MR, et al. Fungal endophthalmitis after a single intravenous administration of presumably contaminated dextrose infusion fluid. Retina 2000;20:262–8.
254. Tarani L, Costantino F, Notheis G, et al. Long-term posaconazole treatment and follow-up of rhino-orbital-cerebral mucormycosis in a diabetic girl. Pediatr Diabetes 2009;10:289–93.
255. Pelton RW, Peterson EA, Patel BC, Davis K. Successful treatment of rhino-orbital mucormycosis without exenteration: the use of multiple treatment modalities. Ophthal Plast Reconstr Surg 2001;17:62–6.
256. Seiff SR, Choo PH, Carter SR. Role of local amphotericin B therapy for sino-orbital fungal infections. Ophthal Plast Reconstr Surg 1999;15:28–31.
256a. Gupta P, Sachdev N, Kaur J, et al. Endogenous mycotic endophthalmitis in an immunocompetent patient. Int Ophthalmol. 2009 Aug;29(4):315–8. Epub 2008 Jun 5.
257. Klintworth GK, Hollingsworth AS, Lusman PA, Bradford WD. Granulomatous choroiditis in a case of disseminated histoplasmosis; histologic demonstration of Histoplasma capsulatum in choroidal lesions. Arch Ophthalmol 1973;90:45–8. [Correspondence 1974;91:237.]
258. Macher A, Rodriguez MM, Kaplan W, et al. Disseminated bilateral chorioretinitis due to Histoplasma capsulatum in a patient with the acquired immunodeficiency syndrome. Ophthalmology 1985;92:1159–64.
259. Acers TE. Toxoplasmic retinochoroiditis: a double blind therapeutic study. Arch Ophthalmol 1964;71:58–62.
260. Asbell PA, Vermund SH, Hofeldt AJ. Presumed toxoplasmic retinochoroiditis in four siblings. Am J Ophthalmol 1982;94:656–63.
261. Awan KJ. Congenital toxoplasmosis: chances of occurrence in subsequent siblings. Ann Ophthalmol 1978;10:459–65.
262. Braunstein RA, Gass JDM. Branch artery obstruction caused by acute toxoplasmosis. Arch Ophthalmol 1980;98:512–3.
263. Culbertson WW, Tabbara KF, O'Connor GR. Experimental ocular toxoplasmosis in primates. Arch Ophthalmol 1982;100:321–3.
264. Doft BH, Gass JDM. Punctate outer retinal toxoplasmosis. Arch Ophthalmol 1985;103:1332–6.
265. Fine SL, Owens SL, Haller JA, et al. Choroidal neovascularization as a late complication of ocular toxoplasmosis. Am J Ophthalmol 1981;91:318–22.
266. Folk JC, Lobes LA. Presumed toxoplasmic papillitis. Ophthalmology 1984;91:64–7.
267. Gass JDM. Fluorescein angiography in endogenous intraocular inflammation. In: Aronson SB, Gamble CN, Goodner EK, O'Connor GR, editors. Clinical methods in uveitis: the Fourth Sloan Symposium on Uveitis. St Louis: CV Mosby; 1968. p. 202–29.
268. Gass JDM. Stereoscopic atlas of macular diseases: diagnosis and treatment, 2nd ed. St Louis: CV Mosby; 1977. p. 296–97.
269. Gass JDM. Stereoscopic atlas of macular diseases: diagnosis and treatment, 3rd ed. St Louis: CV Mosby; 1987. p. 465–67.
270. Gaynon MW, Boldrey EE, Strahlman ER, Fine SL. Retinal neovascularization and ocular toxoplasmosis. Am J Ophthalmol 1984;98:585–9.
271. Ghartey KN, Brockhurst RJ. Photocoagulation of active toxoplasmic retinochoroiditis. Am J Ophthalmol 1980;89:858–64.
272. Gilbert HD. Unusual presentation of acute ocular toxoplasmosis. Albrecht von Graefes Arch Klin Exp Ophthalmol 1980;215:53–8.
273. Hogan MJ. Ocular toxoplasmosis: clinical and laboratory diagnosis; evaluation of immunologic tests; treatment. Arch Ophthalmol 1956;55:333–45.
274. Kennedy JE, Wise GN. Retinochoroidal vascular anastomosis in uveitis. Am J Ophthalmol 1971;71:1221–5.
275. Kyrieleis W. Über atypische Gefässtuberkulose der Netzhaut (Periarteriitis 'nodosa' tuberculosa). Arch Augenheilkd 1933;107:182–90.
276. La Hey E, Rothova A, Baarsma GS, et al. Fuchs' heterochromic iridocyclitis is not associated with ocular toxoplasmosis. Arch Ophthalmol 1992;110:806–11.
277. Lou P, Kazdan J, Basu PK. Ocular toxoplasmosis in three consecutive siblings. Arch Ophthalmol 1978;96:613–4.
278. Manschot WA, Daamen CBF. Connatal ocular toxoplasmosis. Arch Ophthalmol 1965;74:48–54.
279. Morgan CM, Gragoudas ES. Photo essay: branch retinal artery occlusion associated with recurrent toxoplasmic retinochoroiditis. Arch Ophthalmol 1987;105:130–1.
280. Nicholson DH, Wolchok EB. Ocular toxoplasmosis in an adult receiving long-term corticosteroid therapy. Arch Ophthalmol 1976;94:248–54.
281. O'Connor GR, Frenkel JK. Dangers of steroid treatment in toxoplasmosis: periocular injections and systemic therapy. Arch Ophthalmol 1976;94:213.
282. Owens PL, Goldberg MF, Busse BJ. Prospective observation of vascular anastomoses between the retina and choroid in recurrent toxoplasmosis. Am J Ophthalmol 1979;88:402–5.
283. Rothova A. Ocular involvement in toxoplasmosis. Br J Ophthalmol 1993;77:371–7. [correction p. 683.]
284. Ryan Jr SJ, Smith RE. Ocular toxoplasmosis. In: Ryan Jr SJ, Smith RE, editors. Selected topics on the eye in systemic disease. New York: Grune and Stratton; 1974. p. 259–73.
285. Saari M, Vuorre I, Neiminen H, Räisänen S. Acquired toxoplasmic chorioretinitis. Arch Ophthalmol 1976;94:1485–8.
286. Sabates R, Pruett RC, Brockhurst RJ. Fulminant ocular toxoplasmosis. Am J Ophthalmol 1981;92:497–503.
287. Schlaegel Jr TF, Weber JC. The macula in ocular toxoplasmosis. Arch Ophthalmol 1984;102:697–8.
288. Schwartz PL. Segmental retinal periarteritis as a complication of toxoplasmosis. Ann Ophthalmol 1977;9:157–62.
289. Scott EH. New concepts in toxoplasmosis. Surv Ophthalmol 1974;18:255–74.
290. Spalter HF, Campbell CJ, Noyori KS, et al. Prophylactic photocoagulation of recurrent toxoplasmic retinochoroiditis: a preliminary report. Arch Ophthalmol 1966;75:21–31.
291. Webb RM, Tabbara KF, O'Connor GR. Retinal vasculitis in ocular toxoplasmosis in nonhuman primates. Retina 1984;4:182–8.
292. Willerson Jr D, Aaberg TM, Reeser F, Meredith TA. Unusual ocular presentation of acute toxoplasmosis. Br J Ophthalmol 1977;61:693–8.
293. Tetz M, Holz FG, Gallasch G, Völcker HE. Segmentale retinale Arteriitis und Retinochorioiditis. Ophthalmologe 1992;89:71–6.
294. Kasp E, Whiston R, Dumonde D, et al. Antibody affinity to retinal S-antigen in patients with retinal vasculitis. Am J Ophthalmol 1992;113:697–701.
295. Matthews JD, Weiter JJ. Outer retinal toxoplasmosis. Ophthalmology 1988;95:941–6.
296. Fish RH, Hoskins JC, Kline LB. Toxoplasmosis neuroretinitis. Ophthalmology 1993;100:1177–82.
297. Rothova A, van Knapen F, Baarsma GS, et al. Serology in ocular toxoplasmosis. Br J Ophthalmol 1986;70:615–22.
298. Chan C-C, Palestine AG, Li Q, Nussenblatt RB. Diagnosis of ocular toxoplasmosis by the use of immunocytology and the polymerase chain reaction. Am J Ophthalmol 1994;117:803–5.
298a. Rothova A, de Boer JH, Ten Dam-van Loon NH, et al. Usefulness of aqueous humor analysis for the diagnosis of posterior uveitis. Ophthalmol 2008;115(2):306–11.
298b. Pencina, D'Agostino, et al. 2009.
299. Weiss MJ, Velazquez N, Hofeldt AJ. Serologic tests in the diagnosis of presumed toxoplasmic retinochoroiditis. Am J Ophthalmol 1990;109:407–11.
300. Aouizerate F, Cazenave J, Poirier L, et al. Detection of Toxoplasma gondii in aqueous humour by the polymerase chain reaction. Br J Ophthalmol 1993;77:107–9.
301. Greven CM, Teot LA. Cytologic identification of Toxoplasma gondii from vitreous fluid. Arch Ophthalmol 1994;112:1086–8.
302. Jampel HD, Schachat AP, Conway B, et al. Retinal pigment epithelial hyperplasia assuming tumor-like proportions; report of two cases. Retina 1986;6:105–12.
303. Saari M, Miettinen R, Nieminen H, Räisänen S. Retinochoroidal vascular anastomosis in toxoplasmic chorioretinitis; report of a case. Acta Ophthalmol 1975;53:44–51.
304. Cotliar AM, Friedman AH. Subretinal neovascularisation in ocular toxoplasmosis. Br J Ophthalmol 1982;66:524–9.
305. de Abreu MT, Belfort Jr R, Hirata PS. Fuchs' heterochromic cyclitis and ocular toxoplasmosis. Am J Ophthalmol 1982;93:739–44.
306. Schwab IR. The epidemiologic association of Fuchs' heterochromic iridocyclitis and ocular toxoplasmosis. Am J Ophthalmol 1991;111:356–62.
307. Silveira C, Belfort Jr R, Nussenblatt R, et al. Unilateral pigmentary retinopathy associated with ocular toxoplasmosis. Am J Ophthalmol 1989;107:682–4.
308. Glasner PD, Silveira C, Kruszon-Moran D, et al. An unusually high prevalence of ocular toxoplasmosis in southern Brazil. Am J Ophthalmol 1992;114:136–44.
309. Silveira C, Belfort Jr R, Burnier Jr M, Nussenblatt R. Acquired toxoplasmic infection as the cause of toxoplasmic retinochoroiditis in families. Am J Ophthalmol 1988;106:362–4.
310. Holland GN. An epidemic of toxoplasmosis: lessons from Coimbatore, India. Arch Ophthalmol 2010;128:126–8.
311. de Moura L, Bahia-Oliveira LM, Wada MY, et al. Waterborne toxoplasmosis, Brazil, from field to gene. Emerg Infect Dis 2006;12:326–9.
312. Bahia-Oliveira LM, Jones JL, Azevedo-Silva J, et al. Highly endemic, waterborne toxoplasmosis in north Rio de Janeiro state, Brazil. Emerg Infect Dis 2003;9:55–62.
313. Burnett AJ, Shortt SG, Isaac-Renton J, et al. Multiple cases of acquired toxoplasmosis retinitis presenting in an outbreak. Ophthalmology 1998;105:1032–7.
314. Fortier B, Coignard-Chatain C, Dao A, et al. Study of developing clinical outbreak and serological rebounds in children with congenital toxoplasmosis and follow-up during the first 2 years of life. Arch Pediatr 1997;4:940–6.
315. Choi WY, Nam HW, Kwak NH, et al. Foodborne outbreaks of human toxoplasmosis. J Infect Dis 1997;175:1280–2.
316. Bowie WR, King AS, Werker DH, et al. Outbreak of toxoplasmosis associated with municipal drinking water. The BC Toxoplasma Investigation Team. Lancet 1997;350:173–7.
317. Palanisamy M, Madhavan B, Balasundaram MB, et al. Outbreak of ocular toxoplasmosis in Coimbatore, India. Indian J Ophthalmol 2006;54:129–31.
318. Balasundaram MB, Andavar R, Palaniswamy M, Venkatapathy N. Outbreak of acquired ocular toxoplasmosis involving 248 patients. Arch Ophthalmol 2010;128:28–32.
319. Holland GN, Crespi CM, ten Dam-van Loon N, et al. Analysis of recurrence patterns associated with toxoplasmic retinochoroiditis. Am J Ophthalmol 2008;145:1007–13.
320. Hogan MJ, Zimmerman LE. Ophthalmic pathology: an atlas and textbook, 2nd ed. Philadelphia: WB Saunders; 1962. p. 488–91.

321. Schuman JS, Weinberg RS, Ferry AP, Guerry RK. Toxoplasmic scleritis. Ophthalmology 1988;95:1399–403.
322. Rao NA, Font RL. Toxoplasmic retinochoroiditis; electron-microscopic and immunofluorescence studies of formalin-fixed tissue. Arch Ophthalmol 1977;95:273–7.
323. Colin J, Harie JC. Choriorétinites présumées toxoplasmiques: étude comparative des traitements par pyriméthamine et sulfadiazine ou clindamycine. J Fr Ophtalmol 1989;12:161–5.
324. Engstrom Jr RE, Holland GN, Nussenblatt RB, Jabs DA. Current practices in the management of ocular toxoplasmosis. Am J Ophthalmol 1991;111:601–10.
325. Opremcak EM, Scales DK, Sharpe MR. Trimethoprim–sulfamethoxazole therapy for ocular toxoplasmosis. Ophthalmology 1992;99:920–5.
326. Perkins ES, Smith CH, Schofield PB. Treatment of uveitis with pyrimethamine (Daraprim). Br J Ophthalmol 1956;40:577–86.
327. Rothova A, Buitenhuis HJ, Meenken C, et al. Therapy of ocular toxoplasmosis. Int Ophthalmol 1989;13:415–9.
328. Rothova A, Meenken C, Buitenhuis HJ, et al. Therapy for ocular toxoplasmosis. Am J Ophthalmol 1993;115:517–23.
329. Sobrin L, Kump LI, Foster CS. Intravitreal clindamycin for toxoplasmic retinochoroiditis. Retina 2007;27:952–7.
330. Kishore K, Conway MD, Peyman GA. Intravitreal clindamycin and dexamethasone for toxoplasmic retinochoroiditis. Ophthalmic Surg Lasers 2001;32:183–92.
331. Berger BB, Egwuagu CE, Freeman WR, Wiley CA. Miliary toxoplasmic retinitis in acquired immunodeficiency syndrome. Arch Ophthalmol 1993;111:373–6.
332. Bottoni F, Gonnella P, Autelitano A, Orzalesi N. Diffuse necrotizing retinochoroiditis in a child with AIDS and toxoplasmic encephalitis. Graefes Arch Clin Exp Ophthalmol 1990;228:36–9.
333. Cochereau-Massin I, LeHoang P, Lautier-Frau M, et al. Ocular toxoplasmosis in human immunodeficiency virus-infected patients. Am J Ophthalmol 1992;114:130–5.
334. Gagliuso DJ, Teich SA, Friedman AH, Orellana J. Ocular toxoplasmosis in AIDS patients. Trans Am Ophthalmol Soc 1990;88:63–86.
335. Grossniklaus HE, Specht CS, Allaire G, Leavitt JA. Toxoplasma gondii retinochoroiditis and optic neuritis in acquired immune deficiency syndrome. Ophthalmology 1990;97:1342–6.
336. Holland GN, Engstrom Jr RE, Glasgow BJ, et al. Ocular toxoplasmosis in patients with the acquired immunodeficiency syndrome. Am J Ophthalmol 1988;106:653–67.
337. Moorthy RS, Smith RE, Rao NA. Progressive ocular toxoplasmosis in patients with acquired immunodeficiency syndrome. Am J Ophthalmol 1993;115:742–7.
338. Parke II DW, Font RL. Diffuse toxoplasmic retinochoroiditis in a patient with AIDS. Arch Ophthalmol 1986;104:571–5.
339. Pauleikhoff D, Messmer E, Beelen DW, et al. Bone-marrow transplantation and toxoplasmic retinochoroiditis. Graefes Arch Clin Exp Ophthalmol 1987;225:239–43.
340. Singer MA, Hagler WS, Grossniklaus HE. Toxoplasma gondii retinochoroiditis after liver transplantation. Retina 1993;13:40–5.
341. Weiss A, Margo CE, Ledford DK, et al. Toxoplasmic retinochoroiditis as an initial manifestation of the acquired immune deficiency syndrome. Am J Ophthalmol 1986;101:248–50.
342. Yeo JH, Jakobiec FA, Iwamoto T, et al. Opportunistic toxoplasmic retinochoroiditis following chemotherapy for systemic lymphoma; a light and electron microscopic study. Ophthalmology 1983;90:885–98.
343. Lewallen S, Taylor TE, Molyneux ME, et al. Ocular fundus findings in Malawian children with cerebral malaria. Ophthalmology 1993;100:857–61.
344. Maude RJ, Hassan MU, Beare NA. Severe retinal whitening in an adult with cerebral malaria. Am J Trop Med Hyg 2009;80:881.
345. Beare NA, Harding SP, Taylor TE, et al. Perfusion abnormalities in children with cerebral malaria and malarial retinopathy. J Infect Dis 2009;199:263–71.
346. Mehta SA, Ansari AS, Jiandani P. Ophthalmoscopic findings in adult patients with severe falciparum malaria. Ocul Immunol Inflamm 2008;16:239–41.
347. Harding SP, Lewallen S, Beare NA, et al. Classifying and grading retinal signs in severe malaria. Trop Doct 2006;36(Suppl. 1):1–13.
348. Beare NA, Taylor TE, Harding SP, et al. Malarial retinopathy: a newly established diagnostic sign in severe malaria. Am J Trop Med Hyg 2006;75:790–7.
349. Beare NA, Lewis DK, Kublin JG, et al. Retinal changes in adults with cerebral malaria. Ann Trop Med Parasitol 2003;97:313–5.
350. Lewallen S. The fundus in severe malaria. Arch Ophthalmol 1998;116:542–3.
351. Amano Y, Ohashi Y, Haruta Y, et al. A new fundus finding in patients with zoster ophthalmicus. Am J Ophthalmol 1986;102:532–3.
352. Dugel PU, Rao NA, Forster DJ, et al. Pneumocystis carinii choroiditis after long-term aerosolized pentamidine therapy. Am J Ophthalmol 1990;110:113–7.
353. Foster RE, Lowder CY, Meisler DM, et al. Presumed Pneumocystis carinii choroiditis; unifocal presentation, regression with intravenous pentamidine, and choroiditis recurrence. Ophthalmology 1991;98:1360–5.
354. Freeman WR, Gross JG, Labelle J, et al. Pneumocystis carinii choroidopathy: a new clinical entity. Arch Ophthalmol 1989;107:863–7.
355. Holland GN, MacArthur LJ, Foos RY. Choroidal pneumocystosis. Arch Ophthalmol 1991;109:1454–5.
356. Koser MW, Jampol LM, MacDonell K. Treatment of Pneumocystis carinii choroidopathy. Arch Ophthalmol 1990;108:1214–5.
357. Rosenblatt MA, Cunningham C, Teich S, Friedman AH. Choroidal lesions in patients with AIDS. Br J Ophthalmol 1990;74:610–4.
358. Sha BE, Benson CA, Deutsch T, et al. Pneumocystis carinii choroiditis in patients with AIDS: clinical features, response to therapy, and outcome. J Acquir Immune Defic Syndr 1992;5:1051–8.
359. Shami MJ, Freeman W, Friedberg D, et al. A multicenter study of Pneumocystis choroidopathy. Am J Ophthalmol 1991;112:15–22.
360. Teich SA, Rosenblatt M, Friedman A. Pneumocystis carinii choroiditis after long-term aerosolized pentamidine therapy. Am J Ophthalmol 1991;111:118.
361. Whitcup SM, Fenton RM, Pluda JM, et al. Pneumocystis carinii and Mycobacterium avium-intracellulare infection of the choroid. Retina 1992;12:331–5.
362. Rao NA, Zimmerman PL, Boyer D, et al. A clinical, histopathologic, and electron microscopic study of Pneumocystis carinii choroiditis. Am J Ophthalmol 1989;197:218–28.
363. Gupta A, Hustler A, Herieka E, Matthews BN. Pneumocystis choroiditis. Eye (Lond) 2010;24:178.
364. Sabri K, Bibby K. Choroiditis and exudative macular detachments in a post transplant leukaemic patient: an unusual presentation of Pneumocystis jiroveci infection. Br J Ophthalmol 2006;90:118–9.
365. Ashton N. Larval granulomatosis of the retina due to Toxocara. Br J Ophthalmol 1960;44: 129–48.
366. Bird AC, Smith JL, Curtin VT. Nematode optic neuritis. Am J Ophthalmol 1970;69:72–7.
367. Duguid IM. Chronic endophthalmitis due to Toxocara. Br J Ophthalmol 1961;45:705–17.
368. Duguid IM. Features of ocular infestation by Toxocara. Br J Ophthalmol 1961;45:789–96.
369. Ellis Jr GS, Pakalnis VA, Worley G, et al. Toxocara canis infestation; clinical and epidemiological associations with seropositivity in kindergarten children. Ophthalmology 1986;93:1032–7.
370. Hogan MJ, Kimura SJ, Spencer WH. Visceral larva migrans and peripheral retinitis. JAMA 1965;194:1345–7.
371. Nichols RL. The etiology of visceral larva migrans. I. Diagnostic morphology of infective second-stage Toxocara larvae. J Parasitol 1956;42:349–62.
372. Schantz PM, Glickman LT. Toxocaral visceral larva migrans. N Engl J Med 1978;298:436–9.
373. Shields JA. Ocular toxocariasis: a review. Surv Ophthalmol 1984;28:361–81.
374. Wilder HC. Nematode endophthalmitis. Trans Am Acad Ophthalmol Otolaryngol 1951;55:99–109.
375. Wilkinson CP, Welch RB. Intraocular Toxocara. Am J Ophthalmol 1971;71:921–30.
376. Zimmerman LE. Toxoplasma gondii from Toxocara cati. Arch Ophthalmol 1966;76:159–60.
377. Sorr EM. Meandering ocular toxocariasis. Retina 1984;4:90–6.
378. Bowman DD, Mika-Grieve M, Grieve RB. Toxocara canis: monoclonal antibodies to larval excretory–secretory antigens that bind with genus and species specificity to the cuticular surface of infective larvae. Exp Parasitol 1987;64:458–65.
379. Cox TA, Haskins GE, Gangitano JH, Antonson DL. Bilateral Toxocara optic neuropathy. J Clin Neuro-Ophthalmol 1983;3:267–74.
380. Molk R. Treatment of toxocaral optic neuritis. J Clin Neuro-Ophthalmol 1982;2:109–12.
381. Bloom SM, Snady-McCoy L. Multifocal choroiditis uveitis occurring after herpes zoster ophthalmicus. Am J Ophthalmol 1989;108:733–5.
382. Kelly SP, Rosenthal AR. Chickenpox chorioretinitis. Br J Ophthalmol 1990;74:698–9.
383. Gass JDM. Stereoscopic atlas of macular diseases: a funduscopic and angiographic presentation. St Louis: CV Mosby; 1970. p. 108.
384. McElvanney AM, Murray PI. Multifocal choroidal lesions: a rare complication of herpes zoster ophthalmicus. J Neuro-Ophthalmol 1994;14:12–14.
385. Luxenberg MN. An experimental approach to the study of intraocular Toxocara canis. Trans Am Ophthalmol Soc 1979;77:542–602.
386. Shiono T, Abe S, Horiuchi T. A case of miliary tuberculosis with disseminated choroidal haemorrhages. Br J Ophthalmol 1990;74:317–9.
387. Paul M, Stefaniak J, Twardosz-Pawlik H, Pecold K. The co-occurrence of Toxocara ocular and visceral larva migrans syndrome: a case series. Cases J 2009;2:6881.
388. Pollard ZF. Ocular Toxocara in siblings of two families: diagnosis confirmed by ELISA test. Arch Ophthalmol 1979;97:2319–20.
389. Small KW, McCuen II BW, de Juan Jr E, Machemer R. Surgical management of retinal traction caused by toxocariasis. Am J Ophthalmol 1989;108:10–14.
390. Biglan AW, Glickman LT, Lobes Jr LA. Serum and vitreous Toxocara antibody in nematode endophthalmitis. Am J Ophthalmol 1979;88:898–901.
391. Felberg NT, Shields JA, Federman JL. Antibody to Toxocara canis in the aqueous humor. Arch Ophthalmol 1981;99:1563–4.
392. Pollard ZF, Jarrett WH, Hagler WS, et al. ELISA for diagnosis of ocular toxocariasis. Ophthalmology 1979;86:743–9.
393. Shields JA, Lerner HA, Felberg NT. Aqueous cytology and enzymes in nematode endophthalmitis. Am J Ophthalmol 1977;84:319–22.
394. de Visser L, Rothova A, de Boer JH, et al. Diagnosis of ocular toxocariasis by establishing intraocular antibody production. Am J Ophthalmol 2008;145:369–74.
395. Deegan III WF, Duker JS. Unifocal choroiditis in primary varicella zoster (chicken pox). Arch Ophthalmol 1994;112:735–6.
396. Gonvers M, Mermoud A, Uffer S, et al. Toxocara canis oculaire chez un adulte de 30 ans. Klin Monatsbl Augenheilkd 1992;200:522–4.
397. Maguire AM, Green WR, Michels RG, Erozan YS. Recovery of intraocular Toxicara canis by pars plana vitrectomy. Ophthalmology 1990;97:675–80.
398. Ghafoor SYA, Smith HV, Lee WR, et al. Experimental ocular toxocariasis: a mouse model. Br J Ophthalmol 1984;68:89–96.
399. Belmont JB, Irvine A, Benson W, O'Connor GR. Vitrectomy in ocular toxocariasis. Arch Ophthalmol 1982;100:1912–5.
400. Treister G, Machemer R. Results of vitrectomy for rare proliferative and hemorrhagic diseases. Am J Ophthalmol 1977;84:394–412.
401. Chadha V, Pandey PK, Chauhan D, Das S. Simultaneous intraocular and bilateral extraocular muscle involvement in a case of disseminated cysticercosis. Int Ophthalmol 2005;26:35–7.
402. Aracena T, Perez Roca E. Macular and peripheral subretinal cysticercosis. Ann Ophthalmol 1981;13:1265–7.
403. Yanoff M, editor. Case presentation. Washington DC: Verhoeff Society; 1975.
404. Barsante CF. Cysticercus sub-retinalis. In: Shimizu K, editor. Fluorescein angiography: proceedings of the international symposium on fluorescein angiography (ISFA), Tokyo, 1972. Tokyo: Igaku Shoin; 1974. p. 193–8.
405. Malik SRK, Gupta AK, Choudhry S. Ocular cysticercosis. Am J Ophthalmol 1968;66:1168–71.
406. Martinez-López M, Quiroz y Ferrari F. Cysticercosis. J Clin Neuro-Ophthalmol 1985;5:127–43.

407. Agarwal B, Vemuganti GK, Honavar SG. Intraocular cysticercosis simulating retinoblastoma in a 5-year-old child. Eye 2003;17:447–9.
408. Wei JW. Ultrasonic diagnosis of intraocular cysticercus. Chung-Hua Yen Ko Tsa Chih 1990;26:230–1.
409. Topilow HW, Yimoyines DJ, Freeman HM, et al. Bilateral multifocal intraocular cysticercosis. Ophthalmology 1981;88:1166–72.
410. Madigubba S, Vishwanath K, Reddy G, Vemuganti GK. Changing trends in ocular cysticercosis over two decades: an analysis of 118 surgically excised cysts. Indian J Med Microbiol 2007;25:214–9.
411. Cardenas F, Quiroz H, et al. 1992.
412. Sharma T, Sinha S, Shah N, et al. Intraocular cysticercosis: clinical characteristics and visual outcome after vitreoretinal surgery. Ophthalmology 2003;110:996–1004.
413. Mahendradas P, Biswas J, Khetan V. Fibrinous anterior uveitis due to cysticercus cellulosae. Ocul Immunol Inflamm 2007;15:451–4.
414. Kaliaperumal S, Rao VA, Parija SC. Cysticercosis of the eye in South India – a case series. Indian J Med Microbiol 2005;23:227–30.
415. Hutton WL, Vaiser A, Snyder WB. Pars plana vitrectomy for removal of intravitreous cysticercus. Am J Ophthalmol 1976;81:571–3.
416. Kruger-Leite E, Jalkh AE, Quiroz H, Schepens CL. Intraocular cysticercosis. Am J Ophthalmol 1985;99:252–7.
417. Santos R, Chavarria M, Aguirre AE. Failure of medical treatment in two cases of intraocular cysticercosis. Am J Ophthalmol 1984;97:249–50.
418. Steinmetz RL, Masket S, Sidikaro Y. The successful removal of a subretinal cysticercus by pars plana vitrectomy. Retina 1989;9:276–80.
419. Teekhasaenee C, Ritch R, Kanchanaranya C. Ocular parasitic infection in Thailand. Rev Infect Dis 1986;8:350–6.
420. Gass JDM, Braunstein RA. Further observations concerning the diffuse unilateral subacute neuroretinitis syndrome. Arch Ophthalmol 1983;101:1689–97.
421. Gass JDM, Gilbert Jr WR, Guerry RK, Scelfo R. Diffuse unilateral subacute neuroretinitis. Ophthalmology 1978;85:521–45.
422. Gass JDM, Scelfo R. Diffuse unilateral subacute neuroretinitis. J R Soc Med 1978;71: 95–111.
423. Parsons HE. Nematode chorioretinitis: report of a case, with photographs of a viable worm. Arch Ophthalmol 1952;47:799–800.
424. Price Jr JA, Wadsworth JAC. An intraretinal worm: report of a case of macular retinopathy caused by invasion of the retina by a worm. Arch Ophthalmol 1970;83:768–70.
425. Raymond LA, Gutierrez Y, Strong LE, et al. Living retinal nematode (filarial-like) destroyed with photocoagulation. Ophthalmology 1978;85:944–9.
426. Rubin ML, Kaufman HE, Tierney JP, Lucas HC. An intraretinal nematode (a case report). Trans Am Acad Ophthalmol Otolaryngol 1968;72:855–66.
427. Sivalingam A, Goldberg RE, Augsburger J, Frank P. Diffuse unilateral subacute neuroretinitis. Arch Ophthalmol 1991;109:1028.
428. de Souza EC, Abujamra S, Nakashima Y, Gass JD. Diffuse bilateral subacute neuroretinitis: first patient with documented nematodes in both eyes. Arch Ophthalmol 1999;117:1349–51.
429. Cunha de Souza E, Lustosa da Cunha S, Gass JDM. Diffuse unilateral subacute neuroretinitis in South America. Arch Ophthalmol 1992;110:1261–3.
430. Huff DS, Neafie RC, Binder MJ, et al. The first fatal Baylisascaris infection in humans: an infant with eosinophilic meningoencephalitis. Pediatr Pathol 1984;2:345–52.
431. Rasquin F, Waterschoot MP, Termote H, Carlier Y. Diffuse unilateral subacute neuroretinitis in Africa. Ocul Immunol Inflamm 2006;14:59–62.
432. Venkatesh P, Sarkar S, Garg S. Diffuse unilateral subacute neuroretinitis: report of a case from the Indian subcontinent and the importance of immediate photocoagulation. Int Ophthalmol 2005;26:251–4.
433. Cortez R, Denny JP, Muci-Mendoza R, et al. Diffuse unilateral subacute neuroretinitis in Venezuela. Ophthalmology 2005;112:2110–4.
434. Harto MA, Rodriguez-Salvador V, Avino JA, et al. Diffuse unilateral subacute neuroretinitis in Europe. Eur J Ophthalmol 1999;9:58–62.
435. Naumann GO, Knorr HL. DUSN occurs in Europe. Ophthalmology 1994;101:971–2.
436. Carney MD, Combs JL. Diffuse unilateral subacute neuroretinitis. Br J Ophthalmol 1991;75:633–5.
437. Küchle M, Knorr HLJ, Medenblik-Frysch S, et al. Diffuse unilateral subacute neuroretinitis syndrome in a German most likely caused by the raccoon roundworm, Baylisascaris procyonis. Graefes Arch Clin Exp Ophthalmol 1993;231:48–51.
438. Oppenheim S, Rogell G, Peyser R. Diffuse unilateral subacute neuroretinitis. Ann Ophthalmol 1985;17:336–8.
439. Kelsey JH. Diffuse unilateral subacute neuroretinitis. J R Soc Med 1978;71:303–4.
440. Gass JDM. Stereoscopic atlas of macular diseases: diagnosis and treatment, 3rd ed. St Louis: CV Mosby; 1987. p. 474–75.
441. Kuhnt H. Extraction eines neuen Entozoon zus dem Glaskörper des Menschen. Arch Augenheilkd 1892;24:205–29.
442. Bowman DD. Personal communication. 1996.
443. Nichols RL. The etiology of visceral larva migrans. II. Comparative larval morphology of ascaris Lumbricoides, necator americanus, strongyloides stercoralis, and acylostoma caninum. Parasitology 1956;42:363–99.
444. Fox AS, Kazacos KR, Gould NS, et al. Fatal eosinophilic meningoencephalitis and visceral larva migrans caused by the raccoon ascarid, Baylisascaris procyonis. N Engl J Med 1985;312:1619–23.
445. Goldberg MA, Kazacos KR, Boyce WM, et al. Diffuse unilateral subacute neuroretinitis: morphometric, serologic, and epidemiologic support for Baylisascaris as a causative agent. Ophthalmology 1993;100:1695–701.
446. Kazacos KR, Raymond LA, Kazacos EA, Vestre WA. The raccoon ascarid: a probable cause of human ocular larva migrans. Ophthalmology 1985;92:1735–43.
447. Kazacos KR, Reed WM, Kazacos EA, Thacker HL. Fatal cerebrospinal disease caused by Baylisascaris procyonis in domestic rabbits. J Am Vet Med Assoc 1983;183:967–71.
448. Kazacos KR, Vestre WA, Kazacos EA, Raymond LA. Diffuse unilateral subacute neuroretinitis syndrome: probable cause. Arch Ophthalmol 1984;102:967–8.
449. Kazacos KR, Wirtz WL. Experimental cerebrospinal nematodiasis due to Baylisascaris procyonis in chickens. Avian Dis 1983;27:55–65.
450. Kazacos KR, Wirtz WL, Burger PP, Christmas CS. Raccoon ascarid larvae as a cause of fatal central nervous system disease in subhuman primates. J Am Vet Med Assoc 1981; 179:1089–94.
451. Lewis RA, Discussion of Kazacos KR, Raymond LA, Kazacos EA, Vestre WA. The raccoon ascarid: a probable cause of human ocular larva migrans. Ophthalmology 1985;92:1743–44.
452. John T, Barsky HJ, Donnelly JJ, Rockey JH. Retinal pigment epitheliopathy and neuroretinal degeneration in ascarid-infected eyes. Invest Ophthalmol Vis Sci 1987;28:1583–98.
453. Mets MB, Noble AG, Basti S, et al. Eye findings of diffuse unilateral subacute neuroretinitis and multiple choroidal infiltrates associated with neural larva migrans due to Baylisascaris procyonis. Am J Ophthalmol 2003;135:888–90.
454. Gass JDM, Callanan DG, Bowman B. Oral therapy in diffuse unilateral subacute neuroretinitis. Arch Ophthalmol 1992;110:675–80.
455. Anderson J, Font RL. Ocular onchocerciasis. In: Binford CH, Connor DH, editors. Pathology of tropical and extraordinary diseases. Washington DC: Armed Forces Institute of Pathology; 1976. p. 373–81.
456. Bird AC, Anderson J, Fuglsang H. Morphology of posterior segment lesions of the eye in patients with onchocerciasis. Br J Ophthalmol 1976;60:2–20.
457. Bird AC, El Sheikh H, Anderson J, Fuglsang H. Changes in visual function and in the posterior segment of the eye during treatment of onchocerciasis with diethylcarbamazine citrate. Br J Ophthalmol 1980;64:191–200.
458. Murphy RP, Taylor H, Greene BM. Chorioretinal damage in onchocerciasis. Am J Ophthalmol 1984;98:519–21.
459. Neumann E, Gunders AE. Pathogenesis of the posterior segment lesion of ocular onchocerciasis. Am J Ophthalmol 1973;75:82–9.
460. Newland HS, White AT, Greene BM, et al. Ocular manifestations of onchocerciasis in a rain forest area of West Africa. Br J Ophthalmol 1991;75:163–9.
461. Rodger FC. The pathogenesis and pathology of ocular onchocerciasis. Part IV. The pathology. Am J Ophthalmol 1960;49:327–37.
462. Taylor HR, Greene BM. Ocular changes with oral and transepidermal diethylcarbamazine therapy of onchocerciasis. Br J Ophthalmol 1981;65:494–502.
463. Chan C-C, Nussenblatt RB, Kim MK, et al. Immunopathology of ocular onchocerciasis. 2. Anti-retinal autoantibodies in serum and ocular fluids. Ophthalmology 1987;94:439–43.
464. Van der Lelij A, Rothova A, Stilma JS, et al. Cell-mediated immunity against human retinal extract, S-antigen, and interphotoreceptor retinoid binding protein in onchocercal chorioretinopathy. Invest Ophthalmol Vis Sci 1990;31:2031–6.
465. Semba RD, Murphy RP, Newland HS, et al. Longitudinal study of lesions of the posterior segment in onchocerciasis. Ophthalmology 1990;97:1334–41.
466. Dadzie KY, Bird AC, Awadzi K, et al. Ocular findings in a double-blind study of ivermectin versus diethycarbamazine versus placebo in the treatment of onchocerciasis. Br J Ophthalmol 1987;71:78–85.
467. Deng G, Lin H, Seidman A, et al. A phase I/II trial of a polysaccharide extract from Grifola frondosa (Maitake mushroom) in breast cancer patients: immunological effects. J Cancer Res Clin Oncol 2009;135:1215–21.
468. Taylor HR, Murphy RP, Newland HS, et al. Treatment of onchocerciasis: the ocular effects of ivermectin and diethylcarbamazine. Arch Ophthalmol 1986;104:863–70.
469. Taylor HR. Ivermectin treatment of ocular onchocerciasis. Acta Leidensia 1990;59:201–6.
470. Winter FC. The control of onchocerciasis. Am J Ophthalmol 1989;108:84–5.
471. Boussinesq M, Gardon J, Gardon-Wendel N, Chippaux JP. Clinical picture, epidemiology and outcome of Loa-associated serious adverse events related to mass ivermectin treatment of onchocerciasis in Cameroon. Filaria J 2003;2(Suppl. 1):S4.
472. Padgett JJ, Jacobsen KH. Loiasis: African eye worm. Trans R Soc Trop Med Hyg 2008;102:983–9.
473. Mittal M, Sathish KR, Bhatia PG, Chidamber BS. Ocular dirofilariasis in Dubai, UAE. Indian J Ophthalmol 2008;56:325–6.
474. Juri J, Kuzman T, Stiglmayer N, Tojagic M. A case of lacrimal gland dirofilariasis. Ophthalmologica 2007;221:204–6.
475. Mahesh G, Giridhar A, Biswas J, et al. A case of periocular dirofilariasis masquerading as a lid tumour. Indian J Ophthalmol 2005;53:63–4.
476. Aiello A, Aiello P, Aiello F. A case of palpebral dirofilariasis. Eur J Ophthalmol 2005;15:407–8.
477. Angunawela RI, Ataullah S, Whitehead KJ, Sullivan TJ, Rosser P. Dirofilarial infection of the orbit. Orbit 2003;22:41–6.
478. Frieling E, Fritz E, Schmidt U, et al. Vitreoretinale Dirofilariose. Klins Monatsbl Augenheilkd 1990;196:233–6.
479. Gutierrez Y. Diagnostic pathology of parasitic infections with clinical correlations. Philadelphia: Lea and Febiger; 1990. p. 323–24.
480. Kerkenezov N. Intra-ocular filariasis in Australia. Br J Ophthalmol 1962;46:607–15.
481. Moorhouse DE. Dirofilaria immitis: a cause of human intra-ocular infection. Infection 1978;6:192–3.
482. Vodovozov AM, Jarulin GR, Djakonowa SW. Dirofilaria im Glaskörper des Menschen. Ophthalmologica 1973;166:88–93.
483. Gungel H, Kara N, Pinarci EY, et al. An uncommon case with intravitreal worm. Intravitreal Dirofilaria infection. Br J Ophthalmol 2009;93:573–4. [697.]
484. Yamamoto S, Hayashi M, Takeuchi S. Surgically removed submacular nematode. Br J Ophthalmol 1999;83:1088.
485. Sathyan P, Manikandan P, Bhaskar M, et al. Subtenons infection by Dirofilaria repens. Indian J Med Microbiol 2006;24:61–2.

645. Thompson WS, Culbertson WW, Smiddy WE, et al. Acute retinal necrosis caused by reactivation of herpes simplex virus type 2. Am J Ophthalmol 1994;118:205–11.
646. Uninsky E, Jampol LM, Kaufman S, et al. Disseminated herpes simplex infection with retinitis in a renal allograft recipient. Ophthalmology 1983;90:175–8.
647. Anand R, Font RL, Fish RH, et al. Pathology of cytomegalovirus retinitis treated with sustained release intravitreal ganciclovir. Ophthalmology 1993;100:1032–9.
648. Sanborn GE, Anand R, Torti RE, et al. Sustained-release ganciclovir therapy for treatment of cytomegalovirus retinitis: use of an intravitreal device. Arch Ophthalmol 1992;110:188–95.
649. Smith TJ, Pearson PA, Blandford DL, et al. Intravitreal sustained-release ganciclovir. Arch Ophthalmol 1992;110:255–8.
650. Flores-Aquilar M, Kuppermann BD, Quiceno JI, et al. Pathophysiology and treatment of clinically resistant cytomegalovirus retinitis. Ophthalmology 1993;100:1022–31.
651. Kuppermann BD, Flores-Aguilar M, Quiceno JI, et al. Combination gancyclovir and foscarnet in the treatment of clinically resistant cytomegalovirus retinitis in patients with acquired immunodeficiency syndrome. Arch Ophthalmol 1993;111:1359–66.
652. Lehoang P, Girard B, Robinet M, et al. Foscarnet in the treatment of cytomegalovirus retinitis in acquired immune deficiency syndrome. Ophthalmology 1989;96:865–74.
653. Robinson MR, Teitelbaum C, Taylor-Findlay C. Thrombocytopenia and vitreous hemorrhage complicating ganciclovir treatment. Am J Ophthalmol 1989;107:560–1.
654. Studies of Ocular Complications of AIDS Research Group in Collaboration with the AIDS Clinical Trials Group: Foscarnet-Ganciclovir Cytomegalovirus Trial. 4. Visual outcomes. Ophthalmology 1994;101:1250–61.
655. Orellana J, Teich SA, Lieberman RM, et al. Treatment of retinal detachments in patients with the acquired immune deficiency syndrome. Ophthalmology 1991;98:939–43.
656. Christensen L, Beeman HW, Allen A. Cytomegalic inclusion disease. Arch Ophthalmol 1957;57:90–9.
657. Stevens Jr G, Palestine AG, Rodriguez MM, et al. Failure of argon laser to halt cytomegalovirus retinitis. Retina 1986;6:119–22.
658. Nishi M, Hanashiro R, Mori S, et al. Polymerase chain reaction for the detection of the varicella-zoster genome in ocular samples from patients with acute retinal necrosis. Am J Ophthalmol 1992;114:603–9.
659. Huang J-S, Russack V, Flores-Aguilar M, et al. Evaluation of cytologic specimens obtained during experimental vitreous biopsy. Retina 1993;13:160–5.
660. Martin DF, Chan C-C, deSmet MD, et al. The role of chorioretinal biopsy in the management of posterior uveitis. Ophthalmology 1993;100:705–14.
661. Norris AM, Gentry M, Peehl DM, et al. The elevated expression of a mismatch repair protein is a predictor for biochemical recurrence after radical prostatectomy. Cancer Epidemiol Biomarkers Prev 2009;18:57–64.
662. Cibis GW, Flynn JT, Davis EB. Herpes simplex retinitis. Arch Ophthalmol 1978;96:299–302.
663. Cogan DG, Kuwabara T, Young GF, et al. Herpes simplex retinopathy in an infant. Arch Ophthalmol 1964;72:641–5.
664. Reynolds JD, Griebel M, Mallory S, et al. Congenital herpes simplex retinitis. Am J Ophthalmol 1986;102:33–6.
665. Nahmias AJ, Hagler WS. Ocular manifestations of herpes simplex in the newborn (neonatal ocular herpes). Int Ophthalmol Clin 1972;12:191–213.
666. el Azazi M, Malm G, Forsgren M. Late ophthalmologic manifestations of neonatal herpes simplex virus infection. Am J Ophthalmol 1990;109:1–7.
667. Chu SY, Callaghan WM, Bish CL, et al. Gestational weight gain by body mass index among US women delivering live births, 2004–2005: fueling future obesity. Am J Obstet Gynecol 2009;200:271. [e1–7.]
668. Bloom JN, Katz JI, Kaufman HE. Herpes simplex retinitis and encephalitis in an adult. Arch Ophthalmol 1977;95:1798–9.
669. Grutzmacher RD, Henderson D, McDonald PJ, et al. Herpes simplex chorioretinitis in a healthy adult. Am J Ophthalmol 1983;96:788–96.
670. Partamian LG, Morse PH, Klein HZ. Herpes simplex type 1 retinitis in an adult with systemic herpes zoster. Am J Ophthalmol 1981;92:215–20.
671. Centers for Disease Control B-virus infection in humans: Pensacola, Florida. MMWR Morb Mortal Wkly Rep 1987;36:289–90. [95–96.]
672. Kelly SP, Rosenthal AR, Nicholson KG, et al. Retinochoroiditis in acute Epstein–Barr virus infection. Br J Ophthalmol 1989;73:1002–3.
673. Bartlett RE, Mumma CS, Irvine AR. Herpes zoster ophthalmicus with bilateral hemorrhagic retinopathy. Am J Ophthalmol 1951;34:45–8.
674. Culbertson WW, Blumenkranz MS. The acute retinal necrosis syndrome. In: Blodi FC, editor. Herpes simplex infections of the eye. New York: Churchill Livingstone; 1984. p. 77–89.
675. Edgerton AE. Herpes zoster ophthalmicus: report of cases and review of literature. Arch Ophthalmol 1945;34:114–53.
676. Hesse RJ. Herpes zoster ophthalmicus associated with delayed retinal thrombophlebitis. Am J Ophthalmol 1977;84:329–31.
677. Jensen J. A case of herpes zoster ophthalmicus complicated with neuroretinitis. Acta Ophthalmol 1948;26:551–5.
678. Naumann G, Gass JDM, Font RL. Histopathology of herpes zoster ophthalmicus. Am J Ophthalmol 1968;65:533–41.
679. Schwartz JN, Cashwell F, Hawkins HK, et al. Necrotizing retinopathy with herpes zoster ophthalmicus: a light and electron microscopical study. Arch Pathol Lab Med 1976;100:386–91.
680. Bloom SM, Snady-McCoy L. Multifocal choroiditis uveitis occurring after herpes zoster ophthalmicus. Am J Ophthalmol 1989;108:733–5.
681. Lambert SR, Taylor D, Kriss A, et al. Ocular manifestations of the congenital varicella syndrome. Arch Ophthalmol 1989;107:52–6.
682. Capone Jr A, Meredith TA. Central visual loss caused by chicken pox retinitis in a 2-year-old child. Am J Ophthalmol 1992;113:592–3.
683. Cho N, Han H. Central retinal artery occlusion after varicella. Am J Ophthalmol 1992;113:591–2.
684. Copenhaver RM. Chickenpox with retinopathy. Arch Ophthalmol 1966;75:199–200.
685. Friedberg MA, Micale AJ. Monocular blindness from central retinal artery occlusion associated with chicken pox. Am J Ophthalmol 1994;117:117–8.
686. Hugkulstone CE, Watt LL. Branch retinal arteriolar occlusion with chicken-pox. Br J Ophthalmol 1988;72:78–80.
687. Amanat LA, Cant JS, Green FD. Acute phthisis bulbi and external ophthalmoplegia in herpes zoster ophthalmicus. Ann Ophthalmol 1985;17:46–51.
688. Gilbert GJ. Herpes zoster ophthalmicus and delayed contralateral hemiparesis:relationship of the syndrome to central nervous system granulomatous angiitis. JAMA 1974;229:302–4.
689. Womack LW, Liesegang TJ. Complications of herpes zoster ophthalmicus. Arch Ophthalmol 1983;101:42–5.
690. Mora P, Guex-Crosier Y, Kamberi E, et al. Acute retinal necrosis in primary herpes simplex virus type I infection. Pediatr Infect Dis J 2009;28:163–4.
691. Cottet L, Kaiser L, Hirsch HH, et al. HSV2 acute retinal necrosis: diagnosis and monitoring with quantitative polymerase chain reaction. Int Ophthalmol 2009;29:199–201.
692. Vandercam T, Hintzen RQ, de Boer JH, et al. Herpetic encephalitis is a risk factor for acute retinal necrosis. Neurology 2008;71:1268–74.
693. Moesen I, Khemka S, Ayliffe W. Acute retinal necrosis secondary to herpes simplex virus type 2 with preexisting chorioretinal scarring. J Pediatr Ophthalmol Strabismus 2008;45:59–61.
694. King J, Chung M, DiLoreto Jr DA. A 9-year-old girl with herpes simplex virus type 2 acute retinal necrosis treated with intravitreal foscarnet. Ocul Immunol Inflamm 2007;15:395–8.
695. Chang S, Young LH. Acute retinal necrosis: an overview. Int Ophthalmol Clin 2007;47:145–54.
696. Van Gelder RN, Willig JL, Holland GN, et al. Herpes simplex virus type 2 as a cause of acute retinal necrosis syndrome in young patients. Ophthalmology 2001;108:869–76.
697. Yamamoto S, Nakao T, Kajiyama K. Acute retinal necrosis following herpes simplex encephalitis. Arch Neurol 2007;64:283.
698. Usui Y, Goto H. Overview and diagnosis of acute retinal necrosis syndrome. Semin Ophthalmol 2008;23:275–83.
699. Bando K, Kinoshita A, Mimura Y. Six cases of so called 'Kirisawa type' uveitis. Jpn J Clin Ophthalmol 1979;33:1515–21.
700. Blumenkranz MS, Culbertson WW, Clarkson JG, et al. Treatment of the acute retinal necrosis syndrome with intravenous acyclovir. Ophthalmology 1986;93:296–300.
701. Brown RM, Mendis U. Retinal arteritis complicating herpes zoster ophthalmicus. Br J Ophthalmol 1973;57:344–6.
702. Fisher JP, Lewis ML, Blumenkranz M, et al. The acute retinal necrosis syndrome. Part I: Clinical manifestations. Ophthalmology 1982;89:1309–16.
703. Friberg TR, Jost BF. Acute retinal necrosis in an immunosuppressed patient. Am J Ophthalmol 1984;98:515–7.
704. Gartry DS, Spalton DJ, Tilzey A, et al. Acute retinal necrosis syndrome. Br J Ophthalmol 1991;75:292–7.
705. Gass JDM. Acute herpetic thrombotic retinal angiitis and necrotizing neuroretinitis ('acute retinal necrosis syndrome'). Symposium on Medical and Surgical Diseases of the Retina and Vitreous: Transactions of the New Orleans Academy of Ophthalmology. St Louis: CV Mosby; 1983. p. 97–107.
706. Gorman BD, Nadel AJ, Coles RS. Acute retinal necrosis. Ophthalmology 1982;89:809–14.
707. Hayreh MMS, Kreiger AE, Straatsma BR, et al. Acute retinal necrosis. ARVO Abstracts. Invest Ophthalmol Vis Sci 1980;19(Suppl.):48.
708. Hayreh SS. Acute retinal necrosis. Am J Ophthalmol 1984;97:661–2.
709. Holland GN. Executive Committee of the American Uveitis Society: Standard diagnostic criteria for the acute retinal necrosis syndrome. Am J Ophthalmol 1994;117:663–6.
710. Jampol LM. Acute retinal necrosis. Am J Ophthalmol 1982;93:254–5.
711. Kometani J, Asayama T. A case of specific uveitis occurring acutely in the right eye. Folia Ophthalmol Jpn 1978;29:1397–401.
712. Lightman S. Acute retinal necrosis [editorial]. Br J Ophthalmol 1991;75:449.
713. Martenet A-C. Fréquence et aspects cliniques des complications rétiniennes de l'uvéite intermédiaire. Bull Mem Soc Fr Ophtalmol 1980;92:40–2.
714. Okinami S, Tsukahara I. Acute severe uveitis with retinal vasculitis and retinal detachment. Ophthalmologica 1979;179:276–85.
715. Price Jr FW, Schlaegel Jr TF. Bilateral acute retinal necrosis. Am J Ophthalmol 1980;89:419–24.
716. Rummelt V, Wenkel H, Rummelt C, et al. Detection of varicella zoster virus DNA and viral antigen in the late stage of bilateral acute retinal necrosis syndrome. Arch Ophthalmol 1992;110:1132–6.
717. Saari KM, Böke W, Manthey KF, et al. Bilateral acute retinal necrosis. Am J Ophthalmol 1982;93:403–11.
718. Sternberg Jr P, Knox DL, Finkelstein D, et al. Acute retinal necrosis syndrome. Retina 1982;2:145–51.
719. Topilow HW, Nussbaum JJ, Freeman HM, et al. Bilateral acute retinal necrosis: clinical and ultrastructural study. Arch Ophthalmol 1982;100:1901–8.
720. Urayama A, Yamada N, Sasaki T, et al. Unilateral acute uveitis with retinal periarteritis and detachment. Jpn J Clin Ophthalmol 1971;25:607–19.
721. Willerson Jr D, Aaberg TM, Reeser FH. Necrotizing vaso-occlusive retinitis. Am J Ophthalmol 1977;84:209–19.
722. Young NJA, Bird AC. Bilateral acute retinal necrosis. Br J Ophthalmol 1978;62:581–90.
723. Culbertson WW, Blumenkranz MS, Haines H, et al. The acute retinal necrosis syndrome. Part 2: Histopathology and etiology. Ophthalmology 1982;89:1317–25.
724. Margolis T, Irvine AR, Hoyt WF, et al. Acute retinal necrosis syndrome presenting with papillitis and arcuate neuroretinitis. Ophthalmology 1988;95:937–40.

725. Regillo CD, Sergott RC, Ho AC, et al. Hemodynamic alterations in the acute retinal necrosis syndrome. Ophthalmology 1993;100:1171–6.
726. Amano Y, Ohashi Y, Haruta Y, et al. A new fundus finding in patients with zoster ophthalmicus. Am J Ophthalmol 1986;102:532–3.
727. Matsuo T, Nakayama T, Koyama T, et al. A proposed mild type of acute retinal necrosis syndrome. Am J Ophthalmol 1988;105:579–83.
728. Matsuo T, Morimoto K, Matsuo N. Factors associated with poor visual outcome in acute retinal necrosis. Br J Ophthalmol 1991;75:450–4.
729. Rabinovitch T, Nozik RA, Varenhorst MP. Bilateral acute retinal necrosis syndrome. Am J Ophthalmol 1989;108:735–6.
730. Palay DA, Sternberg Jr P, Davis J, et al. Decrease in the risk of bilateral acute retinal necrosis by acyclovir therapy. Am J Ophthalmol 1991;112:250–5.
731. Culbertson WW, Blumenkranz MS, Pepose JS, et al. Varicella zoster virus is a cause of the acute retinal necrosis syndrome. Ophthalmology 1986;93:559–69.
732. Culbertson WW, Brod RD, Flynn Jr HW, et al. Chickenpox-associated acute retinal necrosis syndrome. Ophthalmology 1991;98:1641–5.
733. Jabs DA, Schachat AP, Liss R, et al. Presumed varicella zoster retinitis in immunocompromised patients. Retina 1987;7:9–13.
734. Kelly SP, Rosenthal AR. Chickenpox chorioretinitis. Br J Ophthalmol 1990;74:698–9.
735. Matsuo T, Koyama M, Matsuo N. Acute retinal necrosis as a novel complication of chicken pox in adults. Br J Ophthalmol 1990;74:443–4.
736. Yeo JH, Pepose JS, Stewart JA, et al. Acute retinal necrosis syndrome following herpes zoster dermatitis. Ophthalmology 1986;93:1418–22.
737. el Azaza M, Samuelsson A, Linde A, et al. Intrathecal antibody production against viruses of the herpesvirus family in acute retinal necrosis syndrome. Am J Ophthalmol 1991;112:76–82.
738. Matsuo T, Date S, Tsuji T, et al. Immune complex containing herpesvirus antigen in a patient with acute retinal necrosis. Am J Ophthalmol 1986;101:368–71.
739. Pepose JS, Flowers B, Stewart JA, et al. Herpesvirus antibody levels in the etiologic diagnosis of the acute retinal necrosis syndrome. Am J Ophthalmol 1992;113:248–56.
740. Soushi S, Ozawa H, Matsuhashi M, et al. Demonstration of varicella-zoster virus antigens in the vitreous aspirates of patients with acute retinal necrosis syndrome. Ophthalmology 1988;95:1394–8.
741. Linnemann Jr CC, Alvira MM. Pathogenesis of varicella-zoster angiitis in the CNS. Arch Neurol 1980;37:239–40.
742. Gass JDM. Giant cell reaction surrounding Bruch's membrane and internal limiting membrane. East Ophthalmic Pathol Soc Meet 1991.
743. Green WR, Zimmerman LE. Granulomatous reaction to Descemet's membrane. Am J Ophthalmol 1967;64:555–8.
744. Hedges III TR, Albert DM. The progression of the ocular abnormalities of herpes zoster: histopathologic observations of nine cases. Ophthalmology 1982;89:165–77.
745. Reese LT, Shafer DM, Zweifach P. Acute acquired toxoplasmosis. Ann Ophthalmol 1981;13:467–70.
746. Freeman WR, Thomas EL, Rao NA, et al. Demonstration of herpes group virus in acute retinal necrosis syndrome. Am J Ophthalmol 1986;102:701–9.
747. Freeman WR, Wiley CA, Gross JG, et al. Endoretinal biopsy in immunosuppressed and healthy patients with retinitis: indications, utility, and techniques. Ophthalmology 1989;96:1559–65.
748. Taylor D, Day S, Tiedemann K, et al. Chorioretinal biopsy in a patient with leukaemia. Br J Ophthalmol 1981;65:489–93.
749. Holland GN, Cornell PJ, Park MS, et al. An association between acute retinal necrosis syndrome and HLA-DQw7 and phenotype Bw62,DR4. Am J Ophthalmol 1989;108:370–4.
750. Grossniklaus HE, Aaberg TM, Purnell EW, et al. Retinal necrosis in X-linked lymphoproliferative disease. Ophthalmology 1994;101:705–9.
751. Blumenkranz MS, Kaplan HJ, Clarkson JG, et al. Acute multifocal hemorrhagic retinal vasculitis. Ophthalmology 1988;95:1663–72.
752. Balansard B, Bodaghi B, Cassoux N, et al. Necrotising retinopathies simulating acute retinal necrosis syndrome. Br J Ophthalmol 2005;89:96–101.
753. Diddie KR, Schanzlin DJ, Mausolf FA, et al. Necrotizing retinitis caused by opportunistic virus infection in a patient with Hodgkin's disease. Am J Ophthalmol 1979;88:668–73.
754. Knox DL, King Jr J. Retinal arteritis, iridocyclitis, and giardiasis. Ophthalmology 1982;89:1303–8.
755. Peyman GA, Goldberg MF, Uninsky E, et al. Vitrectomy and intravitreal antiviral drug therapy in acute retinal necrosis syndrome; report of two cases. Arch Ophthalmol 1984;102:1618–21.
756. Kawaguchi T, Spencer DB, Mochizuki M. Therapy for acute retinal necrosis. Semin Ophthalmol 2008;23:285–90.
757. Huynh TH, Johnson MW, Comer GM, et al. Vitreous penetration of orally administered valacyclovir. Am J Ophthalmol 2008;145:682–6.
758. Lau CH, Missotten T, Salzmann J, et al. Acute retinal necrosis features, management, and outcomes. Ophthalmology 2007;114:756–62.
759. Garner HR, Latkany P. Oral drugs for viral retinitis. Ophthalmology 2007;114:2367. [author reply 2367–8.]
760. Han DP, Lewis H, Williams GA, et al. Laser photocoagulation in the acute retinal necrosis syndrome. Arch Ophthalmol 1987;105:1051–4.
761. Sternberg Jr P, Han DP, Yeo JH, et al. Photocoagulation to prevent retinal detachment in acute retinal necrosis. Ophthalmology 1988;95:1389–93.
762. Blumenkranz M, Clarkson J, Culbertson WW, et al. Visual results and complications after retinal reattachment in the acute retinal necrosis syndrome. The influence of operative technique. Retina 1989;9:170–4.
763. Blumenkranz M, Clarkson J, Culbertson WW, et al. Vitrectomy for retinal detachment associated with acute retinal necrosis. Am J Ophthalmol 1988;106:426–9.
764. Carney MD, Peyman GA, Goldberg MF, et al. Acute retinal necrosis. Retina 1986;6:85–94.
765. Clarkson JG, Blumenkranz MS, Culbertson WW, et al. Retinal detachment following the acute retinal necrosis syndrome. Ophthalmology 1984;91:1665–8.
766. McDonald HR, Lewis H, Kreiger AE, et al. Surgical management of retinal detachment associated with acute retinal necrosis syndrome. Br J Ophthalmol 1991;75:455–8.
767. Han DP, Abrams GW, Williams GA. Regression of disc neovascularization by photocoagulation in the acute retinal necrosis syndrome. Retina 1988;8:244–6.
768. Sergott RC, Anand R, Belmont JB, et al. Acute retinal necrosis neuropathy: clinical profile and surgical therapy. Arch Ophthalmol 1989;107:692–6.
769. Duker JS, Shakin EP. Rapidly progressive outer retinal necrosis in the acquired immunodeficiency syndrome. Am J Ophthalmol 1991;111:255–6.
770. Engstrom Jr RE, Holland GN, Margolis TP, et al. The progressive outer retinal necrosis syndrome: a variant of necrotizing herpetic retinopathy in patients with AIDS. Ophthalmology 1994;101:1488–502.
771. Forster DJ, Dugel PU, Frangieh GT, et al. Rapidly progressive outer retinal necrosis in the acquired immunodeficiency syndrome. Am J Ophthalmol 1990;110:341–8.
772. Johnston WH, Holland GN, Engstrom Jr RE, et al. Recurrence of presumed varicella-zoster virus retinopathy in patients with acquired immunodeficiency syndrome. Am J Ophthalmol 1993;116:42–50.
773. Margo CE. (PORN) Progressive outer retinal necrosis syndrome. Presented at the Verhoeff Society Meeting, 1994.
774. Shinoda K, Inoue M, Ishida S, et al. Progressive outer retinal necrosis in a patient with nephrotic syndrome. Ophthalmic Surg Lasers 2001;32:67–72.
775. Foster RE, Petersen MR, Neuss MN, et al. Progressive outer retinal necrosis syndrome in a lymphoma patient with good visual outcome. Am J Ophthalmol 2001;132:117–20.
776. Kashiwase M, Sata T, Yamauchi Y, et al. Progressive outer retinal necrosis caused by herpes simplex virus type 1 in a patient with acquired immunodeficiency syndrome. Ophthalmology 2000;107:790–4.
777. Yang CM, Wang WW, Lin CP. Progressive outer retinal necrosis syndrome as an early manifestation of human immunodeficiency virus infection. J Formos Med Assoc 1999;98:141–4.
778. Laby DM, Nasrallah FP, Butrus SI, et al. Treatment of outer retinal necrosis in AIDS patients. Graefes Arch Clin Exp Ophthalmol 1993;231:271–3.
779. Vrabec TR. Posterior segment manifestations of HIV/AIDS. Surv Ophthalmol 2004;49:131–57.
780. Holland GN. AIDS and ophthalmology: the first quarter century. Am J Ophthalmol 2008;145:397–408.
781. Welch K, Finkbeiner W, Alpers CE, et al. Autopsy findings in the acquired immune deficiency syndrome. JAMA 1984;252:1152–9.
782. Schuman JS, Friedman AH. Retinal manifestations of the acquired immune deficiency syndrome (AIDS): Cytomegalovirus, Candida albicans, Cryptococcus, toxoplasmosis, and Pneumocystis carinii. Trans Ophthalmol Soc UK 1983;103:177–90.
783. Rosenberg PR, Uliss AE, Friedland GH, et al. Acquired immunodeficiency syndrome: ophthalmic manifestations in ambulatory patients. Ophthalmology 1983;90:874–8.
784. Rodrigues MM, Palestine A, Nussenblatt R, et al. Unilateral cytomegalovirus retinochoroiditis and bilateral cytoid bodies in a bisexual man with the acquired immunodeficiency syndrome. Ophthalmology 1983;90:1577–82.
785. Qavi HB, Green MT, SeGall GK, et al. Demonstration of HIV-1 and HHV-6 in AIDS-associated retinitis. Curr Eye Res 1989;8:379–87.
786. Pepose JS, Holland GN, Nestor MS, et al. Acquired immune deficiency syndrome: pathogenic mechanisms of ocular disease. Ophthalmology 1985;92:472–84.
787. Palestine AG, Rodrigues MM, Macher AM, et al. Ophthalmic involvement in acquired immunodeficiency syndrome. Ophthalmology 1984;91:1092–9.
788. Newsome DA, Green WR, Miller ED, et al. Microvascular aspects of acquired immune deficiency syndrome retinopathy. Am J Ophthalmol 1984;98:590–601.
789. Mansour AM, Jampol LM, Logani S, et al. Cotton-wool spots in acquired immunodeficiency syndrome compared with diabetes mellitus, systemic hypertension, and central retinal vein occlusion. Arch Ophthalmol 1988;106:1074–7.
790. Lifson AR, Rutherford GW, Jaffe HW. The natural history of human immunodeficiency virus infection. J Infect Dis 1988;158:1360–7.
791. Kwok S, O'Donnell JJ, Wood IS. Retinal cotton-wool spots in a patient with Pneumocystis carinii infection. N Engl J Med 1982;307:184–5.
792. Khadem M, Kalish SB, Goldsmith J, et al. Ophthalmologic findings in acquired immune deficiency syndrome (AIDS). Arch Ophthalmol 1984;102:201–6.
793. Kestelyn P, Van de Perre P, Rouvroy D, et al. A prospective study of the ophthalmologic findings in the acquired immune deficiency syndrome in Africa. Am J Ophthalmol 1985;100:230–8.
794. Jensen OA, Gerstoft J, Thomsen HK, et al. Cytomegalovirus retinitis in the acquired immunodeficiency syndrome (AIDS); light-microscopical, ultrastructural and immunohistochemical examination of a case. Acta Ophthalmol 1984;62:1–9.
795. Jabs DA, Green WR, Fox R, et al. Ocular manifestations of acquired immune deficiency syndrome. Ophthalmology 1989;96:1092–9.
796. Hummer J, Gass JDM, Huang AJW. Conjunctival Kaposi's sarcoma treated with interferon alpha-2a. Am J Ophthalmol 1993;116:502–3.
797. Holland GN, Pepose JS, Pettit TH, et al. Acquired immune deficiency syndrome; ocular manifestations. Ophthalmology 1983;90:859–72.
798. Holland GN, Gottlieb MS, Foos RY. Retinal cotton-wool patches in acquired immunodeficiency syndrome. N Engl J Med 1982;307:1704.
799. Gal A, Pollack A, Oliver M. Ocular findings in the acquired immunodeficiency syndrome. Br J Ophthalmol 1984;68:238–41.
800. Fujikawa LS, Salahuddin SZ, Ablashi D, et al. Human T-cell leukemia/lymphotropic virus type III in the conjunctival epithelium of a patient with AIDS. Am J Ophthalmol 1985;100:507–9.
801. Freeman WR, Lerner CW, Mines JA, et al. A prospective study of the ophthalmologic findings in the acquired immune deficiency syndrome. Am J Ophthalmol 1984;97:133–42.
802. Drew WL, Buhles W, Erlich KS. Herpesvirus infections (cytomegalovirus, herpes simplex virus, varicella-zoster virus): how to use ganciclovir (DHPG) and acyclovir. Infect Dis Clin North Am 1988;2:495–509.

803. Dennehy PJ, Warman R, Flynn JT, et al. Ocular manifestations in pediatric patients with acquired immunodeficiency syndrome. Arch Ophthalmol 1989;107:978–82.
804. Boyer DS, Discussion of paper by Holland GN, Pepose JS, Pettit TH, et al. Acquired immune deficiency syndrome: ocular manifestations. Ophthalmology 1983;90:872–73.
805. Broder S, Gallo RC. A pathogenic retrovirus (HTLV-III) linked to AIDS. N Engl J Med 1984;311:1292–7.
806. Brodie SE, Friedman AH. Retinal dysfunction as an initial ophthalmic sign in AIDS. Br J Ophthalmol 1990;74:49–51.
807. Brooks Jr HL, Downing J, McClure JA, et al. Orbital Burkitt's lymphoma in a homosexual man with acquired immune deficiency. Arch Ophthalmol 1984;102:1533–7.
808. Cantrill HL, Henry K, Jackson B, et al. Recovery of human immunodeficiency virus from ocular tissues in patients with acquired immune deficiency syndrome. Ophthalmology 1988;95:1458–62.
809. Centers for Disease Control Kaposi's sarcoma and Pneumocystis pneumonia among homosexual men – New York City and California. MMWR Morb Mortal Wkly Rep 1981;30:305–8.
810. Centers for Disease Control Guidelines for prophylaxis against Pneumocystis carinii pneumonia for adults and children infected with human immunodeficiency virus. MMWR Morb Mortal Wkly Rep 1992;41(RR-4):1–11.
811. Centers for Disease Control Pneumocystis pneumonia – Los Angeles. MMWR Morb Mortal Wkly Rep 1981;30:250–2.
812. Centers for Disease Control Provisional Public Health Service inter-agency recommendations for screening donated blood and plasma for antibody to the virus causing acquired immunodeficiency syndrome. MMWR Morb Mortal Wkly Rep 1985;34:1–5.
813. Cole EL, Meisler DM, Calabrese LH, et al. Herpes zoster ophthalmicus and acquired immune deficiency syndrome. Arch Ophthalmol 1984;102:1027–9.
814. Tanenbaum M, Russell S, Richmond P, et al. Calcified cytoid bodies in acquired immunodeficiency syndrome. Retina 1987;7:84–8.
815. Engstrom Jr RE, Holland GN, Hardy WD, et al. Hemorheologic abnormalities in patients with human immunodeficiency virus infection and ophthalmic microvasculopathy. Am J Ophthalmol 1990;109:153–61.
816. Freeman WR, Chen A, Henderly DE, et al. Prevalence and significance of acquired immunodeficiency syndrome-related retinal microvasculopathy. Am J Ophthalmol 1989;107:229–35.
817. Nussenblatt RB, Palestine AG. Human immunodeficiency virus, herpes zoster, and the retina [editorial]. Am J Ophthalmol 1991;112:206–7.
818. Palestine AG, Frishberg B. Macular edema in acquired immunodeficiency syndrome-related microvasculopathy. Am J Ophthalmol 1991;111:770–1.
819. Tenhula WN, Xu S, Madigan MC, et al. Morphometric comparisons of optic nerve axon loss in acquired immunodeficiency syndrome. Am J Ophthalmol 1992;113:14–20.
820. Glascow BJ, Weisberger AK. A quantitative and cartographic study of retinal microvasculopathy in acquired immunodeficiency syndrome. Am J Ophthalmol 1994;118:46–56.
821. Quiceno JI, Capparelli E, Sadun AA, et al. Visual dysfunction without retinitis in patients with acquired immunodeficiency syndrome. Am J Ophthalmol 1992;113:8–13.
822. Winward KE, Hamed LM, Glaser JS. The spectrum of optic nerve disease in human immunodeficiency virus infection. Am J Ophthalmol 1989;107:373–80.
823. Croxatto JO, Mestre C, Puente S, et al. Nonreactive tuberculosis in a patient with acquired immune deficiency syndrome. Am J Ophthalmol 1986;102:659–60.
824. Pepose JS, Hilborne LH, Cancilla PA, et al. Concurrent herpes simplex and cytomegalovirus retinitis and encephalitis in the acquired immune deficiency syndrome (AIDS). Ophthalmology 1984;91:1669–77.
825. Raymond LA, Wilson CA, Linnemann Jr CC, et al. Punctate outer retinitis in acute Epstein–Barr virus infection. Am J Ophthalmol 1987;104:424–6.
826. Purtilo DT. Epstein–Barr virus: The spectrum of its manifestations in human beings. South Med J 1987;80:943–7.
827. Tiedeman JS. Epstein–Barr viral antibodies in multifocal choroiditis and panuveitis. Am J Ophthalmol 1987;103:659–63.
828. Wong KW, D'Amico DJ, Hedges III TR, et al. Ocular involvement associated with chronic Epstein–Barr virus disease. Arch Ophthalmol 1987;105:788–92.
829. Nakao K, Ohba N. Human T-cell lymphotropic virus type 1-associated retinal vasculitis in children. Retina 2003;23:197–201.
830. Levy-Clarke GA, Buggage RR, Shen D, et al. Human T-cell lymphotropic virus type-1 associated T-cell leukemia/lymphoma masquerading as necrotizing retinal vasculitis. Ophthalmology 2002;109:1717–22.
831. Nakao K, Ohba N, Uemura A, et al. Gray-white, spherical deposition on retinal vessel associated with acute retinal necrosis and diabetic retinopathy in HTLV-I carriers. Jpn J Ophthalmol 1998;42:490–4.
832. Mochizuki M, Tajima K, Watanabe T, et al. Human T lymphotropic virus type 1 uveitis. Br J Ophthalmol 1994;78:149–54.
833. Nakao K, Ohba N. Clinical features of HTLV-I associated uveitis. Br J Ophthalmol 1993;77:274–9.
834. Mochizuki M, Watanabe T, Yamaguchi K, et al. Uveitis associated with human T-cell lymphotropic virus type I. Am J Ophthalmol 1992;114:123–9.
835. Ohba N, Matsumoto M, Sameshima M, et al. Ocular manifestations in patients infected with human T-lymphotropic virus type I. Jpn J Ophthalmol 1989;33:1–12.
836. Sasaki K, Morooka I, Inomata H, et al. Retinal vasculitis in human T-lymphotropic virus type I associated myelopathy. Br J Ophthalmol 1989;73:812–5.
837. Spalton DJ, Nicholson F. Mini review: HTLV-I infection in human disease. Br J Ophthalmol 1991;75:174–5.
838. Goto K, Sato K, Kurita M, et al. The seroprevalence of HTLV-I in patients with ocular diseases, pregnant women and healthy volunteers in the Kanto district, central Japan. Scand J Infect Dis 1997;29:219–21.
839. Ohba N, Nakao K, Isashiki Y. HTLV-I associated retinochoroidal degeneration. Jpn J Ophthalmol 1996;40:71–8.
840. Sasaki K, Morooka I, Inomata H, et al. Retinal vasculitis in human T-lymphotropic virus type I associated myelopathy. Br J Ophthalmol 1989;73:812–5.
841. Ohba N, Matsumoto M, Sameshima M, et al. Ocular manifestations in patients infected with human T-lymphotropic virus type I. Jpn J Ophthalmol 1989;33:1–12.
842. Merle H, Donnio A, Gonin C, et al. Retinal vasculitis caused by adult T-cell leukemia/lymphoma. Jpn J Ophthalmol 2005;49:41–5.
843. Shibata K, Shimamoto Y, Nishimura T, et al. Ocular manifestations in adult T-cell leukemia/lymphoma. Ann Hematol 1997;74:163–8.
844. Matsumura N, Sawa M, Ohguro N, et al. Chorioretinitis with late pigmentary changes in a carrier of human T-lymphotropic virus 1. Arch Ophthalmol 2007;125:1436.
845. Kumar SR, Gill PS, Wagner DG, et al. Human T-cell lymphotropic virus type I-associated retinal lymphoma. A clinicopathologic report. Arch Ophthalmol 1994;112:954–9.
846. Alfano JE. Ocular aspects of the maternal rubella syndrome. Trans Am Acad Ophthalmol Otolaryngol 1966;70:235–66.
847. Boniuk M, Zimmerman LE. Ocular pathology in the rubella syndrome. Arch Ophthalmol 1967;77:455–72.
848. Collis WJ, Cohen DN. Rubella retinopathy: a progressive disorder. Arch Ophthalmol 1970;84:33–5.
849. Deutman AF, Grizzard WS. Rubella retinopathy and subretinal neovascularization. Am J Ophthalmol 1978;85:82–7.
850. Franceschetti A, Dieterle P, Schwarz A. Rétinite pigmentaire à virus: relation entre tableau clinique et électrorétinogramme (ERG). Ophthalmologica 1958;135:545–54.
851. Frank KE, Purnell EW. Subretinal neovascularization following rubella retinopathy. Am J Ophthalmol 1978;86:462–6.
852. Gass JDM. Stereoscopic atlas of macular diseases: diagnosis and treatment, 2nd ed. St Louis: CV Mosby; 1977. p. 40, 92, 210.
853. Givens KT, Lee DA, Jones T, et al. Congenital rubella syndrome: ophthalmic manifestations and associated systemic disorders. Br J Ophthalmol 1993;77:358–63.
854. Gregg NM, Discussion of Marks EO. Pigmentary abnormality in children congenitally deaf following maternal German measles. Trans Ophthalmol Soc Aust 1946;6:124.
855. Hertzberg R. Twenty-five-year follow-up of ocular defects in congenital rubella. Am J Ophthalmol 1968;66:269–71.
856. Krill AE. The retinal disease of rubella. Arch Ophthalmol 1967;77:445–9.
857. Krill AE. Retinopathy secondary to rubella. Int Ophthalmol Clin 1972;12:89–103.
858. Menser MA, Dods L, Harley JD. A twenty-five-year follow-up of congenital rubella. Lancet 1967;2:1347–50.
859. Slusher MM, Tyler ME. Rubella retinopathy and subretinal neovascularization. Ann Ophthalmol 1982;14:292–4.
860. Wolff SM. The ocular manifestations of congenital rubella. Trans Am Ophthalmol Soc 1972;70:577–614.
860a. Hirano K, Tanikawa A, Miyake Y. Neovascular Maculopathy Associated with Rubella Retinopathy. Jpn J Ophthalmol 2000;44(6):697.
860b. Fortes Filho JB. Spontaneous involution of choroidal neovascularization secondary to rubella retinopathy: reply to Veloso, Costa, Orefice, and Orefice. Eye (Lond) 2008;22(7):978.
861. Goldberg N, Chou J, Moore A, et al. Autofluorescence imaging in rubella retinopathy. Ocul Immunol Inflamm 2009;17:400–2.
862. Gagnon A, Bouchard RW. Fulminating adult-onset subacute sclerosing panencephalitis in a 49-year-old man. Arch Neurol 2003;60:1160–1.
863. d'Elia G, Di Giacomo A, D'Alessandro P, et al. Traumatic anterior glenohumeral instability: quantification of glenoid bone loss by spiral CT. Radiol Med 2008;113:496–503.
864. Cochereau IM, Gaudric A, Reinert P, et al. Altérations du fond d'oeil au cours de la panencéphalite sclérosante subaiguë. J Fr Ophtalmol 1992;15:255–61.
865. Gravina RF, Nakanishi AS, Faden A. Subacute sclerosing panencephalitis. Am J Ophthalmol 1978;86:106–9.
866. Green SH, Wirtschafter JD. Ophthalmoscopic findings in subacute sclerosing panencephalitis. Br J Ophthalmol 1973;57:780–7.
867. Haltia M, Tarkkanen A, Vaheri A, et al. Measles retinopathy during immunosuppression. Br J Ophthalmol 1978;62:356–60.
868. Schulz E. Ophthalmologische Frühmanifestation einer subakuten sklerosierenden Panencephalitis: diagnostische und mögliche therapeutische Aspekte. Ophthalmologica 1980;180:281–7.
869. Landers III MB, Klintworth GK. Subacute sclerosing panencephalitis (SSPE): a clinicopathologic study of the retinal lesions. Arch Ophthalmol 1971;86:156–63.
870. Nelson DA, Weiner A, Yanoff M, et al. Retinal lesions in subacute sclerosing panencephalitis. Arch Ophthalmol 1970;84:613–21.
871. Nguyen NQ, Lee AG, McClure CD, et al. Subretinal lesions in subacute sclerosing panencephalitis. J AAPOS 1999;3:252–4.
872. Whitcup SM, Butler KM, Caruso R, et al. Retinal toxicity in human immunodeficiency virus-infected children treated with 2′,3′-dideoxyinosine. Am J Ophthalmol 1992;113:1–7.
873. Green HJ, Burnett M, Duhamel TA, et al. Abnormal sarcoplasmic reticulum Ca2+-sequestering properties in skeletal muscle in chronic obstructive pulmonary disease. Am J Physiol Cell Physiol 2008;295:C350–7.
874. Hayasaka S, Takatori Y, Noda S, et al. Retinal vasculitis, in a mother and her son with human T-lymphotropic virus type 1 associated myelopathy. Br J Ophthalmol 1991;75:566–7.
875. Zako M, Kataoka T, Ohno-Jinno A, et al. Analysis of progressive ophthalmic lesion in a patient with subacute sclerosing panencephalitis. Eur J Ophthalmol 2008;18:155–8.
876. Font RL, Jenis EH, Tuck KD. Measles maculopathy associated with subacute sclerosing panencephalitis: immunofluorescent and immuno-ultrastructural studies. Arch Pathol 1973;96:168–74.

877. Bakri SJ, Kaiser PK. Ocular manifestations of West Nile virus. Curr Opin Ophthalmol 2004;15:537–40.
878. Anninger W, Lubow M. Visual loss with West Nile virus infection: a wider spectrum of a 'new' disease. Clin Infect Dis 2004;38:e55–6.
879. Bains HS, Jampol LM, Caughron MC, et al. Vitritis and chorioretinitis in a patient with West Nile virus infection. Arch Ophthalmol 2003;121:205–7.
880. Anninger WV, Lomeo MD, Dingle J, et al. West Nile virus-associated optic neuritis and chorioretinitis. Am J Ophthalmol 2003;136:1183–5.
881. Adelman RA, Membreno JH, Afshari NA, et al. West Nile virus chorioretinitis. Retina 2003;23:100–1.
882. Khairallah M, Ben Yahia S, Attia S, et al. Linear pattern of West Nile virus-associated chorioretinitis is related to retinal nerve fibres organization. Eye 2007;21:952–5.
883. Khairallah M, Ben Yahia S, Attia S, et al. Indocyanine green angiographic features in multifocal chorioretinitis associated with West Nile virus infection. Retina 2006;26:358–9.
884. Khairallah M, Ben Yahia S, Ladjimi A, et al. Chorioretinal involvement in patients with West Nile virus infection. Ophthalmology 2004;111:2065–70.
885. Yahia SB, Khairallah M. Ocular manifestations of West Nile virus infection. Int J Med Sci 2009;6:114–5.
886. Chan CK. Ocular manifestation of West Nile virus: a vanishing disease in North America? Can J Ophthalmol 2007;42:195–8.
887. Chan CK, Limstrom SA, Tarasewicz DG, et al. Ocular features of West Nile virus infection in North America: a study of 14 eyes. Ophthalmology 2006;113:1539–46.
888. Garg S, Jampol LM. Systemic and intraocular manifestations of West Nile virus infection. Surv Ophthalmol 2005;50:3–13.
889. Teitelbaum BA, Newman TL, Tresley DJ. Occlusive retinal vasculitis in a patient with West Nile virus. Clin Exp Optom 2007;90:463–7.
890. Lim WK, Mathur R, Koh A, et al. Ocular manifestations of dengue fever. Ophthalmology 2004;111:2057–64.
891. Cruz-Villegas V, Berrocal AM, Davis JL. Bilateral choroidal effusions associated with dengue fever. Retina 2003;23:576–8.
892. Gupta A, Srinivasan R, Setia S, et al. Uveitis following dengue fever. Eye 2009;23:873–6.
893. Loh BK, Bacsal K, Chee SP, et al. Foveolitis associated with dengue fever: a case series. Ophthalmologica 2008;222:317–20.
894. Kanungo S, Shukla D, Kim R. Branch retinal artery occlusion secondary to dengue fever. Indian J Ophthalmol 2008;56:73–4.
895. Beral L, Merle H, David T. Ocular complications of dengue fever. Ophthalmology 2008;115:1100–1.
896. Tan SY, Kumar G, Surrun SK, et al. Dengue maculopathy: a case report. Travel Med Infect Dis 2007;5:62–3.
897. Pek DC, Teoh SC. Ocular manifestations in dengue fever. Can J Ophthalmol 2007;42:755. [author reply 755–56]
898. Nah G, Tan M, Teoh S, et al. Maculopathy associated with dengue fever in a military pilot. Aviat Space Environ Med 2007;78:1064–7.
899. Bacsal KE, Chee SP, Cheng CL, et al. Dengue-associated maculopathy. Arch Ophthalmol 2007;125:501–10.
900. Kapoor HK, Bhai S, John M, et al. Ocular manifestations of dengue fever in an East Indian epidemic. Can J Ophthalmol 2006;41:741–6.
901. Mehta S. Ocular lesions in severe dengue hemorrhagic fever (DHF). J Assoc Physicians India 2005;53:656–7.
902. Siqueira RC, Vitral NP, Campos WR, et al. Ocular manifestations in dengue fever. Ocul Immunol Inflamm 2004;12:323–7.
903. Sanjay S, Wagle AM, Au Eong KG. Optic neuropathy associated with dengue fever. Eye 2008;22:722–4.
904. Kannan M, Rajendran R, Sunish IP, et al. A study on chikungunya outbreak during 2007 in Kerala, south India. Indian J Med Res 2009;129:311–5.
905. Mahendradas P, Ranganna SK, Shetty R, et al. Ocular manifestations associated with chikungunya. Ophthalmology 2008;115:287–91.
906. Murthy KR, Venkataraman N, Satish V, et al. Bilateral retinitis following chikungunya fever. Indian J Ophthalmol 2008;56:329–31.
907. Mittal A, Mittal S, Bharati MJ, et al. Optic neuritis associated with chikungunya virus infection in South India. Arch Ophthalmol 2007;125:1381–6.
908. Lalitha P, Rathinam S, Banushree K, et al. Ocular involvement associated with an epidemic outbreak of chikungunya virus infection. Am J Ophthalmol 2007;144:552–6.
909. Chanana B, Azad RV, Nair S. Bilateral macular choroiditis following Chikungunya virus infection. Eye (Lond) 2007;21:1020–1.
910. Foster RE, Lowder CY, Meisler DM, et al. Mumps neuroretinitis in an adolescent. Am J Ophthalmol 1990;110:91–3.
911. Riffenburgh RS. Ocular manifestations of mumps. Arch Ophthalmol 1961;66:739–43.
912. Al-Hazmi A, Al-Rajhi AA, Abboud EB, et al. Ocular complications of Rift Valley fever outbreak in Saudi Arabia. Ophthalmology 2005;112:313–8.
913. Cohen C, Luntz MH. Rift-Valley-Fieber und Rickettsianretinitis einschliesslich Fluoresceinangiographie. Klin Monatsbl Augenheilkd 1976;169:685–99.
914. Deutman AF, Klomp HJ. Rift Valley fever retinitis. Am J Ophthalmol 1981;92:38–42.
915. Freed I. Rift Valley fever in man complicated by retinal changes and loss of vision. S Afr Med J 1951;25:930–2.
916. Schrire L. Macular changes in Rift Valley fever. S Afr Med J 1951;25:926–30.
917. Siam AL, Meegan JM, Gharbawi KF. Rift Valley fever ocular manifestations: observations during the 1977 epidemic in Egypt. Br J Ophthalmol 1980;64:366–74.
918. Avila MP, Jalkh AE, Feldman E, et al. Manifestations of Whipple's disease in the posterior segment of the eye. Arch Ophthalmol 1984;102:384–90.
919. Durant WJ, Flood T, Goldberg MF, et al. Vitrectomy and Whipple's disease. Arch Ophthalmol 1984;102:848–51.
920. Font RL, Rao NA, Issarescu S, et al. Ocular involvement in Whipple's disease: light and electron microscopic observations. Arch Ophthalmol 1978;96:1431–6.
921. Gärtner J. Whipple's disease of the central nervous system, associated with ophthalmoplegia externa and severe asteroid hyalitis: a clinicopathologic study. Doc Ophthalmol 1980;49:155–87.
922. Knox DL, Bayless TM, Yardley JH, et al. Whipple's disease presenting with ocular inflammation and minimal intestinal symptoms. Johns Hopkins Med J 1968;123:175–82.
923. Krücke W, Stochdroph O. Über Veränderungen im Zentralnervensystem bei Whipple'scher Krankheit. Verh Dtsch Ges Pathol 1962;46:198–202.
924. Leland TM, Chambers JK. Ocular findings in Whipple's disease. South Med J 1978;71:335–7.
925. Margo CE, Pavan PR, Groden LR. Chronic vitritis with macrophagic inclusions: a sequela of treated endophthalmitis due to a coryneform bacterium. Ophthalmology 1988;95:156–61.
926. Rickman LS, Freeman WR, Green WR, et al. Brief report: Uveitis caused by Tropheryma whippelii (Whipple's bacillus). N Engl J Med 1995;332:363–6.
927. Selsky EJ, Knox DL, Maumenee AE, et al. Ocular involvement in Whipple's disease. Retina 1984;4:103–6.
928. Switz DM, Casey TR, Bogaty GV. Whipple's disease and papilledema: an unreported presentation. Arch Intern Med 1969;123:74–7.
929. Malinowski SM, Pulido JS, Goeken NE, et al. The association of HLA-B8, B51, DR2, and multiple sclerosis in pars planitis. Ophthalmology 1993;100:1199–205.
930. Maumenee AE. Clinical entities in 'uveitis': an approach to the study of intraocular inflammation. Am J Ophthalmol 1970;69:1–27.
931. Mieler WF, Will BR, Lewis H, et al. Vitrectomy in the management of peripheral uveitis. Ophthalmology 1988;95:859–64.
932. Nissenblatt MJ, Masciulli L, Yarian DL, et al. Pars planitis – a demyelinating disease? Arch Ophthalmol 1981;99:697.
933. Nussenblatt RB, Palestine AG. Cyclosporin (Sandimmun) therapy: experience in the treatment of pars planitis and present therapeutic guidelines. Dev Ophthalmol 1992;23:177–84.
934. Pederson JE, Kenyon KR, Green WR, et al. Pathology of pars planitis. Am J Ophthalmol 1978;86:762–74.
935. Porter R. Uveitis in association with multiple sclerosis. Br J Ophthalmol 1972;56:478–81.
936. Pruett RC, Brockhurst RJ, Letts NF. Fluorescein angiography of peripheral uveitis. Am J Ophthalmol 1974;77:448–53.
937. Shorb SR, Irvine AR, Kimura SJ, et al. Optic disk neovascularization associated with chronic uveitis. Am J Ophthalmol 1976;82:175–8.
938. Smith RE, Godfrey WA, Kimura SJ. Chronic cyclitis. I. Course and visual prognosis. Trans Am Acad Ophthalmol Otolaryngol 1973;77:OP760–OP768.
939. Welch RB, Maumenee AE, Wahlen HE. Peripheral posterior segment inflammation, vitreous opacities, and edema of the posterior pole: pars planitis. Arch Ophthalmol 1960;64:540–9.
940. Razonable RR, Pulido JS, Deziel PJ, et al. Chorioretinitis and vitreitis due to Tropheryma whipplei after transplantation: case report and review. Transpl Infect Dis 2008;10:413–8.
941. Ferrari Mde L, Vilela EG, Faria LC, et al. Whipple's disease. Report of five cases with different clinical features. Rev Inst Med Trop Sao Paulo 2001;43:45–50.
942. Schaller J, Carlson JA. Erythema nodosum-like lesions in treated Whipple's disease: signs of immune reconstitution inflammatory syndrome. J Am Acad Dermatol. 2009;60:277–88.
943. Cunha de Souza E, Nakashima Y. Diffuse unilateral subacute neuroretinitis: report of transvitreal surgical removal of a subretinal nematode. Ophthalmology 1995;102:1183–6.
944. Margolis TP, Lowder CY, Holland GN, et al. Varicella-zoster virus retinitis in patients with the acquired immunodeficiency syndrome. Am J Ophthalmol 1991;112:119–31.
945. Dublin AB, Philips HE. Computer tomography of disseminated coccidiodomycosis. Radiology 1980 May;135(2):361-8.
946. Gupta P, Sachdev N, Kaur J, et al. Endogenous mycotic endophthalmitis in an immunocompetent patient. Int Ophthalmol. 2009 Aug;29(4):315–8. Epub 2008 Jun 5.

CHAPTER 11

Inflammatory Diseases of the Retina

Noninfectious inflammatory diseases of the retina can be isolated to the retina or be contiguous with its underlying structures, choroid and sclera, or with adjacent structures, optic nerve, vitreous, and the anterior segment of the eye. These diseases can be idiopathic, autoimmune, or possibly an altered immune response to an infectious agent. A majority of them are isolated to the eye but some have systemic associations.

RETINAL VASCULITIS AND PERIVASCULITIS

The terms "retinal vasculitis" and "retinal perivasculitis" are used interchangeably as clinical names to describe the fundoscopic picture of exudative gray-white sheathing of the major retinal blood vessels. The retinal veins or arteries or both may be primarily affected. Fluorescein angiography shows evidence of perivenous or periarterial staining and may show evidence of vascular obstruction. In using these terms, we recognize that the primary cause of the fundus and angiographic findings may be immune-induced damage rather than inflammatory cell damage to the permeability and patency of the retinal blood vessels. Retinal vasculitis and perivasculitis may occur as part of well-defined ocular diseases of known cause (toxoplasmosis, pp. 848–852; diffuse subacute neuroretinitis, pp. 864–872; cytomegalovirus retinitis, pp. 892-896; syphilis, pp. 818–828) or well-defined syndromes of unknown cause (sarcoidosis, pp. 1022–1026; Behçet's disease, pp. 1026–1028; acute posterior multifocal placoid pigment epitheliopathy (APMPPE), p. 954; acute zonal occult outer retinopathy (AZOOR), p. 980; pars planitis, p. 1036; multiple sclerosis,[1,2] p. 1038; idiopathic recurrent branch retinal artery occlusion, pp. 474–478; and Eales' disease, pp. 564–568). Other more recently described or less well-defined clinical syndromes associated with retinal vasculitis and perivasculitis are retinal phlebitis and panuveitis associated with viral-like upper respiratory disease,[3] frosted-branch retinal angiitis and acute multifocal hemorrhagic retinal vasculitis.[4–10]

11.01 Acute retinal periphlebitis and panuveitis.

A–D: This 9-year-old boy complained of blurred vision while recovering from an acute respiratory infection. Visual acuity was 20/25. There were cells in the anterior chamber and vitreous. Note the retinal striae in the macular region (A). The left eye showed identical changes. Adenovirus was cultured from his throat, and spinal fluid examination revealed pleo-cytosis. Angiography revealed leakage of dye from the optic disc and the major retinal veins (B). Six weeks later visual acuity, the fundi, and fluorescein angiography were normal (D).

E–L: Frosted-branch angiitis occurred in this 25-year-old woman who noted blurred vision as she was recovering from an upper respiratory infection. Her visual acuity was 20/40, right eye and 20/25, left eye. She had vitreous cells, sheathing of the retinal veins, and mild optic disc edema bilaterally (E and F). She was treated with 80 mg daily of prednisone orally. Two weeks later her visual acuity was finger counting at 1 foot (30 cm), right eye, and at 5 feet (1.50 m), left eye. She had severe hemorrhagic retinopathy that was more marked in the right eye (G–I). Angiography (J–L) showed marked closure of the peripheral retinal vasculature. She subsequently developed severe proliferative retinopathy that required panretinal photocoagulation and vitrectomy.

Acute Retinal Periphlebitis and Panuveitis Associated With Viral-Like Upper Respiratory Disease

Acute bilateral visual blurring associated with inflammatory cellular infiltration of the anterior and posterior ocular chambers and fluorescein angiographic evidence of periphlebitis may occur in some patients during or immediately following an upper respiratory or flulike illness (Figure 11.01A–D).[3,11–14] Visual blurring usually disappears in 1–2 weeks in association with return of the fundus and angiographic findings to normal. An adenovirus was cultured from the stool of one such patient (Figure 11.01A–D).

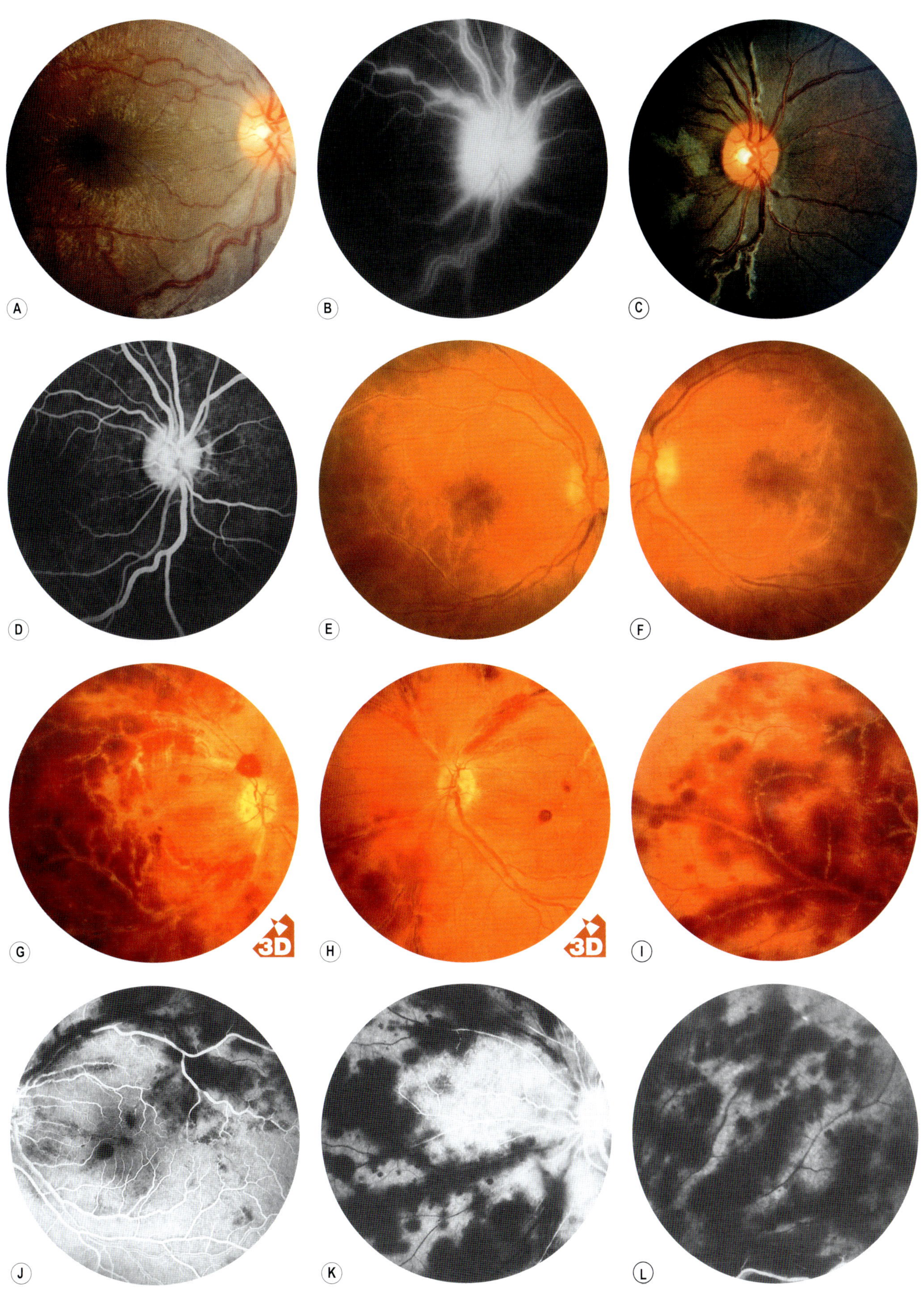
A
B
C
D
E
F
G
3D
H
3D
I
J
K
L

Idiopathic Frosted-Branch Angiitis

Patients with idiopathic frosted-branch angiitis present with visual symptoms associated with a striking ophthalmoscopic picture in one or both eyes of widespread prominent perivascular infiltration that in most patients is confined to the major retinal veins (Figures 11.01E–L and 11.02A–F).[9] About one-third report a flulike illness as a prodrome. Visual loss can be severe, to include macular or peripheral exudative retinal detachment (Figure 11.02A, C and D). The disorder is more common amongst Japanese individuals (70%)[15–17]; children are more often affected than adults, though age distribution ranges from 2 to 42 years.[18] Frosted-branch angiitis responds to systemic steroids very often, though several cases have been known to resolve without treatment. Secondary causes have to be ruled out prior to starting steroids. The disease burns out over weeks to months. Although the visual prognosis is generally good, some patients may develop retinal vein or artery occlusion, extensive retinal vascular closure, retinitis proliferans, vitreous hemorrhage, and rubeosis of the iris, macular epiretinal membrane, macular scarring, diffuse retinal fibrosis, retinal tear, optic atrophy, peripheral atrophic retinal lesions, and severe perivascular hemorrhages (Figure 11.01G–L).[7] These latter patients become indistinguishable from patients with acute multifocal hemorrhagic retinal vasculitis (see following discussion).

Secondary Frosted-Branch Angiitis

Frosted-branch angiitis can be a feature of several retinal diseases, including cytomegalovirus retinitis, Behçet's disease, lupus erythematosus (Figure 11.02G to J), Epstein–Barr virus retinitis, syphilis, toxoplasmosis, herpetic retinitis, human immunodeficiency virus (HIV) positivity, Hodgkin's disease, rapidly progressive glomerulonephritis, staphylococcal and streptococcal endophthalmitis.[19–27]

11.02 Frosted-branch angiitis.

A–F: A 9-year-old boy lost vision painlessly in both eyes to the hand motions level over 4 days. He had 3+ cells in both anterior chambers with fine keratic precipitates. Both retina showed widespread frosted-branch angiitis involving the arteries and veins, and large inferior exudative retinal detachments (A–C). The vessels showed mild leakage from the involved vessels (D). He was afebrile. Systemic workup for collagen vascular disease, sarcoid, tuberculosis, peri-nuclear antineutrophil cytoplasmic antibodies, classical antineutrophil cytoplasmic antibodies, complete blood count, renal function, and chest X-ray was all negative. His white count was slightly elevated to 12 800 cells/ml. He received intravenous methylprednisone for 5 days followed by oral steroids. The vision began to improve subjectively after 2 days, and to count fingers by 4 days. The exudative retinal detachment resolved by day 8. By week 5, the perivascular infiltrates had disappeared in the right eye and were present over some of the small vessels in the left eye (E and F). Over the next 6 months his vision gradually returned to 20/25 and 20/20 with eventual clearing of all perivascular infiltrate. Mild pigment mottling remained in the macula.

Periarteriolar plaques associated with systemic lupus erythematosus.

G–J: This 41-year-old woman had 20/20 and 20/25 vision in each eye. At age 14 she was diagnosed with juvenile rheumatoid arthritis and Still's disease. Since then a diagnosis of systemic lupus erythematosus with immune hepatitis, nephropathy, pleuropericarditis, abdominal serositis, splenic arteritis, and pancreatic vascular lesion was made. Occlusive vasculopathy with multiple-branch retinal artery occlusions, neovascularization of the disc and retina with recurrent vitreous hemorrhages requiring scatter laser, vitrectomy, and cataract surgery was managed. The periarterial white plaques were noted in 2002 (G and I) and remained unchanged until her last evaluation 4 years later (H and J).

(A–F, courtesy of Dr. Peter Sonkin; G–J, courtesy of Dr. Michael Goldbaum.)

Acute Multifocal Hemorrhagic Retinal Vasculitis

Otherwise healthy patients with acute multifocal hemorrhagic retinal vasculitis develop loss of vision associated with mild anterior uveitis, multifocal areas of retinal vasculitis (predominantly venular) with marked intraretinal hemorrhage, retinal capillary nonperfusion, retinal neovascularization, optic disc swelling, and vitritis.[4] Retinal necrosis is not a prominent part of this syndrome. Oral prednisone appears to be of some benefit in treatment of this disorder, which is unresponsive to treatment with acyclovir. Photocoagulation of the neovascular complications may be necessary. The etiology of this disorder, which shares some features with Behçet's disease, Eales' disease, and acute retinal necrosis, is unknown.

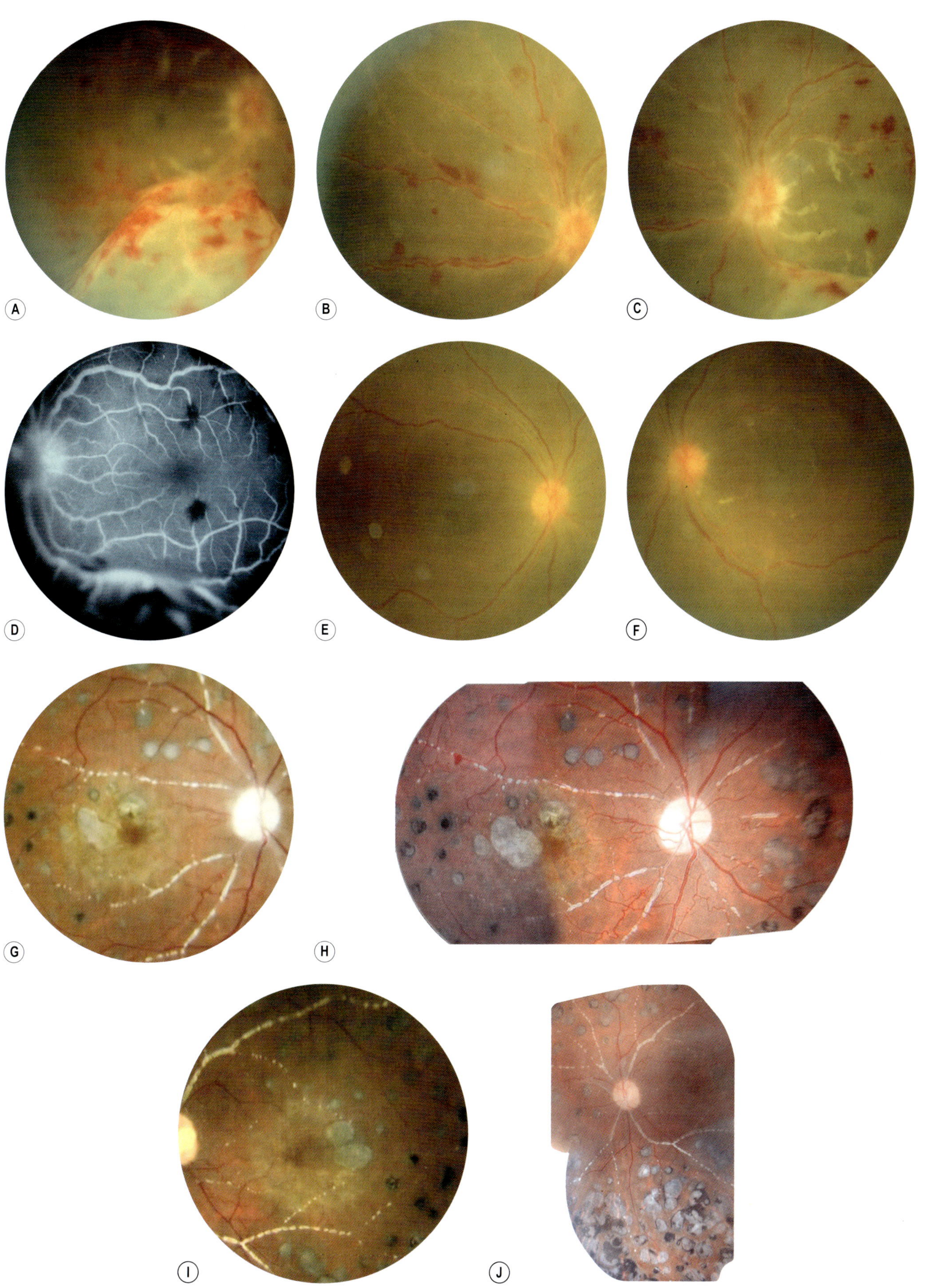
A
B
C
D
E
F
G
H
I
J

RETINOCHOROIDAL DEGENERATION ASSOCIATED WITH PROGRESSIVE IRIS NECROSIS

Margo et al. described progressive pigment epithelial and retinal atrophy that began in the macula and juxtapapillary retina (Figure 11.03A–D, H, I, K, L, and N), mild iritis, elevated intraocular pressure, severe pain, progressive iris atrophy (Figure 11.03E and J), progressive decrease in electroretinography amplitudes, and complete blindness within 3 years in a healthy 34-year-old man whose extensive medical workup was negative.[28] Histopathology revealed pigment granules and pigment-laden macrophages in the anterior chamber, severe ischemic necrosis of the iris (Figure 11.03F), chronic inflammatory cells in the uveal tract, and marked chorioretinal atrophy, with only a thin strand of glial tissue resting on an atrophic choroid. There were patchy areas of preservation of the inner retina posteriorly (Figure 11.03G) and some preservation of the retina and choroid peripherally, where thrombi were found in some of the choroidal blood vessels. Electron microscopy revealed no viral particles or evidence of a storage disease. The authors found no clues as to the pathogenesis of the disorder. A similar patient was seen by Dr. Jampol (Figure 11.03H–O). Note the deep trenchlike chorioretinal atrophy on the angiogram (Figure 11.03M and O).

11.03 Retinochoroidal degeneration associated with progressive iris necrosis.

A–G: This healthy 34-year-old man became bilaterally blind within 3 years of the onset of an unusual retinochoroidal degenerative disease. Within 5 months of the onset of symptoms his visual acuity declined to 20/300. There was severe mottling of the retinal pigment epithelium in the macula bilaterally (A and B). Dark adaptation studies, visual evoked potentials, and electroretinogram were normal. Eighteen months later there was extensive degeneration of the retina, counting fingers visual acuity, and severe ocular pain bilaterally (C and D). The third year of his illness was characterized by severe retinal vascular narrowing, mild iritis, progressive iris atrophy (E), modest elevation of the intraocular pressure, and blindness. Both eyes were enucleated because of severe pain. Histopathologic examination revealed severe ischemic necrosis of the iris (F), mild nongranulomatous uveitis, and marked chorioretinal atrophy and degeneration postequatorially. There were a few areas of preservation of the inner retina posteriorly (G). Electron microscopy revealed no viral particles.
H–O: This male was first seen elsewhere in 2004 with vitelliform lesions in both eyes and vision of count fingers in both eyes (H and I). His visual fields were constricted and electroretinogram revealed decreased rod and cone function in both eyes. In May 2005 he developed bilateral uveitis for the first time. Uveitis workup was negative for human leukocyte antigen (HLA) B27, fluorescent treponemal antibody absorption, Lyme, human immunodeficiency virus, angiotensin-converting enzyme, complete blood count, rheumatoid factor, antinuclear antibody, and erythrocyte sedimentation rate. He suffered several episodes of uveitis that were treated elsewhere and was known to develop steroid-induced glaucoma. By 2006 he had developed iris atrophy and atrophic lesions in both macula. He was first examined by Dr. Jampol in April 2008 with further decrease in vision in the right eye, when both irises were necrotic (J) and both macula showed widespread chorioretinal atrophy (K and L). Extensive choriocapillaris and choroidal atrophy was seen on angiography (M). The right eye had a cloudy cornea and traction retinal detachment. A pars plana vitrectomy, membrane peel, and retinal detachment repair with silicone oil placement in the right eye did not improve his vision. Vitreous and retinal samples showed mixed inflammatory infiltrate and were negative for varicella-zoster, herpes simplex, cytomegalovirus, and Epstein–Barr virus. The macula was very thin on optical coherence tomography imaging. A year later the inflammation stabilized with a clear media and extensive atrophic chorioretinal scar (N and O). The clinical features are similar to the case reported by Curtis Margo.

(A–G, From Margo et al.[28] H–O, courtesy of Dr. Lee Jampol.)

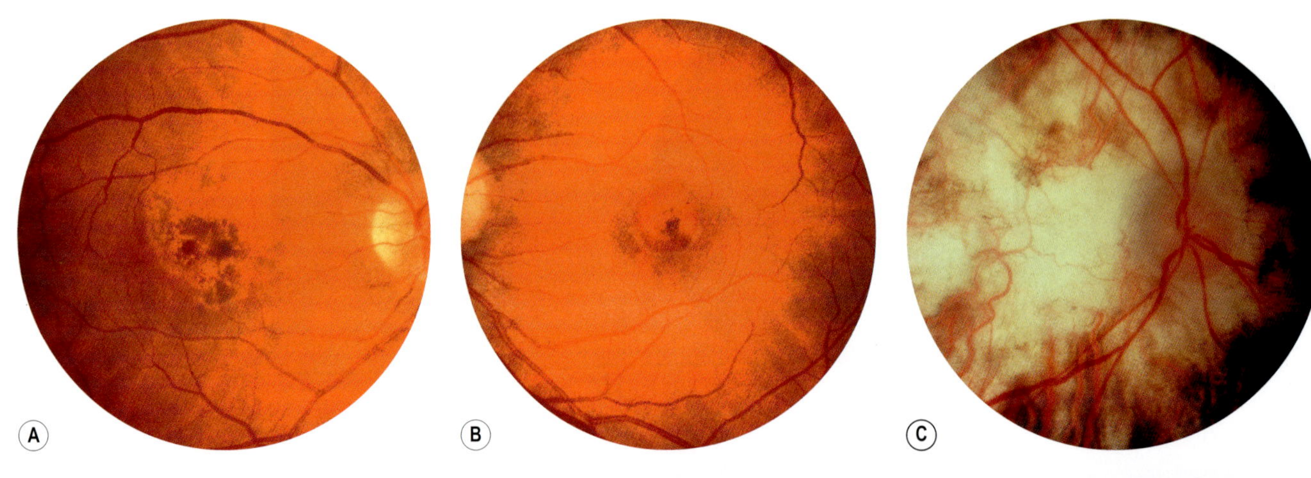

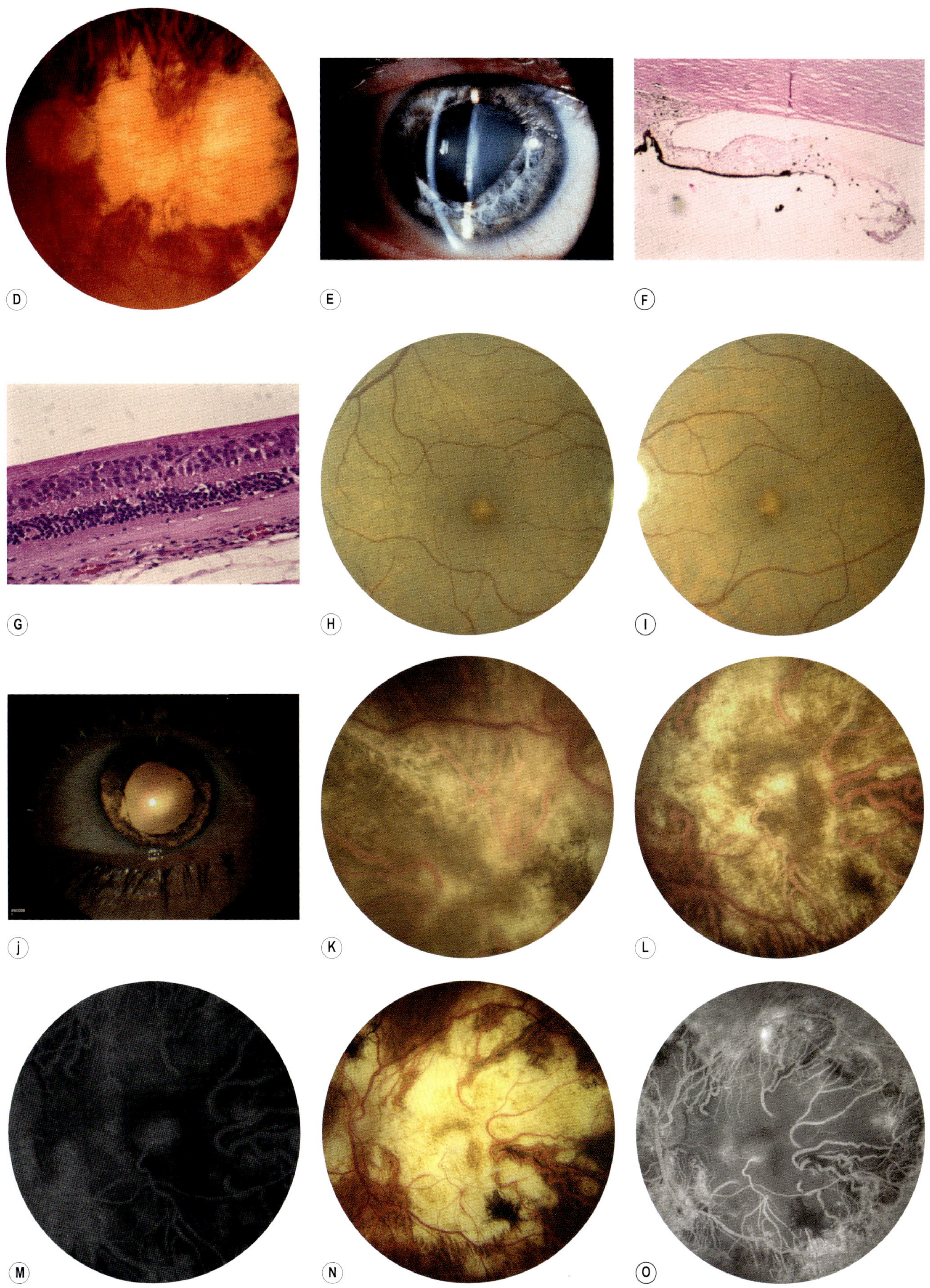
D
E
F
G
H
I
j
K
L
M
N
O

ACUTE POSTERIOR MULTIFOCAL PLACOID PIGMENT EPITHELIOPATHY

APMPPE typically affects young healthy male or female patients (average age approximately 25 years), who develop rapid loss of vision in one or both eyes secondary to multiple postequatorial, circumscribed, flat, gray-white, subretinal lesions involving the retinal pigment epithelium (RPE) (Figures 11.04–11.06).[29–57] These lesions are rarely associated with clinically apparent retinal detachment or with retinal hemorrhage (Figure 11.05B and C).[39,42] The overlying retina usually appears normal. Inflammatory cells in the vitreous may be present in 50% of patients. Approximately one-third of patients give a history of a flulike syndrome antedating the onset of visual symptoms.[30,37,39,42,52,58] In one case it followed a mild hypersensitivity reaction to swine flu vaccine[41] and varicella-zoster vaccination in another.[59] APMPPE has occurred in patients with thyroiditis,[43] cerebrovasculitis,[42,45,54,60–67] adenovirus type 5 infection,[30] lymphadenopathy,[39] hepatomegaly (Figure 11.04K and L),[39] erythema nodosum,[35,39,55] regional enteritis,[39] sarcoidosis,[68,69] acute nephritis,[70] lupus erythematosus,[71] serologic evidence of Lyme disease,[72,73] Wegener's granulomatosis,[74] systemic necrotizing vasculitis,[75] ulcerative colitis,[76] and spinal fluid pleocytosis and elevated protein.[32,36,37,42,54] Two patients with evidence of central nervous system (CNS) vasculitis died within several weeks of onset of APMPPE as systemic corticosteroids were being tapered.[67,77] Autopsy in one case revealed evidence of granulomatous arteritis in the leptomeninges.[67] These cases suggest that APMPPE may be the initial manifestation of primary CNS angiitis, which is associated with a high mortality rate of approximately 95% if untreated, 46% if treated with corticosteroids, and 8% if treated with corticosteroids and cytotoxic agents.[78]

Other ocular findings include perivenous exudation in the retina,[38,41] perichoroidal venous infiltration,[63] and dilation and tortuosity of the retinal veins, papilledema,[40] papillitis, optic neuritis,[40,43–45,53–55,79] episcleritis (Figure 11.05A),[39] iridocyclitis,[37,39] and central retinal vein occlusion (Dr. Lawrence A. Yannuzzi, personal communication). This latter may develop as a result of vasculitis and swelling within the optic nerve.

Infrequently, APMPPE occurs unilaterally. The second eye is usually involved within a few days or weeks after the first. In 2 patients the interval was 30 and 36 months (Figure 11.04G–J).[39] Recurrences are infrequent and usually occur in the first 6 months following the onset of symptoms (Figure 11.04A–F). Characteristic features of the disease are the rapid resolution of the fundus lesions and the delayed remarkable return of visual function, usually to the level of approximately 20/30 or better (Figure 11.04A–D).[39] Within a few days of the onset of symptoms the acute gray-white lesions begin to fade centrally. Within 7–12 days they are completely replaced by areas of partly depigmented RPE (Figure 11.04D and E). Irregular clumping of pigment occurs, and day-to-day changes in its pattern develop over a period of months. The acute and subacute lesions superficially resemble those seen after photocoagulation.

11.04 Acute posterior multifocal placoid pigment epitheliopathy (APMPPE).

A–F: This healthy 22-year-old woman developed blurred vision in both eyes 5 days before admission. Her past history was unremarkable. Visual acuity in the right eye was 20/200 and in the left eye was 20/20. Note the multifocal, flat, white lesions involving the retinal pigment epithelium (RPE) (A). The lesion superiorly had undergone partial resolution, and some details of the underlying choroid were visible. Note absence of serous detachment of the overlying retina. Early angiograms revealed absence of background fluorescence in the region of the active lesions (B). Some background fluorescence is visible in the partly resolved lesion superiorly. One hour after injection, the angiogram showed fluorescein staining of all lesions (C). Nine days later, her visual acuity had returned to 20/50. There was focal depigmentation of the RPE following the rapid resolution of the placoid lesions in both eyes (D and E). Seven months later, visual acuity was 20/20. Thirteen months after the onset of her disease she had recurrence of symptoms in the left eye with transient loss of vision. These lesions healed, and when last seen 40 months after the onset of her disease, visual acuity was 20/20. Note evidence of the more recent lesion superiorly (F).

G–J: This 45-year-old woman developed rapid loss of vision (10/200) in the left eye. Note the large centrally located lesion (G). Angiography revealed other lesions, all of which were nonfluorescent in the early phases of angiography (H) and which stained later (I). Twelve months later, her vision had returned to 20/20 (J). Thirty months after the onset of her disease she developed a similar large central lesion in the right eye and experienced an identical clinical course in that eye.

K and **L:** Severe bilateral APMPPE in a 19-year-old woman who noted the onset of visual loss several days after an upper respiratory infection. Note the evidence of early resolution of the macular lesion (K). Vitreous cells were present. The patient's visual acuity was 20/200. A liver scan revealed hepatomegaly and abnormal uptake of radioisotopes in the left lobe. Her electro-oculographic findings were normal. Her electro-retinographic findings were subnormal. Six months later the visual acuity was 20/50 in the right eye and 20/25 in the left eye, despite the widespread alterations in the RPE throughout the posterior pole of both eyes (L).

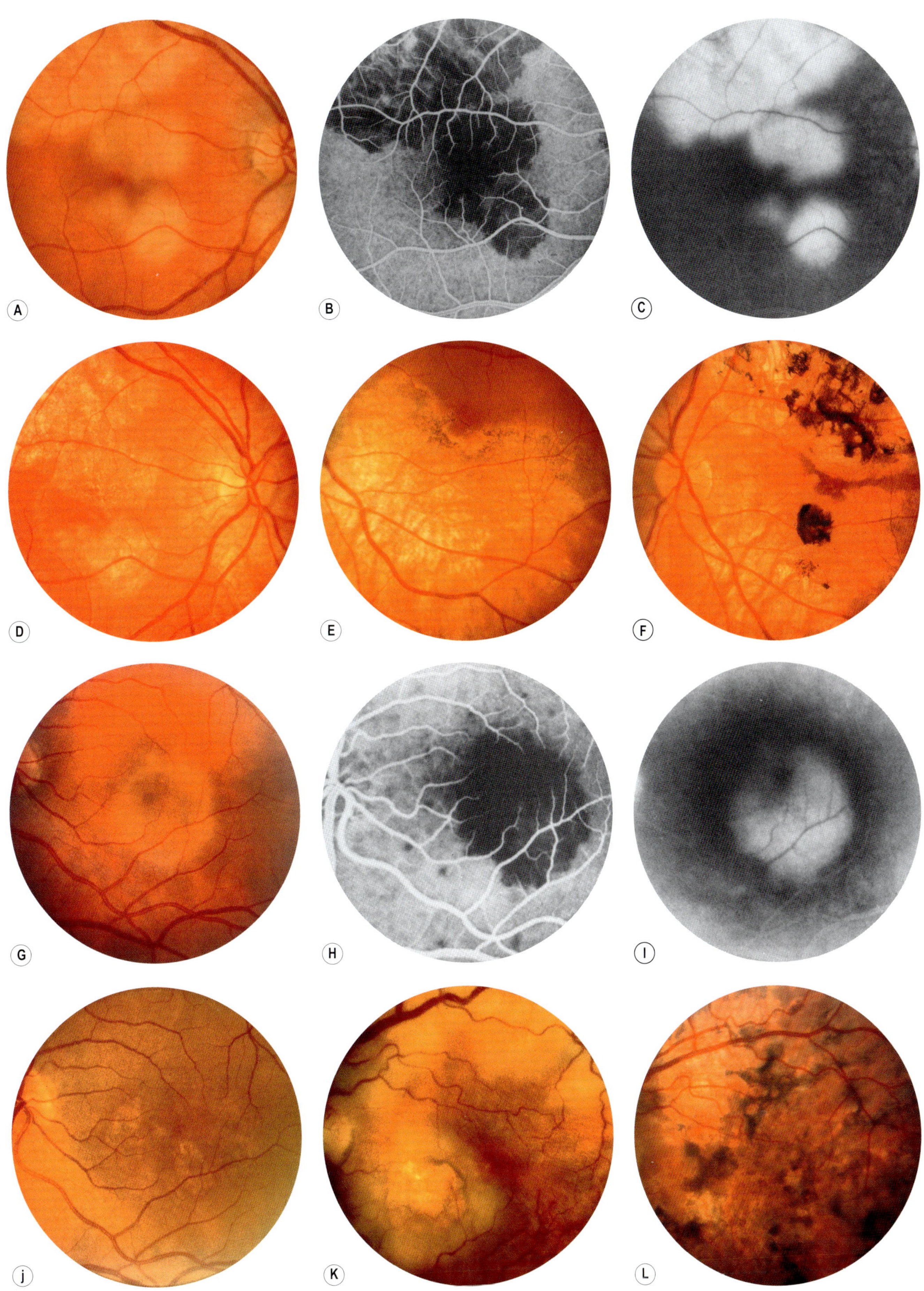
A
B
C
D
E
F
G
H
I
j
K
L

During the acute phase of APMPPE the subretinal lesions block out most of the background choroidal fluorescence (Figures 11.04B and H, 11.05C, and 11.06D). Mid- and late-phase angiograms demonstrate diffuse, even staining of the acute lesions (Figures 11.04B, C, H, and I, and 11.06E). During the course of early resolution of these lesions, angiography demonstrates large choroidal vessels coursing through the center of the partly faded gray lesions before the development of staining in the later pictures (Figure 11.04B). During the later course of resolution, angiography demonstrates extensive alterations in the background choroidal fluorescence caused by changes in the content of the RPE but shows relatively little evidence of occlusion of the choriocapillaris. Indocyanine green (ICG) angiography shows dark spots (Figure 11.06L) corresponding to the placoid lesions and these do not stain late, unlike fluorescein.[80] The lesions appear to involve the RPE and the adjacent photoreceptors on optical coherence tomography (OCT), which shows disruption of these structures during the active phase and recovery when the lesions heal. Very occasionally, shallow subretinal fluid has been seen overlying the placoid lesions on OCT; exudative retinal detachment is not the norm in APMPPE. Microperimetry can demonstrate the involved areas and recovery of function in those areas once the lesions heal.[81] Subnormal electro-oculographic findings have been reported during the acute stage of the disease. Most patients tested during the acute phases of the disease have normal electro-oculograms and electroretinograms (ERGs). One patient with severe involvement had normal electro-oculographic findings with subnormal cone and rod electroretinographic findings (Figure 11.04K and L).

The prognosis for visual recovery is good. Visual recovery can occur up to as long as 6 months. In an average follow-up of over 5 years in 30 patients seen at the Bascom Palmer Eye Institute, all but two eyes had 20/30 or better visual acuity at the last examination.[39] Many patients will identify small residual paracentral scotomata when carefully tested. Recurrences and the development of choroidal neovascularization occur infrequently (Figure 11.05D and E).[39,40,48,82]

The cause of this disease, which in many instances is associated with evidence of systemic involvement, is unknown. In the eye it appears to be an acute, self-limited disease, initially causing multifocal areas of color change in the RPE and perhaps retinal receptor cells. The cell cytoplasm apparently becomes sufficiently cloudy that it blocks out all background choroidal fluorescence. The course and nature of the disease suggest the possibility of viral infection. Figure 11.05 (F–I) illustrates schematically some of the presumed anatomic changes in this disease. Despite the extensive alterations in the pigment content, the RPE cells and most of the retinal receptors apparently recover and visual acuity usually returns to near normal. The end-stage of this disease is similar in this respect to rubella.

Many authors have favored choriocapillaris occlusion as the cause of the color change in the RPE and the early angiographic findings.[34,35,46,55,57,69,83] The following are difficult, however, to explain on the basis of choroidal vascular occlusion: (1) the variability in the size and shape of the lesions, which appear to have no relationship to the anatomy of the choriocapillaris; (2) the failure of the acute lesions to stain with fluorescein from the periphery inward, as would be expected to occur from neighboring normally perfused choriocapillaris; and (3) the frequency of recovery of visual function.[39] Demonstration of large fluorescent choroidal vessels coursing through the area of partly resolved acute lesions (Figure 11.04B) does not necessarily mean there is nonperfusion of the choriocapillaris in these areas. The RPE cells, which undoubtedly are still present in these areas, may be sufficiently opaque to attenuate the fluorescence arising from the choriocapillaris but not that in the large choroidal vessels. The findings with ICG angiography are similar to that with fluorescein and in the author's opinion do not shed further light on the pathophysiology of APMPPE.[83]

Wolf et al. reported HLA-B7 antigens in 40% and HLA-DR2 antigens in 57% of patients with APMPPE versus 17% and 28%, respectively, in controls.[84]

11.05 Acute posterior multifocal placoid pigment epitheliopathy (APMPPE).

A: Episcleritis in a patient presenting with bilateral APMPPE.
B and **C:** APMPPE associated with a small subretinal hemorrhage (arrow).
D and **E:** Choroidal neovascularization (arrows) occurring several years after the patient recovered near-normal visual acuity after bilateral APMPPE.
F–I: Schematic diagrams depicting probable histopathologic changes and fluorescein staining pattern in APMPPE. The acute yellow-white focal lesion is probably composed of swollen retinal pigment epithelial (RPE) cells and damaged outer retinal segments between the arrows in F–H. In the early-phase angiograms the fluorescein (black stippling) has perfused the choroidal circulation (F), and quickly stains the choroid (ch), and is beginning to move into the base of the swollen RPE cells with cloudy cytoplasm (G). Loss of transparency of the RPE and outer retinal receptors totally obscures the fluorescein in the choroid. In the late stage of angiography (H) the dye has stained the affected cells, choroid (ch), and sclera (S), causing the acute lesion to appear hyperfluorescent. Healed stage of APMPPE, late phase of angiography (I) shows restoration of the outer retinal–blood barrier, patchy areas of depigmentation and hyperpigmentation of the RPE cells, and regrowth of the retinal outer segments, but some loss of receptor cells.

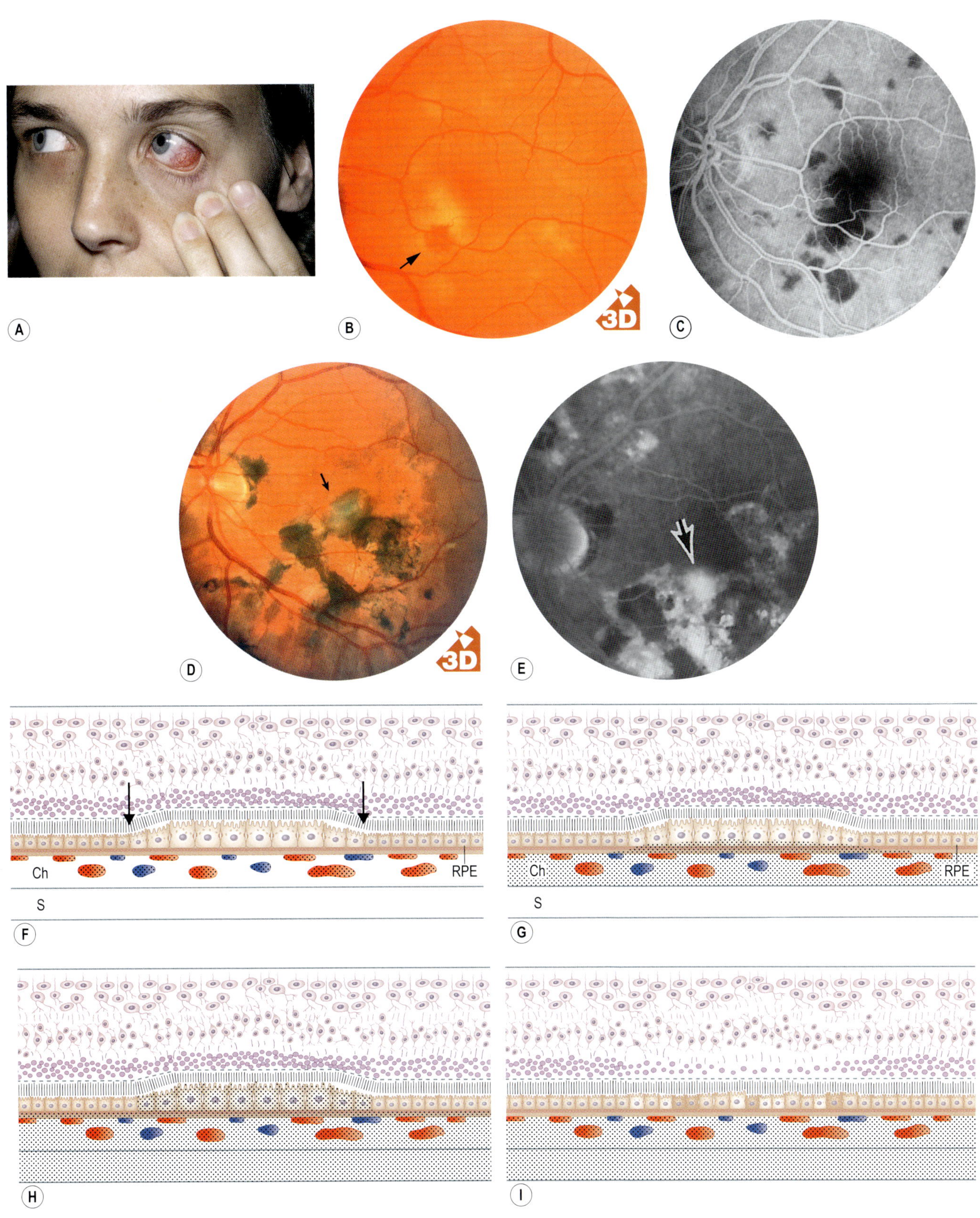
A
B
3D
C
D
3D
E
Ch
RPE
S
F
Ch
RPE
S
G
H
I

There is no information concerning the relative value of systemic treatment with corticosteroids compared to no treatment of patients with APMPPE. The natural course of the disease suggests that the visual prognosis is favorable without treatment. Some might argue that corticosteroids should be given, if for no other reason than to reduce the potential of CNS complications. It is unknown, however, whether this treatment is beneficial or harmful in this regard. Patients and their families should be alerted to the relatively low possibility of CNS complications and of the importance of promptly reporting any symptoms or signs suggesting CNS involvement. There is evidence that patients with idiopathic CNS angiitis benefit from corticosteroid and cytotoxic therapy.[78]

It is important to differentiate APMPPE from serpiginous (geographic) choroiditis. Although the acute lesions in both diseases appear similar ophthalmoscopically and angiographically, the lesions of serpiginous choroiditis resolve more slowly and leave in their wake ophthalmoscopic and angiographic evidence of marked atrophy of the underlying choriocapillaris and larger choroidal vessels (see pp. 962–964). Some patients reported as having APMPPE with atypical features, such as branch vein occlusion, may have had serpiginous choroiditis.[48,85] Serpiginous choroiditis is a chronic, recurring, often severe disease that may leave the patient with severe visual disability in one or both eyes. Table 11.1 outlines some of the important differences in these two diseases.

The multifocal white lesions in APMPPE must be differentiated from other causes of multifocal deep retinitis (e.g., diffuse unilateral subacute neuroretinitis) (see Figure 10.29A–G), multiple evanescent white-dot syndrome (MEWDS) (Figures 11.15 and 11.16), focal inflammatory cell infiltrates of the choroid (e.g., multifocal choroiditis with panuveitis (MCP), pseudo-presumed ocular histoplasmosis syndrome (POHS)), sarcoidosis,[68,69] secondary syphilis (Figures 10.07B and G, 10.10H, and 10.11I), diffuse choroidal infiltration in Harada's disease that may be associated with multifocal ill-defined lesions at the level of the pigment epithelium (see Figure 11.26A),[86] sympathetic uveitis (see Figure 11.29D), multifocal zones of occlusion of the choriocapillaris (e.g., toxemia of pregnancy; see Figure 3.59D), primary or metastatic neoplastic infiltrates of the choroid or sub-RPE space (see Figures 13.31G and H and 14.31D and E), and multifocal areas of depigmentation of the choroid, such as occurs in vitiliginous (birdshot) chorioretinitis (see Figure 11.45A and B). Focal inflammatory cell infiltrates of the choroid are often smaller and slightly elevated, frequently persist for several weeks or more, and often cause secondary detachment of the overlying retina. They may completely resolve without leaving significant changes in the overlying RPE, or they may cause varying degrees of atrophy of the choroid and RPE. The author believes that the patients reported as having retinal detachment secondary to APMPPE showed features more typical of a diffuse underlying choroiditis, probably Harada's disease, rather than APMPPE (see Figure 11.26A).[31,87]

11.06 Acute posterior multifocal placoid pigment epitheliopathy.

A–I: This 17-year-old Caucasian male presented with a 6-day history of decreased vision in both eyes. He had had a low-grade fever and malaise 1 week before the onset of visual symptoms. Visual acuity was 20/200 in both eyes. The right eye showed several placoid gray-white lesions in the posterior pole, and the midperiphery of both eyes (A–C). A fluorescein angiogram showed early hypofluorescence of the active lesions and late diffuse hyperfluorescence consistent with a diagnosis of acute posterior placoid pigment epitheliopathy (D and E). His visual acuity 2 weeks later was 20/400 in both eyes. The acute lesions had faded with significant pigment mottling (F and G). Six months after onset, visual acuity improved to 20/60 in the right and 20/30 on the left, with extensive hyperpigmentary response. Two years later visual acuity was 20/80 on the right and 20/300 on the left with no active lesions. He developed a choroidal neovascular membrane (H and I, arrows) in the left eye, which was treated with photodynamic therapy, and the visual acuity improved to 20/60.
J–L: This patient with bilateral multifocal placoid lesions of acute posterior multifocal placoid pigment epitheliopathy (J and K) shows choroidal nonperfusion on indocyanine green (L).

(A–I, courtesy of Dr. Eric Holtz; J–L, courtesy of Dr. Richard Spaide.)

Table 11.1 Differential diagnostic features of acute posterior multifocal placoid pigment epitheliopathy (APMPPE) and serpiginous choroiditis

	APMPPE	Serpiginous choroiditis
Age of onset	Second and third decades	Beyond third decade
Associated systemic disease	Upper respiratory infection, erythema nodosum, regional enteritis, hepatitis, episcleritis, cerebral vasculitis	None
Visual complaints at onset	Bilateral	Unilateral most often
Acute lesions	Flat, gray-white, retinal pigment epithelial lesions	Same
Lesion distribution	Postequatorial	Peripapillary
Lesion shape	Usually isolated	Usually contiguous
Vitritis	±	±
Choroidal atrophy	Minimal	Maximal
Proliferative subretinal scarring	None	Frequent
Visual recovery	Excellent	Poor
Recurrence	Rare	Typical
Choroidal neovascularization	Rare	30% of patients

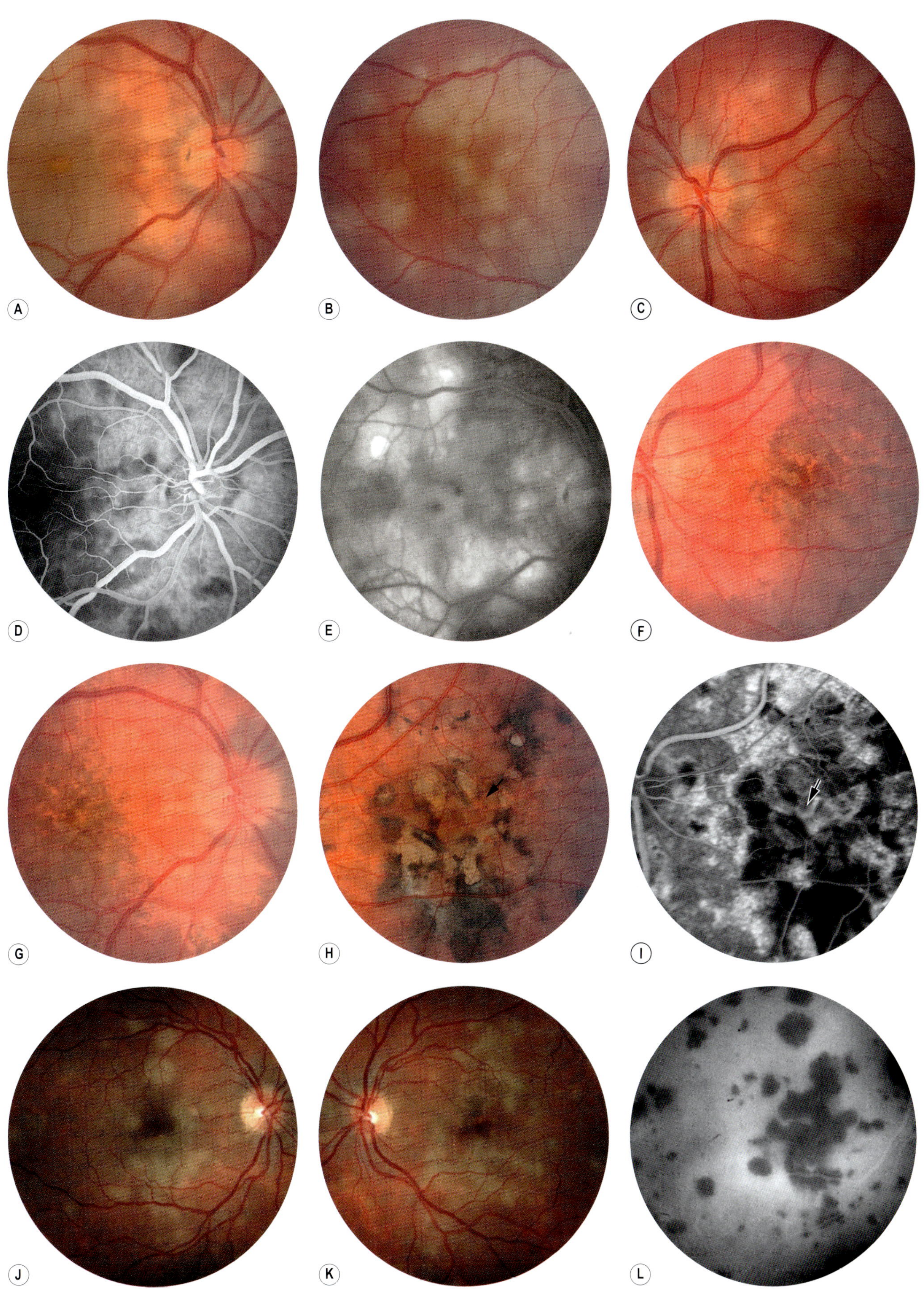
A
B
C
D
E
F
G
H
I
J
K
L

The syndrome of acute retinal pigment epitheliitis is characterized by the development of clusters of small pigment spots surrounded by halos of depigmentation in young patients with a recent history of visual loss. These patients experience rapid recovery of vision (see p. 974). In general, however, the lesions in APMPPE are much larger than can be accounted for on the basis of the RPE findings in acute retinal pigment epitheliitis.

Extensive pigmentary changes remaining during the late stages of APMPPE (Figure 11.04L) may be mistaken for a widespread tapetoretinal dystrophy. The clinical history of rapid loss and recovery of vision, the normal-appearing retinal vessels and optic nerve head, and usually normal electrophysiologic findings should differentiate retinal dystrophies from the late stages of APMPPE.

Priluck and associates have demonstrated the presence of urinary casts in 3 patients during the active phase of APMPPE.[50] The significance of this observation is unknown.

Although most patients with APMPPE present with multiple one-disc diameter-size white lesions randomly scattered in the posterior fundus, the size, shape, and distribution of the lesions may be variable (Figure 11.04G). In some cases the lesions are small, are confluent, and may show some persistence of nonfluorescence into the late stage of angiography. In several of these cases the lesions were uniformly small and closely spaced, similar to those which occurred in a 35-year-old man described as having diffuse punctate pigment epitheliopathy by Blinder et al.[88] Their patient failed to recover central vision. More recently, Taich and Johnson[89] analyzed 6 older patients ranging from 58 to 82 years of age (average age 72.5) with a few placoid lesions in the macula, who had several features differing from APMPPE: older age group, lesions mostly confined to the macula, late fluorescein showing patchy hyperfluorescence unlike the even staining of APMPPE, recurrences, late geographic atrophy, poor visual recovery and choroidal neovascularization in a significant number of them. This group is best considered a separate entity at this time. Description of additional cases in the future and expansion of the spectrum may help understand their pathogenesis. Two other conditions that resemble APMPPE in certain aspects are persistent placoid maculopathy and relentless placoid choroidopathy, described next.

PERSISTENT PLACOID MACULOPATHY

In 2006, 6 patients with bilateral macular placoid lesions superficially resembling macular serpiginous choroidopathy followed variably up to 20 years were described from five centers.[90] They were in their sixth to seventh decade, had bilateral involvement, the white macular lesions persisted for several months to years before fading, and they showed a propensity to choroidal neovascularization, often multiple, resulting in disciform scars. In spite of foveal involvement and persistent lesions, the visual acuity remains good till choroidal neovascularization develops. On fluorescein angiography the lesions remain non- or hypofluorescent till late and show minimal fluorescence in the late frames (Figure 11.07). Several small choroidal neovascular membranes (CNVMs) are seen. On ICG angiography the lesions appear nonfluorescent throughout the study. No evidence of vitritis or anterior-chamber inflammation has been seen. The relatively good vision (unless complicated by CNVM) argues against persistent choriocapillary nonperfusion as the reason for the persistent hypofluorescence on ICG and fluorescein angiography. The etiology is so far unknown. Treatment included systemic/periocular steroids at some time with improvement in vision. The loss of vision is mainly from choroidal neovascularization.[91,92]

11.07 Persistent placoid maculopathy (pigment epitheliopathy).

A–H: This 59-year-old previously healthy male presented with 20/40 and 20/50 vision. Placoid yellow lesions were present in the macula bilaterally. The lesion remained hypofluorescent and stained mildly very late in the angiogram. A classic small choroidal neovascular membrane was present juxtafoveally. He underwent photodynamic therapy and the lesion involuted. But it returned much larger 3 months later (H) and was resistant to treatment.

I–L: This 60-year-old male developed a placoid lesion in the right macula that soon developed evidence of choroidal neovascularization and subretinal hemorrhage (I and J). Angiogram showed persistent hypofluorescence and late mild patchy hyperfluorescence typical of persistent placoid pigment epitheliopathy, except for the early lacy hyperfluorescence of the choroidal neovascular membrane (K and L).

(Courtesy of Dr. Lawrence Yannuzzi. H, Also, Yannuzzi Lawrence J., The Retinal Atlas, Saunders 2010, 978-0-7020-3320-9, p.260.)

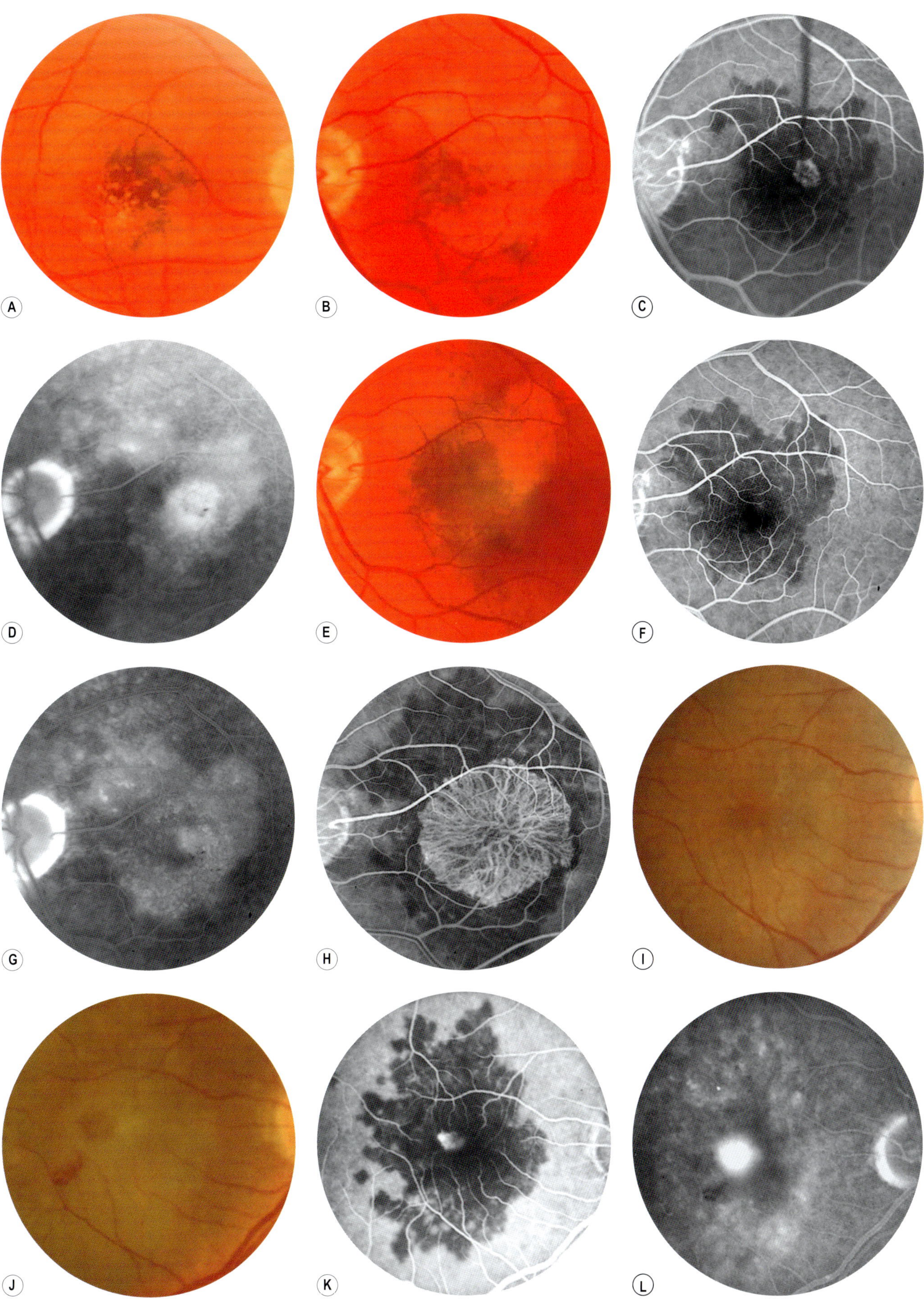
A
B
C
D
E
F
G
H
I
J
K
L

RELENTLESS PLACOID CHOROIDOPATHY

Six patients, aged 17 through 51 years, exhibiting some features of APMPPE and serpiginous choroidopathy were seen at six different centers from 1984 to 1997.[93] The acute placoid retinal lesions were multifocal, confluent, or serpiginous in nature with initial hypo- and late hyperfluorescence on angiography resembling both APMPPE and serpiginous choroidopathy. These patients in addition had numerous posterior and peripheral retinal lesions predating or occurring simultaneously with macular involvement. Older, healing pigmented lesions were often accompanied by the appearance of new active white placoid lesions. Additionally, all cases demonstrated prolonged periods of activity with several crops of new lesions, 50 and sometimes hundreds of them scattered throughout the fundus. Growth of subacute lesions and the appearance of new lesions continued for 5–24 months after initial examination, and relapses were common. Relentless placoid choroidopathy may represent a variant of serpiginous choroiditis or a new entity.[93–97]

One 20-year-old patient has been reported with associated hyperintense lesions on magnetic resonance imaging in the temporal lobe, found during evaluation of persistent headache. He received mycophenolate mofetil in addition to steroids and remained stable with resolution of the brain lesions.[94] Etiologically this condition is probably related to APMPPE, but much needs to be learnt. The condition has to be differentiated from APMPPE, serpiginous choroidopathy, serpiginous-like tuberculous choroiditis (see Chapter 10), persistent placoid choroidopathy, multifocal choroiditis, placoid syphilis, sarcoidosis, and lymphoma.

SERPIGINOUS CHOROIDITIS (GEOGRAPHIC CHOROIDITIS, HELICOID PERIPAPILLARY CHOROIDOPATHY)

Serpiginous choroiditis is an acute and chronic recurrent multifocal inflammatory disease that appears to affect primarily the inner half of the choroid, the RPE, and secondarily the retina.[98–109]

11.08 Serpiginous choroiditis.

A–F: This 43-year-old woman had a 3-week history of loss of central vision in the right eye. Visual acuity was counting fingers in the right eye and 20/25 in the left eye. Note the inactive chorioretinal scar surrounding the optic disc of both eyes and the active gray lesion at the level of the retinal pigment epithelium in the temporal and inferior portions of the right macula (arrows, A). Early angiograms showed obstruction of the background choroidal fluorescence in the area of the acute lesion and early staining of the chorioretinal scar (C). One-hour angiograms showed staining of the acute lesion as well as the chorioretinal scar (D). Seven months later there was pigmentation in the central portion of the active lesion (E). Three years later there was formation of an atrophic chorioretinal scar in the area of the previously active lesion (F). Visual acuity in the right eye was 20/200.

G–J: Active stage of serpiginous choroiditis (G–I). Note jigsaw-puzzle pattern of the lesions. Same eye 7 months later (J) shows evidence of additional lesions all of which are inactive. Haze is caused by vitreous cells.

K and **L:** Simultaneous development of serpiginous choroiditis and herpes zoster ophthalmicus in a 66-year-old man.

It usually begins in the peripapillary area and spreads centrifugally over a period of months or years by means of recurrent episodes of patchy choroiditis in a serpiginous or jigsaw puzzle-like distribution outward from the optic disc to involve the macula and peripheral fundus (Figures 11.08–11.11).

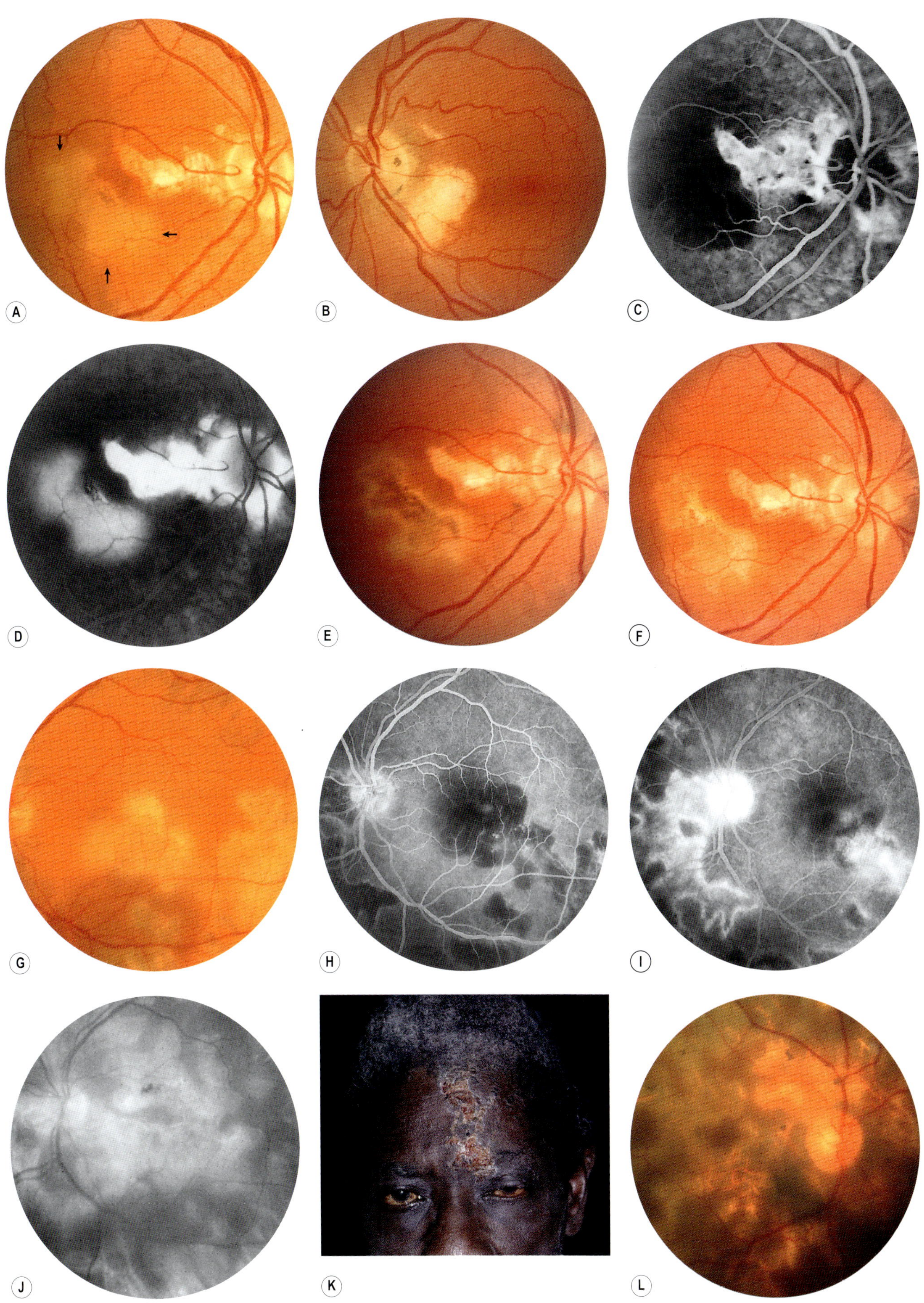
A
B
C
D
E
F
G
H
I
J
K
L

The patient is typically a healthy young or middle-aged individual when he or she first notices the rapid onset of paracentral or central scotomata in one eye. If the center of the macula is involved, the acuity is often 20/40 or less. Biomicroscopic and ophthalmoscopic examination within the first several weeks after the onset of symptoms reveals a well-circumscribed geographic zone of gray-white discoloration of the RPE in the macular area (Figures 11.08A and G, and 11.11I). Serous detachment of the retina is infrequently present. Although an occasional patient has a solitary active lesion in one macula,[106] usually the active lesion is in continuity with a zone of RPE and choroidal atrophy that extends nasally to surround all or a portion of the optic disc. Inflammatory cell reaction is present in the posterior vitreous in approximately one-third of cases during the active phase of the disease. Examination of the opposite asymptomatic eye often reveals an area of chorioretinal scarring adjacent to the optic disc (Figure 11.08B). Over a period of weeks, the acute gray-white lesions, which may appear identical to the acute stage of APMPPE, are partly replaced by mottling and depigmentation of the RPE (Figure 11.08A and F). The peripheral edge of the lesion often maintains a grayish-white active appearance for a month or longer (Figures 11.08E, and 11.09C). Over a period of months, varying degrees of atrophy of the underlying choroid develop within the discrete zone of previous activity. In some cases the atrophy involves the large as well as the small choroidal vessels and produces a trench-like area of choroidal atrophy (Figure 11.08F). In approximately one-half of patients varying amounts of gray-white tissue (fibrous metaplasia of the RPE) develop within the area of chorioretinal atrophy (Figure 11.11A–G). The patient usually develops a permanent dense absolute scotoma corresponding with most of the involved areas. The retinal vessels and optic nerve head are usually normal. At intervals varying from weeks to years, the patient is subject to recurring episodes of activity that each time involve a new and usually contiguous area of the fundus.[99,101,109] This process may spread widely into the far periphery of the fundus in one eye before a similar process begins in the second eye months or many years later. The disease frequently involves the macular area, but in many cases it skirts the edge of the foveola, leaving the patient with good acuity. Although there is a great tendency for the lesions to be contiguous, noncontiguous lesions occur commonly. Some patients will show centripetal spread of the disease.[109] There is some tendency for concentric enlargement of the jigsaw-puzzle zones of chorioretinal atrophy to occur over a period of months or years. An important cause of late loss of central vision is the development of choroidal neovascularization at the edge of an old area of chorioretinal atrophy (Figure 11.11A and B).[98–101,104,105,110–112] This occurs in as many as 25% of these patients. Care must be used to avoid mistaking the gray exudation associated with subretinal neovascularization for that caused by a recurrence of an active inflammatory lesion. Likewise, it is important not to mistake a gray active lesion for a subretinal new-vessel membrane. Fluorescein angiography is helpful in this regard.

11.09 Serpiginous choroiditis – response to treatment.

This 48-year-old woman was seen for mild visual disturbance in her left eye of 4 weeks' duration associated with nasal stuffiness and congestion in 2003. Her visual acuity was 20/20 in each eye, the lesions were inactive (A and B) and a diagnosis of possible atypical acute posterior multifocal placoid pigment epitheliopathy was made. She returned in 2007 with changes in her vision and new scotoma in her left eye. The right eye remained unchanged, while the left eye had developed several new lesions with active outer edges (C). The active edges were hypofluorescent early and became hyperfluorescent in the late stage on the angiogram typical of serpiginous choroidopathy (D and E). Viral titers for varicella-zoster virus were drawn and she was started on oral prednisone 60 mg a day. By 9 days the lesions were less active (F), the viral titers returned low and she was continued on oral steroid that was tapered over 4 months. While she was on 10 mg prednisone, 3 months later she developed new activity at the nonfoveal edges (G). Prednisone was increased to 40 mg and oral methotrexate 15 mg/week was started. She responded with no further recurrences, steroids were tapered off in 4 months, and she remained on methotrexate for 16 months when it was tapered off. The left eye 2 years later shows inactive scars with geographic edges (H); most atrophic areas show decreased autofluorescence with increased autofluorescence in the healthy adjacent retinal pigment epithelium (I).

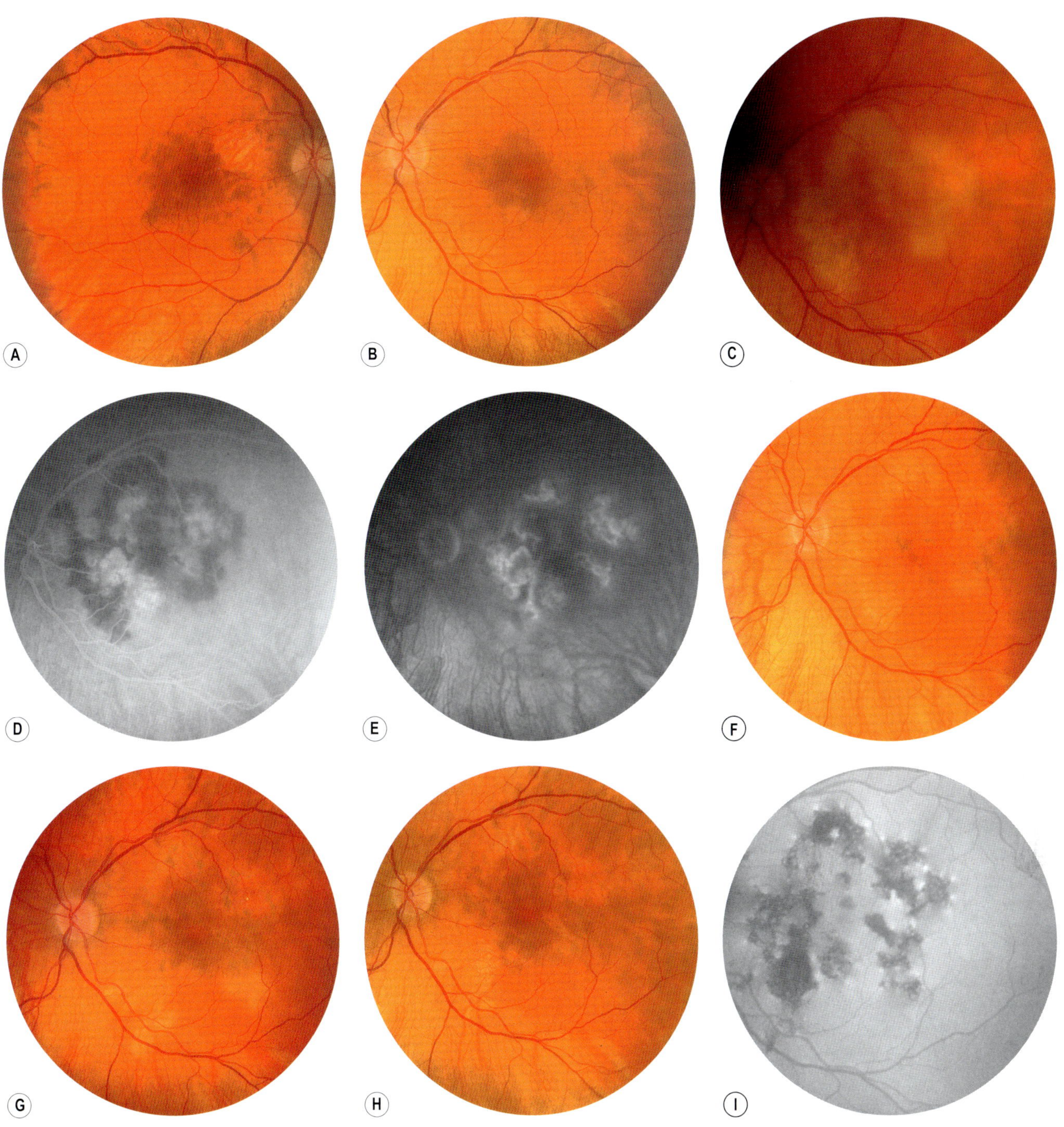
A
B
C
D
E
F
G
H
I

Unusual findings in patients with serpiginous choroiditis include focal retinal phlebitis, branch vein occlusion (Figure 11.10),[98,107,110,113] optic disc neovascularization,[112] retinal neovascularization (Figure 11.10D–K), and a striking predilection in a few patients for the choroidal lesions to correspond with the distribution of the major retinal veins. One or more sites of focal gray retinitis and overlying periphlebitis may be present (Figure 11.10). These foci may be associated with evidence of branch venous obstruction locally or elsewhere in the same or opposite eye (Figure 11.10E–L). Gass has seen one patient who because of widespread venous obstruction developed a picture of Eales' disease with extensive zones of retinal capillary nonperfusion, retinitis proliferans, and vitreous hemorrhage requiring pars plana vitrectomy bilaterally (Figure 11.10G–L). Although there is a strong predilection for this disease to affect the juxtapapillary choroid early in the course of the disease, in some cases this area is spared until later.

11.10 Atypical presentations of serpiginous choroiditis.

A–C: Active retinitis and periphlebitis and focal area of retinitis proliferans (arrows, B and C) at the margin of old area of branch retinal vein occlusion in patient with serpiginous choroiditis.

D–F: Bilateral multiple branch retinal vein occlusions in a 20-year-old black man with acute loss of vision in both eyes caused by active serpiginous choroiditis (D and E). Six years later the patient had severe bilateral loss of central and peripheral vision. Note the extensive scarring (F).

G–L: A healthy 23-year-old man presented with floaters in both eyes associated with bilateral scattered active serpiginous choroiditis lesions, overlying and widely scattered areas of retinal phlebitis (G, arrows), areas of peripheral capillary nonperfusion (J and K), retinitis proliferans (arrows, I–K), and vitreous hemorrhage (H). Bilateral panretinal photocoagulation and pars plana vitrectomy in the left eye were required to control the proliferative retinopathy. Five years after his presentation his visual acuity was 20/15 in both eyes (L).

Fluorescein Angiography

The acute gray-white lesions appear nonfluorescent during the early phases of angiography, and later they show evidence of staining that usually begins at the margin of the lesion and spreads centrally (Figure 11.08C and D).

The subacute and chronic lesions show angiographic evidence of destruction of the choriocapillaris and RPE. Failure of the atrophic areas to fluoresce during the early stages of angiography is indicative of choriocapillary atrophy. As fluorescein diffuses from the neighboring choriocapillaris, the atrophic lesions show progressive staining from the margins centrally. When focal areas of retinal phlebitis are present, angiography shows evidence of staining of the vein wall and may show evidence of branch vein occlusion peripheral to the area of phlebitis (Figure 11.10E).[110] Angiography is useful in detecting and localizing areas of choroidal as well as retinal neovascularization (Figures 11.10 and 11.11B). ICG angiography shows dark areas that correspond to the visible chorioretinal lesions, and sometimes larger than them. The hypofluorescence persists even after the acute lesions involute, suggesting continued activity in the choroid or persistent cellular infiltrate that blocks ICG fluorescence.[114] The acute lesion is hypoautofluorescent with a hyperautofluorescent edge, the subacute lesion becomes hyperautofluorescent and the inactive atrophic lesion shows hypoautofluorescence.[115] OCT in the subacute and inactive stage shows thinning of the outer retina and increased backscattering from the choroidal layers.[115] The electro-oculogram and ERG are usually normal.

Differential Diagnosis

When serpiginous choroiditis is advanced in both eyes, it has been mistaken for various dystrophies affecting the choroid, RPE, and retina.[99,101] The history of episodic and permanent loss of segments of the paracentral visual field, the lack of family history, the jigsaw-puzzle pattern of chorioretinal atrophy, the asymmetry of the disease, and the frequent presence of marginal gray-white edges of activity of the more peripherally located lesions are clues to the true nature of the disease. The color and early-phase angiographic appearance of the acute lesions resemble those seen in APMPPE. In this latter disease, however, the shape of the lesions is more likely to be round or oval, their distribution is more likely to be randomly scattered in the posterior fundus, they resolve usually within 7–14 days, and they leave minimal evidence of choroidal atrophy or loss of visual function. Table 11.1 summarizes the differences between these two diseases. Relentless placoid choroidopathy is the disease that closely resembles serpiginous choroiditis given that recurrences are its feature. Serpiginous choroiditis may simulate any of the diseases causing peripapillary chorioretinal scarring and neovascularization, for example, POHS, age related macular degeneration, angioid streaks, drusen of the optic nerve head, and idiopathic choroidal neovascularization. Clinical and angiographic evidence of juxtapapillary subretinal neovascularization is less likely to be present in patients with serpiginous choroiditis. On the other hand, patients with only minimal peripapillary scarring caused by serpiginous choroiditis may be seen initially with macular detachment caused by juxtapapillary subretinal neovascularization before developing any signs of the typical jigsaw pattern of choroidal involvement.

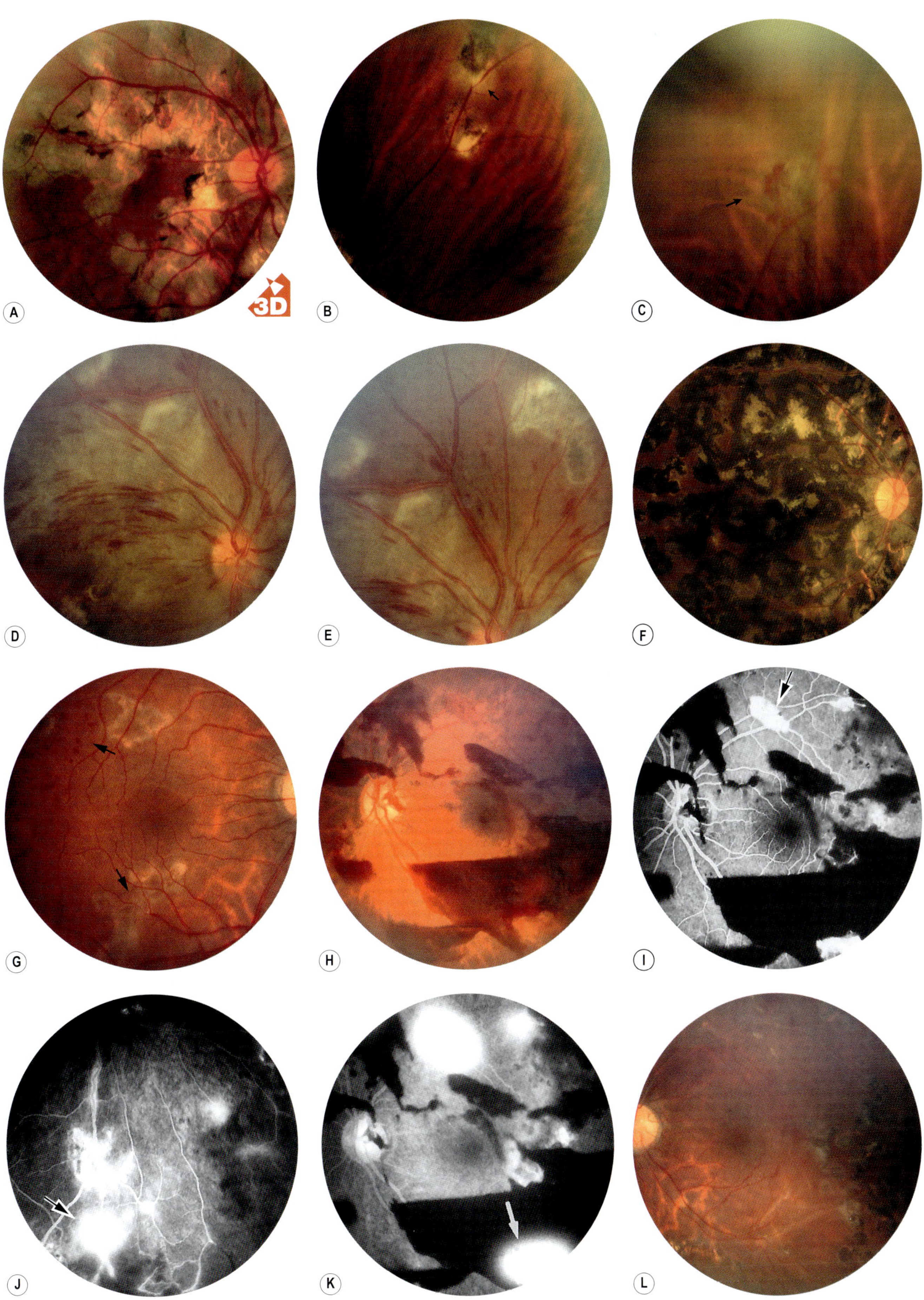
3D
A
B
C
D
E
F
G
H
I
J
K
L

An acute lesion in the paracentral region, particularly in a patient with inactive lesions elsewhere (Figure 11.08A and B), may be mistaken biomicroscopically and angiographically for exudation overlying a CNVM. Likewise, a gray plaque of subretinal exudation caused by subretinal neovascularization may be mistaken for recurrence of the choroiditis. The disease that closely resembles serpiginous choroiditis in its initial presentation and subsequent course is tubercular serpignous like choroiditis (see Chapter 10). When patients with a clinical picture of serpiginous choroiditis do not respond promptly to oral steroids or continue to develop new lesions while on adequate doses of steroids, and if they are from high prevalent countries such as India, tubercular serpignous should be suspected. An exaggerated response to tuberculin skin test, with or without evidence of systemic tuberculosis, calls for a prompt establishment of tissue diagnosis of TB with PCR of the vitreous fluid or needle biopsy of a choroidal lesion.

Pathogenesis and Etiology

The histopathologic findings in 2 patients suggest that serpiginous choroiditis is primarily a nongranulomatous choroiditis (Figure 11.11G and H).[100,101,110] There is no clue, however, as to its cause. There is minimal evidence that it is part of a systemic disease.[116,117] Figure 11.08 (K and L) demonstrates typical serpiginous chorioiditis that developed bilaterally in a patient associated with herpes zoster ophthalmicus. King et al. found elevated factor VIII–von Willebrand factor antigen in 8 patients with serpiginous choroiditis and concluded that occlusive choroidal vascular disease may be important in its pathogenesis.[117] Broekhuyse et al. found immune reactivity to retinal S-antigen in patients with serpiginous choroiditis but not in patients with APMPPE.[118] Serpiginous-like choroidopathy is a common manifestation of tubercular choroiditis.[119] Given the various infectious or noninfectious association, it is likely that serpignous choroiditis is a common morphological manifestation to several antigenic stimulation. Though worldwide in distribution, the disorder is more common in India.

Treatment

Systemic corticosteroids have proved moderately effective in serpiginous choroiditis. Their use in those patients with active lesions threatening the center of the macula is advisable.[103] The value of other agents, such as chlorambucil, cyclosporine A, azathioprine, methotrexate or a combination of these agents, is unpredictable.[120–122] Because of the possibility of a viral etiology, Gass treated one patient with acute loss of central vision in his second eye with a combination of oral acyclovir and prednisone for 6 weeks. The results of treatment in this patient and four others with acute serpiginous choroiditis at the Bascom Palmer Eye Institute suggest that acyclovir may be of some benefit in preserving vision (Figure 11.11J and K). Despite the fact that these patients regained excellent visual acuity after treatment, one of the patients continued to develop new active choroidal lesions peripherally while receiving the combined treatment. The jury is still out on the benefits of acyclovir. Oral steroid as the initial treatment with addition of immunosuppressives if the patient has recurrences is probably the best strategy at the present time.[123–126] Photocoagulation for active choroidal neovascularization that does not extend inside the capillary-free zone is of value. Intravitreal bevacizumab is useful in those cases threatening the fovea.

Prognosis

Good statistics concerning long-term follow-up of this disorder are not available. Generally it is a chronic, recurrent ocular disease that over a period of many years may cause severe visual loss in some patients. Many patients, however, maintain good central and peripheral function in at least one eye.

11.11 Serpiginous choroiditis causing choroidal neovascularization.

A and **B:** Note the subretinal blood (arrow, A) caused by a choroidal neovascular membrane (arrow, B).
C–H: A 17-year-old boy during a period of 3.5 years developed progressive loss of central and paracentral vision in both eyes secondary to a serpiginous pattern of spread of choroiditis. Juxtapapillary subretinal scarring was present in the left eye in August 1964 (C). By January 1965 the lesion had extended and was associated with subretinal neovascularization and blood (D). By November 1967 the disease had progressed into the macular area (E) as well as into the peripheral fundus. Note the subretinal scarring (arrow, E). Between 1963 and 1967 a similar pattern of progressive subretinal choroiditis and scarring occurred in the right eye. Note the tongue of subretinal fibrovascular tissue (arrow) extending into the right macula (F and G). The patient was killed in a motorcycle accident soon after the photographs in E and G. Histopathologic examination of the right macula (H) revealed extensive infiltration of the choroid with lymphocytes underlying a double layer of retinal pigment epithelium and a thick layer of fibrovascular tissue (type II subretinal neovascularization). No organisms were demonstrated by either light or electron microscopy.

Treatment of serpiginous choroiditis with prednisone and acyclovir.

I–K: A 34-year-old woman from India with a 2-year history of widespread serpiginous choroiditis and poor vision of 2 years' duration in the right eye presented because of acute visual loss in the left eye. She was taking prednisone, 80 mg daily, by mouth. Active chorioretinal lesions had extended into the macula of the left eye (I and J). Her visual acuity was 20/60. Acyclovir, 4 g daily, was added to the prednisone. Two weeks later the acuity declined to 20/100 but thereafter improved within 3 months to 20/20 in spite of the presence of subfoveal pigmentary scarring (K).

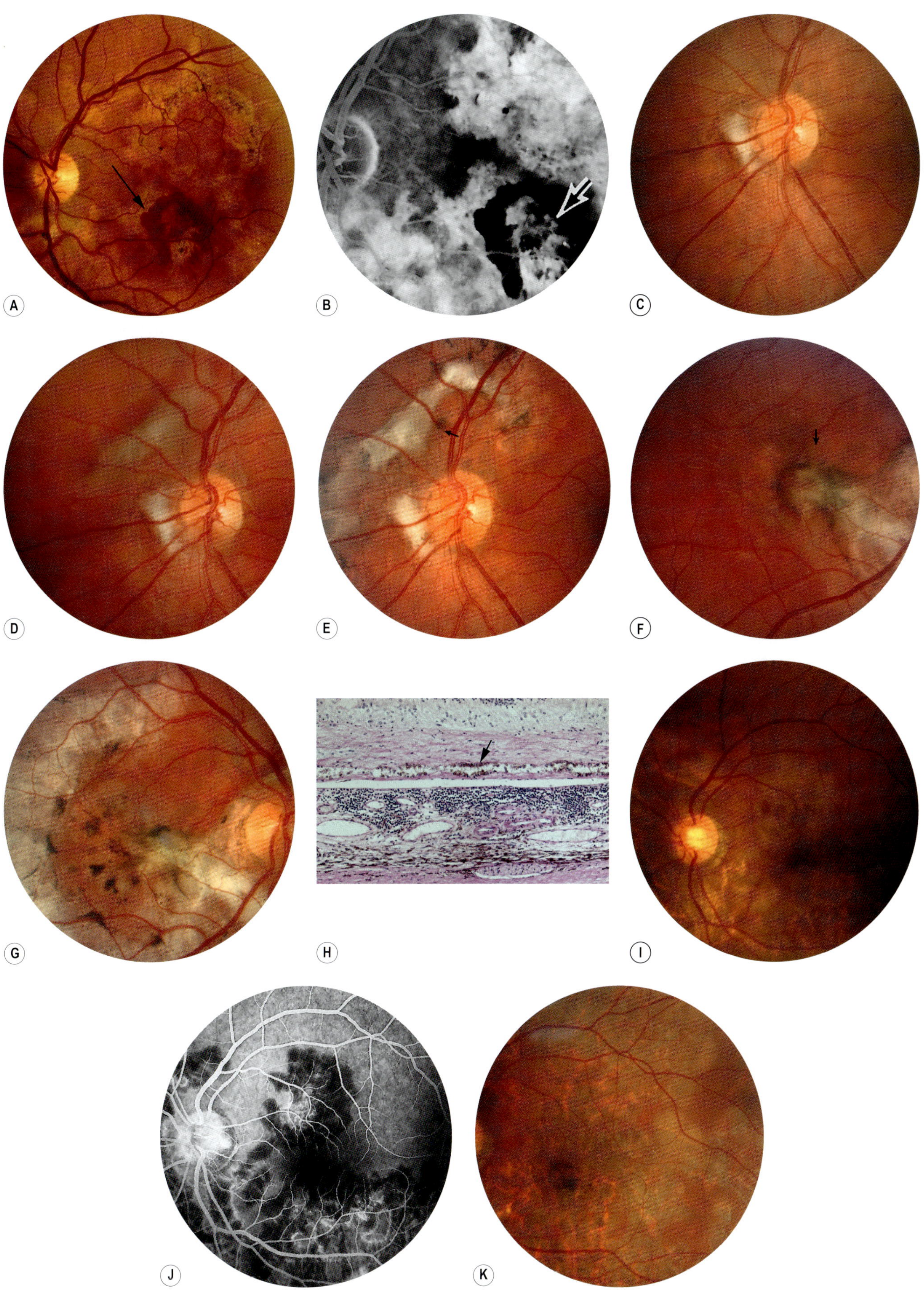
A
B
C
D
E
F
G
H
I
J
K

ACUTE IDIOPATHIC MACULOPATHY

Yannuzzi and coworkers reported 9 patients who after a flulike illness developed sudden severe unilateral central visual loss associated with vitreous cells; neurosensory macular detachment; retinal hemorrhages; an irregular white, gray, or yellow thickening of the RPE that was consistent with a subretinal infiltrate beneath a portion of the retinal detachment; and a neovascular process or acute swelling of the RPE cells (Figure 11.12).[127] A peculiar pseudopodal extension of the subretinal exudation and subretinal hemorrhages were present in some cases (Figure 11.12A). Irregular staining of the subretinal thickening angiographically simulated that occurring with subretinal neovascularization (Figure 11.12C). Complete staining occurred in late pictures. In spite of the appearance, the subretinal exudate disappeared and visual acuity returned to nearly normal. A characteristic "bull's-eye" pattern of pigment epithelial atrophy in the macula persisted (Figure 11.12L). No patient had a recurrence. One patient had late development of subretinal neovascularization. Fish and coworkers presented a similar case that in addition showed evidence of a pseudohypopyon in the macula during the acute phase of the disease.[128] Yannuzzi's group broadened the spectrum of this disorder to include eccentric macular lesions, subretinal exudate, fellow eye involvement, papillitis, and an association of the disorder with pregnancy and acquired immunodeficiency syndrome (AIDS).[129]

In 2004, Beck et al. reported 2 patients with acute idiopathic maculopathy following hand, foot, and mouth disease with the characteristic sore throat, fever, and erythematosus papules on the palms of hands, caused by coxsackievirus.[130] They demonstrated elevated acute and convalescent A16 and B6 titers for the virus. Both patients' children were also diagnosed with hand, foot, and mouth disease. Multifocal ERG shows transient outer retinal dysfunction that recovers over time.[131] Other rare associations have been a macular hole, recurrence at the same site, and transient electro-oculogram impairment.[132–134] ICG may show involvement of the inner choroid, likely from contiguous spread of pathology.[135] Spectral domain OCT shows thickening of the RPE and photoreceptor layers in the acute phase (Figure 11.12D) and restoration of most of the photoreceptors late (Figure 11.12F). The central part of the lesion is hyperautofluorescent and the outer ring hypoautofluorescent, corresponding to the bull's-eye pattern. No specific treatment has been attempted as most cases have shown improvement in vision, including the eye with two recurrences.[132]

11.12 Acute idiopathic maculopathy.

A–G: This 31-year-old woman had a sudden painless decline in vision to 6/200 in her left eye. Vision in the right eye was 20/20. Right fundus was normal. A solitary distinct flat yellow placoid lesion was seen in the macula with a few flecks of retinal hemorrhage (A). Angiogram showed brilliant staining of the retinal pigment epithelium (B and C). Optical coherence tomography (OCT) revealed thickening and disturbance in the photoreceptor layer (D). By history she had lesions in her mouth and her coxsackie titers returned elevated. Rapid plasma reagin was negative. Her vision began to improve after 3 weeks of onset, the OCT showed gradual recovery of photoreceptors at 5 and 9 weeks (E and F), and final vision improved to 20/25 by 10 weeks. Faint pigmentary changes remained in the macula (G).

H–J: A 28 year old Hispanic male had an acute drop of vision in his left eye to 20/400 over 5 days. A solitary yellow gray placoid lesion with minimal overlying subretinal fluid (H) that stained late on the angiogram was seen (I and J). He recalled having a sore throat 1 week prior and was told by his PCP that he had contracted 'hand, foot and mouth ' disease from his children. A week later his vision had improved spontaneously to 20/40 and by 3 weeks to 20/20 with minimal pigmentation.

K and L: This 21-year-old woman complained of acute loss of vision in the right eye upon awakening. She noticed an initial bright light in the center of her vision that progressed to a black central scotoma over the next few days. This was preceded by a upper respiratory infection, high fever, and headache 1 week prior. Past medical history was unremarkable. She was a smoker. Visual acuity was 20/150 in the right eye and 20/20 in the left eye. Color vision was 5 out of 14 on the right and 14 out of 14 on the left. Amsler grid showed a large central scotoma. A ring-shaped yellow-white lesion was present in the fovea. Fluorescein angiogram showed a window defect corresponding to the lesion and late staining. Visual acuity at 3 weeks remained at 20/150. At 11 weeks, the vision had improved spontaneously to 20/30.

(A–G, courtesy of Dr. Kaushik Hazariwala; H to J, courtesy of Dr. Mark Daily; K and L, courtesy of Dr. Calvin Mein.)

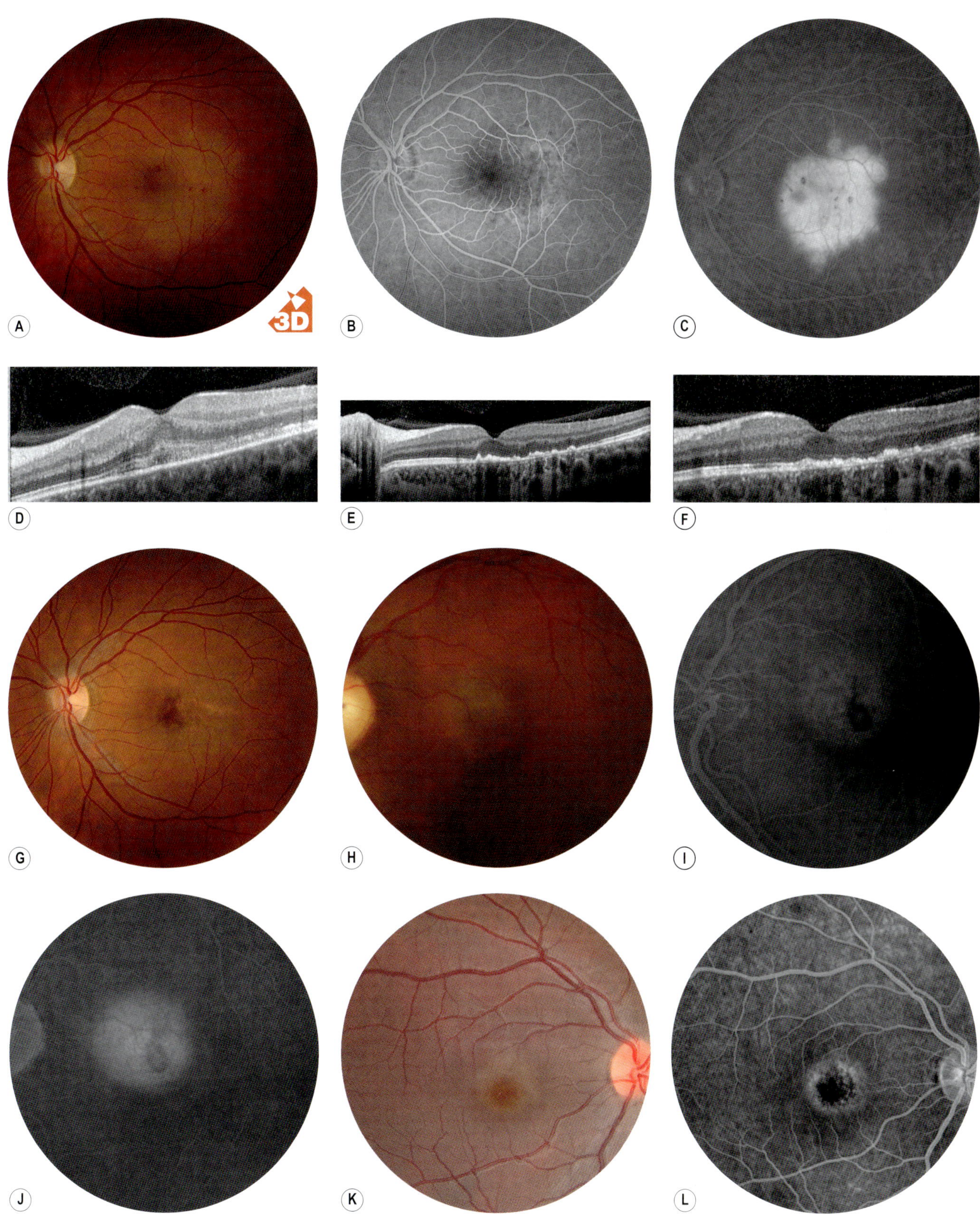
A
3D
B
C
D
E
F
G
H
I
J
K
L

ACUTE RETINAL PIGMENT EPITHELIITIS

Krill and Deutman[138] described the syndrome of acute retinal pigment epitheliitis, which is characterized by the rapid onset of visual disturbances in one or both eyes of young adults followed by gradual and almost complete recovery in 7–10 weeks.[139–142] One to 2 weeks after the onset of symptoms, these patients had multiple clusters of discrete, round, dark spots surrounded by depigmented halolike zones present at the level of the RPE in the macula and paramacular area (Figure 11.14E). These were usually one-fourth disc diameter in size. The fundus findings during the first week after the onset of symptoms were not described. Fluorescein angiography demonstrates a halo of hyperfluorescence surrounding the dark spot seen ophthalmoscopically (Figure 11.14B, C, and L). In some cases, angiography may be essentially normal. The loss of visual function is out of proportion to the changes seen in the macula. After recovery of central vision the RPE changes may be barely visible. The cause of this self-limited disorder is unknown.

Since the original description by Deutman and colleagues, few reports of this condition surfaced till 2007.[143,144] Chittum and Kalina reported 8 patients with acute retinal pigment epitheliitis associated with a fine pattern of pigment stippling confined largely to the foveolar area.[139] It was mostly believed to be a nonspecific finding secondary to a variety of circumstances, including idiopathic central serous chorioretinopathy, drusen, adult-onset vitelliform foveomacular (pattern) dystrophy, and occult choroidal neovascularization, and in asymptomatic patients.

Since the availability of OCT, case reports of acute retinal pigment epitheliitis have re-emerged.[145–147] OCT shows hyperreflectivity at the level of the outer nuclear layer, photoreceptors, and RPE (Figure 11.14D and G). The disease is self-limited with near-complete visual recovery in 10–12 weeks (Figure 11.14I).

11.14 Acute retinal pigment epitheliitis.

A–I: This is a 20-year-old woman with a paracentral "gray spot" in her right eye without associated pain, redness, or photopsia. She had had a diarrheal illness and flu 3 weeks previously and had returned from South America and Peru 6 months before. Her vision was 20/25– on the right and 20/20 on the left. There was a 500-μm-size yellow lesion superior to fixation with indistinct margins (A) that was hyperfluorescent early and the surrounding retina stained late (B and C). Optical coherence tomography revealed mild changes in the photoreceptor layer (D). A week later her vision dropped to 20/70 and the lesion became more distinct (E). Angiogram showed it was made up of several small dots, with disruption and possible inflammation in the photoreceptor and retinal pigment epithelial layers (F and G). Viral titers for coxsackie A and B, hepatitis, dengue, and rapid plasma reagin were negative. A diagnosis of acute retinal pigment epitheliitis was made and she elected to be treated with oral prednisone 60 mg/day, tapered over 2.5 weeks. Her vision improved to 20/25 3 weeks post prednisone therapy; the lesion became smaller and inactive (H) with restoration of most of the photoreceptor layer (I).

J and K: This 25-year-old woman noted photopsia, blurred vision, and multiple paracentral scotomata in the right eye 12 days before her examination at the Bascom Palmer Eye Institute. When examined by her local physician several days after the onset her acuity was 20/20 and the fundus was described as normal. One week later her acuity was 20/30 and some "yellow material was noted in the right macula." At the Bascom Palmer Eye Institute her acuity was 20/25. Multiple paracentral scotomata were demonstrable on the Amsler grid in the right eye. There were no vitreous cells. There were multiple, small, pigmented lesions surrounded by depigmented halos at the level of the RPE (arrow, J). The left fundus was normal. Angiography revealed small halos of hyperfluorescence corresponding with the lesions (arrows, K). She was last seen by her local physician 8 months after the onset of symptoms. Visual acuity was 20/20, and the fundus was normal.

(A–I, courtesy of Dr. Mark Johnson.)

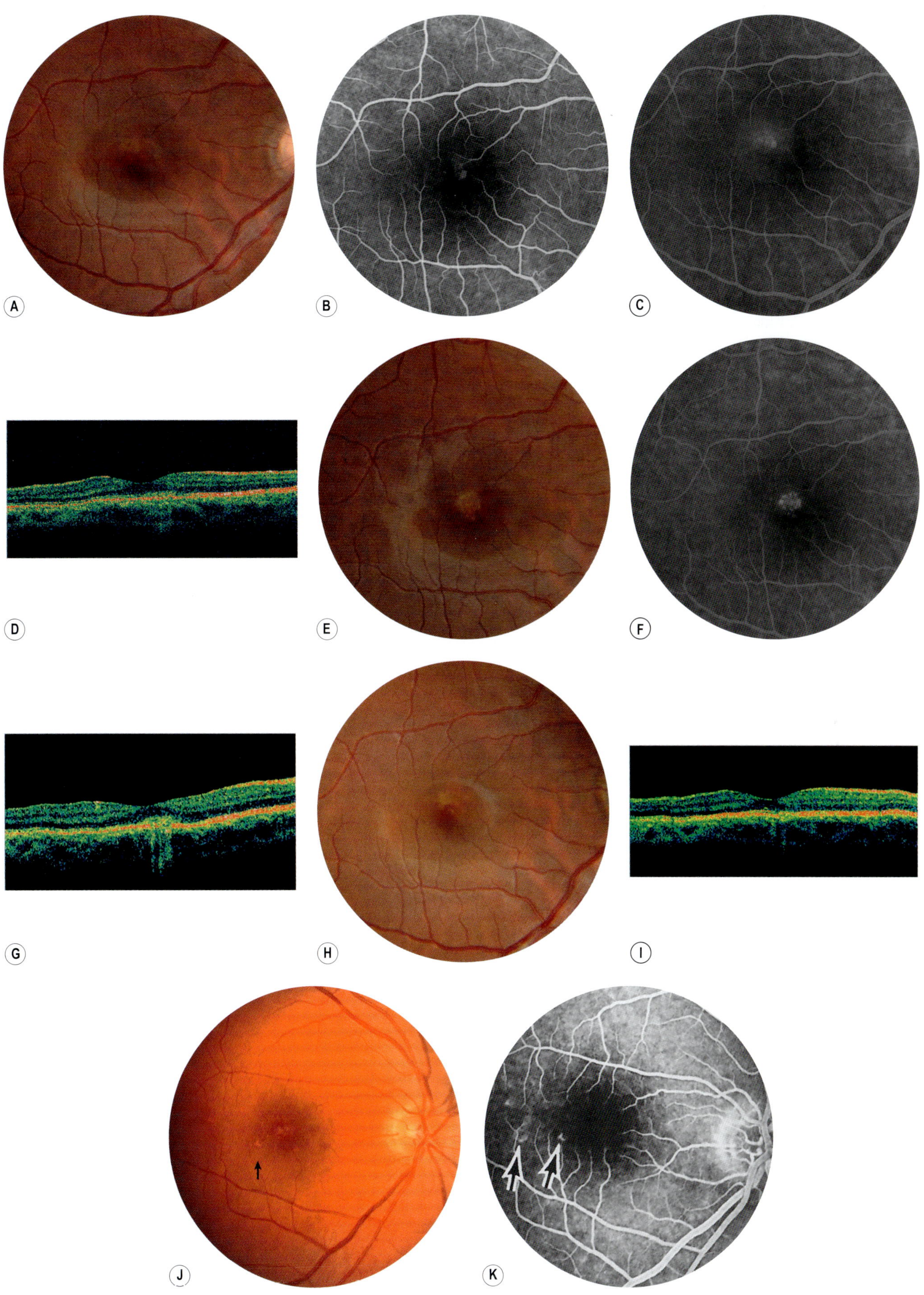
A
B
C
D
E
F
G
H
I
J
K

MULTIPLE EVANESCENT WHITE-DOT SYNDROME

The following features characterize MEWDS, which typically affects one eye of young females: (1) blurred vision, multiple paracentral scotomata, usually including a temporal scotoma, and photopsia occurring in approximately one-half of patients soon after a flulike illness; (2) vitreous cells; (3) multiple small, often poorly defined, gray-white patches at the level of the RPE and outer retina (Figures 11.15 and 11.16); (4) a cluster of tiny white or light-orange dots in the foveola (Figure 11.15A); (5) early punctate hyperfluorescence of the gray-white patches, which often show a cluster or wreath-shaped pattern (Figure 11.15G and H); (6) late fluorescein staining of these lesions, and in some cases staining of the optic nerve head; (7) blind-spot enlargement; (8) decrease in the ERG a-wave and early receptor potential amplitudes; and (9) spontaneous recovery of visual function, normalization of the electroretinographic findings, and return of the ophthalmoscopic and angiographic findings toward normal in 7–10 weeks (Figure 11.16G–I).[148–165] The white spots in MEWDS, which are often small, ill defined, and located in the extramacular area, are easily overlooked. It is probable that most patients reported as having the acute idiopathic blind-spot enlargement syndrome[166] probably had MEWDS, and that the white lesions were either overlooked or had faded at the time of their examination.[167–172]

11.15 Multiple evanescent white-dot syndrome (MEWDS).

A 34-year-old moderately myopic woman noted several small blind spots in her right central field associated with photopsias of 5 days' duration. Her vision was 20/40 on the right and 20/20 on the left. Several gray spots were seen scattered in the right fundus (A–D) and orange dots in the fovea (A). Autofluorescence imaging showed hypoautofluorescence corresponding to the lesions (E), optical coherence tomography showed loss of photoreceptors in the affected gray spots (F). An enlarged blind spot was found on Humphrey field testing. Fluorescein angiography showed ring of hyperfluorescent dots consistent with "wreathlike" spots. A diagnosis of MEWDS was made and she was kept under observation. By 3 weeks her vision had improved to 20/20, the photopsias had resolved and most of the gray spots had disappeared, orange dots were still present. The lesion inferior to fovea appeared to be whiter and inactive. She moved to Seattle and called 3 years later complaining of new metamorphopsia superior to fixation. She had developed a choroidal neovascular membrane at the site of the persistent scar (arrow A) and received intravitreal antivascular endothelial growth factor injections.

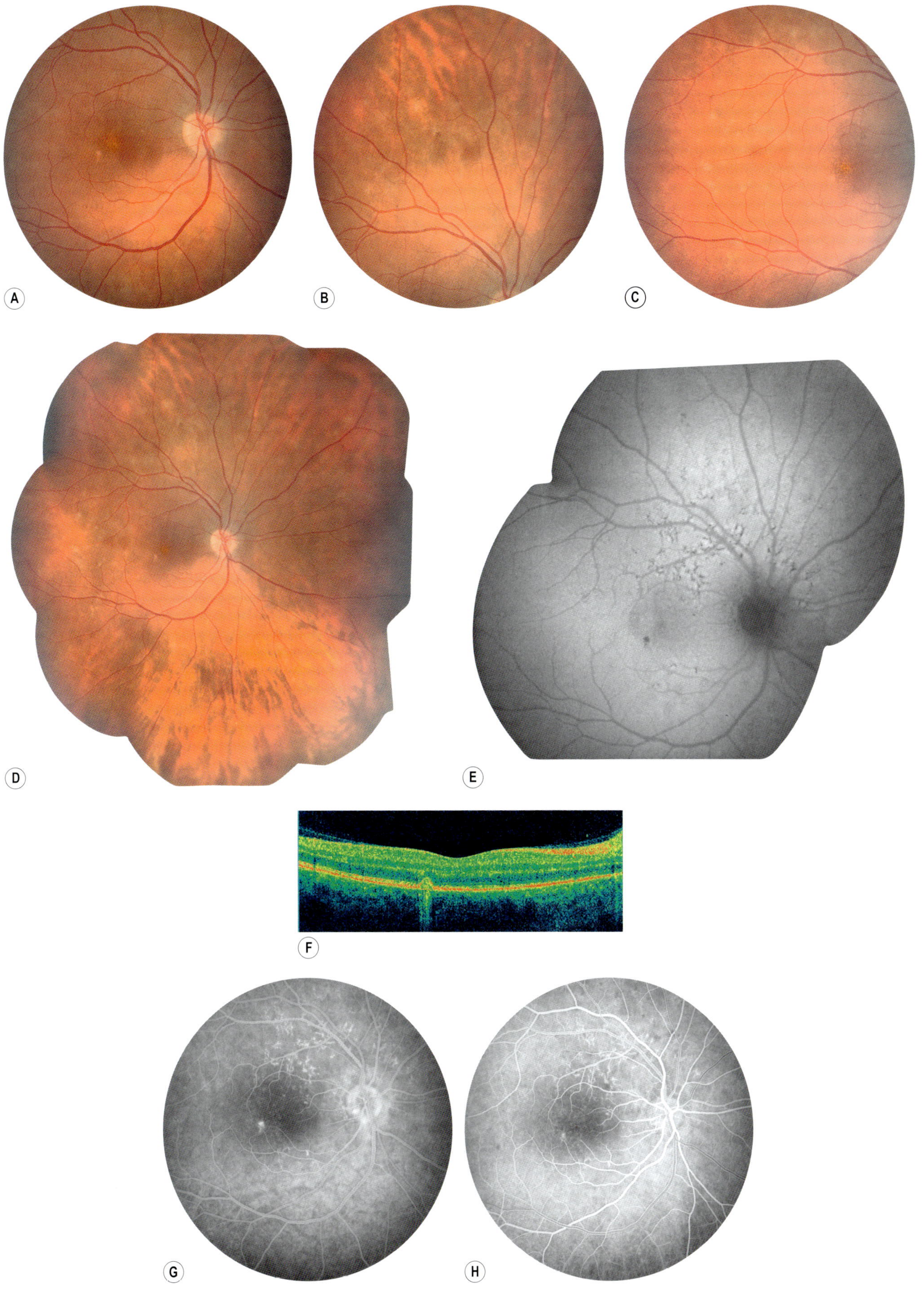
A
B
C
D
E
F
G
H

ICG angiography demonstrates patchy hyperfluorescence at the level of the RPE as well as multiple, small, round, hypofluorescent lesions, some of which occur in the absence of fundus changes.[173] Although fluorescein angiography often shows some staining of the optic disc during the acute phases of the disease, there is minimal evidence that damage to the retinal ganglion cells and optic nerve is responsible for visual loss.[168] Later in the course of the disease a zone of RPE depigmentation and hyperfluorescence corresponding with their enlarged blind spot or other field defect may develop.[169,172] Subretinal neovascularization may occasionally occur.[174,175] Scanning laser densitometry demonstrates evidence of a focal defect in the visual pigment kinetics of the receptor cells in the macular area.[176,177] Evaluation for evidence of systemic disease is usually negative. Some visual field loss and color vision defect may persist.[178] The cause of the disease is unknown. Males may be affected, the disorder may occasionally affect both eyes, and late recurrences may occasionally occur.[153,159,161,179,180] In some cases the visual field defects do not resolve.[151]

Before or following MEWDS some patients develop evidence of pseudo-POHS, acute macular neuroretinopathy, and acute onset of large visual field defects unassociated with visible changes in the fundi.[170,174,181,182] There is evidence that MEWDS may be part of a spectrum of one disease or closely related diseases that include acute idiopathic blind-spot enlargement,[148,163,166,181,183,184] AZOOR (see discussion to follow), pseudo-POHS,[163,175,181,185–187] and acute macular neuroretinopathy.[163,170,188] All of the disorders affect predominantly young women and all may present with photopsia and zones of visual field loss caused by retinal receptor damage unexplained by biomicroscopic changes in the ocular fundi.[189]

11.16 Multiple evanescent white-dot syndrome.

This 24-year-old woman complained of temporal floaters and occasional flashes of light in her right eye of 5 days' duration. She had history of migraine. Her vision was 20/20 in each eye; no visual field defect could be demonstrated on formal testing. A few white spots in the macula, orange dots in the foveal center, and several spots in the midperiphery were seen (A, B, and G). Angiogram showed wreathlike hyperfluorescence of the macular lesions and hyperfluorescence of the extramacular lesions (C and D). On autofluorescence imaging the lesions were hypoautofluorescent (E and F). A week later some of the white lesions had disappeared (H) and by 3 months the fundus was back to normal without evidence of any lesion (I).

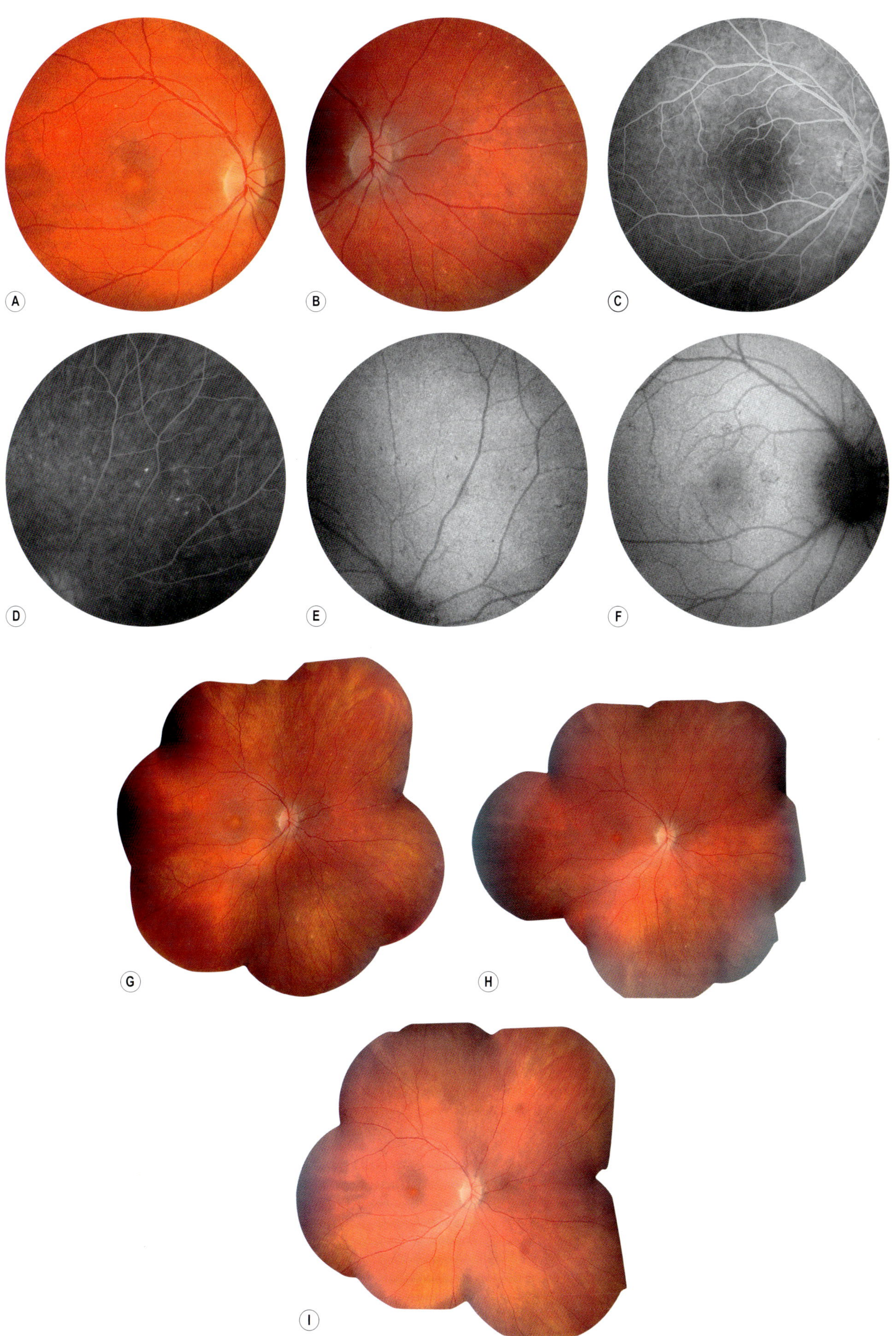
A
B
C
D
E
F
G
H
I

ACUTE ZONAL OCCULT OUTER RETINOPATHY

In 1994 Gass reported 13 patients, predominantly young women, with a syndrome characterized by rapid loss of one or more large zones of outer retinal function, photopsia, minimal fundoscopic changes, usually mild vitritis, and electroretinographic abnormalities affecting one or both eyes (Figure 11.17).[189] Progression of visual field loss occurred over a period of several weeks or months before either improving or stabilizing. Involvement of the second eye may be delayed for at least as long as 2 years (Figure 11.17A–I). All patients on follow-up examination had persistent visual field defects, and most had chronic photopsia and zones of pigment epithelial atrophy and retinal vascular narrowing, which in some cases mimicked that seen in retinitis pigmentosa and cancer-associated retinopathy (Figure 11.17J–L). In some patients large, permanent, visual field defects were unassociated with any visible changes in either the fundus or in fluorescein angiograms.

Most patients with AZOOR are young or middle-aged adults with the predominance of women, who present with an acute onset of visual field loss in one or both eyes. The fundus examination reveals no abnormalities at onset. More than 90% of patients have antecedent or associated photopsias, which are projected to the zone of visual deficit. The photopsias have been described variously as "fireworks, blinking lights, movement of microbes under a microscope, the TV screen being off signal, flashes of light, heat waves coming off the road, and other visual phenomena." A characteristic finding is the description of "movements" associated with these photopsias. Patients often move their fingers or hands while describing the symptom. Unlike in posterior vitreous separation, the photopsias are more noticeable in bright light and patients have been known to come into the doctor's office wearing sunglasses. The photopsias can predate, appear simultaneous, or antedate the field loss. Some patients may have had an antecedent viral illness. Those eyes with large areas of field loss, signifying involvement of a large zone of photoreceptors, may have vitreous cells. However, vitreous cells may be a later phenomenon, seen when photoreceptors die. The visual field defect is variable; it can be small or large, and often is connected to the blind spot. Sometimes the field loss is in the periphery.

The subtle nature of this presumed inflammatory disorder, which causes acute damage to broad zones of the outer retina without producing noticeable ophthalmoscopic changes, is responsible for the diagnostic confusion that usually results in extensive fruitless neurologic, medical, and ophthalmologic consultations and laboratory investigations. Demonstration of electroretinographic abnormalities during the early course of the disease is helpful in this regard. The ERGs in these patients show a pattern of visual dysfunction that is photoreceptor in origin, patchy in distribution, and asymmetric in the two eyes.[190] If the field loss is small and unilateral, the ERG in the affected eye may be reduced compared to the fellow normal eye. If the field loss is extensive the ERG is below normal in the affected eye(s). Either the rod or the cone function, or both, may be affected based on the location of the visual dysfunction. Bilateral involvement causes ERG depression in both eyes. Interocular asymmetry was a prominent feature in the 24 patients studied by Jacobson et al.[190] Multifocal ERG if available is useful in documenting the extent and location of the field loss and is diagnostic of the condition when associated with a normal fundus. However, since multifocal ERG tests cone function only, it will not be able to pick up subtle rod defects.

11.17 Acute zonal outer retinopathy, occult type.

A–C: This 24-year-old woman, while recovering from an upper respiratory infection, experienced rapid severe loss of vision overnight in both eyes. Visual acuity in the right eye was 20/200, left eye 20/20. She had severe constriction of the visual field bilaterally. Both fundi and angiograms appeared normal (A and B). Seven months later she had bilateral photopsia; persistent, severe visual field defects; narrowing of the retinal vessels; and widespread hypopigmentation of the retinal pigment epithelium (RPE) more pronounced anterior to the arcades (C). The visual field loss remained stable but she developed migration of pigment into the retina in a bone corpuscle pattern peripherally over the next year.

D–I: Over a period of several months this 36-year-old woman developed progressive loss of peripheral vision, photopsia, vitreous cells, narrowing of the retinal vessels, nonstaining cystoid macular edema (arrow, D), depigmentation of the RPE in the juxtapapillary area, and electroretinogram changes in the right eye (D and E). Visual field loss stabilized within 8 months. Twenty-six months after the onset of symptoms in the right eye she developed the same symptoms and signs in the left eye that previously was normal except for one focal scar (arrow, F). Compare F and G at the time of onset of symptoms in the left eye with H and I 1 year later, and note development of retinal vessel narrowing and depigmentation of the juxtapapillary RPE (arrowheads, I). The visual field stabilized in the left eye within 6 months. Both eyes have been unchanged for the past 3 years. Her visual acuity is 20/25 right eye and 20/20 left eye. She has mild macular edema bilaterally.

J–L: This 29-year-old woman noted the acute onset of photopsia and "shimmering heatwave" involving the superonasal field of the right eye. The fundi were normal. Medical and neurologic examinations were unremarkable. Her visual acuity was 20/20 in both eyes. Within 1 month she developed a zone of depigmentation and several foci of perivenous sheathing and staining (arrows, J and K) inferotemporally in the right eye. An electroretinogram showed subnormal rod and cone amplitudes in the right eye. The fundi and visual fields remained unchanged over the subsequent 6 years except for migration of pigment into the retina (L) in the right eye and the development of several foci of perivascular sheathing in the left eye nasally. She is still troubled by the photopsia.

(A–L from Gass.[189])

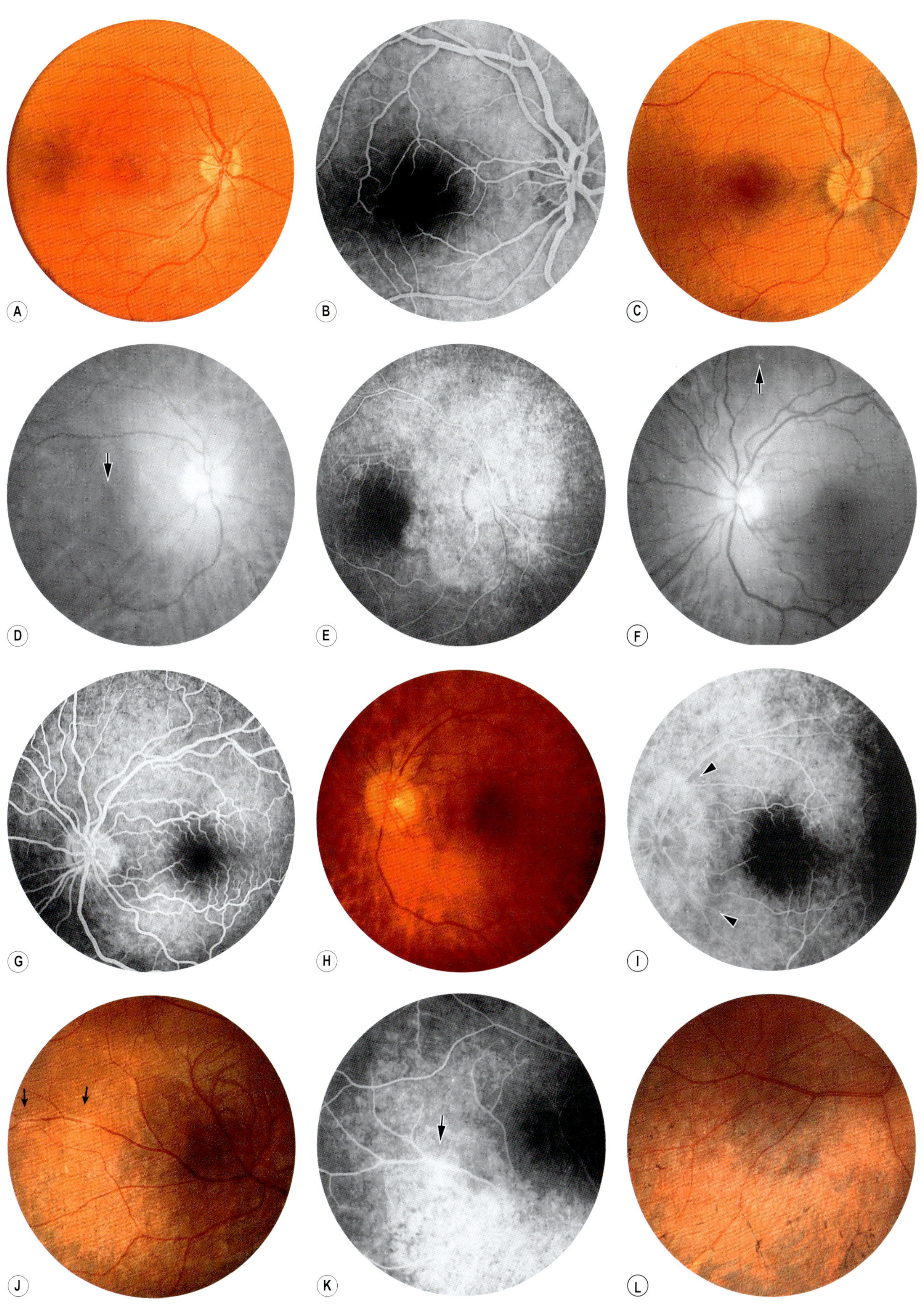
A
B
C
D
E
F
G
H
I
J
K
L

The field loss does not conform to the loss seen with glaucoma or a vascular defect. Goldmann visual field mapping is important in demonstrating the complete field deficit, often associated with an enlarged blind spot. Visual field defects stabilize within 6 months. A small percentage of patients show improvement in field defect if treated early with antivirals and systemic corticosteroids. Fluorescein angiography when the fundus shows no changes is normal (Figure 11.17A and B) and shows transmission hyperfluorescence in those areas of RPE change (Figure 11.17E, I, and K). Autofluorescence imaging of the normal fundus shows no abnormality; however, once RPE atrophy is seen, the areas appear hypoautofluorescent (Figure 11.18G), and occasionally show a rim of increased autofluorescence.[191]

The cause of the acute damage to sharply defined zones of the retinal receptor cells in the absence of visible fundus changes in patients with AZOOR is unknown. There is patchy evidence to date for autoantibodies to any retinal cell type in patients with AZOOR.[190,192] Gass postulated the possibility of an inciting viral or other infectious agent within the photoreceptors. He has hypothesized a "silent preclinical phase," where cell-to-cell spread of the virus occurs, with retention of normal photoreceptor function. In the "acute symptomatic phase," the infected cell dysfunction is triggered by the host immune response. Either a change in the antigenicity of the infective agent or a local auto-immune reaction to the receptors laden with this infective agent may cause loss of photoreceptor function.[2] The finding that over 90% of eyes with AZOOR have visual field defects that include one or both blind spots, and/or the peripheral isopters, suggests that the ora serrata and optic disc margin are possible sites for invasion of a virus into the receptor cells. These are two sites where the retinal receptors anatomically are not isolated from the systemic circulation by surrounding neuroepithelium. In approximately half the patients with AZOOR, the immune response to the intracellular virus results in inactivation of function but preservation of the receptor cell. No biomicroscopic or ophthalmoscopic evidence of inflammation of acute or long-term retinal cell damage is evident. In most cases the retinal cell dysfunction appears to be permanent. Although most instances of recovery occur during the first 6 months after onset of symptoms, at least 2 patients demonstrated improvement in the visual field after several years. Likewise, while stabilization of visual field loss typically occurs within 6 months of the onset of field loss, a few patients, particularly those who show evidence of some recovery early, may develop a gradual increase in visual field loss many months or years later. This delayed loss may occur as a result of resetting of the cells' apoptotic clock during the initial acute phase of AZOOR.

In the other half of patients with AZOOR, the immune response results in early receptor cell death, development of a variable degree of inflammation including vitreous cells, perivascular exudation, and occasionally optic disc edema. These inflammatory signs typically develop within several weeks following the onset of AZOOR, appear to be proportional to the size of the affected retinal zones, and probably result from an inflammatory response to the dead retinal receptor cells.[193]

Weeks or months later, narrowing of the retinal vessels, particularly the retinal arteries, perivascular sheathing, and reactive changes in the RPE occur (Figure 11.18A and F). The loss of interaction of the microvilli of the RPE with the photoreceptors causes migration of the RPE into the inner retina to line up along the blood vessel wall, giving the typical bone spicule appearance.

Similar acute occult zones of visual field loss that are accompanied by ERG changes may occur in patients with MEWDS,[181,189] MCP and punctate inner choroiditis (PIC), (pseudo-POHS),[163,181,182,189,194] and less often in patients with, or who previously had, acute macular neuroretinopathy.[163,170] The authors have seen at least 50 other patients with evidence of overlap between MEWDS, pseudo-POHS, AZOOR, and acute idiopathic blind-spot enlargement syndrome. Whereas occult visual field loss resulting from receptor cell damage is a common link among all these syndromes, we do not know the cause of any of these disorders or, to what degree they are related pathogenetically and etiologically.

11.18 Acute zonal occult outer retinopathy.

A-E: This 40-year-old woman presented with a history of rapidly progressive visual loss in her right eye over 1–2 years approximately 10 years prior, and a recent temporal blind spot associated with photopsias in her left eye. Her symptoms began with photopsias and rapid progressive loss of visual field in her right eye. When I first examined her, the vision in her right eye was hand motions to count fingers. The left eye was 20/20 with a large temporal blind spot. The fundus in the right eye showed widespread pigment alteration with diffusely narrowed retinal vessels, patchy bone spicules (A), while the left fundus was normal (B and C). Optical coherence tomography through the left macula revealed loss of photoreceptors in the peripapillary area (D and E arrow) in spite of a normal-appearing retina. Her electroretinogram showed a significant asymmetry with almost flat waves on the right. The left eye continued to have further field loss, though the fundus remained normal. She was started on oral steroids and valacyclovir for 6 weeks and this seemed to control further progression. However on discontinuation of steroids she felt subjective worsening of her field. She was started on methotrexate and mycophenolate mofetil, and is being monitored.

F to I: Late appearance of the right and left fundus and autofluorescence images of a 48-year-old woman with extensive bitemporal field defect that has remained stable over the past 10 years. Note the asymmetry between the nasal and temporal retina.

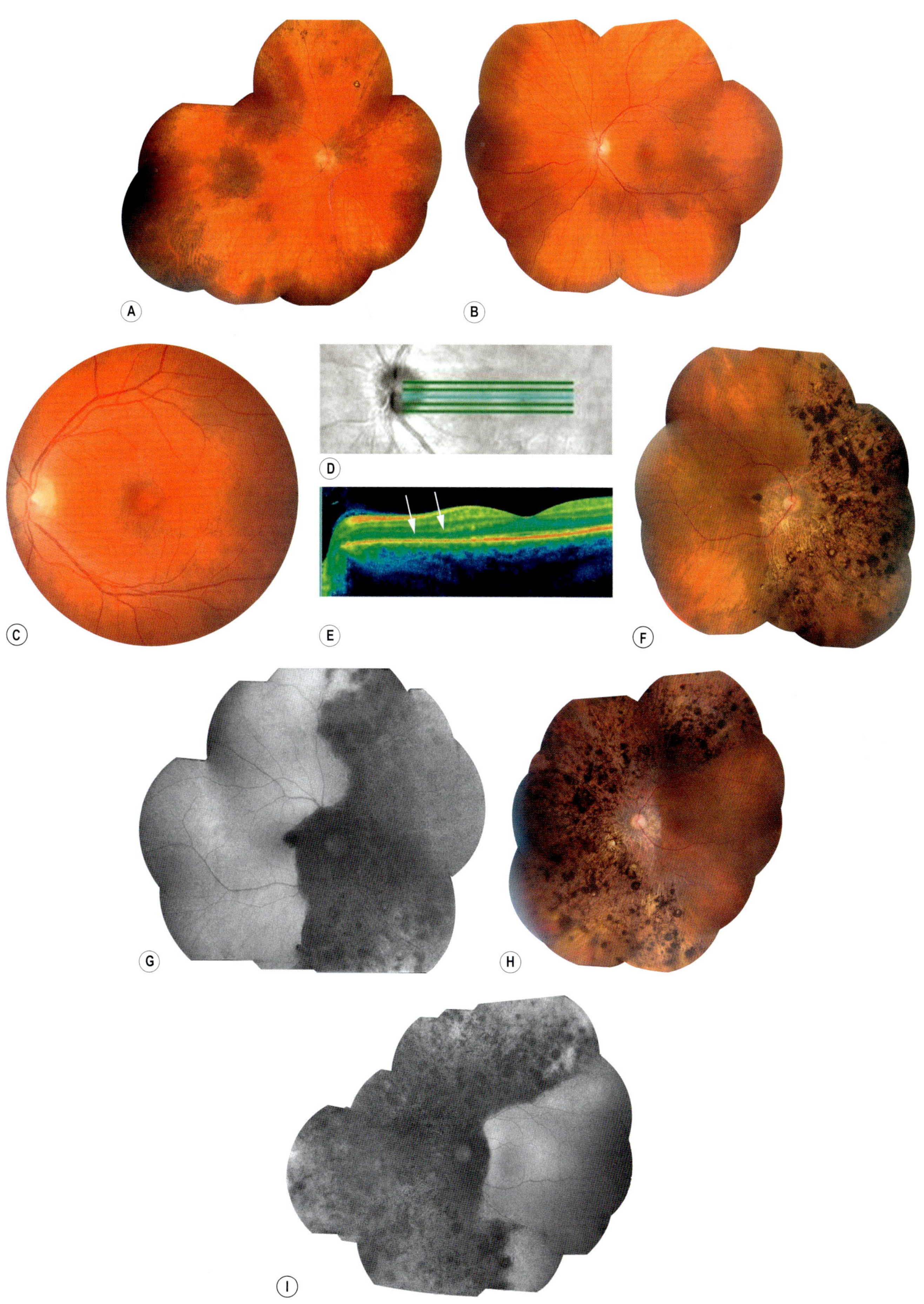
A
B
C
D
E
F
G
H
I

ACUTE ANNULAR OCCULT OUTER RETINOPATHY

In the third edition of this book the author presented the findings in an otherwise healthy young adult patient who presented with acute loss of a large zone of visual field associated with an unique fundoscopic picture consisting of a large-diameter, thin, gray-white ring occupying most of the superior temporal fundus of the left eye (Figure 11.19A–F).[195] Except for slight narrowing of the retinal arteries within this zone, the retina and pigment epithelium had a normal ophthalmoscopic and fluorescein angiographic appearance (Figure 11.19G). There were no vitreous cells. There was a left afferent pupillary defect. For a period of approximately 3 weeks the ring and absolute visual field defect enlarged before stabilizing (Figure 11.19C–F). The ring disappeared. The visual acuity was normal throughout the course. The absence of angiographic changes suggested that the occult destructive process was affecting primarily the inner retina within the area of the ring and the disorder was termed "acute progressive zonal inner retinitis and degeneration." During follow-up over the following months and years, however, the patient developed, within the zone of visual field loss, depigmentation and migration of pigment epithelium into the overlying retina in a bone-corpuscular pattern, indicating that the original damage had in fact involved primarily the outer retinal receptors (Figure 11.19H and I).[196] During the 6 years of follow-up his visual acuity has remained 20/20 and the visual field loss is unchanged. Of interest, he no longer has an afferent pupillary defect.

Luckie and coworkers reported a young woman with the identical findings and early clinical course in one eye.[197] She had serologic evidence of cytomegalovirus infection and they attributed her stabilization of field loss to treatment with acyclovir. The fact that their patient was immunocompetent suggests that her retinitis and clinical course may be unrelated to cytomegalovirus and her therapy.

Except for the presence of the gray ring and the absence of a history of photopsia during the acute phase of the disease, the findings and course of the disease in these 2 patients are the same as those with AZOOR.[198–200] The cause of the zones of acute occult outer retinal damage in both groups of patients is unknown. An attractive, yet unsubstantiated, explanation for the fundus changes is that of a latent viral infection of selective zones of the outer retina that is somehow triggered into activity, causing acute inactivation of function and in some cases death of the retinal receptors within those zones without affecting retinal transparency (except for the ring) and without affecting either the outer or the inner blood–retinal barrier to fluorescein during the acute phase of the disease. The evanescent ring of retinal opacity occurs at the interface of the affected and unaffected outer retina and probably at the level of the outer plexiform layer and receptor cell nuclear layer, where it causes no angiographic abnormality. The ring may be the result of loss of transparency of the most recently affected retina, similar to that which may be seen in immune-suppressed patients with cell-to-cell spread of cytomegalovirus retinopathy.[201] The ring may also be caused by a mild immune reaction taking place at the interface between the normal vascularized inner retina and the leading edge of the advancing infection in the outer avascularized retina, similar to that which may be observed in the cornea (Wesley ring). Neither explanation is completely satisfactory in view of the absence of detectable abnormality in either the inner or the outer blood–retinal barrier. Antiretinal antibodies to inner nuclear layer and ganglion cell layer, and in another case to outer nuclear layer additionally, suggests autoimmunity may play a role.[202] However, it is not known whether the antibodies are primarily involved, or develop as an epiphenomenon. The lesions appear nonfluorescent on ICG angiography once RPE changes have ensued.[203]

11.19 Acute zonal outer retinopathy, annular occult type.

A–I: A healthy 23-year-old man noticed the rapid onset of a large inferonasal scotoma in his left eye. His visual acuity was 20/20. When seen by his local ophthalmologist, the right eye was normal. The anterior chamber and vitreous were clear. In the left fundus there was a sharply defined, thin, gray, circular ring (arrows, A and B) occupying most of the superotemporal quadrant. The gray ring appeared to be within the retina but was external to the retinal vessels. It extended out to the equator but did not reach the ora serrata. The retina within the ring appeared normal. Visual field examination revealed a dense scotoma corresponding to the zone within the ring. Over the next week the scotoma progressively enlarged. When examined in Miami the gray ring was barely visible (arrows, C–E). The zone within the ring had enlarged (compare arrows, A and B, with C and D) but did not reach the center of the macula. The diagram (F) illustrates the change in size of the ring. The retinal vessels within this zone were narrowed, and the surface retinal reflexes were attenuated. The retinal pigment epithelium (RPE) was unaffected. Fluorescein angiography confirmed the attenuation of the retinal vessels and the normality of the RPE (G). Over the subsequent several weeks the scotoma enlarged slightly and then stabilized. Within several years he developed depigmentation of the RPE and migration of pigment into the retina within the zone of visual field loss (arrows, H and I). His visual acuity 6.5 years later was 20/20. The right eye was normal.

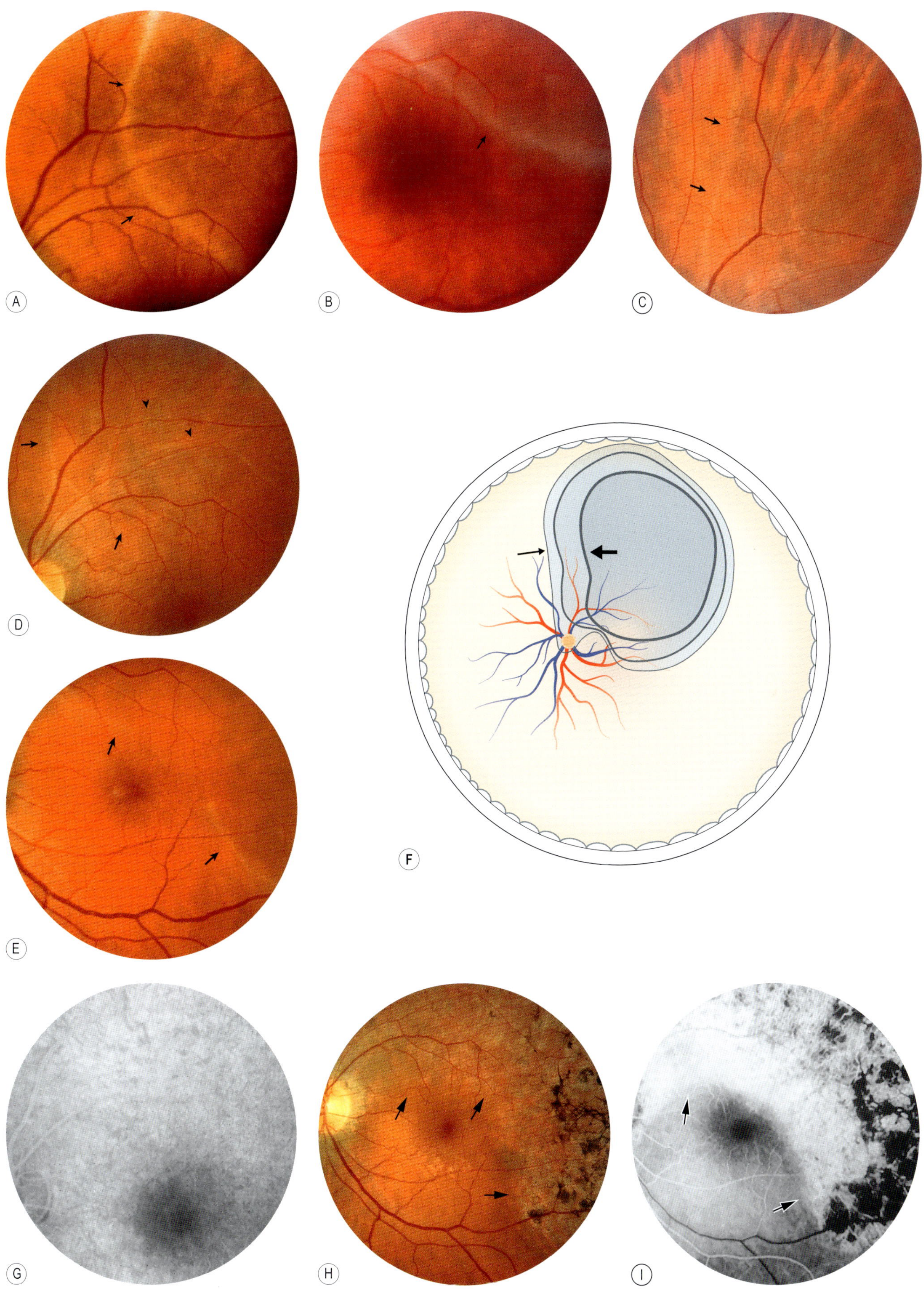
A
B
C
D
E
F
G
H
I

Figure 11.20 illustrates what may be a further variant of AZOOR (annular overt type) in which the affected zone is associated with acute disruption of the RPE and variable degree of whitening of the outer retina and RPE.

11.20 Acute zonal outer retinopathy, annular type.

A–E: This 50-year-old woman with chronic fatigue syndrome noted the sudden onset of a large nasal scotoma in the left eye. Visual acuity was 20/20, right eye and 20/400, left eye. She had a dense scotoma corresponding with a large superotemporal zone of retinal pigment epithelium (RPE) depigmentation surrounded by a border of outer retinal whitening (A and B). This was associated with 2 + vitritis. Angiography revealed early nonfluorescence of the rim of the lesion and hyperfluorescence corresponding to its center (C), and late fluorescence of the entire lesion. Medical evaluation, including titers for syphilis and herpes viruses, was negative except for mild thrombocytosis and granulocytosis. She was hospitalized and received oral prednisone, acyclovir, and doxycycline. Visual acuity improved to 20/70 within 1 week. Over the following 5 weeks it decreased to 20/400 and the zone of RPE destruction continued to enlarge in a nasal direction (D). Five months after the onset of symptoms almost the entire fundus was affected (E), but visual acuity had improved to 20/200 and continued to improve over the next year to 20/30. Four years later her condition was unchanged. The right eye was normal.

Acute zonal outer retinopathy, overt type.

F–L: Soon after developing a sore throat this otherwise healthy 60-year-old man complained of progressive loss of the temporal field of vision in the left eye associated with "shimmering light" of 2 weeks' duration. Nine months previously he noted a similar but more peripheral temporal scotoma in the right eye associated with "shimmering." The symptoms in the right eye resolved spontaneously after several months. His visual acuity was 20/20 bilaterally. There was a 3 + afferent pupillary defect in the left eye. Visual field examination revealed a dense scotoma involving most of the peripheral and almost all of the temporal visual field of the left eye, and an enlarged blind spot in the right eye. In the right eye there were 2 + vitreous cells and a large well-demarcated zone of RPE atrophy involving the juxtapapillary and inferior and nasal areas out as far as the equator (F). This area was far larger than the zone of visual field loss. The optic disc and retinal vessels were normal bilaterally. Fundoscopic examination of the left eye revealed 3 + vitreous cells and a sharply defined zone of disruption of the RPE involving most of the fundus but sparing much of the macular area (G). There was no gray-white demarcation line at the border of the RPE change. Temporal to the macula, however, there were several ill-defined areas of gray-white at the level of the RPE (H). In the left eye fluorescein angiography showed evidence of acute RPE damage but no evidence of involvement of the choriocapillaris (J and K). In the right eye there was mottled hyperfluorescence corresponding to the large area of old RPE damage (I). He received prednisone, 60 mg, and acyclovir, 4 g, daily by mouth. There was some progression of the visual loss and RPE changes in the left eye for several weeks before stabilization occurred (L) as seen on this fundus photograph.

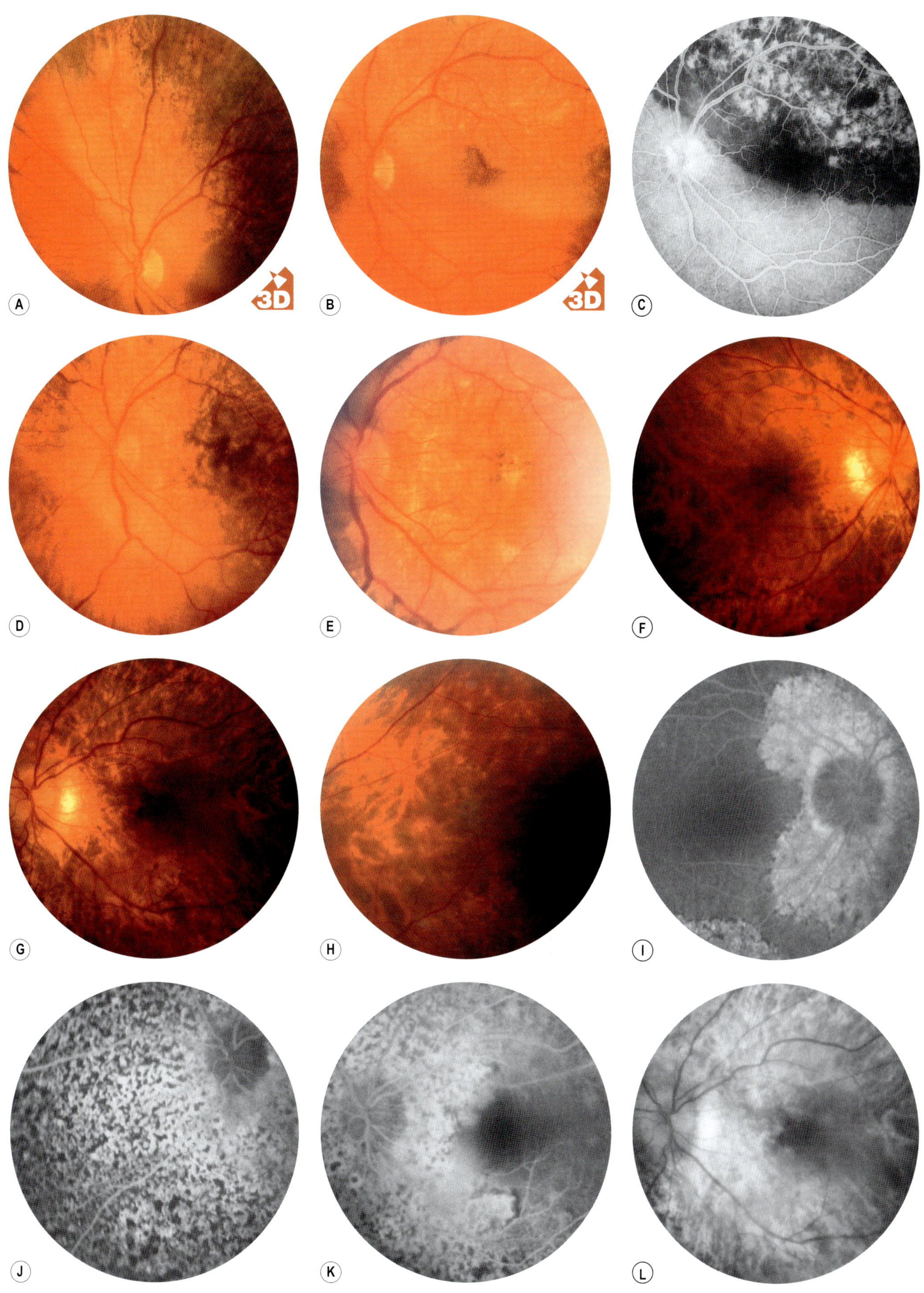
3D
3D
A
B
C
D
E
F
G
H
I
J
K
L

DISORDERS SIMULATING THE PRESUMED OCULAR HISTOPLASMOSIS SYNDROME (PSEUDO-POHS)

The clinical features of POHS are described in Chapter 3. In recent years it has become apparent that there are other disorders, unrelated to infection with *Histoplasma*, that during their inactive stages may cause a pattern of chorioretinal scarring similar to POHS. Collectively referred to as pseudo-POHS, there are at least two groups of patients that may simulate POHS.[163,185–187,204–212] They may or may not be pathogenetically related and are termed multifocal choroiditis with panuveitis (MCP) and punctate inner choroiditis (PIC).

MULTIFOCAL CHOROIDITIS AND PANUVEITIS

Nozik and Dorsch[208] and later, Dreyer and Gass[185] and Tessler and Deutsch[212] described a syndrome of MCP that simulates POHS with the following exceptions: (1) vitreous inflammation is present in one or both eyes; (2) anterior uveitis occurs in 50% of cases; (3) yellow and gray active choroidal lesions that angiographically may be nonfluorescent early and stain later are often observed or may develop during follow-up (Figure 11.21A–C); (4) the inactive lesions are in general smaller than those in the POHS (Figures 11.21A–C and 11.22); (5) most patients come from areas nonendemic for histoplasmosis and have a negative histoplasmin skin test; (6) approximately one-half of eyes demonstrate subnormal electroretinographic findings (Figures 11.21D–F and 11.22); (7) some patients develop acutely large visual field defects that are not explained on the basis of fundus findings and subsequently may develop large areas of RPE depigmentation, which may be associated with retinal vessel narrowing and migration of pigment epithelium into the retina; (8) patients with monocular involvement (25%) may develop severe involvement of the second eye months or years later (Figure 11.22); (9) there is a female sex predilection; (10) the disorder may affect children or adults of any age; (11) lack of HLA-DR2 specificity, which is often present in POHS;[213] and (12) appearance of new lesions over time in several patients. The reader should realize that the presence of vitritis or iritis has been an important requirement for inclusion of patients in reports concerning MCP in order to exclude patients with POHS, and that some patients with MCP and with active choroidal lesions as well as multifocal scars may have no vitreous cells.

11.21 Multifocal choroiditis and panuveitis (pseudo-presumed ocular histoplasmosis syndrome).

A–C: This 31-year-old woman had a 6-year history of loss of vision in the right eye caused by subfoveal neovascularization and recent blurring of vision in the left eye. In addition to widespread multifocal chorioretinal scars and vitritis in both eyes, there were active-appearing focal choroidal lesions in the macula, narrowing of the retinal vessels, and optic disc edema and pallor in the left eye (A and B). Angiography revealed that some of the chorioretinal lesions were nonfluorescent early (C) and stained later. Her visual fields were markedly constricted and the electroretinogram revealed severely abnormal rod and cone responses. Her father had subnormal vision that was attributed to working in a coal mine. Her fluorescent treponemal antibody absorption test was negative. It is of interest that, coincident with the onset of visual symptoms, the patient had a jejunoileostomy for obesity and as a consequence lost 200 lb (91 kg). It is not known whether or not vitamin A deficiency played any role in her tapetoretinal dystrophy-like fundus changes.
D–F: This 30-year-old, healthy, mildly myopic woman noted blurred vision in the left eye of 1 week's duration. Visual acuity in the right eye was 20/20 and in the left eye was 20/200. There was a 1 + afferent pupillary reaction in the left eye. The right fundus was normal. A few vitreous cells were present in the left eye. There were multifocal active gray lesions in the macula and juxtapapillary area (D) as well as a few in the peripheral fundus. Angiography revealed late staining of many of these lesions. Medical evaluation for evidence of systemic disease including histoplasmosis was negative. The diagnosis was chorioretinitis and optic neuritis of unknown cause. Systemic and sub-Tenon's steroids were given. Two months later visual acuity had improved to 20/70. Most of the lesions appeared less active (E). Fourteen months later she returned because of visual loss in the left eye caused by serous detachment of the macula that resolved spontaneously. Nine years later the right eye was normal. The acuity in the left eye was 20/200. There was enlargement and hyperpigmentation of the chorioretinal scars, and several atrophic scars (arrow, F) were evident in areas of previously normal retina.
G–L: This young woman experienced rapid onset of loss of temporal field and photopsia in her right eye. The fundi were normal (G). The gray spot (arrow) in G is an artifact. The scotoma partly resolved within several months, prior to her developing loss of central vision and an enlarged blind spot in the left eye that was associated with multiple active chorioretinal lesions (H and I). The diagnosis was punctate inner choroiditis. Six months later she developed blurred vision in the right eye associated with multiple foci of paracentral chorioretinitis (J). She soon developed evidence of subretinal neovascularization in the macular area of both eyes (K and L).

(D and E from Gass.[205])

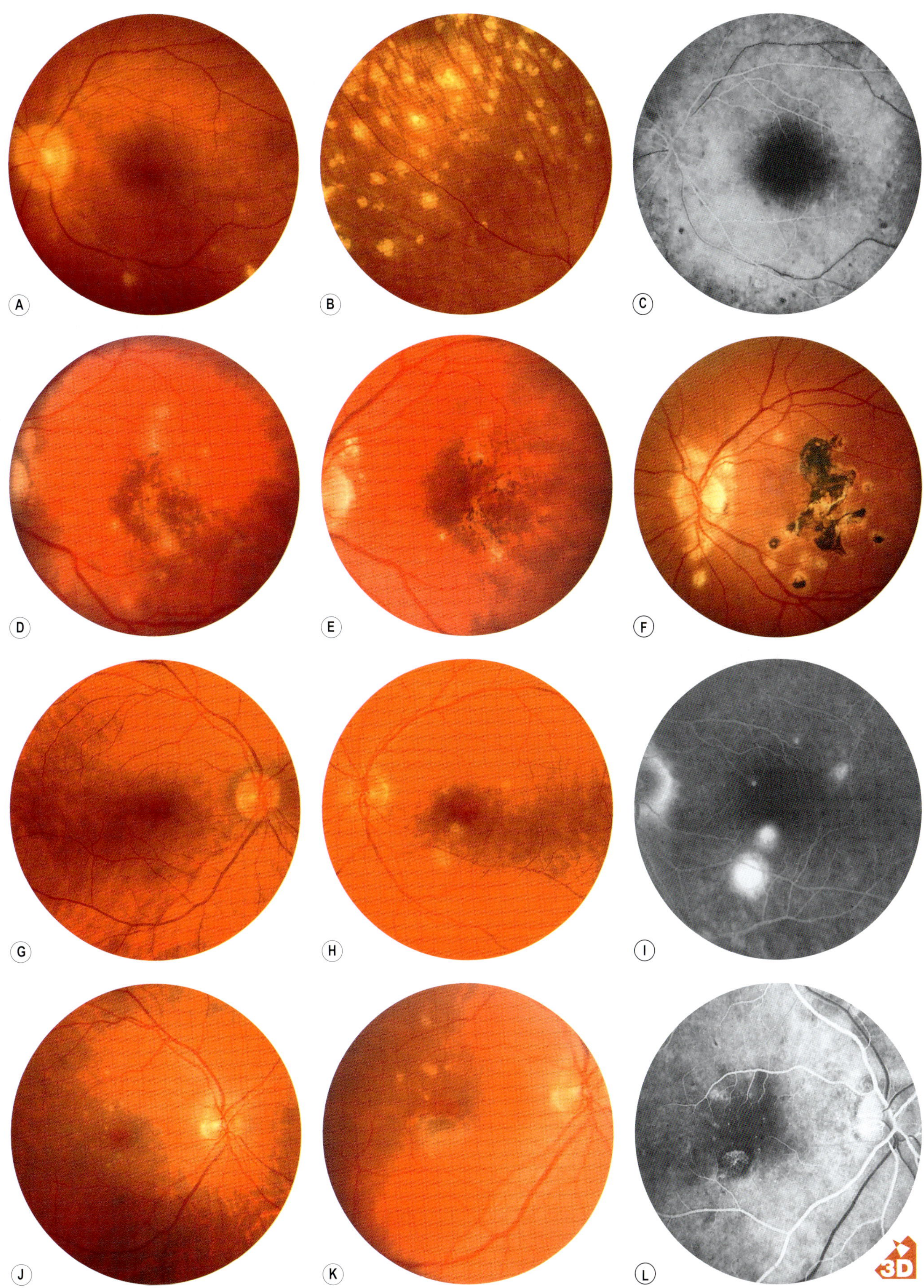
A
B
C
D
E
F
G
H
I
J
K
L
3D

Features of MCP similar to POHS include punched-out peripheral and posterior pole chorioretinal scars that are occasionally arranged in a curvilinear pattern at the equator, juxtapapillary scarring, and the frequent development of juxtapapillary and macular subretinal neovascularization (Figures 11.21 and 11.22).[205,214,215] Gass has seen three children with MCP in association with bilateral pars plana snow-bank exudation (see Figure 11.43J–L).[205] The cause of MCP is unknown. Features of MCP different from vitiliginous retinochoroiditis include: (1) the punched-out nature of chorioretinal scars; (2) a lower median age (33 years); (3) a greater frequency of unilateral disease; (4) a greater frequency of panuveitis; (5) a lower incidence of optic disc pallor, nyctalopia, color vision deficit, and electroretinographic abnormalities; (6) a greater incidence of visual loss caused by choroidal neovascularization; and (7) lack of HLA-A29 specificity. The fundus of patients with unilateral involvement in MCP may simulate that in patients with diffuse unilateral subacute neuroretinitis (see pp. 864–872). Visual loss in the latter disorder is usually unassociated with subretinal neovascularization and is more frequently accompanied by pallor of the optic disc, narrowing of the retinal vessels, and a markedly abnormal ERG. Multifocal choroiditis may occasionally be a manifestation of sarcoidosis. Hershey et al. found focal granulomas on blind biopsy of the conjunctiva in a group of patients over 50 years of age with a fundus picture of pseudo-POHS and no other manifestations of sarcoidosis.[216]

11.22 Multifocal choroiditis and panuveitis (pseudo-presumed ocular histoplasmosis syndrome).

A–I: This healthy 39-year-old woman experienced floaters and blurred vision in the right eye. Her visual acuity was 20/200. There were 1+ cells in the anterior chamber and 2+ cells in the vitreous. There was mild papilledema and cystoid macular edema (A). In the equatorial area for 360° there were hundreds of variably sized, round, chorioretinal scars (B and C). Angiography revealed cystoid macular edema and papilledema (D). There was late staining around some of the peripheral lesions (E and F). The left eye was normal. The scotopic electroretinographic responses were moderately abnormal in the right eye and borderline normal in the left eye. Over the next 6 1/2 years she experienced further loss of vision in the right eye related to subretinal neovascularization, before noting floaters in the left eye. At that time visual acuity in the right eye was 20/200 and in the left eye was 20/15. There were vitreous cells in both eyes. She had a disciform scar in the right macula (G). There were many focal chorioretinal lesions, some of which appeared active in the periphery of the left eye (H and I). Angiography revealed leaky capillaries in the optic disc and retina of both eyes.

J–L: This 31-year-old woman had a 1-year history of episodes of blurred vision and photophobia in the left eye. Visual acuity in the right eye was 20/20 and in the left eye was 20/300. The right fundus and vitreous were normal except for mild peripapillary scarring (J). In the left eye there were 2+ vitreous cells; multiple focal chorioretinal scars, some of which were stellate; and a subfoveal neovascular membrane (K). Ten months later, the visual acuity in the left eye was counting fingers, and there was massive subretinal fibrosis (L). The right eye was unchanged.

PUNCTATE INNER CHOROIDOPATHY

Watzke and associates[187] and Morgan and Schatz[186] reported a syndrome characterized by the following: (1) moderate myopia, blurred vision, photopsia, and scotomata in women; (2) multiple, yellow-white lesions of the inner choroid and retina that are largely confined to the posterior pole, and that after resolution leave atrophic pigmented scars simulating those in POHS (Figures 11.21D–L); (3) frequent serous detachment of the retina that resolves spontaneously; (4) no signs of vitritis or anterior uveitis; (5) both eyes affected in most patients; (6) negative histoplasmin skin test (70%); (7) choroidal neovascularization in 40% of eyes; and (8) relatively good visual prognosis, with one-half of eyes retaining normal acuity. Doran and Hamilton[204] presented four similar cases. The macular lesions tend to be arranged in a linear or branching pattern in some cases (Figure 11.23H–L). Figure 11.21 (D) depicts such a pattern in the left eye of a 30-year-old myopic woman who also had mild vitritis and a few peripheral chorioretinal scars in the right eye.[205] The left eye was normal. This patient, and others seen by the author, suggests that the two syndromes (PIC and MCP) are probably the same disorder or have a similar pathogenesis.[211] The presence or absence of vitreous cells in these patients is probably a function of the size of the area of the fundus affected. Those with lesions confined to the posterior pole (PIC) are less likely to have vitreous cells than those with widespread lesions (MCP). Once the active lesions in both of these syndromes become inactive, and the vitritis and iritis resolve in the case of MCP, the fundus picture in many of these patients becomes indistinguishable from those with POHS. Just as the absence of vitreous cells does not entirely exclude the diagnosis of MCP, likewise, the presence of vitreous cells probably does not completely exclude POHS. Subretinal/choroidal neovascularization can occur during the active phase of choroiditis (Figure 11.23A–G)[217] or in a scar. Systemic steroids used to treat the acute lesions may cause regression of the neovascularization (Figure 11.23A–G). In those eyes with choroidal neovascularization occurring in inactive scars, intravitreal bevacizumab is successful in causing regression. Photodynamic therapy was used prior to intravitreal antivascular endothelial growth factor agents and was reasonably successful.

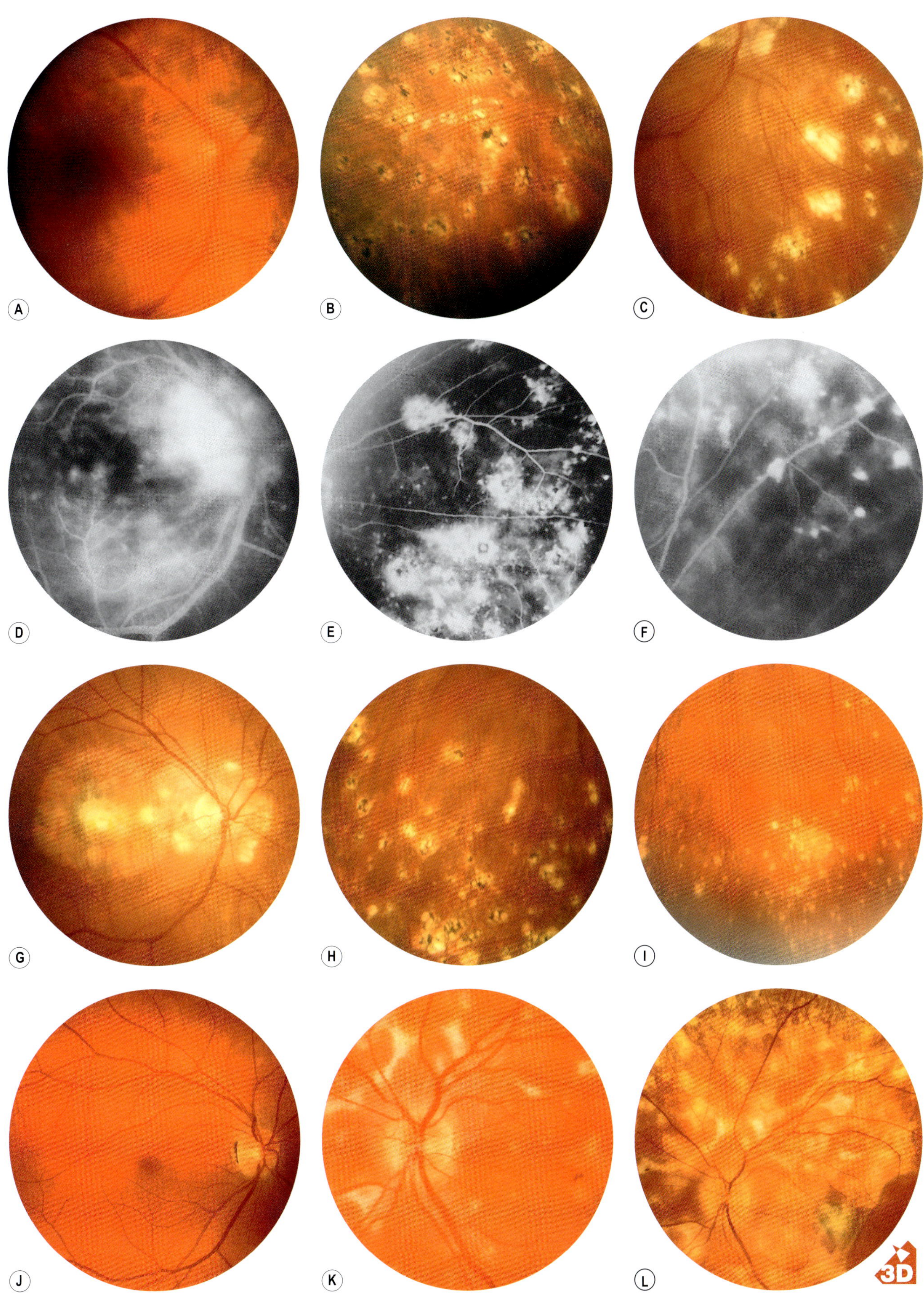
A
B
C
D
E
F
G
H
I
J
K
L
3D

Some patients with MCP and PIC develop prominent subretinal fibrosis in the vicinity of the focal choroiditis (Figure 11.22J–L). This process of reactive fibrosis may be limited to small isolated areas around individual choroidal lesions or may form a large confluent interlacing network or plaque of subretinal fibrous tissue, either in the macula or in the peripheral fundus. Still others may develop massive widespread fibrous tissue mounds and severe visual loss. (See Figure 11.32 and discussion of massive SRF.)[179,218] The etiology, pathogenesis, and natural course of MCP and PIC are not known. Tiedeman found serologic evidence to suggest that Epstein–Barr virus might be a causative factor.[219] This could not be confirmed by others.[220]

The multifocal features of these pseudo-POHS disorders have obscured the fact that some of these patients develop large visual field defects that are usually overlooked, and that are not explained during the early stage of the disease by fundus changes (Figure 11.21G–L). These defects are probably caused by acute damage to zones of the retinal receptors that may or may not recover function. This loss of function may be confined to one or more small zones, particularly surrounding the optic disc, or to large peripheral zones. Loss of retinal receptors in large areas of the fundus is responsible for the narrowing of the retinal blood vessels and alterations in the RPE that may simulate retinitis pigmentosa in some of these patients. This occult phase of these pseudo-POHS disorders is similar to that which occurs in patients with AZOOR, MEWDS, and acute idiopathic blind-spot enlargement and is collectively termed AZOOR complex disorder.[221] (See previous discussion of MEWDS and AZOOR.)

Uncertain at this time is the frequency with which patients who have pseudo-POHS develop recurrent episodes of new lesions or visual loss (H to L), other than that which may occur from delayed development of subretinal neovascularization at the site of a focal scar. Although the author has observed delayed involvement of the second eye for up to 10 years, most of these patients experience a single acute or subacute event lasting for several months in one or both eyes, and they are unlikely to have a recurrence of active disease in the same eye thereafter.

The predilection for pseudo-POHS, AZOOR, MEWDS, and acute idiopathic blind-spot enlargement to occur primarily in women; the primary locus of the disease in these disorders at the level of the retinal receptors and pigment epithelium; and the similarity of the pathologic changes in eyes of patients with multifocal choroiditis and massive SRF to experimental uveitis induced in primates by interphotoreceptor retinoid-binding protein suggest that autoimmunity plays an important role in the pathogenesis of these disorders[207,222] (see Figure 11.32). The experimental model of Hirose and coworkers[222] demonstrates some of the clinical features of pseudo-POHS, including multifocal choroidal lesions, that histologically were focal granulomas associated with widespread retinal receptor changes. Their model demonstrates that antigen localized specifically in the retina may cause widespread changes in the retinal receptors and also may initiate immunopathogenetic changes in the choroid as well (see discussion later) (Figure 11.32D–J).

11.23 Punctate inner choroidopathy.

A–G: A 23-year-old otherwise healthy soldier presented with metamorphopsia and visual decline to 20/50 in his right eye. Several punctate white lesions were present in both foveas associated with a fleck of retinal hemorrhage in his right eye (A and B). Angiogram revealed several hyperfluorescent dots that stained late and a small subfoveal choroidal neovascular membrane consistent with active punctuate inner choroiditis lesions (C–E). Oral steroids at 50 mg were started, the vision gradually improved, the lesions turned inactive (F), and over the next 3 months the choroidal neovascular membrane had regressed (G) and the vision recovered to 20/25.

H–L: This 29-year-old recently pregnant myopic woman developed metamorphopsia in her right eye and a vision change to 20/30 right eye and 20/20– left eye. A few vitreous cells were present in her right eye associated with two yellow white choroidal/outer retinal lesions on the right and one on the left (H and I). A diagnosis of punctuate inner choroiditis was made and she received oral steroids after an angiogram confirmed absence of choroidal neovascularization. Her vision improved to 20/20 in both eyes. Over the next 2 years she developed several new macular lesions (J) every time her prednisone was reduced to the 20-mg range. Oral methotrexate was added after advising against further pregnancies. She continued her follow-up elsewhere and returned 3 years later with several more lesions in both eyes (K and L). She was maintained on mycophenolate mofetil and methotrexate and has remained stable. Fluorescein angiograms at no stage revealed choroidal neovascularization in either eye.

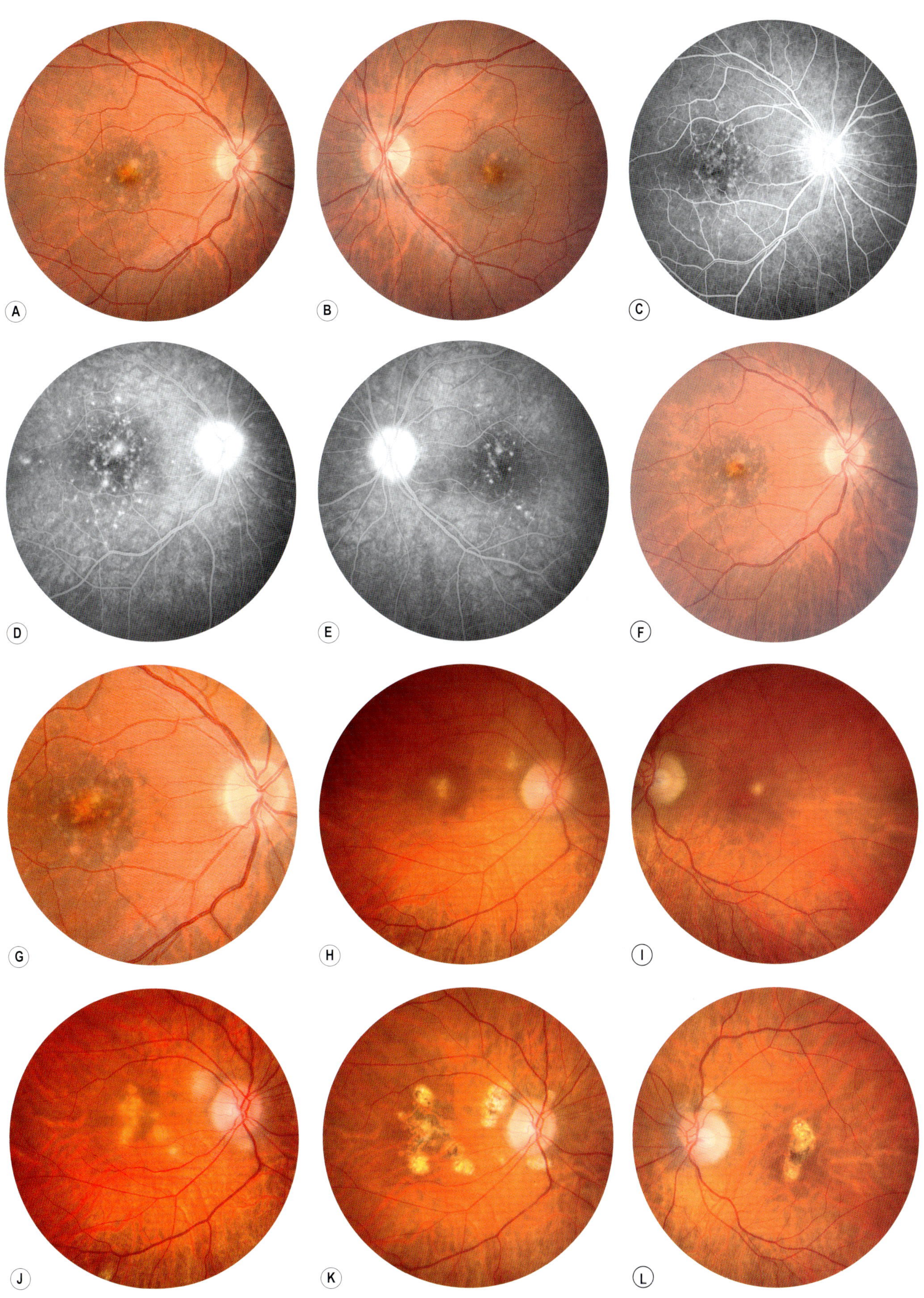
A
B
C
D
E
F
G
H
I
J
K
L

ACUTE MACULAR NEURORETINOPATHY

Bos and Deutman[188] described peculiar cloverleaf, wedge-shaped lesions that develop in the macular region of both eyes of young patients who complain of rapid loss of central and paracentral vision, usually following a flulike syndrome (Figure 11.24A–C).[188,223–233] The color of the fundus lesions is dependent upon the pigmentation of the fundus and varies from grayish to reddish brown. Visual acuity is usually reduced to 20/30–20/40. These patients can outline precisely on the Amsler grid negative scotomata corresponding with the fundus lesions (Figure 11.24G). In patients with the full-blown disease, dark, flower petal-shaped lesions are present in the central macular region (Figure 11.24A, B, and H). In other patients, however, the lesions are less prominent and may consist of multiple oval to round, faintly pinkish patches in the central or paracentral region (Figure 11.24D and E). They are seen better with red-free light but most easily with scanning laser ophthalmoscope (Figure 11.25H).[234–237] These lesions appear to lie at the level of the outer retinal layers,[223,227,228,232] rather than the superficial retina, as suggested by Bos and Deutman. OCT and multifocal ERG demonstrate involvement of the photoreceptors and outer nuclear area. The inner segment–outer segment junction is disrupted with thinning of the corresponding outer nuclear area (Figure 11.25I).[234,238,239] Averaged waveforms from the affected areas are reduced compared to adjacent areas of normal function.[235] Only one eye may be involved. One or two small superficial, flame-shaped retinal hemorrhages may be present (Figure 11.24B).[223,227] The retinal vessels and optic disc are normal. There are no cells in the vitreous. Fluorescein angiography in well-developed cases shows a faint hypofluorescence corresponding with the lesions (Figure 11.24C and I). Transient choroidal ischemia may have a role in some cases (Figure 11.25). Autofluorescence imaging shows no changes corresponding to the lesion (Figure 11.25G). Resolution of the lesions and improvement in acuity and field loss occur slowly over a matter of weeks or months (Figure 11.24F).[229] The scotomas in some cases may be prolonged for many months or years.[224] OCT shows sharp loss of photoreceptors (Figure 11.25). Lesions identical to acute macular neuroretinopathy have occurred in patients with MEWDS and acute blind-spot enlargement.[163,170]

Although most of these patients have noted the onset of symptoms within a week or two following a flulike illness, others develop identical-appearing lesions and acute visual loss after receiving intravenous injections of sympathomimetics[240] or iodine-containing contrast agents,[241] or following anaphylactic shock after a bee sting (Figure 11.24G–I).[157] If examined immediately after the visual loss following the injections the lesions may have a gray-white appearance that is difficult to discern, and later become darker in color similar to Figure 11.25. Acute macular neuroretinopathy has also been reported in association with oral contraceptives, trauma, history of headache or migraine and postpartum hypotension.

11.24 Acute macular neuroretinopathy.

A–C: This 31-year-old black woman gave a 2-week history of a flulike syndrome before the onset of blurred vision and paracentral scotomata in both eyes. She had some pain on ocular movement. Her visual acuity was 20/50 bilaterally. Note the petaloid dark areas in the macular region of both eyes (A and B) and the superficial retinal hemorrhage superior to the macula in the left eye (arrow, B). Angiography revealed only mild dilation of the retinal capillaries superior to the macula. There were no other changes in the fundi. Five months later visual acuity improved to 20/30 and J-1. The appearance of the macula had remained essentially unchanged. The patient was lost to follow-up.

D–F: This 26-year-old white woman noted multiple paracentral scotomata and photopsia in the left eye unassociated with a viral-like illness. The visual acuity was 20/25. She had multiple, small, variably sized, dark, round spots at the level of the outer retina (D and E). These corresponded with dense scotomata evident on the Amsler grid. Angiography, electroretinography, and electro-oculography were normal. These spots and the scotomata faded over a period of many months. Visual acuity 7 years later was 20/25 (F).

G–I: In October 1988 this healthy 27-year-old woman noted multiple paracentral negative scotomas in the right eye. An optometrist noted multiple "hemorrhages" in the right macula. Five months later the scotomas persisted and were evident on Amsler grid testing (G). Visual acuity was 20/15 bilaterally. Fundoscopic examination revealed a pattern of outer retinal red-orange lesions (H) that corresponded with the Amsler grid changes. The left eye was normal. Angiography revealed minimal changes (I). When she returned 6 years later the scotomas and visual acuity were unchanged but the fundus lesions were no longer present.

J and K: This healthy 28-year-old white woman had uterine bleeding after an elective cesarean delivery. She received 10 units of oxytocin (Pitocin) and epinephrine by intravenous push. She experienced severe headache, elevation of blood pressure, and extra systoles that were controlled with intravenous lidocaine and Sodium Pentothal anesthesia. On awakening she noted central scotomata and her visual acuity was 20/200. A "cherry-red spot and macular edema" were described. Her vision improved over the next few days. Six weeks later her visual acuity was 20/20. She had paracentral scotomata and the typical picture of acute macular neuroretinopathy in both macular areas (J). The reddish lesions involved the outer retina and they were slightly hypofluorescent angiographically (K). These lesions faded and were associated with subtle retinal pigment epithelial changes, but they and their corresponding scotomas were still evident 5 years later.

L: This 24-year-old woman had an abdominal computed tomography scan performed with injection of 20 cc of iothalamate because of enlarged abdominal lymph nodes, probably caused by infectious mononucleosis. Because of development of urticaria, palpitations, and severe headache she was given an intravenous injection of 0.2 cc of epinephrine 1:1000 and 50 mg of Benadryl. Ten hours later, on awakening, she noted scotomas centrally. Macular abnormalities were noted. Three weeks later her visual acuity was 20/25, right eye, and 20/30, left eye. Similar reddish outer retinal lesions and corresponding scotomas were present in both maculas. These lesions were associated with slight hypofluorescence angiographically. Three months later the visual acuity and fundi were unchanged. The scotomata were similar but less dense.

(J and K from O'Brien et al.[240]; L from Guzak et al.[241])

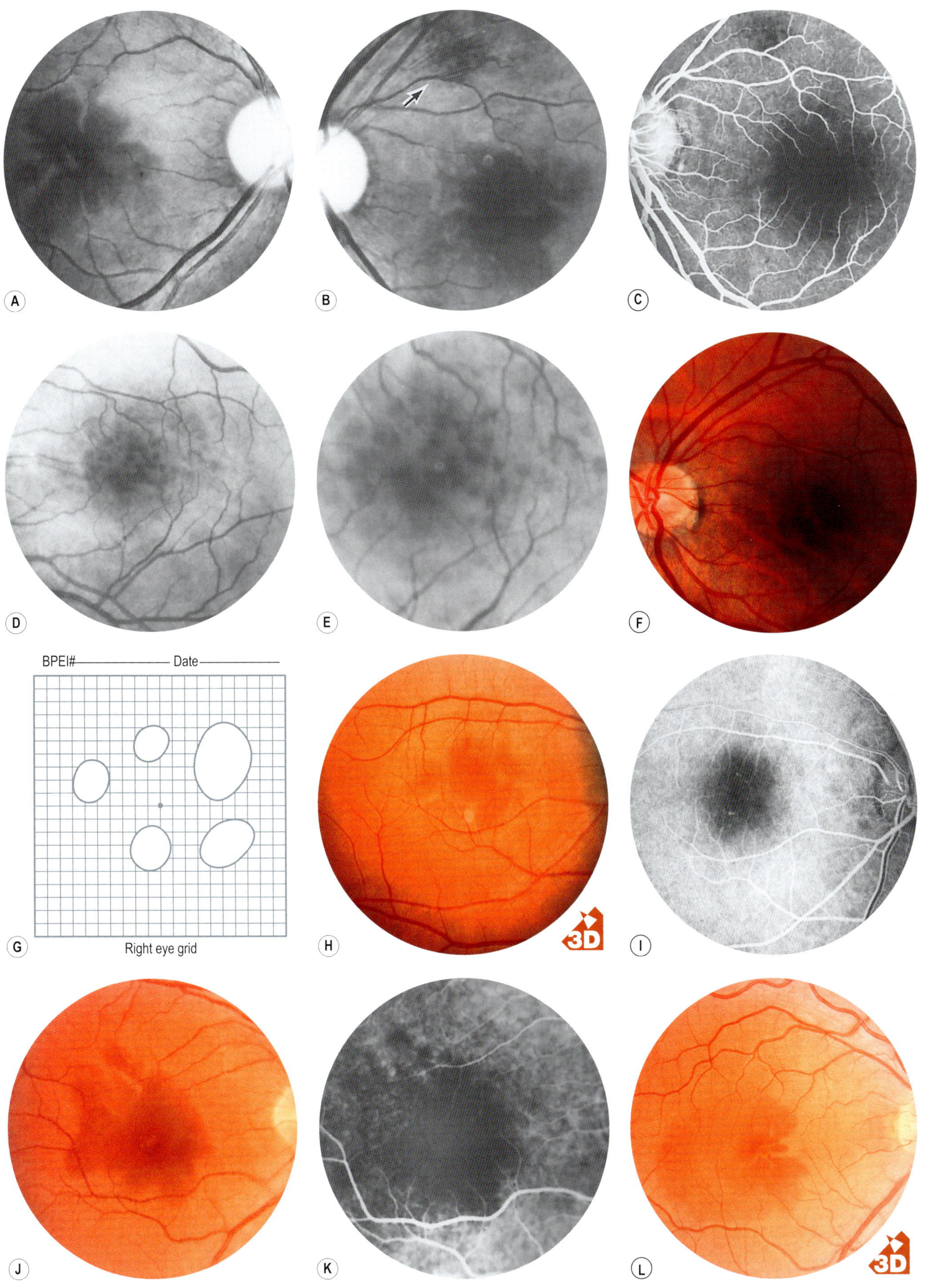
A
B
C
D
E
F
BPEI# Date
Right eye grid
G
H
3D
I
J
K
L
3D

The fundus lesions, when they are reddish in color, may be mistaken for subretinal blood. This may have happened in the case reported by Weinberg and Nerney.[242] The milder forms of this disease (Figure 11.24D–F) may be misdiagnosed as acute retinal pigment epitheliitis since both diseases cause temporary loss of central vision, usually in young individuals (see p. 874). Early receptor potential changes may be evident electroretinographically and may persist for many months.[232] The pathology, pathogenesis, and course of these peculiar macular lesions are unknown. Cases of MEWDS and acute macular neuroretinopathy occurring in the same eye of 2 young women, a few weeks apart in one, and 5 years later in the other, suggest that they may share a common etiologic agent. Furthermore, photoreceptor involvement in these, and in acute idiopathic blind-spot enlargement and AZOOR, suggests they may be related in their etiopathogenesis.[243,244] The sharply demarcated reddish lesions corresponding rather precisely to the visual field loss suggest that acute loss of the retinal outer receptor elements and to some degree the inner receptor elements in sharply delineated zones is responsible for well-demarcated zones of outer retinal thinning that cause the reddish appearance of the lesions. OCT demonstrates loss of photoreceptors corresponding to the lesion (Figure 11.25 I) The mechanism of this focal damage is probably different in the patients who develop this disorder following a viral-like disorder than in the patients who develop it after intravenous injections that usually contain sympathomimetic drugs. In the latter patients, either transient choroidal ischemia (Figure 11.25B–E) or a toxic interaction between the drug and the receptor cells is a possible explanation for the damage. Other causes of sharply defined areas of retinal thinning, e.g., atrophy of the outer retina after resolution of Berlin's edema,[245,246] sickle-cell hemoglobin macular infarcts,[170] cotton-wool infarcts,[247] and inner lamellar macular holes, may produce reddish lesions biomicroscopically.[170,245]

11.25 Acute macular neuroretinopathy (AMN).

This 23-year-old otherwise healthy woman woke up with a superior paracentral defect in her right eye. On Amsler grid testing the lines were absent in the area of the field defect, measuring approximately 2 × 3°. Fundus appeared normal (A), but the retinal and choroidal circulations were slow (B–E). She was on oral contraceptives that were discontinued. The field defect persisted when seen a month later. Now a "bronze" discoloration was noted in her fundus corresponding to the scotoma (F), which is best seen on infrared imaging (H, arrow) and invisible on autofluorescence imaging (G). Optical coherence tomography showed loss of photoreceptors in the affected area (I arrow).

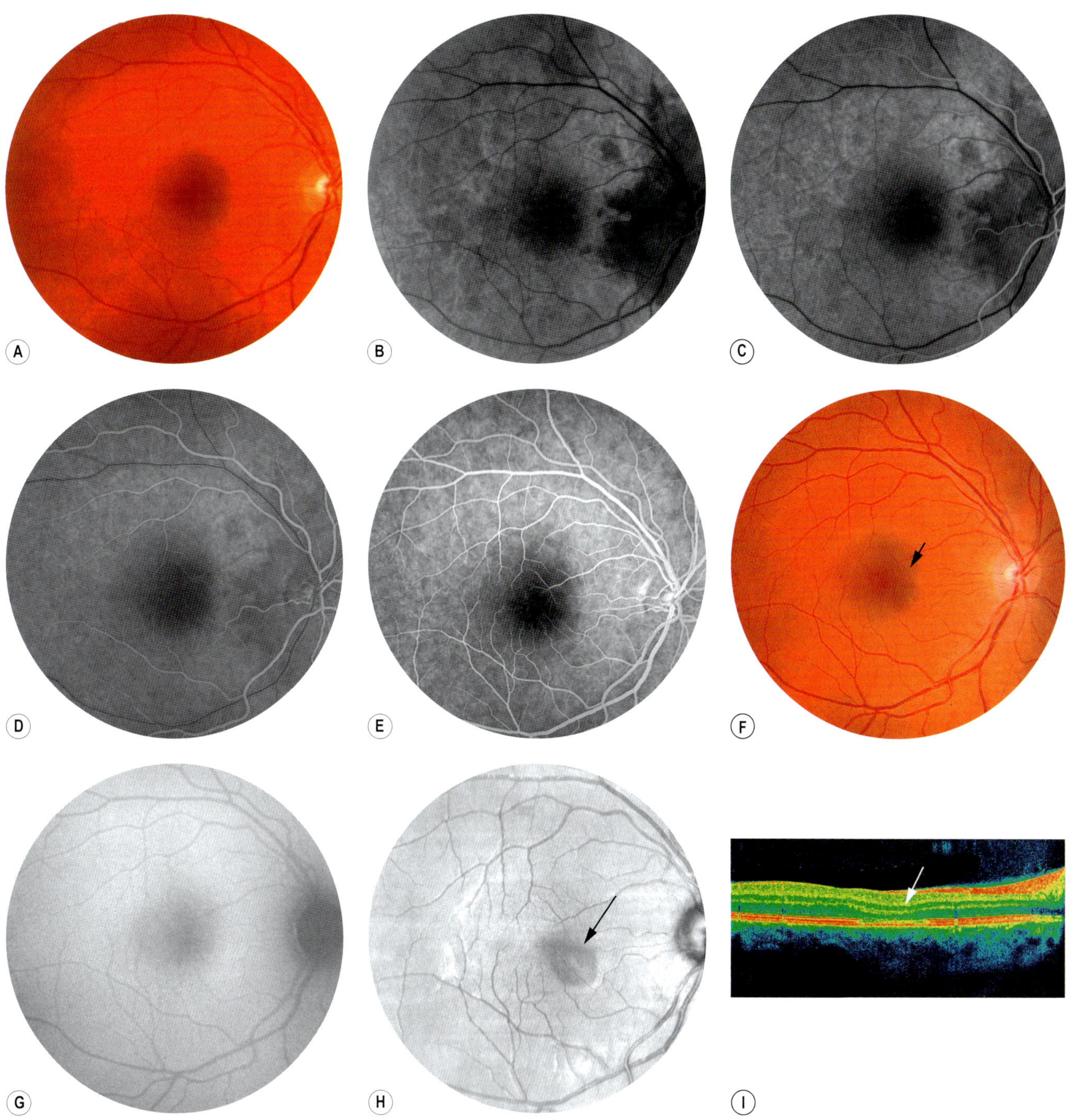
A
B
C
D
E
F
G
H
I

HARADA'S DISEASE

Patients with Harada's disease, who typically are heavily pigmented individuals, may experience rapid loss of vision in one or both eyes caused by serous retinal detachment.[248–257] The disease by definition is bilateral; occasionally involvement of the second eye may be delayed by a few days to a week. Subtle choroidal folds may be the only finding in the fellow eye. These may be detectable by OCT as corrugations of the RPE/choroid and choroidal thickening if not evident clinically. There is some evidence that many affected blacks in the USA have Native American ancestry, which links them to an Oriental ancestry.[254,258–260] There is no sex predilection. Systemic manifestations such as headache, malaise, vomiting, and occasionally focal neurologic signs and symptoms may precede the onset of visual loss.[261] Initially, nondescript, yellow-white areas of either exudate or color change in the RPE occur beneath one or more isolated zones of serous retinal detachment (Figure 11.26A and B). These zones often become confluent to form an extensive bullous serous retinal detachment that shifts with positioning of the patient. In a few patients, multifocal, gray-white patches at the level of the RPE similar to, but less well defined than, those seen in patients with APMPPE, occur (Figures 11.26D and 11.27G). The choroid may appear thickened and in some cases is associated with broad chorioretinal folds (Figure 11.26G–I).[262] The optic disc typically appears hyperemic and swollen. This swelling may be severe and accompanied by hemorrhages and a macular star in some cases (Figures 11.26G and 11.27J).[263] Inflammatory cells are invariably present in the vitreous. Iridocyclitis may be present in some cases. Inflammatory infiltration of the anterior choroid and ciliary body may cause some narrowing of the anterior chamber and, in a rare case, angle closure glaucoma.[264–266] Ultrasonography usually demonstrates diffuse low to medium reflective thickening of the posterior choroid-scleral wall.[267,268] T1-weighted sagittal surface coil magnetic resonance imaging of the orbit is capable of determining that this thickening in Vogt–Koyanagi–Harada (VKH) syndrome is caused by choroidal and not scleral thickening.[250,269]

11.26 Vogt–Koyanagi–Harada (VKH) syndrome.

A-I: This 28-year-old African American woman presented with headaches, neck pain, and loss of vision in both eyes. Bilateral pockets of subretinal fluid and choroidal folds were seen (A, B, and H). Pinpoint hyperfluorescent dots that leaked dye under the retina were seen on the angiogram, typical of VKH syndrome (C–E). Optical coherence tomography confirmed the presence of subretinal fluid in both eyes (F and G). She responded to oral steroids with resolution of the exudative detachments in both eyes (I). Note the change in the color of the fundus to an orange sunset glow (I).

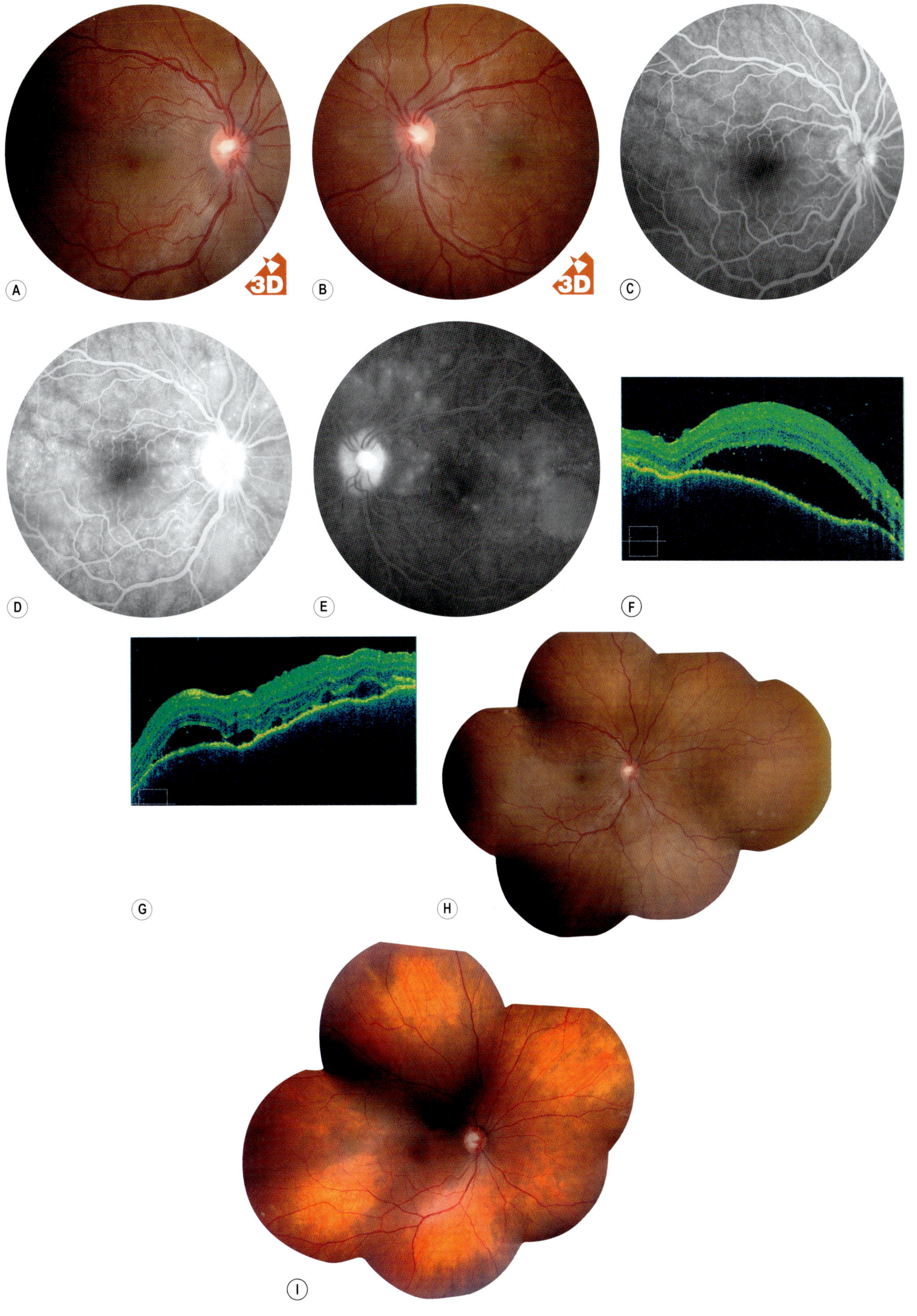

A
3D
B
3D
C
D
E
F
G
H
I

Fluorescein angiography may demonstrate focal or patchy areas of delay in choroidal perfusion (Figure 11.27H). Many pinpoint and irregular areas of fluorescein staining develop at the level of the RPE (Figures 11.26B, C, E, F, K, and L, and 11.27B, E, and F, 11.28C and D). These areas of fluorescence gradually increase in size and in some cases form large placoid areas of hyperfluorescence that sometimes resemble cobblestones at the level of the RPE (Figures 11.26C and 11.27B). The subretinal exudate stains with fluorescein during the late stages of angiography. OCT demonstrates the subretinal fluid, occasionally loculation of fluid due to high fibrin content, may be seen (Figure 11.28E). Spinal fluid examination usually reveals evidence of pleocytosis and elevation of the protein level. Although in a few cases the retinal detachment may resolve spontaneously within several weeks or less, usually the course is prolonged. Intensive systemic corticosteroid therapy appears to shorten the duration of the retinal detachment.[270–272] Use of immunosuppressive agents may be required in patients with severe chronic disease. Varying degrees of visual loss accompany the RPE changes that remain after resolution of the detachment. Most patients regain excellent visual acuity following their first episode. Recurrences are common, but the overall visual prognosis is good.[270,273]

A variety of fundus pictures may develop following resolution of the retinal detachment. Patchy loss of pigment from the underlying choroidal melanocytes as well as the RPE may be evident after resolution of the detachment. An irregular pattern of pigmented demarcation lines caused by the choroidal thickening may radiate out away from the optic disc and be scattered in the peripheral fundus after resolution of choroidal infiltration and prolonged retinal detachment (Figure 11.26H and I). In some patients multifocal atrophic chorioretinal scars simulating that in vitiliginous (birdshot) chorioretinopathy and POHS occur. These lesions may occasionally be confluent and arranged in a curvilinear equatorial pattern similar to that seen in POHS and pseudo-POHS.[274] In other patients a diffuse depigmentation of the choroidal melanocytes occurs and the fundus may change from brunette to blonde or present a "setting-sun, reddish glow" appearance (Figures 11.27A and C, and 11.28H and K). Subretinal choroidal neovascularization and optic disc neovascularization may occasionally occur as a late complication.[254,275–277] Scleromalacia presumably caused by autoimmune attack on the intrascleral melanocytes may occur.[278] A small choroidal osteoma developed in one patient seen by Gass (Figure 11.27D).

The serous detachment in Harada's disease is caused by diffuse granulomatous inflammation of the uveal tract, with a preponderance of lymphocytes, plasma cells, epithelioid cells, and occasional giant cells with evidence of pigment phagocytosis.[252,255,261,279–281] The inflammatory cell reaction usually involves the choriocapillaris. Subpigment epithelial plaques of inflammatory cellular exudate may be the cause of the yellowish subretinal lesions and the placoid areas of late staining that occur in some patients with this disease. In one patient's eye with the active stages of the disease the choroidal infiltrate was composed of predominantly T lymphocytes and HLA-DR + macrophages and, in addition, nondendritic-appearing CD1-(leu-6)-positive cells.[280] A T-cell-mediated immune reaction to ocular antigens seems to play a major role in VKH as well as sympathetic uveitis.[279,282] Inomata and Sakamoto studied the histopathology and immunopathology of two eyes of 2 patients with "sunset" fundus 32 months and 7 years after resolution of the subretinal fluid.[283] They found marked loss of the choroidal melanocytes and scattered infiltration of the choroid with T (70%) and B lymphocytes. Although a few patients may have patchy, gray, subretinal lesions that have suggested to some authors an etiologic relationship to APMPPE, Gass believes there is little evidence that they are manifestations of the same disease.[284,285]

A few patients with Harada's disease eventually develop severe anterior uveitis, alopecia, poliosis, cutaneous as well as perilimbal vitiligo, and dysacousis (VKH syndrome).[255,286–289] The similarity of the clinical and histopathologic findings in this disease, sympathetic uveitis, and experimentally induced uveitis suggest that autoimmunity to melanin is important in the pathogenesis of all three.[222,252,290,291] VKH has occurred in siblings and monozygotic twins.[292,293]

11.27 Harada's disease.

A–C: This 30-year-old Latin woman with headaches and stiff neck had bilateral bullous retinal detachment (A). Note pinpoint as well as placoid areas of late staining (B). C, Seven months after resolution of the detachment. Both fundi had changed from a brunette to a relatively blonde, red-orange ("sunset glow") color (C).

D–F: This 11-year-old Latin girl experienced bilateral retinal detachments secondary to Harada's disease and an orange subretinal lesion that ultrasonographically appeared to be a choroidal osteoma (arrows, D). Angiography revealed multiple pinpoint leaks and fluorescein staining of the subretinal fluid in both eyes (E and F). The detachments resolved after corticosteroid treatment. When she returned several years later her visual acuity was normal. The osteoma in the left eye appeared to have decreased in size.

G–L: Unusual presentation of Harada's disease in a 34-year-old black man who presented with headache and mild visual loss associated with optic disc swelling, macular star, serous retinal detachment that was largely confined to the macula, and multiple ill-defined white spots (arrows) at the level of the retinal pigment epithelium (RPE) (G). Ultrasonography revealed diffuse thickening of the choroid and no abnormality of the optic disc. Angiography showed that the white spots blocked choroidal fluorescence (arrows) and stained late (H and I). Several weeks later there was increased swelling of the optic discs and further retinal detachment (J–L). Neurologic evaluation was normal. After treatment with prednisone, 80 mg daily, the optic disc and retinal changes resolved but irregular RPE atrophy remained.

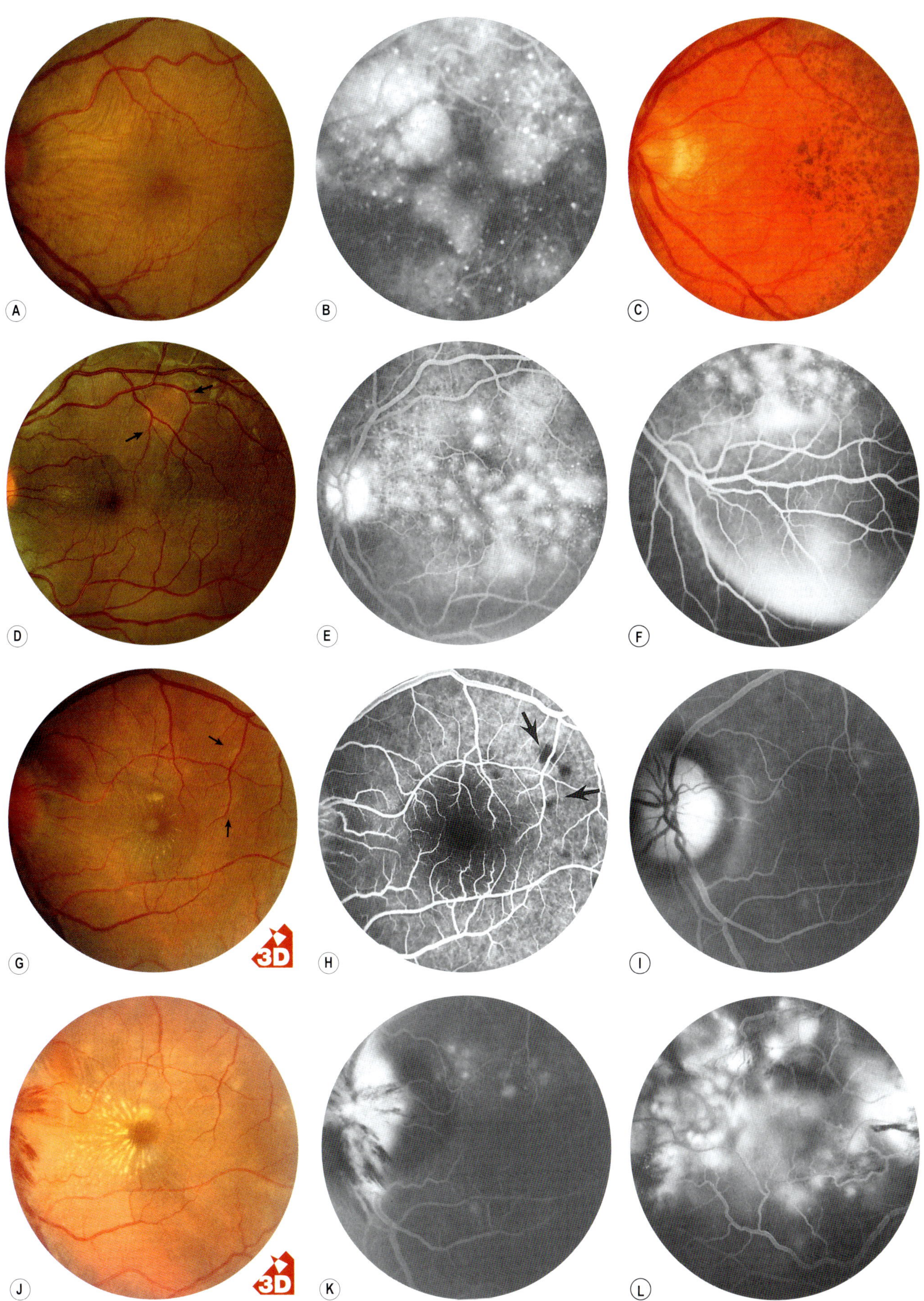
A
B
C
D
E
F
G
3D
H
I
J
3D
K
L

The Revised Diagnostic Criteria for VKH disease was established at the First International Workshop on Vogt-Koyanagi-Harada disease. According to this criteria, VKH disease is divided into two subgroups, incomplete VKH and complete VKH disease; incomplete VKH disease involves ocular findings and either neurological/auditory or integumentary findings, while complete VKH disease includes ocular, neurological/auditory, and integumentary findings.[294]

Corticosteroids are the first line of treatment; they should be started at a fairly high dose of 1–1.5 mg/kg body weight depending on the severity of the disease. Immunusuppressives are added if there is difficulty in tapering the steroids, or in those eyes that show recurrences.[295,296] Steroids should be tapered very slowly and a low dose maintained for up to 6 months or longer. Early withdrawal causes recurrences and secondary complications such as angle closure and pupillary block glaucoma.

The differential diagnosis in Harada's disease includes severe idiopathic central serous chorioretinopathy (Figures 3.10 and 3.11), acute leukemia (Figure 14.35A–L), metastatic carcinoma, uveal melanocytic proliferation associated with systemic carcinoma, idiopathic uveal effusion syndrome (see Figures 3.64–3.66), and benign reactive lymphoid hyperplasia of the uveal tract. Echography in Harada's disease shows low-reflective thickening of the choroid that may be helpful in differentiating it from more highly reflective thickening caused by idiopathic uveal effusion and diffuse metastatic carcinoma, or thickening of the choroid caused by choroiditis as a result of posterior sclerochoroiditis, which is typically associated with an echolucent zone in the episcleral area (see p. 1016).

Orientals with HLA-DR4, -DRw53, and -DQw7 and racially diverse American patients, often with Native American descent, and with HLA-DR4 and -DQw3 and -DRw53 are susceptible to VKH.[258,297,298]

Harada's-Like Syndrome in Children

Bilateral secondary retinal detachment in relatively young and brunette adults is the hallmark of Harada's disease. In some cases, however, children are affected and only one eye may be involved.[299,300] Serous retinal detachment confined to the posterior pole of one or both eyes of children may be associated with mild ocular pain, thickening of the posterior choroid, anterior-chamber and vitreous inflammatory cells, and fluorescein angiographic evidence of multiple pinpoint leaks at the level of the RPE.[299,301] They may or may not have systemic signs or symptoms. The localized detachment may resolve spontaneously or respond rapidly to oral corticosteroid therapy. It is the author's clinical impression that children with this clinical picture in the absence of evidence of systemic disease respond quickly to therapy and have less chance of experiencing a recurrence than adults with Harada's disease. It is possible this is a mild, self limiting posterior scleritis in one or both eyes of some of these children.

11.28 Vogt–Koyanagi–Harada syndrome – asymmetric presentation.

A–G: This patient presented with symptoms in the right eye, which showed several pockets of subretinal fluid (A), while the left fundus showed mild choroidal thickening and superficial chorioretinal folds (B). Angiogram revealed hyperfluorescent dots that leaked fluid (C and D). Optical coherence tomography showed pockets of subretinal and intraretinal fluid on the right and almost normal retinal contour on the left (E and F). Following oral prednisone the serous detachment resolved with mild choroidal folds (G).

H–J: This 17-year-old Latin woman with bilateral bullous retinal detachments presented with multiple ill-defined white lesions (arrows, H) at the level of the RPE. Angiography revealed evidence of multiple pinpoint areas of leakage in both eyes (I and J) and a focal area of serous detachment of the RPE in the left eye (arrow). The detachment in both eyes cleared promptly after systemic corticosteroid treatment.

K–M: Bilateral bullous retinal detachment in 39-year-old woman with Harada's disease associated with ultrasonographic evidence of thickening of the choroid. Note pinpoint leaks in stereo angiograms (L and M).

(A–G, courtesy of James Vander.)

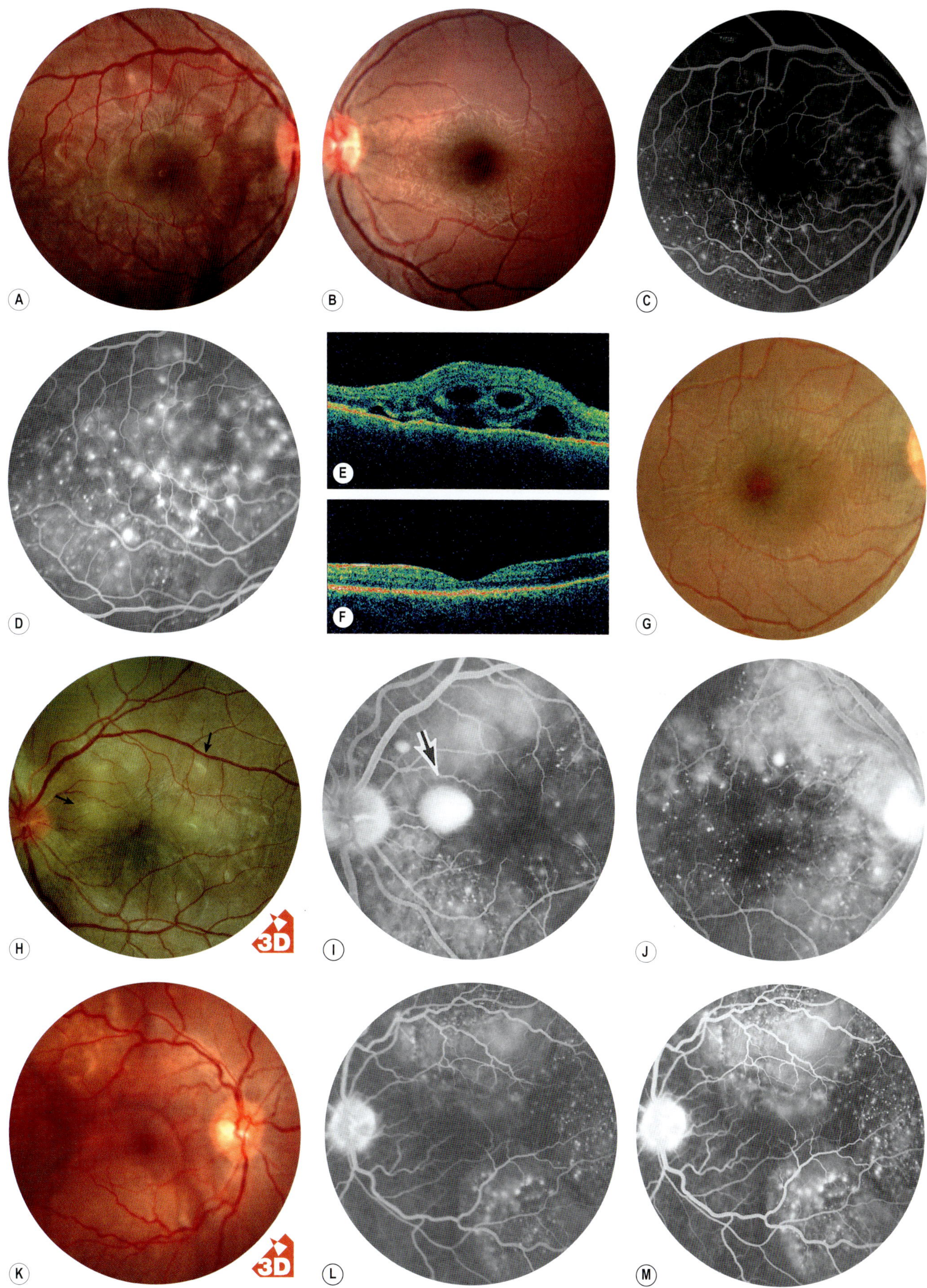
A
B
C
D
E
F
G
H
3D
I
J
K
3D
L
M

SYMPATHETIC UVEITIS

Patients who have sustained a previous penetrating ocular injury, whether accidental or postoperative, affecting the uveal tract of one eye may experience visual symptoms caused by either diffuse or multifocal areas of granulomatous choroiditis in the second eye.[302–310] This is often accompanied by evidence of iridocyclitis. Sympathetic uveitis occasionally occurs following unusual circumstances such as proton beam, plaque, and helium ion irradiation treatment of choroidal melanomas,[311] and cyclodiode laser photocoagulation.[302,309,311–313] The posterior form of sympathetic uveitis, in which the earliest changes are confined to the posterior uveal tract, probably occurs less frequently than the anterior or more diffuse form of the disease.[303–305,314–316]

The onset of symptoms in the sympathizing eye usually occurs between 2 weeks and 6 months following injury to the inciting eye, though it has been reported even 50 years from the time of injury. The incidence is highest in the first year after injury. Light sensitivity, transient obscurations of vision, and lacrimation are frequent prodromal symptoms. The previously traumatized eye usually shows signs of inflammation. Patients with predominantly posterior-segment disease may show evidence of either diffuse (Figure 11.29A–C) or multifocal choroidal involvement (Figure 11.29D–G). In the former there may be one or more areas of localized serous detachment of the retina. These detachments soon become confluent and often result in bullous retinal detachment. Fluorescein angiography may show evidence of multifocal areas of choriocapillaris hypoperfusion and multiple pinpoint areas of fluorescein staining that enlarge during the course of the study (Figure 11.29B, C, E, and F).[273,314,317,318]

Patients with multifocal choroiditis may show scattered, gray-white, slightly elevated subretinal nodules (Figure 11.29D) that may extend throughout the fundus. The clinical and angiographic picture of multifocal granulomas in sympathetic uveitis simulates closely that seen in APMPPE (Figure 11.29D–G).[303,305,315] The lesions in sympathetic uveitis appear slightly elevated, whereas in APMPPE they are flat. The early-phase angiographic picture is identical in both disorders, but in the later phases the central portion of lesions stains less well in sympathetic uveitis (Figure 11.29E and F). The posterior form resembles VKH disease closely with pockets of subretinal fluid that show pinpoint hyperfluorescence early, and leak dye into the SRF late on the angiogram (Figure 11.29 L–O). Some patients may also develop hearing loss, tinnitus, and vitiligo similar to patients with complete VKH syndrome.[319–321]

Histopathologically, the uveal tract is infiltrated by either diffuse or multifocal areas of granulomatous inflammation (Figure 11.29J–L). The lymphocytic infiltration is composed of predominantly T-activated lymphocytes. The T-helper to suppressor ratio is approximately 3:1:4:1.[322,323] The underlying immune pathogenesis in sympathetic uveitis is probably a delayed hypersensitivity to ocular antigens, melanin or related antigen, and/or a soluble fraction from the outer segments of the receptor cells similar to that found in VKH syndrome.[282]

In the diffuse form of sympathetic uveitis the inflammatory reaction may spare the choriocapillaris, but in the nodular form of the disease it causes occlusion of the choriocapillaris and inflammatory cellular detachments of the RPE (Dalen–Fuchs nodules) (Figure 11.29K and L).[303,305,308,310,315,324–330] These latter nodules correspond with the multifocal gray lesions that show delayed central staining with fluorescein.

11.29 Posterior sympathetic uveitis.

A–C: Early posterior sympathetic uveitis and minimal serous retinal detachment in the right eye of a 10-year-old boy 2 months after surgical repair of an anterior scleral rupture of the left eye caused by a firecracker injury. He noted the recent onset of blurred vision in the right eye. Visual acuity was 20/70 right eye and hand movements only left eye. There were 2 + cells and flare in the anterior chamber of the right eye. Note the multiple confluent light-gray lesions at the level of the retinal pigment epithelium (A). These lesions, which are caused by multifocal choroidal granulomas, obstruct the choriocapillaris and appear nonfluorescent early. Histopathologic examination of the left eye confirmed the diagnosis of sympathetic uveitis.

D–K: Posterior sympathetic uveitis simulating acute posterior multifocal placoid pigment epitheliopathy in a 32-year-old man with photophobia, floaters, and paracentral scotomata in the right eye 6 months after penetrating injury to the left eye and 2 months after a trans pars plana vitrectomy in the same eye. Visual acuity in the right eye was 20/15 and in the left eye was no light perception. The left eye was phthisical. Note the multiple gray-white, slightly elevated, subretinal lesions that were also present in the peripheral fundus (D). There were a few inflammatory cells in the vitreous and aqueous humor. There was no serous detachment of the retina. Early angiograms showed that the subretinal lesions were nonfluorescent (E). Later angiograms showed that the lesions stained initially at their edges (F). Four years later the patient had experienced progressive loss of peripheral and central vision in spite of corticosteroid and chlorambucil treatment. Note multiple chorioretinal scars and narrowing of the retinal vessels (G and H). Gross examination of the patient's left eye, which was enucleated 1 day after photographs in D–F, revealed multiple gray-white lesions (arrows) in the choroid (I). The retina was totally detached. Histopathologic examination revealed multiple choroidal granulomas and Dalen–Fuchs nodules (arrows, J and K) corresponding with the gray lesions noted in J. High-power view of choroidal granulomas and Dalen–Fuchs nodules (arrows, K) revealed obliteration of the choriocapillaris beneath the nodules.

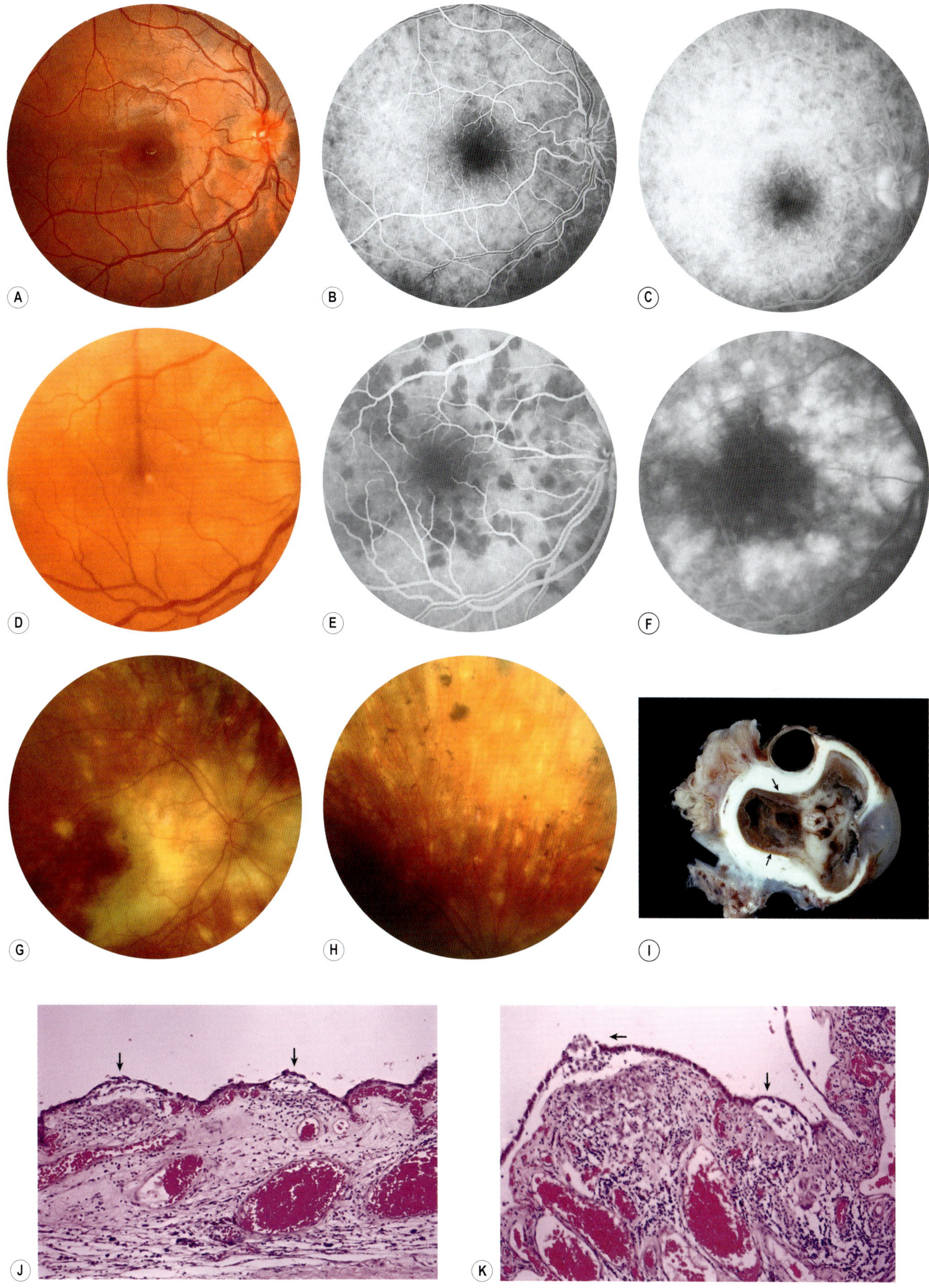
A
B
C
D
E
F
G
H
I
J
K

Rao and his group experimentally induced a granulomatous disease that closely mimics sympathetic ophthalmia by using 5–10 μg of retinal S antigen. In their study of experimental allergic uveitis in guinea pigs, they found varying the dose of S antigen induced varying severity of uveitis; 50 μg produced a massive panophthalmitis containing polymorphonuclear leukocytes, eosinophils, and mononuclear cells, 25 μg produced a less severe panuveitis, 5–10 μg produced a granulomatous uveitis made up of epithelioid and mononuclear cells, and 1 μg produced nongranulomatous uveitis. Lowering the dose eliminated polymorphonuclear leukocytes and eosinophils, suggesting higher antigen dosages may either superimpose immune complex response, or replace a cell-mediated immune disease.[331]

Both the diffuse and the multifocal choroidal lesions of sympathetic ophthalmia will respond promptly to systemic corticosteroid therapy, and they often leave multiple focal areas of RPE atrophy and depigmentation of the choroidal melanocytes (Figure 11.29H and I). Exacerbation, however, is common. Immunosuppressives such as antimetabolites – methotrexate and cytoxan – and immunomodulating drugs such as mycophenolate mofetil are necessary in severe and recurrent cases. High-dose initial treatment followed by a low-dose maintenance therapy is necessary. Placement of an intravitreal steroid implant may be used for selected cases where the inciting eye may be enucleated or phthisical. Subretinal neovascularization may occasionally arise in one of the macular scars.[332] Severe chronic inflammation may cause marked proliferation of subretinal fibrous tissue, widespread degenerative changes in the RPE, narrowing of the retinal vessel, night blindness, and eventually total blindness.[333] The value of enucleating the inciting eye after sympathetic ophthalmia has set in is open to question.[306,308,310,327,334–336]

11.29 Continued

L–O: This 48-year-old male from India developed exudative retinal detachment in his left eye (L) a few years after the right eye had a penetrating injury. His vision was 20/400 in his only eye that showed early hypofluorescent spots in the temporal macula (M), with appearance of tiny pinpoint dots later in the angiogram that eventually leaked fluorescein that pooled in the subretinal space (N and O).

(L–O, courtesy of Dr. Vishali Gupta.)

An increased frequency of HLA-A11 antigens in patients with sympathetic uveitis suggests that a genetic factor may play a role in its pathogenesis.[337]

Sympathetic ophthalmia may rarely occur in the setting of bacterial endophthalmitis or other infections.[338–340] In patients with exogenous postoperative bacterial endophthalmitis or endophthalmitis following trauma, signs of inflammation in the fellow eye should alert the ophthalmologist about the possibility of sympathetic ophthalmia. In a series by Rathinam and Rao, of 26 patients with sympathetic ophthalmia, 4 also had bacterial endophthalmitis, most of them postoperative.[340] It was believed previously that an infection would destroy the antigens that induce sympathetic ophthalmia; however, the infection may not be as severe and some antigens may persist that can incite sympathetic response. It is also possible for patients with sympathetic ophthalmia to present only with posterior-segment findings when termed posterior sympathetic ophthalmia.[341] These patients may show evidence of anterior-segment involvement or vitritis only at the time of recurrence and not at the first episode of sympathetic ophthalmia. Any signs of uveitis, especially associated with exudative retinal detachment in a fellow eye, should alert the ophthalmologist about the likelihood of posterior sympathetic ophthalmia.[137]

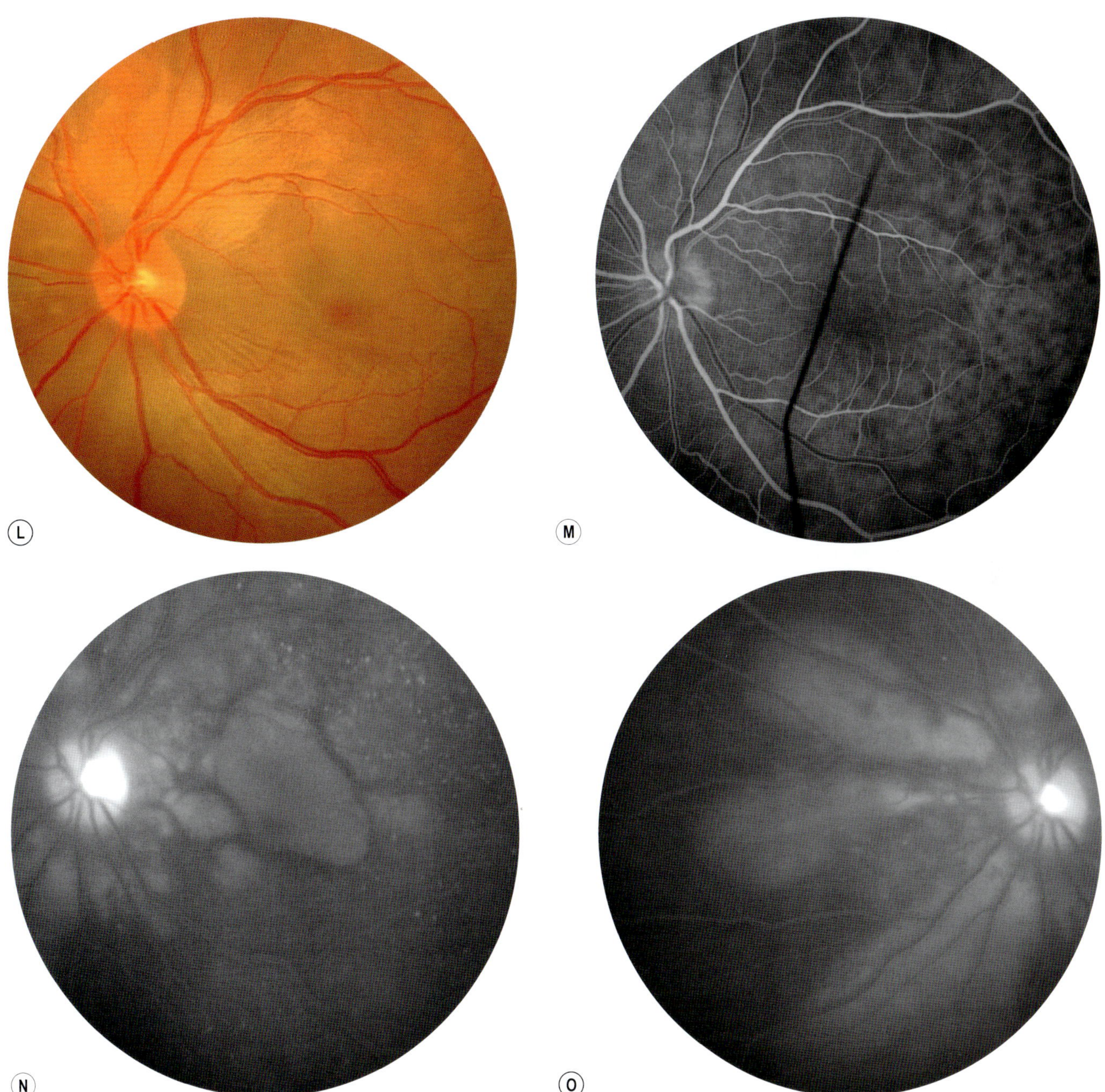
L
M
N
O

ACUTE EXUDATIVE POLYMORPHOUS VITELLIFORM MACULOPATHY

Gass and coworkers reported two young lightly pigmented white adult males who presented because of the acute onset of headaches and visual loss associated with multiple yellow-white ill-defined subretinal lesions and serous retinal detachment in the macular area of both eyes (Figure 11.30A, B, and H).[342] The focal lesions demonstrated early hyperfluorescence and mild late staining (Figure 11.30C, D, and I). One patient had a few vitreous cells. Both patients were treated with oral corticosteroids. Over the following weeks gradual improvement of visual acuity was associated with development of prominent polymorphous deposits of subretinal yellow pigment that tended to gravitate to form a meniscus, giving an appearance similar to that in Best's vitelliform dystrophy (Figure 11.30E, F, J, and K). The visual acuity returned to normal levels and incomplete resolution of the yellow pigment occurred in both patients. It is probable that the yellow pigment is a product of damaged pigment epithelium and/or photoreceptors and not a result of lipoproteins escaping from the choroidal vasculature. Both patients had subnormal electro-oculographic findings, but neither had a family history of eye disease. The peculiar fundoscopic and angiographic findings during the early stage of this disease are similar to those which occur in patients who present with bilateral acute visual loss and retinal detachment caused by bilateral uveal melanocytic proliferation associated with an occult carcinoma (see p. 1202).

11.30 Acute exudative polymorphous vitelliform maculopathy.

A–G: In June 1982 this 24-year-old man presented with a 2-day history of headaches and progressive loss of vision in both eyes. His visual acuity was 20/50, right eye and 20/40, left eye. There was exudative detachment of the retina centrally, and numerous oval, round, and curvilinear yellow-white lesions underlying confluent blisterlike areas of serous retinal detachment bilaterally (A and B). Note the striking early hyperfluorescence of the yellow-white lesions (C) and minimal late staining (D). He received prednisone 80 mg daily and 1 week later visual acuity was 20/20, right eye, and 20/25, left eye. Accompanying resolution of the subretinal fluid was the development of large amounts of yellow subretinal material that showed a tendency to gravitate inferiorly (E, December 1982, and F, June 1983). When last seen in June 1984, visual acuity was 20/20 bilaterally and most of the yellow material had disappeared (G).

H–L: This 30-year-old presented with a 1-month history of visual loss and severe headaches. His findings and clinical course were similar to those of the previous patient. H and I, August 1984; J and K, April 1985; L, October 1985.

(A–L from Gass et al.[342])

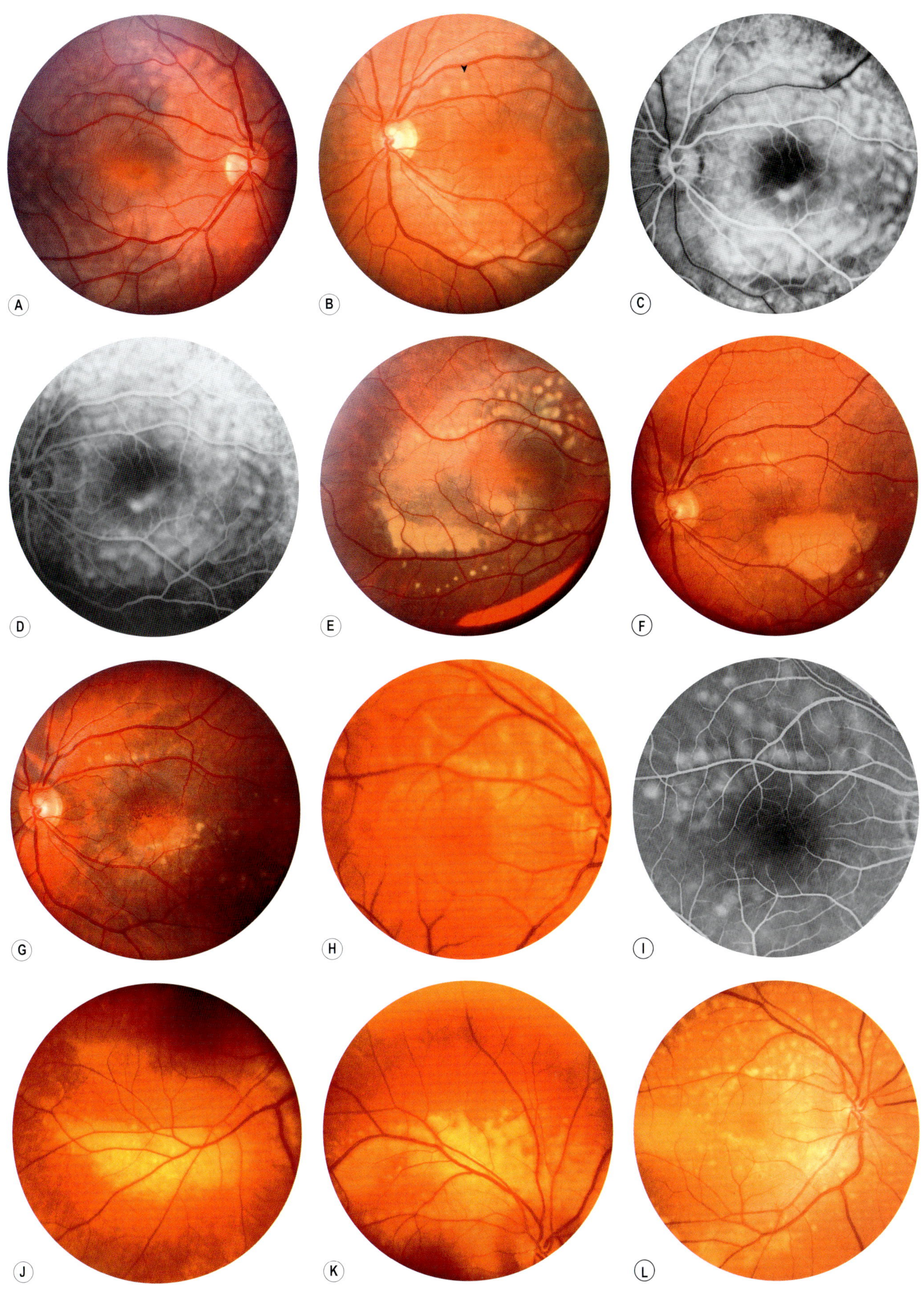
A
B
C
D
E
F
G
H
I
J
K
L

Since the original description of two men by Gass in 1988, there have been several isolated reports of acute exudative polymorphous vitelliform maculopathy that have been described, including women, and even in a child at age 11.[343–347] The majority of patients show a decrease in EOG function, which may recover. Multifocal ERG has shown decreased cone function in the acute phase, sometimes persisting even after visual recovery has occurred.[344] The yellow material hangs around in the subretinal space for several months, even up to 1 or 2 years. A few patients show complete resolution of the yellow material with no residual macular changes; however, many of them show focal irregular pigment epithelial atrophy and changes. On ICG, the material shows gradual hyperfluorescence and staining similar to the appearance on fluorescein angiography (Figure 11.31O).[345] There is increased autofluorescence of the yellow material,[343] suggesting these fluorophores are byproducts possibly of photoreceptors (Figure 11.31P and Q).[348] Headache is a persistent finding in most of these patients. There has been a variable response to steroids and generally the yellow material and the serous detachment resolve over several months to 1–2 years. OCT shows that the yellow material lies between the RPE and the photoreceptors and is also characterized by several isolated or confluent serous detachments.[346]

11.31 Acute idiopathic exudative polymorphous vitelliform maculopathy.

A–I: On June 30, 1982, this previously healthy 24-year-old man presented with a 2-day history of acute headaches and loss of vision in both eyes. Visual acuity, right eye was 20/50 and left eye 20/40. In both eyes there was an oval serous retinal detachment surrounded by radiating retinal folds in the central macula, and numerous oval, round, and irregular yellow-white lesions underlying confluent blisterlike areas of serous retinal detachment that extended throughout the macular and juxtapapillary areas (A and B). Early-phase angiography revealed marked hyperfluorescence corresponding with the yellow-white lesions (C). Later angiograms showed staining of these lesions, but minimal extension of the dye into the subretinal fluid (D). He received oral prednisone and experienced a rapid return of visual acuity to near normal. Over the subsequent 8 months, however, he developed an unusual polymorphous pattern of vitelliform exudative subretinal deposits (E and F, October 1982; G and H, December 1982). These deposits cleared slowly but were still evident 2 years later in both eyes (I).
J–L: This 24-year-old man developed headaches and bilateral visual loss 2 weeks after a motor vehicle accident. His visual acuity was 20/50, right eye and 20/30, left eye. Both eyes showed an ophthalmoscopic and angiographic picture identical to that in A–D. Over the following 2 weeks the patient spontaneously became asymptomatic. He refused further examination until 1 year later when he returned with 20/20 visual acuity and multiple vitelliform lesions scattered in the peripheral macular areas.

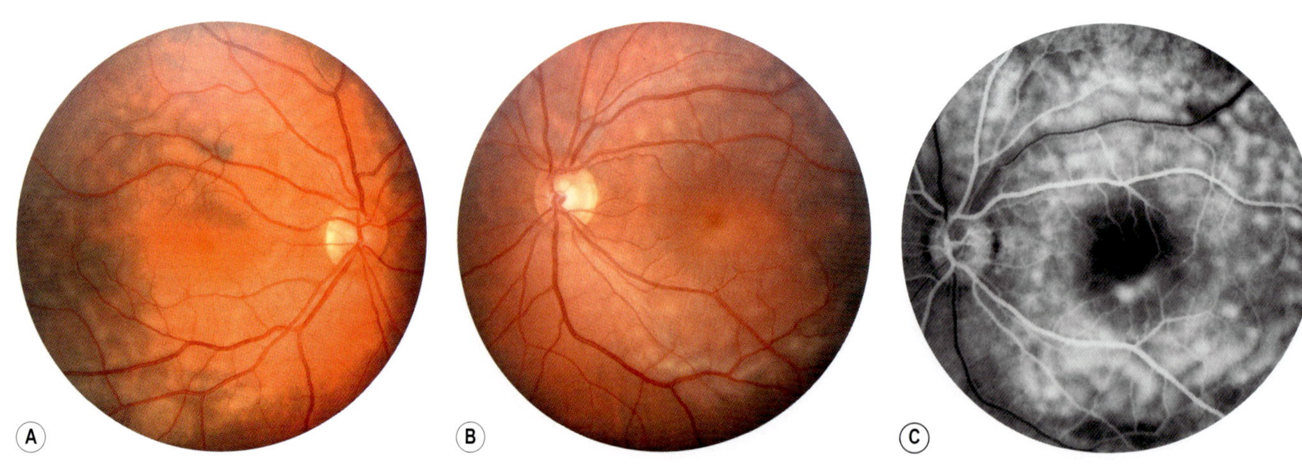

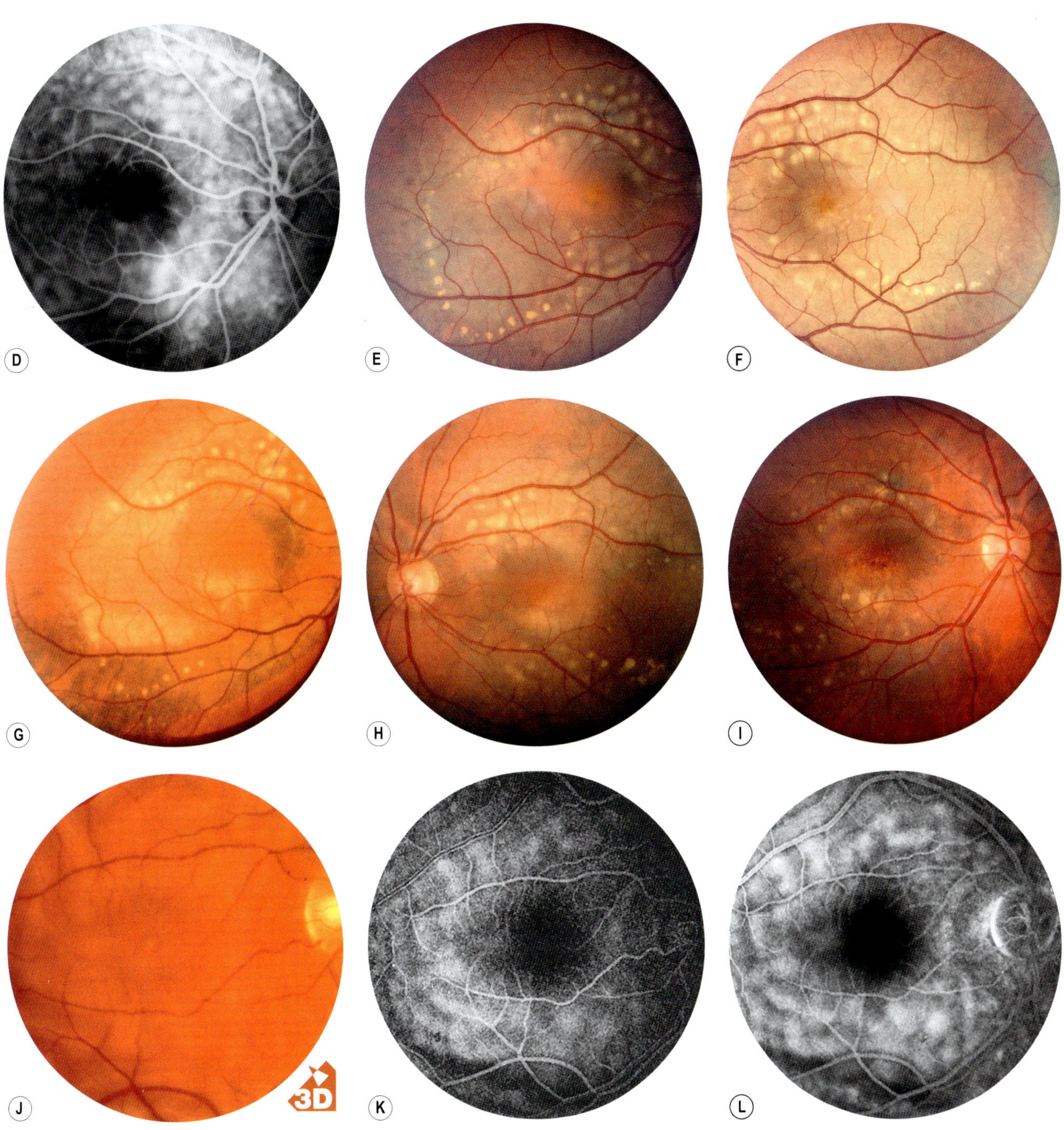
D
E
F
G
H
I
J
3D
K
L

A similar appearance has been seen as a paraneoplastic manifestation in patients with metastatic cutaneous and choroidal melanoma. Some of these cases have been unilateral.[349,350] Eksandh et al. reported positive anti-bestrophin antibodies in a patient with a solitary macular vitelliform lesion with a history of metastatic choroidal melanoma (see Chapter 13).[351] It is not known whether acute exudative polymorphous vitelliform maculopathy is an acquired inflammatory disease or an unusual manifestation of a genetically determined disorder, such as Best's disease or some other as-yet poorly defined RPE dystrophy.

11.31 Continued

M–R: A 38-year-old healthy male physician presented with headaches that worsened towards the end of the day for 2–3 months. His vision could be corrected with a mild hyperopic astigmatic correction to 20/20– in each eye. There were several small vitelliform lesions in the posterior pole and a larger pocket of subretinal fluid with yellow material at its bottom in both foveas (M and N). Indocyanine angiography showed late hyperfluorescence of the yellow lesions in both eyes (O). The vitelliform material was brilliantly autofluorescent in both eyes (P and Q). Subretinal fluid pocket could be seen on optical coherence tomography imaging in both eyes (R). He was kept under observation initially. No change in the lesions after 4 weeks prompted a course of systemic steroids for a couple of months. He did not return for follow-up but when contacted by phone revealed stabilization of vision and resolution of headache.

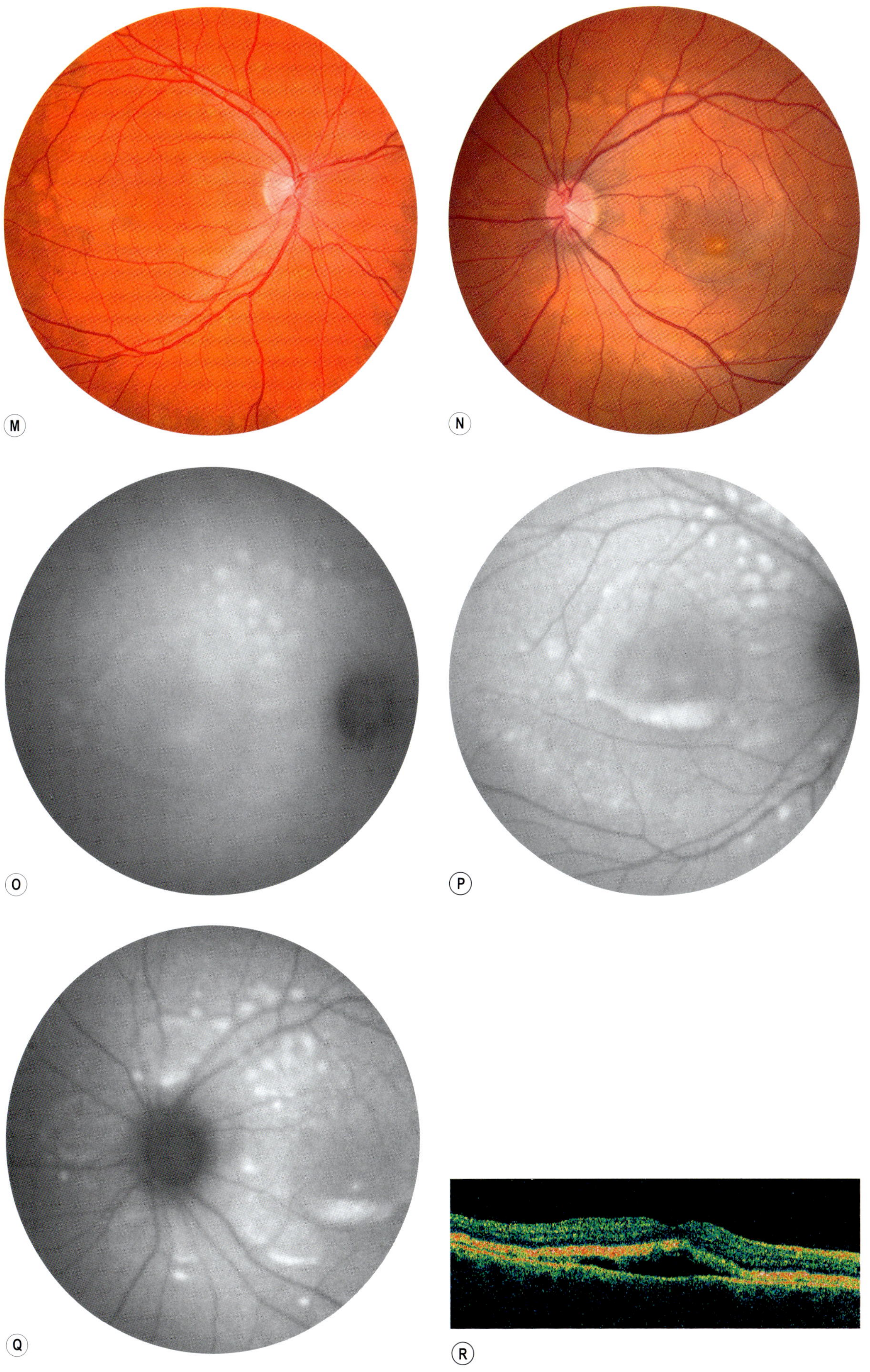
M
N
O
P
Q
R

PROGRESSIVE SUBRETINAL FIBROMATOSIS

Ophthalmoscopic evidence of varying amounts of white fibrous metaplasia of the RPE occurs in a wide variety of diseases causing retinal detachment, including idiopathic central serous chorioretinopathy, senile macular degeneration, large choroidal nevi (see Figure 14.01G), melanomas, serpiginous choroiditis (Figure 11.13D–H), sarcoidosis (see Figure 11.36J and L), and POHS.[218,352] In some cases, particularly patients with MCP, this reactive metaplastic reaction may be massive and mask the underlying cause (Figure 11.32A–C).[218,352–357] Gass has seen two such patients, who, without a recognizable cause, developed multifocal choroiditis and severe loss of vision associated with progressive growth of a thick plaque of white subretinal fibrous tissue, presumably metaplastic RPE from the juxtapapillary areas, throughout the macula and into the peripheral fundus (Figure 11.32D–J). The profound visual loss in both cases was not fully explained on the basis of the fundus findings. Histopathologic examination in one eye of each of two elderly patients who became blind in both eyes within several years of the onset of the disorder (Figure 11.32G–J) revealed widespread destruction of the retinal receptors and pigment epithelium and massive subretinal proliferation of fibrous tissue (presumably metaplasia of the RPE) overlying a diffuse lymphocytic, plasmacytic, and granulomatous choroiditis that was centered around fragmented, degenerated, and calcified Bruch's membrane.[354,356]

Kim et al. reported similar histopathologic findings of a 24-year-old woman who rapidly became blind because of progressive subretinal fibromatosis.[358] They described electron microscopic evidence that the subretinal fibrous tissue was derived from metaplastic pigment epithelium. They also found that the retinal Müller cells expressed class II antigens of the major histocompatibility complex. These authors and Palestine et al.[357] theorize that the histopathologic changes may be caused by an autoimmune antibody-mediated inflammation in which local antibody production to the RPE occurs. The clinical and histopathological findings in the two patients described previously suggest that the immune reaction may have been directed to the photoreceptors as well. The granulomatous component of the inflammatory reaction may be a late response to the immune reaction-damaged and devitalized Bruch's membrane, similar to that seen around Bruch's membrane in eyes of primates with experimentally induced autoimmune uveitis to interphotoreceptor retinoid-binding protein,[222] inflammation surrounding Bruch's membrane and the internal limiting membrane of the retina after herpes zoster chorioretinitis,[355] around degenerated Descemet's membrane after herpes simplex keratitis,[359] and in the vicinity of calcified and degenerated internal elastic lamina of large arteries in giant cell arteritis.

11.32 Massive subretinal fibromatosis.

A–C: A healthy young black woman noted progressive loss of vision in both eyes. Note the thick plaque of white fibrous tissue surrounding the optic disc and extending throughout most of the posterior fundus. Medical evaluation failed to reveal a cause for this process.

D–J: A healthy 68-year-old white woman developed granulomatous uveitis in both eyes and experienced progressive loss of vision in the left eye to no light perception, and in the right eye to light perception only, within 3 years. The left fundus was obscured by a cataract. There were widespread areas of peripheral and peripapillary subretinal fibrous tissue proliferation in the right fundus (D–F). The optic disc was pale. Neurologic and medical examination was negative. The left eye was enucleated. Histopathologic examination revealed extensive subretinal fibrous metaplasia of the retinal pigment epithelium (arrows, G and H) overlying a granulomatous reaction centered around a fragmented and degenerated Bruch's membrane throughout the eye (H–J). Note giant cells, some of which are engulfing pieces of calcified Bruch's membrane (arrow, J).

(A–C, courtesy of Dr. William R. Rimm.)

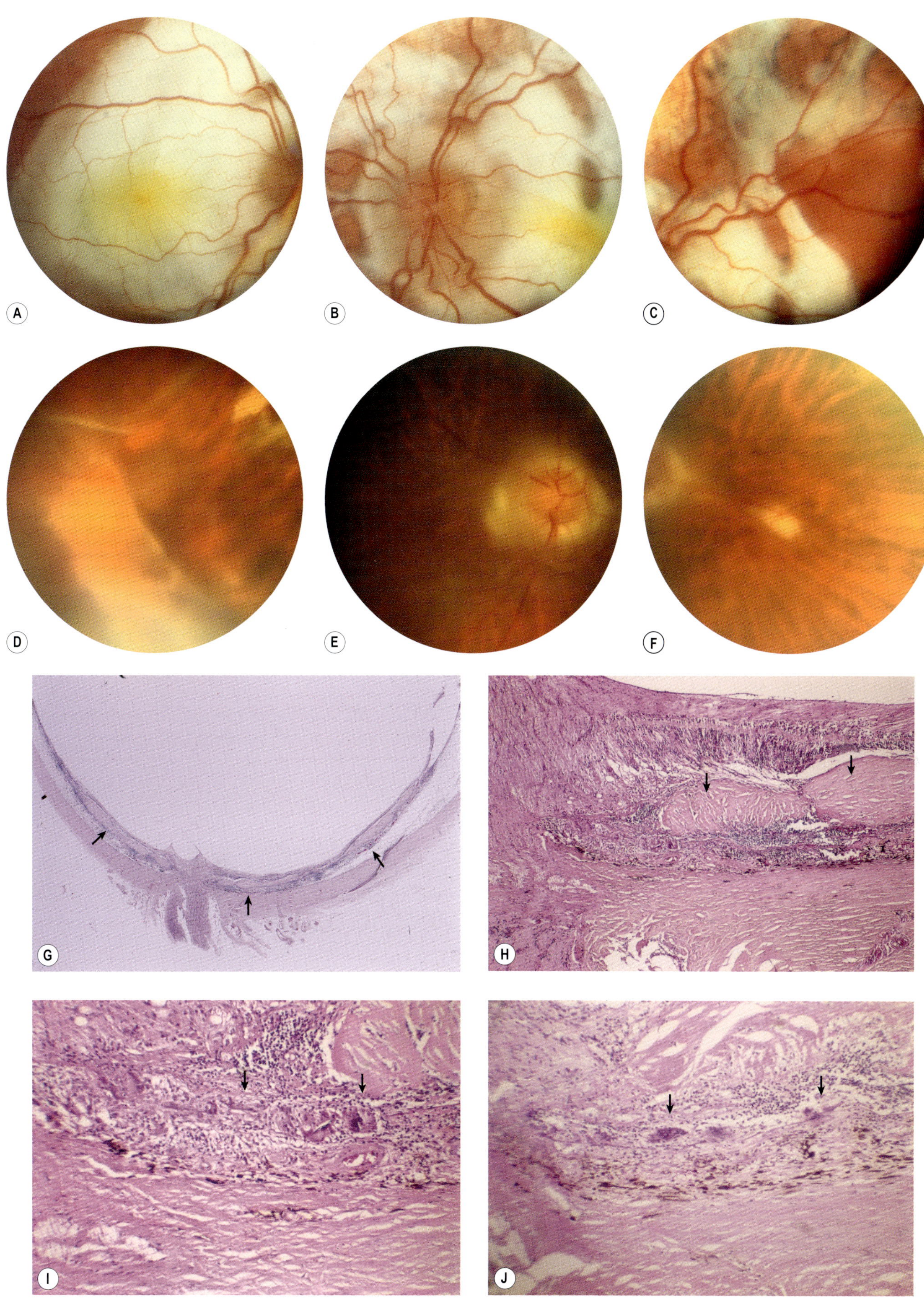
A
B
C
D
E
F
G
H
I
J

POSTERIOR SCLERITIS

Rheumatoid scleritis is an inflammatory disease that may involve the sclera, either diffusely or in a circumscribed fashion. The intensity of the inflammatory reaction varies from that of an acute necrotizing granuloma at one end of the spectrum to a very low-grade chronic sclerosing granulomatous inflammatory reaction.[360] Although most patients have involvement of the sclera anteriorly, in approximately 10–15% of cases the focus of scleritis and overlying uveitis may be confined to the posterior portions of the globe and produce a retinal detachment with or without a subretinal tumefaction (Figures 11.33, 11.34H–J, and 11.35).[360–371] In the latter patients, ocular pain or tenderness, injection of the conjunctival and episcleral vessels, evidence of intraocular inflammation, and a history of rheumatoid arthritis (present in only 50% or fewer of the patients) are features that should arouse suspicion of scleritis. Acute posterior scleritis may cause multifocal areas of white subretinal exudation and serous retinal detachment (Figure 11.33A, E, and G). In some patients an acute inflammatory reaction surrounding the focus of necrotic sclera is sufficiently violent that a posterior scleral abscess occurs and produces a subretinal hypopyon (Figure 11.33G) or a rapidly expanding subretinal mass, retinal whitening, and exudative retinal detachment and vitritis (Figure 11.33K and L).[360] This is accompanied by severe pain and in some cases proptosis.

11.33 Posterior scleritis.

A–D: Unilateral posterior scleritis in a 24-year-old woman complaining of pain and loss of vision in the left eye. Note the ill-defined white areas (arrows) beneath the localized serous retinal detachment in the macula (A). Angiograms (stereoangiograms B–D) show multifocal leaks at the level of the retinal pigment epithelium (RPE) in the area of choroidoscleral thickening.

E and **F:** This 41-year-old black woman noted blurred vision and pain in the right eye. She had injection of the right eye and mild proptosis. There was juxtapapillary serous retinal detachment and the whitish subretinal exudate (E).

G–I: This woman noted acute onset of pain, redness, and a superior scotoma in the left eye. She had episcleritis, and posterior scleritis associated with a localized exudative detachment of the retina (arrowheads, G) inferiorly. Note the intense whitening and flecks of subretinal blood at the focus of sclerochoroiditis (white arrow) and the subretinal hypopyon (black arrow). Angiography showed staining initially in the area of RPE damage and later staining of the subretinal exudate (H). Ultrasound (I) revealed focal thickening of the choroidoscleral layer and an echolucent zone overlying this area posteriorly. Her symptoms and ocular changes responded promptly to systemic corticosteroid treatment.

J–L: An acute posterior rheumatoid scleral abscess developed in the left fundus of a 19-year-old woman with severe intractable pain and visual loss in the left eye (K). Note the white subretinal exudate overlying an elevated sclerochoroidal mass. She had a past history of acute necrotizing scleritis in the left eye (J), thrombocytopenic purpura, polyarthritis, and pneumonia. The ocular pain and abscess failed to respond to systemic corticosteroid and azathioprine therapy. Surgical drainage of the scleral abscess resulted in prompt resolution of the exudative mass, retinal detachment, and pain (L). Several years later this patient died because of widespread unclassified collagen vascular disease.

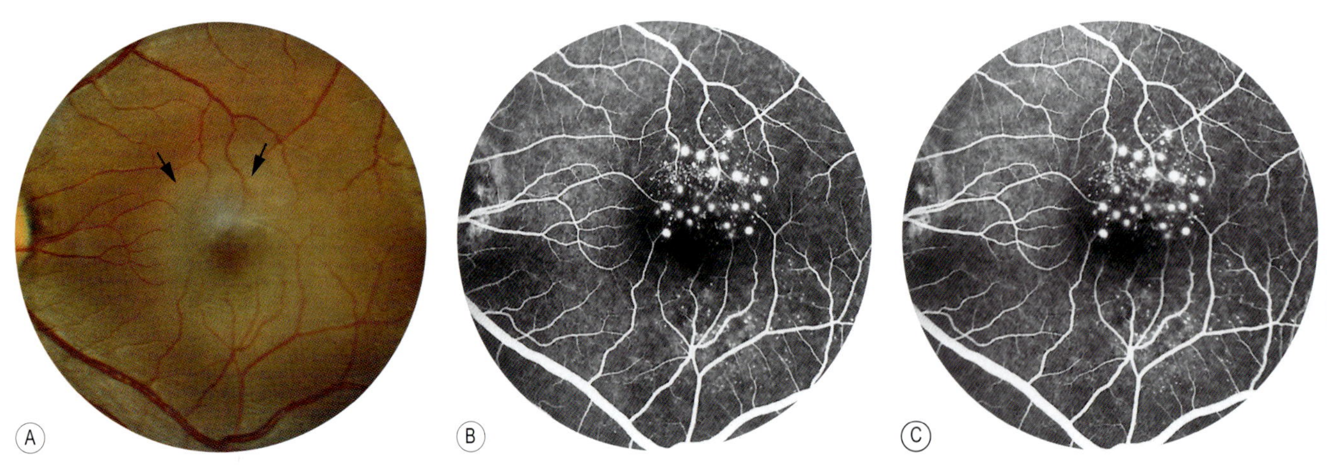

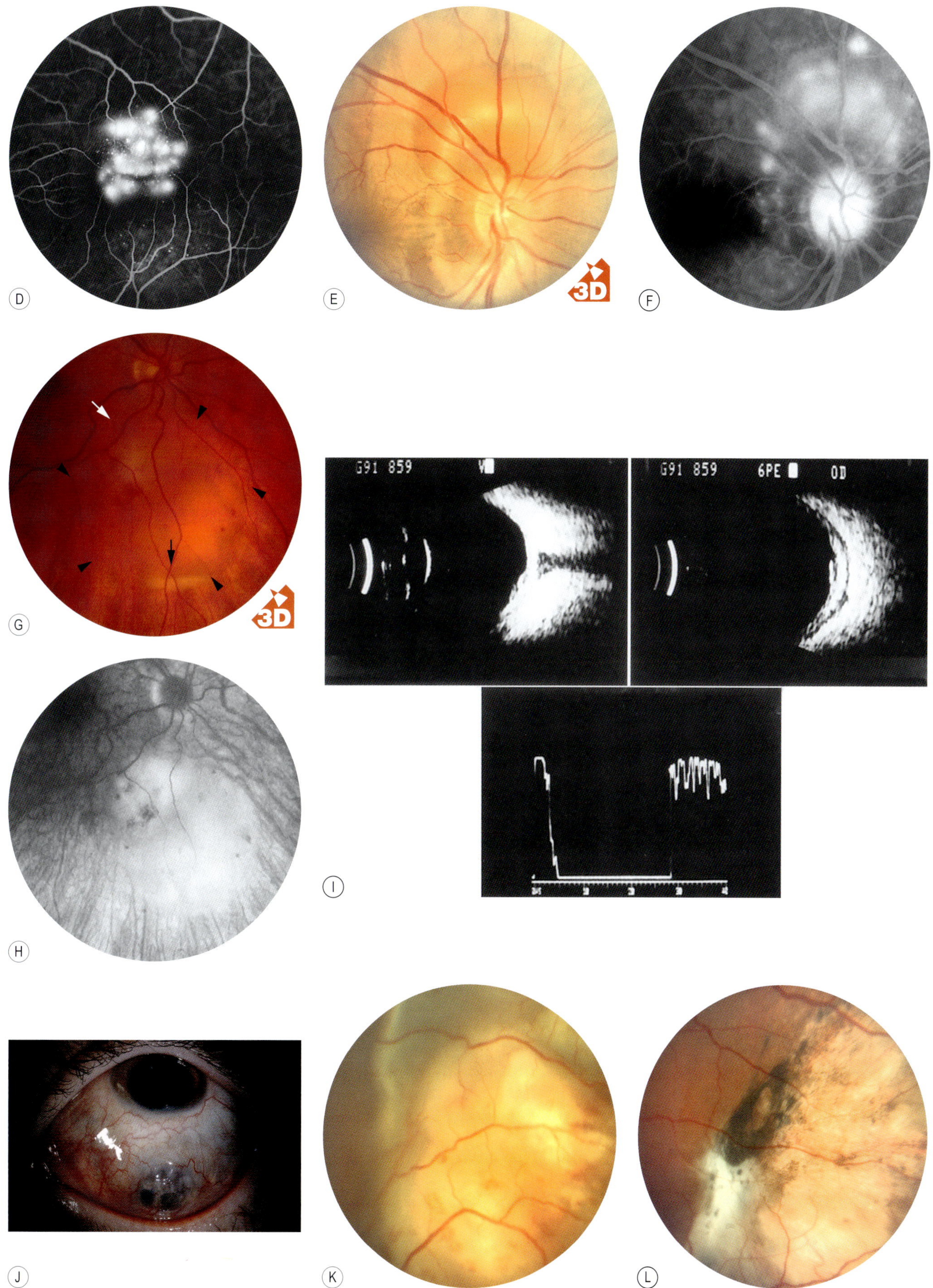
D
E
3D
F
G
3D
G91 859
G91 859 6PE OD
H
I
J
K
L

In other patients the inflammatory reaction is subacute and fewer inflammatory signs accompany the development of a subretinal mass and retinal detachment. In still other patients there may be no clinical history or findings to suggest the presence of an underlying chronic granulomatous mass lesion that is largely confined to the sclera (Figure 11.35A–F).[360,367] In patients with minimal signs of inflammation elevation of the relatively intact choroid and RPE produces an intraocular mass that is orange-colored. The presence of focal lymphoid follicles in the choroid may cause scattered yellow-white nodules on the surface of the tumor (Figure 11.35A, B, and D–G). Chorioretinal folds are frequently evident ophthalmoscopically and angiographically at the edge of these tumors (Figure 11.35C).[360,361] Focal areas of scleritis, when located anywhere in the fundus, may be associated with cystoid macular edema (Figure 11.35J). Chronic scleritis may occasionally be the underlying cause of uveal effusion.[372] Branch retinal artery occlusion and simultaneous central retinal artery and vein occlusions have been described in severe cases.[373,374]

Fluorescein angiography in patients with acute and subacute posterior scleritis and localized exudative detachment typically shows multiple small foci of leaking at the level of the RPE (Figures 11.33B, C, D, and F, and 11.35H and I). In chronic scleritis angiography often demonstrates evidence of folding of the inner choroid (Figure 11.35C). Angiography is of little value in differentiating either the acute or the chronic nodular scleritis from melanomas. The characteristic histopathologic lesion in rheumatoid scleritis is a zonal type of granulomatous inflammatory reaction of variable intensity around a focus of necrotic sclera.

The acute and subacute lesions usually respond to systemic or intraorbital injections of corticosteroids. Nonsteroidal anti-inflammatory agents used alone or combined with corticosteroids, as well as intravenous pulse corticosteroid therapy, may have some advantages over orally administered corticosteroids alone.[375–378] The large brawny lesions containing much fibrous tissue respond poorly to corticosteroid therapy (Figure 11.35A–F). Cyclosporine and mycophenolate mofetil therapy may be helpful in severe scleritis refractory to other treatment.[379]

Ultrasonography is useful in differentiating these lesions from uveal melanomas (Figure 11.33I). Scleral thickening, producing moderately high internal reflectivity, with an adjacent echolucent area caused by edema in Tenon's space is characteristic of posterior scleritis (Figure 11.34I).[363] Computed tomography may also be useful in the differential diagnosis of posterior scleritis.[380] The physician must be aware, however, of the occasional association of placoid choroidal melanomas and posterior scleritis.[381] These patients may present with ocular pain, blurred vision, and anterior-chamber and vitreous inflammatory cell reaction that respond to corticosteroid therapy. Occasionally eyes have been enucleated with a mistaken diagnosis of choroidal melanoma. Severe pain and lack of anterior scleritis led to a mistaken diagnosis of plateau iris and gonioplasty in the patient shown in Figure 11.34 (H–J).

11.34 Posterior scleritis – systemic associations.

A–D: This 73-year-old white male had recurrent episodes of scleritis. The first episode occurred 8 months previously and was treated with oral prednisone. His medical history was significant for type 2 diabetes, hyperlipidemia, and mild arthralgia. Visual acuity was 20/30 in the right eye and 20/60 in the left eye. Intraocular pressure was 13 mmHg on the right and 26 mmHg on the left. The left fundus showed 2+ vitreous cells and mild nonproliferative diabetic retinopathy. The right eye also had nonproliferative diabetic retinopathy. The left eye revealed diffuse scleritis and he was started on a high dose of oral steroids, topical Cosopt, and topical steroids. One month later he developed night sweats and a low-grade fever with intermittent throbbing discomfort in his right ankle joint. His visual acuity was 20/25 on the right and 20/80 in the left. The left fundus showed cystoid macular edema that was visible on the angiogram (B and C). He complained of ear pain over the last year. At his third episode, recurrent left-ear pain and swelling (D) helped make the diagnosis of relapsing polychondritis.
E–G: A 72-year-old woman with rheumatoid arthritis and history of recurrent scleritis. She was stable with 20/40 vision till she came off steroids about 10 days before. She returned with severe pain, redness (E), and loss of vision. Diffuse scleritis with extensive exudative detachment (F and G). Ultrasound B scan shows choroidal thickening and fluid in the sub-Tenon space demonstrating the T sign. She received intravenous Solu-Medrol and was restarted on prednisone and the serous retinal detachment resolved.
H–J: This 19-year-old woman had a history of recurrent deep, boring pain in her left eye for 2+ years previously. The pain often woke her up from sleep. She had been diagnosed as plateau iris for this and received gonioplasty (J) previously. Note the peripheral iris spots from the gonioplasty (J). The pain and inflammation from the scleritis made her unable to open her eye (H). Fundus examination showed retinal folds in the macula. An ultrasound B scan (I) showed sub-Tenon fluid confirming posterior scleritis, which responded to oral steroids with resolution of her symptoms.

(A to D, courtesy of Dr. Ranjeet Dhaliwal. A-C, Also, Yannuzzi Lawrence J., The Retinal Atlas, Saunders 2010, 978-0-7020-3320-9, p.293.)

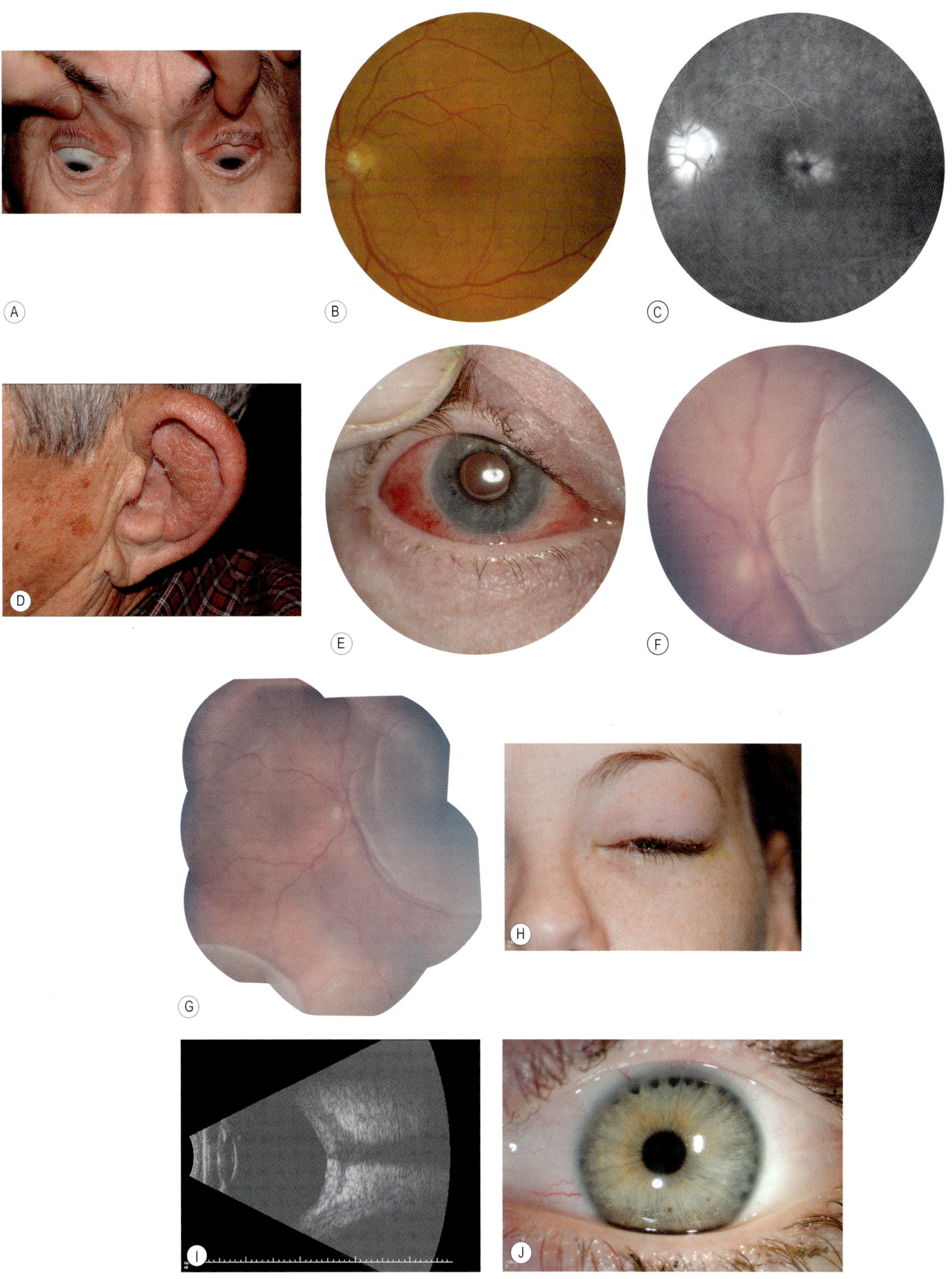
A
B
C
D
E
F
G
H
I
J

Gass has seen posterior scleritis in 2 patients with typical psoriatic arthritis (Figure 11.35G–I) Posterior scleritis has also been reported in association with Wegener's granulomatosis,[382–387] relapsing polychondritis,[388,389] procainamide-induced lupus,[390] systemic idiopathic fibrosis,[391] toxoplasmosis retinochoroiditis,[392] and malignant melanoma of the choroid.[381] Wegener's granulomatosis is a necrotizing granulomatous vasculitis that causes sinusitis, necrotizing lung granulomas, glomerular nephritis, and involvement of other organs, including the eye. In the latter case, it may cause proptosis, orbital cellulitis, scleritis, keratitis, marginal corneal scleral ulceration, and optic nerve vasculitis. A few patients may present early in the course of the disease with loss of central vision as a result of a combined uveal and retinal detachment caused by an area of sclerouveitis.[382–387] Jensen et al. reported an unusual association of an epibulbar granuloma and a massive nodular scleritis in a 5-year-old boy with no evidence of systemic disease.[368] Relapsing inflammation of the cartilage of the other ear with nonerosive polyarthritis and chondritis of the nasal cartilage, tracheobronchial chondritis, and lesions in the inner ear is a feature of relapsing polychondritis. The ocular findings have been reported with proptosis, lid edema, lacrimal pseudotumor, episcleritis, scleritis (Figure 11.34A–D), choroidal infiltrates, uveitis, and optic neuritis. High-dose steroid therapy along with cyclophosphamide, and dapsone have been used. Plasmapheresis can be used for severe relapses.

Most patients with posterior scleritis are adults and there is a slight preponderance of females. Wald et al. reported 4 boys with diminished visual acuity, mild ocular pain, lack of systemic disease, exudative retinal detachment, multiple pinpoint leaks angiographically, and b-scan ultrasonographic evidence of scleral and choroidal thickening.[301] The latter was accompanied by evidence of episcleral edema in only 2 patients. They all recovered good visual function after treatment with corticosteroids and noncorticosteroid medications. Wald et al. attributed this syndrome to posterior scleritis but could not exclude the possibility of Harada's disease.

Occult posterior scleritis has been implicated in the causation of idiopathic chorioretinal folds (see Chapter 4).[393,394] Whereas chorioretinal folds are a frequent manifestation of acute and chronic posterior nodular scleritis, it is not known whether inflammation of the sclera is a precursor of the shrinkage and flattening of the posterior sclera that are characteristically evident ultrasonographically in patients with idiopathic chorioretinal folds.

Surgically Induced Necrotizing Scleritis

SINS is a progressive scleral melt associated with inflammation occurring at previously operated scleral sites, most often after pterygum surgery with mitomycin and less often after strabismus surgery or at sclerotomy sites (Figure 11.35J–L). Judicious use of local and systemic steroids with immunosuppressives such as tacrolimus may be necessary to treat the condition.

11.35 Posterior scleritis.

A–F: Hypertrophic posterior granulomatous scleritis simulating malignant melanoma of the choroid in a healthy 54-year-old Cuban woman complaining of decreased vision unassociated with pain in the right eye of uncertain duration. Her acuity in the right eye was 20/50 and in the left eye was 20/20. She was wearing a hyperopic correction of 4.5 D in the right eye and 2.5 D in the left eye. There was a large, nonpigmented, orange subretinal mass (A and B) in the superior temporal quadrant. The mass extended posteriorly into the macular area. Oblique chorioretinal folds extended through the macular area. A number of fine, very lightly pigmented lines and scattered small white nodules (arrow, B) were present on the surface of the lesion. Angiography showed evidence of chorioretinal folds on the nasal side of the mass (C). A diagnosis of melanoma was made, and the eye was enucleated. Vertical sagittal section of the eye revealed subretinal tumor with an orange inner surface studded with multiple yellow-white nodules (arrow, D). Cut section revealed that the tumor was white and was caused by massive thickening of the sclera. The nodules on the anterior surface of the tumor were lying within the choroid, which was displaced anteriorly by the scleral tumor. Low-power photomicrographs showed extensive thickening of the posterior sclera with scattered foci of granulomatous inflammation (E). There were scattered lymphoid follicles in the choroid and episcleral region (arrow). These large follicles in the choroid were responsible for the nodules noted on the tumor surface ophthalmoscopically and grossly. High-power view of the choroid overlying the scleral mass showed a focal collection of lymphocytes and a ridgelike elevation of the pigment epithelium (arrow, F), which is believed to correspond with the fine pigmented lines noted ophthalmoscopically.

G–I: A 26-year-old woman with typical arthritis associated with psoriasis noted loss of paracentral vision in the right eye. An elevated, five-disc diameter, orange, subretinal tumor was found inferior to the macula (G). There were several gray-white nodules (arrow) on its surface. Angiography revealed staining of the tumor surface and dilated, leaking retinal capillaries as well as cystoid macular edema and optic disc staining (H). Note swelling and redness of the distal finger joints (arrows, I). This distribution of joint involvement and pitting of the fingernails that was partly obscured by the nail polish are typical of psoriatic arthritis. Ultrasonography was compatible with posterior scleritis. The lesion did not change over a 4-year period of follow-up.

Surgically induced necrotizing scleritis (SINS).

J–L: This 20-year-old male developed severe panuveitis with vitritis in his left eye. Failure of resolution of the vitritis following high doses of steroids and immunosuppressives prompted a vitrectomy. He continued to show inflammation of his sclera, in spite of improvement of vitreous inflammation, especially around the sclerotomy sites for almost a year (J-L). He was treated with methotrexate and mycophenolate mofetil, which stabilized the scleritis after almost a year.

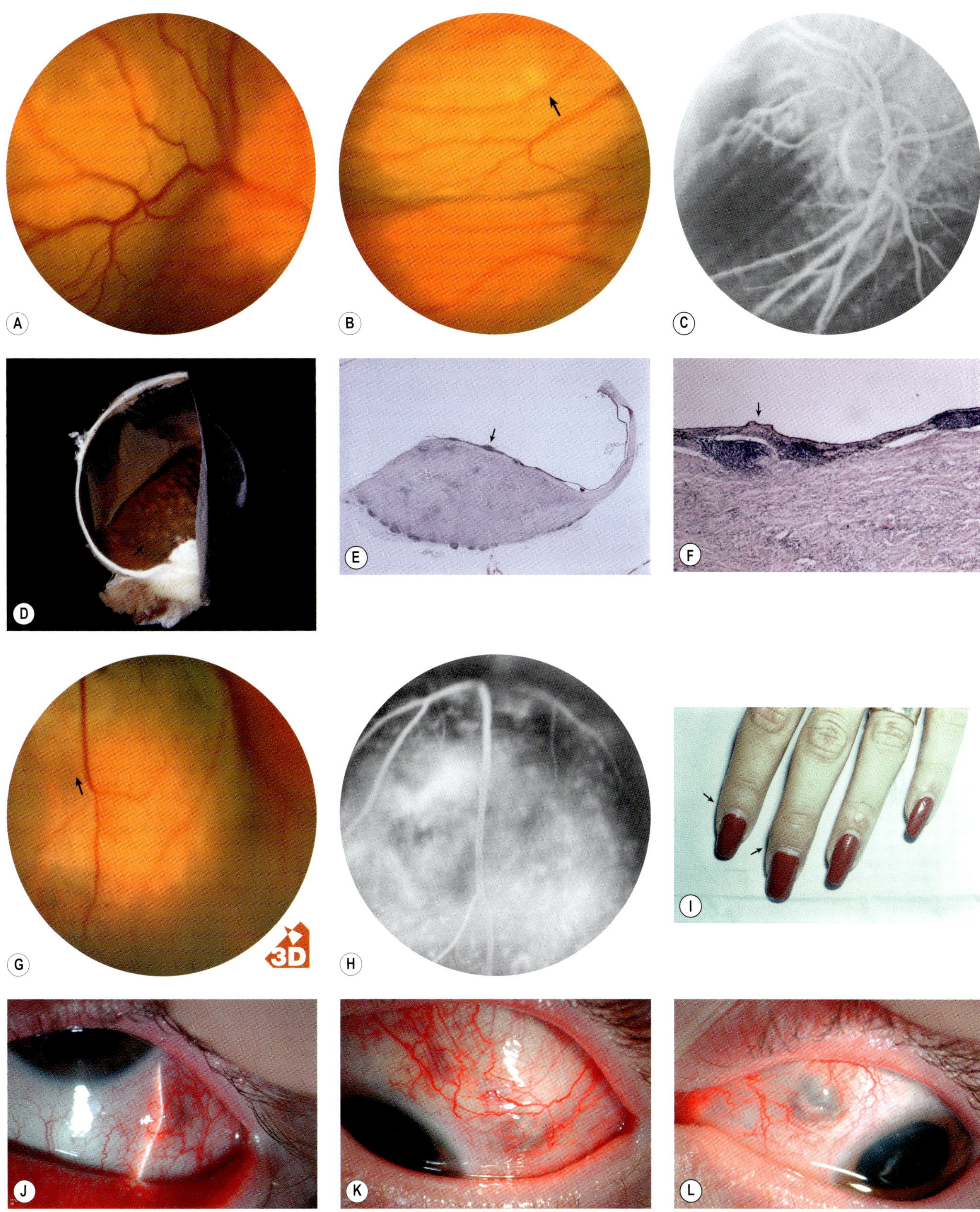
A
B
C
D
E
F
G
3D
H
I
J
K
L

CHOROIDAL SARCOIDOSIS

In the ocular fundus, sarcoidosis most frequently involves the optic nerve head, retina, and vitreous. Some patients, however, may develop one or more focal sarcoid choroidal granulomas, usually in the vicinity of the macular region. Some of these patients, who are typically young, often black individuals, have other clinical evidence of sarcoidosis.[395] They experience blurred vision secondary to a retinal detachment overlying a nonpigmented, usually slightly elevated, yellowish white choroidal mass that simulates closely that of an amelanotic melanoma, metastatic carcinoma, tuberculoma, or other choroidal masses, including choroidal osteomas (Figure 11.36).[396–399] Patients with such masses, particularly young adults, should be evaluated for other evidence of sarcoidosis. These lesions usually respond rather promptly to moderately high doses of corticosteroids systemically (Figure 11.38G–I). A 56-year-old black woman observed at the Bascom Palmer Eye Institute clinic with biopsy-proven sarcoidosis and minimal evidence of uveitis became legally blind because of progressive choroidal neovascularization and subretinal fibrosis (Figure 11.36J–L).

11.36 Sarcoid choroiditis.

A and **B:** Multifocal choroidal granulomas in a 29-year-old black woman with a 1-month history of blurred vision and photopsia and a 2-year history of dyspnea and lymphadenopathy.
D–F: Multifocal choroidal granulomas in a 25-year-old woman with biopsy-proven sarcoidosis. Note the large lesion superior to the optic disc (E) and the two small lesions (arrows, D and F). All of the lesions responded promptly to systemic corticosteroid treatment.
G–I: This 40-year-old woman developed blurred vision in the right eye associated with multiple choroidal granulomas. Note that some appear nonfluorescent (white arrows, I). She had a large area of capillary nonperfusion temporally secondary to an old branch retinal vein occlusion (arrow, H).
J–L: Progressive choroidal neovascularization and subretinal fibrosis in both eyes of a black patient with biopsy-proven sarcoidosis. Loss of vision in the left eye (K) occurred 8 years before her presentation with visual loss in the right eye (J). Angiography revealed juxtapapillary choroidal neovascularization (L). In spite of photocoagulation, she became legally blind because of progressive subretinal fibrosis.

(G–I, courtesy of Dr. David Poer.)

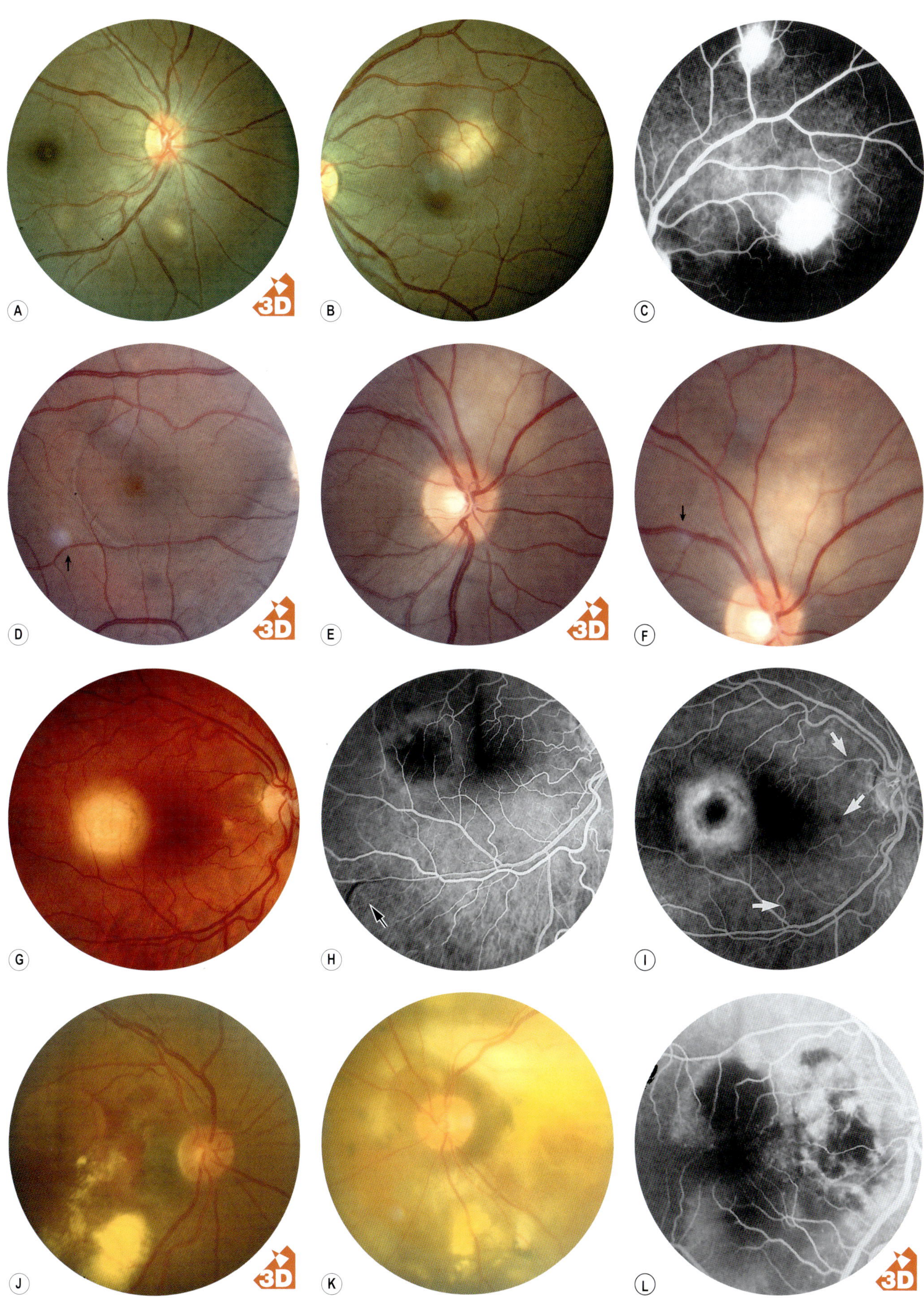
A
B
C
D
E
F
G
H
I
J
K
L

RETINAL AND OPTIC NERVE SARCOIDOSIS

Sarcoidosis is a systemic noncaseating granulomatous disease of unknown cause. Although it has protean clinical manifestations it affects the pulmonary lymph nodes and eye most often.[400–405] Ocular involvement occurs in approximately 40% of patients with sarcoidosis and is more frequent in blacks than in whites. Anterior uveitis is more common than posterior fundus involvement. Fundus lesions more frequently involve the retina than the choroid and may occur in the absence of anterior uveitis and in patients with minimal or no other evidence of systemic disease. Characteristic fundoscopic findings include perivenous exudation (Figure 11.37A, C, E, and G) with candle wax-dripping exudate,[406–409] preretinal and intravitreal white nodules often arranged in a "string of pearls,"[407,408] focal superficial and deep retinal white nodules,[407,408] papilledema, nodular papillitis, optic neuritis, and occasionally large white masses on the inner surface of the retina and optic nerve head (Figures 11.38 and 11.39).[410–417] All of these lesions are caused by epithelioid cell proliferation (Figure 11.39).[406,407,410,418,419] Branch vein occlusion,[407,420,421] central retinal vein occlusion,[415] large areas of capillary nonperfusion, retinal neovascularization,[422–425] vitreous hemorrhage, and optic disc neovascularization[419,426] may occur as complications of the granulomatous periphlebitis and phlebitis (Figure 11.39A). The neovascularization may resolve after treatment with anti-inflammatory agents.[426]

Focal granulomas may occur under the RPE (Figure 11.39C and D) and within the choroid. The predominance of T-helper lymphocytes in the choroid and retinal infiltration suggests that sarcoidosis is a disease of heightened cellular immune response, particularly at the sites of organ and tissue involvement.[427,428] Patients with sarcoidosis confined to the choroid often experience loss of central vision caused by a solitary yellow-white choroidal mass in the paracentral region that may simulate metastatic carcinoma or an amelanotic melanoma (see Figure 11.36A–I). Patients with multifocal sarcoid choroiditis may simulate patients with MCP (pseudo-POHS) and birdshot chorioretinitis.[216,429] Subretinal neovascularization and macular detachment occasionally complicate sarcoid choroiditis.[430] Sarcoidosis may cause widespread chorioretinal degeneration[431] and massive subretinal fibrosis. (see Figure 11.36J and K).

11.37 Sarcoidosis with phlebitis.

A–I: This 35-year-old African American woman was admitted for respiratory distress from presumed fungal pneumonia. Her vision was 20/20 in each eye, and the left fundus showed multifocal perivenous cuffing (A and C). Fluorescein angiogram showed focal endothelial decompensation at the sites of perivenous cuffing (B and D). Two weeks later further diffuse involvement of the veins with several retinal hemorrhages was seen (E). The right eye was now similarly involved (G) with nonperfusion of the venous tributaries (F). A chest computed tomography scan revealed bilateral mediastinal and hilar adenopathy with, calcification and angiotensin-converting enzyme returned mildly elevated at 57 μg/l (normal 8–52). Oral prednisone 60 mg resulted in improvement of her respiratory status and resolution of the phlebitis (H and I) and she was maintained on 10 mg of prednisone.

(Courtesy of Dr. William Mieler and Dr. Joseph Benevento. E and I, Also, Yannuzzi Lawrence J., The Retinal Atlas, Saunders 2010, 978-0-7020-3320-9, p.275.)

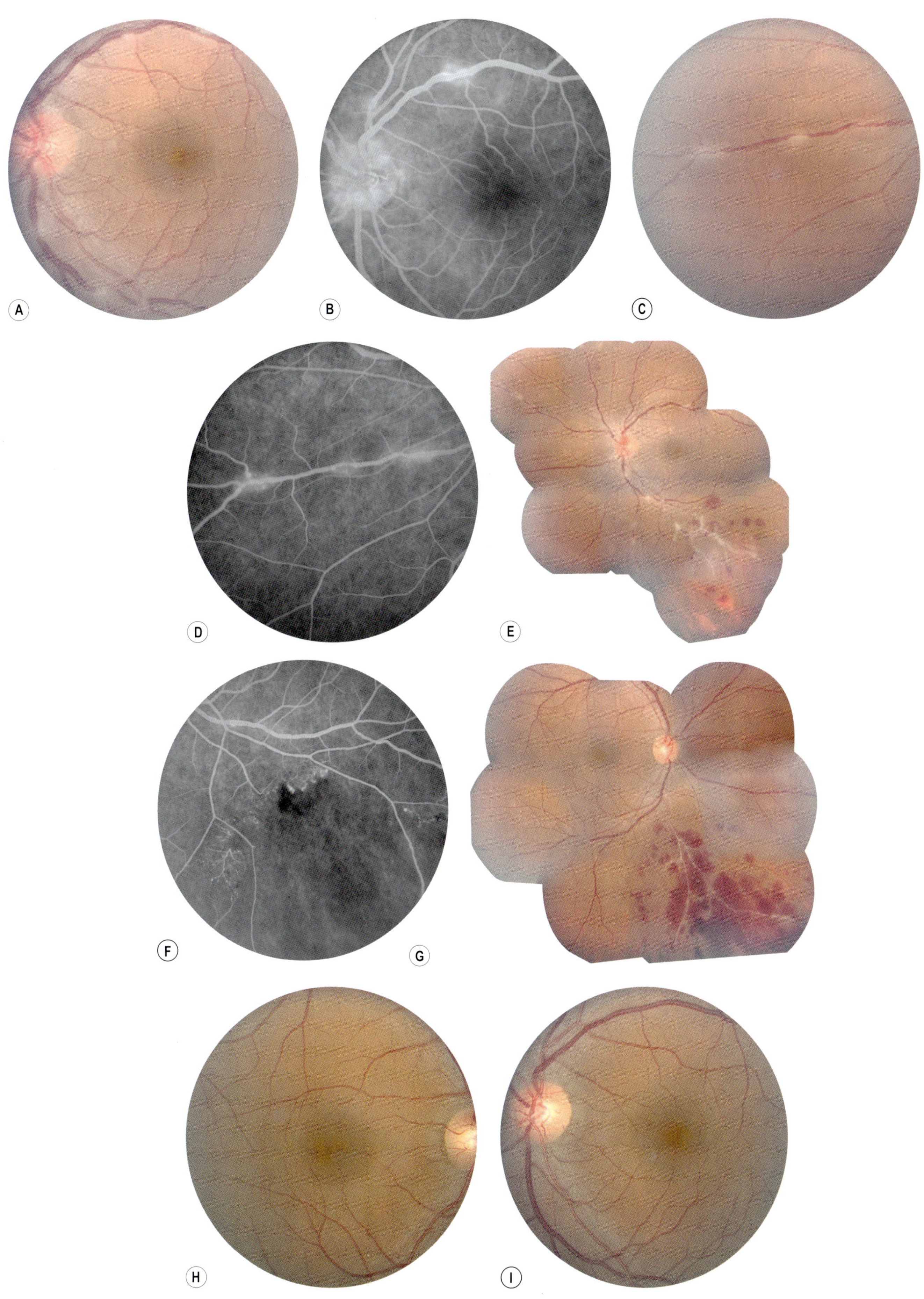
A
B
C
D
E
F
G
H
I

Approximately 20–30% of patients with retinal manifestations of sarcoidosis will have evidence of CNS involvement (Figure 11.39).[407,408,432–434]

Candle wax-dripping exudation, usually accompanied by preretinal white exudates over the inferior fundus (Figures 11.38A and D, and 11.39A, C, and D), and nodular papillitis (Figures 11.38E, F, and J, and 11.39A, G, and H)) are two signs that should strongly suggest the diagnosis of sarcoidosis. The diagnosis can be confirmed by biopsy of affected lymph nodes, conjunctiva,[435–437] salivary glands,[438] and lacrimal gland. Fewer than 5% of patients with sarcoidosis show cutaneous reaction to tuberculin protein. The chest roentgenogram or CT scan shows evidence of sarcoidosis in over 90% of cases. There is a high incidence of elevation of angiotensin-converting enzyme in patients with sarcoidosis.[405,439,440] Gallium citrate uptake studies may be helpful in confirming the diagnosis. Demonstrating noncaseating granuloma in a tissue biopsy is the only confirmatory test for sarcoid. These tests may return negative if the patient has already been empirically started on systemic steroids, and sometimes even topical steroids. Hence it is important to order the investigations prior to starting therapy.

All of the lesions of sarcoidosis usually respond to treatment with corticosteroids. The steroid dose required is not very high and 0.5 mg/kg body weight is usually sufficient. Because of the chronic nature of the disease, corticosteroids should be employed judiciously, primarily for an immediate threat to loss of visual or other vital organ function. Occasionally, use of other agents such as cyclosporine and methotrexate is required to control the inflammation.[441] Low-dose methotrexate once a week works very well in patients with long standing low-grade activity. Mycophenolate mofetil and minocycline have been used.[442,443] Neovascularization of the optic disc may show dramatic resolution following treatment with corticosteroids.[419] Photocoagulation may be helpful in controlling retinal neovascularization in the peripheral fundus. Multiple mechanism glaucoma often accompanies ocular sarcoidosis, due to trabeculitis or nodules in the angle in the early stages, and peripheral anterior synechiae, pupillary block from posterior synechiae and steroid induced glaucoma in the chronic stages of the disease. Severe/chronic cases require judicious use of steroids and immunosuppressive agents, and management of secondary cataract and glaucoma with medications and surgery.[422]

11.38 Sarcoidosis of the retina, optic nerve, skin, and conjunctiva.

A–C: Macular star, optic disc swelling, and perivenous "candle wax-dripping" exudates in a 25-year-old black man with biopsy-proven sarcoidosis (A). Angiography revealed evidence of perivenous leakage of dye in both eyes (B and C).
D: Perivenous exudation and macular star in a 32-year-old black man with biopsy-proven sarcoidosis.
E and **F:** Typical sarcoid nodules of the right optic disc in a 21-year-old black man with biopsy-proven sarcoidosis. Visual acuity in the left eye was 20/200. He was treated with systemic corticosteroids, and 6 months later most of the optic nerve head granulomas (E) had disappeared (F).
G: Preretinal nodules in a patient with sarcoidosis.
H: Sarcoid granulomas of the lid.
I: Sarcoid granuloma of the conjunctiva.
J and **K:** Sarcoidosis of the optic nerve head associated with prominent neovascularization.
L: Sarcoid periphlebitis and papillitis in a patient with sarcoid meningitis.

(L, courtesy of Dr. William F. Crosswell.)

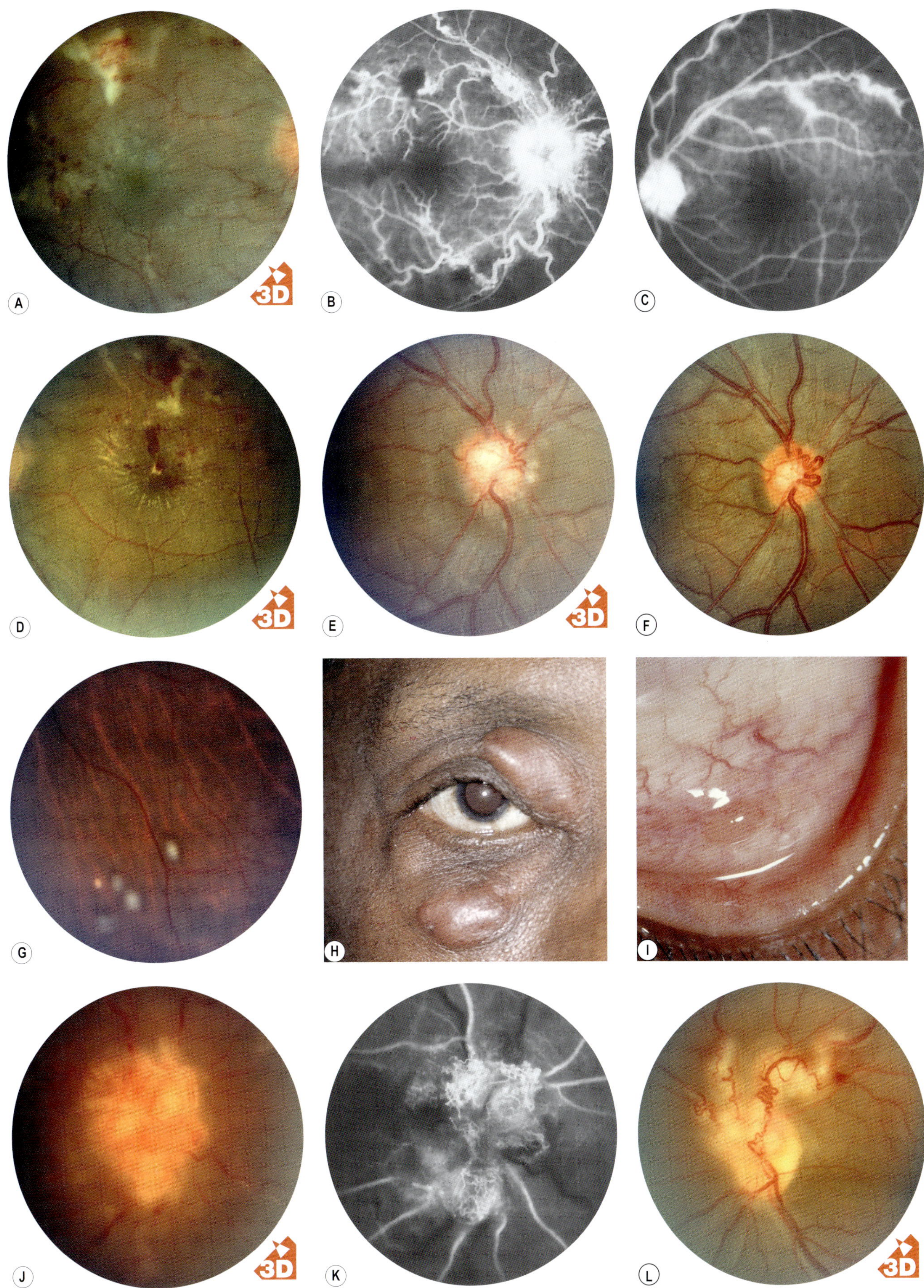
A
3D
B
C
D
3D
E
3D
F
G
H
I
J
3D
K
L
3D

ACUTE IDIOPATHIC MULTIFOCAL INNER RETINITIS AND NEURORETINITIS

These patients are typically children or young adults who soon after a viral-like illness develop loss of vision usually in one eye associated with one or more white foci of acute retinitis and neuroretinitis in one or both eyes.[14,444–449] The acute retinal lesions primarily involve the inner half of the retina and show some predilection for occurring adjacent to major retinal arteries and veins. In this latter location they may cause branch retinal artery or vein obstruction, which, together with optic nerve head involvement, are the major causes of symptoms in these patients (Figure 10.04). At the time of eye examination the patient is usually afebrile. Blood cultures and medical evaluation are usually unremarkable. Some of these patients have a clinical history of a cat scratch and serologic evidence of cat-scratch disease.[450–463] (See discussion on pp. 890 and 1290 and Figures 10.04 and 15.11.) One patient had serologic evidence of influenza A infection.[14] *Leptospira* organisms were cultured from the spinal fluid of another patient.[463]

Within a week of involvement of the optic nerve head, a macular star figure usually becomes evident. Those presenting with branch retinal artery occlusion usually have a permanent scotoma, but most patients with retinal and optic nerve head involvement recover normal or nearly normal visual acuity spontaneously. A few may develop evidence of optic atrophy. The value of corticosteroid and antibiotic treatment is uncertain.

The fundus picture in patients with acute idiopathic multifocal inner retinitis and neuroretinitis may simulate that seen in patients with retinitis and neuroretinitis caused by pyogenic bacteria (Figure 10.01), fungi, syphilis, and toxoplasmosis. Patients with evidence of branch retinal artery occlusion may simulate patients with bilateral idiopathic recurrent branch retinal artery occlusion (see Figures 6.19–6.21).

11.39 Ocular and central nervous system sarcoidosis; clinicopathologic correlation.

A–F: This 38-year-old black man had central nervous system sarcoidosis associated with bilateral retinal and optic nerve sarcoidosis. Fundus painting (A) showed granulomas on the optic disc, along the retinal veins, and in the vitreous inferiorly (inset). There was a branch vein occlusion in the inferotemporal quadrant. The patient died several months later, and histopathologic examination revealed multiple perivenous granulomas with extension of the granulomatous reaction into the overlying vitreous in the juxtapapillary area (B) and the peripheral retina (C and E). Note the granulomatous reaction surrounding the retinal veins (arrows, C and D) and extension of the granulomatous reaction beneath the retinal pigment epithelium (C and D). There were multiple granulomas in the pre- and postlaminar parts of the optic nerve (F) and throughout the central nervous system.

G–L: This 45-year-old Indian woman suffered a sudden-onset painless progressive loss of vision associated with headache for 20 days in both eyes. She was diabetic and hypertensive. Her vision was 20/400 in both eyes. She had 2+ cell and flare in both eyes with posterior synechiae and pigment on the anterior lens surface. She had bilateral nodular elevation of the optic discs and peripapillary hemorrhages, areas of decreased axoplasmic flow, and a macular star with macular subretinal fluid (G and H). Review of systems was positive for malaise, body ache, and shortness of breath. She denied fever, rash, unprotected sex, tuberculosis, and ischemic heart disease. She had no pets. Systemic examination revealed bilateral fine crepitations and hepatosplenomegaly. Her tuberculosis skin test was negative, sedimentation rate was 24 mm, and angiotensin-converting enzyme level was 35.5 μg/l (normal 8–52). Chest X-ray revealed hilar lymphadenopathy and nodular opacities in the parenchyma. Computed tomography scan revealed pleural and interstitial thickening, and enlarged hilar lymph nodes (I). A transbronchial lymphnode biopsy showed noncaseating granuloma suggesting sarcoidosis (J). Abdominal ultrasound revealed hepatosplenomegaly with areas of fatty change in the liver. She received oral prednisone 60 mg and topical steroids and cycloplegics in both eyes. By 4 months her vision had improved to 20/25 in both eyes, and the iridocyclitis and disc edema had resolved with a few resolving exudates (K and L).

(A–F, From Gass and Olson.[407] G to L, courtesy of Dr. Vishali Gupta and Dr. Arnod Gupta).

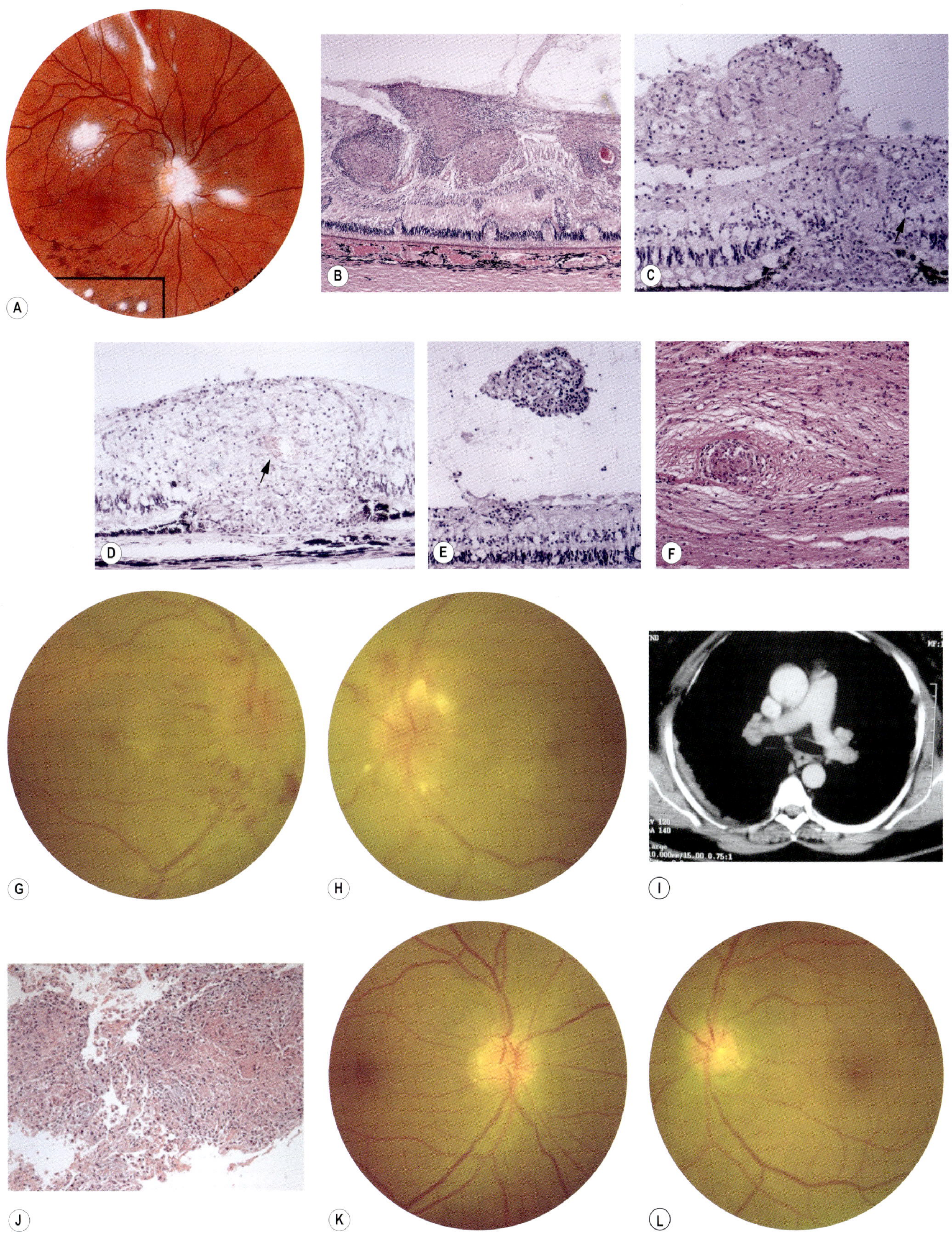
A
B
C
D
E
F
G
H
I
J
K
L

BEHÇET'S DISEASE

Behçet's disease is a chronic systemic disease of unknown cause characterized clinically by aphthous ulcers of the mouth and genitalia (Figure 11.40A and D), intraocular inflammation, nondestructive seronegative arthritis, and cutaneous vasculitis including erythema nodosum (Figure 11.40B).[464–482] The criteria for diagnosis include oral aphthae or genital ulcers in association with any other two of the six major manifestations of the disease. The disease occurs most frequently in people of the Mediterranean basin and Japan. In approximately 80% of patients the ocular disease is bilateral, and it is twice as frequent in men.[473] Behçet's disease has been reported with less frequency in the USA, where the sex difference in regard to ocular involvement has been less pronounced.[467] Iritis and vitreous inflammatory cell infiltration are present in nearly all patients with ocular involvement. In most cases the iritis is nongranulomatous. Hypopyon occurs occasionally (Figure 11.40C). Edema of the macula and optic disc, patches of gray thickened retina, focal accumulations of yellow-white deep retinal exudates (Figure 11.41A–C and H), scattered areas of delicate pigment clumping, perivasculitis, central and branch venous and arterial occlusions (Figure 11.42), papilledema, papillitis, and optic atrophy may occur (Figures 11.40E, F, G, and L and 11.41). Visual loss is usually caused by long-standing retinitis, retinal infarction, retinal arterial attenuation, cystoid macular edema, and, in some cases, retinitis proliferans and vitreous hemorrhage.[424,483] Whereas progressive optic atrophy may accompany the retinal changes, acute loss of vision caused by optic neuropathy without retinal involvement rarely occurs in patients with Behçet's disease.[484]

During an acute attack the erythrocyte sedimentation rate, acute-phase proteins, and circulating immune complexes may be elevated along with dramatic alterations of serum complement levels.[474,485,486] Elevation of serum concentration of interleukin-2 receptor, C9, and complement-reactive protein may occur in all forms of the disease.[469,473,483,487,488] Antibodies against the vascular endothelial cells and mucosa can be demonstrated in some patients with Behçet's disease.[483,486,488–490] Antibody affinity to retinal S antigen is lowered.[13]

A generalized vasculitis is responsible for the multiplicity of clinical manifestations. Neurological manifestations can be seen in Neuro Behcet's. Activated T lymphocytes and hyalinized thickening are found in association with the retinal and optic nerve perivasculitis.[221] Although a virus was implicated early in the history of Behçet's disease,[491] the disease's cause is unknown. The increased incidence of HLA-B5 or -Bw51 antigens in patients with Behçet's disease in the Middle East and Japan suggests that susceptibility genes to the disease may have been spread by the old nomadic tribes or Turks via the silk route.[492,493] These antigens are found less frequently in patients in the United States with Behçet's disease.

11.40 Behçet's disease.

A: Aphthous ulcer (arrow).
B: Erythema nodosum of lower legs.
C: Hypopyon.
D–I: This 31-year-old woman with Behçet's disease had aphthous ulcers (arrow, D), multiple foci of retinitis causing branch retinal artery occlusion (arrow, E), and branch retinal vein occlusion (arrow, F) when she initially presented. One week later she developed another branch retinal artery occlusion (arrow, G–I) in the left eye.
J–L: This 31-year-old man with aphthous stomatitis and hypopyon (C) in the right eye had bilateral vitritis, multiple retinal ischemic patches, and hemorrhages (J). His visual acuity was counting fingers in the right eye and 20/25 in the left eye. Angiography revealed perivascular leakage of fluorescein (K). Forty-two months later his acuity was 7/200. Note the pallor of the optic disc, marked narrowing and sheathing of the retinal vessels, and a macular scar (L).

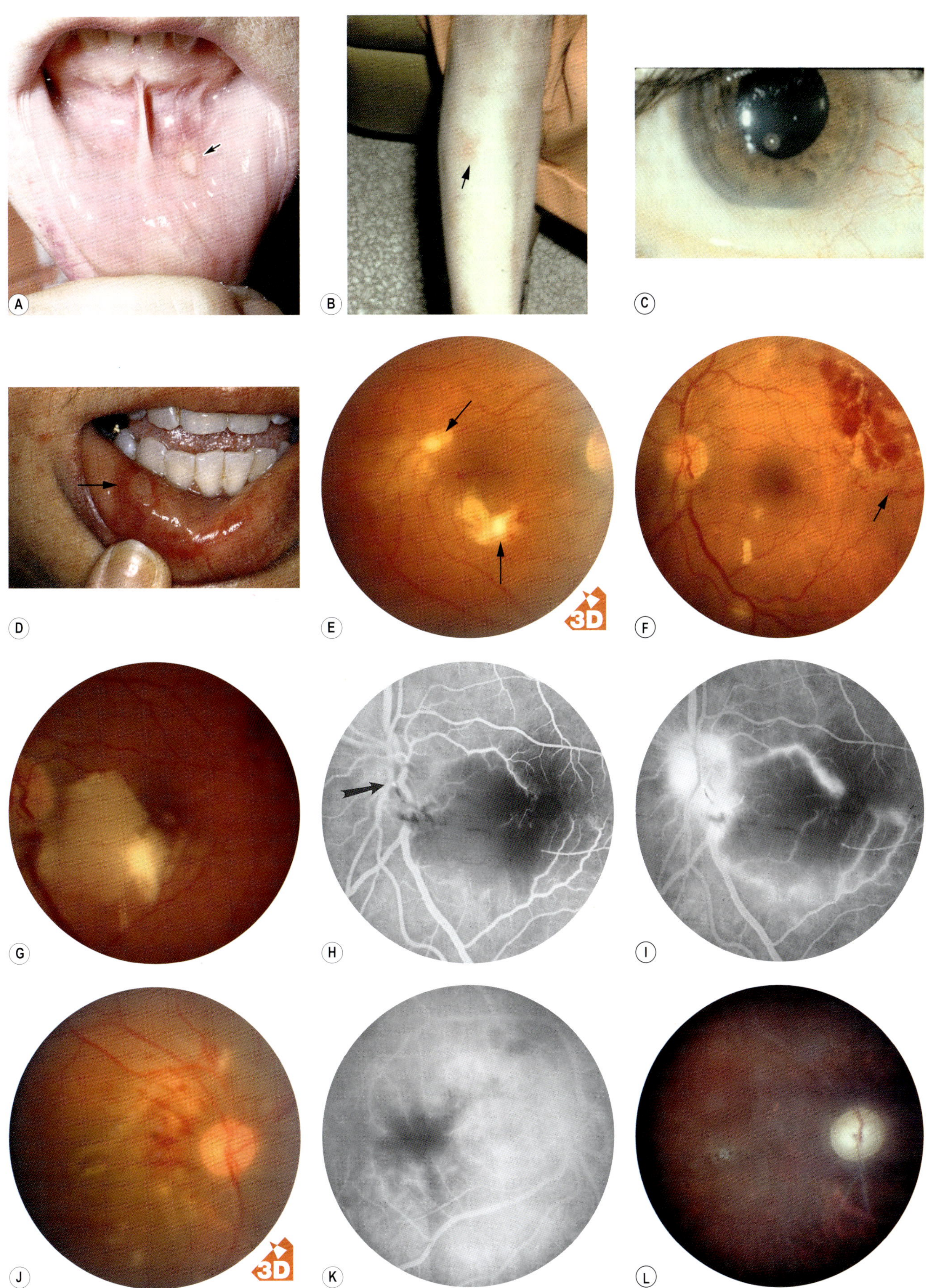
A
B
C
D
E
3D
F
G
H
I
J
3D
K
L

DIFFUSE, CHRONIC NONNECROTIZING RETINITIS, VITRITIS, AND CYSTOID MACULAR EDEMA

The permeability of the retinal capillaries, particularly those in the macular region, may be affected by chronic diffuse inflammation involving the retina and vitreous. Although these patients may be categorized into several different syndromes, in none is the cause known, nor can it be established whether the primary tissue involved is the retina or the vitreous. The clinical features shared by these patients include complaints of floaters caused by inflammatory cell infiltration of the vitreous and loss of central vision caused by cystoid macular edema in eyes that externally show no signs of inflammation. Some degree of papilledema may be present. Bilateral involvement is the rule. A few retinal hemorrhages often occur peripherally. Evidence of peripheral retinal degeneration with some disturbance of the underlying RPE is seen eventually. Narrowing of the retinal vessels and pallor of the optic disc along with complaints of night blindness may occur in some cases. Retinal holes, retinal detachment, and preretinal vitreous membrane formation occur occasionally. The vitreous inflammation and cystoid macular edema often respond poorly to corticosteroids or other therapy.

These patients may be subdivided into three major clinical syndromes: (1) pars planitis; (2) idiopathic vitritis; and (3) vitiliginous (birdshot) chorioretinitis.

11.42 Severe asymmetric Behçet's disease.

A 43-year-old woman with past history of oral and vaginal ulcers, arthritis, and skin ulceration previously controlled with colchicine and steroids, developed right optic neuritis (A) and a positive fluorescent treponemal antibody absorption. The left eye was uninvolved (B). Nine months later vision in the right eye dropped to no light perception and was associated with phlebitis of the left leg. Complete massive infarction of her right optic nerve and diffuse retinal hemorrhages were noted (C). Poor perfusion of the right fundus was seen by angiography (D and E); 100 mg prednisone and 15 mg methotrexate were added. The right optic nerve and vessels turned white over the next 2 months (F and G). The left eye remained uninvolved (H). Neovascularization of the optic disc occurred over time (G).

(Courtesy of Dr. David Fischer.)

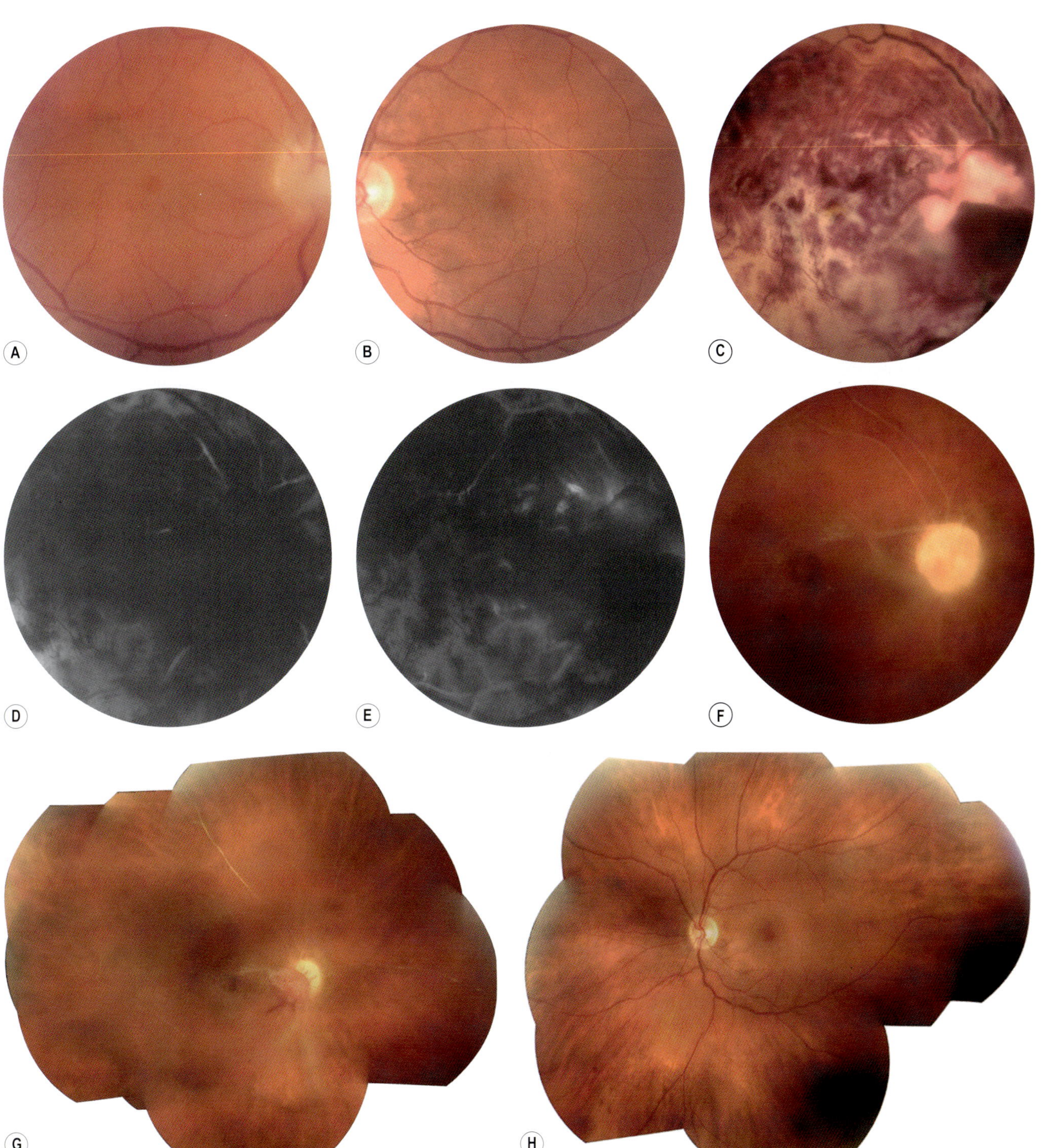
A
B
C
D
E
F
G
H

RETINITIS AND VITRITIS WITH VITREOUS BASE ORGANIZATION (PARS PLANITIS, PERIPHERAL UVEITIS, OR CHRONIC CYCLITIS)

The term "pars planitis" has been used to describe patients with chronic vitritis who develop snow-bank exudates and vitreous condensation overlying the peripheral retina and pars plana, usually inferiorly in both eyes (Figure 11.43).[11,512–537] These patients are typically children or young adults of both sexes in excellent general health when they develop floaters and blurred vision. The eyes are white. A few patients may have fine keratitic precipitates. Fine and coarse vitreous floaters are present and may be responsible for moderate loss of visual acuity. Snowball preretinal aggregates similar to those seen in sarcoidosis may be present (Figure 11.43H). Macular edema is the most common complication of the disease, and it may persist despite vigorous corticosteroid therapy (Figure 11.43B and C). Dilation of the major retinal vessels, particularly the veins; sheathing of the retinal veins; and varying degrees of papilledema often accompany the macular edema (Figure 11.43B and C). Other complications include secondary cataract, secondary glaucoma, sheathing and narrowing of the peripheral retinal vessels, traction and rhegmatogenous detachment of the peripheral retina,[519] retinoschisis,[518] subretinal neovascularization,[538] neovascularization of the optic disc[539] and retina (Figure 11.43E–G),[524] pseudogliomatous angioma formation,[524] vitreous hemorrhage, rhegmatogenous retinal detachment,[519] heterochromia irides, band keratopathy, and rarely phthisis bulbi. The disease is chronic but is subject to remissions and exacerbations. The amount of pars plana exudate generally correlates with the severity of vitreous inflammation and cystoid macular edema.[540] Most patients maintain useful vision in one or both eyes. Eyes with complete posterior vitreous separation may have a better visual prognosis.[541] There is some tendency for the disease to lessen in severity over a period of many years.[537]

Fluorescein angiography demonstrates a variable degree of permeability alterations of the capillaries of the retina and optic disc (Figure 11.43C).[11,535] In patients with macular edema there is usually angiographic evidence of widespread retinal edema, papilledema, and in some patients late staining of the larger retinal veins and venules (Figure 11.43C and G). Most patients have electroretinographic abnormalities, such as delayed b-wave implicit time, abnormal response to flicker, and reduced b-wave oscillations.[521]

The limited histopathologic data available suggest that this disease is a chronic nongranulomatous inflammation involving primarily the retina and vitreous.[517,525,531,534,542] The fluffy snow-bank opacities peripherally are probably caused primarily by cellular infiltrate within the vitreous. Later this fluffy appearance may be replaced by less elevated, white, organized scar tissue, which may be derived from glial elements of the peripheral retina.[542] Prominent perivenous and venous infiltration occurs with lymphocytes that are predominantly T-helper lymphocytes.[542] The uveal tract is relatively free of inflammation.[534]

The pathogenesis of pars planitis is unknown. The development of a migrating corneal endothelial rejection line (autoimmune endotheliopathy) in some patients with pars planitis suggests the possibility that the disorder may be an autoimmune process directed toward the vitreous.[543]

Some of these patients show improvement in visual function following oral corticosteroid therapy. Many others, however, fail to respond to this therapy, which should be used sparingly because of the disease's chronic nature and its tendency to undergo remissions and exacerbations. In the presence of useful central vision it is probably unwise to treat these patients with long-term corticosteroids. The value of cyclodiathermy and cyclocryotherapy in treating the pars plana and peripheral retina is controversial.[515,528,544] These cyclodestructive procedures appear to be of most benefit in those patients unresponsive to corticosteroid therapy and who in addition have neovascularization in the region of the vitreous base.[544,545] The reason for accumulation of exudate over the pars plana predominantly in the inferior fundus is unknown; it is probably more a function of gravitational forces than locus of the disease. The value of vitrectomy in treating cystoid macular edema is also uncertain.[546] Although some success has been reported utilizing combination therapy of corticosteroids with antimetabolites, the value of this treatment in the long-term management of these patients is

11.43 Pars planitis.

A: Fundus drawing showing usual distribution of snow-bank exudates over the pars plana inferiorly.

B–D: This 17-year-old woman with pars planitis noted loss of vision because of cystoid macular edema (B and C). Four months later, after systemic corticosteroid therapy, the edema had resolved (D).

E–G: Retinitis proliferans (arrows) in the macular area of a 31-year-old man with pars planitis. Angiography demonstrated leakage of fluorescein from these vessels and cystoid macular edema (F and G).

H and **I:** Preretinal nodules (H) and cystoid macular edema (I) were present bilaterally in this 52-year-old woman with snow-bank exudates on the pars plana.

J–L: Pars planitis associated with multifocal choroiditis, macular edema, papilledema, vitritis, and anterior uveitis in a 13-year-old male with 3-year history of photophobia, floaters, and visual loss. General physical examination was negative except for axillary lymphadenopathy. Biopsy of the nodes revealed granulomatous inflammation of unknown cause. Serologic tests for toxoplasmosis, syphilis, and Lyme disease were negative. Treatment with systemic corticosteroids and doxycycline produced minimal improvement.

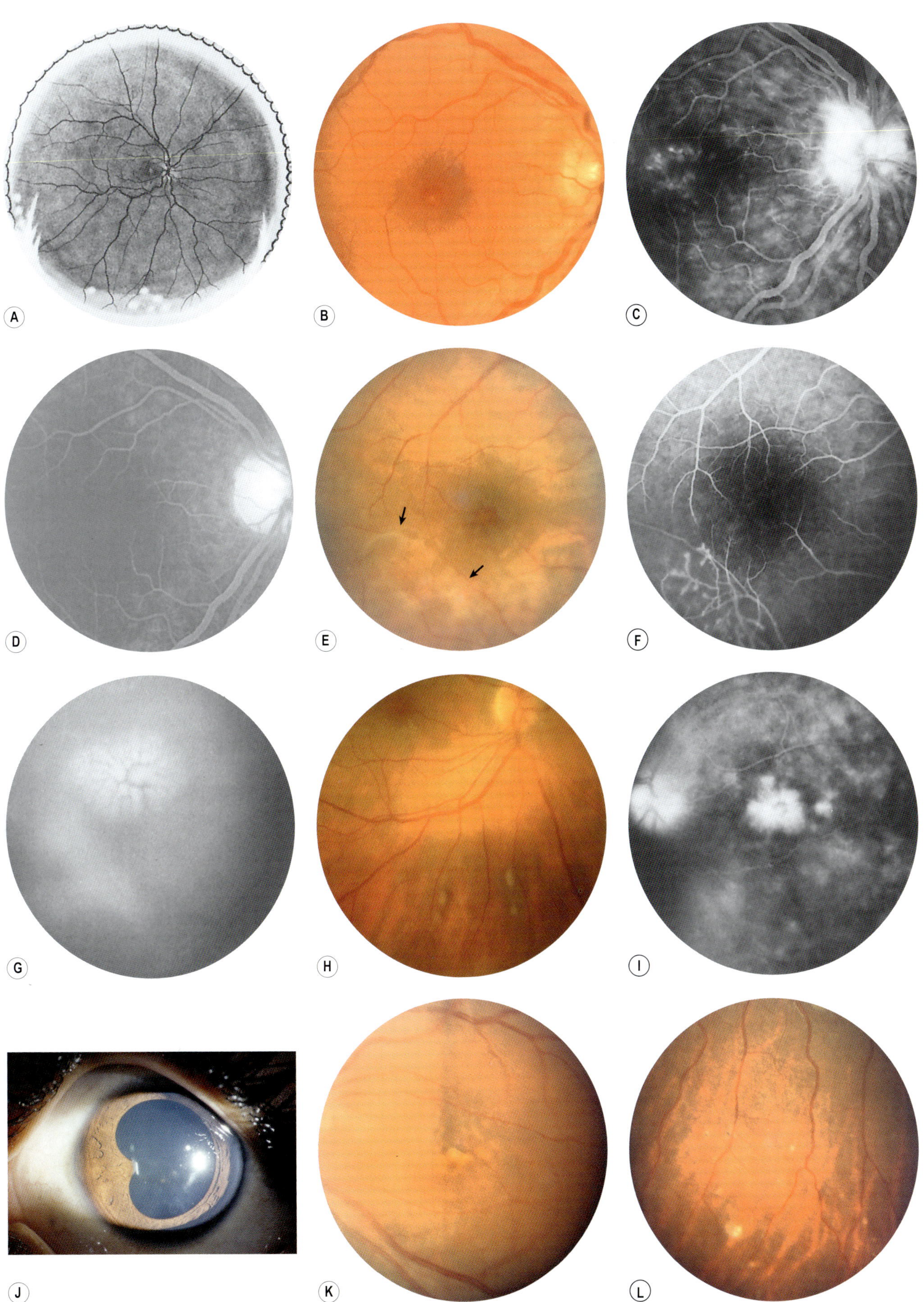
A
B
C
D
E
F
G
H
I
J
K
L

uncertain.[528–530,547] There are significant risks in such treatment, and therefore it should be employed only in patients with severe involvement.

The differential diagnosis includes sarcoidosis, peripheral toxoplasmosis, Behçet's syndrome, *Toxocara canis*, acute recurring cyclitis, and the pseudo-POHS. Gass has seen 3 children with this latter syndrome who in addition had dense white pars plana exudate and who developed loss of macular function secondary to choroidal neovascularization and disciform detachment.[11,548] Lyme disease may be associated with pars planitis and anterior uveitis (see Figure 10.06A–F).

Pars planitis has occurred in multiple members of at least eight families.[516,522,523,527,542] Pars planitis has occurred in patients developing evidence of demyelinating disease.[526,533,549–553] A long-term follow-up of patients with pars planitis revealed that optic neuritis developed in 4 patients (7.4%) and multiple sclerosis in an additional 8 patients (14.8%).[551] This same group found an association of HLA-DR2 in 67.5% of patients with pars planitis (28% controls), and they cited others who had found HLA-DR2 in 50–75% of North Americans and Europeans with multiple sclerosis (20–25% controls).[550,552]

IDIOPATHIC DIFFUSE NONNECROTIZING RETINITIS WITHOUT VITREOUS BASE ORGANIZATION (IDIOPATHIC AGE-RELATED VITRITIS)

The most frequently encountered group of patients with floaters or loss of vision secondary to chronic vitritis and diffuse retinitis are healthy middle-aged or elderly patients, most frequently women, who develop cystoid macular as well as diffuse retinal edema, in some cases papilledema, and cellular infiltrate of the vitreous without any evidence of snow-bank pars plana deposits (Figure 11.44).[554,555] Cellophane maculopathy caused by an epiretinal membrane is frequently present in the macular areas. Externally the eyes are quiet. The peripheral fundi often show evidence of narrowing and sheathing of the retinal vessels as well as irregular derangement of the RPE. Retinal edema and vitritis often respond poorly to corticosteroids or other therapy. The cause is unknown. Gass has seen idiopathic vitritis in identical twins (Figure 11.44E–I).[555] Bennett and coworkers reported a large family with autosomal-dominant adult-onset vitreous inflammation, selective loss of the ERG b-wave, mild anterior-chamber inflammation, and later retinal scarring, pigmentation, peripheral retinal vascular closure, peripheral retinal neovascularization, vitreous hemorrhage, and cystoid macular edema.[556]

Patients with idiopathic vitritis share many features in common with patients with vitiliginous chorioretinitis

11.44 Diffuse nonnecrotizing retinitis, vitritis, and cystoid macular edema without pars plana exudation (idiopathic age-related vitritis).

A–D: This 70-year-old woman noted floaters and visual loss in both eyes at 65 years of age. Visual acuity was 20/200 in the right eye and 20/50 in the left eye. She had bilateral vitritis, cystoid macular edema, and diffuse retinal edema. Note angiographic evidence of irregular focal scars in the periphery and the multiloculated fluorescein staining pattern in the extramacular as well as the macular area (B–D). She has been observed for 22 years, and her acuity and findings are unchanged.
E and **F:** Cystoid macular edema, mild papilledema, and vitritis in a 59-year-old woman whose visual acuity was 20/40 in the right eye and 20/400 in the left eye.
G–I: The identical twin sister of the patient illustrated in E and F with the same condition in both eyes. Note the marked retinal capillary dilation (H) and the extramacular and macular polycystic edema (I). Both twins noted the onset of floaters and blurred vision at 50 years of age. Both have markedly subnormal rod and cone electroretinographic responses.

(see next subsection). Differentiating patients with idiopathic vitritis from patients with genetically determined retinitis pigmentosa sine pigmenti is difficult. The electroretinographic abnormalities are usually less severe in patients with idiopathic vitritis. Other disorders that may simulate idiopathic vitritis include Whipple's disease (see p. 930), large-cell non-Hodgkin's lymphoma (see p. 1150), metastatic carcinoma and melanoma to the vitreous (see Chapter 13), and lymphocytic infiltration of the vitreous associated with X-linked immunodeficiency with increased immunoglobulin M.[557]

VITILIGINOUS CHORIORETINITIS AND BIRDSHOT RETINOCHOROIDOPATHY

The syndrome of birdshot retinochoroidopathy or vitiliginous chorioretinitis is characterized by: (1) onset, in apparently healthy patients, both men and women in the fifth to seventh decade of life, of floaters, photopsia, and blurred vision, often followed later by night blindness and color blindness; (2) vitreous inflammation; (3) multifocal patches of depigmentation first occurring in the choroid and later the RPE in the postequatorial fundi; (4) varying degrees of retinal edema and papilledema, and narrowing of the retinal vessels and mild optic atrophy; (5) moderate to severe electroretinographic abnormalities; (6) a variable rate of progression and severity but with a tendency toward stabilization and preservation of good central vision in at least one eye; and (7) strong association with HLA-A29.[558–568]

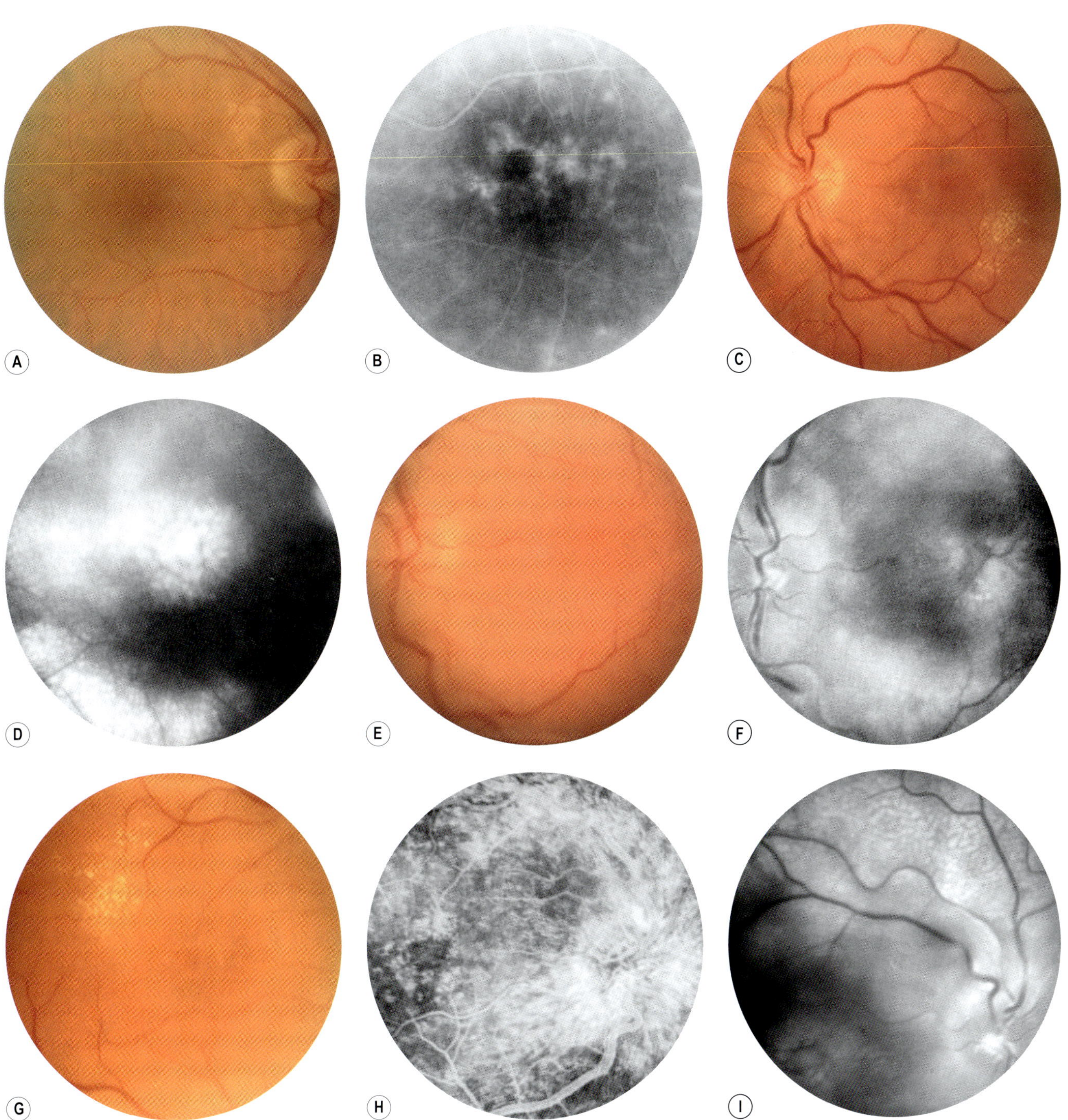
A
B
C
D
E
F
G
H
I

Before the initial publication of this syndrome, called birdshot retinochoroidopathy by Ryan and Maumenee,[569] the name "vitiliginous chorioretinitis" had been used at the Bascom Palmer Eye Institute to describe patients with this syndrome. The author chose this name for this syndrome because of the similarity in the appearance and evolution of the patches of choroidal depigmentation to those occurring in the skin of patients with vitiligo.[560] These orange or yellow ill-defined patches, which may not be present when the patient is seen initially with vitreous cells and macular edema, are typically scattered in the postequatorial portion of the fundus (Figures 11.45 and 11.46). They are most numerous in a broad area surrounding the nasal two-thirds of the optic disc and early in the course of the disease are often absent in the macular area. The patches vary in size and shape. Many of the patches are round to oval. Some are irregular or elongated, often in a pattern that radiates toward the peripheral fundus (Figure 11.45A and B). Striking and characteristic features of these patches are the absence of hyperpigmentation within or at their margins and the absence of slit-lamp evidence of thinning of either the retina or the choroid in the area of depigmentation. Large choroidal blood vessels are often visible within these lesions, and the overlying retinal vessels appear normal. During the early stages of depigmentation, particularly when associated with severe vitreous inflammation, absence of visible choroidal vessels within these lesions may then give the appearance of nonelevated choroidal inflammatory infiltrates. Angiographically in their early evolution these patches show no abnormality (Figure 11.45C). The lesions are usually symmetrically distributed in both eyes. In time the patches enlarge and may be associated with biomicroscopic and angiographic evidence of depigmentation and atrophy of the overlying RPE and retina. Hyperpigmentation may occur in some lesions in the late stages of the disease. Loss of central vision may be caused by cystoid macular edema (Figure 11.45E), by atrophy of the retina associated with the depigmentation of the RPE and choroid (Figure 11.45F), and occasionally by serous macular detachment (Figure 11.45G and H) or by choroidal neovascularization (Figure 11.46H and I).[558,569] Proliferation of new vessels from the optic disc and retina may occasionally occur and cause vitreous hemorrhage (Figure 11.46J–L, and 11.47). Rare associations with vitiliginous chorioretinitis include hearing loss[562] and Lyme disease.[570]

Fluorescein angiography may show evidence of delay in the retinal artery appearance time, increased retinal circulation time, and varying degrees of unexplained quenching of fluorescence of the retinal vessels during the course of angiography.[560] Mild vascular leakage, more from the veins than arteries, and cystoid macular edema can be seen in eyes with active inflammation and vitritis. Dark choroidal patches are seen on ICG angiography; their significance is not completely understood. It is likely the fluorescein is blocked by choroidal lymphocytic infiltrates and inflammation rather than choroidal vascular insufficiency. Early in the course of the disease electroretinography may be normal. Later, it shows moderate to severe abnormality in rod and cone function in both eyes of most patients.[571,572] The rod function is affected first. The electro-oculogram may be either normal or subnormal. Dark adaptation studies may show subnormal rod function. OCT over the choroidal lesions is usually normal unless the RPE is atrophic; then the photoreceptors may also be disrupted.[573] Enhanced depth imaging OCT may offer some insight into choroidal involvement. Autofluorescence imaging is variable depending on the severity of RPE involvement. The oval choroidal lesions do not show abnormal autofluorescence. However the areas where the overlying RPE is disturbed will show decreased autofluorescence. Sometimes these spots are along the retinal vessels, especially the large veins, giving it an appearance of perivenous atrophy (Figure 11.48A and B).

Histopathology of a 49-year-old male with at least a 6-year history of birdshot choroiditis not previously treated with steroids or immunosuppressives showed multiple foci of lymphocytes at different levels of the choroid, occasionally associated with hemorrhage, plasma cells, and epithelioid cells. Some foci were adjacent to choroidal vascular channels. There was no necrosis. The RPE, ciliary body, and iris did not appear to be involved. Other foci of lymphocytes were found around some of the retinal blood vessels and in the prelaminar optic disc. The lymphocytes were primarily CD81 T lymphocytes, with fewer CD41 T and B lymphocytes.[574,575]

11.45 Vitiliginous chorioretinitis.

A–C: This 58-year-old woman complained of floaters and had a visual acuity of 20/20. There were 2 + vitreous cells. A similar pattern of multifocal areas of yellowish depigmentation of the choroid was present in both eyes (A and B). Note relative sparing of the macular areas, and elongation of the more peripheral lesions. Early phases of angiography showed no abnormality in the region of these patches (compare B and C).

D–F: This 50-year-old man experienced floaters and mild loss of vision. Only a few small vitiliginous patches were evident in the juxtapapillary area (D). He had angiographic evidence of cystoid macular edema (E). Two years later, his visual acuity was 20/400 and he had many large vitiliginous patches throughout both fundi (F).

G and H: This 49-year-old woman complained of floaters, blurred vision, and metamorphopsia in both eyes when she was initially examined in February 1980. Bilateral serous detachment of the macula was present. This resolved spontaneously. When seen at Bascom Palmer Eye Institute 2 years later she complained of nyctalopia and loss of color vision. She had vitreous cells, pigment mottling of the macula, and widespread vitiliginous patches throughout the postequatorial fundi with relative sparing of the macular areas (G and H).

(A–F, from Gass[560])

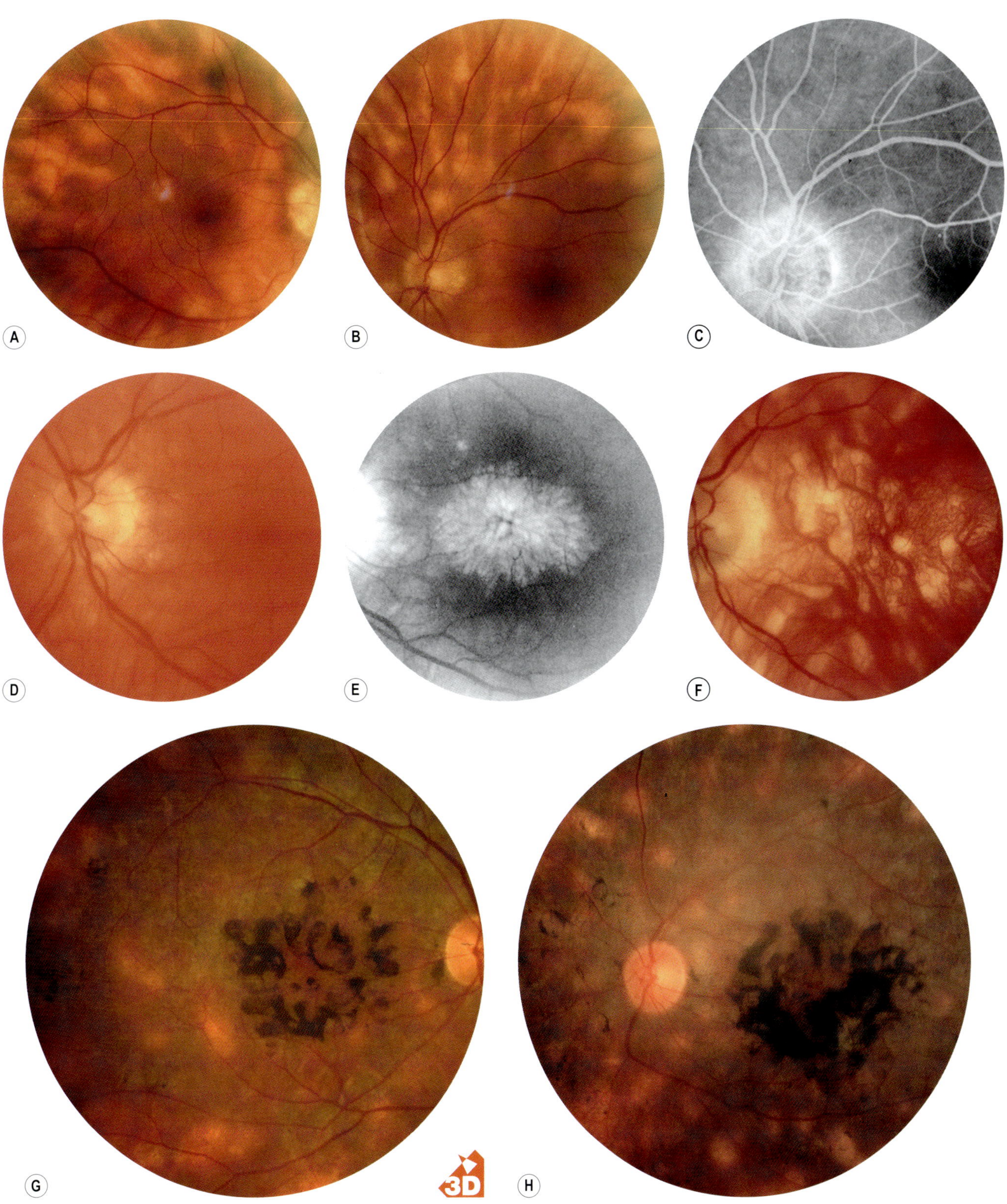
A
B
C
D
E
F
G
3D
H

Although Gass observed multiple depigmented spots on the arms and legs of several patients with vitiliginous chorioretinitis, these appear to be more closely related to idiopathic guttate hypomelanosis than vitiligo. This former disease is a common skin change of unknown origin and similar in both its clinical and histopathologic appearance to vitiligo.[576] Albert and associates[286] observed 5 patients with cutaneous vitiligo and a fundus picture that appeared similar to vitiliginous chorioretinitis. Depigmentation of the choroid and RPE similar to that seen in vitiliginous choroiditis may occur in patients with other ocular diseases that may be associated with vitiligo (VKH disease, sympathetic uveitis, and acute VKH-like uveitis caused by metastatic cutaneous melanoma). This suggests the possibility of a common autoimmune mechanism.[286,577–580] Progressive degeneration of the peripheral retina, retinal artery narrowing, and optic disc pallor and night blindness are features that may occur in all four diseases. Vitiliginous chorioretinitis is usually a chronic, slowly progressive disease that is subject to remissions and exacerbations. Most patients retain useful central vision in at least one eye for many years.

Treatment includes systemic steroids along with, or followed by, immunosuppressives based on the severity of the disease at presentation. If the disease is active with vitritis, cystoid macular edema, and retinal vascular breakdown, systemic steroids at approximately 0.75 mg/kg are recommended. Simultaneous institution of immunosuppressives, such as methotrexate starting at 10 mg once a week and gradually increasing to 15 or 20 mg based on response, is also recommended such that it becomes effective by the time the steriod taper begins. Mycophenolate mofetil is an alternative if methotrexate is not effective or not tolerated. Low-dose cyclosporine (2.5–5 mg/kg daily), with or without other corticosteroid-sparing immunosuppressive agents, has been used as an alternative to long-term corticosteroids.[581] A recent report of use of daclizumab in those refractory to mycophenolate and traditional immunosuppressive therapy needs further exploration.[582] If the disease is relatively inactive and the patient is asymptomatic or only mildly symptomatic, low-dose immunosuppression alone is recommended to slow its progression. Acute exacerbations may need periodic systemic steroids. These patients should be monitored by baseline Goldmann visual fields and ERG and yearly Goldmann visual fields and, less frequently, ERG.

Antigen HLA-A29 is found in approximately 90% of patients with vitiliginous chorioretinitis.[564,583–585] The author believes HLA-A29 is positive in 100% of cases. If a patient suspected of birdshot choroiditis is HLA A-29-negative, diagnosis such as sarcoid or other granulomatous disease should be sought.[586] Vitiliginous chorioretinitis has occurred in monozygotic twins.[587] Over 50% of patients may demonstrate evidence of an in vitro mitotic immune response to purified retinal S-antigen.[583] These findings suggest that this disease has a genetic predisposition and that retinal autoimmunity plays a role in its manifestations.

11.46 Vitiliginous chorioretinitis and choroidal and retinal neovascularization

A–E: This healthy middle-aged man was referred in for postbevacizumab endophthalmitis of the left eye. He had received two intravitreal injections for neovascular AMD in this eye. Following a vitrectomy and lensectomy, both eyes were noted to have several drusen, and a partly active juxtafoveal choroidal neovascular membrane with subretinal hemorrhage in the left eye. In addition, several oval depigmented choroidal lesions of birdshot chorioretinitis were found in both eyes (A and B, and E). The drusen lit up early in the angiogram and stained late, along with the choroidal neovascular membrane (C and D). He continued to receive ranibizumab and the vision stabilized at 20/50 following secondary intraocular lens placement.
F and G: Irregular dilation of retinal veins and retinal hemorrhages in this 51-year-old man who had only a few depigmented patches in his left eye when initially examined (E). Three years later he had developed prominent vitiliginous patches in both eyes (F).
H and I: This 54-year-old woman with vitiliginous chorioretinitis developed loss of central vision in both eyes because of choroidal neovascularization.
J and K: This man with vitiliginous chorioretinitis developed retinal and optic disc neovascularization that required panretinal photocoagulation and vitrectomy.

(E and F, from Gass[560])

The differential diagnosis before the development of the typical hypopigmented fundus lesions includes pars planitis, idiopathic vitritis, reticulum cell sarcoma, papillitis, and papilledema. Irregular dilation of the retinal veins and scattered retinal hemorrhages suggested a diagnosis of macroglobulinemia in one case. Several patients with papilledema were thought initially to have an intracranial tumor (Figure 11.46G). Once the typical hypopigmented fundus lesions develop, the appearance and course of this disease differentiate it from other diseases that have white spots in the fundus associated with vitreous inflammation, such as serpiginous choroiditis, APMPPE, diffuse unilateral subacute neuroretinitis, sarcoidosis, Behçet's disease, reticulum cell sarcoma, combined variable immunodeficiency,[586] and Whipple's disease.

Vitiliginous chorioretinitis shares some features in common with the MCP (pseudo-POHS) (see p. 988–990). Unlike the latter syndrome, vitiliginous chorioretinitis rarely affects children and young adults; is infrequently associated with anterior uveitis, punched-out chorioretinal scars, or choroidal neovascularization; and is associated with HLA-A29.

The relationship of patients with vitiliginous chorioretinitis and the more frequently encountered chronic vitritis and macular edema more often in middle aged or older women but without evidence of the typical vitiliginous lesions, is unknown (see p. 1038).

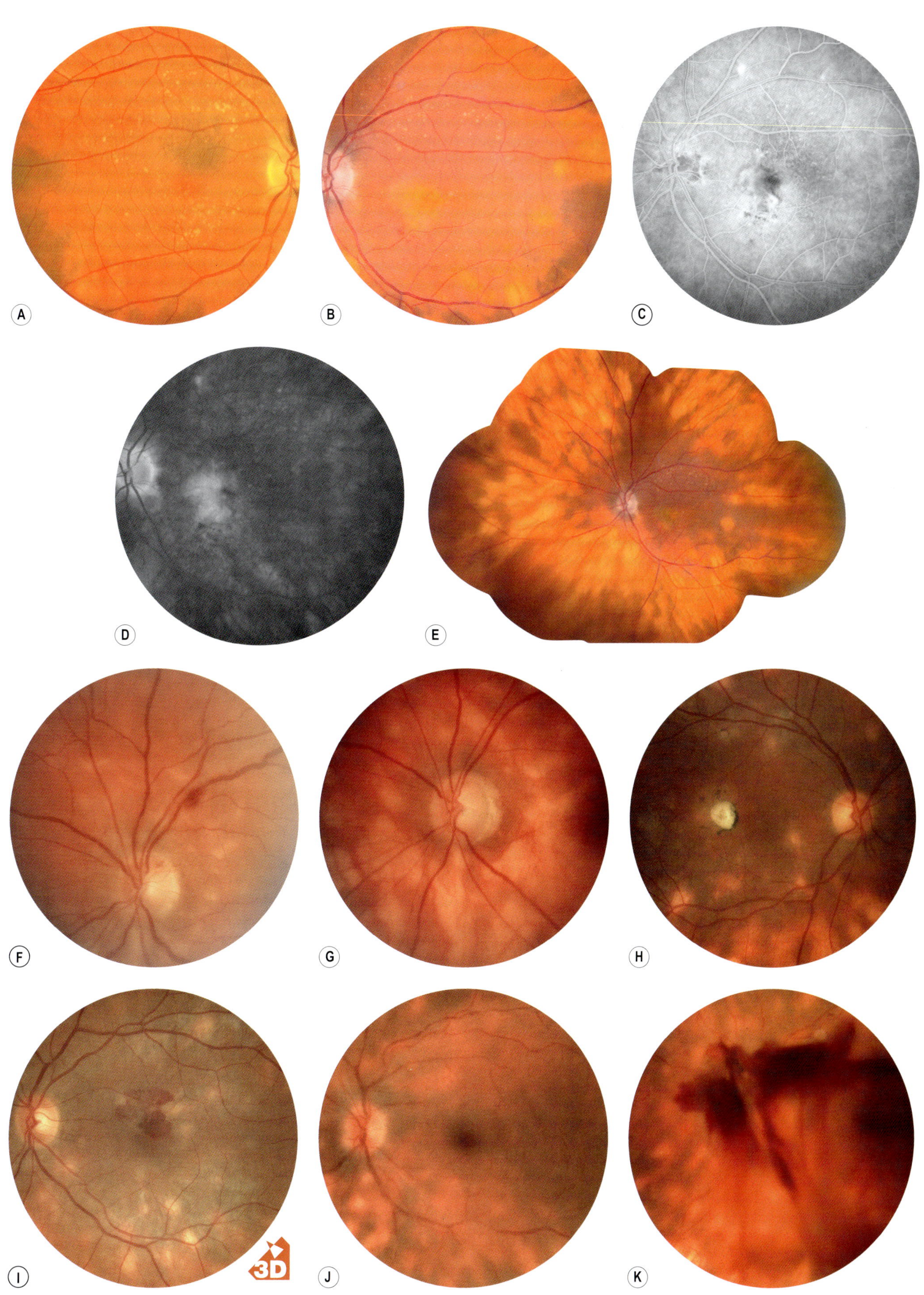
A
B
C
D
E
F
G
H
I
3D
J
K

BLAU SYNDROME

Blau in 1985 described a large family whose members were affected by a disease resembling infantile sarcoidosis.[588] Granulomatous inflammation of three organs resulting in uveitis, arthritis, and skin rash with an autosomal-dominant inheritance was noted. The symptoms begin early in childhood, with the skin rash being observed as early as age 4 months. The rash is composed of painless tiny red dots and often resolves spontaneously. Occasionally more visible flat-topped papules and ichthyosis-like rash have been reported.[588–591] Sometimes the rash can be so mild and may be missed.[591] The joint anomalies always appear before age 10. It begins insidiously with painless cysts on the back of the feet and wrist (Figure 11.48F) and mild boutonnière deformity of the fingers, a characteristic finding in this condition (Figure 11.48F). The cysts over the joints progress to camptodactyly and cystic swelling of the wrists, ankles, knees, and sometimes the elbows. The affected joint is mostly painless and the condition does not lead to severe handicap until the fourth or fifth decade. However camptodactyly may interfere with fine finger movements in early childhood. Narrowing of some of the joint spaces and enlargement of metaphysis are rare.[592] The eye findings are the most severe aspect of the syndrome. It can begin anywhere in early childhood or in adulthood and could be an anterior uveitis or panuveitis presenting with conjunctival erythema, subepithelial corneal opacities, cells and flare in the anterior chamber, and posterior synechiae. Recurrent episodes result in cataract, peripheral anterior synechiae, and secondary glaucoma. Progressive involvement of the posterior segment with multifocal choroiditis (Figure 11.48D and E), optic disc edema, cystoid macular edema, vitreous membranes, anterior ischemic optic neuropathy, and an epiretinal membrane can occur.[593]

The histopathological examination of the skin shows noncaseating granulomas in the dermis and multiple epitheliodal, multinucleated giant cells similar to that seen in sarcoidosis. However, on electron microscopy, comma-shaped bodies are seen within the epithelioid cells, a finding not found in sarcoidosis, which helps differentiate pathologically Blau syndrome from sarcoid. Synovial biopsy reveals granulomatous inflammation with giant multinucleated cells.[592]

Jabs et al. in 1985 described an additional family with disease resembling Blau syndrome with dominant inheritance, granulomatous synovitis, and bilateral recurrent uveitis. This family had associated cranial neuropathies, including hearing loss and sixth-nerve palsy without skin involvement. It is likely that the skin involvement was mild and went unnoticed.[591] Blau syndrome is differentiated clinically from early-onset or infantile sarcoidosis by lack of visceral involvement and familial occurrence. The expressivity can be variable in family members with the same mutation. The susceptibility locus for the Blau syndrome is on chromosome 16 at 16p12-16q21, in close proximity to the inflammatory bowel disease 1 (*IBD1*) locus, and has been identified as the nucleotide-binding oligomerization domain 2 gene (*NOD2*).[593–596] A 9-month-old infant has been described with disseminated systemic granulomatosis, the triad of uveitis, skin rash, and arthritis, and gastrointestinal tract granulomas – features of early-onset sarcoidosis, Blau syndrome and Crohn's disease.[597] His family history was negative and he carried a susceptibility polymorphism of *NOD2* previously described in Crohn's disease and not in early-onset infantile sarcoidosis or Blau syndrome.

11.47 Birdshot chorioretinopathy and retinal neovascularization.

A–G: This 45-year-old male presented with floaters and vitreous hemorrhage in his right eye. He had several areas of flat neovascularization in the right eye in addition to oval pale yellow choroidal lesions all over the fundus in both eyes (A, B, and D). An angiogram confirmed the areas of neovascularization (C and E) and in addition revealed late cystoid macular edema in both eyes. He received intravitreal injections of bevacizumab in this eye and was started on immunosuppressives. The new vessels regressed completely (F and G); he then developed new vessels in his left eye that also responded to bevacizumab.

(Courtesy of Dr. David Sarraf.)

TUBULOINTERSTITIAL NEPHRITIS AND UVEITIS SYNDROME (TINU)

Dobrin et al. first described this anterior uveitis associated with acute interstitial nephritis and immune-mediated process.[598] A female predominance and bimodal age distribution, the first occurring between 8 and 15 years and the second between 30 and 35 years, have been noted, although the disease can present from age 9 to 74. It tends to occur earlier in males, with a median age of onset of 14 (range 9–52 years), and a median age of onset of 17 years (range from 9 to 74 years) in females.[599] HLA-A2 and HLA-A24 are the most commonly reported HLA types. In Japan, about 75% of patients were identified with HLA-A24.

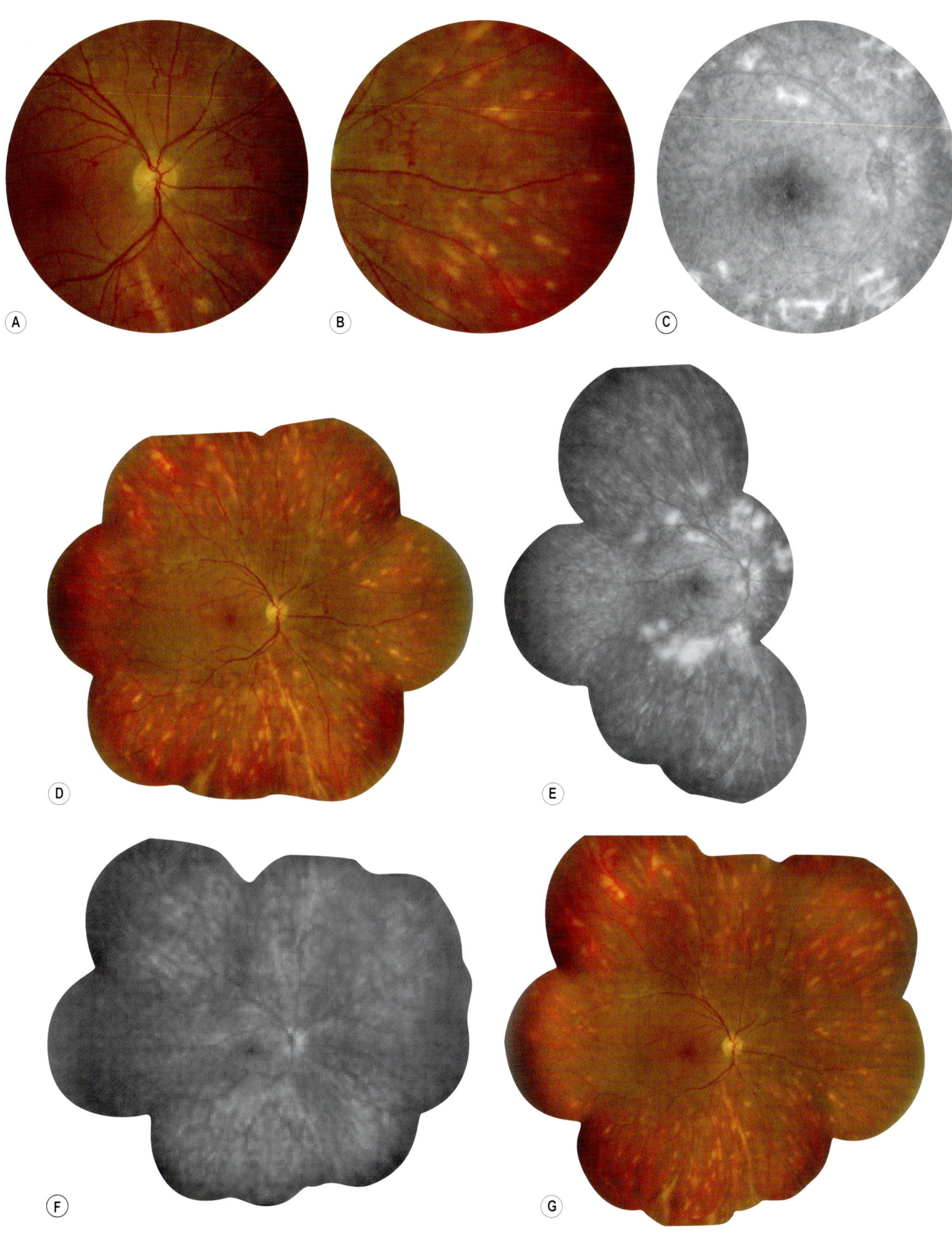
A
B
C
D
E
F
G

Risk factors for development of acute interstitial nephritis are a wide variety of drugs, predominantly anti infectious agents, infections, toxins and autoimmune diseases. No precipitating factor has been found in some patients. It is not known whether patients having an infection or drug-induced renal disease are at an equal risk of developing uveitis as patients with idiopathic renal nephritis. About one-half of the patients have no reported risk factors for acute interstitial nephritis, antibiotic use was documented in 24% of patients, and prior use of nonsteroidal anti-inflammatory drugs was reported in 18% of patients. Some patients with TINU have been found to have serological evidence of autoantibodies such as antinuclear antibody, rheumatoid factor, anti-DNA antibodies, anticardiolipin antibodies, and cytoplasmic antineutrophil cytoplasmic antibodies, that is, c-ANCA. One patient presented with TINU and Sjögren's syndrome. One patient developed nodular scleritis 10 years prior to development of TINU.[600] There have been reports of family members with other autoimmune diseases, such as a patient's father had VKH syndrome, and a sister who had ulcerative colitis. There have been monozygotic twins who developed TINU approximately 1 year apart.[601] A mother and son with TINU have been reported.[602] There have been cases of TINU presenting with uveoretinitis along with Fanconi's anemia, and two sisters being affected in Japan.[601,603–606]

The systemic features associated with TINU are fever, weight loss, fatigue, malaise, anorexia, weakness, abdominal flank pain, arthralgias, and myalgias. One patient reported a red rash, likely drug-induced.

The ocular features are mostly acute, almost always bilateral anterior uveitis (Figure 11.48G). There has been only 1 case with unilateral anterior uveitis. Patients have been described with retinal vasculitis, retinal hemorrhages, optic disc edema, uveoretinitis (Figure 11.48H), retinal vascular sheathing, dilated retinal vessels, and lipid exudates. Pars plana exudates and cells in the anterior vitreous have been noted. In some, this may be a spill-over from the anterior uveitis.

A recurrence of the uveitis can be seen and it is quite common, occurring in about 41% of patients; the recurrences are usually more severe than the initial episode.[607] The recurrence is defined as development of ocular inflammation after a period of disease quiescence. Younger patients less than 20 years of age are more likely to have a chronic course of uveitis, with persistent inflammation lasting greater than 3 months, than older patients. Intraocular complications include posterior synechiae, optic disc edema, cystoid macular edema, macular pucker, chorioretinal scar formation, and 1 patient with a rhegmatogenous retinal detachment. Elevated intraocular pressure can be secondary to the uveitis and synechiae. Secondary cataracts both from the uveitis and with corticosteroid use in the treatment are also seen. Visual acuity as good as 20/25 or better is seen in both eyes in the majority of patients if treated promptly with topical and systemic steroids.

11.48 Autofluorescence in birdshot chorioretinopathy.

A and B: This 65-year-old woman with moderately advanced birdshot chorioretinopathy had extensive oval depigmented lesions in both eyes (A). Some of the lesions showed loss of overlying retinal pigment epithelial (RPE) cells. The areas of RPE loss were hypoautofluorescent. Several of these were along the large retinal veins, suggesting primary or secondary retinal venous changes causing RPE atrophy in their vicinity.

Blau (Jabs) syndrome.

C–F: This 28-year-old Caucasian female with a long history of arthritis and uveitis, previously treated with steroids, cyclosporine, and methotrexate, complained of slow, progressive decrease in vision in the left eye. The arthritis involved joints of the right hand with mild involvement of joints of the left hand and wrist. Her father, paternal grandfather, and brother had similar symptoms. Her visual acuity was 20/20 in her right and 20/40 in the left. She had 1+ cell and flare in the right eye and 2+ cell and flare in the left eye. There were nongranulomatous old keratitic precipitates on both corneal epithelia. The right fundus showed several old chorioretinal scars in the periphery (D and E) and the left cystoid macular edema. Examination of the hand showed a typical boutonnière deformity of the index finger and the little finger on both sides (F). Her diagnosis is consistent with familial juvenile systemic granulomatosis, also known as Jabs syndrome or Blau syndrome.

Tubulointerstitial nephritis with uveitis (TINU).

G–J: A 12-year-old Caucasian girl was seen for red eyes and decreased vision, right more than left. Her vision was 20/30 on the right and 20/20 on the left. Nongranulomatous anterior uveitis with keratic precipitates (G) and deep punched-out scars (H) were seen in the inferior retina. There was a prior history of low-grade fever and weight loss. Blood urea nitrogen was 35 mg/dl, creatinine was 2.4, and urine examination showed 10 white blood cells per high-power field, red blood cells, and hyaline casts. p- and c-ANCA and anti-glomerular basement membrane (GBM) antibodies were negative. Kidney biopsy showed no granulomas, but mixed inflammatory infiltrate (I and J) consistent with TINU.

(C–F, courtesy of Dr. Timothy Olsen; G–J, courtesy of Dr. Jose Pulido.)

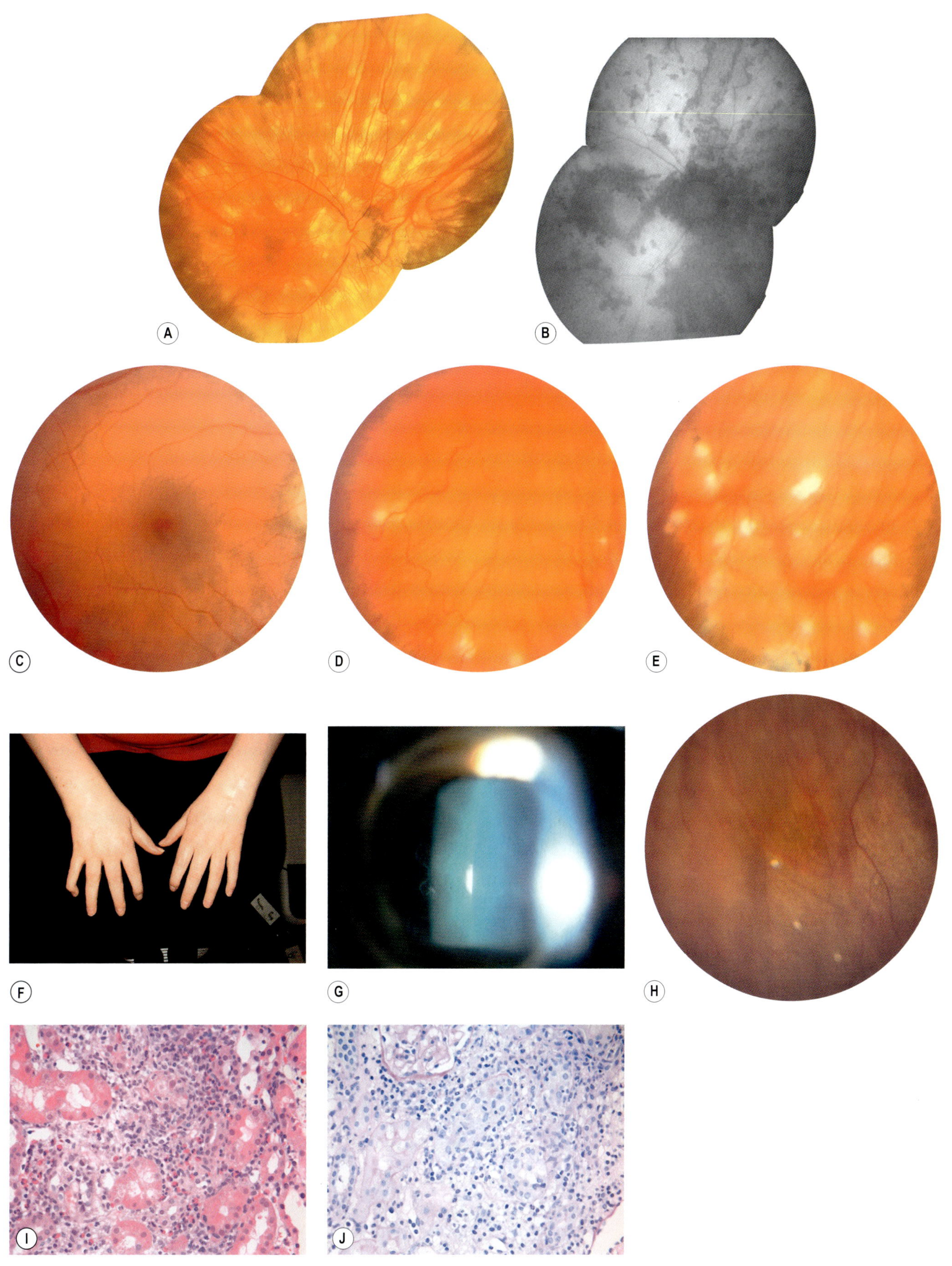
A
B
C
D
E
F
G
H
I
J

The pathology of the disease is not completely understood; it is believed to be autoimmune. The renal diagnosis is established by a kidney biopsy, which shows interstitial edema and infiltration by inflammatory cells of the kidney (Figure 11.48I and J). The glomerular vascular structures were relatively unaffected. The inflammatory infiltrate in the kidneys is composed of mononuclear cells, including lymphocytes, plasma cells, histiocytes, sometimes mast cells, eosinophils and neutrophils. Elevated serum beta-2 microglobulin is seen in more than 60% of patients and urinary beta-2 microglobulin is seen in more than 90% of patients; this is a marker for the presence of the disease and the disease activity. Nonrenal findings have been occasionally described in the gastrointestinal tract, bladder, and lymph nodes. Laboratory investigations include urinalysis with low-grade proteinuria, glycosuria, urinary leukocytes, and beta-2 microglobulin levels. Elevated sedimentation rate is seen in majority of patients. The serum IgG is also elevated in about 80% of patients; anemia is a common finding. Treatment involves the use of systemic and topical steroids along with cycloplegic agents and any pressure-lowering agents if needed. Immunosuppressive drugs are reserved for refractory uveitis or multiple recurrences. Uveitis sometimes predates the interstitial nephritis, but most often the interstitial nephritis is the first presenting feature with flank pain, fever, nausea, malaise and other findings. The T lymphocytes appear to be activated, as evidenced by interleukin-2 receptors on the cell surface.[608]

The diagnostic criteria for the acute interstitial nephritis include histopathological findings consistent with the classic interstitial nephritis on renal biopsy. Clinical diagnosis is based on abnormal renal function and abnormal urinalysis and a systemic illness lasting more than 2 weeks characterized by fever, weight loss, anorexia, malaise, fatigue, rash, abdominal flank pain, arthralgias and myalgias and a sedimentation rate above 40 mmHg, evidence of anemia, abnormal liver function, and eosinophilia.[609] The diagnostic criteria for uveitis include bilateral anterior uveitis with or without intermediate or posterior uveitis. Onset of uveitis is less than 2 months before, or less than 12 months after, acute interstitial nephritis. Unilateral uveitis is rare. In Japan, 50% of children with uveitis seemed to have TINU; the other 50% sarcoid in several series.[603,607,609]

CROHN'S DISEASE

Crohn's disease (regional ileitis) is a granulomatous enterocolitis of unknown etiology that usually affects young adults. Approximately 10% of patients develop ocular complications.[610] These include corneal infiltrates, conjunctivitis, corneal ulceration, episcleritis, scleritis, choroidal folds, acute anterior nongranulomatous and, less often, chronic posterior granulomatous uveitis, acute iritis, macular edema, central serous chorioretinopathy, proptosis, papilledema, retinal vasculitis, and neuroretinitis.[610–616] Gass has seen 1 patient with Crohn's disease associated with erythema nodosum and typical APMPPE.[617] Others have reported multifocal choroidal infiltrates similar to APMPPE but associated with serous retinal detachment in Crohn's disease.[618] Systemic manifestations include low-grade fever, abdominal pain, diarrhea, anemia, weight loss, arthritis, psoriasis, erythema nodosum, and hepatitis. Ocular complications are more likely to occur during the active phase of the disease, and at least 50% of these patients will have evidence of arthritis.[610,619] Patients with colitis and ileocolitis are more likely to have ocular involvement than patients with only small-bowel involvement.[619] There is a higher than normal prevalence of HLA-B27-type leukocytes in patients with Crohn's disease.[620] *CARD15/NOD2* mutations have been implicated in the causation of an autosomal-dominant inherited disease, called Blau syndrome (see above). The gene *CARD15*, also called *NOD2*, has also been implicated in other granulomatous diseases, including Crohn's disease, and in early-onset sarcoidosis. *NOD2* normally controls both innate and adaptive immune responses through the regulation of cytokines, chemokines, and antimicrobial peptide production.[621–624] Strong evidence suggests an initiating and promoting effect of intestinal microbes in the gastrointestinal tract of *NOD2*-predisposed individuals. This could be the underlying mechanism for pathogenesis of Crohn's disease in the susceptible individual.

COLLAGEN VASCULAR DISEASES

Throughout this textbook, various ocular manifestations of collagen vascular diseases have been illustrated relevant to the context, given the protean manifestations of some of them. IgA nephropathy, systemic lupus erythematosus, and Churg–Strauss syndrome are illustrated in Figures 11.49–11.51.

11.49 Immunoglobulin A (IgA) nephropathy.

A–L: A 21-year-old woman complained of abdominal pain, vomiting and shortness of breath associated with visual blurring for 1–2 days. There were several purpuric rashes all over her body (I2) and she was known to have end-stage renal disease requiring hemodialysis. She was found to be anemic with an elevated potassium, blood urea nitrogen, and creatinine. Vision was count fingers on the right and 20/30 on the left. Exudative retinal detachment of the right eye and choroidal thickening of the left were seen (A–C). Pinpoint hyperfluorescent dots that leaked progressively were noted on angiography (D–G). An ultrasound (H) and optical coherence tomography (OCT) confirmed the subretinal fluid. The OCT showed multiloculated fluid due to subretinal fibrin strands (I1). She was known to have biopsy-proven IgA nephropathy. Aggressive peritoneal dialysis followed by hemodialysis, correction of her anemia and control of blood pressure improved her ocular status with visual return to 20/20 in both eyes. The serous detachment resolved and Elschnig spots and a few retinal hemorrhages remained (J–L).

(Courtesy of Dr. Ranjit Dhaliwal and Dr. Oksana Demediuk.)

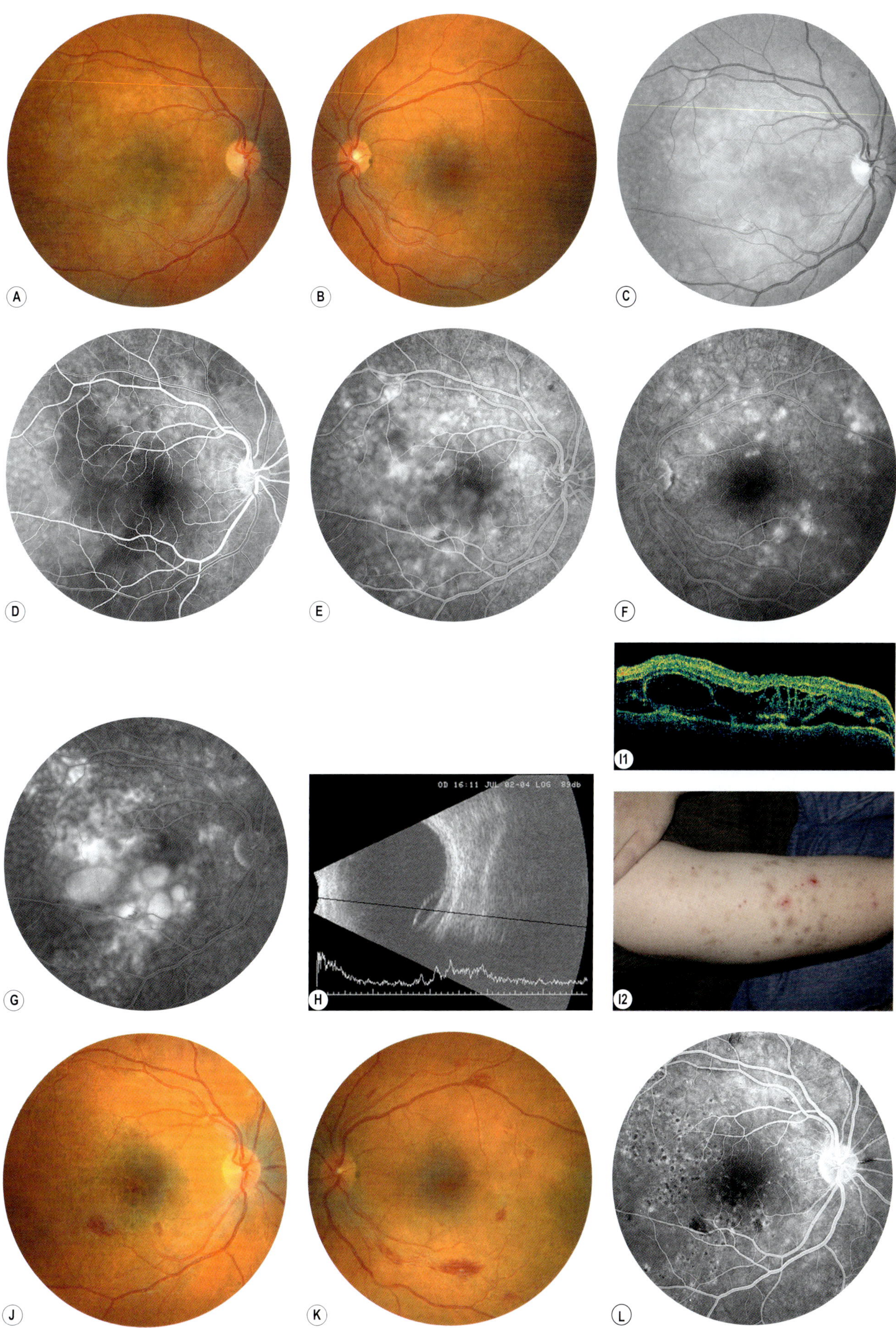
A
B
C
D
E
F
I1
OD 16:11 JUL 02-04 LOG 89db
G
H
I2
J
K
L

IgA Nephropathy

Patients present with malignant hypertension, fluid retention, and generalized anasarca.[625] Kidney biopsy shows IgA nephropathy with focal and segmental mesangiopathic changes and immunoreactivity to IgA with deposits of IgA in the mesangium. Both circulating immune complexes and in situ production of immune complexes with complement activation are involved in the pathogenesis.[626] Figures 11.49 and 11.50A–E illustrate two women, one of whom (Figure 11.50) also suffered abruption of her placenta with a stillborn child and subsequent mild disseminated intravascular coagulation; she presented with hypertensive choroidopathy, retinopathy, and exudative retinal detachments. The women responded to combined treatment with antihypertensives, systemic steroids and immunosuppression, with complete resolution of retinal findings.

Systemic Lupus Erythematosus

Figure 11.50F-H illustrates a patient who developed bilateral exudative retinal and choroidal detachments (Figure 11.50F) with secondary angle closure glaucoma due to forward displacement of the lens iris diaphragm. Renal biopsy helped make the diagnosis of lupus nephropathy. Treatment with systemic steroids alone did not help; addition of azathioprine caused resolution. She later developed spontaneous peripheral vascular occlusion in her left eye with vascular remodeling (Figure 11.50G and H).

Ocular manifestations of lupus include isolated cotton wool spots, retinal vasculitis with or without subsequent non perfusion, Purtscher like retinopathy (see chapter 6), serous retinal detachment resembling VKH disease and secondary hypertensive retinopathy.

11.50 Immunoglobulin A (IgA) nephropathy and eclampsia.

A–E: A 28-year-old Indonesian woman complained of blurred vision in both eyes. Visual acuity was 20/400 in each eye with a small myopic refractive error. Anterior-segment examination was normal. Dilated fundus examination showed detachments of the macula with subretinal fibrin (arrow A and B) and several yellow lesions at the level of the pigment epithelium in both eyes. There were bilateral extensive inferior exudative retinal detachments (A, B, D, and E). Fluorescein angiogram showed pinpoint hyperfluorescence corresponding to the yellow lesions that leaked in the mid and late frames of the angiogram with collection of dye in the subretinal space (C). Optical coherence tomography showed serous detachment with fibrinous strands in both eyes. Five weeks previously, the patient had been admitted for a ruptured placenta and had delivered a stillborn baby at 22 weeks' gestation. She was diagnosed with elevated blood pressure, proteinuria, and elevated creatinine at 19 weeks' gestational age. Her blood pressure was up to 176/111 mmHg. She had 3+ pedal edema, a weight gain of 14 lb (6 kg) in 2 weeks, and a creatinine that went up to 2.7 from 1.7. A renal biopsy confirmed IgA nephropathy with rapidly progressive nephritis, and no findings suggestive of pre-eclampsia. This patient developed hypertensive choroidopathy and IgA nephropathy-associated choroidopathy with exudative retinal detachment. Her clinical course was also complicated by anemia and disseminated intravascular coagulation. She was treated with oral prednisone at 60 mg/day, azathioprine 100 mg/day, and antibiotics levofloxacin and Bactrim along with antihypertensives. Her visual acuity improved over the next 2 months to 20/60 on the right and 20/40 on the left with resolution of the exudative retinal detachment leaving behind pigmentary changes of chronic Elschnig's spots.

Systemic lupus erythematosus and vasculopathy.

F–H: This 24-year-old woman with native American, African American, and Caucasian ancestry recently diagnosed with lupus nephropathy developed sudden loss of vision in both eyes secondary to bilateral choroidal effusions and exudative retinal detachments (A). Her intraocular pressures were elevated due to forward movement of the iris lens diaphragm from the ciliary detachments. Treatment with oral steroids alone did not help, but her findings resolved once azathioprine was added. Her vision and fundus changes returned to normal in 2 months. Three years later she was seen to develop asymptomatic peripheral vasculopathy in the left eye with retinal hemorrhages and vascular occlusions (G, arrow and H), that eventually stabilized in 1 year without specific treatment. She was on systemic treatment for the lupus throughout.

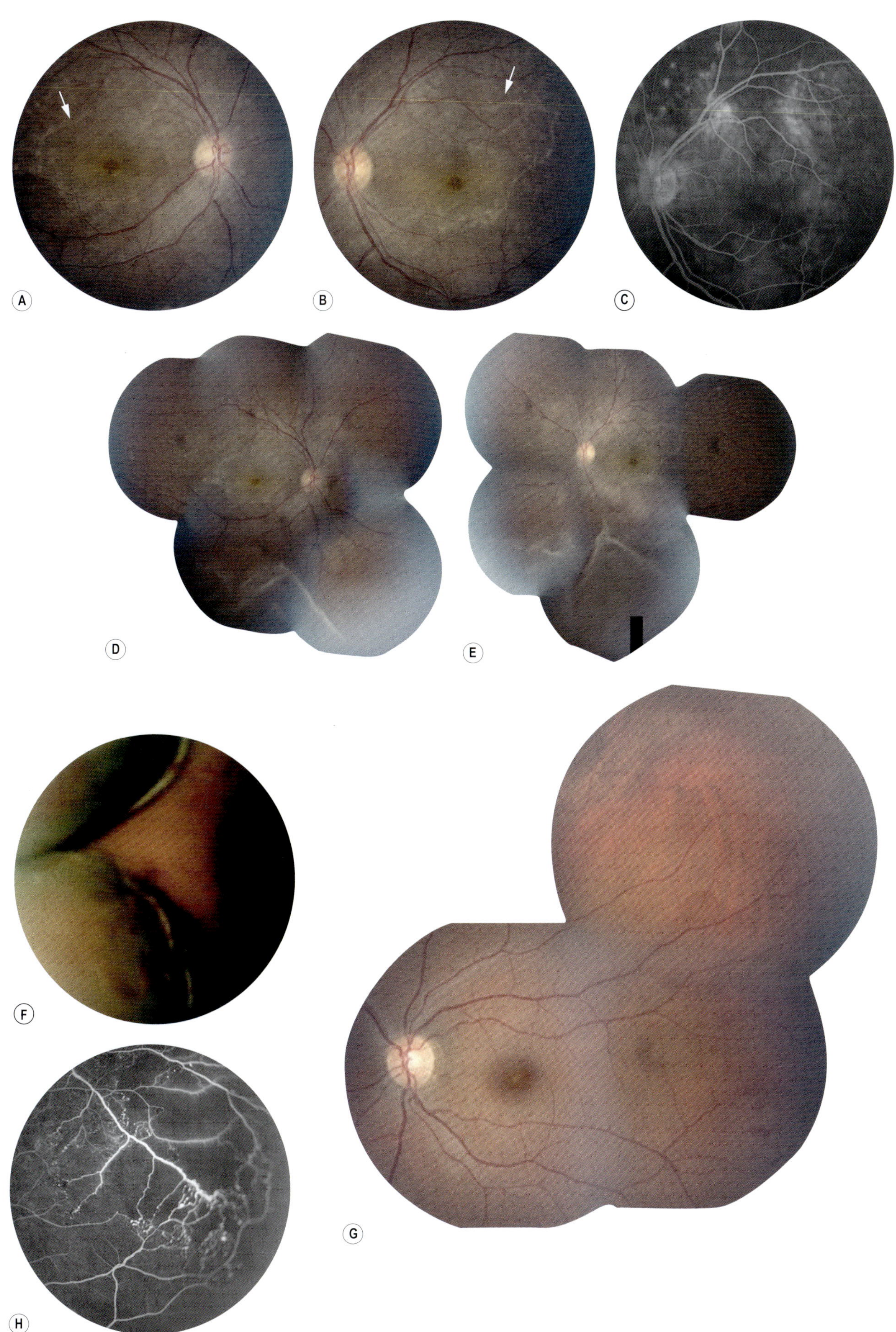
A
B
C
D
E
F
G
H

AQ17

Churg–Strauss Syndrome

Churg–Strauss syndrome is an allergic disease characterized by eosinophilic granulomatous inflammation affecting the respiratory tract and necrotizing vasculitis involving the small and medium-sized vessels. Four of six criteria, which include asthma, hypereosinophilia, mononeuropathy or polyneuropathy, paranasal sinus abnormality, pulmonary infiltrates (Figure 11.51G), and extravascular eosinophilic infiltration (Figure 11.51I), should be met to establish the diagnosis. The heart, skin (Figure 11.51F), and gastrointestinal tract can be involved occasionally. Ocular involvement is very rare and includes conjunctival granuloma, uveitis, corneal ulceration, amaurosis fugax, ischemic optic neuropathy, branch and central retinal artery and vein occlusion, and orbital pseudotumor.[627–640] The patient illustrated in Figure 11.51 shows progressive surgically induced necrotizing scleritis (SINS, see also page 1020) and retinal hemorrhages and vasculitis. He had skin involvement with necrotizing vasculitis, pulmonary infiltrates, biopsy-proven eosinophilic inflammation, and extensive retinal vasculitis, fulfilling the criteria for the diagnosis of Churg–Strauss syndrome. Treatment involves high-dose intravenous and/or oral steroids, immunosuppressives such as cyclophosphamide, and supportive therapy with platelets.[634]

11.51 Churg–Strauss syndrome and surgically induced necrotizing scleritis.

A–I: A 50-year-old Asian physician underwent extracapsular cataract surgery in his left eye in 1994. A year later glaucoma was diagnosed and Xalatan eye drops was begun. Eleven years later his corneal wound began to melt with movement of the iris to wound and dislocation of the posterior-chamber intraocular lens. The corneal melt was covered by conjunctivoplasty. His vision declined to 3/200. Five months later his intraocular lens was exchanged for an anterior-chamber lens via a pars plana vitrectomy. Chronic red eye and eye pain persisted, (A) and was treated with high-dose ibuprofen and topical prednisone acetate for the next several months. He also developed a choroidal neovascular membrane in his left eye requiring ranibizumab injections (B and C). Over the next month he developed progressive thinning and necrotic scleritis extending from the limbal wound consistent with surgically induced necrotizing scleritis (D and E). A chest X-ray revealed right middle and left upper-lobe opacification (G), increased blood urea nitrogen and eosinophilia (15%). He fulfilled the American Rheumatological Society's criteria for Churg–Strauss syndrome with asthma, paranasal sinus abnormality, hypereosinophilia, and pulmonary infiltrates. Systemic findings included retinal vasculitis (H), skin papules (F), and eosinophilic vasculitis (I).

(Courtesy of Drs. J. Michael Jumper, Robert Wong, H. Richard McDonald, and Emmett T. Cunningham.)

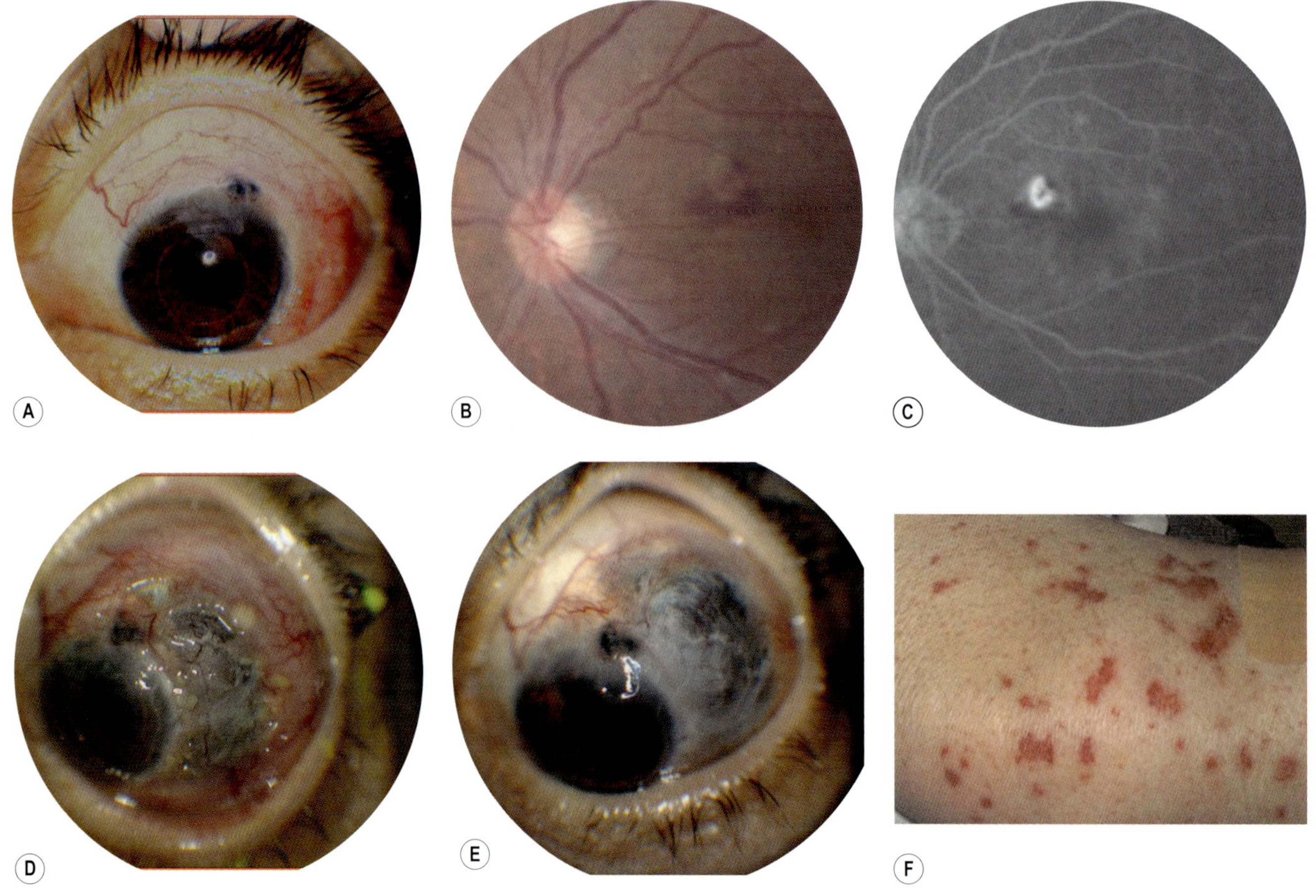

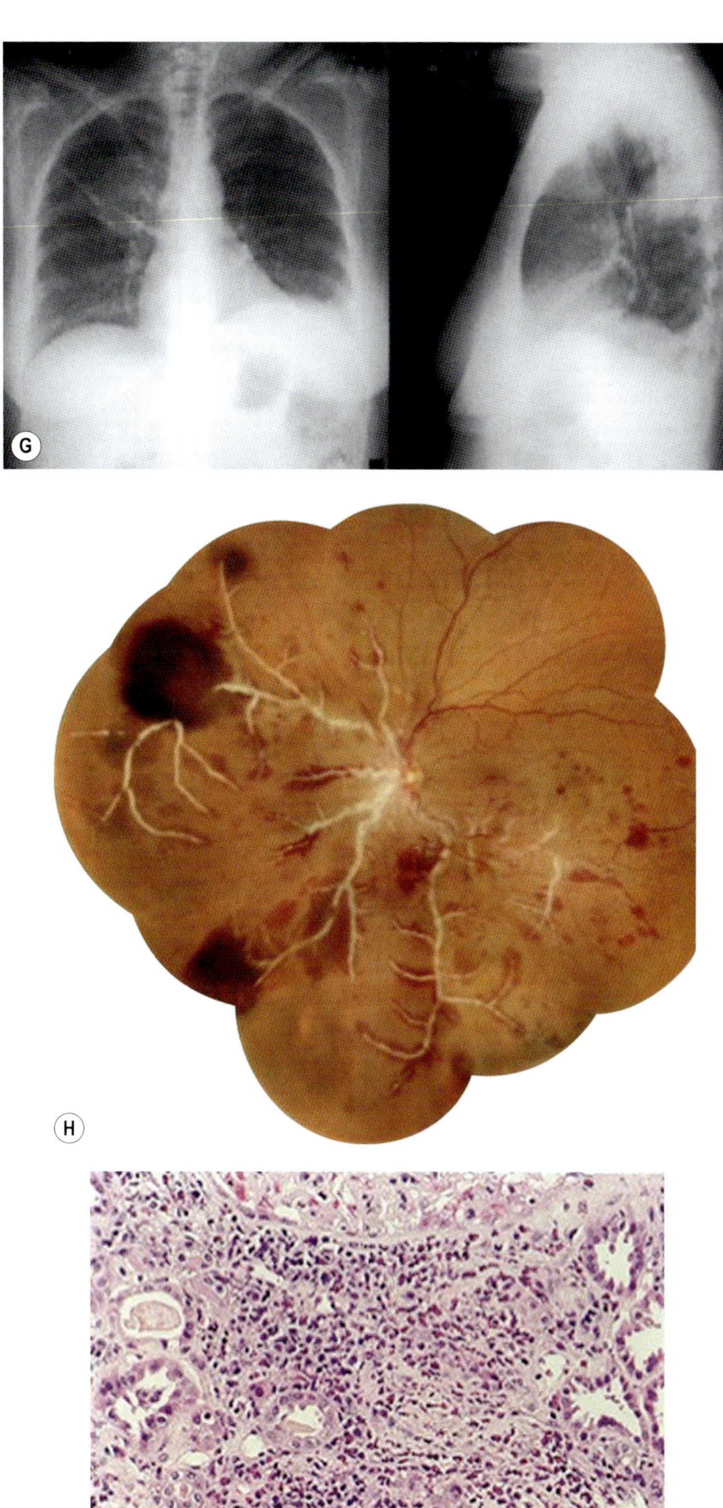

FAMILIAL CHRONIC GRANULOMATOUS DISEASE OF CHILDHOOD

Chronic granulomatous disease of childhood is a genetically determined disorder characterized by relentless succession of chronic granulomatous and suppurative lesions of many organs caused by a defect in the ability of the leukocytes to kill certain microorganisms after phagocytosis.

The disease affects primarily young males, manifests in infancy, and frequently results in death in early childhood.[641–643] Young male patients present with chorioretinal lesions or scars associated with recurrent systemic infections such as pneumonia, suppurative abscesses of various organs and osteomyelitis. These lesions are usually picked up on dilated retinal examinations performed on hospitalized children in the ICU. The active lesions appear yellow gray and the inactive are pigmented punched out scars varying in size from 500 microns to large confluent lesions.[644–647] The more often seen inactive lesions sometimes resemble the lacunae described in female patients with Aicardi's syndrome. They are frequently present in the peripapillary area, and tend to follow the distribution of the retinal vessels out toward the periphery, often sparing the macular region (Figure 11.52 A-D). Optic atrophy may be present. Occasionally patients present with significant vitritis and suppuration, often, vitreous biopsy does not yield an organism. Women are X linked carriers and are usually asymptomatic. However, some women may manifest some of the systemic features of the disease and have deep chorioretinal scars usually distributed along blood vessels. The scars resemble those seen in multifocal choroiditis (Figure 11.52 C-F).

Chronic granulomatous disease is an inherited immuno deficiency disorder of the neutrophil NADPH oxidase complex featured by its inability to produce reactant super oxide and its metabolites such as hydrogen peroxide, hydroxyl anion and hypohalous acid. The neutrophils are able to phagocytose microbes, but are unable to generate superoxide and hydrogen peroxide that is needed to kill the microbe.[648] Hence these patients suffer from recurrent and chronic bacterial and fungal infection in the form of pneumonia, lymphadenitis, eczematoid dermatitis, osteomyelitis, hepatosplenomegaly and abscesses from saprophytic organisms.

There are 2 patterns of inheritance; the more common X linked recessive in 70–80 % and the less common autosomal recessive inheritance in 20–30% of patients. Within each mode of inheritance there are 2 separate genetic types – cytochrome b558 negative CGD and b558 positive CGD. The X- linked cytochrome b558-negative CGD comprises 60% of cases. Autosomal recessive CGD is milder and may present only in adolescence.

Phagocytosis initiates a biochemical chain reaction called respiratory burst in neutrophils resulting in a variety of microbicidal reduced oxygen metabolites such as superoxide and hydrogen peroxide. Neutrophils in CGD lack the respiratory burst and thereby cannot kill certain bacteria. However organisms that themselves produce hydrogen peroxide such as Streptococcus groups B and D, Streptococcus pneumonia, and Clostridium difficile are killed by CGD neutrophils. Catalase positive organisms such as Staphylococcus aureus, pseudomonas, Candida, Aspergillus, E. coli remain viable after phagocytosis by CGD neutrophils.

Aspergillus is the commonest organism causing disseminated pulmonary infection, which is the leading cause of death in these patients. Staphylococcus aureus liver infections are next most common. Recurrent skin abscesses, perianal abscess, osteomyelitis are frequent. Some patients develop strictures or obstruction from granuloma in the esophagus, gastric antrum and genitourinary tract. Women carriers can develop a milder form of the disease and often suffer from enterocolitis that is often misdiagnosed as Crohn's disease.[649] They have a dual population of circulating neutrophils based on random X-chromosome inactivation(lyonization). Recurrent antigenic stimulation leading to autoantibody formation may explain the apparently increased frequency of discoid lupus in female carriers of CGD.[650]

Long-term prophylaxis with antimicrobials with trimethoprim and sulfamethoxazole, itraconazole and gamma-interferon has positively modified the course of CGD and improved the duration and quality of life. Trimethoprim-sulfamethoxazole has reduced the rate of severe infections by 50%, interferon gamma (generates H_2O_2) by 70% and itraconazole has reduced Aspergillus infection by 50%. Granulocyte transfusions can be used in life threatening infections.[651] Active multifocal choroidal lesions that disappeared after systemic treatment with vincristine, prednisone, and cyclophosphamide have been observed.[643] It is believed that the H_2O_2 generated by the normal neutrophils can diffuse into defective CGD neutrophils and produce hypohalous acid and hydroxyl anion thus killing the microbes. Granulocyte transfusions are generally well tolerated, but adverse effects include fevers,

11.52 Carrier state of chronic granulomatous disease

A–F: This 23 year old woman carried a diagnosis of 'Crohn's disease' for 10 years. She was found to have the lesions in the fundus on an examination for floaters that she noted whenever the Crohn's disease flared up. She had failed multiple therapies for Crohn's including methotrexate, mercaptopurine, humira, remicade and was currently on 40 mg prednisone/day. Her vision was 20/25 in each eye, the anterior segment and vitreous were quiet. There were several round chorioretinal scars, many along blood vessels in both eyes, with peripapillary scar in the right eye (A-D). Fluorescein angiogram revealed staining of the chronic lesions (E and F). Her uncle died of chronic granulomatous disease as a child, an aunt carried a diagnosis of 'ulcerative colitis' and was found to be a carrier of CGD and two of her grandmother's brothers died of CGD as children. The patient was also found to be a carrier of CGD.

Courtesy: Dr. Steven Bennett

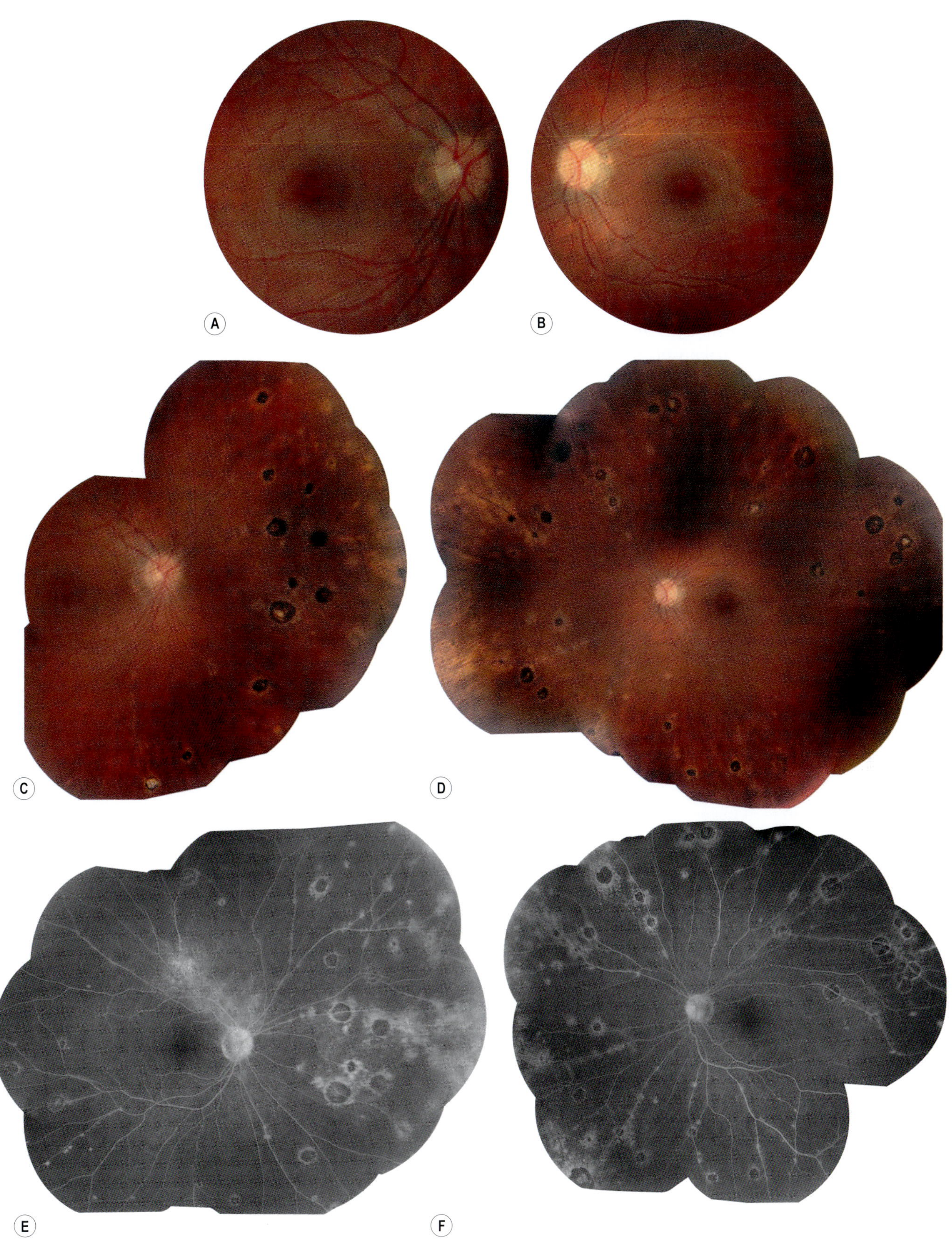
A
B
C
D
E
F

pulmonary leukostasis and development of leuko-agglutinins that lead to rapid loss of transfused neutrophils. Pulmonary leukostasis is common if Amphotericin and granulocyte transfusions are given at the same time hence should be administered several hours apart.

CGD results from mutations in genes coding gp91 phox, p22 phox, p47 phox, or p67 phox. X linked CGD results from defects in gp91 phox and the remaining mutations result in autosomal recessive CGD.

Laboratory tests to detect CGD rely on demonstration of defective NADPH oxidase function. The nitroblue tetrazolium test depends on the capability of normal neutrophils to reduce the colorless NBT dye to blue formazan during phagocytosis, while in CGD this is not possible and hence a negative test is diagnostic.

Transduction of bone marrow and peripheral blood stem-cell progenitors with corrected gene using retroviral vectors has shown improved NADPH oxidase activity. Stem cell gene therapy in animal models has shown increased resistance to experimental infection.[652]

References

1. Lim JI, Tessler HH, Goodwin JA. Anterior granulomatous uveitis in patients with multiple sclerosis. Ophthalmology 1991;98:142–5.
2. Rucker CW. Sheathing of the retinal veins in multiple sclerosis. JAMA 1945;127:970–3.
3. Gass JDM. Stereoscopic atlas of macular diseases; diagnosis and treatment, 2nd ed. St. Louis: CV Mosby; 1977. p. 310–11.
4. Blumenkranz MS, Kaplan HJ, Clarkson JG, et al. Acute multifocal hemorrhagic retinal vasculitis. Ophthalmology 1988;95:1663–72.
5. Browning DJ. Mild frosted branch periphlebitis. Am J Ophthalmol 1992;114:505–6.
6. Ito Y, Nakano M, Kyu N, et al. Frosted-branch angiitis in a child. Jpn J Clin Ophthalmol 1976;30:797–803.
7. Kleiner RC, Kaplan HJ, Shakin JL, et al. Acute frosted retinal periphlebitis. Am J Ophthalmol 1988;106:27–34.
8. Sugin SL, Henderly DE, Friedman SM, et al. Unilateral frosted branch angiitis. Am J Ophthalmol 1991;111:682–5.
9. Vander JF, Masciulli L. Unilateral frosted branch angiitis. Am J Ophthalmol 1991;112:477–8.
10. Watanabe Y, Takeda N, Adachi-Usami E. A case of frosted branch angiitis. Br J Ophthalmol 1987;71:553–8.
11. Gass JDM. Fluorescein angiography in endogenous intraocular inflammation. In: Aronson SB, Gamble CN, Goodner EK, editors. Clinical methods in uveitis: the Fourth Sloan Symposium on Uveitis. St. Louis: CV Mosby; 1968. p. 202–29.
12. Karel I, Peleska M, Divisová G. Fluorescence angiography in retinal vasculitis in children's uveitis. Ophthalmologica 1973;166:251–64.
13. Kasp E, Whiston R, Dumonde D, et al. Antibody affinity to retinal S-antigen in patients with retinal vasculitis. Am J Ophthalmol 1992;113:697–701.
14. Rabon RJ, Louis GJ, Zegarra H, et al. Acute bilateral posterior angiopathy with influenza A viral infection. Am J Ophthalmol 1987;103:289–93.
15. Kaburaki T, Nakamura M, Nagasawa K, et al. Two cases of frosted branch angiitis with central retinal vein occlusion. Jpn J Ophthalmol 2001;45:628–33.
16. Seo MS, Woo JM, Jeong SK, et al. Recurrent unilateral frosted branch angiitis. Jpn J Ophthalmol 1998;42:56–9.
17. Nakai A, Saika S. A case of frosted-branch retinal angiitis in a child. Ann Ophthalmol 1992;24:415–7.
18. Walker S, Iguchi A, Jones NP. Frosted branch angiitis: a review. Eye (Lond) 2004;18:527–33.
19. Jackson TE, Pathak S, Doran RM. Behçet disease presenting with frosted branch angiitis. Ocul Immunol Inflamm 2011;19:65–6.
20. Kono H, Ikewaki J, Kimoto K, et al. Frosted branch angiitis associated with streptococcal infection: optical coherence tomography as a follow-up tool. Acta Ophthalmol 2009;87:909–11.
21. Hua MT, Blaise P, De Leval L, et al. Frosted branch angiitis with undiagnosed Hodgkin lymphoma. Eur J Ophthalmol 2009;19:310–3.
22. Chen E, Ho AC, Garg SJ, et al. *Streptococcus mitis* endophthalmitis presenting as frosted branch angiitis after intravitreal pegaptanib sodium injection. Ophthalmic Surg Lasers Imaging 2009;40:192–4.
23. Reynders S, Dewachter A, de Vriese AS. A case of secondary frosted branch angiitis in Behçet's disease. Bull Soc Belge Ophtalmol 2005;298:41–4.
24. Gupta A, Narang S, Gupta V, et al. Frosted branch angiitis associated with rapidly progressive glomerulonephritis. Indian J Ophthalmol 2002;50:317–9.
25. Shenoy R, Elagib EN, Al-Siyabi H. Frosted retinal branch angiitis in an immunocompetent adult due to herpes simplex virus. Indian J Ophthalmol 2001;49:56–7.
26. Fine HF, Smith JA, Murante BL, et al. Frosted branch angiitis in a child with HIV infection. Am J Ophthalmol 2001;131:394–6.
27. Ysasaga JE, Davis J. Frosted branch angiitis with ocular toxoplasmosis. Arch Ophthalmol 1999;117:1260–1.
28. Margo CE, Friedman SM, Purdy EP, et al. Retinochoroidal degeneration associated with progressive iris necrosis. Arch Ophthalmol 1990;108:989–92.
29. Annesley WH, Tomer TL, Shields JA. Multifocal placoid pigment epitheliopathy. Am J Ophthalmol 1973;76:511–8.
30. Azar Jr P, Gohd RS, Waltman D, et al. Acute posterior multifocal placoid pigment epitheliopathy associated with an adenovirus type 5 infection. Am J Ophthalmol 1975;80:1003–5.
31. Bird AC, Hamilton AM. Placoid pigment epitheliopathy presenting with bilateral serous retinal detachment. Br J Ophthalmol 1972;56:881–6.
32. Bullock JD, Fletcher RL. Cerebrospinal fluid abnormalities in acute posterior multifocal placoid pigment epitheliopathy. Am J Ophthalmol 1977;84:45–9.
33. DeLaey JJ. Fluoro-angiographic study of the choroid in man. Doc Ophthalmol 1978;45:113–39.
34. Deutman AF, Lion F. Choriocapillaris nonperfusion in acute multifocal placoid pigment epitheliopathy. Am J Ophthalmol 1977;84:652–7.
35. Deutman AF, Oosterhuis JA, Boen-Tan TN, et al. Acute posterior multifocal placoid pigment epitheliopathy; pigment epitheliopathy or choriocapillaritis. Br J Ophthalmol 1972;56:863–74.
36. Fishman GA, Rabb MF, Kaplan J. Acute posterior multifocal placoid pigment epitheliopathy. Arch Ophthalmol 1974;92:173–7.
37. Fitzpatrick PJ, Robertson DM. Acute posterior multifocal placoid pigment epitheliopathy. Arch Ophthalmol 1973;89:373–6.
38. Gass JDM. Acute posterior multifocal placoid pigment epitheliopathy. Arch Ophthalmol 1968;80:177–85.
39. Gass JDM. Acute posterior multifocal placoid pigment epitheliopathy: a long-term follow-up study. In: Fine SL, Owens SL, editors. Management of retinal vascular and macular disorders. Baltimore: Williams & Wilkins; 1983. p. 176–81.
40. Gass JDM. Stereoscopic atlas of macular diseases; diagnosis and treatment, 3rd ed. St. Louis: CV Mosby; 1987. p. 504–10.
41. Hector RE. Acute posterior multifocal placoid pigment epitheliopathy. Am J Ophthalmol 1978;86:424–5.
42. Holt WS, Regan CDJ, Trempe C. Acute posterior multifocal placoid pigment epitheliopathy. Am J Ophthalmol 1976;81:403–12.
43. Jacklin HN. Acute posterior multifocal placoid pigment epitheliopathy and thyroiditis. Arch Ophthalmol 1977;95:995–7.
44. Jenkins RB, Savino PJ, Pilkerton AR. Placoid pigment epitheliopathy with swelling of the optic disks. Arch Neurol 1973;29:204–5.
45. Kirkham TH, Ffytche TJ, Sanders MD. Placoid pigment epitheliopathy with retinal vasculitis and papillitis. Br J Ophthalmol 1972;56:875–80.
46. Laatikainen LT, Erkkilä H. Clinical and fluorescein angiographic findings of acute multifocal central subretinal inflammation. Acta Ophthalmol 1973;51:645–55.
47. Lewis RA, Martonyi CL. Acute posterior multifocal placoid pigment epitheliopathy; a recurrence. Arch Ophthalmol 1975;93:235–8.
48. Lyness AL, Bird AC. Recurrences of acute posterior multifocal placoid pigment epitheliopathy. Am J Ophthalmol 1984;98:203–7.
49. McGuinness R, Mitchell P. A case of acute posterior multifocal placoid pigment epitheliopathy associated with erythema nodosum. Aust J Ophthalmol 1977;5:48–51.
50. Priluck IA, Robertson DM, Buettner H. Acute posterior multifocal placoid pigment epitheliopathy; urinary findings. Arch Ophthalmol 1981;99:1560–2.
51. Reuscher A. Zur Pathogenese der sogenannten akuten hinteren multifokalen placoiden Pigmentepitheliopathie. Klin Monatsbl Augenheilkd 1974;165:775–84.
52. Ryan SJ, Maumenee AE. Acute posterior multifocal placoid pigment epitheliopathy. Am J Ophthalmol 1972;74:1066–74.
53. Savino PJ, Weinberg RJ, Yassin JG, et al. Diverse manifestations of acute posterior multifocal placoid pigment epitheliopathy. Am J Ophthalmol 1974;77:659–62.
54. Sigelman J, Behrens M, Hilal S. Acute posterior multifocal placoid pigment epitheliopathy associated with cerebral vasculitis and homonymous hemianopia. Am J Ophthalmol 1979;88:919–24.
55. Van Buskirk EM, Lessell S, Friedman E. Pigmentary epitheliopathy and erythema nodosum. Arch Ophthalmol 1971;85:369–72.
56. Williams DF, Mieler WF. Long-term follow-up of acute multifocal posterior placoid pigment epitheliopathy. Br J Ophthalmol 1989;73:985–90.
57. Young NJA, Bird AC, Sehmi K. Pigment epithelial diseases with abnormal choroidal perfusion. Am J Ophthalmol 1980;90:607–18.
58. Wolf MD, Alward WLM, Folk JC. Long-term visual function in acute posterior multifocal placoid pigment epitheliopathy. Arch Ophthalmol 1991;109:800–3.
59. Fine HF, Kim E, Flynn TE, et al. Acute posterior multifocal placoid pigment epitheliopathy following varicella vaccination. Br J Ophthalmol 2010;94:282–3, 363.
60. Althaus C, Unsöld R, Figge C, et al. Cerebral complications in acute posterior multifocal placoid pigment epitheliopathy. Ger J Ophthalmol 1993;2:150–4.
61. Fishman GA, Baskin M, Jednock N. Spinal fluid pleocytosis in acute posterior multifocal placoid pigment epitheliopathy. Ann Ophthalmol 1977:33–6.
62. Smith CH, Savino PJ, Beck RW, et al. Acute posterior multifocal placoid pigment epitheliopathy and cerebral vasculitis. Arch Neurol 1983;40:48–50.
63. Spaide RF, Yannuzzi LA, Slakter J. Choroidal vasculitis in acute posterior multifocal placoid pigment epitheliopathy. Br J Ophthalmol 1991;75:685–7.
64. Stoll G, Reiners K, Schwartz A, et al. Acute posterior multifocal placoid pigment epitheliopathy with cerebral involvement. J Neurol Neurosurg Psychiatr 1991;54:77–9.
65. Tönjes W, Mielke U, Schmidt HJ, et al. Akute multifokale plakoide Pigmentepitheliopathie mit entzündlichem Liquorbefund; sonderform einer Borreliose? Dtsch Med Wochenschr 1989;114:793–5.
66. Weinstein JM, Bresnick GH, Bell CL, et al. Acute posterior multifocal placoid pigment epitheliopathy associated with cerebral vasculitis. J Clin Neuro-Ophthalmol 1988;8:195–201.

67. Wilson CA, Choromokos EA, Sheppard R. Acute posterior multifocal placoid pigment epitheliopathy and cerebral vasculitis. Arch Ophthalmol 1988;106:796–800.
68. Bodiguel E, Benhamou A, Le Hoang P, et al. Infarctus cerebral, epitheliopathie en plaques et sarcoidose. Rev Neurol 1992;148:746–51.
69. Dick DJ, Newman PK, Richardson J, et al. Acute posterior multifocal placoid pigment epitheliopathy and sarcoidosis. Br J Ophthalmol 1988;72:74–7.
70. Laatikainen LT, Immonen IJR. Acute posterior multifocal placoid pigment epitheliopathy in connection with acute nephritis. Retina 1988;8:122–4.
71. Kawaguchi Y, Hara M, Hirose T, et al. A case of systemic lupus erythematosus complicated with multifocal posterior pigment epitheliopathy. Ryumachi 1990;30:396–400.
72. Bodine SR, Marino J, Camisa TJ, et al. Multifocal choroiditis with evidence of Lyme disease. Ann Ophthalmol 1992;24:169.
73. Wolf MD, Folk JC, Nelson JA, et al. Acute, posterior, multifocal, placoid, pigment epitheliopathy and Lyme disease. Arch Ophthalmol 1992;110:750.
74. Kinyoun JL. APMPPE associated with Wegener's granulomatosis. Retina 2000;20:419–20.
75. Hsu CT, Harlan JB, Goldberg MF, et al. Acute posterior multifocal placoid pigment epitheliopathy associated with a systemic necrotizing vasculitis. Retina 2003;23:64–8.
76. Di Crecchio L, Parodi MB, Saviano S, et al. Acute posterior multifocal placoid pigment epitheliopathy and ulcerative colitis: a possible association. Acta Ophthalmol Scand 2001;79:319–21.
77. Hammer ME, Grizzard WS, Travies D. Death associated with acute posterior multifocal placoid pigment epitheliopathy. Arch Ophthalmol 1989;107:170–1.
78. Calabrese LH, Mallek JA. Primary angiitis of the central nervous system; report of 8 new cases, review of the literature, and proposal for diagnostic criteria. Medicine 1988;67:20–39.
79. Wolf MD, Folk JC, Goeken NE. Acute posterior multifocal pigment epitheliopathy and optic neuritis in a family. Am J Ophthalmol 1990;110:89–90.
80. Dhaliwal RS, Maguire AM, Flower RW, et al. Acute posterior multifocal placoid pigment epitheliopathy. An indocyanine green angiographic study. Retina 1993;13:317–25.
81. Souka AA, Hillenkamp J, Gora F, et al. Correlation between optical coherence tomography and autofluorescence in acute posterior multifocal placoid pigment epitheliopathy. Graefes Arch Clin Exp Ophthalmol 2006;244:1219–23.
82. Espinasse-Berrod MA, Gotte D, Parent de Cruzon H, et al. Un cas d'épithéliopathie en plaques associé à des néovaisseaux sous-rétiniens. J Fr Ophtalmol 1988;11:191–4.
83. Dhaliwal RS, Maguire AM, Flower RW, et al. Acute posterior multifocal placoid pigment epitheliopathy; an indocyanine green angiographic study. Retina 1993;13:317–25.
84. Wolf MD, Folk JC, Panknen CA, et al. HLA-B7 and HLA-DR2 antigens and acute posterior multifocal placoid pigment epitheliopathy. Arch Ophthalmol 1990;108:698–700.
85. Charteris DG, Khanna V, Dhillon B. Acute posterior multifocal placoid pigment epitheliopathy complicated by central retinal vein occlusion. Br J Ophthalmol 1989;73:765–8.
86. Charteris DG, Lee WR. Multifocal posterior uveitis: Clinical and pathological findings. Br J Ophthalmol 1990;74:688–93.
87. Wright BE, Bird AC, Hamilton AM. Placoid pigment epitheliopathy and Harada's disease. Br J Ophthalmol 1978;62:609–21.
88. Blinder KJ, Peyman GA, Paris CL. Diffuse posterior punctate pigment epitheliopathy. Retina 1994;14:31–5.
89. Taich A, Johnson MW. A syndrome resembling acute posterior multifocal placoid pigment epitheliopathy in older adults. Trans Am Ophthalmol Soc 2008;106:56–62. [discussion 63.]
90. Golchet PR, Jampol LM, Wilson D, et al. Persistent placoid maculopathy: a new clinical entity. Trans Am Ophthalmol Soc 2006;104:108–20.
91. Khairallah M, Ben Yahia S. Persistent placoid maculopathy. Ophthalmology 2008;115:220–1.
92. Golchet PR, Jampol LM, Wilson D, et al. Persistent placoid maculopathy: a new clinical entity. Ophthalmology 2007;114:1530–40.
93. Jones BE, Jampol LM, Yannuzzi LA, et al. Relentless placoid chorioretinitis: a new entity or an unusual variant of serpiginous chorioretinitis? Arch Ophthalmol 2000;118:931–8.
94. Yeh S, Lew JC, Wong WT, et al. Relentless placoid chorioretinitis associated with central nervous system lesions treated with mycophenolate mofetil. Arch Ophthalmol 2009;127:341–3.
95. Chen E. Relentless placoid chorioretinitis. Ophthalmic Surg Lasers Imaging 2009 January;40:87–8.
96. Amer R, Florescu T. Optical coherence tomography in relentless placoid chorioretinitis. Clin Experiment Ophthalmol 2008;36:388–90.
97. Orihara T, Wakabayashi T, Okada AA, et al. A young Japanese man with relentless placoid chorioretinitis. Jpn J Ophthalmol 2005;49:539–42.
98. Blumenkranz MS, Gass JDM, Clarkson JG. Atypical serpiginous choroiditis. Arch Ophthalmol 1982;100:1773–5.
99. Chisholm IH, Gass JDM, Hutton WL. The late stage of serpiginous (geographic) choroiditis. Am J Ophthalmol 1976;82:343–51.
100. Gass JDM. Stereoscopic atlas of macular diseases; a fundoscopic and angiographic presentation. St. Louis: CV Mosby; 1970. p. 66.
101. Gass JDM. Stereoscopic atlas of macular diseases; diagnosis and treatment, 2nd ed. St. Louis: CV Mosby; 1977. p. 112.
102. Hamilton AM, Bird AC. Geographical choroidopathy. Br J Ophthalmol 1974;58:784–97.
103. Hardy RA, Schatz H. Macular geographic helicoid choroidopathy. Arch Ophthalmol 1987;105:1237–42.
104. Laatikainen L, Erkkilä H. Serpiginous choroiditis. Br J Ophthalmol 1974;58:777–83.
105. Laatikainen L, Erkkilä H. Subretinal and disc neovascularization in serpiginous choroiditis. Br J Ophthalmol 1982;66:326–31.
106. Mansour AM, Jampol LM, Packo KH, et al. Macular serpiginous choroiditis. Retina 1988;8: 125–31.
107. Masi RJ, O'Connor GR, Kimura SJ. Anterior uveitis in geographic or serpiginous choroiditis. Am J Ophthalmol 1978;86:228–32.
108. Schatz H, Maumenee AE, Patz A. Geographic helicoid peripapillary choroidopathy: Clinical presentation and fluorescein angiographic findings. Trans Am Acad Ophthalmol Otolaryngol 1974;78:OP747–OP761.
109. Weiss H, Annesley Jr WH, Shields JA, et al. The clinical course of serpiginous choroidopathy. Am J Ophthalmol 1979;87:133–42.
110. Gass JDM. Stereoscopic atlas of macular diseases; diagnosis and treatment, 3rd ed. St. Louis: CV Mosby; 1987. p. 136–45.
111. Jampol LM, Orth D, Daily MJ, et al. Subretinal neovascularization with geographic (serpiginous) choroiditis. Am J Ophthalmol 1979;88:683–869.
112. Wojno T, Meredith TA. Unusual findings in serpiginous choroiditis. Am J Ophthalmol 1982;94:650–5.
113. Friberg TR. Serpiginous choroiditis with branch vein occlusion and bilateral periphlebitis. Arch Ophthalmol 1988;106:585–6.
114. Giovannini A, Ripa E, Scassellati-Sforzolini B, et al. Indocyanine green angiography in serpiginous choroidopathy. Eur J Ophthalmol 1996;6:299–306.
115. Cardillo Piccolino F, Grosso A, Savini E. Fundus autofluorescence in serpiginous choroiditis. Graefes Arch Clin Exp Ophthalmol 2009;247:179–85.
116. Richardson RR, Cooper IS, Smith JL. Serpiginous choroiditis and unilateral extrapyramidal dystonia. Ann Ophthalmol 1981;13:15–19.
117. King DG, Grizzard WS, Sever RJ, et al. Serpiginous choroidopathy associated with elevated factor VIII–von Willebrand factor antigen. Retina 1990;10:97–101.
118. Broekhuyse RM, Van Herck M, Pinckers AH, et al. Immune responsiveness to retinal-S antigen and opsin in serpiginous choroiditis and other retinal diseases. Doc Ophthalmol 1988;69:83–93.
119. Gupta V, Gupta A, Arora S, et al. Presumed tubercular serpiginouslike choroiditis: clinical presentations and management. Ophthalmology 2003;110:1744–9.
120. Hooper PL, Kaplan HJ. Triple agent immunosuppression in serpiginous choroiditis. Ophthalmology 1991;98:944–52.
121. Laatikainen L, Tarkkanen A. Failure of cyclosporin A in serpiginous choroiditis. J Ocular Ther Surg 1984;3:280–2.
122. Secchi AG, Tognon MS, Maselli C. Cyclosporine-A in the treatment of serpiginous choroiditis. Int Ophthalmol 1990;14:395–9.
123. Vianna RN, Ozdal PC, Deschenes J, et al. Combination of azathioprine and corticosteroids in the treatment of serpiginous choroiditis. Can J Ophthalmol 2006;41:183–9.
124. Markomichelakis NN, Halkiadakis I, Papaeythymiou-Orchan S, et al. Intravenous pulse methylprednisolone therapy for acute treatment of serpiginous choroiditis. Ocul Immunol Inflamm 2006;14:29–33.
125. Akpek EK, Baltatzis S, Yang J, et al. Long-term immunosuppressive treatment of serpiginous choroiditis. Ocul Immunol Inflamm 2001;9:153–67.
126. Secchi AG, Tognon MS, Maselli C. Cyclosporine-A in the treatment of serpiginous choroiditis. Int Ophthalmol 1990;14:395–9.
127. Yannuzzi LA, Jampol LM, Rabb MF, et al. Unilateral acute idiopathic maculopathy. Arch Ophthalmol 1991;109:1411–6.
128. Fish RH, Territo C, Anand R. Pseudohypopyon in unilateral acute idiopathic maculopathy. Retina 1993;13:26–8.
129. Freund KB, Yannuzzi LA, Barile GR, et al. The expanding clinical spectrum of unilateral acute idiopathic maculopathy. Arch Ophthalmol 1996;114:555–9.
130. Beck AP, Jampol LM, Glaser DA, et al. Is coxsackievirus the cause of unilateral acute idiopathic maculopathy? Arch Ophthalmol 2004;122:121–3.
131. Aggio FB, Farah ME, Meirelles RL, et al. STRATUSOCT and multifocal ERG in unilateral acute idiopathic maculopathy. Graefes Arch Clin Exp Ophthalmol 2006;244:510–6.
132. Xu H, Lin P. Unilateral recurrent acute idiopathic maculopathy. Graefes Arch Clin Exp Ophthalmol 2011;249(6):941–944.
133. Lam BL, Lopez PF, Dubovy SR, et al. Transient electro-oculogram impairment in unilateral acute idiopathic maculopathy. Doc Ophthalmol 2009;119:157–61.
134. Ghazi NG, Daccache A, Conway BP. Acute idiopathic maculopathy: report of a bilateral case manifesting a macular hole. Ophthalmology 2007;114:e1–e6.
135. Haruta H, Sawa M, Saishin Y, et al. Clinical findings in unilateral acute idiopathic maculopathy: New findings in acute idiopathic maculopathy. Int Ophthalmol 2010;30:199–202.
136. Hong PH, Jampol LM, Dodwell DG, et al. Unifocal helioid choroiditis. Arch Ophthalmol 1997;115:1007–13.
137. Shields JA, Shields CL, Demirci H, et al. Solitary idiopathic choroiditis: the Richard B. Weaver lecture. Arch Ophthalmol 2002;120:311–9.
138. Krill AE, Deutman AF. Acute retinal pigment epitheliitis. Am J Ophthalmol 1972;74:193–205.
139. Chittum ME, Kalina RE. Acute retinal pigment epitheliitis. Ophthalmology 1987;94:1114–9.
140. Deutman AF. Acute retinal pigment epitheliitis. Am J Ophthalmol 1974;78:571–8.
141. Eifrig DE, Knobloch WH, Moran JA. Retinal pigment epitheliitis. Ann Ophthalmol 1977;9:639–42.
142. Friedman MW. Bilateral recurrent acute retinal pigment epitheliitis. Am J Ophthalmol 1975;79:567–70.
143. Luttrull JK. Acute retinal pigment epitheliitis. Am J Ophthalmol 1997;123:127–9.
144. Luttrull JK, Chittum ME. Acute retinal pigment epitheliitis. Am J Ophthalmol 1995;120:389–91.
145. Loh BK, Chee SP. Optical coherence tomography findings in acute retinal pigment epitheliitis. Am J Ophthalmol 2007;143:1071. [author reply.]
146. Hsu J, Fineman MS, Kaiser RS. Optical coherence tomography findings in acute retinal pigment epitheliitis. Am J Ophthalmol 2007;143:163–5.
147. Blanco-Rivera C, Campos-Garcia S. Acute retinal pigment epitheliitis: a case report. Arch Soc Esp Oftalmol 2007;82:451–3.
148. Aaberg TM. Multiple evanescent white dot syndrome. Arch Ophthalmol 1988;106:1162–3.
149. Borruat F-X, Othenin-Girard P, Safran AB. Multiple evanescent white dot syndrome. Klin Monatsbl Augenheilkd 1991;198:453–6.
150. Chung Y-M, Yeh T-S, Liu J-H. Increased serum IgM and IgG in the multiple evanescent white-dot syndrome. Am J Ophthalmol 1987;104:187–8.
151. Hamed LM, Glaser JS, Gass JDM, et al. Protracted enlargement of the blind spot in multiple evanescent white dot syndrome. Arch Ophthalmol 1989;107:194–8.
152. Jampol LM, Sieving PA, Pugh D, et al. Multiple evanescent white dot syndrome. I. Clinical findings. Arch Ophthalmol 1984;102:671–4.

153. Jost BF, Olk RJ, McGaughey A. Bilateral symptomatic multiple evanescent white-dot syndrome. Am J Ophthalmol 1986;101:489–90.
154. Laatikainen L, Immonen I. Multiple evanescent white dot syndrome. Graefes Arch Clin Exp Ophthalmol 1988;226:37–40.
155. Lefrançois A, Hamard H, Corbe C, et al. A propos d'un cas de MEWDS. Syndrome des taches blanches rétiniennes fugaces. J Fr Ophtalmol 1989;12:103–9.
156. Leys A, Leys M, Jonckheere P, et al. Multiple evanescent white dot syndrome (MEWDS). Bull Soc Belge Ophtalmol 1990;236:97–108.
157. Leys M, Van Slycken S, Koller J, et al. Acute macular neuropathy after shock. Bull Soc Belge Ophtalmol 1991;241:95–104.
158. Mamalis N, Daily MJ. Multiple evanescent white-dot syndrome; a report of eight cases. Ophthalmology 1987;94:1209–12.
159. Meyer RJ, Jampol LM. Recurrences and bilaterality in the multiple evanescent white-dot syndrome. Am J Ophthalmol 1986;101:388–9.
160. Nakao K, Isashiki M. Multiple evanescent white dot syndrome. Jpn J Ophthalmol 1986;30:376–84.
161. Noske W, Danisevskis M, Priesnitz M, et al. Multiple evanescent white dot-syndrome. Klin Monatsbl Augenheilkd 1992;201:107–9.
162. Sieving PA, Fishman GA, Jampol LM, et al. Multiple evanescent white dot syndrome. II. Electrophysiology of the photoreceptors during retinal pigment epithelial disease. Arch Ophthalmol 1984;102:675–9.
163. Singh K, de Frank MP, Shults WT, et al. Acute idiopathic blind spot enlargement; a spectrum of disease. Ophthalmology 1991;98:497–502.
164. Slusher MM, Weaver RG. Multiple evanescent white dot syndrome. Retina 1988;8:132–5.
165. Takeda M, Kimura S, Tamiya M. Acute disseminated retinal pigment epitheliopathy. Folia Ophthalmol Jpn 1984;35:2613–20.
166. Fletcher WA, Imes RK, Goodman D, et al. Acute idiopathic blind spot enlargement; a big blind spot syndrome without optic disc edema. Arch Ophthalmol 1988;106:44–9.
167. Cooper ML, Lesser RL. Prolonged course of bilateral acute idiopathic blind spot enlargement. J Clin Neuro-Ophthalmol 1992;12:173–7.
168. Dodwell DG, Jampol LM, Rosenberg M, et al. Optic nerve involvement associated with the multiple evanescent white-dot syndrome. Ophthalmology 1990;97:862–8.
169. Gass JDM. Editorial: Retinal causes of the big blind spot syndrome. J Clin Neuro-Ophthalmol 1989;9:144–5.
170. Gass JDM, Hamed LM. Acute macular neuroretinopathy and multiple evanescent white dot syndrome occurring in the same patients. Arch Ophthalmol 1989;107:189–93.
171. Hamed LM, Schatz NJ, Glaser JS, et al. Acute idiopathic blind spot enlargement without optic disc edema. Arch Ophthalmol 1988;106:1030–1.
172. Wakakura M, Furuno K. Bilateral slowly progressive big blind spot syndrome. J Neuro-Ophthalmol 1989;9:141–3.
173. Ie D, Glaser BM, Murphy RP, et al. Indocyanine green angiography in multiple evanescent white-dot syndrome. Am J Ophthalmol 1994;117:7–12.
174. McCollum CJ, Kimble JA. Peripapillary subretinal neovascularization associated with multiple evanescent white-dot syndrome. Arch Ophthalmol 1992;110:13–15.
175. Wyhinny GJ, Jackson JL, Jampol LM, et al. Subretinal neovascularization following multiple evanescent white-dot syndrome. Arch Ophthalmol 1990;108:1384.
176. Keunen JEE, van Norren D. Foveal densitometry in the multiple evanescent white-dot syndrome. Am J Ophthalmol 1988;105:561–2.
177. van Meel GJ, Keunen JEE, van Norren D, et al. Scanning laser densitometry in multiple evanescent white dot syndrome. Retina 1993;13:29–35.
178. Nishimuta M, Kubota M, Kandatsu A, et al. Color vision defect in multiple evanescent white dot syndrome. Folia Ophthalmol Jpn 1988;39:211–7.
179. Aaberg TM, Campo RV, Joffe L. Recurrences and bilaterality in the multiple evanescent white-dot syndrome. Am J Ophthalmol 1985;100:29–37.
180. Tsai L, Jampol LM, Pollock SC, et al. Chronic recurrent multiple evanescent white dot syndrome. Retina 1994;14:160–3.
181. Callanan D, Gass JDM. Multifocal choroiditis and choroidal neovascularization associated with the multiple evanescent white dot and acute idiopathic blind spot enlargement syndrome. Ophthalmology 1992;99:1678–85.
182. Khorram KD, Jampol LM, Rosenberg MA. Blind spot enlargement as a manifestation of multifocal choroiditis. Arch Ophthalmol 1991;109:1403–7.
183. Kimmel AS, Folk JC, Thompson HS, et al. The multiple evanescent white-dot syndrome with acute blind spot enlargement. Am J Ophthalmol 1989;107:425–6.
184. Laatikainen L, Mustonen E. Asymmetry of retinitis pigmentosa-related to initial optic disc vasculitis. Acta Ophthalmol 1992;70:543–8.
185. Dreyer RF, Gass JDM. Multifocal choroiditis and panuveitis; a syndrome that mimics ocular histoplasmosis. Arch Ophthalmol 1984;102:1776–84.
186. Morgan CM, Schatz H. Recurrent multifocal choroiditis. Ophthalmology 1986;93:1138–47.
187. Watzke RC, Packer AJ, Folk JC, et al. Punctate inner choroidopathy. Am J Ophthalmol 1984;98:572–84.
188. Bos PJM, Deutman AF. Acute macular neuroretinopathy. Am J Ophthalmol 1975;80:573–84.
189. Gass JDM. Acute zonal occult outer retinopathy. J Clin Neuro-Ophthalmol 1993;13:79–97.
190. Jacobson SG, Morales DS, Sun XK, et al. Pattern of retinal dysfunction in acute zonal occult outer retinopathy. Ophthalmology 1995;102:1187–98.
191. Spaide RF. Collateral damage in acute zonal occult outer retinopathy. Am J Ophthalmol 2004;138:887–9.
192. Heckenlively JR, Ferreyra HA. Autoimmune retinopathy: a review and summary. Semin Immunopathol 2008;30:127–34.
193. Gass JD, Agarwal A, Scott IU. Acute zonal occult outer retinopathy: a long-term follow-up study. Am J Ophthalmol 2002;134:329–39.
194. Zweifel SA, Engelbert M, Laud K, et al. Outer retinal tubulation: a novel optical coherence tomography finding. Arch Ophthalmol 2009;127:1596–602.
195. Gass JDM. Stereoscopic atlas of macular diseases; diagnosis and treatment, 3rd ed. St. Louis: CV Mosby; 1987. p. 514–15.
196. Gass JDM, Stern C. Acute annular outer retinopathy as a variant of acute zonal occult outer retinopathy. Am J Ophthalmol 1995;119:330–4.
197. Luckie A, Ai E, Del Piero E. Progressive zonal outer retinitis. Am J Ophthalmol 1994;118:583–8.
198. Mitamura Y, Ito H, Nakamura Y, et al. Acute annular outer retinopathy. Clin Experiment Ophthalmol 2005;33:545–8.
199. Cheung CM, Kumar V, Saeed T, et al. Acute annular outer retinopathy. Arch Ophthalmol 2002;120:993.
200. Fekrat S, Wilkinson CP, Chang B, et al. Acute annular outer retinopathy: report of four cases. Am J Ophthalmol 2000;130:636–44.
201. Salem M, Ismail L. Immune complex deposition lines in a case of retinal vasculitis. Graefes Arch Clin Exp Ophthalmol 1993;231:56–7.
202. Tang J, Stevens RA, Okada AA, et al. Association of antiretinal antibodies in acute annular outer retinopathy. Arch Ophthalmol 2008;126:130–2.
203. Harino S, Nagaya C, Matsuda S, et al. Indocyanine green angiographic findings in a case of acute annular outer retinopathy. Retina 2004 Oct;24(5):796–9.
204. Doran RML, Hamilton AM. Disciform macular degeneration in young adults. Trans Ophthalmol Soc UK 1982;102:471–80.
205. Gass JDM. Stereoscopic atlas of macular diseases; diagnosis and treatment, 2nd ed. St Louis: CV Mosby; 1977. p. 220, 360.
206. Gass JDM. Stereoscopic atlas of macular diseases; diagnosis and treatment, 3rd ed. St. Louis: CV Mosby; 1987. p. 534–49.
207. Gass JDM, Margo CE, Levy MH. Progressive subretinal fibrosis and blindness in patients with multifocal granulomatous chorioretinitis. Am J Ophthalmol 1996;122:76–85.
208. Nozik RA, Dorsch W. A new chorioretinopathy associated with anterior uveitis. Am J Ophthalmol 1973;76:758–62.
209. Saraux H, Pelosse B, Guigui A. Choroïdite multifocale interne: Pseudohistoplasmose. Forme européenne de l'histoplasmose présumée américaine. J Fr Ophtalmol 1986;9:645–51.
210. Scheider A. Multifocal inner choroiditis. Ger J Ophthalmol 1993;2:1–9.
211. Singerman LJ. Discussion of Morgan CM, Schatz H: Recurrent multifocal choroiditis. Ophthalmology 1986;93:1143–7.
212. Tessler HH, Deutsch TA. Multifocal choroiditis (inflammatory pseudo-histoplasmosis). In: Saari KM, editor. Uveitis update: proceedings of the First International Symposium on Uveitis held in Hanasaari, Espoo, Finland on May 16–19, 1984. Amsterdam: Excerpta Medica; 1984. p. 221–6.
213. Spaide RF, Skerry JE, Yannuzzi LA, et al. Lack of the HLA-DR2 specificity in multifocal choroiditis and panuveitis. Br J Ophthalmol 1990;74:536–7.
214. Bottoni FG, Deutman AF, Aandekerk AL. Presumed ocular histoplasmosis syndrome and linear streak lesions. Br J Ophthalmol 1989;73:528–35.
215. Spaide RF, Yannuzzi LA, Freund KB. Linear streaks in multifocal choroiditis and panuveitis. Retina 1991;11:229–31.
216. Hershey JM, Pulido JS, Folberg R, et al. Non-caseating conjunctival granulomas in patients with multifocal choroiditis and panuveitis. Ophthalmology 1994;101:596–601.
217. Machida S, Fujiwara T, Murai K, et al. Idiopathic choroidal neovascularization as an early manifestation of inflammatory chorioretinal diseases. Retina 2008;28:703–10.
218. Palestine AG, Nussenblatt RB, Parver LM, et al. Progressive subretinal fibrosis and uveitis. Br J Ophthalmol 1984;68:667–73.
219. Tiedeman JS. Epstein–Barr viral antibodies in multifocal choroiditis and panuveitis. Am J Ophthalmol 1987;103:659–63.
220. Spaide RF, Sugin S, Yannuzzi LA, et al. Epstein–Barr virus antibodies in multifocal choroiditis and panuveitis. Am J Ophthalmol 1991;112:410–3.
221. Charteris DG, Champ C, Rosenthal AR, et al. Behçet's disease: Activated T lymphocytes in retinal perivasculitis. Br J Ophthalmol 1992;76:499–501.
222. Hirose S, Kuwabara T, Nussenblatt RB, et al. Uveitis induced in primates by interphotoreceptor retinoid-binding protein. Arch Ophthalmol 1986;104:1698–702.
223. Gass JDM. Stereoscopic atlas of macular diseases; diagnosis and treatment, 2nd ed. St. Louis: CV Mosby; 1977. p. 304.
224. Miller MH, Spalton DJ, Fitzke FW, et al. Acute macular neuroretinopathy. Ophthalmology 1989;96:265–9.
225. Nagasawa N, Hommura S. A case of acute macular neuroretinopathy – an optical consideration on the peculiar features of fundus oculi. Acta Soc Ophthalmol Jpn 1982;86:2044–9.
226. Neetens A, Burvenich H. Presumed inflammatory maculopathies. Trans Ophthalmol Soc UK 1978;98:160–6.
227. Priluck IA, Buettner H, Robertson DM. Acute macular neuroretinopathy. Am J Ophthalmol 1978;86:775–8.
228. Putteman A, Toussaint D, Deutman AF. Neuroretinopathie maculaire aigue. Bull Soc Belge Ophtalmol 1982;199–200:35–41.
229. Rait JL, O'Day J. Acute macular neuroretinopathy. Aust NZ J Ophthalmol 1987;15:337–40.
230. Rush JA. Acute macular neuroretinopathy. Am J Ophthalmol 1977;83:490–4.
231. Sanders MD. Diagnostic difficulties in optic nerve disease and in papilloedema and disc oedema. Trans Ophthalmol Soc UK 1976;96:386–94.
232. Sieving PA, Fishman GA, Salzano T, et al. Acute macular neuroretinopathy: Early receptor potential change suggests photoreceptor pathology. Br J Ophthalmol 1984;68:229–34.
233. Van Herck M, Leys A, Missotten L. Acute macular neuroretinopathy. Bull Soc Belge Ophtalmol 1984;210:119–25.
234. Hughes EH, Siow YC, Hunyor AP. Acute macular neuroretinopathy: anatomic localisation of the lesion with high-resolution OCT. Eye 2009;23:2132–4.
235. Browning AC, Gupta R, Barber C, et al. The multifocal electroretinogram in acute macular neuroretinopathy. Arch Ophthalmol 2003;121:1506–7.
236. Gandorfer A, Ulbig MW. Scanning laser ophthalmoscope findings in acute macular neuroretinopathy. Am J Ophthalmol 2002;133:413–5.

237. Mirshahi A, Scharioth GB, Klais CM, et al. Enhanced visualization of acute macular neuroretinopathy by Heidelberg Retina Tomography. Clin Experiment Ophthalmol 2006;34:596–9.
238. Monson BK, Greenberg PB, Greenberg E, et al. High-speed, ultra-high-resolution optical coherence tomography of acute macular neuroretinopathy. Br J Ophthalmol 2007;91:119–20.
239. Shukla D, Arora A, Ambatkar S, et al. Optical coherence tomography findings in acute macular neuroretinopathy. Eye 2005;19:107–8.
240. O'Brien DM, Farmer SG, Kalina RE, et al. Acute macular neuroretinopathy following intravenous sympathomimetics. Retina 1989;9:281–6.
241. Guzak SV, Kalina RE, Chenoweth RG. Acute macular neuroretinopathy following adverse reaction to intravenous contrast media. Retina 1983;3:312–7.
242. Weinberg RJ, Nerney JJ. Bilateral submacular hemorrhages associated with an influenza syndrome. Ann Ophthalmol 1983;15:710–2.
243. Singh K, de Frank MP, Shults WT, et al. Acute idiopathic blind spot enlargement. A spectrum of disease. Ophthalmology 1991;98:497–502.
244. Gass JD, Hamed LM. Acute macular neuroretinopathy and multiple evanescent white dot syndrome occurring in the same patients. Arch Ophthalmol 1989;107:189–93.
245. Campo RV, Flindall RJ. Traumatic macular atrophy. Ocular Ther 1985;2:2–7.
246. Gillies M, Sarks J, Dunlop C, et al. Traumatic retinopathy resembling acute macular neuroretinopathy. Aust N Z J Ophthalmol 1997;25:207–10.
247. Goldbaum MH. Retinal depression sign indicating a small retinal infarct. Am J Ophthalmol 1978;86:45–55.
248. Belfort Jr R, Nishi M, Hayashi S, et al. Vogt–Koyanagi–Harada's disease in Brazil. Jpn J Ophthalmol 1988;32:344–7.
249. Beniz J, Forster DJ, Lean JS, et al. Variations in clinical features of the Vogt–Koyanagi–Harada syndrome. Retina 1991;11:275–80.
250. Ibanez HE, Grand MG, Meredith TA, et al. Magnetic resonance imaging findings in Vogt–Koyanagi–Harada syndrome. Retina 1994;14:164–8.
251. Ohno S, Char DH, Kimura SJ, et al. Vogt–Koyanagi–Harada syndrome. Am J Ophthalmol 1977;83:735–40.
252. Perry HD, Font RL. Clinical and histopathologic observations in severe Vogt–Koyanagi–Harada syndrome. Am J Ophthalmol 1977;83:242–54.
253. Shimizu K. Harada's, Behçet's, Vogt–Koyanagi syndromes – are they clinical entities? Trans Am Acad Ophthalmol Otolaryngol 1973;77:OP281–OP290.
254. Snyder DA, Tessler HH. Vogt–Koyanagi–Harada syndrome. Am J Ophthalmol 1980;90:69–75.
255. Sugiura S. Vogt–Koyanagi–Harada disease. Jpn J Ophthalmol 1978;22:9–35.
256. Tagawa Y, Sugiyura S, Yakura H, et al. The association between major histocompatibility antigens (HLA) and Vogt–Koyanagi–Harada syndrome. Acta Soc Ophthalmol Jpn 1976;80:486–90.
257. Yoshioka H. Fluorescence fundus angiographic findings in early stage of Harada's syndrome. Acta Soc Ophthalmol Jpn 1968;72:2298–306.
258. Davis JL, Mittal KK, Freidlin V, et al. HLA associations and ancestry in Vogt–Koyanagi–Harada disease and sympathetic ophthalmia. Ophthalmology 1990;97:1137–42.
259. Martinez JA, Lopez PF, Sternberg Jr P, et al. Vogt–Koyanagi–Harada syndrome in patients with Cherokee ancestry. Am J Ophthalmol 1992;114:615–20.
260. Nussenblatt RB. Clinical studies of Vogt–Koyanagi–Harada's disease at the National Eye Institute, NIH, USA. Jpn J Ophthalmol 1988;32:330–3.
261. Lubin JR, Loewenstein JI, Frederick Jr AR. Vogt–Koyanagi–Harada syndrome with focal neurologic signs. Am J Ophthalmol 1981;91:332–41.
262. Zhao C, Zhang M, Wen X, et al. Choroidal folds in acute Vogt–Koyanagi–Harada disease. Ocul Immunol Inflamm 2009;17:282–8.
263. Lane CM, Jones CA, Bird AC. Optic disc swelling in sympathetic ophthalmitis and Harada's disease. Trans Ophthalmol Soc UK 1986;105:667–73.
264. Kimura R, Sakai M, Okabe H. Transient shallow anterior chamber as initial symptom in Harada's syndrome. Arch Ophthalmol 1981;99:1604–6.
265. Shirato S, Hayashi K, Masuda K. Acute angle closure glaucoma as an initial sign of Harada's disease--report of two cases. Jpn J Ophthalmol 1980;24:260–6.
266. Tomimori S, Uyama M. Shallow anterior chamber and transient myopia as initial signs of Harada's disease. Jpn J Clin Ophthalmol 1977;31:1271–3.
267. Forster DJ, Cano MR, Green RL, et al. Echographic features of the Vogt–Koyanagi–Harada syndrome. Arch Ophthalmol 1990;108:1421–6.
268. Nagaya T. Use of the electro-oculogram for diagnosing and following the development of Harada's disease. Am J Ophthalmol 1972;74:99–109.
269. Johnson CA, Teitelbaum CS. Magnetic resonance imaging in Vogt–Koyanagi–Harada syndrome. Arch Ophthalmol 1990;108:783–4.
270. Rubsamen PE, Gass JDM. Vogt–Koyanagi–Harada syndrome; clinical course, therapy, and long-term visual outcome. Arch Ophthalmol 1991;109:682–7.
271. Sasamoto Y, Ohno S, Matsuda H. Studies on corticosteroid therapy in Vogt–Koyanagi–Harada disease. Ophthalmologica 1990;201:162–7.
272. Shimizu K. Zur Symptomatologie und Therapie der Harada'schen Krankheit. Dtsch Ophthalmol Ges 1968;69:245–7.
273. Wilson P. Sympathetic ophthalmitis simulating Harada's disease. Br J Ophthalmol 1962; 46:626–8.
274. Chung Y-M, Yeh T-S. Linear streak lesions of the fundus equator associated with Vogt–Koyanagi–Harada syndrome. Am J Ophthalmol 1990;109:745–6.
275. Carlson MR, Kerman BM. Hemorrhagic macular detachment in the Vogt–Koyanagi–Harada syndrome. Am J Ophthalmol 1977;84:632–5.
276. Moorthy RS, Chong LP, Smith RE, et al. Subretinal neovascular membranes in Vogt–Koyanagi–Harada syndrome. Am J Ophthalmol 1993;116:164–70.
277. To KW, Nadel AJ, Brockhurst RJ. Optic disc neovascularization in association with Vogt–Koyanagi–Harada syndrome. Arch Ophthalmol 1990;108:918–9.
278. Tabbara KF. Scleromalacia associated with Vogt–Koyanagi–Harada syndrome. Am J Ophthalmol 1988;105:694–5.
279. Chan C-C, Palestine AG, Kuwabara T, et al. Immunopathologic study of Vogt–Koyanagi–Harada syndrome. Am J Ophthalmol 1988;105:607–11.
280. Kahn M, Pepose JS, Green WR, et al. Immunocytologic findings in a case of Vogt–Koyanagi–Harada syndrome. Ophthalmology 1993;100:1191–8.
281. Sakamoto T, Murata T, Inomata H. Class II major histocompatibility complex on melanocytes of Vogt–Koyanagi–Harada disease. Arch Ophthalmol 1991;109:1270–4.
282. Chan C-C. Relationship between sympathetic ophthalmia, phacoanaphylactic endophthalmitis, and Vogt–Koyanagi–Harada disease. Ophthalmology 1988;95:619–24.
283. Inomata H, Sakamoto T. Immunohistochemical studies of Vogt–Koyanagi–Harada disease with sunset sky fundus. Curr Eye Res 1990;9(Suppl.):35–40.
284. Bird AC, Hamilton AM. Placoid pigment epitheliopathy presenting with bilateral serous retinal detachment. Br J Ophthalmol 1972;56:881–6.
285. Wright BE, Bird AC, Hamilton AM. Placoid pigment epitheliopathy and Harada's disease. Br J Ophthalmol 1978;62:609–21.
286. Albert DM, Nordlund JJ, Lerner AB. Ocular abnormalities occurring with vitiligo. Ophthalmology 1979;86:1145–58.
287. Friedman AH, Deutsch-Sokol RH. Sugiura's sign; perilimbal vitiligo in the Vogt–Koyanagi–Harada syndrome. Ophthalmology 1981;88:1159–65.
288. Manger III CC, Ober RR. Retinal arteriovenous anastomoses in the Vogt–Koyanagi–Harada syndrome. Am J Ophthalmol 1980;89:186–91.
289. Ohno S, Minakawa R, Matsuda H. Clinical studies of Vogt–Koyanagi-Harada's disease. Jpn J Ophthalmol 1988;32:334–43.
290. Chan C-C, Palestine AG, Nussenblatt RB, et al. Anti-retinal auto-antibodies, in Vogt–Koyanagi–Harada syndrome, Behçet's disease, and sympathetic ophthalmia. Ophthalmology 1985;92:1025–8.
291. Hammer H. Cellular hypersensitivity to uveal pigment confirmed by leucocyte migration tests in sympathetic ophthalmitis and the Vogt–Koyanagi–Harada syndrome. Br J Ophthalmol 1974;58:773–6.
292. Itho S, Kurimoto S, Kouno T. Vogt–Koyanagi–Harada disease in monozygotic twins. Int Ophthalmol 1992;16:49–54.
293. Ashkenazi I, Gutman I, Melamed S, et al. Vogt–Koyanagi–Harada syndrome in two siblings. Metab Pediatr Syst Ophthalmol 1991;14:64–7.
294. Read RW, Holland GN, Rao NA, et al. Revised diagnostic criteria for Vogt-Koyanagi-Harada disease. Report of an international committee on nomenclature. Am J Ophthalmol 2001;131:647–652.
295. Liu X, Yang P, Lin X, et al. Inhibitory effect of cyclosporin A and corticosteroids on the production of IFN-gamma and IL-17 by T cells in Vogt–Koyanagi–Harada syndrome. Clin Immunol 2009;131:333–42.
296. Kawaguchi T, Horie S, Bouchenaki N, et al. Suboptimal therapy controls clinically apparent disease but not subclinical progression of Vogt–Koyanagi–Harada disease. Int Ophthalmol 2010;30:41–50.
297. Zhang XY, Wang X-M, Hu T-S. Profiling human leukocyte antigens in Vogt–Koyanagi–Harada syndrome. Am J Ophthalmol 1992;113:567–72.
298. Zhao M, Jiang Y, Abrahams IW. Association of HLA antigens with Vogt–Koyanagi–Harada syndrome in a Han Chinese population. Arch Ophthalmol 1991;109:368–70.
299. Forster DJ, Green RL, Rao NA. Unilateral manifestations of the Vogt–Koyanagi–Harada syndrome in a 7-year-old child. Am J Ophthalmol 1991;111:380–2.
300. Kremer I, Yassur Y. Unilateral atypical retinal pigment epitheliopathy associated with serous retinal detachment. Ann Ophthalmol 1992;24:75–7.
301. Wald KJ, Spaide R, Patalano VJ, et al. Posterior scleritis in children. Am J Ophthalmol 1992;113:281–6.
302. Fries PD, Char DH, Crawford JB, et al. Sympathetic ophthalmia complicating helium ion irradiation of a choroidal melanoma. Arch Ophthalmol 1987;105:1561–4.
303. Gass JDM. Correlation of fluorescein angiography and histopathology. Doc Ophthalmol Proc Ser 1976;9:359–65.
304. Gass JDM. Sympathetic ophthalmia following vitrectomy. Am J Ophthalmol 1982;93:552–8.
305. Lewis ML, Gass JDM, Spencer WH. Sympathetic uveitis after trauma and vitrectomy. Arch Ophthalmol 1978;96:263–7.
306. Liddy BStL, Stuart J. Sympathetic ophthalmia in Canada. Can J Ophthalmol 1972;7:157–9.
307. Maisel JM, Vorwerk PA. Sympathetic uveitis after giant tear repair. Retina 1989;9:122–6.
308. Makley Jr TA, Azar A. Sympathetic ophthalmia; a long-term follow-up. Arch Ophthalmol 1978;96:257–62.
309. Margo CE, Pautler SE. Granulomatous uveitis after treatment of a choroidal melanoma with proton-beam irradiation. Retina 1990;10:140–3.
310. Shimizu K, Yokochi K, Kobayashi Y. Inflammations of the choroid. Doc Ophthalmol Proc Ser 1976;9:385–90.
311. Ahmad N, Soong TK, Salvi S, et al. Sympathetic ophthalmia after ruthenium plaque brachytherapy. Br J Ophthalmol 2007;91:399–401.
312. Bechrakis NE, Müller-Stolzenburg NW, Helbig H, et al. Sympathetic ophthalmia following laser cyclocoagulation. Arch Ophthalmol 1994;112:80–4.
313. Lam S, Tessler HH, Lam BL, et al. High incidence of sympathetic ophthalmia after contact and noncontact neodymium: YAG cyclotherapy. Ophthalmology 1992;99:1818–22.
314. Bec P, Arne JL, Aubry JP, et al. Angiographie fluoresceinique du fond d'oeil au cours d'une ophthalmie sympathique. Doc Ophthalmol Proc Ser 1976;9:401–6.
315. Gass JDM. Stereoscopic atlas of macular diseases; diagnosis and treatment, 2nd ed. St. Louis: CV Mosby; 1977. p. 120.
316. McPherson Jr SD, Dalton HT. Posterior form sympathetic ophthalmia. Trans Am Ophthalmol Soc 1975;73:251–63.
317. Dreyer Jr WB, Zegarra H, Zakov ZN, et al. Sympathetic ophthalmia. Am J Ophthalmol 1981;92:816–23.
318. Spitznas M. Fluoreszenzangiographie der sympathischen Ophthalmie. Klin Monatsbl Augenheilkd 1976;169:195–200.

319. Jain IS, Gangwar DN, Kaul RL, et al. Sympathetic ophthalmitis simulating Vogt–Koyanagi-Harada's disease after retinal detachment surgery. Ann Ophthalmol 1979;11:1121–3.
320. Rao NA, Marak GE. Sympathetic ophthalmia simulating Vogt–Koyanagi-Harada's disease: a clinico-pathologic study of four cases. Jpn J Ophthalmol 1983;27:506–11.
321. Albert DM, Nordlund JJ, Lerner AB. Ocular abnormalities occurring with vitiligo. Ophthalmology 1979;86:1145–60.
322. Chan C-C, Benezra D, Rodrigues MM, et al. Immunohistochemistry and electron microscopy of choroidal infiltrates and Dalen-Fuchs nodules in sympathetic ophthalmia. Ophthalmology 1985;92:580–90.
323. Chan C-C, Nussenblatt RB, Fujikawa LS, et al. Sympathetic ophthalmia; immunopathological findings. Ophthalmology 1986;93:690–5.
324. Font RL, Fine BS, Messmer E, et al. Light and electron microscopic study of Dalén-Fuchs nodules in sympathetic ophthalmia. Ophthalmology 1982;90:66–75.
325. Ishikawa T, Ikui H. The fine structure of the Dalen-Fuchs nodule in sympathetic ophthalmia. Report 1. Changes of the pigment epithelial cells within the Dalen-Fuchs nodule. Jpn J Ophthalmol 1972;16:254–65.
326. Jakobiec FA, Marboe CC, Knowles II DM, et al. Human sympathetic ophthalmia; an analysis of the inflammatory infiltrate by hybridoma-monoclonal antibodies, immunochemistry, and correlative electron microscopy. Ophthalmology 1983;90:76–95.
327. Lubin JR, Albert DM, Weinstein M. Sixty-five years of sympathetic ophthalmia; a clinicopathologic review of 105 cases (1913–1978). Ophthalmology 1980;87:109–21.
328. Müller-Hermelink HK, Kraus-Mackiw E, Daus W. Early stage of human sympathetic ophthalmia; histologic and immunopathologic findings. Arch Ophthalmol 1984;102:1353–7.
329. Rao NA, Xu S, Font RL. Sympathetic ophthalmia; an immunohistochemical study of epithelioid and giant cells. Ophthalmology 1985;92:1660–2.
330. Segawa K, Matsuoka N. Sympathetic ophthalmia: A comparative fluorographic and electronmicroscopic study. Jpn J Ophthalmol 1971;15:81–7.
331. Rao NA, Wacker WB, Marak Jr GE. Experimental allergic uveitis: clinicopathologic features associated with varying doses of S antigen. Arch Ophthalmol 1979;97:1954–8.
332. Chew EY, Crawford J. Sympathetic ophthalmia and choroidal neovascularization. Arch Ophthalmol 1988;106:1507–8.
333. Wang RC, Zamir E, Dugel PU, et al. Progressive subretinal fibrosis and blindness associated with multifocal granulomatous chorioretinitis: a variant of sympathetic ophthalmia. Ophthalmology 2002;109:1527–31.
334. Jennings T, Tessler HH. Twenty cases of sympathetic ophthalmia. Br J Ophthalmol 1989;73:140–5.
335. Kaplan HJ, Waldrep JC, Chan WC, et al. Human sympathetic ophthalmia; immunologic analysis of the vitreous and uvea. Arch Ophthalmol 1986;104:240–4.
336. Reynard M, Riffenburgh RS, Maes EF. Effect of corticosteroid treatment and enucleation on the visual prognosis of sympathetic ophthalmia. Am J Ophthalmol 1983;96:290–4.
337. Reynard M, Shulman IA, Azen SP, et al. Histocompatibility antigens in sympathetic ophthalmia. Am J Ophthalmol 1983;95:216–21.
338. Buller AJ, Doris JP, Bonshek R, et al. Sympathetic ophthalmia following severe fungal keratitis. Eye 2006;20:1306–7.
339. Androudi S, Theodoridou A, Praidou A, et al. Sympathetic ophthalmia following postoperative endophthalmitis and evisceration. Hippokratia 2010;14:131–2.
340. Rathinam SR, Rao NA. Sympathetic ophthalmia following postoperative bacterial endophthalmitis: a clinicopathologic study. Am J Ophthalmol 2006;141:498–507.
341. Gupta V, Gupta A, Dogra MR. Posterior sympathetic ophthalmia: a single centre long-term study of 40 patients from North India. Eye 2008;22:1459–64.
342. Gass JDM, Chuang EL, Granek H. Acute exudative polymorphous vitelliform maculopathy. Trans Am Ophthalmol Soc 1988;86:354–63.
343. Vaclavik V, Ooi KG, Bird AC, et al. Autofluorescence findings in acute exudative polymorphous vitelliform maculopathy. Arch Ophthalmol 2007;125:274–7.
344. Kozma P, Locke KG, Wang YZ, et al. Persistent cone dysfunction in acute exudative polymorphous vitelliform maculopathy. Retina 2007;27:109–13.
345. Vianna RN, Muralha A, Muralha L. Indocyanine-green angiography in acute idiopathic exudative polymorphous vitelliform maculopathy. Retina 2003;23:538–41.
346. Cruz-Villegas V, Villate N, Knighton RW, et al. Optical coherence tomographic findings in acute exudative polymorphous vitelliform maculopathy. Am J Ophthalmol 2003;136:760–3.
347. Chan CK, Gass JD, Lin SG. Acute exudative polymorphous vitelliform maculopathy syndrome. Retina 2003;23:453–62.
348. Spaide R. Autofluorescence from the outer retina and subretinal space: hypothesis and review. Retina 2008;28:5–35.
349. Nieuwendijk TJ, Hooymans JM. Paraneoplastic vitelliform retinopathy associated with metastatic choroidal melanoma. Eye (Lond) 2007;21:1436–7.
350. Sotodeh M, Paridaens D, Keunen J, et al. Paraneoplastic vitelliform retinopathy associated with cutaneous or uveal melanoma and metastases. Klin Monbl Augenheilkd 2005;222:910–4.
351. Eksandh L, Adamus G, Mosgrove L, et al. Autoantibodies against bestrophin in a patient with vitelliform paraneoplastic retinopathy and a metastatic choroidal malignant melanoma. Arch Ophthalmol 2008;126:432–5.
352. Cantrill HL, Folk JC. Multifocal choroiditis associated with progressive subretinal fibrosis. Am J Ophthalmol 1986;101:170–80.
353. Calixto N. Histopathologic and immunohistopathologic features of subretinal fibrosis and uveitis syndrome. Am J Ophthalmol 1988;105:220–1.
354. Gass JDM, Margo CE, Levy MH. Progressive subretinal fibrosis and blindness in patients with multifocal granulomatous chorioretinitis. Am J Ophthalmol 1996;122:76–85.
355. Gass JDM, editor. Giant-cell reaction surrounding Bruch's membrane and internal limiting membrane of the retina after herpes zoster ophthalmicus and acute retinal necrosis. Presented Eastern Ophthalmic Pathology Club 1991.
356. Gass JDM. Stereoscopic atlas of macular diseases; diagnosis and treatment, 3rd ed. St. Louis: CV Mosby; 1987. p. 146–47.
357. Palestine AG, Nussenblatt RB, Chan CC, et al. Histopathology of the subretinal fibrosis and uveitis syndrome. Ophthalmology 1985;92:838–44.
358. Kim MK, Chan CC, Belfort Jr R, et al. Histopathologic and immunohistopathologic features of subretinal fibrosis and uveitis syndrome. Am J Ophthalmol 1987;104:15–23.
359. Green WR, Zimmerman LE. Granulomatous reaction to Descemet's membrane. Am J Ophthalmol 1967;64:555–8.
360. Gass JDM. Differential diagnosis of intraocular tumors; a stereoscopic presentation. St. Louis: CV Mosby; 1974. p. 180, 200.
361. Benson WE, Shields JA, Tasman W, et al. Posterior scleritis; a cause of diagnostic confusion. Arch Ophthalmol 1979;97:1482–6.
362. Berger B, Reeser F. Retinal pigment epithelial detachments in posterior scleritis. Am J Ophthalmol 1980;90:604–6.
363. Brod RD, Saul RF. Nodular posterior scleritis. Arch Ophthalmol 1990;108:1170–1.
364. Calthorpe CM, Watson PG, McCartney AC. Posterior scleritis: a clinical and histological survey. Eye 1988;2:267–77.
365. Cleary PE, Watson PG, McGill JI, et al. Visual loss due to posterior segment disease in scleritis. Trans Ophthalmol Soc UK 1975;95:297–300.
366. Feldon SE, Sigelman J, Albert DM, et al. Clinical manifestations of brawny scleritis. Am J Ophthalmol 1978;85:781–7.
367. Finger PT, Perry HD, Packer S, et al. Posterior scleritis as an intraocular tumour. Br J Ophthalmol 1990;74:121–2.
368. Jensen JE, Fledelius HC, Prause JU, et al. An unusual ophthalmic tumour in a 5-year-old boy. Acta Ophthalmol Suppl 1992;204:110–2.
369. Sears ML. Choroidal and retinal detachments associated with scleritis. Am J Ophthalmol 1964;58:764–6.
370. Tuft SJ, Watson PG. Progression of scleral disease. Ophthalmology 1991;98:467–71.
371. Watson PG. The diagnosis and management of scleritis. Ophthalmology 1980;87:716–20.
372. Leitch RJ, Bearn MA, Watson PG. Exudative retinal detachment and posterior scleritis associated with massive scleral thickening and calcification treated by scleral decompression. Br J Ophthalmol 1992;76:109–12.
373. Shukla D, Agrawal D, Dhawan A, et al. Posterior scleritis presenting with simultaneous branch retinal artery occlusion and exudative retinal detachment. Eye (Lond) 2009;23:1475–7.
374. Shukla D, Mohan KC, Rao N, et al. Posterior scleritis causing combined central retinal artery and vein occlusion. Retina 2004;24:467–9.
375. McClusky P, Wakefield D. Intravenous pulse methylprednisolone in scleritis. Arch Ophthalmol 1987;105:793–7.
376. Medway DC, Donzis DM, Donzis PB. Ketoprofen in the treatment of scleritis. Am J Ophthalmol 1991;111:249–50.
377. Mondino BJ, Phinney RB. Treatment of scleritis with combined oral prednisone and indomethacin therapy. Am J Ophthalmol 1988;106:473–9.
378. Rosenbaum JT, Robertson Jr JE. Recognition of posterior scleritis and its treatment with indomethacin. Retina 1993;13:17–21.
379. Wakefield D, McClusky P. Cyclosporin therapy for severe scleritis. Br J Ophthalmol 1989;73:743–6.
380. Johnson MH, DeFilipp GJ, Zimmerman RA, et al. Scleral inflammatory disease. Am J Neuroradiol 1987;8:861–5.
381. Yap E-Y, Robertson DM, Buettner H. Scleritis as an initial manifestation of choroidal malignant melanoma. Ophthalmology 1992;99:1693–7.
382. Bullen CL, Liesegang TJ, McDonald TJ, et al. Ocular complications of Wegener's granulomatosis. Ophthalmology 1983;90:279–90.
383. Cassan SM, Coles DT, Harrison Jr EG. The concept of limited forms of Wegener's granulomatosis. Am J Med 1970;49:366–79.
384. Jaben SL. Norton EWD. Exudative retinal detachment in Wegener's granulomatosis: case report. Ann Ophthalmol 1982;14:717–20.
385. Leveille AS, Morse PH. Combined detachments in Wegener's granulomatosis. Br J Ophthalmol 1981;65:564–7.
386. Spalton DJ, Graham EM, Page NG, et al. Ocular changes in limited forms of Wegener's granulomatosis. Br J Ophthalmol 1981;65:553–63.
387. Vogiatzis KV. Bilateral blindness due to necrotizing scleritis in a case of Wegener's granulomatosis. Ann Ophthalmol 1983;15:185–8.
388. Hoang-Xuan T, Foster CS, Rice BA. Scleritis in relapsing polychondritis; response to therapy. Ophthalmology 1990;97:892–8.
389. Magargal LE, Donoso LA, Goldberg RE, et al. Ocular manifestations of relapsing polychondritis. Retina 1981;1:96–9.
390. Turgeon PW, Slamovits TL. Scleritis as the presenting manifestation of procainamide-induced lupus. Ophthalmology 1989;96:68–71.
391. Ellis Jr GS, Pakalnis VA, Worley G, et al. *Toxocara canis* infestation; clinical and epidemiological associations with seropositivity in kindergarten children. Ophthalmology 1986;93:1032–7.
392. Schuman JS, Weinberg RS, Ferry AP, et al. Toxoplasmic scleritis. Ophthalmology 1988;95:1399–403.
393. Kalina RE, Mills RP. Observations on long-term follow-up of posterior scleritis. Am J Ophthalmol 1986;102:671–2.
394. Singh G, Guthoff R, Foster CS. Observations on long-term follow-up of posterior scleritis. Am J Ophthalmol 1986;101:570–5.
395. Hoover DL, Khan JA, Giangiacomo J. Pediatric ocular sarcoidosis. Surv Ophthalmol 1986;30:215–28.
396. De Potter P, Shields JA, Shields CL, et al. Unusual MRI findings in metastatic carcinoma to the choroid and optic nerve: a case report. Int Ophthalmol 1992;16:39–44.
397. Merritt JC, Ballard DJ, Checkoway H, et al. Ocular sarcoidosis; a case-control study among black patients. Ann NY Acad Sci 1986;465:619–24.
398. Olk RJ, Lipmann MJ, Cundiff HC, et al. Solitary choroidal mass as the presenting sign in systemic sarcoidosis. Br J Ophthalmol 1983;67:826–9.
399. Tingey DP, Gonder JR. Ocular sarcoidosis presenting as a solitary choroidal mass. Can J Ophthalmol 1992;27:25–9.
400. Aaberg TA. Editorial: The role of the ophthalmologist in the management of sarcoidosis. Am J Ophthalmol 1987;103:99–100.

401. Jabs DA, Johns CJ. Ocular involvement in chronic sarcoidosis. Am J Ophthalmol 1986;102:297–301.
402. Karma A. Ophthalmic changes in sarcoidosis. Acta Ophthalmol Suppl 1979:141.
403. Ohara K, Okubo A, Sasaki H, et al. Intraocular manifestations of systemic sarcoidosis. Jpn J Ophthalmol 1992;36:452–7.
404. Spalton DJ, Sanders MD. Fundus changes in histologically confirmed sarcoidosis. Br J Ophthalmol 1981;65:348–58.
405. Weinreb RN, Tessler H. Laboratory diagnosis of ophthalmic sarcoidosis. Surv Ophthalmol 1984;28:653–64.
406. Franceschetti A, Babel J. La chorio-rétinite en "taches de bougie," manifestation de la maladie de Besnier-Boeck. Ophthalmologica 1949;118:701–10.
407. Gass JDM, Olson CL. Sarcoidosis with optic nerve and retinal involvement; a clinicopathologic case report. Trans Am Acad Ophthalmol Otolaryngol 1973;77:OP739–OP750.
408. Gould HL, Kaufman HE. Boeck's sarcoid of the ocular fundus; historical review and report of a case. Am J Ophthalmol 1961;52:633–7.
409. Letocha CE, Shields JA, Goldberg RE. Retinal changes in sarcoidosis. Can J Ophthalmol 1975;10:184–92.
410. Brownstein S, Jannotta FS. Sarcoid granulomas of the optic nerve and retina; report of a case. Can J Ophthalmol 1974;9:372–8.
411. DeBroff BM, Donahue SP. Bilateral optic neuropathy as the initial manifestation of systemic sarcoidosis. Am J Ophthalmol 1993;116:108–11.
412. Galetta S, Schatz NJ, Glaser JS. Acute sarcoid optic neuropathy with spontaneous recovery. J Clin Neuro-Ophthalmol 1989;9:27–32.
413. Krohel GB, Charles H, Smith RS. Granulomatous optic neuropathy. Arch Ophthalmol 1981;99:1053–5.
414. Laties AM, Scheie HG. Evolution of multiple small tumors in sarcoid granuloma of the optic disk. Am J Ophthalmol 1972;74:60–7.
415. Lustgarten JS, Mindel JS, Yablonski ME, et al. An unusual presentation of isolated optic nerve sarcoidosis. J Clin Neuro-Ophthalmol 1983;3:13–18.
416. Mansour AM. Sarcoid optic disc edema and optociliary shunts. J Clin Neuro-Ophthalmol 1986;6:47–52.
417. Noble KG. Ocular sarcoidosis occurring as a unilateral optic disk vascular lesion. Am J Ophthalmol 1979;87:490–3.
418. Chumbley LC, Kearns TP. Retinopathy of sarcoidosis. Am J Ophthalmol 1972;73:123–31.
419. Doxanas MT, Kelley JS, Prout TE. Sarcoidosis with neovascularization of the optic nerve head. Am J Ophthalmol 1980;90:347–51.
420. Denis P, Nordmann J-P, Laroche L, et al. Branch retinal vein occlusion associated with a sarcoid choroidal granuloma. Am J Ophthalmol 1992;113:333–4.
421. Kimmel AS, McCarthy MJ, Blodi CF, et al. Branch retinal vein occlusion in sarcoidosis. Am J Ophthalmol 1989;107:561–2.
422. Asdourian GK, Goldberg MF, Busse BJ. Peripheral retinal neovascularization in sarcoidosis. Arch Ophthalmol 1975;93:787–91.
423. Duker JS, Brown GC, McNamara JA. Proliferative sarcoid retinopathy. Ophthalmology 1988;95:1680–6.
424. Graham EM, Stanford MR, Shilling JS, et al. Neovascularisation associated with posterior uveitis. Br J Ophthalmol 1987;71:826–33.
425. Madigan Jr JC, Gragoudas ES, Schwartz PL, et al. Peripheral retinal neovascularization in sarcoidosis and sickle cell anemia. Am J Ophthalmol 1977;83:387–91.
426. Kelly PJ, Weiter JJ. Resolution of optic disk neovascularization associated with intraocular inflammation. Am J Ophthalmol 1980;90:545–8.
427. Chan C-C, Wetzig RP, Palestine AG, et al. Immunohistopathology of ocular sarcoidosis; report of a case and discussion of immunopathogenesis. Arch Ophthalmol 1987;105:1398–402.
428. Karma A, Taskinen E, Kainulainen H, et al. Phenotypes of conjunctival inflammatory cells in sarcoidosis. Br J Ophthalmol 1992;76:101–6.
429. Brod RD. Presumed sarcoid choroidopathy mimicking birdshot retinochoroidopathy. Am J Ophthalmol 1990;109:357–8.
430. Pellegrini V, Ohno S, Hirose S, et al. Subretinal neovascularisation and snow banking in a case of sarcoidosis: case report. Br J Ophthalmol 1986;70:474–7.
431. Fiore PM, Friedman AH. Unusual chorioretinal degeneration associated with sarcoidosis. Am J Ophthalmol 1988;106:490–1.
432. Obenauf CD, Shaw HE, Sydnor CF, et al. Sarcoidosis and its ophthalmic manifestations. Am J Ophthalmol 1978;86:648–55.
433. Sanders MD, Shilling JS. Retinal, choroidal, and optic disc involvement in sarcoidosis. Trans Ophthalmol Soc UK 1976;96:140–4.
434. Tang RA, Grotta JC, Lee KF, et al. Chiasmal syndrome in sarcoidosis. Arch Ophthalmol 1983;101:1069–73.
435. Karcioglu ZA, Brear R. Conjunctival biopsy in sarcoidosis. Am J Ophthalmol 1985;99:68–73.
436. Spaide RF, Ward DL. Conjunctival biopsy in the diagnosis of sarcoidosis. Br J Ophthalmol 1990;74:469–71.
437. Weinreb RN. Diagnosing sarcoidosis by transconjunctival biopsy of the lacrimal gland. Am J Ophthalmol 1984;97:573–6.
438. Nessan VJ, Jacoway JR. Biopsy of minor salivary glands in the diagnosis of sarcoidosis. N Engl J Med 1979;301:922–4.
439. Baarsma GS, La Hey E, Glasius E, et al. The predictive value of serum angiotensin converting enzyme and lysozyme levels in the diagnosis of ocular sarcoidosis. Am J Ophthalmol 1987;104:211–7.
440. Weinreb RN, Kimura SJ. Uveitis associated with sarcoidosis and angiotensin converting enzyme. Am J Ophthalmol 1980;89:180–5.
441. Bielory L, Frohman LP. Low-dose cyclosporine therapy of granulomatous optic neuropathy and orbitopathy. Ophthalmology 1991;98:1732–6.
442. Bhat P, Cervantes-Castaneda RA, Doctor PP, et al. Mycophenolate mofetil therapy for sarcoidosis-associated uveitis. Ocul Immunol Inflamm 2009;17:185–90.
443. Miyazaki E, Ando M, Fukami T, et al. Minocycline for the treatment of sarcoidosis: is the mechanism of action immunomodulating or antimicrobial effect? Clin Rheumatol 2008;27:1195–7.
444. Carroll DM, Franklin RM. Leber's idiopathic stellate retinopathy. Am J Ophthalmol 1982;93:96–101.
445. Cohen SM, Davis JL, Gass JDM. Branch retinal arterial occlusions in multifocal retinitis with optic nerve edema. Arch Ophthalmol 1995;113:1271–6.
446. Foster RE, Gutman FA, Meyers SM, et al. Acute multifocal inner retinitis. Am J Ophthalmol 1991;111:673–81.
447. Gass JDM. Fluorescein angiography in endogenous intraocular inflammation. In: Aronson SB, Gamble CN, Goodner EK, editors. Clinical methods in uveitis: the Fourth Sloan Symposium on Uveitis. St. Louis: CV Mosby; 1968. p. 214–5.
448. Goldstein BG, Pavan PR. Retinal infiltrates in six patients with an associated viral syndrome. Retina 1985;5:144–50.
449. Maitland CG, Miller NR. Neuroretinitis. Arch Ophthalmol 1984;102:1146–50.
450. Bar S, Segal M, Shapira R, Savir H. Neuroretinitis associated with cat scratch disease. Am J Ophthalmol 1990;110:703–5.
451. Carithers HA, Margileth AM. Cat-scratch disease; acute encephalopathy and other neurologic manifestations. Am J Dis Child 1991;145:98–101.
452. Chrousos GA, Drack AV, Young M, et al. Neuroretinitis in cat scratch disease. J Clin Neuro-Ophthalmol 1990;10:92–4.
453. Dalton MJ, Robinson LE, Cooper J, et al. Use of *Bartonella* antigens for serologic diagnosis of cat-scratch disease at a national referral center. Arch Intern Med 1995;155:1670–6.
454. Fish RH, Hogan RN, Nightingale SD, et al. Peripapillary angiomatosis associated with cat-scratch neuroretinitis. Arch Ophthalmol 1992;110:323.
455. Gass JDM. Stereoscopic atlas of macular diseases; diagnosis and treatment, 2nd ed. St. Louis: CV Mosby; 1977. [p. 376.]
456. Golnik KC, Marotto ME, Fanous MM, et al. Ophthalmic manifestations of Rochalimaea species. Am J Ophthalmol 1994;118:145–51.
457. Grossniklaus HE. The cat scratch disease-bacillary angiomatosis puzzle. Am J Ophthalmol 1994;118:246–8.
458. LeBoit PE, Berger TG, Egbert BM, et al. Epithelioid haemangioma-like vascular proliferation in AIDS: Manifestation of cat scratch disease or bacillus infection? Lancet 1988;1:960–3.
459. Schlossberg D, Morad Y, Krouse TB, et al. Culture-proved disseminated cat-scratch disease in acquired immunodeficiency syndrome. Arch Intern Med 1989;149:1437–9.
460. Ulrich GG, Waecker Jr NJ, Meister SJ, et al. Cat scratch disease associated with neuroretinitis in a 6-year-old girl. Ophthalmology 1992;99:246–9.
461. Wear DJ, Margileth AM, Hadfield TL, et al. Cat scratch disease: a bacterial infection. Science 1983;221:1403–5.
462. Dreyer RF, Hopen G, Gass JDM, et al. Leber's idiopathic stellate neuroretinitis. Arch Ophthalmol 1984;102:1140–5.
463. Gass JDM. Stereoscopic atlas of macular diseases; diagnosis and treatment, 3rd ed. St. Louis: CV Mosby; 1987. p. 746–51.
464. Atmaca LS. Fundus changes associated with Behçet's disease. Graefes Arch Clin Exp Ophthalmol 1989;227:340–4.
465. Barra C, Belfort Jr R, Abreu MT, et al. Behçet's disease in Brazil – a review of 49 cases with emphasis on ophthalmic manifestations. Jpn J Ophthalmol 1991;35:339–46.
466. BenEzra D, Cohen E. Treatment and visual prognosis in Behçets disease. Br J Ophthalmol 1986;70:589–92.
467. Colvard DM, Robertson DM, O'Duffy JD. The ocular manifestations of Behçet's disease. Arch Ophthalmol 1977;95:1813–7.
468. D'Alessandro LP, Forster DJ, Rao NA. Anterior uveitis and hypopyon. Am J Ophthalmol 1991;112:317–21.
469. Graham EM, Stanford MR, Sanders MD, et al. A point prevalence study of 150 patients with idiopathic retinal vasculitis: 1. Diagnostic value of ophthalmological features. Br J Ophthalmol 1989;73:714–21.
470. International Study Group for Behçet's disease: criteria for diagnosis of Behçet's disease. Lancet. 1990;335:1078–80.
471. James DG. Editorial: Behçet's syndrome. N Engl J Med 1979;301:431–2.
472. James DG. 'Silk route disease' (Behçet's disease). West J Med 1988;148:433–7.
473. James DG, Spiteri MA. Behçet's disease. Ophthalmology 1982;89:1279–84.
474. Levinsky RJ, Lehner T. Circulating soluble immune complexes in recurrent oral ulceration and Behçet's syndrome. Clin Exp Immunol 1978;32:193–8.
475. Mamo JG. Treatment of Behçet disease with chlorambucil; a follow-up report. Arch Ophthalmol 1976;94:580–3.
476. Mamo JG, Baghdassarian A. Behçet's disease; a report of 28 cases. Arch Ophthalmol 1964;71:4–14.
477. Mishima S, Masuda K, Izawa Y, et al. Behçet's disease in Japan: ophthalmologic aspects. Trans Am Ophthalmol Soc 1979;77:225–79.
478. O'Duffy JD, Carney JA, Deodhar S. Behçet's disease; report of 10 cases, 3 with new manifestations. Ann Intern Med 1971;75:561–70.
479. Shimizu K. Fluorescein fundus angiography in Behçet's syndrome. Mod Probl Ophthalmol 1972;10:224–8.
480. Shimizu T. Clinical and immunological studies on Behçet's syndrome. Folia Ophthalmol Jpn 1971;22:801–10.
481. Shimizu T. Clinicopathological studies on Behçet's disease 29–30 September 1977, 1979, p. 9–43. In: DillAcsen N, Koniçe M, Övül C, editors. Behçet's disease: proceedings of an International Symposium on Behçet's Disease, Istanbul, 29–30 September 1977. Amsterdam: Excerpta Medica; 1979. p. 9–43.
482. Smulders FM, Oosterhuis JA. Treatment of Behçet's disease with chlorambucil. Ophthalmologica 1975;171:347–52.
483. Michelson JB, Michelson PE, Chisari FV. Subretinal neovascular membrane and disciform scar in Behçet's disease. Am J Ophthalmol 1980;90:182–5.
484. Kansu T, Kirkali P, Kansu E, et al. Optic neuropathy in Behçet's disease. J Clin Neuro-Ophthalmol 1989;9:277–80.
485. Adinolfi M, Lehner T. Acute phase proteins and C9 in patients with Behçet's syndrome and aphthous ulcers. Clin Exp Immunol 1976;25:36–9.

Chapter 12

Tumors of the Retinal Pigment Epithelium (RPE)

The terms "hamartoma," "choristoma," "phacoma (mother spot)," and "nevus" are used to describe benign developmental tumors or placoid lesions. *Stedman's Medical Dictionary* defines a hamartoma as: "a focal malformation that resembles a neoplasm grossly and even microscopically, but results from faulty development in an organ; it is composed of an abnormal mixture of tissue elements, or an abnormal proportion of a single element, normally present at that site, which develops and grows at virtually the same rate as normal components, and is not likely to result in compression of the adjacent tissue (in contrast to neoplastic tissue)." A choristoma is defined as a "mass formed by maldevelopment of tissue of a type not normally found at that site." Phacoma is defined as "a hamartoma found in phacomatosis," a group of hereditary diseases characterized by hamartomas of multiple tissues. A nevus is a "birthmark; a circumscribed malformation of the skin, especially if colored by hyperpigmentation or increased vascularity; it may be predominantly epidermal, adnexal, melanocytic, vascular, or mesodermal, or a localized overgrowth of melanin-forming cells arising in the skin early in life." Ophthalmologists have adopted the term "nevi" to refer to developmental melanocytic lesions of the uveal tract, and it has been suggested as an appropriate term to describe developmental placoid lesions of the RPE.[1] Developmental uveal melanocytic nevi have been described in Chapter 14.

It is important to realize that reactive proliferation of RPE, retinal glial cells, and retinal vascular endothelial cells can occasionally duplicate the clinical and histopathologic changes of all of the RPE hamartomatous lesions discussed in this chapter.

12.01 Congenital hypertrophy of the retinal pigment epithelium (CHRPE).

A: Multiple areas of CHRPE simulating large animal tracks.
B and **C**: Large area of CHRPE mistaken for a malignant melanoma in a 59-year-old woman who was asymptomatic. Note several areas of thinning of the RPE within the central portion of the lesion (arrows, B). There was an absolute field defect corresponding with the lesion. Angiography revealed obstruction of the background choroidal fluorescence except in the areas of thinning of the RPE (arrow, C).
D: A jet black CHRPE with small fenestrations (arrow) and absolute scotoma in the paramacular region of a young woman.
E: CHRPE associated with multiple fenestrations (arrows) and a peripheral nonpigmented ring.
F: CHRPE showing generalized hypopigmentation and a nonpigmented peripheral ring.
G: CHRPE showing generalized hypopigmentation that extends out to and includes a poorly defined, nonpigmented ring and a well-defined, pigmented ring.
H and **I**: Growth of CHRPE in a 47-year-old woman between January 1978 (H) and June 1985 (I).
J–L: Growth of CHRPE into the central macular area of the left eye.

(A–D from Gass[72]; E and F from Buettner[4]; J–L, courtesy of Dr. Richard Dreyer.)

MELANOTIC NEVI OF THE RETINAL PIGMENT EPITHELIUM

Solitary-Type Congenital Hypertrophy of the Retinal Pigment Epithelium (CHRPE)

Solitary-type CHRPEs are well-demarcated, slightly elevated, gray-brown to black, oval, round, or occasionally geographic lesions with smooth or scalloped margins (Figures 12.01–12.03). They are usually solitary but may be multiple and grouped in a pattern suggesting animal tracks (Figure 12.01A). A CHRPE may occur anywhere in the fundus.[9] However, CHRPE in macula and juxtapapillary location are rare.[9–12] There is often a halo of depigmentation just inside the outer edge of these lesions (Figure 12.01E and F). Although most CHRPE are between one and two disc diameters, some may occupy an area equal to one quadrant of the fundus (Figure 12.01B). They have been observed in newborns.[13] Hypopigmented or depigmented lacunae within these lesions are frequently evident, particularly in older patients (Figures 12.01B, D, E, and I, and 12.03G and H). These lacunae may show progressive enlargement, and eventually the entire lesion may become depigmented (Figure 12.01G). Although most of these lesions remain rather stationary, concentric enlargement has been demonstrated in up to 74–83% of cases (Figure 12.01H and I).[3,5,9,14] Occasionally, linear depigmented streaks and localized zones of mild hyperpigmentation occur at the anterior margin of these lesions.[5] Uncommonly, nodular growth may develop within CHRPE[15] with histological confirmation of malignant transformation into adenocarcinoma of the RPE.[16–18]

Many CHRPE are associated with either a relative or an absolute scotoma corresponding to the site of the lesion.[12] CHRPE are hypoautofluorescent exhibiting mild hyperautofluoresence of the lacunae.[19] Fluorescein angiography in patients with lightly pigmented fundi shows obstruction of the background choroidal fluorescence in the area of the lesion except in the fenestrated areas of hypopigmentation (Figure 12.01C). Angiographic evidence of alterations in the structure and permeability of the retinal vessels overlying these lesions may occasionally occur.[20–22] This includes capillary nonperfusion, capillary leakage, and chorioretinal anastomosis. Optical coherence tomography (OCT) reveals thinning of overlying retina with overall thickening of RPE layer, except in the region of lacunae, where RPE thinning is expected (Figure 12.02I and J).[23]

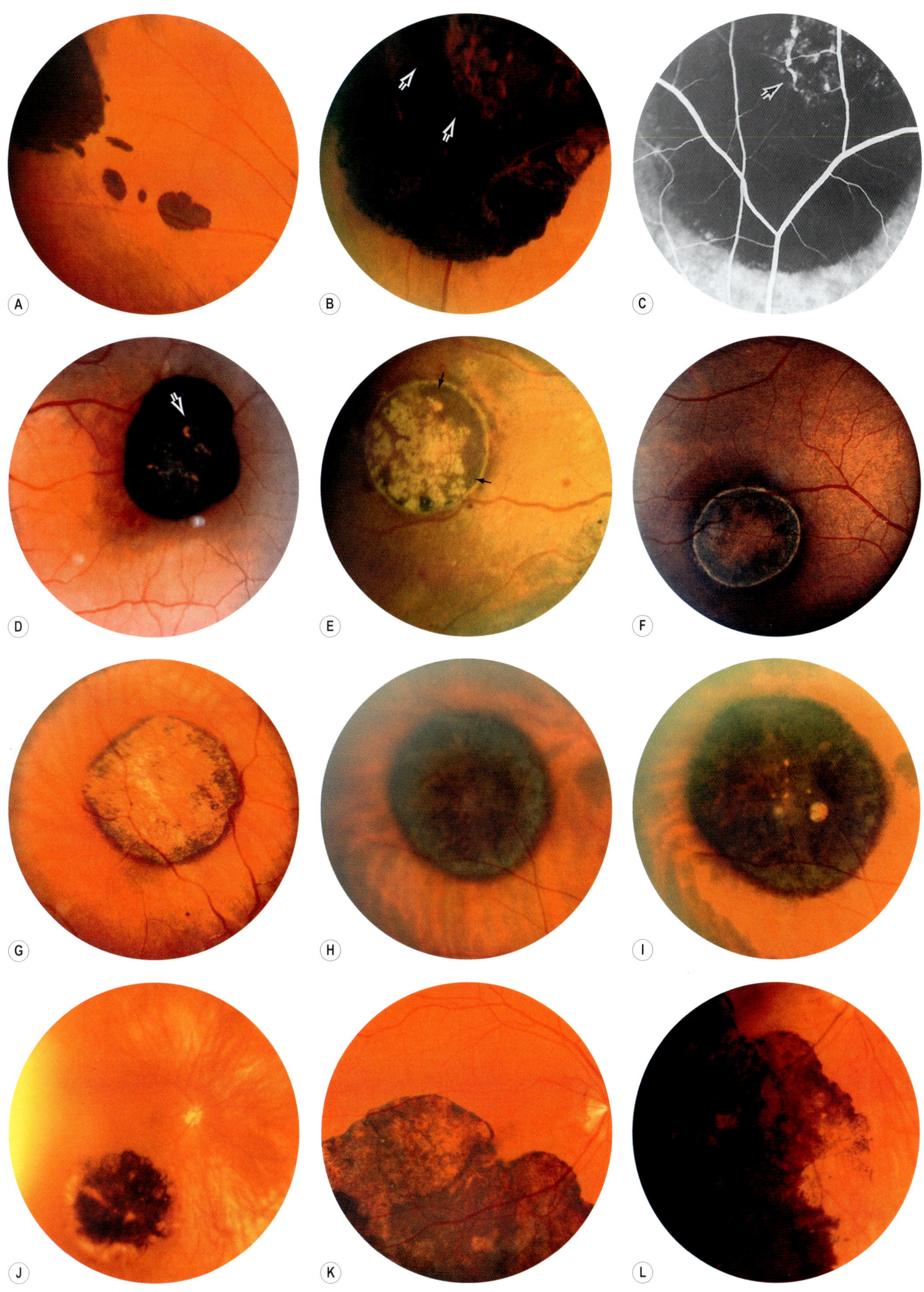
A
B
C
D
E
F
G
H
I
J
K
L

Histopathologically, CHRPE lesions are characterized by a single layer of enlarged RPE cells containing macromelanin granules that may be associated with varying degrees of degeneration of the overlying outer retinal layers (Figure 12.02).[4,13,24–26] Some degree of RPE hyperplasia may also be evident.[27] Absence of lipofuscin in the hypertrophied RPE cells suggests that their incapacity to phagocytose and digest photoreceptor outer segments may be responsible for the receptor cell degeneration so often present overlying these lesions.[25] This may explain the thinning of the overlying neurosensory retina seen on OCT (Figure 12.02I and J). The structure of the macromelanosomes in CHRPE is similar to that described in X-linked ocular albinism.[25,28]

The differential diagnosis of CHRPE includes choroidal melanocytic nevi, secondary and primary hyperplasia of the RPE, pigmented hypertrophic chorioretinal scars, and geographic dark fundus patches that are probably caused by subretinal bleeding and hemosiderin deposits, usually occurring in patients with sickle-cell disease (see Figures 6.59C and D and 6.58I).[8] The large lesions, if not viewed binocularly, may be mistaken for malignant melanomas of the choroid (Figure 12.01B).

These lesions are similar histopathologically to lesions referred to as congenital grouped pigmentation of the RPE (see next subsection). Hypertrophy of the RPE has been identified histopathologically as being part of combined RPE and retinal hamartomas (see Figures 12.08K and 12.10E).

12.02 Histopathologic findings in congenital hypertrophy of the retinal pigment epithelium (CHRPE).

A–D: Clinicopathologic correlation of a coin-shaped, flat, pigmented lesion noted on gross examination of an autopsy eye (A). Note the nonpigmented halo just inside the margins of the pigmented lesion. Histopathologic examination revealed a pigmented tumor to be composed of a single layer of large RPE cells (right half of photomicrograph, B). The main body of the lesion was separated from the normal surrounding RPE by a halo of partly depigmented RPE (arrows, B). There was extensive degeneration of the outer layers of retina overlying the entire lesion. A high-power view of the lesion revealed large RPE cells packed with large, round melanin granules (C). (Compare with the normal surrounding RPE in D.)

E: Electron microscopic view of the normal RPE (left side) and CHRPE RPE (right side) in the same case illustrated in A–D. Note thickening of the basement membrane (bm) of the RPE.

F and G: Clinicopathologic correlation of CHRPE associated with a large central fenestrated area noted on gross examination of an autopsy eye (F). Photomicrograph of the margin (arrow, G) of the hypertrophied RPE to the left of the arrow and the central fenestrated area showed loss of RPE in the fenestrated area and proliferation of glial cells along the inner surface of Bruch's membrane (G).

H: Histopathologic condition of another patient with CHRPE showing a sharp line of junction (arrow) separating the normal RPE on the left side of the photomicrograph and the hypertrophy of the RPE on the right side. Note that Bruch's membrane appears thickened and there is atrophy of the underlying choriocapillaris.

I and J: Fundus appearance of asymptomatic solitary CHRPE detected on a routine examination (I). Optical coherence tomography shows thinning of the overlying retina and prominence of the RPE layer (J).

(A–C and F–H from Buettner.[4])

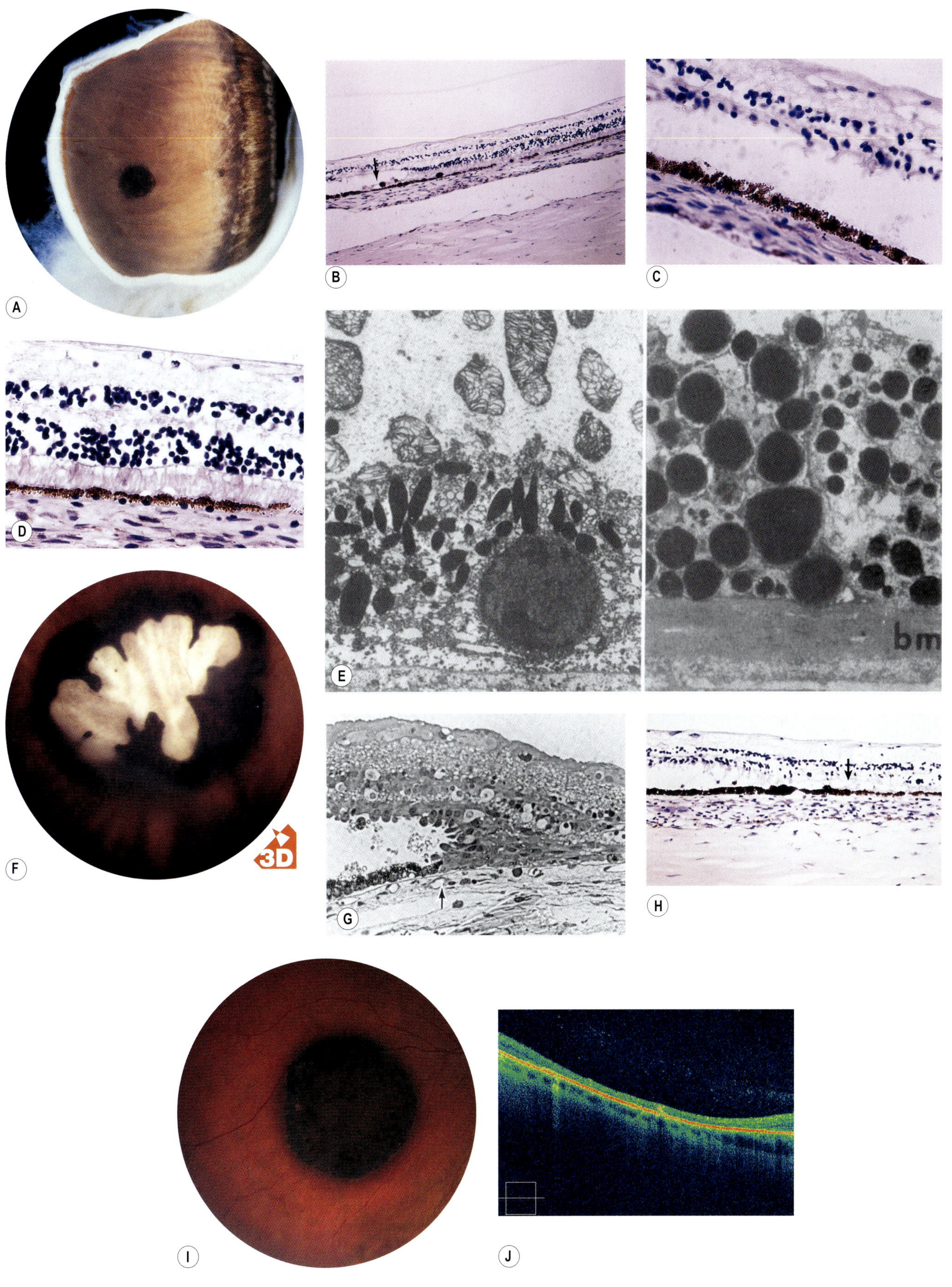
A
B
C
D
E
bm
F
3D
G
H
I
J

Multiple CHRPE Associated with Familial Adenomatous Polyposis and Gardner's Syndrome

Multiple isolated CHRPE lesions occur usually in both eyes of a high percentage of patients with this dominantly inherited familial cancer syndrome that includes intestinal polyposis, osteomas of the skull, and various soft-tissue tumors, including fibromas, lipomas, and epidermal and sebaceous cysts.[1,6,22,28–43] The risk for intestinal malignancy during adult life is virtually 100%. The soft-tissue tumors tend to occur during the first two decades, the bony tumors in the second decade, and the polyps in adulthood (mean age 30 years). Osteomas of the orbit may occur.[43] Approximately 50% of patients will develop adenocarcinoma of the colon by 35 years of age. There is a disproportionate risk of other cancers (carcinoma of ampulla of Vater, adrenal gland, thyroid gland, and bladder), a variety of sarcomas, and neuroepithelial tumors (Turcot syndrome) (Figure 12.03G–I).[6] Multiple CHRPE affecting both eyes is a reliable marker for Gardner's syndrome. Multiple CHRPE appears to be specific for Gardner's syndrome and is not found in the other familial intestinal polyposis syndromes (familial polyposis without extraintestinal manifestations, Peutz–Jeghers syndrome) or in patients with familial nonpolyposis colorectal cancers.[28] The CHRPE lesions in Gardner's syndrome often show a peculiar oval shape with a fishtail-like change at one or both poles (Figure 12.03C, E, and F).[44] In some cases the lesions appear to be located in close approximation to the major retinal vessels and may be associated with abnormalities in the overlying retinal vessels.[40] Histopathologically, some of the lesions appear similar to solitary CHRPE. Others show in addition hamartomatous malformations of the RPE featuring cellular hypertrophy, hyperplasia, and retinal invasion, and formation of a mushroom-shaped tumor (Figure 12.03K and L).[34,42]

12.03 Familial multifocal congenital hypertrophy of the retinal pigment epithelium (CHRPE).

A–F: Multiple, oval areas of flat CHRPE were present bilaterally in the 30-year-old mother (A), the 8-year-old son (B–D), and the 10-year-old daughter (E and F). Note the depigmented halo near the margin of the lesions, their radial orientation in respect to the posterior pole, and the fish-tail-shaped hypopigmented area at one or both ends of the lesions (arrows). The lesions showed varying degrees of pigmentation. The eye examinations were otherwise normal in these patients. Medical evaluation failed to find evidence of intestinal polyposis or other disease.
G–I: Turcot's syndrome with multiple CHRPE (G); adenomatous polyps of the stomach, duodenum, and colon (I); and a cerebellar medulloblastoma (arrow, H) occurred in this 20-year-old man, who presented with nausea, headaches, and vomiting after head trauma.
J and **K**: Histopathology of CHRPE lesions found in the eyes of a patient with Gardner's syndrome. Hypertrophy of RPE (J). Hyperplasia and hypertrophy of RPE (K).
L: Hypertrophy and hyperplasia of RPE with extension through the full thickness of the retina.

(G–I from Munden et al.[6]; J and K from Traboulsi et al.[42])

Patients with bilateral lesions, multiple lesions (more than 4), or both are specific (specificity, 0.95) and sensitive (sensitivity, 0.78) markers for Gardner's syndrome.[45] A review of published studies regarding genotype–phenotype correlation suggests that CHRPE is associated with mutations between codons 311 and 1444 of the adenomatous polyposis coli (APC) gene.[46] The gene for adenomatous polyposis of the colon (*APC*) was found to be on 5q21-22 by Bodmer et al.[47] There is no evidence that typical solitary or grouped CHRPE lesions represent a marker for Gardner's syndrome.[22] Multifocal CHRPE lesions have occurred in a family with microcephaly and hyperreflexia[48] and in one family in Miami without any other abnormalities (Figure 12.03).[44]

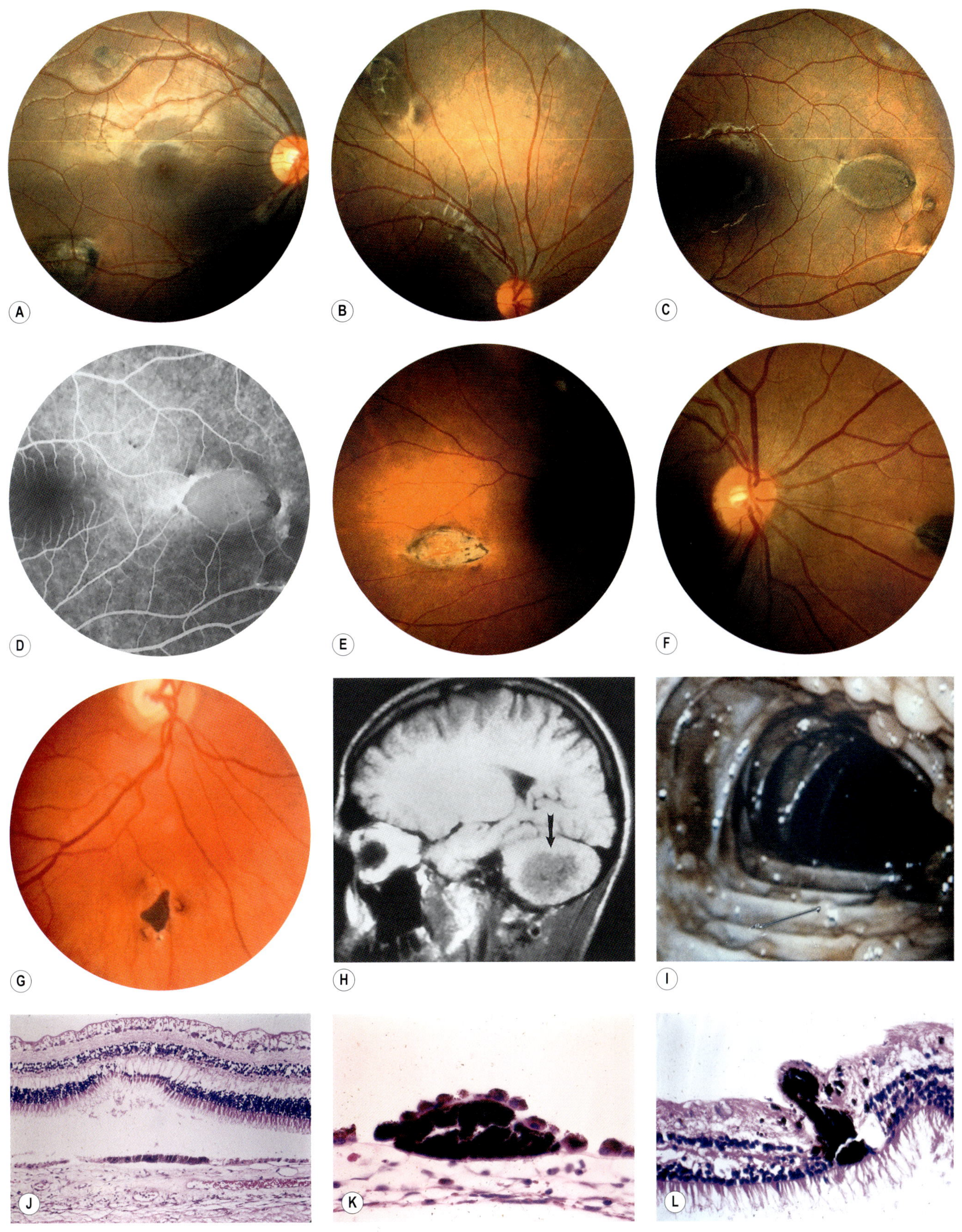
A
B
C
D
E
F
G
H
I
J
K
L

Grouped-Type Congenital Pigmented Nevi of the Retinal Pigment Epithelium, "Bear Tracks"

This is a rare congenital anomaly first described in 1868 by Mauthner.[49] It is characterized by sharply circumscribed, small, variably sized, pigment spots that are often arranged in groups to resemble the footprints of animals (Figure 12.04).[50–53] They are usually grouped in one sector of the fundus with the smaller spots located at the apex directed toward the optic disc.[54] They infrequently are present in the macular area. Extensive areas of the fundus may be affected and be associated with bilateral involvement (Figure 12.04D and E).[55–58] The lesions can occasionally be quite large and simulate "elephant tracks or grizzly bear tracks" (Figure 12.04H–L), a finding that has been noted as early as 1926.[54] Familial cases involving two successive generations are reported.[59–61] Two sisters, one with pigmented bear tracks and the other with albinotic spots, have been seen.[62] Whether the grouped pigmentation and the other associations in a patient with microcephaly, mild mental retardation, and deletions of 13q33.3-q34 and 11p15.4 are causally related cannot be established.[63] The retina overlying "bear tracks" appears normal bio-microscopically and angiographically.[51] Electro-oculographic findings are normal. These lesions are believed to be stationary, but long-term follow-up studies have not been done. Grouped nevi have infrequently occurred in association with other anomalies or disorders including retinoblastoma and skin hyperpigmentation.[57,64–66]

These lesions histopathologically are similar to CHRPE with increased number of pigment granules in normal-sized RPE cells.[52,67] Unlike CHRPE most of the melanin granules retain their ellipsoidal shape and hypertrophy and hyperplasia of the RPE are less prominent.[67] Clinically, some patients may show lesions typical of both grouped nevi and CHRPE (Figures 12.01A and 12.04G).

12.04 Congenital grouped pigmentation of the retinal pigment epithelium (RPE).

A–C: Uniocular involvement in three patients. Each showed lesions in one quadrant or less. None had macular involvement. All had normal visual function.
D and **E**: Marked peripheral involvement in both eyes of this patient with normal visual function.
F: Higher-power view of the upper nasal quadrant of the right fundus.
G: Several large peripheral zones of hypertrophy of the RPE accompanied grouped pigmentation in this patient.
H–J: A 36-year-old asymptomatic African American woman with large lesions resembling "elephant tracks."
K and **L**: a 3-year-old boy with large lesions in nasal retina.

(K and L, courtesy of Dr. David Morrison.)

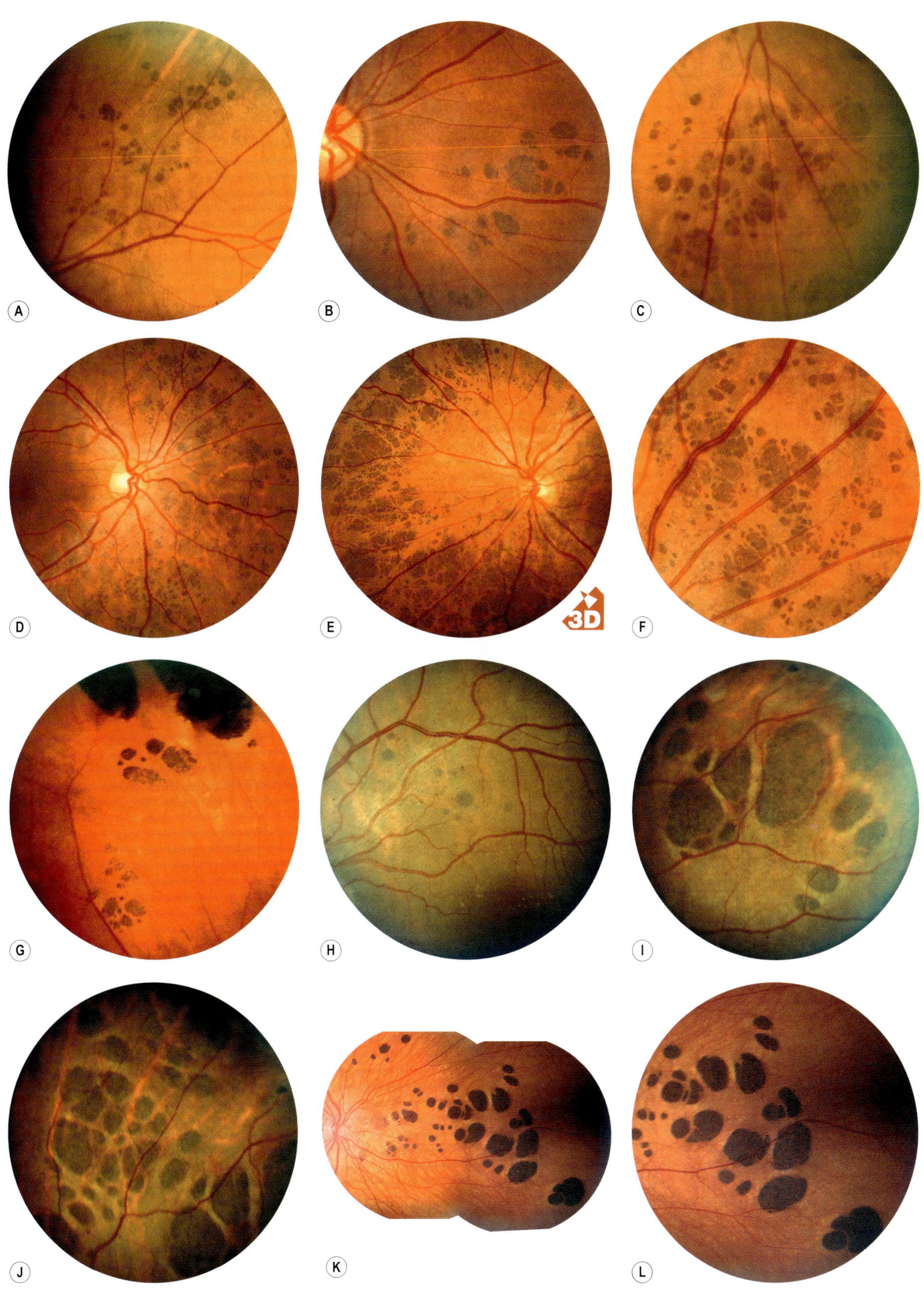
A
B
C
D
E
3D
F
G
H
I
J
K
L

ALBINOTIC AND NONPIGMENTED NEVI OF THE RETINAL PIGMENT EPITHELIUM

Grouped-Type Congenital Albinotic and Hypomelanotic Nevi of the Retinal Pigment Epithelium, "Polar Bear Tracks"

Congenital grouped albinotic nevi are multiple, white, variably sized spots involving the RPE in a pattern similar to that in congenital grouped pigmentation of the RPE (Figure 12.05).[1,44,48,68] They may occur in one or both eyes and may be mistaken for other flecked retina diseases (e.g., drusen, fundus flavimaculatus, pattern dystrophy, fundus albipunctatus, and Gaucher's disease). Like pigmented "bear tracks," these albinotic spots occur rarely and tend to be more numerous and larger in the peripheral fundus, and they usually do not involve the macular area. They appear to represent focal thickening of the RPE that is filled with a white material. This white material may be diffusely distributed or may be more concentrated in the periphery of the lesion (Figure 12.05A and C). In some cases the spots appear to be devoid of white material, and the underlying choroidal vessels are visible. In other cases, some of the spots may appear to contain dark gray pigment. The overlying retina appears normal, except that larger retinal vessels may appear to be locally narrowed (Figure 12.05C and D). The lesions are probably relatively stable, but further long-term follow-up studies are required to document this. Although considered to be functionally of no significance, one patient with macular as well as peripheral lesions developed neovascularization (Figure 12.05G and H).

Fluorescein angiography shows variable degrees of transmission of the choroidal fluorescence through these lesions (Figure 12.05B).

Although longer follow-up of these rarely encountered patients is required, it is probable that the albinotic spots represent a congenital anomaly of the RPE closely akin to congenital grouped hyperpigmentation of the RPE. In the case of the albinotic spots, the RPE cells appear to be stuffed with a white material, possibly an abnormal precursor of melanin rather than enlarged melanin granules as in grouped hyperpigmentation of the RPE.

Dr. Gass believed that these albinotic RPE spots are identical to those reported by Kandori and associates[69–71] in association with stationary night blindness that was manifest primarily by abnormal dark adaptation. None of the four patients seen at the Bascom Palmer Eye Institute had nyctalopia. Studies, including dark adaptation, electroretinography, and electro-oculography, were normal in the two patients illustrated in Figure 12.05A–C, G, and H. Parke et al.[48] reported similar white spots in one of two siblings with pigmented RPE lesions, microcephaly, mental retardation, and autosomal-dominant hyperreflexia.

12.05 Congenital grouped retinal pigment epithelium albinotic nevi.

A–C: Except for the albinotic spots the results of an eye examination that included color vision testing, electroretinography, electro-oculography, and dark-adaptation studies were normal in this healthy 15-year-old girl. Note the peripheral distribution of white material in some of the larger spots (arrows, A) and slight narrowing of a retinal artery overlying one spot (arrow, C). Angiography showed variable transmission of the choroidal fluorescence through the spots (B).

D and E: Albinotic spots in one eye of a 40-year-old asymptomatic woman. Note narrowing of retinal vein (arrow) overlying a large spot.

F: Albinotic spots in one eye of an asymptomatic young man.

G and H: This healthy 14-year-old girl was observed for 3 years with grouped albinotic spots in both eyes before she was seen because of loss of central vision in the left eye associated with choroidal neovascularization (arrow, H). Her electroretinographic and electro-oculographic findings were normal.

(D and E, courtesy of Dr. Alvaro Rodriguez; G and H, courtesy of Dr. Harry W. Flynn.)

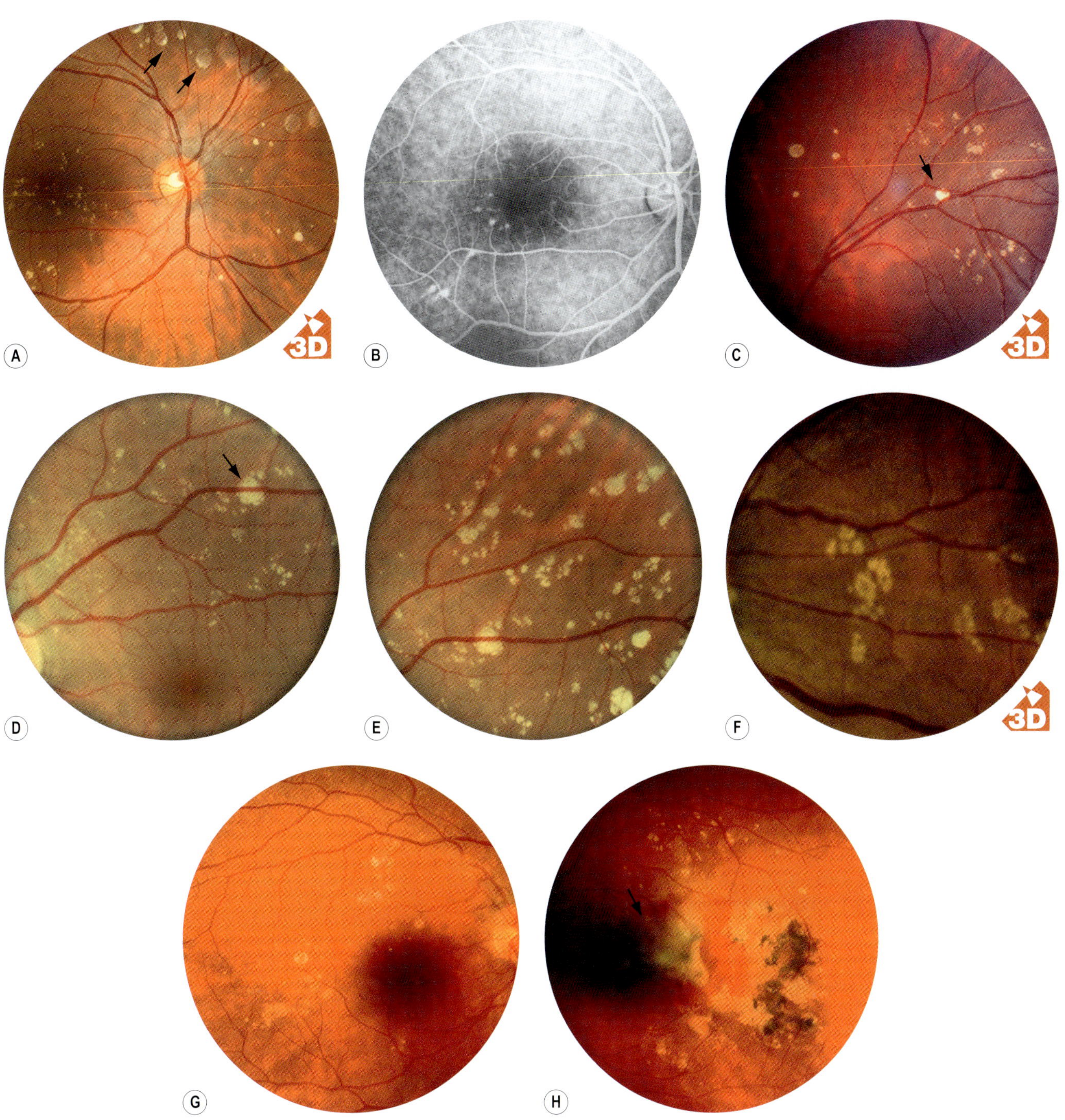
3D
3D
3D

Solitary-Type Hypomelanotic and Albinotic Nevi (Torpedo Maculopathy)

These solitary, sharply circumscribed, hypopigmented reddish-orange or white lesions of the RPE, which have been previously referred to as "congenital hypomelanotic freckle" or "retinal albinotic spots," are most frequently observed in the peripheral fundus and in the temporal half of the macula.[1,72–75] These latter lesions often have an oval or fish-shaped appearance similar to that seen in the CHRPE lesions associated with Gardner's syndrome (Figure 12.06A and D–F).[74] They are often discovered on routine eye examination in children. They may[76] or may not be associated with a demonstrable visual field defect. Although they may show a slight milky white color, they are rarely as densely white as the grouped albinotic RPE nevi. Unlike most acquired atrophic lesions of the RPE, hypopigmented RPE nevi typically have no margin or irregular hyperpigmentation. Angiographically the choriocapillaris underlying these lesions appears to be normal (Figure 12.06B and C). OCT done on two patients by Golchet et al. has shown thin RPE with increased signal transmission in the choroid.[76] Both patients showed a "cleft" in the outer retina associated with loss of photoreceptors, irregular edges of the residual photoreceptors, and thinning of the outer plexiform layer. The OCT finding remained unchanged over 6 years of follow-up in one patient. The authors inferred that "something occupied the cleft, the nature of which is unknown." It is likely that this space is empty due to loss of the overlying photoreceptors; both patients had an absolute scotoma corresponding to the lesion. The OCT appearance has led to speculation that the lesion may not be a nevus, but rather a localized congenital thin or atrophic RPE.[76]

Why this bears the same shape as a torpedo or fish-shaped CHRPE (Figure 12.03A–F) as seen in patients with intestinal polyposis (Gardner's) is unclear, if it indeed is not a CHRPE. It is likely the same trigger causes the lesions in both these conditions, but the pigment epithelium is devoid of melanosomes here while the Gardner's eyes develop an excess of them. Choroidal neovascularization arising at the edge of a lesion is rare but reported (Figure 12.06J–L). Microscopically, hypopigmented RPE nevi show a sharp transition from normal RPE to flat nonpigmented epithelium (Figure 12.06G and H).[14,72,75] Unlike the presentation in most cases of congenital hypertrophy of the RPE, the overlying retina is normal. The underlying choroid is also unaffected. So far there are no histopathologic studies of solitary nevi that clinically appear white.

12.06 Large solitary amelanotic spot or nevus of the retinal pigment epithelium (RPE).

A–C: Amelanotic RPE nevus first noted on a routine eye examination 6 years previously in an asymptomatic 51-year-old black woman with 20/15 visual acuity bilaterally. She had only a faint relative scotoma to 3/1000 color test objects. Note the relatively intact choriocapillaris (B and C).
D: Amelanotic nevus in a 12-year-old boy with normal acuity, Amsler grid, and Goldmann visual field examinations.
E: Paired amelanotic nevi in an asymptomatic patient.
F: Hypopigmented RPE nevus with focus of RPE hyperplasia and atrophy.
G–I: Amelanotic nevus or freckle noted on gross examination of a fresh eye removed at autopsy (G). Histopathologic examination revealed a focal area of depigmentation of the artifactitiously detached RPE (arrows, H). A high-power view showed a sharp transition (arrows) between the nonpigmented, flattened RPE cells and the relatively normal, surrounding RPE cells (arrows, I).
J–L: A 17-year-old male with a known history of a spot in the left eye presented with vision of 20/200. An oval hypopigmented lesion under the fovea is partly covered by a thin layer of subretinal blood adjacent to a circular pigmented type 2 CNVM, temporal to which is a crescent of subretinal fluid. The angiogram shows hyperfluorescence of the partly obscured torpedo lesion, the lacy CNVM, and the surrounding SRF. The patient received three injections of monthly intravitreal bevacizumab resulting in involution of the CNVM, resolution of the SRF, and return of his vision to 20/20.
M–N: A 17 year old with an atypical shape and location of an amelanotic spot that was first seen 10 years previously. Note the visible choroidal vessels under the thinned out/depigmented RPE (M). Hypo autofluorescence of the lesion implies lack of pigment granules within the RPE that renders the lesion amelanotic, corroborating the histology seen in H and I (N).

(D from Roseman and Gass[74] © 1992, American Medical Association. All rights reserved. E, F, J–L, courtesy of Dr. Mark J. Daily; G–I from Gass.[72]).

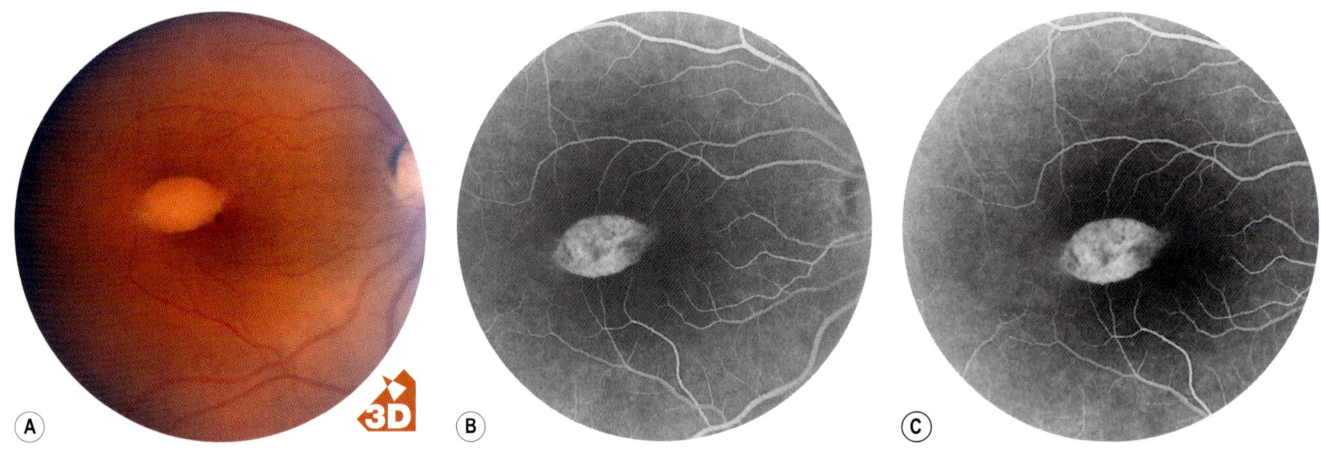

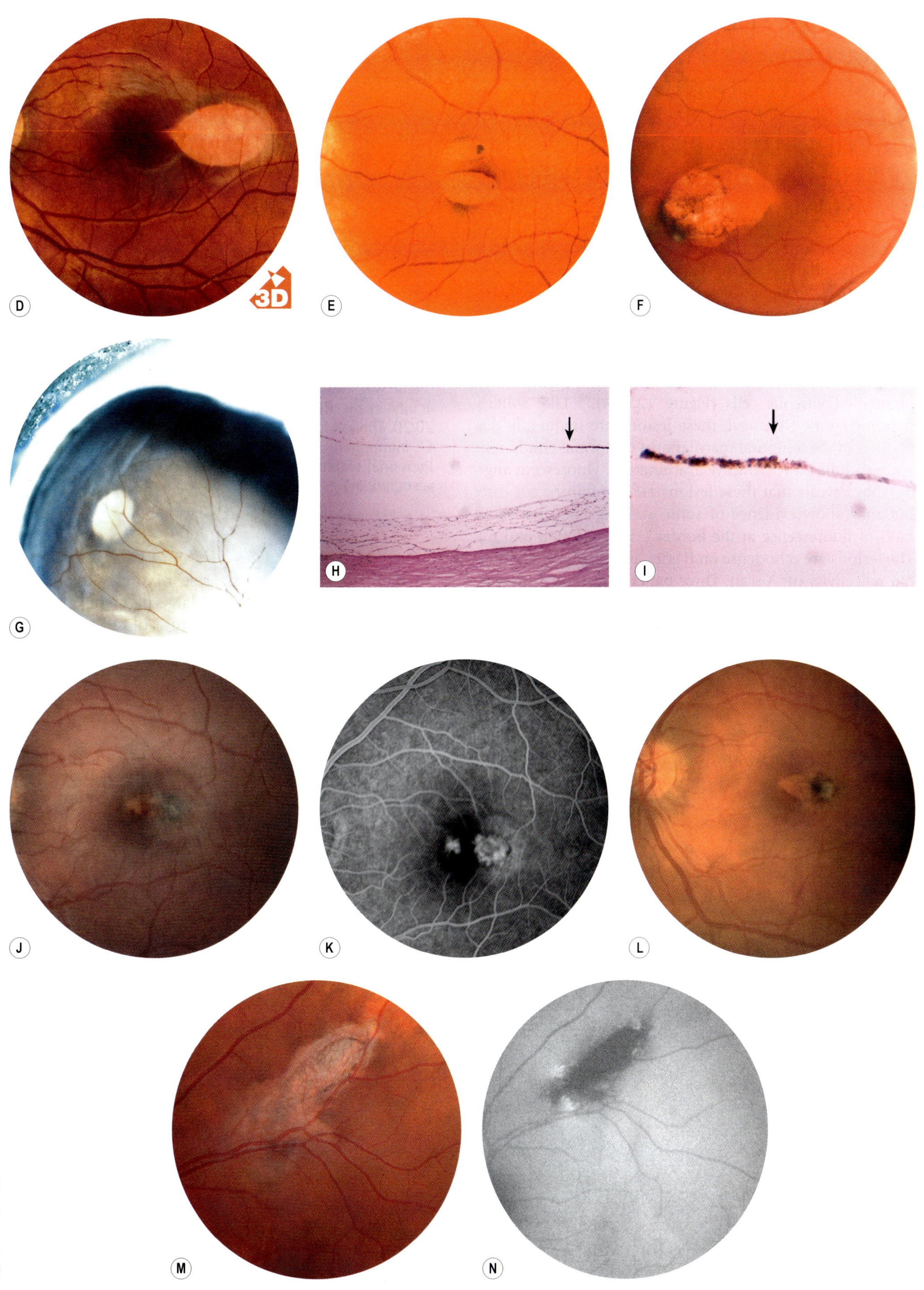
D
3D
E
F
G
H
I
J
K
L
M
N

COMBINED PIGMENT EPITHELIAL AND RETINAL HAMARTOMA

Combined pigment epithelial and retinal hamartomas are peculiar, slightly elevated, partly pigmented lesions, which may be mistaken for a postinflammatory scar or a malignant melanoma, and which may be present anywhere in the fundus.[72,84–94] The clinical history, appearance of the tumor, and its structure vary with its location.

Combined Pigment Epithelial and Retinal Hamartoma Involving the Optic Disc

Patients with tumors that involve the optic nerve head and juxtapapillary retina typically are seen in young adults because of blurred and distorted vision in one eye. The visual acuity is usually 20/100 or better. Biomicroscopic examination reveals an ill-defined, slightly elevated, partly pigmented tumor involving part of the optic nerve head and adjacent retina (Figure 12.08). The tumor is composed of a fine granular distribution of pigment, giving it a charcoal-gray filigree appearance.[72,80,84–88,94–100] The presence of many fine capillaries within the tumor may be partly obscured from view by a semitranslucent gray membrane that is always present on the inner retinal surface. Patients become symptomatic either because of metamorphopsia caused by contraction of this membrane that produces traction folds in the retina that extend into the central macular area (Figure 12.08A), or less frequently because of subretinal and intraretinal exudation derived from the capillary component of the tumor (Figure 12.08D). This exudation may reabsorb spontaneously and leave atrophic changes in the RPE surrounding the tumor. Other complications that may occur infrequently include choroidal neovascularization, retinal hemorrhages, and vitreous hemorrhages.[101,102] The early phases of angiography demonstrate dilated, multiple, fine blood vessels within the tumor, and later phases show evidence of leakage of dye from these vessels (Figure 12.08B, C, E, F, H, and I).[72,87,94] The clinical appearance and fluorescein angiogram features are enough to make the diagnosis in most cases. OCT is useful in distinguishing lesions that are not very thick from epiretinal membranes by detecting disorganized underlying retina.[103] Vitreous traction if present may also be detected, and thus help in selecting cases that may have a potential for visual improvement with vitrectomy and membrane peel to relieve traction.

Histopathologically, the optic disc tumors show evidence of a hamartomatous malformation involving hyperplasia of the RPE, glial cells, and blood vessels (Figure 12.08J and K).[72,84,85,87,92,94,100] Many of these lesions remain stable. Some may develop exudative changes and show an increase in opacification of the glial component of the tumor. The surface glial membrane causing the retinal folding is an integral part of the tumor and accounts for the fact that surgical stripping of the membrane is difficult and has little chance of restoring central vision.[104,105]

12.08 Combined retinal pigment epithelium and retinal hamartoma (CRPE-RH) of the juxtapapillary retina and optic disc head.

A–C: A circumscribed, slightly elevated, finely mottled, pigmented lesion was noted in a 21-year-old man with a 1-year history of progressive distortion of the vision in his left eye. Two years previously his visual acuity had been 20/20. He had multiple flat pigmented lesions on the buttocks and arms. His past medical history was otherwise negative. Visual acuity in the left eye was 20/50. Flecks of pigmented tissue extended anteriorly into the thickened retina and optic nerve tissue and partly covered the major retinal vessels as they entered the optic nerve head (A). This was associated with an epiretinal glial membrane. Prominent retinal traction folds extended from this membrane into the macula. There were many fine, dilated, tortuous capillaries within the tumor. These were best seen angiographically (B). There was slight leakage of dye from vessels in the later angiograms (C).
D–F: Serous detachment of the macula and circinate retinopathy caused by a juxtapapillary retinal and RPE hamartoma in a 55-year-old woman (D). Angiography revealed a capillary angiomatous component of this lesion (E and F, stereo).
G–I: Small hypopigmented combined RPE and retinal hamartoma in a 66-year-old asymptomatic man who was suspected of having ischemic optic neuropathy (G). An epiretinal membrane on the surface of the lesion partly obscured the retinal vessels and the mottled pigmentation within the tumor (G). Angiography revealed evidence of the capillary angiomatous nature of this lesion as well as some dilation of the retinal capillaries in the papillomacular bundle (H and I).
J and K: Clinicopathologic correlation of a juxtapapillary CRPE-RH in a 29-year-old man with an 8-week history of blurred vision in his left eye (J). Melanoma was suspected, and the eye was enucleated. Histopathologic examination revealed disorganization of the normal architecture of the optic nerve head and retina associated with hyperplasia of the retinal blood vessels, RPE, and glial tissue (K). Cords and sheets of RPE proliferation extended throughout the tumor and surrounded blood vessels (arrows, K). Note the proliferation of fibrous tissue near the surface of the retina.

(A–C from Vogel et al.[94]; J and K from Machemer.[100])

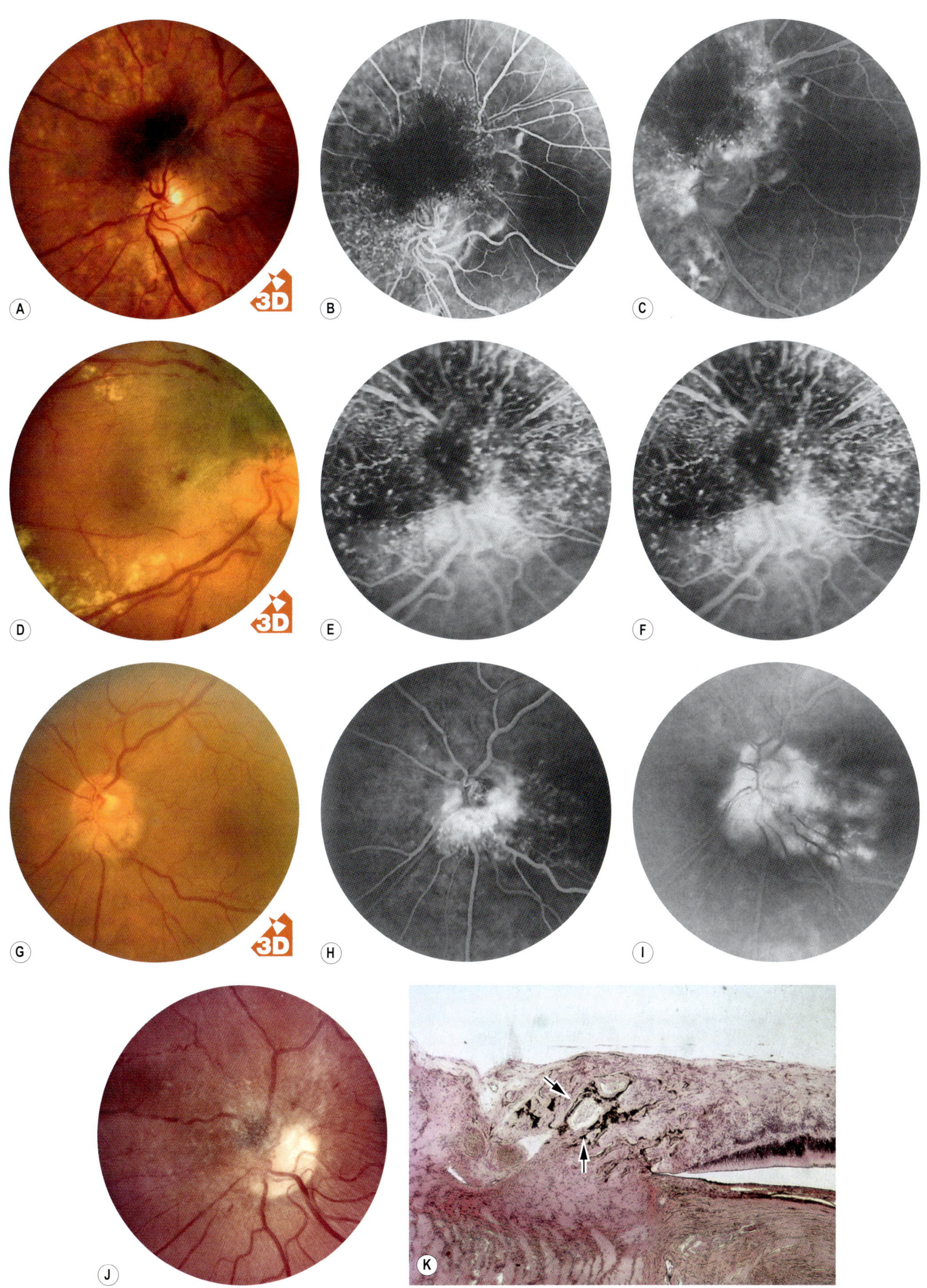
A
3D
B
C
D
3D
E
F
G
3D
H
I
J
K

These tumors, particularly if lightly pigmented, when discovered in infants or young children may be mistaken for retinoblastoma and *Toxocara canis*. In patients with more heavily pigmented tumors, the differential diagnosis includes melanocytoma, malignant melanoma, and reactive hyperplasia of the RPE. The optic disc tumors with minimal pigmentation may be difficult or impossible to differentiate from capillary angiomas, astrocytic hamartoma or from epipapillary and juxtapapillary epiretinal membranes associated with other causes.[106] One patient's hypopigmented tumor was misdiagnosed as ischemic optic neuropathy (Figure 12.08G–I). Reactive proliferation of retinal endothelial, glial, and RPE cells may duplicate any of the retinal and RPE hamartomas. Spontaneous development of lesions indistinguishable from a juxtapapillary and a peripheral combined pigment epithelial and retinal hamartoma in two adult patients where previously there was no lesion has been reported (see Figure 12.13G and H, below).[107] Development of similar tumors in children with previous optic disc edema has been seen and the authors speculate that the lesion may not be a hamartoma, but rather an acquired glial response.[108]

Shields et al. in their recent review of 77 patients found the mean age at diagnosis to be 7 months for macular and 8 months for extramacular lesions, and the youngest child was 2 weeks of age.[72,87,97,109–111] It is likely that the trigger for development of this disorganized tumor occurs in utero or very soon postnatally and the tumor continues to grow and remodel after birth (C Shields, personal communication). Surgical intervention with vitrectomy and epiretinal membrane peel has shown a minimal to modest visual improvement in few cases.[104,112–115] These cases should be selected carefully; full-thickness macular holes have occurred when the membrane is intrinsically woven into the lesion.

Figure 12.09 Combined retinal pigment epithelium and retinal hamartomas (CRPE-RH) without intrinsic involvement of the optic disc head.

A: CRPE-RH in the macula of the left eye of an otherwise healthy 7-year-old girl with amblyopia in the left eye.
B–D: CRPE-RH in the macular region of an 8-year-old boy (A). His right fundus was normal. Fluorescein angiography demonstrated tortuosity, dilation, and abnormal permeability of the retinal vessels in the region of the tumor (B–D). Arrows indicate the temporal border of the flat pigmented portion of the tumor (C).
E and F: Peripheral CRPE-RH simulating a retinoblastoma and malignant melanoma of the choroid in a 19-month-old girl who was the product of an uncomplicated full-term pregnancy and delivery. Her birth weight was 8 lb (3.63 kg). At age 5 months intermittent exotropia was noted. There was dragging of the retinal vessels and displacement of the macula (arrow, F) in a superotemporal direction by a slightly elevated, partly pigmented tumor that was located near the equator superotemporally (E). Much of the central portion of the pigmented lesion was obscured by gray-white, semitranslucent, thickened retinal tissue and an epiretinal membrane (E). Note the dilation and tortuosity of the retinal vessels and the feathery appearance of the flat pigmented portion of the tumor (arrows, E) where it blended imperceptibly into the normal RPE. By the age of 40 months the child's visual acuity in the affected eye was counting fingers only and the lesion was unchanged.
G–J: Mid peripheral CRPE-RH (H) associated with heterotopia of the macula and congenital optic disc pit (I). Note the dilated capillaries and leakage of fluorescein (I and J).
K and L: Healthy 4-year-old boy referred for possible retinoblastoma discovered during evaluation of poor vision in the right eye. He had anisometropic amblyopia with 20/60 vision, right eye, and 20/30 vision, left eye. There was a slightly elevated pigmented lesion covered by gray-white retinal tissue and tortuous retinal vessels near the superotemporal border of the left macula (L).

(A–F from Gass.[72])

Combined Pigment Epithelial and Retinal Hamartoma Without Optic Disc Involvement

These tumors, which are often only slightly elevated, are usually discovered in one eye of an infant or child with strabismus and subnormal visual acuity.[72,87,97,109–111] They are associated with increased number, dilation, and tortuosity of the retinal vessels, evidence of gray epiretinal fibrous tissue, and hyperpigmentation confined to the level of the RPE. This pigmentation is greatest at the border of the lesion, where its feathery edges blend imperceptibly into the surrounding normal RPE. Unlike tumors involving the optic disc, these show no evidence of RPE cells or capillary angiomatous tissue near their inner surface. These tumors may involve the peripapillary area (see Figure 12.10, below), the macula (Figures 12.09 and 12.11), or the peripheral fundus (Figure 12.09H–L). Those in the temporal half of the eye peripherally are often associated with displacement of the macula toward the lesion (Figure 12.09G–L). Fluorescein angiography usually shows marked tortuosity and leakage of dye from the retinal vessels within these macular and peripheral tumors (Figures 12.09A–D and 12.11D–G). These patients, most of whom are children, have no history of prematurity and have none of the changes in the far periphery of the fundus typical of retinopathy of prematurity. Subretinal exudation may occasionally occur from the tumor vessels, resulting in progressive detachment of the retina, rubeotic glaucoma, and loss of the eye (Figure 12.11A–C).

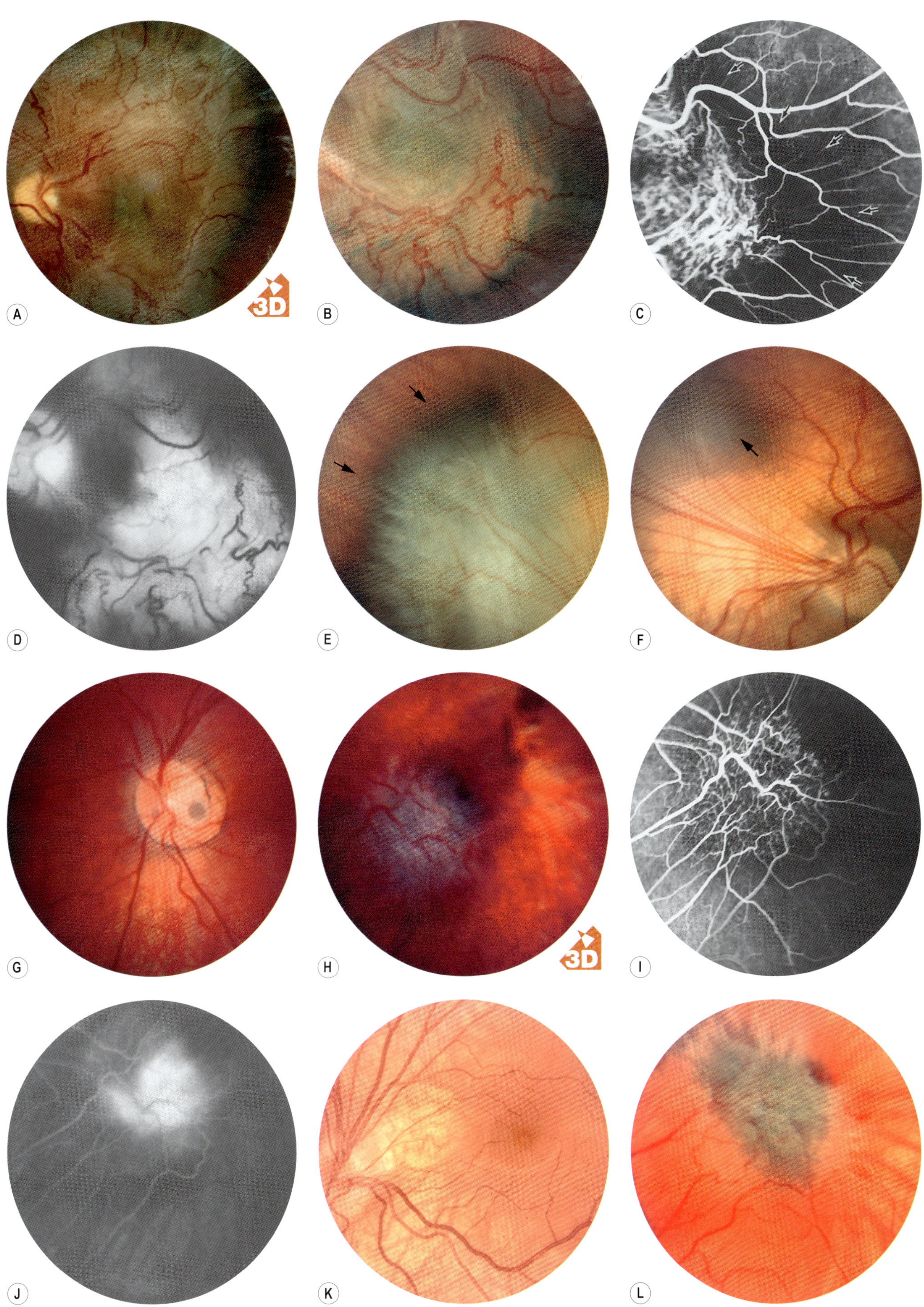
3D
A
B
C
D
E
F
G
H
3D
I
J
K
L

The histopathologic findings in the peripheral lesions differ from those involving the optic disc in that they show less disorganization of the retina, absence of RPE migration, and less evidence of capillary proliferation within the retina, and evidence of hypertrophy of the RPE (Figure 12.10D and E).[109]

12.10 Peripapillary combined retinal pigment epithelium and retinal hamartoma (CRPE-RH).

A–C: CRPE-RH surrounding the right optic disc (arrows, A and B) in an infant. Within several years there was further condensation of the fibrous tissue on the tumor surface (C).
D and E: Large peripapillary RPE and retinal hamartoma in a 16-year-old boy. Melanoma was suspected, and the eye was enucleated. Histopathologic examination revealed hypertrophy of the RPE (arrows, E), mild dysplasia of the retina, and epiretinal fibrous tissue.

(A–C, courtesy of Dr. John P. Shock, Jr; D and E from Laqua and Wessing.[109] Published with permission from the American Journal of Ophthalmology, copyright The Ophthalmic Publishing Co.)

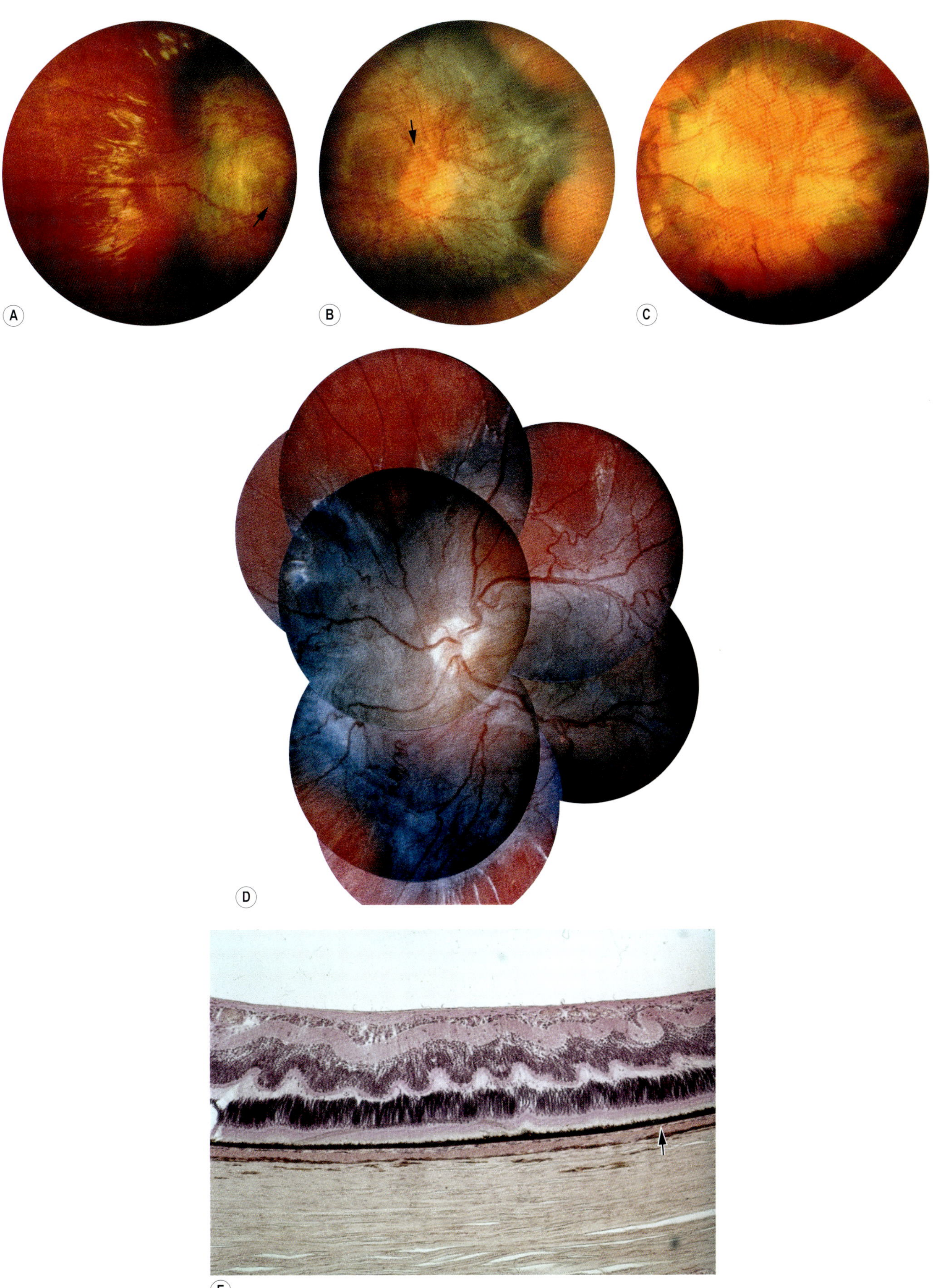
A
B
C
D
E

Dr. Gass had seen these hamartomas, or lesions simulating them, occur in patients with cutaneous hemangiomas, X-linked juvenile retinoschisis, a congenital pit of the optic disc in the opposite eye, and in patients with neurofibromatosis (Figures 12.09G–J and 12.11).[44] The association of these hamartomas with neurofibromatosis is now well established.[1,44,98,116–125] Neurofibromatosis has been subdivided into at least two major disorders, NF-1 and NF-2, with gene defects on two different chromosomes.[116,124] The combined pigment epithelial and retinal hamartomas in patients with neurofibromatosis usually involve the macula (Figure 12.11), may be bilateral, and have occurred most commonly in neurofibromatosis type 2.[118,121,123,126]

12.11 Combined retinal and retinal pigment epithelium hamartomas occurring in patients with neurofibromatosis.

A–C: A combined RPE and retinal hamartoma of the macular region in a 30-month-old girl with suspected retinoblastoma or malignant melanoma (A and B). Left exotropia was noted at 2 months of age. There was inferotemporal displacement of the optic nerve head and retinal vessels by a large (eight disc diameters), elevated, partly pigmented mass in the macular and paramacular areas. The central portion of the pigmented lesion was obscured by thickened translucent retinal tissue and a gray preretinal membrane. The patient had several prominent café-au-lait spots on the abdomen (C). Several years later she developed an exudative retinal detachment and rubeotic glaucoma, and the eye was enucleated.
D–G: Bilateral hypopigmented combined retinal and RPE hamartomas in an infant with neurofibromatosis.
H–J: Bilateral hypopigmented combined retinal and RPE hamartomas in a child with neurofibromatosis.

(A and B from Gass[87]; D–G from Palmer et al.[137]; H–J, courtesy of Dr. Lanning B. Kline.)

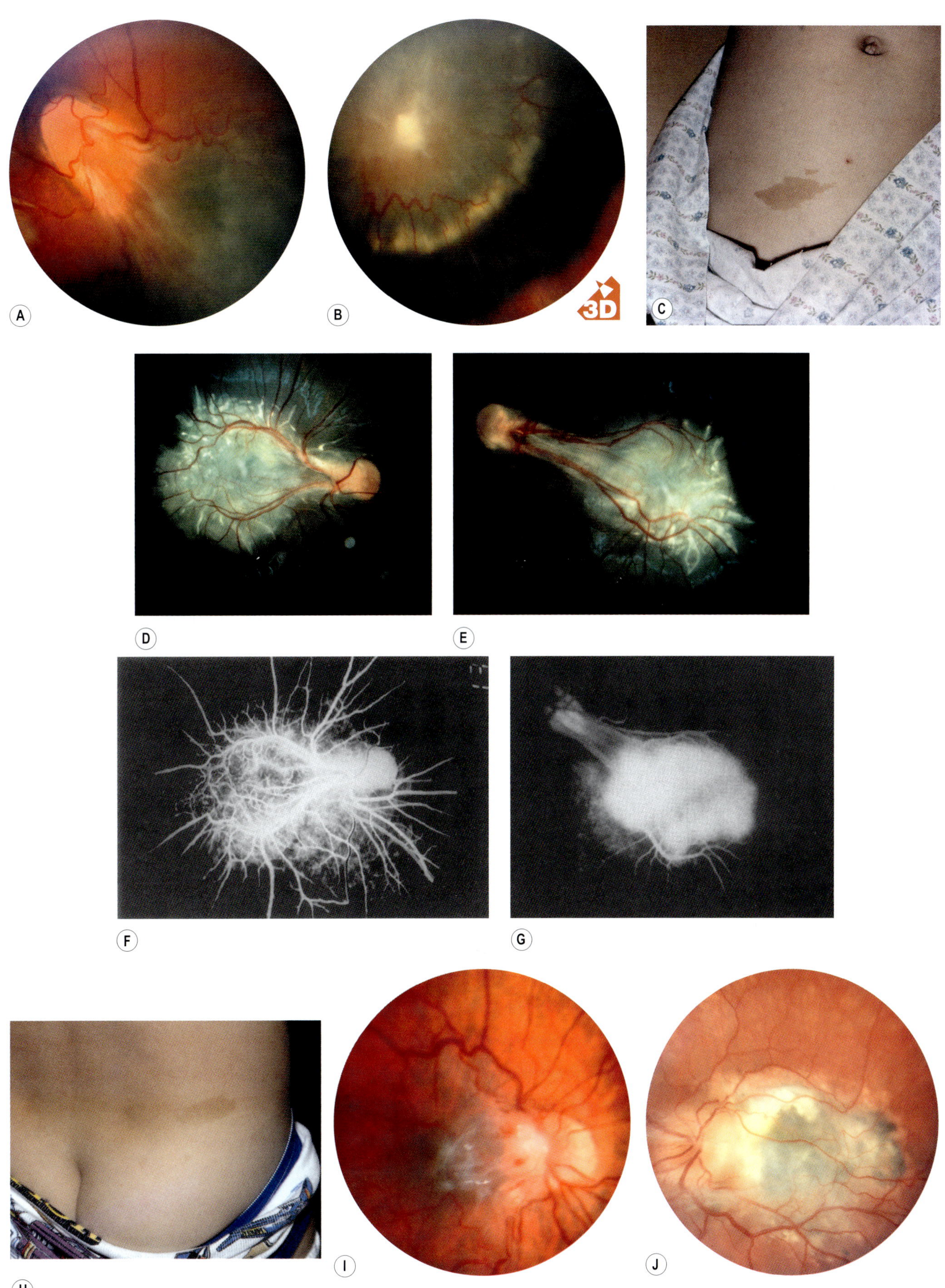
A
B
3D
C
D
E
F
G
H
I
J

UNILATERAL RETINAL PIGMENT EPITHELIAL DYSGENESIS

Variant of Combined Hamartoma of the Retinal Pigment Epithelium and Retina

In 2002, Cohen et al. reported a condition they named unilateral leopard-spot lesion of the RPE,[127] and later renamed it unilateral RPE dysgenesis.[128] The lesion is unilateral, continuous with the optic disc, and characterized by hyperpigmentation of the RPE at the edges with several uniform mid-lesion patches of hypopigmented RPE (lacunae) and a characteristic scalloped margin (Figure 12.12A, C, E, and G). A few patients also show retinal vascular telangiectasia, mild fibrous proliferation, and retinal folds (Figure 12.12C–J) that likely make this condition a forme fruste of combined hamartoma of the RPE and retina. The hyperpigmented RPE is hypofluorescent and the lacunae show transmission hyperfluorescence on angiography. On autofluorescence imaging the lacunae are hypoautofluorescent. The authors used the term "RPE hyperplasia and lacunae" in describing this lesion; on careful examination of the cases illustrated in Figure 12.12, it appears that all cases do not have excess pigment (Figure 12.12G–L) and in some instances the hyperpigmented appearance may appear exaggerated from the contrast of the hypopigmented center (Figure 12.12A and C). Several of the eyes have 20/20 vision in spite of the center being within the "lacunae," implying that the RPE cells here are intact but lightly pigmented (Figure 12.12C, D, K, and L). The lesions are known to progress minimally; choroidal neovascularization can occur similar to combined hamartoma. Overlying serous retinal detachment and fibrous tissues have been seen, which are evidence suggesting that at least some of these are a milder version of combined hamartoma. The dominant feature however, is the " leopard spot appearance" of the hyperpigmented RPE with its lacunae and scalloped margins.[127,129] Visual acuities range from 20/20 to 20/400 depending on the degree of foveal RPE atrophy or overlying retinal changes, including sensory retinal detachment, cystoid macular edema, chorioretinal folds, vitreomacular traction, and choroidal neovascularization. Age at presentation is variable depending on the severity of foveal involvement; often it is detected as an incidental finding.

Sanderson Grizzard had a similar patient who was reviewed by Gass in 1999 (personal communication: Figure 12.12C and D), showing the typical appearance, including a mild vascular and fibrous component. Why all sporadic combined hamartomas and RPE dysgenesis are unilateral and monofocal is unknown. Bilateral and multifocal lesions have only been described in patients with neurofibromatosis, (see Figure. 12.11D-G and H-J)

12.12 Unilateral retinal pigment epithelium (RPE) dysgenesis (variant of combined hamartoma of the RPE and retina).

A and B: This 17-year-old Caucasian girl's macula has a flat lesion with several patches of hypopigmented, thin RPE with finger-like projections at the margin. Islands of normal-appearing and hyperpigmented RPE are seen between the hypomelanotic patches. No overlying retinal vascular or fibrotic abnormalities are seen. She was seen previously at age 10 with the lesion but not photographed. Angiogram shows window defects corresponding to the hypopigmented RPE. Her visual acuity was 20/50 in this eye and 20/20 in the normal fellow eye.

C and D: This patient has a large patch of hypomelanotic RPE in the macula and superotemporal quadrant with typical scalloped edge of hyperpigmented RPE. Overlying mild vascular telangiectasia and fibrous tissue that has contracted causing retinal folds is seen (arrows), hinting that the anomaly may not be limited to the RPE. Visual acuity was 20/25, thus signifying hypopigmented, but intact RPE.

E and F: Another female patient with the typical RPE lesion and clearly evident fibrovascular tissue in the retinal substance (arrow) that shows vascular telangiectasia on angiography.

G–J: Almost no hyperpigmentation seen at the margins of this lesion with a mild fibrovascular component and subtle retinal folds (G). Fluorescein angiogram shows vascular remodeling (arrows, I and J).

K and L: Another example of a 47-year-old male with 20/20 vision and a flat, mostly hypopigmented lesion with the typical scalloped margins.

(A, B, E, F, K and L, courtesy of Dr. H. Richard McDonald; C and D, courtesy of Dr. Sanderson Grizzard; E and F, courtesy of Dr. Craig Morgan.)

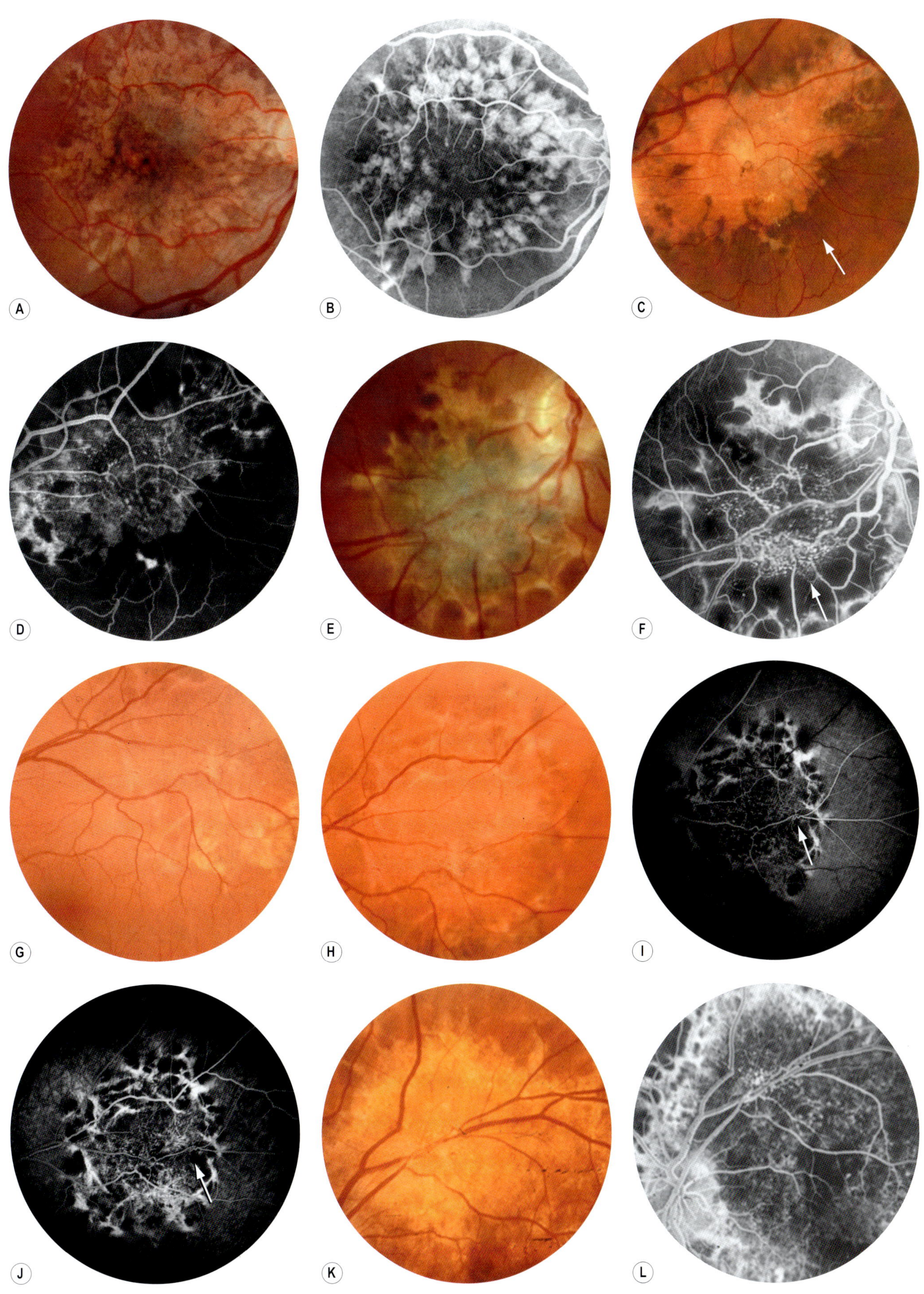
A
B
C
D
E
F
G
H
I
J
K
L

REACTIVE HYPERPLASIAS OF THE RETINAL PIGMENT EPITHELIUM SIMULATING HAMARTOMAS AND NEOPLASIAS

A variety of stimuli are capable of exciting the highly reactive RPE to proliferate to form mass lesions that may simulate RPE and uveal hamartomatous and neoplastic lesions (Figures 12.13 and 12.14).[81,83,130–135] One of these stimuli is recurrent and chronic focal choroiditis occurring at the site of chorioretinal scars in patients with the presumed ocular histoplasmosis syndrome (Figure 12.14F–L). The lesions may be pigmented or nonpigmented and they may be difficult to distinguish from choroidal melanomas biomicroscopically, angiographically, or ultrasonographically.[82] Histopathologically, some of the lesions may demonstrate cytologic features suggestive of RPE neoplasia (Figure 12.14H–L). These highly reactive lesions may be locally destructive but are apparently incapable of metastasis. Histopathologically, the index of suspicion of reactive hyperplasia should be high if the lesion arises within or adjacent to a chorioretinal scar, particularly in the juxtapapillary area. Figure 12.14A–E demonstrates the unusual development of mass lesions presumed to be reactive RPE hyperplasia arising within congenital familial macular colobomata.

12.13 Vitreoretinal traction causing lesions simulating combined retinal pigment epithelium and retinal hamartoma (CRPE-RH).

A–F: Vitreoretinal traction was associated with an elevated gray retinal lesion with dilated retinal vessels surrounded by a zone of RPE darkening in the inferior fundus of this boy with bilateral X-linked foveomacular schisis (A and B). Angiography showed dilated, distorted, and partly occluded retinal vessels (C). One year later lipid exudate extended into the macular area (D and E) and there was increased vitreous condensation and band formation (F).

G and H: This patient developed loss of vision associated with vitreomacular traction in the left eye. Note the tenting of the retina by a vitreous band (arrow, G). Four months later the juxtapapillary retina was tented anteriorly by further vitreous condensation and traction. Note the darkening of the RPE (arrow, H) that surrounds the mass and caused it to simulate CRPE-RH.

I and J: Focal vitreoretinal traction caused an elevated pigmented lesion associated with distortion of the retinal vessels and a gray epiretinal membrane simulating CRPE-RH (I). Four years later the vitreous and part of the epiretinal membrane (arrow, J) spontaneously detached from the retina.

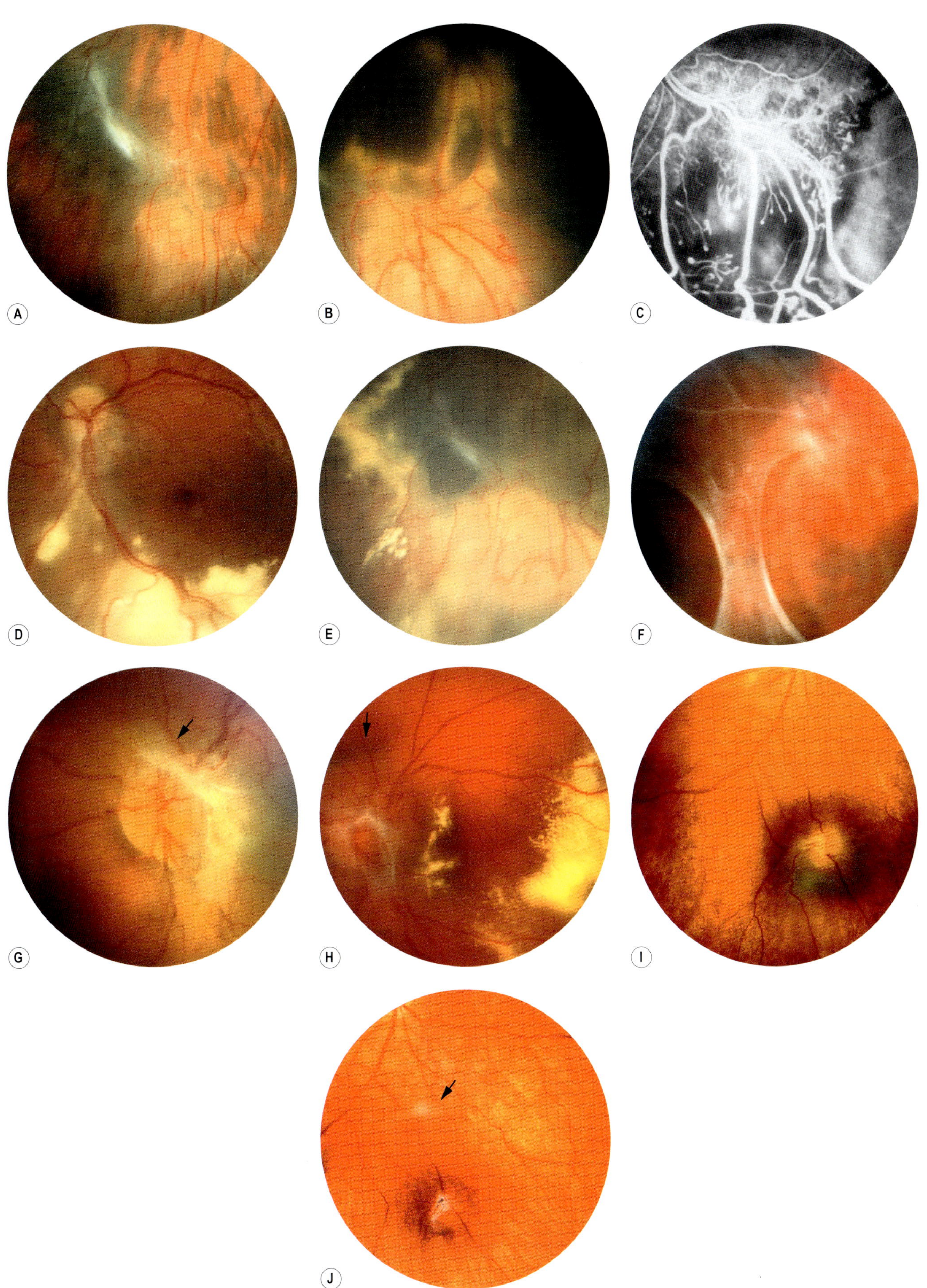
A
B
C
D
E
F
G
H
I
J

12.14 Reactive hyperplasia of the retinal pigment epithelium (RPE) simulating RPE hamartomas and choroidal melanomas.

A–E: A nodule of RPE hyperplasia (arrows, A and B) developed within congenital macular staphylomas of this 25-year-old woman. Visual acuity was 20/400 bilaterally. Over a period of several years the RPE nodule in the left eye enlarged and a melanoma was suspected (C). Angiography revealed the presence of blood vessels within the nodule (arrow, D) and late staining (E). Bilateral macular scars noted in early childhood in the patient and her brother were attributed to toxoplasmosis. Her grandfather had macular degeneration.

F and G: A small pigmented nodule (arrow, F) developed on the right optic disc of this patient with multifocal chorioretinal and juxtapapillary scars typical of the presumed ocular histoplasmosis syndrome (POHS). Angiography showed dilation of the capillaries in the surface of the nodule (G) and late staining.

H–L: This 64-year-old woman with bilateral POHS developed a slowly enlarging mass on the left optic disc (H) that for a period of 8 years was unassociated with loss of visual acuity, before development of an extension of lipid exudate into the macula (J). Because of concern of a melanoma a needle biopsy was done. The results were equivocal and the eye was enucleated. Histopathologically the tumor was composed of large hypopigmented RPE cells showing minimal mitotic activity (K and L). The tumor was interpreted as a low-grade adenocarcinoma of the RPE by Shields et al.[133] but in the author's opinion represents reactive RPE hyperplasia.

(H–L from Shields et al.[133])

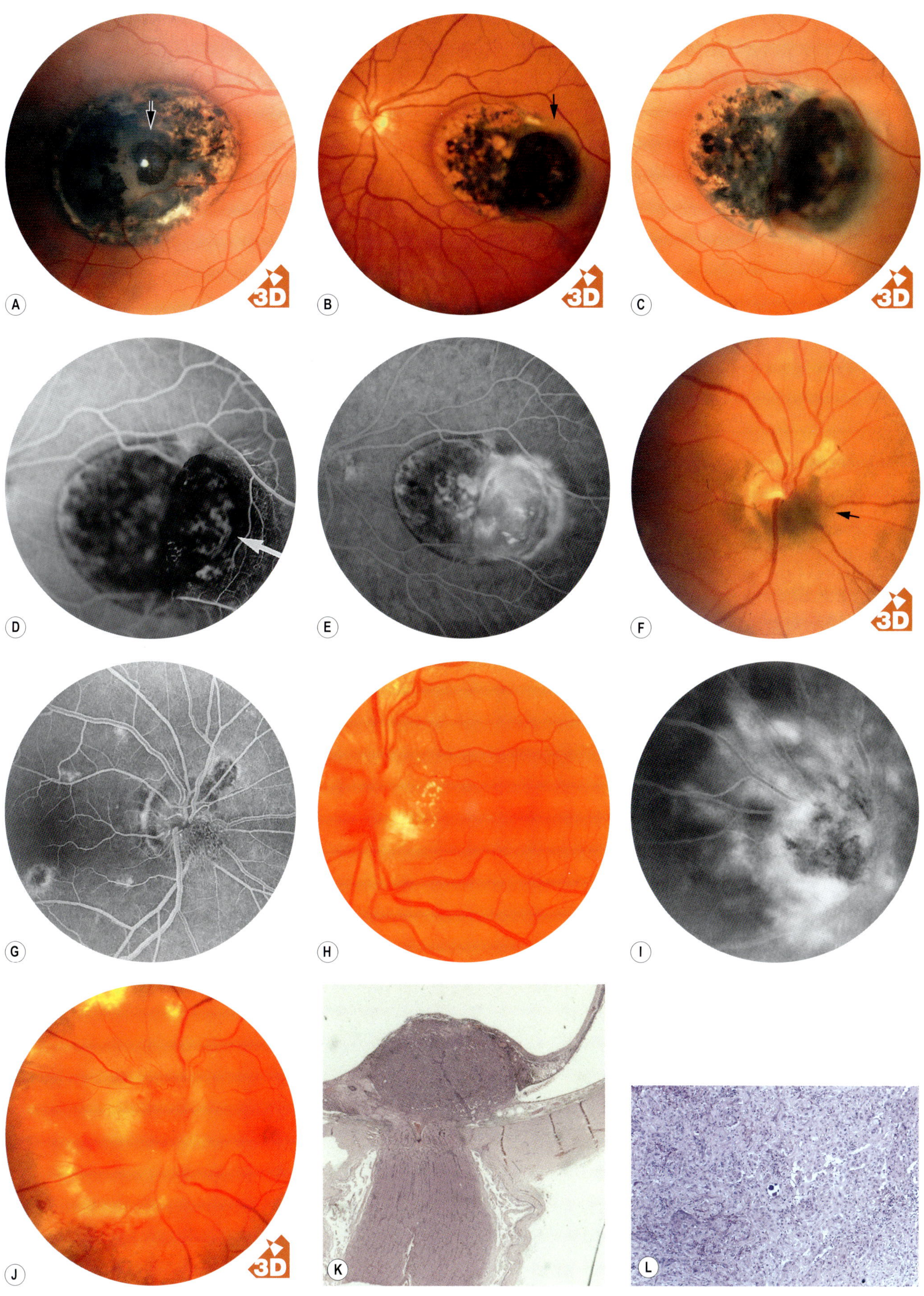
A
3D
B
3D
C
3D
D
E
F
3D
G
H
I
J
3D
K
L

ADENOCARCINOMA (MALIGNANT EPITHELIOMA) OF THE RETINAL PIGMENT EPITHELIUM

Adenocarcinoma of the RPE is an extremely rare tumor and often the diagnosis is made after enucleation. Finger reviewed the literature in 1996[136] and found 12 cases, the majority of them in women (10/12, 82%), often associated with uveitis/inflammation (58%), resistant to plaque radiation or other treatment and resulting eventually in a painful blind eye. A few more cases have since been described, some de novo, and others arising from a CHRPE lesion.[16–18] It should be suspected in women with a hyperpigmented tuberous-appearing mass associated with large feeder vessels, lipid exudation, and inflammatory signs (Figure 12.15A–C). The mass becomes highly elevated, invades the sensory retina, and produces a progressive exudative retinal detachment (Figure 12.15A–F). Cystoid macular edema, epiretinal gliosis, and vitreous membranes are often seen over time. Ultrasonogram shows the elevated lesion and associated retinal detachment. Plaque radiotherapy, intravitreal steroids, photodynamic therapy, vitrectomy, or other therapy does not control the growth and the eye becomes painful or phthisical. Sections of the enucleated eye show large sinusoidal feeder vessels around a diffusely pigmented tumor (Figure 12.15G and H). Pathological examination reveals cords of RPE cells on a basement membrane (Figure 12.15J), some of which are anaplastic, where the adenoma has turned into a malignant epithelioma (Figure 12.15K). Shields et al. have seen this in two African American women where the affected eye became phthisical.[18] To date, the tumor is locally destructive and distant metastasis has not been seen.

12.15 Malignant epithelioma of the retinal pigment epithelium (RPE) (adenocarcinoma of the RPE).

A–K: This 60-year-old asymptomatic woman was found to have a raised pigmented mass in the inferotemporal periphery with a feeding arteriole, surface retinal hemorrhages, and surrounding lipid exudates during a routine exam. Her vision was 20/20 in each eye (A). A year later the exudation had increased and was associated with subretinal fluid (B). Over the next 4 years the tumor enlarged with surface wrinkling, progressive exudation, cystoid macular edema, vitreous cells, and fibrosis (C and D). B scan reveals an ovoid tumor and adjacent retinal detachment (E). During the subsequent 3 years she received various treatments including topical and sub-Tenon's steroids, nonsteroidal agents, photodynamic therapy, vitrectomy, and laser photocoagulation. Overall, during this time the tumor progressed very little, but the complications progressed relentlessly. The eye became painful and vision decreased to hand motions. She underwent enucleation. Gross section reveals a diffusely pigmented tumor and adjacent retinal detachment. Note the large sinusoidal vessels feeding the tumor at its base (G and H). Hematoxylin and eosin stain shows rows of RPE cells arranged over its basement membrane (J). The inner RPE cells show anaplastic features with larger nuclei (K).

(Courtesy of Dr. Jerry Shields and Dr. Carol Shields.)

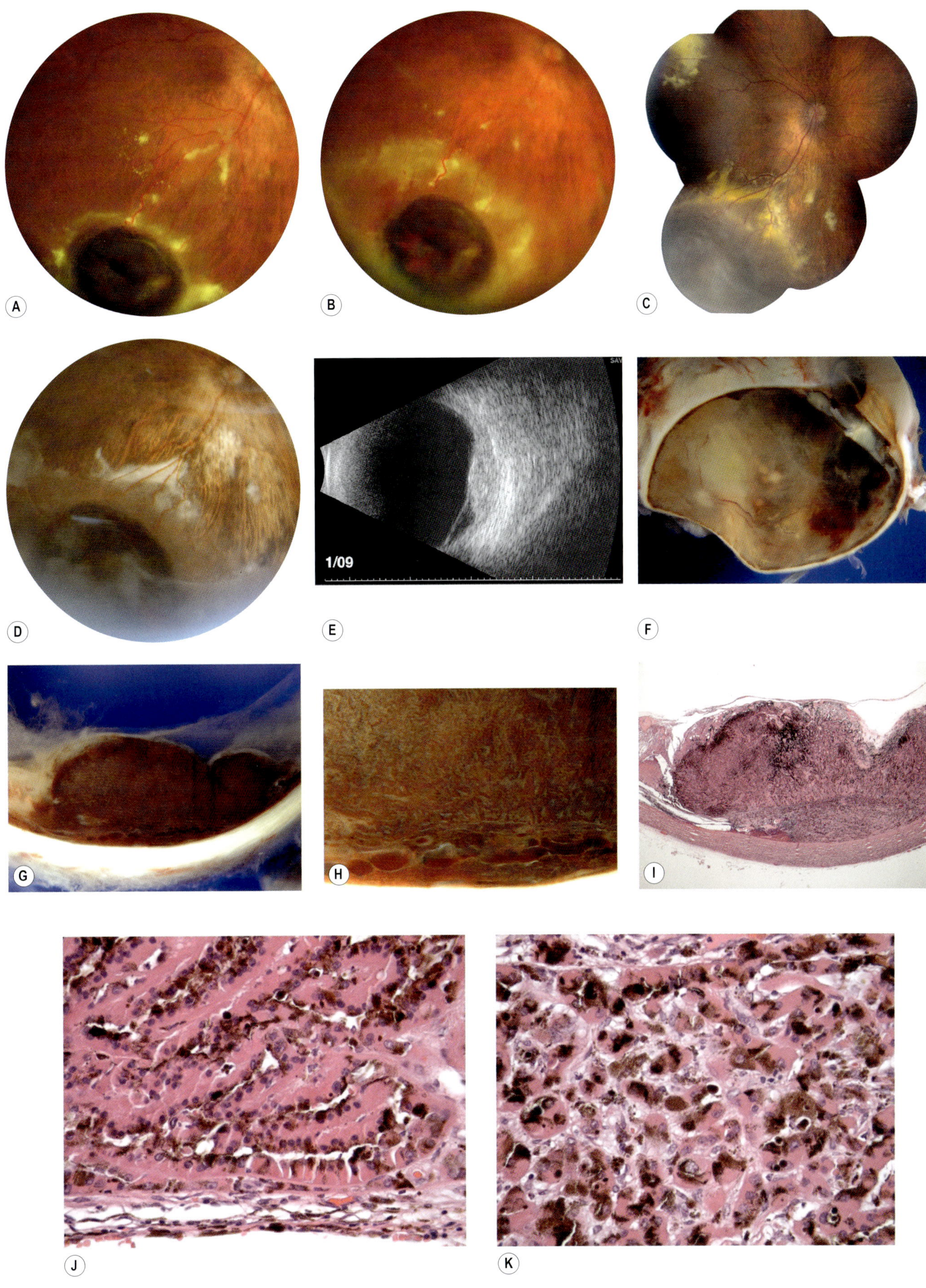
A
B
C
D
1/09
E
F
G
H
I
J
K

References

1. Gass JDM. Focal congenital anomalies of the retinal pigment epithelium. Eye 1989;3:1–18.
2. Blair NP, Trempe CL. Hypertrophy of the retinal pigment epithelium associated with Gardner's syndrome. Am J Ophthalmol 1980;90:661–7.
3. Boldrey EE, Schwartz A. Enlargement of congenital hypertrophy of the retinal pigment epithelium. Am J Ophthalmol 1982;94:64–6.
4. Buettner H. Congenital hypertrophy of the retinal pigment epithelium. Am J Ophthalmol 1975;79:177–89.
5. Chamot L, Zografos L, Klainguti G. Fundus changes associated with congenital hypertrophy of the retinal pigment epithelium. Am J Ophthalmol 1993;115:154–61.
6. Munden PM, Sobol WM, Weingeist TA. Ocular findings in Turcot syndrome (glioma-polyposis). Ophthalmology 1991;98:111–4.
7. Reese AB, Jones IS. Benign melanomas of the retinal pigment epithelium. Am J Ophthalmol 1956;42:207–12.
8. Sugar HS, Wolff L. Geographic dark posterior fundus patches. Am J Ophthalmol 1977;83: 847–52.
9. Shields CL, Mashayekhi A, Ho T, et al. Solitary congenital hypertrophy of the retinal pigment epithelium: clinical features and frequency of enlargement in 330 patients. Ophthalmology 2003;110:1968–76.
10. Nishikatsu H, Shiono T. Congenital hypertrophy of the retinal pigment epithelium in the macula. Ophthalmologica 1996;210:126–8.
11. Augsburger JJ, Henson GL, Hershberger VS, et al. Topographical distribution of typical unifocal congenital hypertrophy of retinal pigment epithelium. Graefes Arch Clin Exp Ophthalmol 2006;244:1412–4.
12. Zucchiatti I, Battaglia Parodi M, Pala M, et al. Macular congenital hypertrophy of the retinal pigment epithelium: a case report. Eur J Ophthalmol 2010;20:621–4.
13. Champion R, Daicker BC. Congenital hypertrophy of the pigment epithelium: light microscopic and ultrastructural findings in young children. Retina 1989;9:44–8.
14. Norris JL, Cleasby GW. An unusual case of congenital hypertrophy of the retinal pigment epithelium. Arch Ophthalmol 1976;94:1910–1.
15. Shields JA, Shields CL, Singh AD. Acquired tumors arising from congenital hypertrophy of the retinal pigment epithelium. Arch Ophthalmol 2000;118:637–41.
16. Shields JA, Shields CL, Eagle Jr RC, et al. Adenocarcinoma arising from congenital hypertrophy of retinal pigment epithelium. Arch Ophthalmol 2001;119:597–602.
17. Trichopoulos N, Augsburger JJ, Schneider S. Adenocarcinoma arising from congenital hypertrophy of the retinal pigment epithelium. Graefes Arch Clin Exp Ophthalmol 2006;244: 125–8.
18. Shields JA, Eagle Jr RC, Shields CL, et al. Malignant transformation of congenital hypertrophy of the retinal pigment epithelium. Ophthalmology 2009;116:2213–6.
19. Shields CL, Pirondini C, Bianciotto C, et al. Autofluorescence of congenital hypertrophy of the retinal pigment epithelium. Retina 2007;27:1097–100.
20. Cleary PE, Gregor Z, Bird AC. Retinal vascular changes in congenital hypertrophy of the retinal pigment epithelium. Br J Ophthalmol 1976;60:499–503.
21. Cohen SY, Quentel G, Guiberteau B, et al. Retinal vascular changes in congenital hypertrophy of the retinal pigment epithelium. Ophthalmology 1993;100:471–4.
22. Shields JA, Shields CL, Shah PG, et al. Lack of association among typical congenital hypertrophy of the retinal pigment epithelium, adenomatous polyposis, and Gardner syndrome. Ophthalmology 1992;99:1709–13.
23. Shields CL, Materin MA, Walker C, et al. Photoreceptor loss overlying congenital hypertrophy of the retinal pigment epithelium by optical coherence tomography. Ophthalmology 2006;113: 661–5.
24. Kurz GH, Zimmerman LE. Vagaries of the retinal pigment epithelium. Int Ophthalmol Clin 1962;2:441–64.
25. Lloyd III WC, Eagle RCJR, Shields JA, et al. Congenital hypertrophy of the retinal pigment epithelium; electron microscopic and morphometric observations. Ophthalmology 1990;97:1052–60.
26. Parsons MA, Rennie IG, Rundle PA, et al. Congenital hypertrophy of retinal pigment epithelium: a clinico-pathological case report. Br J Ophthalmol 2005;89:920–1.
27. Wirz K, Lee WR, Coaker T. Progressive changes in congenital hypertrophy of the retinal pigment epithelium; an electron microscopic study. Graefes Arch Clin Exp Ophthalmol 1982;219:214–21.
28. Traboulsi EI, Maumenee IH, Krush AJ, et al. Pigmented ocular fundus lesions in the inherited gastrointestinal polyposis syndromes and in hereditary nonpolyposis colorectal cancer. Ophthalmology 1988;95:964–9.
29. Aiello LP, Traboulsi EI. Pigmented fundus lesions in a preterm infant with familial adenomatous polyposis. Arch Ophthalmol 1993;111:302–3.
30. Diaz-Llopis M, Menezo JL. Congenital hypertrophy of the retinal pigment epithelium in familial adenomatous polyposis. Arch Ophthalmol 1988;106:412–3.
31. Gardner EJ, Richards RC. Multiple cutaneous and subcutaneous lesions occurring simultaneously with hereditary polyposis and osteomatosis. Am J Hum Genet 1953;5:139–47.
32. Giardiello FM, Offerhaus GJ, Traboulsi EI, et al. Value of combined phenotypic markers in identifying inheritance of familial adenomatous polyposis. Gut 1991;32:1170–4.
33. Heinemann M-H, Baker RH, Miller HH, et al. Familial polyposis coli: the spectrum of ocular and other extracolonic manifestations. Graefes Arch Clin Exp Ophthalmol 1991;229:213–8.
34. Kasner L, Traboulsi EI, Delacruz Z, et al. A histopathologic study of the pigmented fundus lesions in familial adenomatous polyposis. Retina 1992;12:35–42.
35. Lewis RA, Crowder WE, Eierman LA, et al. The Gardner syndrome; significance of ocular features. Ophthalmology 1984;91:916–25.
36. Llopis MD, Menezo JL. Congenital hypertrophy of the retinal pigment epithelium and familial polyposis of the colon. Am J Ophthalmol 1987;103:235–6.
37. Romania A, Zakov ZN, Church JM, et al. Retinal pigment epithelium lesions as a biomarker of disease in patients with familial adenomatous polyposis; a follow-up report. Ophthalmology 1992;99:911–3.
38. Romania A, Zakov ZN, McGannon E, et al. Congenital hypertrophy of the retinal pigment epithelium in familial adenomatous polyposis. Ophthalmology 1989;96:879–84.
39. Santos A, Morales L, Hernandez-Quintela E, et al. Congenital hypertrophy of the retinal pigment epithelium associated with familial adenomatous polyposis. Retina 1994;14:6–9.
40. Schmidt D, Jung CE, Wolff G. Changes in the retinal pigment epithelium close to retinal vessels in familial adenomatous polyposis. Graefes Arch Clin Exp Ophthalmol 1994;232:96–102.
41. Stein EA, Brady KD. Ophthalmologic and electro-oculographic findings in Gardner's syndrome. Am J Ophthalmol 1988;106:326–31.
42. Traboulsi EI, Murphy SF, de la Cruz ZC, et al. A clinicopathologic study of the eyes in familial adenomatous polyposis with extracolonic manifestations (Gardner's syndrome). Am J Ophthalmol 1990;110:550–61.
43. Whitson WE, Orcutt JC, Walkinshaw MD. Orbital osteoma in Gardner's syndrome. Am J Ophthalmol 1986;101:236–41.
44. Gass JDM. Stereoscopic atlas of macular diseases; diagnosis and treatment, 3rd ed. St. Louis: CV Mosby; 1987. p. 606–11.
45. Traboulsi EI, Krush AJ, Gardner EJ, et al. Prevalence and importance of pigmented ocular fundus lesions in Gardner's syndrome. N Engl J Med 1987;316:661–7.
46. Nieuwenhuis MH, Vasen HF. Correlations between mutation site in APC and phenotype of familial adenomatous polyposis (FAP): a review of the literature. Crit Rev Oncol Hematol 2007;61: 153–61.
47. Bodmer WF, Bailey CJ, Bodmer J, et al. Localization of the gene for familial adenomatous polyposis on chromosome 5. Nature 1987;328:614–6.
48. Parke JT, Riccardi VM, Lewis RA, et al. A syndrome of microcephaly and retinal pigmentary abnormalities without mental retardation in a family with coincidental autosomal dominant hyperreflexia. Am J Med Genet 1984;17:585–94.
49. Mauthner L. Lehrbuch der Ophthalmoscopie. Vienna: Tendler; 1868. p. 388.
50. Höeg N. Die gruppierte Pigmentation des Augengrundes. Klin Monatsbl Augenheilkd 1911;49:49–77.
51. Morse PH. Fluorescein angiography of grouped pigmentation of the retina. Ann Ophthalmol 1973;5:27–30.
52. Shields JA, Tso MOM. Congenital grouped pigmentation of the retina; histopathologic description and report of a case. Arch Ophthalmol 1975;93:1153–5.
53. Silvan Lopez F. Pigmentación agrupada retiniana. Arch Soc Oftalmol Hisp-Am 1948;8:448–56.
54. Blake EM. Congenital grouped pigmentation of the retina. Trans Am Ophthalmol Soc 1926;24:223–33.
55. Loewenstein A, Steel J. Special case of melanosis fundi: bilateral congenital group pigmentation of the central area. Br J Ophthalmol 1941;25:417–23.
56. McGregor IS. Macular coloboma with bilateral grouped pigmentation of the retina. Br J Ophthalmol 1945;29:132–6.
57. Schwarz GT. Case report of congenital grouped pigmentation of the retina with maculocerebral degeneration. Am J Ophthalmol 1943;26:72–4.
58. Welter SL. Naevus pigmentosus des Augenhintergrundes. Klin Monatsbl Augenheilkd 1927;78:682–7.
59. De Jong PTVM, Delleman JW. Familial grouped pigmentation of the retinal pigment epithelium. Br J Ophthalmol 1988;72:439.
60. Gasparová D, Szedélyová L. Familial occurrence of grouped pigmentation of the ocular fundus. Cesk Oftalmol 1980;36:406–8.
61. Renardel de Lavalette VW, Cruysberg JRM, Deutman AF. Familial congenital grouped pigmentation of the retina. Am J Ophthalmol 1991;112:406–9.
62. Kadoi C, Hayasaka S, Hayasaka Y, et al. Bilateral congenital grouped pigmentation of the retina in one girl and bilateral congenital albinotic spots of the retina in her sister. Retina 1999;19:571–2.
63. Siddiqui AM, Everman DB, Rogers RC, et al. Microcephaly and congenital grouped pigmentation of the retinal pigment epithelium associated with submicroscopic deletions of 13q33.3-q34 and 11p15.4. Ophthalmic Genet 2009;30:136–41.
64. Collier M. Les manifestations oculaires associées à la dyschondroplasie d'Ollier (à propos d'un cas comportant une pigmentation congénitale de la rétine. Bull Soc Ophtalmol Fr 1961;4:161–9.
65. Meyer CH, Freyschmidt-Paul P, Happle R, et al. Unilateral linear hyperpigmentation of the skin with ipsilateral sectorial hyperpigmentation of the retina. Am J Med Genet A 2004;126A:89–92.
66. Regillo CD, Eagle Jr RC, Shields JA, et al. Histopathologic findings in congenital grouped pigmentation of the retina. Ophthalmology 1993;100:400–5.
67. Regillo CD, Eagle Jr RC, Shields JA, et al. Histopathologic findings in congenital grouped pigmentation of the retina. Ophthalmology 1993;100:400–5.
68. Fuhrmann C, Bopp S, Laqua H. Congenital grouped albinotic spots: a rare anomaly of the retinal pigment epithelium. Ger J Ophthalmol 1992;1:103–4.
69. Kandori F. Very rare case of congenital nonprogressive night blindness with fleck retina. Clin Ophthalmol 1959;13:384–6.
70. Kandori F, Setogawa T, Tamai A. Electroretinographical studies on fleck retina with congenital nonprogressive night blindness. Acta Soc Ophthalmol Jpn 1966;70:1311–25.
71. Kandori F, Tamai A, Kurimoto S, et al. Fleck retina. Am J Ophthalmol 1972;73:673–85.
72. Gass JDM. Differential diagnosis of intraocular tumors; a stereoscopic presentation. St. Louis: CV Mosby; 1974. p. 221–46.
73. Kraupa E. Beiträge zur Morphologie des Augenhintergrundes III. Klin Monatsbl Augenheilkd 1921;67:15–26.
74. Roseman RL, Gass JDM. Solitary hypopigmented nevus of the retinal pigment epithelium in the macula. Arch Ophthalmol 1992;110:1358–9. [correction p. 762.]
75. Schlernitzauer DA, Green WR. Peripheral retinal albinotic spots. Am J Ophthalmol 1971;72: 729–32.
76. Golchet PR, Jampol LM, Mathura Jr JR, et al. Torpedo maculopathy. Br J Ophthalmol 2010;94:302–6.
77. Shields CL, Shields JA, Marr BP, et al. Congenital simple hamartoma of the retinal pigment epithelium: a study of five cases. Ophthalmology 2003;110:1005–11.
78. Blodi FC, Reuling FH, Sornson ET. Pseudomelanocytoma at the optic nerve head; an adenoma of the retinal pigment epithelium. Arch Ophthalmol 1965;73:353–5.

79. Duke JR, Maumenee AE. An unusual tumor of the retinal pigment epithelium in an eye with early open-angle glaucoma. Am J Ophthalmol 1959;47:311–7.
80. Font RL, Zimmerman LE, Fine BS. Adenoma of the retinal pigment epithelium; histochemical and electron microscopic observations. Am J Ophthalmol 1972;73:544–54.
81. Garner A. Tumours of the retinal pigment epithelium. Br J Ophthalmol 1970;54:715–23.
82. Jampel HD, Schachat AP, Conway B, et al. Retinal pigment epithelial hyperplasia assuming tumor-like proportions; report of two cases. Retina 1986;6:105–12.
83. Tso MOM, Albert DM. Pathological condition of the retinal pigment epithelium; neoplasms and nodular non-neoplastic lesions. Arch Ophthalmol 1972;88:27–38.
84. Cardell BS, Starbuck MJ. Juxtapapillary hamartoma of retina. Br J Ophthalmol 1961;45:672–7.
85. Font RL, Moura RA, Shetlar DJ, et al. Combined hamartoma of sensory retina and retinal pigment epithelium. Retina 1989;9:302–11.
86. Friberg TR, Gulledge SL. Hamartomas of the retina and pigment epithelium. Can J Ophthalmol 1982;17:56–60.
87. Gass JDM. An unusual hamartoma of the pigment epithelium and retina simulating choroidal melanoma and retinoblastoma. Trans Am Ophthalmol Soc 1973;71:171–85.
88. Mele A, Cennamo G, Sorrentino V, et al. Fluoroangiographic and echographic study on a juxtapapillary hamartoma of the retinal pigment epithelium. Ophthalmologica 1984;189:180–5.
89. Reynolds WD, Goldstein BG. Retinal pigment epithelial hamartoma. Ophthalmology 1983;90:117–9.
90. Schachat AP, Glaser BM. Retinal hamartoma, acquired retinoschisis, and retinal hole. Am J Ophthalmol 1985;99:604–5.
91. Schachat AP, Shields JA, Fine SL, et al. Combined hamartomas of the retina and retinal pigment epithelium. Ophthalmology 1984;91:1609–14.
92. Theobald GD, Floyd G, Kirk HQ. Hyperplasia of the retinal pigment epithelium simulating a neoplasm: report of two cases. Am J Ophthalmol 1958;45:235–40.
93. Vogel MH, Wessing A. Die Proliferation des juxtapapillären retinalen Pigmentepithels. Klin Monatsbl Augenheilkd 1973;162:736–43.
94. Vogel MH, Zimmerman LE, Gass JDM. Proliferation of the juxtapapillary retinal pigment epithelium simulating malignant melanoma. Doc Ophthalmol 1969;26:461–81.
95. Corcostegui B, Mendez M, Corcostegui G, et al. Éléments diagnostiques des hamartomes de la rétine et de l'épithélium pigmentaire. Bull Mem Soc Fr Ophtalmol 1985;96:152.
96. Cosgrove JM, Sharp DM, Bird AC. Combined hamartoma of the retina and retinal pigment epithelium: the clinical spectrum. Trans Ophthalmol Soc UK 1986;105:106–13.
97. Flood TP, Orth DH, Aaberg TM, et al. Macular hamartomas of the retinal pigment epithelium and retina. Retina 1983;3:164–70.
98. Gass JDM. Combined hamartomas of the retinal and retinal pigment epithelium. Ophthalmology 1984;91:1615.
99. Jabbour O, Payeur G. Malformation congénitale de l'épithélium pigmentaire et de la rétine. J Fr Ophtalmol 1983;6:149–54.
100. Machemer R. Die Primäre retinale Pigmentepithelhyperplasie. Albrecht von Graefes Arch Ophthalmol 1964;167:284–95.
101. Kahn D, Goldberg MF, Jednock N. Combined retinal-retina pigment epithelial hamartoma presenting as a vitreous hemorrhage. Retina 1984;4:40–3.
102. Wang C-L, Brucker AJ. Vitreous hemorrhage secondary to juxtapapillary vascular hamartoma of the retina. Retina 1984;4:44–7.
103. Shields CL, Mashayekhi A, Dai VV, et al. Optical coherence tomographic findings of combined hamartoma of the retina and retinal pigment epithelium in 11 patients. Arch Ophthalmol 2005;123:1746–50.
104. McDonald HR, Abrams GW, Burke JM, et al. Clinicopathologic results of vitreous surgery for epiretinal membranes in patients with combined retinal and retinal pigment epithelial hamartomas. Am J Ophthalmol 1985;100:806–13.
105. Sappenfield DL, Gitter KA. Surgical intervention for combined retinal-retinal pigment epithelial hamartoma. Retina 1990;10:119–24.
106. Rosenberg PR, Walsh JB. Retinal pigment epithelial hamartoma – unusual manifestations. Br J Ophthalmol 1984;68:439–42.
107. Hrisomalos NF, Mansour AM, Jampol LM, et al. "Pseudo"-combined hamartoma following papilledema. Arch Ophthalmol 1987;105:1634–5.
108. Ticho BH, Egel RT, Jampol LM. Acquired combined hamartoma of the retina and pigment epithelium following parainfectious meningoencephalitis with optic neuritis. J Pediatr Ophthalmol Strabismus 1998;35:116–8.
109. Laqua H, Wessing A. Congenital retino-pigment epithelial malformation, previously described as hamartoma. Am J Ophthalmol 1979;87:34–42.
110. McLean EB. Hamartoma of the retinal pigment epithelium. Am J Ophthalmol 1976;82:227–31.
111. Shields CL, Thangappan A, Hartzell K, et al. Combined hamartoma of the retina and retinal pigment epithelium in 77 consecutive patients visual outcome based on macular versus extramacular tumor location. Ophthalmology 2008;115:2246–52.
112. Cohn AD, Quiram PA, Drenser KA, et al. Surgical outcomes of epiretinal membranes associated with combined hamartoma of the retina and retinal pigment epithelium. Retina 2009;29: 825–30.
113. Konstantinidis L, Chamot L, Zografos L, et al. Pars plana vitrectomy and epiretinal membrane peeling for vitreoretinal traction associated with combined hamartoma of the retina and retinal pigment epithelium (CHRRPE). Klin Monbl Augenheilkd 2007;224:356–9.
114. Stallman JB. Visual improvement after pars plana vitrectomy and membrane peeling for vitreoretinal traction associated with combined hamartoma of the retina and retinal pigment epithelium. Retina 2002;22:101–4.
115. Mason III JO. Visual improvement after pars plana vitrectomy and membrane peeling for vitreoretinal traction associated with combined hamartoma of the retina and retinal pigment epithelium. Retina 2002;22:824–5. [author reply 5–6.]
116. Aoki S, Barkovich AJ, Nishimura K, et al. Neurofibromatosis types 1 and 2; cranial MR findings. Radiology 1989;172:527–34.
117. Bouzas EA, Parry DM, Eldridge R, et al. Familial occurrence of combined pigment epithelial and retinal hamartomas associated with neurofibromatosis 2. Retina 1992;12:103–7.
118. Bouzas EA, Parry DM, Eldridge R, et al. Visual impairment in patients with neurofibromatosis 2. Neurology 1993;43:622–3.
119. Cotlier E. Café-au-lait spots of the fundus in neurofibromatosis. Arch Ophthalmol 1977;95:1990–2.
120. Destro M, D'Amico DJ, Gragoudas ES, et al. Retinal manifestations of neurofibromatosis; diagnosis and management. Arch Ophthalmol 1991;109:662–6.
121. Good WV, Brodsky MC, Edwards MS, et al. Bilateral retinal hamartomas in neurofibromatosis type 2. Br J Ophthalmol 1991;75:190.
122. Kaye LD, Rothner AD, Beauchamp GR, et al. Ocular findings associated with neurofibromatosis type II. Ophthalmology 1992;99:1424–9.
123. Landau K, Dossetor FM, Hoyt WF, et al. Retinal hamartoma in neurofibromatosis 2. Arch Ophthalmol 1990;108:328–9.
124. Mulvihill JJ, Parry DM, Sherman JL, et al. NIH Conference. Neurofibromatosis 1 (Recklinghausen disease) and neurofibromatosis 2 (bilateral acoustic neurofibromatosis); an update. Ann Intern Med 1990;113:39–52.
125. Sivalingam A, Augsburger J, Perilongo G, et al. Combined hamartoma of the retina and retinal pigment epithelium in a patient with neurofibromatosis type 2. J Pediatr Ophthalmol Strabismus 1991;28:320–2.
126. Grant EA, Trzupek KM, Reiss J, et al. Combined retinal hamartomas leading to the diagnosis of neurofibromatosis type 2. Ophthalmic Genet 2008;29:133–8.
127. Cohen SY, Massin P, Quentel G. Clinicopathologic reports, case reports, and small case series: unilateral, idiopathic leopard-spot lesion of the retinal pigment epithelium. Arch Ophthalmol 2002;120:512–6.
128. Cohen SY, Fung AE, Tadayoni R, et al. Unilateral retinal pigment epithelium dysgenesis. Am J Ophthalmol 2009;148:914–9.
129. Cohen SY, Fung AE, Tadayoni R, et al. Unilateral retinal pigment epithelium dysgenesis. Am J Ophthalmol 2009;148:914–9.
130. Laqua H. Tumors and tumor-like lesions of the retinal pigment epithelium. Ophthalmologica 1981;183:34–8.
131. Minckler D, Allen Jr AW. Adenocarcinoma of the retinal pigment epithelium. Arch Ophthalmol 1978;96:2252–4.
132. Ramahefasolo S, Coscas G, Regenbogen L, et al. Adenocarcinoma of retinal pigment epithelium. Br J Ophthalmol 1987;71:516–20.
133. Shields JA, Eagle Jr RC, Barr CC, et al. Adenocarcinoma of retinal pigment epithelium arising from a juxtapapillary histoplasmosis scar. Arch Ophthalmol 1994;112:650–3.
134. Shields JA, Eagle Jr RC, Shields CL, et al. Pigmented adenoma of the optic nerve head simulating a melanocytoma. Ophthalmology 1992;99:1705–8.
135. Vogel MH, Wölz U. Malignes Epitheliom des retinalen Pigmentepithels. Klin Monatsbl Augenheilkd 1979;175:592–6.
136. Finger PT, McCormick SA, Davidian M, et al. Adenocarcinoma of the retinal pigment epithelium: a diagnostic and therapeutic challenge. Graefes Arch Clin Exp Ophthalmol 1996;234(Suppl. 1):S22–7.
137. Palmer ML, Carney MD, Combs JL. Combined hamartomas of the retinal pigment epithelium and retina. Retina 1990;10:33–6.

CHAPTER 13

Neoplastic Diseases of the Retina

RETINOBLASTOMA

Presenting signs of retinoblastoma include leukocoria (a white pupil), strabismus, hyphema (blood in the anterior chamber), vitreous hemorrhage, and, rarely, a red painful eye (Figure 13.01A).[1] Parents are usually the first to note a "glazed look," "wandering eye," or "shiny" appearance of the pupil. A prolonged time to diagnosis, advanced disease, and extraocular involvement are more frequently observed in developing countries.[2] The diagnosis of retinoblastoma is made in 90% of patients before 5 years of age.[3] In cases with a family history of retinoblastoma, the diagnosis may be made in the first few days of life at a screening examination. Although most patients with retinoblastoma present as young children, retinoblastoma has been reported in patients as old as 60 years.[4] Approximately 200 cases occur each year in the USA.[5] Bilateral involvement occurs in 20–35% of cases. Second-eye involvement is delayed in approximately 20–25% of cases. The mean age of diagnosis is 13 months for those with bilateral retinoblastoma versus a mean age of 24 months in those with unilateral retinoblastoma.[6] In a recently published study, the mean age-adjusted incidence rate of retinoblastoma in the USA was 11.8 cases per million children aged 0–4 years, similar to rates reported from European countries.[7] Moreover, the age-adjusted incidence rate of retinoblastoma in the USA has remained stable for the last 30 years.[7]

Retinoblastomas are typically globular, white, usually well-circumscribed tumors that may arise anywhere in the fundus (Figure 13.01B and C). They may grow inward toward the vitreous (endophytic) or outward (exophytic) into the subretinal space and may or may not be associated with ophthalmoscopic evidence of focal areas of calcification (Figure 13.01J).[8] Varying degrees of vascularization of the tumor occur, and this is usually seen best with fluorescein angiography (Figure 13.01D, E, K, and L).[9–11] Telangiectasis of the retinal vessels on the surface of exophytic tumors may occur. Biomicroscopic and angiographic evidence of communication of these dilated vessels with blood vessels extending into the depth of the tumor serves to differentiate retinoblastomas from primary retinal telangiectasis associated with underlying exudative detachment (Coats' syndrome) (Figure 13.01A–E).[9] Seeding of the tumor along the inner retinal surface and into the vitreous occurs frequently in advanced cases (Figure 13.01G–I). Extension of retinoblastoma into the anterior chamber may occur.[12]

13.01 Retinoblastoma.

A: Heterochromia irides, the presenting manifestation of retinoblastoma, in the right eye of this infant.

B–F: Large exophytic retinoblastoma. Note dilated tortuous retinal vessels that extend down into the substance of the tumor (B and C) and angiographic evidence of staining (D and E). Large blood vessels (arrows) were evident histopathologically near the surface of the tumor (F).

G–I: Multiple white tumor seeds were evident on the retinal surface posteriorly in this child with a peripherally located retinoblastoma. They showed no angiographic evidence of blood vessels (arrows, H). Note the necrotic center of the tumor seeds (arrow) evident histopathologically (I).

J–L: Small retinoblastoma or retinoma showing calcification (arrow, J) in a 4-year-old Indian child who had enucleation of his left eye 1 month before examination. Histopathologic examination of that eye revealed retinoblastoma with invasion of the optic nerve. He was referred for treatment of this solitary lesion noted in the right eye. He had a 6-year-old brother who had an enucleation of one eye at 6 months of age. His mother (Figure 13-04 A-E) had a retinoma. Fluorescein angiography revealed a fine capillary network within and immediately surrounding the tumor (K and L). There was extensive leakage of dye from these vessels. This patient died of widespread metastasis several months later. The clinical and angiographic appearance of this solitary nodule is quite similar to that of retinal astrocytic hamartomas and retinoma.

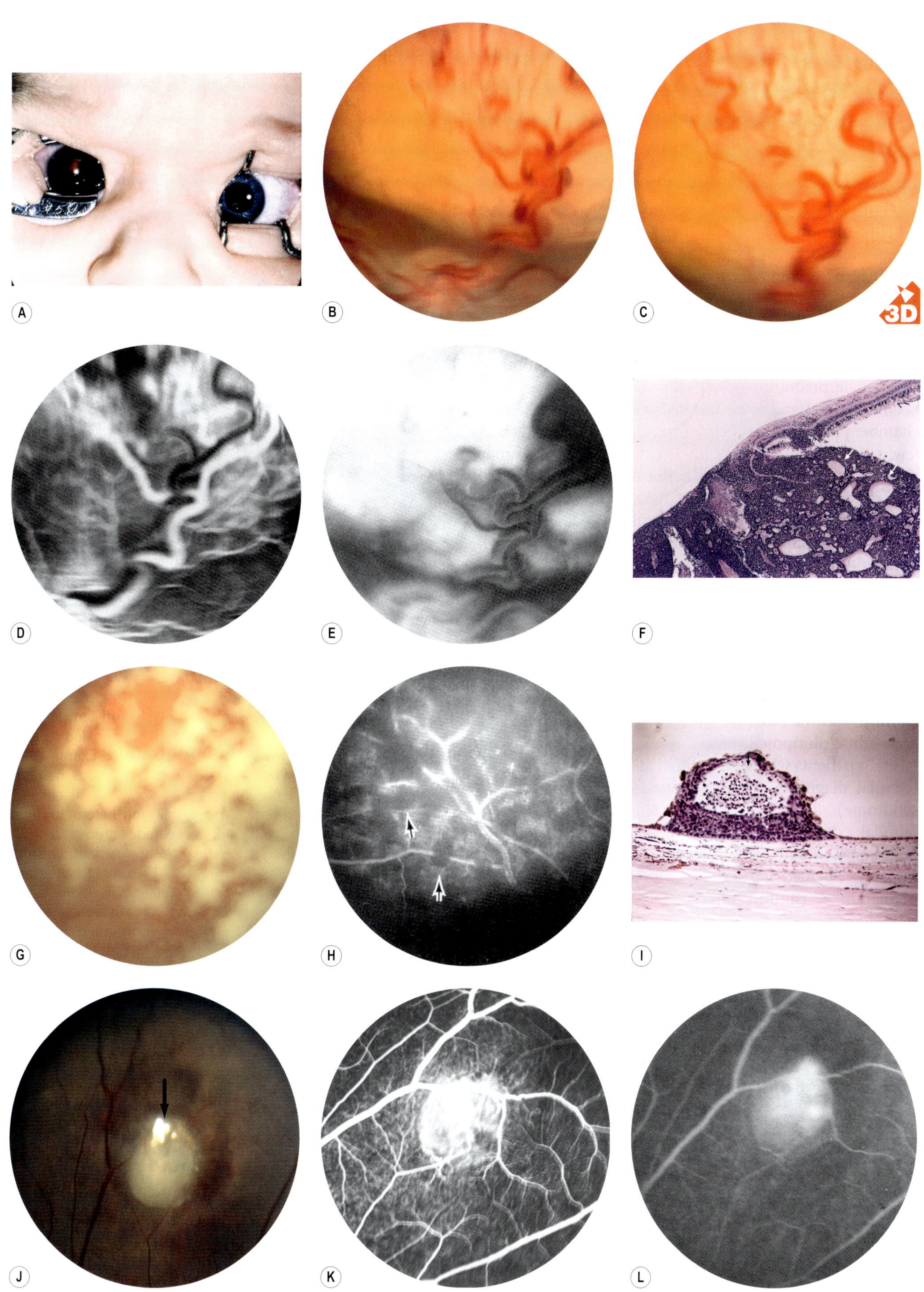
A
B
C
3D
D
E
F
G
H
I
J
K
L

Retinoma/Retinocytoma

Retinocytoma is a benign variant of retinoblastoma, previously referred to as retinoma, spontaneously regressed/arrested retinoblastoma, and retinoblastoma group 0 (Figure 13.04).[35–37] The diagnosis of retinocytoma is based upon its characteristic features of homogeneous translucent retinal mass, calcification, nonspecific retinal pigment epithelial (RPE) alteration, and chorioretinal atrophy.[37] Nearly one-half of patients diagnosed with retinocytoma have a family history of retinoblastoma.[35] Approximately 50% of their offspring will develop retinoblastoma. Malignant transformation of a retinoma has occurred.[38] Fluorescein angiography reveals evidence of a vascular network within retinomas and some evidence of dye leakage (Figure 13.04D, E, H, and I).[9,10,39] There is often evidence of RPE and choriocapillaris atrophy in the area of the retinoma (Figure 13.04D). Anastomosis between the retinal and choroidal vessels may occur.[39] Histopathologically, in contrast to retinoblastoma, retinoma/retinocytoma is composed of well-differentiated, benign-appearing mature retinal cells without evidence of necrosis or mitotic activity.[35] Ophthalmoscopically retinomas appear identical to so-called regressed retinoblastoma following irradiation treatment (Figure 13.05). It has been suggested that this portion of the tumor remaining after treatment may be the result of a coexistent retinoma.[40]

Retinoblastoma can be considered as familial or sporadic, bilateral or unilateral, and heritable or nonheritable. Thus, a case may be unilateral sporadic, bilateral sporadic, unilateral familial, or bilateral familial. About two-thirds of all cases are unilateral and one-third are bilateral. Approximately 10% of newly diagnosed retinoblastoma cases are familial and 90% are sporadic. All patients with familial retinoblastoma are at 50% risk of passing the predisposition for the development of the tumor to their offspring. From a genetic perspective, it is simpler to discuss retinoblastoma as heritable or nonheritable. Heritable cases (ones in which the predisposition to the tumor can be passed on to the next generation) result from a primary mutation in the germ cells (sperm or egg, hence all retinal cells in the individual have a first mutation) and second mutation(s) in retinal cells. Heritable cases include all bilateral cases, all multifocal cases, all familial cases, and all cases in which a second neoplasm developed. About 15% of sporadic unilateral cases (no family history) are also heritable.

13.04 Retinoma/retinocytoma.

A–E: This asymptomatic 23-year-old mother of the patient illustrated in Figure 13.1J–L had three retinomas (A–C). The one in the right macula had club-shaped calcified opacities (arrow, A) within the zone of atrophic retina. Angiography showed perfusion of a network of retinal vessels and underlying large choroidal vessels in the area of the lesion (D). There was some staining of the periphery of the lesion (E).
F: Probable retinoma or astrocytic hamartoma in an asymptomatic 4-year-old child with no other ocular abnormalities and a negative family history.
G–I: Retinoma with calcification (arrow, G) in a 21-year-old asymptomatic mother who had a child with bilateral retinoblastomas. Note the "fish-flesh" tumor (G) and the rich vascular network and localized staining evident angiographically (H and I).

(F, courtesy of Dr. Bernard H. Doft.)

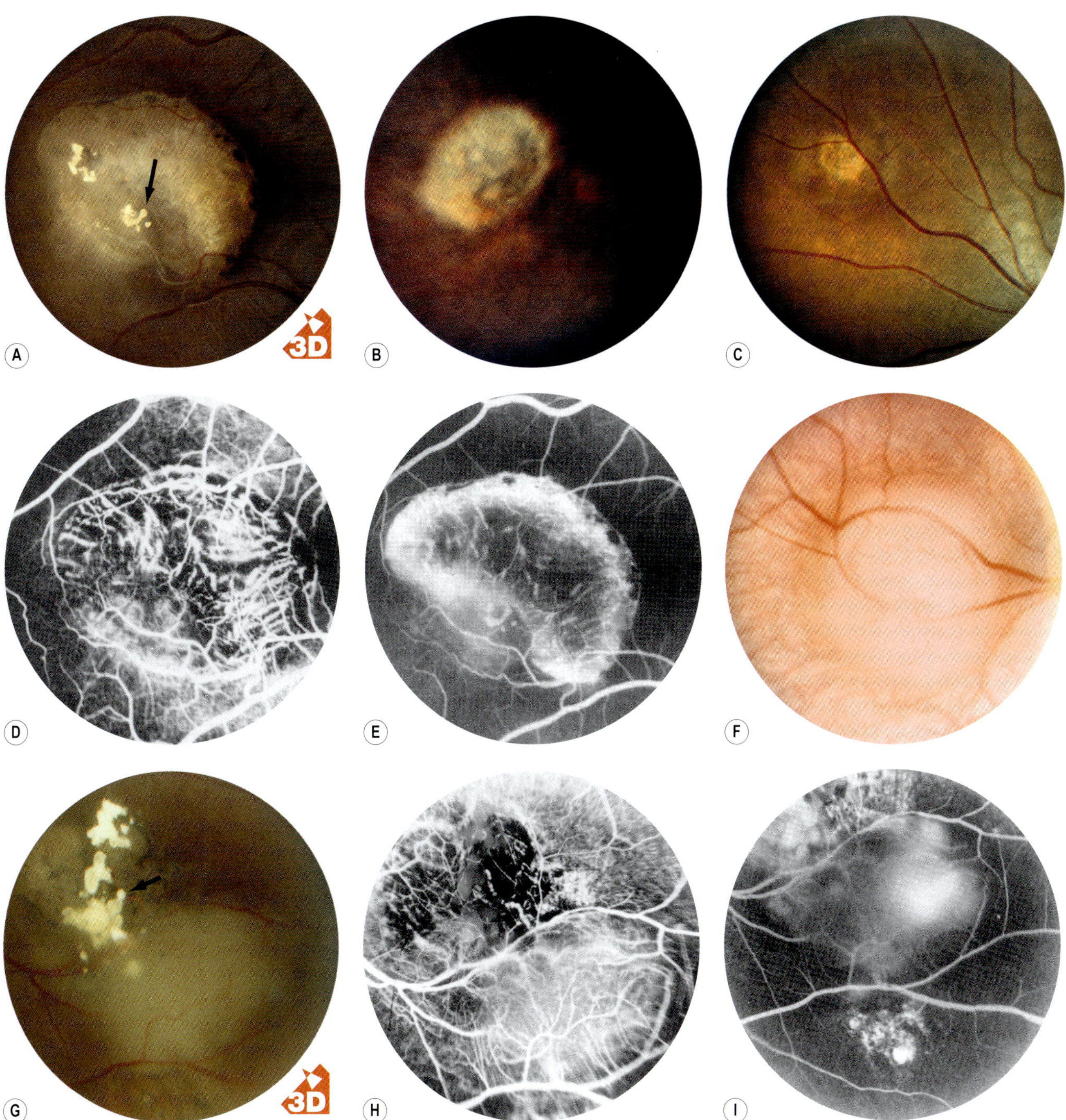
A
3D
B
C
D
E
F
G
3D
H
I

In about 10% of families, reduced penetrance can be seen in individuals (absence of retinoblastoma) who are determined to be *RB1* mutation carriers, either through molecular diagnosis or obligate carrier status in a family. Mechanisms of reduced penetrance and variable expressivity include mutations that lead to reduced expression of retinoblastoma protein expression or production of partially inactive protein.[25–27]

The human retinoblastoma susceptibility gene (*RB1*) was sequenced in 1993, allowing for development of molecular techniques for mutation detection and diagnosis.[28] *RB1* is located on chromosome 13 region q13–14.[29,30] It is relatively large, with 180 kilobases and 27 exons. Analysis of a large number of germline mutations in patients with hereditary retinoblastoma has revealed that about 15% are large deletions, of which ~5–6% are cytogenetically detectable, 26% small-length alterations including small insertions and deletions, and 42% base substitutions.[31] *RB1* mutation analysis is appropriate in any case of retinoblastoma when the results will affect future treatment or surveillance.[32] In patients with a known or suspected family history of retinoblastoma, *RB1* analysis will detect a mutation in ~90% of families. If *RB1* mutation has been identified in a family, then the individual is tested for the specific known family mutation. In this manner, unaffected at-risk children with a family history of hereditary retinoblastoma can undergo predictive testing. Prenatal and preimplantation genetic diagnoses are also available when an *RB1* mutation is known in a parent or sibling.[33,34] Bilateral tumors in the setting of a negative family history also indicate a high probability of a germline *RB1* mutation (~90%) and therefore *RB1* testing is recommended. In sporadic cases, it is recommended that both peripheral blood and tumor tissue (if available) should be analyzed. In all situations, a positive result clearly establishes a diagnosis of hereditary retinoblastoma but a negative result does not rule it out completely.

13.05 Retinoma/retinocytoma.

A–D: A 32-year-old Caucasian man was examined because his two children were diagnosed with bilateral multifocal retinoblastoma before the age of 1 (A). He reported a history of "amblyopia" in the right eye with a visual acuity of 20/40. Dilated fundoscopy showed two circumscribed chorioretinal atrophic lesions in the temporal region of the macula (B). Nonspecific retinal pigment epithelium (RPE) change of the margins and minimal intrinsic calcification were evident. Fluorescein angiogram showed transmission defects indicative of RPE and choroidal atrophy (C). Optical coherence tomography confirmed marked retinal atrophy within the lesions (D). No retinal tumor was identified.

The patient, his second daughter, and her biological mother underwent genetic testing. A heterozygous G to C substitution in the final base position of exon 19 of the *RB1* gene (c.1960G→C (V654L)) was identified in the patient and his daughter on sequence analysis of peripheral blood. This mutation caused missplicing and out-of-frame skipping of exon 19 that resulted in a subsequent termination codon, and unstable mRNA with subsequent reduction of the retinoblastoma protein. The mother did not have the mutation.

Teratoma simulating retinoblastoma.

E–K: Two gray elevated tumors in the right fundus of this 2-month-old girl born at 32 weeks by cesarean section. Note the absence of large feeder vessels dipping into the tumor (E). Visual acuity was no light perception; the left eye was normal. Fluorescein angiography showed increased vascularity within the mass and late hyperfluorescence (F). The tumors grew in size over the next 2 months, and subsequently developed a total retinal detachment (G), neovascularization of the iris, and buphthalmos. Enucleation (H) and histology revealed cartilage, muscle, respiratory epithelium, glandular, and brain tissue consistent with a teratoma (I and J). The child had been delivered by elective cesarean section at 32 weeks for a sacral teratoma (K) that was operated upon soon after birth.

(E–K, courtesy of Dr. David Abramson; E and F, also from Yannuzzi, Lawrence J., The Retinal Atlas, Saunders 2010, 978-0-7020-3320-9, p.211.)

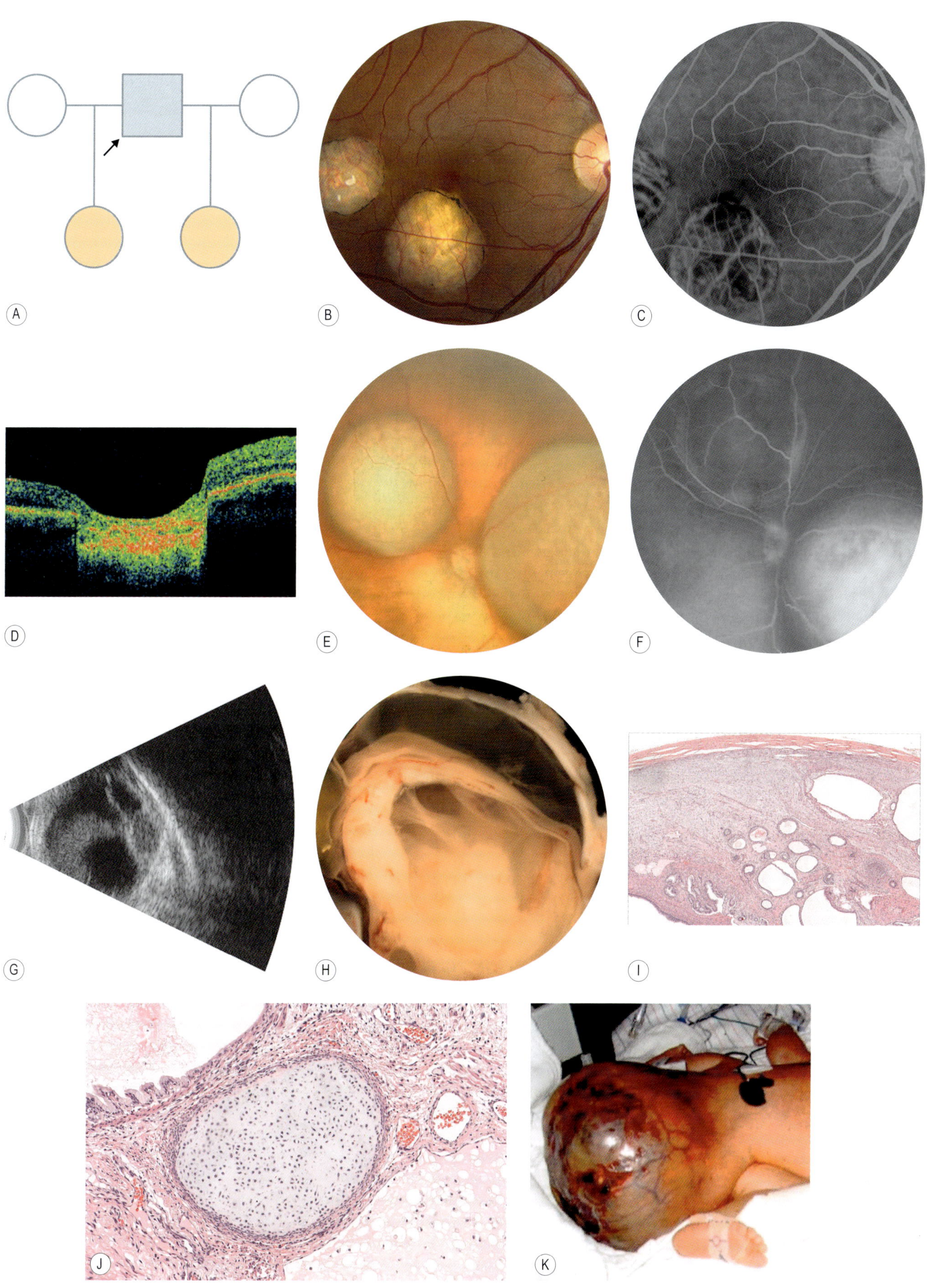
A
B
C
D
E
F
G
H
I
J
K

In recent years there has been a trend away from enucleation and from external-beam radiotherapy with the increasing use of alternative globe-conserving methods of treatment, including laser photocoagulation, cryotherapy, transpupillary thermotherapy, plaque radiotherapy, and chemotherapy.[41–44] Laser photocoagulation or transpupillary thermotherapy is used to treat very small tumors located posterior to the equator.[41,45,46] Cryotherapy is used to treat very small tumors located anterior to the equator.[41,47] Transpupillary thermotherapy may be used for small tumors either primarily or in conjunction with chemotherapy.[41,46,48] Plaque radiotherapy is highly effective in treating medium-sized tumors either as primary treatment or as secondary treatment for recurrent tumors (Figure 13.06).[41,49] External-beam radiotherapy is less frequently used for large and multiple tumors associated with vitreous seeding.[50,51] Enucleation continues to be the main therapeutic option for advanced unilateral retinoblastoma.[24]

Since the 1990s chemoreduction has been increasingly used for the management of retinoblastoma to avoid external-beam radiotherapy or enucleation.[52–54] Chemotherapy is delivered intravenously to reduce the volume of intraocular retinoblastoma to make it amenable to focal therapy, such as cryotherapy, thermotherapy, or brachytherapy (Figure 13.07). Six-cycle chemoreduction using three agents (vincristine, etoposide, and carboplatin) is generally prescribed.[55–57] Based on the available (noncomparative series) data it can be concluded that chemoreduction combined with adjuvant focal therapy offers about 50–100% probability of avoiding enucleation or external-beam radiotherapy depending upon the severity of disease at initial presentation.[56–58] It must be realized that chemoreduction is not without its problems. Recurrence of the neoplasm while on chemotherapy has been observed.[59,60] Immediate complications related to transient bone marrow suppression requiring hospital admissions and intravenous antibiotics with consequent delay in examinations under anesthesia are frequent. Risk of late complications such as drug-induced leukemia cannot yet be excluded.[61] It is recommended that chemoreduction therapy for retinoblastoma should only be offered at a specialist center.

13.06 Retinoblastoma treated with iodine episcleral plaque.

A 6-month-old girl with a familial unilateral retinoblastoma of the macular region. The tumor was 9 × 9 mm in basal dimension and was 4 mm in height.
A: Associated subretinal fluid and seeding (vitreous and subretinal were absent). The tumor was treated with iodine-125-notched episcleral plaque.
B: Fundus appearance 4 weeks later. The tumor has remained regressed over a period of 3 years.

13.07 Retinoblastoma treated with systemic chemotherapy.

A: A 6-month-old girl presented with bilateral retinoblastoma (group D, right eye; group E, left eye). She was treated with chemoreduction and sub-Tenon carboplatin (cycles 2–4). She also received adjuvant focal therapy (cryotherapy and transpupillary thermotherapy).
B: Note dramatic reduction in tumor size. Subsequently, there was recurrence of the macular tumor, which failed to respond to iodine-125 plaque. The left eye was eventually enucleated.

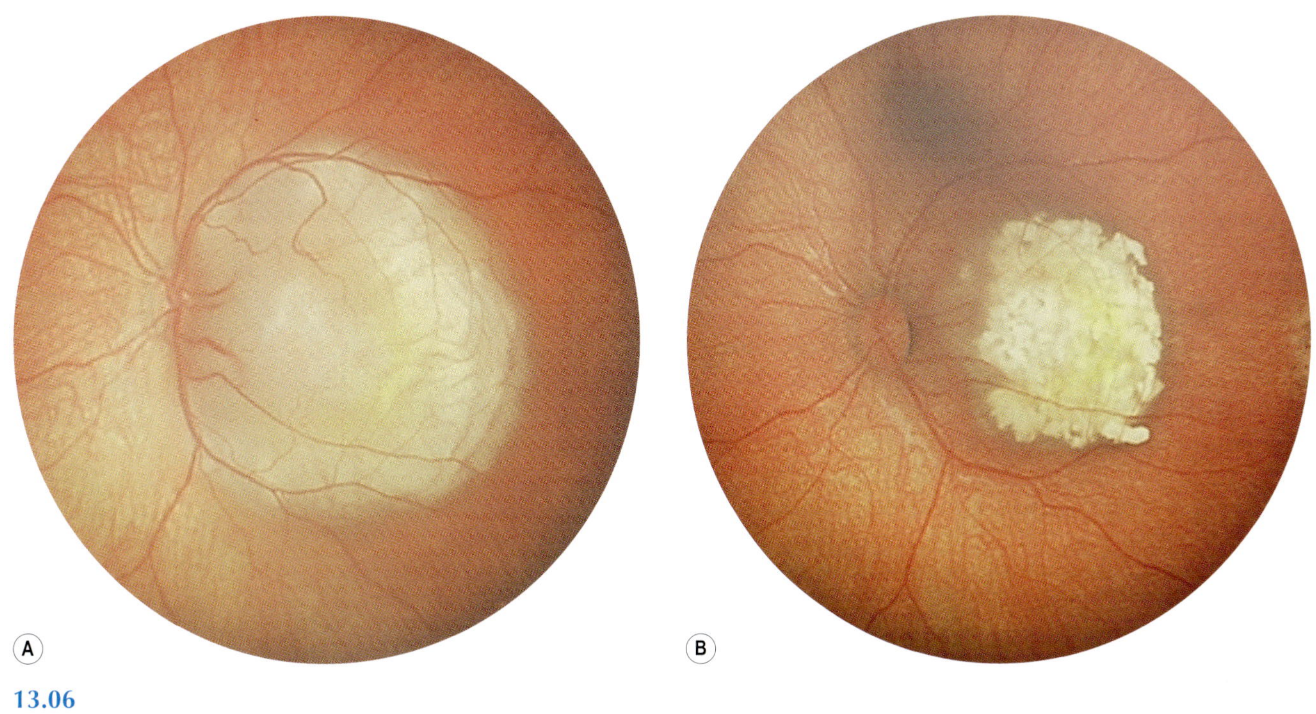

13.06

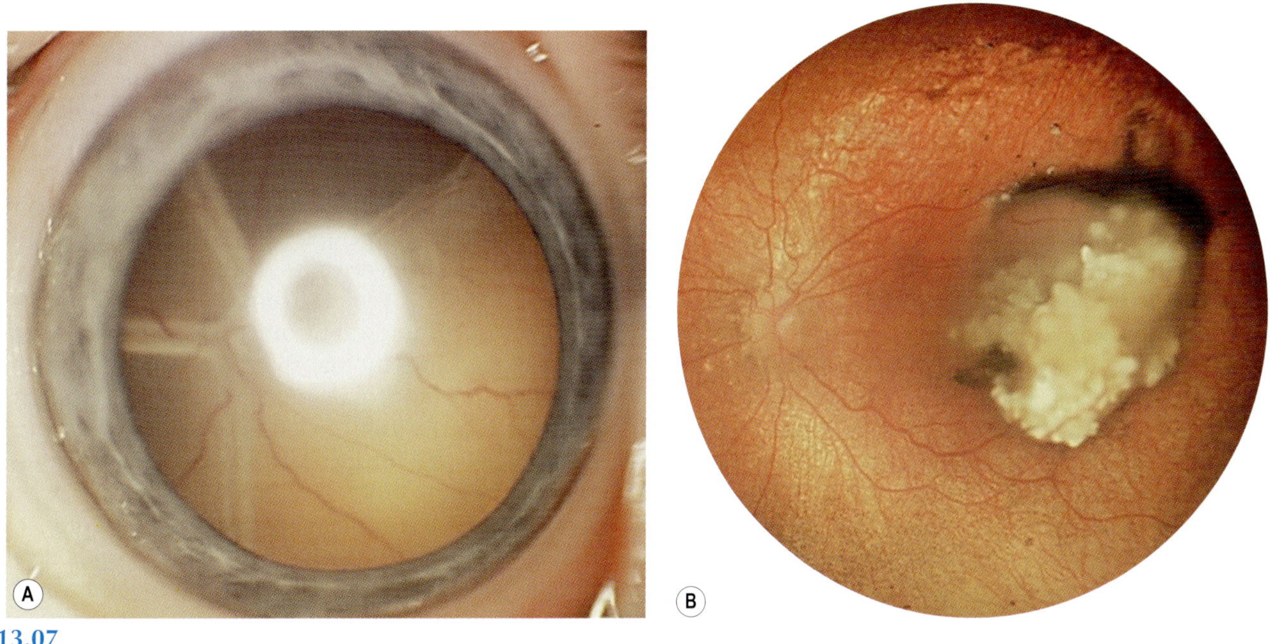

13.07

International group classification of retinoblastoma, a newer system of classification of retinoblastoma, is most suited for the present-day management of retinoblastoma compared to the traditional Reese–Ellsworth classification.[58,62] Eyes are classified according to the extent of disease and dissemination of intraocular tumor defined by the most advanced tumor in each eye. Moreover, the international group classification of retinoblastoma forms the basis of Children Oncology Group trials currently underway.[63]

More recently, there is a trend towards superselective delivery of chemotherapy (melphalan) via cannulation of the ophthalmic artery.[64,65] The aim of such an approach is to avoid the systemic complications and to achieve higher drug levels within the vitreous cavity. Although the initial results are encouraging, such treatments should only be conducted within a framework of a clinical trial in a specialized center (Figure 13.08).[66] The procedure involves three 1-weekly injections of 1 cc/5 mg melphalan (diluted in 30 ml of normal saline), an alkylating agent, directly into the ophthalmic artery via selective percutaneous catheterization via the femoral artery. An approximately 450-µm (1.5–1.7 French)-size catheter is used; an arteriogram is first performed by injecting contrast into the ophthalmic artery to ensure good blood supply to the eye, following which the medication is infused (Figure 13.08C–E). Since the drug is injected into the arterial supply of the tumor, a very small dose of one chemotherapeutic agent has proven sufficient. The procedure is done by skilled interventional neuroradiologists and has a learning curve. The drug is injected in a pulsatile fashion so as to deliver the drug uniformly. In bilateral cases (Figure 13.08G–J), after the chemotherapy is infused through one ophthalmic artery, the catheter is withdrawn into the aorta and threaded into the opposite internal carotid artery and on to the ophthalmic artery and delivered to the second eye. Complications outside the difficulties with catheterization include complete vascular obstruction of the arterial supply leading to total blindness if the catheter is wedged tightly into the lumen of the ophthalmic artery. The procedure is successfully performed at the Memorial Sloan Kettering by Dr. David Abramson and his team (USA) and in some centers in Europe.[67–70]

About 8% of patients with heritable retinoblastoma may develop an associated pinealoblastoma, a tumor that is identical to retinoblastoma.[71] This association of midline intracranial pineal tumors and suprasellar/parasellar neuroblastic tumors with bilateral retinoblastoma has been termed trilateral retinoblastoma.[72] Unlike other second tumors mentioned below, pinealoblastoma usually occurs during the first 4 years of life.[71] Prospective screening by periodic neuroimaging is generally recommended.[73] The possibility of pinealoblastoma should be included in the genetic counseling of patients with hereditary retinoblastoma. Newer evidence suggests that recent treatment methods of systemic chemotherapy.[74] A total of 95% of trilateral retinoblastoma patients have bilateral retinoblastomas and in most cases the disease is fatal.[71] Most patients present with symptoms of increased intracranial pressure caused by obstructive hydrocephalus.

13.08 Intra-arterial chemotherapy for retinoblastoma.

A–J: This 10-month-old girl, one of a nonidentical set of twins with unilateral retinoblastoma, had a large mass with a total retinal detachment and a flat electroretinogram (ERG) (A and B). She received 1 cc of melphalan intra-arterially once a week for 3 weeks. The catheter that is 450 µm in diameter is threaded up the internal carotid artery into the ophthalmic artery (C–E). Melphalan is injected in a pulsed manner so as not to obstruct the blood flow through the artery. The retinal detachment disappeared, the tumor showed cottage-cheese type of regression, and 60% of her ERG amplitudes returned (F).

G–J: Another child with bilateral multiple tumors (G and H) shows complete regression (I and J).

Medulloepithelioma.

K: A 3-year-old white girl was evaluated for a white pupillary reflex in her right eye. Examination revealed a pigmented ciliary body mass with a fibrovascular membrane surrounding the lens. Following initial resection, the eye was enucleated because of tumor recurrence.

(A–J, courtesy of Dr. David Abramson; H, also from Abramson et al.[450] © 2010, American Medical Association. All rights reserved. A, F, G, H, I, and J, also from Yannuzzi, Lawrence J., The Retinal Atlas, Saunders 2010, 978-0-7020-3320-9, p. 212; K, from Shields et al.[98] © 2002 American Medical Association. All rights reserved.)

An important aspect concerns the development of unrelated cancers in survivors of bilateral or heritable retinoblastoma. The mean latency period for the appearance of the second malignant neoplasm (SMN) is approximately 13 years.[75,76] There is a 5% chance of developing SMN during the first 10 years of follow-up, 18% during the first 20 years, and 26% within 30 years.[75,77] The 30-year cumulative incidence of SMN is about 35% for those patients who receive radiation therapy (external-beam therapy) as compared to an incidence rate of 6% for those patients who do not.[78] Osteogenic sarcoma, often involving the femur, is most common, but other tumors such as cutaneous malignant melanoma, spindle cell sarcoma, chondrosarcoma, rhabdomyosarcoma, neuroblastoma, glioma, leukemia, sebaceous cell carcinoma, squamous cell carcinoma, and lung and bladder carcinomas as SMN have also been recognized.[79,80]

Several studies have evaluated histopathologic prognostic factors for metastasis, including choroidal, optic nerve, and extrascleral extension.[81–84] Choroidal involvement by the retinoblastoma is a risk for metastasis, especially if it is associated with any degree of optic nerve involvement.[85] Mortality increases with increasing extent of optic nerve involvement.[3] However, it is generally agreed that prelaminar involvement of the optic nerve does not increase the risk of metastasis.[86] The impact of laminar involvement on metastasis is debatable. Retrolaminar involvement is a poor prognostic factor and optic nerve involvement by retinoblastoma cells up to the line of transection predicts the worst prognosis.[3]

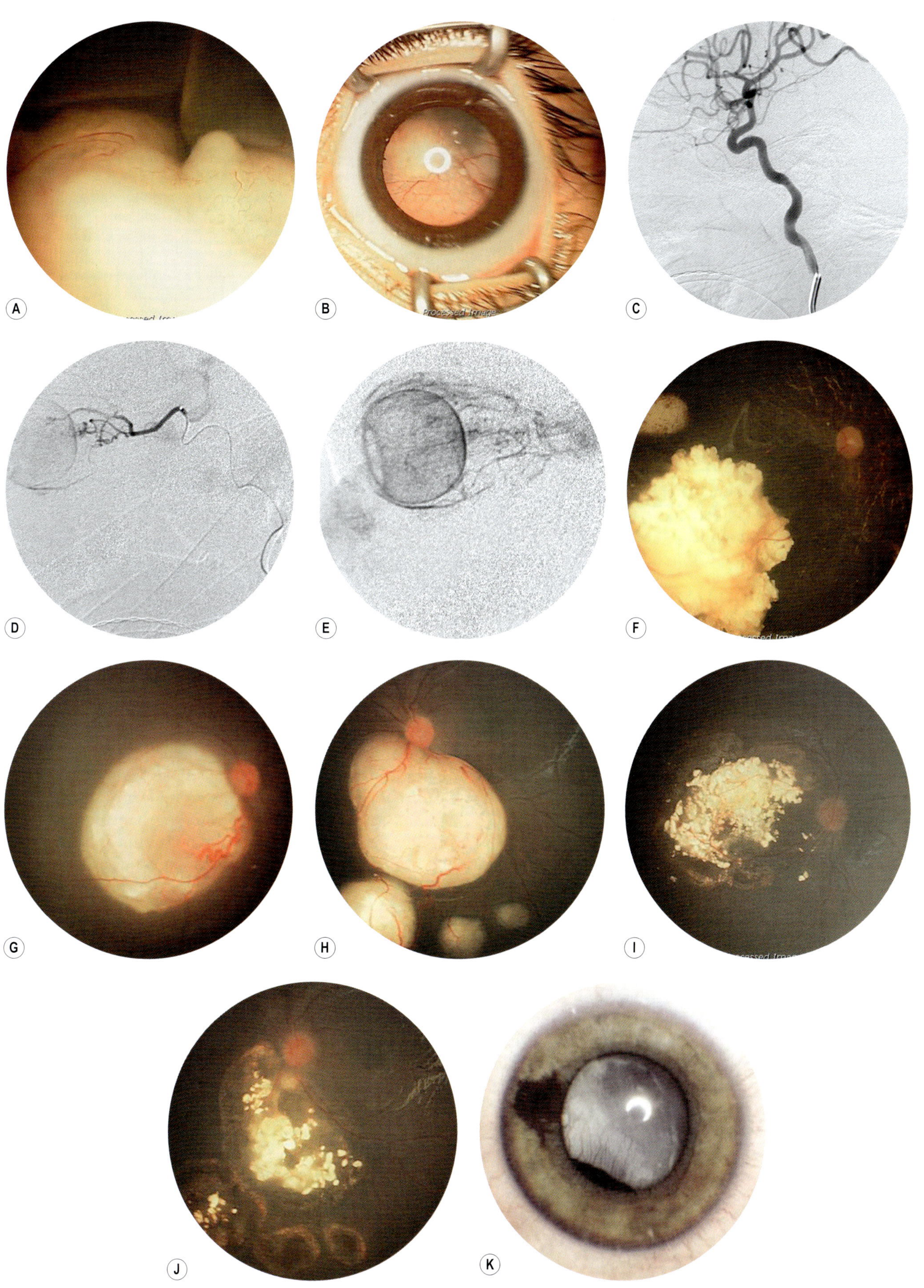
A
B
Processed Image
C
D
E
F
G
H
I
J
K

It must be realized that retinoblastoma-related mortality could be due to one of three distinct causes: (1) metastases; (2) trilateral retinoblastoma; and (3) SMN. Metastases in retinoblastoma usually occur within 1 year of diagnosis. Metastatic retinoblastoma is observed infrequently in the USA[87] and other developed nations.[88,89] However, metastases continue to be a challenge in developing nations.[90–92] Therefore, bone scans, lumbar puncture, and bone marrow aspirations at initial presentation are generally not performed in the USA.[93] If there is no metastatic disease within 5 years of retinoblastoma diagnosis, the child is usually considered cured.[81,94] Metastases usually involve the central nervous system (CNS), bones, and bone marrow.[94,95] The prognosis of metastatic retinoblastoma is poor, with death usually occurring within 6 months.[81,94] In the USA, over a period of 30 years (1975–2004), the 5-year observed actuarial survival rate increased from 92.3% (1975–1984) to 96.5% (1995–2004).[44]

MEDULLOEPITHELIOMA

Intraocular medulloepithelioma is an embryonal neoplasm of the ciliary epithelium. It may contain cartilage, skeletal muscle, and brain tissue (teratoid medulloepithelioma).[96,97] Medulloepithelioma typically presents during the first decade of life with poor vision, pain, leukocoria, and iris vascularization associated with a mass or cyst appearing behind the pupillary area (Figure 13.08K).[96–98] Children with neovascularization of the iris of unknown cause should be evaluated to exclude underlying medulloepithelioma.[99] Recently, an association with pleuropulmonary blastoma has been reported.[100] Therapeutic options include local excision or enucleation depending upon the size, location, and secondary effects of the tumor.[96,97,101]

ASTROCYTIC HAMARTOMAS

Retinal and optic disc astrocytic hamartomas may occur as a solitary finding in normal patients, in patients with dominantly inherited tuberous sclerosis complex (TSC) (Bourneville's disease), or, rarely, in patients with neurofibromatosis (von Recklinghausen's disease).[9,102–123] The intraocular tumors are typically globular, white, well-circumscribed, elevated lesions arising from the inner surface of the retina or optic nerve head (Figures 13.09–13.11). Multiple lesions are common in patients with TSC (Figure 13.09A–F). Early in life the tumors may be semitranslucent, free of calcification, and mistaken for retinoblastoma (Figures 13.09A and D, and 13.10F).[9,115,119,122,124,125] In infants and children they may occasionally arise where earlier no lesion was present. Later in life they assume a more densely white color and may develop multiple nodular areas of calcification, taking on a mulberry appearance (Figures 13.09A and D, 13.10E, and 13.11A). Clear cystic spaces may be present within the tumor (Figure 13.09D). The tumors may show varying degrees of vascularization that are more evident angiographically than ophthalmoscopically (Figures 13.09B and C, and 13.11E and F). The tumor's blood vessels are usually permeable to fluorescein. In addition to nodular retinal tumors, flat or slightly elevated, white, circular or oval astrocytic hamartomas of the inner retinal layers are common (Figure 13.09D). These sessile tumors show less tendency to undergo calcific degeneration. In general, retinal astrocytic hamartomas show minimal evidence of growth and no treatment is indicated. Occasionally, however, particularly in younger individuals, progressive enlargement and calcification of these tumors may be demonstrated (Figure 13.10G to J, 13.11J–L).[118] Visual loss may be caused by tumor growth, vitreous hemorrhage, or intraretinal and subretinal exudation (Figure 13.12D–F).[102,104,111,120,126–128] The exudative complications of astrocytic hamartomas can be self-limited, and cases of spontaneous resolution within a few weeks have been observed (Fig. 13.10K to N)[129,130]; however, some cases are persistent, progressive, and vision-threatening, and for these cases various treatments have been attempted, including laser photocoagulation (Figure 13.12D–F),[104] brachytherapy, transpupillary thermotherapy, and endoresection.[131,132] More aggressive cases exhibiting progressive growth, tumor seeding, and neovascular glaucoma have been managed by enucleation.[133] Recently, photodynamic therapy using the photosensitizing dye verteporfin (Visudyne) has been used in the treatment of a few cases of exudative astrocytic hamartomas, with encouraging results (Figure 13.13).[134,135]

13.09 Retinal astrocytic hamartoma associated with tuberous sclerosis.

A–C: Multiple astrocytic hamartomas of the optic nerve head and retina in a 35-year-old woman with tuberous sclerosis (A). She had a lifelong history of generalized seizures. She had five mentally retarded children. Examination revealed sebaceous adenoma and subungual fibromas of the fingers and toes (Figure 10.15B). Multiple endophytic astrocytic hamartomas of the retina were present in the left fundus. The lesions were elevated, globular, and semitranslucent. Retinal vessels could be seen within some of these tumors. Several of the tumefactions showed evidence of early calcification (arrow, A). Angiography revealed a capillary network within the hamartomas (B and C). These capillaries were permeable to fluorescein dye, and there was evidence of diffusion of the dye into the vitreous (C).

D–F: A partly calcified cystic astrocytic hamartoma in a 9-year-old girl with tuberous sclerosis. She had a history of seizures but was not mentally retarded. Note the mulberry-like areas of calcification within the large cystic lesions. Two smaller hamartomas were present within the optic nerve head (arrow) and inferior to the papillomacular bundle. Fluorescein angiography demonstrated dilation of the capillary network and staining within these tumors (E and F).

G–I: Large astrocytic hamartoma of the left macula of an 8-year-old boy with tuberous sclerosis. He had sebaceous adenoma and a large fibroma of the left lower lid (G).

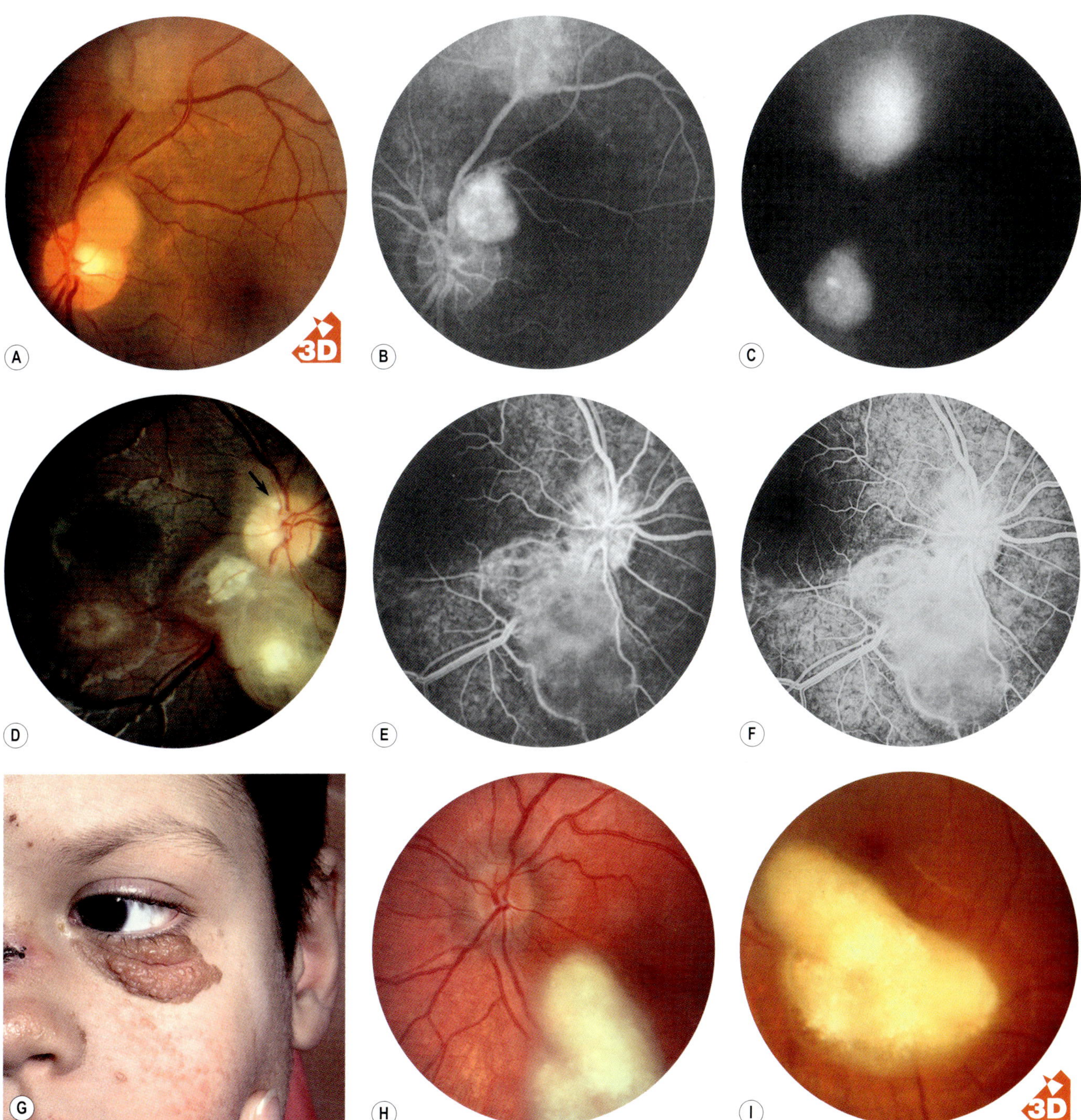
A
3D
B
C
D
E
F
G
H
I
3D

In some, the rapid growth and necrosis may be mistaken for a nonpigmented melanoma (Figure 13.11J–L).[116,127,128,136–138] In other patients the highly vascular component of the tumor may simulate a retinal angioma (Figures 13.10G-J, 13.11G–I and 13.12A–C).[139] In the case of spontaneous necrosis astrocytomas may simulate necrotizing retinochoroiditis.[124] The fossilized mulberry tumors involving the optic nerve head should be distinguished from hyaline bodies of the optic nerve head. These latter are calcified masses of extracellular material unrelated to astrocytic hamartomas. When calcified astrocytic hamartomas of the optic disc are small, they may be difficult or impossible to distinguish from hyaline bodies.[106] Demonstration of growth of these small lesions in patients with retinitis pigmentosa has suggested that these lesions in patients with retinitis pigmentosa are astrocytic hamartomas.[107,140,141] Retinal telangiectasis, retinitis proliferans, and retinal exudation developed in one eye of a patient with familial TSC but no evidence of a retinal astrocytoma.[142]

13.10 Retinal astrocytic hamartoma associated with tuberous sclerosis.

A–D: Sebaceous adenoma of the nose and cheeks and a solitary hamartoma of the forehead (A). Subungual fibroma (arrow, B). Skull X-ray film of patient shown in (A) showed multiple calcified astrocytic hamartomas (arrows) characteristic of tuberous sclerosis (C). Enhanced computed tomography scan showed multiple astrocytic hamartomas in the paraventricular system of a patient with tuberous sclerosis (D).
E and **F**: Photomicrograph of calcified astrocytic hamartoma of the optic disc and adjacent retina of a 17-year-old boy with sebaceous adenoma. The calcified central portion of the tumor was lost in sectioning (E). Endophytic noncalcified astrocytic hamartoma of the peripheral retina of the same patient in E (F).

Growth of astrocytic hamartoma

G–J: In 1978, this 9 year old male patient was evaluated at Wilmer with a calcified astrocytic hamartoma in the right eye (G) and 4 lesions in the left eye consisting of 2 atrophic patches above the ST arcade, 1 calcified and another non calcified hamartoma along the IT arcade (H). The optic nerve was swollen with blurred margins suggesting presence of abnormal tissue within its substance. He presented to Vanderbilt in 1997 with a vitreous hemorrhage in his left eye from a large partly calcified and partly fibrous hamartoma that had grown from the optic disc (J). Note the previously non calcified tumor inferior to the optic disc was now calcified (arrow). The calcified astrocytoma in the right eye was unchanged (I). The left eye needed a vitrectomy a year later for further vitreous hemorrhage.

Spontaneous regression of astrocytic hamartoma

K–N: This 11 year old boy with known history of tuberous sclerosis presented with an inferior scotoma in his right eye. He was found to have a circumscribed gelatinous appearing vascular lesion superonasal to the disc associated with lipid and blood (K). Fluorescein angiogram showed vascularity of the lesion without evidence of retinal nonperfusion elsewhere (L). The lesion began to regress spontaneously 2 months later with gradual resolution of the scotoma. By 4 months the lipid, blood and vascularity of the lesion had regressed considerably (M and N).

(E and F, from Zimmerman and Walsh.[122] K-N, Dr. Affortit)

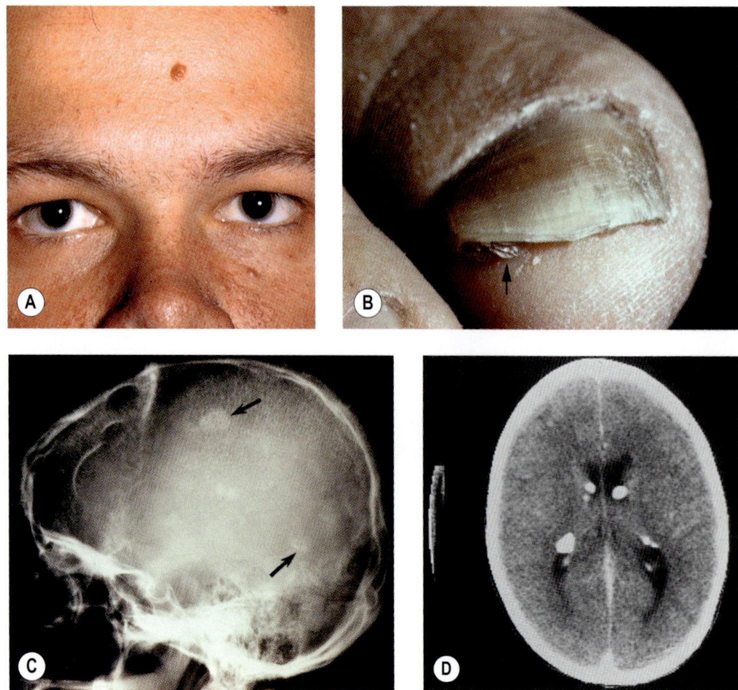

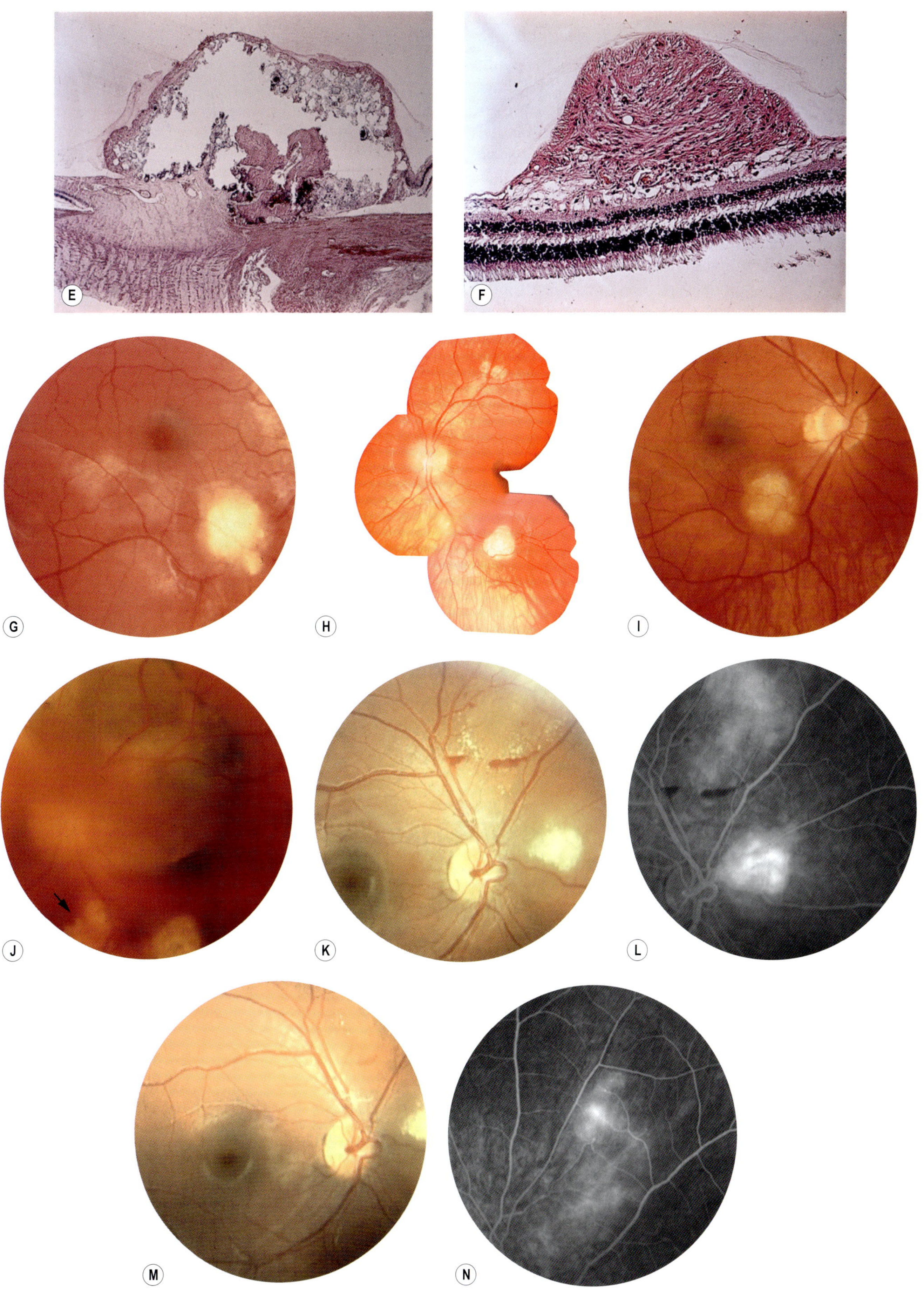
E
F
G
H
I
J
K
L
M
N

Histopathologically, these tumors are typically composed of spindle-shaped fibrous astrocytes, some of which are elongated and contain small oval nucleoli (Figures 13.10F and 13.11L). Other tumors are composed of large, bizarre, pleomorphic astrocytic cells, that in at least one case showed ultrastructural and histochemical similarities to Müller cells.[115] Cystic areas containing serous exudate and blood, as well as areas of calcified degeneration, may be present. Some of these tumors may be of Müller cell origin.[115]

Retinal achromic patches have also been observed in published series, ranging from 8% to 39% of TSC patients.[143,144] Some authors have described these lesions as diffusely hypopigmented, while others have noted them to be surrounded by some degree of pigment proliferation (Figure 13.14).[143,145] Clinically, these lesions bear a striking resemblance to the solitary-type hypomelanotic nevi described by Dr. Gass.[146] While retinal achromic patches appear in increased frequency in individuals with TSC, the underlying mechanism explaining their existence is unknown.

13.11 Retinal astrocytic hamartomas not associated with tuberous sclerosis.

A–C: Large calcified exophytic astrocytic hamartoma of the retina in a 15-year-old boy without other evidence of tuberous sclerosis (A). He gave an 8-year history of defective vision in the right eye first noted while firing a gun. The family history and past medical history were negative. Visual acuity in the affected eye was 20/300. Angiography (B and C) revealed an extensive capillary network that extended down into the tumor. There was leakage of dye from this network and pooling of dye within the cystic areas of the tumor (arrow, C).

D–F: Cystic astrocytic hamartoma of the retina in a 10-year-old girl without other evidence of tuberous sclerosis (D). This was an incidental finding, and her eye examination was otherwise normal. Note the white, finely polycystic tumor arising from the inner retinal layers just superior to the left macular region (D). Note that most of the retinal vessels are hidden within this cottony tumor. Fluorescein angiography revealed a network of retinal vessels within the tumor and late leakage of the dye (E and F).

G–I: Elevated, vascularized, partly calcified retinal mass in a healthy 17-year-old boy with no family history of tuberous sclerosis or retinoblastoma.

J–L: Nonpigmented, pedunculated, vascularized astrocytic hamartoma in the juxtapapillary region of a 41-year-old man with a 3-week history of blurred vision in the right eye (J and K). This was misinterpreted as a melanoma because of an increased phosphorus-32 uptake test (100%). Histopathologic examination of the enucleated eye revealed a retinal astrocytic hamartoma (L).

(J–L, from Ramsay et al.[451])

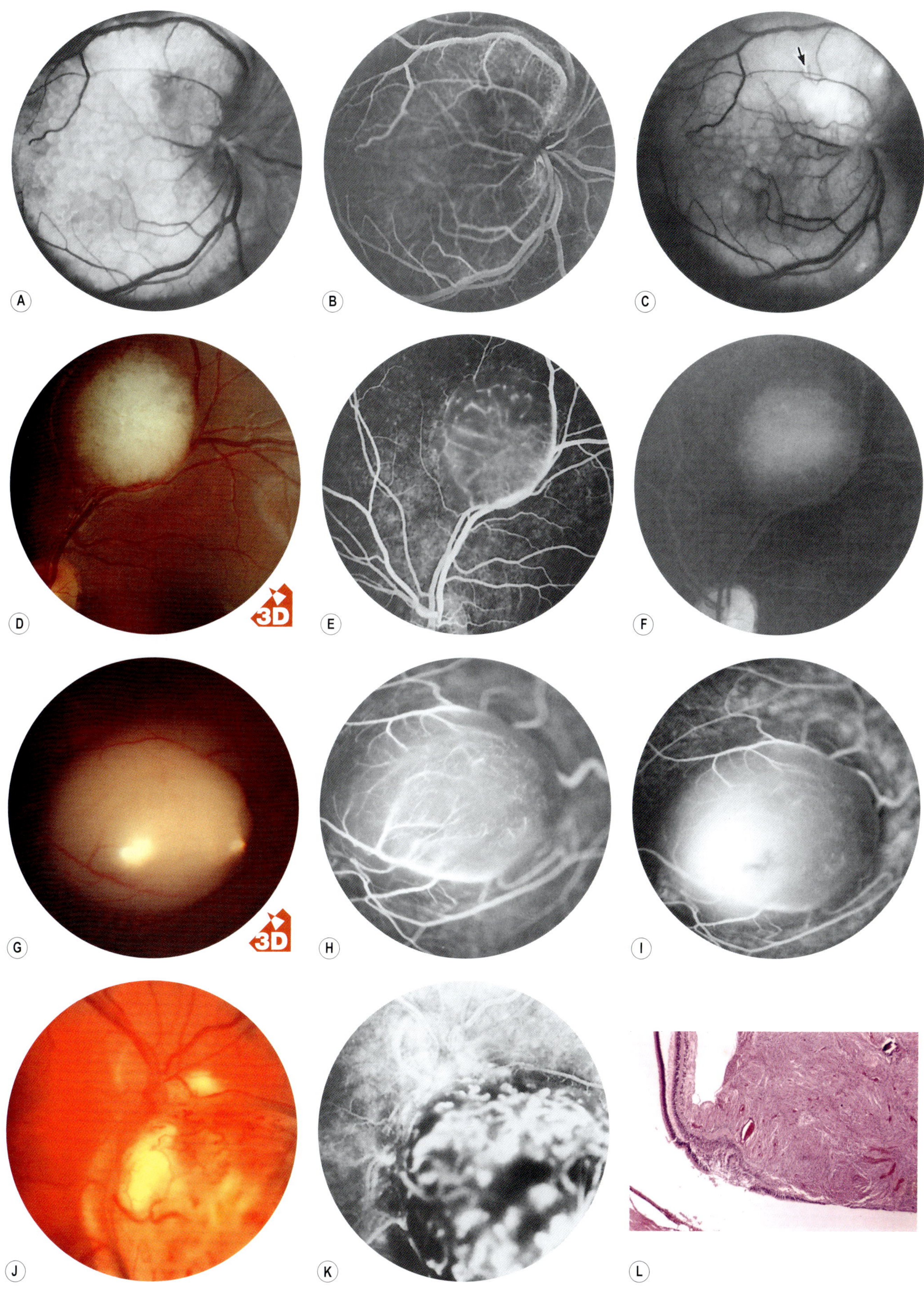
A
B
C
D
3D
E
F
G
3D
H
I
J
K
L

A careful search should be made for the various manifestations of TSC in any patient with a white retinal tumor. These include the classic triad of seizures, mental deficiency, and sebaceous adenoma (fibroangiomas) as well as other manifestations, including white ash-leaf spots on the skin and iris, soft yellow-brown cutaneous fibromas (Figures 13.09G and 13.10A), subungual fibromas (Figure 13.10B), renal hamartomas, cardiac rhabdomyomas, calcified cerebral astrocytic hamartomas (Figure 13.10C and D), cystic lung disease, and bony changes, including cystic changes of the phalanges and cortical thickening of the metatarsal and metacarpal bones.[117] In 1998, at the Tuberous Sclerosis Complex Consensus Conference, a revised set of clinical diagnostic criteria based upon major and minor features of the disease was firmly established.[147]

CT and roentgenographic techniques are useful in the detection of intraocular tumors.[106] In infants and children these tumors can appear identical to retinoblastoma or may mimic necrotizing retinochoroiditis.[105] In older patients they may be confused with regressed retinoblastoma or retinoma (Figure 13.11G–I), capillary hemangiomas of the retina, or a localized retinal scar secondary to previous hemorrhage or inflammation.

More recently, genetic mutational analysis has uncovered two distinct variants of TSC resulting from mutations is the *TSC1* gene located on chromosome 9q34 and the *TSC2* gene on chromosome 16p13.[148,149] These genes encode for hamartin and tuberin respectively, both of which are involved in regulation of the cellular growth cycle.[150] *TSC2* mutations are more frequent than *TSC1* mutations in patients with atsrocytic hamartoma or retinal achromic patches.[151]

13.12 Lesions of uncertain etiology simulating retinal astrocytic hamartomas.

A–C: Endophytic retinal tumor in a 38-year-old woman with a 3-month history of blurred vision in her left eye (A). Her past history revealed convulsions unassociated with fever at 1 year of age. It was otherwise unremarkable. There were many dilated blood vessels present within the tumor, which was located in the retina inferior to the left macula (A). Angiography demonstrated an extensive vascular network within the tumor and late leakage of dye (B and C). Medical evaluation failed to reveal other evidence of tuberous sclerosis. The patient was re-examined 10 months later, and there was no change in the appearance of the lesion. Examination 3 years after her initial visit revealed that the lesion had disappeared, leaving only a minor disturbance in the retina in the area of the tumor. Because of its spontaneous disappearance, it is doubtful that it was an astrocytic hamartoma.
D–F: Sessile presumed astrocytic hamartoma in a healthy 42-year-old man with a recent history of blurred vision in the left eye. He had a small angioma and a pigmented nevus of the conjunctiva in the same eye. His visual acuity was 20/25, left eye, and 20/20, right eye. Note the ill-defined gray-whitening of the retina in the inferonasal macular area (arrowheads, D) and the cystoid macular edema (arrow, D). Angiography revealed evidence of a capillary network within the lesion and evidence of intraretinal edema (E and F). Two months following laser photocoagulation the vision had improved to 20/20. He had no other findings of tuberous sclerosis.
G–I: This 28-year-old woman complained of blurred vision in the left eye. Examination of the right eye was normal. In the left eye she had a gray, slightly elevated retinal tumor that straddled the major retinal vascular arcades in the superior macular area (G). Angiography showed evidence of the vascular nature of this lesion (H and I). There were no other stigmata of tuberous sclerosis. Several months later she had developed extensive exudative maculopathy. She was lost to follow-up.
J–L: An elevated, vascularized, and partly calcified tumor developed in this 17-year-old boy who when he was first examined at 10 years of age had the typical findings of bilateral pars planitis and no evidence of an intraocular mass. Stereo angiograms (H and I) revealed the highly vascular nature of this exophytic mass, which probably was the result of a reactive proliferation of the retinal vasculature and glial cells in response to the intraocular inflammatory disease.

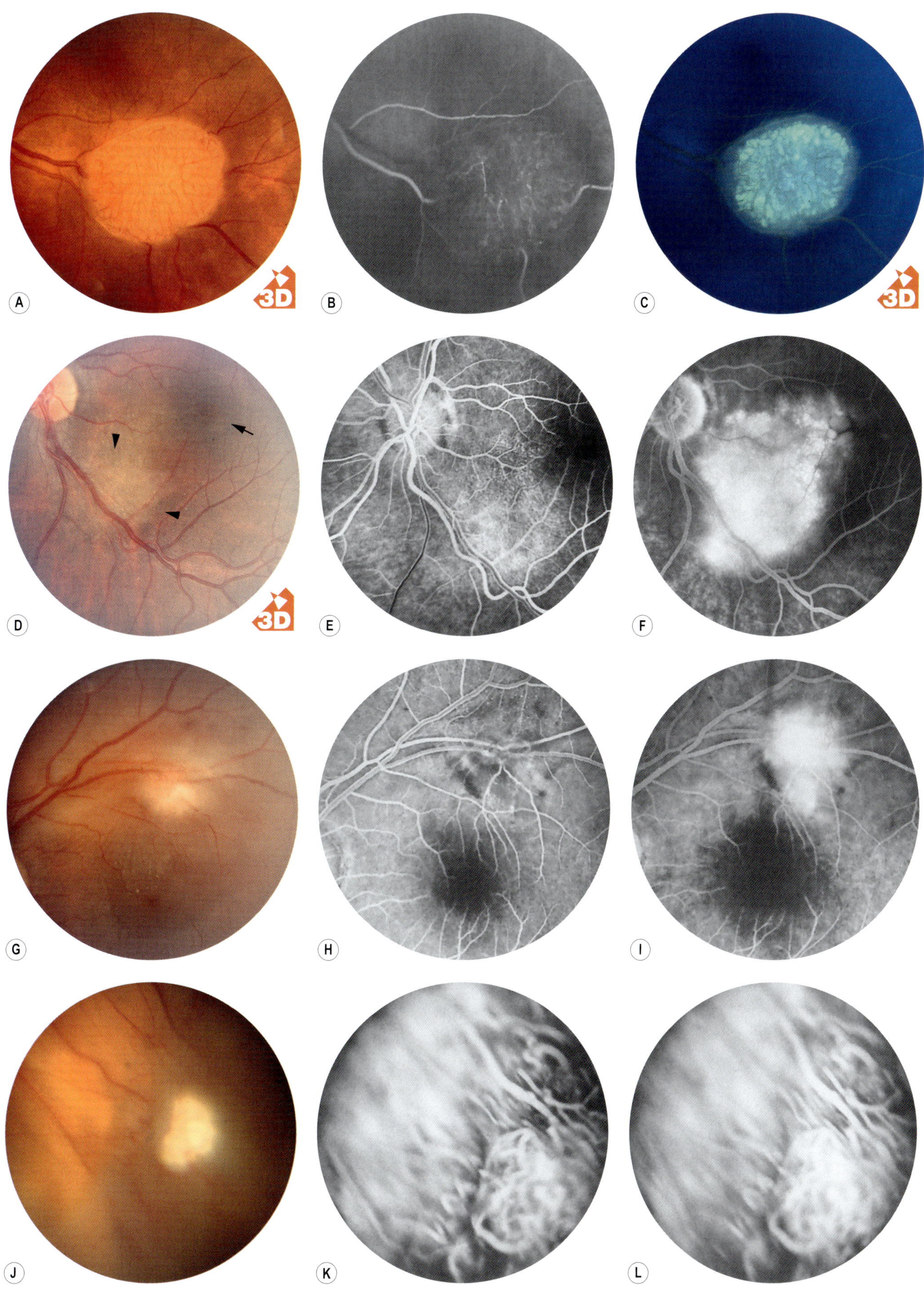
3D
3D
3D
A
B
C
D
E
F
G
H
I
J
K
L

REACTIVE ASTROCYTIC HYPERPLASIA SIMULATING AN ASTROCYTIC HAMARTOMA

Dr. Gass had observed four healthy adult patients with focal vascularized retinal masses that appeared similar to astrocytic hamartomas. In two cases the lesions subsequently disappeared spontaneously (Figure 13.12A–C).[9] In one boy with bilateral pars planitis an exophytic vascularized white retinal mass developed during observation (Figure 13.12J and K). It is probable that most of these lesions and some of those reported in the literature as sporadic astrocytomas are products of reactive proliferation of the retinal glial cells caused by focal retinitis, focal retinal vascular leakage, chorioretinitis, vitreoretinal traction, and, less often, subretinal neovascularization. (See discussion in Chapter 10, p. 812 and Figure 10.04I-L.)

RETINAL VASCULAR HAMARTOMAS

There are two distinct retinal vascular hamartomas, both of which may be associated with similar hamartomas elsewhere in the body.

13.13 Retinal astrocytoma treated with photodynamic therapy.

A–D: A 45-year-old Caucasian female with an unremarkable past medical history was referred for evaluation of a peripapillary tumor associated with a scotoma in the right eye (A). On initial evaluation, visual acuities (VA) were 20/20 in both eyes. An ill-defined, translucent, yellow-white superficial mass along the superotemporal margin of the optic disc and extending into the retina was observed (B). Prominent intrinsic vessels as well as dilated collateral vessels were present. The macula was flat; however, lipid exudates were present superonasal to the fovea, and a few retinal striae were noted in the papillomacular area. Based on morphological characteristics, the diagnosis of retinal astrocytoma was made with a decision to observe for progression. At a 6-month visit, VA remained 20/20; however, the lipid exudates were noted to be approaching the foveola (C). Four months after two sessions of standard-fluence photodynamic therapy (TAP; 1.5-mm spot covering the entire tumor up to the superotemporal edge of the optic disc), VA remained 20/15, the lipid exudates were diminished, and some gliosis of the tumor could be appreciated (D).

13.14 Retinal achromic patch of tuberous sclerosis.
A: Fundus photograph of a retinal achromic patch.

(From Turell et al.,[151] with permission.)

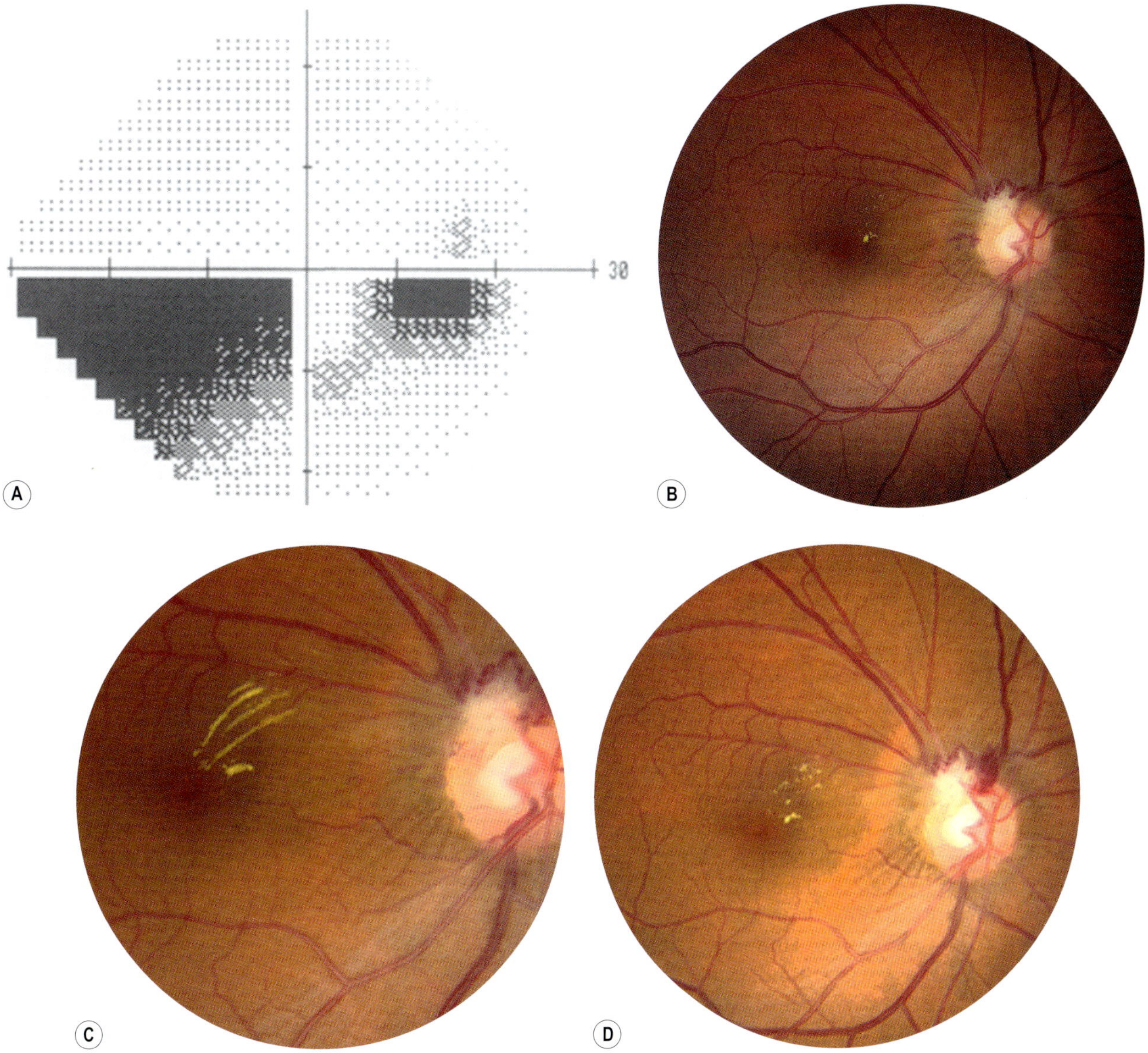

13.13

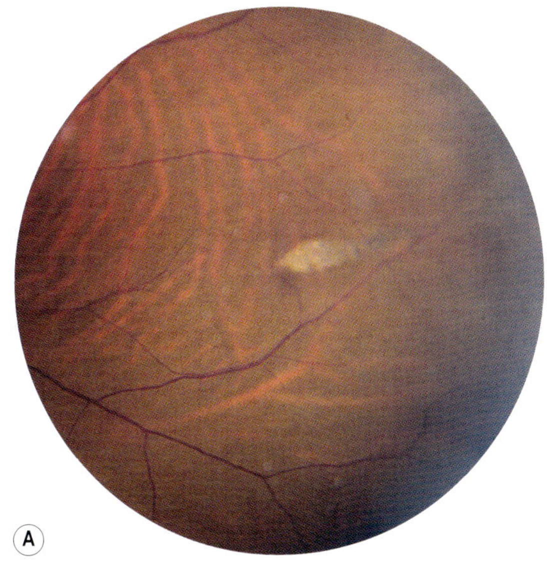

13.14

Whereas most retinal and optic nerve cavernous hemangiomas occur sporadically, there is evidence that some patients may have a dominantly inherited neurocutaneous syndrome that includes cavernous hemangiomas of the optic nerves, chiasm, optic tracts, the prerolandic area of the cerebral cortex, the midbrain, brainstem, and cerebellum (Figure 13.17F), as well as the skin (Figure 13.17E).[9,157,161,168,169,171,172,175–185]

Familial cavernous hemangioma has been linked to three loci on chromosomes 3q, 7p, and 7q.[186,187] Familial cases of cerebral cavernous malformation (FCCM)[187] are associated with mutations in *KRIT1* (CCM1), *MGC4607* (CCM2), and *PDCD10* (CCM3) genes. CCM1 is located at chromosome locus 7q11–q22 and was the first one identified with the familial form of CCMs. CCM1 mutation is involved in 40 – 53% of familial CCMs and nearly half these patients have neurological manifestations before 25 years of age. CCM2 is located at 7p15–13 and mutations in this gene are involved in up to 25-40% of familial CCMs. The numbers of lesions increase less rapidly with age in patients with CCM2 than with CCM1 disease. CCM3 is localized at 3q25.2–q27 and is the least common of mutations (10%), but has near 100% penetrance and patients are more likely to present with hemorrhage and become symptomatic before 15 years of age.[188]

The angiomas of the brain may cause seizures or subarachnoid hemorrhages. Twin retinal vessels, defined as a pair of vessels, separated by less than one venule width, that run a parallel course for more than 1 disc diameter, located at least 2 disc areas distant from the optic disc, have been described in carriers as well as affected members of families with cavernous hemangiomas of the eye and brain, as well as in family members of patients with von Hippel–Lindau (VHL) disease.[189] Cavernous hemangiomas do not increase in size. The amount of fibrous tissue on the anterior surface increases over a period of time and is associated with partial obliteration of the tumor.

Histopathologically, the tumor is composed of multiple thin-walled interconnecting aneurysms of variable size, occupying the inner half of the retina and in some patients the optic nerve (Figure 13.17A–D).[155,157,162,183,190] The endothelial lining of the large vascular channels ultrastructurally appears normal.[190] The gray membrane that overlies part of the angiomas in some cases is of glial origin.[190]

Photocoagulation has been used to obliterate these lesions but is unnecessary as long as the patient shows no signs of developing vitreous hemorrhage.[159,162,163] In one case of severe vitreous hemorrhage, the tumor was partly excised during a pars plana vitrectomy.[191] Some of the cerebral cortical angiomas causing seizures or subarachnoid hemorrhage may be resectable.[192]

13.16 Retinal cavernous hemangioma.

A–C: Cavernous hemangioma discovered in a 27-year-old woman who was hospitalized because of a generalized seizure. An electroencephalogram revealed low voltage in the left cerebral hemisphere. A skull roentgenogram and a carotid arteriogram were normal. Her father died at 49 years of age with status epilepticus. Autopsy of the father revealed a focal cavernous hemangioma in the midbrain, pons, and cerebellum (Figure 10.20F). The woman's eye examination was normal except for the presence of a slightly elevated sessile cavernous hemangioma involving the inferonasal quadrant of the right eye (A). A small subretinal and deep retinal hemorrhage was present (arrow, A). Angiography revealed delayed and incomplete perfusion of the cavernous hemangioma (B and C). Note evidence of plasma layering (arrows) and minimal evidence of extravascular escape of dye. A general physical examination revealed a stellate angiomatous hamartoma of the right chin and several cherry angiomas of the thigh.

D and E: This 45-year-old otherwise healthy male suffered constant severe headache for 5 months associated with occasional dizziness and nausea. He had no visual complaints. Magnetic resonance imaging of his head to evaluate headache revealed more than 50 small vascular malformations in various parts of his brain (E). There was a family history of spine and neck lesions in his sister, a cousin with brain and abdominal tumors, an uncle with a brain lesion, and a son with epilepsy. His vision was 20/20 in each eye. He had 3–4 aneurysmal dilations in the far temporal periphery of his left fundus (D). The right eye was normal. Both he and his sister, who was evaluated at the Mayo Clinic, were positive for *CCM1* gene at the 7q locus that codes for KRIT1 protein. He tested negative for the *VHL* gene.

F–K: This 13-year-old girl presented with floaters secondary to spontaneous vitreous hemorrhage from thin-walled saccular malformations in her left eye (F, H, J, and K). The lesions were extensive, involving the superior half of the fundus. Several of the aneurysmal walls were made up of glial tissue alone; these did not fill with fluorescein (arrows, F and G). Typical separation of blood cells and plasma was seen in some of them in the late angiograms (I). Of significance is the involvement of the larger vein walls with the malformation (arrow heads, F and G), which is unusual since these aneurysms are believed to occur at the capillary level (see Figure 13.16L). She was kept under observation and the vitreous hemorrhage cleared over 5 months without treatment (K). She had an ipsilateral cavernous malformation of the corpus callosum. Gene testing is underway.

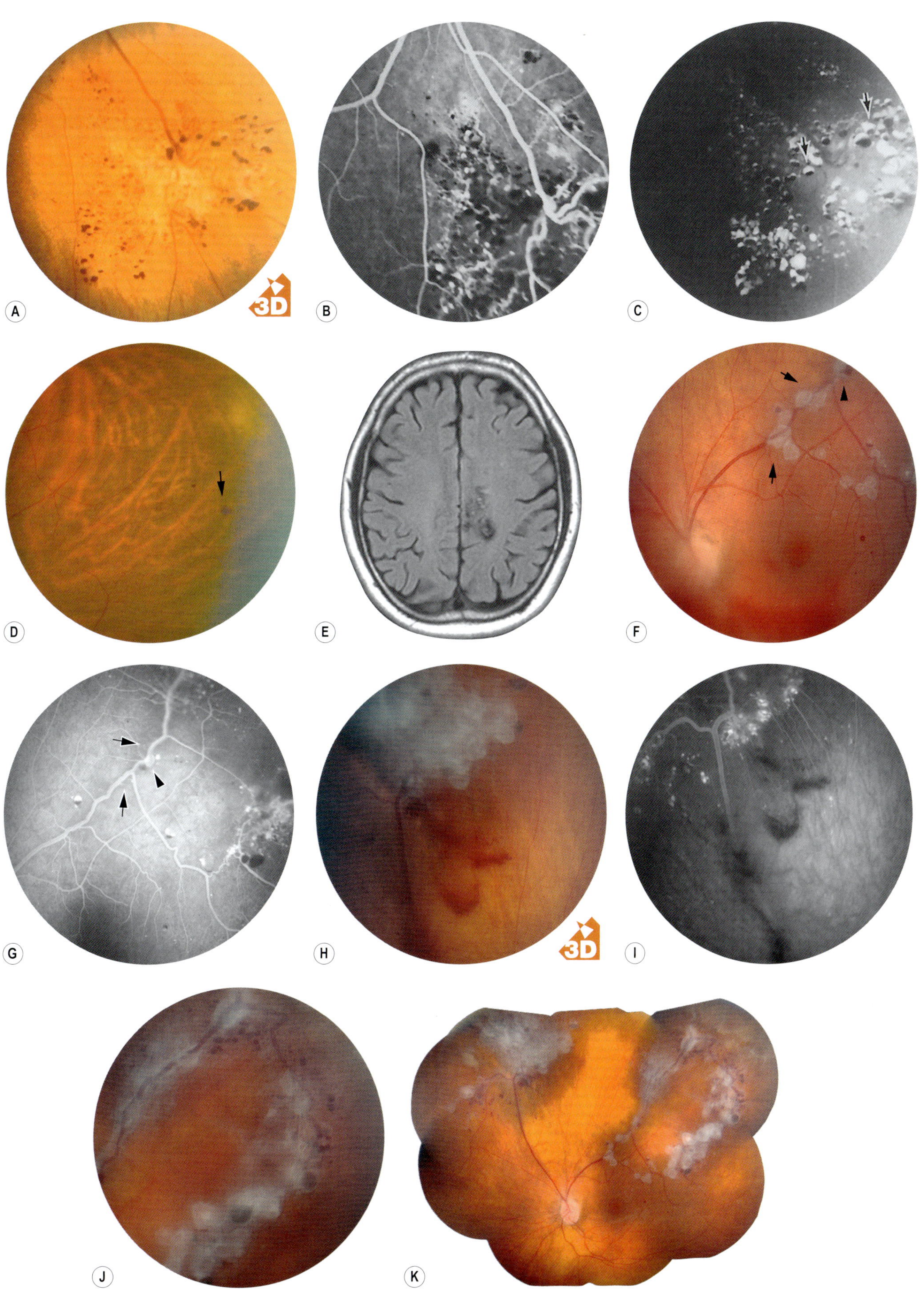
A
3D
B
C
D
E
F
G
H
3D
I
J
K

In the past, retinal cavernous hemangioma was not recognized as a distinct retinal vascular hamartoma. The more sessile and smaller lesions (Figure 13.16A) were often misdiagnosed as congenital retinal telangiectasis.[193] Figure 13.16D diagrammatically indicates the basic structural difference between retinal telangiectasis, which is a congenital anomaly affecting the structure and integrity of the intrinsic retinal vasculature, and a retinal cavernous hemangioma, which is a localized vascular tumefaction composed of cavernous vascular channels that are partly isolated from normal retinal circulation. Some of the more globular retinal cavernous hemangiomas have been reported in the older literature as angiomatosis retinae.[167]

It is uncertain whether the retinal vascular lesion reported in one patient with CNS symptoms and the dermatologic disorder angioma serpiginosum is related to retinal cavernous hemangioma.[194] A lesion that angiographically was similar to a retinal cavernous hemangioma was observed in an infant with blue rubber bleb nevus syndrome.[195] The fact that the lesion spontaneously disappeared over a 4-month period suggests that it may not have been a cavernous hemangioma.

13.16 Continued

L: Diagram showing structural differences of: (1) normal retinal vessels; (2) diffuse and focal vascular dilation and permeability alteration in retinal telangiectasis; and (3) localized vascular malformation (hamartoma) arising from the capillary bed in cavernous hemangioma.

(A and B, from Gass[157]; F–K, courtesy of Dr. Stephen J. Kim.)

13.17 Retinal cavernous hemangioma.

A and B: Histopathologic condition of cavernous hemangioma of the retina in a 2-year-old girl whose eye was enucleated with the mistaken diagnosis of retinoblastoma. The sessile retinal tumor was composed of multiple, thin-walled, dilated blood vessels that replaced the inner half of the retina (A). The arrow indicates pigment-laden macrophages in the subretinal space. The retinal detachment was artifactitious. A high-power view of the lesion revealed dilated, endothelium-lined aneurysms interconnected by narrow channels (arrows, B). These relatively isolated vascular saccules account for the sluggish circulation and plasma–erythrocytic separation demonstrated angiographically in these lesions.
C: Histologic condition of cavernous hemangioma of the optic nerve and adjacent retina.
D: Histopathologic condition of a retrobulbar cavernous hemangioma of the optic nerve head. This was an incidental finding in the optic nerve of a 3-month-old white girl who was born prematurely with a birth weight of 2 lb 14 oz (1.3 kg).
E: A slightly raised cutaneous cavernous hemangioma on the arm of a patient with a retinal cavernous hemangioma. This patient had generalized seizures. One son, who had multiple cutaneous angiomas on the face, leg, and foot, died soon after surgical excision of a cavernous hemangioma of the brain.
F: Cavernous hemangioma of the midbrain in the father of the patient illustrated in Figure 13.16 A-C.

(A, from Hogan and Zimmerman[162]; B, from Gass[157]; C, from Davies and Thumim[155]; D, from Spencer[183]; E, courtesy of Dr. L.L. Calkins; F, from Gass.[157])

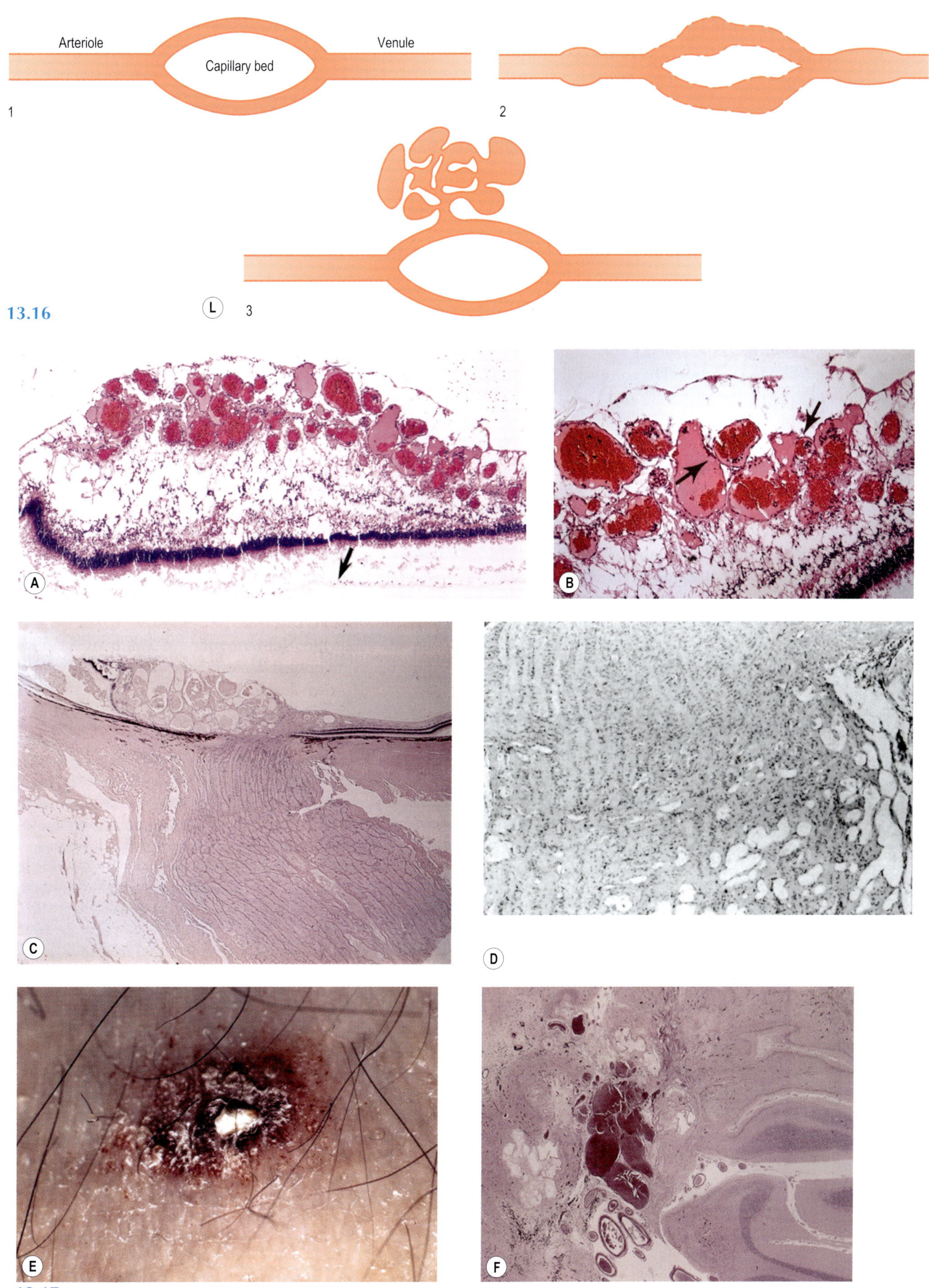

13.16

13.17

Retinal Capillary Hemangioma

The terms "retinal and optic disc capillary hemangiomas," "angiomatosis retinae," and "von Hippel's disease"[196] are used synonymously to refer to congenital hereditary capillary angiomatous hamartomas of the retina and optic nerve head.[196–218] When associated with CNS and other organ involvement the condition is referred to as von Hippel–Lindau disease VHL.[204,205] VHL disease is a dominantly inherited systemic hamartia that includes not only capillary angiomas of the retina, cerebellum, brainstem, and spinal cord, but also angiomas, adenomas, and cysts affecting the kidney, liver, pancreas, epididymis, and mesosalpinx.[219] The diagnosis of VHL is justified when either a retinal angioma or a CNS angioma occurs together with one or more visceral cysts or tumors in one patient or when a single lesion of the VHL complex is found in a relative at risk. Ocular manifestations of VHL are often the first to appear. Retinal angiomas and CNS angioma both eventually occur in approximately 50% of patients with VHL. Pheochromocytomas occur in approximately 10% of patients with VHL.[201,203,206] Approximately 25% of patients with VHL develop clear cell renal carcinomas, typically during the late stages of the disease.[198,206,220] Polycythemia occurs in approximately 15% of patients. Twin retinal vessels, a retinal sign of dominantly inherited retinal cavernous hemangioma (see previous discussion of retinal cavernous hemangioma), occur in approximately 70% of patients with familial VHL disease and in 50% of at-risk family members without ocular angiomas.[221] Since most patients who present with a solitary retinal angioma and a negative family history suggesting VHL fail to show other evidence of the disease, the medical evaluation of these patients with sporadic tumors probably does not need to be as comprehensive as in patients with multiple ocular tumors or other evidence of familial involvement. Identification of the VHL gene on chromosome 3p25–26 has now made it possible for suspected individuals to undergo genetic testing with a high degree of accuracy.[222–224]

Capillary hemangiomas are typically red or pink tumors that may arise from the superficial retina or optic nerve head and protrude inward (endophytic angiomas) (Figures 13.18A-I, A-II, E, 13.19H, and 13.20G–I). When located peripheral to the optic disc, these endophytic tumors are usually associated with arteriovenous shunting between a dilated tortuous feeding artery and a draining vein (Figure 13.19H and I). Capillary hemangiomas may also arise from the outer retinal layers (exophytic capillary hemangiomas) (Figures 13.18B, 13.19A, A-III, A-IV, 13.20A, F, and G, and 13.21A and D–F). These tumors are usually not associated with evidence of arteriovenous shunting, and there is a predilection for them to develop in the juxtapapillary area. When they arise in this area they are frequently sessile and may be misdiagnosed as papilledema or juxtapapillary choroidal neovascularization because of their predilection for causing juxtapapillary serous detachment of the retina and circinate exudation extending into the macular region (Figures 13.18B, 13.20A, F, and G, and 13.21A and E).[199,215] Loss of central vision may occur secondary to the accumulation of yellow, lipid-rich exudate in the macula derived from peripheral retinal angiomas. The mechanism for this accumulation is similar to that in patients with peripheral retinal telangiectasia (see Chapter 6). Loss of vision may also be caused by an epiretinal membrane distorting the macula remote from the site of the angioma (Figure 13.19A–C). There is a striking predilection for these epiretinal membranes to peel spontaneously and for vision to return to near normal after treatment of the peripheral angioma (Figure 13.19A–F).[157,158,225–227] For this reason, vitrectomy for excision of the epiretinal membrane should be considered only after a 4–6-month period of observation following treatment. Floaters and visual loss may also be caused by development of a retinal tear adjacent to an angioma and subsequent rhegmatogenous retinal detachment.[158,228] Vitreous traction developing at the anterior surface of the retinal angioma and adjacent retina is responsible for the retinal tear. Vitreous traction may also be a factor in the development on the tumor surface of proliferative retinopathy, vitreous hemorrhage either spontaneously or following treatment of the tumor, and tractional retinal detachment. A retrobulbar capillary angioma (Figure 13.18A–E) should be considered in patients with angiomatosis and unexplained visual loss.

13.18 Retinal capillary hemangiomas.

A: Diagram showing sites of origin of retinal capillary angiomas. I, Endophytic angioma of the optic nerve head. II, Endophytic peripheral retinal angioma. III, Exophytic juxtapapillary angioma. IV, Exophytic peripheral retinal angioma. V, Intraneural angioma.
B–D: This 36-year-old woman noted blurred vision in the left eye caused by a juxtapapillary capillary hemangioma (arrow, A). She had no other stigmata of von Hippel–Lindau disease. Stereoscopic angiography revealed the sessile capillary angiomatous nature of the lesion (C and D).
E–J: Juxtapapillary (E) and peripheral capillary hemangioma (F) in a 10-year-old girl with no evidence of extraocular involvement with angiomatosis. Angiography revealed the capillary nature of the tumors (G and H), shunting of blood from the arterial to the venous side of the circulation in the region of the peripheral tumor (H), and late staining (I and J).

(A, from Gass.[9])

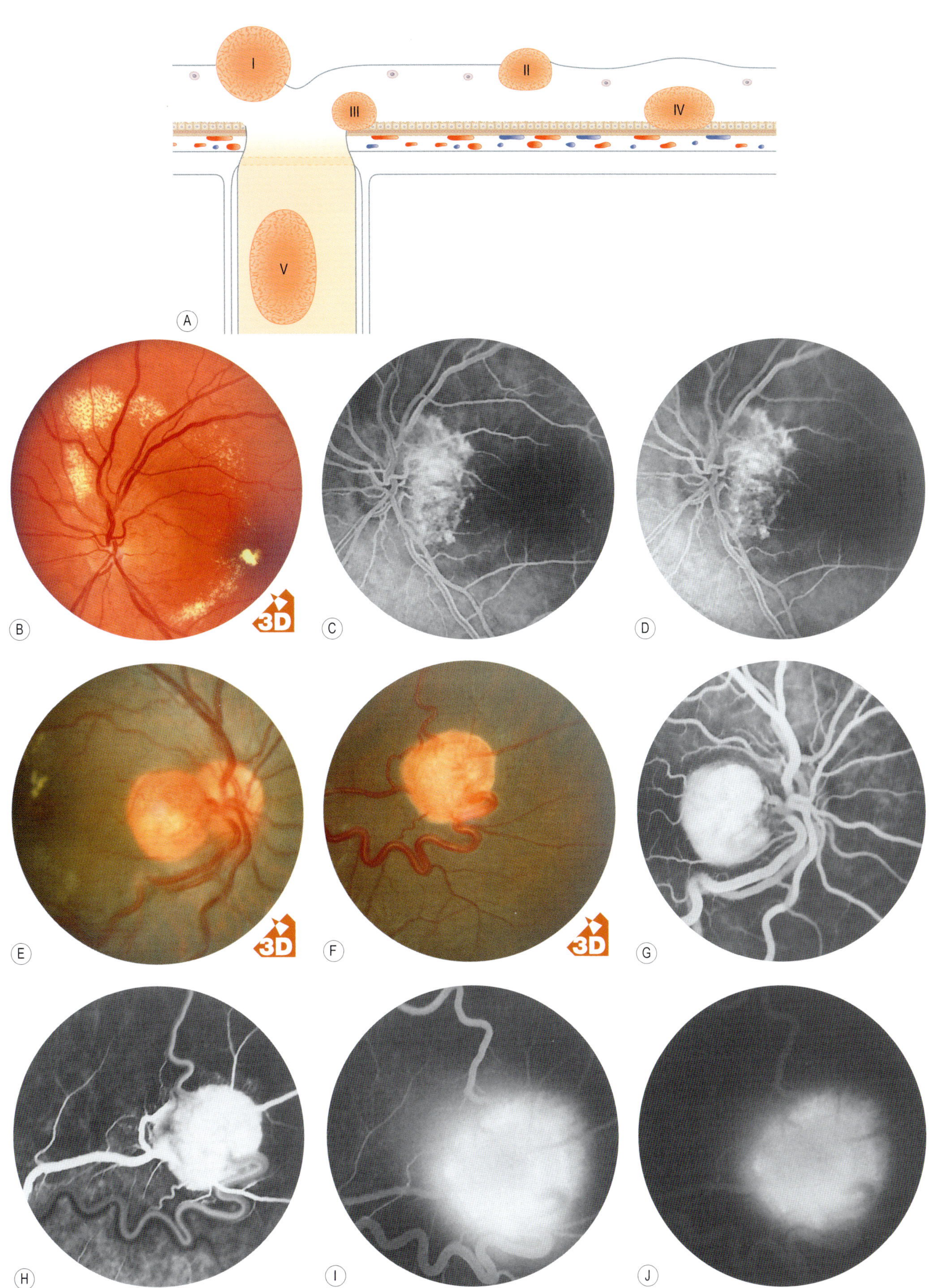
I
II
III
IV
V
A
B
3D
C
D
E
3D
F
3D
G
H
I
J

Stereoscopic fluorescein angiography is invaluable in detecting exophytic sessile juxtapapillary capillary hemangiomas (Figures 13.18B and 13.20).[199] Because these tumors protrude into the subretinal space adjacent to the optic disc and because they frequently arise in the papillomacular bundle area in symptomatic patients, they are difficult to treat with photocoagulation (Figure 13.20A–F and G–L). Fluorescein angiography in peripheral endophytic lesions shows evidence of arteriovenous shunting (Figures 13.18J and 13.19I). Angiography usually shows no evidence of fluorescein staining in the macular region in those patients with lipid-rich accumulations secondary to peripheral angiomas. Angiography is particularly useful in the detection of very small lesions that may be barely visible biomicroscopically (Figure 13.19B and E).[158,215,229–233]

Light and electron microscopy reveals that these tumors are composed of a mass of retinal capillaries, many of which have a normal endothelium, basement membrane, and pericytes (Figure 13.22).[200,234–239]

13.19 Retinal capillary hemangiomas.

A–F: Peripheral retinal capillary angiomas (A and B) and macular pucker (C) in a 23-year-old woman complaining of recent loss of central vision in the right eye. Her past medical history and family history were unremarkable. Visual acuity in the right eye was 20/70 and in the left eye was 20/15. In addition to the solitary angioma in the superotemporal fundus (A), there was a small angioma nasally (arrow, B). Fluorescein angiography demonstrated both lesions (D and E). The retinal tumors were treated with cryopexy and photocoagulation. Soon afterward the preretinal membrane spontaneously detached from the inner surface of the macula and remained attached to the optic nerve head (arrow, F). Her visual acuity improved to 20/25 + 3.

G–K: Exudative maculopathy (G) caused by an endophytic angioma nasal to the right optic disc (H and I) in this 23-year-old woman who presented with a 2-month history of blurred vision in the right eye. Her family history and past medical history were negative. Computed tomography scan of the brain was negative. Visual acuity was 20/70, right eye, and 20/20, left eye. Laser photocoagulation of the feeder artery and tumor resulted in a vitreous hemorrhage (J). Six years later her visual acuity was 20/40. Note the vitreoretinal traction, nasal displacement of the optic disc and foveal center (arrow, K), and resolution of the macular exudation.

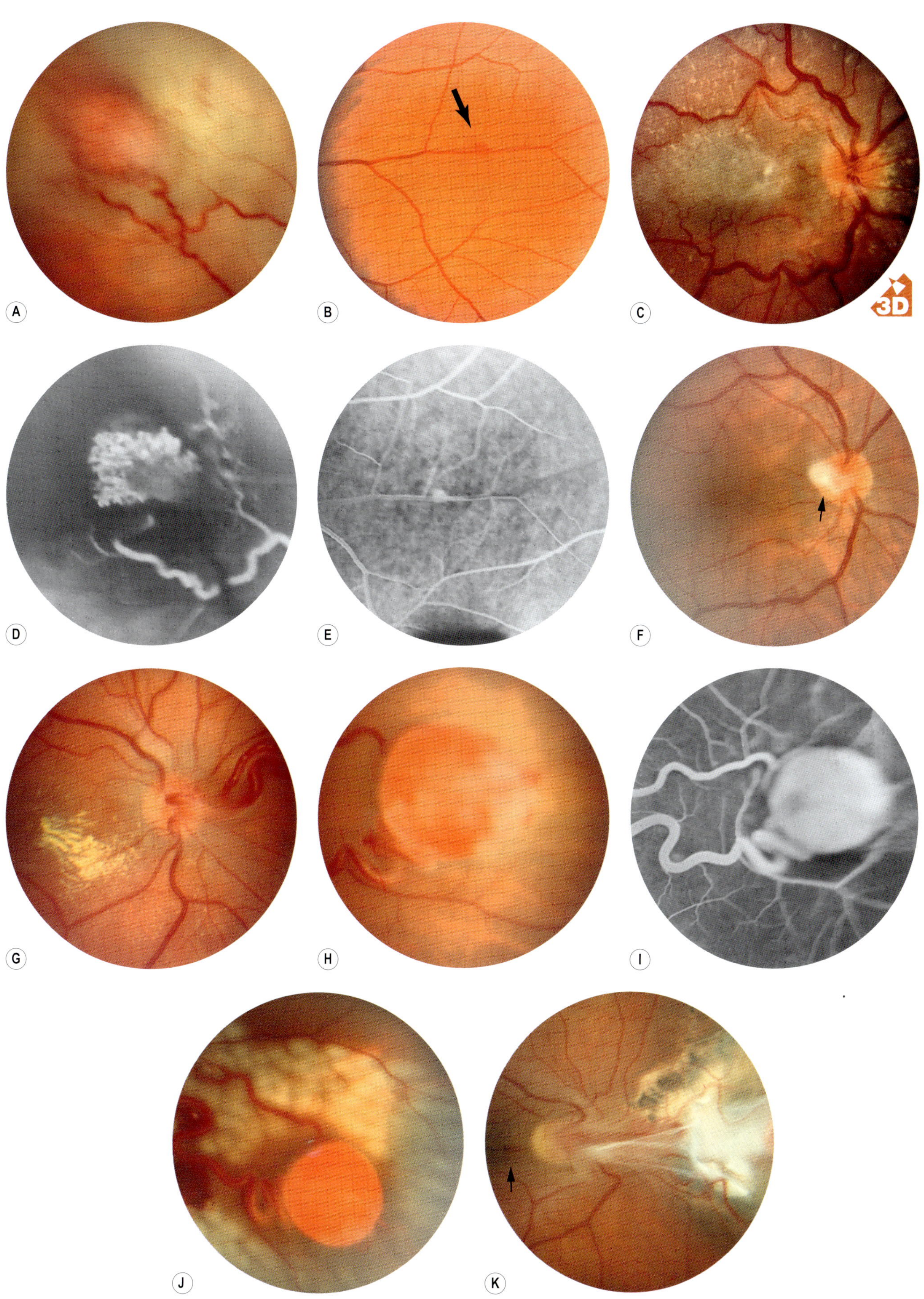
A
B
C
3D
D
E
F
G
H
I
J
K

In some cases, capillaries making up these tumors may show abnormal fenestrations.[235,236] Stromal cells, which some have attributed to astrocytes, separate the vascular channels and frequently contain large lipid-filled vacuoles. It is now believed that the true neoplastic component (i.e., the cells with allelic deletion at the VHL gene locus) are the foamy stromal cells.[240] The VHL protein (pVHL) targets hypoxia-inducible factors for degradation. In the absence of pVHL there is excessive production of vascular endothelial growth factor.[241] New vessels may develop on the anterior surface of these tumors and extend into the vitreous (Figure 13.22D). Exophytic tumors may have vascular communication with the choroid in some cases.

Because of their capillary nature and predilection for the development of arteriovenous fistulas and exudation, these tumors are capable of reactive proliferation and continued growth even into adulthood. Progressive intraretinal and subretinal exudation and detachment are part of the natural course of the disease. Spontaneous fibrotic involution of angiomas, however, occasionally occurs.[213,239] Identification of capillary angiomas ophthalmoscopically and by fluorescein angiography during the early stages is important because treatment with photocoagulation[159,230,242–244] or cryotherapy[159,233,245–247] at this stage of the disease is easier. Treatment of retinal capillary hemangioma is based upon tumor size, location, presence of subretinal fluid or retinal traction, and visual acuity.[248] The sessile exophytic juxtapapillary hemangiomas associated with loss of macular vision are difficult to treat because of the frequency with which they are located in the papillomacular bundle and because laser treatment is ineffective in stopping the exudation derived from the outer portion of the tumor that protrudes into the subretinal space. The use of photocoagulation to create a barrier between juxtapapillary angiomas and the center of the macula before they cause macular detachment and exudation may prove to be of value (Figure 13.21D–I).

13.20 Retinal capillary hemangioma.

A–E: Sessile juxtapapillary retinal angioma (A) misdiagnosed as papilledema in a 31-year-old woman with a 5-month history of intermittent headaches. She had recently been hospitalized for a thorough neurologic evaluation, which was negative. Her visual acuity in both eyes was 20/20. Angiography revealed a capillary angioma, largely confined to the outer two-thirds of the retina (B and C). She developed chronic serous detachment of the macula, and her visual acuity decreased to 20/50 in the right eye. She had two courses of argon laser grid pattern treatment (D) to the tumor that resulted in resolution of the intraretinal and subretinal exudate (E). At the time of her last photograph, made 9 years after her initial treatment, her visual acuity was 20/30.
F–L: This 19-year-old woman had a history of blurred vision and optic disc lesions first noted at age 15 years. She was asymptomatic in the right eye. Visual acuity was 20/30, right eye, and 20/400, left eye. There was exudative maculopathy associated with a juxtapapillary capillary angioma bilaterally (arrows, F and G). The angioma in the left eye was treated with argon green laser (H) and was retreated 4 months later. At that time the acuity in the right eye had decreased to 20/50 and the angioma (J) was treated with laser. One month later the angioma in the right eye (K) was retreated. Forty-two months later her visual acuity in the right eye was 20/40 and the left eye was 20/60. There was improvement in the exudation in both eyes (I and L). At the time of her initial examination magnetic resonance imaging of the brain revealed a left cerebellar hemangioblastoma that was successfully removed. There was no family history of angiomatosis.

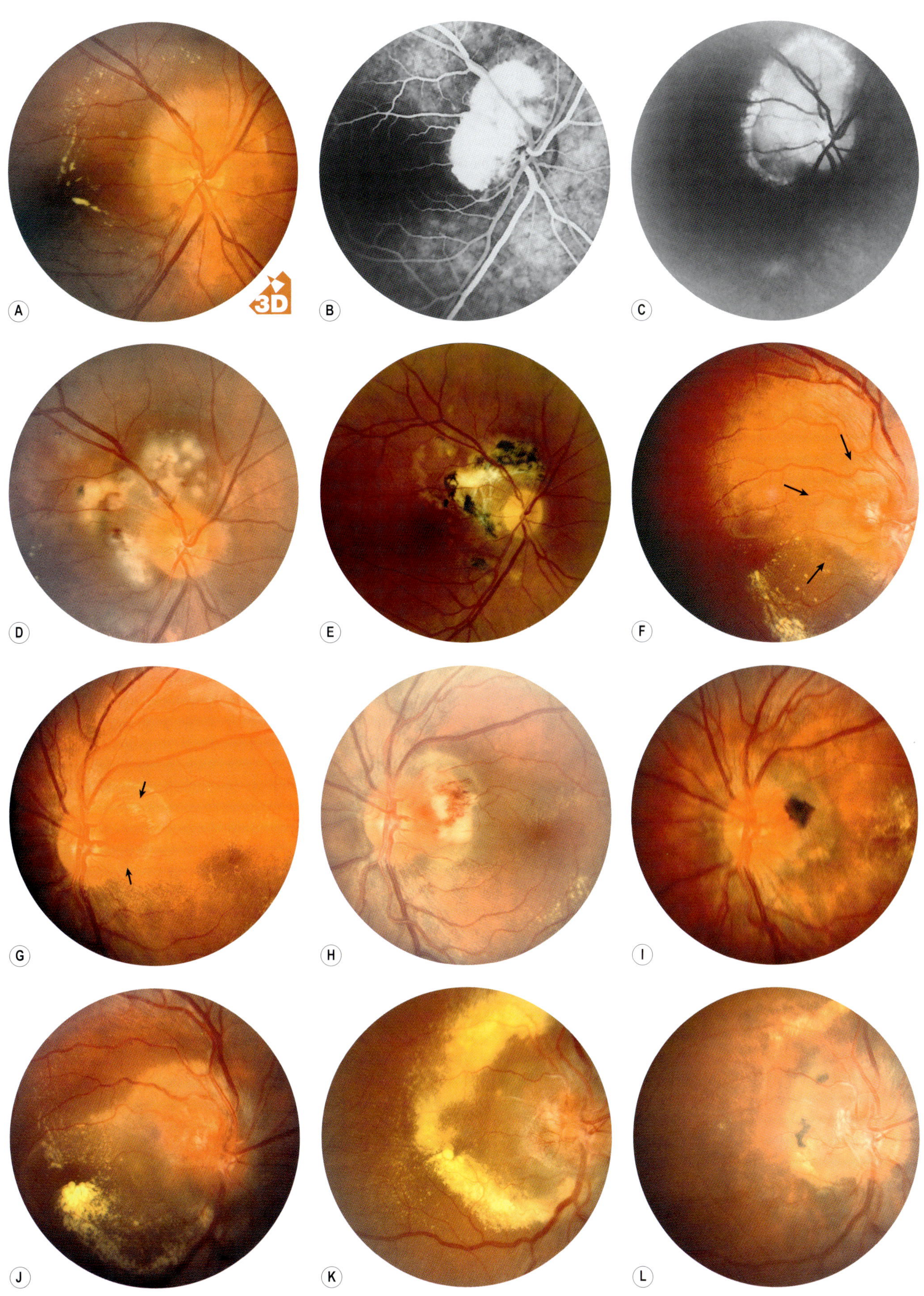
A
3D
B
C
D
E
F
G
H
I
J
K
L

Treatment of the peripheral angiomas with photocoagulation or cryotherapy or both is generally effective in lesions whose diameter does exceed 1 disc diameter. Treatment of larger lesions is complicated by excessive subretinal exudation and a predilection for the development of retinitis proliferans on the surface of these tumors. Techniques for treating large retinal angiomas include repeated applications of laser to the feeding artery to reduce the tumor perfusion before treating the tumor directly, use of transscleral penetrating diathermy, and pars plana vitrectomy and direct diathermy to the tumor.[249,250] The use of a transvitreal arterial clip together with diathermy and removal of the posterior vitreous may prove to be useful in the treatment of large angiomas.[155] Surgical excision of these lesions has been reported.[251]

Photodynamic therapy has been tried with moderate results to induce the occlusion of both juxtapapillary and peripheral retinal capillary hemangiomas (Figure 13.23).[252–255]

13.21 Natural course of retinal capillary hemangiomas.

A–F: Exophytic capillary angioma in a 17-year-old boy complaining of blurred vision in the left eye (arrows, A and B). At that time there were no other lesions in either eye. Medical evaluation for extraocular evidence of angiomatosis was negative. Over the subsequent 10 years he had gradual enlargement of the angiomatous mass that grew through the center of his macula despite laser photocoagulation. During this time he developed a small angioma in the inferior fundus of the same eye and a small angioma on the right optic disc (arrow, C). This remained unchanged from 1979 until 1992, when he returned because he had noticed a paracentral scotoma in the right eye (D). Meanwhile he had developed total retinal detachment and had no light perception in the left eye. Laser treatment along the temporal margin of the tumor was advised and was refused. He returned in 1995 complaining of difficulty reading. His acuity was 20/15 but he had a large cecocentral scotoma associated with exudative retinal detachment and further enlargement of the angioma (E). In an effort to isolate the tumor from the center of the macula a row of krypton red laser burns was placed near the temporal margin of the tumor (arrow, F). Nine months later the exudate was gone and he was asymptomatic.
G–I: Gradual enlargement of juxtapapillary angioma occurred in this patient. G, March 1983. H, March 1985. I, September 1996. Several years later the patient had severe loss of central vision because of exudative retinal detachment. Use of a barrier-type laser treatment and direct treatment of the angioma early (G and H) may have prevented or delayed the loss of central vision.
J–L: A juxtapapillary angioma (arrows, K) developed 5 years later at the site of a choroidal rupture (arrow, J) in this 19-year-old woman with Stargardt's disease. Her sister had Stargardt's disease, but her family history was negative otherwise. This tumor may be a secondary angioma resulting from reactive glial vascular proliferation at the site of chorioretinal scarring.

(G–I, courtesy of Dr. Arnold Patz; J–L, from Retsas et al.[455])

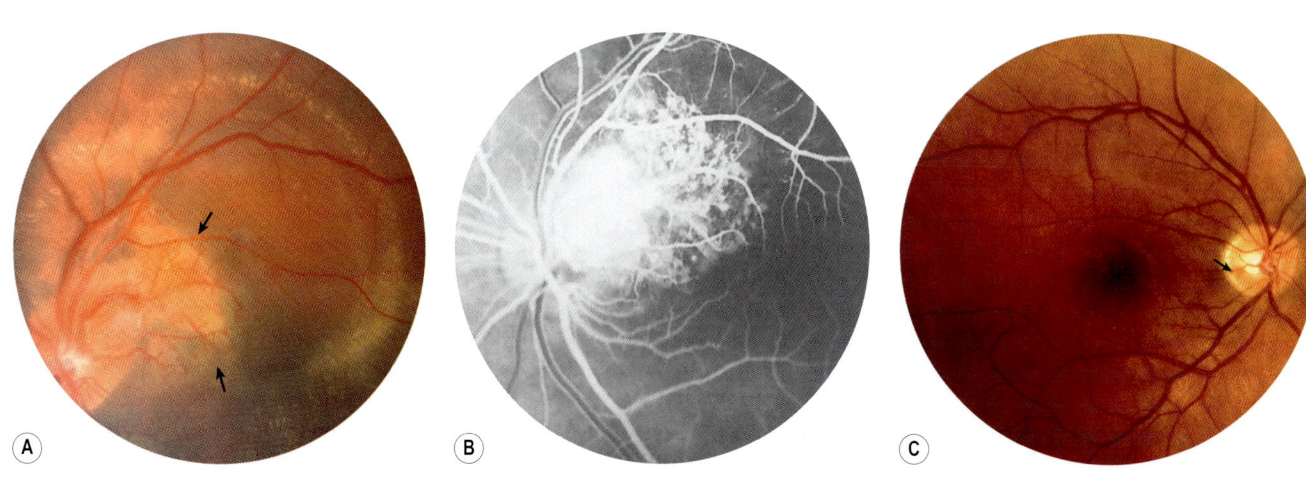

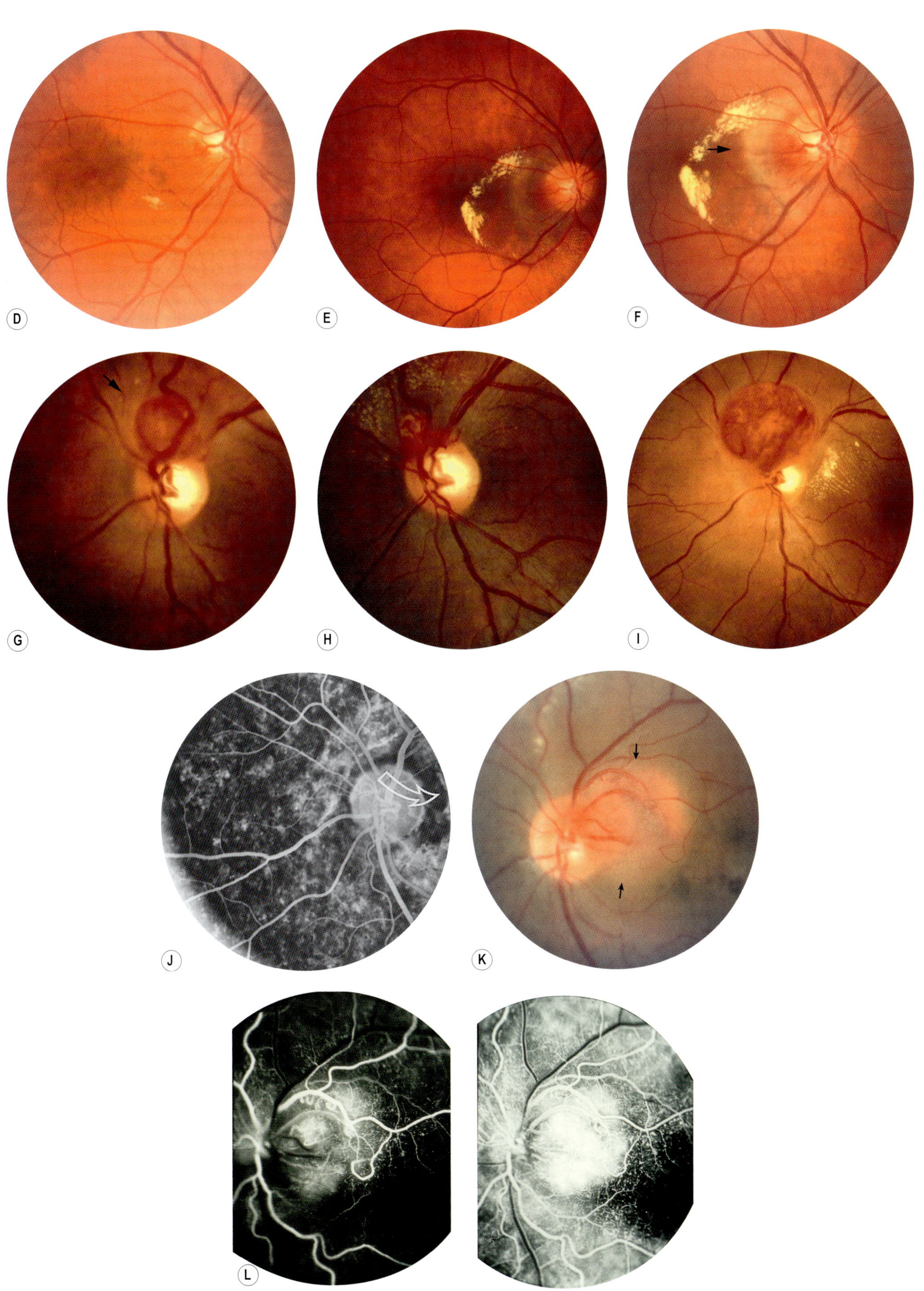
D
E
F
G
H
I
J
K
L

Most recently, systemic and intravitreal administration of inhibitors of vascular endothelial growth factor have demonstrated mixed treatment outcomes, suggesting that the general efficacy of antiangiogenic agents in VHL is uncertain.[256–258]

The differential diagnosis for juxtapapillary capillary angiomas includes juxtapapillary choroidal neovascularization, hypopigmented combined retinal and RPE hamartoma, papilledema,[259,260] juxtapapillary choroidal hemangiomas and osteomas, and reactive retinal glial and vascular proliferation (see discussion in the next section). Stereoscopic fluorescein angiography is the most important study in the differential diagnosis. The diagnosis of peripheral capillary hemangiomas is not difficult in the presence of a dilated, tortuous retinal artery and vein extending from the optic disc to the tumor. Vasoproliferative tumor can be mistaken for a peripheral retinal angioma.

13.22 Histopathology of retinal capillary hemangioma.

A–D: Histopathologic condition of pre-exudative phase of retinal angioma in a 48-year-old man who complained of paresthesias of the arms and legs. His mother had died of a brain tumor at 40 years of age. His neurologic examination was normal. His cerebrospinal fluid protein was 300 mg/dl. A myelogram revealed a block at the first cervical vertebra, and a right brachial arteriogram revealed a large vascular tumor at the level of the brainstem. A cerebellar hemangioblastoma was found at the time of craniotomy. The patient died soon afterward. An autopsy revealed multiple cysts of the right kidney and pancreas. Gross examination of the right eye revealed two nodular retinal angiomas. The larger one (arrow, A) measured 1.5 mm. The retinal vessels leading to both angiomas were dilated. Histopathologic examination revealed dilated feeder vessels (arrow, B) supplying the capillary tumor, which replaced the normal retinal architecture and protruded into the vitreous cavity. A high-power view of the tumor showed that it was composed of capillary-sized blood vessels lined by flattened endothelial cells (C). Strands of fibroglial tissue and capillaries were present on the surface of the tumor and extended into the vitreous (arrow, D).
E and **F**: Clinicopathologic correlation of an exophytic capillary angioma of the optic nerve head and peripapillary retina simulating chronic papilledema in a 29-year-old man who first noted blurred vision in his right eye in 1959. He had similar swelling of both optic discs associated with exudative detachment of the surrounding retina (E). Over the subsequent 3 years he had progressive loss of vision in both eyes, and because of the uncertainty of the diagnosis the left eye was enucleated. His family history was positive for an angioblastic meningioma in his mother, a pheochromocytoma in a niece and a nephew, and bilateral optic nerve lesions similar to those in the patient in a nephew. Histopathologic examination revealed an exophytic capillary hemangioma involving the juxtapapillary retina and optic nerve head (arrows, F).

(A–D, from Nicholson et al.[237]; E and F, from Darr et al.[260]

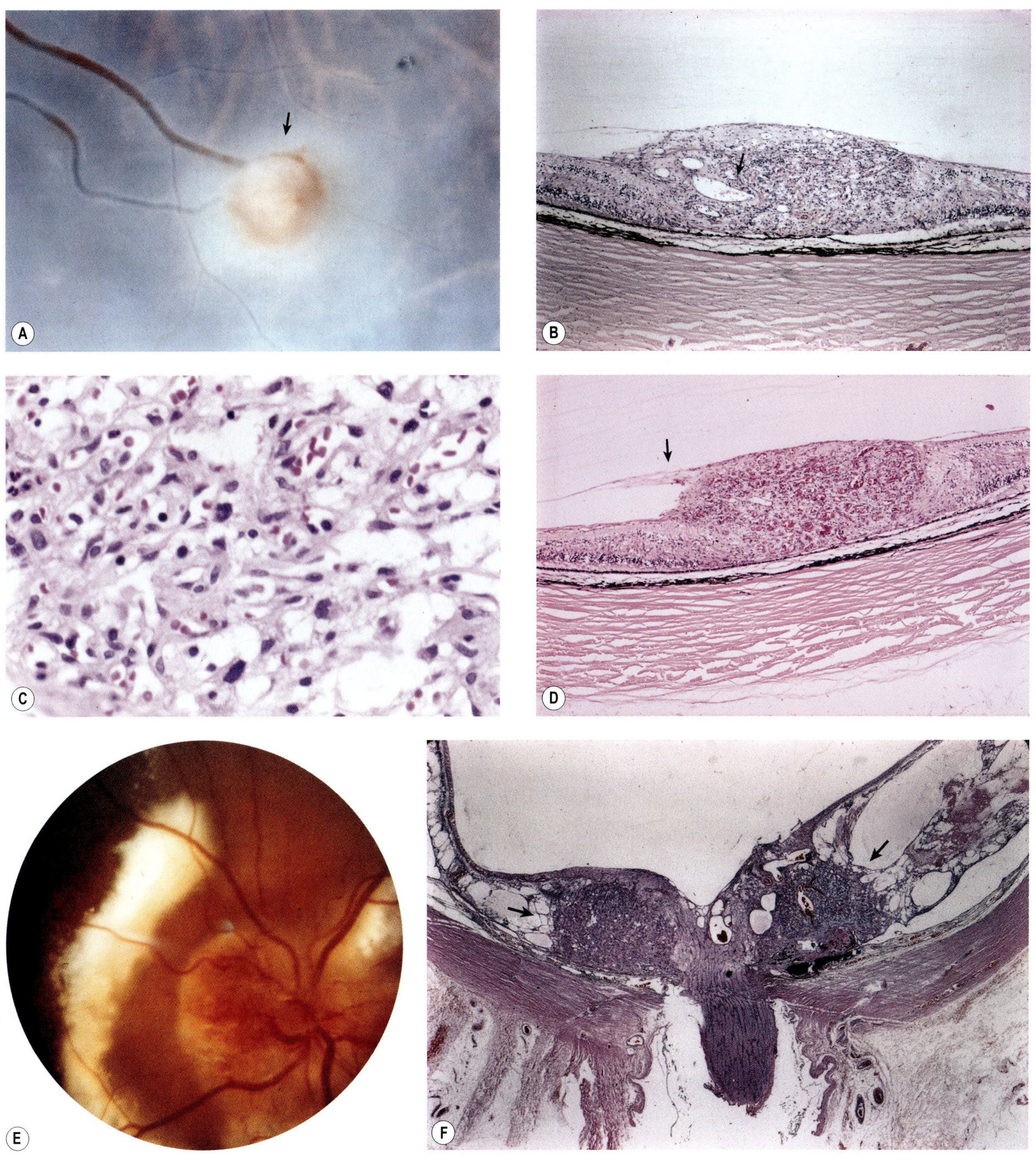
A
B
C
D
E
F

RETINAL TELANGIECTASIS AND ARTERIOVENOUS ANEURYSM

Retinal telangiectasias, macrovessels, arteriovenous aneurysms, and arteriovenous communications are not true tumors and are discussed in Chapter 6.

13.23 Retinal capillary hemangioma treated with photodynamic therapy.

A–F: A 20-year-old man with solitary retinal capillary hemangioma with extensive exudation involving the macula (A and B). In addition to the hemangioma there are several small microaneurysms beyond the tumor suggesting associated retinal telangiectasia. In addition to the tumor vasculature filling up, fluorescein angiogram shows dilated capillary bed, peripheral nonperfusion and microaneurysms, suggesting associated Coats'-like vascular malformation (C). Family history, systemic evaluation, and genetic testing were negative for von Hippel–Lindau disease. Note shrinkage and gliosis with resolution of subretinal fluid and hard lipid exudation 3 months following treatment with a single session of standard-fluence photodynamic therapy (E and F).

G–M: A 76-year-old woman was observed for at least 10 years for a "retinal lesion." Her vision decreased to 20/30– in this eye and a HVF showed paracentral scotoma. A strawberry-shaped capillary hemangioma was seen obscuring most of the optic disc (G and H). Angiogram showed that the vessels within the mass filled and leaked mildly, appearing like a smoke stack emanating from the superior pole of the tumor (I). There were lipid exudates inferior to the disc that extended to the fovea. Optical coherence tomography revealed cystic swelling of the inner retina in the vicinity of the tumor (J) and mild thickening of the fovea (K). She had no family history suggestive of von Hippel–Lindau and gene testing for von Hippel–Lindau returned negative. She underwent a reduced-fluence photodynamic therapy, which shrank the tumor considerably to reveal the underlying optic disc (L), lipid exudates gradually disappeared, and the foveal cysts resolved. Her vision remained at 20/30 eccentrically. However, the lesion regained some size at 13-month follow-up (M), and it has remained stable at 3 years. The vision returned to 20/20.

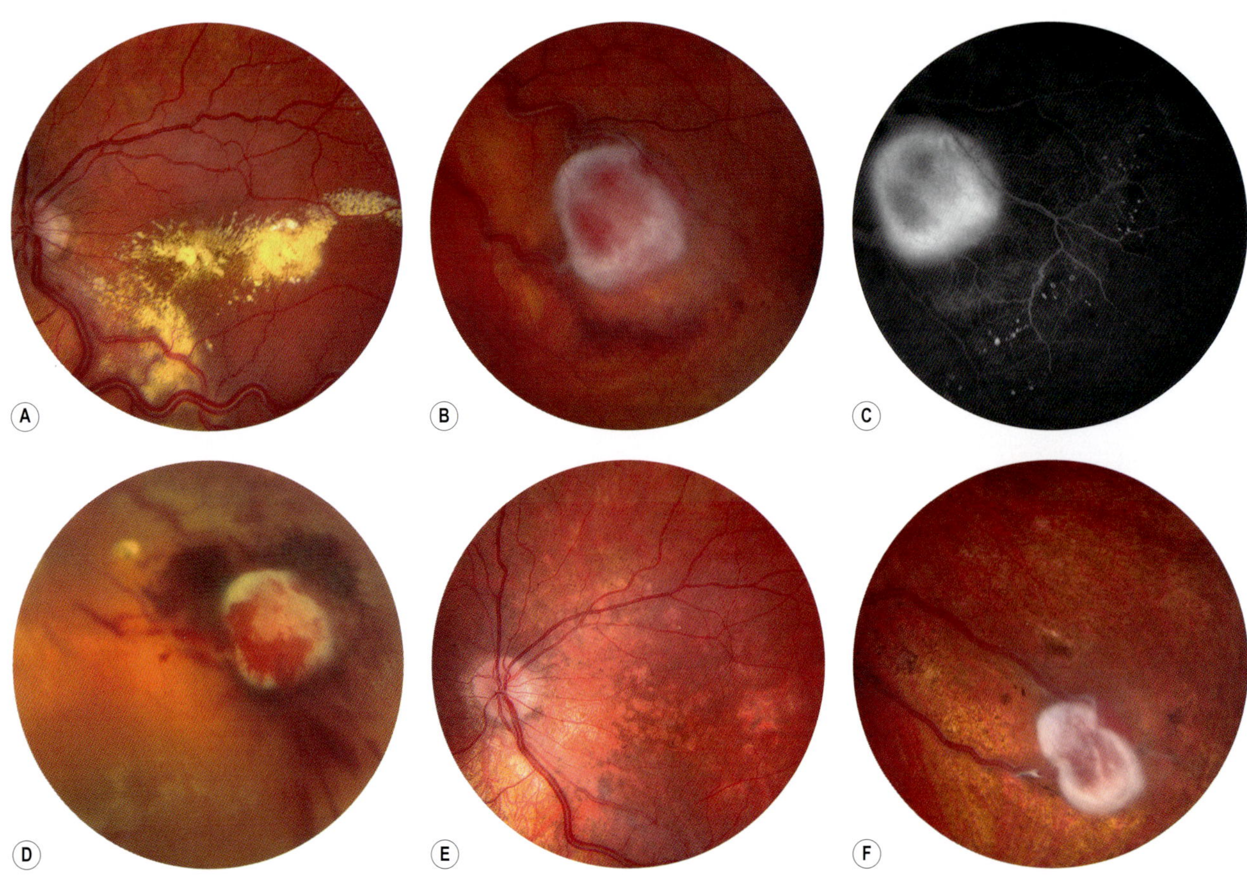

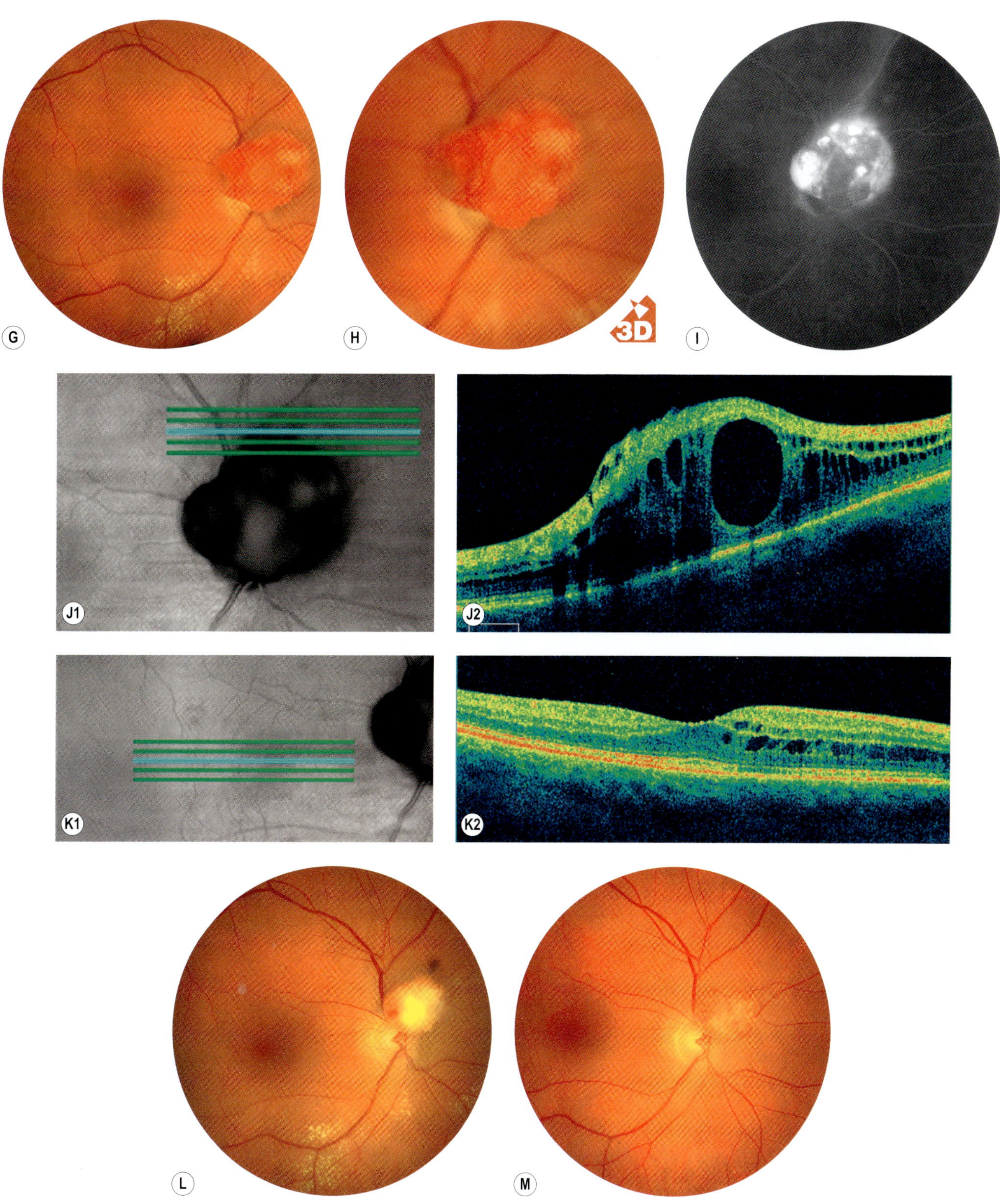
G
H
3D
I
J1
J2
K1
K2
L
M

VASOPROLIFERATIVE RETINAL TUMOR (REACTIVE RETINAL VASCULAR PROLIFERATION)

There may be some difficulty in differentiating peripheral exophytic angiomas from retinal telangiectasis or pseudoangiomatous masses caused by reactive vascular proliferation in patients with retinopathy of prematurity, branch vein occlusion, diabetic retinopathy, familial exudative vitreoretinopathy, pars planitis, X-linked juvenile retinoschisis, chronic rhegmatogenous retinal detachment, and retinitis proliferans (Figures 13.21J–L and 13.24).[225,261–265]

13.24 Vasoproliferative tumor.

A 15-year-old female with neurofibromatosis type-1 was referred for evaluation of painless floaters in her right eye of 1 month's duration. Vision was absence of light perception in the left eye as a result of a left optic nerve glioma that had been treated with chemotherapy. In the right eye, visual acuity was 20/30 and intraocular pressure (IOP) was 12 mmHg. Anterior-segment examination revealed numerous Lisch nodules, florid neovascularization of the iris, and 360° neovascularization of the angle (A). Dilated fundus examination of the right eye revealed 1–2+ anterior vitreous cells and an inferiorly located pink, elevated vascular mass with areas of surrounding subretinal fluid and lipid accumulation (B). Dilated tortuous feeder vessels, as seen with retinal capillary hemangioma, were not observed. The patient had just completed a tapering course of oral steroids (starting dose 60 mg QD, tapered by 20 mg/week) that had been prescribed by the referring physician. Patient was treated with double freeze–thaw transconjunctival cryotherapy and simultaneous intravitreal injection of bevacizumab (1.25 mg in 0.05 ml).

One week later, the NVI was nearly completely resolved and the IOP was 13 mmHg. One month after treatment the retinal detachment overlying the vasoproliferative tumor had resolved and the tumor appeared less vascular with fibrotic changes. A second injection of intravitreal bevacizumab was given for persistent NVI. Over the course of the next 6 months the NVI resolved and the tumor underwent fibrotic changes with chorioretinal atrophy and hyperpigmentation at the posterior margin (C). At 36 months after initial treatment, clinical findings were stable, with vision of 20/30.

(From Hood et al.,[456] with permission.)

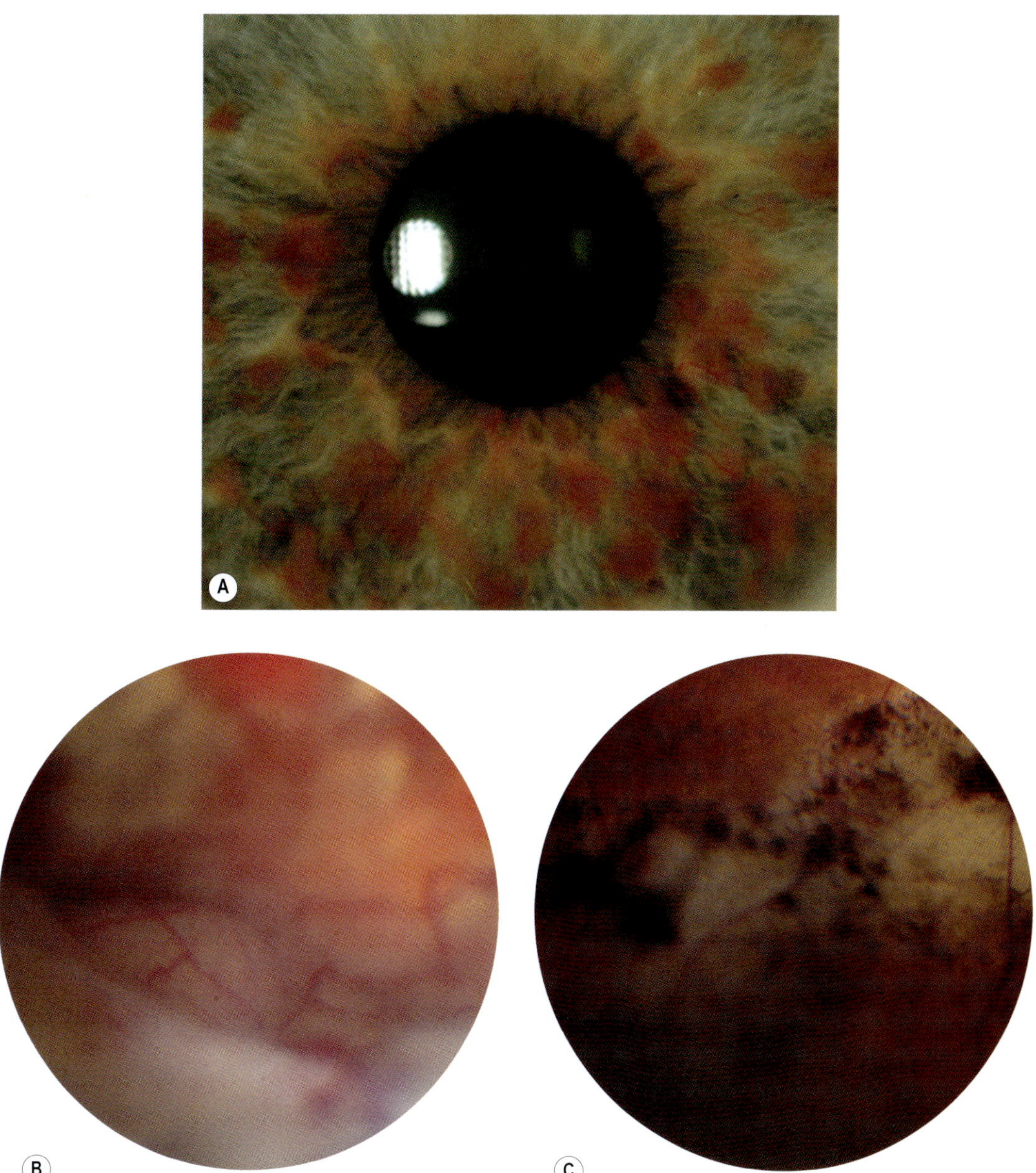
A
B
C

LEUKEMIC RETINOPATHY AND OPTIC NEUROPATHY

Loss of central vision in patients with either acute or chronic leukemia may be caused either by direct leukemic invasion of the uveal tract, retina, vitreous, or optic nerve or by other associated hematologic abnormalities, including anemia and hyperviscosity or a combination of both. Previous studies have described an overall ocular involvement in 9–90% of cases based on clinical examination or autopsy findings.[266–268] A figure of about 40% based on prospective clinical studies is more realistic.[266,269] However, previously published reports have been biased towards acute leukemia, suggesting that ocular involvement in more common chronic leukemia is infrequent.[266,270]

13.25 Hemorrhagic retinopathy associated with acute leukemia.

A–E: This man with acute myelogenous leukemia developed bilateral loss of vision. Five months later after chemotherapy his vision had improved and there was marked improvement in the retinopathy.
F–H: This man with acute lymphatic leukemia experienced bilateral loss of vision. Note the white-centered hemorrhages and superficial retinal hematoma (arrow, G).
I and J: Before death this patient with chronic granulocytic leukemia had extensive perivascular infiltration and nodular white and hemorrhagic masses in the retina. Histopathologic examination of the eyes revealed massive perivascular leukemic infiltration and hemorrhagic nodular leukemic tumefactions lying beneath the internal limiting membrane (arrow).

(From Kuwabara et al. © 1964, American Medical Association. All rights reserved.[284])

Leukemic Retinopathy

The most striking fundus pictures associated with leukemia involve the retina and they typically occur in patients with acute leukemia, frequently during a period of relapse and frequently associated with severe and coexisting anemia (Figure 13.25).[158,266,271–281] These patients may develop dilation, tortuosity, and beading of the retinal veins; retinal vascular sheathing; cotton-wool patches; superficial flame-shaped hemorrhages; deep, round hemorrhages; white-centered hemorrhages; and subhyaloid and subinternal limiting membrane hemorrhages (Figure 13.25). These changes are similar to those seen in patients with severe anemia from any cause as well as dysproteinemias (see Figure 6.84A–F).[269,282,283] Some patients may develop grayish-white nodular leukemic retinal infiltrations and perivascular retinal infiltration (Figure 13.26).[284,285] Patients, particularly with chronic myelogenous leukemia, may develop peripheral retinal microaneurysms,[275,286] retinal vascular closure,[287–289] and retinal and optic disc neovascularization.[266,287,290–293] Increased blood viscosity and reduced blood flow associated with prolonged and marked leukocytosis[290,292,293] and thrombocytosis[291] are probably the cause of these latter changes. Fluorescein angiography is helpful in detecting these alterations. Leopard-spot RPE alterations seen in these patients, often during the stage of remission, are probably caused by choroidal infiltration (Figure 13.27 G–I).[268,294–296] Pigment epithelial and retinal degeneration may occur in one or both eyes and occasionally may be accompanied by development of a macular hole.[295,296]

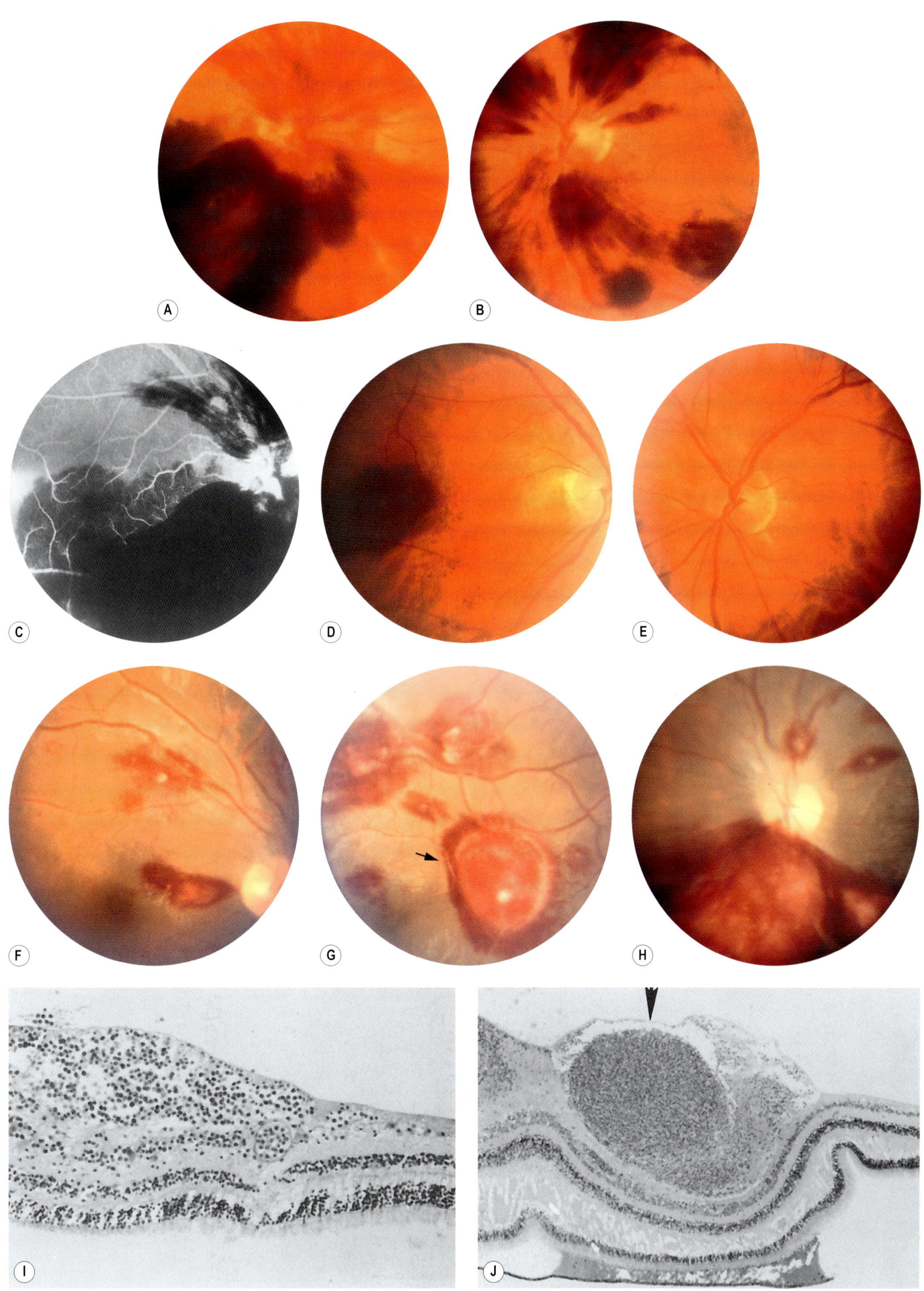
A
B
C
D
E
F
G
H
I
J

Leukemic Optic Neuropathy

Acute visual loss may be caused by leukemic invasion of the optic nerve, usually in children with acute lymphocytic leukemia (Figures 13.26A–F and 13.28A and B). In some patients the infiltration may be confined to the retrobulbar area or may involve the optic nerve head.[278,297–301] Visual loss in these latter patients may be minimal, and the swollen optic nerve may be mistaken for papilledema associated with increased intracranial pressure (Figure 13.28A). These patients show a dramatic response to antimetabolite, corticosteroid, or orbital irradiation therapy, which should be instituted promptly after a CT study and lumbar puncture to exclude papilledema.[302] Infiltration of the optic nerve may be associated with occlusion of the central retinal artery (Figure 13.28C–H) and vein.[266,303] Progressive visual loss and optic atrophy may occasionally occur coincident with a worsening of chronic lymphocytic leukemia[304] or blast crisis in chronic myeloid leukemia (Figure 13.28I–K).

Leukemic Infiltration of the Vitreous

An occasional patient with acute leukemia may lose vision because of vitreous cellular infiltration, and vitrectomy may be of value in making the diagnosis as well as improving the vision.[279] Other unusual causes of visual loss in patients with leukemia include iris infiltration,[305] anterior-segment ischemia,[273] open-angle glaucoma,[306] and corneal ring ulcer.[280]

13.26 Leukemic infiltration of the retina and optic nerve.

A–F: This 6-year-old girl developed lymphocytic leukemia in December 1966. She was treated with vincristine, prednisone, and methotrexate. Because of visual loss she was seen at the Bascom Palmer Eye Institute on November 8, 1967. Visual acuity in the right eye was finger counting and in the left eye was hand movements. The optic nerve head in both eyes was obscured by a massive cellular infiltration that extended into the retina in the peripapillary region (A and B). There was pronounced perivenous infiltration. By December 3, 1967, the degree of infiltration in the right eye had improved (C). There was further improvement by March 13, 1968 (D). On June 11, 1968, her visual acuity had returned to 20/20 in this eye. By November 14, 1968, the patient was quite well and was attending school. Her vision in the right eye was 20/20. Most of the perivascular infiltration had disappeared (E). The optic nerve head was pale, and its margins were blurred. The visual acuity in the left eye was 20/200, and there was still evidence of perivascular infiltration (F).
G–J: Leukemic infiltration of the retina. This 8-year-old girl with acute leukemia developed loss of central vision in the left eye. The optic nerve head was blurred, and there were scattered retinal hemorrhages in the macula and elsewhere in the fundus (G). In the periphery there was pronounced perivascular sheathing, presumed to be secondary to leukemic infiltration (H). Fluorescein angiography revealed dilation and microaneurysmal formation in the retinal capillary bed and widespread leakage of dye from the capillaries and veins (I and J).

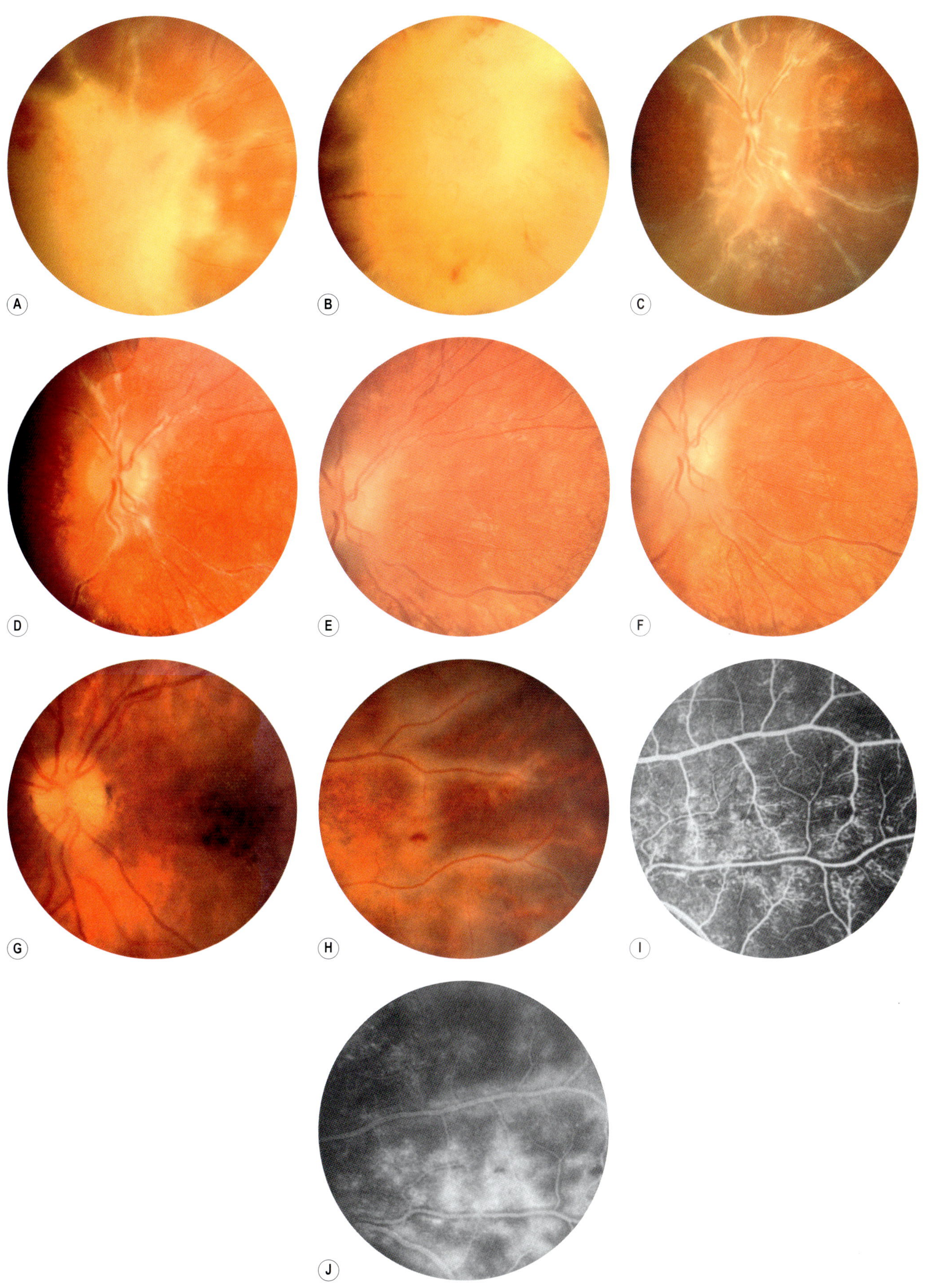
A
B
C
D
E
F
G
H
I
J

13.27 Leukemic retinopathy.

A–F: This 16-year-old African American male woke up with sudden painless loss of vision in both eyes to hand motion. He had mild pulsating eye pain bilaterally. The anterior segment was quiet. The right eye revealed massive retinal, preretinal, and subretinal hemorrhages in the posterior pole (A–C). The mid-retina showed targetlike intraretinal hemorrhage with white center. Fluorescein angiogram revealed blockage of choroidal fluorescence from the blood (D). His laboratory investigations revealed hemoglobin of 3.4 with a hematocrit of 9.6, a platelet count of 4000, and a white blood cell count of 4000, suggesting severe pancytopenia. Computed tomography of the head was normal. Bone marrow biopsy confirmed acute lymphocytic leukemia of T-cell lineage. He was treated with intrathecal methotrexate weekly, vincristine, 6-thioguanine, and Bactrim and received several blood transfusions and platelet transfusions. The visual acuity improved to 20/50 in the right eye and 20/100 in the left eye. Two months later hemorrhages resolved with some pallor to the optic disc and residual pigmentary changes in the macula (E, F).

(Courtesy of Dr. William Mieler.)

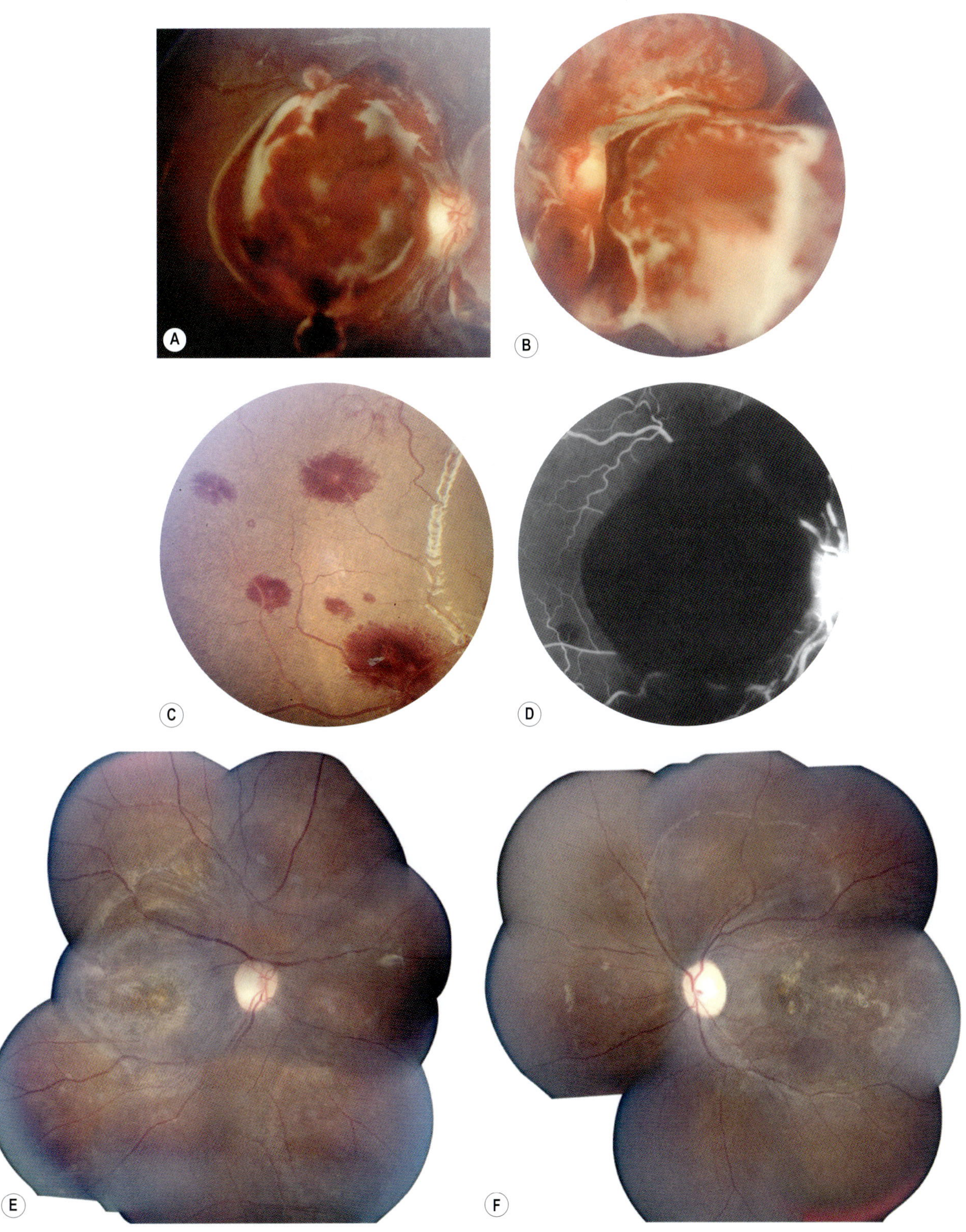
A
B
C
D
E
F

13.28 Leukemic infiltration of the optic nerve.

A and **B**: This 6-year-old girl developed leukemic transformation of a lymphosarcoma of the mediastinum. In June 1970 she was treated with a regimen of vincristine, methotrexate, and prednisone. Remission was achieved, but by September the child developed signs and symptoms of central nervous system involvement. Intrathecal methotrexate was given on September 1, 1970. On September 10, 1970, her vision in the right eye was light perception with projection and the left eye was 20/20. The right optic nerve head and peripapillary retina (K) were swollen and white in color. This was presumed to be related to leukemic infiltration. The optic disc in the left eye was normal. A subconjunctival injection of triamcinolone was given, and a course of oral prednisone, 20 mg three times per day, was begun. On October 15, 1970 visual acuity was 20/20 in each eye. The swelling of the right optic disc had largely disappeared (L). There was loss of pigment from the retinal pigment epithelium associated with multiple black clumps of pigment surrounding the optic disc. Her general condition deteriorated, and she died on December 27, 1970.

C–H: This 37-year-old male with T-cell acute lymphocytic leukemia, diagnosed 6 months earlier, had received five cycles of hypercentral venous access device chemotherapy that consisted of cyclophosphamide, vincristine, Adriamycin, and daunorubicin 4 months ago. He had suffered sudden loss of vision in his right eye 6 days previously that he described as "vision with dark sunglasses" that was intermittent for a day, then remained permanently dark thereafter. He had a similar episode in the left eye 4 months previously and did not recover vision. He received intravenous steroids but ophthalmic examination was not sought. His vision was light perception on the right and no light perception on the left. The optic nerve was pale and swollen with peripapillary and macular whitening, cherry-red spot and boxcarring of the blood column in the arteries. There were several retinal hemorrhages in the posterior pole (C–E). The left optic nerve was pale and cupped with an artery-to-artery collateral superior to the disc. A fluorescein angiogram revealed almost no blood flow through the branches of the central retinal artery at the disc both early and late (G and H). He received radiation to the optic nerve and chemotherapy via an Ommaya reservoir, but his vision did not improve.

I–K: This 20-year-old mentally challenged male with chronic myeloid leukemia went into blast crisis and noted loss of vision in both eyes. The left eye had a dense vitreous hemorrhage while the right eye had leukemic infiltration of the optic nerve (I). He received 24 Gy external-beam radiation to both orbits over 2.5 weeks. The infiltrates thinned out over 8 weeks (J and K) but vision did not improve subjectively. An accurate assessment of his visual acuity could not be made due to his mental status.

(I–K, courtesy of Dr. Franco Recchia.)

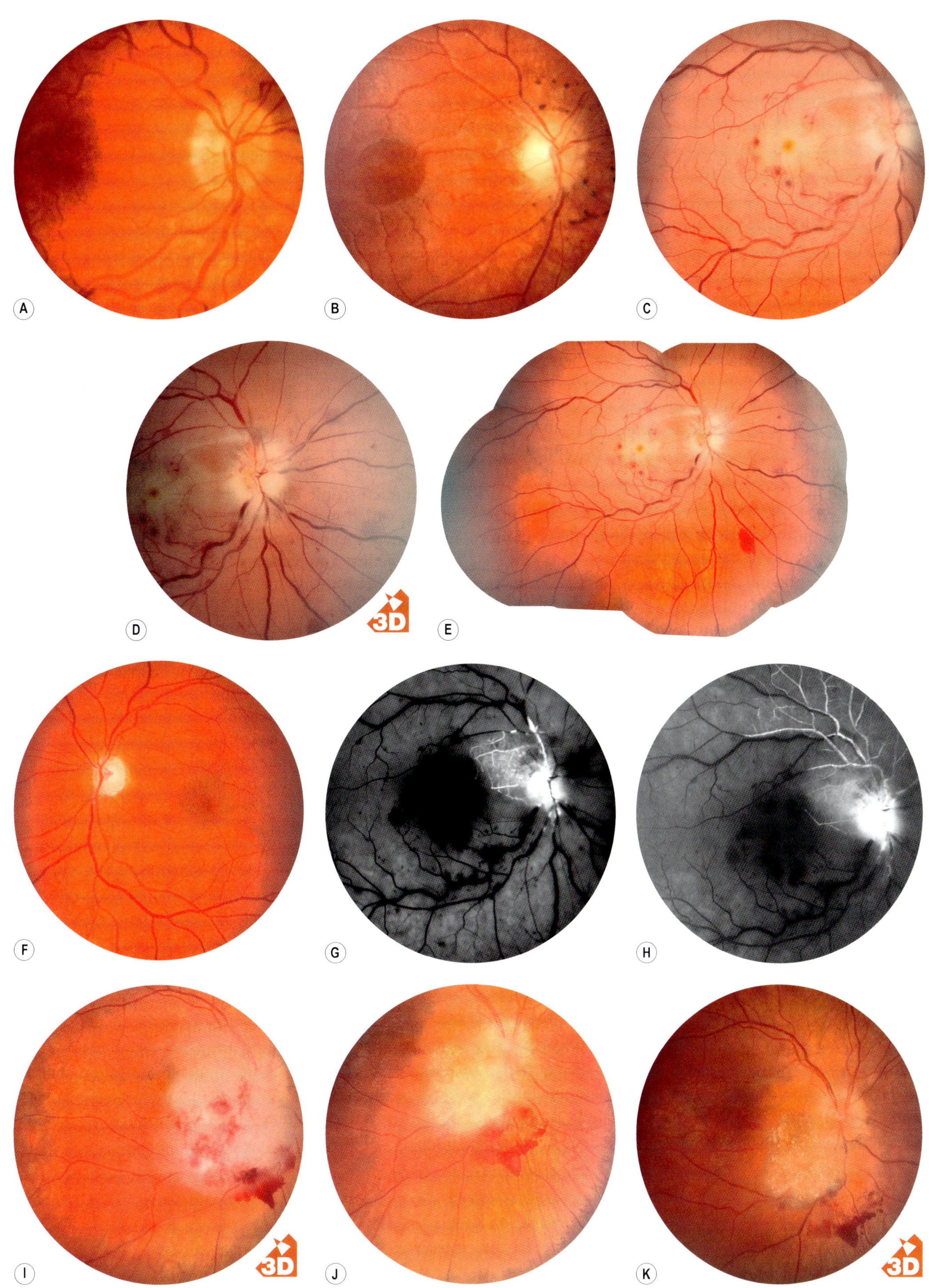
A
B
C
D
3D
E
F
G
H
I
3D
J
K
3D

If large cell lymphoma is suspected the patient should have a general medical evaluation, including neurologic examination, MRI scan, and lumbar puncture. In most cases this evaluation will be negative. Examination of the cerebrospinal fluid in some patients may demonstrate lymphocytosis but infrequently demonstrates the presence of malignant cells. Vitreous biopsy may be necessary to confirm the diagnosis.[329–337] This should be done only when an experienced team for cytologic evaluation is available. Even under the best of circumstances, after obtaining the vitreous specimen, proper concentrating and staining of the vitreous cells, and examination by a skilled cytologist, a definitive diagnosis may not be possible. In some patients cytologic examination of the vitreous aspirant may reveal only inflammatory cells.[333] Direct biopsy of the choroid–RPE complex in the area of a visible lesion offers the best chance for a definitive diagnosis but the procedure has a higher morbidity.[338] If the evaluation of the patient reveals evidence of a CNS lesion, a CT-guided stereotactic biopsy is an effective means of arriving at a diagnosis.[339,340] Cytologic examination is more important than lymphocyte surface markers in arriving at the correct diagnosis of large-cell lymphoma.[331,341] Irregular nuclear contours, lobation of nuclei, coarse irregular chromatin, and the presence of nucleoli are cytologic features of large-cell lymphoma (Figure 13.30J). Ancillary techniques include immunohistochemistry and flow cytometry to determine the immunophenotypes of lymphocytes, gene rearrangement studies, and measurement of interleukin levels.[342–344]

Histopathologically patients with ocular–CNS large cell lymphoma typically show multiple areas of lymphomatous infiltration of the sub-RPE space (Figure 13.30F–H).[9,307,336,345,346] The large sub-RPE lesions are composed primarily of necrotic tumor that is separated from Bruch's membrane by a thin layer of viable hyperchromatic tumor cells (Figure 13.30F–H). In most patients the uveal tract is free of tumor but is infiltrated with lymphocytes, mostly reactive T lymphocytes, and plasma cells (Figure 13.30H). In some cases the tumor may extend into the underlying choroid or the overlying retina and vitreous (Figure 13.31G–L). Histopathologic examination of eyes after spontaneous resolution of the lymphoma shows multiple geographic areas of RPE atrophy or placoid disciform scars that may simulate either postinflammatory scars or a diffuse chorioretinal dystrophy.[9,307]

13.30. Primary central nervous system lymphoma confined to vitreous/retinal pigment epithelium (RPE)/retina (PCNS-O lymphoma).

A–H: This 60-year-old woman was seen in December 1968 with widespread areas of solid yellow-white detachments of the RPE in her left eye (A, B, and D). Angiographically these lesions were largely nonfluorescent (C). Medical evaluation was negative. These lesions disappeared spontaneously and the patient had 20/20 vision (E). When she returned 4 years later there were widespread RPE atrophic changes in the left eye. In the right eye she had the same picture, illustrated in the left eye in D. Ten weeks later she died after experiencing jacksonian seizures. Gross examination of the right eye revealed multiple necrotic white tumors beneath the detached RPE (arrows, F). Note detachment of the thinned and clumped RPE (upper arrow, G) and liquefactive necrosis of tumor between the RPE and viable tumor lying along the inner surface of Bruch's membrane (lower arrow, G). Viable reticulum cell sarcoma (arrow) was lying along the inner surface of Bruch's membrane (H). Note chronic inflammatory cells in the choroid.

I–K: Subpigment epithelial lymphoma in a 62-year-old man after vitrectomy. Note tumor (arrow, I) breaking through the RPE. Vitreous aspirate showed cells with enlarged hyperchromatic indented nuclei and minimal cytoplasm (arrow, J) characteristic of reticulum cell sarcoma. Resolution of tumor occurred 5 months after external-beam irradiation (K).

(A–K, from Gass et al.[307])

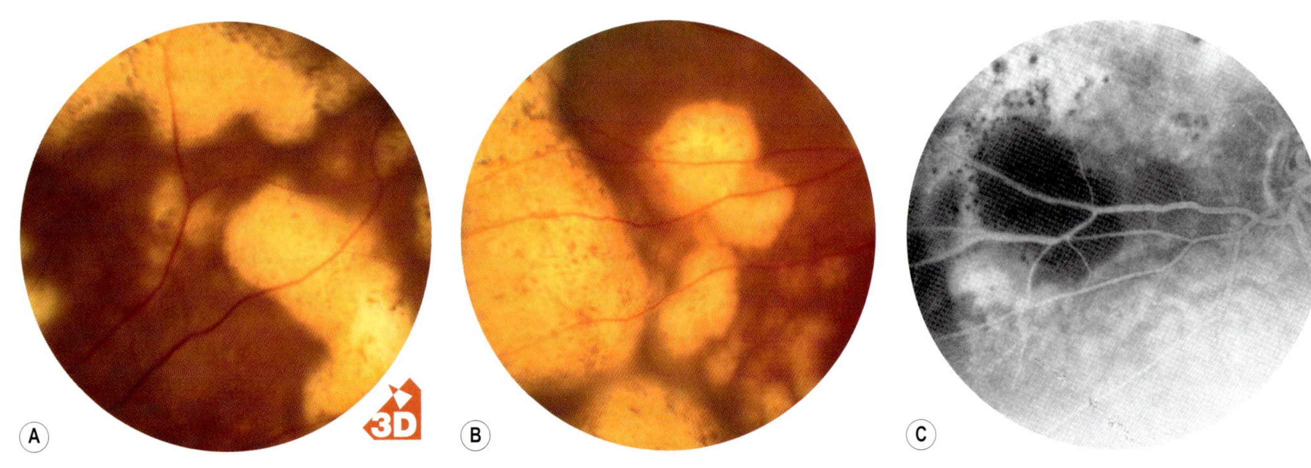

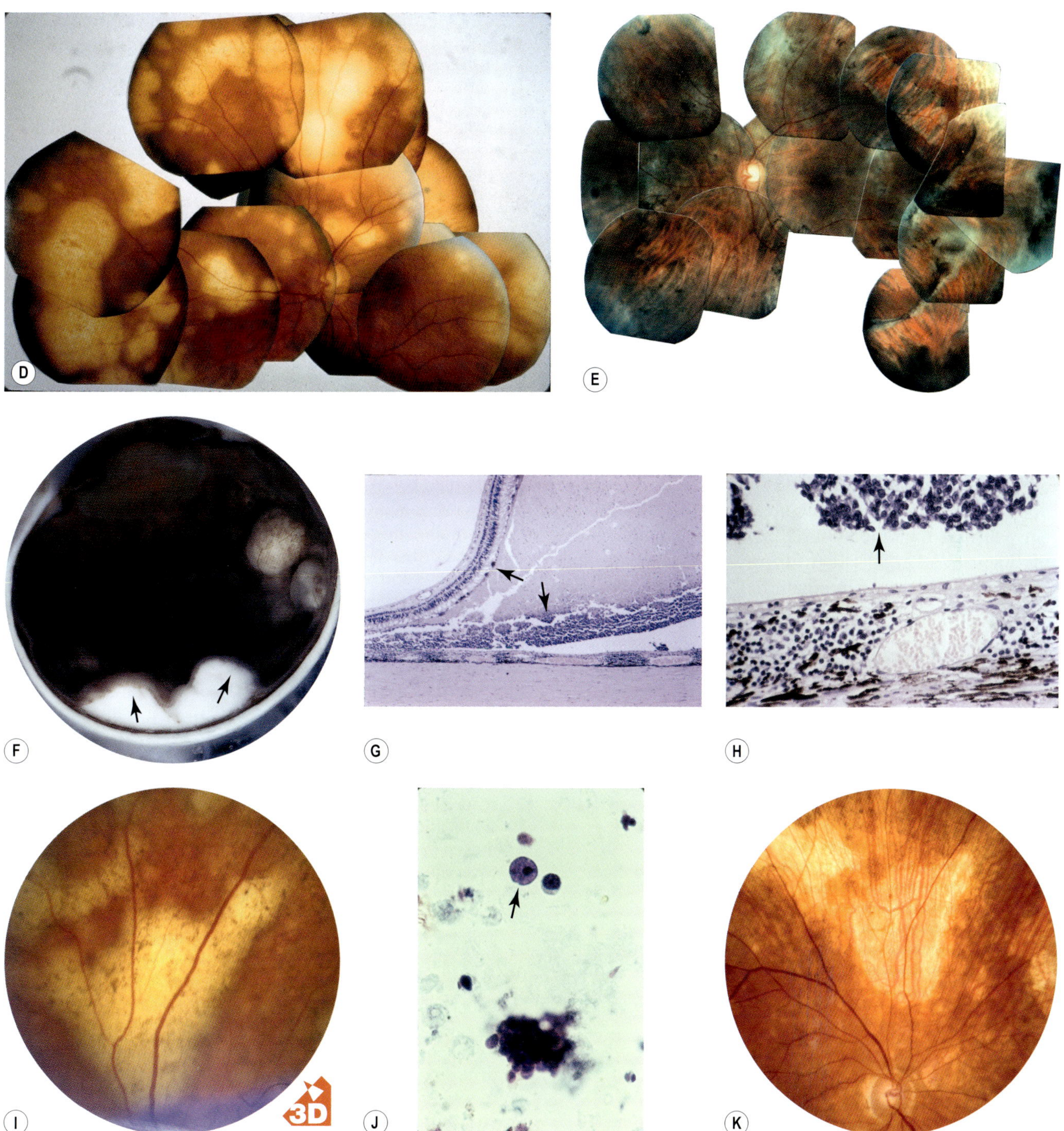
D
E
F
G
H
I
3D
J
K

Management of PCNSL-O with ocular radiation (40 Gy in divided doses) controls ocular involvement in the majority of cases, but most progress to develop CNS disease.[328] Because radiation therapy to the brain may have significant side-effects, its use for prophylaxis in patients without proven CNS involvement is not advisable. Systemic therapy may not be sufficient for treatment of PCNSL-O.[347] Intravitreal methotrexate (400 µg/0.1 ml) given over a period of 1 year according to a standard induction–consolidation–maintenance regimen appears to provide excellent control rates with minimal toxicity.[348] Intravitreal injections of rituximab (anti-CD20 antibody; 1 mg/0.1 ml) are under investigation.[349,350]

For CNS involvement, high-dose methotrexate is usually considered.[351,352] As the blood–brain barrier is a limiting factor that restricts drug entry into the CNS, intrathecal drug delivery, intraventricular drug delivery by a reservoir, and disruption of the blood–brain barrier with mannitol infusion are generally used.[309,353] Disruption of the blood–brain barrier with mannitol infusion may inadvertently disrupt the blood–retinal barrier causing maculopathy (Figure 13.32).[354] The treatment of PCNSL is evolving within a framework of international multidisciplinary collaborative studies.[355]

13.31 Primary central nervous system lymphoma confined to vitreous/retinal pigment epithelium (RPE)/ retina (PCNS-O lymphoma).

A–F: This 56-year-old woman noted blurred vision and floaters in the right eye. Vitritis and multiple small white or gray-white subretinal lesions confined to the right eye were interpreted as multiple evanescent white-dot syndrome (arrows, A). When examined 1 month later her visual acuity was 5/200, right eye, and 20/20, left eye. She had developed a sub-RPE mass (arrow, B) and a Swiss cheeselike subretinal infiltration in the right eye. Angiography showed evidence of RPE changes centrally as well as staining in the area of the infiltrate. The right eye was normal. The diagnosis was large-cell lymphoma with probable involvement of the retrobulbar optic nerve. Medical evaluation was negative. Four months later the tumor had resolved temporally but had extended nasally (C). Repeated evaluations for evidence of lymphoma were negative. She refused vitreous biopsy. The lesions in the right eye resolved spontaneously and over the subsequent 40 months she developed similar lesions in the left eye. Vitreous biopsy was positive for lymphoma. Three years after her onset of symptoms she developed evidence of lymphoma in the brain. She received irradiation treatment to the eyes and brain. When last examined her visual acuity was 20/200, right eye, and 20/400, left eye. There was widespread evidence of degeneration of the RPE but no evidence of tumor in either eye (E and F). Five years after her initial visit she was alive and tumorfree. Forgetfulness and depression were attributed to postirradiation changes.

G–L: This apparently healthy 71-year-old woman developed a superotemporal branch retinal artery occlusion caused by intraretinal invasion of a sub-RPE lymphoma in the right eye (G). At the time of initial presentation she had vitreous cellular infiltration and multiple atrophic chorioretinal scars in the right eye. The left eye was normal except for a single focal scar and lesions in the macula interpreted as drusen. Six weeks later the retinal whitening extended into other quadrants (H) and multiple yellow plaques (arrows) had developed in the formally occluded retinal artery. Angiographically there was evidence of narrowing of the artery caliber in the area of these plaques (arrows, I). She subsequently developed the clinical picture of acute retinal necrosis and rubeotic glaucoma in the right eye that was enucleated. Histopathologic examination revealed large mounds of necrotic lymphoma beneath the RPE, extensive retinal necrosis, tumor invasion of the retinal arteries, and occlusion of the artery (arrow, K) on the optic disc and narrowing of the retinal artery (arrows, L) by tumor and atheromatous deposits. Medical evaluation for other evidence of lymphoma was negative. She developed multiple focal lesions simulating choroiditis in the left eye (J). Note that some were hypofluorescent (arrows, J). Fourteen months after her initial presentation she developed hemiparesis and brain scan evidence of a lymphoma.

(G–L, from Gass and Trattler.[322])

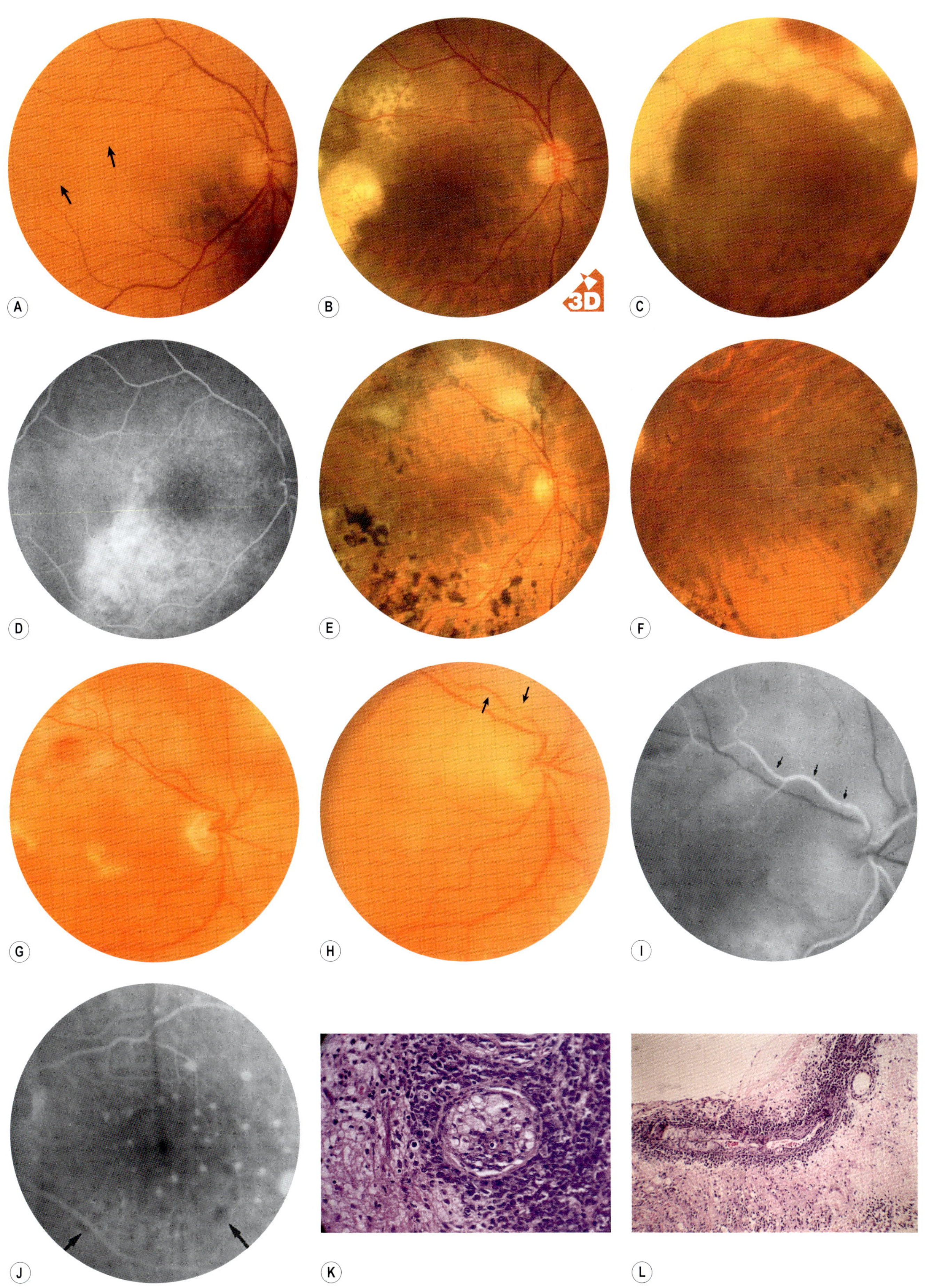
A
B
3D
C
D
E
F
G
H
I
J
K
L

Mycosis Fungoides

Mycosis fungoides, a malignant lymphomatous disease derived from T lymphocytes, arises in the skin and may be confused with psoriasis. Later it may involve other body organs. It infrequently affects the CNS and eye.[362–365] Infiltration of the iris,[366] vitreous,[363,367,368] choroid,[369] sub-RPE space,[368,370] optic nerve, and retina[362,363,367] has been reported.

Lymphocytic Lymphoma

Lymphocytic lymphoma only rarely involves the eye (Figure 13.34J–L).[326,371] Lewis and Clark[371] reported a peculiar pattern of widespread retinal infiltration in a 48-year-old woman with a well-differentiated lymphocytic lymphoma involving the abdominal, cervical, and submandibular areas. Retinal infiltration cleared within 1 month following treatment with cyclophosphamide, vincristine, and oral prednisone.

13.32 Blood–brain barrier disruption maculopathy.

A–F: A 66-year-old Caucasian woman was diagnosed with central nervous system lymphoma after presenting with confusion and headache. She began blood–brain barrier disruption therapy 2 months later and underwent 23 treatments (divided into 12 cycles); five were given through the right internal carotid artery, 8 through the left internal carotid artery, and the remaining through the vertebral artery system. One cycle was aborted early after an arterial dissection was seen on angiography. Baseline examination revealed best-corrected visual acuity of 20/30 in the right eye and 20/25 in the left eye; no retinal pigment epithelium (RPE) changes were found on fundus examination. The patient first noted visual disturbances in the form of "spots of gray clouds" after four treatments; acute exacerbations in these subjective visual complaints occurred during each treatment and then returned to baseline. These disturbances remained stable throughout and were still present 1 year after completion of therapy. Macular RPE changes in the form of speckled hyperpigmentation were first documented after completion of therapy, at which time best-corrected visual acuity was 20/40, right eye, and 20/50, left eye (A). Humphrey visual field testing revealed an inferior right-sided homonymous hemianopia secondary to the patient's brain tumor and a small paracentral scotoma in the right eye. Four months later, visual acuity was stable in the right eye (20/40) and decreased in the left eye (20/200) with increasing atrophy and proliferation of the RPE noted on clinical examination (B). Fluorescein angiogram revealed bilateral early focal hyperfluorescence which faded in late phase and focal hypofluorescence in the maculas (C, D). Optical coherence tomography was consistent with mild cystoid macular edema in the right eye and irregular thickening of the RPE in the left eye (E, F).

Primary central nervous system lymphoma confined to vitreous/RPE/retina (PCNS-O lymphoma) lymphoma simulating multifocal choroiditis and acute retinal necrosis.

G–L: This 53-year-old male was observed for gradual onset of low-grade vitreous cells and a few deep flat choroidal lesions over 9 months in his right eye. He became symptomatic with floaters and photopsias when the vitreous cells increased. At that time he was noted to have in addition a few flat new deep choroidal lesions in the left eye and had a visual acuity of 20/40 on the right and 20/20 on the left (G and H). A diagnosis of multifocal choroiditis was made and started on oral steroids after ensuring he was negative for rapid plasma reagin, chest X-ray, and other infectious causes. His symptoms improved and vitreous cells cleared over 3 weeks, but by 6 weeks the number of choroidal lesions increased in both eyes. Discontinuing steroids and a diagnostic vitrectomy yielded a "reactive lymphoid population of cells." He was started on intravenous acyclovir with a presumed diagnosis of herpetic retinitis; the right eye lesions stabilized and became pigmented postvitrectomy; however, the left eye continued to progress with inner retinitis and hemorrhages resembling acute retinal necrosis (I and J). Seeing continued progression of the left-eye lesions, antifungal voriconazole was added. Further progression of inner retinitis (K) and hemorrhages prompted a vitrectomy and retinal biopsy of the left eye, which was diagnostic of primary ocular lymphoma. Systemic evaluation for central nervous system involvement was negative for 2.5 years, after which he developed a lesion in the pons. He received systemic chemotherapy, supplemental intraocular methotrexate, and is negative for cells in his cerebrospinal fluid and eye for the past 5 years. Both retinas now show pigmented punched-out scars simulating multifocal choroiditis (L). His final visual acuity is 20/20 on the right and 20/30– on the left following cataract surgery and stabilization of the lesions.

(A–F, from Galor et al.,[354] with permission.)

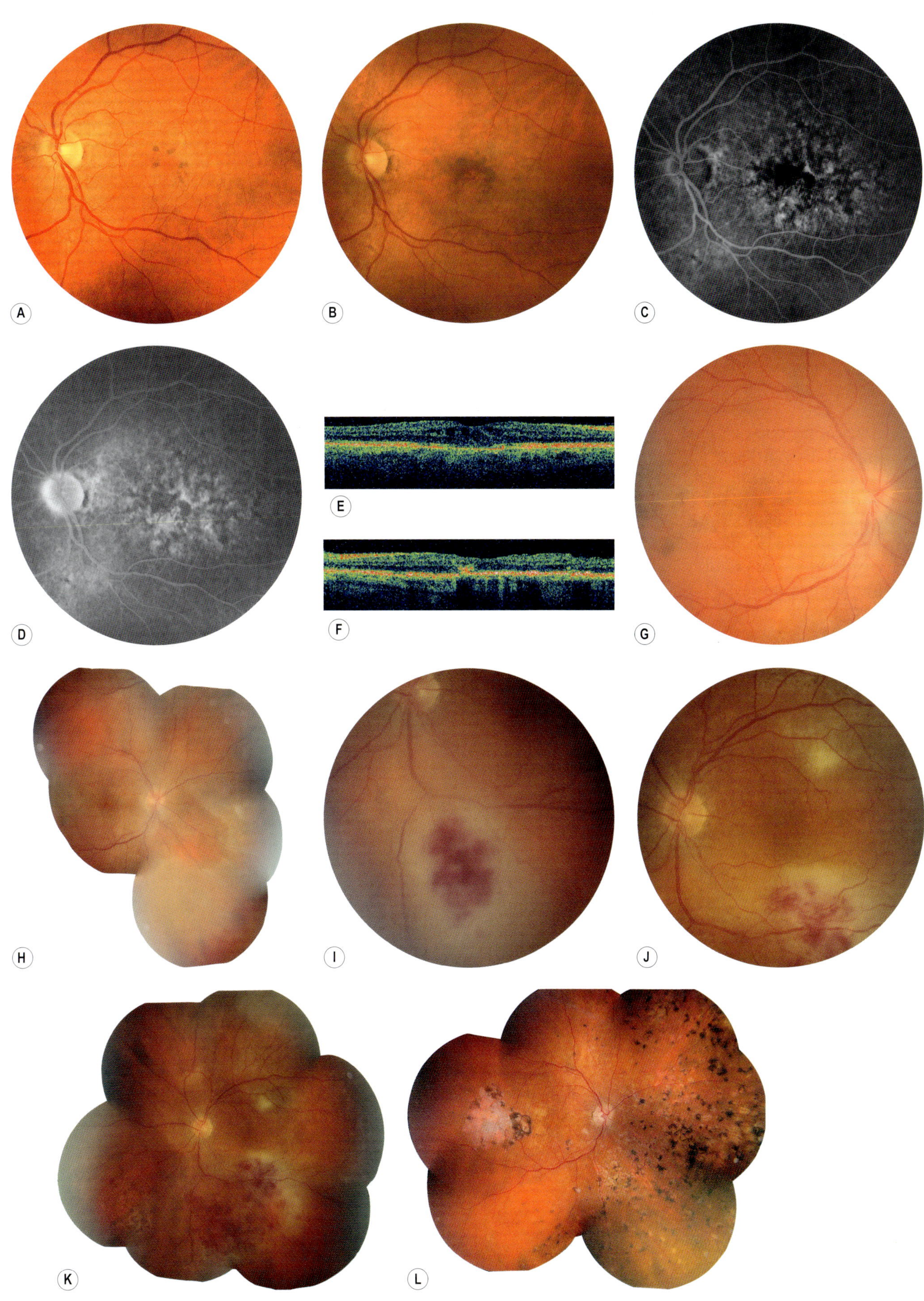
A
B
C
D
E
F
G
H
I
J
K
L

OTHER LYMPHOMAS AND RELATED CONDITIONS

Adult T-Cell Leukemia/Lymphoma

Adult T-cell leukemia/lymphoma is a recently described clinicopathologic entity characterized by an extremely aggressive course, a leukemic or lymphomatous proliferation of hyperlobated peripheral T cells, and an association with infection by a retrovirus, human T-lymphotropic virus type 1 (HTLV-1).[356,357] These patients develop infiltration of multiple organ systems, which may include a pattern of intraocular involvement similar to that in patients with ocular–CNS non-Hodgkin's lymphoma[358] and acute retinal necrosis (Figure 13.33).[359–361] The latter presents with retinal and perivascular infiltrates affecting both arteries and veins, resembling frosted-branch angiitis, retinal vasculitis, cytomegalovirus retinitis, and acute retinal necrosis. Hemorrhages around the infiltrates are not a prominent feature, unlike cytomegalovirus and herpetic retinitis (Figure 13.33B, C, G, and H). Poor response to antivirals, or a patient from an endemic area for HTLV-1 virus such as Japan, South America, the Caribbean islands and French West Indies and tropical Africa, should alert the clinician to consider HTLV-1 retinitis/adult T-cell leukemia/lymphoma in the diagnosis.

The virus also causes a myelopathy called HTLV-associated myelopathy. The provirus HTLV-1 integrates randomly in the genome of the host cell without a preferential insertion site. The integration is monoclonal in adult T-cell leukemia/lymphoma patients and polyclonal in the lymphoid cells of the peripheral blood of patients with HTLV-associated myelopathy. Most ocular lymphomas are of B-cell origin. HTLV-1-induced intraocular lymphoma is a rare cause of T-cell lymphoma: the others spread to the eye from mycosis fungoides, peripheral T-cell lymphoma, and Sézary syndrome (see Chapter 14).

13.33 Adult T-cell leukemia/lymphoma (human T-lymphotrophic virus: HTLV).

A–L: This 39-year-old Caucasian woman presented with gradual, painless decrease in vision in her right eye over 2 months, not associated with redness, photophobia, or photopsias. She had received a stem cell transplant 3 years previously for adult T-cell leukemia/lymphoma and was presently in remission. She had had several infectious complications over the previous 3 years, including *Pseudomonas* and *Streptococcus* bacteremia, cytomegalovirus reactivation, *Alternaria/Moraxella* sinusitis, mucocutaneous graft-versus-host disease, bronchiolitis obliterans, and hypertension. She was receiving Ceftin for a recent sinusitis and fever to 102.8°F (39.3°C), Combivent, prednisone 15 mg, azithromycin, and Advair. Visual acuity was 20/70 right eye and 20/20 left eye with a moderate afferent papillary defect on the right, 3/11 color plates on the right, and 11/11 on the left. The vitreous was full of debris and membranes (A) and obscured some of the retinal changes that consisted of a swollen optic nerve with infiltrates within it, retinitis, and perivascular whitish infiltrates with feathery borders resembling frosted-branch angiitis (B and C). The left fundus was normal with no vitreous cells (D). Angiogram revealed breakdown of the blood–retinal barrier with diffuse leakage from the vessels in the posterior fundus and staining of the optic disc and areas of retinitis (E and F). She was started on intravenous ganciclovir; aqueous sample returned negative for cytomegalovirus (CMV), herpes simplex virus (HSV), and herpes zoster virus by polymerase chain reaction (PCR). Serum toxoplasma and rapid plasma reagin were negative. Multiple cerebrospinal fluid samples were negative for malignant cells and infection. Magnetic resonance imaging of the brain and orbits revealed no new pathology. After no response to systemic valganciclovir and equivocal response to 60 mg prednisone for 2 weeks each, a diagnostic vitrectomy was performed. Vitreous samples were negative for viral, fungal, bacterial cultures, negative PCR for parvo B19, HSV-1 and -2, varicella-zoster virus, CMV, human immunodeficiency virus, H6D and H7D. PCR for HTLV1 and 2 was not available. The vitreous cytology was read as: "mixed inflammatory infiltrate, with weak CD3-positive and CD20-negative lymphocytes, likely reactive and not diagnostic of a lymphoid malignancy." Postvitrectomy the media cleared, and there was a hint of reduction in the extent of the perivascular infiltrates (G). The vision gradually decreased to 20/100, and the patient left on a cross-country trip on an empiric treatment of 15 mg of weekly methotrexate. She returned 6 weeks later with further decrease in vision to count fingers at 1 foot (30 cm) and increase in the extent of the retinal changes (H). A repeat vitrectomy and a touch prep of a retinal biopsy revealed cells consistent with T-cell leukemia/lymphoma (I, J). Flow cytology showed large CD3+ T cells that coexpressed CD4 and CD25. In the meanwhile the left optic disc became swollen (K) and she developed small "snowballs" in the inferior vitreous. An aggressive chemotherapy regimen with high-dose methotrexate via the Ommaya reservoir over the next 3 months resolved the optic disc infiltrates and she has remained disease-free in her left eye (L) with a visual acuity of 20/20 for 2 + years. The right-eye vision remains at light perception.

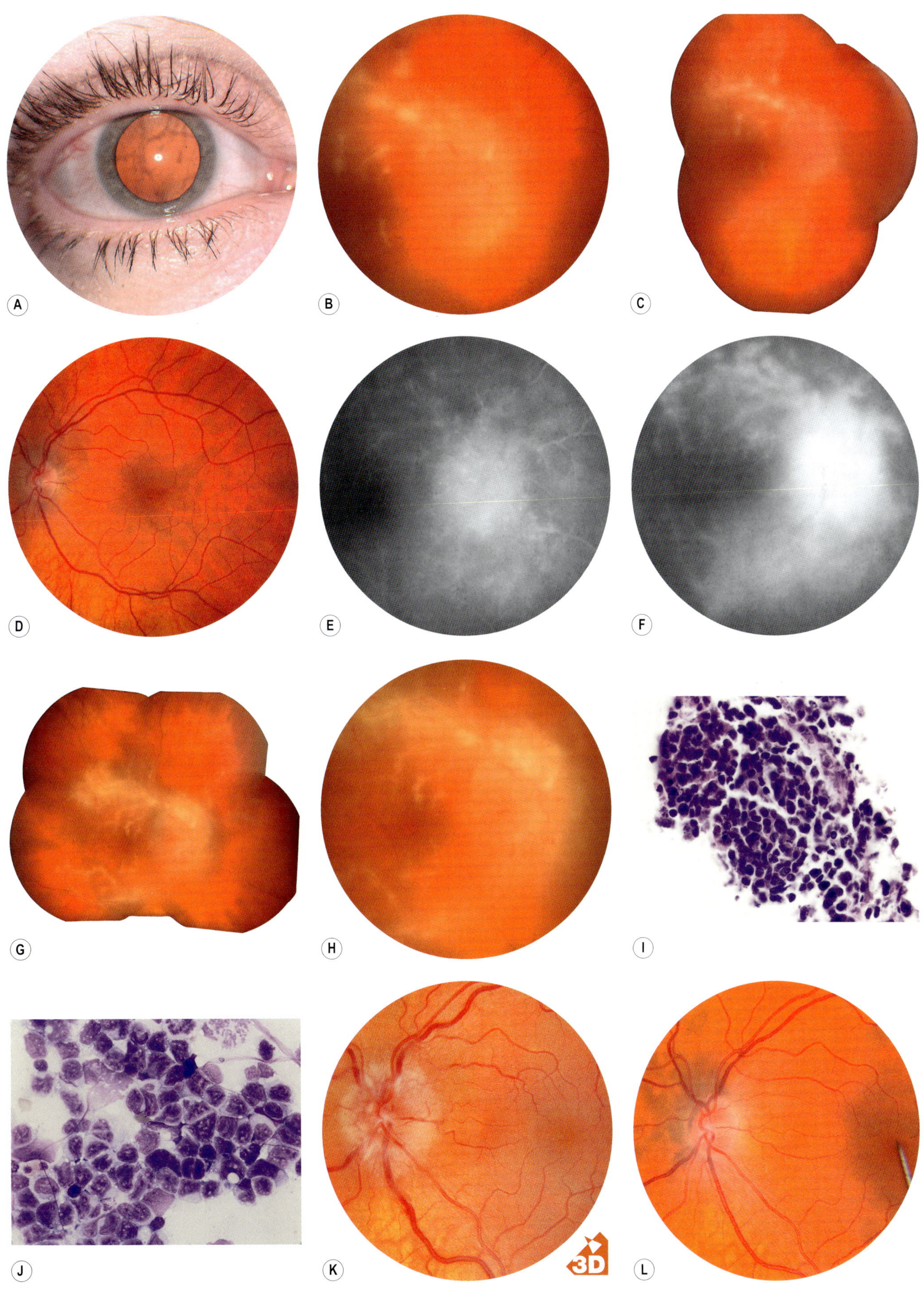
A
B
C
D
E
F
G
H
I
J
K
L
3D

Richter Transformation

Richter transformation is development of high-grade non-Hodgkin lymphoma or Hodgkin lymphoma in patients with chronic lymphocytic leukemia or small lymphocytic lymphoma.[378] Bilateral vitreous cells in a patient with large B-cell lymphoma representing Richter transformation have also been observed.[379]

Angioendotheliomatosis

Neoplastic angioendotheliomatosis is a rare form of extranodal large cell lymphoma characterized by multifocal proliferation of neoplastic mononuclear cells within the lumen of blood vessels. It is a rare, fatal disease characterized by widespread intravascular proliferations of malignant cells of putative endothelial origin. Clinically, fever of unknown origin and dermatologic and bizarre neurologic manifestations predominate. Ocular changes include iridocyclitis, keratic precipitates, vitritis, papilledema, and retinal vascular alterations, including hemorrhages and retinal artery occlusion.[380–382] Infiltration of the choroid producing a clinical picture simulating Harada's disease may occur occasionally. Histologically, there is panuveal involvement with granulomatous iridocyclitis in addition to vascular and secondary pigmentary changes resembling somewhat hypertensive choroidopathy. The vascular endothelial cells show signs of malignant transformation.

13.34 Retinal involvement simulating fundus flavimaculatus in systemic large-cell non-Hodgkin's lymphoma.

A–C: This healthy 53-year-old woman noted recent blurring of vision in the right eye. Her visual acuity was 20/25 in the right eye and 20/15 in the left eye. Amsler grid testing revealed paracentral scotomata in the right eye. In the right eye there were 2+ vitreous cells and the fundus showed a reticular pattern of yellowish clumping of pigment simulating fundus flavimaculatus at the level of the retinal pigment epithelium (RPE) throughout the macula and juxtapapillary area (A). There were several areas of subretinal white infiltration superonasally (B). The left eye was normal. Early angiograms revealed the pigment clumps to be hypofluorescent on a background of greater than normal choroidal fluorescence (C). There was late staining in the area of the white infiltrate. Angiograms of the left eye were normal. Medical evaluation for inflammatory and neoplastic disease was negative. Her visual blurring gradually improved, and 7 weeks later her visual acuity was 20/20. She still noted slight loss of light and color sensitivity. Six months after the onset of visual symptoms she noted axillary lymphadenopathy. Tumors were discovered in the left supraclavicular area, retroperitoneal area, and left breast. Biopsy revealed a histiocytic, non-Hodgkin's lymphoma (reticulum cell sarcoma). She received systemic corticosteroid and antimetabolite therapy, and 14 months after the onset of visual symptoms she was apparently in remission. She has not returned for eye examination but can read the newspaper with the right eye and is still asymptomatic in the left eye.
D–I: This apparently healthy 67-year-old man developed blurred vision in the left eye in association with a fundus picture simulating fundus flavimaculatus (D). Angiography (E and F) was similar to that in (C). His visual acuity was 20/20. Medical evaluation was negative. Six weeks later his acuity had declined to 20/80. There was an increase in the damage to the RPE (G–I). Several months later he developed lymphadenopathy. Biopsy revealed a large-cell lymphoma.

Retinal involvement in lymphocytic lymphoma.
J–L: Rapid visual loss occurred in both eyes of a 48-year-old woman caused by well-differentiated lymphocytic lymphoma. There was marked retinal perivascular and optic disc infiltration in both eyes. This infiltration cleared within a month of cobalt irradiation treatment, and visual acuity improved from counting fingers to 20/60 in both eyes.

(A–I, from Gass et al.[457]; J–L, from Lewis and Clark[371] published with permission from The American Journal of Ophthalmology; copyright by The Ophthalmic Publishing Co. J and K also, Yannuzzi, Lawrence J., The Retinal Atlas, Saunders 2010, 978-0-7020-3320-9, p.706.)

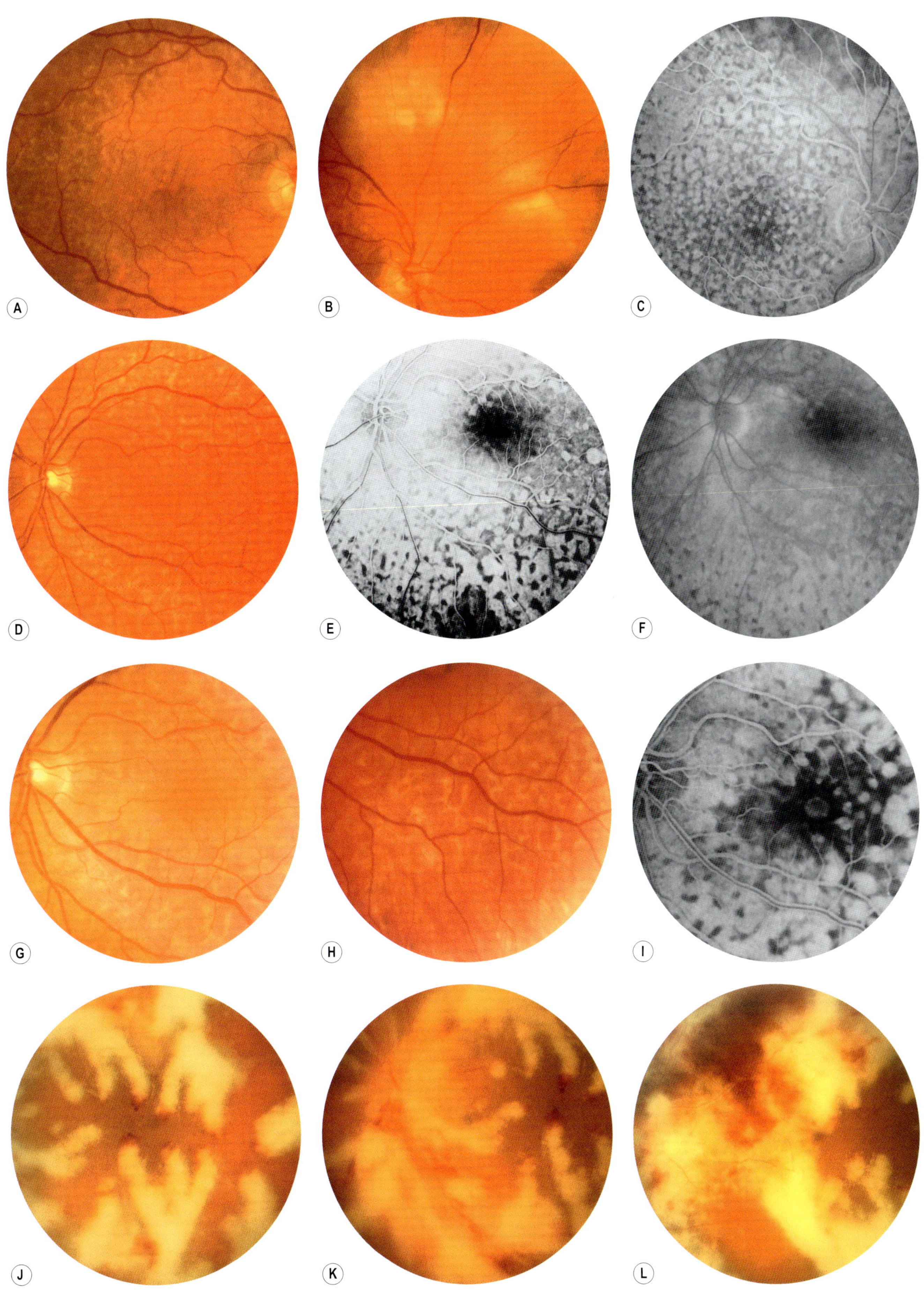
A
B
C
D
E
F
G
H
I
J
K
L

Multiple Myeloma

Multiple myeloma is a neoplastic disease of plasma cells that in its advanced stages produces osteoporosis, punched-out bony lesions, multiple fractures, and bone tumors. Proptosis caused by bony involvement may be the first sign of the disease.[372] Rarely, the optic nerve may be infiltrated and cause a picture of optic neuritis and, in some cases, central retinal artery occlusion.[373,374] One patient seen at Bascom Palmer Eye Institute with optic nerve involvement responded promptly to external-beam irradiation (Figure 13.35).[9] Ciliary body plasmacytoma,[375] choroidal plasmacytoma,[376] and even vitritis and retinal vasculitis as manifestations of multiple myeloma have been observed.[377] More often patients with multiple myeloma and Waldenström's macroglobulinemia present with clinical features secondary to hypercoagulation. Serous retinal detachments due to their osmotic properties of absorbing fluid are seen, when high-molecular-weight immunoglobulins enter the subretinal space. They characteristically do not leak fluorescein dye since the outer blood–retinal barrier is not broken (see Chapter 3). Anemic retinopathy with deep inkblot-like retinal hemorrhages occurs when the bone marrow is infiltrated with myeloma cells (see Chapter 6).

Lymphomatoid Granulomatosis

Lymphomatoid granulomatosis is an angiocentric and angiodestructive lymphoproliferative disorder that predominantly affects lungs. Epstein–Barr virus RNA can be detected in most cases. In advanced cases, there is an overlap with large B-cell lymphoma.[383] Most ophthalmic manifestations of the disease are the result of cranial nerve involvement. Intraocular involvement, however, may manifest as granulomatous posterior uveitis,[384] or fundus picture simulating acute posterior multifocal placoid pigment epitheliopathy.[385] A case with bilateral exudative retinal detachments that responded to oral steroids has also been reported.[386]

Posttransplant Lymphoproliferative Disorder

Posttransplant immunosuppression can be associated with Epstein–Barr virus-induced lymphoproliferative disorder which may manifest as intraocular lymphoma.[387–389] Demols et al.[389] reported a 59-year-old man with single-lung transplant who developed a chorioretinal lesion that was initially suspected to be cytomegalovirus retinitis or toxoplasmic retinochoroiditis. Vitreous biopsy revealed monoclonal proliferation of B lymphocytes. Immunoglobulin gene rearrangement and Epstein–Barr virus were detected by polymerase chain reaction. Reduction of immunosuppression led to regression of the lesion.[389]

13.35 Hemorrhagic optic neuropathy and visual loss caused by multiple myeloma.

A–D: This 67-year-old woman reported blurred vision in the left eye of 1 week's duration. Visual acuity was 20/30 in the right eye and counting fingers at 8 foot (2.44 meters) in the left eye. The right fundus was normal. There were some cells in the vitreous of the left eye. Note cotton-wool patches and opacification (arrows, A) of the optic nerve head posterior to the hemorrhages. Angiography showed minimal capillary dilation and staining of the optic disc (B and C). The clinical impression was myeloma infiltration of the optic nerve. She had a total dose of 2000 rad of cobalt-60 to the posterior pole over a 2-week period. Three months later her visual acuity was 20/70 and the optic disc was slightly pale (D).

Metastasis of systemic tumor to the retina and optic nerve.

E–L: A 55-year-old African American woman suffered a rapid progressive visual change in the left eye over 3 weeks. Her visual acuity was 20/20 in the right eye and 20/400 in the left eye. The right fundus was normal. The left fundus showed a white disc and full-thickness necrosis of the surrounding retina associated with hemorrhages and a serous detachment extending to the macula (E and F). The vessels on the disc and surrounding retina showed focal endothelial decompensation, aneurysm formation, and leakage (G and H). Her serum antibodies to *Toxoplasma*, herpes simplex virus-1 and -2, and varicella-zoster virus were within normal range. Repeated 2-weekly intravitreal ganciclovir injections over 6 weeks did not improve the retinal findings. She suffered a seizure during this time, which led to a computed tomography scan detection of a central nervous system lesion, hilar adenopathy, and a lung biopsy, confirmatory for adenocarcinoma of the lung. A diagnostic vitrectomy, retinal detachment repair and retinal biopsy with silicone oil placement (I) revealed metastatic adenocarcinoma. Hematoxylin and eosin and electron microscopy of the lung lesion (J and L) showed large malignant cells with high nuclear cytoplasmic ratio. Toluidine blue staining of the retinal biopsy revealed tumor cells (K).

(E to L, Courtesy of Dr. Jon Adleberg.)

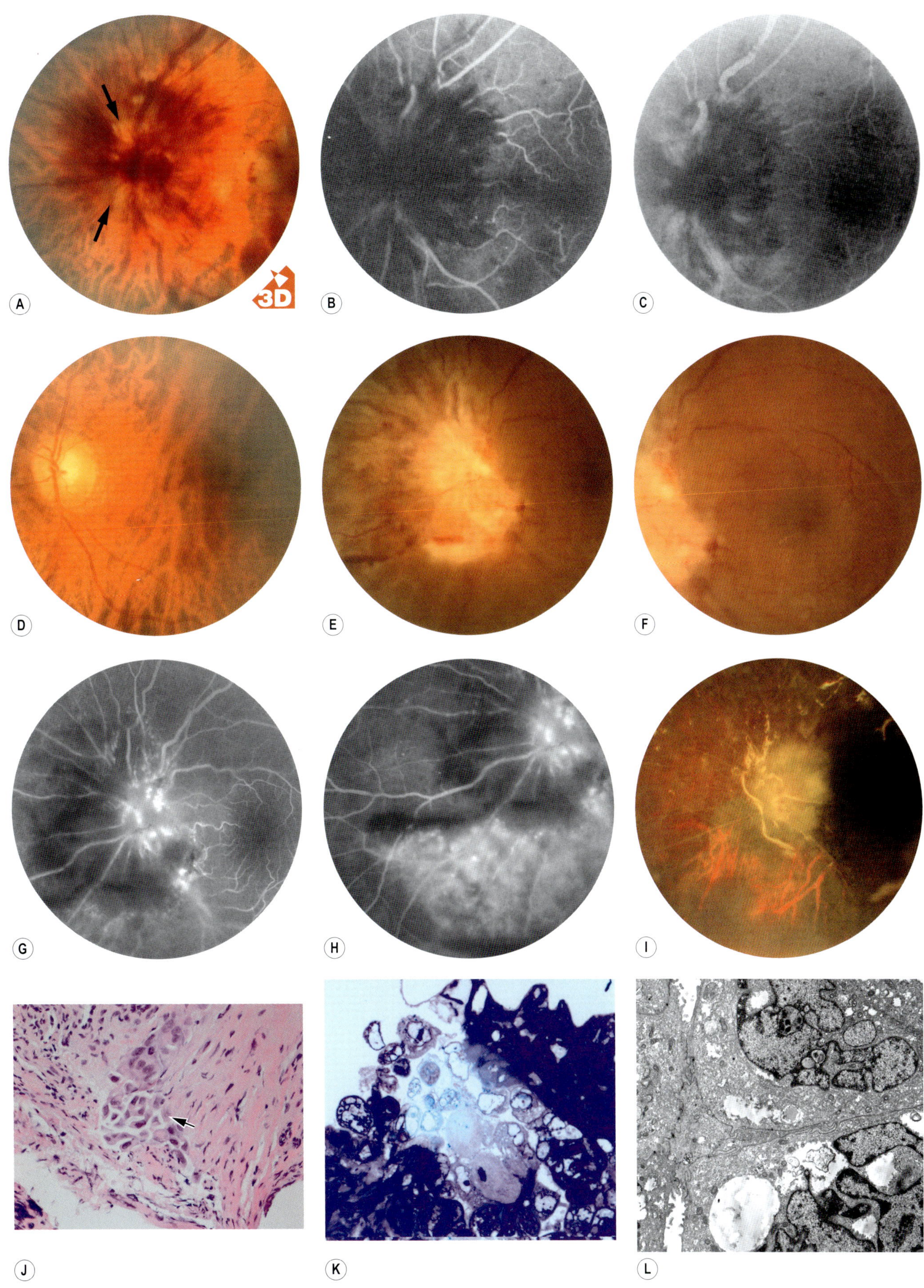
A
3D
B
C
D
E
F
G
H
I
J
K
L

METASTATIC CARCINOMA TO THE RETINA

Metastatic carcinoma to the retina occurs infrequently.[390–402] It usually occurs in one eye but may affect both eyes.[403] Initially the retinal metastasis may be indistinguishable from an ischemic infarct of the retina (Figure 13.36A). As the tumor enlarges, it produces a denser, whitish opacification of the retina that may simulate necrotizing retinitis caused by toxoplasmosis, cytomegalovirus, or other infections (Figure 13.36E). Overlying vitreous cells may or may not be present.[390,391,402] Cytologic examination of the vitreous in such cases may establish the diagnosis.[402,404,405] The borders of metastatic lesions in the retina are more irregular than in choroidal metastasis. In approximately one-half of reported cases, choroidal involvement was also present. Multiple perivascular white infiltrates may accompany the main tumor mass.[402]

13.36 Metastatic carcinoma to the retina and vitreous.

A–D: This 42-year-old woman who had received treatment for metastatic breast carcinoma complained of floaters. Examination revealed coarse vitreous opacities near the surface of the retina (A and B). Fluorescein angiography revealed patchy areas of leaking retinal vessels (C and D). Vitreous biopsy revealed metastatic breast carcinoma.

E–I: This 49-year-old man complained of dizziness, headaches, dysarthria, and right hemiparesis. Examination revealed a solitary white retinal lesion in the left eye (E). Computed tomography and magnetic resonance imaging of the brain revealed multiple nodular lesions (F). Chest roentgenogram revealed enlarged mediastinal nodes and a nodular density in the right middle lobe (G). Postmortem examination of the eyes revealed a solitary metastatic oat cell carcinoma lesion in the retina (H and I). Note that the choroid (arrow, H) is unaffected.

(A–I, from Leys et al.[396])

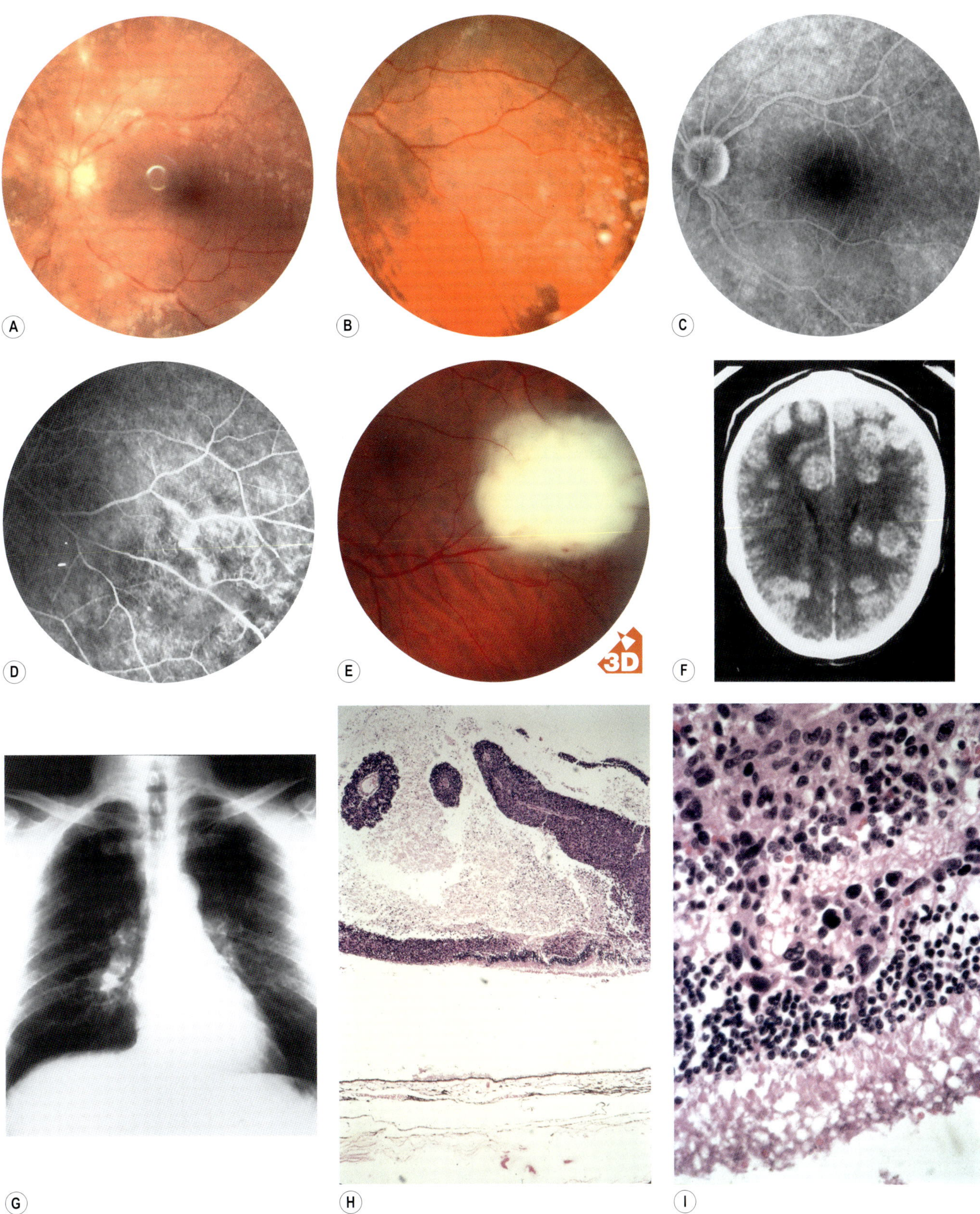
A
B
C
D
E
3D
F
G
H
I

Cutaneous melanoma may occasionally metastasize to the eye, and in approximately 20% of such cases it does so to the retina rather than to the uveal tract (Figure 13.37).[401,402,406–410] In some cases it may metastasize to the vitreous and cause the patient to complain of vitreous floaters that are the result of brown, cellular, spherical clumps of melanoma cells suspended in the vitreous cavity (Figure 13.37A). These cell clumps are sufficiently characteristic and different from the irregular clumps of proliferating RPE cells (tobacco dust) that the diagnosis of metastatic melanoma should be suspected. The vitreous infiltration may be accompanied by superficial gray-brown infiltrates arranged in a dendritic pattern with feathery edges infiltrating the nerve fiber layer of the retina surrounding the optic nerve head (Figure 13.37B). Large, beige-colored plaques or clusters of the tumor cells in the vitreous may partly obscure the fundus from view. In other cases there may be localized irregular plaques of melanoma cells within the retina (Figure 13.37C and D). In spite of subconjunctival injection and systemic treatment with antimetabolites, the tumor in the eye may proliferate and cause rubeosis and secondary glaucoma.[410]

The reasons for the rarity of metastatic cancer to the retina compared to the uveal tract are uncertain. Differences in blood flow (turbulent flow in the choroid versus laminar flow in the retina), absence of fenestrations in the retinal vascular endothelium, and inhibitory factors present in the vitreous are possibly important.[411]

13.37 Metastatic cutaneous melanoma to the retina and vitreous.

A and **B**: A 43-year-old woman noted floaters in the left eye. Three years previously she had a cutaneous melanoma excised. Cobalt treatment was given because of a positive lymph node biopsy. Visual acuity was 20/20. Slit-lamp examination of the left eye revealed golden-brown spherules in the anterior vitreous cavity (A) and pigmented cells emanating from the region of the optic disc (B). Angiography revealed some staining of the optic disc. The patient died 4 months later in spite of antimetabolite therapy.
C and **D**: Retinal metastasis in a 44-year-old man 3 years after excision of a cutaneous melanoma.

(A and B, from Robertson et al.[458]; C and D, from Letson and Davidorf.[404] E and I also, Yannuzzi, Lawrence J., The Retinal Atlas, Saunders 2010, 978-0-7020-3320-9, p.275.)

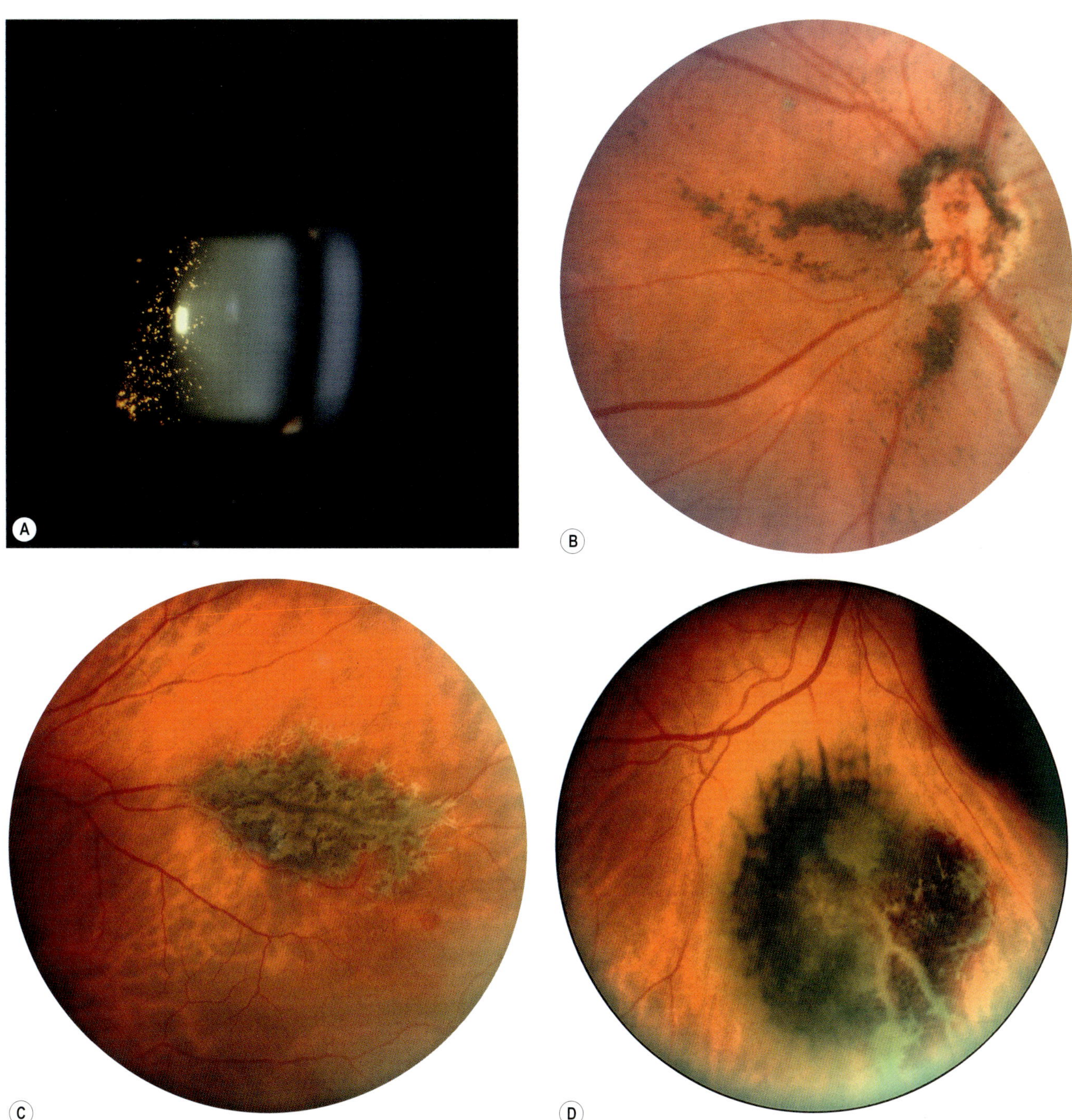
A
B
C
D

PARANEOPLASTIC RETINOPATHY ASSOCIATED WITH CARCINOMA (CANCER-ASSOCIATED RETINOPATHY OR CAR SYNDROME)

The rapid development of visual loss associated with bizarre visual sensations, nyctalopia, ring scotoma, flat electroretinographic response, progressive retinal arterial narrowing, and no or minimal changes in the RPE and optic disc may occur as a remote effect of a systemic carcinoma, most frequently a small cell carcinoma of the lung (Figure 13.38A).[412–425] A few vitreous cells were noted in one case,[417] and aqueous cells in another.[418] Fluorescein angiography in two cases showed evidence of mottled hyperfluorescence in both eyes.[417,418] Blindness may occur within 4 months. The visual symptoms may antedate the discovery of the carcinoma. Histopathologic examination shows severe degeneration and loss of the receptor cells and, unlike retinitis pigmentosa, minimal damage to the RPE and normal choriocapillaris.[412,413,417,421,422] In one case there was loss of ganglion cells.[415] Electron microscopy in one patient revealed immature melanin granules with melanolysosomes, suggesting abnormal melanin synthesis and resorption.[412] This suggested to the authors that increased melanin synthesis and melanin content within the RPE in response to a hormonelike substance produced by the cancer may compromise its ability to phagocytose and maintain normal turnover of receptor outer segments. This in turn may cause photoreceptor cell degeneration.

13.38 Cancer-associated retinopathy.

A: Cancer-associated retinopathy in an elderly man who noted the rapid progression of loss of peripheral vision and nyctalopia. Note the narrowed retinal vessels and absence of evidence of retinal pigment epithelial changes other than the juxtapapillary atrophy that was present in both eyes.

B and C: A 72-year-old-woman developed total achromatopsia, bilateral central scotomas, predominant suppression of cone response by electroretinogram, and narrowing of the retinal arteries. She died 9 months later from metastatic carcinoma. Histopathologic examination revealed loss of photoreceptors most marked in the macular areas (B and C) and selective loss of cones elsewhere.

Acute Vogt–Koyanagi–Harada-like syndrome in a patient with metastatic cutaneous melanoma.

D–I: This 71-year-old woman had had a melanoma of the dorsum of her foot removed 3 years previously. Two weeks before admission she had noted headache, progressive vitiligo of the skin of the face and arms (D and E), deafness, floaters, and progressive loss of vision in both eyes. Her visual acuity was light perception with poor projection in both eyes. She had 2+ aqueous cells and flare and keratic precipitates, 3+ vitreous cells, and large areas of depigmentation of the choroid and posterior fundus (F and G). Her general physical examination revealed inguinal lymphadenopathy but no other evidence of metastatic disease. The nodes were positive for melanoma. Computed tomography of the brain and abdomen was negative, and electroretinographic responses were extinguished in both eyes. Lumbar puncture revealed 130 lymphocytes and spinal fluid protein of 90 mg/dl. Treatment with systemic corticosteroids resulted in rapid return of visual function to 20/50 in the right eye and 20/70 in the left eye. Ten months after the onset of visual symptoms, the vitreous inflammation was minimal and there were scattered focal areas of depigmentation of the choroid in both eyes (H and I). The patient led an active life and was able to read until the time of her death, caused by metastatic melanoma 15 months later.

(B and C, from Cogan et al.[413]; D–I, from Gass.[434])

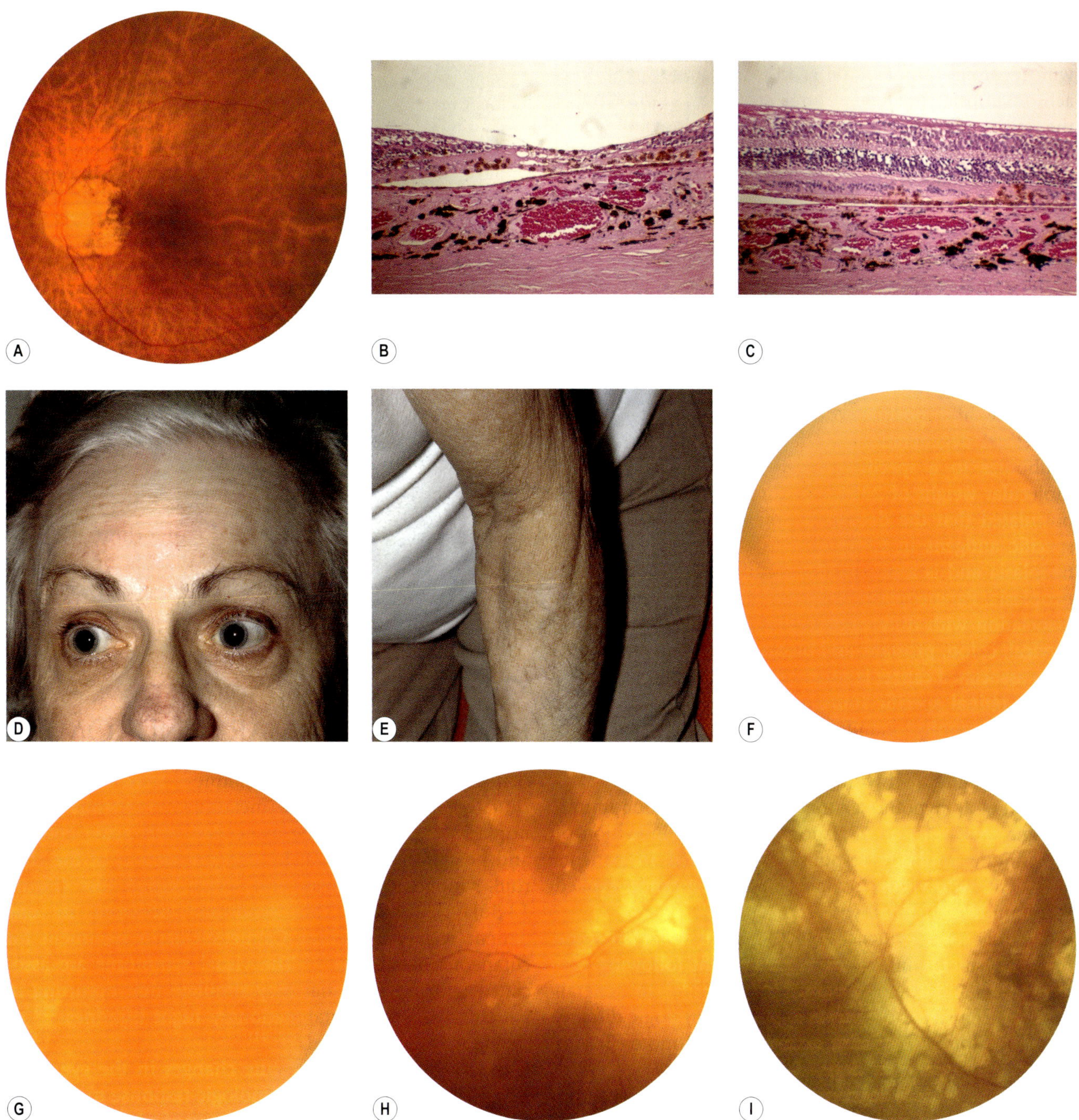
A
B
C
D
E
F
G
H
I

Patients with MAR, unlike those with CAR, experience primarily central visual loss rather than ring scotomas and, early, their ERG does not show the severely depressed or absent a-wave indicative of photoreceptor dysfunction.[437] Vitiligo has been reported in association with cutaneous melanomas in as many as 20% of cases. In a few patients it may be accompanied by intraocular inflammation.[421,442] Other diseases linking vitiligo and intraocular inflammation, particularly chorioretinitis and patchy depigmentation of the fundus, include sympathetic uveitis[442] and vitiliginous chorioretinitis (birdshot chorioretinitis).[443] The frequent association of nyctalopia in vitiliginous chorioretinitis, its occasional occurrence in association with sympathetic uveitis, and its occurrence in the patient illustrated in Figure 7.39 indicate that the receptor cells as well as the melanocytes may be the target of the immunologic reaction.

Paraneoplastic Vitelliform Retinopathy

Acute-onset bilateral multifocal RPE detachments that resemble vitelliform retinopathy have been recently recognized (Figure 13.40). Sotodeh and associates reported 3 cases, 1 with choroidal melanoma and 2 with cutaneous melanoma.[444] Autoantibodies against a 120-kDa photoreceptor protein, bestrophin, and bipolar cells have been isolated. ERG and electro-oculogram results have been variable.[444–446] It is quite likely that previously reported cases of multiple RPE detachments in patients with skin or uveal melanoma fall within the spectrum of paraneoplastic vitelliform retinopathy.[446–449]

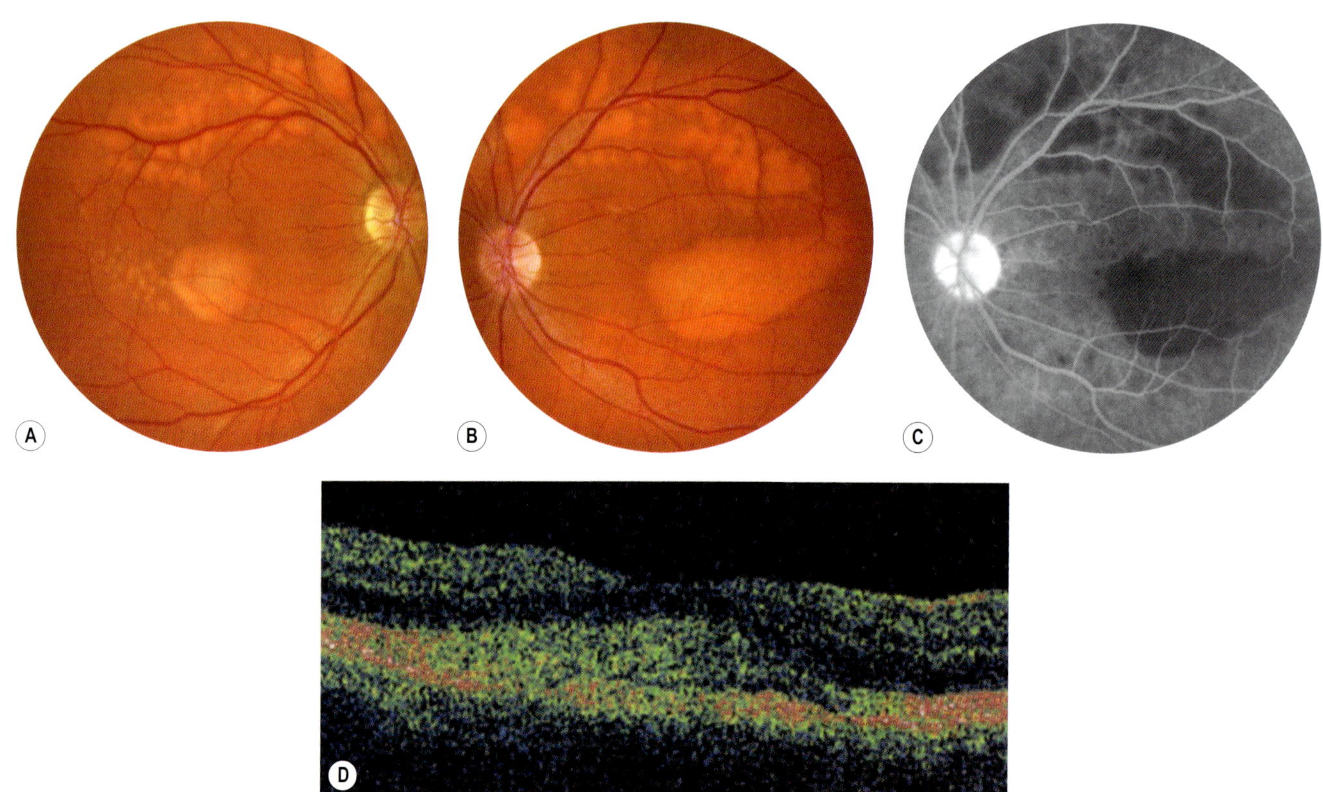

13.40 Paraneoplastic vitelliform dystrophy.

A–D: This is a 58-year-old white male who complained of worsening vision in both eyes and noticed after images with lights and television screen and photopsias and a triangle of blur on the left side. He had left axillary node resected for a malignant melanoma. No primary cutaneous lesion was found. He was treated with interferon alpha 2B, which was completed a month prior. His visual acuity was 20/20 in the right eye and 20/25 in the left eye.

(Courtesy of Dr. Peter J. Kertes.)

References

1. Abramson DH, Frank CM, Susman M, et al. Presenting signs of retinoblastoma. J Pediatr 1998;132:505–8.
2. Chantada GL, Dunkel IJ, de Davila MT, et al. Retinoblastoma patients with high risk ocular pathological features: who needs adjuvant therapy? Br J Ophthalmol 2004;88:1069–73.
3. Magramm I, Abramson DH, Ellsworth RM. Optic nerve involvement in retinoblastoma. Ophthalmology 1989;96:217–22.
4. Smith JLS. Histology and spontaneous regression of retinoblastoma. Trans Ophthalmol Soc UK 1974;94:953–67.
5. Devesa SS. The incidence of retinoblastoma. Am J Ophthalmol 1975;80:263–5.
6. Rubenfeld M, Abramson DH, Ellsworth RM, et al. Unilateral vs. bilateral retinoblastoma; correlations between age at diagnosis and stage of ocular disease. Ophthalmology 1986;93:1016–9.
7. Broaddus E, Topham A, Singh A. Incidence of Retinoblastoma in the United States: 1975–2004. Br J Ophthalmol 2009;93:24–7.
8. Chévez-Barrios P, Eagle RC, Marback EF. Histopathologic features and prognostic factors. In: Singh AD, Damato BE, Pe'er J, editors. Clinical ophthalmic oncology. Philadelphia: Saunders-Elsevier; 2007. p. 468–76.
9. Gass JDM. Differential diagnosis of intraocular tumors; a stereoscopic presentation. St. Louis: CV Mosby; 1974. p. 331.
10. Ohnishi Y, Yamana Y, Minei M, et al. Application of fluorescein angiography in retinoblastoma. Am J Ophthalmol 1982;93:578–88.
11. Shields JA, Sanborn GE, Augsburger JJ, et al. Fluorescein angiography of retinoblastoma. Retina 1982;2:206–14.
12. Haik BG, Dunleavy SA, Cooke C, et al. Retinoblastoma with anterior chamber extension. Ophthalmology 1987;94:367–70.
13. Bullock JD, Campbell RJ, Waller RR. Calcification in retinoblastoma. Invest Ophthalmol Vis Sci 1977;16:252–5.
14. Mafee MF, Goldberg MF, Cohen SB, et al. Magnetic resonance imaging versus computed tomography of leukocoric eyes and use of in vitro proton magnetic resonance spectroscopy of retinoblastoma. Ophthalmology 1989;96:965–76.
15. Shields JA, Shields CL. Differentiation of Coats' disease and retinoblastoma. J Pediatr Ophthalmol Strabismus 2001;38:262–6. [quiz 302–303.]
16. Bhatnagar R, Vine AK. Diffuse infiltrating retinoblastoma. Ophthalmology 1991;98:1657–61.
17. Shields JA, Shields CL, Eagle RC, et al. Spontaneous pseudohypopyon secondary to diffuse infiltrating retinoblastoma. Arch Ophthalmol 1988;106:1301.
18. Sachdeva R, Schoenfield L, Traboulsi ET, et al. Retinoblastoma with autoinfarction presenting as orbital cellulitis. J POS 2011. [in press.]
19. Shields JA, Shields CL, Suvarnamani C, et al. Retinoblastoma manifesting as orbital cellulitis. Am J Ophthalmol 1991;112:442–9.
20. Shields JA, Shields CL, Parsons HM. Differential diagnosis of retinoblastoma. Retina 1991;11:232–43.
21. Howard GM. Erroneous clinical diagnoses of retinoblastoma and uveal melanoma. Trans Am Acad Ophthalmol Otolaryngol 1969;73:199–202.
22. Robertson DM, Campbell RJ. Analysis of misdiagnosed retinoblastoma in a series of 726 enucleated eyes. Mod Probl Ophthalmol 1977;18:156–9.
23. Shields JA, Shields CL, Eagle RC, et al. Calcified intraocular abscess simulating retinoblastoma. Am J Ophthalmol 1992;114:227–9.
24. Shields CL, Shields JA. Recent developments in the management of retinoblastoma. J Pediatr Ophthalmol Strabismus 1999;36:8–18. [quiz 35–36.]
25. Harbour JW. Molecular basis of low penetrance retinoblastoma. Arch Ophthalmol 2001;119:1699–704.
26. Ahmad NN, Melo MB, Singh AD, et al. A possible hot spot in exon 21 of the retinoblastoma gene predisposing to a low penetrant retinoblastoma phenotype? Ophthalmic Genet 1999;20:225–31.
27. Dryja TP, Rapaport J, McGee TL, et al. Molecular etiology of low-penetrance retinoblastoma in two pedigrees. Am J Hum Genet 1993;52:1122–8.
28. Toguchida J, McGee TL, Paterson JC, et al. Complete genomic sequence of the human retinoblastoma susceptibility gene. Genomics 1993;17:535–43.
29. Friend SH, Bernards R, Rogelj S, et al. A human DNA segment with properties of the gene that predisposes to retinoblastoma and osteosarcoma. Nature 1986;323:643–6.
30. Lee WH, Bookstein R, Hong F, et al. Human retinoblastoma susceptibility gene: cloning, identification, and sequence. Science 1987;235:1394–9.
31. Lohmann DR, Brandt B, Hopping W, et al. The spectrum of RB1 germ-line mutations in hereditary retinoblastoma. Am J Hum Genet 1996;58:940–9.
32. Clark RD, Mansfield NC. Retinoblastoma: genetic testing and counseling. In: Singh AD, Damato BE, Pe'er J, editors. Clinical ophthalmic oncology. Philadelphia: Saunders-Elsevier; 2007. p. 441–6.
33. Singh AD, Black SH, Shields CL, et al. Prenatal diagnosis of retinoblastoma. J Pediatr Ophthalmol Strabismus 2003;40:222–4.
34. Xu K, Rosenwaks Z, Beaverson K, et al. Preimplantation genetic diagnosis for retinoblastoma: the first reported liveborn. Am J Ophthalmol 2004;137:18–23.
35. Gallie BL, Ellsworth RM, Abramson DH, et al. Retinoma: spontaneous regression of retinoblastoma or benign manifestation of the mutation? Br J Cancer 1982;45:513–21.
36. Abramson DH. Retinoma, retinocytoma, and the retinoblastoma gene. Arch Ophthalmol 1983;101:1517–8.
37. Singh AD, Santos MCM, Shields CL, et al. Observations on 17 patients with retinocytoma. Arch Ophthalmol 2000;118:199–205.
38. Eagle Jr CR, Shields JA, Donoso L, et al. Malignant transformation of spontaneously regressed retinoblastoma, retinoma/retinocytoma variant. Ophthalmology 1989;96:1389–95.
39. Gallie BL, Phillips RA, Ellsworth RM, et al. Significance of retinoma and phthisis bulbi for retinoblastoma. Ophthalmology 1982;89:1393–9.
40. Dimaras H, Khetan V, Halliday W, et al. Retinoma underlying retinoblastoma revealed after tumor response to 1 cycle of chemotherapy. Arch Ophthalmol 2009;127:1066–8.
41. Murphree AL. Local therapy, brachytherapy, and enucleation. In: Singh AD, Damato BE, Pe'er J, editors. Clinical ophthalmic oncology. Philadelphia: Saunders-Elsevier; 2007. p. 454–61.
42. Melamud A, Palekar R, Singh A. Retinoblastoma. Am Fam Physician 2006;73:1039–44.
43. Shields JA, Shields CL, Sivalingam V. Decreasing frequency of enucleation in patients with retinoblastoma. Am J Ophthalmol 1989;108:185–8.
44. Broaddus E, Topham A, Singh A. Survival with Retinoblastoma in the United States: 1975–2004. Br J Ophthalmol 2009;93:21–3.
45. Shields JA, Shields CL, Parsons H, et al. The role of photocoagulation in the management of retinoblastoma. Arch Ophthalmol 1990;108:205–8.
46. Abramson DH, Schefler AC. Transpupillary thermotherapy as initial treatment for small intraocular retinoblastoma: technique and predictors of success. Ophthalmology 2004;111:984–91.
47. Shields JA, Parsons H, Shields CL, et al. The role of cryotherapy in the management of retinoblastoma. Am J Ophthalmol 1989;108:260–4.
48. Shields CL, Santos MC, Diniz W, et al. Thermotherapy for retinoblastoma. Arch Ophthalmol 1999;117:885–93.
49. Shields JA, Shields CL, De Potter P, et al. Plaque radiotherapy for residual or recurrent retinoblastoma in 91 cases. J Pediatr Ophthalmol Strabismus 1994;31:242–5.
50. Hernandez JC, Brady LW, Shields JA, et al. External beam radiation for retinoblastoma: results, patterns of failure, and a proposal for treatment guidelines. Int J Radiat Oncol Biol Phys 1996;35:125–32.
51. Merchant TE. Teletherapy: indications, risks, and new delivery options. In: Singh AD, Damato BE, Pe'er J, editors. Clinical ophthalmic oncology. Philadelphia: Saunders-Elsevier; 2007. p. 462–7.
52. Ferris FL, Chew EY. A new era for the treatment of retinoblastoma. Arch Ophthalmol 1996;114:1412.
53. Murphree AL, Villablanca JG, Deegan III WF, et al. Chemotherapy plus local treatment in the management of intraocular retinoblastoma. Arch Ophthalmol 1996;114:1348–56.
54. Kingston JE, Hungerford JL, Madreperla SA, et al. Results of combined chemotherapy and radiotherapy for advanced intraocular retinoblastoma. Arch Ophthalmol 1996;114:1339–43.
55. Friedman DL, Himelstein B, Shields CL, et al. Chemoreduction and local ophthalmic therapy for intraocular retinoblastoma. J Clin Oncol 2000;18:12–17.
56. Jubran RF, Villablanca JG, Meadows AT. Chemotherapy for retinoblastoma: an overview. In: Singh AD, Damato BE, Pe'er J, editors. Clinical ophthalmic oncology. Philadelphia: Saunders-Elsevier; 2007. p. 449–53.
57. Chan HS, Gallie BL, Munier FL, et al. Chemotherapy for retinoblastoma. Ophthalmol Clin North Am 2005;18:55–63. viii.
58. Shields CL, Mashayekhi A, Au AK, et al. The International Classification of Retinoblastoma predicts chemoreduction success. Ophthalmology 2006;113:2276–80.
59. Scott IU, Murray TG, Toledano S, et al. New retinoblastoma tumors in children undergoing systemic chemotherapy. Arch Ophthalmol 1998;12:1685–6.
60. Benz MS, Scott UI, Murray TG, et al. Complications of systemic chemotherapy as treatment of retinoblastoma. Arch Ophthalmol 2000;118:577–8.
61. Gombos DS, Hungerford J, Abramson DH, et al. Secondary acute myelogenous leukemia in patients with retinoblastoma: is chemotherapy a factor? Ophthalmology 2007;114:1378–83.
62. Murphree AL, Chantada GL. Staging and grouping of retinoblastoma. In: Singh AD, Damato BE, Pe'er J, editors. Clinical Ophthalmic Oncology. Philadelphia, Saunders-Elsevier; 2007. p. 422–7.
63. Meadows AT, Chintagumpala M, Dunkel IJ, et al. Children's Oncology Group (COG) Trials for Retinoblastoma. In: Singh AD, Damato BE, Pe'er J, editors. Clinical ophthalmic oncology. Philadelphia: Saunders-Elsevier; 2007. p. 491–5.
64. Yamane T, Kaneko A, Mohri M. The technique of ophthalmic arterial infusion therapy for patients with intraocular retinoblastoma. Int J Clin Oncol 2004;9:69–73.
65. Abramson DH. Super selective ophthalmic artery delivery of chemotherapy for intraocular retinoblastoma: 'chemosurgery': the first Stallard lecture. Br J Ophthalmol 2010;94:396–9.
66. Shields CL, Shields JA. Intra-arterial chemotherapy for retinoblastoma: the beginning of a long journey. Clin Experiment Ophthalmol 2010;38:638–43.
67. Abramson DH. Super selective ophthalmic artery delivery of chemotherapy for intraocular retinoblastoma: 'chemosurgery': the first Stallard lecture. Br J Ophthalmol 2010;94:396–9.
68. Abramson DH, Dunkel IJ, Brodie SE, et al. A phase I/II study of direct intraarterial (ophthalmic artery) chemotherapy with melphalan for intraocular retinoblastoma initial results. Ophthalmology 2008;115:1398–404.
69. Abramson DH, Dunkel IJ, Brodie SE, et al. Superselective ophthalmic artery chemotherapy as primary treatment for retinoblastoma (chemosurgery). Ophthalmology 2010;117:1623–9.
70. Brodie SE, Pierre Gobin Y, Dunkel IJ, et al. Persistence of retinal function after selective ophthalmic artery chemotherapy infusion for retinoblastoma. Doc Ophthalmol 2009;119:13–22.
71. Kivela T. Trilateral retinoblastoma: a meta-analysis of hereditary retinoblastoma associated with primary ectopic intracranial retinoblastoma. J Clin Oncol 1999;17:1829–37.
72. Bader JL, Miller RW, Meadows AT, et al. Trilateral retinoblastoma. Lancet 1982;2:582–3.
73. Singh AD, Shields CL, Shields JA. New insights into trilateral retinoblastoma. Cancer 1999;86:3–5.
74. Shields CL, Meadows AT, Shields JA, et al. Chemoreduction for retinoblastoma may prevent intracranial neuroblastic malignancy (trilateral retinoblastoma). Arch Ophthalmol 2001;119:1269–72.
75. Abramson DH, Ronner HJ, Ellsworth RM. Nonocular cancer in nonirradiated retinoblastoma. Am J Ophthalmol 1979;87:624–7.
76. Abramson DH, Ellsworth RM, Kitchin FD, et al. Second nonocular tumors in retinoblastoma survivors; are they radiation-induced? Ophthalmology 1984;91:1351–5.
77. Kleinerman RA, Tucker MA, Tarone RE, et al. Risk of new cancers after radiotherapy in long-term survivors of retinoblastoma: an extended follow-up. J Clin Oncol 2005;23:2272–9.

78. Wong FL, Boice Jr JD, Abramson DH, et al. Cancer incidence after retinoblastoma. Radiation dose and sarcoma risk. Jama 278:1262–1267.
79. Moll AC, Imhof SM, Bouter LM, et al. Second primary tumors in patients with retinoblastoma. A review of the literature. Ophthalmic Genet 1997;18:27–34.
80. Woo KI, Harbour JW. Review of 676 second primary tumors in patients with retinoblastoma: association between age at onset and tumor type. Arch Ophthalmol 2010;128:865–70.
81. Kopelman JE, McLean IW, Rosenberg SH. Multivariate analysis of risk factors for metastasis in retinoblastoma treated by enucleation. Ophthalmology 1987;94:371–7.
82. Singh AD, Shields CL, Shields JA. Prognostic factors in retinoblastoma. J Pediatr Ophthalmol Strabismus 2000;37:134–41. quiz 68–69
83. Messmer EP, Heinrich T, Höpping W, et al. Risk factors for metastases in patients with retinoblastoma. Ophthalmology 1991;98:136–41.
84. Khelfaoui F, Validire P, Auperin A, et al. Histopathologic risk factors in retinoblastoma: a retrospective study of 172 patients treated in a single institution. Cancer 1996;77:1206–13.
85. Shields CL, Shields JA, Baez KA, et al. Choroidal invasion of retinoblastoma: metastatic potential and clinical risk factors. Br J Ophthalmol 1993;77:544–8.
86. Hungerford J. Factors influencing metastasis in retinoblastoma. Br J Ophthalmol. 1993;77:541.
87. Young J., Smith MA, Roffers SD, et al. In: Ries LAG, Smith MA, Linet M, et al. editors. Cancer incidence and survival among children and adolescents: United States SEER Program 1975–1995. SEER Program. NIH Pub. No. 99-4649. Bethesda, MD: National Cancer Institute 1999.
88. Sanders BM, Draper GJ, Kingston JE. Retinoblastoma in Great Britain 1969–80: incidence, treatment, and survival. Br J Ophthalmol 1988;72:576–83.
89. Sant M, Capocaccia R, Badioni V, et al. Survival for retinoblastoma in Europe. Eur J Cancer 2001;37:730–5.
90. Senft S, al-Kaff A, Bergqvist G, et al. Retinoblastoma: the Saudi Arabian experience. Ophthalmic Paediatr Genet 1988;9:115–9.
91. Ajaiyeoba IA, Akang EE, Campbell OB, et al. Retinoblastomas in Ibadan: treatment and prognosis. West Afr J Med 1993;12:223–7.
92. Nandakumar A, Anantha N, Appaji L, et al. Descriptive epidemiology of childhood cancers in Bangalore, India. Cancer Causes Control 1996;7:405–10.
93. Mohney BG, Robertson DM. Ancillary testing for metastasis in patients with newly diagnosed retinoblastoma. Am J Ophthalmol 1994;118:707–11.
94. McCay CJ, Abramson DH, Ellsworth RM. Metastatic patterns of retinoblastoma. Arch Ophthalmol 1984;102:391–6.
95. Honavar SG, Singh AD, Shields CL, et al. Postenucleation adjuvant therapy in high-risk retinoblastoma. Arch Ophthalmol 2002;120:923–31.
96. Broughton WL, Zimmerman LE. A clinicopathologic study of 56 cases of intraocular medulloepitheliomas. Am J Ophthalmol 1978;85:407–18.
97. Shields JA, Eagle Jr RC, Shields CL, et al. Congenital neoplasms of the nonpigmented ciliary epithelium (medulloepithelioma). Ophthalmology 1996;103:1998–2006.
98. Shields JA, Eagle Jr RC, Shields CL, et al. Pigmented medulloepithelioma of the ciliary body. Arch Ophthalmol 2002;120:207–10.
99. Singh A, Singh AD, Shields CL, et al. Iris neovascularization in children as a manifestation of underlying medulloepithelioma. J Pediatr Ophthalmol Strabismus 2001;38:224–8.
100. Priest JR, Williams GR, Jenkinson H, et al. Pleuropulmonary blastoma family tumor and dysplasia syndrome – A Report from the International Pleuropulmonary Blastoma Registry. Br J Ophthalmol 2011 [in press]
101. Canning CR, McCartney AC, Hungerford J. Medulloepithelioma (diktyoma). Br J Ophthalmol 1988;72:764–7.
102. Atkinson A, Sanders MD, Wong V. Vitreous haemorrhage in tuberous sclerosis; report of two cases. Br J Ophthalmol 1973;57:773–9.
103. Barksy D, Wolter JR. The retinal lesion of tuberous sclerosis: An angiogliomatous hamartoma? J Pediatr Ophthalmol 1971;8:261–5.
104. Bloom SM, Mahl CF. Photocoagulation for serous detachment of the macula secondary to retinal astrocytoma. Retina 1991;11:416–22.
105. Coppeto JR, Lubin JR, Albert DM. Astrocytic hamartoma in tuberous sclerosis mimicking necrotizing retinochoroiditis. J Pediatr Ophthalmol Strabismus 1982;19:306–13.
106. Daily MJ, Smith JL, Dickens W. Giant drusen (astrocytic hamartoma) of the optic nerve seen with computerized axial tomography. Am J Ophthalmol 1976;81:100–1.
107. De Bustros S, Miller NR, Finkelstein D, et al. Bilateral astrocytic hamartomas of the optic nerve heads in retinitis pigmentosa. Retina 1983;3:21–3.
108. Destro M, D'Amico DJ, Gragoudas ES, et al. Retinal manifestations of neurofibromatosis; diagnosis and management. Arch Ophthalmol 1991;109:662–6.
109. Eng LF, Rubinstein LJ. Contribution of immunohistochemistry to diagnostic problems of human cerebral tumors. J Histochem Cytochem 1978;26:513–22.
110. Font RL, Ferry AP. The phakomatoses. Int Ophthalmol Clin 1972;12:1–50.
111. Foos RY, Straatsma BR, Allen RA. Astrocytoma of the optic nerve head. Arch Ophthalmol 1965;74:319–26.
112. Garron LK, Spencer WH. Retinal glioneuroma associated with tuberous sclerosis. Trans Am Acad Ophthalmol Otolaryngol 1964;68:1018–21.
113. Gutman I, Dunn D, Behrens M, et al. Hypopigmented iris spot: an early sign of tuberous sclerosis. Ophthalmology 1982;89:1155–9.
114. Harley RD, Grover WD. Tuberous sclerosis; description and report of 12 cases. Ann Ophthalmol 1970;1:477–81.
115. Jakobiec FA, Brodie SE, Haik B, et al. Giant cell astrocytoma of the retina; a tumor of possible Mueller cell origin. Ophthalmology 1983;90:1565–76.
116. Jordano J, Galera H, Toro M, et al. Astrocytoma of the retina: Report of a case. Br J Ophthalmol 1974;58:555–9.
117. Jozwiak S. Diagnostic value of clinical features and supplementary investigations in tuberous sclerosis in children. Acta Paediatr Hung 1992;32:71–88.
118. Nyboer JH, Robertson DM, Gomez MR. Retinal lesions in tuberous sclerosis. Arch Ophthalmol 1976;94:1277–80.
119. Shami MJ, Benedict WL, Myers M. Early manifestation of retinal hamartomas in tuberous sclerosis. Am J Ophthalmol 1993;115:539–40.
120. Wang C-L, Brucker AJ. Vitreous hemorrhage secondary to juxtapapillary vascular hamartoma of the retina. Retina 1984;4:44–7.
121. Wolter JR, Mertus JM. Exophytic retinal astrocytoma in tuberous sclerosis; report of a case. J Pediatr Ophthalmol 1969;6:186–91.
122. Zimmerman LE, Walsh FB. Clinical pathologic conference. Am J Ophthalmol 1956;42:737–47.
123. Gass JDM. The phakomatoses. In: Smith JL, editor. Neuro-ophthalmology; symposium of the University of Miami and the Bascom Palmer Eye Institute. St. Louis: CV Mosby; 1965. p. 223–68.
124. Cleasby GW, Fung WE, Shekter WB. Astrocytoma of the retina; report of two cases. Am J Ophthalmol 1967;64:633–7.
125. McLean JM. Glial tumors of the retina in relation to tuberous sclerosis. Am J Ophthalmol 1956;41:428–32.
126. Kroll AJ, Ricker DP, Robb RM, et al. Vitreous hemorrhage complicating retinal astrocytic hamartoma. Surv Ophthalmol 1981;26:31–8.
127. Ramsay RC, Kinyoun JL, Hill CW, et al. Retinal astrocytoma. Am J Ophthalmol 1979;88:32–6.
128. Reeser FH, Aaberg TM, Van Horn DL. Astrocytic hamartoma of the retina not associated with tuberous sclerosis. Am J Ophthalmol 1978;86:688–98.
129. Panzo GJ, Meyers SM, Gutman FA, et al. Spontaneous regression of parafoveal exudates and serous retinal detachment in a patient with tuberous sclerosis and retinal astrocytomas. Retina 1984;4:242–5.
130. Sahli O, Sickenberg M, Piguet B. [Exudative parafoveal astrocytic hamartoma associated with Bourneville tuberous sclerosis: spontaneous evolution.] Klin Monbl Augenheilkd 1997;210: 332–3.
131. Drummond SR, Kemp EG. Retinal astrocytoma managed by brachytherapy. Ophthalmology 2009;116(597):e1.
132. Vilaplana D, Castilla M, Poposki V, et al. Acquired retinal astrocytoma managed with endoresection. Retina 2006;26:1081–2.
133. Shields JA, Eagle Jr. RC, Shields CL, et al. Aggressive retinal astrocytomas in 4 patients with tuberous sclerosis complex. Arch Ophthalmol 2005;123:856–63.
134. Eskelin S, Tommila P, Palosaari T, et al. Photodynamic therapy with verteporfin to induce regression of aggressive retinal astrocytomas. Acta Ophthalmol 2008;86:794–9.
135. Mennel S, Hausmann N, Meyer CH, et al. Photodynamic therapy for exudative hamartoma in tuberous sclerosis. Arch Ophthalmol 2006;124:597–9.
136. Bornfeld N, Messmer EP, Theodossiadis G, et al. Giant cell astrocytoma of the retina; clinicopathologic report of a case not associated with Bourneville's disease. Retina 1987;7: 183–9.
137. Margo CE, Barletta JP, Staman JA. Giant cell astrocytoma of the retina in tuberous sclerosis. Retina 1993;13:155–9.
138. Sahel JA, Frederick Jr AR, Pesavento R, et al. Idiopathic retinal gliosis mimicking a choroidal melanoma. Retina 1988;8:282–7.
139. Schwartz PL, Beards JA, Maris PJG. Tuberous sclerosis associated with a retinal angioma. Am J Ophthalmol 1980;90:485–8.
140. Pillai S, Limaye SR, Saimovici L-B. Optic disc hamartoma associated with retinitis pigmentosa. Retina 1983;3:24–6.
141. Robertson DM. Hamartomas of the optic disk with retinitis pigmentosa. Am J Ophthalmol 1972;74:526–31.
142. Jost BF, Olk RJ. Atypical retinitis proliferans, retinal telangiectasis, and vitreous hemorrhage in a patient with tuberous sclerosis. Retina 1986;6:53–6.
143. Rowley SA, O'Callaghan FJ, Osborne JP. Ophthalmic manifestations of tuberous sclerosis: a population based study. Br J Ophthalmol 2001;85:420–3.
144. Au KS, Williams AT, Roach ES, et al. Genotype/phenotype correlation in 325 individuals referred for a diagnosis of tuberous sclerosis complex in the United States. Genet Med 2007;9:88–100.
145. Robertson DM. Ophthalmic manifestations of tuberous sclerosis. Ann N Y Acad Sci 1991;615:17–25.
146. Gass JDM. Stereoscopic atlas of macular diseases: diagnosis and treatment, 4th ed. St Louis: Mosby; 1997.
147. Roach ES, Gomez MR, Northrup H. Tuberous Sclerosis Complex Consensus Conference: revised clinical diagnostic criteria. J Child Neurol 1998;13:624–8.
148. van Slegtenhorst M, de Hoogt R, Hermans C, et al. Identification of the tuberous sclerosis gene TSC1 on chromosome 9q34. Science 1997;277:805–8.
149. European Chromosome 16 Tuberous Sclerosis Consortium. Identification and characterization of the tuberous sclerosis gene on chromosome 16. Cell 1993;75:1305–1315.
150. Catania MG, Johnson MW, Liau LM, et al. Hamartin expression and interaction with tuberin in tumor cell lines and primary cultures. J Neurosci Res 2001;63:276–83.
151. Turell ME, Traboulsi ET, Gupta A, et al. Tuberous sclerosis complex: Genotype/phenotype correlation of retinal findings. Opthalmology 2011. [in press.]
152. Amalric P, Biau C. L'angiographie fluorescéinique chez l'enfant. Arch Ophtalmol (Paris) 1968;28:55–60.
153. Augsburger JJ, Shields JA, Goldberg RE. Classification and management of hereditary retinal angiomas. Int Ophthalmol 1981;4:93–106.
154. Colvard DM, Robertson DM, Trautmann JC. Cavernous hemangioma of the retina. Arch Ophthalmol 1978;96:2042–4.
155. Davies WS, Thumim M. Cavernous hemangioma of the optic disc and retina. Trans Am Acad Ophthalmol Otolaryngol 1956;60:217–8.
156. Drummond JW, Hall DL, Steen Jr WH, et al. Cavernous hemangioma of the optic disc. Ann Ophthalmol 1980;12:1017–8.
157. Gass JDM. Cavernous hemangioma of the retina; a neuro-oculo-cutaneous syndrome. Am J Ophthalmol 1971;71:799–814.

158. Gass JDM. Fluorescein angiography: an aid to the retinal surgeon. In: Pruett RC, Regan CDJ, editors. Retina Congress; 25th anniversary meeting of the Retina Service Massachusetts Eye and Ear Infirmary. New York: Appleton-Century-Crofts; 1974. p. 181–201.
159. Gass JDM. Treatment of retinal vascular anomalies. Trans Am Acad Ophthalmol Otolaryngol 1977;83:OP432–OP442.
160. Gislason I, Stenkula S, Alm A, et al. Cavernous haemangioma of the retina. Acta Ophthalmol 1979;57:709–17.
161. Goldberg RE, Pheasant TR, Shields JA. Cavernous hemangioma of the retina; a four-generation pedigree with neurocutaneous manifestations and an example of bilateral retinal involvement. Arch Ophthalmol 1979;97:2321–4.
162. Hogan MJ, Zimmerman LE. Ophthalmic pathology; an atlas and textbook. Philadelphia: WB Saunders; 1962. p. 492.
163. Klein M, Goldberg MF, Cotlier E. Cavernous hemangioma of the retina: report of four cases. Ann Ophthalmol 1975;7:1213–21.
164. Krause U. A case of cavernous haemangioma of the retina. Acta Ophthalmol 1971;49:221–31.
165. Lewis RA, Cohen MH, Wise GN. Cavernous haemangioma of the retina and optic disc; a report of three cases and a review of the literature. Br J Ophthalmol 1975;59:422–34.
166. Mansour AM, Jampol LM, Hrisomalos NF, et al. Cavernous hemangioma of the optic disc. Arch Ophthalmol 1988;106:22.
167. Niccol W, Moore RF. A case of angiomatosis retinae. Br J Ophthalmol 1934;18:454–7.
168. Pancurak J, Goldberg MF, Frenkel M, et al. Cavernous hemangioma of the retina; genetic and central nervous system involvement. Retina 1985;5:215–20.
169. Schwartz AC, Weaver Jr RG, Bloomfield R, et al. Cavernous hemangioma of the retina, cutaneous angiomas, and intracranial vascular lesion by computed tomography and nuclear magnetic resonance imaging. Am J Ophthalmol 1984;98:483–7.
170. Turut P, François P. Hémangiome caverneux de la rétine. J Fr Ophtalmol 1979;2:393–404.
171. Weskamp C, Cotlier I. Angioma del cerebro y de la retina con malformaciones capilares de la piel. Arch Oftalmol Buenos Aires 1940;15:1–10.
172. Yen M-Y, Wu C-C. Cavernous hemangioma of the retina and agenesis of internal carotid artery with bilateral oculomotor palsies. J Clin Neuro-Ophthalmol 1985;5:258–62.
173. Messmer E, Laqua H, Wessing A, et al. Nine cases of cavernous hemangioma of the retina. Am J Ophthalmol 1983;95:383–90.
174. Gass JDM. Stereoscopic atlas of macular diseases; diagnosis and treatment, 3rd ed. St. Louis: CV Mosby; 1987. p. 606–11.
175. Corboy JR, Galetta SL. Familial cavernous angiomas manifesting with an acute chiasmal syndrome. Am J Ophthalmol 1989;108:245–50.
176. Dobyns WB, Michels VV, Groover RV, et al. Familial cavernous malformations of the central nervous system and retina. Ann Neurol 1987;21:578–83.
177. Giuffrè G. Cavernous hemangioma of the retina and retinal telangiectasis; distinct or related vascular malformations? Retina 1985;5:221–4.
178. Hassler W, Zentner J, Wilhelm H. Cavernous angiomas of the anterior visual pathways. J Clin Neuro-Ophthalmol 1989;9:160–4.
179. Malik S, Cohen BH, Robinson J, et al. Progressive vision loss; a rare manifestation of familial cavernous angiomas. Arch Neurol 1992;49:170–3.
180. McCormick WF, Hardman JM, Boulter TR. Vascular malformations ("angiomas") of the brain, with special reference to those occurring in the posterior fossa. J Neurosurg 1968;28:241–51.
181. Neame H. Angiomatosis retinae, with report of pathological examination. Br J Ophthalmol 1948;32:677–89.
182. Roberson GH, Kase CS, Wolpow ER. Telangiectases and cavernous angiomas of the brainstem: "Cryptic" vascular malformations; a report of a case. Neuroradiology 1974;8:83–9.
183. Spencer WH. Primary neoplasms of the optic nerve and its sheaths: clinical features and current concepts of pathogenetic mechanisms. Trans Am Ophthalmol Soc 1972;70:490–528.
184. Voigt K, Yasargil MG. Cerebral cavernous haemangiomas or cavernomas; incidence, pathology, localization, diagnosis, clinical features and treatment; review of the literature and report of an unusual case. Neurochirurgia 1976;19:59–68.
185. Wallner Jr EF, Moorman LT. Hemangioma of the optic disc. Arch Ophthalmol 1955;53:115–7.
186. Davenport WJ, Siegel AM, Dichgans J, et al. CCM1 gene mutations in families segregating cerebral cavernous malformations. Neurology 2001;56:540–3.
187. Couteulx SL, Brezin AP, Fontaine B, et al. A novel KRIT1/CCM1 truncating mutation in a patient with cerebral and retinal cavernous angiomas. Arch Ophthalmol 2002;120:217–8.
188. D'Angelo R, Marini V, Rinaldi C, et al. Mutation Analysis of CCM1, CCM2 and CCM3 genes in a cohort of italian patients with cerebral cavernous malformation. Brain Pathol 2011;21:215–24.
189. Bottoni F, Canevini MP, Canger R, et al. Twin vessels in familial retinal cavernous hemangioma. Am J Ophthalmol 1990;109:285–9.
190. Messmer E, Font RL, Laqua H, et al. Cavernous hemangioma of the retina; immunohistochemical and ultrastructural observations. Arch Ophthalmol 1984;102:413–8.
191. Haller JA, Knox DL. Vitrectomy for persistent vitreous hemorrhage from a cavernous hemangioma of the optic disk. Am J Ophthalmol 1993;116:106–7.
192. Simard JM, Garcia-Bengochea F, Ballinger Jr WE, et al. Cavernous angioma: A review of 126 collected and 12 new cases. Neurosurgery 1986;18:162–72.
193. Frenkel M, Russe HP. Retinal telangiectasia associated with hypogammaglobulinemia. Am J Ophthalmol 1967;63:215–20.
194. Gautier-Smith PC, Sanders MD, Sanderson KV. Ocular and nervous system involvement in angioma serpiginosum. Br J Ophthalmol 1971;55:433–43.
195. Crompton JL, Taylor D. Ocular lesions in the blue rubber bleb naevus syndrome. Br J Ophthalmol 1981;65:133–7.
196. Hippel E von. Über eine sehr seltene Erkrankung der Natzhaut; Klinische Beobachtungen. Albrecht von Graefes Arch Ophthalmol 1904;59:83–106.
197. Annesley Jr WH, Leonard BC, Shields JA, et al. Fifteen year review of treated cases of retinal angiomatosis. Trans Am Acad Ophthalmol Otolaryngol 1977;83:OP446–OP453.
198. Benson M, Mody C, Rennie I, et al. Haemangioma of the optic disc. Graefes Arch Clin Exp Ophthalmol 1990;228:332–4.
199. Gass JDM, Braunstein R. Sessile and exophytic capillary angiomas of the juxtapapillary retina and optic nerve head. Arch Ophthalmol 1980;98:1790–7.
200. Goldberg MF, Duke JR. von Hippel–Lindau disease; histopathologic findings in a treated and an untreated eye. Am J Ophthalmol 1968;66:693–705.
201. Hagler WS, Hyman BN, Waters III WC. von Hippel's angiomatosis retinae and pheochromocytoma. Trans Am Acad Ophthalmol Otolaryngol 1971;75:1022–34.
202. Haining WM, Zweifach PH. Fluorescein angiography in von Hippel–Lindau disease. Arch Ophthalmol 1967;78:475–9.
203. Hardwig T, Robertson DM. von Hippel–Lindau disease: A familial, often lethal, multi-system phakomatosis. Ophthalmology 1984;91:263–70.
204. Lindau A. Studien über Kleinhirncysten; Bau, Pathogenese und Beziehungen zur Angiomatosis Retinae. Acta Pathol Microbiol Scand Suppl 1926;1:77.
205. Lindau A. Zur Frage der Angiomatosis retinae und ihrer Hirnkomplikationen. Acta Ophthalmol 1926;4:193–226.
206. Machemer R, Williams Sr JM. Pathogenesis and therapy of traction detachment in various retinal vascular diseases. Am J Ophthalmol 1988;105:170–81.
207. Maher ER, Moore AT. von Hippel–Lindau disease. Br J Ophthalmol 1992;76:743–5.
208. Melmon KL, Rosen SW. Lindau's disease; review of the literature and study of a large kindred. Am J Med 1964;36:595–617.
209. Nerad JA, Kersten RC, Anderson RL. Hemangioblastoma of the optic nerve; report of a case and review of literature. Ophthalmology 1988;95:398–402.
210. Oosterhuis JA, Rubinstein K. Haemangioma at the optic disc. Ophthalmologica 1972;164:362–74.
211. Ridley M, Green J, Johnson G. Retinal angiomatosis: the ocular manifestations of von Hippel–Lindau disease. Can J Ophthalmol 1986;21:276–83.
212. Schindler RF, Sarin LK, MacDonald PR. Hemangiomas of the optic disc. Can J Ophthalmol 1975;10:305–18.
213. Schmidt D, Neumann HPH. Atypische retinale Veränderungen bei v. Hippel–Lindau-Syndrom. Fortschr Ophthalmol 1987;84:187–9.
214. Schmidt D, Neumann HPH, Witschel H. Mikroläsionen der Retina bei Patienten mit v. Hippel–Lindau-Syndrom. Fortschr Ophthalmol 1986;83:233–5.
215. Takahashi T, Wada H, Tani E, et al. Capillary hemangioma of the optic disc. J Clin Neuro-Ophthalmol 1984;4:159–62.
216. Thomas JV, Gragoudas ES, Blair NP, et al. Correlation of epinephrine use and macular edema in aphakic glaucomatous eyes. Arch Ophthalmol 1978;96:625–8.
217. Yimoyines DJ, Topilow HW, Abedin S, et al. Bilateral peripapillary exophytic retinal hemangioblastomas. Ophthalmology 1982;89:1388–92.
218. Singh AD, Nouri M, Shields CL, et al. Retinal capillary hemangioma: a comparison of sporadic cases and cases associated with von Hippel–Lindau disease. Ophthalmology 2001;108:1907–11.
219. Singh AD, Shields CL, Shields JA. von Hippel–Lindau disease. Surv Ophthalmol 2001;46: 117–42.
220. Fritch CD. Multiple carcinomatosis and von Hippel–Lindau disease requiring bilateral nephrectomy. Ann Ophthalmol 1980;12:1307–9.
221. de Jong PTVM, Verkaart RJF, van de Vooren MJ, et al. Twin vessels in von Hippel–Lindau disease. Am J Ophthalmol 1988;105:165–9.
222. Latif F, Tory K, Gnarra J, et al. Identification of the von Hippel–Lindau disease tumor suppressor gene. Science 1993;260:1317–20.
223. Stolle C, Glenn G, Zbar B, et al. Improved detection of germline mutations in the von Hippel–Lindau disease tumor suppressor gene. Hum Mutat 1998;12:417–23.
224. Singh AD, Ahmad NN, Shields CL, et al. Solitary retinal capillary hemangioma: lack of genetic evidence for von Hippel–Lindau disease. Ophthalmic Genet 2002;23:21–7.
225. Laatikainen L, Immonen I, Summanen P. Peripheral retinal angiomalike lesion and macular pucker. Am J Ophthalmol 1989;108:563–6.
226. Schwartz PL, Fastenberg DM, Shakin JL. Management of macular puckers associated with retinal angiomas. Ophthalmic Surg 1990;21:550–6.
227. Schwartz PL, Trubowitsch G, Fastenberg DM, et al. Macular pucker and retinal angioma. Ophthalmic Surg 1987;18:677–9.
228. Nicholson DH, Anderson LS, Blodi C. Rhegmatogenous retinal detachment in angiomatosis retinae. Am J Ophthalmol 1986;101:187–9.
229. Imes RK, Monteiro MLR, Hoyt WF. Incipient hemangioblastoma of the optic disk. Am J Ophthalmol 1984;98:116.
230. Jesberg DO, Spencer WH, Hoyt WF. Incipient lesions of von Hippel–Lindau disease. Arch Ophthalmol 1968;80:632–40.
231. Magnússon L, Törnquist R. Incipient lesions in angiomatosis retinae. Acta Ophthalmol 1973;51:152–8.
232. Salazar FG, Lamiell JM. Early identification of retinal angiomas in a large kindred with von Hippel–Lindau disease. Am J Ophthalmol 1980;89:540–5.
233. Welch RB. von Hippel–Lindau disease: The recognition and treatment of early angiomatosis retinae and the use of cryosurgery as an adjunct to therapy. Trans Am Ophthalmol Soc 1970;68:367–424.
234. Grossniklaus HE, Thomas JW, Vigneswaran N, et al. Retinal hemangioblastoma; a histologic, immunohistochemical, and ultrastructural evaluation. Ophthalmology 1992;99:140–5.
235. Jakobiec FA, Font RL, Johnson FB. Angiomatosis retinae: an ultrastructural study and lipid analysis. Cancer 1976;38:2042–56.
236. Mottow-Lippa L, Tso MOM, Peyman GA, et al. von Hippel angiomatosis; a light, electron microscopic, and immunoperoxidase characterization. Ophthalmology 1983;90:848–55.
237. Nicholson DH, Green WR, Kenyon KR. Light and electron microscopic study of early lesions in angiomatosis retinae. Am J Ophthalmol 1976;82:193–204.
238. Souders BF. Juxtapapillary hemangioendothelioma of the retina; report of a case. Arch Ophthalmol 1949;41:178–82.
239. Whitson JT, Welch RB, Green WR. Von Hippel–Lindau disease: case report of a patient with spontaneous regression of a retinal angioma. Retina 1986;6:253–9.

240. Chan CC, Vortmeyer AO, Chew EY, et al. VHL gene deletion and enhanced VEGF gene expression detected in the stromal cells of retinal angioma. Arch Ophthalmol 1999;117:625–30.
241. Kaelin WG, Iliopoulos O, Lonergan KM, et al. Functions of the von Hippel–Lindau tumour suppressor protein. J Intern Med 1998;243:535–9.
242. Apple DJ, Goldberg MF, Wyhinny GJ. Argon laser treatment of von Hippel–Lindau retinal angiomas. II. Histopathology of treated lesions. Arch Ophthalmol 1974;92:126–30.
243. Blodi CF, Russell SR, Pulido JS, et al. Direct and feeder vessel photocoagulation of retinal angiomas with dye yellow laser. Ophthalmology 1990;97:791–5.
244. Goldberg MF, Koenig S. Argon laser treatment of von Hippel–Lindau retinal angiomas. I. Clinical and angiographic findings. Arch Ophthalmol 1974;92:121–5.
245. Amoils SP, Smith TR. Cryotherapy of angiomatosis retinae. Arch Ophthalmol 1969;81:689–91.
246. Watzke RC. Cryotherapy for retinal angiomatosis; a clinicopathologic report. Arch Ophthalmol 1974;92:399–401.
247. Watzke RC, Weingeist TA, Constantine JB. Diagnosis and management of von Hippel–Lindau disease. In: Peyman GA, Apple DJ, Sanders DR, editors. Intraocular tumors. New York: Appleton-Century-Crofts; 1977. p. 199–217.
248. Singh AD, Nouri M, Shields CL, et al. Treatment of retinal capillary hemangioma. Ophthalmology 2002;109:1799–806.
249. Cardosa RD, Brockhurst RJ. Perforating diathermy coagulation for retinal angiomas. Arch Ophthalmol 1976;94:1702–15.
250. Johnson MW, Flynn Jr HW, Gass JDM. Pars plana vitrectomy and direct diathermy for complications of multiple retinal angiomas. Ophthalmic Surg 1992;23:47–50.
251. Peyman GA, Rednam KRV, Mottow-Lippa L, et al. Treatment of large von Hippel tumors by eye wall resection. Ophthalmology 1983;90:840–7.
252. Atebara NH. Retinal capillary hemangioma treated with verteporfin photodynamic therapy. Am J Ophthalmol 2002;134:788–90.
253. Schmidt-Erfurth UM, Kusserow C, Barbazetto IA, et al. Benefits and complications of photodynamic therapy of papillary capillary hemangiomas. Ophthalmology 2002;109:1256–66.
254. Schmidt D, Natt E, Neumann HP. Long-term results of laser treatment for retinal angiomatosis in von Hippel–Lindau disease. Eur J Med Res 2000;5:47–58.
255. Sachdeva R, Dadgostar H, Kaiser PK, et al. Verteporfin photodynamic therapy of six eyes with retinal capillary haemangioma. Acta Ophthalmol 2010;88:e334–40.
256. Dahr SS, Cusick M, Rodriguez-Coleman H, et al. Intravitreal anti-vascular endothelial growth factor therapy with pegaptanib for advanced von Hippel–Lindau disease of the retina. Retina 2007;27:150–8.
257. Wong WT, Liang KJ, Hammel K, et al. Intravitreal ranibizumab therapy for retinal capillary hemangioblastoma related to von Hippel–Lindau disease. Ophthalmology 2008;115:1957–64.
258. Wong WT, Chew EY. Ocular von Hippel–Lindau disease: clinical update and emerging treatments. Curr Opin Ophthalmol 2008;19:213–7.
259. Dabezies OH, Walsh FB, Hayes GJ. Papilledema with hamartoma of hypothalmus. Arch Ophthalmol 1961;65:174–80.
260. Darr JL, Hughes Jr RP, McNair JN. Bilateral peripapillary retinal hemangiomas; a case report. Arch Ophthalmol 1966;75:77–81.
261. Campochiaro PA, Conway BP. Hemangiomalike masses of the retina. Arch Ophthalmol 1988;106:1409–13.
262. De Laey JJ, Heintz B, Pollet L. Retinal angioma and juvenile sex-linked retinoschisis. Ophthalmic Paediatr Genet 1992;13:73–6.
263. Gottlieb F, Fammartino JJ, Stratford TP, et al. Retinal angiomatous mass; a complication of retinal detachment surgery. Retina 1984;4:152–7.
264. Medlock RD, Shields JA, Shields CL, et al. Retinal hemangioma-like lesions in eyes with retinitis pigmentosa. Retina 1990;10:274–7.
265. Retsas C, Sarks J, Shanahan J. Angiomatose rétinienne associée à une maladie de Stargardt. A propos d'un cas clique. J Fr Ophtalmol 1989;12:857–62.
266. Schachat AP, Markowitz JA, Guyer DR, et al. Ophthalmic manifestations of leukemia. Arch Ophthalmol 1989;107:697–700.
267. Kincaid MC, Green WR. Ocular and orbital involvement in leukemia. Surv Ophthalmol 1983;27:211–32.
268. Leonardy NJ, Rupani M, Dent G, et al. Analysis of 135 autopsy eyes for ocular involvement in leukemia. Am J Ophthalmol 1990;109:436–44.
269. Guyer DR, Schachat AP, Vitale S, et al. Leukemic retinopathy; relationship between fundus lesions and hematologic parameters at diagnosis. Ophthalmology 1989;96:860–4.
270. Buchan J, McKibbin M, Burton T. The prevalence of ocular disease in chronic lymphocytic leukaemia. Eye (Lond) 2003;17:27–30.
271. Allen RA, Straatsma BR. Ocular involvement in leukemia and allied disorders. Arch Ophthalmol 1961;66:490–508.
272. Culler AM. Fundus changes in leukemia. Trans Am Ophthalmol Soc 1951;49:445–73.
273. Cullis CM, Hines DR, Bullock JD. Anterior segment ischemia: classification and description in chronic myelogenous leukemia. Ann Ophthalmol 1979;11:1739–44.
274. De Juan E, Green WR, Rice TA, et al. Optic disc neovascularization associated with ocular involvement in acute lymphocytic leukemia. Retina 1982;2:61–4.
275. Duke JR, Wilkinson CP, Sigelman S. Retinal microaneurysms in leukaemia. Br J Ophthalmol 1968;52:368–74.
276. Holt JM, Gordon-Smith EC. Retinal abnormalities in diseases of the blood. Br J Ophthalmol 1969;53:145–60.
277. Mahneke A, Videbaek A. On changes in the optic fundus in leukaemia; aetiology, diagnostic and prognostic role. Acta Ophthalmol 1964;42:201–10.
278. Rosenthal AR, Egbert PR, Wilbur JR, et al. Leukemic involvement of the optic nerve. J Pediatr Ophthalmol 1975;12:84–93.
279. Swartz M, Schumann GB. Acute leukemic infiltration of the vitreous diagnosed by pars plana aspiration. Am J Ophthalmol 1980;90:326–30.
280. Wood WJ, Nicholson DH. Corneal ring ulcer as the presenting manifestation of acute monocytic leukemia. Am J Ophthalmol 1973;76:69–72.
281. Mehta P. Ophthalmologic manifestations of leukemia. J Pediatr 1979;95:156–7.
282. Karesh JW, Goldman EJ, Reck K, et al. A prospective ophthalmic evaluation of patients with acute myeloid leukemia: correlation of ocular and hematologic findings. J Clin Oncol 1989;7:1528–32.
283. Ohkoshi K, Tsiaras WG. Prognostic importance of ophthalmic manifestations in childhood leukaemia. Br J Ophthalmol 1992;76:651–5.
284. Kuwabara T, Aiello L. Leukemic miliary nodules in the retina. Arch Ophthalmol 1964;72:494–7.
285. Robb RM, Ervin LD, Sallan SE. A pathological study of eye involvement in acute leukemia of childhood. Trans Am Ophthalmol Soc 1978;76:90–101.
286. Jampol LM, Goldberg MF, Busse B. Peripheral retinal microaneurysms in chronic leukemia. Am J Ophthalmol 1975;80:242–8.
287. Delaney Jr WV, Kinsella G. Optic disk neovascularization in leukemia. Am J Ophthalmol 1985;99:212–3.
288. Minnella AM, Yannuzzi LA, Slakter JS, et al. Bilateral perifoveal ischemia associated with chronic granulocytic leukemia. Arch Ophthalmol 1988;106:1170–1.
289. Wiznia RA, Rose A, Levy AL. Occlusive microvascular retinopathy with optic disc and retinal neovascularization in acute lymphocytic leukemia. Retina 1994;14:253–5.
290. Frank RN, Ryan Jr SJ. Peripheral retinal neovascularization with chronic myelogenous leukemia. Arch Ophthalmol 1972;87:585–9.
291. Leveille AS, Morse PH. Platelet-induced retinal neovascularization in leukemia. Am J Ophthalmol 1981;91:640–3.
292. Little HL. The role of abnormal hemorrheodynamics in the pathogenesis of diabetic retinopathy. Trans Am Ophthalmol Soc 1976;74:573–636.
293. Morse PH, McCready JL. Peripheral retinal neovascularization in chronic myelocytic leukemia. Am J Ophthalmol 1971;72:975–8.
294. Hofman P, Le Tourneau A, Negre F, et al. Primary uveal B immunoblastic lymphoma in a patient with AIDS. Br J Ophthalmol 1992;76:700–2.
295. Inkeles DM, Friedman AH. Retinal pigment epithelial degeneration, partial retinal atrophy and macular hole in acute lymphocytic leukemia. Albrecht von Graefes Arch Clin Exp Ophthalmol 1975;194:253–61.
296. Verbraak FD, van den Berg W, Bos PJM. Retinal pigment epitheliopathy in acute leukemia. Am J Ophthalmol 1991;111:111–3.
297. Brown DM, Kimura AE, Ossoinig KC, et al. Acute promyelocytic infiltration of the optic nerve treated by oral trans-retinoic acid. Ophthalmology 1992;99:1463–7.
298. Ellis W, Little HL. Leukemic infiltration of the optic nerve head. Am J Ophthalmol 1973;75:867–71.
299. Horton JC, Garcia EG, Becker EK. Magnetic resonance imaging of leukemic invasion of the optic nerve. Arch Ophthalmol 1992;110:1207–8.
300. Nikaido H, Mishima H, Ono H, et al. Leukemic involvement of the optic nerve. Am J Ophthalmol 1988;105:294–8.
301. Zimmerman LE, Thoreson HT. Sudden loss of vision in acute leukemia; a clinicopathologic report of two unusual cases. Surv Ophthalmol 1964;9:467–73.
302. Rosenthal AR. Ocular manifestations of leukemia; a review. Ophthalmology 1983;90:899–905.
303. Badelon I, Chaine G, Tolub O, et al. Occlusion de la veine et de l'artère centrale de la rétine par infiltration du nerf optique au cours d'une leucémie aigue lymphoblastique. Bull Soc Ophtalmol Fr 1986;86:261–4.
304. Currie JN, Lessell S, Lessell IM, et al. Optic neuropathy in chronic lymphocytic leukemia. Arch Ophthalmol 1988;106:654–60.
305. Johnston SS, Ware CF. Iris involvement in leukaemia. Br J Ophthalmol 1973;57:320–4.
306. Glaser B, Smith JL. Leukaemic glaucoma. Br J Ophthalmol 1966;50:92–4.
307. Gass JDM, Sever RJ, Grizzard WS, et al. Multifocal pigment epithelial detachments by reticulum cell sarcoma; a characteristic fundoscopic picture. Retina 1984;4:135–43.
308. Chan CC, Gonzales JA, Hidayat AA. Intraocular lymphoproliferations simulating uveitis. In: Albert DM, Miller JW, editors. Principles and practice of ophthalmology, 3rd ed. New York: Saunders-Elsevier; 2008. p. 1255–80.
309. Singh AD, Lewis H, Schachat AP, et al. Lymphoma of the retina and CNS. In: Singh AD, Damato BE, Pe'er J, editors. Clinical ophthalmic oncology. Philadelphia: Saunders-Elsevier; 2007. p. 372–7.
310. Bardenstein DS. Intraocular lymphoma. Cancer Control 1998;5:317–25.
311. Eby NL, Grufferman S, Flannelly CM, et al. Increasing incidence of primary brain lymphoma in the US. Cancer 1988;62:2461–5.
312. Corn BW, Marcus SM, Topham A, et al. Will primary central nervous system lymphoma be the most frequent brain tumor diagnosed in the year 2000? Cancer 1997;79:2409–13.
313. Schabet M. Epidemiology of primary CNS lymphoma. J Neurooncol 1999;43:199–201.
314. Deangelis LM, Hormigo A. Treatment of primary central nervous system lymphoma. Semin Oncol 2004;31:684–92.
315. Peterson K, Gordon KB, Heinemann MH, et al. The clinical spectrum of ocular lymphoma. Cancer 1993;72:843–9.
316. Akpek EK, Ahmed I, Hochberg FH, et al. Intraocular-central nervous system lymphoma: clinical features, diagnosis, and outcomes. Ophthalmology 1999;106:1805–10.
317. Rockwood EJ, Zakov ZN, Bay JW. Combined malignant lymphoma of the eye and CNS (reticulum-cell sarcoma). Report of three cases. J Neurosurg 1984;61:369–74.
318. Chan CC. Primary intraocular lymphoma: clinical features, diagnosis, and treatment. Clin Lymphoma 2003;4:30–1.
319. Wender A, Adar A, Maor E, et al. Primary B-cell lymphoma of the eyes and brain in a 3-year-old boy. Arch Ophthalmol 1994;112:450–1.
320. Givner I. Malignant lymphoma with ocular involvement; a clinico-pathologic report. Am J Ophthalmol 1955;39:29–32.
321. Goder G, Klein S, Königsdörffer E. Klinische und pathologische Besonderheiten des malignen Lymphoms der Netzhaut. Klin Monatsbl Augenheilkd 1990;197:514–8.
322. Gass JDM, Trattler HL. Retinal artery obstruction and atheromas associated with non-Hodgkin's large cell lymphoma (reticulum cell sarcoma). Arch Ophthalmol 1991;109:1134–9.
323. Ridley ME, McDonald HR, Sternberg Jr P, et al. Retinal manifestations of ocular lymphoma (reticulum cell sarcoma). Ophthalmology 1992;99:1153–61.

324. Gray RS, Abrahams JJ, Hufnagel TJ, et al. Ghost-cell tumor of the optic chiasm; primary CNS lymphoma. J Clin Neuro-Ophthalmol 1989;9:98–104.
325. Guyer DR, Green WR, Schachat AP, et al. Bilateral ischemic optic neuropathy and retinal vascular occlusions associated with lymphoma and sepsis; clinicopathologic correlation. Ophthalmology 1990;97:882–8.
326. Kattah JC, Suski ET, Killen JY, et al. Optic neuritis and systemic lymphoma. Am J Ophthalmol 1980;89:431–6.
327. Lang GK, Surer JL, Green WR, et al. Ocular reticulum cell sarcoma; clinicopathologic correlation of a case with multifocal lesions. Retina 1985;5:79–86.
328. Margolis L, Fraser R, Lichter A, et al. The role of radiation therapy in the management of ocular reticulum cell sarcoma. Cancer 1980;45:688–92.
329. Whitcup SM, de Smet MD, Rubin BI, et al. Intraocular lymphoma; clinical and histopathologic diagnosis. Ophthalmology 1993;100:1399–406.
330. Blumenkranz MS, Ward T, Murphy S, et al. Applications and limitations of vitreoretinal biopsy techniques in intraocular large cell lymphoma. Retina 1992;12(Suppl.):S64–70.
331. Char DH, Ljung B-M, Deschenes J, et al. Intraocular lymphoma: immunological and cytological analysis. Br J Ophthalmol 1988;72:905–11.
332. Kaplan HJ, Meredith TA, Aaberg TM, et al. Reclassification of intraocular reticulum cell sarcoma (histiocytic lymphoma); immunologic characterization of vitreous cells. Arch Ophthalmol 1980;98:707–10.
333. Kennerdell JS, Johnson BL, Wisotzkey HM. Vitreous cellular reaction; association with reticulum cell sarcoma of brain. Arch Ophthalmol 1975;93:1341–5.
334. Michels RG, Knox DL, Erozan YS, et al. Intraocular reticulum cell sarcoma; diagnosis by pars plana vitrectomy. Arch Ophthalmol 1975;93:1331–5.
335. Michelson JB, Michelson PE, Bordin GM, et al. Ocular reticulum cell sarcoma; presentation as retinal detachment with demonstration of monoclonal immunoglobulin light chains on the vitreous cells. Arch Ophthalmol 1981;99:1409–11.
336. Minckler DS, Font RL, Zimmerman LE. Uveitis and reticulum cell sarcoma of brain with bilateral neoplastic seeding of vitreous without retinal or uveal involvement. Am J Ophthalmol 1975;80:433–9.
337. Parver LM, Font RL. Malignant lymphoma of the retina and brain; initial diagnosis by cytologic examination of vitreous aspirate. Arch Ophthalmol 1979;97:1505–7.
338. Kirmani MH, Thomas EL, Rao NA, et al. Intraocular reticulum cell sarcoma: diagnosis by choroidal biopsy. Br J Ophthalmol 1987;71:748–52.
339. DeAngelis LM. Primary central nervous system lymphoma: a new clinical challenge. Neurology 1991;41:619–21.
340. Neuwelt EA, Frenkel EP, Gumerlock MK, et al. Developments in the diagnosis and treatment of primary CNS lymphoma; a prospective series. Cancer 1986;58:1609–20.
341. Wilson DJ, Braziel R, Rosenbaum JT. Intraocular lymphoma; immunopathologic analysis of vitreous biopsy specimens. Arch Ophthalmol 1992;110:1455–8.
342. White VA, Gascoyne RD, Paton KE. Use of the polymerase chain reaction to detect B- and T-cell gene rearrangements in vitreous specimens from patients with intraocular lymphoma. Arch Ophthalmol 1999;117:761–5.
343. Coupland SE, Bechrakis NE, Anastassiou G, et al. Evaluation of vitrectomy specimens and chorioretinal biopsies in the diagnosis of primary intraocular lymphoma in patients with Masquerade syndrome. Graefes Arch Clin Exp Ophthalmol 2003;241:860–70.
344. Chan CC, Whitcup SM, Solomon D, et al. Interleukin-10 in the vitreous of patients with primary intraocular lymphoma. Am J Ophthalmol 1995;120:671–3.
345. Barr CC, Green WR, Payne JW, et al. Intraocular reticulum-cell sarcoma: clinicopathologic study of four cases and review of the literature. Surv Ophthalmol 1975;19:224–39.
346. Vogel MH, Font RL, Zimmerman LE, et al. Reticulum cell sarcoma of the retina and uvea; report of six cases and review of the literature. Am J Ophthalmol 1968;66:205–15.
347. Batchelor TT, Kolak G, Ciordia R, et al. High-dose methotrexate for intraocular lymphoma. Clin Cancer Res 2003;9:711–5.
348. Frenkel S, Hendler K, Siegal T, et al. Intravitreal methotrexate for treating vitreoretinal lymphoma: 10 years of experience. Br J Ophthalmol 2008;92:383–8.
349. Itty S, Pulido JS. Rituximab for intraocular lymphoma. Retina 2009;29:129–32.
350. Yeh S, Wilson DJ. Combination intravitreal rituximab and methotrexate for massive subretinal lymphoma. Eye (Lond) 2010;24:1625–7.
351. Sandor V, Stark-Vancs V, Pearson D, et al. Phase II trial of chemotherapy alone for primary CNS and intraocular lymphoma. J Clin Oncol 1998;16:3000–6.
352. Hormigo A, DeAngelis LM. Primary ocular lymphoma: clinical features, diagnosis, and treatment. Clin Lymphoma 2003;4:22–9.
353. Ahluwalia MS, Peereboom DM. Primary Central Nervous System Lymphoma. Curr Treat Options Neurol 2010;12:347–59.
354. Galor A, Ference SJ, Singh AD, et al. Maculopathy as a complication of blood–brain barrier disruption in patients with central nervous system lymphoma. Am J Ophthalmol 2007;144:45–9.
355. Angelov L, Doolittle ND, Kraemer DF, et al. Blood–brain barrier disruption and intra-arterial methotrexate-based therapy for newly diagnosed primary CNS lymphoma: a multi-institutional experience. J Clin Oncol 2009;27:3503–9.
356. Kohno T, Uchida H, Inomata H, et al. Ocular manifestations of adult T-cell leukemia/lymphoma; a clinicopathologic study. Ophthalmology 1993;100:1794–9.
357. Kumar SR, Gill PS, Wagner DG, et al. Human T-cell lymphotropic virus type I-associated retinal lymphoma; a clinicopathologic report. Arch Ophthalmol 1994;112:954–9.
358. Kumar SR, Gill PS, Wagner DG, et al. Human T-cell lymphotropic virus type I-associated retinal lymphoma. A clinicopathologic report. Arch Ophthalmol 1994;112:954–9.
359. Merle H, Donnio A, Gonin C, et al. Retinal vasculitis caused by adult T-cell leukemia/lymphoma. Jpn J Ophthalmol 2005;49:41–5.
360. Levy-Clarke GA, Buggage RR, Shen D, et al. Human T-cell lymphotropic virus type-1 associated t-cell leukemia/lymphoma masquerading as necrotizing retinal vasculitis. Ophthalmology 2002;109:1717–22.
361. Brown SM, Jampol LM, Cantrill HL. Intraocular lymphoma presenting as retinal vasculitis. Surv Ophthalmol 1994;39:133–40.
362. Hogan MJ, editor. A case of intraocular mycosis fungoides. Read before the Verhoeff Society meeting, April 11, 1972, Washington, DC.
363. Keltner JL, Fritsch E, Cykiert RC, et al. Mycosis fungoides; intraocular and central nervous system involvement. Arch Ophthalmol 1977;95:645–50.
364. Wolter JR, Leenhouts TM, Hendrix RC. Corneal involvement in mycosis fungoides. Am J Ophthalmol 1963;55:317–22.
365. Cook Jr. BE, Bartley GB, Pittelkow MR. Ophthalmic abnormalities in patients with cutaneous T-cell lymphoma. Ophthalmology 1999;106:1339–44.
366. Ralli M, Goldman JW, Lee E, et al. Intraocular involvement of mycosis fungoides. Arch Ophthalmol 2009;127:343–5.
367. Leitch RJ, Rennie IG, Parsons MA. Ocular involvement in mycosis fungoides. Br J Ophthalmol 1993;77:126–7.
368. Foerster HC. Mycosis fungoides with intraocular involvement. Trans Am Acad Ophthalmol Otolaryngol 1960;64:308–13.
369. Gärtner J. Mycosis fungoides mit Beteiligung der Aderhaut. Klin Monatsbl Augenheilkd 1957;131:61–9.
370. Erny BC, Egbert PR, Peat IM, et al. Intraocular involvement with subretinal pigment epithelium infiltrates by mycosis fungoides. Br J Ophthalmol 1991;75:698–701.
371. Lewis RA, Clark RB. Infiltrative retinopathy in systemic lymphoma. Am J Ophthalmol 1975;79:48–52.
372. Clarke E. Ophthalmological complications of multiple myelomatosis. Br J Ophthalmol 1955;39:233–6.
373. Gudas Jr. PP. Optic nerve myeloma. Am J Ophthalmol 1971;71:1085–9.
374. Langdon HM. Multiple myeloma with bilateral sixth nerve paralysis and left retrobulbar neuritis. Trans Am Ophthalmol Soc 1939;37:223–8.
375. Shields CL, Chong WH, Ehya H, et al. Sequential bilateral solitary extramedullary plasmacytoma of the ciliary body. Cornea 2007;26:759–61.
376. Palamar M, Shields CL, Ghassemi F, et al. Choroidal plasmacytoma in a patient with multiple myeloma. Diagnosis by fine-needle aspiration biopsy. Graefes Arch Clin Exp Ophthalmol 2008;246:1195–7.
377. Chan TY, Hodge WG. Vitritis and retinal vasculitis as presenting signs of monoclonal gammopathy of unknown significance with progression to multiple myeloma. Can J Ophthalmol 2010;45: 82–3.
378. Omoti CE, Omoti AE. Richter syndrome: a review of clinical, ocular, neurological and other manifestations. Br J Haematol 2008;142:709–16.
379. Hattenhauer MG, Pach JM. Ocular lymphoma in a patient with chronic lymphocytic leukemia. Am J Ophthalmol 1996;122:266–8.
380. Antle CM, White VA, Horsman DE, et al. Large cell orbital lymphoma in a patient with acquired immune deficiency syndrome; case report and review. Ophthalmology 1990;97:1494–8.
381. Al-Hazzaa SAF, Green WR, Mann RB. Uveal involvement in systemic angiotropic large cell lymphoma; microscopic and immunohistochemical studies. Ophthalmology 1993;100: 961–5.
382. Elner VM, Hidayat AA, Charles NC, et al. Neoplastic angioendotheliomatosis; a variant of malignant lymphoma immunohistochemical and ultrastructural observations of three cases. Ophthalmology 1986;93:1237–45.
383. Katzenstein AL, Doxtader E, Narendra S. Lymphomatoid granulomatosis: insights gained over 4 decades. Am J Surg Pathol 2010;34:e35–48.
384. Tse DT, Mandelbaum S, Chuck DA, et al. Lymphomatoid granulomatosis with ocular involvement. Retina 1985;5:94–7.
385. Kinyoun LJ, Kalina RE, Klein ML. Choroidal involvement in systemic necrotizing vasculitis. Arch Ophthalmol 1987;105:939–42.
386. Cameron JR, Cackett P. Lymphomatoid granulomatosis associated with bilateral exudative retinal detachments. Arch Ophthalmol 2007;125:712–3.
387. Ziemianski MC, Godfrey WA, Lee KY, et al. Lymphoma of the vitreous associated with renal transplantation and immunosuppressive therapy. Ophthalmology 1980;87:596–601.
388. Kheterpal S, Kirkby GR, Neuberger JM, et al. Intraocular lymphoma after liver transplantation. Am J Ophthalmol 1993;116:507–8.
389. Demols PF, Cochaux PM, Velu T, et al. Chorioretinal post-transplant lymphoproliferative disorder induced by the Epstein-Barr virus. Br J Ophthalmol 2001;85:93–5.
390. Duke JR, Walsh FB. Metastatic carcinoma to the retina. Am J Ophthalmol 1959;47:44–8.
391. Flindall RJ, Fleming KO. Metastatic tumour of the retina. Can J Ophthalmol 1967;2:130–2.
392. Kennedy RJ, Rummel WD, McCarthy JL, et al. Metastatic carcinoma of the retina; report of a case and the pathologic findings. Arch Ophthalmol 1958;60:12–18.
393. Klein R, Nicholson DH, Luxenberg MN. Retinal metastasis from squamous cell carcinoma of the lung. Am J Ophthalmol 1977;83:358–61.
394. Koenig RP, Johnson DL, Monahan RH. Bronchogenic carcinoma with metastases to the retina. Am J Ophthalmol 1963;56:827–9.
395. Levy RM, de Venecia G. Trypsin digest study of retinal metastasis and tumor cell emboli. Am J Ophthalmol 1970;70:778–82.
396. Leys AM, Van Eyck LM, Nuttin BJ, et al. Metastatic carcinoma to the retina; clinicopathologic findings in two cases. Arch Ophthalmol 1990;108:1448–52.
397. Smoleroff JW, Agatston SA. Metastatic carcinoma of the retina; report of a case, with pathologic observations. Arch Ophthalmol 1934;12:359–65.
398. Striebel-Gerecke SU, Messmer EP, Landolt U. Retinale and vitreale Metastase eines kleinzelligen Bronchuskarzinoms. Klin Monatsbl Augenheilkd 1992;20:535–6.
399. Tachinami K, Katayama T, Takeda N, et al. A case of metastatic carcinoma to the retina. Acta Soc Ophthalmol Jpn 1992;96:1336–40.
400. Takagi T, Yamaguchi T, Mizoguchi T, et al. A case of metastatic optic nerve head and retinal carcinoma with vitreous seeds. Ophthalmologica 1989;199:123–6.
401. Uhler EM. Metastatic malignant melanoma of the retina. Am J Ophthalmol 1940;23:158–62.

402. Young SE, Cruciger M, Lukeman J. Metastatic carcinoma to the retina: case report. Ophthalmology 1979;86:1350–4.
403. Font RL, Naumann G, Zimmerman LE. Primary malignant melanoma of the skin metastatic to the eye and orbit; report of ten cases and review of the literature. Am J Ophthalmol 1967;63:738–54.
404. Letson AD, Davidorf FH. Bilateral retinal metastases from cutaneous malignant melanoma. Arch Ophthalmol 1982;100:605–7.
405. Piro P, Pappas HR, Erozan YS, et al. Diagnostic vitrectomy in metastatic breast carcinoma in the vitreous. Retina 1982;2:182–8.
406. De Bustros S, Augsburger JJ, Shields JA, et al. Intraocular metastases from cutaneous malignant melanoma. Arch Ophthalmol 1985;103:937–40.
407. Liddicoat DA, Wolter JR, Wilkinson WC. Retinal metastasis of malignant melanoblastoma; a case report. Am J Ophthalmol 1959;48:172–7.
408. Pollock SC, Awh CC, Dutton JJ. Cutaneous melanoma metastatic to the optic disc and vitreous. Arch Ophthalmol 1991;109:1352–4.
409. Riffenburgh RS. Metastatic malignant melanoma to the retina. Arch Ophthalmol 1961;66:487–9.
410. Robertson DM, Wilkinson CP, Murray JL, et al. Metastatic tumor to the retina and vitreous cavity from primary melanoma of the skin; treatment with systemic and subconjunctival chemotherapy. Ophthalmology 1981;88:1296–301.
411. Friedman AH. Discussion of three papers. Ophthalmology 1979;86:1355–8.
412. Buchanan TAS, Gardiner TA, Archer DB. An ultrastructural study of retinal photoreceptor degeneration associated with bronchial carcinoma. Am J Ophthalmol 1984;97:277–87.
413. Cogan DG, Kuwabara T, Currie J, et al. Paraneoplastische Retinopathie unter dem klinischen Bild einer Zapfendystrophie mit Achromatopsie. Klin Monatsbl Augenheilkd 1990;197:156–8.
414. Grunwald GB, Klein R, Simmonds MA, et al. Autoimmune basis for visual paraneoplastic syndrome in patients with small-cell lung carcinoma. Lancet 1985;1:658–61.
415. Grunwald GB, Kornguth SC, Towfighi J, et al. Autoimmune basis for visual paraneoplastic syndrome in patients with small cell lung carcinoma; retinal immune deposits and ablation of retinal ganglion cells. Cancer 1987;60:780–6.
416. Jacobson DM, Thirkill CE, Tipping SJ. A clinical triad to diagnose paraneoplastic retinopathy. Ann Neurol 1990;28:162–7.
417. Keltner JL, Roth AM, Chang RS. Photoreceptor degeneration; possible autoimmune disorder. Arch Ophthalmol 1983;101:564–9.
418. Klingele TG, Burde RM, Rappazzo JA, et al. Paraneoplastic retinopathy. J Clin Neuro-Ophthalmol 1984;4:239–45.
419. Kornguth SE, Kalinke T, Grunwald GB, et al. Anti-neurofilament antibodies in the sera of patients with small cell carcinoma of the lung and with paraneoplastic syndrome. Cancer Res 1986;46:2588–95.
420. Matsui Y, Mehta MC, Katsumi O, et al. Electrophysiological findings in paraneoplastic retinopathy. Graefes Arch Clin Exp Ophthalmol 1992;230:324–8.
421. Rizzo III JF, Gittinger Jr. JW. Selective immunohistochemical staining in the paraneoplastic retinopathy syndrome. Ophthalmology 1992;99:1286–95.
422. Sawyer RA, Selhorst JB, Zimmerman LE, et al. Blindness caused by photoreceptor degeneration as a remote effect of cancer. Am J Ophthalmol 1976;81:606–13.
423. Thirkill CE, FitzGerald P, Sergott RC, et al. Cancer-associated retinopathy (CAR syndrome) with antibodies reacting with retinal, optic-nerve, and cancer cells. N Engl J Med 1989;321:1589–94.
424. Van Der Pol BAE, Planten JT. A non-metastatic remote effect of lung carcinoma. Doc Ophthalmol 1987;67:89–94.
425. Thirkill CE. Cancer-induced, immune-mediated ocular degenerations. Ocul Immunol Inflamm 2005;13:119–31.
426. Thirkill CE, Roth AM, Keltner JR. Cancer-associated retinopathy. Arch Ophthalmol 1987;105:372–5.
427. Thirkill CE, Keltner JL, Tyler NK, et al. Antibody reactions with retina and cancer-associated antigens in 10 patients with cancer-associated retinopathy. Arch Ophthalmol 1993;111:931–7.
428. Thirkill CE, Tait RC, Tyler NK, et al. Intraperitoneal cultivation of small-cell carcinoma induces expression of the retinal cancer-associated retinopathy antigen. Arch Ophthalmol 1993;111:974–8.
429. Keltner JL, Thirkill CE, Tyler NK, et al. Management and monitoring of cancer-associated retinopathy. Arch Ophthalmol 1992;110:48–53.
430. Brain RL, Norris Jr. FH. The remote effects of cancer on the nervous system. New York: Grune & Stratton; 1965. p. 24.
431. Malik S, Furlan AJ, Sweeney PJ, et al. Optic neuropathy: a rare paraneoplastic syndrome. J Clin Neuro-Ophthalmol 1992;12:137–41.
432. Albert DM, Sober AJ, Fitzpatrick TB. Iritis in patients with cutaneous melanoma and vitiligo. Arch Ophthalmol 1978;96:2081–4.
433. Berson EL, Lessell S. Paraneoplastic night blindness with malignant melanoma. Am J Ophthalmol 1988;106:307–11.
434. Gass JDM. Acute Vogt–Koyanagi–Harada-like syndrome occurring in a patient with metastatic cutaneous melanoma. In: Saari KM, editors. Uveitis update: proceedings of the First International Symposium on Uveitis held in Hanasaari, Espoo, Finland on May 16–19, 1984. Amsterdam: Excerpta Medica; 1984, p. 407–408.
435. Hertz KC, Gazze LA, Kirkpatrick CH, et al. Autoimmune vitiligo; detection of antibodies to melanin-producing cells. N Engl J Med 1977;297:634–7.
436. Rush JA. Paraneoplastic retinopathy in malignant melanoma. Am J Ophthalmol 1993;115:390–1.
437. Weinstein JM, Kelman SE, Bresnick GH, et al. Paraneoplastic retinopathy associated with antiretinal bipolar cell antibodies in cutaneous malignant melanoma. Ophthalmology 1994;101:1236–43.
438. Donaldson RC. Canaan Jr SA McLean RB, et al. Uveitis and vitiligo associated with BCG treatment for malignant melanoma. Surgery 1974;76:771–8.
439. Singh AD, Milam AH, Shields CL, et al. Melanoma-associated retinopathy. Am J Ophthalmol 1995;119:369–70.
440. Milam AH, Saari JC, Jacobson SG, et al. Autoantibodies against retinal bipolar cells in cutaneous melanoma-associated retinopathy. Invest Ophthalmol Vis Sci 1993;34:91–100.
441. Keltner JL, Thirkill CE, Yip PT. Clinical and immunologic characteristics of melanoma-associated retinopathy syndrome: eleven new cases and a review of 51 previously published cases. J NeuroOphthalmol 2001;21:173–87.
442. Duke-Elder S. System of ophthalmology, vol. 9. Diseases of the uveal tract. St. Louis: CV Mosby; 1966. p. 373.
443. Gass JDM. Vitiliginous chorioretinitis. Arch Ophthalmol 1981;99:1778–87.
444. Sotodeh M, Paridaens D, Keunen J, et al. Paraneoplastic vitelliform retinopathy associated with cutaneous or uveal melanoma and metastases. Klin Monbl Augenheilkd 2005;222:910–4.
445. Eksandh L, Adamus G, Mosgrove L, et al. Autoantibodies against bestrophin in a patient with vitelliform paraneoplastic retinopathy and a metastatic choroidal malignant melanoma. Arch Ophthalmol 2008;126:432–5.
446. Borkowski LM, Grover S, Fishman GA, et al. Retinal findings in melanoma-associated retinopathy. Am J Ophthalmol 2001;132:273–5.
447. Palmowski AM, Haus AH, Pfohler C, et al. Bilateral multifocal chorioretinopathy in a woman with cutaneous malignant melanoma. Arch Ophthalmol 2002;120:1756–61.
448. Jampol LM, Kim HH, Bryar PJ, et al. Multiple serous retinal detachments and subretinal deposits as the presenting signs of metastatic melanoma. Retina 2004;24:320–2.
449. Zacks DN, Pinnolis MK, Berson EL, et al. Melanoma-associated retinopathy and recurrent exudative retinal detachments in a patient with choroidal melanoma. Am J Ophthalmol 2001;132:578–81.
450. Abramson DH, Dunkel IJ, Brodie SE, et al. Bilateral superselective ophthalmic artery chemotherapy for bilateral retinoblastoma: tandem therapy. Arch Ophthalmol 2010;128:370–2.
451. Ramsay RC, Kinyoun JL, Hill CW, et al. Retinal astrocytoma. Am J Ophthalmol 1979;88:32–6.
455. Retsas C, Sarks J, Shanahan L. [Retinal angiomatosis in association with Stargardt's disease. A case report.] J Fr Ophtalmol 1989;12:857–62.
456. Hood CT, Janku L, Lowder CY, et al. Retinal vasoproliferative tumor in association with neurofibromatosis type 1. J Pediatr Ophthalmol Strabismus 2009 Jun;25:1–3.
457. Gass JDM, Weleber RG, Johnson DR. Non-Hodgkin's lymphoma causing fundus picture simulating fundus flavimaculatus. Retina 1987;7:209–14.
458. Robertson DM, Wilkinson CP, Murray JL, et al. Metastatic tumor to the retina and vitreous cavity from primary melanoma of the skin: treatment with systemic and subconjunctival chemotherapy. Ophthalmology 1981;88:1296–301.

CHAPTER 14

Neoplastic Diseases of the Choroid

A variety of tumors, including hamartomas and neoplastic tumors of the choroid, may lead to serous and less often to hemorrhagic detachment of the macula. Examples used in this text are presented to illustrate how these choroidal tumors may cause a clinical picture that can be confused with degenerative or inflammatory diseases of the choroid and retina affecting the macular area.

CHOROIDAL NEVI

Choroidal nevi are developmental tumors composed of benign melanocytes.[1] These tumors are usually not evident at birth. Their maximum period of growth occurs before puberty.[2] However, up to 6.5% of the adult white population may have choroidal nevi.[3,4] Although most do not achieve a size greater than one disc diameter, some reach a size that may simulate that of a medium-size or even large malignant melanoma. It is estimated that the risk of malignant transformation of a choroidal nevus[5] is about 1 in 10 000.[5] Over a period of many years these pigmented or nonpigmented choroidal nevi may cause degenerative changes in Bruch's membrane, drusen deposition (Figures 14.01D and 14.02), serous detachment of the retinal pigment epithelium (RPE) and retina (Figure 14.01A), choroidal neovascularization (Figure 14.01D, G, and J), circinate retinopathy (Figure 14.01J), hemorrhagic detachment of the macula (Figure 14.01J), vitreous hemorrhage, and RPE hyperplasia (Figure 14.03A–C).[2,6–15] Clumps or patches of orange pigment may overlie choroidal nevi, although they are more frequently observed in greater numbers overlying choroidal melanomas. Zones of atrophy of the RPE and a bone corpuscular pattern of pigment migration into the retina may occur at the inferior margin of these nevi, particularly those that are elevated and greater than two disc diameters in size (Figure 14.01G–I and 14.04F–L).[2,9,16] These areas are caused by prolonged detachment of the retina that previously existed in that area, probably during the growth phase of the tumor in childhood. Similar zones occur inferior to choroidal hemangiomas (see Figure 14.16) and choroidal osteomas and in patients with chronic idiopathic central serous chorioretinopathy (see Figure 3.05) and traumatic chorioretinopathy (see Figure 8.02F).

14.01 Macular detachment caused by choroidal melanocytic nevi.

A–C: Serous detachment of the macula caused by a pigmented choroidal tumor presumed to be a nevus in a 27-year-old woman who was seen in June 1972 with a 2-week history of blurred vision in the right eye. Her visual acuity in the right eye was 20/25. She had a two-disc diameter, slightly elevated, pigmented choroidal tumor (A). Overlying the tumor there was a dumbbell-shaped serous detachment of the retina (arrows) that extended into the foveal area. Angiography demonstrated a focal leak of fluorescein dye into the subretinal space (arrow, B). The focal leak was treated with six 50-mm applications of the argon laser. The serous detachment resolved. Her visual acuity returned to 20/15. Ten years later the tumor appears unchanged (C). Visual acuity is 20/20.
D–F: Serous detachment of the macula secondary to a choroidal nevus with overlying drusen in a 67-year-old woman with visual acuity of 20/25. There are several small elevations of the retinal pigment epithelium (RPE) overlying small choroidal neovascular tufts and blood-stained exudate (arrow, D). Early angiograms demonstrated several choroidal neovascular tufts (arrows, E). Later angiograms showed staining of the drusen and choroidal neovascular membranes (CNVMs) on the surface of the tumor (F).
G–I: This 37-year-old woman had subnormal vision in the right eye for at least 14 years. Note the gray-white plaque of fibrovascular tissue lying on the surface of pigmented choroidal tumor that ultrasonographically was elevated 3.5 mm (G). Angiograms showed a CNVM (arrows, H) and a funnel-shaped area of depigmentation (arrow, I) of the RPE that extends inferiorly from the tumor to the ora serrata. The tumor remained unchanged during 13 years of follow-up.
J–L: Hemorrhagic detachment of the macula caused by a CNVM (arrows, K and L) overlying the inferior surface of an elevated pigmented nevus that has remained unchanged in size during 12 years of follow-up.

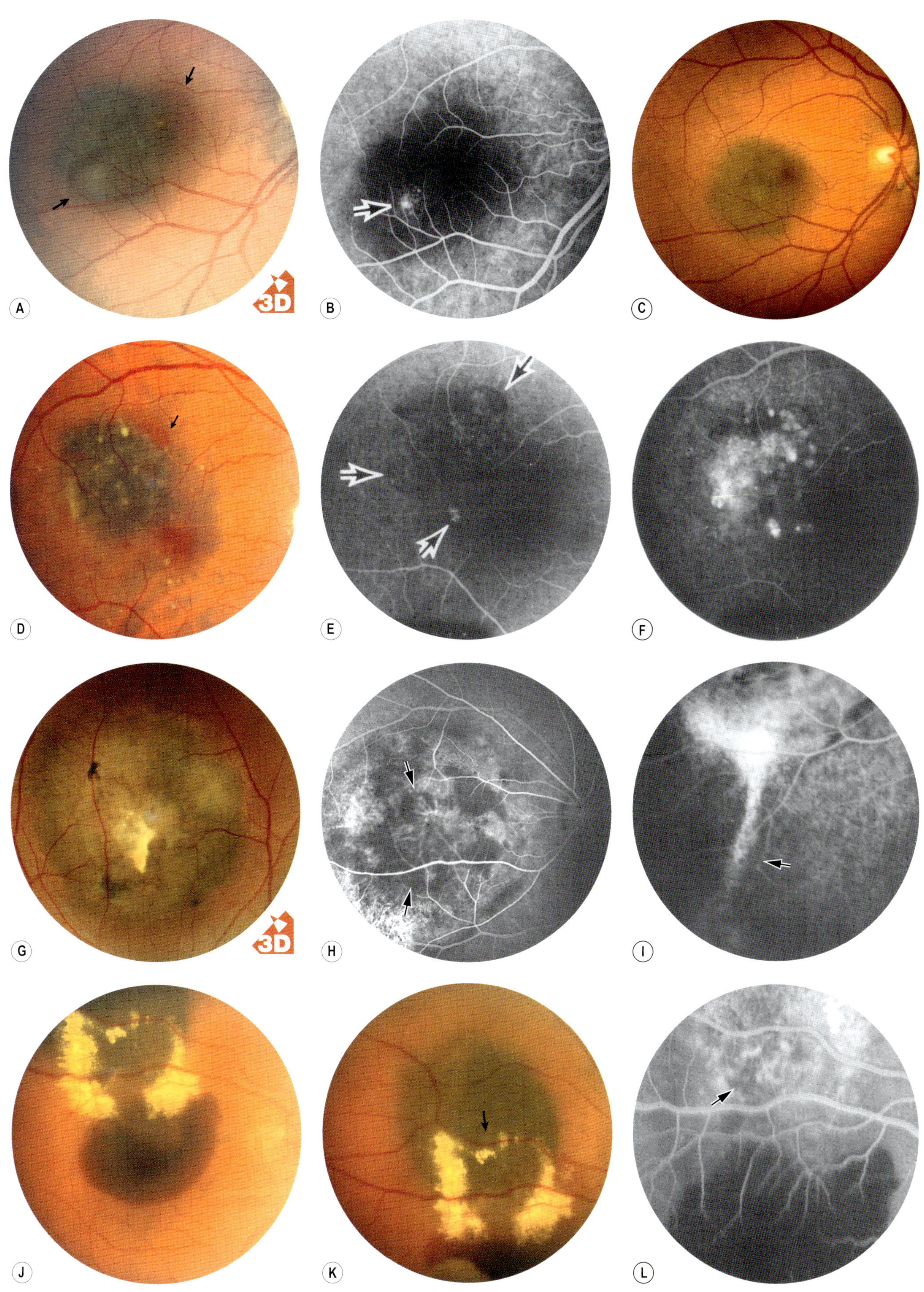
3D
A
B
C
D
E
F
3D
G
H
I
J
K
L

Patients with macular detachments caused by small pigmented choroidal lesions, and those with larger more elevated lesions of uncertain growth potential, should be observed carefully with serial photographs and ultrasonography to exclude the possibility of a malignant melanoma.[16,20] If the lesion is a nevus, particularly in a teenager or young patient, the detachment may resolve spontaneously. In some cases, however, with persistence of the detachment, laser treatment may be necessary (Figure 14.01A–C). The presence of multiple drusen on the surface of a pigmented choroidal tumor, dependent zones of pigment epithelial atrophy adjacent to the tumor, and overlying choroidal neovascularization is highly suggestive that the tumor is a choroidal nevus. While serous retinal detachment may occur overlying a nevus, it is more often a sign of growth potential, particularly if associated with fluorescein angiographic evidence of multiple pinpoint areas of leakage. (See subsection on melanoma for discussion of signs suggesting growth potential of small melanocytic tumors.) Since some choroidal nevi and melanocytomas (one of the cytologic variants of choroidal nevi) may continue to grow beyond adolescence, demonstrable growth, particularly in children or young adults, is not an unequivocal sign of malignancy.[9,16,21–24] It is important to differentiate an increase in size of a nevus caused by an expanding reactive pigment epithelial proliferative and fibrous metaplastic disciform process on the surface of the nevus from growth of the melanocytic tumor itself (Figures 14.03A–C and 14.06).[25,26]

14.03 Long-term follow-up of presumed hypopigmented melanocytic choroidal nevi or tumors of low growth potential.

A–C: In November 1969 this 60-year-old woman presented with visual loss caused by serous macular detachment overlying a submacular elevated hypopigmented choroidal tumor (arrowheads, A). The center of the lesion was hyperpigmented. The diagnosis was melanoma of the choroid. The patient elected to have no treatment. In March 1985 the lesion was unchanged in diameter. Except for a small amount of lipid exudate in the center of the macula, most of the subretinal exudate had resolved (B). Note that the superficial pigmented portion of the tumor was larger. In October 1992 the tumor was unchanged in size (C, wide-angle view). There was no subretinal exudation. It is probable that the pigmented portion of the tumor represents reactive retinal pigment epithelium (RPE) hyperplasia overlying a choroidal nevus.

D and **E**: In 1983 this 65-year-old woman noted a positive central scotoma associated with an elevated nonpigmented choroidal tumor in the right inferior macular area (arrows, D). Note the blood vessels within the tumor. Angiography revealed evidence of RPE depigmentation and clumping as well as staining within and on the surface of the tumor (E). Her visual acuity was 20/40. Ultrasound revealed a 3.2-mm elevated choroidal medium-reflective tumor. Medical evaluation revealed no evidence of metastatic carcinoma. The tumor remained unchanged during 10 years' follow-up. Her visual acuity at last examination was 20/25.

F–L: In December 1968 a small elevated white choroidal tumor (F) was discovered during a routine eye examination in this 46-year-old man. Medical evaluation of evidence of metastatic carcinoma was negative. Over the subsequent 25 years of follow-up the lesion gradually enlarged and the patient remained asymptomatic: August 1973 (G), June 1975 (H), March 1982 (I), and stereo angiograms (J and K), and March 1994 (L). Because of the superficial resemblance to a choroidal osteoma, ultrasonographic examinations were done on three occasions between 1977 and 1994. They, along with orbital roentgenograms, revealed no evidence of calcification.

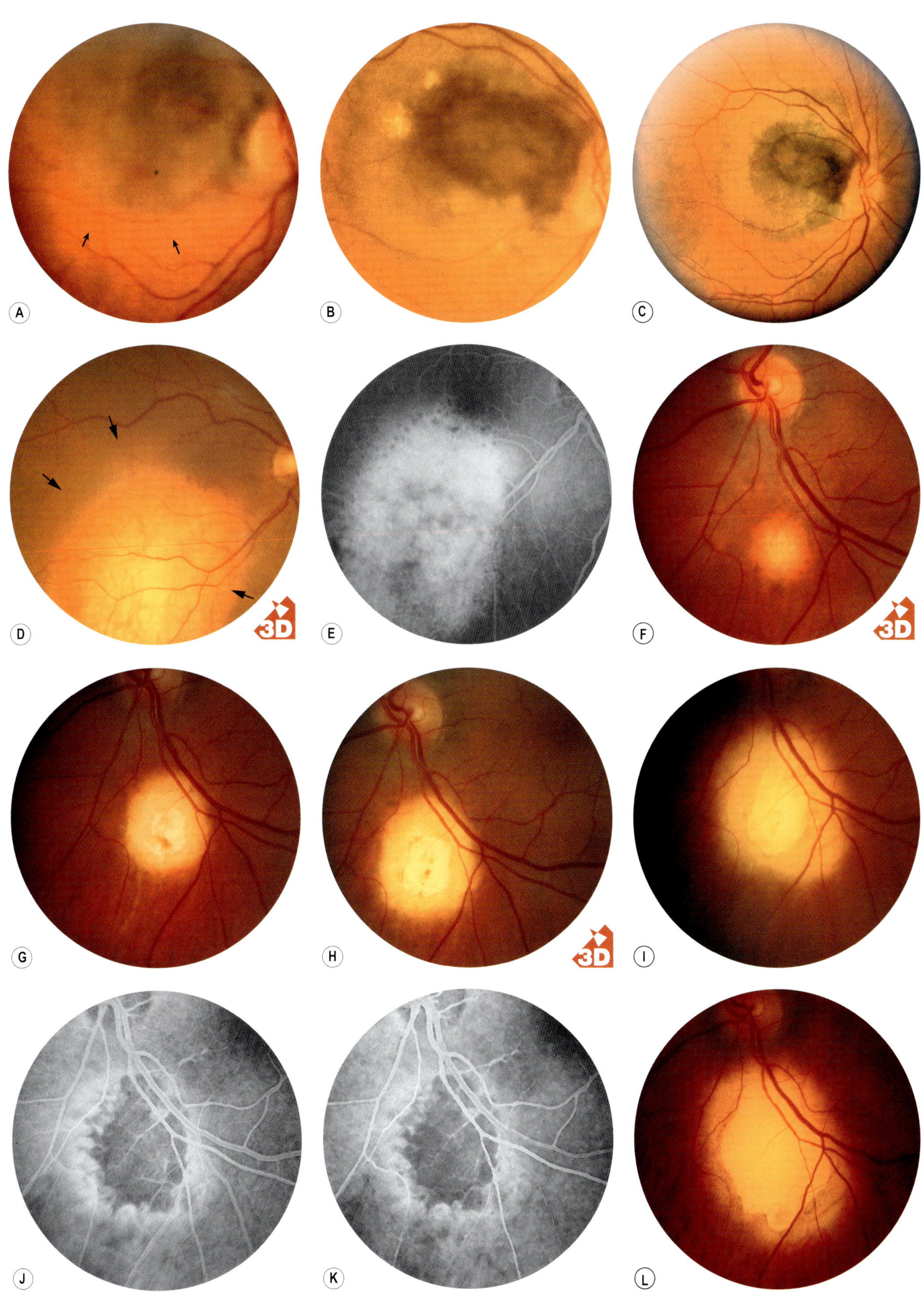
A
B
C
D
3D
E
F
3D
G
H
3D
I
J
K
L

Patients presenting with choroidal neovascularization should be managed using the same guidelines for treatment of neovascularization associated with presumed ocular histoplasmosis and age-related macular degeneration.[16,17,27,28] Those presenting with serous retinal detachment without evidence of neovascularization and with no clear signs of a growth potential can be followed for up to 4 months after onset of symptoms, for evidence of spontaneous resolution of the detachment or growth of the tumor. If no growth occurs after that period and the area of fluorescein leakage is outside the center of the fovea, the author recommends photocoagulation to the area of leakage only, while continuing to monitor the patient for evidence of tumor growth (Figure 14.01A–C). Whereas some of these patients will show evidence of tumor breakthrough Bruch's membrane at the site of photocoagulation, usually many months or several years after treatment, there is no evidence to suggest that this affects the likelihood of extraocular spread of the tumor (Figure 14.04).[7,29] The development of a localized nodule of tumor breakthrough on the surface of these tumors after treatment, particularly if it occurs many months after the treatment, may not necessarily indicate a change in the tumor's growth potential (Figure 14.04). In some cases this extension appears to occur more as mechanical displacement of pliable tissue, rather than growth of tumor, through a focus of laser-damaged Bruch's membrane. Other treatment options include photodynamic therapy,[30] transpupillary thermotherapy,[31] and intravitreal antivascular endothelial growth factor agents.

14.04 Tumor breakthrough Bruch's membrane and minimal growth of presumed melanocytic choroidal nevi following photocoagulation treatment for serous macular detachment.

A–E: In November 1972 this 54-year-old woman presented with metamorphopsia associated with serous retinal detachment surrounding a slightly elevated pigmented choroidal tumor (arrowheads, A). The diagnosis was melanocytic choroidal tumor of uncertain growth potential. When the retinal detachment failed to resolve, focal laser treatment to a site of fluorescein leakage on the tumor surface was done. The detachment resolved but recurred again in March 1973. The tumor was unchanged otherwise. Argon laser treatment was done (B) and the detachment resolved. She was followed at yearly intervals with no change until May 1979. At that time evidence of a small nodularity of the tumor surface was noted (arrow, C). By September 1979 a 2-mm nodule of tumor extending through Bruch's membrane was evident (arrow, D). Medical evaluation for metastatic disease was negative except for chronic lymphatic leukemia that had been diagnosed several years previously. She elected to have no treatment for choroidal tumor. Over the subsequent 6 years of follow-up there was only slight enlargement of the choroidal tumor (arrowheads, E) as well as the overlying tumor nodule (arrow, E).

F–L: On a routine eye examination in April 1983, a five disc diameter elevated pigmented choroidal tumor was discovered temporal to the left macula (F). A gray fibrovascular plaque (arrow, F) was present on its surface. There was a zone of atrophy, hyperplasia, and intraretinal migration of RPE extending from the tumor inferotemporally almost to the equator. Angiography demonstrated evidence of choroidal neovascularization within the gray plaque on the tumor surface. This finding and the zone of dependent retinal pigment epithelial change suggested that the tumor was a large nevus. She was followed at 6-month intervals without any change until March 1985, when she returned because of metamorphopsia in the left eye. At that time there was evidence of reactivation and nasal extension of the new vessels (arrows, G) on the tumor surface. Note the lipid exudate near the center of the macula. The area of the new vessels was treated with argon laser (arrows, H). By October 1986, the exudate was gone (I) and the patient's acuity was 20/20. No further change occurred until May 1991 when two nodules (arrows, J) were noted on the tumor surface within the area of previous laser treatment. These two nodules of tumor, which appeared to extend through Bruch's membrane, enlarged slowly over the subsequent year (arrows, K) although no definite change occurred in the size of the tumor otherwise. At that time she had recently undergone surgery and chemotherapy for ovarian carcinoma that had extended to regional lymph nodes. In May 1992 she experienced a vitreous hemorrhage in the left eye. This cleared and, in October 1993, the choroidal tumor and the foci of extension of tumor through Bruch's membrane showed minimal evidence of enlargement (black arrows, L). The presence of pigment debris in the vitreous overlying the tumor (white arrow, L) suggested that focal necrosis within the tumor nodules may have been responsible for the vitreous hemorrhage. The fundus remained unchanged when she was last examined in December 1994.

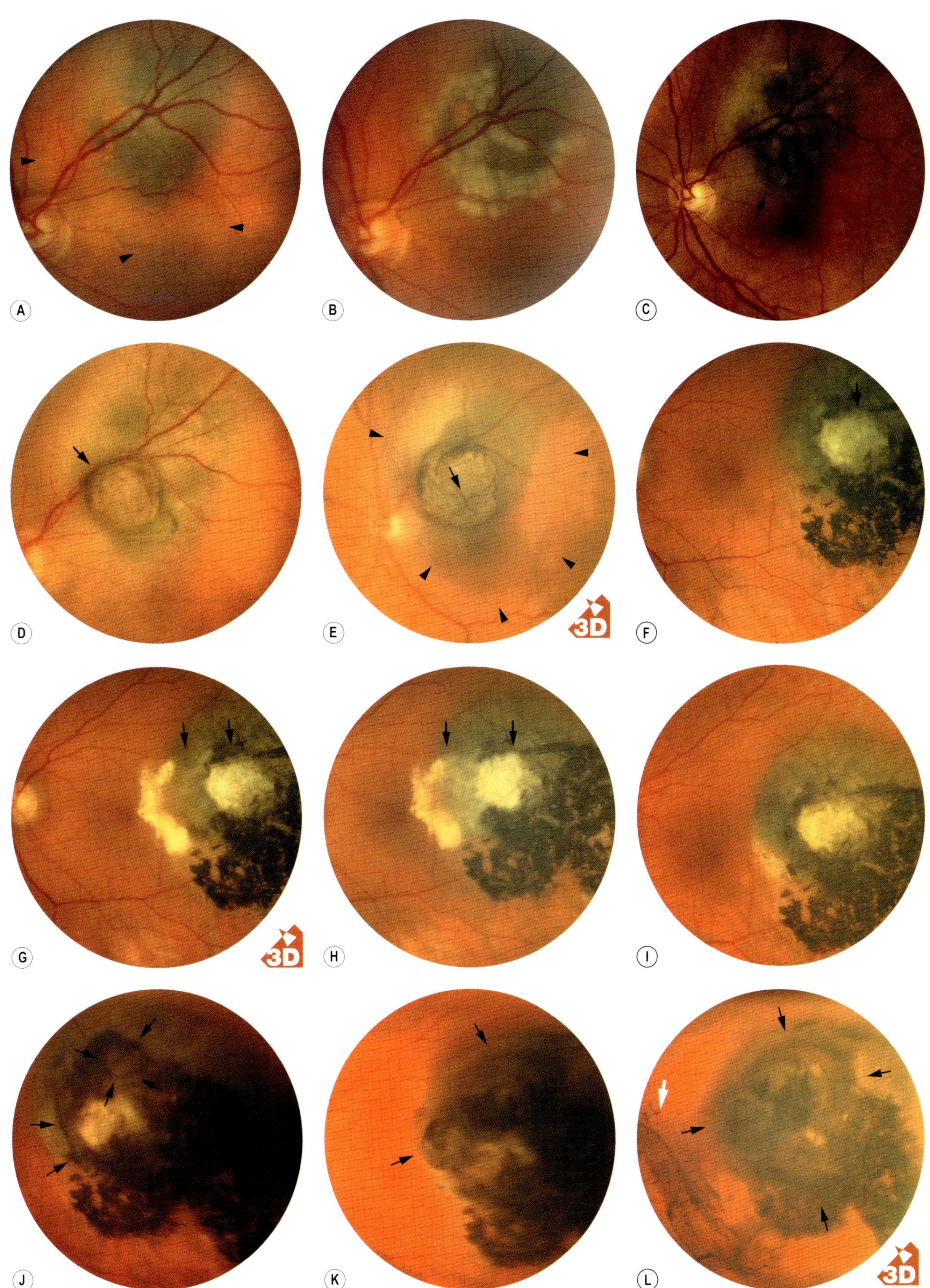
A
B
C
D
E
3D
F
G
3D
H
I
J
K
L
3D

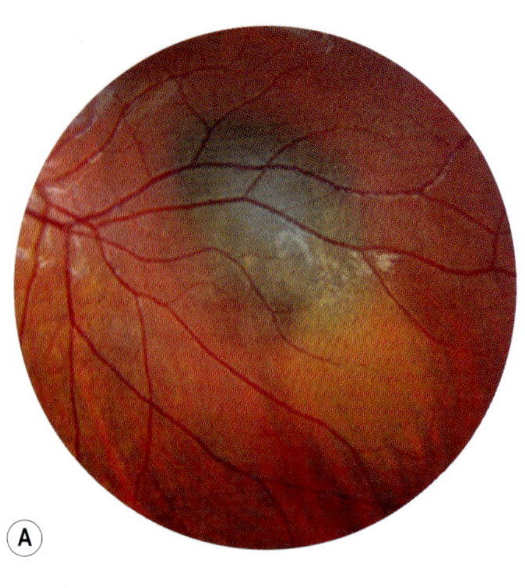

A

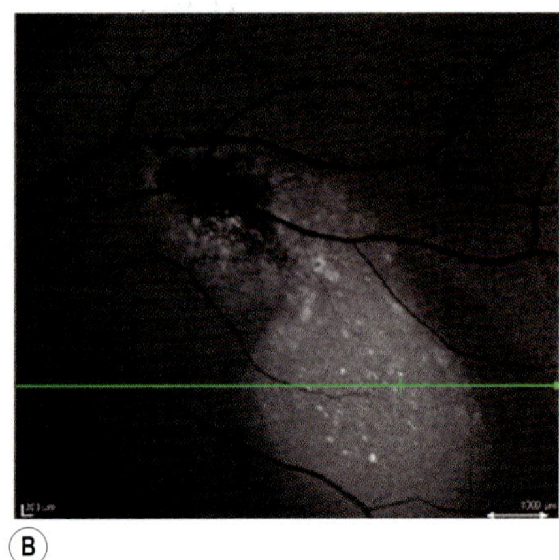

B

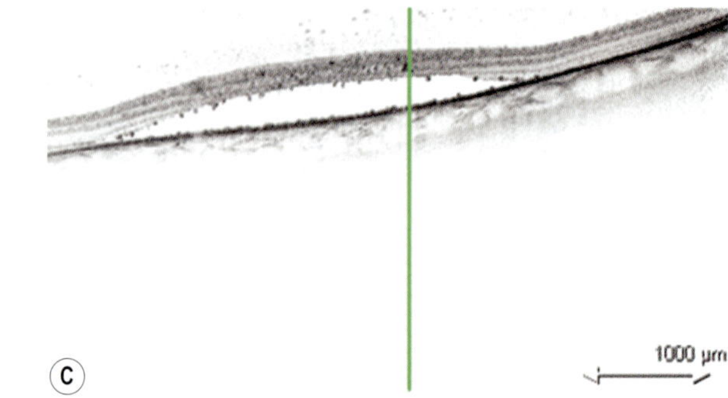

C

14.05

14.05 Extrinsic effects of the nevus.

A: Effects on the surrounding retina retinal pigment epithelium can be readily assessed by optical coherence tomography and fundus autofluorescence. Fundus photograph with orange pigment and subretinal fluid (SRF).
B: On fundus autofluorescence, orange pigment appears as focal hyperautofluorescent spot. In addition there is diffuse dispersion of orange pigment within the SRF imparting diffuse hyperautoflouresence to the SRF.
C: Presumed dispersed lipofuscin (orange pigment) is seen in the subretinal space.

(From Singh et al.,[19] with permission.)

14.06 Optic disc melanocytoma.

A: A 50-year-old white man noted to have optic disc tumor on a routine examination. Patient had no symptoms and his visual acuity was 20/20. Note a melanocytic tumor that is intrinsic to the optic nerve head with fine vitreous pigment dispersion.

Optic disc melanocytosis

B and C: A 35-year-old woman seen for a routine eye examination was found to have pigmentation of the optic disc surface. Her visual fields were normal, ruling out compression.
D–G: This 55-year-old African American diabetic male reported "a wave coming towards the center of my vision" for 3 weeks. His visual acuity was 20/20 on the right and 20/25 on the left. His right fundus was normal. The left fundus had a darkly pigmented mass on the optic disc that extended into the adjacent temporal retina. Two pockets of subretinal fluid, one extending to the foveal center and the other to the inferior equatorial region (arrow E) associated with lipid, and a vascular lesion were seen emanating from the lesion. Fluorescein angiogram showed a lacy network of vessels early that leaked late in the angiogram. Laser photocoagulation of the choroidal neovascular membrane resolved the subretinal fluid and symptoms (H).
H–K: This 50-year-old Indian woman presented with sudden loss of vision in her right eye to count fingers. A darkly pigmented mass covered most of her right optic disc, with some extension into the nerve fiber layer. The macula showed opacification secondary to occlusion of the temporal branches of the central retinal artery (I). An angiogram confirmed poor perfusion of the superior and inferior branch arteries supplying the macula (J and K).

(D–G, courtesy of Dr. Kourus Rezai; H–K, courtesy of Dr. Vishali Gupta and Dr. Amod Gupta.)

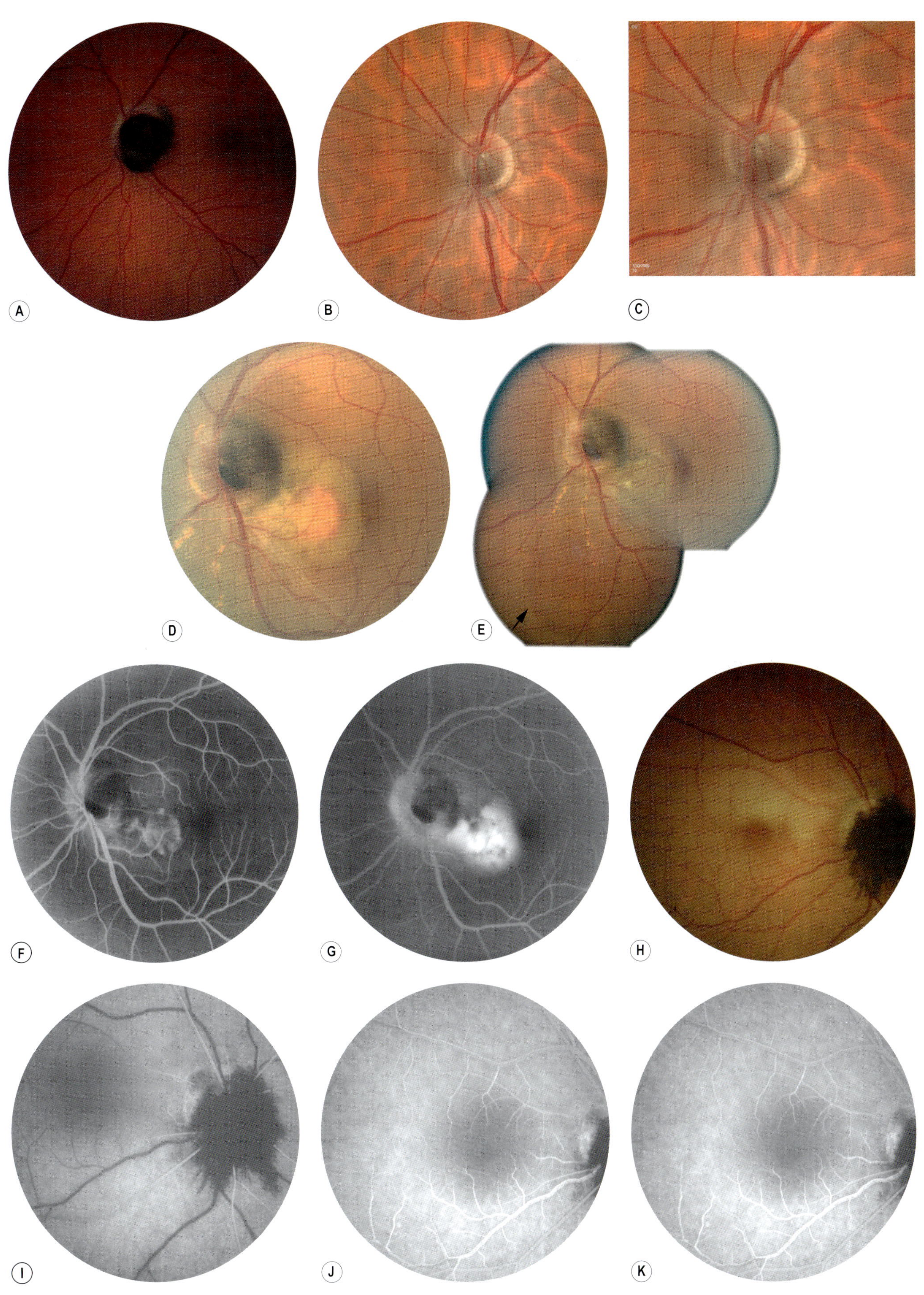

14.06

MELANOCYTOMA

Melanocytoma (Figure 14.06A) and magnocellular nevus are histopathologic names used to describe highly pigmented uveal nevi that are composed of large, round, polygonal, or fusiform melanocytes with small nuclei and occasionally abundant nucleoli. These same cells are the predominant cell type found in eyes with diffuse uveal melanocytosis.[1] Occasionally, melanocytosis of the optic disc without tumefaction can be seen (Figure 14.06B and C). Clinical differentiation of uveal melanocytomas from other highly pigmented nevi composed of spindle and dendritic melanocytes is not possible, except when the tumor involves the optic nerve head. Benign melanocytic tumors that are intrinsic to the optic nerve head and may extend into the surrounding choroid and nerve fiber layer of the retina, histologically are invariably melanocytomas. Features, other than their intense black or greenish-black pigmentation, that to some degree differentiate melanocytomas from other uveal nevi include an apparent greater propensity to exhibit some local growth potential beyond puberty; a greater predilection for undergoing spontaneous necrosis; a greater likelihood of involving adjacent structures, including the sclera as well as the optic nerve head and retina; and perhaps a lower propensity for malignant transformation (Figure 14.06).[1,18,24,26,32–34] The incidence of melanocytoma is equal in all ethnic groups, unlike uveal melanomas that are more common in lightly pigmented individuals. Spontaneous necrosis of a melanocytoma, particularly when it involves the optic nerve head or ciliary body, may cause pigment debris in the vitreous that may be mistaken for vitreous seeding of a melanoma. Necrosis of an iris melanocytoma may cause similar confusion because of a macrophage response to necrotic tumor in the aqueous humor and trabecular meshwork. The reason for their predilection for spontaneous necrosis is unknown. It may be that these cells are more responsive than usual to hormonal and immunologic changes. (See discussion of bilateral diffuse uveal melanocytic proliferation associated with systemic carcinoma, below.) Slow local growth can be documented over years of observation; malignant transformation is rare but known. Complications secondary to compression of the optic nerve fibers resulting in a visual field defect, rarely severe enough to lose light perception, central or branch retinal artery (Figure 14.06H–J) and vein occlusions and choroidal neovascularization, can occur (Figure 14.06D–G).

14.07 Diffuse sclerochoroidal melanocytic nevus/ schwannoma.

A–E: This 9-year-old boy with subnormal vision in the left eye had diffuse thickening and hyperpigmentation of the temporal and inferior fundus, a shallow retinal detachment inferiorly, and blurring of the optic disc margin in the left eye (B). Note the absence of choroidal markings in the left eye (B) compared with the normal right eye (A). The left eye was enucleated. Histopathologic examination revealed diffuse thickening of the choroid and sclera, which were infiltrated with benign spindle melanocytic cells in the macula and inferior fundus (low-power, C, and higher-powers, D and E). Note the posterior bowing of the thickened choroid and sclera in the macular region (arrows, C and D).

E–J: A 14-year-old girl presented in January 1985 because of a recent change in the vision in the right eye, which had always been amblyopic. The fundus appeared almost identical to the left eye of the patient in B. In addition to the thickened and darkened choroid posteriorly and inferiorly there was a localized serous retinal detachment and a gray subretinal neovascular complex (arrow, F) in the macular area. There were some inflammatory cells in the vitreous. There was blurring of the optic disc margins. The left fundus was normal. Angiography revealed a choroidal neovascular membrane (arrow, G), a large zone of depigmentation of the retinal pigment epithelium extending temporally to the macula, and some staining of the optic disc. Ultrasonography revealed a diffuse choroidal tumor posteriorly in an area of posterior bowing and thickening of the sclera (H). The clinical diagnosis was diffuse sclerochoroidal melanocytic nevus. Because of suspected growth of the lesion the eye was enucleated in 1993. Histopathologic examination revealed a highly vascular benign melanocytic mass involving the choroid and sclera posteriorly and inferiorly (I and higher-power, J). The tumor was classified microscopically as a melanotic schwannoma.

(A–H, from Gass[280]; I and J, from Shields et al.[281])

Diffuse Sclerochoroidal Melanocytic Nevus

Diffuse choroidal hyperpigmentation and thickening may be observed either as an isolated finding (Figure 14.08) or in association with episcleral pigmentation (ocular melanocytosis) that may extend to involve ipsilateral skin in the distribution of branches of the trigeminal nerve (oculodermal melanocytosis: nevus of Ota).[35] The lifetime risk of developing uveal melanoma in a Caucasian with ocular melanocytosis is estimated to be about 1 in 400 (Figure 14.09).[36] The risk in nonwhites may also be higher but has not been quantified.[37]

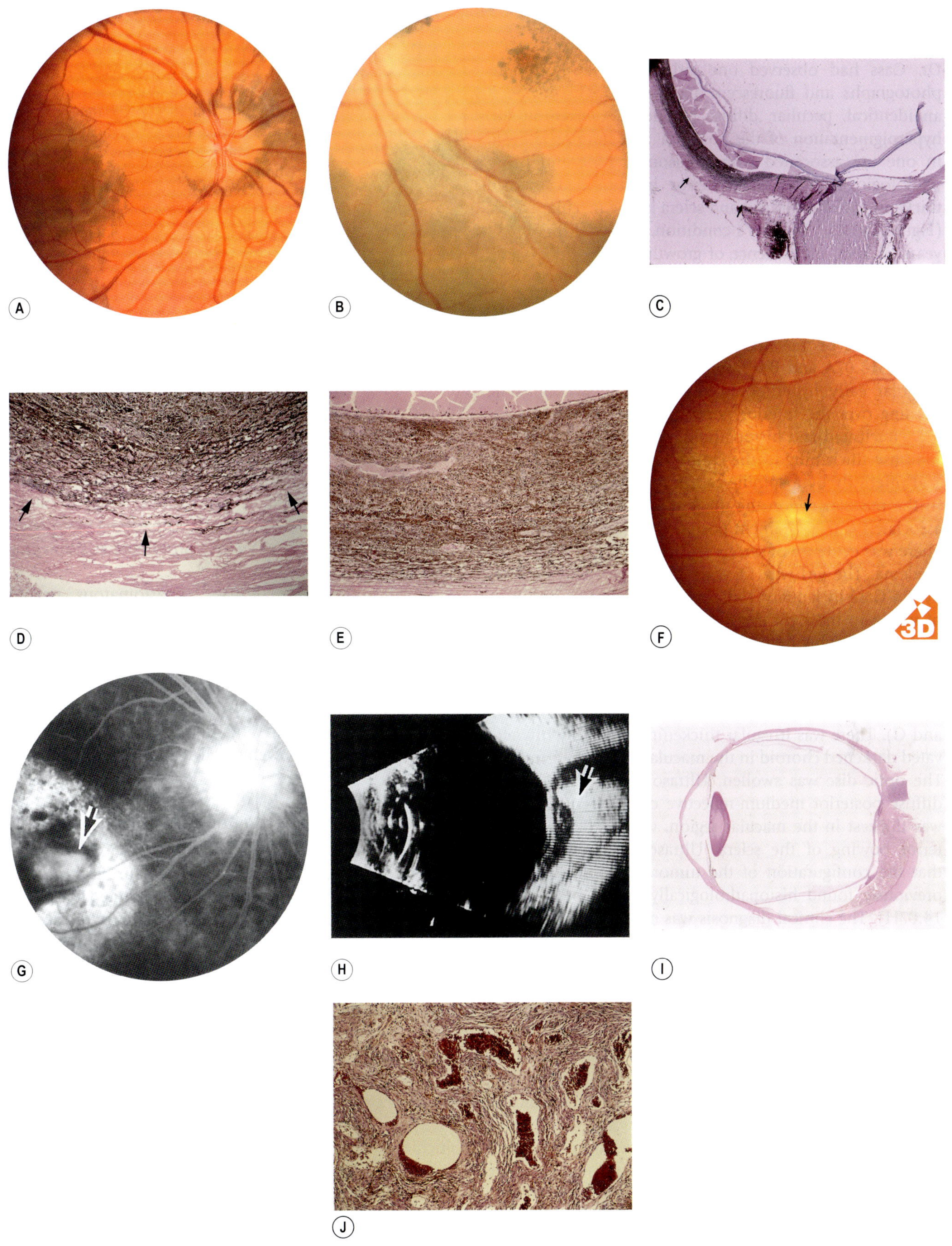
A
B
C
D
E
F
3D
G
H
I
J

14.09 Oculodermal melanocytosis with choroidal melanoma.

A–D: A 54-year-old white man presented with blurred vision. External examination revealed left eyelids, forehead, and episcleral hyperpigmentation (A). Fundus was dark in color with a dome-shaped choroidal mass suggestive of choroidal melanoma (B) that was confirmed by Ultrasonography B-scan (C). Enucleation confirmed amelanotic choroidal melanoma (D).

14.10 Choroidal nevus with neurofibromatosis type 1 (NF1).

A and **B**: A 10-year-old girl with NF1. Note diffuse choroidal nevus (melanocytosis) (A) which resembles café-au-lait lesions of the skin (B).

14.11 Uveal melanoma with neurofibromatosis type 1 (NF1).

A–D: A 15-year-old white male with NF1 was found to have unilateral juvenile glaucoma. He was managed medically initially followed by trabeculectomy. A pigmented iris lesion that had increased in size was reported. The patient had numerous café-au-lait spots on his skin (A), and cutaneous neurofibromas on his left forearm and right leg. His visual acuity was 20/20 in each eye. Intraocular pressures were 30 mmHg in the right eye and 11 mmHg in the left eye (A). In addition to prominent corneal nerves and numerous Lisch nodules in both eyes, an ill-defined pigmented iris mass, extending from 2 o' clock to 4 o' clock and measuring 5 × 4 × 3 mm, was observed (B). The entire surface of the iris stroma was diffusely seeded with tumor. Gonioscopy showed heavy pigmentation of the trabecular meshwork. Enucleation was performed in view of diffuse seeding of the iris melanoma with secondary glaucoma (C). The sectioned globe showed the darkly pigmented iris lesion extending into the nasal angle, heavily pigmented trabecular meshwork, and tumor infiltrating the temporal angle (D).

(Reproduced with permission from Honavar et al.[41])

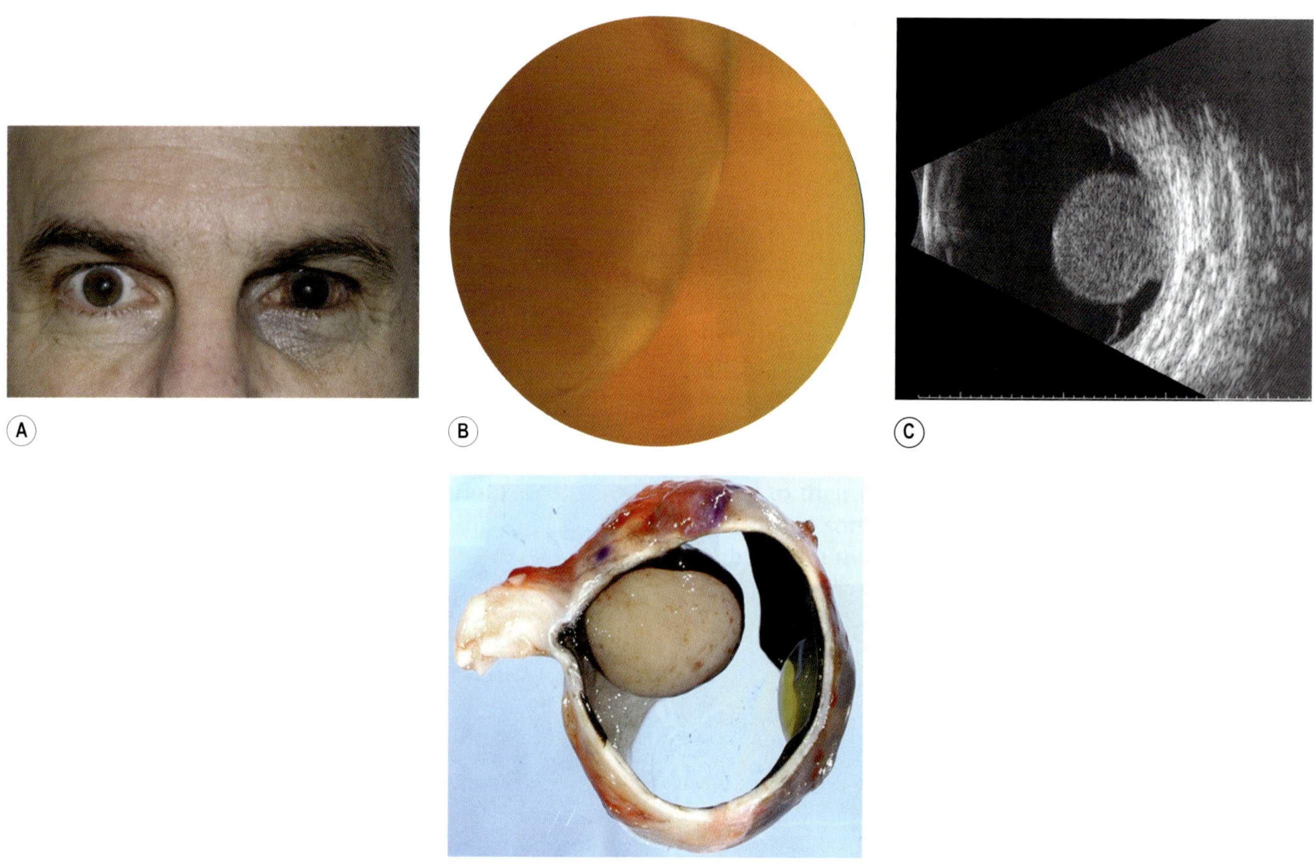

14.09

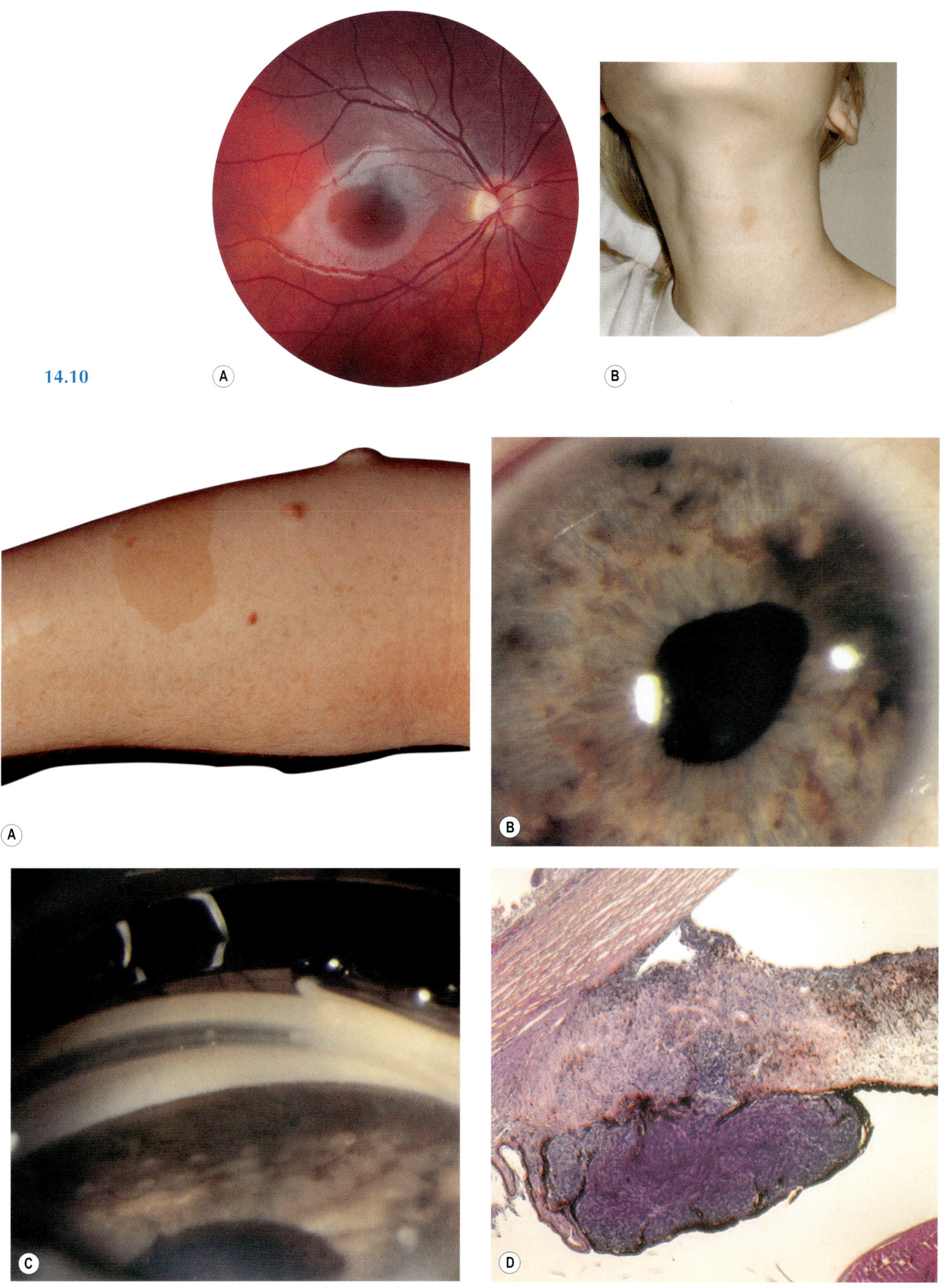
A
B
14.10
A
B
C
D
14.11

CHOROIDAL MALIGNANT MELANOMA

A melanoma in its earlier stages of development is most likely to be observed clinically when it arises in or near the macular area. There it may cause a scotoma and photopsia produced by invasion of the retina or loss of vision caused by serous retinal detachment. The clinician who discovers a small pigmented choroidal lesion associated with a macular detachment should not, however, conclude that the lesion is a malignant melanoma, since, as mentioned previously, macular detachment may occur overlying a choroidal nevus. The most helpful signs that distinguish a small choroidal melanoma from a nevus are: (1) globular elevation of the lesion of 3 mm or more; (2) multiple areas of orange pigment deposition over the tumor surface (Figure 14.12D); (3) serous retinal detachment in the absence of drusen or evidence of choroidal neovascularization; (4) evidence of tumor breaking through Bruch's membrane; and (5) fluorescein angiographic evidence of multiple pinpoint leaks that increase in size during the course of angiography on the surface of the tumor (Figure 14.12B, C, and F).[2,9,16,42]

Analysis of Collaborative Ocular Melanoma Study (COMS) data suggests that the majority of tumors enrolled in the observational small-melanoma study were choroidal nevi rather than true melanoma, as more than 60% of such tumors did not grow (without treatment) over a period of 5 years.[43] It is preferable to classify small choroidal melanoma (COMS size definition of 5–16 mm in basal diameter and less than 2.5 mm in height) as indeterminate melanocytic tumor[44] rather than small melanoma, large nevus, suspicious nevus, or dormant melanoma.[29,45] It can be assumed that the size category of indeterminate lesions (IML) includes an as-yet undetermined proportion of large choroidal nevus, small choroidal melanoma, or even true intermediate lesions.[45] Several authors have tried to identify qualitative surface features that predict the likelihood of growth suggestive of melanoma.[42,46,47] Reappraisal of the published COMS data has revealed that the presence of orange pigmentation significantly predicts risk of growth.[45] Abnormal intrinsic choroidal vasculature, as observed by indo cyanine green, may also be predictive of growth risk.[48,49]

14.12 Submacular choroidal melanomas.

A–C: Small malignant melanoma of the choroid in a 22-year-old woman who noted photopsia and mild blurring of vision. Note the ring of pinpoint subretinal leaks and late staining (B and C). The tumor showed evidence of enlargement within a few months and the eye was enucleated. Histopathologically it was a spindle B melanoma.

D–F: Localized serous detachment of the retinal pigment epithelium (RPE) caused by small choroidal melanoma that might be confused with a hemorrhagic detachment of the RPE and retina. Note absence of halo of blood at the margins of the lesion and the presence of the patches of orange pigment scattered over the surface of the lesion and surrounding the base of the small RPE detachment (arrows, D). There is some serous detachment of the retina surrounding the melanoma. Angiography shows intense fluorescein staining of the sub-RPE exudate (E and F). The patches of orange pigment appear as nonfluorescent spots on the angiogram. Note the small pinpoint-sized hyperfluorescent spots (arrows) on the surface of the tumor. (Compare with histopathology in Figure 14.13 A and B.)

Laser photocoagulation treatment of small choroidal melanoma.

G–I: In November 1983 this 53-year-old man noted a paracentral scotoma associated with exudative retinal detachment caused by a partly pigmented choroidal melanoma that had extended through Bruch's membrane in two areas (arrows, G). To produce choroidal atrophy around the tumor, intense, 0.5- and 1-second argon green 500- and 1000-mm applications were used to surround the margin of the tumor (H). Two weeks later similar laser applications were used to treat the entire surface of the tumor. Forty-three months later a placoid, irregularly pigmented scar remained. Eleven years later there had been no further recurrence of the tumor, the patient had no evidence of metastasis, and the visual acuity in the left eye was 20/20.

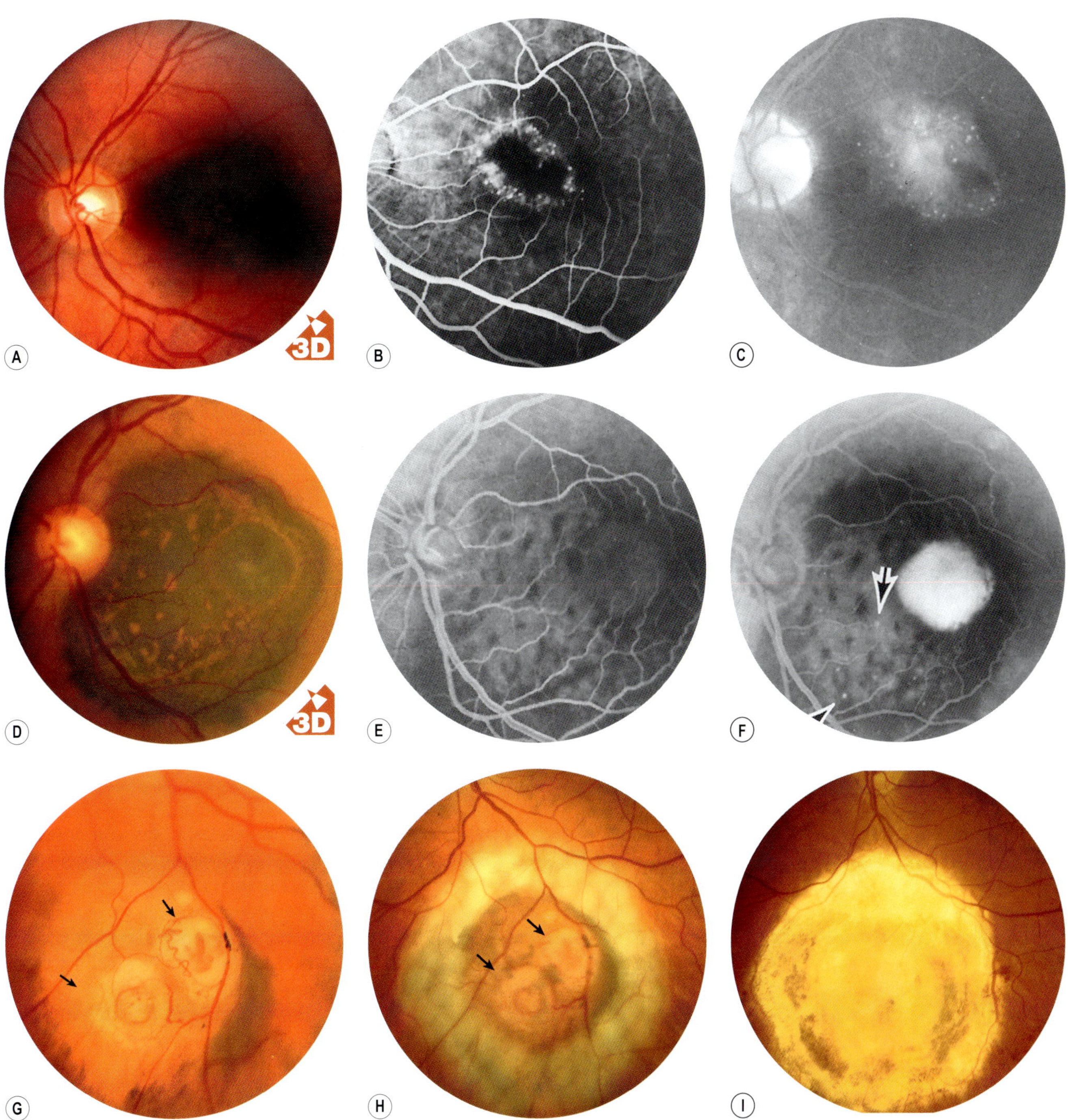
A
3D
B
C
D
3D
E
F
G
H
I

At present, the management of IML (small choroidal melanoma) remains controversial in the absence of data from a randomized clinical trial.[50–52] It must be emphasized that one can only attribute an estimated risk to a given IML depending upon the presence of "risk factors" predictive of growth.[45] Therefore, caution should be exercised in making a diagnosis of a small choroidal melanoma in the absence of documented growth. The treatment options of prompt treatment versus observation to document growth prior to treatment should be clearly discussed with the patient. With few exceptions, the growth rate of a melanoma is constant but the growth rate of different melanomas varies widely. Some will demonstrate growth within a few months (Figure 14.12A), but 3 years or longer may be required to detect the growth of some melanomas.[21,53,54] As mentioned in the previous section, the demonstration of growth, although the single most reliable sign of malignancy, may occasionally occur in a benign choroidal nevus in children and young adults.[16] If the macular detachment persists and the choroidal lesion remains unchanged, low- to moderate-intensity argon photocoagulation applied to the area of fluorescein leakage usually causes resolution of the subretinal fluid. Only the leaking area should be treated; no attempt should be made to destroy the tumor. (See previous discussion concerning treatment of choroidal nevi with retinal detachment.) During pregnancy there is some evidence that benign nevi or low-grade melanomas may be stimulated to grow (Figure 14.13E–J).[55] Large nevi, like choroidal hemangiomas and osteomas, may be first detected during the course of pregnancy because of development of an overlying serous retinal detachment (see Figures 14.15J–L, and 14.20J–L). Figure 14.13 (E–K) illustrates a patient who during the third trimester of pregnancy developed blurred vision caused by a localized serous macular detachment caused by 10 × 10 × 6 mm partly pigmented choroidal tumor that was associated with a focal area suggesting extension of the tumor through Bruch's membrane. The ultrasound was atypical in that the lesion appeared moderately reflective with evidence of prominent vascularity (Figure 14.13H). The presence of a large zone of RPE atrophy and bone corpuscular intraretinal migration of RPE that extended from the inferior edge of the tumor to the ora serrata inferiorly suggested that the tumor had been previously associated with a long-standing retinal detachment that had spontaneously resolved. In spite of these atypical features for a melanoma, the eye was enucleated. The tumor contained many large dilated blood vessels and was composed of benign-appearing melanocytes showing no evidence of mitotic activity (Figure 14.13I and J).

Histopathologically the retina inferior to the tumor was markedly degenerated and showed migration of RPE into the retina around blood vessels (Figure 14.13K). Presumably the pregnancy played a role in causing increased tumor vascular engorgement and macular detachment.[55] If it had not been enucleated, it is likely that the retina would have spontaneously reattached after delivery of the infant. This case and two other cases illustrated in Figure 14.04 demonstrate that biomicroscopic evidence of tumor extension through Bruch's membrane alone is not necessarily a sign of high growth potential or malignancy. In this case it is probable that the extension through Bruch's membrane occurred many years previously during the active growth phase of the tumor.

14.13 Clinicopathologic correlations of melanomas.

A and B: Compare with Figure 14.12 D–F. Note serous detachment of the retinal pigment epithelium (RPE) (black arrow, A) and clump of orange pigment (black and white arrows, A and B) composed of either macrophages filled with epithelial cell pigment or hyperplastic pigment epithelium overlying a spindle B melanoma.

C and D: Nonpigmented juxtapapillary melanoma simulating benign subretinal fibrovascular proliferation or choroidal osteoma. It grew and the eye was enucleated. Histopathologic examination revealed a spindle cell melanoma that extended posteriorly through the sclera (D).

E–K: This healthy 31-year-old woman who was in her last trimester of pregnancy noted metamorphopsia and a central scotoma in the right eye. She had a prominent pigmented tumor of the right caruncle since childhood. Examination revealed a localized serous macular detachment (upper arrow, E) at the superior margin of a large elevated hypopigmented choroidal tumor (small arrows, F) inferior to the right macula. There was a bone-corpuscular pattern of migration of pigment into the retina over the peripheral aspect of the tumor and in a broad zone along the inferior border of the tumor extending to the ora serrata (lower arrow, E, and G). There was a focal nodular area of extension of the tumor through Bruch's membrane (large arrow, F, and white arrows, G). Ultrasound revealed a medium-reflective choroidal tumor with prominent vascularity (H). Histopathologic examination revealed a highly vascular tumor composed of relatively benign spindle cells showing no mitotic activity (I and J). Note extension of the tumor through Bruch's membrane (arrow, I). Overlying and surrounding the tumor

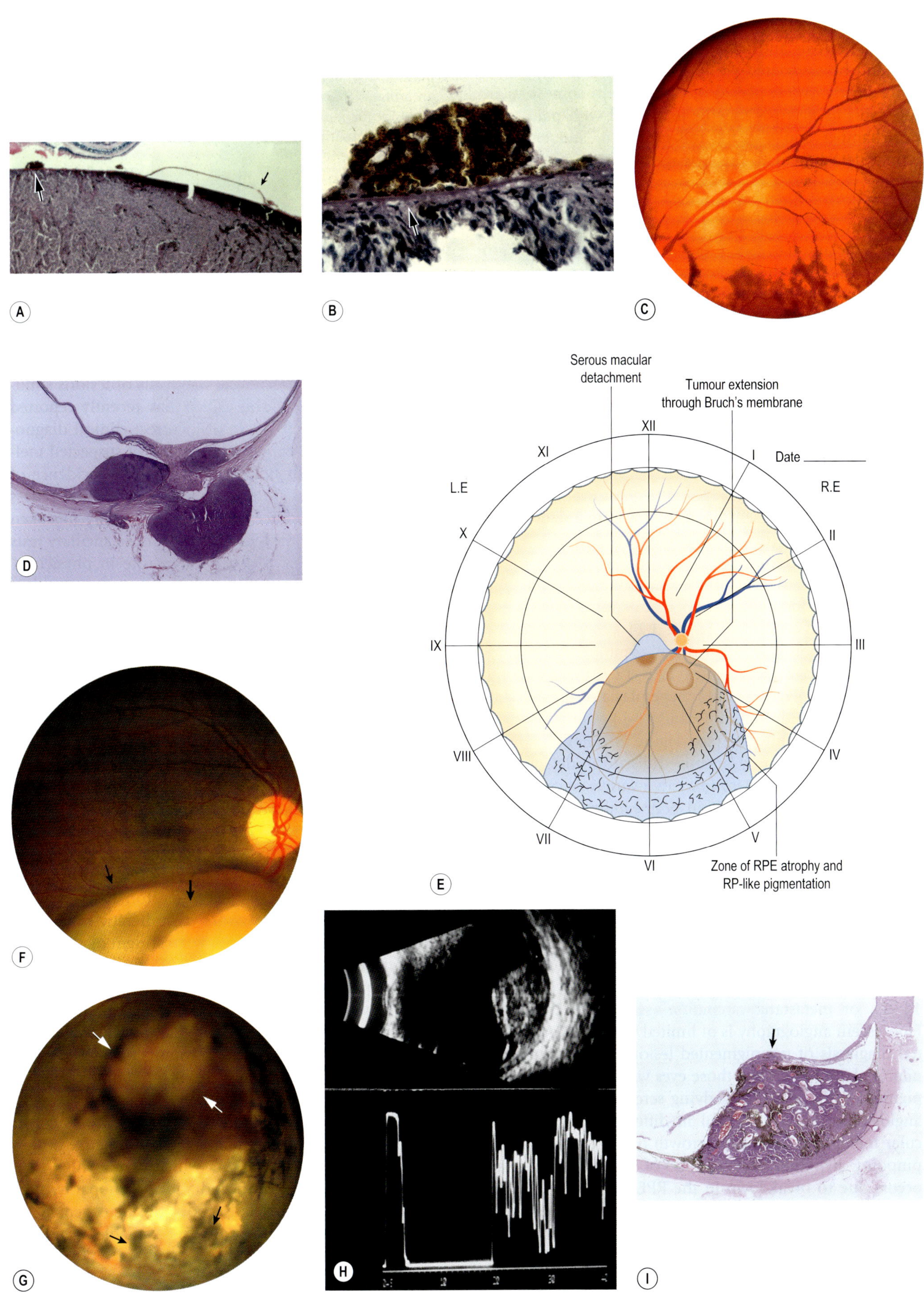
A
B
C
D
Serous macular detachment
Tumour extension through Bruch's membrane
XII
XI
I
Date
L.E
R.E
X
II
IX
III
VIII
IV
VII
V
VI
Zone of RPE atrophy and RP-like pigmentation
E
F
G
H
I

Despite improvements in diagnosis and local tumor control using eye-sparing techniques, improvement in uveal melanoma survival has not been observed.[92] This current situation underlines the need for effective methods to predict and address microscopic metastatic disease. The cytologic classification of Callender has undergone considerable modification and amplification during the past decade in an effort to provide better prognostic information regarding these tumors.[2,85–90] More recently, prognostication of uveal melanoma based upon tumor cytogenetic and molecular assays has become feasible.[93] Karyotype abnormalities, including loss of chromosome 3 (monosomy 3), loss of 6q, and gain of chromosome 8q, have a statistically significant association with increased risk of metastatic death.[93–96] Gene expression profiling by microarray can also be used to sort tumors into one of two subgroups: less aggressive class 1 tumors and class 2 tumors with a higher risk of metastasis.[97,98] Such techniques are applicable to tumor sample obtained after enucleation or resection and even after fine-needle aspiration biopsy.[99–100] The ultimate goal is to develop targeted adjuvant therapies for patients at high risk of metastasis.[101]

Rapid resolution of melanomas following either brachytherapy or ionizing irradiation usually indicates a more rapidly growing melanoma and is associated with a higher mortality.[20,73] Similarly, a tumor that shows minimal decrease in size after irradiation is more likely to have been a slow-growing melanoma and is associated with a more favorable prognosis.

BILATERAL DIFFUSE UVEAL MELANOCYTIC PROLIFERATION ASSOCIATED WITH SYSTEMIC CARCINOMA

Bilateral diffuse uveal melanocytic proliferation (BDUMP) is an unusual syndrome occurring in predominantly elderly patients who have diffuse uveal thickening that has been attributed to proliferating, predominantly spindle-type benign melanocytes in both eyes associated with a carcinoma elsewhere in the body.[102–116] The onset of visual symptoms may antedate or follow those caused by the systemic carcinoma. Visual loss is associated with either or both rapidly progressing cataract and loss of retinal function. This latter may be caused either by direct nutritional or toxic damage to the overlying retina and RPE or by bilateral secondary retinal detachment. The diffuse usually mild uveal thickening may be overlooked and may be difficult to detect with ultrasonography. There may be multiple faint orange spots or patches scattered throughout the posterior fundus (Figure 14.14B, M, and N).[103,107] At the time of presentation or soon afterward these patients develop the sine qua non of the syndrome: multiple, slightly elevated, pigmented choroidal tumors suggesting multiple nevi or metastatic melanomas scattered throughout the fundus (Figure 14.14A, K, L–N). Focal pigmented and nonpigmented tumors may develop on the iris. Signs of iridocyclitis may be present.

14.14 Bilateral diffuse uveal melanocytic proliferation.

A–C: This 65-year-old woman experienced blurred vision in both eyes. Two years previously she had an ovarian carcinoma incompletely excised and was treated by irradiation. Visual acuity was 20/25 in both eyes. Fundus examination in both eyes revealed multiple slightly elevated pigmented tumors in the extramacular areas and peculiar orange spots (arrows, B) in the macular areas. Angiography revealed focal areas of early hyperfluorescence corresponding with the orange spots (C). Metastatic evaluation was negative. The patient developed bilateral cataracts and retinal detachments. Both eyes were treated with external-beam irradiation and cataract extractions. Subsequently she had bilateral enucleations. Ten years after the onset of visual symptoms she had no evidence of metastatic disease.

D–F: Histopathologic examination of a patient with benign uveal melanocytic proliferation and a systemic carcinoma. Note enlargement of the ciliary body, mild thickening of the uveal tract by nonpigmented benign melanocytes (F), and focal pigmented tumefactions (arrows, D and E) composed of partly necrotic melanocytes. Note relative sparing of the choriocapillaris (F).

G–L: This 74-year-old man developed progressive focal Peutz–Jeghers-like hyperpigmented spots on the lips (G), penis (H), and mucous membranes of the mouth (I) several months before developing progressive severe loss of vision in both eyes. Examination of the fundi revealed a leopard-spot hyperpigmentation and widespread depigmentation of the retinal pigment epithelium in both eyes (J–L). There were multiple, variably sized, slightly elevated, pigmented lesions scattered in the fundi (J–L). Medical evaluation discovered adenocarcinoma of the sigmoid colon. His visual acuity declined to light perception only in the right eye and counting fingers in the left eye. He had no further evidence of carcinoma until he developed widespread metastatic carcinoma of the skin just before his death 26 months after the onset of symptoms. Histopathologic examination of the eyes confirmed the diagnosis of bilateral diffuse uveal melanocytic proliferation.

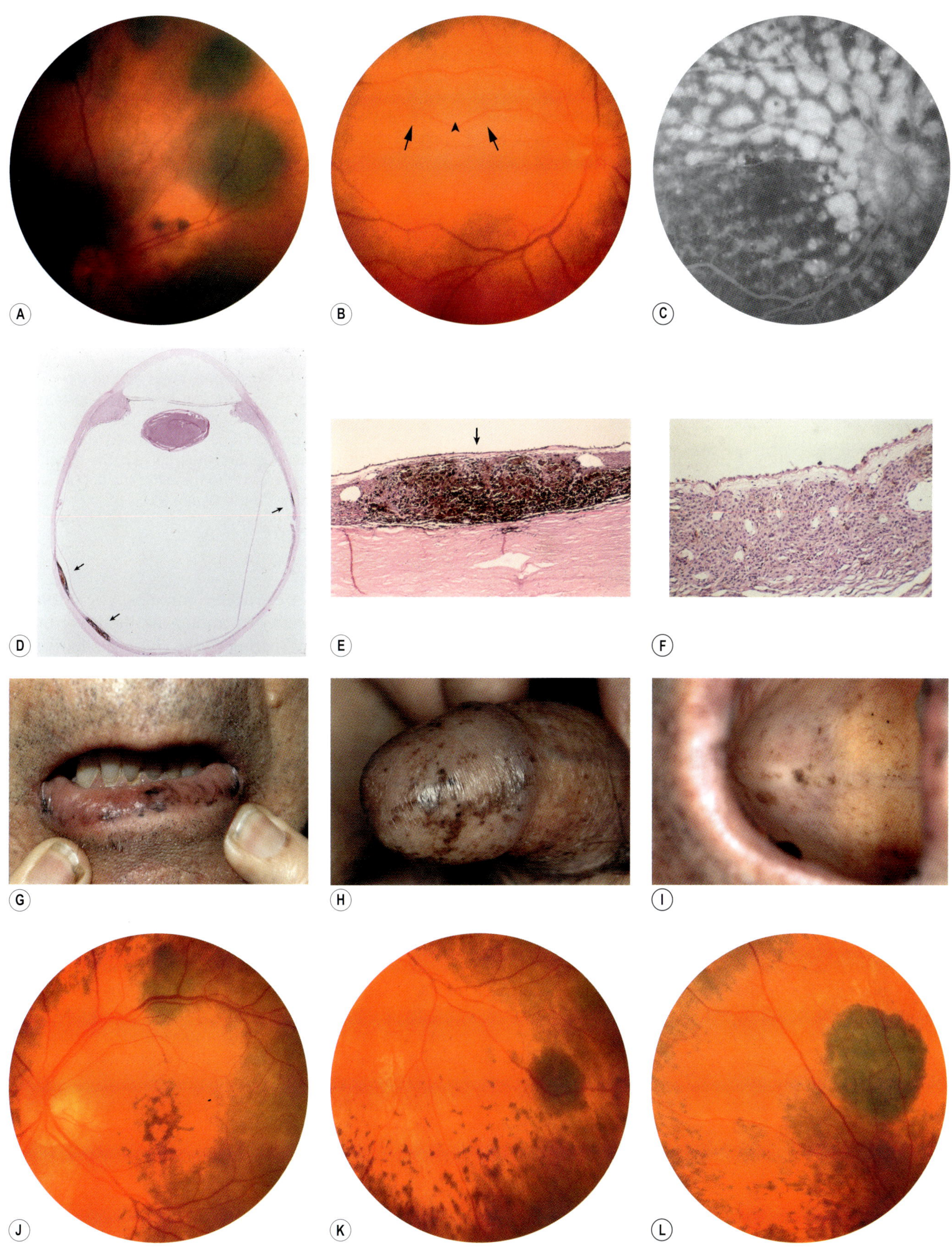

In areas of the posterior fundus that may appear ophthalmoscopically relatively normal, early-phase fluorescein angiography may show a striking, rather widespread pattern of multiple irregularly round areas of hyperfluorescence that correspond with the orange spots seen biomicroscopically, as well as pinpoint and patchy areas of fluorescein staining later during the study (Figure 14.14C, P–R).[107] This dramatic angiographic picture is apparently caused by the patchy depigmentation and destructive changes of the RPE overlying the relatively intact choriocapillaris and diffuse uveal melanocytic infiltration (Figure 14.14F). Autofluorescence shows decreased autofluorescence corresponding to the RPE destruction and increased autofluorescence in the intervening areas (Figure 14.14U and V). The presence of subretinal fluid can be confirmed by OCT (Figure 14.14O). Electroretinography may show severe abnormalities.[103,108] Ultrasonography may show evidence of diffuse, usually mild thickening of the uveal tract. Histopathologically the melanocytic cells responsible for the diffuse uveal thickening are relatively hypopigmented plump spindle cells with a benign appearance. Mitotic figures are rare. Relative sparing of the choriocapillaris and extensive patchy areas of destruction and degeneration of the pigment epithelium and retinal receptor cells are characteristic features (Figure 14.14F). The multifocal more elevated and pigmented choroidal lesions are composed of large round or polygonal melanocytes, small nuclei, and abundant cytoplasm packed with melanin (Figure 14.14D and E). Necrosis is present in most of these lesions. The ciliary body, including the ciliary processes, is thickened by infiltration of melanocytic cells and the lens shows cataractous changes. Although some authors have classified this uveal infiltration as a melanoma, most have favored a benign classification.

These patients usually die because of metastatic carcinoma within 2 years of the onset of visual symptoms. The longest survival to date is 6.5 years for a woman whose primary carcinoma was ovarian and who had bilateral enucleations because of uncontrolled melanocytic proliferation, retinal detachment, and postirradiation complications.[108] Another patient who had bilateral enucleations has survived 5 years without developing evidence of a primary cancer.[115] The primary tumor in women is usually carcinoma of the uterus or ovary and in men is carcinoma of the lungs or a retroperitoneal carcinoma of uncertain origin. None of the patients to date have had evidence of metastatic melanoma.[117] It is not known whether the intraocular proliferation is a response to substances released by the systemic carcinoma or whether they both arise from a common oncogenic stimulus. The cytologic structure of the melanocytes composing the uveal thickening and the relative sparing of the choriocapillaris suggest that diffuse congenital uveal melanocytosis may be a pre-existing requirement for the development of this syndrome. The concept that hormonal substances released by certain carcinomas are responsible for stimulating proliferation, focal melanin production, and necrosis in the uveal melanocytes, as well as causing immune-induced destruction of the RPE and retina, is an attractive but as yet unproven theory.[103,108,116] This cancer-associated melanocytopathy may be associated with severe loss of visual function and severe electroretinographic changes before the development of retinal detachment. This suggests that these patients may share some pathogenetic features in common with those who develop acute loss of retinal receptor elements in the presence of a systemic carcinoma, the so-called cancer-associated retinopathy syndrome (see discussion in Chapter 13).[108,118,119] Stimulation of production of melanin by melanocytes in the skin and mucous membranes of the mouth and genitalia may also occur occasionally in these patients and produce a clinical picture simulating the Peutz–Jeghers syndrome (Figure 14.14G–L).[108,120]

14.14 Continued

M–X: This 72-year-old man with a history of metastatic renal cell carcinoma to the lung noted bilateral dimness in vision over 4 weeks. The lung tumors were shrinking with sorafenib (Nexavar), a kinase inhibitor used to treat renal and hepatic carcinomas. His vision was 20/40 and 20/50. Both eyes showed shallow serous detachments associated with two types of pigmented lesions: some were more pigmented, 1–2 disc areas in size, the others were flat 300–500 μm in size and arranged in a leopard-spot pattern (arrows M and N). The choroid was diffusely thickened on ultrasound. The larger pigmented lesions blocked fluorescence on both fluorescein and indocyanine angiography: while the smaller lesions showed early hyperfluorescence along with several pinpoint hyperfluorescent dots in the adjacent area and leaked dye late (P–T). Autofluorescence showed decreased autofluorescence of the leopard-spot lesions and increased autofluorescence in the intervening areas (U and V). A diagnosis of paraneoplastic lesions of bilateral diffuse uveal melanocytic proliferation was made. He received plasmapheresis three times per week, vision improved to 20/20 and 20/25, and the serous detachments resolved. The larger pigmented lesions now began to resemble the smaller ones with the leopard-spot pattern (arrow W and X).

(M–X, courtesy of Dr. Lee Jampol.)

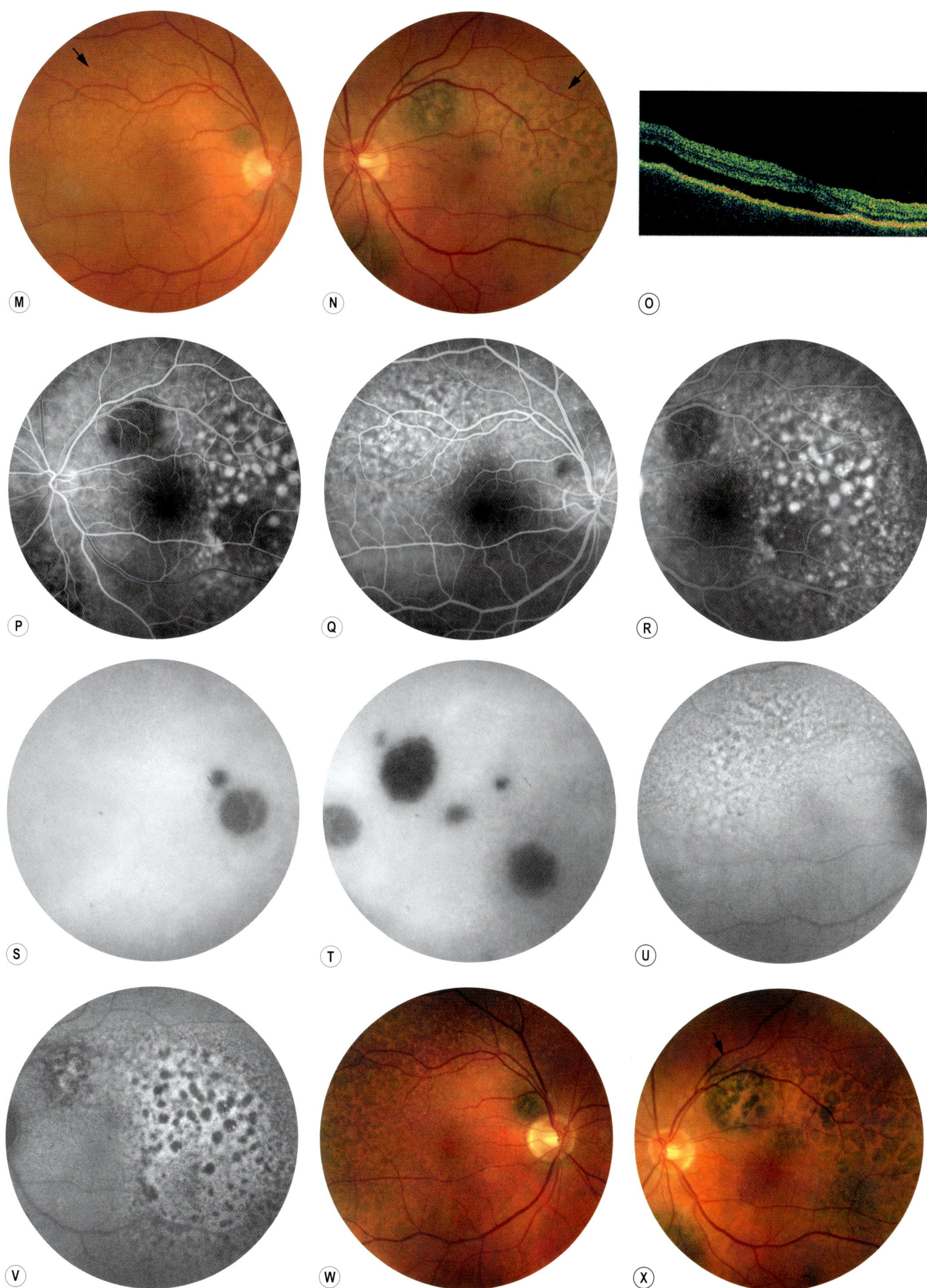
M
N
O
P
Q
R
S
T
U
V
W
X

The term BDUMP does not fully describe extraocular paraneoplastic manifestations of the disease, and given that extraocular manifestations may occur in about 20% of cases, the author has suggested paraneoplastic melanocytic proliferation be used to describe this unique paraneoplastic disease.[120]

The differential diagnosis includes Harada's disease, idiopathic uveal effusion, metastatic carcinoma, metastatic melanoma, reactive lymphoid hyperplasia of the uveal tract, and bilateral multicentric or diffuse primary uveal melanomas.[121]

The retinal detachment in these patients is nonresponsive to corticosteroids, antimetabolites, and irradiation treatment.[103,108] Plasmapheresis may be useful if steroids and antimetabolites do not help. In desperate cases use of pars plana vitrectomy and fluid–silicone exchange to tamponade the retina in place may be successful in restoring ambulatory vision.[108]

CIRCUMSCRIBED CHOROIDAL HEMANGIOMA

Cavernous hemangioma of the choroid is a benign developmental tumor[122] that typically occurs either as a localized tumefaction, usually in patients without other vascular malformation, or as a diffuse thickening of the choroid in patients with Sturge–Weber syndrome (see next subsection).[9,22,123–130] Localized cavernous hemangiomas of the choroid are rarely detected before the third decade of life. They occur nearly always as a solitary tumor in one eye, although bilateral involvement occasionally occurs.[131] Their rate of growth is probably maximal during the normal growth period of the individual. By adulthood the hemangioma may cause secondary degenerative and proliferative changes in the overlying pigment epithelium and cystic edema and degeneration of the retina. These changes as well as the development of some varicosity and congestion of the large vascular channels are probably responsible for the minor enlargement of choroidal hemangiomas demonstrated in later life.[132,133] Unless the tumor is large and is located directly in the macular area, patients are usually asymptomatic until middle or later life (average age approximately 50 years), when they develop serous retinal detachment that spreads from the edge of the tumor into the macular area (Figure 14.15). Less often, these tumors may be discovered as an incidental finding by the physician or by the patient, who on covering the eye, notices a slight distortion of central vision caused by the tumor's presence in the macula before it causes any significant alteration in the overlying RPE and retina.

14.15 Choroidal hemangioma.

A–E: Serous detachment of the macula secondary to choroidal hemangioma in a 47-year-old woman complaining of recent onset of blurred vision in the right eye. Note the mottled, yellowish appearance of the surface of the tumor (arrow, A), which was located superotemporal to the optic disc.

Arteriovenous angiograms showed the presence of multiple blood vessels in this tumor (B). Later-phase angiograms showed staining of the surface of the tumor (C). Argon photocoagulation was placed on the tumor surface (D). Several months later the serous detachment had resolved (E).

F and G: Hemangioma of the choroid with serous and lipid exudative maculopathy in a 46-year-old woman before (F) and after (G) laser photocoagulation. Note the incomplete resolution of the lipid exudate. Her visual acuity improved from 20/200 to 20/25.

H and I, Juxtapapillary choroidal hemangioma (arrows) in a 47-year-old man who was treated unsuccessfully for 10 years for a recurrent serous detachment of the macula of unknown cause. His visual acuity was 20/200. There was extensive cystoid degeneration of the retina but no serous detachment of the macula (H). His visual loss was the result of permanent degenerative changes in the retina secondary to multiple recurrences of serous retinal detachment. Note reddish-orange color of the tumor and small, round, yellow deposits of exudate in the outer cystic spaces of the retina. Venous-phase angiogram showed early staining of the tumor surface. One-hour angiogram showed multiloculated pattern of dye indicative of cystoid degeneration and edema of the retina (I).

J–L: During the eighth month of pregnancy this 32-year-old woman noted metamorphopsia caused by serous macular detachment (black and white arrows, J) and a previously undetected hemangioma of choroid (black arrows, J). Angiography showed evidence of large vascular spaces within the tumor and late staining on its surface (K and L). The retinal detachment resolved and visual function returned to near normal during the early postpartum period.

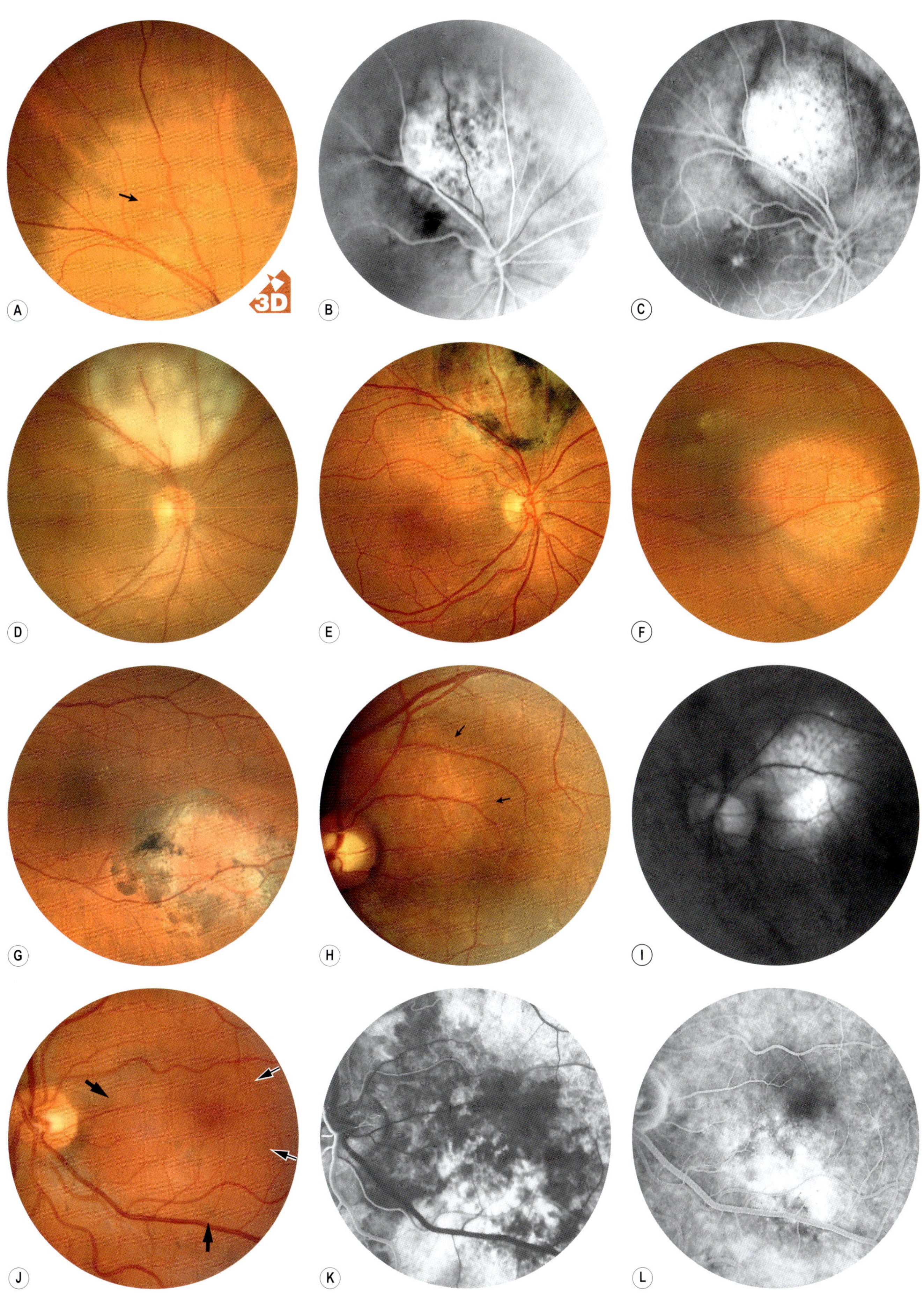
3D
A
B
C
D
E
F
G
H
I
J
K
L

Many of these patients are referred with the incorrect diagnosis of central serous chorioretinopathy, choroiditis, disciform degeneration, metastatic carcinoma, malignant melanoma, or rhegmatogenous detachment. The hemangiomas are typically round or oval, slightly elevated, orange-red tumors with an indistinct border (Figure 14.15A, F, H, and J). They are most easily detected with binocular indirect ophthalmoscopy. They usually measure 2–10 disc diameters in size. Most of the tumors are centered in the paramacular area, but may extend into the edge of the central macular area. Some are juxtapapillary in location. Others may be located on the nasal side of the optic disc.[134] In most cases the retinal detachment extends away from the margins of the tumor. The retina overlying the tumor is usually thickened by cystic degeneration. Complete separation of the tumor from the overlying retina by a serous detachment occurs infrequently. Varying amounts of splotchy yellowish material lie between the tumor and within the cystic spaces of the overlying retina (Figure 14.15A, F, and H). Hyperpigmentation caused by RPE hyperplasia is relatively uncommon but, when prominent, may cause a misdiagnosis of a melanoma or disciform scar. Some patients develop a bullous detachment of the retina inferior to the tumor at the time of presentation. Others will show large flask-shaped areas of atrophy of the RPE with a bone corpuscular pattern of pigmentation in the overlying retina extending inferiorly from the margins of the tumor (Figure 14.16B and C). These areas are indicative of previous long-standing retinal detachment with atrophy of the outer retinal layers permitting migration of pigment epithelial cells into the overlying retina. When the hemangioma is small, the subtle elevation and hyperfluorescence may be missed and a misdiagnosis of chronic idiopathic central serous chorioretinopathy may be made. Stereoscopic imaging helps to detect the elevation of the hemangioma. In addition to retinal detachment, other causes for loss of central vision in these patients include cystoid macular edema, lamellar macular hole formation, and epiretinal membrane changes. Choroidal neovascularization is an uncommon complication in these patients.[135] The maintenance of a high oxygen tension in the vicinity of the hemangiomas may be part of the explanation, if ischemia is important in the pathogenesis of choroidal neovascularization. Retinal and optic disc neovascularization occasionally develops in patients with choroidal hemangiomas.[136] Two patients presented to the Bascom Palmer Eye Institute because of rubeosis iridis and long-standing bullous retinal detachment caused by previously unrecognized solitary choroidal hemangiomas.

14.16 Choroidal hemangioma.

A–F: Loss of central and superior field of vision caused by a previous long-standing retinal detachment extending inferiorly from a choroidal hemangioma. Note marked hyperplasia of the pigment epithelium overlying the tumor (A) as well as dependent zones of pigment epithelial atrophy and intraretinal migration of pigment inferior to the tumor (A–C). Angiogram showed staining of subretinal tissue overlying the hemangioma and a zone of depigmentation (arrow, D) that extend in a flask-like shape to the ora serrata inferiorly. Ultrasonography showed highly reflective tumor typical of hemangioma (E and F).

G and H: Histopathology of cavernous hemangioma of the choroid. Note secondary cystic degeneration of the overlying retina (G). High-power view (H) shows cystic degeneration of the retina and hyperplasia and metaplasia of the retina pigment epithelium on the tumor surface.

Patients with choroidal hemangiomas associated with overlying cystic changes and serous detachment demonstrate field defects corresponding with the site of the tumor and the surrounding detachment. Nerve fiber bundle defects have been reported but are unusual.

The characteristic angiographic findings in choroidal hemangiomas are: (1) a pattern of fluorescence indicative of large vascular channels corresponding to the location of the tumor in the prearterial and arterial phase of angiography (Figure 14.15K); (2) widespread and irregular areas of fluorescence secondary to diffuse leakage of dye from the surface of the tumor; and (3) a diffuse multiloculated pattern of fluorescein accumulation in the outer retina characteristic of polycystic degeneration and edema during the later stages of angiography (Figure 14.15I).[2,9,132,137–139] A circular zone of hypofluorescence corresponding to the peripheral part of the hemangioma is often present during the early and middle stages of angiography. In some cases this corresponds with an area seen ophthalmoscopically in these tumors that may suggest slight pigmentation of the peripheral portion of the tumor. The reasons for this color and angiographic change are unclear. Evidence of cystoid macular edema may be present remote from the area of the tumor. In patients with choroidal hemangiomas without extensive secondary degenerative changes in the overlying RPE and retina, angiography may reveal only an exaggerated background choroidal fluorescence in the area of the tumor during the first few minutes of the study and no abnormalities during the later stages of angiography.

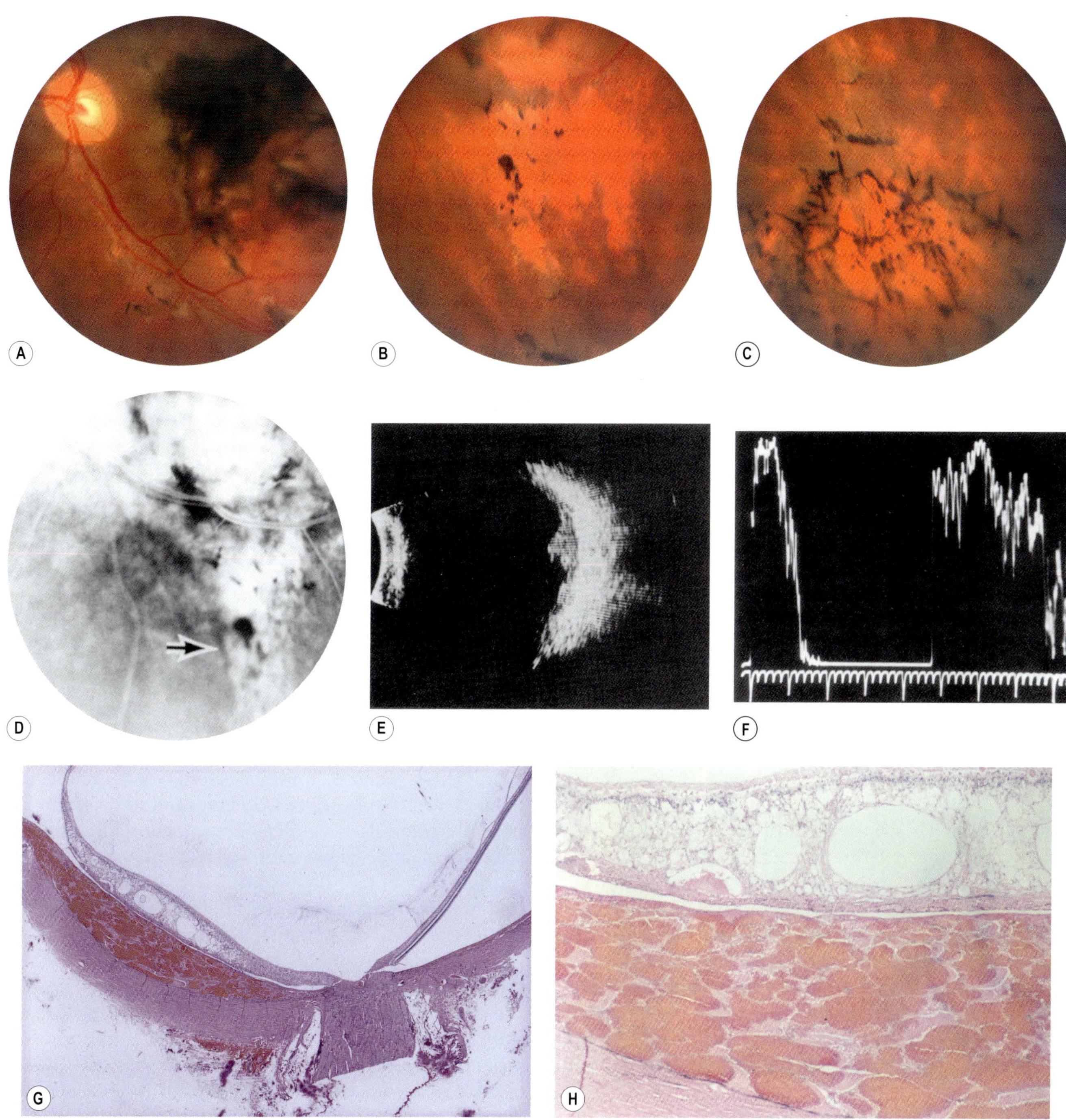
A
B
C
D
E
F
G
H

Indocyanine angiography reveals a diagnostic pattern of early diffuse hyperfluorescence (within 1 minute) with late hypofluorescence (5 minutes) and delayed washout phenomenon (beyond 10 minutes) due to exit of the dye from the tumor (Figure 14.17).[140]

Histopathologically a cavernous hemangioma of the choroid is composed of predominantly large, dilated, thin-walled vessels with minimal stroma. These tumors blend almost imperceptibly into the surrounding normal choroidal tissue (Figure 14.16G and H).[9,22,141] Extensive cystic degeneration of the overlying retina is usually present and in some cases may be associated with extensive fibrous metaplasia of the RPE and, less often, RPE hyperplasia.

Although not pathognomonic for cavernous hemangioma of the choroid, the early pattern of fluorescence caused by the large vascular spaces in the tumor and the late pattern of dye staining caused by the cystic degeneration of the overlying retina are infrequently found in association with other similarly sized tumors. The ^{32}P uptake is usually, but not always, negative in cavernous hemangioma.[125,142] Ultrasonography gives a characteristic pattern of high reflectivity that is helpful in differentiating a choroidal hemangioma from a melanoma (Figure 14.16E and F).[143] In the last analysis, however, the reddish-orange color of choroidal hemangiomas as viewed with a binocular indirect ophthalmoscope is the most important diagnostic sign that differentiates choroidal hemangiomas from white or cream-colored metastatic carcinomas and amelanotic melanomas. Other orange fundus tumors that must be considered in the differential diagnosis include serous or partly organized detachment of the RPE (see Figure 3.21 and 3.23), osteoma of the choroid (see Figure 14.21A), nodular scleritis (see Figure 11.35A), and exophytic retinal capillary hemangioma (see Figure 13.18).

Localized cavernous hemangiomas of the choroid located in the extrafoveal area and associated with serous detachment of the retina may be treated successfully with xenon or intense argon photocoagulation directed to that portion of the tumor surface where the fluorescein angiography shows evidence of diffusion of dye from the surface of the tumor (Figure 14.15D; see p. 1206). Photocoagulation should be sufficiently intense to create prominent whitening of the outer retinal layers. It is successful in collapsing the cystic retina on to the surface of the tumor and causing complete resolution of all subretinal fluid in most cases. It does not alter the size of the tumor. Photodynamic therapy offers the advantage of selective ablation of the tumors while sparing the overlying retina.[144–146] Using standard full-fluence protocol (TAP study) we have been able to achieve excellent tumor response of more than 90% with a single treatment application (Figure 14.17A, D).[147] Repeat treatment may be necessary but it is recommended to wait for about 6 weeks to 3 months to assess full response before embarking on additional treatment. Overall, excellent visual results can be expected over the long term following photodynamic therapy.[148] It is preferable to use a single large spot rather than multiple overlapping spots to avoid damage to overlying RPE that may lead to delayed visual loss.[147]

14.17 Circumscribed choroidal hemangioma.

A–D: A 42-year-old woman presented with reduced vision (20/40). Fundus appearance of an orange-colored circumscribed tumor suggestive of hemangioma (A). Indocyanine angiography reveals a diagnostic pattern of early diffuse hyperfluorescence at 1 minute with C, delayed washout phenomenon (12 minutes). Using standard full-fluence protocol (TAP study) a 6-mm single spot of treatment was applied (B). Six weeks later, note flattening of the choroidal tumor with minimal overlying retinal pigment epithelium alteration (D).

Transscleral cryopexy, microwave thermotherapy, and external-beam and episcleral irradiation have been used to treat choroidal hemangiomas.[130,149–151] Because of the morbidity associated with these latter techniques they should be reserved for use either in those patients for whom photocoagulation or photodynamic therapy is not successful or for patients in whom, because of the large size and central location of the tumor, photocoagulation is unlikely to be successful in restoring or preserving visual function. Treatment is optional in patients with the incidental finding of cavernous hemangioma unassociated with retinal detachment or evidence of previous detachment. These patients, however, should be cautioned to monitor their visual acuity frequently and to be examined at yearly intervals. Treatment of patients with localized detachment and evidence of severe permanent macular damage is optional. Photocoagulation might be considered to prevent further spread of retinal damage caused by further extension of the retinal detachment.

The onset of symptoms in patients with hemangiomas usually is unrelated to any recognized precipitating cause. The first manifestation, however, of a choroidal hemangioma, as well as choroidal osteoma or a large choroidal melanocytic nevus, may be visual loss caused by development of serous retinal detachment in the macula during the latter half of pregnancy. The author has seen this occur in four women, two with choroidal hemangiomas, one each with a choroidal osteoma and large choroidal nevus.[152] In three patients the detachment resolved spontaneously soon after delivery of the infant. The added hemodynamic stress, and perhaps other endocrine changes, occurring during pregnancy are probably responsible for transient decompensation of the altered choriocapillaris and RPE overlying the hamartomas. A similar decompensation may occur during pregnancy in some patients who develop idiopathic central serous chorioretinopathy in the absence of any other choroidal abnormality (see p. 82).

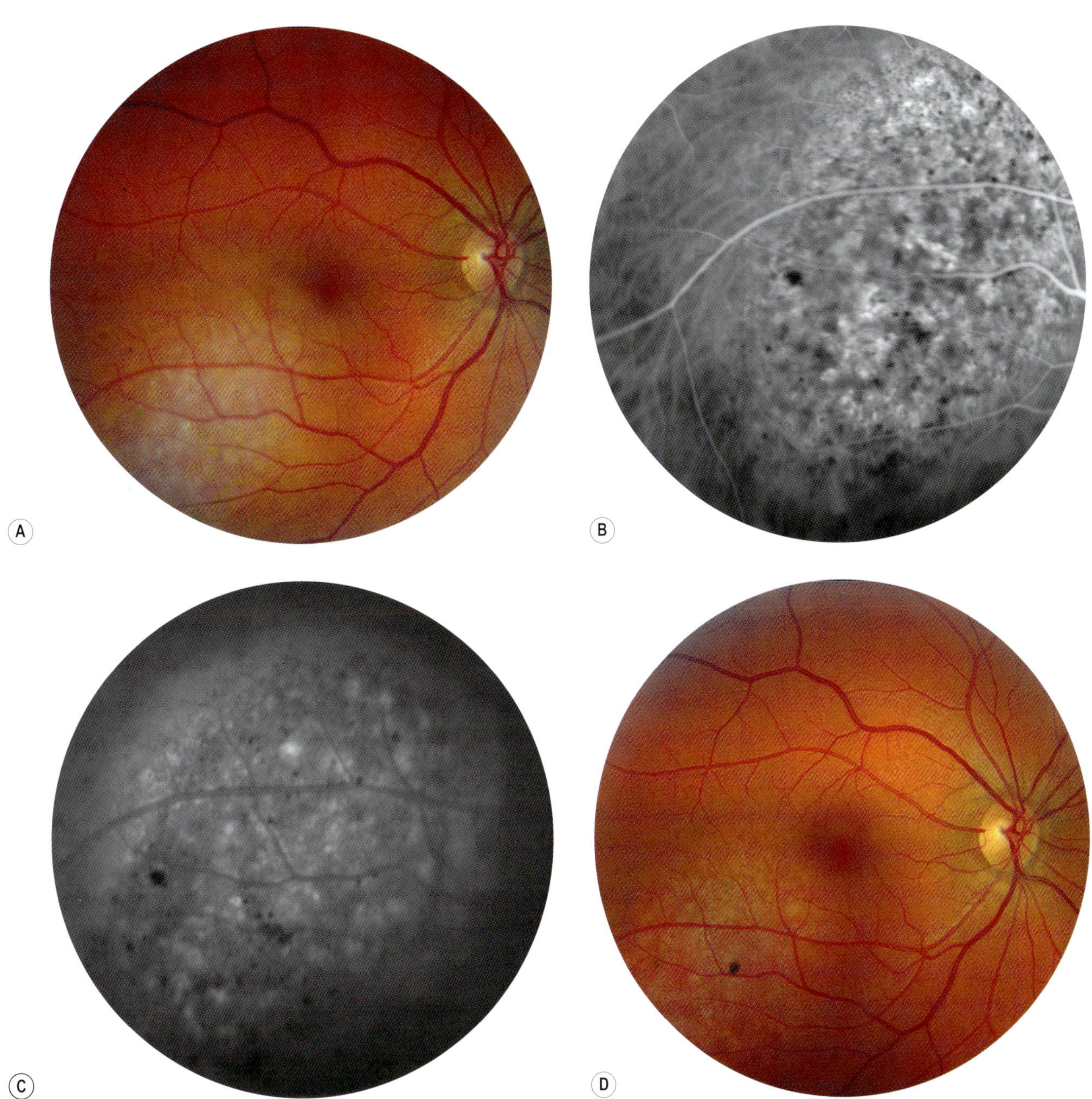
A
B
C
D

Other less common and rare choroidal tumors of vascular origin include capillary angiomas (see following discussion), hemangioendotheliomas, hemangioendotheliosarcomas, leiomyomas, and hemangiopericytomas.[153]

Sturge–Weber Syndrome

Sturge–Weber syndrome is a nonfamilial hamartomatous disease characterized by ipsilateral angiomatous malformation involving the brain, face (nevus flammeus), and uveal tract in a patient who often has seizures, evidence of intracranial calcification, and ipsilateral development of glaucoma (Figure 14.18). Most patients have diffuse hypertrophy of the choroid, eye, and face on the same side of the nevus flammeus and intracranial vascular malformation.[9,130,131,141,151,154,155] In a few cases both eyes may be affected.[151] The choroidal hypertrophy (diffuse angioma) gives the fundus a reddish glow compared to the opposite eye (Figure 14.18A and B).[155] Elevation of the intraocular pressure and glaucomatous cupping of the optic disc may be present. Some patients with Sturge–Weber syndrome have a focal area of angiomatous thickening of the choroid in addition to the diffuse thickening (Figure 14.18C–H). In the author's experience it is these patients who are most likely to develop secondary retinal detachment with shifting of the subretinal fluid, either spontaneously or after filtering operations for glaucoma. In most cases the localized highly elevated portion of the tumor is located somewhere in the posterior fundus in the paramacular area. The retina, which is usually attached to the dome of this localized thickening, shows marked cystic degeneration and some yellowish and gray tissue lying between the retina and the tumor surface. Angiographically, this area in the fundus is usually the only one that shows evidence of staining. Intense xenon or argon photocoagulation to this area may be successful in reattaching the retina (Figure 14.18C–H). Retinal and ciliochoroidal detachment occurring immediately after filtering surgery may reattach without treatment. When elevation of the hemangioma is so abrupt that adequate treatment cannot be applied by the transpupillary route, intravitreal photocoagulation may prove successful. In the absence of evidence of a localized choroidal tumefaction or pigmentary retinal degenerative changes, the use of prophylactic scatter laser treatment to prevent retinal detachment is probably unnecessary. Scatter treatment, however, may prove to be useful in preventing recurrent detachment in patients after successful reattachment of the retina.

14.18 Sturge–Weber syndrome.

A and **B**: Right and left eyes, respectively, of a child with the Sturge–Weber syndrome with nevus flammeus involving the left side of the face and diffuse choroidal vascular hypertrophy of the right eye. The large choroidal vessels in the normal fundus of the left eye were easily seen. The right fundus appeared diffusely red, and no vascular details of the choroid were visible.

C–H: Localized choroidal hemangioma in a 9-year-old boy with nevus flammeus of the right side of his face (C). He was initially examined at age 7, at which time visual acuity in the right eye was 20/40 and in the left eye was 20/20. His local ophthalmologist noted no abnormality at that time. In November 1971 the visual acuity decreased further. His local physician noted a mass in the inferior fundus for the first time. His intraocular pressure was normal, and there was no cupping of the optic discs. The patient was seen initially at the Bascom Palmer Eye Institute in January 1972 with an elevated, reddish tumor involving most of the inferior half of the fundus. It extended up to and bisected the macula. There was serous detachment of the retina overlying the tumor except in one area temporal to the macula where a 4 × 6 disc diameter, oval, gray-white exudative membrane was present between the tumor and overlying retina. The retinal detachment did not extend into the superior fundus. The patient was lost to follow-up until March 1973, when he returned with only light perception in the right eye. At that time he had a total bullous detachment of the retina except in the area of gray-white subretinal membrane (indicated in black in the fundus drawing arrow, D, and by arrows in E). The tumor (stippled area in fundus drawing, D) was unchanged. The retinal pigment epithelium (RPE) appeared to be normal elsewhere over the surface of the tumor. Fluorescein angiography revealed diffusion of dye from the surface of the tumor into the gray-white subretinal membrane temporal to the macula (F). There was no evidence of abnormal choroidal fluorescence elsewhere. Heavy xenon photocoagulation was used to treat the area of the subretinal membrane (G). In May 1973 the retina was completely flat and the visual acuity had returned to 20/400 (H). Note the faint traction lines radiating through the central macular area (arrow) toward the area of photocoagulation temporal to the macula. RE, right eye.

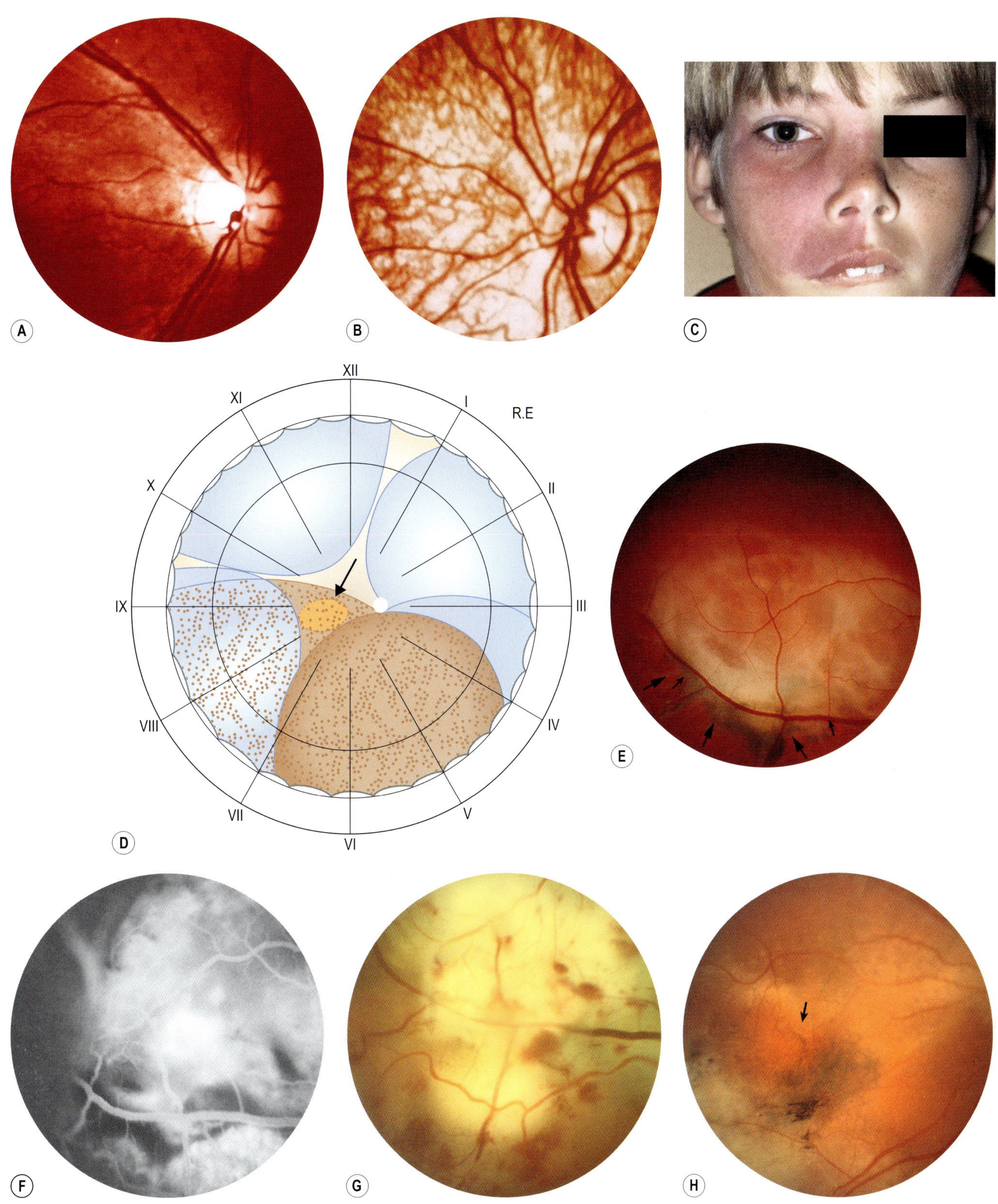
A
B
C
XII
XI
I
R.E
X
II
IX
III
VIII
IV
VII
V
VI
D
E
F
G
H

At the Fluorescein Club Meeting in 1990, Dr. Morton Goldberg reported a patient who, after prophylactic scatter laser treatment in the macula done to prevent retinal detachment before a glaucoma filtering operation, developed loss of central vision caused by choroidal neovascularization occurring at the site of a photocoagulation scar. Photodynamic therapy has also been tried but can cause transient worsening of exudative retinal detachment.[14–19,156] Use of low-dose external-beam irradiation 20 Gy in multiple fractional doses has proved successful in causing retinal reattachment within 6–12 months in patients with Sturge–Weber syndrome.[149,151,157] This treatment was used successfully in the child illustrated in Figure 14.18 (J–K) to cause resolution of bullous retinal detachment overlying massive diffuse uveal hemangiomas.

Forme fruste of Sturge–Weber syndrome may occur, e.g., a child with an ipsilateral solitary choroidal hemangioma and facial angioma without diffuse choroidal angioma, seizures, or evidence of intracranial angioma.

14.18 Continued

I: Skull roentgenogram of a patient with Sturge–Weber syndrome showing the typical railroad-track calcification of the vascular anomaly of the brain.

J–L: This 8-year-old child, with only slight extension of the right facial angioma to her left face (J), developed bilateral retinal detachment associated with massive thickening of the uveal tract in both eyes. This thickening was 6 mm in the right eye and 8 mm in the left eye ultrasonographically (K and L). It was not possible angiographically to define the sites of RPE decompensation. The patient underwent external-beam irradiation using fractional dosages for a total of 1800 cGy to each eye. There was prompt resolution of the subretinal fluid and reduction in the choroidal thickness. Nine months later her visual acuity was 20/300 right eye and 20/40 left eye.

(A and B, from Susac et al.[155])

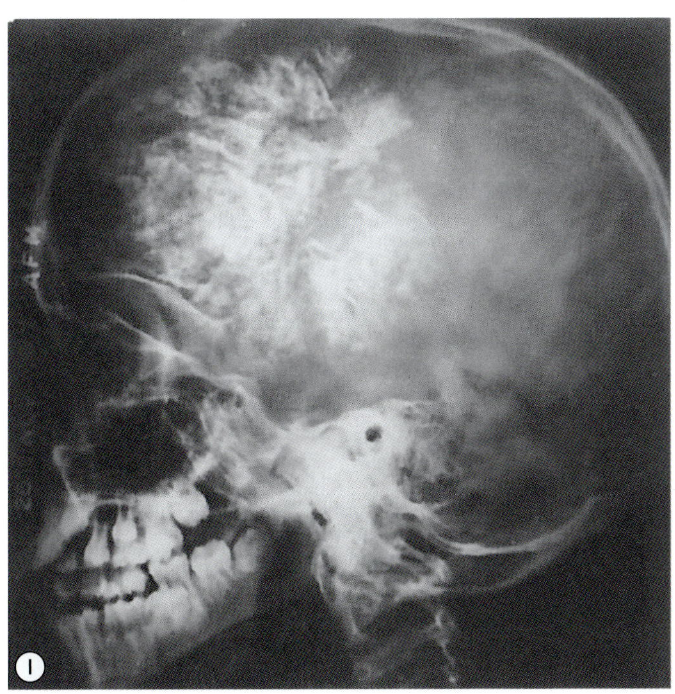

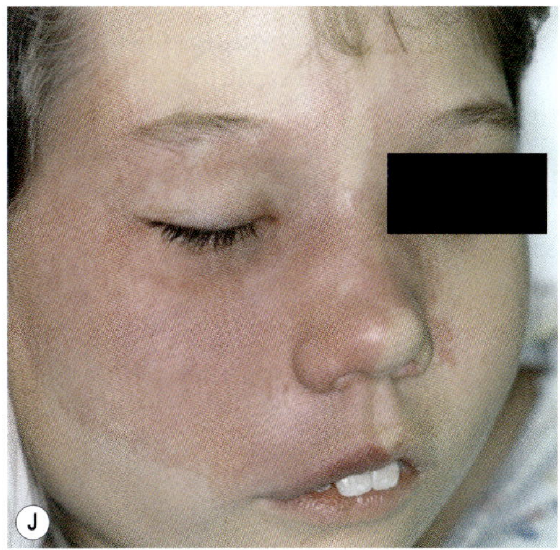

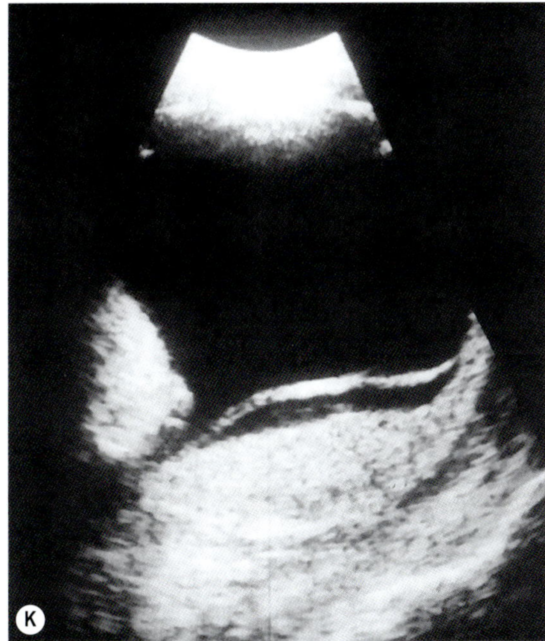

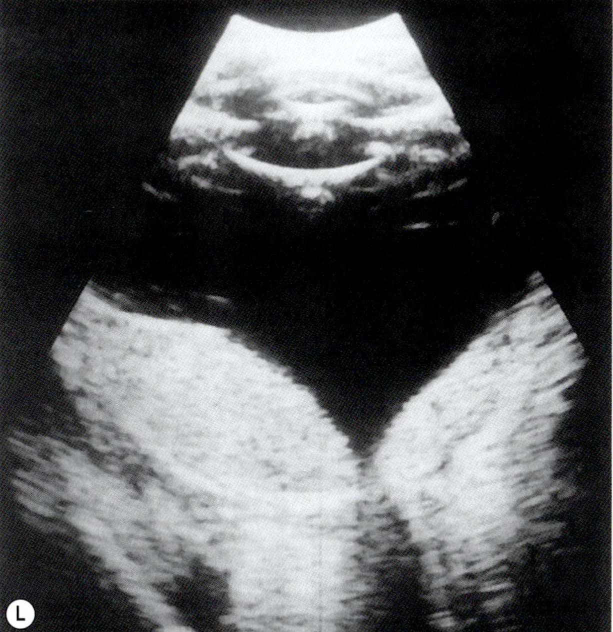

Ipsilateral Facial and Diffuse Uveal Capillary Angioma Associated with Microphthalmos, Heterochromia of the Iris, Chorioretinal Arterial Anastomosis, and Hypotony

Dr. Gass had seen an infant with ipsilateral capillary hemangioma involving the forehead, iris, and choroid associated with mild microphthalmos, hypotony, dilated retinal arteries, retinochoroidal anastomosis, and bullous retinal detachment (Figure 14.19). There was no history of seizures; computed tomography of the brain and her general medical evaluations were normal. At the time of initial examination under general anesthesia at 6 weeks of age, the local retinal specialist noted tortuous dilated retinal arteries extending from the optic disc superiorly to several large white atrophic areas, where they appeared either to anastomose with the choroidal circulation or to exit from the eye. There was no evidence of retinal detachment. The retina appeared thickened, but no evidence of a diffuse choroidal angioma was noted. The intraocular pressure measured 1–2 mmHg. Several months later the patient developed evidence of an inferior retinal detachment and a diffuse reddish color of the fundus suggesting a diffuse choroidal angioma. At 11 months, examination by the author confirmed the previous observations in addition to a total bullous retinal detachment except in the areas of peripheral chorioretinal atrophy superiorly (Figure 14.19C–F). There was no evidence of a retinal hole, and no explanation for the hypotony. The angioma on the forehead showed evidence of some regression (Figure 14.19A). When the patient cried there was evidence of a subcutaneous arteriovenous malformation adjacent to the posterior edge of the cutaneous angioma. Angiography confirmed the arterial nature of the dilated retinal vessels and showed staining primarily confined to the peripheral zones of chorioretinal atrophy (Figure 14.19F). Ultrasound revealed diffuse thickening of the choroid by a highly reflective tumor, whose average elevation was approximately 4 mm (Figure 14.19G and H), as well as dilated orbital blood vessels in the right orbit.

14.19 Ipsilateral capillary angioma of skin and uveal tract associated with aneurysmal dilation of retinal arteries, microphthalmos, heterochromia of the iris, and hypotony.

A: Note elevated partly involuted cutaneous hemangioma on the forehead, microphthalmos, and iris heterochromia in this otherwise healthy 21-month-old girl.
B: Dilated iris vessels (left arrow) and irregular angiomatous mass (right arrow) extending into the anterior-chamber angle of the right eye.
C: Fundus drawing of right eye. Note dilated tortuous retinal arteries that appeared to exit the eye in the peripheral zones of choroidal atrophy.
D–F: Bullous retinal detachment and dilated tortuous superotemporal retinal artery (arrows).
G: B-scan and H, A-scan ultrasonography showing retinal detachment and highly reflective diffuse choroidal mass.
I and J: Photomicrographs of right eye showing closed anterior chamber, calcified lens, funnel-shaped retinal detachment, and diffuse capillary hemangioma of the choroid (arrows, I). High-power view (J) shows details of capillary hemangioma. Note the stroma separating the capillary channels.

The retinal detachment was unresponsive to transscleral cryopexy of the areas of staining but was partly responsive to scleral windows done in the thickened sclera in each quadrant. Several years later the patient lost light perception, but she retained the eye until age 8 years when it was enucleated. The visual acuity in the normal left eye was 20/20.

Gross and microscopic examination of the right eye revealed a microphthalmic eye with a diffuse capillary hemangioma of the choroid except in the peripheral zones of chorioretinal attenuation (Figure 14.19I and J). Extensive atrophy of the iris and ciliary body, a ruptured calcified cataractous lens, and a funnel-shaped detachment of the degenerated retina were present. There were numerous large ciliary arteries and venous channels in the episcleral tissue surrounding the optic nerve.

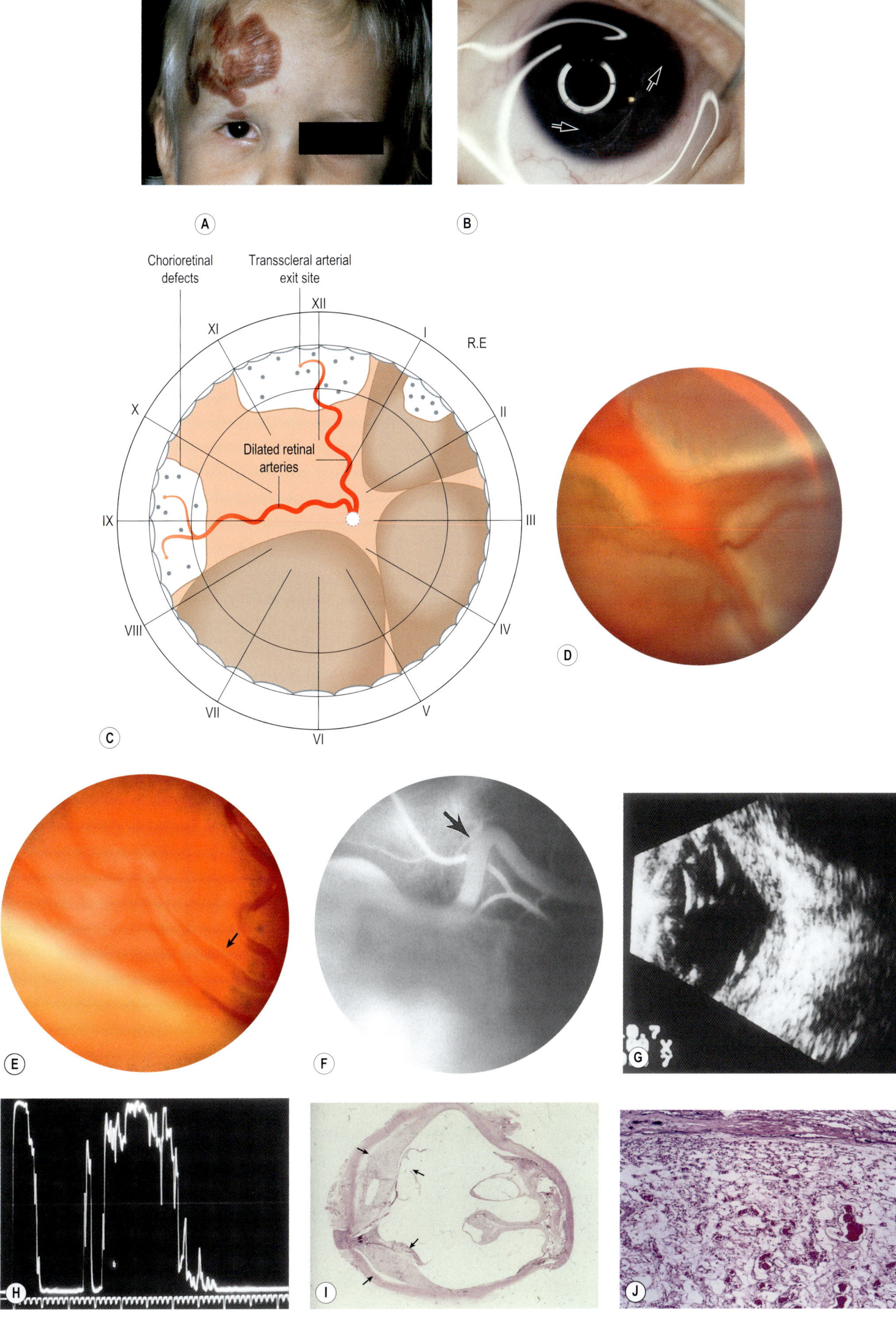
A
B
Chorioretinal defects
Transscleral arterial exit site
XII
XI
I
R.E
X
II
Dilated retinal arteries
IX
III
VIII
IV
VII
V
VI
C
D
E
F
G
H
I
J

This patient, unlike patients with Sturge–Weber syndrome, had oculocutaneous capillary rather than cavernous hemangioma, microphthalmos rather than the ocular hypertrophy that frequently accompanies Sturge–Weber syndrome, and hypotony rather than glaucoma. Unlike patients with Sturge–Weber syndrome and retinal detachment, there was no focal elevation of the diffuse angioma or a well-defined area of RPE decompensation angiographically that would permit us to direct either photocoagulation or cryotherapy. Because of the microphthalmos and the thickened sclera, we elected to try scleral windows despite the absence of ultrasonic evidence of uveal effusion (ciliochoroidal detachment). This was partly successful. Although we knew that facial hemangioma was a typical capillary angioma, we did not consider the possibility that the uveal angioma might also be a capillary angioma. Witschel and Font, in a review of the histopathology of 45 solitary and 17 diffuse hemangiomas of the choroid, found three cases of solitary and no cases of diffuse capillary angiomas.[141] Naidoff et al.[158] and Ruttum et al.[159] reported iris angiomas associated with cutaneous periorbital capillary angiomas. In one case this was associated with diffuse congenital angiomatosis.[158] If faced with another similar case, the author would consider the use of interferon-alpha, which has been effective in the treatment of some cases of systemic capillary angiomatosis. Another option that should be considered is external-beam irradiation.

Some interesting and unanswered questions in this case are: What was the cause of the hypotony that was a consistent finding on every examination, even prior to the development of retinal detachment? How did it relate to the apparent retinochoroidal and retro-orbital arterial anastomosis? Was hypotony important in causing the microphthalmos? Why did the retinal specialist, whose presumptive diagnosis was a variant of Sturge–Weber syndrome, not find evidence of a diffuse choroidal angioma at the time of his initial examination at 6 weeks of age? Could the angioma have developed or enlarged during the neonatal period? Growth of capillary angiomas in systemic congenital angiomatosis may occur during the first few months after birth.[158]

CHOROIDAL OSTEOMA

Choroidal osteomas arise in the juxtapapillary and macular region usually in young females who are seen because of metamorphopsia and a positive scotoma caused by either serous or hemorrhagic detachment of the macula, the latter associated with choroidal neovascularization (Figures 14.20 and 14.21A–C).[106,160–195] Initially, these tumors, which are generally only slightly elevated, may appear orange in color and may simulate a choroidal hemangioma (Figure 14.20A). Usually, however, by the time the patient becomes symptomatic, depigmentation of the RPE has occurred and the tumor has a cream color and well-defined geographic borders (Figures 14.20B–E and I–K, and 3.78A). There is often some mottling of gray pigment on the tumor surface. The orange color of the RPE may still be preserved over the peripheral aspect of the tumor. A dependent zone of RPE atrophy caused by prior long-standing retinal detachment may be present. A characteristic and pathognomonic feature when visible is the presence of numerous small vascular spiders located on the tumor surface in areas where the pigment epithelium is depigmented (Figure 14.20C and D). These are the feeder blood vessels exiting from the holes in the anterior surface of the cancellous bone. They interconnect the modified choriocapillaris on the anterior surface of the tumor with the large choroidal vessels that lie posterior to the tumor (Figure 14.21H). In some cases these vessels form large vascular trunks beneath the retina. Choroidal neovascularization or subretinal fibrous metaplasia may be evident (Figures 14.20C and D, and 14.21A).[168,178,196] The tumor may be multicentric (Figure 14.20E). It may be present or develop later in the opposite eye in approximately 10–20% of cases (Figure 14.20H and I).[175]

14.20 Choroidal osteoma.

A and B: Choroidal osteoma in a 25-year-old woman complaining of blurred vision. There was a circumscribed orange subretinal mass in the macula with minimal changes in the overlying retinal pigment epithelium (RPE) (A). Over a 2-year period there was progressive depigmentation of the RPE overlying the tumor (B). Visual acuity was 20/20. Ultrasonography and computed tomography revealed evidence of a choroidal osteoma. Over the subsequent 19 years of follow-up the tumor enlarged slightly and subretinal fibrovascular proliferation was associated with a decrease in visual acuity to 7/400.
C and D: A 10-year-old girl presented with acute loss of vision in the right eye caused by a subfoveal type II choroidal neovascularization and hemorrhage overlying a large macular and juxtapapillary choroidal osteoma in the right eye. She had a central disciform scar overlying a similar osteoma in the left eye. The blood resolved in the right eye and she regained 20/30 visual acuity, which she retained until age 24 years. During that follow-up period the diameter of the osteoma in both eyes increased slightly and there was extensive depigmentation of the RPE overlying the osteomas (D). Note the vascular trunks (arrows, D) on the tumor surface.
E–I: Growth of a peripapillary choroidal osteoma over a 5-year period in a 19-year-old man (E and F). A frontal-view roentgenogram of left eye shown in F revealed perioptic calcification (arrow, G). Right eye of same patient showing development of an osteoma and choroidal neovascularization (arrow, I) in the initially uninvolved eye (H).
J–L: This 29-year-old woman with a choroidal osteoma developed visual blurring in the right eye during the last trimester of pregnancy (J). Note the spontaneous rapid resolution of subretinal exudation that occurred within several months after delivery (K). Three years later she is asymptomatic. The osteoma is larger (L).

(A and B, from Coston and Wilkinson[281], published with permission from The American Journal of Ophthalmology, copyright by The Ophthalmic Publishing Co. C and D, from Gass et al.[282] © 1978, American Medical Association. All rights reserved. E–I, from Gass.[283])

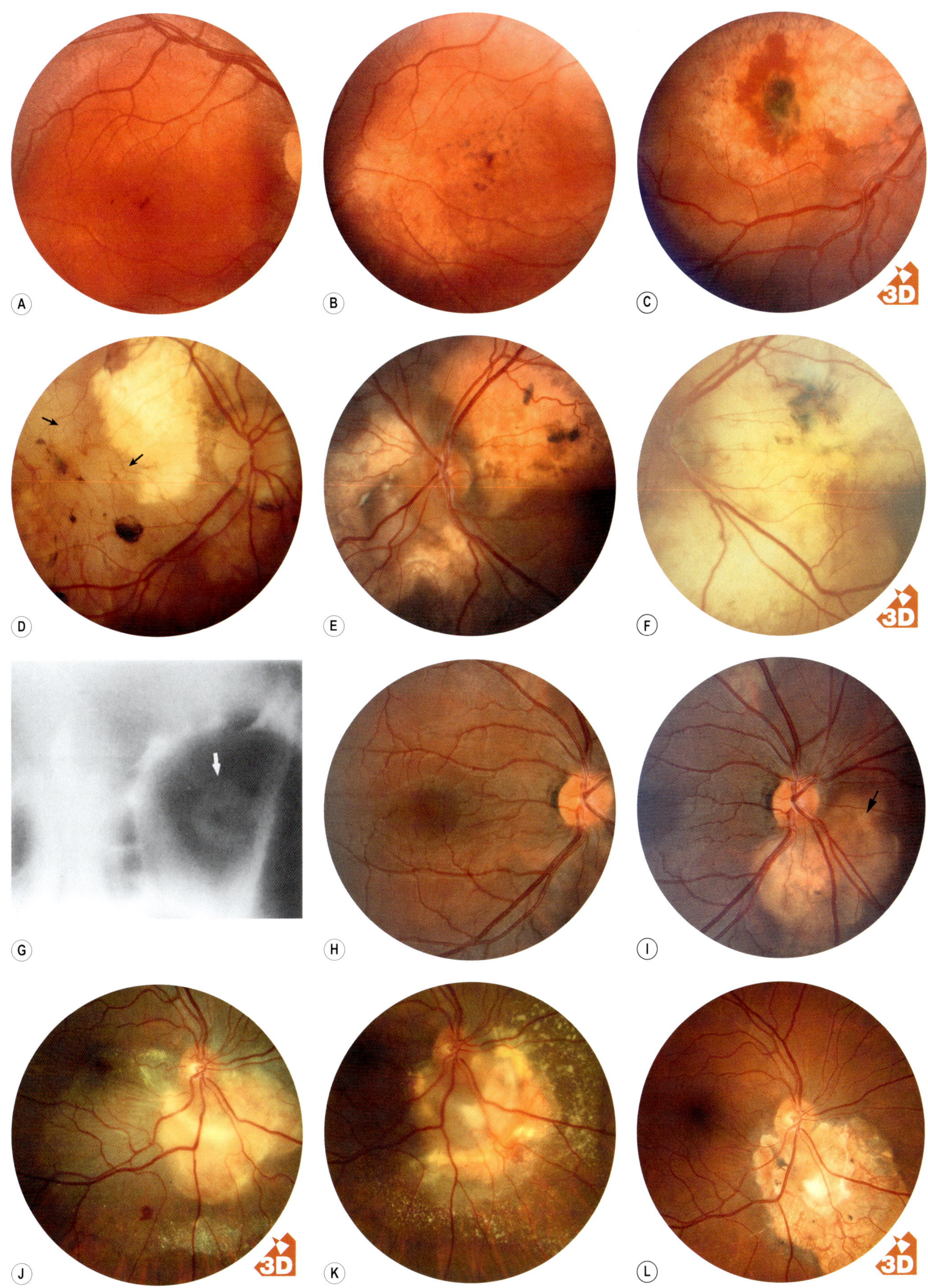
A
B
C
3D
D
E
F
3D
G
H
I
J
3D
K
L
3D

Fluorescein angiography demonstrates an irregular pattern of early hyperfluorescence in those areas where the RPE is thinned and late focal staining in those patients with serous detachment of the retina with or without choroidal neovascularization. Because of sluggish blood flow within the osteoma, the angiographic demonstration of discrete, early perfusion of the vascular spiders on the tumor surface does not occur. In the late phases of the angiogram, however, they are often seen as nonfluorescent structures on a background of fluorescein staining on the tumor surface. Spontaneous reattachment of the macula may occur with or without choroidal neovascularization, and the patient may regain excellent visual acuity. (Figure 14.20C and D).[176]

Dr. Gass had seen rapid resolution of a lipid-rich subretinal exudate caused by choroidal neovascularization overlying a juxtapapillary choroidal osteoma in a woman with rapid visual loss in the ninth month of gestation.[106,197] Disappearance of the exudation and return of vision occurred during the 6 months after delivery (Figure 14.20J–L). Photocoagulation may be indicated for the treatment of subretinal exudation caused by neovascular membranes that are outside the capillary-free zone.[177] Intravitreal bevacizumab can also induce regression of the neovascular membrane.[198] Photodynamic therapy may be preferable for the treatment of extramacular neovascular membrane (Figure 14.22).[199] Incidental decalcification of the osteoma (Figure 14.22F–I) following photodynamic therapy, and even laser, has been reported.[200] There is belief that decalcification may stop further growth of the osteoma; however decalcification under the fovea results in atrophy and loss of vision.

14.21 Choroidal osteoma.

A–C: This 15-year-old girl experienced rapid loss of central vision in the left because of subretinal neovascularization (arrows) complicating a large choroidal osteoma. Note the hyperpigmentation of the neovascular membrane that probably is a type 2 subsensory retinal membrane. She had a similar osteoma in the fellow eye. She has two siblings with bilateral choroidal osteomas.

D: Arrows indicate osteoma in the 9-year-old male sibling of the patient illustrated in A–C.

E and **F**: Several small choroidal osteomas developed during observation of a 10-year-old black girl during multiple episodes of bilateral orbital inflammatory pseudotumor and a transient period of mild hyperparathyroidism. She had no evidence of intraocular inflammation. Computed tomography demonstrated the osteoma (arrow, F) depicted in E.

G: Ultrasonography of another patient with a similar juxtapapillary and macular choroidal osteoma showing absence of echoes posterior to the tumor (arrows).

H: Histopathology of osteoma of the choroid shows plaque of cancellous bones lying between the inner one-third and outer two-thirds of the choroid.

I–K: Bilateral sclerochoroidal osteomas were present in this child with facial linear sebaceous nevus of Jadassohn.

(A–D, from Noble.[284] E and F, from Katz and Gass[285] I and K, from Alfonso et al.[286] J, from Gass et al.[282])

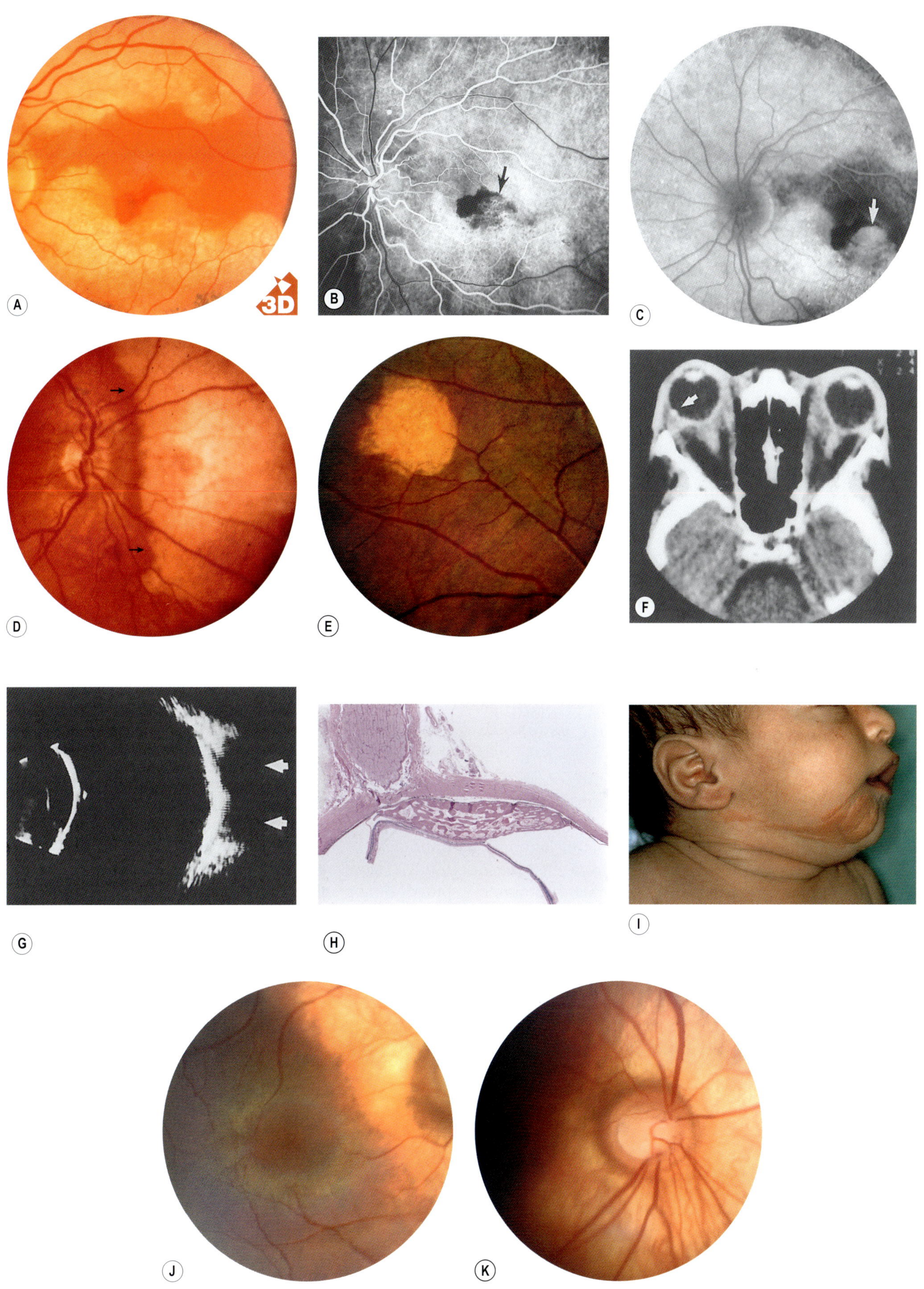
A
3D
B
C
D
E
F
G
H
I
J
K

The fundoscopic picture is usually sufficiently characteristic to permit an accurate diagnosis. The demonstration of marked attenuation of sound by the tumor ultrasonographically or of calcification of the tumor by either orbital roentgenography or computed tomography may be used to confirm the diagnosis (Figures 14.20G and 14.21F and G).[166,175,176] Magnetic resonance imaging shows less specific findings.[172]

Histopathologically these tumors are composed of plaques or mounds of cancellous bone that lie between the altered choriocapillaris and the outer choroidal circulation (Figure 14.21H). The large choroidal blood vessels communicate through the canals within the bone to choriocapillaris.[128,176,195] The RPE overlying these tumors shows varying degrees of degeneration.

The cause of these lesions is uncertain.[176,187] It is unlikely that they represent choristomas, since they have been observed to develop in adults in eyes that were previously unaffected (Figure 14.20H and I).[175] Choroidal osteomas have developed in patients with recurrent bilateral orbital inflammatory pseudotumors (Figure 14.21E and F),[181] uveitis,[190] vitritis,[106] Harada's disease (see Figure 3.60D–F),[176] and in the area of a photocoagulation scar.[163] Osteomas in adults may enlarge during observation (Figure 14.20E and F, J–L). Spontaneous reabsorption of choroidal osteomas may occur.[167,191,192,201] In one case this occurred over an 8-year period after photocoagulation of a subretinal neovascular membrane.[201] Bilateral osteomas have occurred in an 11-year-old black boy who died of a long-term illness that was thought to be either histiocytosis X or some form of systemic reaction to an unidentified infectious or toxic agent.[184] Choroidal osteomas may occasionally occur in siblings (Figure 14.21A–D).[171,173,202]

The differential diagnosis in the early stage of the disease, when the tumor has a red-orange color, includes hemangioma of the choroid, RPE detachment, and posterior scleritis; in the later stages, differential diagnosis includes metastatic melanoma, amelanotic melanoma or nevus, leukemia, sarcoidosis, and disciform detachment and scarring. Lesions that might be confused ultrasonographically and radiologically with choroidal osteomas include focal posterior scleral ossification in patients with hyperparathyroidism[203] and, in elderly patients with no known systemic disease (see discussion of idiopathic sclerochoroidal calcification, next subsection), posterior scleral osseous and cartilaginous choristomas that in some cases may be associated with facial linear sebaceous nevus of Jadassohn.[204–207] One infant with this syndrome had ultrasonographic and ophthalmoscopic evidence of choroidoscleral osteomas extending above and below both optic nerves and extending into the far periphery of the fundi (Figure 14.21I–K).[204] Ultrasonographic and computed tomographic evidence of calcification has been observed in the area of ophthalmoscopically visible small pigmented choroidal nevi in two patients by Basta and associates.[208] In an elderly man who had received laser treatment for a neovascular membrane complicating age-related macular degeneration, I observed the development of a choroidal osteoma adjacent to a laser photocoagulation scar.[163]

14.22 Choroidal osteoma.

A–E: A 50-year-old white woman presented with a recent-onset blurred vision of 2 weeks' duration (20/30). Ophthalmoscopic evaluation of the left eye revealed a solitary amelanotic choroidal lesion in the superior macular region. The lesion was about 6 × 5 mm in basal dimension and was minimally elevated. The margins were scalloped. Overlying retinal hemorrhages and subretinal fluid, which extended into the foveal region, were also observed (A). B-scan ultrasonography demonstrated high reflectivity at the level of the choroid suggestive of calcium deposition. On fluorescein angiography, the lesion revealed early patchy hyperfluorescence and late staining (B). In addition, overlying the posterior aspect of the choroidal lesion, lacy hyperfluorescence indicative of extrafoveal classic choroidal neovascularization was present. A diagnosis of choroidal osteoma with choroidal neovascularization was made. Photodynamic therapy (PDT) according to TAP study protocol (three sessions at 6 weeks' interval under fluorescein angiographic guidance was performed). Following completion of therapy, the vision improved to 20/20 (C). Ophthalmoscopically a grayish subretinal fibrotic membrane was noted in the treated area with total resolution of subretinal fluid and retinal hemorrhages (D). Complete closure of choroidal neovascularization was seen on fluorescein angiogram (E).
G–I: Decalcification of choroidal osteoma following PDT. This 25-year-old asymptomatic woman developed a choroidal neovascular membrane associated with an extramacular choroidal osteoma (G). Ultrasound B scan detected the choroidal bone (H). She underwent PDT and the choroidal neovascular membrane resolved, as did the calcium associated with the osteoma (H and I).

(A–E, from Singh et al[199] with permission; F–I, from Shields et al.[200])

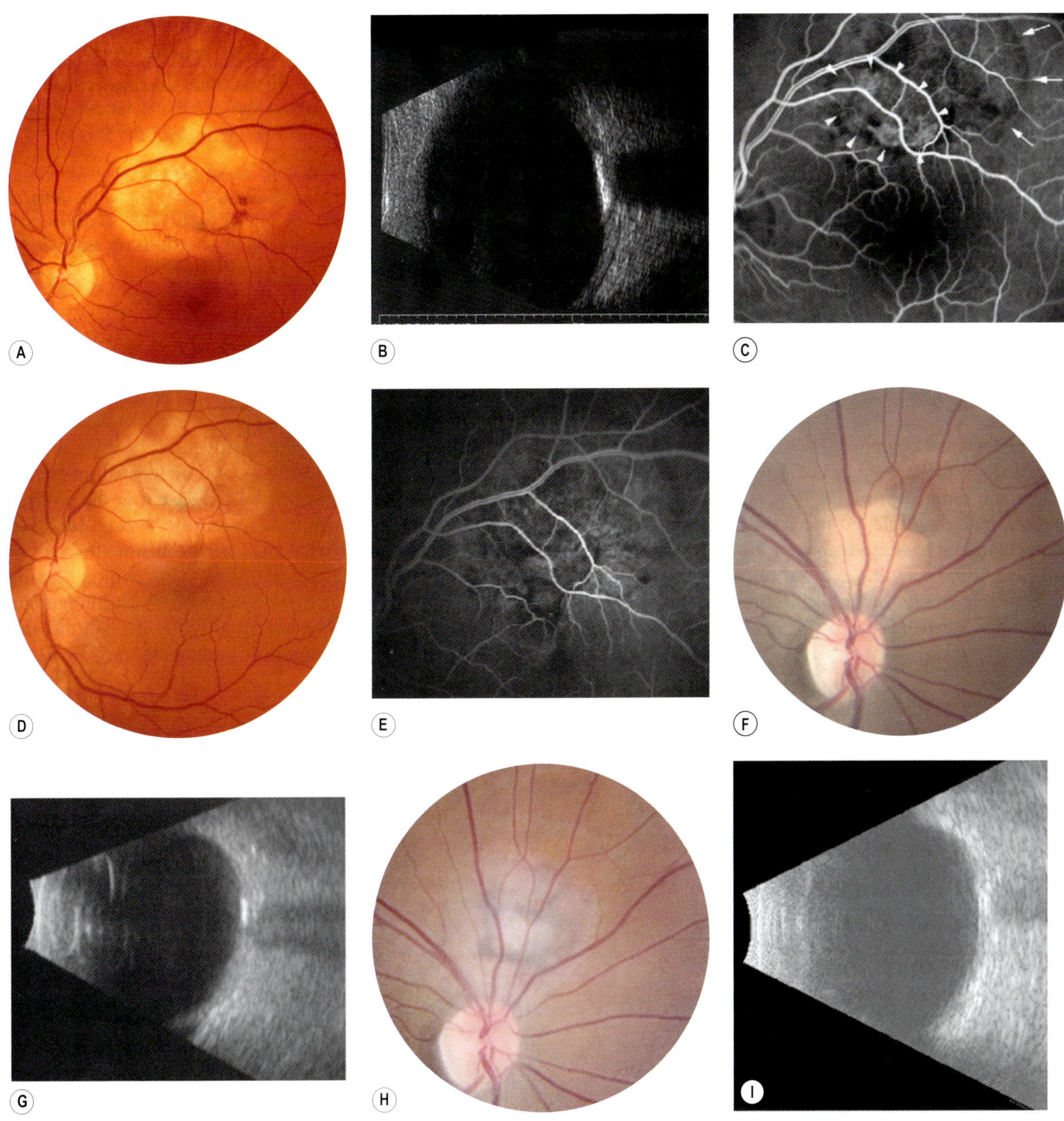
A
B
C
D
E
F
G
H
I

Sclerochoroidal Cartilage

Linear sebaceous nevus of Jadassohn can be associated with anterior epibulbar choristoma.[217] In rare cases, posterior scleral cartilaginous choristomas that resemble choroidal osteoma ophthalmoscopically have been observed.[218]

Choroidal Ciliary Neuromas Associated with Multiple Endocrine Neoplasia Type II-A

Multiple endocrine neoplasia (MEN) type II-A is a syndrome consisting of medullary carcinoma, marfanoid habitus, thickened lips, skeletal abnormalities, and neuromas of the corneal nerves, ciliary nerves, and mucosa, including the conjunctiva and mouth (Figure 14.24).[219] The ropelike enlargement of the long ciliary nerve that is visible temporal to the macula as it courses through the choroid (Figure 14.24G) is unassociated with alteration in visual function. Prophylactic thyroidectomy is recommended to prevent morbidity associated with medullary carcinoma that invariably develops in these patients. Histopathologic examination of the affected branches of the ciliary nerves shows hyperplasia of the perineural and schwannian tissue.[219] Fifty percent of cases of type II-B MEN occur sporadically; 50% are inherited as an autosomal dominant.

14.24 Multiple neuromas associated with the multiple endocrine neoplasia syndrome.

A–G: Note protruding conjunctival neuromas (arrow, A and C) near upper-lid margin, the thickened lips and postthyroidectomy scar (arrow, B), arachnodactyly (D), tongue neuromas (arrow, E), enlarged corneal nerves (F), and ropelike enlargement of the temporal long ciliary nerve (arrow, G).
H and **I**: Histopathology of enlarged long ciliary nerve (low-power view arrow, H) and enlarged conjunctival nerves at the limbus (high-power view, I) in another patient with the same disorder.

(H and I, from Spector et al.[287])

Neurofibroma

Solitary choroidal neurofibroma occurs sporadically and should be considered in the differential diagnosis of an amelanotic choroidal melanoma.[220] Diffuse neurofibromas generally occur in association with neurofibromatosis type 1 presenting as a triad of unilateral buphthalmos, homolateral eyelid plexiform neurofibroma, and homolateral facial hypertrophy (François syndrome).[122]

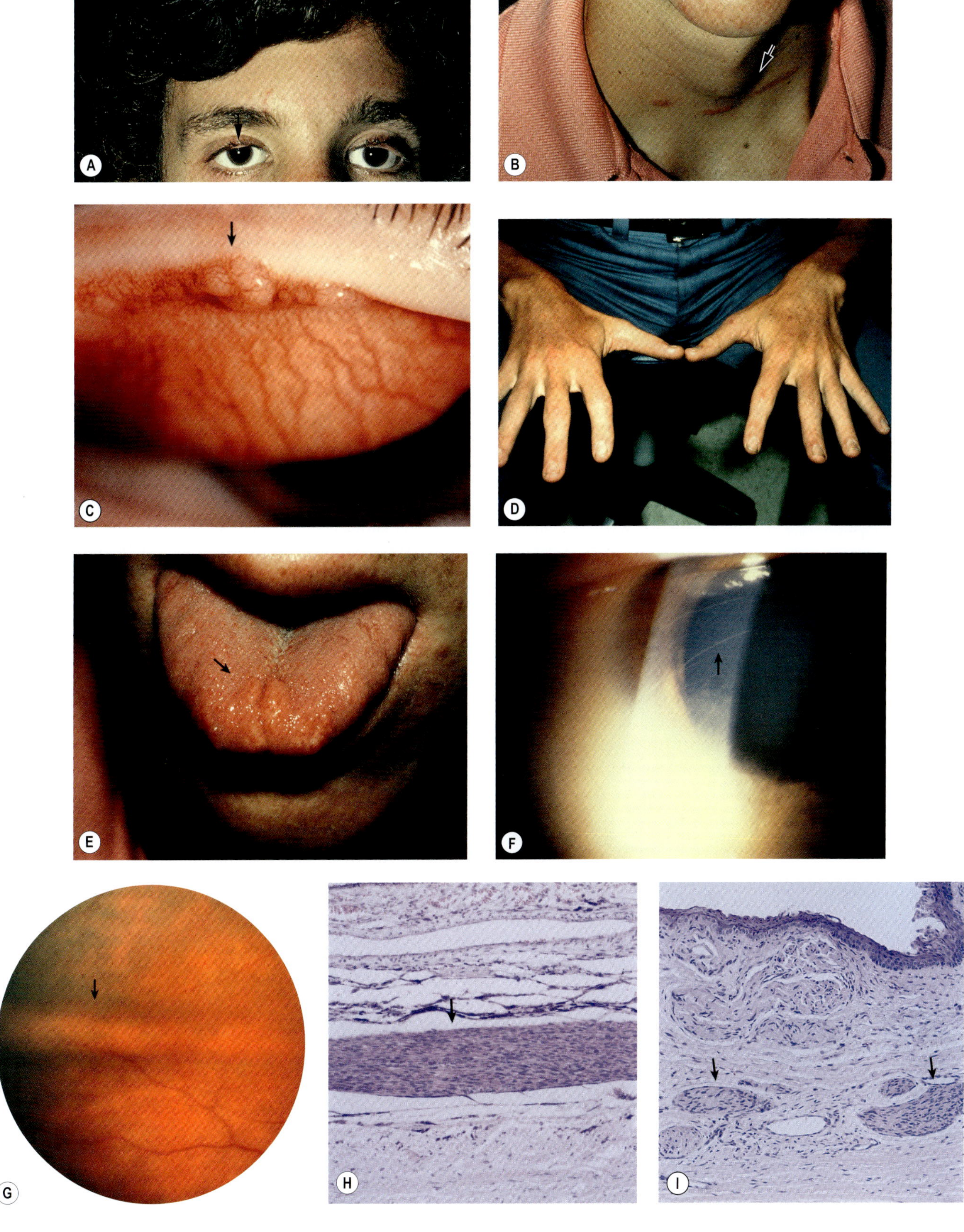
A
B
C
D
E
F
G
H
I

Schwannoma

Uveal schwannoma can present as a solitary tumor in the ciliary body or choroid, or diffusely in the whole uvea.[221] Typically, uveal schwannoma presents as a solitary amelanotic tumor (Figure 14.25).[222] Multifocal plexiform schwannoma has also been reported.[223]

Uveal Leiomyoma

Leiomyoma is a benign, smooth-muscle tumor of the uvea, most often arising in the ciliary body and iris,[38,224–227] and occasionally in the choroid,[228,229] or can extend into it from the ciliary body. It is nonpigmented or amelanotic, and lets more light through on transillumination compared to an amelanotic melanoma. Often it arises in the suprachoroidal aspect and pushes the choroidal stroma inwards when the lesion can appear pigmented. Sentinel blood vessels and extrascleral extension can occur similar to a melanoma. In all, 80–90% occur in females, with preponderance in young adults during reproductive age.[38] It may be associated with uterine leiomyoma in some.[228] A brightly transilluminating, nonpigmented tumor that localizes to the suprauveal space on careful ultrasonography in young adult females suggests a clinical diagnosis of leiomyoma.[38] Fine-needle aspiration biopsy may be helpful. Histologically, the tumor shows bland nonpigmented spindle cells with abundant connective tissue. Positive smooth-muscle antigen and muscle-specific actin help confirm the diagnosis. Some of them may be estrogen receptor-positive.

Small tumors can be observed; larger ones if confirmed by biopsy can be resected through a suprachoroidal approach.[230] The tumor is benign with an excellent prognosis. Dr. Shields has used aromatase inhibitors (anastrozole) in a male patient whose tumor, despite being estrogen receptor-negative, responded with shrinkage (Figure 14.25K–M).

Rhabdomyosarcoma is a malignant mesenchymal tumor of childhood that can rarely arise in the iris and ciliary body, but is never reported in the choroid.

14.25 Uveal schwannoma.

A–J: A 47-year-old white male presented with gradual, progressive blurring of vision in his left eye (20/50). Slit-lamp examination of the left eye revealed a dome-shaped ciliochoroidal mass (A). B-scan ultrasonography determined the dimensions of the dome-shaped lesion to be 17 × 15 mm (base) with a height of 11.4 mm. Definite intrinsic vascularity could not be observed. The lesion also had acoustic void. There was no evidence of extrascleral extension (B). A-scan ultrasonography showed a high initial spike with medium internal reflectivity (C). Following incisional biopsy that confirmed the diagnosis, surgical excision of ciliochoroidal schwannoma from suprachoroidal space was performed (D). Fundus photograph of the left eye taken 3 months following excision showing normal macula with vision of 20/20 (E). Light microscopy showing spindle cells in palisading pattern, immunohistochemical stains of ciliochoroidal mass were negative for (G) HMB-45, (H) SMA, and positive for (I) S-100 (F). Electron microscopy showing spindled cells with elongated nuclei and bland cytoplasm (J).

Leiomyoma

K–M: A Caucasian male presented with a ciliary body mass in the inferonasal quadrant of his right eye (K). The fundus was otherwise normal. A biopsy revealed the mass to be a leiomyoma that was estrogen receptor-negative. He was treated with anastrozole and the tumor shrank in size. Ultrasound B scan of the mass in 2008 before treatment (L) and 2 years following treatment (M) showed reduction in height of the lesion.

(A–J, from Turell et al.,[222] with permission; K–M, courtesy of Dr. Carol Shields and Dr. Jerry Shields.)

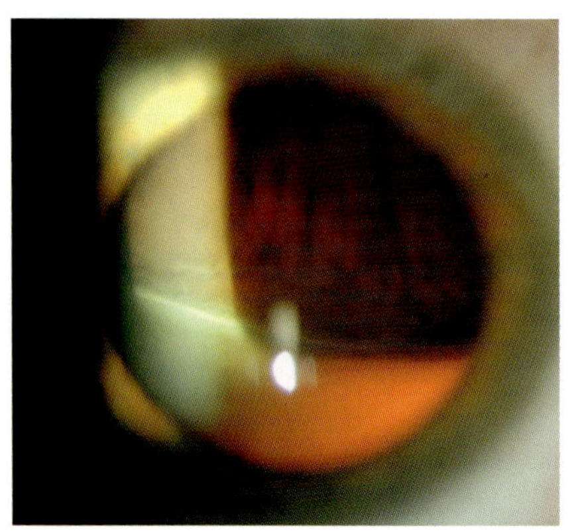

A

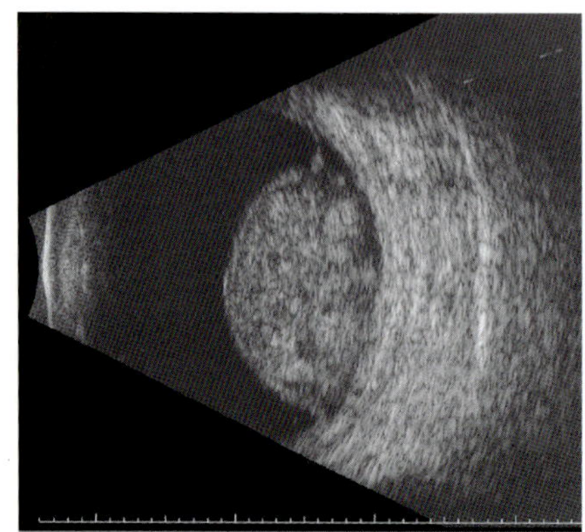

B

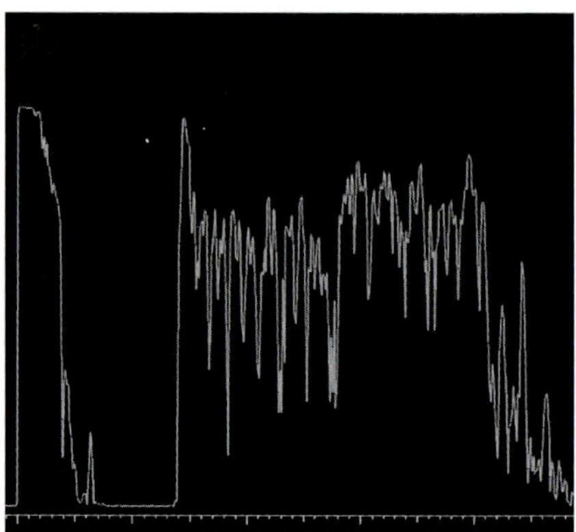

C

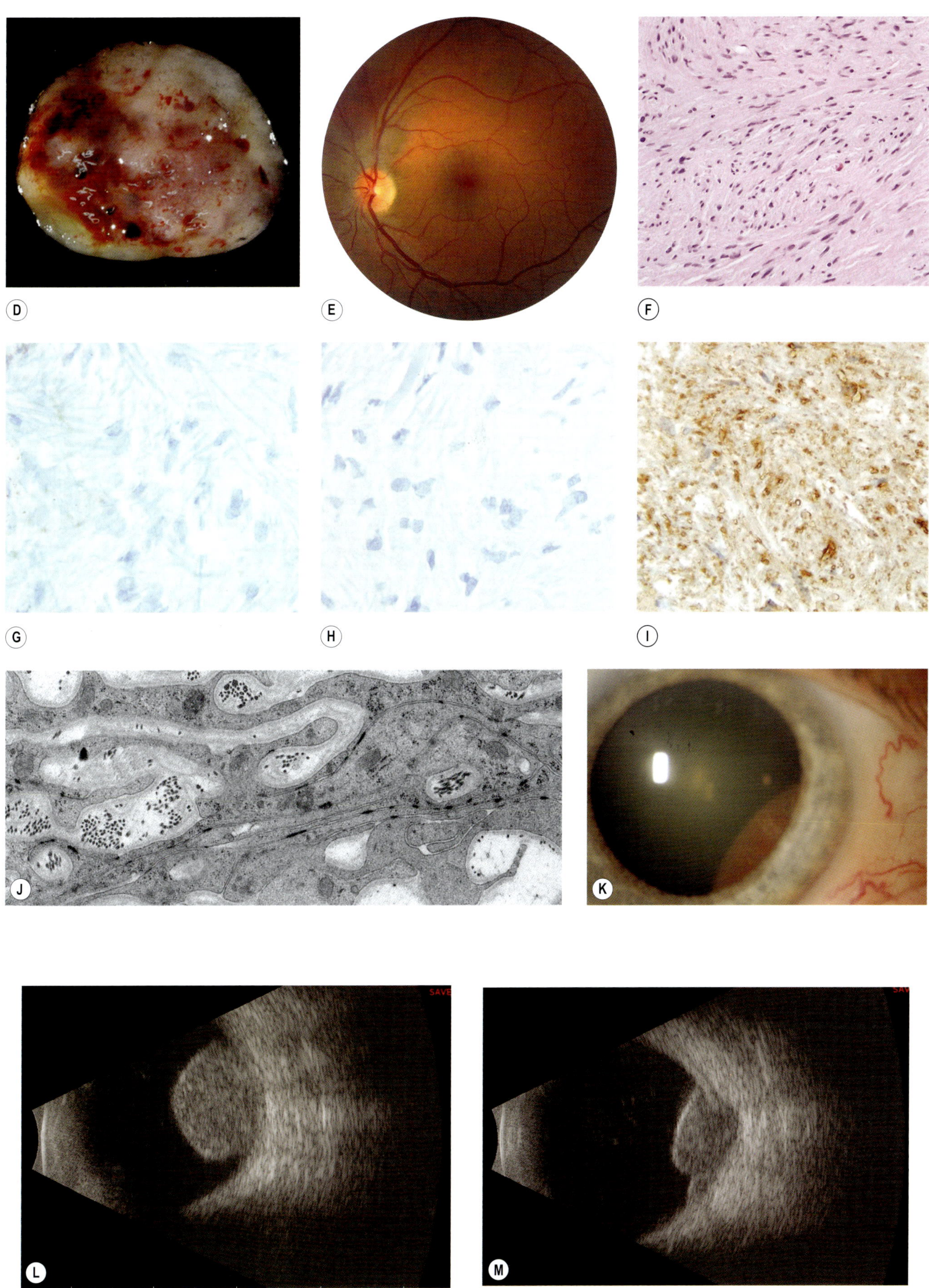
D
E
F
G
H
I
J
K
L
M

REACTIVE LYMPHOID HYPERPLASIA OF THE UVEA

Diffuse benign reactive lymphoid hyperplasia involving the choroid, ciliary body, and iris usually in one eye of otherwise healthy middle-aged or older individuals (mean age 55 years) is a rare clinical syndrome that is difficult to diagnose and may resemble in all respects metastatic carcinoma of the choroid (see p. 1236), diffuse malignant lymphoma of the uveal tract (see p. 1224), diffuse amelanotic melanoma (see p. 1200), or diffuse uveal melanocytic proliferation associated with systemic carcinoma (see p. 1202).[231–237] Patients with benign reactive lymphoid hyperplasia may complain initially of recurrent episodes of blurred vision and metamorphopsia secondary to serous detachment of the macula and be misdiagnosed as having idiopathic central serous chorioretinopathy. Eventually diffuse, occasionally undulating thickening of the uveal tract becomes manifest (Figure 14.26F). The fundus develops a yellowish-gray color with depigmentation and mottling of the RPE, loss of the normal choroidal vascular markings, and formation of linear streaks separating areas of uneven choroidal infiltration (Figure 14.26A, B, F, and G). In some patients the uveal infiltrate begins as multifocal yellow-orange lesions or as multifocal cream-colored lesions superimposed on the diffuse yellowish color change caused by the choroidal infiltration.[238,239] Pink, smooth-surfaced subconjunctival extensions of the lymphocytic infiltration occur in some cases (Figure 14.26E).[233] Small epibulbar nodular extensions of the infiltrate through the posterior emissary scleral canals occur frequently. These nodular extensions are usually unassociated with proptosis, and usually are discovered incidentally during ultrasonography or computerized scanning of the orbit.[240,241] As the ciliary body becomes diffusely involved, the anterior-chamber angle may narrow and cause acute angle closure glaucoma. Extensive retinal detachment may occur. A large tear in the RPE occurred in one elderly patient with polyclonal hypergammaglobulinemia.[242] Early phases of fluorescein angiography reveal irregular mottled areas of hyperfluorescence caused by the changes in the RPE and a series of hyperfluorescent lines demarcating zones of irregular thickening of the choroid (Figure 14.26H and I). Later-phase angiograms show evidence of multifocal areas of staining at the level of the RPE. Computed tomography and ultrasonography demonstrate diffuse thickening of the uveal tract as well as the posterior nodular episcleral extensions of the lymphoid proliferation (Figure 14.26J).[240] Ultrasound typically shows a smooth, low reflective thickening of the uveal tract and one or more epibulbar extensions of the infiltrate (Figure 14.26K and L).

14.26 Reactive lymphoid hyperplasia of the uveal tract simulating diffuse malignant melanoma or metastatic carcinoma.

A–E: A 55-year-old woman gave a 2½-year history of recurrent episodes of unexplained metamorphopsia and blurred vision in the right eye. Vision in the right eye was 20/400 and in the left eye was 20/20. Her exophthalmometer readings were right eye 20 and left eye 19. The extraocular movements were full. The eyes were not inflamed. Gonioscopy revealed a totally occluded angle on the right. The ciliary processes and pars plana were readily visible through an undilated pupil. The intraocular pressure was 35 mmHg in the right eye and 17 mmHg in the left eye before and after pupillary dilation. There was a diffuse yellow discoloration of the fundus attributable to choroidal thickening and alteration of the normal choroidal pigmentary pattern (A and B). There was a serous macular detachment. The fundus of the left eye was normal. The eye was enucleated because of suspected diffuse melanoma. Histopathologic examination revealed that the uveal tract was diffusely thickened and infiltrated with mature lymphocytes and lymphoid follicles (C and D). Note extension of infiltrate into the retrobulbar tissues (arrow, C). Thirty years later she returned because of the slow development of a smooth, elevated, pink subconjunctival infiltrate in the left eye (E) that remained unchanged during 6 months of follow-up. It presumably has the same histopathologic findings as in the uveal tract of the right eye. Her left eye is otherwise normal. She never developed evidence of recurrence of the inflammation in the right orbit.

F–L: Same disease in the right eye (E) of an 84-year-old woman with mild right proptosis and visual acuity of 20/400 in the right eye and 20/20 in the left eye. Note the irregular thickening of the choroid posteriorly and loss of choroidal vascular markings (E) compared to the normal left eye (F). Note irregular pattern of pigment epithelial demarcation lines seen overlying the thickened peripheral choroid (G). Angiograms showed hypofluorescent lines in the valleys separating broad zones of irregular choroidal thickening (H and I). Computed tomography showed diffuse uveal tract thickening and retrobulbar extension of the infiltrate (arrow, J). Comparison of ultrasonograms before and after treatment with systemic corticosteroids revealed reduction of uveal thickening (K and L).

(A–D, from Gass[278] published with permission from The American Journal of Ophthalmology; copyright by The Ophthalmic Publishing Co. E–I, from Desroches et al.[233])

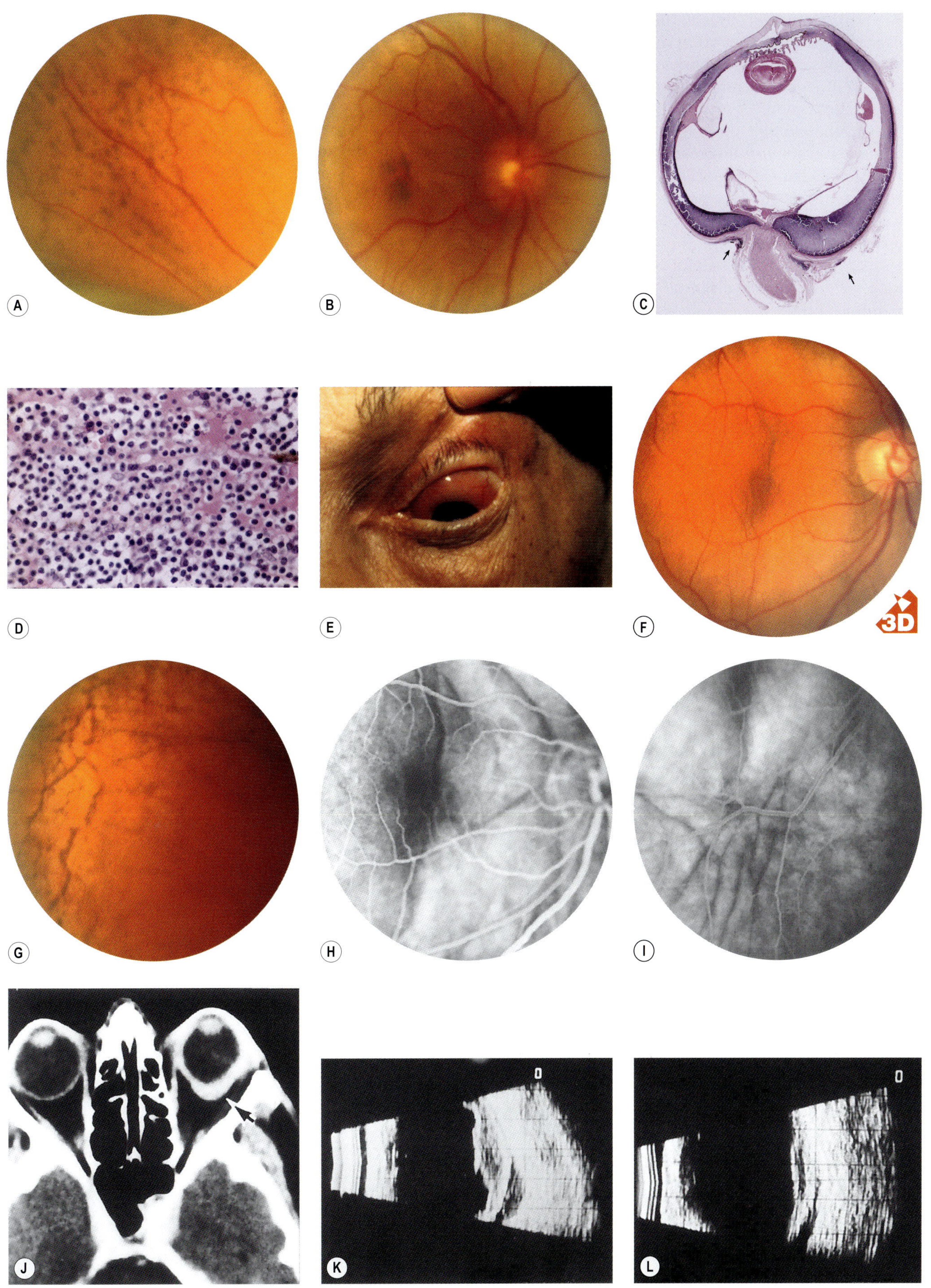
A
B
C
D
E
F
3D
G
H
I
J
K
L

Medical evaluation usually fails to detect evidence of systemic involvement as it is exceptionally rare to have multisystem reactive lymphoid hyperplasia (Figure 14.27).[243] Even if systemic involvement occurs, the prognosis for life is good.[243]

Histopathologically the uveal tract is infiltrated predominantly with well-differentiated lymphocytes, often with residual germinal centers (Figure 14.26C and D). The lymphoid proliferation is polyclonal. Determination of the clonality of the lesion is of little prognostic value.[244] Biopsy of either an anterior or posterior extrascleral nodule or of the choroid is helpful in establishing the diagnosis.[240,241] A correct diagnosis of reactive lymphoid hyperplasia versus follicular lymphoma can be reliably established employing immunohistochemical methods.[243]

If all studies for the presence of metastatic disease are negative, moderately heavy doses of systemic corticosteroids may be successful in causing resolution of the uveal infiltration (Figure 14.26K and L).[233] As the infiltrate resolves, it leaves varying degrees of coarsely mottled degenerative changes in the RPE. Low-dose irradiation may be necessary in some cases to effect resolution of the disorder.

Gittinger[245] reported a similar uveal infiltration with multiple creamy white subretinal lesions and exudative retinal detachment and mild proptosis in a 21-year-old patient with Castleman's disease. This is a lymphoproliferative disorder characterized by a thymoma-like mass with hyperplastic lymphoid follicles with accompanying capillary and endothelial hyperplasia arising in the mediastinum.[245] The uveal lesions responded to 20 Gy given in divided doses.

14.27 Reactive lymphoid hyperplasia.

A–F: External photograph of patient with bilateral fullness of both orbits and cheeks (A). Fundus photograph of the right eye of the same patient reveals creamy choroidal lesions consistent with uveal reactive hyperplasia (B). The left fundus had similar findings (C). Optical coherence tomography demonstrates choroidal thickening (D). Magnetic resonance imaging of the same patient demonstrates bilateral lacrimal gland swelling (E). F (inset), Biopsy exhibited follicles that were separated by wide interfollicular areas with prominent mantle zones. The follicles were composed of a pleomorphic lymphoid cell population, including dendritic cells and tingible body macrophages (arrow). No polykaryocytes (multinucleated dendritic cells) were found. Mitotic figures were readily apparent (F).

(From Stacy et al.[243] with permission.)

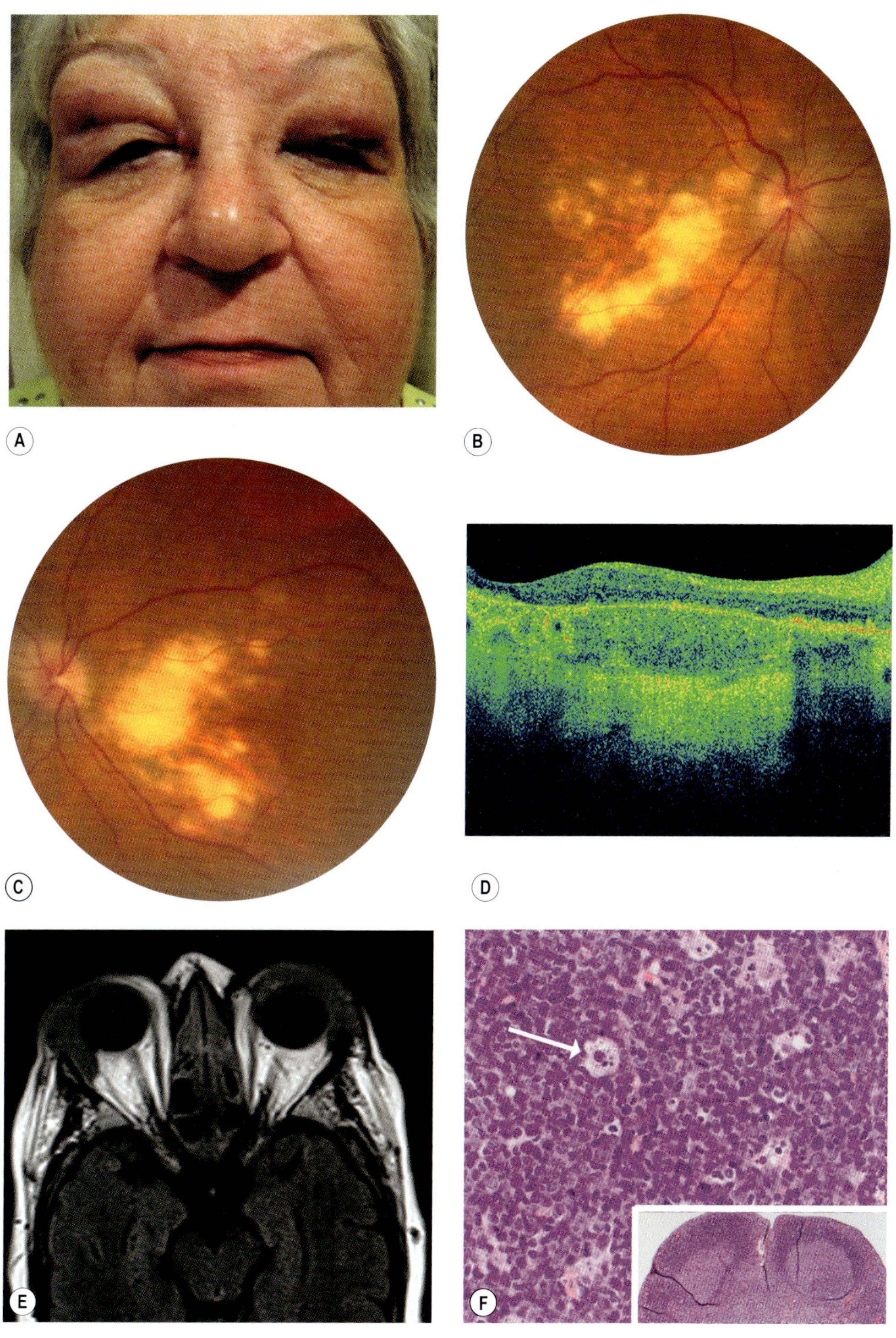
A
B
C
D
E
F

UVEAL LYMPHOMA

Uveal lymphoma (primary or secondary) should be differentiated from vitreoretinal lymphoma.[246] Primary uveal lymphoma is a variant of ocular adnexal lymphoma representing a low-grade non-Hodgkin's B-cell lymphoid malignant neoplasm.[247] The clinical features are similar to that of reactive lymphoid hyperplasia and it is believed that, in the past, a vast majority of cases that were diagnosed to have reactive lymphoid hyperplasia were in fact low-grade lymphoma.[248,249] The ocular involvement can be unilateral or bilateral and may have extrauveal extension such as salmon patch lesion visible in the anterior orbit or small areas of extrascleral extension detected by ultrasonography (Figure 14.28). The pathologic diagnosis is based upon combination of histologic, immunohistochemistry, flow cytometric, and gene rearrangement studies that are used to diagnose and classify lymphomas. A thorough systemic investigation, at initial diagnosis and periodically thereafter, similar to that undertaken for patients with ocular adnexal lymphoma, is mandatory to detect lymphoma elsewhere. Treatment options include low-dose radiation (30 Gy) given in divided doses if only a single site is involved or systemic targeted therapy with CD 20 antibody (rituximab) if lymphoma is multifocal.

Uveal involvement with lymphoma may also occur as a metastatic event in the setting of a progressive high-grade non-Hodgkin's lymphoma (Figures 14.28G–L and 14.29A–F)[250] or Hodgkin's lymphoma (Figure 14.29G–L). Such cases should be evaluated and treated by an oncologist depending on the overall systemic status.

14.28 Primary uveal lymphoma.

A–F: An 85-year-old male underwent uncomplicated cataract surgery in both eyes. Within a month of surgery, he noticed difficulty with the central vision in the right eye. External examination was negative. On fundus examination, small oval-shaped yellow lesions were observed that were scattered throughout the choroid in both eyes with confluence in the macular and temporal regions in the right eye. There were no vitreous cells (A and B). Fluorescein angiography showed early hypofluorescence with late hyperfluorescence corresponding to the distribution of the choroidal lesions (C and D). Optical coherence tomography confirmed significant elevation of the retina with shallow subretinal fluid. Magnetic resonance imaging of the brain and orbits showed no intraorbital mass lesions or abnormal enhancement of adnexal tissues. Complete blood count, CMP and computed tomography of the chest, abdomen, and pelvis were negative for lymphoma. A transvitreal fine-needle aspiration biopsy of the choroidal lesion was performed in the right eye; this was complicated by transient vitreous and subretinal hemorrhage (E). The cytology evaluation along with flow cytometry showed intermediate and small, CD5–, CD19+, CD20+ B cells, expressing predominantly lambda chains. These findings were consistent with a low-grade non-Hodgkin's lymphoma. The patient was treated with bilateral radiation therapy totaling 30 Gy in divided doses. At 3 months posttreatment, there was complete resolution of uveal lymphoma (F).

Metastatic uveal lymphoma.

G–L: A 38-year-old Hispanic male presented with floaters in both eyes of 1 month's duration causing a visual decline to counting fingers 1 foot (30 cm) in the right and 20/200 in the left eye. He underwent a diagnostic and possible therapeutic vitrectomy. His past medical history was significant for testicular natural killer/T-cell non-Hodgkin's lymphoma for which he had had an orchiectomy, and received intravenous and intrathecal chemotherapy and radiation for sinus metastasis. Following vitrectomy the fundus revealed multifocal creamy white choroidal lesions with overlying subretinal fluid in both eyes (G). Flow cytometry revealed CD2 +, CD3ϵ +, and CD56 + T cells; polymerase chain reaction was positive for Epstein–Barr virus and negative for toxoplasmosis, herpes simplex virus, herpes zoster virus, cytomegalovirus, human T-lymphotropic virus, and bacterial and fungal cultures. He received intravitreal methotrexate to both eyes, which progressively resolved the lesions, leaving behind a leopard-spot fundus appearance resembling bilateral diffuse uveal melanocytic proliferation (J–L). The lesions were hypoautofluorescent (H) and showed transmission hyperfluorescence on angiography (I). His vision improved to 20/50 and 20/40.

(A–F, from Fuller et al.[247] with permission; G–L, courtesy of Dr. John Huang.)

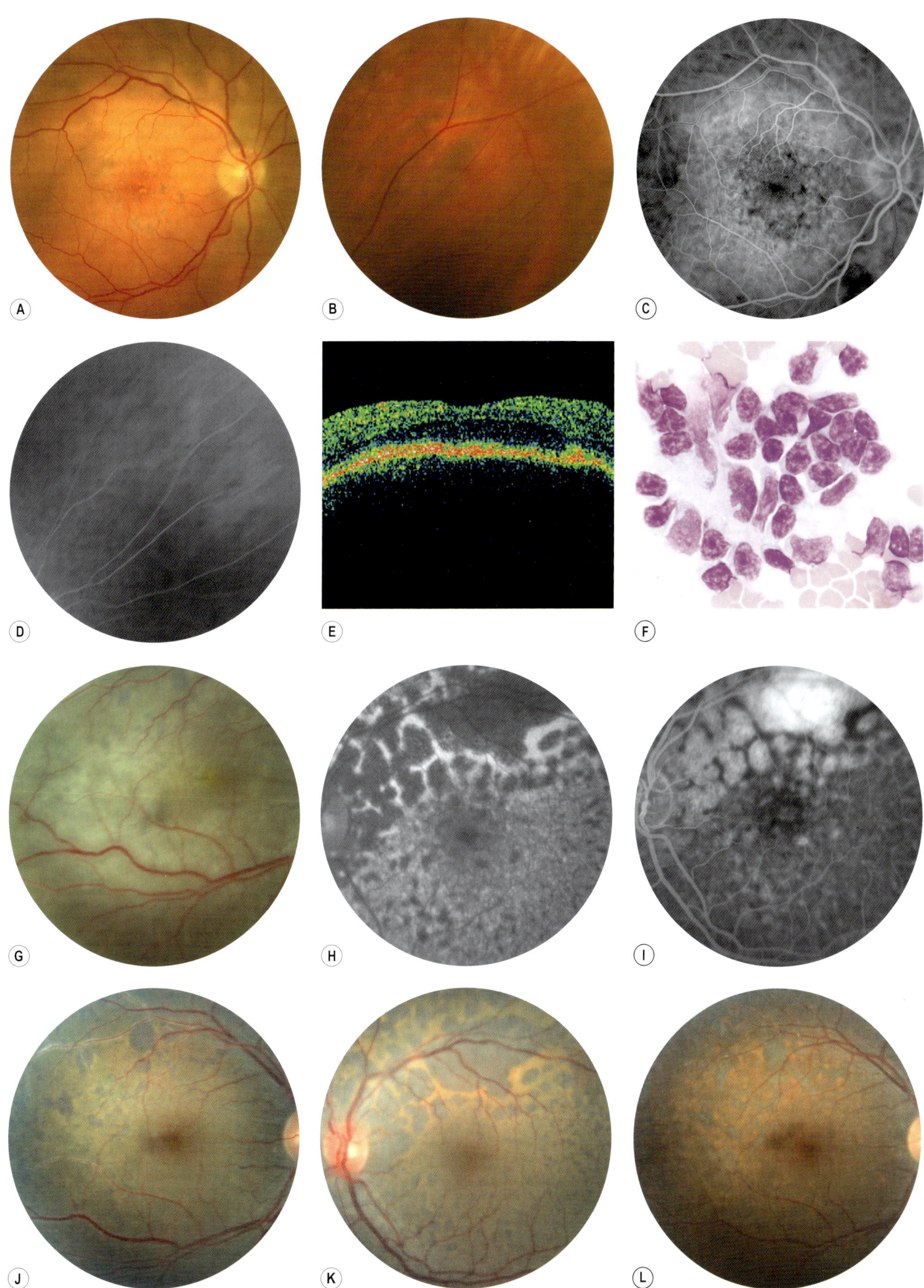
A
B
C
D
E
F
G
H
I
J
K
L

CHOROIDAL METASTATIC TUMORS

Patients with metastatic carcinoma to the choroid may develop serous, and occasionally hemorrhagic, retinal detachment involving the macula (Figure 14.30).[9,251–256] Ophthalmoscopic examination typically reveals a pale white or yellow-white choroidal lesion underlying the serous detachment. Orange-colored choroidal metastasis may localize the primary tumor to thyroid gland, kidneys, or lungs (carcinoid). Many metastatic lesions are only mildly elevated (3 mm or less), but their growth pattern may simulate that of a melanoma in every way. Coarse, mottled depigmentation and clumping of the RPE are frequently present. There may be multiple lesions in one or both eyes (Figure 14.30D and E). Fluorescein angiography usually reveals an irregular, widespread area of fluorescein leakage from the surface of the lesion (Figure 14.30B, C, F, and G). The angiographic pattern is not helpful in distinguishing metastatic carcinoma from choroidal infiltration by a nonpigmented melanoma or by inflammatory cells.[9] Ultrasonography of lesions 3 mm or higher may be helpful in differentiating metastatic tumors, which are usually more highly reflective than melanomas.

14.29 Metastatic uveal lymphoma.

A–F: A 51-year-old female presented with complaints of bilateral red eye of 2 weeks' duration associated with photophobia and blurred vision. She had begun a series of chemotherapy regimens 17 months previously for mantle cell lymphoma that culminated in autologous stem cell transplantation. On presentation, she was receiving rituximab in combination with intrathecal cytarabine for leptomeningeal involvement. Visual acuity was 20/40 in the right eye and count fingers at 1 foot (30 cm) in the left eye. External examination revealed multiple cutaneous eyelid nodules bilaterally and salmon patch in the superior fornix of the right eye (A and B). Slit-lamp examination was significant for pseudohypopyon, irregular stromal thickening of iris, and vitreous cells (left eye more than right) bilaterally. She was placed on hourly prednisone eye drops. In addition, external-beam radiation treatment at a dose of 14 Gy (seven fractions) was administered as a cone down to the area of gross ocular disease, with an additional dose of 16 Gy (eight fractions) to the brain (C and D). One week following initiation of external-beam radiation treatment, ocular signs had dramatically resolved (E and F). This 64-year-old diabetic male presented with 2 years' history of narrow vision in the right eye. He had had unilateral iritis, asteroid hyalosis, and nonproliferative diabetic retinopathy in this eye 2 years previously. There were several yellow subretinal linear lesions in the posterior pole and areas of retinal pigment epithelial atrophy in the midperiphery (G and H). Early-phase fluorescein angiogram showed leopard-spot pigmentary change that persists through all phases of the angiogram (I). A chest X-ray revealed mild pleural effusion (J). A chest computed tomographic scan revealed mediastinal lymphadenopathy, two pulmonary nodules, and pleural effusion (K and L). Open-lung biopsy revealed lymphocyte-rich variant type of Hodgkin's lymphoma. The pleural fluid showed lymphocytosis. Diagnostic vitrectomy was declined by the patient. The patient was started on systemic chemotherapy for the Hodgkin's lymphoma, and his visual symptoms and signs improved.

(A–F, from Chappelow et al.[250] with permission; G–L, courtesy of Dr. Quan D. Nguyen and Dr. John Choi.)

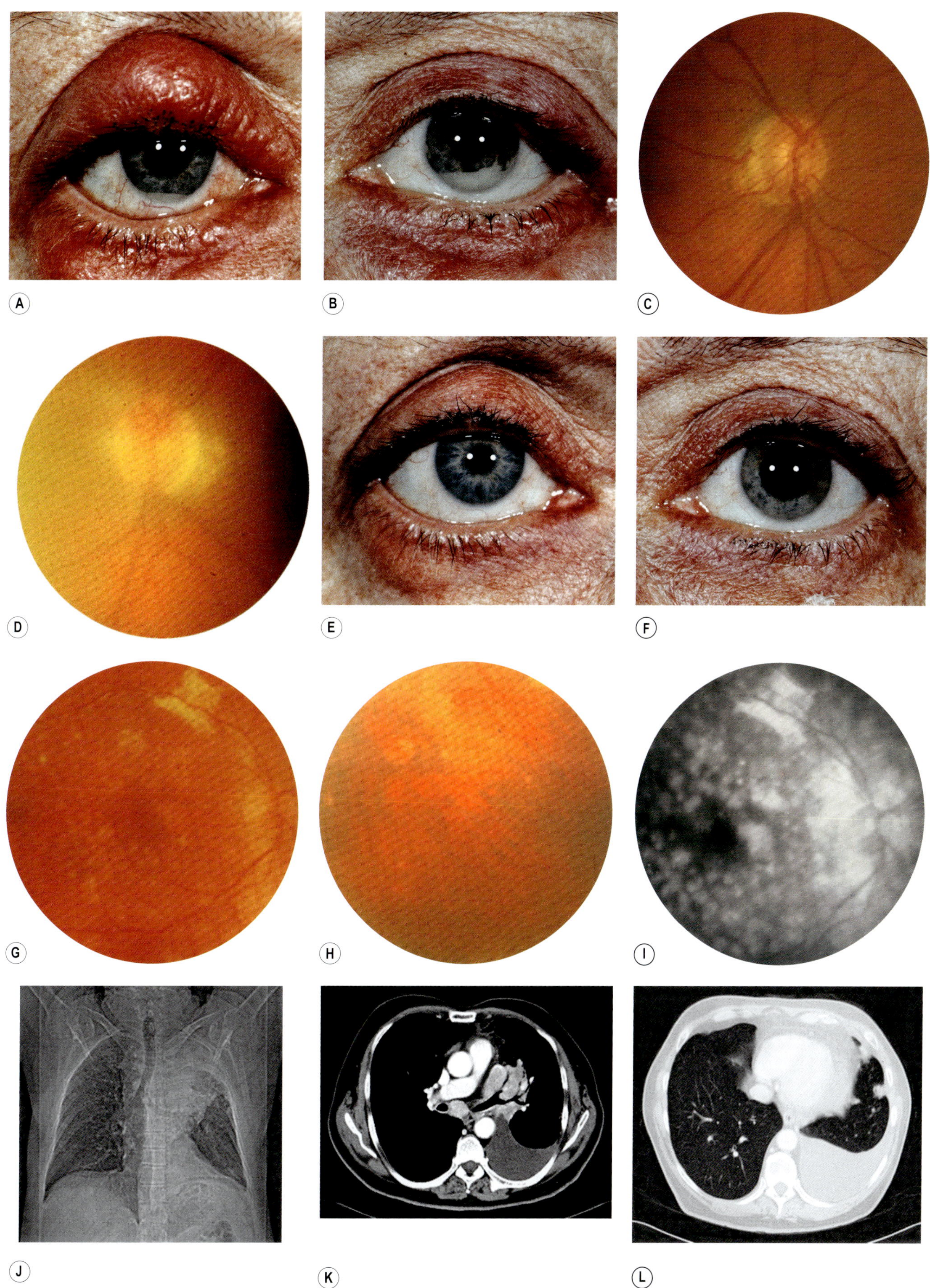
A
B
C
D
E
F
G
H
I
J
K
L

14.30 Choroidal metastasis.

A–C: Occult, small, nonpigmented metastatic breast carcinoma causing retinal detachment and blurred vision in a 29-year-old woman with a history of mastectomy and ductal cell carcinoma. Stereoscopic angiograms demonstrated evidence of a focal choroidal tumor with pinpoint fluorescein leaks overlying its surface in the juxtapapillary area (B and C).
D–G: Multifocal metastatic carcinoma from the lungs simulating acute posterior multifocal placoid pigment epitheliopathy (APMPPE) in a 33-year-old man. The patient was unaware of the lung carcinoma at the time he was initially seen. Angiography, unlike that in APMPPE, showed no evidence of opacification of the retinal pigment epithelium (RPE) but only irregular disruption of the RPE and late staining (F and G).
H and **I**: This woman was seen because of rapid loss of vision in both eyes. It was caused by metastatic breast carcinoma to the choroid and hemorrhagic detachment of the retina in both eyes. Angiography showed extensive leakage of dye from the tumor surface that was partly obscured by the subretinal blood (I).
J–L: This woman experienced bilateral loss of vision and recent development of a nodule on the forehead (arrows, J). There was bullous detachment of the retina in both eyes (K) overlying nonpigmented choroidal tumors. Biopsy of the nodule on the forehead revealed metastatic breast carcinoma. Irradiation of both eyes caused prompt flattening of the metastatic tumor, disappearance of the subretinal fluid, and restoration of vision (L). Note increased mottling of the RPE in the area of the tumor after treatment.

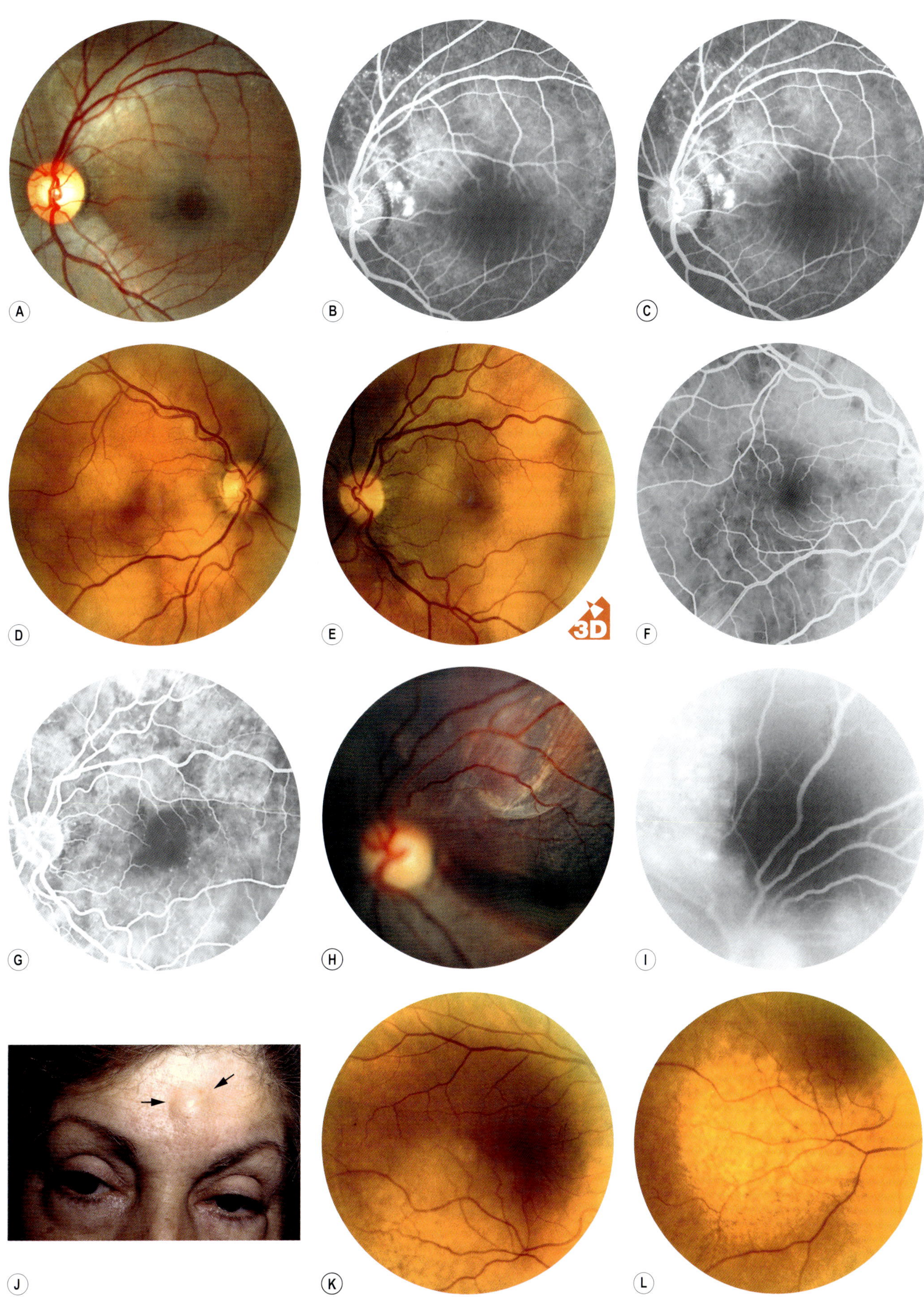
A
B
C
D
E
3D
F
G
H
I
J
K
L

Differential diagnosis includes amelanotic nevus, amelanotic malignant melanoma, leukemia, large cell lymphoma (reticulum cell sarcoma), choroidal osteoma, choroidal hemangioma, choroidal neovascularization with overlying focal exudative detachment, granulomas such as sarcoidosis and tuberculosis, and juxtapapillary exophytic capillary hemangiomas of the retina.[9,257] When the tumor is multifocal in nature, the differential diagnosis may include inflammatory diseases such as acute posterior multifocal placoid pigment epitheliopathy (Figure 14.30D and E). A thorough medical history and evaluation should be done to determine the presence or absence of a primary tumor, which in females most frequently occurs in the breast and in males in the lung.[258] In general, metastasis from breast cancer occurs in the setting of a known primary tumor while ocular presentation may precede the diagnosis of the primary tumor in the lung.[258] In the absence of detectable primary tumor, fine-needle aspiration biopsy of the choroidal tumor may be necessary to establish the diagnosis. X-ray irradiation, hormonal therapy, and chemotherapy may be successful in causing resolution of the detachment and reducing the size of the choroidal tumor (Figure 14.30K and L).[259–262] Metastatic thyroid carcinoma may resolve following systemic ^{131}I therapy.[263] Estrogen and progesterone receptor-positive breast cancer often responds to oral aromatase inhibitors such as anastrazole (Figure 14.31).[264] Most recently, metastatic and primary adenocarcinoma of the lung has shown response to oral erlotinib (Tarceva), an epidermal growth factor receptor inhibitor protein kinase inhibitor (Figure 14.31G–L).

14.31 Choroidal metastasis.

A–F: A 64-year-old woman presented with a progressive macular lesion in her left eye. Her past medical history was significant for breast cancer with spread to two axillary lymph nodes (stage IIA), which was diagnosed 18 years previously and treated with a modified radical mastectomy followed by chemotherapy. As the tumor was estrogen and progesterone receptor-positive, tamoxifen was prescribed for 5 years (approximate total dose 36.5 grams) and the patient had been in remission since. One year ago, she noted blurred vision in her left eye (20/100). A placoid partially amelanotic macular mass was observed, which was continuous with an extrascleral nodule of lower acoustic reflectivity than that of the surrounding orbital tissue. Given the patient's history of breast cancer, a metastatic evaluation was performed (A). Scattered lytic bone lesions were detected by computed tomography, and C, technetium-99 bone scan revealed multiple foci of abnormal uptake (B). Due to these findings, a bone marrow biopsy was performed, which showed adenocarcinoma that was strongly estrogen receptor-positive. The patient was diagnosed with breast cancer metastatic to bone and choroid with transscleral extension. After 6 months of treatment with an aromatase inhibitor (anastrozole 1 mg daily), visual acuity improved to 20/40 (D and E). The macular lesion regressed with concomitant resolution of the extrascleral component (F).

Lung metastasis responding to erlotinib.

G–L: A 49-year-old nonsmoking woman noted a left paracentral scotoma. A solitary creamy white slightly raised lesion without overlying subretinal fluid was seen in her left eye (G–I). Visual acuity was 20/20 in each eye. A systemic workup revealed a primary adenocarcinoma of the lung that was confirmed by biopsy. She received oral erlotinib (Tarceva), an epidermal growth factor receptor inhibitor protein kinase inhibitor. The lesion progressively regressed in thickness (J and K at 6 weeks) with complete flattening over 7 months, along with regression of her lung mass (L). Autofluorescence imaging showed punctate increased autofluorescence, even extending beyond the tumor dimensions, suggesting activity in the surrounding retinal pigment epithelium during the process of regression (K). She has maintained a vision of 20/20 with no further symptoms till date.

(A–F, from Margolis et al.[264] with permission.)

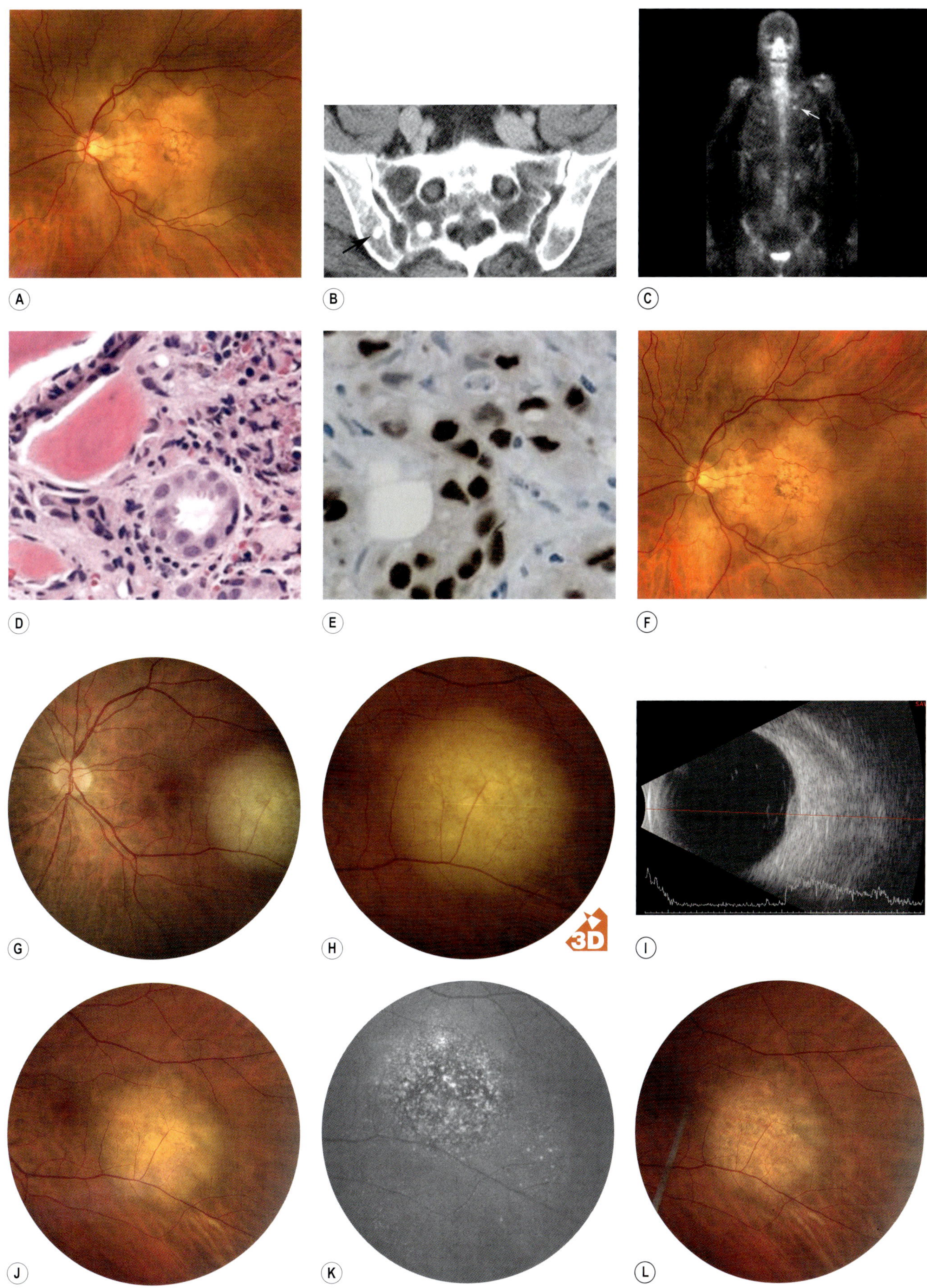
A
B
C
D
E
F
G
H
3D
I
J
K
L

Metastatic Sarcoma

Sarcomas rarely, if ever, metastasize to the eye, with only six previously known cases in the literature, one each from an alveolar soft-part sarcoma of the right lower extremity, congenital fibrosarcoma of the left lower extremity, osteogenic sarcoma of the left lower extremity, gastrointestinal stromal tumor, and Ewing sarcoma of the pelvis and rib. The patient with metastatic liposarcoma to the choroid, retina, and vitreous illustrated in Figure 14.32 mimicked an inflammatory granuloma, and was diagnosed based on cytology of her vitreous fluid obtained at surgery.

14.32 Liposarcoma metastasis to choroid, retina, and vitreous.

A–H: This 67-year-old African American woman presented with painless gradual decrease in vision in the left eye to 20/50 over 6 months. There were a few vitreous cells associated with a white fibrovascular pedunculated mass arising from the retina and hanging in the vitreous cavity (A). She was an avid gardener; a clinical diagnosis of possible *Toxocara* granuloma was made. Positive serum *Toxocara* titer and peripheral blood eosinophilia of 8% corroborated the clinical diagnosis. She was advised oral albendazole and tapering systemic steroids for a month. The patient did not fill her prescription and returned 5 months later with no appreciable change in symptoms. Her vision had decreased to 20/400, the white mass had increased in size, and the peduncle was more vascular (B and C). Ultrasound showed a solid mass with adjacent tractional retinal detachment (D). A diagnostic vitrectomy and a biopsy of the mass yielded only a small piece. The lesion was "rubbery" and difficult to cut into. Vitreous fluid was sent for cytology expecting to find eosinophils, but returned with presence of undifferentiated, anaplastic cells with markedly atypical nuclei and a high nuclear-to-cytoplasmic ratio (E). She gave a history of retroperitoneal sarcoma requiring a nephrectomy 10 years prior. Enucleation of the eye confirmed chorioretinovitreal metastasis from the liposarcoma. The tumor consisted of pleomorphic tumor cells and abundant collagen (F–H). The cells had a high nuclear-to-cytoplasmic ratio with hyperchromatic nuclei and prominent nucleoli (H). The choroid contained a chronic inflammatory cell infiltrate in the area surrounding the mass. The retina displayed outer-layer atrophy and gliosis overlying the base of the lesion. There was no evidence of scleral or optic nerve invasion.

(Reproduced with permission Mehta S, Agarwal A[265].

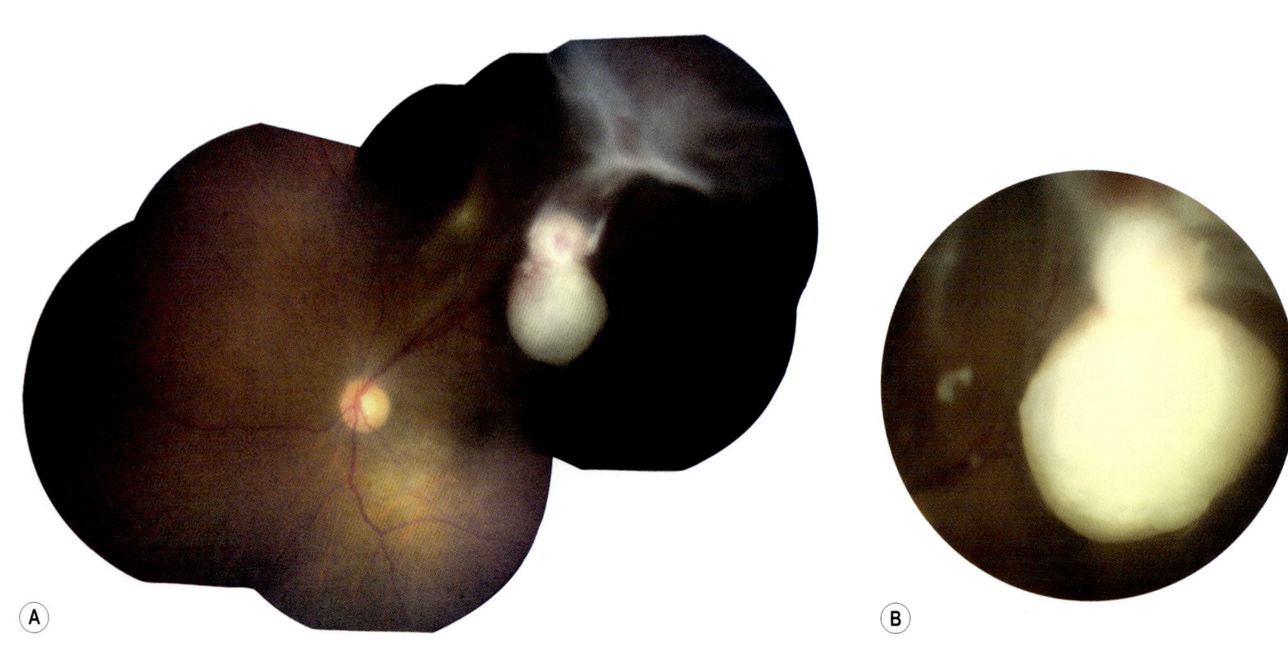

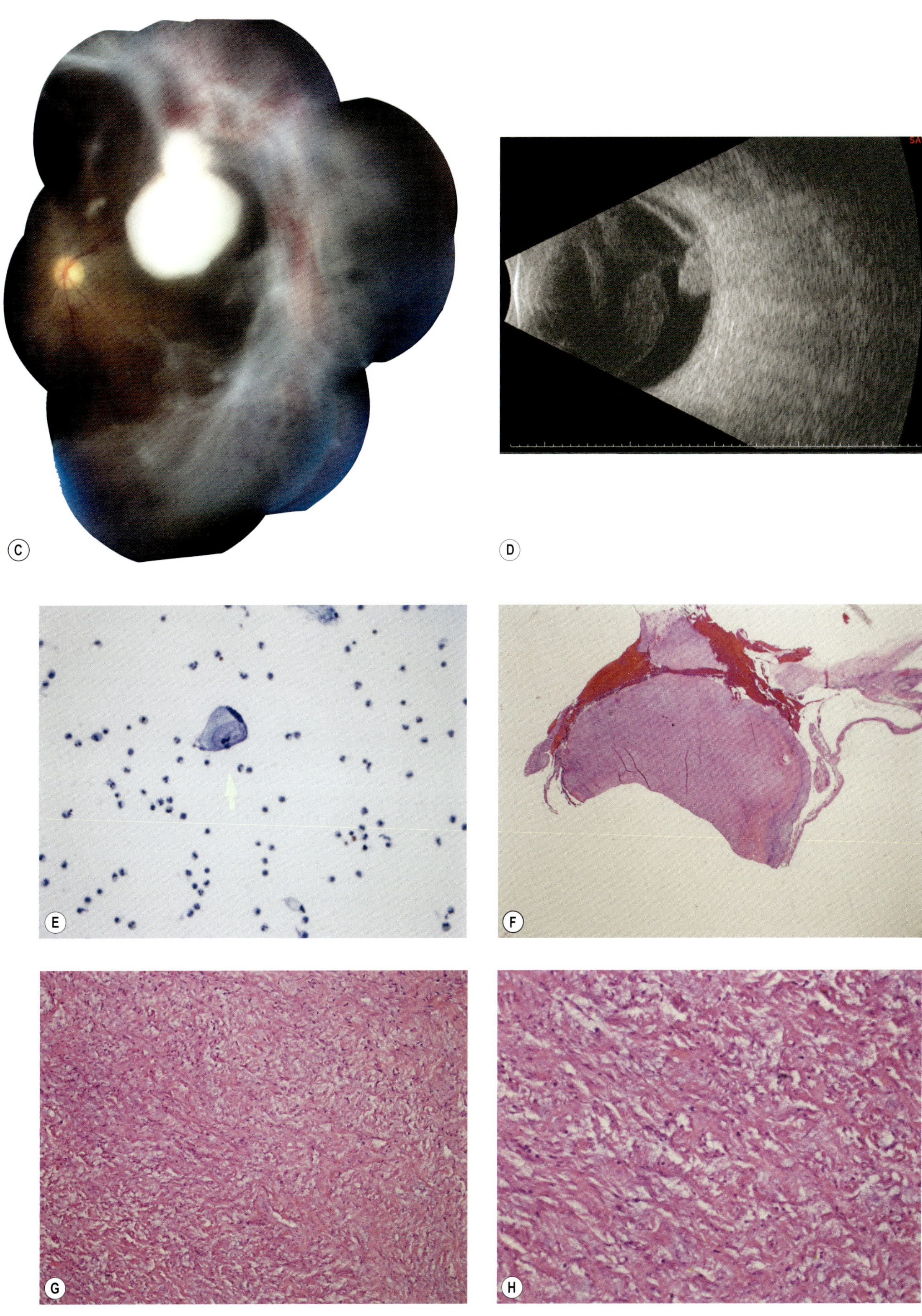
C
D
E
F
G
H

Leukemic Choroidopathy

Postmortem eyes of patients with leukemia demonstrate histopathologically a mild leukemic infiltration of the uveal tract, but most do not show ophthalmoscopic evidence of choroidal involvement during life. In some patients, however, the infiltrate becomes sufficiently intense to cause damage to the overlying RPE and serous retinal detachment.[266–269] Detachment of the RPE may also occur.[270] The clinical picture may be mistaken for central serous chorioretinopathy (Figure 14.33A), or in the case of more widespread retinal detachment, Harada's disease (Figures 14.33D and E and 14.34). Fluorescein angiography is useful in detecting the areas of RPE damage underlying the serous detachment (Figures 14.33B, C, and F and 14.34C). The sites of leakage of dye from the underlying choroid are usually multiple pinpoint areas similar to those seen in Harada's disease and other infiltrative diseases of the choroid. The choroidal infiltrate may occasionally produce a localized or diffuse choroidal tumor. Leukemic tumefactions of the choroid are more frequently associated with acute lymphatic leukemia.

Occasionally, striking leopard-spot changes may occur in the RPE in patients with extensive choroidal involvement with leukemia (Figures 14.33G–J and 14.34H, I, K, and L).[267,270,271] It is likely the extensive RPE necrosis and clumping of pigment that occurs in these cases is caused by the leukemic infiltration of the choriocapillaris, chemotherapy, or a combination of both.

The reader is referred to Chapter 13 for discussion of retinal and vitreous manifestations of leukemia and large cell lymphoma, which may cause a variety of fundoscopic pictures that may simulate metastatic carcinoma, multiple exudative RPE detachments, multifocal choroiditis, retinal artery occlusion, and acute retinitis.

14.33 Macular detachment caused by leukemic infiltration of choroid.

A–C: Choroidal tumor and serous detachment of the macula secondary to leukemia in a 59-year-old white woman who developed blurred vision and metamorphopsia in the left eye. Near the temporal margin of the left optic disc there was a mound-like elevation of the choroid and a shallow serous retinal detachment that extended into the macular region (black arrows, A). A small amount of subretinal blood (black and white arrow) was present. Angiography revealed multiple, small, pinpoint areas of diffusion of dye from the surface of the tumor as well as evidence of leakage of dye from the optic nerve capillaries into the subretinal exudate (B and C). The patient was admitted to the hospital, and bone marrow examination revealed acute myelomonocytic leukemia. The patient died soon afterward.

D–F: Bilateral bullous retinal detachment simulating Harada's disease in a 25-year-old patient with acute leukemia (D and E). His initial medical evaluation revealed leukopenia but no evidence of leukemia. Angiography revealed multiple focal areas of dye leakage from the choroid and later a flagstone pattern of staining beneath the retina (F). Although the cause of the peculiar placoid pattern of late fluorescein staining is unknown, its appearance suggests that there were multiple relatively flat areas of detachment of the retinal pigment epithelium (RPE), which in this patient may have been caused by leukemic infiltration from the choroid into the sub-RPE space. The retinal detachment disappeared after corticosteroid treatment. He died, however, about 6 weeks later, and autopsy revealed myelogenous leukemia.

G–J: Peculiar clumping of the pigment epithelium in a 6-year-old patient treated for acute lymphocytic leukemia. He had been treated with vincristine, prednisone, methotrexate, and cyclophosphamide. He developed alopecia and severe visual loss. The visual loss was more noticeable at night than during the day. He died 3 months later and histopathologic examination revealed multiple clumps of RPE cells (arrow, J) and mild leukemic infiltration of the choroid. It is unknown whether the changes in the RPE were primarily attributable to anoxia secondary to the anemia or leukemic infiltration of the choriocapillaris or to the toxic effects of drugs used in therapy. (G–J, from Clayman et al.[288] published with permission from The American Journal of Ophthalmology; Copyright by The Ophthalmic Publishing Co.)

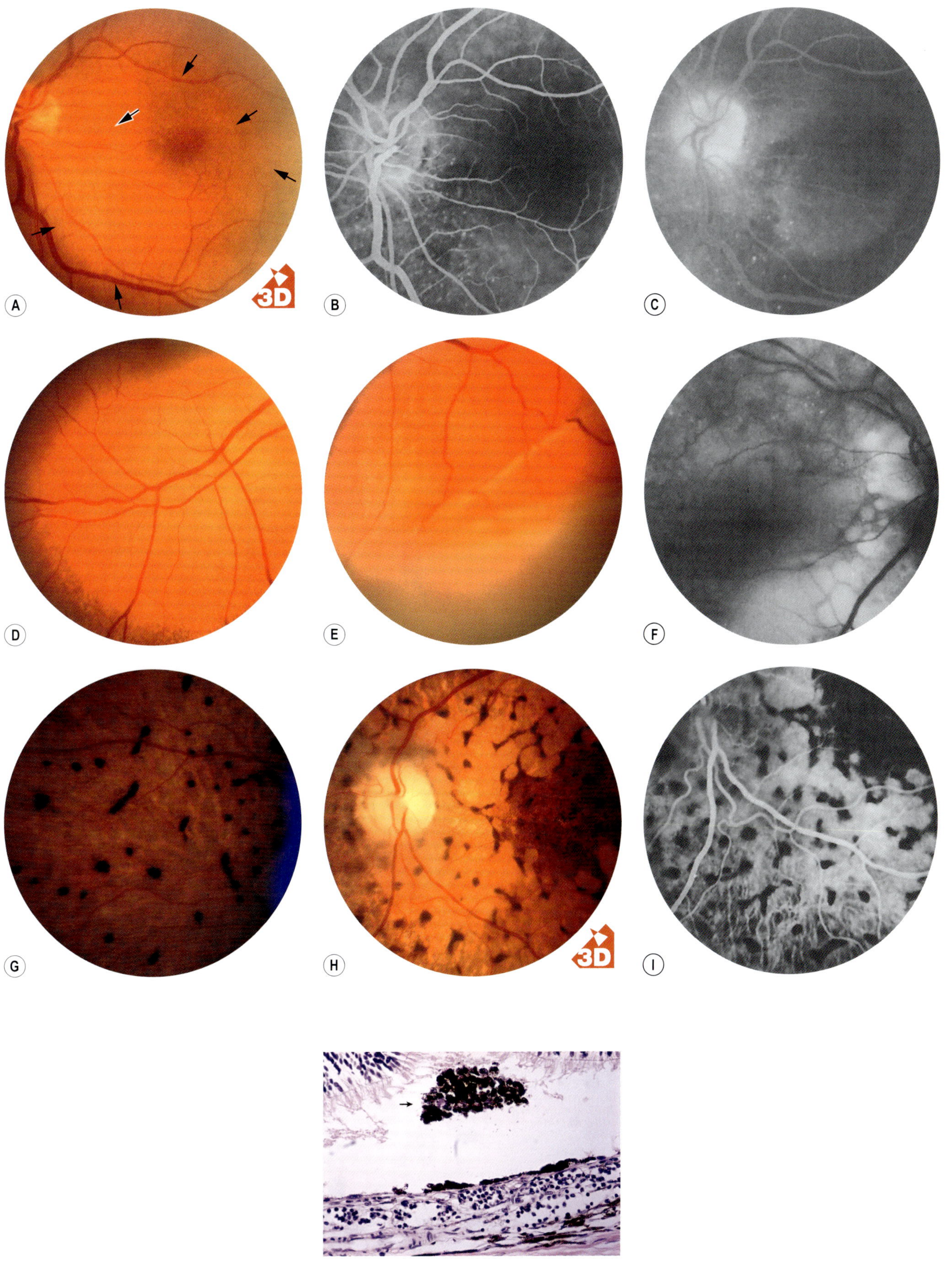
A
3D
B
C
D
E
F
G
H
3D
I
J

14.34 Acute myeloid leukemia with leukemia cutis simulating Vogt–Koyanagi–Harada disease.

A–L: A 55-year-old female on treatment for acute myeloid leukemia developed unilateral rapid loss of vision in her right eye over 6 days to count fingers. The right fundus showed serous retinal detachment involving the posterior pole (A and B). Fluorescein angiogram revealed several pinpoint hyperfluorescent areas that leaked dye into the subretinal space (C). Optical coherence tomography detected several septa within the serous elevation suggesting high fibrin content and in addition, small RPE detachments (D1 and D2 arrows) and at the same time she developed multiple fluctuant blisters over her body (E). She was neutropenic with a white count of 0.3. The skin lesions were diagnosed clinically as leukemia cutis and she was considered to be in end-stage disease. Biopsy of the lesions showed blasts infiltrating the skin (F and G). Short of not doing anything, she was started on oral prednisone 60 mg and given neupogen to improve her white count. Ten days later her vision had improved to 20/100, the exudative detachment had decreased (H and J), the skin lesions began to disappear, and her white count improved. A bone marrow biopsy done at this time showed no blasts. The retina showed mild pigmentation corresponding to the choroidal lobules (arrows, K), which increased over the next visit at 8 weeks. The fundus autofluorescence gradually increased, suggesting ingestion of protein from the subretinal fluid by the retinal pigment epithelial cells, giving it a leopard-spot appearance (I and L). All skin lesions disappeared by 8 weeks.

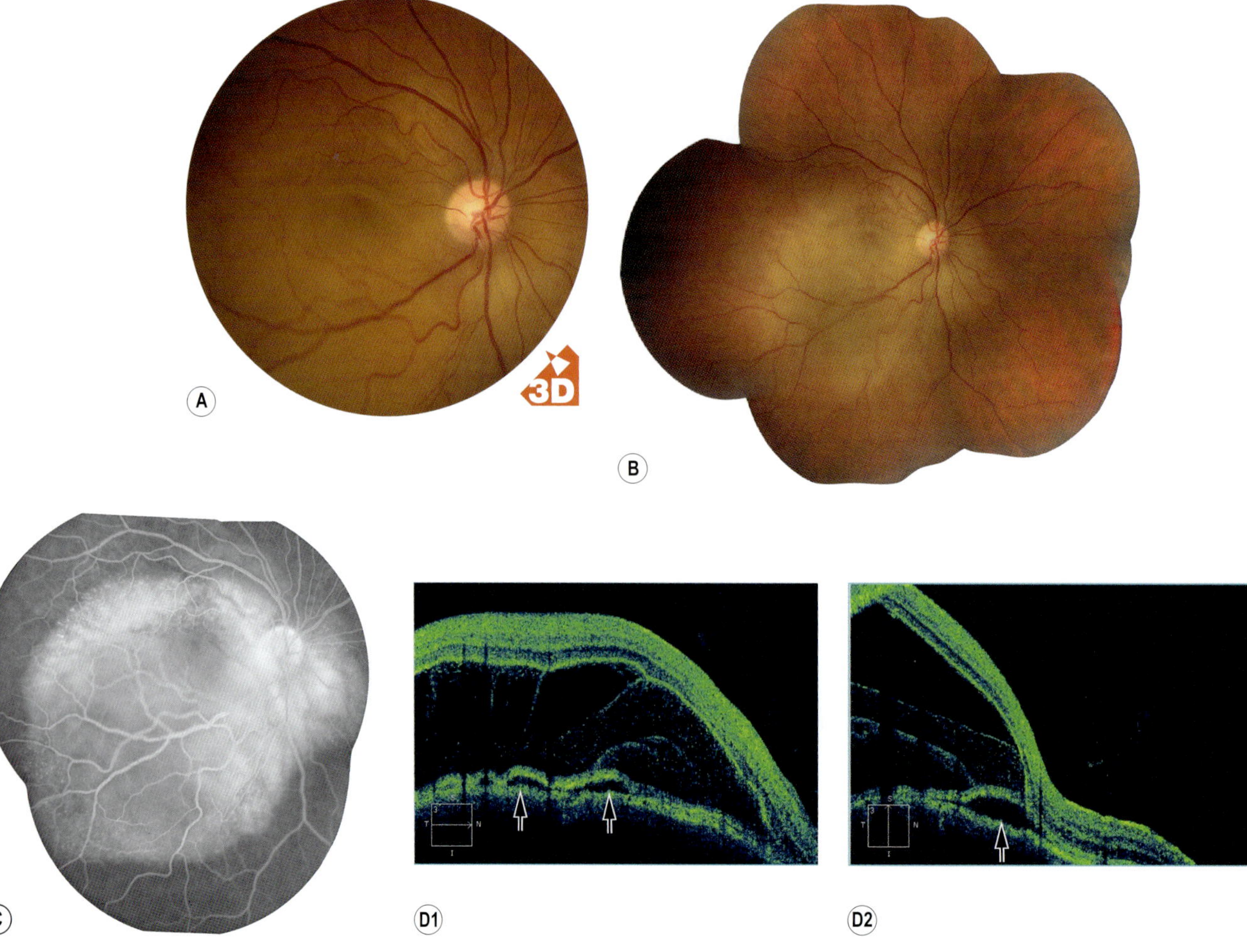

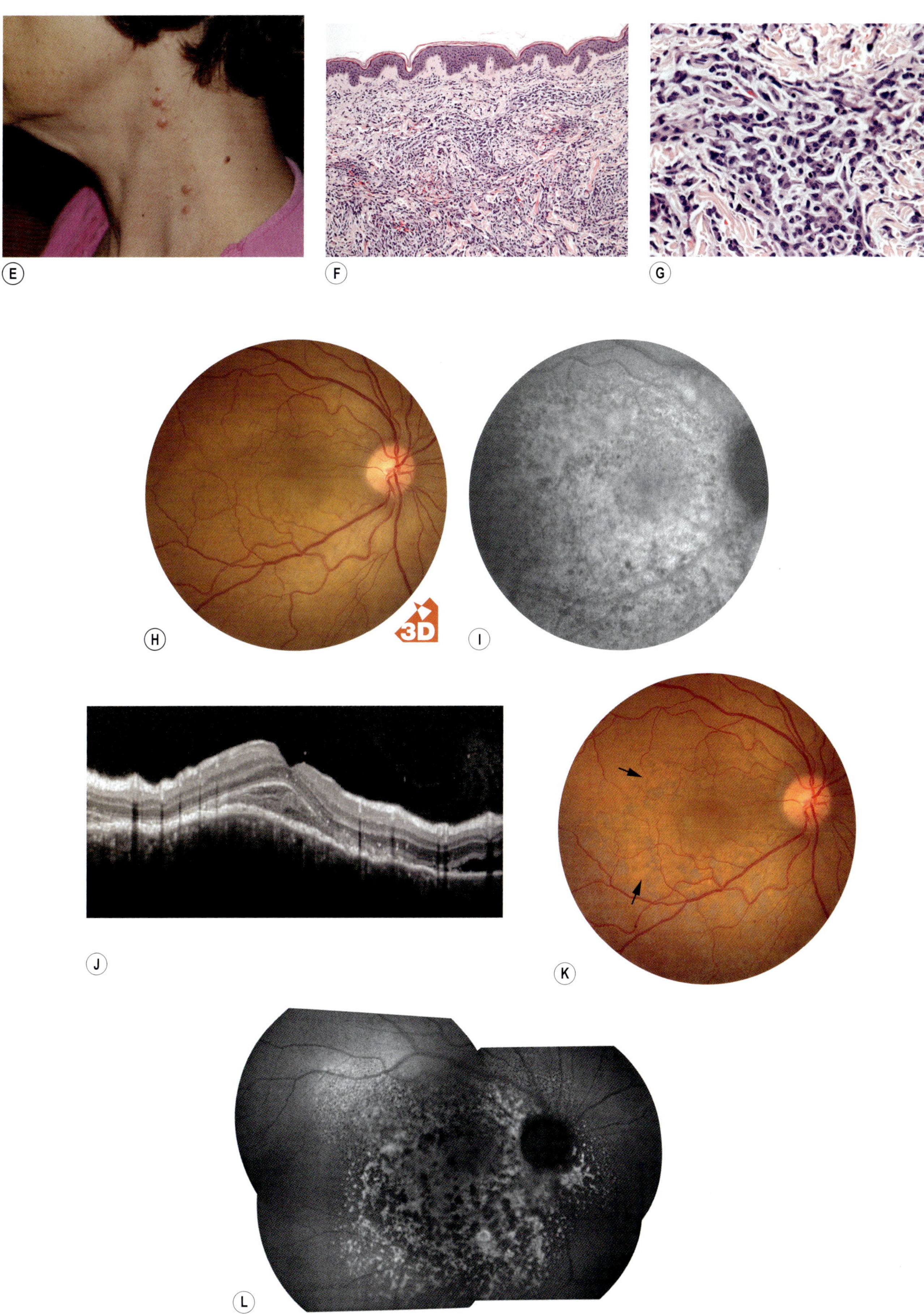
E
F
G
H
3D
I
J
K
L

Histiocytosis (Erdheim–Chester Disease)

Erdheim–Chester disease is a rare, widespread xanthogranulomatous infiltrative disease involving the bones and soft tissue. The exact nature of origin of the disease is poorly understood. Whether it initially manifests in the bone marrow and spreads, or originates in extramedullary sites similar to lymphomas is not known. Histologically, it is composed of sheets of foamy histiocytes associated with Touton-type giant cells, lymphocytes, and plasma cells that infiltrate the soft tissue. The disease affects bones, viscera such as liver, lungs, heart, and subcutaneous tissue. Bilateral symmetrical osteosclerosis of the metaphyseal and diaphyseal regions of long bones is considered a characteristic feature.[272] Ophthalmic manifestations are rare; the orbit and periocular tissue are the most frequent sites of involvement.[273-277] Choroidal infiltration (Figure 14.35) is extremely rare. These patients are diagnosed based on systemic association and biopsy from a suitable site.

Infiltration of the choroid with creamy yellow granulomas mimics a clinical appearance of sarcoidosis. Orbital involvement mimics thyroid orbitopathy and pseudotumor of the orbit. Treatment involves the use of systemic steroids and immunosuppressives.

14.35 Choroidal involvement in Erdheim–Chester disease (histiocytosis).

A–I: A 38-year-old Japanese American with a known diagnosis of Erdheim–Chester disease following a bone biopsy for persistent leg pain for 6 years presented with blurred vision in his left eye for 1 year. Multiple creamy placoid lesions associated with intraretinal lipid exudates were seen at the level of the choroid in both eyes (A and B). Optical coherence tomography of both eyes showed diffuse choroidal thickening (C and D). Fluorescein angiogram showed staining of the lesions bilaterally and a partly involuted choroidal neovascular membrane (CNVM) in the left eye (E–G, arrow). Further worsening of vision to 20/400 from serous fluid (H) over 3 months prompted an intraocular injection of bevacizumab in his left eye with further regression of the CNVM. He remained stable on systemic colchicine and oral steroids (I).

(Courtesy of Dr. Neal Attebara.)

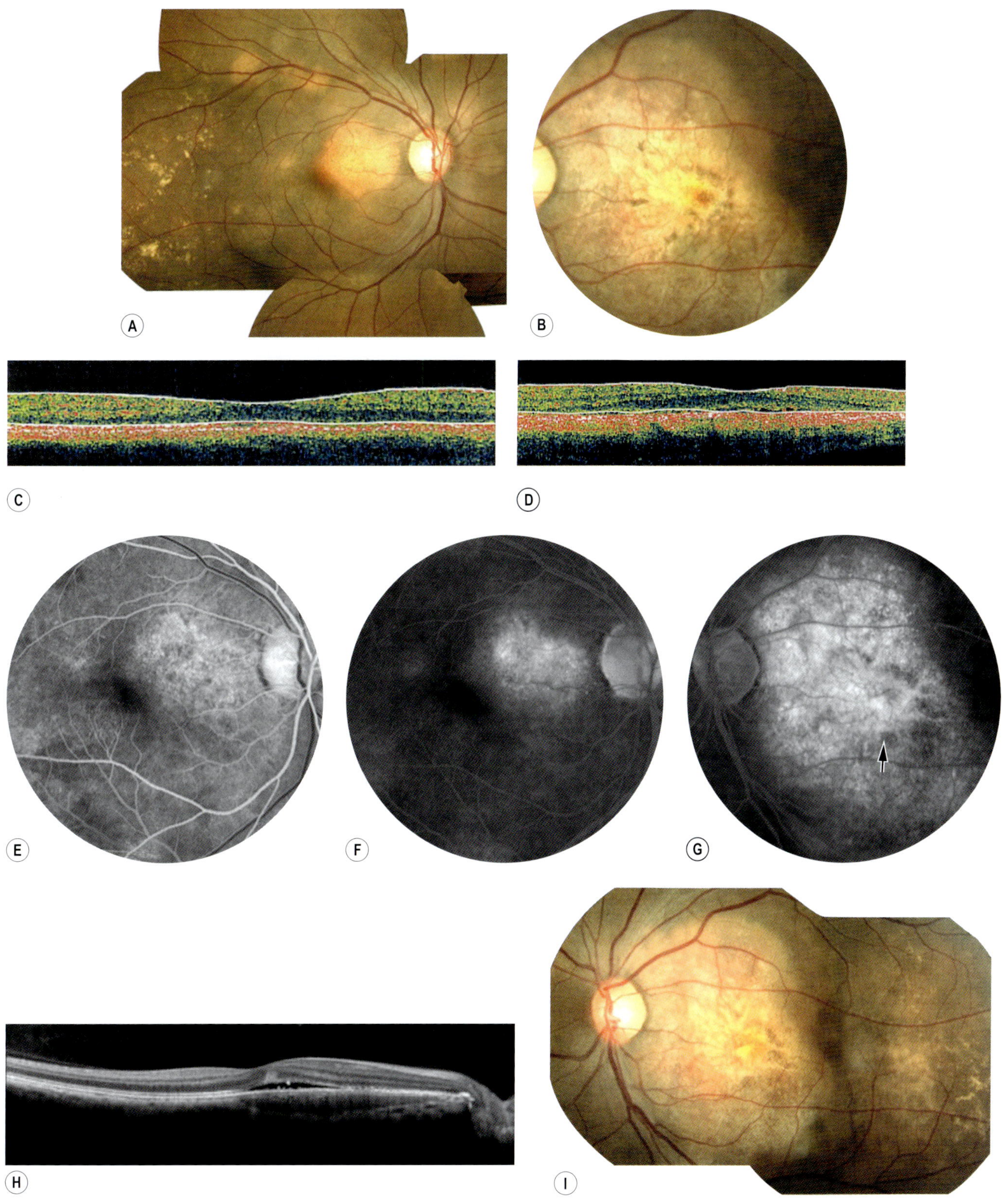
A
B
C
D
E
F
G
H
I

References

1. Zimmerman LE. Melanocytes, melanocytic nevi, and melanocytomas. Invest Ophthalmol 1965;4:11–41.
2. Gass JDM. Problems in the differential diagnosis of choroidal nevi and malignant melanomas. Am J Ophthalmol 1977;83:299–323.
3. Sumich P, Mitchell P, Wang JJ. Choroidal nevi in a white population: the Blue Mountains Eye Study. Arch Ophthalmol 1998;116:645–50.
4. Reese AB. Tumors of the eye. New York: Paul B. Hoeber; 1951. p. 277.
5. Singh AD, Kalyani P, Topham A. Estimating the risk of malignant transformation of a choroidal nevus. Ophthalmology 2005;112:1784–9.
6. Deutsch TA, Jampol LM. Large druse-like lesions on the surface of choroidal nevi. Ophthalmology 1985;92:73–6.
7. Erie JC, Robertson DM, Mieler WF. Presumed small choroidal melanomas with serous macular detachments with and without surface laser photocoagulation treatment. Am J Ophthalmol 1990;109:259–64.
8. Folk JC, Weingeist TA, Coonan P, et al. The treatment of serous macular detachment secondary to choroidal melanomas and nevi. Ophthalmology 1989;96:547–51.
9. Gass JDM. Differential diagnosis of intraocular tumors; a stereoscopic presentation. St. Louis: CV Mosby; 1974. pp. 59–111.
10. Gass JDM. Pathogenesis of disciform detachment of the neuroepithelium. VI. Disciform detachment secondary to heredodegenerative, neoplastic and traumatic lesions of the choroid. Am J Ophthalmol 1967;63:689–711.
11. Gonder JR, Augsburger JJ, McCarthy EF, et al. Visual loss associated with choroidal nevi. Ophthalmology 1982;89:961–5.
12. Pro M, Shields JA, Tomer TL. Serous detachment of the macula associated with presumed choroidal nevi. Arch Ophthalmol 1978;96:1374–7.
13. Slusher MM, Weaver RG. Presumed choroidal naevi and sensory retinal detachment. Br J Ophthalmol 1977;61:414–6.
14. Snip RC, Green WR. Jaegers KR. Choroidal nevus with subretinal pigment epithelial neovascular membrane and a positive P-32 test. Ophthalmic Surg 1978;9:35–42.
15. Waltman DD, Gitter KA, Yannuzzi L, et al. Choroidal neovascularization associated with choroidal nevi. Am J Ophthalmol 1978;85:704–10.
16. Gass JDM. Observation of suspected choroidal and ciliary body melanomas for evidence of growth prior to enucleation. Ophthalmology 1980;87:523–8.
17. Callanan DG, Lewis ML, Byrne SF, et al. Choroidal neovascularization associated with choroidal nevi. Arch Ophthalmol 1993;111:789–94.
18. Gass JDM. Fluorescein angiography; an aid in the differential diagnosis of intraocular tumors. Int Ophthalmol Clin 1972;12:85–120.
19. Singh AD, Belfort RN, Sayanagi K, et al. Fourier domain optical coherence tomographic and auto-fluorescence findings in indeterminate choroidal melanocytic lesions. Br J Ophthalmol 2010;94:474–8.
20. Gosbell AD, Barry WR, Favilla I, et al. Volume measurement of intraocular tumours by cross-sectional ultrasonographic scans. Aust NZ J Ophthalmol 1991;19:327–33.
21. Gass JDM. Comparison of uveal melanoma growth rates with mitotic index and mortality. Arch Ophthalmol 1985;103:924–31.
22. Gass JDM. Stereoscopic atlas of macular diseases; diagnosis and treatment, 2nd ed. St. Louis: CV Mosby; 1977. p. 40.
23. MacIlwaine IV WA, Anderson Jr B, Klintworth GK. Enlargement of histologically documented choroidal nevus. Am J Ophthalmol 1979;87:480–6.
24. Mansour AM, Zimmerman L, La Piana FG, et al. Clinicopathological findings in a growing optic nerve melanocytoma. Br J Ophthalmol 1989;73:410–5.
25. Daicker B. Der 46 jährige Verlauf eines maligne entarteten Aderhautnaevus mit vaskularisierten Flächendrusen. Klin Monastbl Augenheilkd 1991;198:442–4.
26. Rubin ML. Disciform lesion overlying melanocytoma simulating progression of choroidal melanoma. Trans Am Ophthalmol Soc 1976;74:282–94.
27. Gass JDM, Wilkinson CP. Follow-up study of presumed ocular histoplasmosis. Trans Am Acad Ophthalmol Otolaryngol 1972;76:672–94.
28. Mines JA, Freilich DB, Friedman AH, et al. Choroidal (subretinal) neovascularization secondary to choroidal nevus and successful treatment with argon laser photocoagulation; case reports and review of literature. Ophthalmologica 1985;190:210–8.
29. Butler P, Char DH, Zarbin M, et al. Natural history of indeterminate pigmented choroidal tumors. Ophthalmology 1994;101:710–6.
30. Parodi MB, Boscia F, Piermarocchi S, et al. Variable outcome of photodynamic therapy for choroidal neovascularization associated with choroidal nevus. Retina 2005;25:438–42.
31. Parodi MB. Transpupillary thermotherapy for subfoveal choroidal neovascularization associated with choroidal nevus. Am J Ophthalmol 2004;138:1074–5.
32. Lauritzen K, Augsburger JJ, Timmes J. Vitreous seeding associated with melanocytoma of the optic disc. Retina 1990;10:60–2.
33. Shields JA, Shields CL, Eagle Jr RC, et al. Malignant melanoma associated with melanocytoma of the optic disc. Ophthalmology 1990;97:225–30.
34. Shields JA, Demirci H, Mashayekhi A, et al. Melanocytoma of optic disc in 115 cases: the 2004 Samuel Johnson Memorial Lecture. Ophthalmology 2004;111:1739–46.
35. Kovoor TA, Bahl D, Singh AD, et al. Bilateral isolated choroidal melanocytosis. Br J Ophthalmol 2008;92(892):1008.
36. Singh AD, De Potter P, Fijal BA, et al. Lifetime prevalence of uveal melanoma in white patients with oculo(dermal) melanocytosis. Ophthalmology 1998;105:195–8.
37. Infante de German-Ribon R, Singh AD, Arevalo JF, et al. Choroidal melanoma with oculodermal melanocytosis in Hispanic patients. Am J Ophthalmol 1999;128:251–3.
38. Shields JA, Font RL, Eagle Jr RC, et al. Melanotic schwannoma of the choroid; immunohistochemistry and electron microscopic observations. Ophthalmology 1994;101: 843–9.
39. Huson S, Jones D, Beck L. Ophthalmic manifestations of neurofibromatosis. Br J Ophthalmol 1987;71:235–8.
40. Klein RM, Glassman L. Neurofibromatosis of the choroid. Am J Ophthalmol 1985;99:367–8.
41. Honavar SG, Singh AD, Shields CL, et al. Iris melanoma in a patient with neurofibromatosis. Surv Ophthalmol 2000;45:231–6.
42. Augsburger JJ, Schroeder RP, Territo C, et al. Clinical parameters predictive of enlargement of melanocytic choroidal lesions. Br J Ophthalmol 1989;73:911–7.
43. Anonymous. Factors predictive of growth and treatment of small choroidal melanoma: COMS Report No. 5. The Collaborative Ocular Melanoma Study Group. Arch Ophthalmol. 1997;115:1537–1544.
44. Heimler A, Fox JE, Hershey JE, et al. Sensorineural hearing loss, enamel hypoplasia, and nail abnormalities in sibs. Am J Med Genet 1991;39:192–5.
45. Singh AD, Schachat AP, Diener-West M, et al. Small choroidal melanoma. Ophthalmology 2008;115:2319-e3.
46. Shields CL, Demirci H, Materin MA, et al. Clinical factors in the identification of small choroidal melanoma. Can J Ophthalmol 2004;39:351–7.
47. Singh AD, Mokashi AA, Bena JF, et al. Small choroidal melanocytic lesions: features predictive of growth. Ophthalmology 2006;113:1032–9.
48. Mueller AJ, Freeman WR, Schaller UC, et al. Complex microcirculation patterns detected by confocal indocyanine green angiography predict time to growth of small choroidal melanocytic tumors: MuSIC Report II. Ophthalmology 2002;109:2207–14.
49. Singh AD, Bena JF, Mokashi AA, et al. Growth of small tumors. Ophthalmology 2006;113(1061):e1–4.
50. Kupfer C. Discussion: risk factors for growth and metastasis of small choroidal melanocytic lesions. Trans Am Ophthalmol Soc 1995;93:277–8.
51. Murray TG, Sobrin L. The case for observational management of suspected small choroidal melanoma. Arch Ophthalmol 2006;124:1342–4.
52. Shields JA. Treating some small melanocytic choroidal lesions without waiting for growth. Arch Ophthalmol 2006;124:1344–6.
53. Canny CLB, Shields JA, Kay ML. Clinically stationary choroidal melanoma with extraocular extension. Arch Ophthalmol 1978;96:436–9.
54. Friberg TR, Fineberg E, McQuaig S. Extremely rapid growth of a primary choroidal melanoma. Arch Ophthalmol 1983;101:1375–7.
55. Shields CL, Shields JA, Eagle Jr RC, et al. Uveal melanoma and pregnancy; a report of 16 cases. Ophthalmology 1991;98:1667–73.
56. Chong CA, Gregor RJ, Augsburger JJ, et al. Spontaneous regression of choroidal melanoma over 8 years. Retina 1989;9:136–8.
57. Lambert SR, Char DH, Howes Jr E, et al. Spontaneous regression of a choroidal melanoma. Arch Ophthalmol 1986;104:732–4.
58. Williams DF, Mieler WF, Lewandowski M. Resolution of an apparent choroidal melanoma. Retina 1989;9:131–5.
59. Dunn WJ, Lambert HM, Kincaid MC, et al. Choroidal malignant melanoma with early vitreous seeding. Retina 1988;8:188–92.
60. Pavan PR, Margo CE, Drucker M. Malignant melanoma of the choroid with vitreal seeding. Arch Ophthalmol 1989;107:130.
61. Yap E-Y, Robertson DM, Buettner H. Scleritis as an initial manifestation of choroidal malignant melanoma. Ophthalmology 1992;99:1693–7.
62. Augsburger JJ. Fine needle aspiration biopsy of suspected metastatic cancers to the posterior uvea. Trans Am Ophthalmol Soc 1988;86:499–560.
63. Char DH, Miller TR, Crawford JB. Cytopathologic diagnosis of benign lesions simulating choroidal melanomas. Am J Ophthalmol 1991;112:70–5.
64. Fastenberg DM, Finger PT, Chess Q, et al. Vitrectomy retinotomy aspiration biopsy of choroidal tumors. Am J Ophthalmol 1990;110:361–5.
65. Folberg R, Augsburger JJ, Gamel JW, et al. Fine-needle aspirates of uveal melanomas and prognosis. Am J Ophthalmol 1985;100:654–7.
66. Shields JA, Shields CL, Ehya H, et al. Fine-needle aspiration biopsy of suspected intraocular tumors. Ophthalmology 1993;100:1677–84.
67. Sassani JW, Blankenship G. Disciform choroidal melanoma. Retina 1993;14:177–80.
68. Brownstein S, Orton R, Jackson WB. Cystoid macular edema with equatorial choroidal melanoma. Arch Ophthalmol 1978;96:2105–7.
69. Gass JDM, Anderson DR, Davis EB. A clinical, fluorescein angiographic, and electron microscopic correlation of cystoid macular edema. Am J Ophthalmol 1985;100:82–6.
70. Osher RH, Abrams GW, Yarian D, et al. Varix of the vortex ampulla. Am J Ophthalmol 1981;92:653–60.
71. Gass JDM. Drusen and disciform macular detachment and degeneration. Trans Am Ophthalmol Soc 1972;70:409–36.
72. Chang M, Zimmerman LE, McLean I. The persisting pseudomelanoma problem. Arch Ophthalmol 1984;102:726–7.
73. Buettner H. Varix of the vortex ampulla simulating a choroidal melanoma. Am J Ophthalmol 1990;109:607–8.
74. Augsburger JJ, Coats TD, Lauritzen K. Localized suprachoroidal hematomas; ophthalmoscopic features, fluorescein angiography, and clinical course. Arch Ophthalmol. 1990;108:968–72.
75. Augsburger JJ, Golden MI, Shields JA. Fluorescein angiography of choroidal malignant melanomas with retinal invasion. Retina 1984;4:232–41.
76. Farah ME, Byrne SF, Hughes JR. Standardized echography in uveal melanomas with scleral or extraocular extension. Arch Ophthalmol 1984;102:1482–5.
77. Davidorf FH, Chambers RB, Gresak P. False-positive magnetic resonance imaging of a metastatic carcinoma simulating a malignant melanoma. Ann Ophthalmol 1992;24:391–4.
78. Shammas HF, Burton TC, Weingeist TA. False-positive results with the radioactive phosphorus test. Arch Ophthalmol 1977;95:2190–2.
79. Zakov ZN, Smith TR, Albert DM. False-positive ^{32}P uptake tests. Arch Ophthalmol 1978;96:2240–3.

80. Augsburger JJ, Peyster RG, Markoe AM, et al. Computed tomography of posterior uveal melanomas. Arch Ophthalmol 1987;105:1512–6.
81. Bloom PA, Ferris JD, Laidlaw DA, et al. Magnetic resonance imaging; diverse appearances of uveal malignant melanomas. Arch Ophthalmol 1992;110:1105–11.
82. Lieb WE, Shields JA, Cohen SM, et al. Color Doppler imaging in the management of intraocular tumors. Ophthalmology 1990;97:1660–4.
83. Scheidler J, Leinsinger G, Kirsch C-M, et al. Immunoimaging of choroidal melanoma: assessment of its diagnostic accuracy and limitations in 101 cases. Br J Ophthalmol 1992;76:457–60.
84. Collaborative Ocular Melanoma Study Group. Accuracy of diagnosis of choroidal melanomas in the Collaborative Ocular Melanoma Study; COMS report no. 1. Arch Ophthalmol 1990;108:1268–73.
85. Donoso LA, Augsburger JJ, Shields JA, et al. Metastatic uveal melanoma; correlation between survival time and cytomorphometry of primary tumors. Arch Ophthalmol 1986; 104:76–8.
86. Gamel JW, McLean IW. Computerized histopathologic assessment of malignant potential. II. A practical method for predicting survival following enucleation for uveal melanoma. Cancer 1983;52:1032–8.
87. McLean IW, Foster WD, Zimmerman LE. Prognostic factors in small malignant melanomas of choroid and ciliary body. Arch Ophthalmol 1977;95:48–58.
88. McLean IW, Foster WD, Zimmerman LE. Uveal melanoma: location, size, cell type, and enucleation as risk factors in metastasis. Hum Pathol 1982;13:123–32.
89. McLean IW, Foster WD, Zimmerman LE, et al. Modifications of Callender's classification of uveal melanoma at the Armed Forces Institute of Pathology. Am J Ophthalmol 1983;96:502–9.
90. McLean IW, Zimmerman LE, Evans RM. Reappraisal of Callender's spindle A type of malignant melanoma of choroid and ciliary body. Am J Ophthalmol 1978;86:557–64.
91. Damato BE. Management of patients with uveal melanoma. In: Singh AD, Damato BE, Pe'er J, editors. Clinical ophthalmic oncology. Philadelphia: Saunders-Elsevier; 2007. p. 226–31.
92. Singh AD, Topham A. Survival rates with uveal melanoma in the United States: 1973–1997. Ophthalmology 2003;110:962–5.
93. Turell ME, Saunthararajah Y, Triozzi PL, et al. Recent advances in prognostication for uveal melanoma. Intl Ophthalmol 2011. [in press.]
94. Bornfeld N, Prescher G, Horsthemke B, et al. Monosomy-3 is correlated with poor-risk factors in uveal malignant-melanoma. Invest Ophth Vis Sci 1995;36:S393.
95. Prescher G, Bornfeld N, Hirche H, et al. Prognostic implications of monosomy 3 in uveal melanoma. Lancet 1996;347:1222–5.
96. Patel KA, Edmondson ND, Talbot F, et al. Prediction of prognosis in patients with uveal melanoma using fluorescence in situ hybridisation. Br J Ophthalmol 2001;85:1440–4.
97. Tschentscher F, Husing J, Holter T, et al. Tumor classification based on gene expression profiling shows that uveal melanomas with and without monosomy 3 represent two distinct entities. Cancer Res 2003;63:2578–84.
98. Onken MD, Worley LA, Tuscan MD, et al. An accurate, clinically feasible multi-gene expression assay for predicting metastasis in uveal melanoma. J Mol Diagn 2010;12:461–8.
99. Midena E, Bonaldi L, Parrozzani R, et al. In vivo detection of monosomy 3 in eyes with medium-sized uveal melanoma using transscleral fine needle aspiration biopsy. Eur J Ophthalmol 2006;16:422–5.
100. Damato B, Duke C, Coupland SE, et al. Cytogenetics of uveal melanoma: a 7-year clinical experience. Ophthalmology 2007;114:1925–31.
101. http://clinicaltrials.gov/ct2/show/NCT01100528?term = uveal + melanoma + dacarbazine&rank = 1, #3095). 2010.
102. Barr CC, Zimmerman LE, Curtin VT, et al. Bilateral diffuse melanocytic uveal tumors associated with systemic malignant neoplasms; a recently recognized syndrome. Arch Ophthalmol 1982;100:249–55.
103. Borruat FX, Othenin-Girard P, Uffer S, et al. Natural history of diffuse uveal melanocytic proliferation; case report. Ophthalmology 1992;99:1698–704.
104. de Wolff-Rouendall D. Bilateral diffuse benign melanocytic tumours of the uveal tract; a clinicopathological study. Int Ophthalmol 1985;7:149–60.
105. Filipic M, Ambler JS. Bilateral diffuse melanocytic uveal tumours associated with systemic malignant neoplasm. Aust NZ J Ophthalmol 1986;14:293–9.
106. Gass JDM. Stereoscopic atlas of macular diseases; diagnosis and treatment, 3rd ed. St. Louis: CV Mosby; 1987. p. 276–7.
107. Gass JDM, Gieser RG, Wilkinson CT, et al. Bilateral diffuse uveal melanocytic proliferation in patients with occult carcinoma. Arch Ophthalmol 1990;108:527–33.
108. Gass JDM, Glatzer RJ. Acquired pigmentation simulating Peutz–Jeghers syndrome: initial manifestation of diffuse uveal melanocytic proliferation. Br J Ophthalmol 1991;75:693–5.
109. Leys AM, Dierick HG, Sciot RM. Early lesions of bilateral diffuse melanocytic proliferation. Arch Ophthalmol 1991;109:1590–4.
110. Machemer R. Zur Pathogenese des flächenhaften malignen Melanoms. Klin Monatsbl Augenheilkd 1966;148:641–52.
111. Margo CE, Pavan PR, Gendelman D, et al. Bilateral melanocytic uveal tumors associated with systemic non-ocular malignancy; malignant melanomas or benign paraneoplastic syndrome? Retina 1987;7:137–41.
112. Mullaney J, Mooney D, O'Connor M, et al. Bilateral ovarian carcinoma with bilateral melanoma. Br J Ophthalmol 1984;68:261–7.
113. Prause JU, Jensen OA, Eisgart F, et al. Bilateral diffuse malignant melanoma of the uvea associated with large cell carcinoma, giant cell type, of the lung; case report of a newly described syndrome. Ophthalmologica 1984;189:221–8.
114. Prusiner PE, Butler A, Yavitz EQ, et al. Metastatic adenocarcinoma presenting as bilateral blindness. Ann Ophthalmol 1983;15:653–6.
115. Rohrbach JM, Roggendorf W, Thanos S, et al. Simultaneous bilateral diffuse melanocytic uveal hyperplasia. Am J Ophthalmol 1990;110:49–56.
116. Ryll DL, Campbell RJ, Robertson DM, et al. Pseudometastatic lesions of the choroid. Ophthalmology 1980;87:1181–6.
117. Chahud F, Young RH, Remulla JF, et al. Bilateral diffuse uveal melanocytic proliferation associated with extraocular cancers: review of a process particularly associated with gynecologic cancers. Am J Surg Pathol 2001;25:212–8.
118. Klingele TG, Burde RM, Rappazzo JA, et al. Paraneoplastic retinopathy. J Clin Neuro-Ophthalmol 1984;4:239–45.
119. Sawyer RA, Selhorst JB, Zimmerman LE, et al. Blindness caused by photoreceptor degeneration as a remote effect of cancer. Am J Ophthalmol 1976;81:606–13.
120. Singh AD, Rundle PA, Slater DN, et al. Uveal and cutaneous involvement in paraneoplastic melanocytic proliferation. Arch Ophthalmol 2003;121:1637–40.
121. Tsukahara S, Wakui K, Ohzeki S. Simultaneous bilateral primary diffuse malignant melanoma: case report with pathological examination. Br J Ophthalmol 1986;70:33–8.
122. Brownstein S, Little JM. Ocular neurofibromatosis. Ophthalmology 1983;90:1595–9.
123. Anand R, Augsburger JJ, Shields JA. Circumscribed choroidal hemangiomas. Arch Ophthalmol. 1989;107:1338–42.
124. Augsburger JJ, Shields JA, Moffat KP. Circumscribed choroidal hemangiomas: long-term visual prognosis. Retina 1981;1:56–61.
125. Jarrett II WH, Hagler WS, Larose JH, et al. Clinical experience with presumed hemangioma of the choroid: radioactive phosphorus uptake studies as an aid in differential diagnosis. Trans Am Acad Ophthalmol Otolaryngol 1976;81:OP862–OP870.
126. Jones IS, Cleasby GW. Hemangioma of the choroid: a clinicopathologic analysis. Am J Ophthalmol 1959;48:612–28.
127. Pitta CG, Shingleton BJ, Harris PJ, et al. Solitary choroidal hemangioma. Am J Ophthalmol 1979;88:698–701.
128. Reese AB. Tumors of the eye, 2nd ed. New York: Harper & Row; 1963. p. 269.
129. Sanborn GE, Augsburger JJ, Shields JA. Treatment of circumscribed choroidal hemangiomas. Ophthalmology 1982;89:1374–80.
130. Zografos L, Gailloud C, Bercher L. Le traitement des hémangiomes de la choroïde par radiothérapie. J Fr Ophtalmol 1989;12:797–807.
131. Lindsey PS, Shields JA, Goldberg RE, et al. Bilateral choroidal hemangiomas and facial nevus flammeus. Retina 1981;1:88–95.
132. MacLean AL, Maumenee AE. Hemangioma of the choroid. Am J Ophthalmol 1960;50:3–11.
133. Shields JA, Stephens RF, Eagle Jr RC, et al. Progressive enlargement of a circumscribed choroidal hemangioma. Arch Ophthalmol 1992;110:1276–8.
134. Shields CL, Honavar SG, Shields JA, et al. Circumscribed choroidal hemangioma: clinical manifestations and factors predictive of visual outcome in 200 consecutive cases. Ophthalmology 2001;108:2237–48.
135. Ruby AJ, Jampol LM, Goldberg MF, et al. Choroidal neovascularization associated with choroidal hemangiomas. Arch Ophthalmol 1992;110:658–61.
136. Leys AM, Bonnet S. Case report: associated retinal neovascularization and choroidal hemangioma. Retina 1993;13:22–5.
137. Gass JDM. Photocoagulation of macular lesions. Trans Am Acad Ophthalmol Otolaryngol 1971;75:580–608.
138. Norton EWD, Gutman F. Fluorescein angiography and hemangiomas of the choroid. Arch Ophthalmol 1967;78:121–5.
139. Smith JL, David NJ, Hart LM, et al. Hemangioma of the choroid; fluorescein photography and photocoagulation. Arch Ophthalmol 1963;69:51–4.
140. Arevalo JF, Shields CL, Shields JA, et al. Circumscribed choroidal hemangioma: characteristic features with indocyanine green videoangiography. Ophthalmology 2000;107:344–50.
141. Witschel H, Font RL. Hemangioma of the choroid: a clinicopathologic study of 71 cases and a review of the literature. Surv Ophthalmol 1976;20:415–31.
142. Cox Jr. MS. Discussion of the two preceding papers [on ^{32}P uptake test]. Trans Am Acad Ophthalmol Otolaryngol 1975;79:OP307–OP309.
143. Ossoinig KC, Blodi FC. Preoperative differential diagnosis of tumors with echography. III. Diagnosis of intraocular tumors. In: Blodi FC, editor. Current concepts in ophthalmology. St. Louis: CV Mosby; 1974. p. 296–313.
144. Madreperla SA. Choroidal hemangioma treated with photodynamic therapy using verteporfin. Arch Ophthalmol 2001;119:1606–10.
145. Robertson DM. Photodynamic therapy for choroidal hemangioma associated with serous retinal detachment. Arch Ophthalmol 2002;120:1155–61.
146. Schmidt-Erfurth UM, Michels S, Kusserow C, et al. Photodynamic therapy for symptomatic choroidal hemangioma: visual and anatomic results. Ophthalmology 2002;109:2284–94.
147. Singh AD, Kaiser PK, Sears JE, et al. Photodynamic therapy of circumscribed choroidal haemangioma. Br J Ophthalmol 2004;88:1414–8.
148. Michels S, Michels R, Simader C, et al. Verteporfin therapy for choroidal hemangioma: a long-term follow-up. Retina 2005;25:697–703.
149. Greber H, Alberti W, Scherer E. Strahlentherapie der Aderhauthämangiome. Fortschr Ophthalmol 1985;82:450–2.
150. Humphrey WT. Choroidal hemangioma: response to cryotherapy. Ann Ophthalmol 1979;11: 100–4.
151. Scott TA, Augsburger JJ, Brady LW, et al. Low dose ocular irradiation for diffuse choroidal hemangiomas associated with bullous nonrhegmatogenous retinal detachment. Retina 1991;11:389–93.
152. Pitta C, Bergen R, Littwin S. Spontaneous regression of a choroidal hemangioma following pregnancy. Ann Ophthalmol 1979;11:772–4.
153. Papale JJ, Frederick AR, Albert DM. Intraocular hemangiopericytoma. Arch Ophthalmol 1983;101:1409–11.
154. Sullivan TJ, Clarke MP, Morin JD. The ocular manifestations of the Sturge–Weber syndrome. J Pediatr Ophthalmol Strabismus 1992;29:349–56.
155. Susac JO, Smith JL, Scelfo RJ. The "tomato catsup" fundus in Sturge–Weber syndrome. Arch Ophthalmol 1974;92:69–70.
156. Singh AD, Rundle PA, Vardy SJ, et al. Photodynamic therapy of choroidal haemangioma associated with Sturge–Weber syndrome. Eye (Lond) 2005;19:365–7.

157. Grant LW, Anderson C, Macklis RM, et al. Low dose irradiation for diffuse choroidal hemangioma. Ophthalmic Genet 2008;29:186–8.
158. Naidoff MA, Kenyon KR, Green WR. Iris hemangioma and abnormal retinal vasculature in a case of diffuse congenital hemangiomatosis. Am J Ophthalmol 1971;72:633–44.
159. Ruttum MS, Mittelman D, Singh P. Iris hemangiomas in infants with periorbital capillary hemangiomas. J Pediatr Ophthalmol Strabismus 1993;30:331–3.
160. Amalric P. Osteomes choroïdiens. Bull Soc Ophtalmol Fr 1980;80:47–50.
161. Augsburger JJ, Shields JA, Rife CJ. Bilateral choroidal osteoma after nine years. Can J Ophthalmol 1979;14:281–4.
162. Avila MP, El-Markabi H, Azzolini C, et al. Bilateral choroidal osteoma with subretinal neovascularization. Ann Ophthalmol 1984;16:381–5.
163. Aylward, GW, Chang, TS, et al. (1998). A long-term follow-up of choroidal osteoma. Arch Ophthalmol 116(10): 1337–1341.
164. Baarsma GS, Craandijk A. Osteoma of the choroid. Doc Ophthalmol 1981;50:205–12.
165. Baum MD, Pilkerton AR, Berler DK, et al. Choroidal osteoma. Ann Ophthalmol 1979;11: 1849–51.
166. Bloom PA, Ferris JD, Laidlaw A, et al. Appearances of choroidal osteomas with diagnostic imaging. Br J Radiol 1992;65:845–8.
167. Buettner H. Spontaneous involution of a choroidal osteoma. Arch Ophthalmol 1990;108:1517–8.
168. Burke JF, Brockhurst RJ. Argon laser photocoagulation of subretinal neovascular membrane associated with osteoma of the choroid. Retina 1983;3:304–7.
169. Cennamo G, Iaccarino G, de Crecchio G, et al. Choroidal osteoma (osseous choristoma): an atypical case. Br J Ophthalmol 1990;74:700–1.
170. Coston TO, Wilkinson CP. Choroidal osteoma. Am J Ophthalmol 1978;86:368–72.
171. Cunha SL. Osseous choristoma of the choroid; a familial disease. Arch Ophthalmol 1984;102:1052–4.
172. De Potter P, Shields JA, Shields CL, et al. Magnetic resonance imaging in choroidal osteoma. Retina 1991;11:221–3.
173. Eting E, Savir H. An atypical fulminant course of choroidal osteoma in two siblings. Am J Ophthalmol 1992;113:52–5.
174. Fava GE, Brown GC, Shields JA, et al. Choroidal osteoma in a 6-year-old child. J Pediatr Ophthalmol Strabismus 1980;17:203–5.
175. Gass JDM. New observations concerning choroidal osteomas. Int Ophthalmol 1979;1:71–84.
176. Gass JDM, Guerry RK, Jack RL, et al. Choroidal osteoma. Arch Ophthalmol 1978;96:428–35.
177. Grand MG, Burgess DB, Singerman LJ, et al. Choroidal osteoma; treatment of associated subretinal neovascular membranes. Retina 1984;4:84–9.
178. Hoffman ME, Sorr EM. Photocoagulation of subretinal neovascularization associated with choroidal osteoma. Arch Ophthalmol 1987;105:998–9.
179. Jackson WE, Freed S. Unilateral osseous choristoma of the choroid. Ann Ophthalmol 1984;16:134–6.
180. Joffe L, Shields JA, Fitzgerald JR. Osseous choristoma of the choroid. Arch Ophthalmol 1978;96:1809–12.
181. Katz RS. Gass JDM. Multiple choroidal osteomas developing in association with recurrent orbital inflammatory pseudotumor. Arch Ophthalmol 1983;101:1724–7.
182. Kayazawa F, Shimamoto S. Choroidal osteoma: two cases in Japanese women. Ann Ophthalmol 1981;13:1053–6.
183. Kelinske M, Weinstein GW. Bilateral choroidal osteomas. Am J Ophthalmol 1981;92:676–80.
184. Kline LB, Skalka HW, Davidson JD, et al. Bilateral choroidal osteomas associated with fatal systemic illness. Am J Ophthalmol 1982;93:192–7.
185. Laibovitz RA. An unusual cause of intraocular calcification: choroidal osteoma. Ann Ophthalmol 1979;11:1077–9.
186. O'Connor PS. Choroidal osteoma: a new clinicopathologic syndrome. In: Smith JL, editor. Neuro-ophthalmology focus 1980. New York: Masson Publishing; 1979. p. 31–5.
187. Shields CL, Shields JA, Augsburger JJ. Choroidal osteoma. Surv Ophthalmol 1988;33:17–27.
188. Shields JA. Diagnosis and management of intraocular tumors. St. Louis: CV Mosby; 1983. p. 373.
189. Teich SA, Walsh JB. Choroidal osteoma. Ophthalmology 1981;88:696–8.
190. Trimble SN, Schatz H. Choroidal osteoma after intraocular inflammation. Am J Ophthalmol 1983;96:759–64.
191. Trimble SN, Schatz H. Decalcification of a choroidal osteoma. Br J Ophthalmol 1991;75:61–3.
192. Trimble SN, Schatz H, Schneider GB. Spontaneous decalcification of a choroidal osteoma. Ophthalmology 1988;95:631–4.
193. Tsukahara I, Hayashi M. Osseous choristoma of the choroid. Jpn J Ophthalmol 1980;24:90–5.
194. Wilkes SR, Campbell RJ, Waller RR. Ocular malformation in association with ipsilateral facial nevus of Jadassohn. Am J Ophthalmol 1981;92:344–52.
195. Williams AT, Font RL, Van Dyk HJ, et al. Osseous choristoma of the choroid simulating a choroidal melanoma; association with a positive ^{32}P test. Arch Ophthalmol 1978;96:1874–7.
196. Morrison DL, Magargal LE, Ehrlich DR, et al. Review of choroidal osteoma: successful krypton red laser photocoagulation of an associated subretinal neovascular membrane involving the fovea. Ophthalmic Surg 1987;18:299–303.
197. McLeod BK. Choroidal osteoma presenting in pregnancy. Br J Ophthalmol 1988;72:612–4.
198. Narayanan R, Shah VA. Intravitreal bevacizumab in the management of choroidal neovascular membrane secondary to choroidal osteoma. Eur J Ophthalmol 2008;18:466–8.
199. Singh AD, Talbot JF, Rundle PA, et al. Choroidal neovascularization secondary to choroidal osteoma: successful treatment with photodynamic therapy. Eye (Lond) 2005;19:482–4.
200. Shields CL, Materin MA, Mehta S, et al. Regression of extrafoveal choroidal osteoma following photodynamic therapy. Arch Ophthalmol 2008;126:135–7.
201. Rose SJ, Burke JF, Brockhurst RJ. Argon laser photoablation of a choroidal osteoma. Retina 1991;11:224–8.
202. Noble KG. Bilateral choroidal osteoma in three siblings. Am J Ophthalmol 1990;109:656–60.
203. Goldstein BG, Miller J. Metastatic calcification of the choroid in a patient with primary hyperparathyroidism. Retina 1982;2:76–9.
204. Alfonso I, Howard C, Lopez PF, et al. Linear nevus sebaceous syndrome: a review. J Clin Neuro-opthalmol 1987;7:170–7.
205. Campbell SH, Patterson A. Pseudopapilloedema in the linear naevus syndrome. Br J Ophthalmol 1992;76:372–4.
206. Lambert HM, Sipperley JO, Shore JW, et al. Linear nevus sebaceus syndrome. Ophthalmology 1987;94:278–82.
207. Pittke EC, Marquardt R, Mohr W. Cartilage choristoma of the eye. Arch Ophthalmol 1983;101:1569–71.
208. Basta LL, Wilkenson CP, Anderson LS, et al. Focal choroidal calcification. Ann Ophthalmol 1981;13:447–50.
209. Lim JI, Goldberg MF. Idiopathic sclerochoroidal calcification. Arch Ophthalmol 1989;107: 1122–3.
210. Menchini U, Davi G, Pierro L, et al. Ostéome de la choroïde bilatéral chez un sujet agé. J Fr Ophtalmol 1990;13:3–9.
211. Munier F, Zografos L, Schnyder P. Idiopathic sclerochoroidal calcification: new observations. Eur J Ophthalmol 1991;1:167–72.
212. Schachat AP, Robertson DM, Mieler WF, et al. Sclerochoroidal calcification. Arch Ophthalmol 1992;110:196–9.
213. Sivalingam A, Shields CL, Shields JA, et al. Idiopathic sclerochoroidal calcification. Ophthalmology 1991;98:720–4.
214. Wiessner PD, Nofsinger K, Jackson WE. Choroidal osteoma: two case reports in elderly patients. Ann Ophthalmol 1987;19:1923.
215. Jensen OA. Ocular calcifications in primary hyperparathyroidism; histochemical and ultrastructural study of a case: comparison with ocular calcifications in idiopathic hypercalcaemia of infancy and in renal failure. Acta Ophthalmol 1975;53:173–86.
216. Honavar SG, Shields CL, Demirci H, et al. Sclerochoroidal calcification: clinical manifestations and systemic associations. Arch Ophthalmol 2001;119:833–40.
217. Park JM, Kim DS, Kim J, et al. Epibulbar complex choristoma and hemimegalencephaly in linear sebaceous naevus syndrome. Clin Exp Dermatol 2009;34:e686–9.
218. Traboulsi EI, Zin A, Massicotte SJ, et al. Posterior scleral choristoma in the organoid nevus syndrome (linear nevus sebaceus of Jadassohn). Ophthalmology 1999;106:2126–30.
219. Spector B, Klintworth GK, Wells Jr SA. Histologic study of the ocular lesions in multiple endocrine neoplasia syndrome type IIb. Am J Ophthalmol 1981;91:204–15.
220. Shields JA, Sanborn GE, Kurz GH, et al. Benign peripheral nerve tumor of the choroid; a clinicopathologic correlation and review of the literature. Ophthalmology 1981;88:1322–9.
221. Fan JT, Campbell RJ, Robertson DM. A survey of intraocular schwannoma with a case report. Can J Ophthalmol 1995;30:37–41.
222. Turell ME, Hayden BC, McMahon JT, et al. Uveal schwannoma surgery. Ophthalmology 2009;116 163-e6.
223. Saavedra E, Singh AD, Sears JE, et al. Plexiform pigmented schwannoma of the uvea. Surv Ophthalmol 2006;51:162–8.
224. Odashiro AN, Fernandes BF, Al-Kandari A, et al. Report of two cases of ciliary body mesectodermal leiomyoma: unique expression of neural markers. Ophthalmology 2007;114:157–61.
225. Toth J, Bausz M, Imre L. Unilateral Malassezia furfur blepharitis after perforating keratoplasty. Br J Ophthalmol 1996;80:488.
226. Jakobiec FA, Mitchell JP, Chauhan PM, et al. Mesectodermal leiomyosarcoma of the antrum and orbit. Am J Ophthalmol 1978;85:51–7.
227. Blodi FC. Leiomyoma of the ciliary body. Am J Ophthalmol 1950;33:939–42.
228. Miyamoto K, Kashii S, Oishi A, et al. Mesectodermal leiomyoma confined to the posterior choroid. Jpn J Ophthalmol 2007;51:240–3.
229. Perri P, Paduano B, Incorvaia C, et al. Mesectodermal leiomyoma exclusively involving the posterior choroid. Am J Ophthalmol 2002;134:451–4.
230. Shields JA, Shields CL, Eagle Jr RC. Mesectodermal leiomyoma of the ciliary body managed by partial lamellar iridocyclochoroidectomy. Ophthalmology 1989;96:1369–76.
231. Ben-Ezra D, Sahel JA, Harris NL, et al. Uveal lymphoid infiltrates: immunohistochemical evidence for a lymphoid neoplasia. Br J Ophthalmol 1989;73:846–51.
232. Crookes GP, Mullaney J. Lymphoid hyperplasia of the uveal tract simulating malignant lymphoma. Am J Ophthalmol 1967;63:962–7.
233. Desroches G, Abrams GW. Gass JDM. Reactive lymphoid hyperplasia of the uvea; a case with ultrasonographic and computed tomographic studies. Arch Ophthalmol 1983;101:725–8.
234. Gass JDM. Retinal detachment and narrow-angle glaucoma secondary to inflammatory pseudotumor of the uveal tract. Am J Ophthalmol 1967;64:612–21.
235. Ryan SJ, Zimmerman LE, King EM. Reactive lymphoid hyperplasia; an unusual form of intraocular pseudotumor. Trans Am Acad Ophthalmol Otolaryngol 1972;76:652–71.
236. Ryan Jr SJ, Frank RN, Green WR. Bilateral inflammatory pseudotumors of the ciliary body. Am J Ophthalmol 1971;72:586–91.
237. Zimmerman LE. Lymphoid tumors. In: Boniuk M, editor. Ocular and adnexal tumors: new and controversial aspects. St. Louis: CV Mosby; 1964. p. 429–46.
238. Duker JS, Shields JA, Eagle Jr RC. Ocular lymphoid hyperplasia. Arch Ophthalmol 1989;107:446–7.
239. Jakobiec FA, Sacks E, Kronish JW, et al. Multifocal static creamy choroidal infiltrates; an early sign of lymphoid neoplasia. Ophthalmology 1987;94:397–406.
240. Chang TS, Burne F, Gass JDM, et al. Echographic findings in benign reactive lymphoid hyperplasia of the choroid. Arch Ophthalmol 1996;114:669–75.
241. Cheung MK, Martin DF, Chan C-C, et al. Diagnosis of reactive lymphoid hyperplasia by chorioretinal biopsy. Am J Ophthalmol 1994;118:457–62.
242. Matsuo T, Matsuo N, Shiraga F, et al. Retinal pigment epithelial tear in reactive lymphoid hyperplasia of uvea. Ophthalmologica 1990;200:46–54.
243. Stacy RC, Jakobiec FA, Schoenfield L, et al. Unifocal and multifocal reactive lymphoid hyperplasia vs follicular lymphoma of the ocular adnexa. Am J Ophthalmol 2010;150 412-26e1.

244. Gulley ML, Dent GA, Ross DW. Classification and staging of lymphoma by molecular genetics. Cancer 1992;69:1600–6.
245. Gittinger Jr JW. Ocular involvement in Castleman's disease; response to radiotherapy. Ophthalmology 1989;96:1646–9.
246. Coupland SE, Foss HD, Hidayat AA, et al. Extranodal marginal zone B cell lymphomas of the uvea: an analysis of 13 cases. J Pathol 2002;197:333–40.
247. Fuller ML, Sweetenham J, Schoenfield L, et al. Uveal lymphoma: a variant of ocular adnexal lymphoma. Leuk Lymphoma 2008;49:2393–7.
248. Grossniklaus HE, Martin DF, Avery R, et al. Uveal lymphoid infiltration. Report of four cases and clinicopathologic review. Ophthalmology 1998;105:1265–73.
249. Cockerham GC, Hidayat AA, Bijwaard KE, et al. Re-evaluation of "reactive lymphoid hyperplasia of the uvea": an immunohistochemical and molecular analysis of 10 cases. Ophthalmology 2000;107:151–8.
250. Chappelow AV, Singh AD, Perez VL, et al. Bilateral panocular involvement with mantle-cell lymphoma. J Clin Oncol 2008;26:1167.
251. Cibis GW, Freeman AI, Pang V, et al. Bilateral choroidal neonatal neuroblastoma. Am J Ophthalmol 1990;109:445–9.
252. Ferry AP, Font RL. Carcinoma metastatic to the eye and orbit. I. A clinicopathologic study of 227 cases. Arch Ophthalmol 1974;92:276–86.
253. Ferry AP, Font RL. Carcinoma metastatic to the eye and orbit. II. A clinicopathologic study of 26 patients with carcinoma metastatic to the anterior segment of the eye. Arch Ophthalmol 1975;93:472–82.
254. Gonvers M, Zografos L. Choroidal metastasis and rhegmatogenous retinal detachment. Retina 1991;11:426–9.
255. Mames RN, Margo CE. Retinal pigment epithelial tear after treatment of metastatic carcinoma of the choroid. Retina 1991;11:430–2.
256. Stephens RF, Shields JA. Diagnosis and management of cancer metastatic to the uvea: a study of 70 cases. Ophthalmology 1979;86:1336–49.
257. Michelson JB, Stephens RF, Shields JA. Clinical conditions mistaken for metastatic cancer to the choroid. Ann Ophthalmol 1979;11:149–53.
258. Shields CL, Shields JA, Gross NE, et al. Survey of 520 eyes with uveal metastases. Ophthalmology 1997;104:1265–76.
259. Barondes MJ, Hamilton AM, Hungerford J, et al. Treatment of choroidal metastasis from choriocarcinoma. Arch Ophthalmol 1989;107:796–8.
260. Jaeger EA, Frayer WC, Southard ME, et al. Effect of radiation therapy on metastatic choroidal tumors. Trans Am Acad Ophthalmol Otolaryngol 1971;75:94–101.
261. Letson AD, Davidorf FH, Bruce Jr RA. Chemotherapy for treatment of choroidal metastases from breast carcinoma. Am J Ophthalmol 1982;93:102–6.
262. Logani S, Gomez H, Jampol LM. Resolution of choroidal metastasis in breast cancer with high estrogen receptors. Arch Ophthalmol 1992;110:451–2.
263. Anteby I, Pe'er J, Uziely B, et al. Thyroid carcinoma metastasis to the choroid responding to systemic ^{131}I therapy. Am J Ophthalmol 1992;113:461–2.
264. Margolis R, Budd GT, Singh AD. Unusual macular degeneration following breast cancer. Acta Ophthalmol Scand 2007 Sep;85(6):686–7.
265. Sachin Mehta, Anita Agarwal. Metastatic liposarcoma masquerading as an inflammatory granuloma. Retinal Cases and Brief Reports, 2011; 5: 18–21.
266. Blodi FC. The difficult diagnosis of choroidal melanoma. Arch Ophthalmol 1963;69:253–6.
267. Clayman HM, Flynn JT, Koch K, et al. Retinal pigment epithelial abnormalities in leukemic disease. Am J Ophthalmol 1972;74:416–9.
268. Schimmelpfennig W, Aur RJA. Leopardenfleck-Chorioretinopathie; erstes Anzeichen eines Rezidivs einer akuten lymphozytischen Leukämie. Ophthalmologe 1992;89:430–1.
269. Chang GC, Moshfeghi DM, Alcorn DM. Choroidal infiltration in juvenile myelomonocytic leukaemia. Br J Ophthalmol 2006;90:1067.
270. Tang RA, Vila-Coro AA, Wall S, et al. Acute leukemia presenting as a retinal pigment epithelium detachment. Arch Ophthalmol 1988;106:21–2.
271. Jakobiec F, Behrens M. Leukemic pigment epitheliopathy with report of a unilateral case. J Pediatr Ophthalmol 1975;12:10–15.
272. Dickson BC, Pethe V, Chung CT, et al. Systemic Erdheim–Chester disease. Virchows Arch 2008;452:221–7.
273. Karcioglu ZA. Ocular and periocular histiocytoses. Ophthal Plast Reconstr Surg 2007;23: 8–10.
274. Cheung N, Selva D, McNab AA. Orbital Langerhans cell histiocytosis in adults. Ophthalmology 2007;114:1569–73.
275. Valmaggia C, Neuweiler J, Fretz C, et al. A case of Erdheim–Chester disease with orbital involvement. Arch Ophthalmol 1997;115:1467–8.
276. Shields JA, Karcioglu ZA, Shields CL, et al. Orbital and eyelid involvement with Erdheim–Chester disease. A report of two cases. Arch Ophthalmol 1991;109:850–4.
277. Shields JA, Shields CL. Clinical spectrum of histiocytic tumors of the orbit. Trans Pa Acad Ophthalmol Otolaryngol 1990;42:931–47.
278. Gass JD. Retinal detachment and narrow-angle glaucoma secondary to inflammatory pseudotumor of the uveal tract. Am J Ophthalmol 1967;64(Suppl.):612–21.
279. Gass JD. A clinicopathologic study of a peculiar foveomacular dystrophy. Trans Am Ophthalmol Soc 1974;72:139–56.
280. Shields JA, Font RL, Eagle Jr RC, et al. Melanotic schwannoma of the choroid. Immunohistochemistry and electron microscopic observations. Ophthalmology 1994;101: 843–9.
281. Coston TO, Wilkinson CP. Choroidal osteoma. Am J Ophthalmol 1978;86:368–72.
282. Gass JD, Guerry RK, Jack RL, et al. Choroidal osteoma. Arch Ophthalmol 1978;96:428–35.
283. Gass JD. New observations concerning choroidal osteomas. Int Ophthalmol 1979;1:71–84.
284. Noble KG. Bilateral choroidal osteoma in three siblings. Am J Ophthalmol 1990;109:656–60.
285. Katz RS, Gass JD. Multiple choroidal osteomas developing in association with recurrent orbital inflammatory pseudotumor. Arch Ophthalmol 1983;101:1724–7.
286. Alfonso I, Howard C, Lopez PF, et al. Linear nevus sebaceous syndrome. A review. J Clin Neuroophthalmol 1987;7:170–7.
287. Spector B, Klintworth GK, Wells Jr SA. Histologic study of the ocular lesions in multiple endocrine neoplasia syndrome type IIb. Am J Ophthalmol 1981;91:204–15.
288. Clayman HM, Flynn JT, Koch K, et al. Retinal pigment epithelial abnormalities in leukemic disease. Am J Ophthalmol 1972;74:416–9.

Diseases that primarily affect the optic nerve may occasionally involve secondarily the macular area or may be mistaken for retinal diseases. Some of the most frequent of these diseases are discussed in this chapter.

OPTIC DISC ANOMALIES ASSOCIATED WITH SEROUS DETACHMENT OF THE MACULA

Serous detachment of the sensory retina may occur in association with one or a combination of developmental anomalies of the optic nerve head. This spectrum of anomalies includes pit, coloboma, morning glory deformity, and juxtapapillary staphyloma.

CONGENITAL PIT OF THE OPTIC DISC AND SEROUS DETACHMENT OF THE MACULA

Usually between the ages of 20 and 40 years, patients with congenital pit of the optic nerve head may develop serous detachment of the macula (Figures 15.01–15.03).[1–30] The detachment usually extends in a teardrop fashion (Figure 15.01A, I–K) from the disc margin in the vicinity of the optic pit, which in most cases is located along the temporal margin of the optic disc. Pits and detachment are uncommon at the nasal margin of the optic disc (Figure 15.02A–C). The optic disc diameter in the affected eye is usually larger than in the unaffected eye.[5,12] An optic pit may occur bilaterally in 10–15% of cases and may be inherited as an autosomal-dominant abnormality.[5,31–33] Pits may be associated with a coloboma of the optic nerve head, and details of the pit may be difficult or impossible to identify (Figure 15.02H and I). Some patients with severe colobomatous malformation of the optic disc may develop extensive retinal detachment (see discussion below). Optic pits located in the center of the optic disc are not associated with macular detachment. The optic pit is often covered with a gray membrane that frequently has one or more holes within it, particularly in patients with macular detachments. Most authors agree that there typically is no posterior vitreous detachment in eyes with a pit and serous detachment of the macula.[4,5,13,31] Occasionally, condensed vitreous strands may extend from the surface of the optic pit into the anterior vitreous (Figure 15.01M). In some patients a cloudy precipitate may occur on the posterior surface of the detached retina (Figure 15.01A, I, and J). When this occurs, the area of detachment may be misdiagnosed as a solid tumor (Figure 15.03C and D).[10,12] Some patients develop a central area of sharply defined retinal detachment with a surrounding larger, less well-defined area of elevation of the inner retinal surface, suggesting the presence of retinoschisis (Figure 15.01I–L).[20,21] Unlike retinoschisis, however, there is not complete loss of retinal function in the area of pseudoschisis in patients with an optic pit. There has been no satisfactory anatomic explanation for this peculiar configuration of retinal elevation seen biomicroscopically in these patients. With prolonged retinal detachment, depigmentation of the retinal pigment epithelium (RPE) occurs in the area of the detachment (Figures 15.01K and 15.03A and B). Cystic retinal degeneration, schisis-like appearance, marked thinning of the foveolar portion of the retina, and rarely full-thickness macular hole and rhegmatogenous retinal detachment may occur (Figure 15.02D).[3,26,34,35] Subretinal neovascularization may arise near the optic pit.[5,17]

15.01 Congenital pit of the optic disc causing serous macular detachment.

A–D: This 27-year-old woman complained of blurred vision that fluctuated in the right eye for several weeks. Serous detachment of the retina extended to the margin of the optic disc pit (arrow, A and B). Note subretinitic precipitates forming concentric lines of demarcation temporally. The diameter of the optic disc was about twice that of the normal eye. Xenon photocoagulation was placed along the temporal edge of the optic disc as well as in the optic pit (C). Seven months later the detachment had not resolved. Six and one-half years later the patient returned with approximately 20/200 vision in the right eye. There was no longer any serous detachment of the macula (D).
E: Long-standing large serous retinal detachment associated with an optic pit. There was yellow exudate on the posterior surface of the detached retina centrally.
F–H: This 29-year-old woman, who was known to have an optic pit and normal visual function in the right eye since 10 years of age, presented with a 4-month history of blurred vision in the right eye. Visual acuity was 20/50. There was a mound-like elevation of the inner retinal surface (arrowheads) that extended from the optic pit throughout the macular area. There was a smaller sharply circumscribed zone of what appeared to be detachment of the retinal receptors from the pigment epithelium (arrows, F) that did not extend to the optic pit. The patient could see a 50-μm krypton red laser aiming beam throughout the area of inner retinal elevation, including the central area of retinal detachment, both before and even after placement of two rows of krypton red photocoagulations along the temporal edge of the optic pit. Seven months later the elevation of the inner retinal surface and retinal detachment were no longer present. There was a pattern of radiating lines resembling foveomacular schisis centrally (G). Twenty-six months after treatment her visual acuity was 20/20 and the macula appeared normal (H).
I–M: A 17-year-old African American girl with decreased vision in her left eye for 4 years to counting fingers. A central schisis-like defect with surrounding subretinal fluid and precipitates is seen in the left macula emanating from a temporal optic disc pit (I, J). The pit remains nonfluorescent due to capillary nonperfusion, the central schisis shows mottled hyperfluorescence, and dye leaks into the subretinal space on the angiogram (K). The schisis cavity (arrow) present in the central macula, and a full-thickness defect (arrow) at the disc edge is demonstrated on optical coherence tomography (L, M).

(A–C from Gass[12]; I–M, courtesy of Dr. Jonathan Williams.)

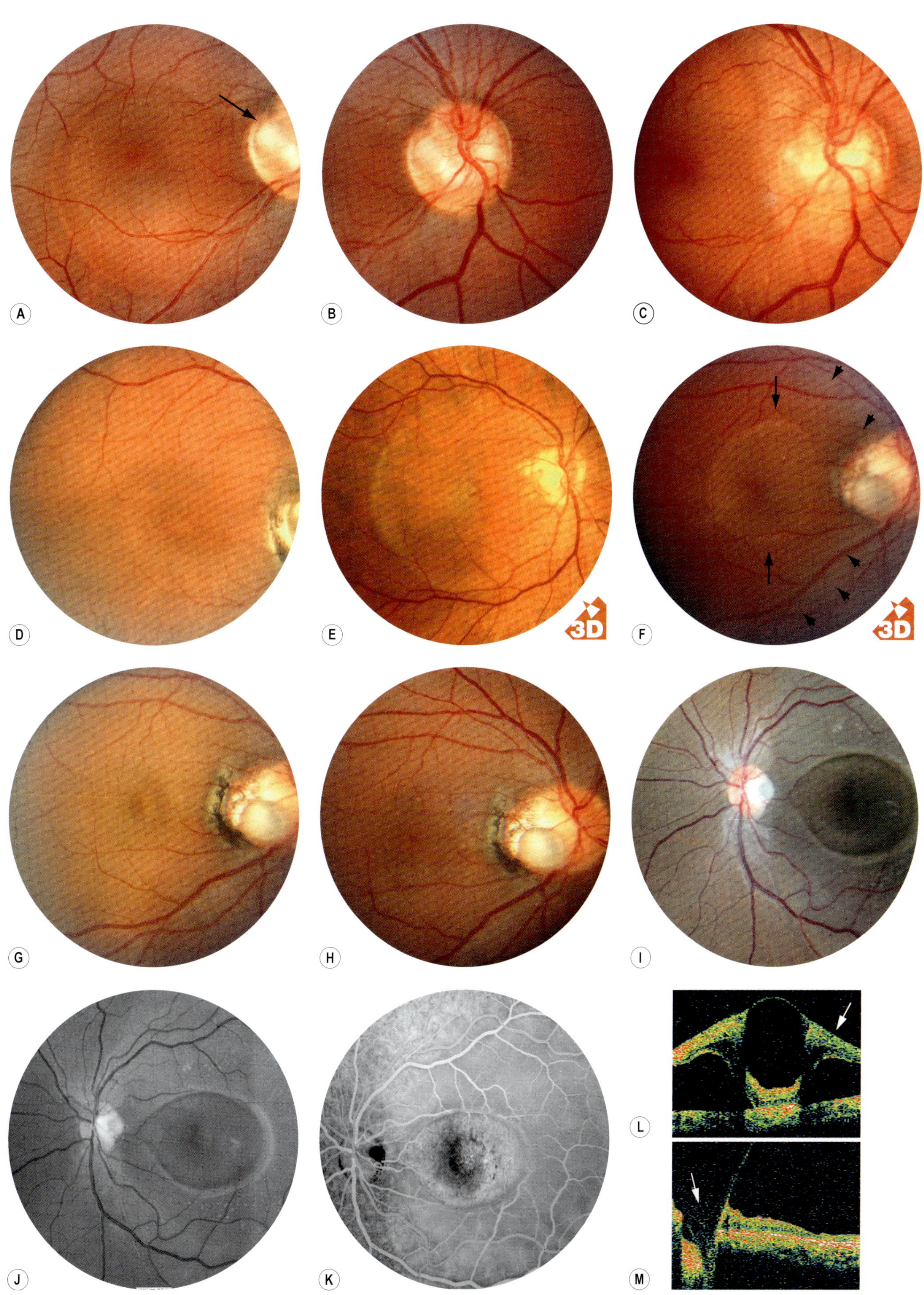
A
B
C
D
E
3D
F
3D
G
H
I
J
K
L
M

In patients with a recent onset of macular detachment, angiography shows no abnormalities in the macular area.[4,12] In early-phase angiograms the pit appears hypofluorescent (Figure 15.01K). In later phases, in most patients, there is evidence of staining in the area of the pit with no evidence of perfusion of dye into the subretinal fluid. Absence of staining of the pit has been associated with absence of retinal detachment, recent macular detachment, and no cilioretinal arteries emanating from the pit.[4,36] Staining of the subretinal fluid occasionally occurs (Figure 15.01K).[5] Patients with loss of pigment in the RPE caused by prolonged retinal detachment show hyperfluorescence corresponding with the areas of depigmentation during the early phases of angiography (Figure 15.01K).[12] This is often seen in the papillomacular bundle region adjacent to the optic disc in patients with no previous history of macular detachment. Angiography shows no evidence of either choroidal or retinal capillary permeability alterations. The failure to demonstrate angiographically either retinal or choroidal permeability alterations in the presence of a serous macular detachment should always alert the clinician to the possibility of an optic pit or a more peripheral lesion to account for the detachment. Optical coherence tomography (OCT) through the pit shows the defect, and any communication with the vitreous and/or the subarachnoid space (Figure 15.01M). OCT through the macula can show either a serous retinal detachment (Figure 15.03H and J) or a schisis or both (Figures 15.01L and 15.03I).[27,37–41]

Presently there is limited information concerning the natural course of eyes with an optic pit before or after development of serous macular detachment.[5,11,26,42] It is probable that only a small percentage of eyes with a pit ever develop serous retinal detachment. Spontaneous reattachment of the macula occurs in 25% or more of patients with optic pits.[4,6,11,42] With a prolonged delay in reattachment, cystic degeneration and partial- or full-thickness hole formation may occur.[3,26] Long-term follow-up of untreated eyes suggests that in approximately 50–75% of eyes the visual acuity will be reduced to 20/100 or worse within 5–9 years.[5,26]

Histopathologically, an optic pit consists of herniation of dysplastic retina into a collagen-lined pocket extending posteriorly through a defect in the lamina cribrosa into the subarachnoid space (Figure 15.03C and D).

The pathogenesis of the detachment appears to involve the passage of fluid from the area of the pit into the subretinal space. The failure of intravascular fluorescein to diffuse into the subretinal fluid in all but a few cases suggests that it is derived from either the cerebrospinal fluid[12,23] or the vitreous (Figure 15.03E).[5,6] Chang and associates[43] reported metrizamide cisternographic evidence of communication of the subretinal and subarachnoid spaces in a child with a colobomatous malformation of the optic nerve and extensive retinal detachment. Other studies involving radioisotope cisternography[32] and intrathecal fluorescein,[18] as well as attempts to displace subretinal fluid into the subarachnoid space by elevating the intraocular pressure,[12] have failed to demonstrate evidence of direct communication between the subarachnoid space and subretinal space. One patient with an optic pit experienced two episodes of increased intracranial pressure caused by pseudotumor cerebri without developing a retinal detachment.[14] Direct communication between the vitreous cavity and subretinal space via the optic pit has been demonstrated in collie dogs (Figure 15.03E).[6] This communication could not be demonstrated in a human eye with an optic pit.[44]

15.02 Congenital pit and juxtapapillary coloboma of the optic disc.

A–D: A congenital pit in the nasal part of the nerve head caused a serous retinal detachment (arrows) nasally (A) that subsequently spread to the macular area (B and C) in this boy. A mid-phase angiogram showed marked hyperfluorescence within the pit (arrows, D).

E and **F**: Serous detachment of the macula and macular hole secondary to a congenital pit (arrow, E) of the optic nerve in a 39-year-old woman with a 2-month history of blurred vision in the right eye. Visual acuity in the right eye was 20/200. Fluorescein angiography showed evidence of depigmentation of the retinal pigment epithelium (arrows, F) in the area of the serous detachment. Note the mottled-background hyperfluorescence apparent in the area of the macular hole. This angiogram suggests the probability that the serous detachment of the right macula had been present much longer than 2 months.

G–I: This 15-year-old boy with a large optic disc pit developed a peculiar vitelliform deposit in the subretinal space over a 6-month period (G and H). He had a positive scotoma, but his visual acuity was 20/20 on both occasions. There was early mottled hyperfluorescence centrally and late staining of the pit (I).

J: Coloboma with "double disc" deformity in a 5-year-old, otherwise normal, child.

K and **L**: Morning glory deformity of the right optic nerve and extensive retinal detachment in the right eye (K) that developed in a 21-year-old woman noted to have the optic disc deformity since age 6 years. Her visual acuity was finger counting only in the right eye. The retina was reattached following a vitrectomy (L). There was no retinal hole, and the source of the subretinal fluid presumably was via a pit-like deformity hidden within the disc anomaly.

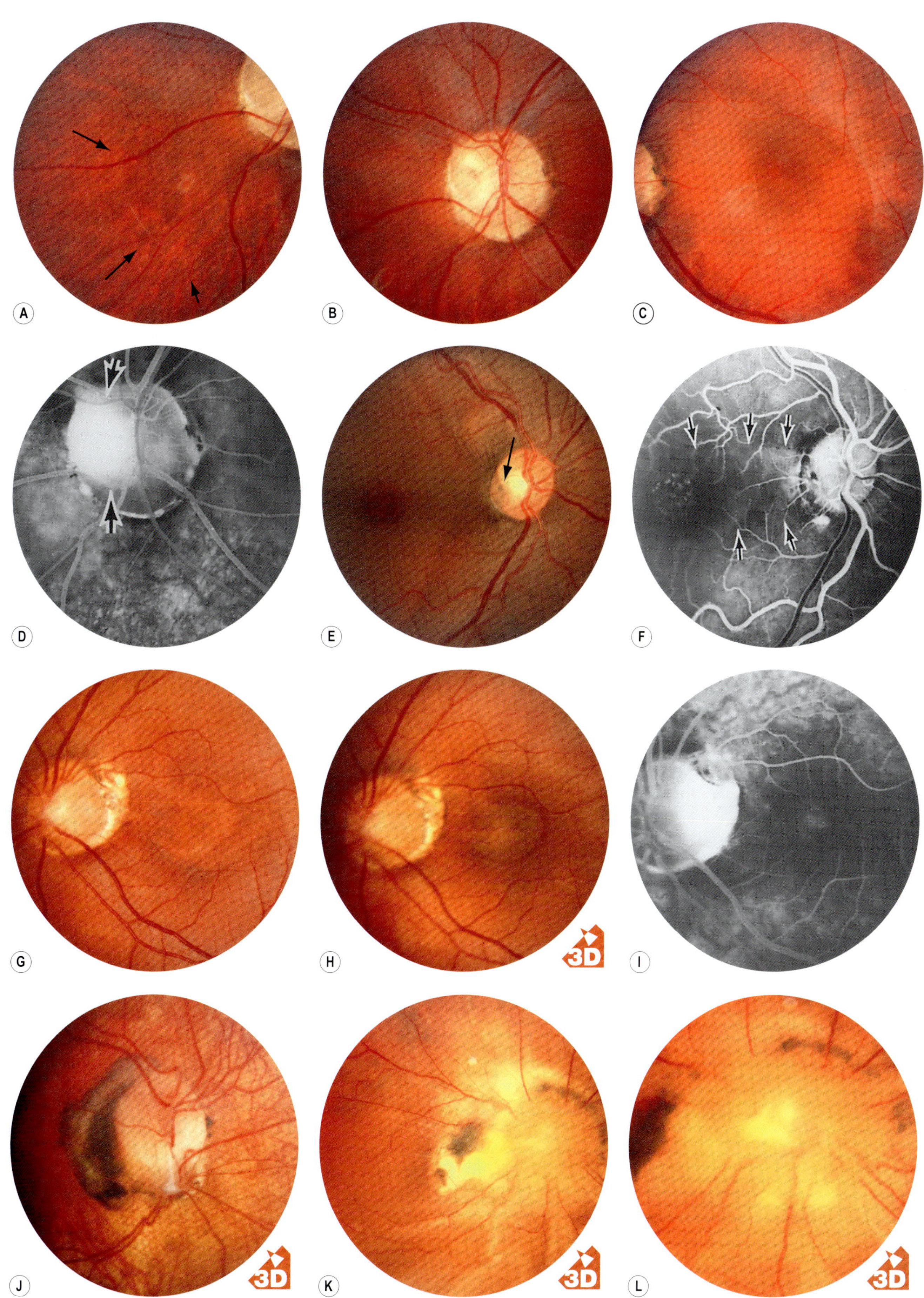
A
B
C
D
E
F
G
H
3D
I
J
3D
K
3D
L
3D

In general, attempts to close the neck of the detachment at the margin of the optic disc with photocoagulation, as well as photocoagulation of the optic pit itself, have been unsuccessful in causing prompt resolution of the macular detachment (Figures 15.01A–C, G, and H and 15.03G–I).[4,12,42,45,46] Several authors have reported resolution that may require several months or longer after photocoagulation.[3,16,45,47,48] Redetachment may occur weeks or months later.[25,49] The absence of posterior vitreous separation in patients with macular detachment suggests that traction of the formed vitreous in these patients on the anterior surface of the retina throughout the macular area may be important in causing the passive movement of either fluid vitreous or of cerebrospinal fluid through a defect within or at the margin of the optic pit into the subretinal space. In older patients whose posterior vitreous is extensively liquefied full-thickness holes in the macula and elsewhere in the posterior fundus do not cause retinal detachment in the absence of biomicroscopic evidence of focal vitreous traction. Some authors have reported successful reattachment of the macula using a combination of one or more of the following: pars plana vitrectomy, intravitreal gas tamponade, and photocoagulation.[2,8,25,31,49–54] No technique of treatment has proved uniformly successful in permanently reattaching the retina. Ocassionally gas and/or emulsified silicone oil can migrate through the pit intracranially. This is especially likely to occur when the gas bubble is smaller than the size of the pit or when the intraocular pressure is too high. A reasonable recommendation is observation for at least a month after the onset of detachment; if no improvement in the detachment occurs, photocoagulation across the neck of the detachment; if no response occurs within 6–8 weeks, repeat the laser treatment; if still no improvement in the detachment, consider intravitreal gas tamponade with or without pars plana vitrectomy. Use of intravitreal tissel tissue glue to cover the pit has been reported. The author has used tissel successfully in a patient with two previous vitrectomy failures. Use of prophylactic treatment either adjacent to the pit or as a coarse scatter pattern of laser in the macula to prevent detachment might be considered in the rare patient with a strong family history of detachment associated with optic nerve pit, and particularly in the second eye if the first eye has permanent loss of acuity from this complication.

ACQUIRED PITS OF THE OPTIC NERVE

Pit-like changes in the optic nerve head may be acquired and may be the cause of unexplained loss of paracentral and occasionally central visual field loss. These pits typically develop in the inferotemporal quadrant in older patients with normal intraocular pressure or glaucoma.[55–58] There is an increased incidence of acquired pits in patients with low-tension glaucoma (74%) versus patients with typical glaucoma (15%).[55] Development of the pit may be preceded by the appearance on one or more occasions of a flame-shaped hemorrhage on the optic disc. The typical field defect in normotensive eyes extends from the blind spot to near fixation in a pistol-shaped configuration and has a steep central margin.

Because patients with acquired pits and with low-tension glaucoma have significantly greater amounts of field loss than those with elevated intraocular pressure without pits, it is probable that optic nerves predisposed to developing pits are more susceptible to damage from the damaging effects of intraocular pressure. Whereas there are structural differences in the lamina cribrosa in patients with and without low-tension glaucoma,[59] the pathogenesis of the acquired pit of the optic disc is still not clear.[60] It is postulated that these patients have cavitatory defects behind the lamina cribrosa, the walls of which collapse with elevated pressure and become confluent to look like a pit or a large cup. Ischemic necrosis in eyes with poor optic nerve head circulation may be responsible in some eyes.[61]

15.03 Congenital pit of the optic disc.

A–C: In 1975 this 21-year-old man presented with blurred vision in the right eye caused by serous macular detachment (arrows, A) associated with an oval pit of the optic disc. His visual acuity was 20/70. Note in the stereoangiogram (BL and BR) the focal thinning of the retina and attenuation of the retinal pigment epithelium at the temporal margin of the optic disc. The retina reattached spontaneously within several years, and 8 years later his visual acuity was 20/30. There are radiating pericentral retinal folds simulating X-linked schisis (C).

D and **E**: Histopathology of serous detachment of the retina in a 29-year-old woman with an optic disc pit. The eye was enucleated because of a misdiagnosis of a choroidal melanoma, presumably caused by some opacification of the subretinal fluid. Note the cystic degeneration of the detached retina (arrow, D). E shows details of the pit, indicating three possible routes (1–3) by which fluid from the vitreous (v) or the subarachnoid space (ss) might pass into the subretinal space (srs). The neuroectodermal portion of the pit (n) is separated from its surrounding fibrous capsule (f) by a multiloculated space (s).

F: Photomicrograph of optic pit in collie dog. Arrows indicate communication of vitreous cavity with subretinal space.

G–I: This 18-year-old noted decrease in vision in his left eye to 20/400 for 4 months. The right eye was normal with 20/20 vision. A temporal optic disc pit with adajacent serous detachment and subretinal precipitates is seen (G). The patient had undergone laser (arrow) to the temporal edge of the disc 4 months previously with no evidence of fluid resorption. Optical coherence tomography showed subretinal fluid beginning beyond the laser scar site (arrow) and extending to the macula (H and I).

J–L: This 21-year-old woman was visually asymptomatic and correctable to 20/20 vision in both eyes. She gave a history of constant headaches 2 years previously that was diagnosed as pseudotumor cerebri. The right optic nerve was normal; the left showed a deep cup with a temporal pit. No macular detachment was present.

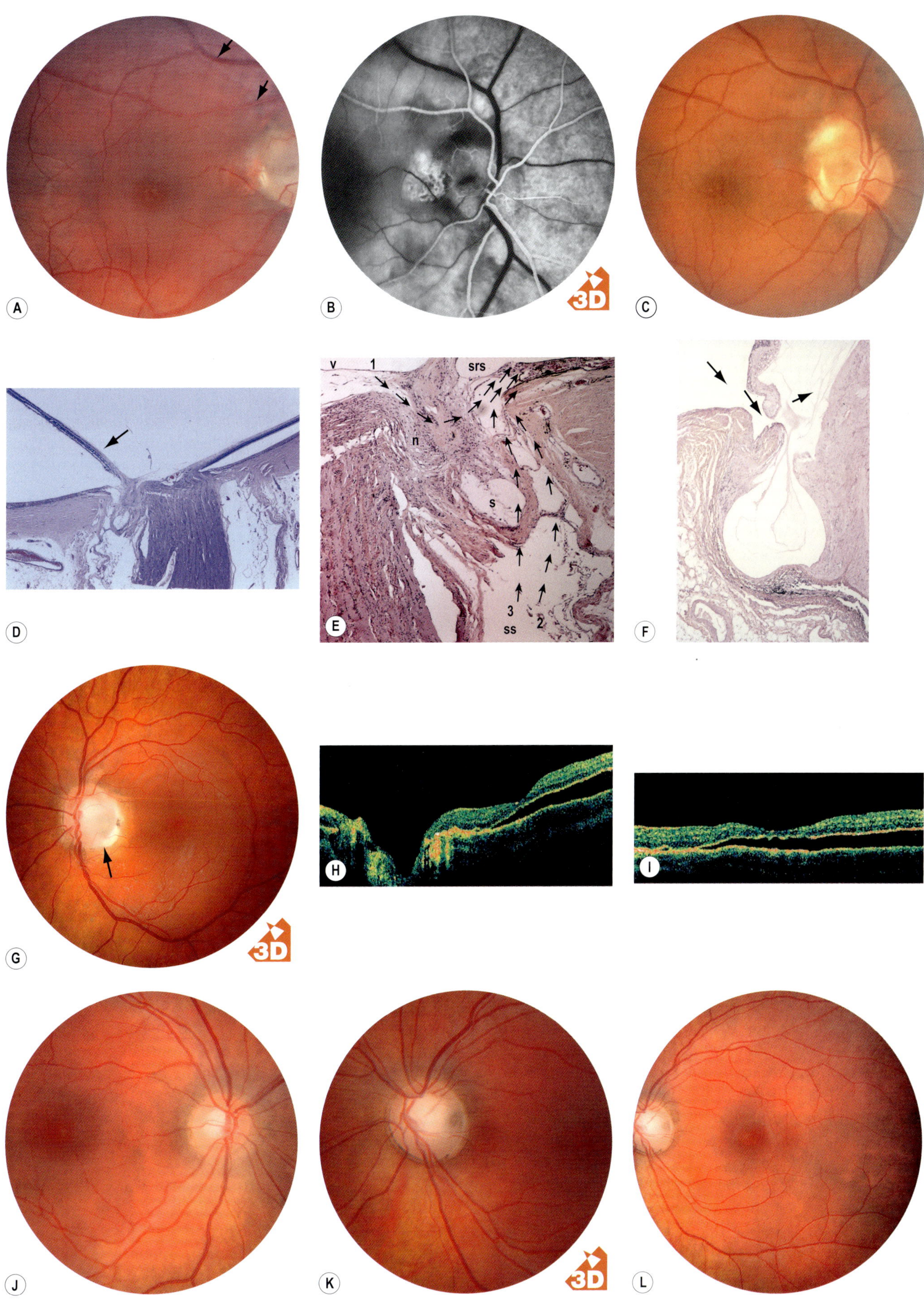
A
B
C
D
v
1
srs
n
s
3
ss
2
E
F
G
H
I
J
K
L

Some of these patients develop macular thickening leading to schisis-like change that can sometimes progress to macular detachment.[62–64] This has been noted in acute angle closure glaucoma, juvenile glaucoma, traumatic and primary open-angle glaucoma. The acute rise or frequent spikes in intraocular pressure may force fluid into the inner retina through small defects at the edge of the disc or cup. The increasing fluid may eventually dissect into the subretinal space in some eyes. Lowering the intraocular pressure with surgery or medications results in resolution of the fluid in some eyes; others require a vitrectomy and gas displacement.[62–64] The schisis may be subtle and may be mistaken for cystoid macular edema secondary to prostaglandin inhibitors or be treated without success with topical nonsteroidal agents.

COLOBOMA, JUXTAPAPILLARY STAPHYLOMA, AND MORNING GLORY DEFORMITY

A coloboma of the optic nerve head involves a defect in its structure occurring as a result of malclosure of the ocular fissure. It may be mild, in which case there is a defect in the optic nerve substance, usually inferiorly. This defect may be more extensive and involve the juxtapapillary choroid and retina. It may be associated with a pit deformity and with a juxtapapillary staphyloma. This latter term refers to an outpouching of the ocular wall around the optic nerve head. This outpouching may occur with little or no abnormality in the structure and function of the eye, or with varying degree of dysplasia of the nerve. If the coloboma or staphyloma is filled with glial tissue, the retinal blood vessels may exit from this tissue in a pattern that has suggested to some a morning glory (Figure 15.02K and L). These more severe anomalies of the optic disc may be associated with serous macular detachment (Figure 15.04D–H); with other ocular abnormalities, including microphthalmos, lens coloboma, persistent primary hyperplastic vitreous, orbital cyst,[32,65–70] and occasionally intracranial abnormalities such as a basal encephalocele (Figure 15.04B and C), and midline defects including pituitary stalk duplication, and moya moya disease.[71–80]

A pit deformity may or may not be present and is often obscured clinically by other anomalies (Figure 15.02K and L). In some cases these anomalies may be combined to form a mass lesion simulating a capillary angioma, astrocytoma, combined retinal–RPE hamartoma, or melanoma (Figure 15.04B) in the region of the optic disc.[81] Some patients may manifest clinical evidence of communication between the vitreous and retrobulbar ocular cysts via the optic disc anomalies.[68,82,83] In patients with these severe disc anomalies the retinal detachment begins in the juxtapapillary area, often on the temporal side.[32,43,65–67,84–93] The detachment, unlike that occurring with a pit alone, may extend to involve most of the fundus (Figure 15.02K and L). These detachments, like those associated with a pit, may resolve spontaneously.[66] The pathogenesis of the detachment occurring with all of these anomalies is probably similar in most cases, although this is controversial. In the morning glory deformity and juxtapapillary staphyloma, the detachment has been attributed to retinal breaks in the vicinity of the anomaly,[84,87,94] to communication between the subarachnoid and subretinal space,[12,43,90] to communication between the vitreous and subretinal space,[87] to communication with both the vitreous and subarachnoid space,[88] to vitreoretinal traction,[86] and to exudation from blood vessels within the anomaly,[89] the orbital tissue,[90] and juxtapapillary choriocapillaris.[90] Vitreoretinal traction is probably important in all cases, and successful repair of the detachment has been accomplished by vitrectomy, intravitreal gas, and thermal treatment at the edge of the anomaly.[84,87] Choroidal neovascularization may occur at the edge of any of these anomalies.[5,17,92,95,96]

Familial cases have been associated with mutations in the *PAX6* gene on chromosome 11p13[97]; however, given the association of morning glory discs with dissimilar anomalies, a more complex genetic influence is likely.[98]

15.04 Morning glory disc.

A: A typical morning glory deformity with a large optic disc and radial vessels arising near its edge. Note the peripapillary atrophy and pigmentation.

B and **C**: Morning glory disc (B) and basal encephalocele seen on T1-weighted noncontrast sagittal magnetic resonance imaging (C, arrow) in an otherwise healthy 18-year-old female with no light perception vision. Note the peripapillary hyperpigmentation. The only association was a wide nasal bridge.

D–H: Disc coloboma associated with a macular detachment in this 31-year-old female. Fluorescein angiogram shows no hyperfluorescence or site of leakage (F). Optical coherence tomography shows subretinal fluid extending from the disc edge and a separate pocket of SRF under the fovea (G, H).

Peripapillary staphyloma.

I and **J**: Peripapillary staphyloma in the right eye of a 31-year-old woman complaining of transient obscurations of vision in this eye. Note the circular area of depigmentation and excavation surrounding the optic disc (I). There was slight narrowing of the retinal vessels adjacent to the optic disc. Visual acuity in the right eye was 20/20 and in the left eye was 20/15. The left fundus was normal (J).

K: Marked peripapillary staphyloma, the walls of which contracted about every minute to form a cavity approximately two-thirds of the diameter shown.

L and **M**: Photomicrographs of a cross-section of the dysplastic optic nerve just behind the eye of a patient with a peripapillary staphyloma. Note the dysplastic nerve surrounded by a ring of smooth muscle (arrows). Contraction of similar atavistic muscle is apparently responsible for the spontaneous contraction noted in the patient (K).

(D and F; Also, Yannuzzi L J., The Retinal Atlas, Saunders 2010, 978-0-7020-3320-9, p. 885.)

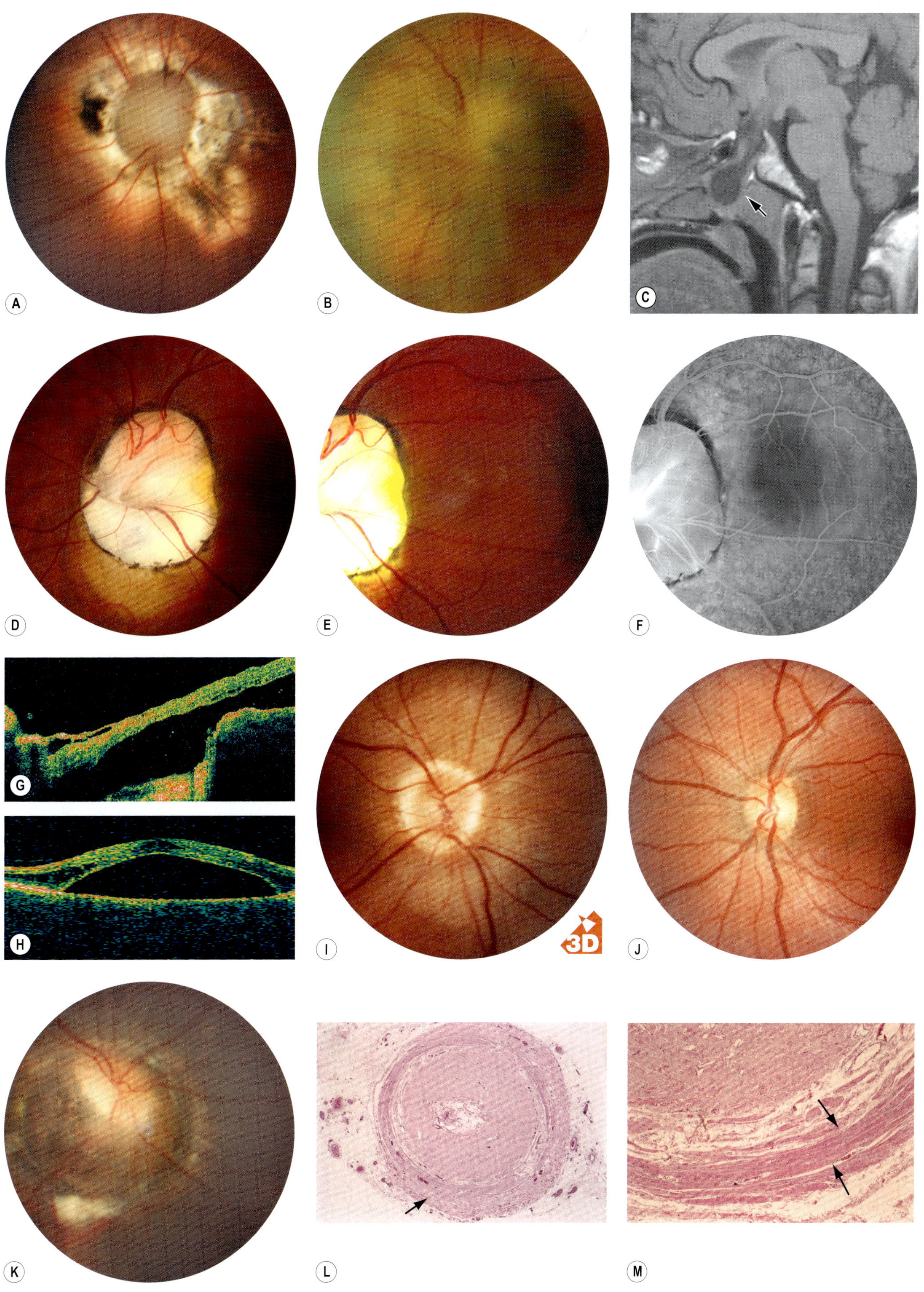
A
B
C
D
E
F
G
H
I
3D
J
K
L
M

TRANSIENT OBSCURATION OF VISION SECONDARY TO PERIPAPILLARY STAPHYLOMA

Peripapillary staphyloma is a rare congenital anomaly in which the normal or nearly normal optic nerve head lies in the depth of an excavation in the fundus (Figure 15.04I, K, and N). It is usually present in only one eye. If the staphyloma does not involve the macula, the visual acuity may be normal (Figure 15.04I and N). In adulthood these patients may complain of transient obscurations of vision that in some cases may be associated with intermittent dilation of the retinal veins.[99–101] Figure 15.04I illustrates a mild degree of peripapillary staphylomatous formation that was initially misinterpreted as a choroidal hemangioma in a young woman with transient obscurations of vision.[101]

Peripapillary staphylomata may occasionally be associated with contractile movements of the walls of the staphyloma (Figure 15.04K).[102,103] These contractions are not associated with the patient's respiration or pulse rate. There is some histopathologic evidence to suggest that the presence of atavistic smooth muscle in and around peripapillary staphylomata may be responsible for this contraction and, further, may be responsible for the transient obscuration of vision (Figure 15.04L and M).[104] Contractile movements have also been described in patients with choroidal coloboma and morning glory syndrome.[81,91,105] In 1962 Longfellow and coworkers reported a young man with unilateral intermittent blindness associated with marked dilation of the retinal veins of undetermined cause.[100] He had minimal abnormality of the optic nerve head, but the clinical findings otherwise suggest the possibility of an anomalous smooth-muscle sphincter around the retrobulbar optic nerve.

PAPILLORENAL (RENAL COLOBOMA) SYNDROME

First described in 1977 by Rieger,[106] it was considered to be a rare autosomal dominant disorder of the optic disc and kidneys. Work by Parsa and colleagues suggests that the highly variable phenotype may be responsible for its underdiagnosis. Initial description was of anomalous optic discs associated with hypoplastic kidneys resulting in hypertension and renal failure. Serous retinal detachment extending to the macula accompanies the disc anomalies in some cases.[107–111]

The extended ophthalmic features of papillorenal syndrome include large optic discs with several cilioretinal arteries with hairpin-like loops emerging at the edge of the disc (Figure 15.04O–S). A large portion of the central part of the disc is devoid of vessels or has rudimentary cilioretinal vessels. Along with multiple cilioretinal vessels, the retinal vasculature is not fully developed, and the choroid is affected to various degrees in certain families (Figure 15.04T-V). It appears that there may be a primary deficiency in the vascular development that compromises growth of substantial portion of the retina and the choroid. Cats and lemurs have a poorly defined central retinal artery and vein and most of the retinal circulation is derived from ciliary vessels in these animals. The eyes with papillorenal syndrome seem to have converted to this feline pattern of circulation. Papillorenal syndrome is likely a hereditary vascular

15.04 Peripapillary staphyloma (Continued)

N: More fully developed peripapillary staphyloma in a 17-year-old girl with a 3-year history of intermittent episodes of complete amaurosis in the left eye.

Papillorenal syndrome (renal coloboma syndrome)

O and P: This 34-year-old graduate student gave a history of undergoing laser treatment to his right optic nerve at age 8. His visual acuity was 20/20 OU. He complained of right flank pain and was known to have small kidneys for the previous 8 years; this was discovered when he was screened as a potential kidney donor for his mother, who had end-stage renal disease for 18 years. His creatinine clearance was decreased and his blood pressure was elevated. A sister and niece were known to have abnormal renal function and renal stones. The vessels come off the disc at its edge and the central area of the disc is "vacant"' (O, P). Laser scar is seen in the temporal juxtapapillary retina. Horizontal striae temporal to the disc likely signify previous SRF. A clinical diagnosis of papillorenal syndrome was made and the patient and the family are being further investigated to confirm the diagnosis.
Q–S: This 37-year-old male had undergone a cadaveric renal transplant for "end-stage renal disease" with hypertension at age 26. He presented with a nonrhegmatogenous retinal detachment in the right eye and changes at the pigment epithelium in both macula (Q and R); this was thought to be related to chronic ICSC/organ transplant retinopathy superimposed on an "anomalous disc." Krypton laser to the temporal edge of the right optic disc failed to resolve the retinal detachment requiring a pars plana vitrectomy and endo drainage (Q, arrow at drainage site). Careful examination shows both optic discs to be "vacant" centrally with vessels arising at the edge, some of which are "hairpin-like," typical of papillorenal syndrome (Q–S).
T–V: The right eye in this 5-month-old Nigerian American girl with pendular nystagmus and hypoplastic kidneys, reveals segmental and simultaneous filling of the superior choroid, retina and disc vessels during the early arterial phase (U). Relative non-perfusion of the inferior choroidal and retinal vasculature is seen that fills in a later angiogram (V). There is a watershed area of retinal and choroidal non-perfusion from the disc that extends inferotemporally (arrows, V). No distinct foveal avascular zone was present. This patient also lacked both retinal and choroidal perfusion in the inferonasal periphery where the retinal vessels end-anastomosed at the edge of retinal perfusion. The left disc had no central retinal vessels (not shown). Her Nigerian father with 20/20 acuity bilaterally had optic discs with hairpin vessels arising at the disc edge.
W–Y: This 49-year-old African American woman suffered recurrent pyleonephritis. Both optic discs had vessels arising at the edge of the disc with rudimentary central disc vessels (W and Y). Mid phase angiogram on the disc reveals very small central retinal vessels.

(B and C, courtesy of Dr. M. Tariq Bhatti; D–H, courtesy of Dr. Edwin H. Ryan Jr, D and F, in Yannuzzi, Lawrence A. The Retinal Atlas. Philadelphia: Saunders/Elsevier, 2010. p.885.; I and J from Seybold and Rosen[101]; K, courtesy of Dr. A.R. Frederick Jr; L and M, courtesy of Dr. William H. Spencer, O and P, courtesy of Dr. Louise Mawn; T to Y, courtesy of Dr. Cameron Parsa, reprinted with permission from Ophthalmology. Elsevier[109].)

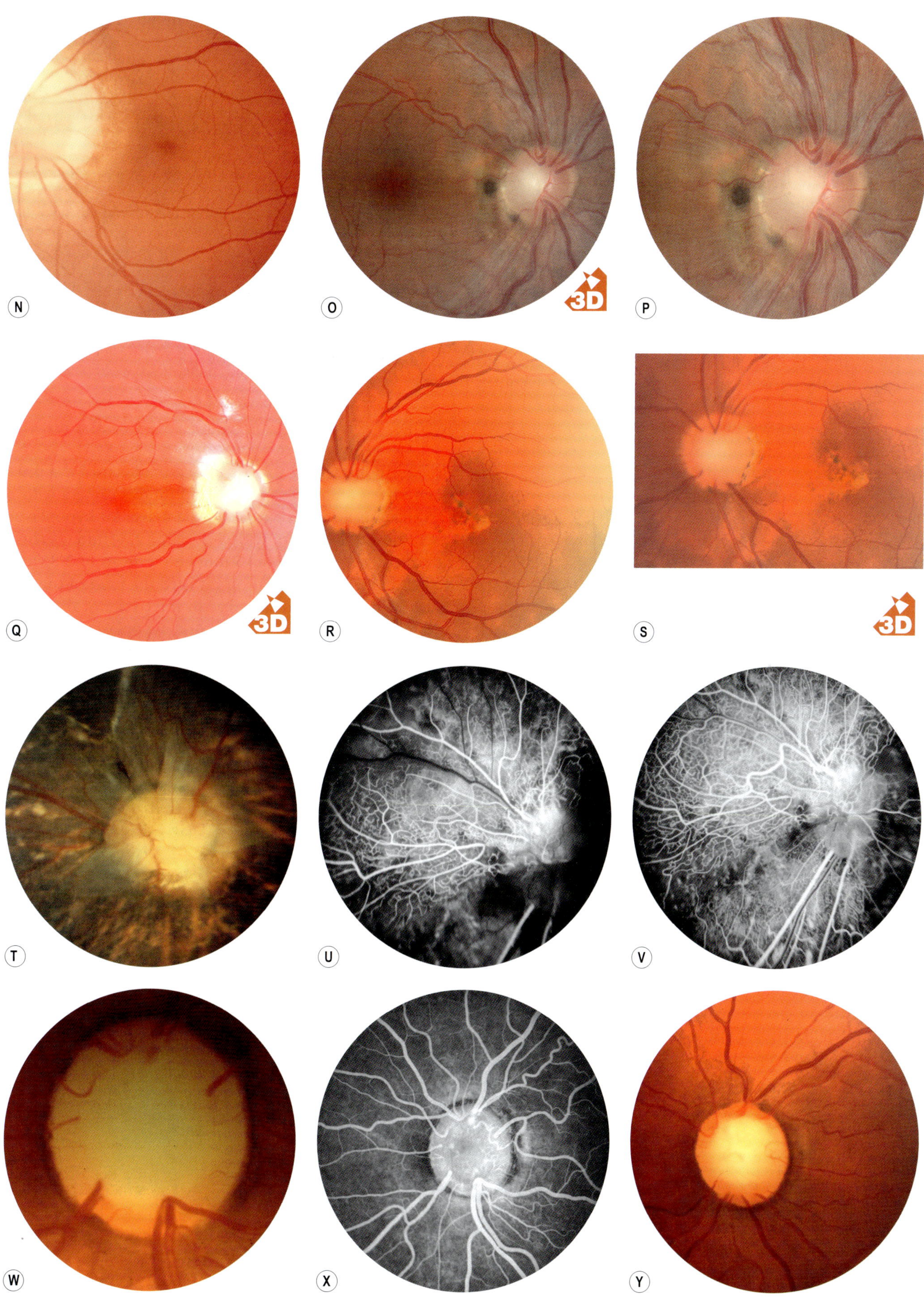
N
O
3D
P
Q
3D
R
S
3D
T
U
V
W
X
Y

dysgenesis that most severely affects the ocular and renal circulation, the most vascular organs. Visual field defects that do not correspond to glaucomatous changes are seen; this is explained by the absence of retinal ganglion cells and decreased retinal thickness as a result of defect in the vasculogenesis of the retina and choroid. Magnetic resonance imaging (MRI) shows hypoplasia of the optic chiasm due to defect in the decussating fibers of the optic nerve.[110] A significant number of these discs may be misdiagnosed as morning glory or normal-tension glaucoma. The associated kidney diseases include renal hypoplasia, renal hypertension, and renal failure. There is extreme resistance to renal blood flow within the renal parenchyma resulting in renal hypertension. The recurrent pyelonephritis and kidney stones is a variant of expression of the renal disease.

There may be several defects in the *PAX2* gene to account for the variable phenotype. In 1995, Sanyanusin et al. discovered mutations in the developmental gene *PAX2* in two families with papillorenal syndrome.[112,113] Schimmenti et al. identified three additional families with ocular and renal abnormalities, including vesicoureteral reflux.[114] Since then five other families with mutations of the *PAX2* gene have been reported.[115–117] However, not all cases can be explained by the *PAX2* mutations.

The features that should alert a diagnosis of papillorenal syndrome include the "vacant discs," presence of multiple ciliary retinal vessels with their abnormal insertion posterior to the globe, peripheral dysgenesis of the retinal vessels, hypoplasia of the optic chiasm on MRI, and visual field defects that do not correspond to glaucoma.[118]

OPTIC DISC HYPOPLASIA AND TILTED-DISC SYNDROME

Mild dysplasia of the optic nerve must be considered in patients with unexplained visual loss.[119–121] There is considerable variation in the size of the normal optic disc. The disc diameter is often directly related to eye size and refractive error. Some anomalies of the disc may be either overlooked or misinterpreted as papilledema. Failure to recognize a disc anomaly in a patient with a visual defect may cause initiation of an unnecessarily extensive evaluation for a retinal, retrobulbar, or intracranial lesion.

Moderate or severe hypoplasia of the optic disc is often associated with a visual defect (Figure 15.05).[122,123] Ophthalmoscopic clues to its presence include reduction in the disc diameter, a low disc/artery ratio, and the peripapillary double-ring sign (Figure 15.05A and B). This sign consists of a yellow-gray peripapillary halo delineated by an outer ring corresponding to the junction between the sclera and lamina cribrosa and an inner ring caused by the termination of the RPE.[122,124] The diagnosis of mild degrees of hypoplasia may be difficult or impossible. Several techniques for measuring and defining optic disc hypoplasia have been described.[122,125,126] Romano, using photogrametric methods, found no overlap between the horizontal diameters of normal and hypoplastic discs.[125]

15.05 Hypoplasia and dysplasia of the optic disc.

A: Marked hypoplasia of the optic disc in an infant.
B: Photomicrograph of severe optic disc hypoplasia.
C and D: Unilateral optic disc hypoplasia in left eye (D) of a young woman who had normal visual acuity in both eyes but an afferent pupillary defect and a peculiar visual field defect in the left eye. Compare with normal right disc (C).
E: Tilted optic disc was present bilaterally in this patient, who had superotemporal visual field defects in both eyes.
F and G: Septo-optic dysplasia in a 17-year-old girl who was the product of full-term normal pregnancy and delivery. She had neonatal jaundice caused by Rh incompatibility. She was of short stature. She had nystagmus and concentric field constriction. Her visual acuity, right eye, was 20/60 and, left eye, no light perception. Magnetic resonance imaging (MRI) showed evidence of aplasia of the septum pellucidum.
H–J: Bilateral optic nerve hypoplasia and absent septum pellucidum seen on coronal MRI in this 10-year-old patient.

(C and D, courtesy of Dr. Joel S. Glaser; H–J, courtesy of Dr. Patrick Lavin.)

He directly measured the horizontal diameter of the discs taken on a standard 30 degree field fundus camera with a x2.5 magnification. The range in diameters for hypoplastic discs was 1.8–3.27 mm, with a mean of 2.64 mm, as compared to a range of 3.44–4.7 mm and a mean of 3.88 mm for normal discs. Zeki and others used the ratio of the distance from the edge of the disc to the center of the fovea to disc diameter to define optic disc hypoplasia; a ratio of 3 to 1 or greater characterizes a hypoplastic optic disc.[126] Disc hypoplasia may be unilateral or bilateral (Figure 15.05C and D). In bilateral cases the eye with the smaller disc often has a better Snellen acuity, indicating that factors other than size determine the visual function, e.g., macular hypoplasia, high refractive error, amblyopia, central scotoma, and optic atrophy.[126] A hypoplastic disc with a large central cup may have a disc diameter of normal size.[127] Hypoplastic optic discs may occasionally be supplied largely by cilioretinal arteries.[128] Disc hypoplasia may be associated with other extraocular or intraocular anomalies (e.g., aniridia)[129]; it may be segmental[119]; and it may be associated with normal visual acuity (Figure 15.05C and D).[130] Superior segmental disc hypoplasia may occur as a sign of maternal diabetes[131,132] and can be diagnosed by finding characteristic inferior visual field defects.[133]

Optic nerve hypoplasia can result from an insult to the embryo at any level of the optic pathway.[134] Evidence for a neuroendocrine disorder should be sought in any child presenting with bilateral optic disc hypoplasia, because of the frequent association of hypothalamic and pituitary dysfunction, partial or complete absence of the septum pellucidum, midbrain abnormalities, hypotonia, hydrocephalus, porencephaly, and orthopedic deformities (de Morsier's syndrome) (Figure 15.05D and F–I).[135–143] Other known associations include aniridia, monocular temporal hemianopsia, contralateral megalopapilla, microphthalmia, achiasmia, polymicrogyria, periodic alternating-gaze nystagmus, intracranial arachnoid cyst, oval cornea and lens duplication, tortuous retinal veins, and mitochondrial cytopathies.[144–153]

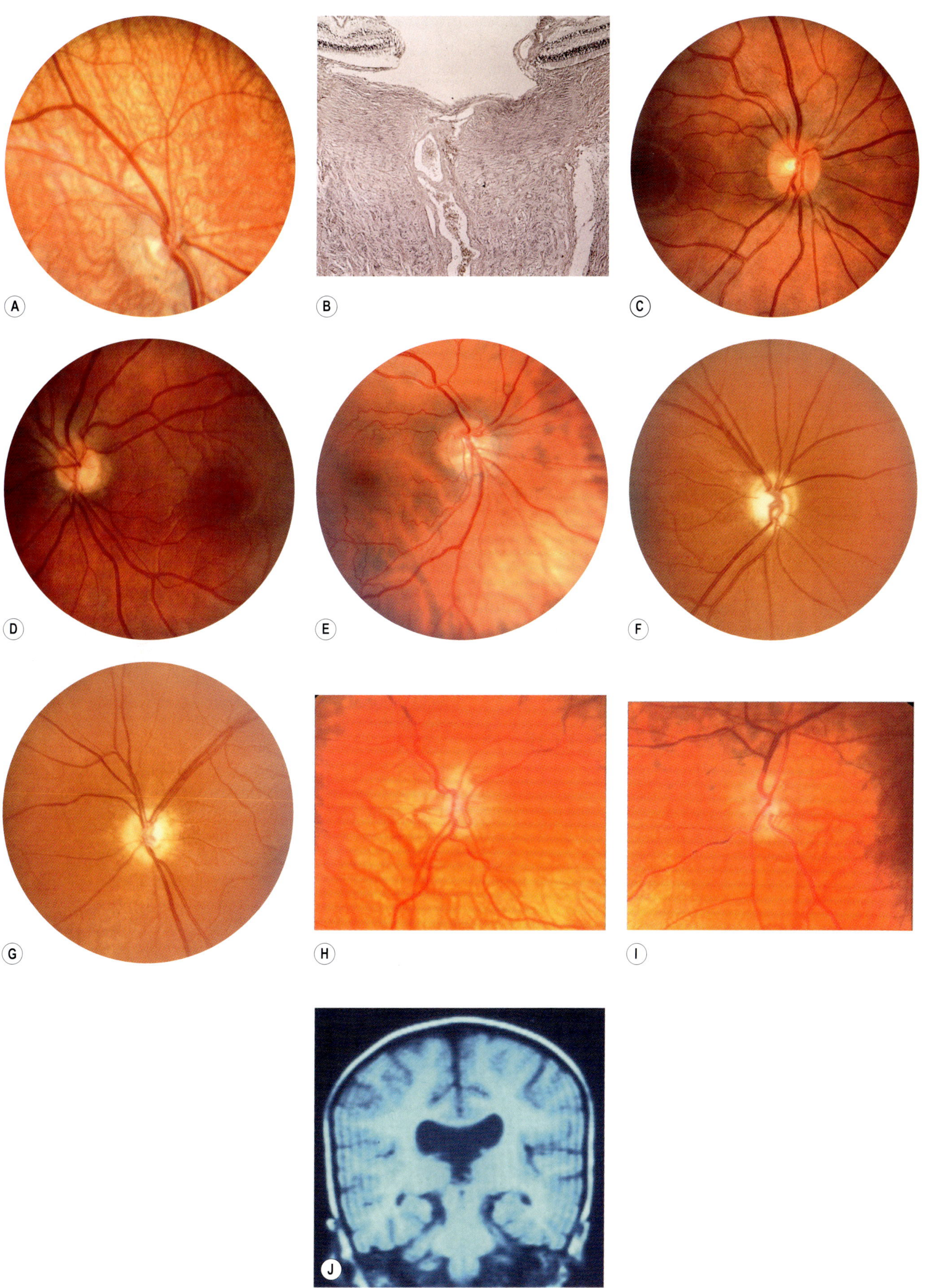
A
B
C
D
E
F
G
H
I
J

In a 100-case series, optic nerve hypoplasia was associated with premature birth (21%), maternal diabetes (6%), fetal alcohol syndrome (9%), and endocrine abnormalities (6%). Thirty-two percent had associated developmental delay, 13% cerebral palsy, and 12% seizures. Sixty percent had abnormal neuroimaging, including ventricular and white- or gray-matter abnormalities, septo-optic dysplasia (Figure 15.05J), corpus callosum abnormalities, and hydrocephalus. Associated clinical neurological deficits were seen in 57% of bilateral and 32% of unilateral cases.[154]

No specific gene defect has been found, though isolated cases have been associated with *PAX6* defect, pericentric inversion of chromosome 9, trisomy 18, 5p deletion (cri du chat syndrome), *SOX2*, *SOX*, and *HESX1* gene mutations.[155]

The tilted-disc syndrome has the following features: the long axis of the oval optic disc is obliquely directed; the upper and temporal portion of the disc lies anterior to the inferonasal portion; the retinal vessels emerge from the disc tissue in the upper and temporal aspect rather than nasally (situs inversus); there is an RPE conus in the direction of the tilt, as well as a large area of hypopigmentation and staphylomatous ectasia inferonasal to the optic disc; myopic astigmatism is present; and visual field depression occurs bitemporally (not truly hemianopic) (Figure 15.05E).[156,157] Central vision may or may not be affected. The asymmetry of the disc elevation with the ill-defined margins superiorly may be mistaken for papilledema. Visual loss may be caused occasionally by choroidal neovascularization.[158] The disc anomaly may occur in association with other, nonocular anomalies.[139]

DRUSEN (HYALINE BODIES) OF THE OPTIC NERVE HEAD

Drusen are discrete, multiple, amorphous, partly calcified extracellular deposits in the prelaminar portion of the optic nerve reported in 2% of population.[159–167] In small numbers they may be present deep within a normal-appearing optic nerve head. In larger numbers in children and young adults, they cause a swollen nerve head that may simulate papilledema (Figure 15.06A and B).[168] As they become larger, more calcified, and associated with atrophy of surrounding nerve fibers, they become visible as discrete crystalline structures later in life (Figure 15.06C and E and 15.07J and K). When buried, they are most easily detected by retroillumination biomicroscopically. Although a "lumpy, bumpy" appearance to a swollen disc suggests the presence of drusen (Figure 15.06E–L), a similar picture occasionally occurs in papilledema.[169] They frequently occur in small discs and may be associated with anomalous branching and tortuosity of the retinal vessels (Figures 15.06A and B and 15.07A and B).[170–173]

15.06 Hyaline bodies of the optic disc.

A and **B**: Asymmetric distribution of optic disc hyaline bodies in a 14-year-old girl whose condition was misdiagnosed as papilledema. Note the congenital tortuosity of the retinal vessels and the relatively small, less involved left optic disc.
C: Subretinal hemorrhage (arrow) caused by calcified hyaline bodies.
D: Photomicrograph of a calcified hyaline body located anteriorly to the lamina cribrosa. Note multiple dilated capillaries (arrows) near the margins of the hyaline body.
E–L: This 17-year-old girl presented with poor vision in the left eye for a year. Her visual acuity was 20/20 in the right and 20/80 in the left eye. Intraocular pressures were 9 and 11 mmHg respectively. Both optic discs were lumpy-bumpy with mild peripapillary fibrosis and subretinal calcification (E, I). The left eye had a disciform scar signifying involuted subretinal neovascularization. Autofluorescence imaging by filters on the fundus camera (F, J) and with barrier and excitation filters (G, K) showed increased autofluorescence in both eyes. Optical coherence tomography showed raised nodular surface with increased reflectance of both discs (H, L).

In some patients drusen may cause slow progressive loss of visual fields (characteristically inferonasal) in a nerve fiber distribution.[174–177] Drusen may be associated with abnormal visual evoked potentials.[177,178] In a few patients drusen of the optic disc may lead to severe loss of central vision.[168,179] Drusen may also cause acute visual loss, presumably resulting from acute swelling of the optic nerve head induced by the drusen interfering with the blood supply of the nerve (Figure 15.07G).[169,178–187] This swelling may be evident ophthalmoscopically and may be accompanied by a few flame-shaped hemorrhages and cotton-wool patches, a picture suggesting anterior ischemic optic neuropathy (AION).[179,182–184,187] In others the swelling of the optic nerve may be less apparent and cause obstruction of the central retinal vessels.[159,180,181,188,189] In those eyes that develop an AION, the prevalence of vascular risk factors, pattern of visual field loss, and incidence of second eye involvement are similar to eyes without disc drusen; however they are younger, enjoy a better prognosis, and more often report transient visual obscurations.[190] Optic disc drusen may also cause loss of vision associated with subretinal exudation and hemorrhage derived from peripapillary choroidal neovascularization (Figure 15.07A–F).[191–196] Bleeding into the subretinal space may occur adjacent to the optic disc in the absence of angiographic evidence of subretinal neovascularization (Figure 15.07A).[191] Very rarely Pulfrich phenomenon is reported, likely from delayed conduction in one eye compared to the other, and this can be minimized by using a tinted lens on the affected side.[197]

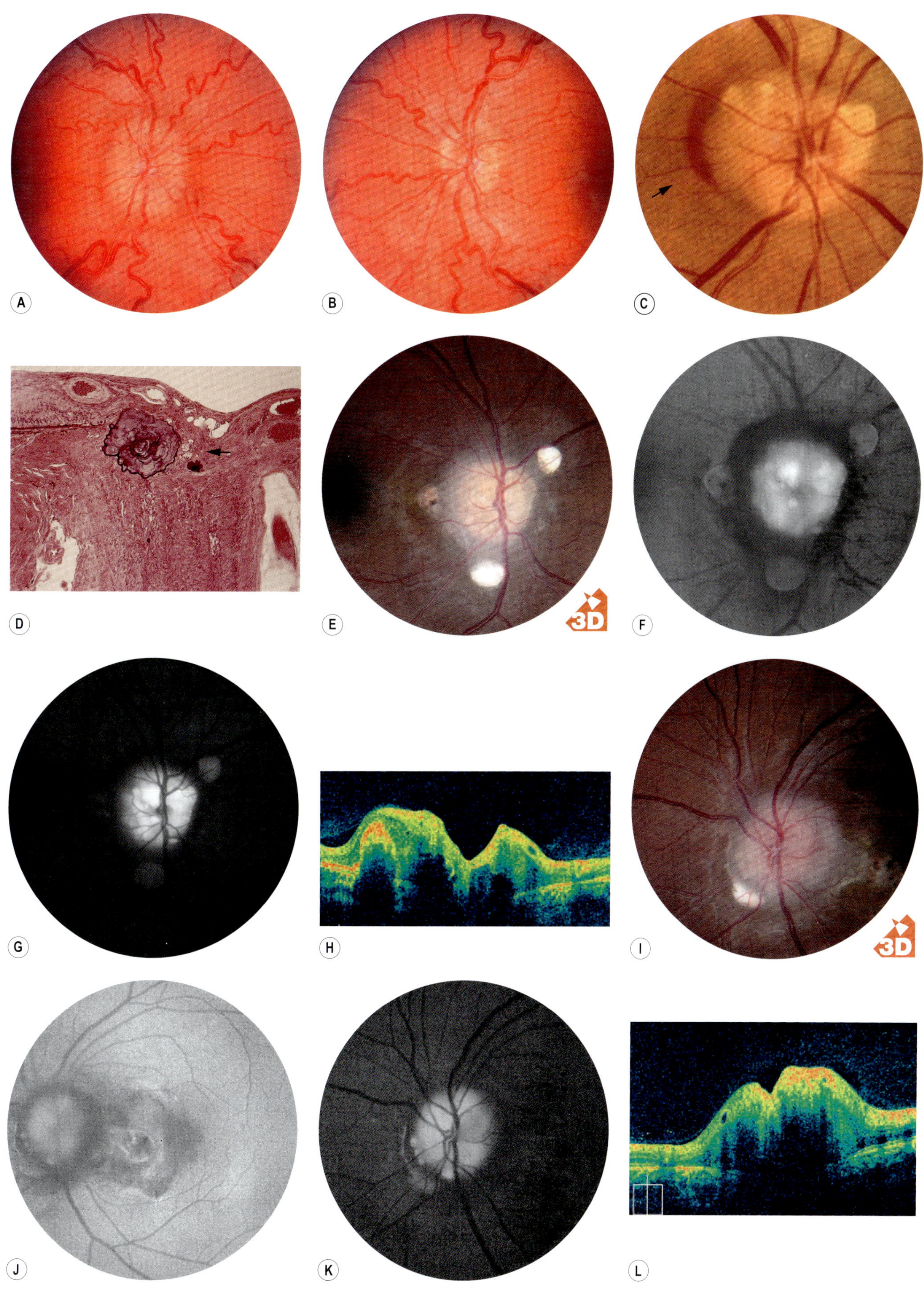
A
B
C
D
E
3D
F
G
H
I
3D
J
K
L

Other fundus findings that have occurred in association with drusen of the optic nerve head include retinitis pigmentosa,[172,198] retinal hemorrhages,[160] angioid streaks in patients with pseudoxanthoma elasticum[199] (see Figure 3.38I and 3.40H to L) subfoveal choroidal neovascularization,[200] chronic papilledema associated with pseudotumor cerebri,[172,201] and chorioretinal folds (see Chapter 4). Disc drusen have been reported in children with primary megacephaly.[202] Drusen bodies of the optic nerve head occur commonly, and therefore many associated findings may be coincidental.[203] The association of drusen and chorioretinal folds probably is not coincidental. Most chorioretinal folds are probably acquired and are caused by some subclinical inflammatory process causing shrinking and flattening of the posterior sclera. This process also causes narrowing of the optic canal and in turn may predispose the optic nerve head to drusen accumulation and other complications such as ischemic optic neuropathy and obstruction of the central retinal vessels. In some patients hyaline bodies are inherited as an autosomal-dominant trait.[173,189,204]

Fluorescein angiography is helpful in identifying alterations in the normal optic nerve vascular pattern as well as in identifying subretinal neovascularization associated with drusen.[182,205] By virtue of their autofluorescence, drusen near the surface of the optic disc can be detected with fundus photography using appropriate filters (Figure 15.06F, G, J, and K). The author has found this technique helpful in detecting drusen that were not visible biomicroscopically. OCT is helpful in monitoring the change in contour of the disc, with changes in the size or anterior movement of the drusen over time (Figure 15.06H and L).

Ultrasonography is also helpful in detecting optic disc drusen, particularly when they are buried in an optic disc that appears normal clinically, or in cases of unexplained optic disc swelling.[180] Failure to demonstrate calcified bodies in the optic nerve head of infants and children with a swollen optic nerve head may not exclude the presence of drusen. It is possible, although not proven histopathologically, that drusen may be relatively noncalcified hyaline structures in young patients.[206] The calcification caused by drusen anterior to the level of the lamina cribrosa should not be confused with that located several millimeters posterior to the lamina cribrosa.[207] The cause of this latter focal calcification is uncertain. In some patients the calcification may be located in the walls or lumen of the central retinal artery, where it may develop as a degenerative change in association with atheromatous disease, or it may be a calcific embolus derived from the aortic valve. These focal retrolaminar calcifications may be found in some eyes with central retinal artery occlusion. Computed tomography (CT) is also capable of detecting buried drusen.[208,209]

Histopathologically, drusen are calcified extracellular bodies located anterior to the lamina cribrosa (Figure 15.06D).[159,162–164,167,173,210,211] They are associated with small scleral canal, crowding of nerve fibers, partial optic atrophy, elevated disc margins, cytoid bodies, dilated capillaries, juxtapapillary subretinal hemorrhage, subretinal neovascularization (Figure 15.07B–F), retinal scarring, and calcification. Histochemically they are composed of a mucoprotein matrix containing acid mucopolysaccharides, ribonucleic acid, and occasionally iron.[159,162,163] Their pathogenesis has been ascribed to RPE migration, hyaline degeneration of the neuroglia, accumulation of degenerative products of axons, and coalescing intracellular deposits of glial cells,[211] transudative vasculopathy,[167] and axoplasmic transport alterations.[173] It is probable that a congenital, and less commonly an acquired, small optic nerve scleral canal that is crowded with nerve fibers is responsible for a local disturbance of axoplasmic transport and drusen formation.[170,173] Tso found ultrastructural evidence to suggest that optic disc drusen are the result of abnormal intracellular metabolism and calcification of mitochondria.[212] The mitochondria are extruded into the extracellular space, where they act as nidi for continued build-up of calcific deposits. Acquired causes of chronic crowding of the optic nerve fibers such as idiopathic chorioretinal folds (see Chapter 4) and pseudotumor cerebri may also be a factor in drusen formation.[172,201]

The long-term visual prognosis for most patients with drusen of the optic disc is probably good. Those with buried drusen have fewer visual field defects than those with visible drusen.[213] Visual field defects may show progression in some patients. The natural course of those patients who develop juxtapapillary subretinal neovascularization is variable, and some patients may retain central vision in spite of peripapillary subretinal hemorrhage.[166,191]

15.07 Hyaline bodies of the optic disc.

A–F: Serous and hemorrhagic disciform detachment of the left macula (B) secondary to hyaline bodies of the optic disc in a 4-year-old boy with a 3-week history of left esotropia. Visual acuity in the right eye was 20/30 and in the left eye was 20/200. Note swollen optic disc in both eyes (A and B) and the gray, type 2, subretinal neovascular membrane (arrows, B) extending temporally from the left optic disc. Fluorescein angiography revealed evidence of perfusion and staining of the neovascular membrane extending from the temporal edge of the left optic disc (C and D). Xenon photo-coagulation was placed over the area of subretinal neovascularization (E). Note that the photocoagulation was not carried into the center of the foveal area. Two months following photocoagulation note the atrophy of the retinal pigment epithelium that extends into the central macular area (F). The patient's visual acuity was approximately 6/200.
G–I: Acute optic neuropathy with disc edema, peripapillary exudation, and exudative macular detachment in the right eye (G) of a 31-year-old man complaining of rapid loss of vision. His left optic disc was small and contained hyaline bodies (arrow, H). Two months later visual acuity had improved and hyaline bodies were evident in the right disc (arrows, I).
J and **K**: Visible calcified drusen on the disc surface in both eyes of a 50-year-old woman.

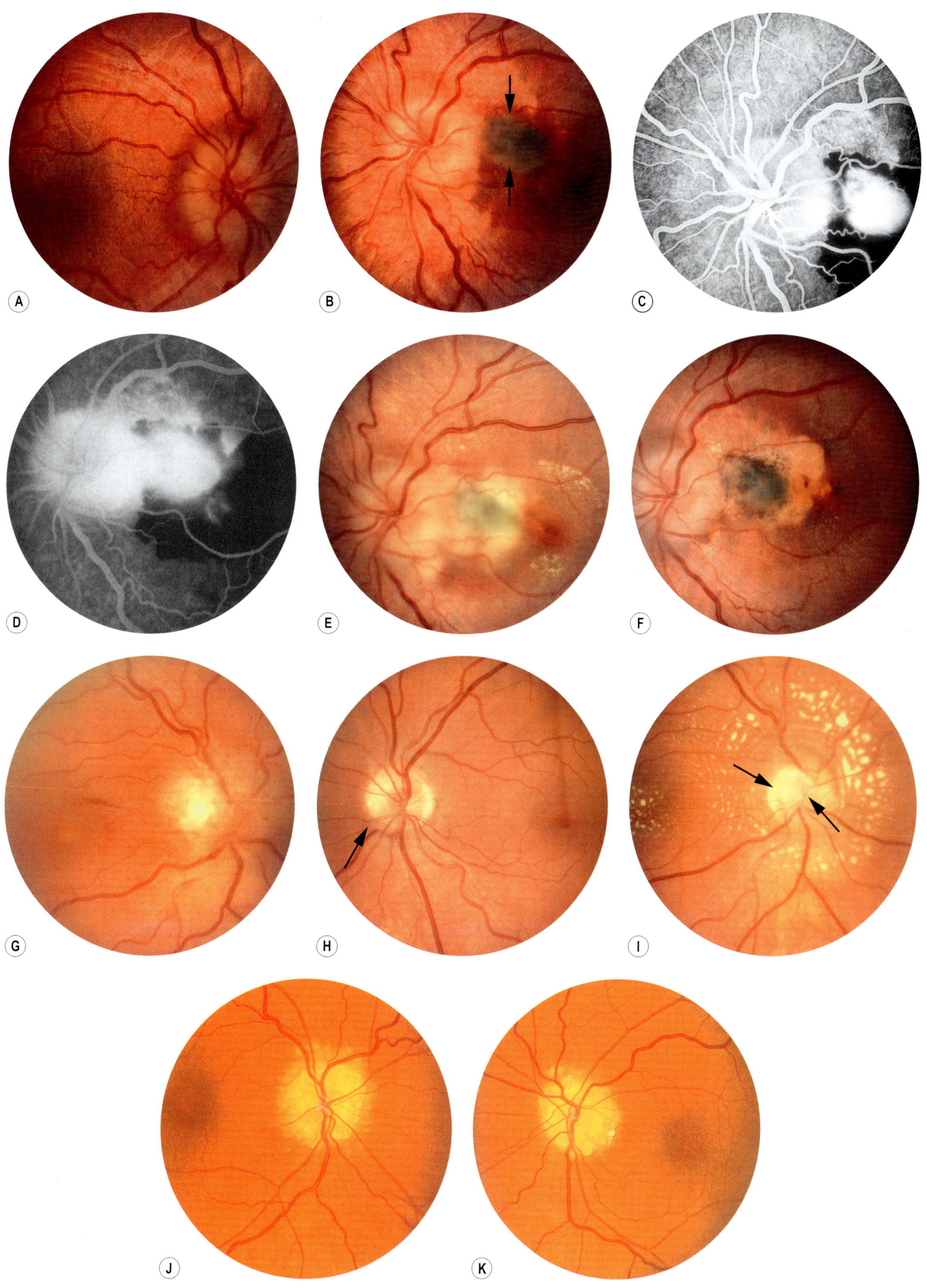
A
B
C
D
E
F
G
H
I
J
K

The biomicroscopic diagnosis of drusen of the optic disc is relatively secure if the calcified bodies are visible within the elevated optic nerve head. Occasionally noncalcified drusen-like changes are caused by papilledema.[169] The differential diagnosis of juxtapapillary choroidal neovascularization associated with a swollen optic disc includes the presumed ocular histoplasmosis syndrome, angioid streaks, idiopathic choroidal neovascularization, sarcoidosis, papilledema with pseudotumor cerebri, and congenital pit of the optic disc.

HEREDITARY OPTIC NEUROPATHIES

The heredodegenerative optic neuropathies must be considered in patients with insidious as well as rapid loss of central vision.

Dominant Optic Atrophy (Kjer Type)

Patients with dominant optic atrophy note the insidious onset of mildly progressive loss of visual acuity, usually beginning before 10 years of age.[214–220] Visual loss is bilateral but may be asymmetric. Many patients are unable to recall the time of onset of the disease, and some may be asymptomatic. Although the optic atrophy is dominantly inherited, a positive family history may not be obtained (Figure 15.08). Interfamilial and intrafamilial variations in acuity loss may occur (range: 20/30–20/400). The characteristic field defect is a cecocentral scotoma. Depression of the temporal isopters may simulate a bitemporal hemianopia. Constriction of peripheral isopters is rare. Tritan (blue) dyschromatopsia is the characteristic color defect in dominant optic atrophy. A generalized dyschromatopsia, however, may be present in some cases. Temporal optic disc pallor, often with a triangular area of temporal excavation, is characteristic (Figure 15.08A and B). Although uncertainties remain concerning the pathogenesis of the frequently encountered West Indian optic atrophy, it is probable that many cases are examples of dominant optic atrophy (Figure 15.08B and C; see discussion of nutritional amblyopia below).

Weleber and Miyake described familial optic atrophy associated with "negative" electroretinograms in two families with loss of central vision occurring in the second and third decades of life, optic atrophy, defective color vision, mild to moderate myopia, and pericentral or central scotomas.[221]

15.08 Familial optic neuropathy.

A: This young girl had mild visual loss and a cecocentral scotoma in both eyes. Her sibling had similar findings. Note the segmental area of optic atrophy temporally.
B: This 49-year-old Jamaican man had poor vision in his left eye since sustaining trauma to that eye at 30 years of age. He was asymptomatic in the right eye but was referred because his best corrected vision in the eye was 20/70. There was a wedge-shaped area of temporal pallor in both optic discs (B) and posttraumatic scarring in the left macula. He had bilateral cecocentral scotomata. It is probable that a familial optic atrophy that developed in early childhood was responsible for subnormal acuity in the right eye.
C–F: Dominant optic atrophy affected four generations of the family of this 8-year-old boy (C and D) and his 25-year-old father (E and F). The son's visual acuity was 20/40 bilaterally. The father gave a history of slow loss of vision since childhood. His visual acuity was 20/200 in both eyes.
G–L: Dominant optic atrophy affecting three generations of this family. Proband is a 12-year-old boy with 20/50 vision in each eye. Both optic discs showed temporal pallor (G and H) and he had bilateral centrocecal scotomas on visual field testing. Optical coherence tomography through both maculas showed normal photoreceptors, but mild thinning of the nasal inner retina (I1 and I2 arrows). His 45-year-old father was asymptomatic with 20/20 vision in both eyes (J). His 74-year-old paternal grandfather complained of slow loss of vision, never correctable beyond 20/40 for the previous 30-plus years, and had temporal pallor of both optic discs (K, L).

The *OPA1* (optic atrophy type 1) gene is localized to a 1.4-cM interval on chromosome 3q28-q29.[222–225] Missense, nonsense, deletion frameshift and splice site alterations accounting for more than 100 mutations have been seen in various pedigrees of patients with dominant optic atrophy. This explains the heterogeneity of the pathophysiology of the disease and the variable phenotype (Figure 15.08G–L). The penetrance of the gene varies from 43 to 89%.[226–228] It is likely that environmental factors also play a role in disease severity in susceptible individuals. The OPA1 protein is anchored to the mitochondrial cristate inner membrane and is believed to prevent cytochrome c release from mitochondria and block organelle fragmentation, thus protecting the cells from apoptosis.[222,229,230] It is likely there are other hitherto unknown gene defects that account for some cases of dominant optic atrophy.

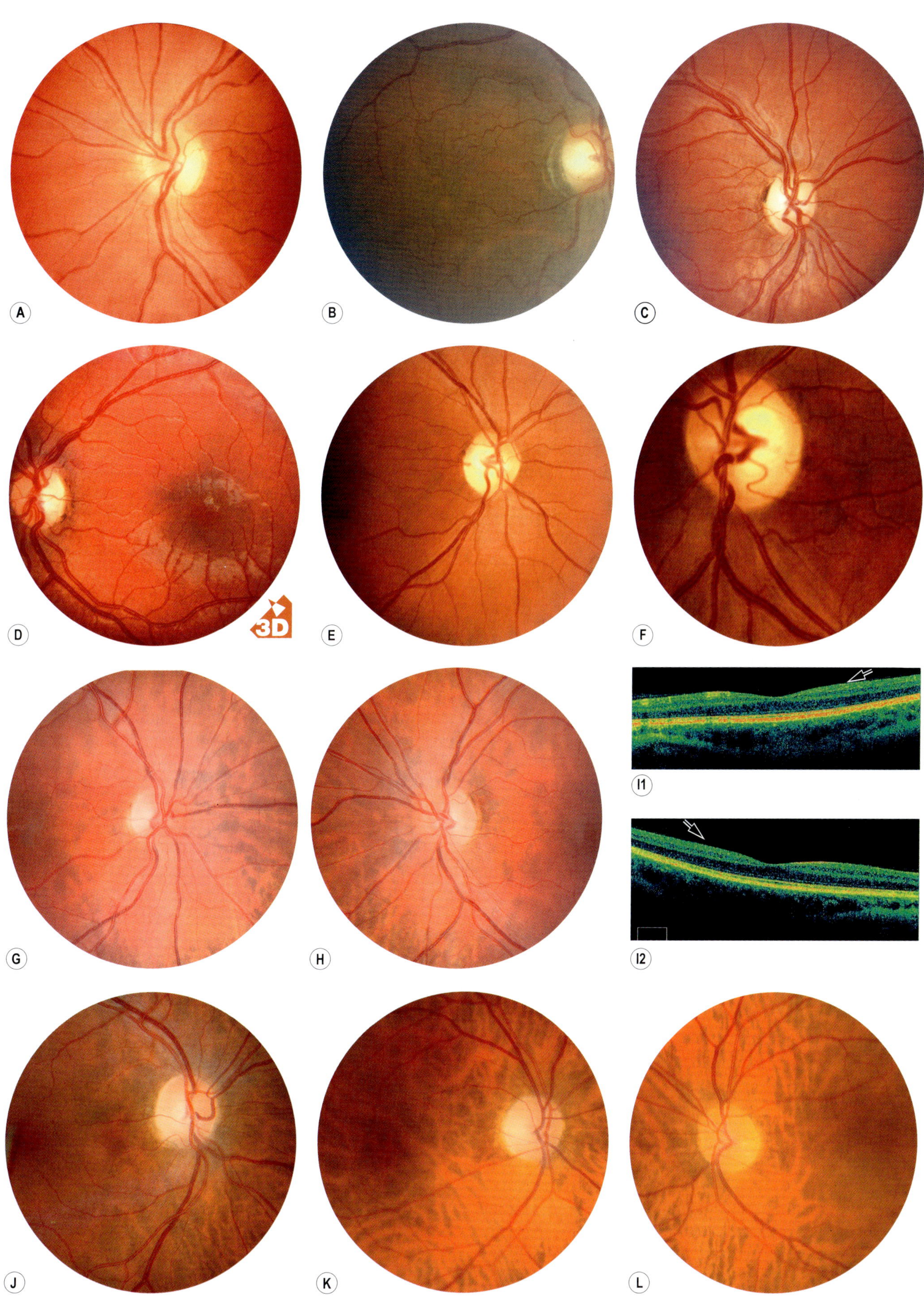
A
B
C
D
3D
E
F
I1
G
H
I2
J
K
L

Leber's Hereditary Optic Neuropathy

Leber's hereditary optic neuropathy (LHON) is a maternally inherited disease that is characterized by acute, severe, bilateral visual loss in healthy young persons (15–35 years), usually males (80–90%).[231–233] The visual loss can occur in younger and older individuals and the age range of onset is 2–80 years. This variability of age at onset can occur in members of the same family.[234–237] The central visual loss is acute or subacute at onset, painless, and accompanied by large cecocentral scotomata and dyschromatopsia. Central vision deteriorates progressively, first in one eye then in the other, typically with an interval of days to weeks. Intervals of as long as 12 years have been reported.[238] Transient worsening with exercise or warming, as occurs in other optic neuropathies (Uhthoff's symptom), may occur.[238–240] All levels of visual acuity loss have been reported ranging from no light perception to 20/20, but it commonly declines to levels worse than 20/200 bilaterally, usually over several weeks to several months.[238,241] Although these patients are typically between the ages of 18 and 30 years at onset, visual loss may not occur until the sixth decade or beyond, when the clinical picture may be mistaken for AION.[238,242–245] Color vision is affected early, and visual field examination reveals a central or cecocentral scotoma.[238,239] Biomicroscopy reveals circumpapillary telangiectatic microangiopathy, swelling of the nerve fiber layer around the disc (pseudo-edema), and absence of fluorescein leakage (Figure 15.09).[240,246,247] Most patients show no improvement but partial or even complete recovery may occur 5–10 years after onset of visual loss.[238,248–251] Environmental triggers such as smoking, trauma, human immunodeficiency virus (HIV) infection can precipitate onset of visual loss in susceptible individuals carrying the genetic defect.[244,252,253] Dilation of the optic nerve sheaths with cerebrospinal fluid has been demonstrated by ultrasonography (30° test) and histopathologically.[254,255] Pathology of the retina and optic nerve is available only for late-stage disease. Ganglion cell atrophy, excavation of the optic disc cup filled with glial and connective tissue, and symmetric destruction of the myelin sheaths in the optic nerve transmitting papillomacular bundle fibers are the findings within the eye. The optic chiasm and tracts also showed loss of myelin sheaths and axis cylinders centrally with relative preservation of peripheral fibers. Shriveled lateral geniculate bodies and demyelination of the optic radiations suggest transsynaptic degeneration.[256]

Visual dysfunction is the only manifestation of LHON in most patients. Although other neurologic disorders are occasionally reported (LHON "plus"), the best-established link is between LHON and cardiac conduction abnormalities.[257–259] Wolff–Parkinson–White and Lown–Ganong–Levine are the most common associations (9%). Prolonged QT interval, syncope, palpitations, and sudden death are seen occasionally. Minor neurological associations include exaggerated reflexes, myoclonus, seizures, muscle wasting, sensory and auditory neuropathy, and migraine. More severe associations include movement disorders, spasticity, psychiatric disturbances, skeletal abnormalities, acute infantile encephalopathic episodes, dystonia, Leigh-like encephalopathy, periaqueductal syndrome, and demyelinating disease resembling multiple sclerosis.[260] A similar optic neuropathy has been reported with skeletal abnormalities,[238] and in association with Charcot–Marie–Tooth (CMT) disease, a hereditary disease of peripheral nerves in at least two families.[261,262] Uemura and coworkers have identified mild but distinct biochemical and electron microscopic changes in muscle biopsy in patients with LHON.[263] Wallace and others, in 1988, identified a mitochondrial replacement mutation in nine of 11 families with members diagnosed with LHON.[264]

When LHON appears for the first time in a family, the diagnosis is often delayed or missed. In the acute stage, circumpapillary telangiectatic microangiopathy, swelling of the nerve fiber layer around the optic disc (pseudo-edema), and absence of staining on fluorescein angiography are characteristic (Figures 15.09 and 15.10B).[239,240] Progressive enlargement of the blind spot until it reaches fixation characterizes the early progression of field loss. Many asymptomatic family members with Leber's disease have peripapillary microangiopathy.[241,246,265] These vascular changes may be evident angiographically and occur years before the acute phase of the disease.[266,267] They include progressive arteriovenous shunting that starts in the inferior arcuate nerve fibers and that may be associated occasionally with preretinal hemorrhages. Acute visual loss is accompanied by dilation of the branches of the central retinal artery and peripapillary telangiectatic capillaries.

15.09 Leber's optic neuropathy.

A–D: One year previously this 18-year-old man developed blurred vision in the right eye. The diagnosis at that time was retrobulbar neuritis. Neurologic evaluation was negative. He gave a 2-week history of blurred vision in the left eye. Visual acuity in the right eye was 6/200 and in the left eye was 20/300. There was segmental atrophy of the right optic disc. There was telangiectasis and tortuosity of the capillaries of the left optic disc and juxtapapillary retina (A). Angiography demonstrated the pattern of these abnormal vessels (arrows, B), which showed no evidence of late staining (C). Fourteen years later visual acuity in the right eye was 20/400 and in the left eye was 20/200. Both optic discs showed temporal pallor (D). The telangiectatic vessels were less apparent.
E and **F**: A 38-year-old man with acute Leber's optic neuropathy. Note the telangiectatic tortuous retinal vessels (arrows).
G–J: This 14-year-old boy, with a family history of Leber's optic neuropathy, presented because of rapid loss of vision of 3 weeks' duration. At age 12 years his visual acuity was 20/20 and genetic analysis of his blood was positive for Leber's disease. His visual acuity at the time of these photographs was 20/200 in the right eye and 9/200 left eye. The right optic disc was hyperemic (G); the left optic disc showed temporal pallor. There was generalized tortuosity of the retinal veins. Note the dilation and tortuosity of the small juxta-papillary venules (arrows, H). Several months later both optic discs showed temporal pallor (I and J) and the visual acuity was 3/200.
K and **L**: Optic atrophy in two siblings of the patient illustrated in G–J.

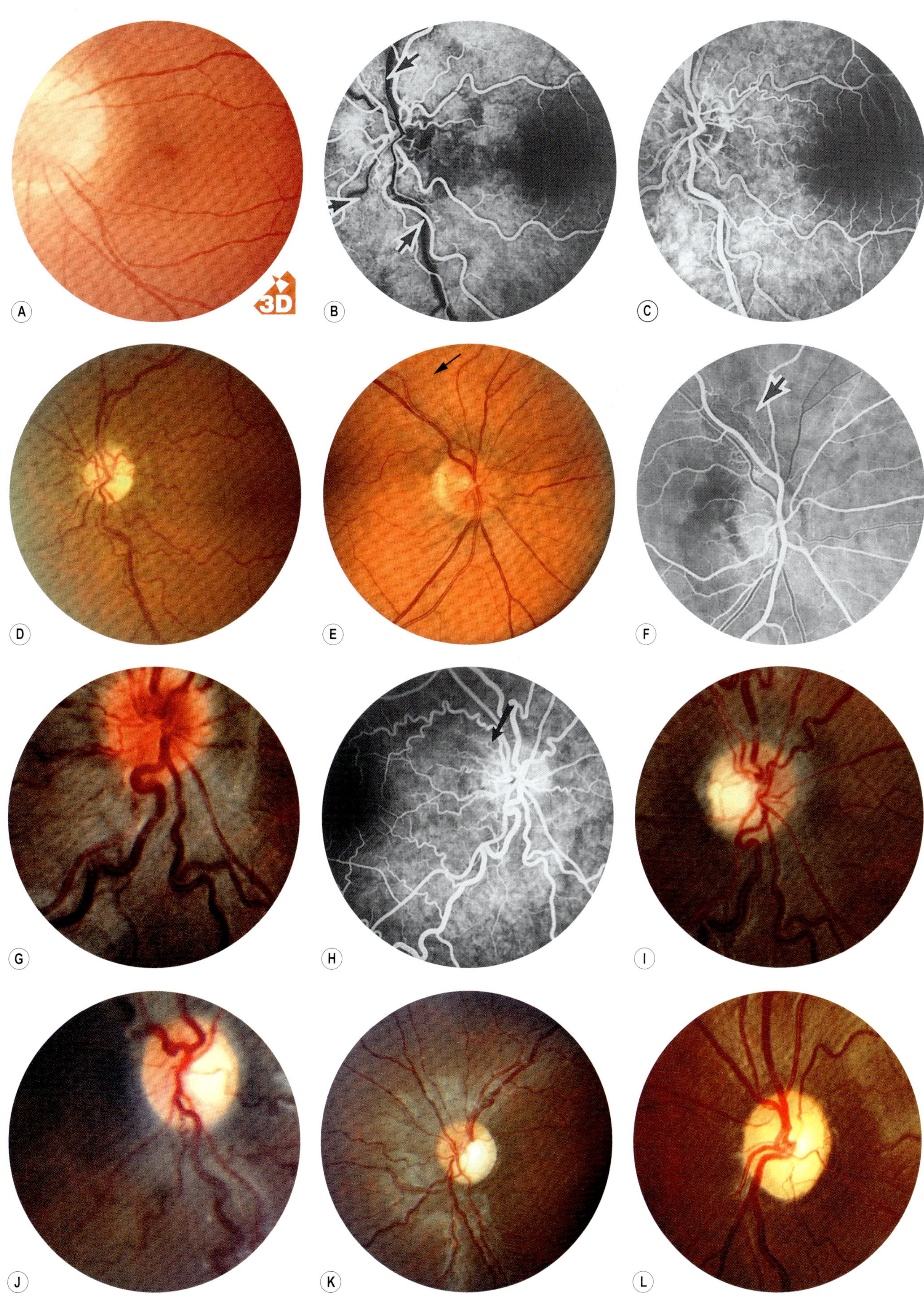
A
3D
B
C
D
E
F
G
H
I
J
K
L

These changes disappear as atrophy of the optic nerve develops (Figure 15.09D). Unlike dominant optic atrophy, the atrophy often progresses to involve the entire optic disc. Retinal arterial narrowing and increased circulation time occur. Angiography is probably useful in excluding Leber's disease in asymptomatic individuals.[266] Acquired red–green deficiency characterized by a deutan-like discrimination defect is characteristic and may be detected in some asymptomatic carriers. Electroretinography and dark adaptation are usually normal in these patients.[218] Visual loss typically stabilizes soon after onset, but some patients may show either improvement or worsening. There is no effective treatment for the disease. Since the primary locus of the disease appears to be in the intraocular rather than the retrobulbar area, Leber's hereditary vascular neuroretinopathy has been suggested as a more appropriate name.[241] LHON is strictly maternally inherited and passes to future generations only through women. An affected male never has affected offspring, whereas a woman may have affected children although she herself is visually normal.

LHON is associated with four different point mutations of mitochondrial DNA that appear to be pathogenetic for the disease.[231,248,254,255,264,268–274] These mutations affect nucleotide positions 11778, 14484, 3460, and 15257 and are located within the genes that code for proteins in the complex I of the respiratory chain. The clinical findings are similar, except that patients with 14484 are more likely to experience visual recovery than patients with the other three mutations.[231] Patients with 15257, who also have an associated mutation at 15812, are less likely to recover vision than those without this association.[275] Patients with the 15257 mutation also have a higher incidence of spinal cord and peripheral neurologic symptoms than patients with the other mutations. Molecular genetic testing is of practical value in confirming the diagnosis of atypical cases or in patients presenting with optic atrophy, in the absence of a family history, and after the characteristic telangiectasis is no longer evident.[270,275] The proportion of mutant mitochondrial DNA molecules was found to shift markedly across generations and within tissues of an individual (heteroplasmy). This explains the variability of expression of the disease in family members. Approximately 20% of men and 4% of women experienced visual loss in an Australian study where a dramatic decline in the penetrance of the disease has been noted.[276–280] Therefore, successful determination of the mitochondrial DNA genotype of a family or patient with LHON requires testing of more than one family member and more than one tissue from each individual.[271] Molecular genetic tests are 100% specific but only 50% sensitive for the diagnosis of LHON. It may be prudent to advise carriers to avoid exposure to toxins such as tobacco smoke and excessive alcohol intake since they may further compromise mitochondrial energy metabolism.[269,281]

15.10 Leber's heredtary optic neuropathy.

A–C: A 20-year-old otherwise healthy man who had painless loss of vision in his left eye to 20/100. Vision in the right eye was 20/20. Redfree photographs and fluorescein angiogram show telangiectasia of small vessels around the disc (arrows). Optical coherence tomography of the left eye shows thickened "nerve fiber layer-pseudoedema" compared to the right eye and is outside the normal range. His maternal male cousins had unexplained loss of vision and he had a genetic mitochondrial point mutation at 11778.

Leber's idiopathic stellate neuroretinitis.

D and E: A 38-year-old woman developed blurred vision in the right eye 11 days after an episode of headaches, vomiting, and diarrhea. Note the oval, yellowish exudate in the center of the macula and the fine macular star, which is more prominent nasally than temporally (D). There is some exudative detachment of the peripapillary retina. The left fundus was normal. Angiography showed definite leakage of dye from the optic disc and no evidence of abnormality in the macular area (E). Angiography of the left eye was normal.

F and G: This 31-year-old man gave a 1-month history of decreased vision in his left eye. Visual acuity was 20/50. Note the faint yellowish material in the center of the macula and the macular star, which is more prominent nasally (F). The optic disc is within normal limits. Angiography of the right eye was normal. Angiography of the left eye (G) showed marked fluorescence of the optic disc.

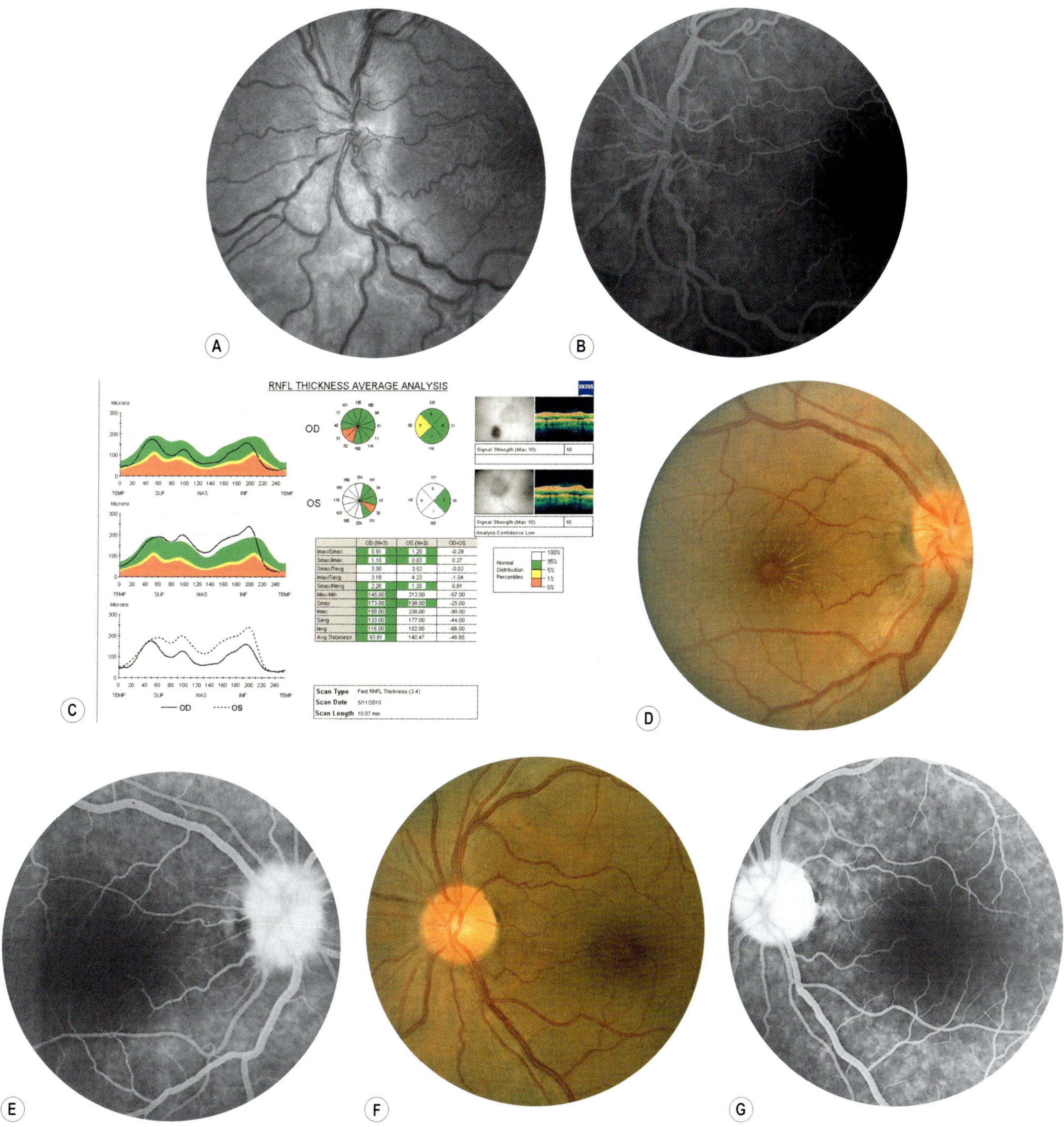
A
B
RNFL THICKNESS AVERAGE ANALYSIS
Microns
TEMP SUP NAS INF TEMP
OD
OS
Signal Strength (Max 10) 10
Analysis Confidence Low
Normal Distribution Percentiles
100%
95%
5%
1%
0%

	OD (N=3)	OS (N=3)	OD-OS
Imax/Smax	0.91	1.20	-0.29
Smax/Imax	1.10	0.83	0.27
Smax/Tavg	3.50	3.52	-0.02
Imax/Tavg	3.18	4.22	-1.04
Smax/Navg	2.26	1.35	0.91
Max-Min	145.00	212.00	-67.00
Smax	173.00	198.00	-25.00
Imax	158.00	238.00	-80.00
Savg	133.00	177.00	-44.00
Iavg	116.00	182.00	-66.00
Avg.Thickness	93.81	140.47	-46.65

Scan Type Fast RNFL Thickness (3.4)
Scan Date 5/11/2010
Scan Length 10.87 mm
C
D
E
F
G

Histopathologically, the macular star is caused by the microglial ingestion of the lipid-rich exudate lying in the outer plexiform layer of Henle. Figure 15.11M depicts diagrammatically the probable pathogenesis of a macular star. A protein- and lipid-rich exudate leaks from the capillaries in the depth of the optic disc and extends beneath the retina in the peripapillary region as well as along the plane of the outer plexiform layer into the macular region.[210,284] With reabsorption of the serous component of the exudate in the macular region the lipid and protein precipitate in the outer plexiform layer and are engulfed by macrophages. This creates the fine stellate pattern of yellow exudate that is characteristic of a macular star. Stellate maculopathy is caused by a variety of diseases affecting the permeability of the capillaries in the depth of the optic nerve head. Retinal vascular diseases usually cause a more irregular and coarser deposition of yellowish exudate in the inner nuclear as well as the outer plexiform layers in the macular region.

The differential diagnosis of patients with an optic disc swelling and a macular star includes hypertensive retinopathy (see Figures 6.25A and 6.26D), diabetic optic neuropathy and diseases associated with optic neuritis, such as sarcoidosis, bacterial septic optic neuritis, Lyme disease, and luetic optic neuritis.[302] A macular star infrequently accompanies diffuse unilateral subacute neuroretinitis and is rarely, if ever, seen in patients with optic neuritis secondary to demyelinating diseases.[283] The possibility of septic retinitis caused by pyogenic bacteria, cat-scratch disease, toxoplasmosis, or fungi is greater in those patients who manifest multifocal retinitis. The differential diagnosis in those presenting with a branch retinal artery or vein inclusion expands to include idiopathic recurrent branch retinal artery disease and Eales' disease (see Chapter 6). Management of these patients depends upon the ocular findings and the presence or absence of signs and symptoms of systemic disease. Many of these patients are afebrile and the antecedent illness has resolved by the time of their eye examination. A general physical examination, routine blood counts, and serology to exclude syphilis may be all that is necessary. Those with multifocal retinitis, and particularly those who are febrile, should have appropriate evaluation including blood cultures to exclude systemic septic disease. Serologic testing for exposure to *Bartonella*, skin test for cat-scratch disease, and biopsy of enlarged lymph nodes may be appropriate in those patients exposed to cats. The *Bartonella* bacillus can be identified with the Warthin–Starry stain. The visual

15.11 Leber's idiopathic stellate neuroretinitis with angiographic evidence of involvement of the asymptomatic eye.

A–D: This 9-year-old girl noted rapid loss of vision in the right eye. Note the macular star and slight swelling and pallor of the optic disc (A). The left fundus appeared normal (B). Visual acuity was 20/200 in the right eye and 20/20 in the left eye. Angiography revealed staining of the temporal half of the right optic disc (C) and the superonasal quadrant of the left optic disc (D).
E–I: This 14-year-old girl had a history of an upper respiratory infection before the onset of visual loss in the left eye. She also had a 6-month history of intermittent fever of unknown origin. Her visual acuity was 20/50 in the left eye. Note swelling of the left optic disc (E) and small white retinal lesions in the left fundus (arrows, E and F) and one that was unnoticed in the asymptomatic right eye until review of her angiographic study (arrows, G and H). The white lesions in the left eye as well as of the optic disc stained (I). Spinal fluid examination revealed pleocytosis. Spinal fluid and blood cultures were negative.
J–L: A 24-year-old female with bilateral asymmetric disc edema secondary to cat-scratch disease. Macular star is seen in the more involved right eye (J). The left fundus shows several focal inner retinitis that is often seen in these patients (L, arrows). Her visual acuity was light perception in the right and 20/20 in the left. There was a functional element to the visual loss in the right eye. One month later her vision had improved to 20/25 in the right and 20/15 in the left eye and the macular star had broken up with resolution of disc swelling bilaterally.
M: The pathogenesis of a macular star. Lipid-rich exudate leaking from capillaries within the depth of the optic nerve head (small arrows) extends into the subretinal space surrounding the optic nerve head as well as along the outer plexiform layer into the macular region. Reabsorption of the serous portion of the exudate leaves a concentrated lipid exudate (large arrows) in the outer plexiform layer of Henle and causes a macular star that is usually more prominent in the nasal half of the macula.

(J–L, courtesy of Dr. Patrick Lavin.)

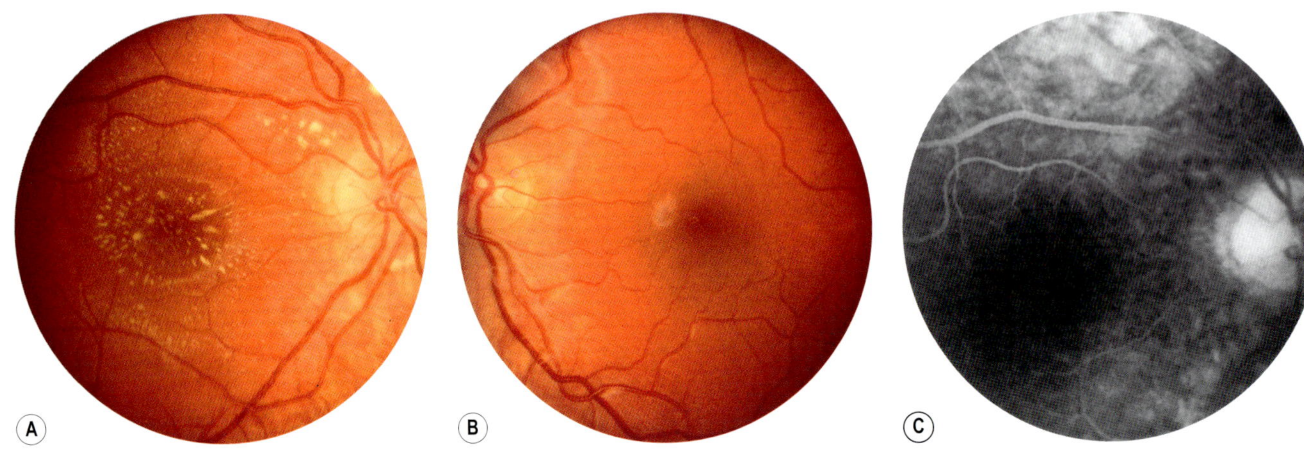

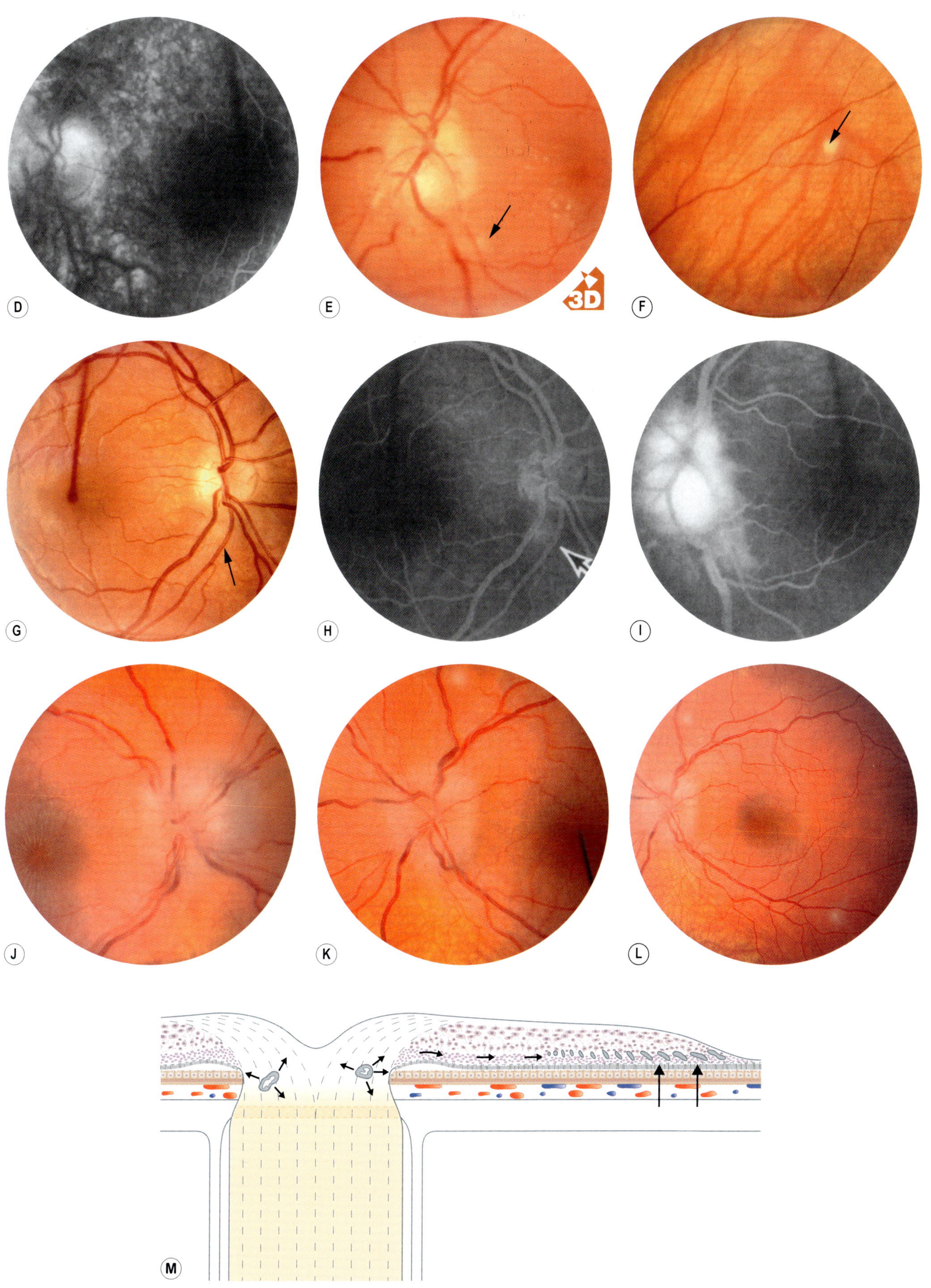
D
E
3D
F
G
H
I
J
K
L
M

prognosis for patients with idiopathic stellate neuroretinitis and multifocal retinitis is good, and no treatment is required. An occasional patient will have a recurrence in the opposite eye months or years later (see Chapter 10).

Purvin and Chioran reported on seven young adults (mean age of 27 years) who developed multiple episodes of monocular neuroretinitis, macular star formation, dense arcuate visual field defects, and in some cases severe permanent visual loss.[303] Both eyes were eventually affected in five patients. Laboratory studies were not revealing and the disorder appeared unresponsive to systemic corticosteroids. Except for the presence of a macular star, their cases seem to share more in common with AION in young patients (see discussion of idiopathic AION in the young, below).

RECURRENT OPTIC NEUROPATHY ASSOCIATED WITH FAMILY HISTORY OF CHARCOT–MARIE–TOOTH DISEASE

Progressive muscular weakness and atrophy that begin in the first two decades of life characterize CMT disease spectrum. CMT is a genetically heterogeneous group of diseases that accounts for almost 90% of hereditary polyneuropathies.[304–306] The commonest form, CMT type 1, is an autosomal-dominantly inherited demyelinating neuropathy mapped most commonly to the short arm of chromosome 17(17p11.2) type 1A, and a few to long arm of chromosome 1(type 1B). Type 2 CMT has a similar clinical phenotype but nerve conduction is normal, suggesting the disease is neuronal rather than demyelinating. It is inherited in a dominant fashion (short arm of chromosome 1) or recessively (long arm of chromosome 8). Type 3 is the most severe form – AD linked to chromosome 1, the same locus as type 1B, and AR to chromosome 17, same as type 1A. X-linked dominant and recessive forms are also seen.

Systemic features begin with foot deformities, pes cavus, and scoliosis, followed by progressive weakening of the muscles of the leg, feet, and hands. Sensory abnormalities are few. Progressive optic atrophy that usually begins in the sixth decade or later has been reported in several pedigrees.[307–310] Subclinical optic neuropathy can be detected by electrophysiologic testing in asymptomatic individuals. CMT type 6 is especially associated with optic atrophy. This 40-year-old woman had a family history of clinically diagnosed CMT disease in her brother, niece, paternal aunt, and father. She had no neurological disease, but presented with recurrent optic neuritis associated with lipid exudation that improved with systemic steroid therapy each time (Figure 15.12).

15.12 Recurrent optic neuropathy associated with family history of Charcot–Marie–Tooth disease.

A–I: This 46-year-old woman presented with decreased vision in the left eye associated with pain on eye movements. She complained of gradual decrease in peripheral vision in both eyes over 2 years. Her father, paternal aunt, brother, and brother's daughter carried a diagnosis of Charcot–Marie–Tooth disease and her sister had "uveitis." Visual acuity was 20/30 in the right eye and count fingers in the left eye. The right optic disc was pale and the left swollen with lipid exudates into the macula (A, B). Optical coherence tomography confirmed macular thickening with intraretinal lipid (C). She received oral steroids followed by cyclophosphamide. The vision in the left eye improved to 20/80 in 2 weeks but the right eye vision dropped to 20/400. She now had a swollen right optic disc and the left macular exudates were clearing (D, E). Four months later visual acuity had improved to 20/50 in the right eye and 20/60– in the left eye (F, G). The optic nerves were pale with no swelling and the lipid exudates were resolving. Two months later all lipid exudates were absorbed with residual optic atrophy and vision of 20/50 in the right and 20/60– in the left eye (H, I). Goldmann visual fields showed severe constriction in both eyes and electroretinogram showed normal rod and cone function. Neurological exam did not reveal neuropathy or myopathy. She was negative for the known mutations for Leber's hereditary optic neuropathy. A biopsy of her normal skin was consistent with autoimmune/connective tissue disease. She has been continued on low-dose immunosuppressives.

FAMILIAL DYSAUTONOMIA

Familial dysautonomia (Riley–Day syndrome) is an autosomal-recessive disorder causing congenital sensory and autonomic dysfunction that affects Ashkenazi Jews exclusively.

The disease is present from birth, manifested as hypotonia and feeding difficulties resulting in frequent aspirations and pneumonias. Autonomic disturbances with lack of emotional tears, defective body temperature control, cold hands and feet, excessive sweating over head and trunk when emotionally excited, skin blotching, blood pressure lability, and orthostatic hypotension are hallmarks of the disease. There is also decreased sensitivity to pain and temperature, hypo- or areflexia, poor corneal sensation, and pupillary abnormalities.[311] Progressive optic atrophy is seen in those patients that survive beyond early childhood.[312–314]

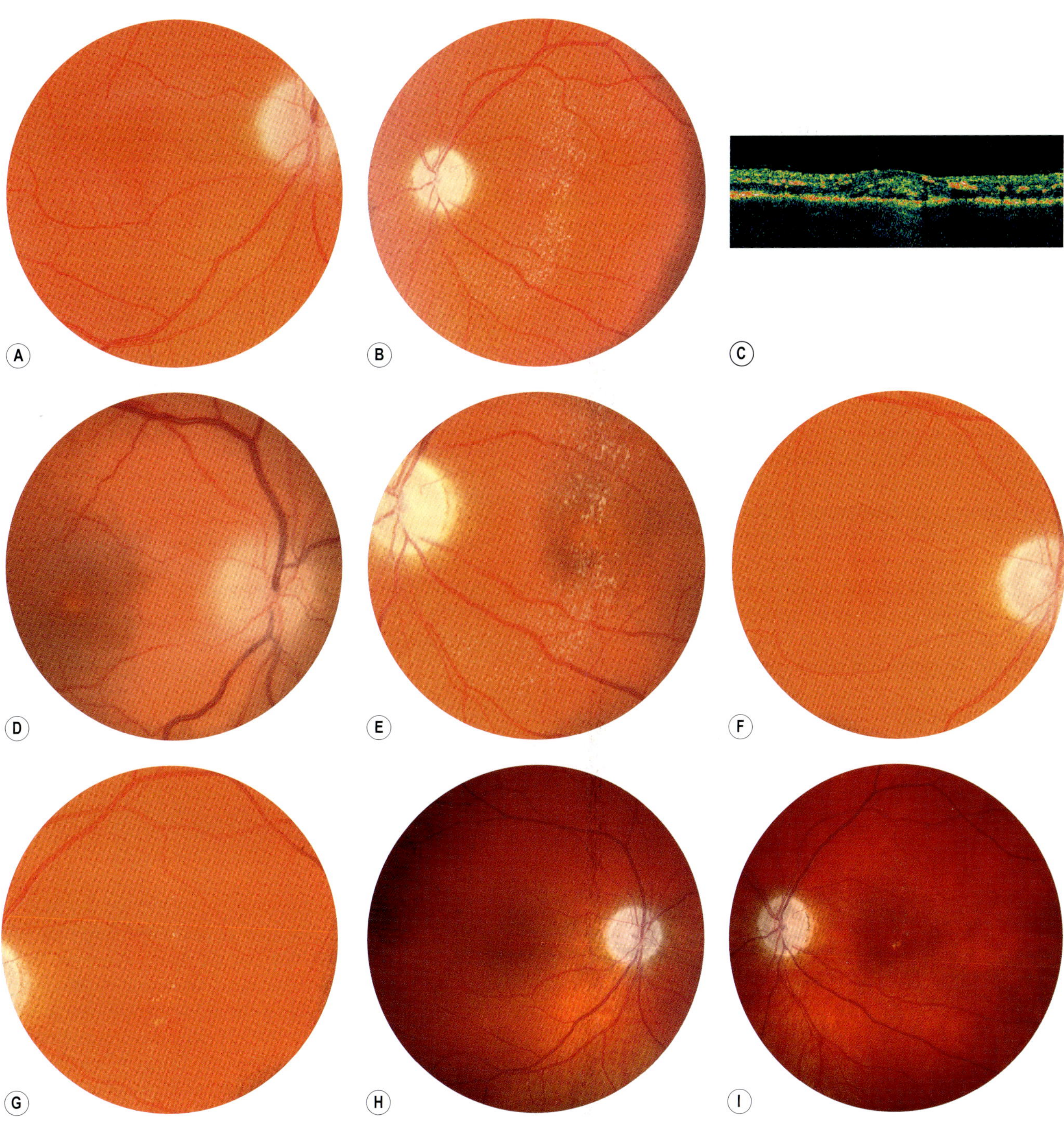
A
B
C
D
E
F
G
H
I

NEURORETINOPATHY AND PROGRESSIVE FACIAL HEMIATROPHY

Progressive facial hemiatrophy (Parry–Romberg syndrome) is a disorder of unknown cause that is characterized by progressive unilateral atrophy of the skin, muscles, and bony structures of the face, usually in preadolescent patients.[217–224,315–322] It may extend down into the neck, shoulders, trunk, and extremities. All of the facial structures on one side may be involved (Figure 15.13D and H), or there may be only a linear depression in the scalp and forehead (coup de sabre) (Figure 15.13A). Vitiligo, poliosis, nevus flammeus, and moles are often present on the affected side. Ptosis, trichiasis, lagophthalmos, ectropion, neuroparalytic keratitis, canalicular obstruction, dacryocystitis, extraocular muscle palsies, enophthalmos, Horner's syndrome, heterochromia of the iris, uveitis, optic atrophy, and pigmentary disturbances of the fundi may occur. The brain may show evidence of hemiatrophy, homolateral migraine, contralateral epilepsy, evidence of encephalitis, intracranial vascular malformations; and occasionally movement disorders may be present.[323–330] This syndrome is not usually associated with visual loss. Visual loss, however, may be caused by either ipsilateral neuroretinopathy characterized by acute visual loss, optic disc swelling, peripapillary exudation, and macular star, or retinal telangiectasis and exudative retinal detachment (Figure 15.13A–I and see Figure 6.40I–L).[217–221,315–319] Ultrasonography may demonstrate some enlargement of the affected optic nerve. The optic foramina are normal radiographically. Optic atrophy may occur as the peripapillary and macular exudation clears, but no patient has demonstrated progressive loss of visual field. Retinal vascular abnormalities have been reported previously in this disorder[316,318,319] (see Chapter 6, Coats' syndrome).

The pathogenesis of the acute neuroretinopathy and retinal vasculopathy is unknown. The pathogenesis of the entire disorder is complex and poorly understood. Autonomic dysfunction secondary to sympathetic abnormality as evidenced by Horner's syndrome[331,332]; autoimmune etiology due to positive autoantibodies to double-stranded DNA, and some features common to scleroderma[333–337]; facial trauma as the inciting factor; trigeminal neuritis as evidenced by hemifacial changes; genetic etiology due to familial occurrence; developmental abnormality; possible encephalitis due to association of Rasmussen encephalitis in some[326,327] have all been considered. None of these hypotheses explains all the manifestations seen in the condition. It is best considered a disorder of clinical heterogeneity likely caused by etiological heterogeneity.

ANTERIOR ISCHEMIC OPTIC NEUROPATHY

The term "anterior ischemic optic neuropathy" is used to describe swelling, ischemia, and varying degrees of infarction of the anterior part of the optic nerve caused by reduction in blood flow to the nerve (Figures 15.14 and 15.15). The optic nerve head, by virtue of its closely arranged nerve fibers within the nonexpansile intrascleral canal, is ideally situated for ischemia to occur. Primary vascular insufficiency or secondary vascular insufficiency caused by any process that promotes stasis of axoplasmic flow and nerve fiber swelling can cause ischemia. AION typically affects older patients, and the acute loss of vision may be mistakenly attributed to a macular disorder, for example, macular degeneration if pigment epithelial changes are present, or to cystoid macular edema in the aphakic patient (Figure 15.14K and L). For pathogenetic as well as therapeutic reasons, these patients can be subdivided into two major subgroups: (1) a nonarteritic group, n-AION (those without evidence of arteritis, 95%) and (2) an arteritic group, a-AION (those with giant-cell arteritis, 5%). The nonarteritic group may be subdivided into an idiopathic group, those with no identifiable cause, and those with a probable cause. Functionally, ophthalmoscopically, and fluorescein angiographically, all subgroups may present similar findings. The visual prognosis, however, is not the same for all groups.

15.13 Acute neuroretinopathy and progressive facial hemiatrophy (Parry–Romberg syndrome).

A–C: This 21-year-old woman, who had developed a linear depression of the forehead and scalp beginning at 4 years of age (A), had a 6-week history of acute visual loss in the ipsilateral eye caused by stellate exudative neuroretinopathy (B). Her visual acuity was 5/200. Optic foramina roentgenograms were normal. Three and one-half years later, the optic disc was pale (C) and her visual acuity was 20/80.

D–G: This 8-year-old boy developed progressive loss of vision in the left eye on the same side that he had facial hemiatrophy (D) that began at 6 years of age. His visual acuity was 10/400. He had a stellate exudative neuroretinopathy (E). Angiography revealed capillary dilation (F) and late staining in the area of the swollen optic disc. It also showed evidence of some dilation and leakage of the peripheral retinal capillaries (G). Computed tomography (CT) revealed normal optic canals. Echography and CT showed some evidence of distention of the left optic nerve sheath.

H and I: This 13-year-old boy with progressive facial hemiatrophy (H), left deafness, congenital bowel defect, and hypospadias developed loss of vision in the right eye because of peripheral retinal telangiectasis and exudative retinal detachment (I). A similar exudative detachment was present in his opposite eye. Cryotherapy was successful in reattaching the retina in both eyes.

(H and I from Gass.[316])

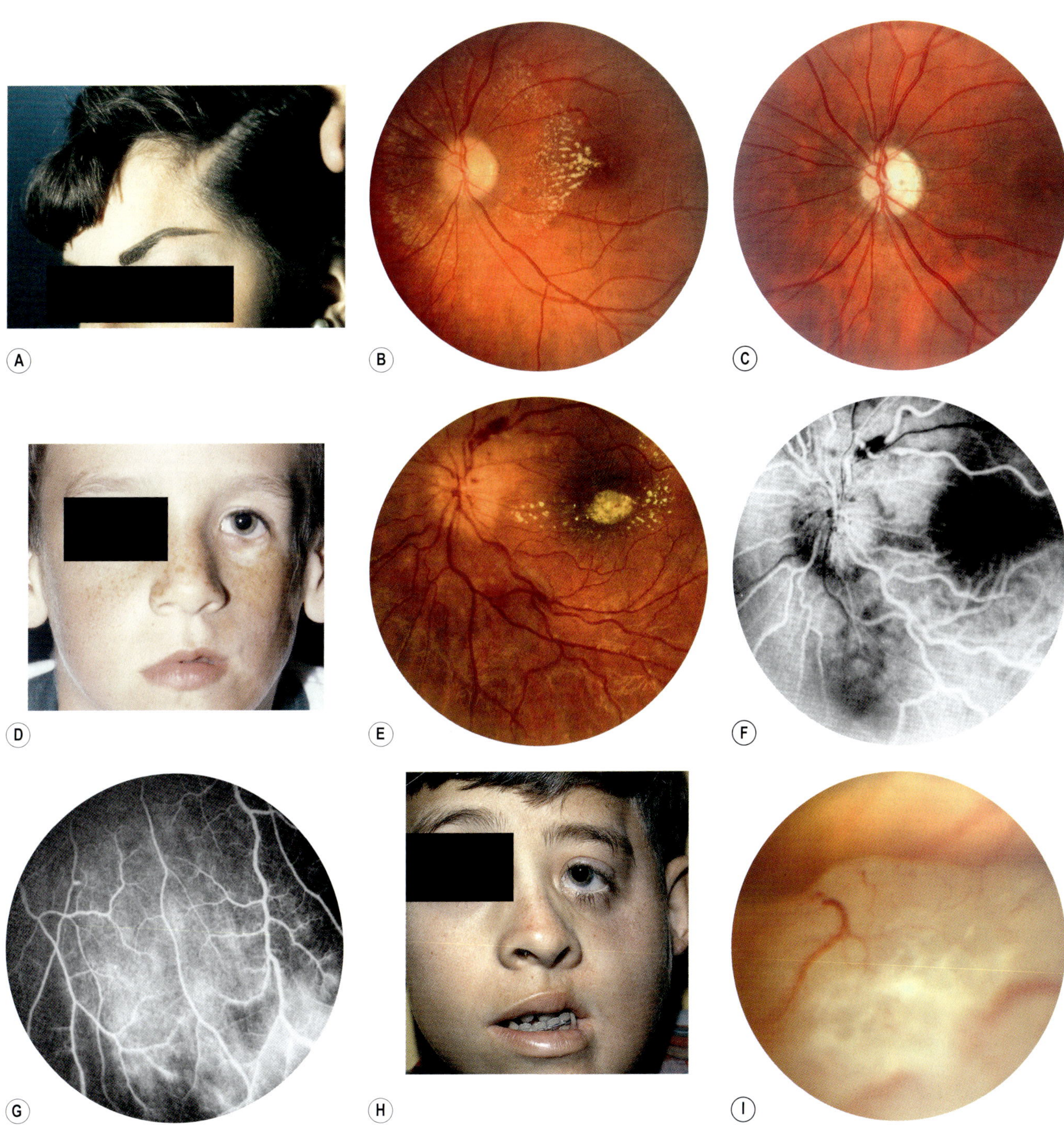
A
B
C
D
E
F
G
H
I

Idiopathic ("Nonarteritic") Anterior Ischemic Optic Neuropathy

Over 50% of patients with n-AION are generally healthy patients whose age is 45 years or older (mean of 57–65 years) and who experience an acute, usually moderate loss of vision in one eye (20/50 to 20/200) over hours to days.[338–346] Unlike patients with optic neuritis or arteritic AION (a-AION), pain and headache are not features. About 10% report a minor discomfort. Less than 5% report prodrome such as intermittent transient visual blurs, shadows, or spots that more often accompany a-AION. Optic disc swelling accompanied by one or several flame-shaped hemorrhages is usually evident (Figure 15.14). The swelling may or may not be pallid. It may be more pronounced in the superior half of the optic disc. A lower altitudinal or arcuate field defect that often is maximum at the time of presentation but that may progress during the first few weeks of the disease is present.[347,348] Occasionally hard exudates and cotton-wool spots are present (7%). Fluorescein angiography usually demonstrates a delay of perfusion of the optic disc blood vessels, minimal alterations of choroidal filling, and staining of the optic disc (Figure 15.14B and C).[349] In some cases there is a delay in the retinal artery appearance time, and an increased retinal circulation time, that presumably is caused by compression of the central retinal vessels by the swollen ischemic nerve fibers in the region of the lamina cribrosa. This compression occasionally may be sufficient to cause a fundus picture of central retinal artery or vein occlusion (Figure 15.14A–C). Occasionally the compression could occlude a cilioretinal artery or a branch retinal artery coming off the disc (Figure 15.14G–I). Focal telangiectatic changes may appear on the surface vessels of the disc within a few days, considered to be luxury perfusion due to autoregulatory response by increased perfusion surrounding an infarct. Sometimes this may be interpreted as a capillary hemangioma or neovascularization when prominent (Figure 15.14K).[350] The disc swelling resolves in several weeks. The disc becomes pale and usually shows minimal cupping. Spontaneous improvement of visual acuity occurs in 10–35% of cases.[351–355] Recurrence of n-AION in the same eye is infrequent.[339,356,357] Possible explanations for the infrequent recurrences in n-AION include loss of nerve fibers after n-AION, providing more space for surviving nerve fibers to swell, and shunting of blood from the area of infarction to the surviving part of the nerve.[345,357,358] Approximately 40% of patients will develop n-AION in the opposite eye.[359] Although it has been presumed that most of these patients probably have an arteriosclerotic disorder, there is minimal evidence to support this view. These patients have no greater incidence of cardiovascular or cerebrovascular disease than a matched group of patients.[346,360–362] Idiopathic or n-AION occurs at a younger age in smokers (mean age 51 years) compared to nonsmokers (mean age 64 years).[363] The frequency of involvement in the upper half of the optic disc,[338,341,346] the rarity of second attacks of AION in the same eye,[339] and the small cup/disc ratio[187,338,339,343,360,364–366] suggest that structural factors are important in the pathogenesis of idiopathic AION.

Associated disorders that may precipitate nonarteritic AION include diabetes, malignant hypertension (Figure 15.15A and B), uremia,[367,368] eclampsia,[369,370] migraine,[357] embolism,[371–373] hemodynamic shock,[374,375] anemia,[376] papilledema, orbital inflammation (Figure 15.14A–C), cataract extraction (Figure 15.13K and L),[377–380] elevation of intraocular pressure,[381–383] congenital anomalies of the optic disc, and optic disc drusen.[184] Subretinal neovascularization occasionally occurs.[384] Familial n-AION has been reported.[385] HLA-A29 may be a risk factor for development of n-AION.[386]

15.14 Nonarteritic anterior ischemic neuropathy.

A–C: This 57-year-old woman with noncongestive thyroid exophthalmos noted rapid loss of vision in the left eye. Her visual acuity was 4/200. The left optic disc was swollen, and a flame-shaped hemorrhage was present at its margin (A). Angiography showed a marked increase in retinal circulation time and late staining of the disc (B and C). She had an inferior attitudinal visual field defect. The acuity remained 20/200 in spite of intensive oral corticosteroid treatment for 2 months. She received X-ray irradiation to the left orbit. Her acuity 1 year later was 20/40.

D and E: Acute visual loss and an inferior attitudinal field defect occurred in the right eye of this healthy elderly patient with optic disc swelling and juxtapapillary hemorrhages (D) and a visual acuity decrease to 20/40. The left eye was normal with 20/20 vision (E).

F: This 67-year-old patient with marked inferior tilting of both optic discs developed acute visual loss and an inferior attitudinal field defect in the right eye. Note the pale swelling of the upper part of the disc (F) and the juxtapapillary subretinal hemorrhage. Several months later the blood resolved and there was remarkably little pallor of the optic disc (G).

G–J: This 61-year-old hypertensive woman experienced visual loss to 20/400 due to a nonarteritic anterior ischemic optic neuropathy 2 years previously in the right eye which eventually improved to 20/80. She developed ischemic optic neuropathy associated with a branch retinal artery occlusion in the left eye, and her vision dropped to 8/200. She also had fine cuticular drusen in both eyes that lit up early on the angiogram (H and I). The vessels on the disc were dilated and the flow through the branch retinal artery was delayed. Her visual acuity in the left eye improved to 20/50– in 2 months. The branch retinal artery showed sheathing and the disc edema had resolved (J).

K and L: This 67-year-old hypertensive patient experienced visual loss caused by ischemic optic neuropathy (K) soon after uneventful cataract extraction. Cystoid macular edema was suspected, but angiography revealed staining of the optic disc and no evidence of retinal capillary leakage in the macula. He subsequently developed optic atrophy (L). A similar course of events occurred in his left eye.

(G–J, courtesy of Dr. Edward Cherney.)

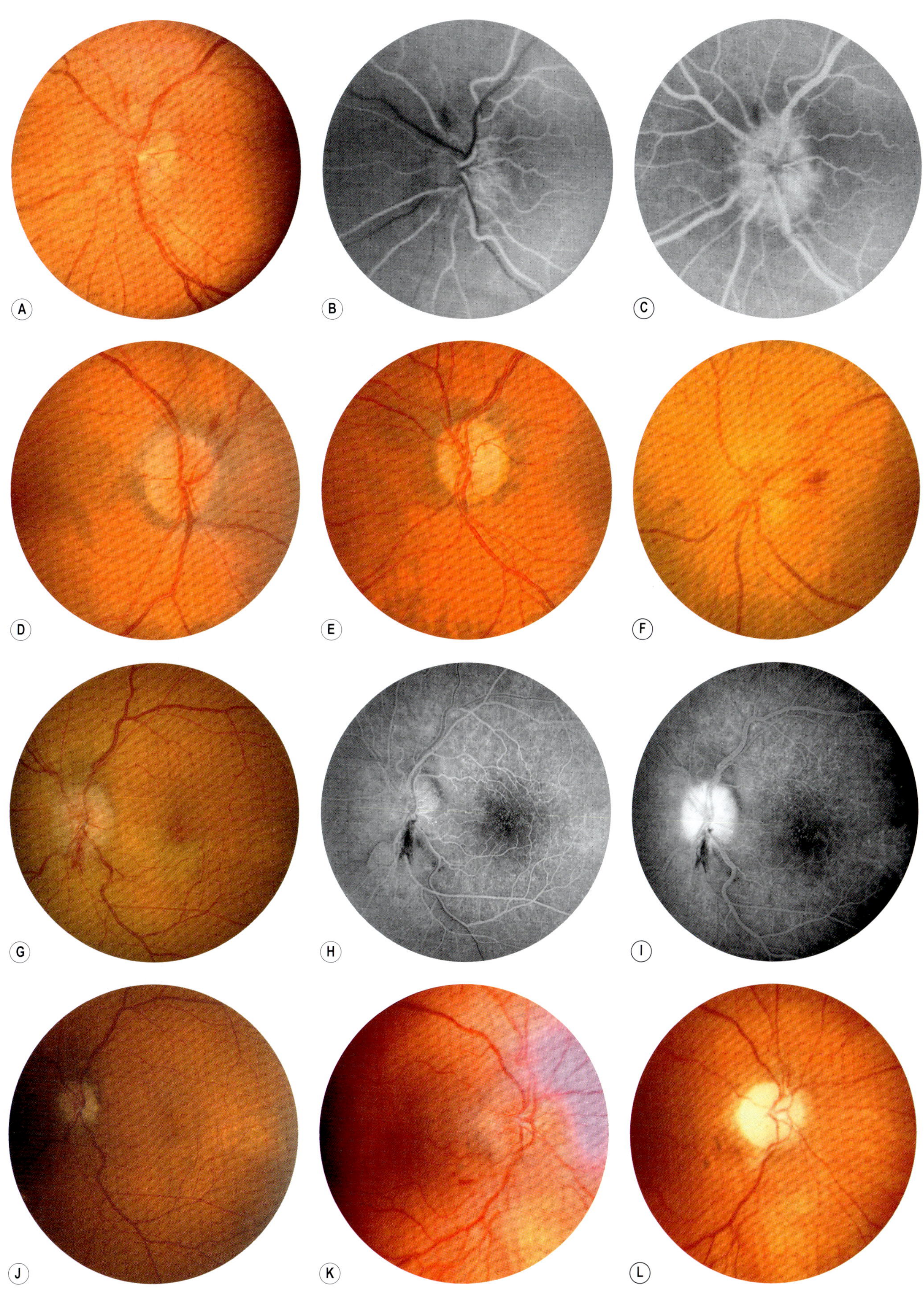
A
B
C
D
E
F
G
H
I
J
K
L

Histopathologic evidence suggests that vascular insufficiency causing acute ischemic swelling of a segment of the nerve fibers immediately posterior to the lamina cribrosa is responsible for the clinical picture of n-AION.[387] Vasculopathy of the paraoptic branches of the short posterior ciliary arteries may play a major role. The reason for the susceptibility of the superior segments of the optic nerve to ischemic damage and the role of nocturnal hypotension and sleep apnea are uncertain.

Additional factors that might affect perfusion such as optic disc drusen, hyperopia, elevated intraocular pressure, migraine, and drugs such as sildenafil and interferon-alpha may have a role in some cases. Amiodarone may itself cause toxic optic neuropathy or trigger an ischemic optic neuropathy in susceptible individuals, hence a history of its use should be sought.[388,389] There is no proven treatment for n-AION; aspirin is recommended for its role in decreasing strokes and myocardial infarctions in this vasculopathic population.[389]

Idiopathic Anterior Ischemic Optic Neuropathy in the Young (AIONY)

Idiopathic AIONY is a rare entity characterized by recurrent episodes of acute visual loss associated with segmental pallid swelling of the optic nerve that frequently causes severe and permanent visual loss in otherwise healthy young adults with a mean age of onset of 25 years.[357,390] The fundus picture and visual field changes during the acute stage are identical to those in n-AION. This similarity includes the small optic disc size. Medical evaluation is negative. The cause is unknown.

It is important therapeutically to differentiate n-AION and AIONY from a-AION. The blood sedimentation rate, acute-phase reactants such as C-reactive proteins, and platelet counts are usually within normal limits in n-AION and AIONY and are usually greatly elevated in most cases of a-AION.

There is no effective treatment for n-AION or AIONY. Optic nerve sheath decompression was suggested as effective in the treatment of the acute progressive stage of n-AION.[391–394] Evidence, however, including the results of a controlled clinical trial, indicates that the procedure is ineffective and may be harmful for the treatment of n-AION.[355,395–401] The rate of operative complications, which include central retinal artery occlusion associated with optic nerve sheath decompression, may be as high as 40%.[402] Treatment of the associated systemic disorders in patients with nonarteritic AION, for example, corticosteroids or X-ray irradiation in orbital inflammatory disease (Figure 15.14A–C), blood transfusion for patients with anemia, or hemodialysis in patients with uremia, may improve the prognosis for return of vision.[367,368] Patients with evidence of a-AION require prompt treatment with high doses of corticosteroids (see next subsection).

15.15 Anterior ischemic optic neuropathy (AION).

A and **B**: Hemorrhagic nonarteritic AION associated with a branch retinal artery occlusion in a severely hypertensive 40-year-old patient. Note ischemic whitening of the retina superotemporally (B).
C: Arteritic AION in a 68-year-old woman with cranial arteritis. She presented because of blurred vision in the left eye. She previously lost vision in the right eye. Note the marked pallor of the swollen optic disc (C). Several months later the optic disc was atrophic.
D and **E**: Nonarteritic ischemic optic neuropathy caused by acute blood loss occurred in this 47-year-old woman who experienced massive extravasation of blood into the body tissues associated with liposuction. On the first postoperative day she noted roaring in the ear and no light perception in the right eye. The right optic disc was swollen and pale (D). The left eye was normal (E). Her hemoglobin was 5.5, and hematocrit was 16. Magnetic resonance imaging of the brain was normal. She was treated with prednisone, 80 mg daily, and received 2 units of blood. Her vision improved to light perception only.
F–L: This 80-year-old woman noticed double vision for 3 days prior to presentation. The double vision was replaced by a superior field loss on the day of presentation in her right eye. Her visual acuity was 20/30 in this eye and 20/20 in the unaffected left eye. The inferior half of the optic disc shows pallid swelling (F). A fluorescein angiogram shows delayed choroidal filling at 25 seconds (G) and up to 77 seconds (H). She was being treated for left temporomandibular joint arthritis for 4–5 months. She denied scalp tenderness and weight loss, but was mildly irritable. She received 1 gram of intravenous solumedrol followed by oral prednisone. A temporal artery biopsy showed thickened arterial wall with infiltration of inflammatory and giant cells (arrow, J) and an extremely narrowed lumen (I and J, arrow heads). Her vision remained at 20/30 with a superior field defect. The optic disc shows pallor in the inferior half at 1 month (K, L (arrow)).

(I and J, courtesy of Dr. Joyce Johnson.)

Arteritic Anterior Ischemic Optic Neuropathy (a-AION)

Giant-cell arteritis (temporal arteritis, cranial arteritis) is a systemic disease that is characterized by arthralgias, headaches, fever, weight loss, jaw claudication, myalgia, and, frequently, acute severe visual loss in one eye that is often followed by severe loss in the second eye in elderly patients, usually 60 years of age or older.[403,404] Ischemic necrosis of the scalp may occur in severe cases; often these patients are also irritable due to the myalgia in the examining chair.[405–409] The visual loss is generally more profound than in n-AION, and the optic disc pallor is usually more striking (Figure 15.15D and F and Figure 6.23L). Cotton-wool patches and flame-shaped hemorrhages may be present. Other findings may include hypotony, extraocular muscle palsies, and central retinal arterial as well as choroidal arterial occlusion (see Figure 6.23). Fluorescein angiography demonstrates delayed perfusion of the choroid and optic disc (Figure 15.15G and H).[410,411]

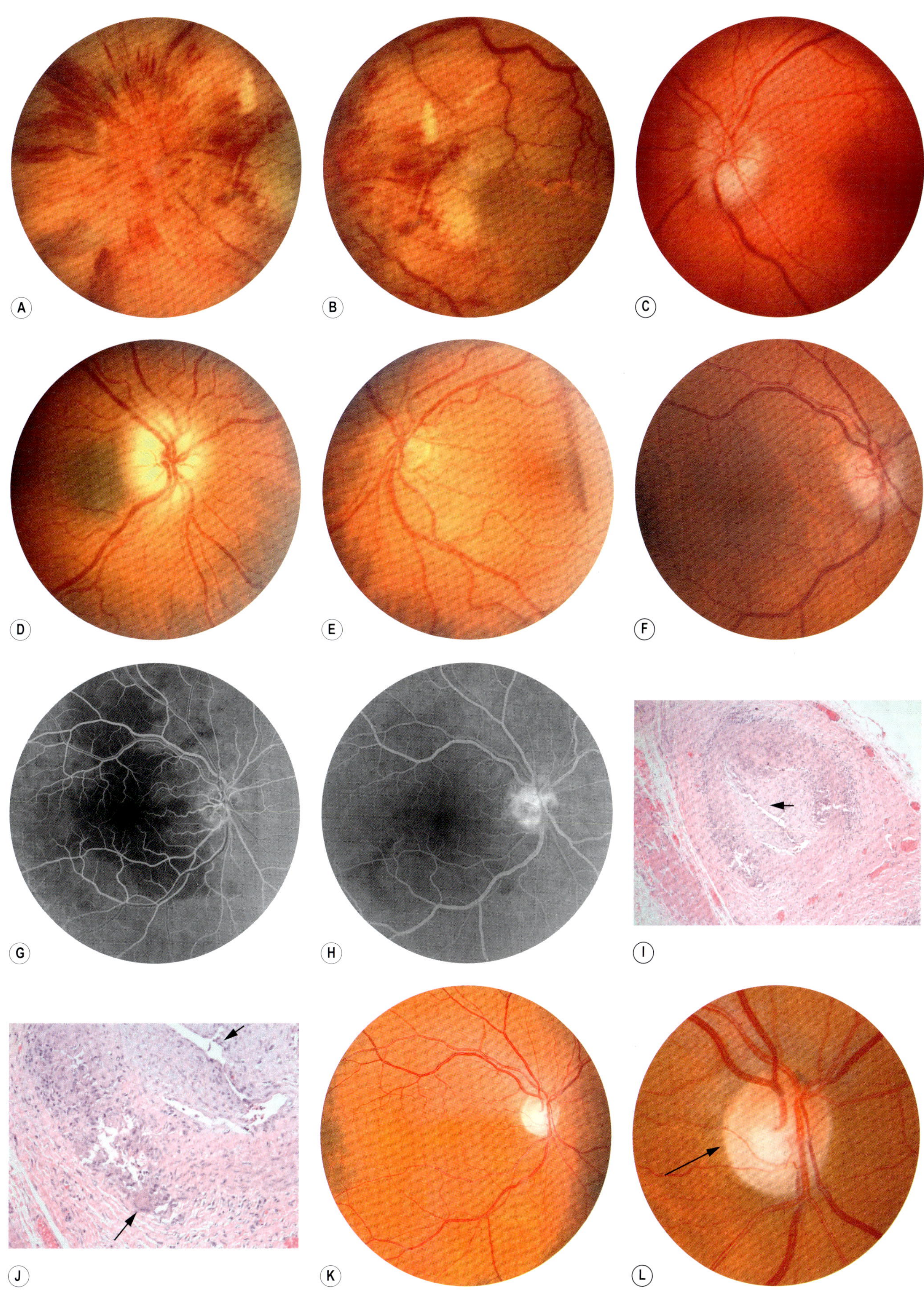
A
B
C
D
E
F
G
H
I
J
K
L

The Westergren sedimentation rate is usually 100 mm or greater; C-reactive proteins and platelets are elevated. Increased plasma viscosity, decreased red cell filterability, and decreased hematocrit are other findings in these patients.[412] The sedimentation rate and temporal artery biopsy findings are important in differentiating a-AION from n-AION.[404,412] Occasionally there may be a delay in the rise of the sedimentation rate, hence a high index of suspicion by positive review of systems warrants a repeat check 1–2 days later. Biopsy of the temporal artery shows infiltration and thickening of the media and proliferation into the lumen thus obliterating it, resulting in vascular insufficiency (Figure 15.15 I and J). Systemic corticosteroids should be instituted promptly if giant-cell arteritis is suspected. Monitoring changes in the blood sedimentation rate or C-reactive protein is used to adjust the corticosteroid dosage,[413] which should be continued for 2 years or more. The goal of steroid therapy is to prevent loss of vision in the fellow eye and involvement of other cranial arteries.

Development or progression of visual loss occurs rarely in patients with giant-cell arteritis after the initiation of glucocorticoid therapy.[359,414] In a retrospective study of 245 patients with giant-cell arteritis seen over a 5-year period at the Mayo Clinic, Aiello and coworkers found that 14% had permanent loss of vision in one or both eyes.[414] In all but two of the patients, visual loss occurred before institution of corticosteroid therapy. Visual loss progressed after corticosteroid therapy in three patients. After 5 years the probability of developing visual loss after initiation of oral glucocorticoid treatment was determined to be 1% (Kaplan–Meier), and the probability of additional loss in patients who had a visual deficit at the time therapy was begun was 13%.

Other rare causes of a-AION are periarteritis nodosa, Churg–Strauss syndrome, Wegener's granulomatosis, systemic lupus erythematosus, rheumatoid arthritis, and relapsing polychondritis. These conditions should be considered in patients who present earlier than 60 years of age or if review of systems points to any of them.

IDIOPATHIC OPTIC NEURITIS AND PAPILLITIS

The results of the Optic Neuritis Treatment Trial, which enrolled 448 patients, indicate that this disorder is characterized by acute visual loss, often associated with pain (90%) worsened by eye movement, in predominantly females (77%) with a mean age of 32 years (20–50 years). The optic disc is swollen in approximately one-third of cases. Macular star figures occur rarely.[415] The patients demonstrate a wide variety of visual field defects. Color vision is almost always abnormal and a relative afferent pupillary defect is seen. MRI of the brain showed evidence of demyelinization in approximately 50% of cases. MRI, serologic studies (antinuclear antibody, fluorescent treponemal antibody-absorbed), chest X-ray examination, and lumbar puncture are of limited value in defining a cause for visual loss other than optic neuritis associated with demyelinating disease.[416] The MRI is more likely to be positive in patients with severe visual loss. The presence of oligoclonal bands in the cerebrospinal fluid correlates with the development of clinically definite multiple sclerosis. Patients with retrobulbar neuritis are more likely to show evidence of multiple sclerosis than those with papillitis. Eliciting either Uhthoff's symptom (transient blurring of vision during exercise, hot shower or bath, or while under emotional stress) or Lhermitte's sign (sudden or transient electric-like shocks radiating down the spine or extremities, particularly with neck flexion) is evidence in patients with unexplained visual loss, suggesting retrobulbar neuritis and multiple sclerosis. If clinical signs and symptoms are typical for optic neuritis, other work-up is unlikely to be fruitful. If the features are atypical, such as progression of visual loss beyond 1 week, evidence of vitritis, presence of a macular star figure or iritis, age more than 45 years, or absence of pain, other diagnoses, such as syphilis, cat-scratch disease, systemic lupus erythematosus, Lyme disease, viral or bacterial optic neuritis should be considered. In most patients the visual acuity and visual field return to normal within a year.[417] In those patients who at the onset of visual symptoms have MRI evidence of multiple sclerosis-like lesions, intravenous therapy with corticosteroids reduces the chances of the patient's developing new clinical signs of multiple sclerosis during the subsequent 2 years.[418,419] This restraining effect of cortisone wears off after 2 years. Oral administration of corticosteroids has no effect on visual outcome and increases the risk of recurrent optic neuritis.[418,420]

15.16 Meningioma of the optic disc.

A–C: Blurred vision, papilledema, and chorioretinal folds in this 46-year-old woman were caused by a meningioma of the left optic nerve (A). Note resolution of the edema and folds and the development of dilated venous loops (arrows, B) that occurred spontaneously over a 32-month period. Angiography showed evidence that venous blood in these loops as well as that in the retina was draining into the central retinal vein. The patient had 3600 R of X-ray irradiation to the right orbit. Note the reduced prominence of the venous loops 18 months later (C). Visual acuity was 20/20.

D and **E**: This 14-year-old boy developed blurred vision 4 months previously after being struck on the chin with a broomstick. He was treated for 4 weeks with 100 mg prednisone daily. His visual acuity was bare hand movements, right eye, and 20/20, left eye. He had 2 mm of right proptosis. Orbital magnetic resonance imaging showed a mass that failed to enhance with gadolinium. Optociliary shunt vessels (arrows, D) suggested a meningioma that was confirmed on biopsy of an enlarged optic nerve. Angiography (E) shows the venous nature of shunt vessels. He received 4500 cGy irradiation. The fundus changes stabilized but there was no visual improvement.

F: Meningioma of the optic nerve in this 56-year-old woman with juxtapapillary chorioretinal folds.

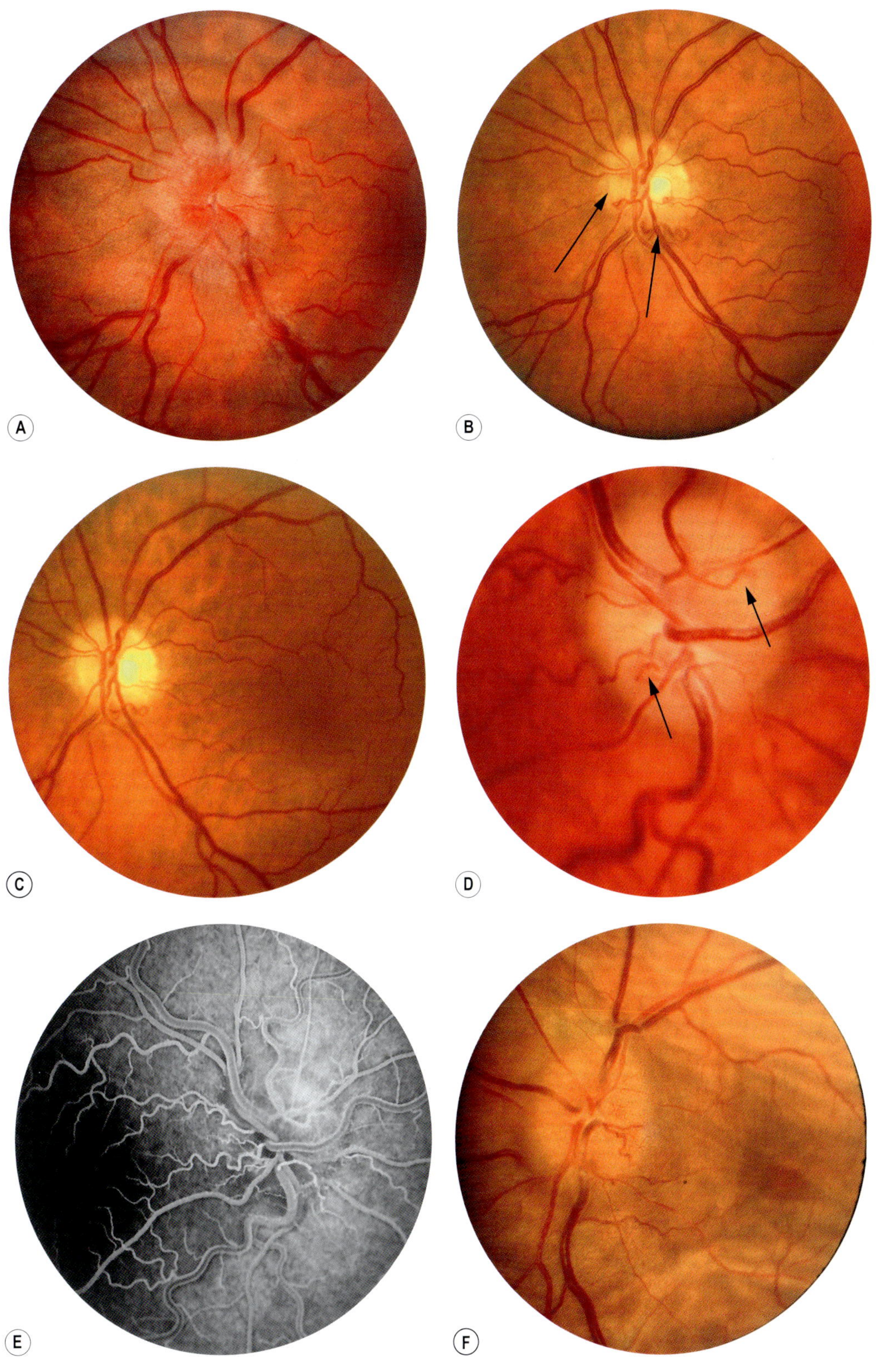
A
B
C
D
E
F

OPTIC NEURITIS IN CHILDREN

Optic neuritis in children is unique in that it is more often anterior, bilateral, known to occur 1–2 weeks after a presumed viral infection, less often associated with development of multiple sclerosis and is steroid-sensitive or steroid-dependent.[421] This should be differentiated from neuroretinitis secondary to cat-scratch disease that is more often unilateral and is characterized by disc swelling, peripapillary exudative detachment, and macular star formation. Those who progress to development of multiple sclerosis are older and have unilateral involvement.[421–424]

TRAUMATIC OPTIC NEUROPATHY

Blunt injuries, particularly to the forehead, may cause loss of vision and no fundoscopic changes as a result of injury to the optic nerve, even when the trauma seems trivial.[401,425,425] The optic nerve is most vulnerable to injury at either end of the optic canal. Shearing forces caused by abrupt deceleration of the skull probably cause injury to small nutrient blood vessels as well as contusion necrosis to the nerve. Immediate loss of vision to no light perception on impact portends a poor prognosis for recovery; a short lucid interval before deterioration suggests a potentially reversible process. Direct injury to the nerve may result from a fracture through the bony canal that severs or compresses the nerve. The value of corticosteroids and surgical decompression in both types of injury is uncertain.[427] Optic disc pallor usually appears several weeks after the injury.

RADIATION-INDUCED OPTIC NEUROPATHY

See Chapter 6.

OPTIC NERVE MENINGIOMAS

Patients with meningiomas confined to the orbital portion of the optic nerve are typically women (70–80%) who are seen between the ages of 35 and 60 years because of transient obscurations of vision or mild visual loss in one eye (Figure 15.16A–I).[428–436] The visual acuity is usually normal or only mildly affected. Mild proptosis is present in 50–75% of cases and is easily overlooked. Ophthalmoscopic examination typically reveals mild optic disc edema and some dilation of the retinal veins (Figure 15.16A). Other evidence of central retinal vein obstruction is infrequently present.[433] Enlargement of the blind spot is the characteristic field defect initially. Over a period of months or years visual loss, increased papilledema (Figure 15.16D and F), refractile bodies and pallor of the optic disc, mild retinal vein dilation, and in 20–40% of cases optic disc shunt or collateral vessels develop (Figure 15.16B and D).[429,437–443] These changes are usually accompanied by contraction of the peripheral isopters. Juxtapapillary retinal and chorioretinal folds may be present (Figure 15.16A, G, and I). Extension of the tumor into the inner eye is rare (Figure 15.16H).[444–447] In the presence of optic disc edema, fluorescein angiography shows capillary dilation and leakage of the optic disc vessels. Later, after optic atrophy has occurred, dilation of the capillaries and leakage are usually no longer apparent. The pattern of dye filling the dilated venous loops on the optic disc suggests, at least in some cases, that these vessels may not be shunting venous blood from the retina into the juxtapapillary venous system but instead are hypertrophied collateral channels transporting venous blood from the retrobulbar meningioma into the central retinal vein.[429] Histopathologic examination in one case demonstrated communication between the retinal veins and the choroidal veins.[440] Primary optic nerve meningiomas occasionally occur bilaterally,[430,435,448] and may be associated with neurofibromatosis type 2 along with cranial nerve schwannomas.[449] Meningiomas as well as acoustic neuromas may be caused by loss of tumor suppressor genes on chromosome 22.[449]

CT and ultrasonography are invaluable in demonstrating the enlargement of the perioptic dural sheaths and in excluding tumor extension into the optic canals. About one-third of patients show calcification on CT scan that appears as bright lines along the length of the nerve; this is called the "tram track" sign. MRI plus fat saturation after gadolinium-diethylenepentaacetic acid is helpful in detecting intracranial extension of optic nerve meningioma that is not easily imaged with MRI alone.[432,436] The differential diagnosis includes optic nerve glioma, papilledema, and optic nerve cysts. In some cases an occult meningioma may be the cause of the cyst.[450] Whereas optic disc pallor and collateral venous channels are highly suggestive of a meningioma, they occasionally are caused by other disorders such as central retinal vein occlusion, hydrocephalus, and perioptic neuritis.[451,452] Visual loss typically occurs slowly over a period of months or years, and surgical extirpation of the meningioma is usually associated with profound visual loss. Therefore, in patients with good

15.16 Continued

G: Photomicrograph of meningioma of the optic nerve. Note compression of the optic nerve (arrows) by the tumor.
H and I: Meningioma of the optic nerve with anterior extension into the subretinal space (arrow, J). Note the evidence of choroidal folds (arrows, I) adjacent to the subretinal tumor.

Optic nerve glioma

J–L: This 28-year-old Caucasian woman presented with proptosis, limited eye movements, optic atrophy (J1) and no light perception vision. T1-weighted axial magnetic resonance imaging with gadolinium showed an irregular fusiform enlargement of the right optic nerve (J), that was sectioned (K). Histology showed Rosenthal fibers typical of juvenile pilocytic astrocytoma (L).

(H from Dunn and Walsh[445], ; J–L, courtesy of Dr. M.Tariq Bhatti.)

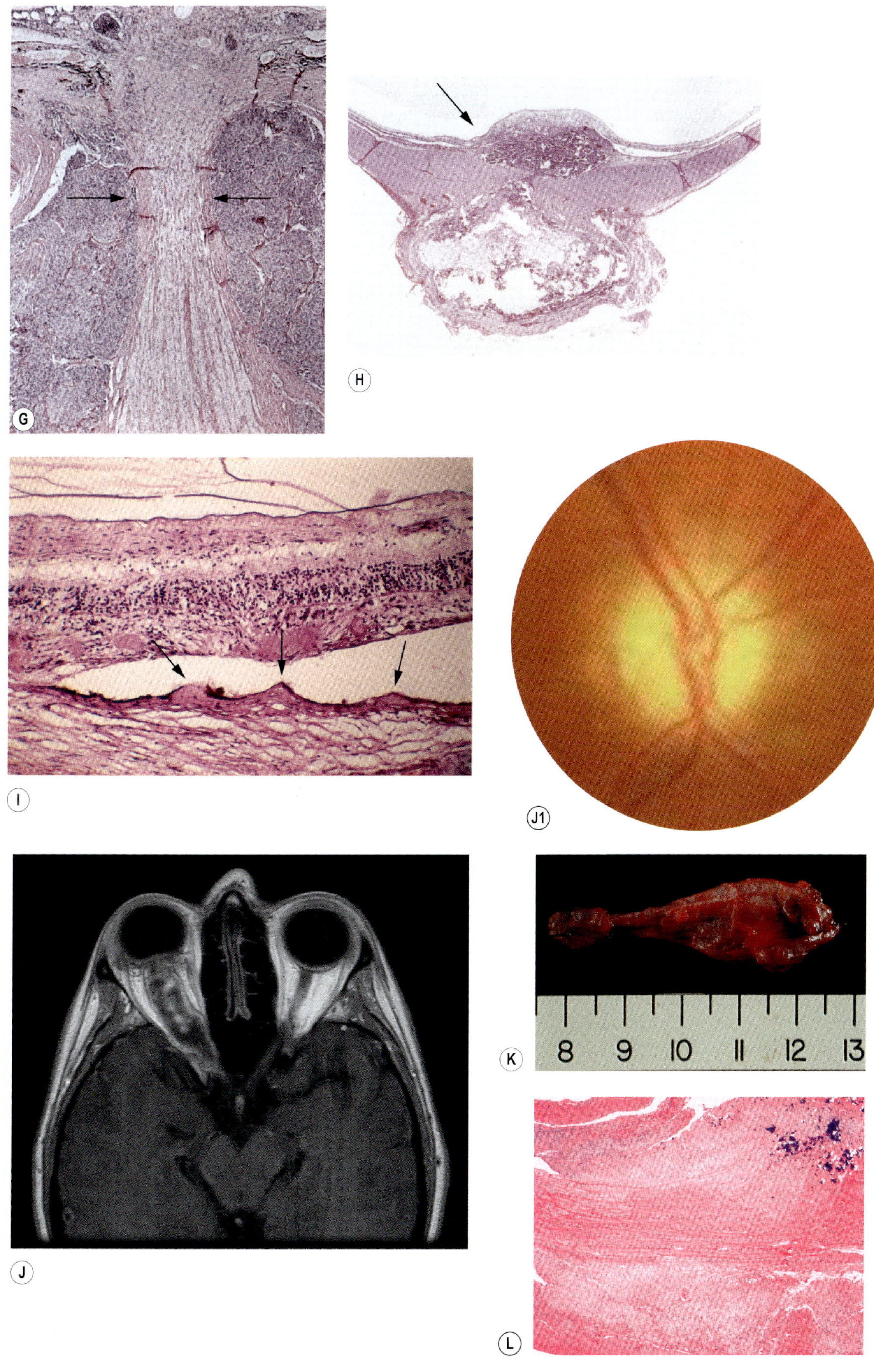
G
H
I
J1
J
8 9 10 11 12 13
K
L

visual function and no evidence of extraorbital extension of the meningioma, observation for evidence of progressive visual loss or extraorbital extension is usually recommended before either surgical or irradiation treatment is considered.[430,431,434,435,453,454] Some patients achieve at least temporary restoration of vision following irradiation treatment.[431,455] Optic nerve meningiomas in children and young adults are more aggressive and these patients require closer follow-up.[435,456,457]

OPTIC NERVE GLIOMAS

Optic nerve gliomas cause insidious loss of vision, proptosis, and optic atrophy (Figure 15.16J inset) that are often discovered in children during a routine eye examination. They represent 1% of all cranial tumors and 1.5–3.5% of orbital tumors. The tumor may involve one or both optic nerves alone (25%) or may involve the chiasm and tract in addition to the optic nerve (75%). When both nerves are affected the patient is likely to have other manifestations of type 1 neurofibromatosis, for example, Leisch iris nodules and bright lesions demonstrated throughout the brain with gadolinium-enhanced MRI.[458–460] The latter lesions have uncertain pathology and consequences. They present with insidious loss of vision and proptosis. Hyperopia and chorioretinal folds may be seen in anterior tumors due to compression of the posteror wall of the eye. Posterior optic nerve gliomas present as a slowly progressive optic neuropathy. Radiologic studies may reveal enlargement of the optic foramen on the affected side or evidence of J-shaped sella turcica in the case of chiasmal involvement. The optic nerve enlargement is fusiform in shape and shows mild enhancement on gadolinium scanning (Figure 15.16J and K). Optic nerve gliomas have a variable histopathologic appearance and growth potential. Most neural tumors of the anterior visual pathways are generally benign and are classified as pilocytic astrocytomas. Some, however, may exhibit aggressive growth and rarely may invade the eye.[461] Those with less growth potential frequently occur in association with other manifestations of neurofibromatosis.[462] The management of these tumors is controversial.[462,463]

15.17 Choroidal folds associated with unilateral disc edema of unknown cause.

A and **B**: This apparently healthy 55-year-old man presented with visual complaints in the left eye. His right eye was normal. In the left eye he had papilledema and horizontally oriented chorioretinal folds (arrows, A). He noted further decline in his acuity and returned 5 days later. His visual acuity was 20/60. The papilledema had lessened. The chorioretinal folds were unchanged. (B) Neurologic evaluation including computed tomography scan was negative.
C: This 34-year-old woman had bilateral swollen optic discs secondary to pseudotumor cerebri. Subretinal hemorrhage was seen at the edge of the swollen disc (C, arrow).

Subretinal neovascularization associated with papilledema secondary to idiopathic intracranial hypertension.

D–H: This 30-year-old woman had papilledema from idiopathic intracranial hypertension (D and E). There was a pigmented type 2 juxtapapillary SRNVM in the left eye at the superotemporal edge of the disc. Thirteen months later she developed a second SRNVM at the inferotemporal disc edge with leakage of fluid, blood, and lipid. Angiogram shows an active SRNVM at the inferotemporal edge of the disc and a spontaneously involuted SRNVM at the superotemporal edge of the disc (arrow). She underwent krypton red laser photocoagulation of the active membrane with gradual resolution of the fluid, blood, and lipid over 3 months. Six years later the nerve swelling has resolved with a small fibrotic scar. The superotemporal membrane was never treated.

Nutritional amblyopia.

I and **J**: Nutritional amblyopia misdiagnosed as macular degeneration in this 66-year-old man, who complained of loss of central vision of over 16 months' duration. His visual acuity was 20/100. There were mild retinal pigment epithelium changes biomicroscopically (I and J). Angiography, however, was normal. He had bilateral cecocentral scotomata. He was treated with oral and intramuscular injections of B-complex vitamins and within several months experienced dramatic improvement of vision to 20/30 and J-1+ in both eyes.
K and **L**: This 73-year-old man, with a history of nontropical sprue and lifelong amblyopia in the left eye, noted the development of a paracentral scotoma in the right eye 6 months previously. He was eating a wheat-free diet. Visual acuity in the right eye was 20/40 and in the left eye 20/400. He had a cecocentral scotoma in the right eye. His pupils and right fundus were normal except for a small, one-clock-hour sector of pallor temporally in the optic disc (arrow, K). The left optic disc was hypoplastic (L). The diagnosis was possible nutritional amblyopia or focal ischemic optic atrophy.

(C, courtesy of Dr. Patrick Lavin.)

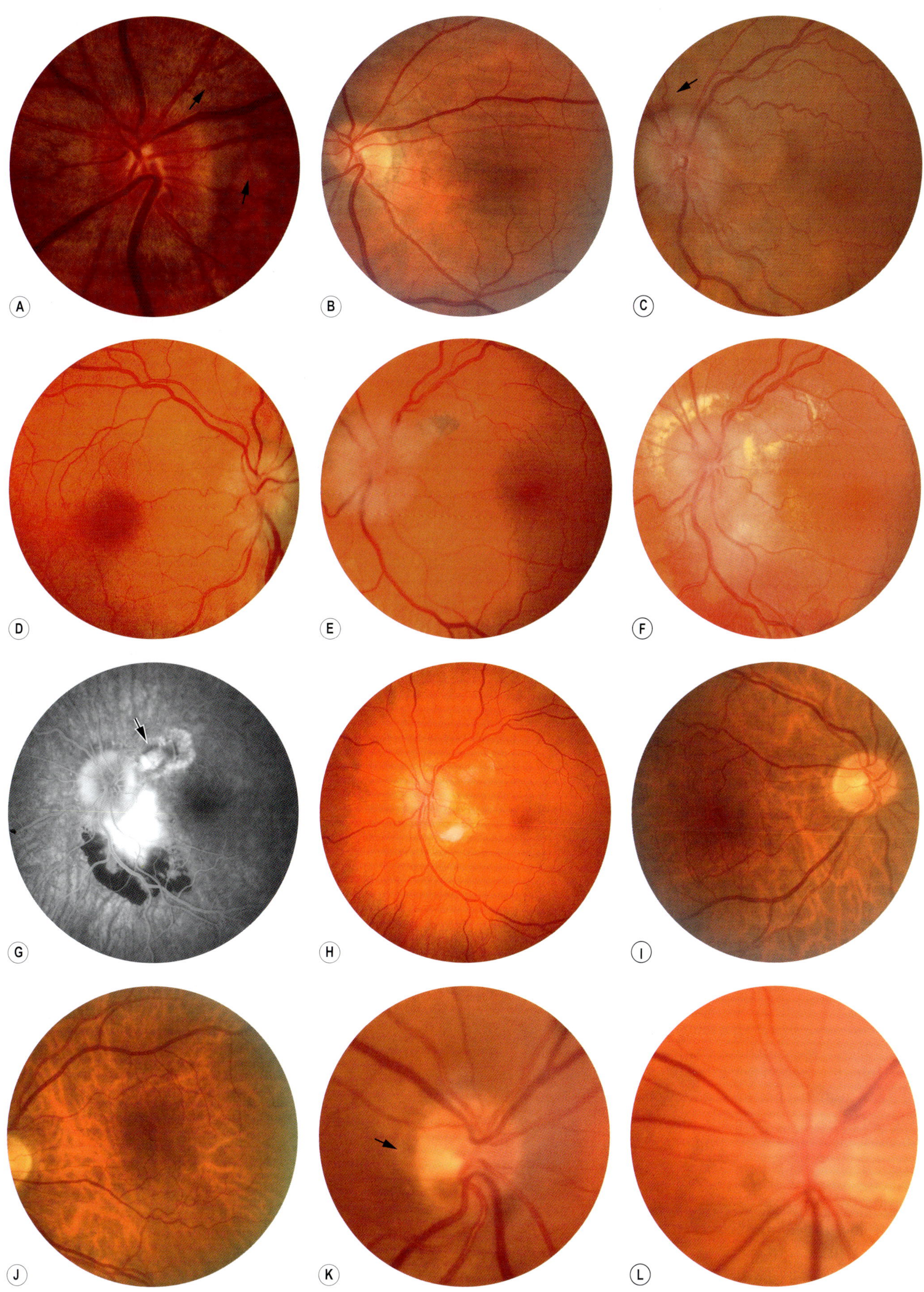
A
B
C
D
E
F
G
H
I
J
K
L

VISUAL LOSS SECONDARY TO PAPILLEDEMA CAUSED BY INCREASED INTRACRANIAL PRESSURE

Although transient obscuration of vision is a frequent complaint of patients with papilledema and increased intracranial pressure, most of them have normal visual acuity during the early stages. Headache, nausea, vomiting, photophobia, and diplopia due to abducens nerve palsy are nonvisual manifestations. Those with chronic papilledema, particularly patients with pseudotumor cerebri, may develop loss of visual field and visual acuity in as many as 50% of cases.[464–466] Nerve fiber layer atrophy with slit-like or diffuse loss is best viewed by using the red-free light at the slit lamp. Persons at high risk of visual loss are those with high-grade or atrophic papilledema, peripapillary subretinal hemorrhage,[467] anemia, high myopia, and old age.[468] The primary cause of visual loss is progressive atrophy and degeneration of the nerve fibers.[469] Other less frequent causes include juxtapapillary subretinal neovascularization,[67,470–474] preretinal hemorrhage that occurs when the rise in intracranial pressure is rapid,[472,475] central retinal vein occlusion,[470] serous macular detachment,[476] macular star,[472,477] macular pigmentation,[478] AION,[476] and chorioretinal folds (Figure 15.17A and C).[464,472,477,479,480] The latter three findings are not usually associated with visual loss when they occur in patients with papilledema. Occasionally the patient may be aware of a temporal scotoma associated with enlargement of the blind spot.[481] In such cases, particularly if the optic disc swelling is unilateral, visual field testing may yield a blind spot enlargement far larger than can be explained on the basis of the papilledema. (See discussion of idiopathic blind spot enlargement syndrome and acute zonal occult outer retinopathy in Chapter 11.)

PSEUDOTUMOR CEREBRI (IDIOPATHIC INTRACRANIAL HYPERTENSION)

Idiopathic intracranial hypertension occurs primarily in young obese women and less often in men, without evidence of underlying disease. In about 10% of patients secondary causes include exogenous substances or other systemic illnesses. Tetracyclines, nalidixic acid, withdrawal of beta-human chorionic gonadotrophin and corticosteroids, cyclosporine, growth hormone, leuprolide acetate, lithium, levenorgestrel implants, vitamin A, and other retinoids are known to be associated. Systemic diseases include obesity, hyperthyroidism, anemia, obstructive sleep apnea, chronic respiratory insufficiency, pickwickian syndrome, and nephrotic syndrome.

In addition to the disc edema, some of these patients develop choroidal folds (Figure 15.17A and B), subretinal hemorrhage (Figure 15.17C), and subretinal neovascularization (Figure 15.17D–G).

The primary goal of treatment is to preserve vision and alleviate secondary symptoms. Treatment consists of oral diuretics, weight loss, lumbar puncture, and occasional use of corticosteroids.[482,483] Correction of the secondary causes such as improving oxyenation and decreasing hypercapnia, treatment of hyperthyroidism, and nephrotic syndrome is necessary when appropriate. In patients with visual loss who fail to respond to medical therapy, optic nerve sheath decompression is an effective form of treatment.[478,484–490] It probably should be done initially in only one eye since in some patients this will result in resolution of papilledema bilaterally.[486] Recurrences may occur.[488] Those with headache as their predominant symptom may undergo ventriculoperitoneal or lumboperitoneal shunt.

NUTRITIONAL AMBLYOPIA (TOXIC/NUTRITIONAL OPTIC NEUROPATHY)

Insidious and slowly progressive loss of central vision associated with central and cecocentral visual field defects may be caused by dietary deficiency of one or several vitamins as well as by exposure to toxins or adverse reaction to pharmaceuticals.[491–493] Initially the visual loss is not usually associated with fundus changes (Figure 15.17I and J). Evanescent dilation and tortuosity of small retinal vessels within the arcuate areas of the nerve fiber layer similar to that described in LHON, however, have been described during the early phase of acute malnutrition optic neuropathy.[492] Temporal disc pallor and atrophy of the papillomacular nerve fiber layer eventually occur (Figure 15.17K). Demonstration of a cecocentral scotoma, particularly to red test objects, with preservation of peripheral fields is the typical finding. Deficiency of the B-complex vitamins (predominantly thiamin) is probably more important than either chronic use of alcohol or tobacco alone in causing visual loss. There are only a few well-documented cases of toxic amblyopia in smokers with no history of alcohol ingestion or nutritional deficiency.[494] A reliable dietary history is often best obtained from a friend or relative of the patient. Most of these patients show improvement of vision following institution of a balanced diet and B-complex vitamin supplementation (Figure 15.17I and J).

A review of published cases of amblyopia among malnourished allied prisoners of the Japanese during World War II and among Cubans showed premonitory keratopathy, rapid onset of visual loss, a high incidence of hearing loss, and the presence of peripapillary retinopathy in some cases. No single causative factor was identified. Genetic susceptibility rarely, if ever, played a role and vitamin deficiency was not important. Protein deficiency, antioxidant deficiency, physical labor, and tobacco smoking likely contributed to the occurrence of amblyopia.[495]

A peculiar optic neuropathy, referred to as West Indian Jamaican optic neuropathy, is characterized by the rapid development of visual loss and optic atrophy in predominantly young West Indian blacks.[496,497] The male-to-female ratio is 2:1.[498] A similar optic neuropathy has been described in West Africans. Vision is usually reduced to 20/200 levels, and dense central scotoma and temporal disc pallor are characteristic. Nerve deafness, ataxia, and spasticity may accompany ocular involvement in a few instances; the pathology is a chronic meningomyelitis with loss of myelin of the nerve roots, including the optic and auditory nerves when involved.[497] It is uncertain whether this amblyopia has an infectious, toxic, hereditary, or nutritional basis. A study of 21 inpatients in London revealed demyelination as a possible mechanism of optic atrophy characterized by increased latency of visual evoked responses in four of them. Consumption of bush tea, cassava, cyanide, syphilis, and vitamin deficiencies were not significantly associated. A small number of patients may show improvement in vision; most remain stable after a period of visual deterioration.[498]

An epidemic of optic neuropathy, characterized by bilateral subacute visual loss, dyschromatopsia, central or cecocentral scotomas, fatigue, weight loss, and in some patients peripheral neuropathy, occurring primarily in men, was identified in Cuba in 1992 (1000 cases) and 1993 (48 000 cases). Cigarette smoking, rum drinking, cassava ingestion (it contains variable amount of cyanide) and vitamin deficiencies, especially folic acid, were identified as risk factors affecting mitochondrial oxidative phosphorylation in this Cuban epidemic optic neuropathy.[499,500] In spite of the features in common with LHON, mitochondrial DNA mutations were found infrequently in these patients.[501,502] However, both may share depletion of mitochondrial adenosine triphosphate in their pathogenesis. Papillomacular bundle (smallest axons with least myelin) and sural nerve (longest axons requiring longest transport) are most vulnerable to the challenges of mitochondrial transport and show the most damage as temporal pallor of the disc.[499]

Experimental cyanide exposure in animals causes demye-lination, and circumstantial clinical and laboratory evidence suggests similarity to several human conditions. Defective cyanide metabolism may be a common path in Leber's and other hereditary optic atrophies (dominant and recessive), retrobulbar neuritis, optic atrophy, and subacute combined degeneration of the spinal cord of vitamin B_{12} deficiency, and in the so-called tobacco–alcohol amblyopia with more complex nutritional deficiencies. In protein-malnourished populations consuming large amounts of cyanide or cyanogens, as in the form of cassava, optic neuropathy is seen. A similar explanation may be plausible for lathyrism.[503] To exclude the diagnosis of LHON, all patients suspected of having nutritional or tobacco–alcohol amblyopia should have mitochondrial testing.[504,505]

DIABETIC PAPILLOPATHY

See Chapter 6.

References

1. Akiba J, Kakehashi A, Hikichi T, et al. Vitreous findings in cases of optic nerve pits and serous macular detachment. Am J Ophthalmol 1993;116:38–41.
2. Alexander TA, Billson FA. Vitrectomy and photocoagulation in the management of serous detachment associated with optic nerve pits. Aust J Ophthalmol 1984;12:139–42.
3. Annesley W, Brown G, Bolling J, et al. Treatment of retinal detachment with congenital optic pit by krypton laser photocoagulation. Graefes Arch Clin Exp Ophthalmol 1987;225:311–4.
4. Bonnet M. Serous macular detachment associated with optic nerve pits. Graefes Arch Clin Exp Ophthalmol 1991;229:526–32.
5. Brown GC, Shields JA, Goldberg RE. Congenital pits of the optic nerve head. II. Clinical studies in humans. Ophthalmology 1980;87:51–65.
6. Brown GC, Shields JA, Patty BE, et al. Congenital pits of the optic nerve head. I. Experimental studies in collie dogs. Arch Ophthalmol 1979;97:1341–4.
7. Calhoun FP. Bilateral coloboma of the optic nerve associated with holes in the disk and a cyst of the optic sheath. Arch Ophthalmol 1930;3:71–9.
8. Cox MS, Witherspoon CD, Morris RE, et al. Evolving techniques in the treatment of macular detachment caused by optic nerve pits. Ophthalmology 1988;95:889–96.
9. Farpour H, Babel J. Les fossettes papillaires; diagnostic différentiel, anomalies vasculaires et cas limites. Ann Oculist 1968;201:1–17.
10. Ferry AP. Macular detachment associated with congenital pit of the optic nerve head; pathologic findings in two cases simulating malignant melanoma of the choroid. Arch Ophthalmol 1963;70:346–57.
11. Gass JDM. Discussion of paper by Brockhurst RJ: Optic pits and posterior retinal detachment. Trans Am Ophthalmol Soc 1975;73:288–9.
12. Gass JDM. Serous detachment of the macula secondary to congenital pit of the optic nervehead. Am J Ophthalmol 1969;67:821–41.
13. Gordon R, Chatfield RK. Pits in the optic disc associated with macular degeneration. Br J Ophthalmol 1969;53:481–9.
14. Grimson BS, Mann JD, Pantell JP. Optic nerve pit during papilledema. Arch Ophthalmol 1982;100:99–100.
15. Hendrikse F, Deutman AF. Central serous detachment with optic pit treated by gas injection and laser coagulation. Lasers Light Ophthalmol 1989;2:249–52.
16. Jack MK. Central serous retinopathy with optic pit treated with photocoagulation. Am J Ophthalmol 1969;67:519–21.
17. Jay WM, Pope Jr J, Riffle JE. Juxtapapillary subretinal neovascularization associated with congenital pit of the optic nerve. Am J Ophthalmol 1984;97:655–8.
18. Kalina RE, Conrad WC. Intrathecal fluorescein for serous macular detachment. Arch Ophthalmol 1976;94:1421.
19. Kranenburg EW. Crater-like holes in the optic disc and central serous retinopathy. Arch Ophthalmol 1960;64:912–24.
20. Lincoff H, Lopez R, Kreissig I, et al. Retinoschisis associated with optic nerve pits. Arch Ophthalmol 1988;106:61–7.
21. Lincoff H, Yannuzzi L, Singerman L, et al. Improvement in visual function after displacement of the retinal elevations emanating from optic pits. Arch Ophthalmol 1993;111:1071–9.
22. Petersen HP. Pits or crater-like holes in the optic disc. Acta Ophthalmol 1958;36:435–43.
23. Regenbogen L, Stein R, Lazar M. Macular and juxtapapillary serous retinal detachment associated with pit of optic disc. Ophthalmologica 1964;148:247–51.
24. Rubinstein K, Ali M. Complications of optic disc pits. Trans Ophthalmol Soc UK 1978;98: 195–200.
25. Schatz H, McDonald HR. Treatment of sensory retinal detachment associated with optic nerve pit or coloboma. Ophthalmology 1988;95:178–86.
26. Sobol WM, Blodi CF, Folk JC, et al. Long-term visual outcome in patients with optic nerve pit and serous retinal detachment of the macula. Ophthalmology 1990;97:1539–42.
27. Doyle E, Trivedi D, Good P, et al. High-resolution optical coherence tomography demonstration of membranes spanning optic disc pits and colobomas. Br J Ophthalmol 2009;93:360–5.
28. Vedantham V, Ramasamy K. Spontaneous improvement of serous maculopathy associated with congenital optic disc pit: an OCT study. Eye (Lond) 2005;19:596–9.
29. Vedantham V. Double optic discs, optic disc coloboma, and pit: spectrum of hybrid disc anomalies in a single eye. Arch Ophthalmol 2005;123:1450–2.
30. Brockhurst RJ. Optic pits and posterior retinal detachment. Trans Am Ophthalmol Soc 1975;73:264–91.
31. Gass JDM. Stereoscopic atlas macular diseases; diagnosis and treatment, 3rd ed. St. Louis: CV Mosby; 1987. p. 728–33.
32. Savell J, Cook JR. Optic nerve colobomas of autosomal-dominant heredity. Arch Ophthalmol 1976;94:395–400.
33. Slusher MM, Weaver Jr RG, Greven CM, et al. The spectrum of cavitary optic disc anomalies in a family. Ophthalmology 1989;96:342–7.
34. Theodossiadis GP, Koutsandrea C, Theodossiadis PG. Optic nerve pit with serous macular detachment resulting in rhegmatogenous retinal detachment. Br J Ophthalmol 1993;77:385–6.
35. Cavarretta S, Salvatore S, Vingolo EM. Use of MP-1 microperimetry in optic disc pit and secondary retinoschisis. Int Ophthalmol 2009;29:423–5.
36. Theodossiadis GP, Kollia AK, Theodossiadis PG. Cilioretinal arteries in conjunction with a pit of the optic disc. Ophthalmologica 1992;204:115–21.

198. Gartner S. Drusen of the optic disk in retinitis pigmentosa. Am J Ophthalmol 1987;103:845.
199. Kelley JS. Autofluorescence of drusen of the optic nerve head. Arch Ophthalmol 1974;92:263–4.
200. Wilhelm JL, Gutman FA. Macular choroidal neovascular membrane with bilateral optic nerve drusen: case report. Ann Ophthalmol 1983;15:48–51.
201. Reifler DM, Kaufman DI. Optic disk drusen and pseudotumor cerebri. Am J Ophthalmol 1988;106:95–6.
202. Hoover DL, Robb RM, Petersen RA. Optic disc drusen and primary megalencephaly in children. J Pediatr Ophthalmol Strabismus 1989;26:81–5.
203. Moisseiev J, Cahane M, Treister G. Optic nerve head drusen and peripapillary central serous chorioretinopathy. Am J Ophthalmol 1989;108:202–3.
204. Walsh FB, Hoyt WF. Clinical neuro-ophthalmology, 3rd ed. Baltimore: Williams & Wilkins; 1974. p. 673.
205. Sanders MD, Ffytche TJ. Fluorescein angiography in the diagnosis of drusen of the disc. Trans Ophthalmol Soc UK 1967;87:457–68.
206. Spencer TS, Katz BJ, Weber SW, et al. Progression from anomalous optic discs to visible optic disc drusen. J Neuroophthalmol 2004;24:297–8.
207. Sadun AA, Green RL, Nobe JR, et al. Papillopathies associated with unusual calcifications in the retrolaminar optic nerve. J Clin Neuro-Ophthalmol 1991;11:175–80.
208. Bec P, Adam P, Mathis A, et al. Optic nerve head drusen; high-resolution computed tomographic approach. Arch Ophthalmol 1984;102:680–2.
209. Frisén L, Schöldström G, Svendsen P. Drusen in the optic nerve head; verification by computerized tomography. Arch Ophthalmol 1978;96:1611–4.
210. Gass JDM. Diseases of the optic nerve that may simulate macular disease. Trans Am Acad Ophthalmol Otolaryngol 1977;83:OP763–OP770.
211. Kamin DF, Hepler RS, Foos RY. Optic nerve drusen. Arch Ophthalmol 1973;89:359–62.
212. Tso MOM. Pathology and pathogenesis of drusen of the optic nervehead. Ophthalmology 1981;88:1066–80.
213. Wilkins JM, Pomeranz HD. Visual manifestations of visible and buried optic disc drusen. J Neuroophthalmol 2004;24:125–9.
214. Berninger TA, Jaeger W, Krastel H. Electrophysiology and colour perimetry in dominant infantile optic atrophy. Br J Ophthalmol 1991;75:49–52.
215. Caldwell JBH, Howard RO, Riggs LA. Dominant juvenile optic atrophy; a study in two families and review of hereditary disease in childhood. Arch Ophthalmol 1971;85:133–47.
216. Glaser JS. Heredofamilial disorders of the optic nerve. In: Goldberg MF, editor. Genetic and metabolic eye disease. Boston: Little, Brown; 1974. p. 463–86.
217. Kjer P. Infantile optic atrophy with dominant mode of inheritance; a clinical and genetic study of 19 Danish families. Acta Ophthalmol Suppl 1959;164(Suppl. 54):1–147.
218. Kline LB, Glaser JS. Dominant optic atrophy; the clinical profile. Arch Ophthalmol 1979;97:1680–6.
219. Krill AE, Smith VC, Pokorny J. Further studies supporting the identity of congenital tritanopia and hereditary dominant optic atrophy. Invest Ophthalmol 1971;10:457–65.
220. Manchester Jr PT, Calhoun Jr FP. Dominant hereditary optic atrophy with bitemporal field defects. Arch Ophthalmol 1958;60:479–84.
221. Weleber RG, Miyake Y. Familial optic atrophy with negative electroretinograms. Arch Ophthalmol 1992;110:640–5.
222. Thiselton DL, Alexander C, Taanman JW, et al. A comprehensive survey of mutations in the OPA1 gene in patients with autosomal dominant optic atrophy. Invest Ophthalmol Vis Sci 2002;43:1715–24.
223. Delettre C, Lenaers G, Griffoin JM, et al. Nuclear gene OPA1, encoding a mitochondrial dynamin-related protein, is mutated in dominant optic atrophy. Nat Genet 2000;26:207–10.
224. Alexander C, Votruba M, Pesch UE, et al. OPA1, encoding a dynamin-related GTPase, is mutated in autosomal dominant optic atrophy linked to chromosome 3q28. Nat Genet 2000;26:211–5.
225. Jonasdottir A, Eiberg H, Kjer B, et al. Refinement of the dominant optic atrophy locus (OPA1) to a 1.4-cM interval on chromosome 3q28-3q29, within a 3-Mb YAC contig. Hum Genet 1997;99:115–20.
226. Liguori M, La Russa A, Manna I, et al. A phenotypic variation of dominant optic atrophy and deafness (ADOAD) due to a novel OPA1 mutation. J Neurol 2008;255:127–9.
227. Cohn AC, Toomes C, Potter C, et al. Autosomal dominant optic atrophy: penetrance and expressivity in patients with OPA1 mutations. Am J Ophthalmol 2007;143:656–62.
228. Han J, Thompson-Lowrey AJ, Reiss A, et al. OPA1 mutations and mitochondrial DNA haplotypes in autosomal dominant optic atrophy. Genet Med 2006;8:217–25.
229. Zanna C, Ghelli A, Porcelli AM, et al. OPA1 mutations associated with dominant optic atrophy impair oxidative phosphorylation and mitochondrial fusion. Brain 2008;131:352–67.
230. Cohn AC, Toomes C, Hewitt AW, et al. The natural history of OPA1-related autosomal dominant optic atrophy. Br J Ophthalmol 2008;92:1333–6.
231. Johns DR, Heher KL, Miller NR, et al. Leber's hereditary optic neuropathy; clinical manifestations of the 14484 mutation. Arch Ophthalmol 1993;111:495–8.
232. Leber T. Ueber hereditäre und congenital-angelegte Sehnervenleiden. Albrecht von Graefes Arch Ophthalmol 1871;17:249–91.
233. van Heuven GJ. Die Diagnose der hereditären Leberschen Sehnervenatrophie (abstract). Klin Monatsbl Augenheilkd 1924;73:252–3.
234. Tong Y, Sun YH, Zhou X, et al. Very low penetrance of Leber's hereditary optic neuropathy in five Han Chinese families carrying the ND1 G3460A mutation. Mol Genet Metab 2010;99: 417–24.
235. Qu J, Zhou X, Zhang J, et al. Extremely low penetrance of Leber's hereditary optic neuropathy in 8 Han Chinese families carrying the ND4 G11778A mutation. Ophthalmology 2009;116:558–64.
236. Kerrison JB. Latent, acute, and chronic Leber's hereditary optic neuropathy. Ophthalmology 2005;112:1–2.
237. Tanaka A, Kiyosawa M, Mashima Y, et al. A family with Leber's hereditary optic neuropathy with mitochondrial DNA heteroplasmy related to disease expression. J Neuroophthalmol 1998;18:81–3.
238. Miller NR. Walsh and Hoyt's clinical neuro-ophthalmology, 4th ed. Baltimore: Williams and Wilkins; 1982. p. 212–26.
239. Nikoskelainen E, Sogg RL, Rosenthal AR, et al. The early phase in Leber hereditary optic atrophy. Arch Ophthalmol 1977;95:969–78.
240. Smith JL, Hoyt WF, Susac JO. Ocular fundus in acute Leber optic neuropathy. Arch Ophthalmol 1973;90:349–54.
241. Nikoskelainen E, Hoyt WF, Nummelin K. Ophthalmoscopic findings in Leber's hereditary optic neuropathy. II. The fundus findings in the affected family members. Arch Ophthalmol 1983;101:1059–68.
242. Borruat F-X, Green WT, Graham EM, et al. Late onset Leber's optic neuropathy: a case confused with ischaemic optic neuropathy. Br J Ophthalmol 1992;76:571–3.
243. Goyal S, Riordan-Eva P, Coakes RL. Late onset of Leber's hereditary optic neuropathy precipitated by anaemia. Eye (Lond) 2004;18:1017–8.
244. Luke C, Cornely OA, Fricke J, et al. Late onset of Leber's hereditary optic neuropathy in HIV infection. Br J Ophthalmol 1999;83:1204–5.
245. Ajax ET, Kardon R. Late-onset Leber's hereditary optic neuropathy. J Neuroophthalmol 1998;18:30–1.
246. Lopez PF, Smith JL. Leber's optic neuropathy; new observations. J Clin Neuro-Ophthalmol 1986;6:144–52.
247. Sanders MD, Riordan-Eva P. Difficulties in interpreting optic disc fluorescein leakage in Leber's hereditary optic neuropathy. J Neuroophthalmol 1997;17:143.
248. Stone EM, Newman NJ, Miller NR, et al. Visual recovery in patients with Leber's hereditary optic neuropathy and the 11778 mutation. J Clin Neuro-Ophthalmol 1992;12:10–14.
249. Barboni P, Carbonelli M, Savini G, et al. Natural history of Leber's hereditary optic neuropathy: longitudinal analysis of the retinal nerve fiber layer by optical coherence tomography. Ophthalmology 2010;117:623–7.
250. Acaroglu G, Kansu T, Dogulu CF. Visual recovery patterns in children with Leber's hereditary optic neuropathy. Int Ophthalmol 2001;24:349–55.
251. Yamada K, Mashima Y, Kigasawa K, et al. High incidence of visual recovery among four Japanese patients with Leber's hereditary optic neuropathy with the 14484 mutation. J Neuroophthalmol 1997;17:103–7.
252. Nagai A, Nakamura M, Kusuhara S, et al. Unilateral manifestation of Leber's hereditary optic neuropathy after blunt ocular trauma. Jpn J Ophthalmol 2005;49:65–7.
253. Redmill B, Mutamba A, Tandon M. Leber's hereditary optic neuropathy following trauma. Eye (Lond) 2001;15:544–7.
254. de Gottrau P, Büchi ER, Daicker B. Distended optic nerve sheaths in Leber's hereditary optic neuropathy. J Clin Neuro-Ophthalmol 1992;12:89–93.
255. Smith JL, Tse DT, Bryne SF, et al. Optic nerve sheath distention in Leber's optic neuropathy and the significance of the "Wallace" mutation. J Clin Neuro-Ophthalmol 1990;10:231–8.
256. Kwittken J, Barest HD. The neuropathology of hereditary optic atrophy (Leber's disease); the first complete anatomic study. Am J Pathol 1958;34:185–207.
257. Nikoskelainen EK, Savontaus M-L, Wanne OP, et al. Leber's hereditary optic neuroretinopathy, a maternally inherited disease; a genealogic study in four pedigrees. Arch Ophthalmol 1987;105:665–71.
258. Ortiz RG, Newman NJ, Manoukian SV, et al. Optic disk cupping and electrocardiographic abnormalities in an American pedigree with Leber's hereditary optic neuropathy. Am J Ophthalmol 1992;113:561–6.
259. Finsterer J, Stollberger C, Kopsa W, et al. Wolff–Parkinson–White syndrome and isolated left ventricular abnormal trabeculation as a manifestation of Leber's hereditary optic neuropathy. Can J Cardiol 2001;17:464–6.
260. Wallace DC. A new manifestation of Leber's disease and a new explanation for the agency responsible for its unusual pattern of inheritance. Brain 1970;93:121–32.
261. McCluskey DAJ, O'Connor PS, Sheehy JT. Leber's optic neuropathy and Charcot–Marie–Tooth disease; report of a case. J Clin Neuro-Ophthalmol 1986;6:76–81.
262. McLeod JG, Low PA, Morgan JA. Charcot–Marie–Tooth disease with Leber optic atrophy. Neurology 1978;28:179–84.
263. Uemura A, Osame M, Nakagawa M, et al. Leber's hereditary optic neuropathy: mitochondrial and biochemical studies on muscle biopsies. Br J Ophthalmol 1987;71:531–6.
264. Wallace DC, Singh G, Lott MT, et al. Mitochondrial DNA mutation associated with Leber's hereditary optic neuropathy. Science 1988;242:1427–30.
265. Nikoskelainen E, Hoyt WF, Nummelin K. Ophthalmoscopic findings in Leber's hereditary optic neuropathy. I. Fundus findings in asymptomatic family members. Arch Ophthalmol 1982;100:1597–602.
266. Nikoskelainen E, Hoyt WF, Nummelin K, et al. Fundus findings in Leber's hereditary optic neuroretinopathy. III. Fluorescein angiographic studies. Arch Ophthalmol 1984;102:981–9.
267. Stehouwer A, Oosterhuis JA, Renger-van Dijk AH, et al. Leber's optic neuropathy. II. Fluorescein angiographic studies. Doc Ophthalmol 1982;53:113–22.
268. Jacobson DM, Stone EM. Difficulty differentiating Leber's from dominant optic neuropathy in a patient with remote visual loss. J Clin Neuro-Ophthalmol 1991;11:152–7.
269. Johns DR. The molecular genetics of Leber's hereditary optic neuropathy. Arch Ophthalmol 1990;108:1405–6.
270. Johns DR, Smith KH, Miller NR. Leber's hereditary optic neuropathy; clinical manifestations of the 3460 mutation. Arch Ophthalmol 1992;110:1577–81.
271. Lott MT, Voljavec AS, Wallace DC. Variable genotype of Leber's hereditary optic neuropathy patients. Am J Ophthalmol 1990;109:625–31.
272. Newman NJ, Lott MT, Wallace DC. The clinical characteristics of pedigrees of Leber's hereditary optic neuropathy with the 11778 mutation. Am J Ophthalmol 1991;111:750–62.
273. Newman NJ, Wallace DC. Mitochondria and Leber's hereditary optic neuropathy. Am J Ophthalmol 1990;109:726–30.
274. Singh G, Lott MT, Wallace DC. A mitochondrial DNA mutation as a cause of Leber's hereditary optic neuropathy. N Engl J Med 1989;320:1300–5.
275. Johns DR, Smith KH, Savino PJ, et al. Leber's hereditary optic neuropathy; clinical manifestations of the 15257 mutation. Ophthalmology 1993;100:981–6.

276. Man PY, Howell N, Mackey DA, et al. Mitochondrial DNA haplogroup distribution within Leber hereditary optic neuropathy pedigrees. J Med Genet 2004;41:e41.
277. Howell N, Mackey DA. Low-penetrance branches in matrilineal pedigrees with Leber hereditary optic neuropathy. Am J Hum Genet 1998;63:1220–4.
278. Howell N, Kubacka I, Halvorson S, et al. Phylogenetic analysis of the mitochondrial genomes from Leber hereditary optic neuropathy pedigrees. Genetics 1995;140:285–302.
279. Mackey DA. Three subgroups of patients from the United Kingdom with Leber hereditary optic neuropathy. Eye (Lond) 1994;8:431–6.
280. Mackey DA, Buttery RG. Leber hereditary optic neuropathy in Australia. Aust N Z J Ophthalmol 1992;20:177–84.
281. Berninger TA, von Meyer L, Siess E, et al. Leber's hereditary optic atrophy: further evidence for a defect of cyanide metabolism? Br J Ophthalmol 1989;73:314–6.
282. Leber T. Die pseudonephritischen Netzhauterkrankungen, die Retinitis stellata; die Purtschersche Netzhautaffektion nach schwerer Schädelverletzung. In: Graefe AC, Saemisch T, editors. Graefe-Saemisch Handbuch der Augenheilkunde, 2nd ed. Leipzig: Englemann; 1916. p. 1349–59.
283. Dreyer RF, Hopen G, Gass JDM, et al. Leber's idiopathic stellate neuroretinitis. Arch Ophthalmol 1984;102:1140–5.
284. Gass JDM. Stereoscopic atlas of macular diseases; diagnosis and treatment, 2nd ed. St. Louis: CV Mosby; 1977. p. 376.
285. Carroll DM, Franklin RM. Leber's idiopathic stellate retinopathy. Am J Ophthalmol 1982;93:96–101.
286. François J, Verriest G, De Laey JJ. Leber's idiopathic stellate retinopathy. Am J Ophthalmol 1969;68:340–5.
287. Glaser JS. Topical diagnosis: prechiasmal visual pathways. In: Glaser JS, editor. Neuro-ophthalmology, 2nd ed. Philadelphia: JB Lippincott; 1990. p. 126.
288. Maitland CG, Miller NR. Neuroretinitis. Arch Ophthalmol 1984;102:1146–50.
289. Miller NR. Walsh and Hoyt's clinical neuro-ophthalmology, 4th ed. Baltimore: Williams & Wilkins; 1982. p. 234.
290. Papastratigakis B, Stavrakas E, Phanouriakis C, et al. Leber's idiopathic stellate maculopathy. Ophthalmologica 1981;183:68–71.
291. Gass JDM. Fluorescein angiography in endogenous intraocular inflammation. In: Aronson SB, Gamble CN, Goodner EK, editors. Clinical methods in uveitis: the Fourth Sloan Symposium on Uveitis. St. Louis: CV Mosby; 1968. p. 214–5.
292. Gass JDM. Stereoscopic atlas of macular diseases; diagnosis and treatment, 3rd ed. St. Louis: CV Mosby; 1987. p. 748–49.
293. Goldstein BG, Pavan PR. Retinal infiltrates in six patients with an associated viral syndrome. Retina 1985;5:144–50.
294. Carithers HA, Margileth AM. Cat-scratch disease; acute encephalopathy and other neurologic manifestations. Am J Dis Child 1991;145:98–101.
295. Foster RE, Gutman FA, Meyers SM, et al. Acute multifocal inner retinitis. Am J Ophthalmol 1991;111:673–81.
296. Bar S, Segal M, Shapira R, et al. Neuroretinitis associated with cat scratch disease. Am J Ophthalmol 1990;110:703–5.
297. Brazis PW, Stokes HR, Ervin FR. Optic neuritis in cat scratch disease. J Clin Neuro-Ophthalmol 1986;6:172–4.
298. Chrousos GA, Drack AV, Young M, et al. Neuroretinitis in cat scratch disease. J Clin Neuro-Ophthalmol 1990;10:92–4.
299. Fish RH, Hogan RN, Nightingale SD, et al. Peripapillary angiomatosis associated with cat-scratch neuroretinitis. Arch Ophthalmol 1992;110:323.
300. Ulrich GG, Waecker Jr NJ, Meister SJ, et al. Cat scratch disease associated with neuroretinitis in a 6-year-old girl. Ophthalmology 1992;99:246–9.
301. Weiss AH, Beck RW. Neuroretinitis in childhood. J Pediatr Ophthalmol 1989;26:198–203.
302. Lesser RL, Kornmehl EW, Pachner AR, et al. Neuro-ophthalmologic manifestations of Lyme disease. Ophthalmology 1990;97:699–706.
303. Purvin VA, Chioran G. Recurrent neuroretinitis. Arch Ophthalmol 1994;112:365–71.
304. de Brouwer AP, van Bokhoven H, Nabuurs SB, et al. PRPS1 mutations: four distinct syndromes and potential treatment. Am J Hum Genet 2010;86:506–18.
305. Chung KW, Kim SB, Park KD, et al. Early onset severe and late-onset mild Charcot–Marie–Tooth disease with mitofusin 2 (MFN2) mutations. Brain 2006;129:2103–18.
306. Ippel EF, Wittebol-Post D, Jennekens FG, et al. Genetic heterogeneity of hereditary motor and sensory neuropathy type VI. J Child Neurol 1995;10:459–63.
307. Katz BJ, Zhao Y, Warner JE, et al. A family with X-linked optic atrophy linked to the OPA2 locus Xp11.4-Xp11.2. Am J Med Genet A 2006;140:2207–11.
308. Sugano M, Hirayama K, Saito T, et al. Optic atrophy, sensorineural hearing loss and polyneuropathy – a case of sporadic Rosenberg–Chutorian syndrome. Fukushima J Med Sci 1992;38:57–65.
309. McCluskey DJ, O'Connor PS, Sheehy JT. Leber's optic neuropathy and Charcot–Marie–Tooth disease. Report of a case. J Clin Neuroophthalmol 1986;6:76–81.
310. Hoyt WF. Charcot–Marie–Tooth disease with primary optic atrophy; report of a case. Arch Ophthalmol 1960;64:925–8.
311. Alvarez E, Ferrer T, Perez-Conde C, et al. Evaluation of congenital dysautonomia other than Riley-Day syndrome. Neuropediatrics 1996;27:26–31.
312. Newman NJ, Biousse V. Hereditary optic neuropathies. Eye (Lond) 2004;18:1144–60.
313. Groom M, Kay MD, Corrent GF. Optic neuropathy in familial dysautonomia. J Neuroophthalmol 1997;17:101–2.
314. Rizzo III JF, Lessell S, Liebman SD. Optic atrophy in familial dysautonomia. Am J Ophthalmol 1986;102:463–7.
315. Garcher C, Humbert P, Bron A, et al. Neuropathie optique et syndrome de Parry–Romberg. A propos d'un cas. J Fr Ophtalmol 1990;13:557–61.
316. Gass JDM. Differential diagnosis of intraocular tumors; a stereoscopic presentation. St. Louis: CV Mosby; 1974. p. 256.
317. Gass JDM, Harbin Jr TS, Del Piero EJ. Exudative stellate neuroretinopathy and Coats' syndrome in patients with progressive hemifacial atrophy. Eur J Ophthalmol 1991;1:2 10.
318. Josten K. Sclérodermie en coup de sabre und Auge. Klin Monatsbl Augenheilkd 1958;133:567–70.
319. Meunier A, Toussaint D. Sclérodermie en "coup de sabre" avec lesion du fond d'oeil. Bull Soc Belge Ophtalmol 1958;118:369–77.
320. Parry CH. Collections from the unpublished medical writings of the late Caleb Hillier Parry, MD, FRS. London: Underwoods; 1825. p. 478.
321. Romberg MH. Klinishe Ergebnisse. Berlin: A. Forstner; 1846. p. 75.
322. Wartenberg R. Progressive facial hemiatrophy. Arch Neurol Psychiatr 1945;54:75–96.
323. Takenouchi T, Solomon GE. Alien hand syndrome in Parry–Romberg syndrome. Pediatr Neurol 2010;42:280–2.
324. Qureshi UA, Wani NA, Altaf U. Parry–Romberg syndrome associated with unusual intracranial vascular malformations and Phthisis bulbi. J Neurol Sci 2010;291:107–9.
325. Menascu S, Padeh S, Hoffman C, et al. Parry–Romberg syndrome presenting as status migrainosus. Pediatr Neurol 2009;40:321–3.
326. Longo D, Paonessa A, Specchio N, et al. Parry–Romberg syndrome and Rasmussen encephalitis: Possible association. Clinical and neuroimaging features. J Neuroimaging 2009 Jun; 23.
327. Shah JR, Juhasz C, Kupsky WJ, et al. Rasmussen encephalitis associated with Parry–Romberg syndrome. Neurology 2003;61:395–7.
328. Pichiecchio A, Uggetti C, Grazia Egitto M, et al. Parry–Romberg syndrome with migraine and intracranial aneurysm. Neurology 2002;59:606–8. [discussion 481.]
329. Miedziak AI, Stefanyszyn M, Flanagan J, et al. Parry–Romberg syndrome associated with intracranial vascular malformations. Arch Ophthalmol 1998;116:1235–7.
330. Catala M. Progressive intracranial aneurysmal disease in a child with progressive hemifacial atrophy (Parry–Romberg disease): case report. Neurosurgery 1998;42:1195–6.
331. Scope A, Barzilai A, Trau H, et al. Parry–Romberg syndrome and sympathectomy – a coincidence? Cutis 2004;73:343–6.
332. Aynaci FM, Sen Y, Erdol H, et al. Parry–Romberg syndrome associated with Adie's pupil and radiologic findings. Pediatr Neurol 2001;25:416–8.
333. Slimani S, Hounas F, Ladjouze-Rezig A. Multiple linear sclerodermas with a diffuse Parry–Romberg syndrome. Joint Bone Spine 2009;76:114–6.
334. Echenne B, Sebire G. Parry–Romberg syndrome and linear scleroderma en coup de sabre mimicking Rasmussen encephalitis. Neurology 2007;69:2274. [author reply.]
335. Carreno M, Donaire A, Barcelo MI, et al. Parry Romberg syndrome and linear scleroderma in coup de sabre mimicking Rasmussen encephalitis. Neurology 2007;68:1308–10.
336. Gonul M, Dogan B, Izci Y, et al. Parry–Romberg syndrome in association with anti-dsDNA antibodies: a case report. J Eur Acad Dermatol Venereol 2005;19:740–2.
337. Buonaccorsi S, Leonardi A, Covelli E, et al. Parry–Romberg syndrome. J Craniofac Surg 2005;16:1132–5.
338. Beck RW, Savino PJ, Repka MX, et al. Optic disc structure in anterior ischemic optic neuropathy. Ophthalmology 1984;91:1334–7.
339. Boghen DR, Glaser JS. Ischaemic optic neuropathy; the clinical profile and natural history. Brain 1975;98:689–708.
340. Eagling EM, Sanders MD, Miller SJH. Ischaemic papillopathy; clinical and fluorescein angiographic review of forty cases. Br J Ophthalmol 1974;58:990–1008.
341. Ellenberger Jr C. Ischemic optic neuropathy as a possible early complication of vascular hypertension. Am J Ophthalmol 1979;88:1045–51.
342. Ellenberger Jr C, Keltner JL, Burde RM. Acute optic neuropathy in older patients. Arch Neurol 1973;28:182–5.
343. Feit RH, Tomsak RL, Ellenberger Jr C. Structural factors in the pathogenesis of ischemic optic neuropathy. Am J Ophthalmol 1984;98:105–8.
344. Hayreh SS. Anterior ischemic optic neuropathy. V. Optic disc edema an early sign. Arch Ophthalmol 1981;99:1030–40.
345. Lavin PJM, Ellenberger Jr C. Recurrent ischemic optic neuropathy. Neuro-Ophthalmol 1983;3:193–8.
346. Repka MX, Savino PJ, Schatz NJ, et al. Clinical profile and long-term implications of anterior ischemic optic neuropathy. Am J Ophthalmol 1983;96:478–83.
347. Kline LB. Progression of visual defects in ischemic optic neuropathy. Am J Ophthalmol 1988;106:199–203.
348. Traustason OI, Feldon SE, Leemaster JE, et al. Anterior ischemic optic neuropathy: classification of field defects by Octopus™ automated static perimetry. Graefes Arch Clin Exp Ophthalmol 1988;226:206–12.
349. Arnold AC, Hepler RS. Fluorescein angiography in acute nonarteritic anterior ischemic optic neuropathy. Am J Ophthalmol 1994;117:220–30.
350. Smith JL. Pseudohemangioma of the optic disc following ischemic optic neuropathy. J Clin Neuro-Ophthalmol 1985;5:81–9.
351. Aiello AL, Sadun AA, Feldon SE. Spontaneous improvement of progressive anterior ischemic optic neuropathy: report of two cases. Arch Ophthalmol 1992;110:1197–9.
352. Barrett DA, Glaser JS, Schatz NJ, et al. Spontaneous recovery of vision in progressive anterior ischemic optic neuropathy. J Clin Neuro-Ophthalmol 1992;12:219–25.
353. Johnson LN, Arnold AC. Incidence of nonarteritic and arteritic ischemic optic neuropathy; population-based study in the state of Missouri and Los Angeles County, California. J Neuro-Ophthalmol 1994;14:38–44.
354. Rizzo III JF, Lessell S. Optic neuritis and ischemic optic neuropathy; overlapping clinical profiles. Arch Ophthalmol 1991;109:1668–72.
355. Wall M, Newman SA. Optic nerve sheath decompression for the treatment of progressive nonarteritic ischemic optic neuropathy. Am J Ophthalmol 1991;112:741.
356. Borchert M, Lessell S. Progressive and recurrent nonarteritic anterior ischemic optic neuropathy. Am J Ophthalmol 1988;106:443–9.
357. Hamed LM, Purvin V, Rosenberg M. Recurrent anterior ischemic optic neuropathy in young adults. J Clin Neuro-Ophthalmol 1988;8:239–46.
358. Burde RM. Optic disk risk factors for nonarteritic anterior ischemic optic neuropathy. Am J Ophthalmol 1993;116:759–64.

Index

A

D

E

F

G

H

I

J

K

L

M

Q

R

S

T

U

V

W

X

Z